W9-BXX-487

PATHOPHYSIOLOGY
Foundations of Disease and Clinical Intervention

PATHOPHYSIOLOGY
Foundations of Disease and Clinical Intervention

Margie Hansen, PhD (Physiology), RN
Clinical Associate Professor
Family Nurse Practitioner Program
College of Nursing
University of North Dakota
Grand Forks, North Dakota

W.B. SAUNDERS COMPANY
A Division of Harcourt Brace & Company
Philadelphia London Toronto Montreal Sydney Tokyo

W.B. SAUNDERS COMPANY
A Division of Harcourt Brace & Company

The Curtis Center
Independence Square West
Philadelphia, Pennsylvania 19106

Library of Congress Cataloging-in-Publication Data

Hansen, Margie.
Pathophysiology: Foundations of disease and clinical intervention/Margie Hansen.

p. cm.

ISBN 0-7216-4465-1

1. Physiology, Pathological. I. Title.
[DNLM: 1. Pathology. QZ 4 H249p 1998]

RB 113.H26 1998 616.07—dc21

DNLM/DLC 96-38014

NOTICE

Nursing is an ever-changing field. Standard safety precautions must be followed, but as new research and clinical experience broaden our knowledge, changes in treatment and drug therapy become necessary or appropriate. The editors of this work have carefully checked the generic and trade drug names and verified drug dosages to ensure that the dosage information in this work is accurate and in accord with the standards accepted at the time of publication. Readers are advised, however, to check the product information currently provided by the manufacturer of each drug to be administered to be certain that changes have not been made in the recommended dose or in the contraindications for administration. This is of particular importance in regard to new or infrequently used drugs. It is the responsibility of the treating clinician, relying on experience and knowledge of the patient, to determine dosages and the best treatment for the patient. The editors cannot be responsible for misuse or misapplication of the material in this work.

THE PUBLISHER

PATHOPHYSIOLOGY: FOUNDATIONS OF DISEASE AND CLINICAL INTERVENTION ISBN 0-7216-4465-1

Printed in the United States of America.

Last digit is the print number: 9 8 7 6 5 4 3 2 1

With love and gratitude

To my father, James Cramer,
for teaching me how to figure things out for myself;

To my mother, Ethel Cramer,
for teaching me compassion for all living things;

To my husband, James Hansen,
for his unflagging support with words of encouragement
and for taking on more than his share of the domestic labor;

To my son, John Hansen, and my daughter, Jennifer Hansen,
for bringing joy and perspective into my life every day;

and

To my students,
for teaching me how to teach
and for always letting me know that it mattered.

PREFACE

Health and disease are subjects of interest to many, as is apparent from the frequent reports in the public media about research findings related to causes of disease and new interventions. For students of the health professions, *pathophysiology,* the study of human physiologic function in disease, is an essential foundation for rational clinical practice. This intermediate-level textbook of pathophysiology is aimed at a target audience of upper-division undergraduates and beginning graduate students in the health-related disciplines. It aims to bridge the gap between textbooks that review physiologic processes and pathophysiologic mechanisms in great detail, yet do not clearly relate this content to clinical practice, and those texts that are superficially descriptive and encyclopedic but that lack explanation and scientific rigor. Drawing from my experiences in clinical practice (in nursing), teaching (in nursing and pharmacy), and scientific research (in physiology), I have tried to create a textbook that is scientifically accurate, clinically relevant, and explanatory rather than merely descriptive.

Potential clinical application of scientific concepts has been integrated throughout the text. The specific diseases emphasized have been carefully screened on the basis of commonality or utility in illustrating important scientific principles. Clinical characteristics of less common disorders are addressed in tables. While it is probable that the reader will have had introductory coursework in chemistry, biology, anatomy, and physiology, sufficient review of basic scientific foundations is included to promote their application to pathophysiologic concepts.

Organization and Teaching Tools

Consistent with the current emphasis on cellular and subcellular mechanisms that characterizes the biologic sciences, Part I of this textbook focuses on these elements, which have broad applicability to pathophysiology of all organ systems. Theoretical perspectives that promote integration of concepts from multiple scientific disciplines and that provide a logical framework for approaching the study of pathophysiology are also introduced. Part II is organized more traditionally on the basis of organ systems, facilitating use of the text as an adjunct to discipline-specific texts, many of which use this approach. This organization of the text is intended to permit flexibility in its use by students, in that those with more background in the basic sciences could begin with Part II. Cross-references within the systems chapters direct the learner back to specific concepts in foundations chapters for review, if necessary.

Pedagogic tools have been used extensively. Each chapter begins with a

Chapter Outline, Learning Objectives, and a list of **Key Terms** whose definitions are found in the **Glossary** (Appendix A). A consistent format is employed in discussion of specific diseases, including the definition, epidemiology, etiology, pathophysiology, clinical manifestations, prevention/treatment, and prognosis/outcome for each disorder. At the end of each chapter is a **Summary of Key Points,** a list of **References** cited in the chapter, and an extensive **Selected Bibliography** emphasizing recent original research and professional reviews. The straightforward writing style is augmented by approximately 400 tables to illustrate examples, relationships, and classification systems. More than 500 illustrations are used (75% original to this text). Illustrations are typically simplified yet referenced to realistic anatomy rather than to abstract schematics. An eight-page full-color insert illustrates visible clinical manifestations of many disorders of hematology, immunity, hemostasis, sensory function, the gastrointestinal system, the reproductive systems, and dermatology. In addition to the Glossary, the appendices include **Abbreviations, Laboratory Values of Clinical Importance** and **AHCPR Guidelines,** all of which should be of use in clinical studies.

Clinical Application, Developmental Variables, and Research

The emphasis in this book upon clinical integration, developmental variables in disease, and current research is evident not only in the text but also in highlighted special features. In each chapter, **Clinical Scenarios** provide brief vignettes with questions intended to personalize concepts and to promote critical thinking. **Developmental Perspective** boxes are introduced in Chapter 8 and are used in each of the remaining chapters to identify factors pertaining to the embryonic and fetal periods, infancy and childhood, adolescence and young adulthood, and middle and older adulthood. Each chapter includes a **Focus of Current Research** box that provides a synopsis of representative basic, epidemiologic, and clinical research related to chapter topics.

Consistency and Efficiency

The fact that this book is a single-author text is its most distinguishing feature. I have made every attempt to be consistent throughout with regard to format, writing style, and reading level and to be as efficient as possible in coverage of content to avoid the duplications and gaps that are more likely to occur when multiple authors contribute to the writing of a text. In writing this book, I have tried to teach, rather than merely to impart information. After 30 years of clinical practice, teaching, and research, my fascination with the subject of pathophysiology continues to grow. If this book "infects" readers with this same interest, promotes their understanding of the subject, and fosters development of a scientific foundation for the practice of their professions, it will have achieved its aims.

ACKNOWLEDGMENTS

The talents and generosity of so many people made this book possible. I am very grateful to all, including the designers and copy editors whose names I may never know but whose work I greatly admire and appreciate. Others are well known to me, and I want to specifically acknowledge their essential contributions to this work. At W.B. Saunders Company, Ilze S. Rader, formerly Senior Editor, first approached me with the idea for the book and convinced me that I could write it. Barbara Nelson Cullen, formerly Senior Editor, distilled our initial ideas into a specific template for the manuscript. Robin Levin Richman, Senior Developmental Editor, dealt with the details, providing the gentle but tenacious direction that saw the book to its completion. The work of Karen Gulliver, of Karen Gulliver Productions, Bethesda, Maryland, was invaluable in synthesizing reviewer comments and in applying her considerable expertise to the critique of the manuscript and development of the art program. I am very fortunate to have had the opportunity to work with, and learn from, these outstanding professionals.

The feedback provided by the scientific and clinical experts who reviewed sections of the manuscript was of tremendous value in making decisions about content and approach and in making the text as current and clinically accurate as possible. I sincerely appreciate their careful scrutiny and practical suggestions.

The Clinical Scenarios in the text are based on actual case histories documented by sixth-year students in the Doctor of Pharmacy Program at North Dakota State University. I am thankful to them and to their clinical professors, Dr. Mary Kuzel, Dr. Diann Clarens-Hoedl, Dr. Donald Miller, Dr. Harvey Hanel, and Dr. Robert Sylvester, for their generosity in sharing these materials.

My student assistants, Jamie Zacher and Jenny Hansen, worked closely with me for 2 years, doing the "legwork" of locating and photocopying research and professional articles. Their energy and reliability were critical in providing the primary literature upon which the text is based and enabled the extensive referencing of the text. Diana Kowalski of the Pharmacy Library at North Dakota State University was helpful to them and to me countless times. I am indebted to all three of these young women.

With love and many thanks, I recognize my colleagues and students in nursing and pharmacy who have been consistently supportive during this 5-year project. I am especially grateful to Professors Agnes Harrington, Carla Gross, Dean Gross, and Martha Vorvick and to Dr. Edward Magarian, who so often provided encouragement in both word and deed. Finally, and most important, the responses of my students to my teaching efforts, whether as verbal or written feedback or as demonstrated learning, have been of tremendous benefit to me in shaping this work.

MARGIE CRAMER HANSEN
September, 1997

REVIEWERS

Anita Dupre Althans, MSN, RN, C
Our Lady of Holy Cross College
New Orleans, Louisiana

Linda Becker, MSN, RN, C
St. Clair Community College
Point Huron, Michigan

Wendy Blackburn, RN, BAA, MA, PG, MNI, CCN(c)
Fanshawe College, London, Ontario
St. Michael's Hospital, Toronto, Ontario, Canada

Claire M. Chee, RN
Children's Hospital of Philadelphia
Philadelphia, Pennsylvania

Sara E. Connor, MSN, EdD, RN
Armstrong State College
Savannah, Georgia

Lawrence Cornett, PhD
University of Arkansas for Medical Sciences
Little Rock, Arkansas

Luann M. Daggett, MSN, RN
University of Southern Mississippi
Meridian, Mississippi

Ellen Duke, MSN, RN, CCRN
Angelina Community College
Lufkin, Texas

Geraldine Flaherty, MSN, RN
Wayne State University
Detroit, Michigan

Mary Kay Flynn, MA, DNSc, RN, CCRN
Grand Canyon University
Samaritan College of Nursing
Phoenix, Arizona

Carol Fountain, MN, RN, ONC
Boise State University
Boise, Idaho

Mary Jo Gay, MSN, RN
Missouri Western State University
St. Joseph, Missouri

Michele A. Gerwick, MSN, RN
Indiana University of Pennsylvania
Indiana, Pennsylvania

JoAnn M. Gordon, PhD, RN
Southwest Missouri State University
Springfield, Missouri

Joan S. Grant, DSN, RN, CS
University of Alabama at Birmingham
Birmingham, Alabama

Mary Gray, RN, CS
Peara Hospice of Montana
Great Falls, Montana

Karen Hammond, MS, RN, CCRN
Washington County Hospital
Hagerstown, Maryland

Shirley Hemminger, MSN, RN, CCRN
Kent State University, Kent, Ohio
University Hospitals of Cleveland, Cleveland, Ohio

Barbara Herlihy, PhD, MA, BSN
University of the Incarnate Word
San Antonio, Texas

Susan R. Herman, MSN, RN, CNS
Caffey College, Alta Loma, California
Azusa Pacific University, Azusa, California

REVIEWERS

Wendy Hillman, MSN, RN
Kirtland Community College
Roscommon, Michigan

Ruthellyn H. Hinton, MS, MN, RN, CS, ARNP
Pittsburg State University
Pittsburg, Kansas

Sharon Leech Hofland, PhD, RN
South Dakota State University
Brookings, South Dakota

Christopher J. Hubbard, PhD
Northern Illinois University
De Kalb, Illinois

Donald J. Jacobs, MSN, MEd, RN
Cardiology of Tulsa
Tulsa, Oklahoma

Ruth Kleinpell, PhD, RN, CCRN
Rush University, Chicago, Illinois
Rush Presbyterian St. Luke's Medical Center,
Chicago, Illinois

Joan Klemballa, PhD, MA, BS, RN
The College of West Virginia
Beckley, West Virginia

Nancy Kupper, MSN, RN
Tarrant County Junior College
Fort Worth, Texas

Larry E. Lancaster, MSN, EdD, RN
Vanderbilt University
Nashville, Tennessee

Priscilla LeMone, DSN, RN
University of Missouri
Columbia, Missouri

Nancy Ryan Macklin, PhD, RN
Maryville University
St. Louis, Missouri

Bonnie A. Nelson, MSN, RN
Medical College of Ohio
Toledo, Ohio

Sara G. Parkerson, MSN, RN, OCN
Johns Hopkins Hospital
Baltimore, Maryland

Marilyn Nelsen Pase, MSN, RN
New Mexico State University
Las Cruces, New Mexico

Phyllis G. Peterson, MN, RN
Our Lady of Holy Cross College
New Orleans, Louisiana

Kimberly Quinn, MSN, RN, CCRN
Johns Hopkins Hospital
Baltimore, Maryland

Christine Rosner, MSN, RN
Holy Family College
Philadelphia, Pennsylvania

Mary Sampel, MSN, RN
St. Louis University
St. Louis, Missouri

Mariakutty Samuel, MSN, RN, CCRN, CNS
Wharton County Junior College
Wharton, Texas

Olive Santavenere, PhD, MSN, MSOB, RN
Southern Connecticut State University
New Haven, Connecticut

Lisa Anderson Shaw, MSN, MA, RN, C
University of Illinois at Chicago
University of Illinois Medical Center
Chicago, Illinois

William A. Sodeman, Jr., MD
Medical College of Ohio
Toledo, Ohio

Gary L. Soderberg, PhD, PT, FAPTA
University of Central Arkansas
Conway, Arkansas

Christopher Steidle, MD
Northeast Indiana Urology P.C.
Fort Wayne, Indiana

Janice Sylakowski, MS, RN
State University of New York College at Buffalo
Buffalo, New York

Karen L. Then, MN, RN
University of Calgary
Calgary, Alberta, Canada

Roselena Thorpe, PhD, RN
Community College of Allegheny County
Pittsburgh, Pennsylvania

Jane Brocksmith Tiek, MSN, RN
Vincennes University
Good Samaritan Hospital
Vincennes, Indiana

REVIEWERS

Kuei-Shen Tu, MSN, RN
University of Alabama at Birmingham
Birmingham, Alabama

Patricia E.H. Vermeersch, PhD, RN
University of North Dakota
Grand Forks, North Dakota

Carole J. Petrosky Vozel, PhD, MSN, RN, C
The Western Pennsylvania Hospital
Pittsburgh, Pennsylvania

Kathleen S. Whalen, MN, RN, CCRN
Community College of Denver
Denver, Colorado

Ann H. White, MSN, MBA, RN, CNA
University of Southern Indiana
Evansville, Indiana

Marge Whitman, MSN, RN, OCN
Utah Valley Regional Medical Center
Provo, Utah

Diana O. Williams, MSN, RN, CCRN
Johns Hopkins Hospital
Baltimore, Maryland

Deborah Wojak, MS, RN
Eastern Arizona College
Thatcher, Arizona

Gladys M. Word, MSN, EdM, EdD, RN
The College of New Jersey
Trenton, New Jersey

CONTENTS-Brief

APPENDICES

CONTENTS-Detailed

PART ONE

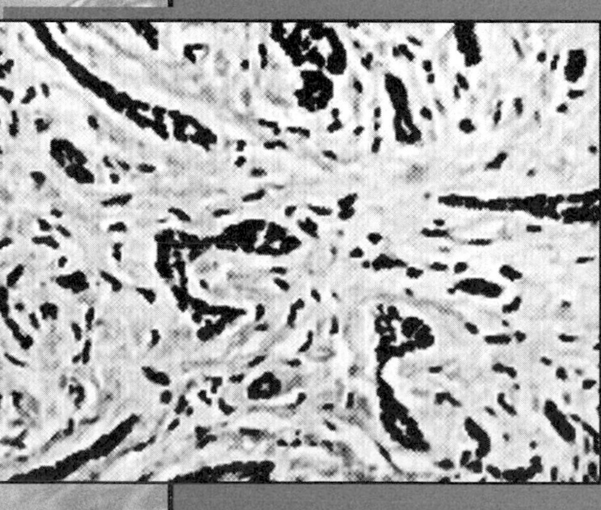

FOUNDATIONS OF PATHOPHYSIOLOGY

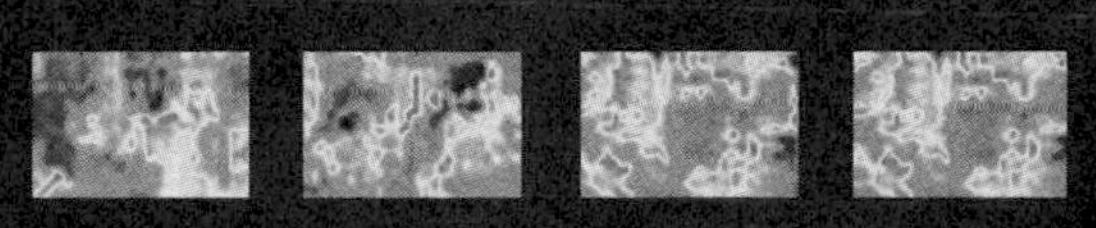

UNIT I
Theoretical Perspective

UNIT II
Cellular Perspective

UNIT III
The Cellular Environment

Unit I

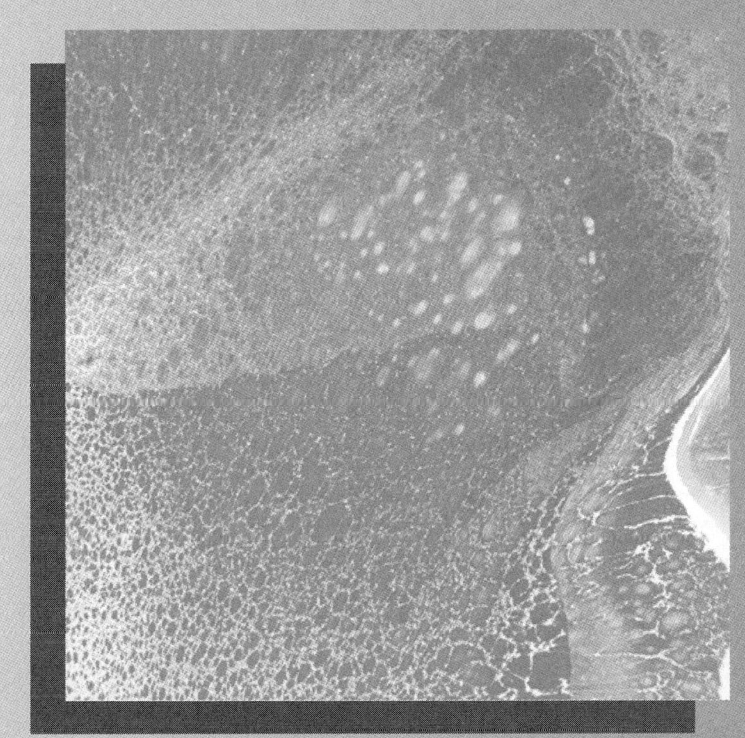

Chapter 1
Concepts and Theories of Pathophysiology

THEORETICAL PERSPECTIVE

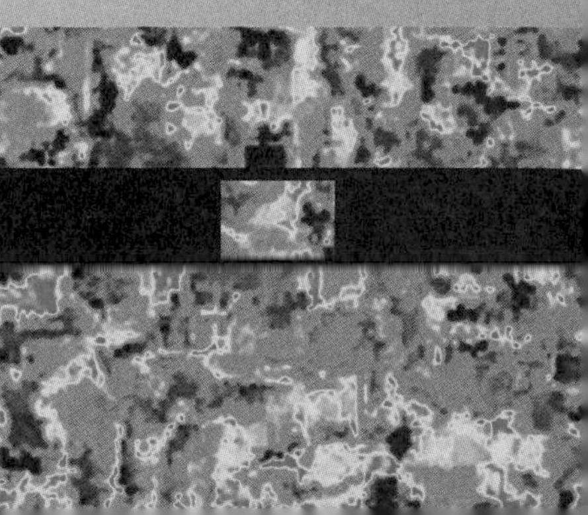

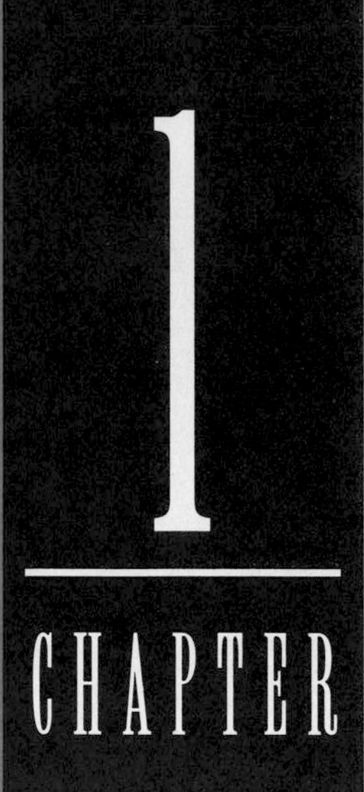

Concepts and Theories of Pathophysiology

LEARNING OBJECTIVES

1. Differentiate among pathophysiology and other biomedical sciences.
2. Discuss the concept of mechanism of disease.
3. Characterize the relationships among health, wellness, and disease.
4. Relate clinical intervention models to concepts of health, wellness, and disease.
5. Define each of the five components of the disease process: epidemiology, etiology, pathophysiology, clinical manifestations, and outcome.
6. Compare and contrast disease classifications based on anatomy, development, and etiology.
7. Discuss general modes of prevention and treatment of disease.
8. Identify the relevance of general systems theory to the science of pathophysiology.
9. Discuss the evolution of contemporary stress theory.
10. Relate the phases and clinical manifestations of the physiologic stress response (Selye's general adaptation syndrome) to the underlying neuroendocrine regulatory mechanisms and resulting systemic effects.
11. Identify the relationship between adaptation and homeostasis.
12. Differentiate between negative and positive feedback responses.
13. Differentiate among the three levels of regulation of physiologic adaptation.

key terms

adaptation
clinical intervention
clinical manifestation
cortisol
cure
cytokine
definitive therapy
disease
epidemiology
epinephrine
etiology
feedback
general adaptation syndrome
health
heat shock protein
holism
homeostasis
hormone
iatrogenic
idiopathic
incidence
mechanism (of disease)
morbidity
morphology
mortality
negative feedback loop
neurotransmitter
norepinephrine
open system
palliation
pathogenesis
pathophysiology
positive feedback loop
prevalence
prognosis
psychoneuroimmunology
remission
risk factor
sign (of disease)
stress
stressor
symptom
system
systems theory
wellness

INTRODUCTION TO PATHOPHYSIOLOGY

Pathophysiology is the study of human physiologic function in disease. It is an integrative science that draws on concepts from many basic and clinical sciences, including anatomy, physiology, pathology, biochemistry, genetics, pharmacology, cell and molecular biology, and biophysics. Unlike its sister science pathology, which emphasizes the measurable aspects of disease such as structural changes and laboratory findings, pathophysiology focuses on the **mechanisms** of disease. These mechanisms are the dynamic processes that (1) cause disease, (2) give rise to **signs** and **symptoms**, and (3) signify the body's attempts to overcome disease.

Understanding the mechanisms of disease is essential to health practitioners because it enables the design and implementation of **clinical interventions**. These are actions that aim to interrupt causative mechanisms, relieve signs and symptoms, and support the body's efforts to resist and compensate for disease.

Pathophysiology is founded on a theoretical basis that provides the framework for organizing knowledge gained through research. Some theories are applicable to more specific aspects of disease, such as etiologic theories, proposed mechanisms of disease, or postulated mechanisms by which clinical interventions are effective in treatment of disease. The theories discussed in this chapter provide the foundation for the discipline as a whole in that they are generally applicable to disease and its treatment. **Systems theory**, **stress**, and the related concepts of **adaptation** and **homeostasis** form the general theoretical framework of pathophysiology.

CONCEPTS OF HEALTH, DISEASE, AND CLINICAL INTERVENTION

Definitions and Models

Health

The best-known definition of **health**, attributed to the World Health Organization, affirms that health is "more than the absence of disease," but rather a state of "complete physical, mental, and social well-being."[1] This definition sets a lofty goal for patients seeking health as well as for health care professionals.

Disease and Illness

Disease (literally, "lack of ease") can be defined at several levels, from cellular injury to loss of system equilibrium. Defining disease as absence of health is not particularly useful because many patients with well-managed chronic diseases are appropriately defined by themselves and by society as healthy. Clinical definitions of disease usually include two aspects: (1) a process disrupting physiologic function (although the precise nature of the process or mechanism may be unknown), and (2) a characteristic set of signs and symptoms.

The terms disease and illness are used interchangeably in most clinical settings, although *illness* technically refers to a subjective state that is experienced by the individual as the presence of symptoms, whereas disease is understood to be an objective state that is demonstrated by an observable structural or functional abnormality.[2] A person may feel ill whether or not disease is present, and, conversely, disease may be present in a person who does not have symptoms.

Wellness and the Health Continuum

It is clinically useful to view health and disease in relation to each other if the two states are seen as opposite directions on a continuum rather than as mutually exclusive conditions. As described in the work of Dunn[3] and others, the polar extreme in the direction of disease is death; the opposite extreme is the state of optimal **wellness**. The term wellness connotes a state characterized not only by absence of disease or its manifestations but also by minimization of modifiable **risk factors** for disease.

Intervention Models

Acceptance of these definitions and the relationships among health, wellness, and disease has resulted in the evolution of clinical practice models. The traditional biomedical, or treatment, model in which the individual seeks clinical intervention when signs and symptoms of illness become noticeable (or intolerable), has largely given way to modern preventive, or wellness, models, in which the individual may seek intervention at any point on the continuum (Fig. 1–1). Access to health care is sought not only for treatment of disease but also for identification and modification of lifestyle choices, environmental exposures, and other factors that may contribute to disease risk. In the traditional model, the impetuses for practice in the health professions are treatment of disease and restoration of health; the intervention models have extended the clinical practice arena to include prevention (often referred to as *health maintenance* or *health promotion*).

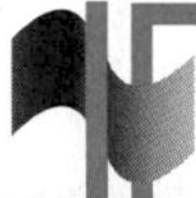

Clinical Scenario

J.R. was diagnosed with insulin-dependent diabetes mellitus at 7 years of age. He is now 16 years of age and is a starting pitcher on his high school baseball team. He monitors his blood glucose levels twice each day and self-injects insulin each morning and evening. J.R.'s diet consists mainly of fast foods. He reports that he lives a "normal life" and that he has no symptoms related to his diabetes.

1. Is J.R. healthy? Is he ill?
2. Is J.R.'s diabetes being managed optimally from the perspective of the wellness model? What interventions might be considered?

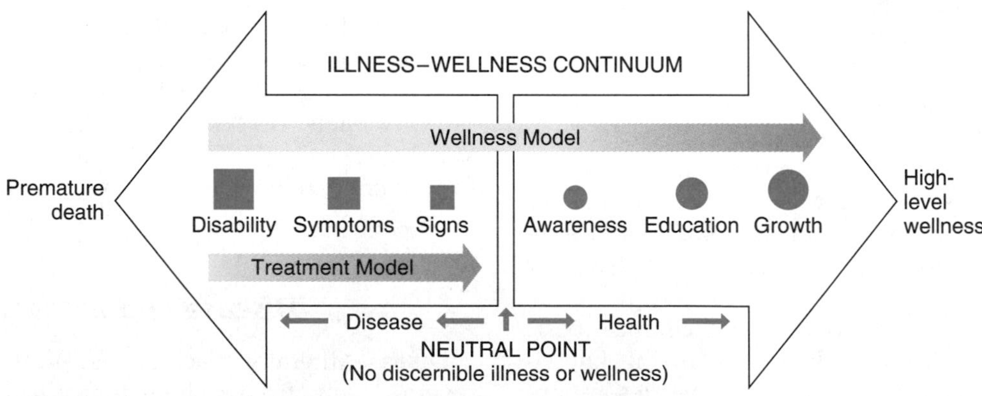

FIGURE 1–1

Illness–wellness continuum and intervention models. Health and disease are viewed as opposite directions on a continuum in which high-level wellness and premature death represent extreme outcomes. Superimposed on this continuum are the traditional *treatment model* of intervention, in which the individual seeks health care when manifestations of disease become apparent, and the contemporary *wellness model*, in which intervention is sought at any point for preventive measures (risk reduction or health promotion) as well as for treatment of manifest disease. (Modified from Travis, L.W., and Ryan, R.S. [1988]. *Wellness Workbook*. Berkeley, CA: Ten Speed Press.)

Components of the Disease Process

The disease process consists of five components: epidemiology, etiology, pathophysiology, clinical manifestations, and outcome. As illustrated in Figure 1–2, each component may be the basis for the development and evaluation of clinical interventions.

Epidemiology

Epidemiology is the study of the cause and distribution of disease in populations. Derived from the term *epidemic*, this science had its origins in the study of infectious diseases but now focuses more broadly on all diseases that have a significant impact on public health. Epidemiologic research is primarily concerned with the outcome measures of **mortality** and **morbidity** and with their antecedent or associated conditions (possible causes or risk factors).

Morbidity, or disease occurrence, is quantified in two ways: as **incidence** (the rate of disease, or number of new cases occurring during a given time period) and **prevalence** (the density of disease, or total number of cases present at a given point in time). Morbidity statistics are derived from varied sources, such as records of hospitalization, clinic visits, patient interviews, and reported absences from work or school. Because of inherent risk to public health, reporting of the occurrence of some diseases is mandated by state or federal law (Table 1–1).

In the United States, acute and chronic diseases of the respiratory system account for most morbidity.[4] Cardiovascular disease has been the leading cause of mortality for several decades, with cancer a close second (Fig. 1–3).

Etiology

Etiology is the identified cause of a disease. It may refer to a specific agent, such as a microorganism or a traumatic event, or to a mechanism that describes an interaction between individual (host or patient) factors and environmental factors, culminating in disease.

The three broad categories of etiology are as follows:

Genetic—disease that originates from a spontaneous or inherited defect in the genetic control of cellular development.

Acquired—disease that originates from harmful effects of environmental agents in a host who may or may not be compromised.

Multifactorial—disease that results from a combination of genetic and environmental factors.

Examples of each category are listed in Table 1–2.

In many cases, the exact cause of disease cannot

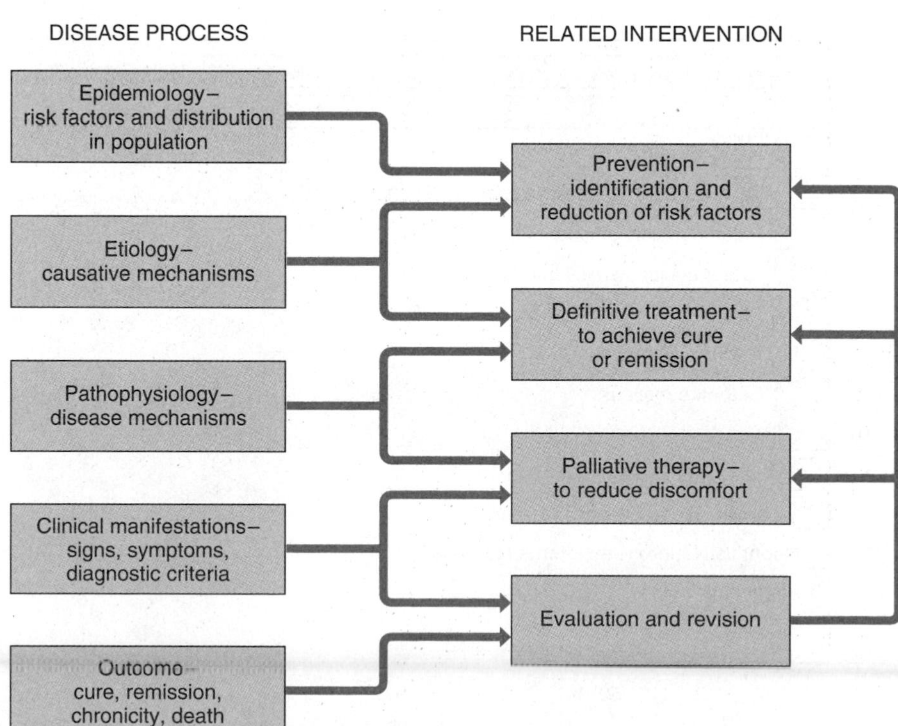

FIGURE 1–2

Components of disease process and related interventions. Each component of the disease process potentially gives rise to modes of clinical intervention. Clinical evaluation of signs, symptoms, diagnostic findings, and disease outcomes facilitates appropriate revision of interventions.

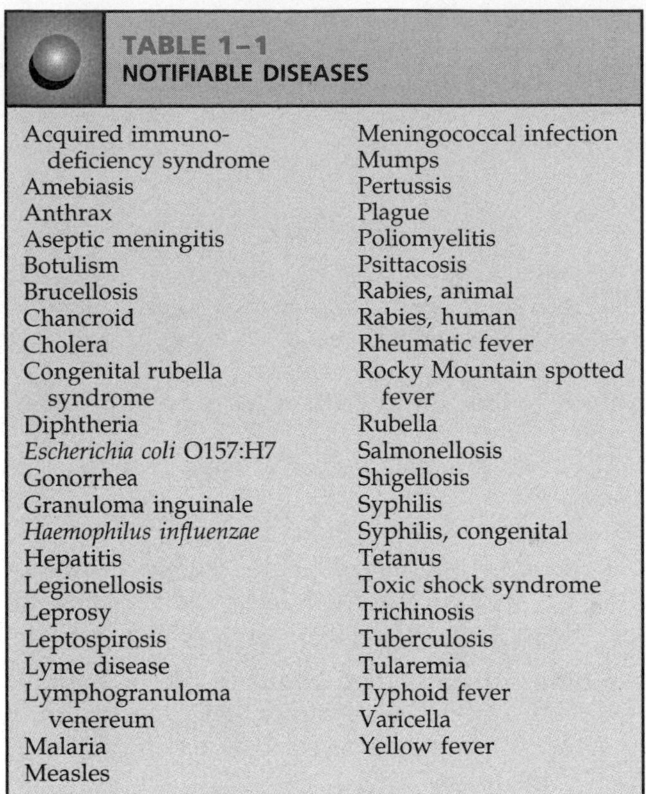

TABLE 1–1
NOTIFIABLE DISEASES

Acquired immunodeficiency syndrome	Meningococcal infection
Amebiasis	Mumps
Anthrax	Pertussis
Aseptic meningitis	Plague
Botulism	Poliomyelitis
Brucellosis	Psittacosis
Chancroid	Rabies, animal
Cholera	Rabies, human
Congenital rubella syndrome	Rheumatic fever
Diphtheria	Rocky Mountain spotted fever
Escherichia coli O157:H7	Rubella
Gonorrhea	Salmonellosis
Granuloma inguinale	Shigellosis
Haemophilus influenzae	Syphilis
Hepatitis	Syphilis, congenital
Legionellosis	Tetanus
Leprosy	Toxic shock syndrome
Leptospirosis	Trichinosis
Lyme disease	Tuberculosis
Lymphogranuloma venereum	Tularemia
Malaria	Typhoid fever
Measles	Varicella
	Yellow fever

From Centers for Disease Control and Prevention. (1994). National notifiable diseases reporting—United States, 1994. *Morbidity and Mortality Weekly Report* 43(43), 800–801.

be identified. Most diseases have multifactorial etiologies, although the relative contribution of genetic and environmental factors (nature versus nurture) is often debatable. Adding to the controversy is the difficulty of establishing a clear cause-and-effect relationship between factors that may precede disease and its subsequent development. Establishment of such a relationship requires experimental research on humans, and such studies often have ethical constraints. A statistically significant association between antecedent factors and disease can often be established based on epidemiologic data. The associations between hypertension and stroke and between cigarette smoking and lung cancer are well-known examples. Such associated factors are called risk factors, and risk reduction is a critical aspect of clinical intervention for many diseases.

Pathophysiology

The focus of pathophysiology is on the mechanisms of disease: the disruption of normal physiologic processes that occurs as a result of etiologic factors. With reference to a specific disease, pathophysiology includes descriptive aspects, such as **pathogenesis** (the clinical course of the disease) and **morphology** (structural changes). The principal aim of pathophysiology is explanatory rather than descriptive, however. Pathophysiology explains structural and functional changes attributable to disease, including both the mechanisms of the disease and the resultant responses of the body.

Clinical Manifestations

The presence of disease is suspected and confirmed on the basis of patient-reported effects and

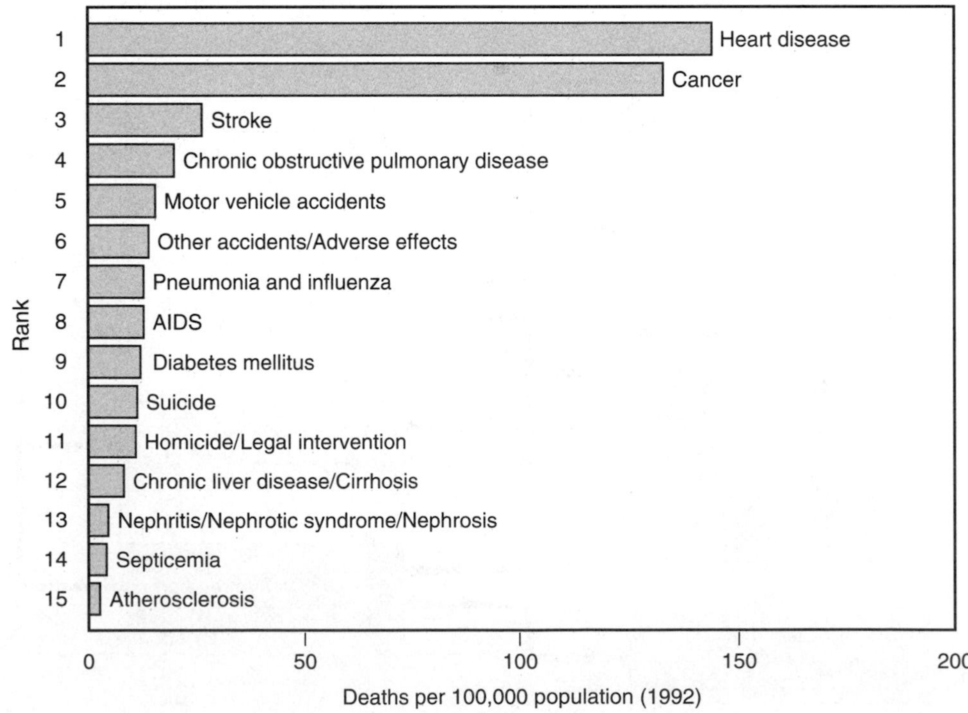

FIGURE 1–3
Major causes of mortality in the United States. (Data from Centers for Disease Control and Prevention. [1994]. Mortality patterns—United States, 1992. *Morbidity and Mortality Weekly Report* 43(49), 916–920.)

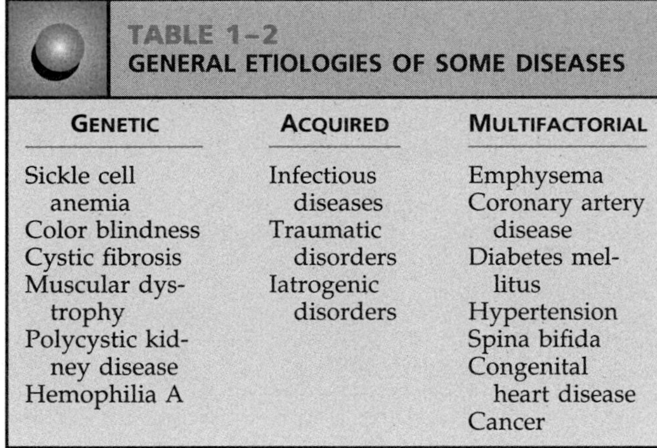

TABLE 1–2
GENERAL ETIOLOGIES OF SOME DISEASES

GENETIC	ACQUIRED	MULTIFACTORIAL
Sickle cell anemia	Infectious diseases	Emphysema
Color blindness	Traumatic disorders	Coronary artery disease
Cystic fibrosis	Iatrogenic disorders	Diabetes mellitus
Muscular dystrophy		Hypertension
Polycystic kidney disease		Spina bifida
Hemophilia A		Congenital heart disease
		Cancer

physical evidence resulting from etiologic and pathophysiologic processes. **Clinical manifestations** may include physical signs (observable phenomena such as skin rashes, cough, joint deformity, or elevated temperature) or symptoms (subjective feelings expressed by the patient such as pain, difficulty breathing, fatigue, or anxiety). Signs are noted by health care professionals during the physical examination, whereas symptoms are discerned during the patient interview. Clinical manifestations may also be detected through specific laboratory and diagnostic testing procedures.

Outcome

Prognosis refers to the *expected* outcome of a disease. The *actual* outcome, ideally, is **cure** (the complete eradication of disease). In some diseases, notably some cancers, cure can be physically confirmed only by postmortem examination (autopsy), so cure is instead defined statistically as a period of survival during which overt signs of disease are absent.

Many diseases have no known cure. The desired outcome of treatment in these cases is the induction of **remission**, that is, the eradication of any clinical manifestations of disease. Achievement of extended remission is a positive outcome in many cancers as well as in degenerative neurologic conditions, such as multiple sclerosis.

Other conditions that cannot be cured leave the patient with chronic disease or disability. In these cases, manifestations of disease are always present to some degree, and the goal of treatment is to manage the disease by minimizing signs and symptoms and by slowing disease progression. Finally, when the manifestations of disease are such that neither the body's adaptive mechanisms nor the aid of clinical interventions can prevent lethal damage to critical body systems, death is the outcome.

Classification of Disease

The classification of disease based on anatomy, development, or etiology gives rise to specialized areas of knowledge and practice within the health care professions. Disease is commonly categorized according to the organ system affected. Cardiovascular disease, for example, is the focus of the medical practice of cardiology, of specialized coronary care units in hospitals, and of cardiac rehabilitation centers.

Disease may also be classified on the basis of the age of the patient. Neonatology (newborn care), pediatrics (care of children), adolescent medicine, adult medicine, and gerontology (elder care) are examples of specialties derived from this developmental basis.

An etiology-based classification system for diseases is illustrated in Table 1–3. These etiologic categories are not mutually exclusive. Diabetes mellitus, for example, might be classified as immunologic, metabolic, nutritional, or in some cases, inherited. Included among the etiologic categories are **iatrogenic**, or treatment-induced, disorders, such as Cushing's syndrome induced by steroid therapy or aplastic anemia resulting from radiation therapy. The category of **idiopathic** disorders, in which the etiologic agents or mechanisms are unknown, is still an extensive one despite ongoing research.

The *International Classification of Diseases*, Ninth Revision, with Clinical Modifications (ICD-9 CM)[5] represents a combination of anatomic, developmental,

TABLE 1–3
ETIOLOGIC CLASSIFICATION OF DISEASE

CATEGORY	DEFINITION
Congenital	Present at birth
Inherited	Multifactorial or genetic
Metabolic	Abnormal body chemistry
Degenerative	Progressive loss of normal structure and function
Neoplastic	Benign or malignant tumor growth
Immunologic	Abnormality of specific immune response
Infectious	Due to microorganism
Nutritional	Abnormality of dietary intake or nutrient use
Physical agent–induced	Accidental or intentional trauma or toxicity
Iatrogenic	Therapy-induced
Psychogenic	Related to psychological or functional state
Idiopathic	Unknown etiology

Adapted from Purtilo, D.T., and Purtilo, R.B. (1989). *A Survey of Human Diseases*. (2nd ed.). Boston: Little, Brown, and Co.

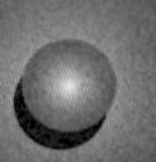

TABLE 1–4
CATEGORIES OF DISEASES FROM THE INTERNATIONAL CLASSIFICATION OF DISEASES

Infectious and parasitic diseases	Diseases of the genitourinary system
Neoplasms	Complications of pregnancy, childbirth, and the puerperium
Endocrine, nutritional, and metabolic diseases, and immunity disorders	Diseases of the skin and subcutaneous tissues
Diseases of the blood and blood-forming organs	Diseases of the musculoskeletal system and connective tissue
Mental disorders	Congenital anomalies
Diseases of the nervous system and sense organs	Certain conditions originating in the perinatal period
Diseases of the circulatory system	Symptoms, signs, and ill-defined conditions
Diseases of the respiratory system	Injury and poisoning
Diseases of the digestive system	

From United States Department of Health and Human Services. (1991). *The International Classification of Diseases (9th Revision)—Clinical Modifications.* (4th ed.). Volume 2. Disease Index. Hyattsville, MD: USDHHS.

and etiologic approaches (Table 1–4). The ICD system was initiated in the 1920s by the World Health Organization in an effort to facilitate health-related research and statistical analyses. Revisions have been useful in standardizing costs of care and reimbursement. Initial components of a tenth revision (ICD-10) were released in 1993.[6] Full transition to ICD-10 is expected to take several years.

Clinical Intervention

Clinical intervention in disease is the responsibility of members of the health professions—medicine, nursing, pharmacy, physical therapy, nutrition therapy, respiratory therapy, and other allied health fields. The individual and collective actions of these professionals encompass prevention as well as diagnosis and treatment of disease.

Prevention

Prevention includes (1) identification of risk factors for disease through health screening interviews, physical examination, and diagnostic testing, and (2) reduction of risk through advocacy and education pertaining to lifestyle and behavioral changes or through more specialized interventions such as drug therapy, exercise programs, or dietary regimens.

Treatment

Treatment, or therapy, is intervention aimed at achieving the optimal outcome of disease for each patient. **Definitive therapy** is designed to achieve cure or remission. When this is not possible, **palliation** of symptoms is the goal of treatment. Palliative measures are undertaken to alleviate clinical manifestations, such as pain and discomfort, nausea, breathing difficulty, and anxiety, and when possible, to minimize progression of disease. Palliative interventions may thus be targeted against signs and symptoms (e.g., pain-relieving or antinausea drugs) or against the disease process (e.g., surgery or radiation therapy to reduce tumor mass). In general, patient comfort is the overriding goal of palliative therapy.

In cases in which the mechanism of disease and the mechanism of clinical intervention are well understood, the treatment is said to be *rational,* or clearly based on scientific knowledge. For example, diseases caused by bacterial infections are rationally treated with specific antibiotic therapy. In other situations, however, one or both of these mechanisms is unknown or uncertain, and treatment is then *empiric.* The treatment is employed because it works, or appears to work. Such interventions may have been discovered accidentally or on a trial and error basis. The administration of gold salts to relieve joint inflammation in rheumatoid arthritis is an example of an empiric therapy. Medical history is replete with examples of treatments that were used empirically for many years (even centuries) before their rational bases were identified. A notable example is the use of digitalis in the treatment of heart failure. Establishing the rational basis for clinical intervention is the overriding goal of comprehensive research programs in laboratory and clinical settings.

THEORY AND SCIENCE

As a science, pathophysiology is built on a foundation of factual knowledge derived from disciplinary research. This knowledge base is continuously evolving as new research methodologies are developed and as more is learned about the function of the human body in health and disease. In pathophysiology, theory provides a means of organizing scientific facts into frameworks that may be useful in integrating multiple research findings, in explaining clinical phenomena, and in predicting the course of disease and outcomes of interventions.

General systems theory, stress theory, and the related concepts of adaptation and homeostasis are three areas of theory that facilitate the understanding of pathophysiology. Although these theories have diverse origins, their interrelatedness is evident. Systems theory provides a way of conceptualizing the human body, its components, and the environmental context in which it functions. Stress theories clarify the nature of forces that may perturb the human system as well as the typical physiologic responses to such forces. Adaptation describes the specific physiologic processes by which the body attempts to achieve, maintain, or regain a state of optimal system function, or homeostasis.

General Systems Theory

General systems theory has been described by von Bertalanffy, its founder, as "a general science of wholeness."[7] The concepts of this theory attempt to simplify and unify all of science and to facilitate interdisciplinary approaches to scientific problems.

The Nature of Systems

General systems theory defines a **system** as a whole composed of interrelated, interacting parts. As illustrated in Figure 1–4, the human body may be conceptualized as a system composed of hierarchic subsystems (organ systems, organs, tissues, cells, subcellular elements). Alteration in the function of any subsystem affects other subsystems as well as the system as a whole.

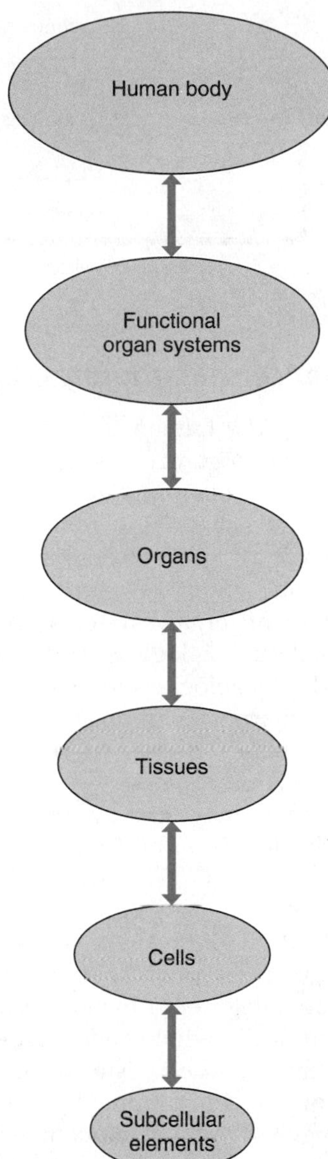

FIGURE 1–4
Hierarchy of body subsystems. Consistent with general systems theory, the human body can be conceptualized as a system composed of subsystems that have a hierarchic order. Disruption of any subsystem affects the subsystems above and below it as well as the system as a whole.

Systems may be open or closed to their environments. As an **open system**, the human receives input from the environment (energy, information, or matter), processes that input, and generates output to the environment (Fig. 1–5). In energy metabolism, for example, nutrients generated by the environment are ingested by the human system, which processes these into forms in which they can be used for the production of work and heat, yielding carbon dioxide and water as metabolic by-products (see Chapter 3). These by-products are released into the environment, where they in turn affect the human system.

The body thus operates within the environment on which it depends for its survival (i.e., for sensory stimuli, oxygen, and nutrients). The environment also constitutes a potential threat to the system, in that some inputs (e.g., toxins and microorganisms) may be harmful. Humans depend on the environment for removal of system by-products or wastes. The output of the human system thus affects the environment as well. System output in any form may be redirected back into the system as information or **feedback**, which again affects the system in a cyclic manner.

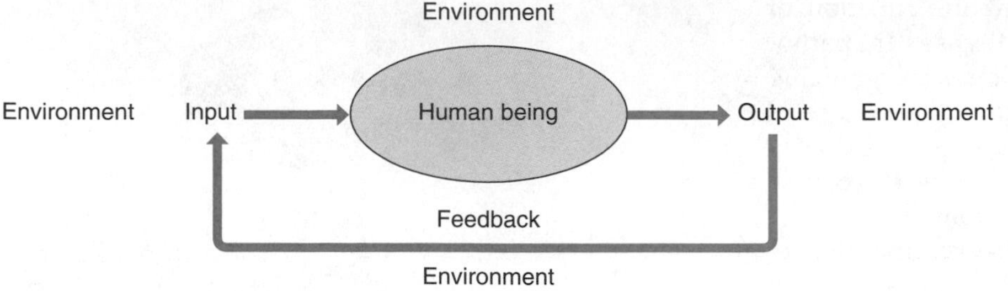

FIGURE 1–5
Elements of an open system. As an open system, the human body interacts with its environment. The body receives input from the environment, processes this input, and generates output to the environment. System output may be directed back into the human system as feedback, which influences system operation.

Relevance to Pathophysiology

Conceptualizing the human body as a system is a convenient way to organize disease processes and their effects into a coherent field of study. Organ systems are logical subsystems around which to organize the science of pathophysiology. Organs, tissues, cells, and subcellular elements may be considered subsystems of organ systems. Although the emphasis of pathophysiology is on the physical environment and physiologic subsystems, the critical importance of interpersonal, societal, cultural, and spiritual subsystems and environmental factors must be appreciated. These factors, beyond the scope of this text, may greatly influence maintenance of health, definition and incidence of disease, and the nature of and responses to clinical interventions.

In the application of general systems theory to pathophysiology, care must be taken not to focus too narrowly on subsystem function to the exclusion of consideration of the whole and of all environmental influences. Such reductionism in thinking, or superspecialization in clinical practice, may be detrimental to achieving optimal outcomes. Among the most difficult diseases to diagnose and treat are those that, at their onset, affect tissues of multiple organ systems (e.g., systemic lupus erythematosus). General systems theory may also attribute more predictability to human systems than actually exists. In research studies in which the effects of age, gender, genetic factors, culture, and social support are held constant, findings indicate that humans are still highly variable in their physiologic responses. When used within the context of **holism** (viewing the individual as an integrated whole or totality), however, general systems theory is a useful framework for the study of disease.

Stress

Stress is a term borrowed from physics in the 1930s by Hans Selye, a Canadian endocrinologist, to describe "the nonspecific results of any demand on the body."[8] Such a demand, or **stressor**, could originate from outside the body or from within, and would elicit a stereotypic, three-stage response, which Selye referred to as the **general adaptation syndrome** (Table 1–5). In systems terminology, stress could be seen as a disturbance of system func-

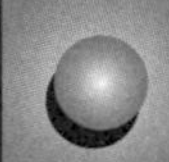

TABLE 1–5
GENERAL ADAPTATION SYNDROME

ALARM REACTION

Primary Regulation
Sympathetic–adrenomedullary system

Primary Responses
1. Hypothalamus signals sympathetic nervous system.
2. Sympathetic nervous system neurons release norepinephrine (NE) and trigger release of epinephrine (EPI) from adrenal medulla.
3. NE and EPI initiate increased vigilance and cardiovascular responses that serve organ systems critical to defense.
4. Parasympathetic nervous system suppresses growth and restorative functions.

STAGE OF RESISTANCE

Primary Regulation
Hypothalamic–pituitary–adrenocortical system

Primary Responses
1. Effects of EPI are sustained.
2. Hypothalamus releases corticotropin-releasing hormone (CRH)
3. CRH stimulates release of adrenocorticotropic hormone (ACTH) from the anterior pituitary.
4. ACTH stimulates release of cortisol from adrenal cortex.
5. Cortisol mobilizes energy stores to support continued defense and suppresses inflammatory and immune responses.

STAGE OF EXHAUSTION

Primary Regulation
Positive feedback loops

Primary Responses
1. Stress-related diseases
2. Multiple organ system failure
3. Death

tion arising from any force from within a subsystem or from the external environment.

Evolution of Stress Response Theories

Walter Cannon. In the 1920s, Walter Cannon, an American physician, published his first works describing a "fight or flight" reaction to emotional arousal or anxiety.[9] This response typically included increases in alertness, muscle tone, heart rate and contractile force, pupil dilation, rate and depth of respiration, and sweating. These physiologic responses were appropriate in primitive times when fighting and fleeing were the only survival options available to humans in the face of environmental hazards such as predatory animals. Cannon correctly attributed regulation of these responses to the sympathetic division of the autonomic nervous system, which mediates reflex, or automatic, adjustments in the function of internal organs in response to a variety of stimuli (see Chapter 22).

Hans Selye. Selye broadened the concept of fight or flight to incorporate responses to physical as well as psychological stimuli. He also described effects beyond the immediate period of confrontation with a stressor and characterized their regulation by the endocrine system. While a medical student in Austria, Selye worked as a laboratory assistant, conducting research on ovarian hormones. During his research, which called for injection of blenderized cow ovaries into rats, he noted a consistent response to injection of this impure substance: adrenal gland enlargement, shrinking of the thymus gland (an immune system organ), and ulceration of the gastrointestinal tract. At first, Selye attributed these effects to specific hormone actions, but later he noted these same responses to many other injected materials as well as to pain or other unpleasant stimuli.

In the course of his medical studies, Selye also observed similar clinical manifestations in hospitalized patients, despite their varied diagnoses. He at first referred to these findings as the "syndrome of just being sick,"[10] and later incorporated them into the general adaptation syndrome.

Selye concluded that the stress response was nonspecific—an automatic response to a stressor, whether psychological or physiologic, pleasant or unpleasant, mild or severe, real or imagined, present or anticipated. His characterization of the nature of stressors and the phases of the stress response is still widely accepted. The *nonspecific* aspect of his definition of stress, however, has been called into question by the more recent research of Mason, Lazarus, and others, discussed in the following sections.

John Mason. Mason's work with fasting and nonfasting monkeys revealed the presence of contextual (or cultural) variables influencing the stress response.[11] Fasting, an obvious physiologic stressor, elicited a stress response in monkeys that were denied food while housed with other monkeys that were fed. Fasting did *not* elicit a stress response when all monkeys housed together were treated equally. Mason also measured levels of "stress hormones," specifically **epinephrine, norepinephrine**, and **cortisol**, in varying conditions of stress in humans.[12] He noted differences in hormone levels that depended on the nature of the stressor, the coping state of the person (sleep-deprived versus rested), and whether the person had previously encountered the stressor.

Thomas Holmes. Thomas Holmes, an internist who practiced psychiatry for most of his medical career, also explored the relationship between stress and disease.[13] It had long been observed that not all people exposed to microorganisms are equally susceptible to development of infectious disease. Holmes' work with tuberculosis patients led him to believe that people who had experienced stressful situations, such as death of a spouse, divorce, or job loss, are more likely to develop tuberculosis and less likely to recover from it.

The Social Readjustment Rating Scale developed by Holmes and Rahe (Table 1–6) is perhaps the best-known example of early efforts to quantify the magnitude of the stress response and the likelihood of subsequent illness on the basis of the number and nature of stressors affecting an individual.[14] This instrument demonstrates the wide variety of life events (both positive and negative by societal definition) that may constitute stressors that can culminate in illness. In the years following publication of the scale, prospective studies demonstrated that 80% of patients who had a score of more than 300 points developed a serious illness within 2 years, compared with 30% of those who scored less than 150 points.[13] Subsequent research has validated the additional importance of the meaning of such events to the affected person as well as the numerous factors influencing that person's ability to cope. Also, the impact of chronic minor stressors may be as significant as that of isolated major events.

Richard Lazarus and Susan Folkman. The work of Lazarus and Folkman, of particular importance to the field of psychology, also refuted the nonspecific nature of the stress response.[15] Their *transaction theory* holds that the nature of the stress response and whether it occurs depend on the outcome of a person's appraisal of the stressor (as a threat, challenge, or opportunity) and that person's adequacy to cope with the stressor.

TABLE 1–6
SOCIAL READJUSTMENT RATING SCALE

Rank	Life Event	Mean Value
1	Death of spouse	100
2	Divorce	73
3	Marital separation	65
4	Jail term	63
5	Death of close family member	63
6	Personal injury or illness	53
7	Marriage	50
8	Fired at work	47
9	Marital reconciliation	45
10	Retirement	45
11	Change in health of family member	44
12	Pregnancy	40
13	Sexual difficulties	39
14	Gain of new family member	39
15	Business adjustment	39
16	Change in financial state	38
17	Death of close friend	37
18	Change to different line of work	36
19	Change in number of arguments with spouse	35
20	Mortgage or loan more than $10,000	31
21	Foreclosure of mortgage or loan	30
22	Change in responsibilities at work	29
23	Son or daughter leaving home	29
24	Trouble with in-laws	29
25	Outstanding personal achievement	28
26	Wife beginning or stopping work	26
27	Beginning or ending school	26
28	Change in living conditions	25
29	Revision of personal habits	24
30	Trouble with boss	23
31	Change in work hours or conditions	20
32	Change in residence	20
33	Change in school	20
34	Change in recreation	19
35	Change in church activities	19
36	Change in social activities	18
37	Mortgage or loan less than $10,000	17
38	Change in sleeping habits	16
39	Change in number of family get-togethers	15
40	Change in eating habits	15
41	Vacation	13
42	Christmas	12
43	Minor violations of the law	11

Adapted from Holmes, T. H., and Rahe, R. H. (1967). The Social Readjustment Rating Scale. *Journal of Psychosomatic Research* 11(2), 213–218. Used with permission. Copyright 1967 by Elsevier Science Inc.

Summary. Current stress theories, then, describe a typical physiologic response. Although predictable manifestations are seen, the stress response is not identical among all individuals and across all stressors. Rather, it is a *graded* response, variable in its intensity and duration, depending on numerous individual and environmental factors. Furthermore, there is a psychological intermediary between stressor and response. Examples of studies of the impact of stress on physiologic function and disease are summarized in the Focus of Current Research.

Physiologic Stress Response

Selye's general adaptation syndrome provides a framework for examining the typical stages of the stress response. The response is regulated by neural, endocrine, and local mechanisms (Fig. 1–6).

Stage 1: Alarm Reaction. When confronted with a stressor, a fight or flight response occurs within 2 to 3 seconds and typically persists for 5 to 10 minutes, during which the body prepares to either confront or escape. The stressor may be first perceived by association areas in the cerebral cortex of the brain through input from various sensors, such as the eyes, ears, or internal sensory receptors. Activation of the immune system also initiates a signal to the brain, presumably through release of **cytokines** (regulatory molecules) from immune cells.[16] The cortex may then signal the hypothalamus, a group of nerve cell bodies located deep in the brain in an area known as the *limbic system*. Alternatively, the hypothalamus may receive sensory input directly from internal receptors or cells, without cortical involvement. The hypothalamus, in reciprocal communication with nerve cells in the locus ceruleus of the brain stem, coordinates the stereotyped, or automatic, portion of the stress response by both neural and endocrine mechanisms.

During the alarm reaction, the hypothalamus activates the autonomic nervous system. The sympathetic division of this system is most important to the fight or flight aspect of the stress response, but the opposing parasympathetic nervous system is also active in stress. By suppressing less critical vegetative (basal or restorative) functions such as eating, digestion, and reproduction, the parasympathetic nervous system diverts energy to systems involved in combatting the stressor.

The sympathetic nervous system (SNS) secretes primarily norepinephrine from its nerve endings and triggers the secretion of both norepinephrine and epinephrine (adrenaline) from the adrenal medullae (see Chapter 22). Norepinephrine and epinephrine, known as *catecholamines* because of their chemical structures, may act locally as **neurotrans-**

Focus of Current Research

Study	Objective and Findings
Gillis (1993) Determinants of a health-promoting lifestyle: An integrative review.	*Objective:* To identify determinants of a health-promoting lifestyle *Findings:* Self-efficacy was the strongest predictor, followed by social support, perceived benefits, self-concept, perceived barriers, and health definition.
Berlin, et al. (1994) Suspected postprandial hypoglycemia is associated with β-adrenergic hypersensitivity and emotional distress.	*Objective:* To quantify sympathetic nervous system responsiveness and emotional distress in patients with low serum glucose after eating compared with control subjects *Findings:* Patients with symptoms of hypoglycemia had normal glucose tolerance when compared with controls but demonstrated increased sympathetic reactivity and emotional distress.
Yang, et al. (1995) Clinical significance of admission hyperglycemia and factors related to it in patients with acute severe head injury.	*Objective:* To assess the clinical importance of catecholamine levels and serum glucose levels during the period immediately after acute head injury *Findings:* Hyperglycemia and increased serum catecholamine levels were seen in head injury patients compared with controls. Levels of elevation correlated with injury severity and were predictive of outcome.
Lanuza (1995) Postoperative circadian rhythms and cortisol stress response to two types of cardiac surgery.	*Objective:* To compare patterns and magnitudes of cortisol stress responses in patients undergoing two types of surgery *Findings:* Cortisol levels increased significantly during the latter part of both operations. No significant differences in levels were found between groups. Circadian rhythms for cortisol, heart rate, and temperature were disturbed.
Boyce, et al. (1995) Psychobiologic reactivity to stress and childhood respiratory illnesses: Results of two prospective studies.	*Objective:* To investigate the relationships among environmental stressors, psychobiologic reactivity to stress, and infection in children *Findings:* Environmental stress was not an independent risk factor. Incidence of illness was associated with an interaction between childcare stress and sympathetic reactivity in one study and between stressful life events and immune reactivity in another.

Box continued on following page

Box continued from previous page

Hinds, et al. (1994) A comparison of the stress-response sequence in new and experienced pediatric oncology nurses.	*Objective:* To identify the specific components of the stress-response sequence in new and experienced pediatric oncology nurses *Findings:* New and experienced nurses have notably different stressors, reactions, and consequences.
Jiang, et al. (1996) Mental stress-induced myocardial ischemia and cardiac events.	*Objective:* To assess the clinical significance of mental stress-induced myocardial ischemia in patients with coronary artery disease. *Findings:* Ischemia induced by psychological stress is associated with increased incidence of fatal and nonfatal cardiac events, independent of patient age, left ventricular function, and previous myocardial infarction.

mitters to produce effects in organs directly innervated by the sympathetic nervous system, or they may enter the blood as **hormones** and produce effects by combining with receptors on organs not directly innervated (see Chapter 2).

Table 1–7 summarizes effects of catecholamines and other major mediators of the stress response. Norepinephrine causes constriction of blood vessels to organs such as the kidneys, gastrointestinal tract, and skin, thus diverting more blood to the skeletal

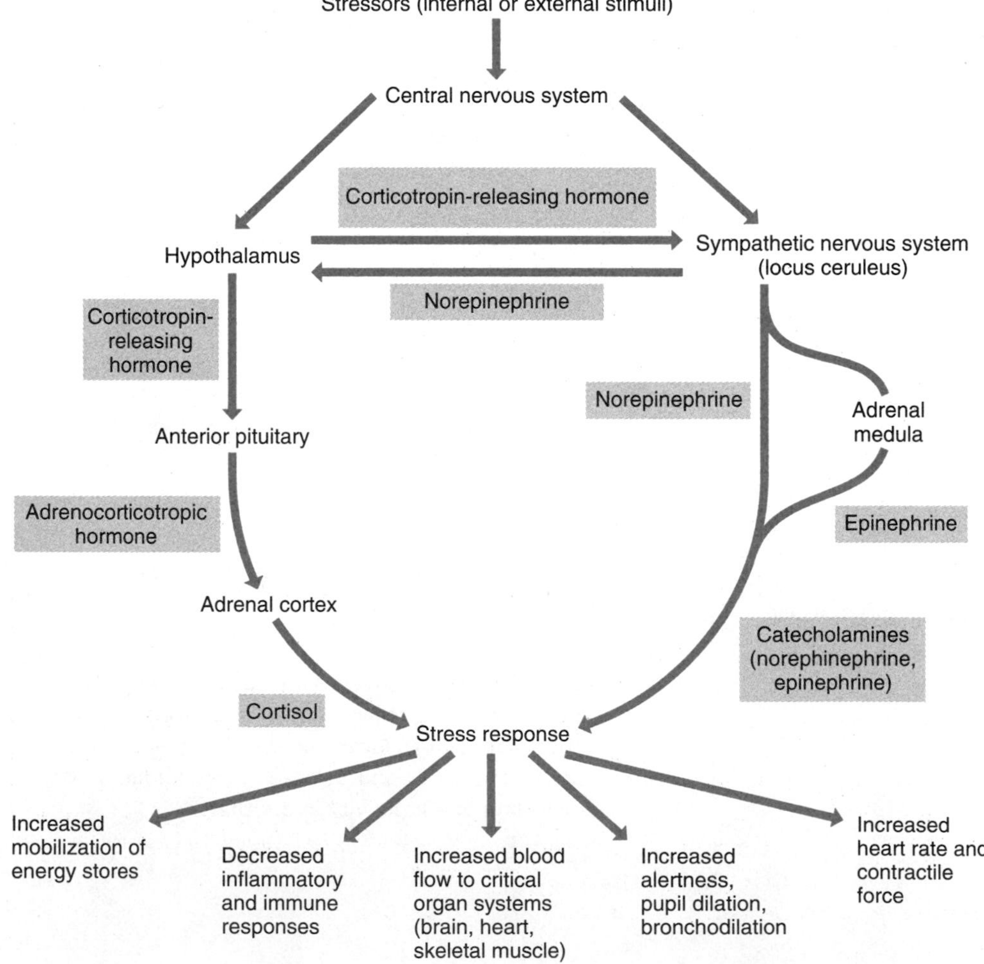

FIGURE 1–6
Neuroendocrine regulation of the stress response. The typical stress response is mediated by a complex interaction between neural effects, particularly sympathetic nervous system effects, and endocrine effects, primarily due to the "stress hormones" norepinephrine, epinephrine, and cortisol.

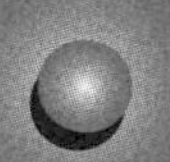

TABLE 1–7
PHYSIOLOGIC RESPONSES TO STRESS MEDIATORS AND ASSOCIATED CLINICAL MANIFESTATIONS

Physiologic Response	Clinical Manifestations
Catecholamine Effects (Epinephrine, Norepinephrine)	
Venous constriction to shunt pooled blood into central circulation; renin release	Bounding pulse; palpitations; elevated blood pressure
Increased heart rate and contractility	Rapid, bounding pulse; elevated blood pressure
Selective arteriolar vasoconstriction to distribute blood to critical systems (heart, brain, muscle)	Cool, clammy skin; decreased urine output; increased alertness; increased muscle strength; tremors; decreased appetite; difficulty swallowing; tension headache
Bronchodilation	Increased alveolar ventilation
Pupil dilation	Increased visual acuity; dilated but light-responsive pupils
Increased sweating	Damp skin, sweaty palms
Increased metabolic rate	Elevated temperature
Release of glucagon	Glucagon effects (see later section)
Corticotropin-Releasing Hormone Effects	
Activation of sympathetic nervous system	Catecholamine effects (see previous section)
Increased subjective fear	Anxiety; restlessness, insomnia; shortness of breath; hyperventilation
Release of adrenocorticotropic hormone (ACTH) and β-endorphin	ACTH effects (see next section); decreased pain perception
Adrenocorticotropic Hormone Effects	
Release of cortisol	Cortisol effects (see next section)
Stimulation of aldosterone and antidiuretic hormone release	Fluid retention
Cortisol Effects	
Increased glycogen breakdown	Energy surge; elevated blood glucose level
Increased catabolism of tissue proteins	Increased energy in the short term; fatigue and muscle wasting in the long term
Suppression of growth hormone and insulin action	Elevated blood glucose level
Inhibition of thyroid and gonadal function	Decreased sexual desire; absence of menstruation
Suppression of inflammatory and immune responses	Decreased pain perception; delayed wound healing; susceptibility to infection in the short term and possibly to cancer and autoimmune disorders in the long term
Glucagon Effects	
Increased glycogen breakdown and gluconeogenesis in the liver	Increased muscle strength; elevated temperature; elevated blood glucose level
Increased cardiac contractility	Bounding pulse; elevated blood pressure

muscles, heart, and brain—critical systems for fight or flight. Norepinephrine also mediates pupil dilation, bronchodilation, and sweating. Increased alertness occurs as a result of activation of the locus ceruleus of the brain stem by a norepinephrine stimulus.

Epinephrine influences these same responses; in addition, it causes increased heart rate and force of contraction and stimulates the pancreas to release the hormone glucagon. Glucagon promotes release of stored glucose from the liver, raising blood glucose and making "quick energy" available to the critical organ systems. Immune system cells have receptors for catecholamine hormones, but the predominant effect of stress on immune function (suppression of the immune response) is believed to be mediated by cortisol during the second stage of stress (see subsequent section and Chapter 13).

Stage 2: Stage of Resistance. The longer-term responses of the body to a persistent stressor are regulated in part by the catecholamines, which sustain, to some degree, the responses of the alarm reaction. Of greater importance during chronic stress, however, are the endocrine effects mediated by the hypothalamus. In its endocrine function, the hypothalamus signals release of *corticotropin-releasing hormone*, which (1) signals the locus ceruleus of the brain stem, influencing autonomic nervous system responses, and (2) stimulates the release of *adrenocorticotropic hormone* (ACTH) from the anterior pituitary gland. ACTH then triggers the secretion of cortisol from the adrenal cortex, the outer portion of the adrenal gland. This sequential stimulation of the hypothalamus, the anterior pituitary, and target endocrine organs is critical to endocrine system regulation and is discussed in detail in Chapter 27. In addition to cortisol secretion, activation of this hypothalamic–pituitary axis results in the secretion of a number of other hormones (e.g., thyroid hormones, sex hormones, growth hormone). Although all of these hormones and others may play a role in the stress response, cortisol-mediated effects are of greatest importance during the stage of resistance.

The primary effect of cortisol in stress is to mobilize energy stores from body tissues to the blood (see detailed discussion in Chapter 29), thus maintaining fuel for critical organ systems over a longer period. Cortisol promotes increased gluconeogenesis (glucose formation from protein and fat) in the liver and also suppresses cellular uptake of glucose except by exercising muscle. A secondary effect of cortisol is suppression of the inflammatory and immune responses, presumably to conserve energy and to decrease pain and swelling during active resistance to stress.

Circulating blood volume is maintained or enhanced by other hormones, including antidiuretic hormone (arginine vasopressin), renin, angiotensin II, and aldosterone (see Chapter 8). β-Endorphin, a hormone derived from the same molecule as ACTH, acts on opioid receptors in the brain to suppress pain (see Chapter 23). In addition to these hormones, several substances (typically peptides) are locally produced by specific cells, on which they exert their primary effects. These local mediators include protein-derived cytokines and lipid-derived mediators and are involved in tissue-level defense against cell injury (see Chapter 13).

Within cells, stress induces increased synthesis of specific proteins, often referred to as **heat shock proteins** because of the conditions under which they were discovered.[17] The importance of these stress proteins is becoming increasingly apparent. Heat shock proteins are known to be critical in mediating the cellular response to cortisol and may constitute the cellular link between prolonged stress and physiologic diseases (particularly autoimmune diseases) as well as psychiatric disorders (particularly clinical depression).[18]

Stage 3: Stage of Exhaustion. The ability of the body to withstand stress is limited. The neuroendocrine effects that are beneficial in the short term are detrimental in the long term. A sustained increase in heart rate and force of contraction, for example, consumes much energy. Because the heart must pump against increased resistance in constricted vessels, its workload is increased. Patients who have limited cardiovascular reserve function owing to cardiac disease are prone to cardiac failure under these conditions (see Chapter 16). Prolonged blood vessel constriction deprives noncritical organ systems of adequate oxygen, nutrients, and waste removal, eventually damaging these tissues. Stress ulceration of the gastrointestinal tract and acute renal failure are examples of conditions that may result from prolonged vasoconstriction (see Chapters 15 and 20).

As discussed in Chapter 29, cortisol-mediated mobilization of energy stores contributes to elevated blood glucose levels (hyperglycemia), which may damage the basement membranes of blood vessels and cause capillary fragility. Diversion of metabolism from anabolic (tissue-building) to catabolic (tissue-breakdown) processes leads, in the long term, to muscle wasting and redistribution of body fat (see Chapter 3). The anti-inflammatory and immunosuppressive effects of cortisol may increase the risk of infection, tumor growth, or autoimmune disorders and may aggravate existing tissue injury. The immune system may be involved in linking the stress response to both physiologic and psychological disorders. The relatively new science of **psychoneuroimmunology**, the study of interactions among behavior, the brain, and the immune system, focuses on the relationship between psychological states, such as anxiety and depression, and the immune system.[19] Regulation of the immune response is discussed in detail in Chapter 13.

In prolonged stress, then, the stress response may contribute to organ system failure, disease, and even death. Examples of disorders in which stress is a probable risk factor are listed in Table 1–8.

Adaptation and Homeostasis

Origin of the Concepts

The first writings that espoused a view of health as a harmonious balance of forces within the body, and disease as a disharmony of these elements, are centuries old. Early Greek physicians, including Hippocrates, proposed that imbalance, or disease, was due to natural, rather than supernatural, forces, and that counterbalancing forces were also natural—originating within the individual.[20] The concept of internal harmony as a dynamic equilibrium was proposed by Claude Bernard in the 19th century. Walter Cannon coined the term homeostasis to describe this state of internal (physiologic and psychological) balance or organization of function.

Adaptation refers to processes by which a system seeks to restore or maintain homeostasis. Adaptive

TABLE 1–8
EXAMPLES OF STRESS-RELATED DISORDERS

SYSTEM	DISEASE OR SYNDROME	CHAPTER
Immune	Neoplasia	7
	Autoimmune diseases	13
	Infectious diseases	13
Cardiovascular	Hypertension	15
	Vasovagal syncope	15
	Stress ulceration	15
	Coronary artery disease	16
	Cardiac dysrhythmias	17
Respiratory	Bronchial asthma	18
	Upper respiratory infection	18
	Tuberculosis	19
Renal and urinary	Interstitial cystitis	20
Neurologic	Clinical depression	21
	Sleep disorders	21
	Multiple sclerosis	22
	Headache	23
Gastrointestinal	Diarrhea	24
	Irritable bowel syndrome	24
	Eating disorders	25
Endocrine	Hyperthyroidism	28
	Diabetes mellitus	29
Reproductive	Amenorrhea	31
	Infertility	32
Musculoskeletal	Rheumatoid arthritis	34
	Systemic lupus erythematosus	34
	Chronic fatigue syndrome	35
Integumentary	Eczema	36
	Acne	36
	Urticaria	36
	Herpesvirus infection	36

mechanisms may also be referred to as *compensatory mechanisms, homeostatic mechanisms, control systems*, or *regulatory systems*. Although physiologic adaptive mechanisms are emphasized in this chapter, adaptation may be physiologic, psychological, or behavioral.

Feedback Loops

In systems terminology, adaptive mechanisms are examples of feedback to the system and may be represented by either negative or positive feedback loops. Nearly all physiologic adaptive responses are **negative feedback loops**. These processes act to restore homeostasis by inducing changes in the opposite direction of a force perturbing the system. For example, if injury with hemorrhage causes a decrease in blood pressure, sensors in blood vessels activate a neural response that causes increased cardiac pumping and constriction of blood vessels. These changes cause an increase in blood pressure—a change that negates the original disruption, closing the feedback loop and restoring the steady state. Other examples of negative feedback are shown in Figure 1–7.

In **positive feedback loops**, the response to a disruptive force is in the same direction as the force, thus tending to increase the instability of the system (Fig. 1–8). Positive feedback loops are almost always *maladaptive*, or harmful and are often termed *vicious cycles, downward spirals*, or *decompensation states*. These states can lead to death if not interrupted by treatment. In advanced shock, for example, the increased rate and pumping force of the heart eventually increase the demand of the heart muscle for oxygenated blood. The gap between oxygen supply and demand widens, and cardiac failure results. There are a few examples of *adaptive* positive feedback in humans (e.g., blood clotting, ovarian cycles), but these are always limited amplification effects that are part of a larger negative feedback loop.

Regulation of Adaptation

Physiologic adaptive responses act to restore system homeostasis that has been disrupted by environmental or behavioral changes, stress, or disease. These adaptive responses are regulated at three physiologic levels: (1) by the nervous system, which mediates rapid but short-acting responses; (2) by the endocrine system, which responds more slowly but with longer-lasting effects; and (3) by local, tissue-specific mechanisms mediated by cytokines and other secreted mediators or by intracellular proteins influencing genetic processes. As illustrated by the stress response, the interdependence of these regulatory systems facilitates fine control of physiologic processes. This complexity, however, also introduces multiple levels of possible system deregulation, constituting a potential basis for disease.

Limits of Adaptation

Adaptive mechanisms are essential to human function and in many cases are sufficient to overcome disrupting forces, including disease (i.e., natural healing, innate immunity). In other cases, however, adaptive responses may not completely restore homeostasis unless the disrupting force is removed (e.g., with definitive treatment or aversive behavior). Furthermore, adaptive mechanisms consume energy, and not all are equally efficient and effective. When disease is present, the function of one or more regu-

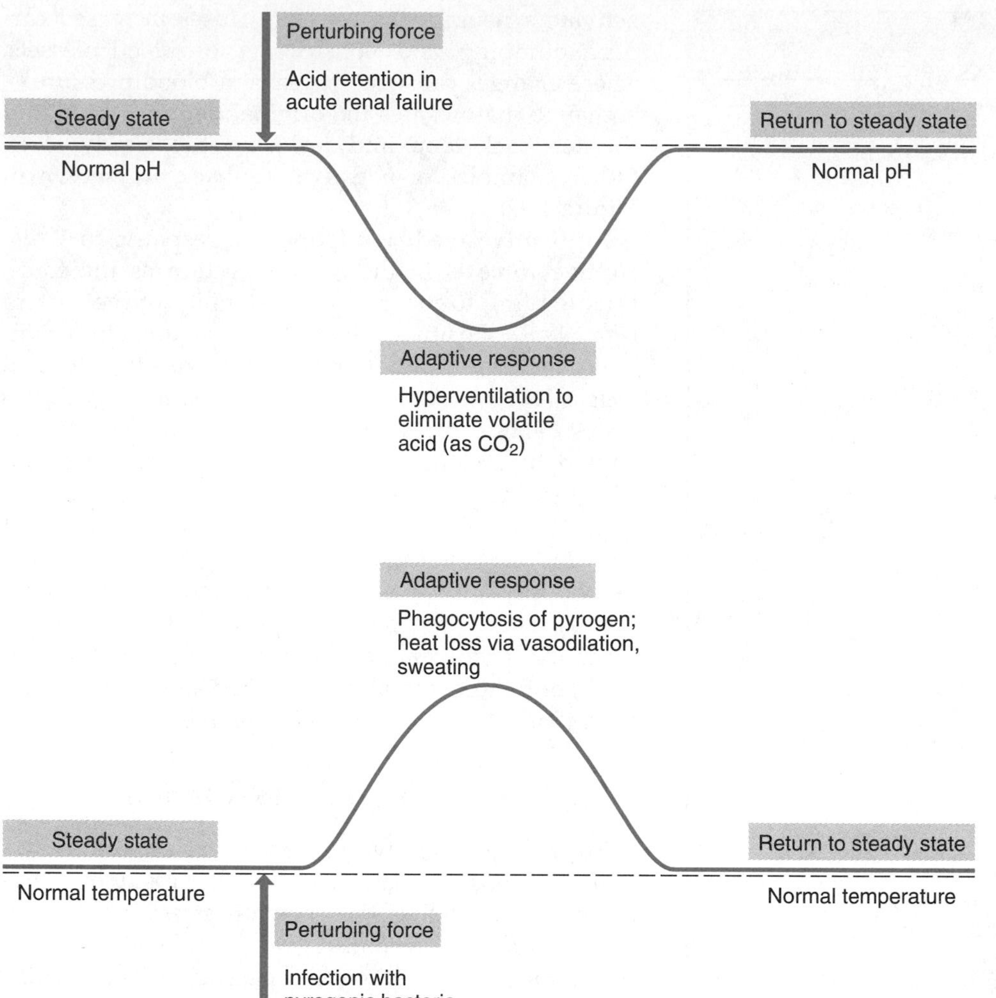

FIGURE 1–7

Negative feedback. Nearly all adaptive responses are negative feedback loops, which act to restore the steady state by inducing changes in the *opposite direction* of a force perturbing the system. Examples of processes regulating the pH of body fluids and body temperature are used to illustrate this concept.

latory systems may be compromised, resulting in "overshoot" or oscillation of negative feedback loops. Slowed blood flow in severe congestive heart failure, for example, results in delays between sensor and response within the major respiratory control system. This causes an abnormal, exaggerated waxing and waning pattern of breathing called *Cheyne-Stokes respirations* (Fig. 1–9).

As illustrated by the stress response, temporal factors affect adaptation as well. Responses that are initially adaptive may, if prolonged, create positive feedback loops, contributing to disease. Many of the clinical manifestations of disease are due to adaptive responses rather than to etiology. Rapid heart rate, elevated blood glucose, and fluid retention are common adaptive responses to the stressor of surgery, for example.

Developmental Factors

Adaptive processes and resulting clinical manifestations vary among individuals at different stages of physiologic development. For example, the dependence of the fetus on maternal systems for input and processing of nutrients and for elimination of wastes limits the range of independent fetal adaptation and imposes vulnerability to potentially harmful effects of external stressors (see Chapters 7 and 33). The fetus may respond to stressors such as labor with unique signs such as slowing of the heart rate and elimination of meconium (feces) into the amniotic fluid. Infants and young children have more limited adaptive capacity because of immature development of organ systems, notably the immune system (see Chapter 13). The growth and development of infants and children may be impeded by chronic stress because energy fuels are diverted to the stress response instead of to tissue building. Adolescents may also exhibit growth impairment, and onset of puberty may be delayed as a consequence of stress-induced hormonal alterations.

Adults of all ages are subject to different categories of occupational and other situational stressors as

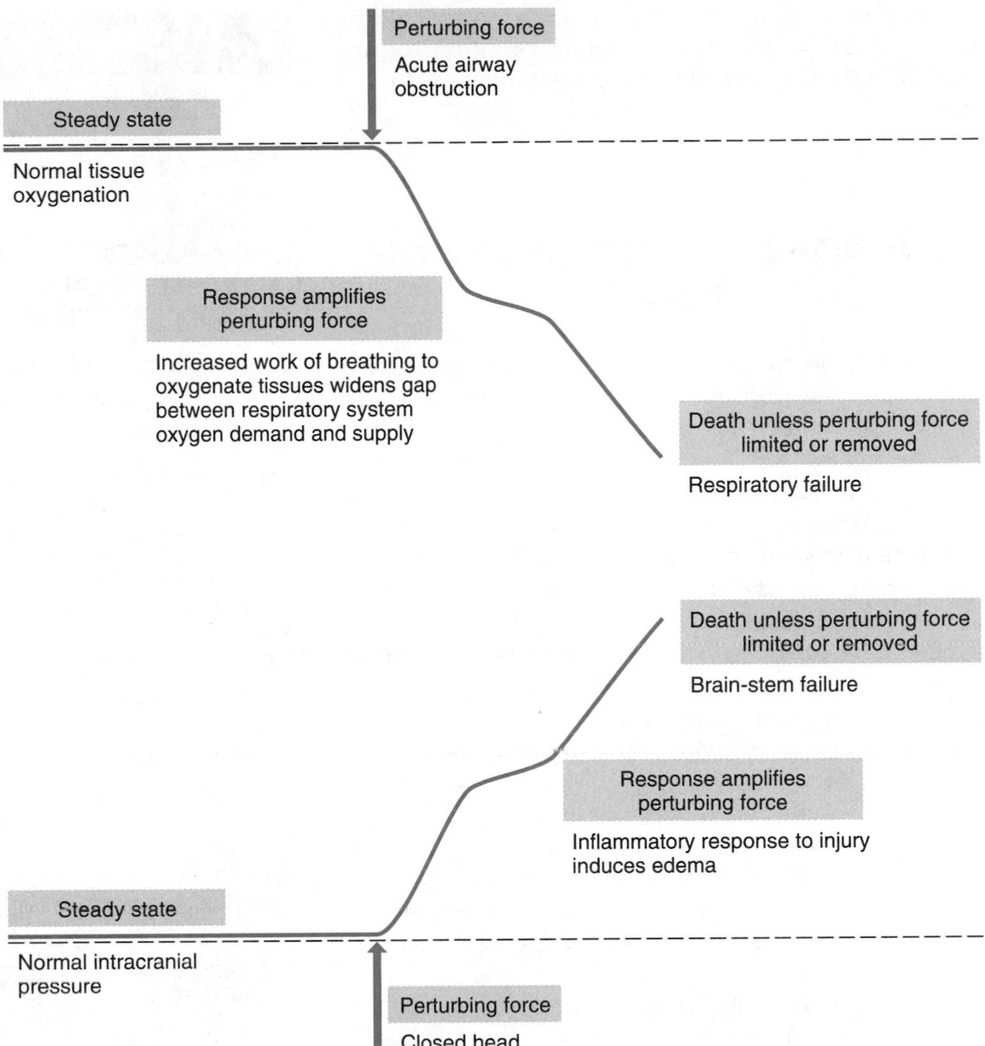

FIGURE 1–8
Positive feedback. Positive feedback loops usually represent maladaptive responses, in which the response to a perturbing force is in the *same direction* as this force, tending to increase the instability of the system. Maladaptive positive feedback loops lead to death unless interrupted by intervention. Examples related to the disrupting forces of acute airway obstruction and closed head injury are shown.

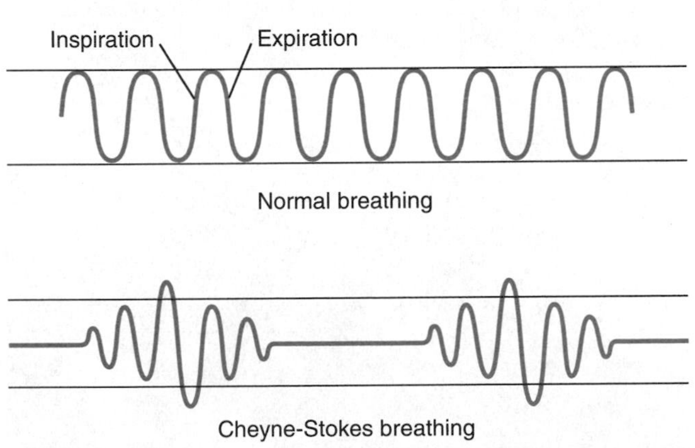

FIGURE 1–9
Oscillation in a negative feedback loop. Disease or dysfunction of regulatory systems may compromise adaptive responses, leading to clinical manifestations. In congestive heart failure, for example, slowed blood flow impairs signaling between peripheral sensors and the respiratory control center in the brain stem, resulting in an abnormal waxing and waning breathing pattern known as *Cheyne-Stokes respiration.*

well as to developmental stressors such as childbearing. Variation in physical fitness contributes to differing capacities for response to such stressors (see Chapter 35). The adaptive capacity of elderly people is limited by normal tissue changes with aging (see Chapter 6). The immune response, for example, declines with advancing age, increasing the risk of infection, autoimmune disorders, and neoplasia in the elderly. In many elderly people, the presence of chronic disease of the cardiovascular, respiratory, and other systems also limits adaptation.

Homeostatic end points also vary widely among individuals. Clinical reference points, or norms, for measurable physiologic parameters are statistically derived from group means but must often be adjusted on the basis of age, sex, height, or weight. Clinical norms may also vary owing to genetic, nutritional, or environmental factors. In addition, some parameters, such as temperature and circulating hormone levels, display natural cyclic variation (intrinsic biorhythms); thus, time of measurement also is a variable.

APPROACH TO THE STUDY OF DISEASE

Systems theory, stress, and adaptation provide a foundation for conceptual understanding of health and disease. Much of the language of clinical practice originates from these theoretical formulations. Effects of disease that disrupt total human function are referred to as *systemic*, and the physiologic adaptation that is seen in disease constitutes feedback to the system. Disease and its treatment are viewed as stressors, and stress is a contributing factor in many diseases. Disease may also be viewed as homeostatic imbalance or adaptive failure. The term homeostasis is commonly employed in reference to regulation of specific body constituents, for example, calcium homeostasis. Much clinical evidence of disease results not from specific etiologies but from more general stress responses and from specific neurologic, endocrine, and local adaptive responses. Understanding of the complexity of specific disease mechanisms is enhanced when viewed within this general theoretical context.

This textbook employs a general to specific approach to the study of disease. An overall framework for conceptualizing disease and its effects on human physiologic function has been introduced in this chapter and is used to describe specific disorders throughout the text. The remainder of Part One reviews basic physiologic and biochemical processes at the level of the cell and its environment. Abnormalities of these cellular processes and tissue responses constitute the most basic mechanisms of disease.

Beginning with Part Two, the study of disease within specific body systems is facilitated by a consistent format. Normal system structure and function are reviewed before a discussion of common disorders that illustrate all components of the disease process. Clinical interventions in each disorder are specifically related to the mechanisms of disease. In addition, developmental factors influencing diseases of each system are discussed, and examples of current research are included to illustrate advances in the understanding of the causes of system diseases as well as the rational basis of their clinical interventions.

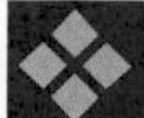

Summary of Key Points

- Pathophysiology is the study of human physiologic function in disease. It differs from other biomedical sciences in its focus on the mechanisms of disease.
- Mechanisms of disease are the dynamic processes that cause disease and give rise to signs and symptoms.
- Health and disease can be conceptualized as opposite directions on a continuum between the extremes of optimal wellness and death.
- Traditional intervention models treat the individual from the point of onset of clinical manifestations of disease, whereas more recent wellness models interact with the individual at any point on the health continuum.
- The five components of the disease process are epidemiology (risk factors and distribution in populations), etiology (causative mechanisms), pathophysiology (disease mechanisms), clinical manifestations (signs, symptoms, and diagnostic criteria), and outcome (cure, remission, chronicity, or death).
- Disease may be classified on the basis of anatomy (e.g., cardiovascular disease), development (e.g., pediatric disease), or etiology (e.g., infectious disease).
- Clinical intervention encompasses prevention (risk reduction) and treatment (definitive or palliative therapies).
- Conceptualization of the human body as a system is a convenient way of organizing disease processes and their effects into a coherent field of study.
- Stress theory has evolved over 75 years to encompass both physiologic and psychological stressors and both short- and long-term neuroendocrine responses. The stress response is stereotypic but not entirely nonspecific. Clinical manifestations of disease include manifestations of stress and adaptation as well as those responses due to the disease itself.
- Catecholamines mediate the initial alarm reaction during stress, whereas cortisol is the primary mediator during the stage of resistance. The stage of exhaustion is character-

ized by development of positive feedback loops.

- Homeostasis is the goal of adaptive responses.
- Negative feedback loops are aimed at restoration of the steady state, whereas positive feedback loops amplify disturbances in homeostasis.
- Adaptive responses are mediated by nervous, endocrine, and local autoregulatory signals.

REFERENCES

1. World Health Organization. (1946). Constitution of the World Health Organization. *Public Health Reports* 61(12), 1268.
2. Justice, B. (1994). Critical life events and the onset of illness. *Comprehensive Therapy* 20(4), 232–238.
3. Dunn, H.L. (1961). *High Level Wellness*. Arlington, VA: R.W. Beatty.
4. United States Department of Health and Human Services. (1992). Vital and health statistics: Current estimates from the National Health Interview Survey, 1991. Hyattsville, MD: USDHHS. (p. 14).
5. United States Department of Health and Human Services. (1991). *The International Classification of Diseases, Ninth Revision—Clinical Modifications*. (4th ed.). Volume 2. Diseases Index. Hyattsville, MD: USDHHS.
6. World Health Organization. (1992). *International Statistical Classification of Diseases and Related Health Problems, Tenth Revision*. Volume 1. Geneva: WHO.
7. von Bertalanffy, L. (1968). *General System Theory: Foundations, Development, Applications*. (Revised ed.). New York: George Braziller. (p. 37).
8. Selye, H.A. (1982). History and present status of the stress concept. In: Goldberger, L., and Breznitz, S. (Eds.). *Handbook of Stress: Theoretical and Clinical Aspects*. New York: The Free Press. (p. 7).
9. Cannon, W.B. (1932). *The Wisdom of the Body*. New York: W.W. Norton.
10. Selye, H. (1956). *The Stress of Life*. New York: McGraw-Hill Book Co. (p. 16).
11. Mason, J.W., Mangan, G.F., Brady, J.V., *et al.* (1961). Concurrent plasma epinephrine, norepinephrine, and 17-hydroxycorticosteroid levels during conditioned emotional disturbances in monkeys. *Psychosomatic Medicine* 23, 344–353.
12. Mason, J.W. (1975). A historical view of the stress field. Part I. *Journal of Human Stress* 1(1), 6–12.
13. Lerner, B.H. (1996). Can stress cause disease? Revisiting the tuberculosis research of Thomas Holmes, 1949–1961. *Annals of Internal Medicine* 124(7), 673–680.
14. Holmes, T.H., and Rahe, R.H. (1967). The Social Readjustment Rating Scale. *Journal of Psychosomatic Research* 11(2), 213–218.
15. Lazarus, R.S., and Folkman, S. (1984). *Stress, Appraisal, and Coping*. New York: Springer Publishing Co.
16. Black, P.H. (1994). Central nervous system-immune system interactions: Psychoneuroendocrinology of stress and its immune consequences. *Antimicrobial Agents and Chemotherapy* 38(1), 1–6.
17. Welch, W.J. (1992). Mammalian stress response: Cell physiology, structure/function of stress proteins, and implications for medicine and disease. *Physiological Reviews* 72(4), 1063–1081.
18. Minowada, G., and Welch, W.J. (1995). Clinical implications of the stress response. *Journal of Clinical Investigations* 95(1), 3–12.
19. Maier, S.F., Watkins, L.R., and Fleshner, M. (1994). Psychoneuroimmunology: The interface between behavior, brain, and immunity. *American Psychologist* 49(2), 1004–1017.
20. Langley, L.L. (1965). *Homeostasis*. New York: Van Nostrand Reinhold Co.

SELECTED BIBLIOGRAPHY

Armentrout, G. (1993). A comparison of the medical model and the wellness model: The importance of knowing the difference. *Holistic Nursing Practice* 7(4), 57–62.

Berlin, I., Grimaldi, A., Landault, C., *et al.* (1994). Suspected postprandial hypoglycemia is associated with β-adrenergic hypersensitivity and emotional distress. *Journal of Clinical Endocrinology and Metabolism* 79(5), 1428–1433.

Boyce, W.T., Chesney, M., Alkon, A., *et al.* (1995). Psychobiologic reactivity to stress and childhood respiratory illnesses: Results of two prospective studies. *Psychosomatic Medicine* 57(5), 411–422.

Bryan, R.M. Jr. (1990). Cerebral blood flow and energy metabolism during stress. *American Journal of Physiology*. 259(2 Pt. 2), H269–H280.

Cacioppo, J.T. (1994). Social neuroscience: Autonomic, neuroendocrine, and immune responses to stress. *Psychophysiology* 31(2), 113–128.

Centers for Disease Control and Prevention. (1994). Mortality patterns—United States, 1992. *Morbidity and Mortality Weekly Report* 43(49), 916–920.

Centers for Disease Control and Prevention. (1994). National notifiable diseases reporting—United States, 1994. *Morbidity and Mortality Weekly Report* 43(43), 800–801.

Chrousos, G.P., and Gold, P.W. (1992). The concepts of stress and stress system disorders: Overview of physical and behavioral homeostasis. *Journal of the American Medical Association* 267(9), 1244–1252.

Cohen, S. (1995). Psychological stress and susceptibility to upper respiratory infections. *American Journal of Respiratory Critical Care Medicine* 152(4 Pt. 2), S53–S58.

Collier, J.H. (1990). Developmental and systems perspectives on chronic illness. *Holistic Nursing Practice* 5(1), 1–9.

Deshpande, S., Platt, M.P.W., and Aynsley-Green, A. (1993). Patterns of metabolic and endocrine stress response to surgery and medical illness in infancy and childhood. *Critical Care Medicine* 21(9 suppl.), S359–S361.

Dorn, L.D., and Chrousos, G.P. (1993). The endocrinology of stress system disorders in adolescence. *Endocrinology and Metabolism Clinics of North America* 22(3), 685–700.

Elder, J.P., Geller, E.S., Hovell, M.F., *et al.* (1994). *Motivating Health Behavior*. Albany, NY: Delmar Publishers Inc.

Epstein, R.S., and Sherwood, L.M. (1996). From outcomes research to disease management: A guide for the perplexed. *Annals of Internal Medicine* 124(9), 832–837.

Gillis, A.J. (1993). Determinants of a health-promoting lifestyle: An integrative review. *Journal of Advanced Nursing* 18(3), 345–353.

Goodman, A. (1991). Organic unity theory: The mind-body problem revisited. *American Journal of Psychiatry* 148(5), 553–563.

Herd, J.A. (1991). Cardiovascular response to stress. *Physiological Reviews* 71(1), 305–330.

Hinds, P.S., Quargnenti, A.G., Hickey, S.S., *et al.* (1994). A comparison of the stress-response sequence in new and experienced pediatric oncology nurses. *Cancer Nursing* 17(1), 61–71.

Jiang, W., Babyak, M., Krantz, D.S., *et al.* (1996). Mental stress-induced myocardial ischemia and cardiac events. *Journal of the American Medical Association* 275(21), 1651–1656.

Kiecolt-Glaser, J.K., and Glaser, R. (1995). Psychoneuroimmunology and health consequences: Data and shared mechanisms. *Psychosomatic Medicine* 57(3), 269–274.

Lanuza, D.M. (1995). Postoperative circadian rhythms and cortisol stress response to two types of cardiac surgery. *American Journal of Critical Care* 4(3), 212–220.

LaPerriere, A., Ironson, G., Antoni, M.H., *et al.* (1993). Exercise and psychoneuroimmunology. *Medicine and Science in Sports and Exercise* 26(2), 182–190.

Leape, L.L. (1994). Error in medicine. *Journal of the American Medical Association* 272(23), 1851–1857.

Leutwyler, K. (1995). The price of prevention. *Scientific American* 272(4), 124–129.

Lewis-Fernandez, R., and Kleinman, A. (1995). Cultural psychiatry: Theoretical, clinical, and research issues. *The Psychiatric Clinics of North America* 18(3), 433–448.

Maddox, J. (1993). Has nature overwhelmed nurture? (Editorial.) *Nature* 366(6451), 107.

Marcucilli, C.J., and Miller, R.J. (1994). CNS stress response: Too hot to handle? *Trends in Neurosciences* 17(4), 135–138.

McDaniel, J.S. (1992). Psychoimmunology: Implications for future research. *Southern Medical Journal* 85(4), 388–402.

McGinnis, J.M., and Foege, W.H. (1993). Actual causes of death in the United States. *Journal of the American Medical Association* 270(18), 2207–2212.

Nazarro, P., Merlo, M., Manzari, M., *et al.* (1993). Stress response and antihypertensive treatment. *Drugs* 46(suppl. 2), 133–141.

Perrin, E.C., Newacheck, P., Pless, I.B., *et al.* (1993). Issues involved in the definition and classification of chronic health conditions. *Pediatrics* 91(4), 787–793.

Porges, S.W. (1992). Vagal tone: a physiologic marker of stress vulnerability. *Pediatrics* 90(3), 498–504.

Pruessner, H.T., Hensel, W.A., and Rasco, T.L. (1992). The scientific basis of generalist medicine. *Academic Medicine* 67(1992), 232–235.

Purtilo, D.T., and Purtilo, R.B. (1989). *A Survey of Human Diseases.* (2nd ed.). Boston: Little, Brown & Co.

Robinson, L. (1990). Stress and anxiety. *Nursing Clinics of North America* 25(4), 935–943.

Sadler, J.Z., and Hulgus, Y.F. (1992). Clinical problem solving and the biopsychosocial model. *American Journal of Psychiatry* 149(10), 1315–1323.

Schneiderman, N., and McCabe, P.M. (1985). Biobehavioral responses to stressors. In: Field, T.M., McCabe, P.M., and Schneiderman, N. (Eds.). *Stress and Coping*. Hillsdale, NJ: Lawrence Erlbaum Associates, Publishers.

Selye, H.A. (1956). *The Stress of Life*. New York: McGraw-Hill Book Co.

Selye, H.A. (1974). *Stress Without Distress*. New York: Signet (New American Library, Inc.).

Stanford, G.C. (1994). The stress response to trauma and critical illness. *Critical Care Nursing Clinics of North America* 6(4), 693–702.

Sternberg, E.M., Chrousos, G.P., Wilder, R.L., *et al.* (1992). The stress response and the regulation of inflammatory disease. *Annals of Internal Medicine* 117(10), 854–866.

Taubes, G. (1995). Epidemiology faces its limits. *Science* 269(5221), 164–169.

Taylor, E. (1992). New international disease classification. *Health Reports* 4(3), 331–333.

Travis, J.W., and Ryan, R.S. (1988). *Wellness Workbook*. Berkeley, CA: Ten Speed Press.

U.S. Department of Health and Human Services. (1992). *Vital and Health Statistics: Current Estimates from the National Health Interview Survey, 1991*. Hyattsville, MD: USDHHS.

Udelsman, R., and Holbrook, N.J. (1994). Endocrine and molecular responses to surgical stress. *Current Problems in Surgery* 31(8), 658–720.

von Bertalanffy, L. (1975). *Perspectives on General System Theory: Scientific-Philosophical Studies*. New York: George Braziller.

Wilson, I.B., and Cleary, P.D. (1995). Linking clinical variables with health-related quality of life: A conceptual model of patient outcomes. *Journal of the American Medical Association* 273 (1), 59–65.

World Health Organization. (1946). Constitution of the World Health Organization. *Public Health Reports* 61(12), 1268.

Yang, S., Zhang, S., and Wang, M. (1995). Clinical significance of admission hyperglycemia and factors related to it in patients with acute severe head injury. *Surgical Neurology* 44(4), 373–377.

Unit II

Chapter 2
Cell Structure and Intercellular Communication

Chapter 3
Cellular Nutrition and Energy Metabolism

Chapter 4
Electrophysiology: Action Potentials and Conduction

Chapter 5
Cellular Mechanism of Muscle Contraction

Chapter 6
Cellular Development: Genetic Regulation, Embryology, and Aging

Chapter 7
Cellular Development: Congenital Defects and Neoplasia

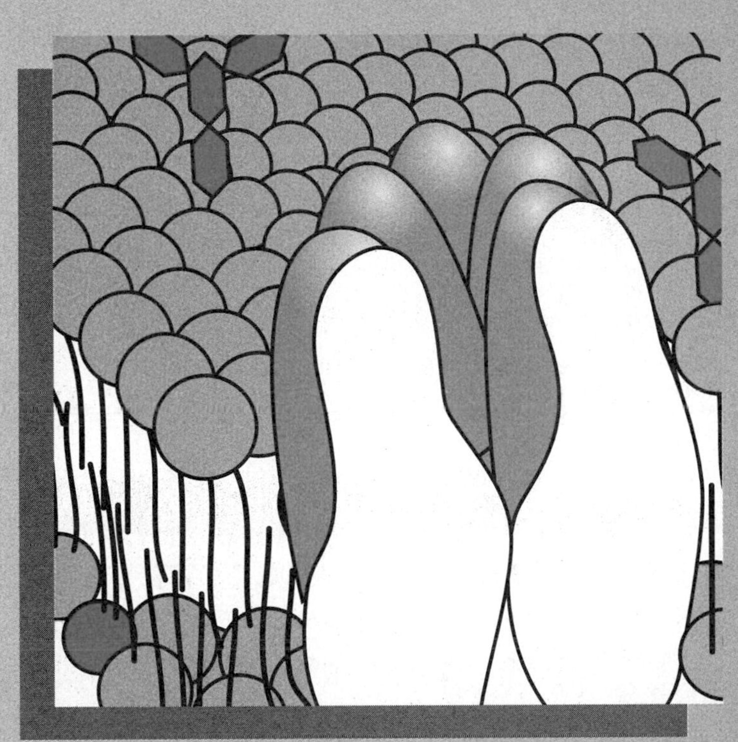

CELLULAR PERSPECTIVE

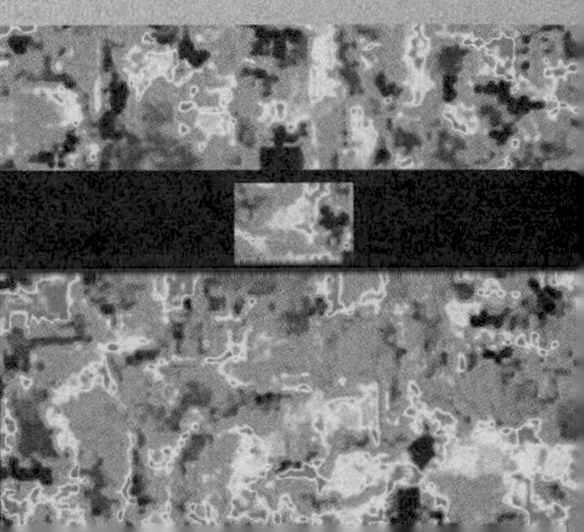

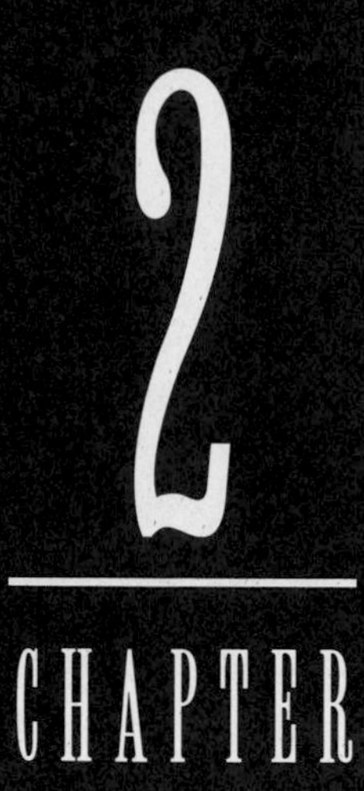

Cell Structure and Intercellular Communication

LEARNING OBJECTIVES

1. Describe the structure and general function of the cell and its components.
2. Relate concepts of molecular adhesion to selective membrane permeability and transport.
3. Compare and contrast mechanisms of gradient-related and gradient-independent membrane transport.
4. Discuss categories and examples of endogenous and exogenous signaling molecules.
5. Differentiate among receptor types on the basis of location, structure, and function.
6. Identify the four principal mechanisms of signal transduction.
7. Differentiate between short-term and long-term cellular responses to receptor-mediated signals.
8. Discuss mechanisms by which receptor function may be regulated.
9. Discuss general mechanisms through which abnormal intercellular communication may cause or result from disease.

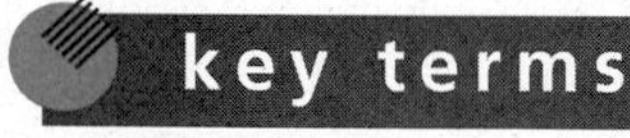

key terms

active transport
adhesion molecule
adhesive junction
agonist
antagonist
autocrine
bulk flow
cadherin
concentration gradient
cotransport
countertransport
electrical gradient
endocrine
endocytosis
epithelial transport
exocytosis
facilitated diffusion
gap junction
G protein
hydrostatic pressure
immunoglobulin superfamily
integrin
intercellular adhesion molecule (I-CAM)
intermediate filament
ligand-gated channel
mechanically gated channel
microfilament
microtubule
neural cell adhesion molecule (N-CAM)
osmotic pressure
paracrine
passive transport
phagocytosis
pinocytosis

pressure gradient
receptor
receptor-mediated endocytosis
receptor tyrosine kinase
secondary active transport
selectin
simple diffusion
solvent drag
tight junction
vesicle
voltage-gated channel

The dynamic processes of life take place within and between an estimated 100 trillion cells, the basic functional units of the body. Many normal and adaptive processes, as well as mechanisms of disease and clinical intervention, are best understood by examining them at the cellular level. Consistent with systems theory, dysfunction at the cellular and subcellular levels manifests as disruption of both organ system function and total human function.

Organization of individual cells into functional systems requires some means of interaction between them. Intercellular communication depends on structural characteristics of cells and on the operation of biochemical and molecular pathways that are responsive to a variety of signals. Alteration of these communication mechanisms is a common denominator in many disorders, whether as a component of the etiology or a result of pathophysiologic processes.

Body cells vary in their structure and function. Characteristics of the *typical* cell are described in this chapter, along with intercellular communication processes and their regulation. The relationships between altered communication and disease are also examined, as are potential applications of these concepts to clinical intervention.

OVERVIEW OF CELLULAR STRUCTURE AND FUNCTION

The two general classes of cells in the biologic world are relevant to the study of disease in human systems. Because they contain nuclei at some stage of their development, human cells are classified as *eukaryotes*. Bacteria, in contrast, are non-nucleated and are classified as *prokaryotes*. Most eukaryotes are composed of (1) an outer boundary, or *plasma membrane*; (2) an interior fluid matrix, or *cytoplasm*; (3) a nucleus; (4) several membrane-bound compartments, or *organelles*; and (5) a protein scaffold, the *cytoskeleton*. Figure 2–1 depicts a typical human cell.

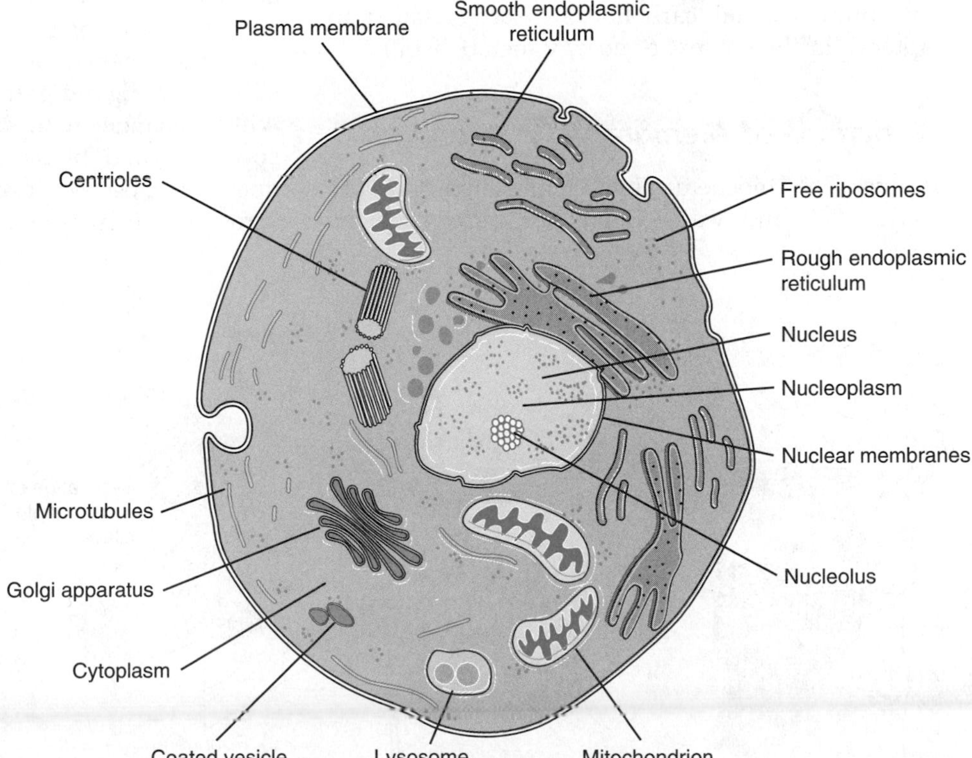

FIGURE 2–1
Typical eukaryotic cell. Body cells vary widely depending on their function; however, all human cells are bounded by a plasma membrane and contain a fluid cytoplasm with specialized organelles. All eukaryotes, including human cells, have nuclei at some stage of their development. A protein cytoskeleton composed of microtubules and other fibers provides structural support and organization of the cytoplasm.

Plasma Membrane

General Structure

The human plasma membrane has a fluid mosaic structure, first described by Singer and Nicholson in 1972.[1] The membrane is composed of a double layer of *phospholipids*, molecules composed of phosphorus and fatty acid–containing lipids (Fig. 2–2). Membrane phospholipids are *amphipathic*, that is, they have distinct polar and nonpolar segments. *Polarity* refers to a separation of electrical charge derived from the configuration of chemical bonds within the molecule. Polar molecules are more soluble in water, whereas nonpolar molecules are more soluble in lipid. Membrane phospholipids are arranged so that their polar, *hydrophilic* (water-loving), phosphorus-containing "heads" are oriented toward the watery exterior and interior of the cell. Their nonpolar, *hydrophobic* (water-hating), hydrocarbon "tails," which could also be described as *lipophilic*, or fat-loving, are oriented toward the interior of the membrane.

Embedded within these membrane lipids are *integral* proteins, while additional *peripheral* proteins are associated with the membrane at its intracellular surface. Integral proteins are important to the transport of substances across the membrane, whereas peripheral proteins are components of signaling pathways, discussed later in this chapter. Many membrane proteins and lipids have attached carbohydrate groups, forming a loose network or cell coat known as the *glycocalyx*. (The chemical structures of lipids, proteins, and carbohydrates are detailed in Chapter 3, in the context of energy metabolism.)

Functions of Membrane Components

Lipids. The biochemical principle stated in lay terms as "oil and water don't mix" underlies the principal function of the lipid bilayer: to serve as a barrier between the watery extracellular and intracellular compartments. The plasma membrane permits some substances, particularly gases (e.g., oxygen and carbon dioxide) and small, electrically neutral, lipid-soluble particles (e.g., urea and ethanol) to enter the cell. At the same time, it selectively excludes large, charged, or water-soluble particles (e.g., glucose, ions, and amino acids). Membrane lipids are also important in intercellular communication, serving as signaling molecules and components of certain biochemical pathways, as discussed later in this chapter.

Proteins. Membrane proteins may form watery channels through the membrane, allowing selective entry of polar molecules, or they may act as transporters or pumps, facilitating entry of molecules that bind to them. Membrane **receptors**, an essential component of most communication mechanisms, are usually proteins or glycoproteins (protein–carbohydrate molecules). Protein channels, transporters, and pumps are essential to the transport of most substances across biologic membranes. Binding of a substance (ligand) to a receptor is the initiating event in most pathways, mediating intercellular communication and regulation of physiologic function. These functions of membrane proteins are detailed subsequently.

Membrane Channels. Channel proteins are interspersed within membrane lipids and may or may not move freely within the membrane. As shown in cross-section in Figure 2–3, membrane channels may be either leak channels (continuously open) or gated channels (opened or closed, depending on specific stimuli). A **ligand-gated channel** may open or close with a change in the shape of the protein when a specific ligand binds to it. **Voltage-gated channels** open or close with changes in electrical voltage across the membrane, whereas **mechanically gated**

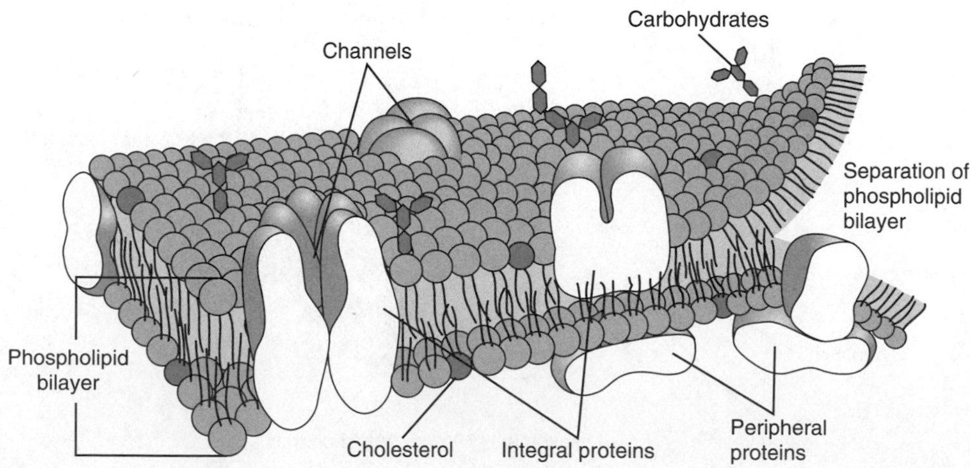

FIGURE 2–2
Fluid mosaic model of the plasma membrane. When viewed from above, the plasma membrane appears to be a composition of individual pieces, analogous to tiles in a mosaic. The components are the polar heads of membrane phospholipids and the embedded membrane proteins. Membrane lipids separate the watery intracellular and extracellular compartments, while proteins mediate selective transport and intercellular signaling pathways.

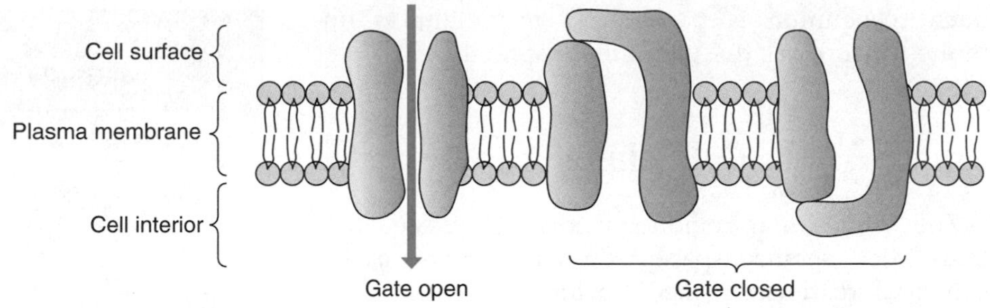

FIGURE 2–3
Membrane protein channels. Integral membrane proteins may form watery channels through the membrane, permitting passage of polar substances such as ions. Channels may be continuously open *(leak channels)* or intermittently open or closed in response to stimuli that change the shape of the protein subunits *(gated channels).*

channels open in response to deforming forces, such as pressure or friction.

Leak channels are important structural components of *pacemaker cells* in cardiac tissue as well as in some neural tissues and smooth muscle. As discussed in Chapter 4, continuous transport of charged particles (ions) through these channels is critical to the ability of pacemaker cells to generate an electrical signal. In the heart, this mechanism is the basis of the origin of the heartbeat. In the central nervous system, it governs the rate of entry of ascending electrical signals to the cerebral cortex. In the smooth muscle of the intestine, pacemaker activity permits mixing and propulsive movements in the absence of neural stimuli.

Voltage-gated channels are essential to intercellular signaling in "excitable" tissues, that is, nervous tissue and the three types of muscle: cardiac, skeletal, and smooth. As discussed in Chapters 4 and 5, transport of ions across the membranes of these cells is the basis of generation of the electrical signal in neurotransmission, cardiac conduction, and muscle contraction.

Ligand-gated channels are also classified as a receptor type. Binding of a ligand (e.g., hormone, neurotransmitter, or drug) to a channel protein induces opening or closing of the channel, altering ion flux and resulting in a change in cellular function. Function of channel-associated receptors is discussed in more detail later in this chapter.

Mechanically gated channels are important components of pressure sensors in blood vessels (baroreceptors), tactile receptors in the skin, and other specialized endings of sensory nerves. These sensory receptors initiate an electrical signal on deformation by physical stimuli (see Chapter 23).

Transport Proteins. Membrane proteins may also serve as transport proteins (transporters or pumps). Binding of molecules to these proteins induces a conformational change (protein refolding or reshaping), which moves the bound substance into or out of the cell. Transport proteins are classified as follows: *uniports* move one substance in one direction; *symports* move two or more different substances in one direction; and *antiports* move different substances in opposite directions simultaneously (Figure 2–4). **Cotransport** mechanisms use symport proteins, whereas **countertransport** mechanisms use antiports.

Receptors. Except in the context of sensory nerve function, the term *receptor* refers to specialized regions of proteins or glycoproteins located on the plasma membrane, on organelle membranes, on genetic material in the nucleus, or in the cytoplasm. Receptors contain binding sites (specific chemical sequences) that recognize and bind certain ligands, setting in motion a chain of events that culminates in either short-term or long-term alterations in cell function. The structures of ligand and receptor must be highly compatible in terms of molecular shape, surface charges, and binding groups.

Carbohydrates. As has been stated, some membrane lipids and proteins have carbohydrate groups attached, forming a glycocalyx. These surface glycolipids and glycoproteins serve as recognition sites or cellular markers that may facilitate receptor binding.

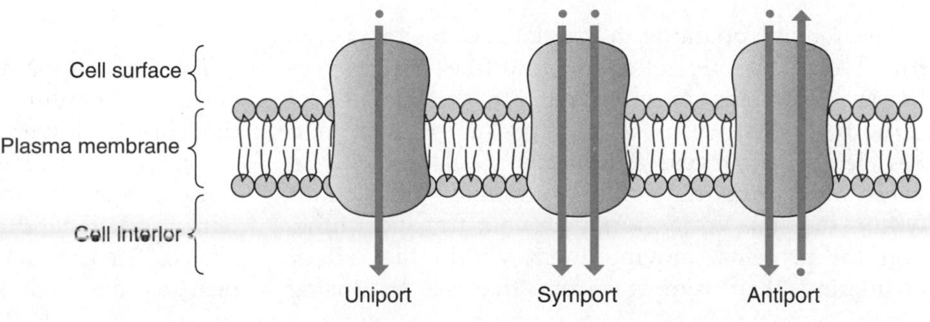

FIGURE 2–4
Classes of transport proteins. *Uniports* move one substance in a single direction, while *symports* move two or more different substances in a single direction. *Antiports* move two or more different substances in opposite directions.

Such recognition is particularly important to immune function, as discussed in Chapter 13.

Cytoplasm

The intracellular region outside the nucleus contains thick, semitransparent fluid that serves as the solvent and transport medium for substances within the cell. The cytoplasm is 75% to 90% water, containing carbohydrates, soluble proteins, and inorganic molecules. Advances in electron microscopy have revealed that the cytoplasm is not merely a "soup" with randomly scattered components, but rather a highly organized medium, with functional networks defined by membrane-enclosed organelles and the protein cytoskeleton.[2] The term *cytosol* refers to the part of the cytoplasm that is not contained within organelles.

Organelles

The cytoplasm is subdivided structurally and functionally by organelles—membrane-bound structures that serve specialized functions within the cell (Table 2–1). The largest of the organelles is the nucleus, discussed separately later. Others include the endoplasmic reticulum, Golgi apparatus, lysosomes, peroxisomes, ribosomes, and mitochondria.

TABLE 2–1
ORGANELLES AND THEIR FUNCTIONS

Organelle	Primary Functions
Endoplasmic reticulum	
Smooth	Site of synthesis of membrane lipids; calcium reservoir
Rough	Site of protein synthesis
Golgi apparatus	Modification of newly synthesized proteins; packaging of proteins into vesicles for transport
	Processing of newly synthesized lipids for dispersion or discharge from the cell
Lysosome	Isolation and degradation of damaged or aged cellular components
	Digestion of foreign substances (phagocytosis)
Peroxisome	Metabolism of fatty acids, producing heat but no ATP
Ribosome	
Free ribosome	Synthesis of proteins destined for use within the cell
Attached to endoplasmic reticulum	Synthesis of proteins destined for transport from the cell
Mitochondrion	Oxidative energy metabolism
Nucleus	Genetic regulation of cell structure and function

Endoplasmic Reticulum

Most cells have two types of endoplasmic reticulum: smooth and rough. The smooth type serves as the site of synthesis of new membrane lipids in most cells. In muscle cells, the smooth endoplasmic reticulum functions as a calcium reservoir and is called the *sarcoplasmic reticulum*. The rough appearance of the rough endoplasmic reticulum is due to attached ribosomes. The rough type is attached to the nuclear membrane and is the site of protein synthesis in cells, a process detailed in Chapter 6.

Golgi Apparatus

The Golgi apparatus, a specialized region of the rough endoplasmic reticulum, modifies newly synthesized proteins by glycosylation (attachment of carbohydrate molecules) and packages them into **vesicles**. This process apparently labels proteins in ways that determine their ultimate destinations within the cell. Vesicles may serve a transport function for proteins, moving them within the cell or facilitating their removal from the cell by fusing with the cell membrane in a process known as exocytosis, discussed later in this chapter. Lipids synthesized by the smooth endoplasmic reticulum also pass through the Golgi apparatus, which may disperse them as droplets within the cytoplasm or package them for discharge from the cell. Not surprisingly, secretory cells such as those of the endocrine system and gastrointestinal tract have the most highly developed Golgi complexes.

Lysosomes

The Golgi apparatus also manufactures lysosomes, vesicles containing hydrolytic (digestive) enzymes that break down complex molecules into smaller subunits. Lysosomes isolate and degrade damaged cellular components, such as membrane lipids, proteins, and genetic material, as well as foreign substances, such as bacterial toxins. Lysosomes also attach to aged or defective organelles, degrading them. Lysosomal enzymes work only in an acidic environment, maintained within the lysosome by a hydrogen pump in its membrane. Lysosome storage diseases are rare genetic disorders in which lysosomal function is abnormal, causing accumulation of some substance that is normally cleared from the cell by lysosomes (Table 2–2).

Peroxisomes

Smaller vesicles, called *peroxisomes*, are the principal sites of fatty acid breakdown in cells, although the mitochondria in liver tissue may also metabolize fatty acids for energy (see Chapter 3). Peroxisomes contain oxidase enzymes, which break down lipids and amino acids to a corrosive substance, hydrogen peroxide (H_2O_2). Another peroxisomal enzyme, catalase, then metabolizes hydrogen peroxide to water and oxygen. Unlike mitochondrial oxidation, no energy in the form of adenosine triphosphate (ATP) is produced by this reaction. Heat produced during peroxisomal oxidation is released to the cytoplasm.

A rare genetic disorder, adrenoleukodystrophy, results in severe neurologic dysfunction and death. This disorder is caused by absence of a membrane transport protein that normally facilitates uptake of a critical enzyme into peroxisomes.

TABLE 2–2
LYSOSOME STORAGE DISEASES

Disorder	Clinical Features
Tay-Sachs disease	Gangliosides accumulate in nerve and retinal cells. Motor and mental retardation become evident at 6 months of age, with death at 2 to 3 years of age. One in 30 Ashkenazi Jews is a carrier of the defect.
Niemann-Pick disease	Sphingomyelin and cholesterol accumulate in tissue macrophages in the spleen, liver, lymph nodes, bone marrow, tonsils, gastrointestinal tract, and lungs. Cells of the brain and eyes may also be involved. Severity varies from organ enlargement with no nervous system involvement to death within the first 3 years of life.
Gaucher's disease	Glucocerebroside accumulates in phagocytic cells and, in some cases, in nervous system cells. Severity and course are variable.
Mucopolysaccharidoses	Glycosaminoglycans accumulate in phagocytic cells, endothelial cells, intimal smooth muscle cells, and fibroblasts throughout the body. Seven types are recognized that vary in severity and course.

Data from Cotran, R.S., Kumar, V., and Robbins, S.L. (1994). *Robbins Pathologic Basis of Disease.* (5th ed.). Philadelphia: W.B. Saunders (pp. 138–145).

Ribosomes

Ribosomes are small cytoplasmic granules composed of ribosomal ribonucleic acid and several proteins. Ribosomes synthesize specific proteins as directed by the genetic code (see Chapter 6). Ribosomes exist in two forms: free in the cytoplasm and attached to the rough endoplasmic reticulum. Free ribosomes synthesize proteins for use within the cell, whereas attached ribosomes synthesize proteins destined for transport out of the cell.

Mitochondria

The intracellular organelles that are most important in energy metabolism are the mitochondria. These elongated, oval structures are surrounded by double-layered membranes and contain their own genetic material (mitochondrial DNA). Mitochondria also contain the enzymes necessary for the oxygen-dependent reactions involved in the production of energy from ingested nutrients or catabolism of body tissues (see Chapter 3).

Nucleus

With the exception of mature red blood cells, every body cell has at least one nucleus. This oval or spheric structure contains its own fluid matrix (nucleoplasm) and protein scaffold (core filaments) as well as the hereditary factors (genes and chromosomes) that direct the structure, function, and potential growth and reproduction of the cell (see Chapter 6). One or more round nucleoli are also found within the nucleus. These are known to be essential to the synthesis of ribosomes. The nucleus is surrounded by a porous, double-layered nuclear membrane that acts as a selective barrier to transport between the nucleus and the cytoplasm.

Cytoskeleton

Within the cytoplasm are extensive networks of interconnected protein fibers known collectively as the *cytoskeleton*. Three types of fibers are seen; from smallest to largest they are the **microfilaments, intermediate filaments**, and **microtubules**. These proteins provide structural support to the cell and its components, mediate cell motility, and are the basis of an intercellular communication process known as *tissue matrix signaling*, discussed later in this chapter.

Microfilaments

Microfilaments are involved in the two mechanisms that permit cells to move: motor protein actions and cytoskeletal rearrangements. Motor protein actions are regulated by specialized enzymes that use the energy from hydrolysis of ATP to slide the microfilaments *actin* and *myosin* past each other (as in muscle contraction) or to move cellular components along tracks composed of microfilaments or microtubules (as in cell division). The molecular mechanism of muscle contraction is discussed in detail in Chapter 5. Cell division is discussed in Chapter 6.

Cellular locomotion refers to changes in cell shape and ameboid movements of individual cells that result from cytoskeletal rearrangements. Actin is the most abundant microfilament within the cytoskeleton, and it may rapidly assemble and disassemble through changes in the length of fibers and through protein cross-linking of fibers into bundles and networks. Processes by which these rearrangements are regulated are still incompletely understood but are known to involve a number of regulatory proteins (actin-binding proteins), many of which are dependent on calcium. Examples of cellular locomotion include the squeezing of white blood cells through vessel walls in inflammation (see Chapter 13), motility of sperm (see Chapter 30), and the rhythmic "beating" of cilia, membrane projections found in a variety of cells, including those lining the airways (see Chapter 18).

Actin–myosin interaction is also important to cell division, mediating the final phase in which the membrane of the dividing cell constricts at the center, "pinching off" the cytoplasm and forming two daughter cells (see Chapter 6). Along with microtubular proteins, myosin is known to be involved in transport of vesicles from place to place within cells. The transport of vesicles containing neurotransmitters from the neuron cell body to the axon terminal is a notable example (see Chapter 21).

Actin is also important in stiffening and strengthening the plasma membrane as well as in stabilizing the position of certain membrane proteins, such as ion channels. Actin bundles, known as *stress fibers*, lie beneath the intracellular surface of the plasma membrane. Stress fibers have specialized ends that participate in molecular adhesion, or attachment of cells to adjacent cells and to extracellular substrate. Molecular adhesion is an important component of intercellular communication, as discussed later. The actin skeleton runs both radially and axially within the cell, providing continuity between the three components of the tissue matrix: the extracellular matrix, the cytoplasmic cytoskeleton, and the nuclear core filaments. This continuity is essential to tissue matrix signaling.

Intermediate Filaments

Although microfilaments and microtubules are important to cell motility, intermediate filaments are believed to play a role only in cell structure. These fibers provide mechanical support to the plasma membrane where it comes into contact with other cells or with the extracellular matrix. The best-known intermediate filament is keratin, which lends strength to epithelial cells (keratinocytes) of the skin, hair, and nails (see Chapter 36).

Microtubules

Microtubules are composed of *tubulin*, protein subunits arranged in a cylindric tube. Microtubules are much stiffer than microfilaments or intermediate fibers and may vary greatly in length. Some microtubules are unstable and short-lived, such as those which form spindle fibers during cell division, whereas others are very stable. Examples of the latter include those within cilia and sperm and within the axons of neurons. Short-lived microtubules assemble and disassemble similarly to actin microfilaments, mediated by calcium-dependent regulatory proteins known as *microtubule-associated proteins*. The centrioles are paired cylindric structures in the cytoplasm, each composed of nine sets of triplet microtubules. The centrioles act as organizing centers for assembly of microtubular tracks.

Transport of membrane-bound proteins and vesicles to specific sites within the cell may occur along microtubular tracks, and such transport depends on motor proteins, similar to those regulating microfilament motility. The motor proteins involved in microtubular transport include *kinesin* and *dynein*. As with myosin, microtubules are important to the transport of neurotransmitter vesicles along axons, a process known as *fast axonal transport* or *axoplasmic flow*. Microtubules are associated with the Golgi apparatus and the endoplasmic reticulum, serving to transport the products of these organelles to targeted sites.

Beating of cilia and swimming movements of sperm depend on sliding of adjacent microtubules past each other, similar to the microfilament processes of muscle contraction. Chromosomal separation during cell division is also mediated by microtubules, which attach to sister chromatids and pull them to opposite poles of the cell. Some anticancer drugs, such as vinblastine (Velban) and paclitaxel (Taxol), bind selectively to the microtubules, inhibiting mitosis (see Chapter 7).

MECHANISMS OF INTERCELLULAR COMMUNICATION

Organization of cells into functional organ systems requires interaction between cells. Four general categories of intercellular communication are recognized: tissue matrix signaling, molecular adhesion, membrane transport, and ligand–receptor interactions. These mechanisms are interdependent.

Tissue Matrix Signaling

The cytoskeleton is part of a tissue matrix system that forms a structural bridge from the genetic material in the nucleus of the cell to the cell membrane and beyond, to the extracellular matrix and to other cells.[3] The importance of this system to intercellular communication has only recently been appreciated and is under intense study.[4] Many enzymes regulating cell functions are associated with the cytoskeleton, and changes in cell structure alter cellular processes and energy requirements. Cancer cells, for example, are characterized by alteration of the actin cytoskeleton as well as the nuclear membrane. Whether structure affects function, or vice versa, remains unknown.

Extracellular matrix components vary among different tissues but usually include collagen proteins, multiadhesive (laminin) proteins, complex carbohydrate (hyaluronan) molecules, and protein–carbohydrate molecules (proteoglycans and glycosaminoglycans). Many adjacent cells that form biologic barriers (e.g., skin, linings and coverings of organs) are organized into tissues by virtue of their common binding to a thin sheet of matrix components known as the *basal lamina*, or *basement membrane*. Presence of an intact basement membrane is important in limiting the responses of intercellular signals to the intended target tissues.

Information flow among the extracellular matrix, the plasma membrane, and the genetic material in the cell nucleus regulates many processes critical to embryologic development (see Chapter 6). Certain tissue changes, such as those occurring during pregnancy and lactation, are also triggered by signals generated in the extracellular matrix. This communication occurs as a result of a dynamic, complex system that depends on tissue architecture, molecular adhesion, and ligand–receptor interactions.

The extracellular matrix contains receptors for many regulatory ligands, such as hormones and cytokines. After binding these signaling molecules, the matrix may either prevent them from influencing cells or facilitate their interaction with cells. Interaction between the extracellular matrix and the plasma membrane is mediated at first by structural contacts or adhesions involving **integrins**, membrane proteins that bind one or more types of ligand in the matrix (or to other **adhesion molecules** on adjacent cells, as discussed later).

The adhesion complex establishes a physical link with the cytoskeleton, inducing actin rearrangement, which alters cell shape. Changes in the tension of the cytoskeleton constitute a signal that is transmitted to the core filaments in the nucleus by both mechanical and receptor-mediated processes. In the nucleus, alteration in core filaments changes the compartmentalization of soluble proteins known as *transcription factors*. These, in turn, bind to DNA, influencing genetic regulation of cellular structure and function (see Chapter 6).

Molecular Adhesion

Adhesion Molecules

Adhesion molecules are cell surface proteins that act as ligands or receptors in mediating stable or transient contacts between cells.[5, 6] They may bind either to signaling molecules or to other adhesion molecules. There are four major categories of adhesion molecules: (1) integrins (introduced earlier); (2) **immunoglobulin superfamily** members, including **neural cell adhesion molecules** (N-CAMs) and **intercellular adhesion molecules** (I-CAMs); (3) **cadherins**; and (4) **selectins** (Table 2–3).

N-CAMs and cadherins mediate cell–cell contacts, which generally remain stable for the life of the cells. N-CAMs, which have an immunoglobulin-like or antibody-like structure (see Chapter 13), are found predominantly in nervous tissue. N-CAMs bind like cells together and may also induce nerve fiber growth by binding cytokine growth factors. Cadherins are integral membrane glycoproteins that are important in establishing stable intercellular

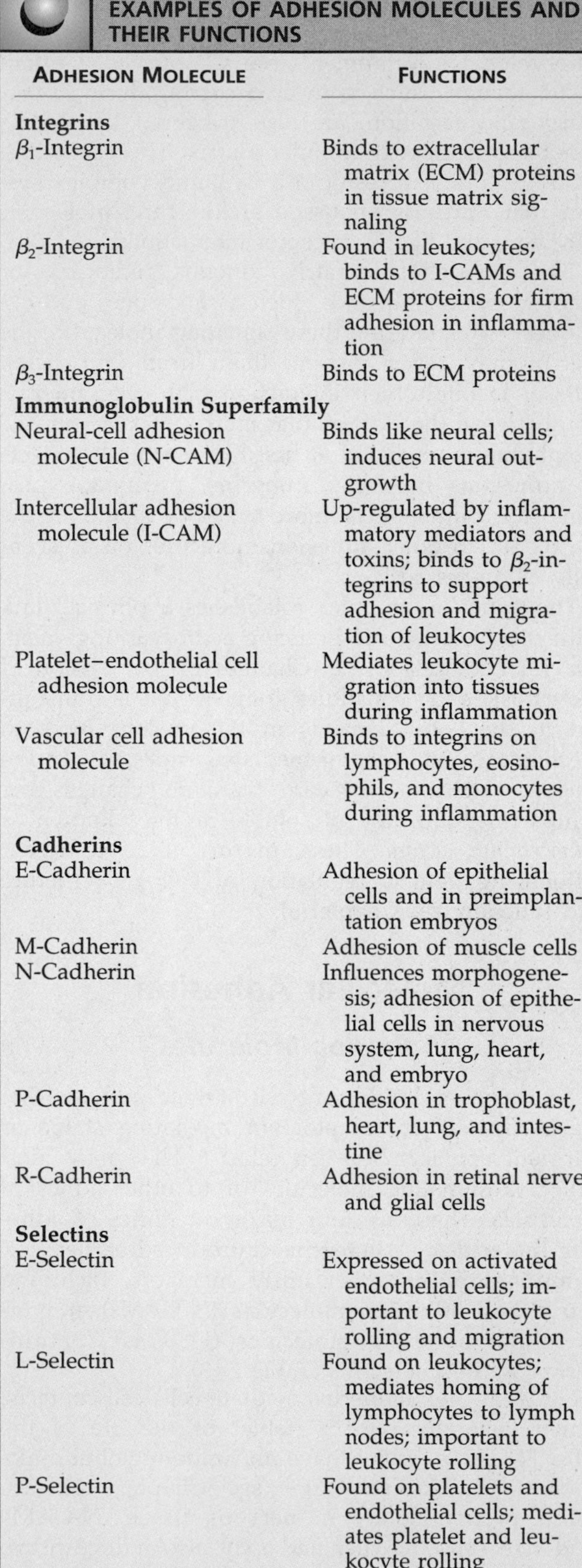

TABLE 2–3
EXAMPLES OF ADHESION MOLECULES AND THEIR FUNCTIONS

Adhesion Molecule	Functions
Integrins	
β_1-Integrin	Binds to extracellular matrix (ECM) proteins in tissue matrix signaling
β_2-Integrin	Found in leukocytes; binds to I-CAMs and ECM proteins for firm adhesion in inflammation
β_3-Integrin	Binds to ECM proteins
Immunoglobulin Superfamily	
Neural-cell adhesion molecule (N-CAM)	Binds like neural cells; induces neural outgrowth
Intercellular adhesion molecule (I-CAM)	Up-regulated by inflammatory mediators and toxins; binds to β_2-integrins to support adhesion and migration of leukocytes
Platelet–endothelial cell adhesion molecule	Mediates leukocyte migration into tissues during inflammation
Vascular cell adhesion molecule	Binds to integrins on lymphocytes, eosinophils, and monocytes during inflammation
Cadherins	
E-Cadherin	Adhesion of epithelial cells and in preimplantation embryos
M-Cadherin	Adhesion of muscle cells
N-Cadherin	Influences morphogenesis; adhesion of epithelial cells in nervous system, lung, heart, and embryo
P-Cadherin	Adhesion in trophoblast, heart, lung, and intestine
R-Cadherin	Adhesion in retinal nerve and glial cells
Selectins	
E-Selectin	Expressed on activated endothelial cells; important to leukocyte rolling and migration
L-Selectin	Found on leukocytes; mediates homing of lymphocytes to lymph nodes; important to leukocyte rolling
P-Selectin	Found on platelets and endothelial cells; mediates platelet and leukocyte rolling

junctions (see later) and thus in holding multicellular biologic membranes together. As is true of all proteins, expression of cadherins on the plasma membrane is genetically regulated. During embryologic development, cell contacts form and break as a consequence of cells gaining and losing cadherins under genetic direction.

Transient adhesive contacts between cells are important for maintenance of blood vessel integrity and for movement of cells into tissues during inflammatory and immune responses. These contacts are mediated by selectins, integrins, and I-CAMs. Selectins are found in endothelial cells, the cells lining blood vessels. They are normally intracellular and inactive. On stimulation by inflammatory cytokines, however, selectins are transported by **exocytosis** to the plasma membrane. Activated selectins bind loosely to carbohydrate ligands on white blood cells, causing these cells to roll and decelerate in the inflamed area. A phospholipid mediator, platelet-activating factor, is also released from activated endothelium and induces expression of integrins on immune cells (T lymphocytes). Integrins bind to I-CAMs, which are normally expressed on endothelial cell membranes. Attraction, or homing, of inflammatory and immune cells to the injured area occurs as a result of these molecular adhesion processes. Molecular adhesion is thus critical to appropriate location and limitation of inflammatory and immune responses, discussed in detail in Chapter 13.

Molecular adhesion also plays an important role in hemostasis, or blood clot formation. Disruption of the blood vessel wall stimulates endothelial cells in the area to express selectin. Binding of selectin to circulating platelets slows them down, facilitating their more permanent binding by means of integrins and initiating platelet plug formation (see Chapter 14).

Membrane Junctions

Membrane junctions are areas of physical or functional communication between cells (Fig. 2–5). **Adhesive junctions** are zipper-like contacts that hold cells together firmly, maintaining their position despite mechanical stress and forming connections between the cytoskeletons of adjacent cells. Adhesive junctions are found primarily in the epithelial cells of the skin and in the linings of body cavities, and are mediated by cadherins and related adhesion molecules. Adhesive junctions in epithelial tissues are characterized by points of contact known as *desmosomes,* which serve as anchoring sites for intermediate filaments of the cytoskeleton.

Tight junctions are areas in which the membrane proteins of adjacent cells are fused, restricting move-

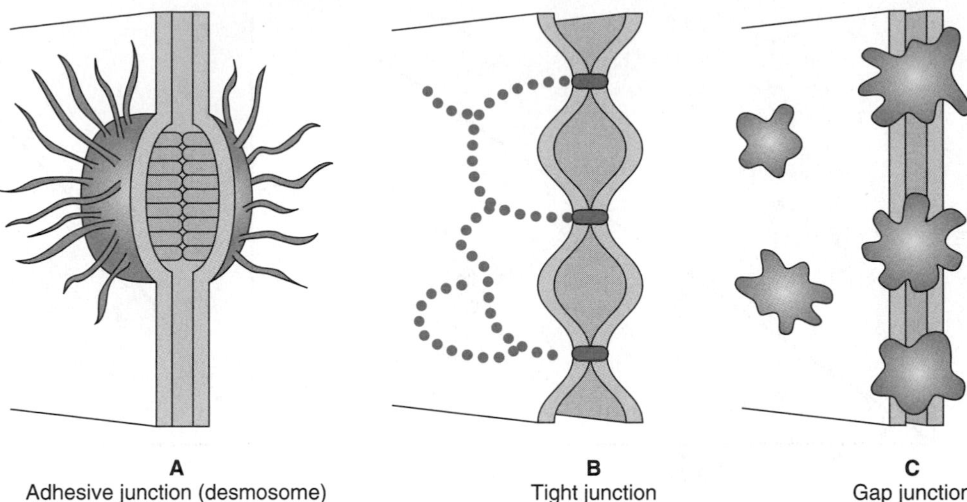

FIGURE 2-5
Membrane junctions. *A, Adhesive junctions* are zipper-like points of contact that hold cells together and connect the cytoskeletons of adjacent cells. Adhesive junctions in epithelial tissues are known as *desmosomes. B, Tight junctions* are areas where the membranes of adjacent cells are fused, restricting transport. *C, Gap junctions* connect cells through protein channels that traverse both membranes, permitting transport of molecules between cells.

ment of molecules between the cells. Tight junctions are found in biologic membranes of tissues where separation of compartments is desirable, such as between the blood and the intestinal lumen, and between the blood and brain tissue (blood–brain barrier). Conversely, **gap junctions** facilitate transport of molecules from one cell to another because cell membranes are close together and connected by protein channels that traverse both cell membranes. Gap junctions are found primarily in smooth muscle and cardiac tissues, which are dependent on *syncytial function*, or function of several individual cells as a coordinated unit.

Membrane Transport Processes

Membrane transport refers to the multiple processes by which molecules are transferred across biologic membranes. These processes are the basis of the transfer of fluid and particles between body cells and compartments and the exchange of matter between the human system and the environment. Biologic membranes consist of either single membranes (e.g., plasma membranes or organelle membranes) or multicellular membranes composed of adjacent cells adherent to each other and to a basement membrane.

Selective Membrane Permeability

Biologic membranes are often characterized as selectively permeable filters, a characteristic that is central to the regulation of physiologic function. The selective permeability of the intact skin and mucous membranes, for example, allows the human system to eliminate waste products while preventing some harmful environmental agents from entering the system. Selective permeability also governs the degree and type of transport of fluid and particles between subsystems of the body. Selective permeability originates from anatomic variability of membrane junctions and from functional variability of transport processes in different tissues and organs.

Selective permeability is also influenced by regulatory processes that induce opening and closing of gated protein channels as well as insertion and deletion of channel proteins. As discussed later in this chapter, protein-dependent transport processes are subject to stimuli that may increase (up-regulate) or decrease (down-regulate) numbers of channels, receptors, or transport proteins. Furthermore, any transport process involving protein transporters or pumps is *saturable*, that is, it has a maximal rate regardless of the magnitude of the gradient (see next section) or the amount of available ligand. The reason for this is that the number of transport proteins or receptors present at a given point in time is finite. When all available sites are bound, the addition of more ligand cannot induce further transport or receptor-mediated effect (Fig. 2–6).

Biologic Gradients

Transport processes in the body may be categorized as gradient-related or gradient-independent. A *gradient* is a driving force for movement of fluid or particles across a biologic membrane. Gradients are quantified in terms of direction and magnitude and as such may be conceptualized as vectors.

Three types of gradients are found in human systems: **concentration gradients, electrical gradients**, and **pressure gradients** (Fig. 2–7). Transport of small, nonpolar, or uncharged substances is typically determined by concentration gradients. A concentration gradient exists when the density of particles on one side of a membrane differs from that on the

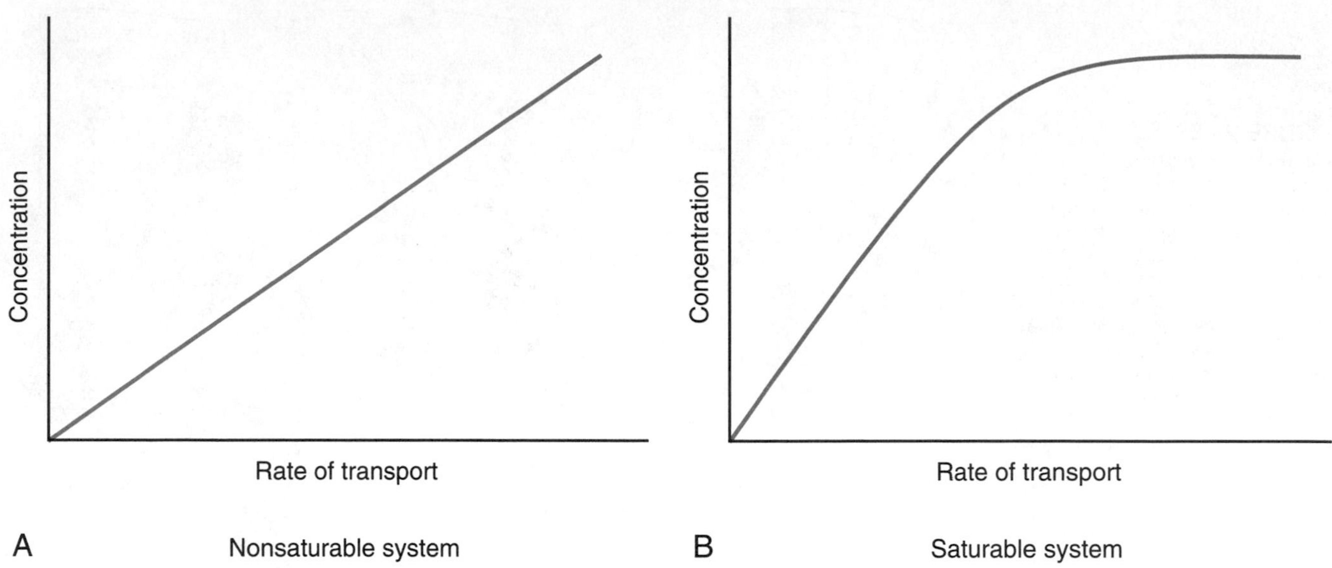

FIGURE 2–6
Membrane transport in nonsaturable and saturable systems. *A*, Transport in nonsaturable systems is not protein-mediated and thus depends only on the gradient and the permeability of the membrane to the transported particle. *B*, Transport in saturable systems requires protein transporters or pumps, which are finite in number. The system is *saturated* when all transporters are occupied. At this point, an increase in the gradient does not result in further increase in the rate of transport.

other side. Particles are continuously mobile owing to their random kinetic or thermal activity. If the membrane is permeable to the particle, net movement of particles occurs from the side of higher concentration to that of lower concentration, until the concentrations are equal in both compartments, and the gradient is exhausted.

Transport of polar or charged molecules is determined by both concentration and electrical gradients. Electrical gradients are derived from the attractive forces between particles of unlike or opposite charge, and the repellant forces between particles of like charge. The negative charge on many intracellular proteins tends to attract positively charged ions, such as sodium and potassium, from the extracellular fluid.

Although movement of particles across membranes is primarily dependent on concentration and electrical gradients, movement of fluid depends on two types of pressure gradients. **Osmotic pressure** determines movement of water molecules across a membrane that is freely permeable to water but not to particles. As shown in Figure 2–8, water moves from the side of lesser concentration of particles (greater concentration of water molecules or more dilute solution) to that of greater concentration of particles (lesser concentration of water molecules or more concentrated solution). Osmosis may thus be conceptualized as a pulling force exerted by particles on water.

Movement of fluid is also governed by **hydrostatic pressure**, a pushing force derived from the force of gravity or mechanical pumping (Fig. 2–7). As a result of gravitational force, water tends to concentrate in the lowest or most dependent areas of the body, as evidenced by swelling in the ankles and feet with prolonged standing (see Chapter 8). The heart is the primary mechanical pump in the circulatory system, although circulation of blood occurs as a result of secondary pumps as well, such as elastic recoil of blood vessels and compression of veins by skeletal muscle contraction with activity or diaphragmatic movement during respiration (see Chapter 15). Forces influencing movement and pressure of blood are collectively known as *hemodynamic forces*.

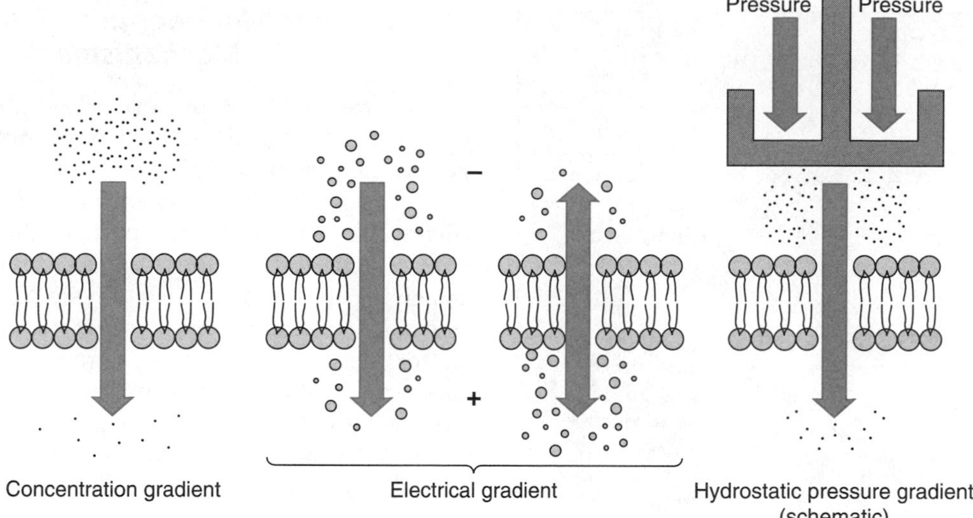

FIGURE 2–7

Three types of biologic gradients. *Concentration gradients* move particles from an area of greater concentration to one of lesser concentration of particles. *Electrical gradients* are derived from attraction of particles of unlike charge and repulsion of particles of like charge. Assuming that all the particles shown are negatively charged, a gradient exists for their movement toward the more positive side of the membrane, as shown in the left diagram. Accumulation of these particles is limited by the concentration gradient which then develops (right diagram). *Hydrostatic pressure gradients* move fluid as a consequence of gravitational or mechanical pumping forces, carrying particles along by solvent drag, as illustrated here. (The other type of pressure gradient, *osmotic pressure*, is illustrated in Figure 2–8.)

In addition to its movement through the plasma membrane as a consequence of osmotic or hydrostatic forces, water may be transported through pores between cells composing multicellular membranes. This **bulk flow** generally carries with it dissolved and suspended particles by a process known as **solvent drag**.

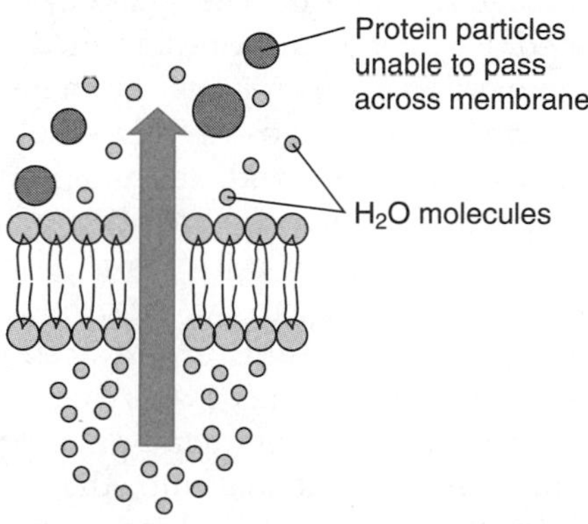

FIGURE 2–8

Osmosis. Osmotic pressure drives the movement of water across membranes that restrict the movement of particles. Water moves from an area of greater concentration of water (more dilute solution of particles) to one of lesser concentration of water (more concentrated solution of particles). Nondiffusible proteins are the source of osmotic pressure in this illustration.

Gradient-Related Transport Mechanisms

Gradient-related transport processes are classified as **passive transport**, if movement of particles occurs along a biologic gradient, or **active transport** if movement is against a gradient. Passive transport requires no energy infusion, whereas active transport consumes energy in the form of ATP. An intermediate form, **secondary active transport,** has aspects of both in that a gradient is first established by active transport of one particle, allowing a second particle to be transported passively along this gradient. Table 2–4 illustrates modes of transport of selected substances.

Passive Transport. Simple diffusion is the movement of particles or fluid along a concentration or electrical gradient. The larger the gradient, the more rapid the rate of diffusion. Lipophilic (nonpolar or uncharged) molecules diffuse easily through membrane lipids, particularly if the particles are of low molecular weight. Water also moves easily across membrane lipids by a process that is not well understood but that is thought to involve transport through both membrane lipids and transmembrane channels.[7] Hydrophilic (polar or charged) molecules other than water generally must diffuse through protein channels in the cell membrane. Again, smaller particles diffuse more rapidly.

TABLE 2–4
MODES OF TRANSPORT OF SELECTED ENDOGENOUS SUBSTANCES

Transport Mechanism	Substance Transported
Simple diffusion through membrane lipids	Oxygen Carbon dioxide Glycerol Urea Ethanol Water
Simple diffusion through protein channels	Sodium ions Potassium ions Calcium ions Hydrogen ions Water
Facilitated diffusion	Glucose Amino acids Nucleotides
Active transport	Sodium ions Potassium ions Calcium ions Hydrogen ions
Receptor-mediated endocytosis	Cholesterol
Regulated exocytosis	Neurotransmitters Hormones

Facilitated diffusion (mediated transport) is the movement of particles with the assistance of membrane transporter proteins. These proteins may be uniports, symports, or antiports, as previously described, and are generally restricted to specific particles or classes of particles. Larger molecules and charged particles often require transporters.

Active Transport. Active transport is driven by energy-consuming processes involving membrane pumps. Gradient-related active transport moves particles against existing gradients and often serves to restore resting state conditions in physiologic processes consisting of sequential steps, such as muscle contraction and action potential generation. The most widely distributed membrane pump is the Na^+-K^+-ATPase system, shown in Figure 2–9. An example of an antiport, this system consumes the energy released with hydrolysis of one molecule of ATP in moving three sodium ions out of the cell and two potassium ions in. Ion movement in both cases is against concentration gradients.

Another important example of active transport in plasma membranes and mitochondrial membranes is calcium pumping, which is critical to energy metabolism and muscle contraction (see Chapters 3 and 5). Active transport of sodium by kidney tubule cells is important in establishing gradients for secondary active transport of other particles. Renal regulation of glucose, ions, acids, and bases is highly dependent on active transport of sodium (see Chapter 20).

Gradient-Independent Transport Mechanisms

Exocytosis. The transport of nondiffusible particles (typically large proteins or complex molecules) across the plasma membrane occurs through energy-consuming processes that are not dependent on gradients. Movement of large particles from the interior to the exterior of the cell occurs by exocytosis, which is the basis of such physiologic processes as hormone secretion, mucus secretion, and neurotransmitter release. As shown in Figure 2–10, the cellular product to be secreted is first enclosed within a vesicle, which is transported along cytoskeletal tracks to the plasma membrane. The vesicle then "docks" at a specific membrane site by a receptor-mediated process. Although the precise mechanism is poorly understood, it is widely believed that protein–protein interactions result in fusion of the vesicle with the membrane. A *fusion pore* then forms and widens, releasing the vesicular product to the exterior of the cell.

Exocytosis is said to be *constitutive* if it occurs without apparent extracellular signaling and if it is not affected by changes in intracellular calcium levels. Neurotransmitter secretion is an example of *regulated* exocytosis, which requires a stimulatory signal and is mediated by a rise in intracellular calcium.[8]

Endocytosis. Endocytosis is the general process by which large molecules are taken into cells. Three specific types of endocytosis are **phagocytosis, pinocytosis,** and **receptor-mediated endocytosis** (Fig. 2–11). Phagocytosis ("eating of cells") occurs in specialized white blood cells of the inflammatory and immune systems and serves to destroy bacterial products or cellular debris. The phagocytic cell enters inflamed tissue by an adhesion-mediated process, then expands and surrounds the material to be removed, forming a phagosome. Lysosomes from the cell interior then fuse with the phagosome, and lysosomal enzymes destroy the engulfed material.

Pinocytosis ("drinking of cells") is a process similar to phagocytosis that occurs in most body cells. In this process, a small amount of extracellular fluid containing dissolved particles is surrounded by an invaginated part of the cell membrane, forming a vesicle, which is then taken into the cytoplasm. Pinocytosis is the process by which many nutrient molecules are absorbed from the gastrointestinal tract.

Phagocytosis and pinocytosis are nonspecific processes; that is, they are not selective for specific molecules. In contrast, receptor-mediated endocytosis is highly selective in that it is activated by the binding of specific ligands for which the cell has membrane receptors. Both the receptor and the ligand are en-

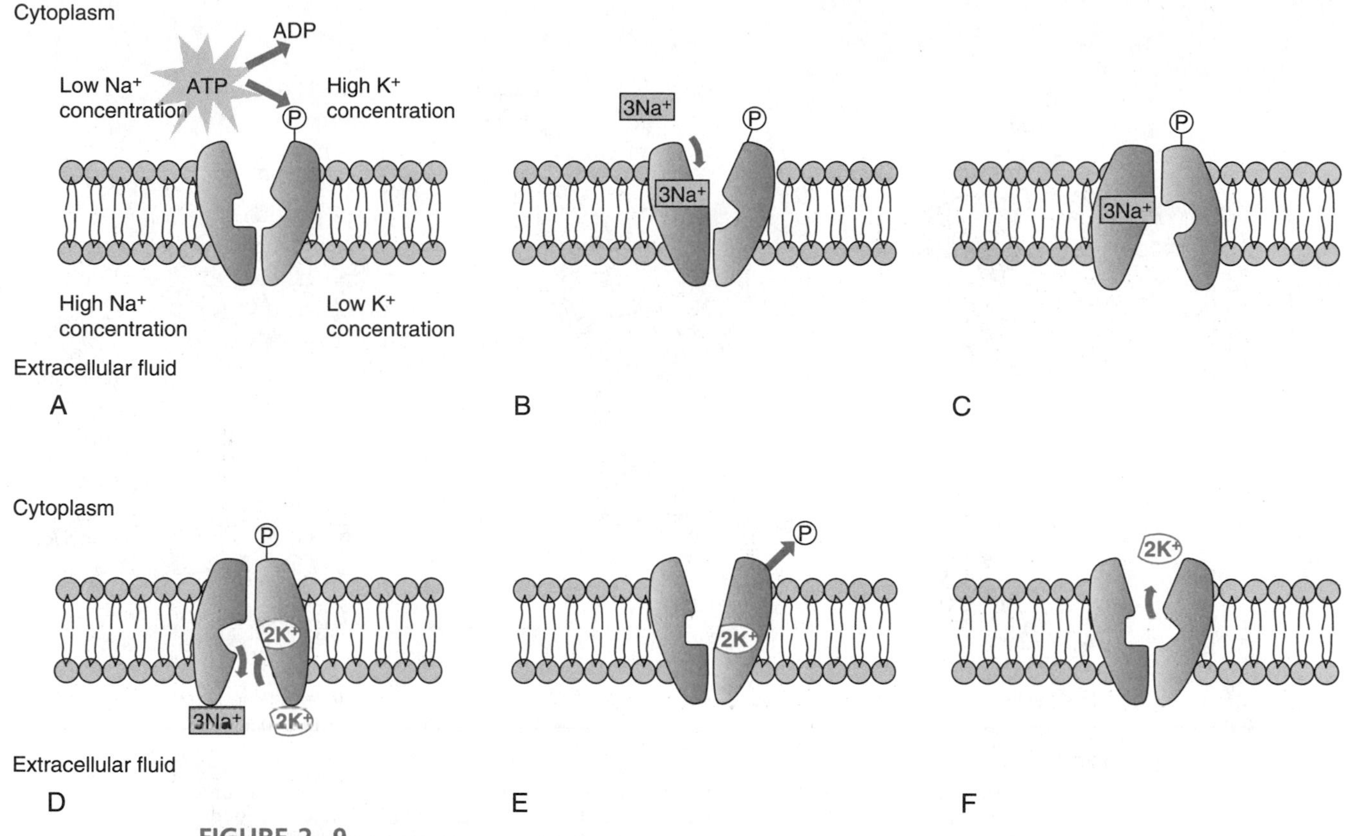

FIGURE 2–9

Na^+-K^+-ATPase pump. This widely distributed membrane pump represents active transport and antiport functions. The energy in one molecule of ATP is consumed in moving three sodium ions out of the cell and two potassium ions into the cell. *A,* Hydrolysis of ATP transfers phosphate to the pump, inducing a high-affinity state for Na^+. *B,* Three Na^+ ions bind (from cytoplasmic side). *C,* Na^+ binding induces a conformational change, which exposes Na^+ to extracellular fluid and reduces Na^+ affinity while increasing affinity for K^+. *D,* Three Na^+ ions are released into extracellular fluid, and two K^+ ions bind (from extracellular side). *E,* K^+ binding induces a conformational change, which exposes K^+ to cytoplasm and releases the phosphate group. *F,* Two K^+ ions are released into cytoplasm.

gulfed by the cell membrane, forming a vesicle called a *coated pit* because of its surface characteristics. Insulin, cholesterol, and iron are among the ligands that are transported into cells by receptor-mediated endocytosis. Plasma membrane components consumed during endocytosis are processed by lysosomes, and the resulting products are then reincorporated into the plasma membrane.

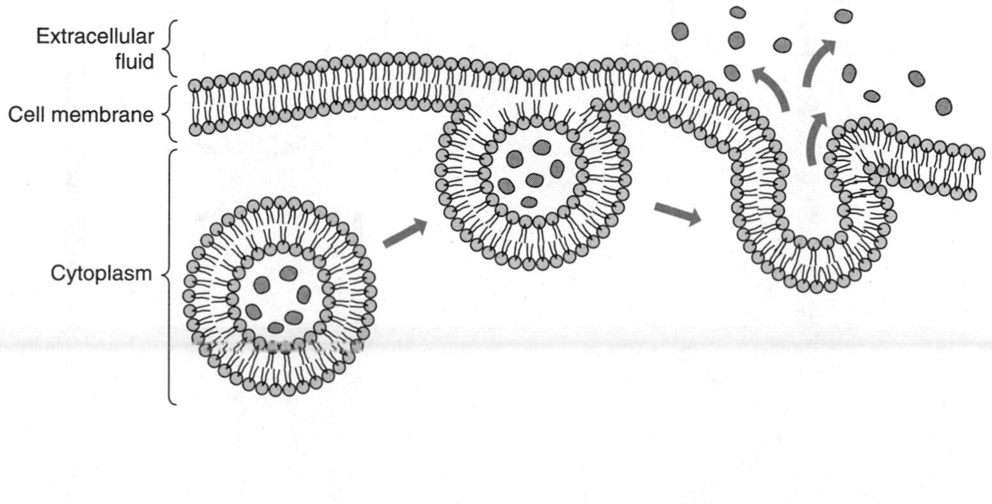

FIGURE 2–10

Exocytosis. This energy-dependent mechanism moves large particles from the cell. Particles are first enclosed in vesicles, which dock at specific membrane sites. A fusion pore then forms and widens, releasing the particles to the exterior.

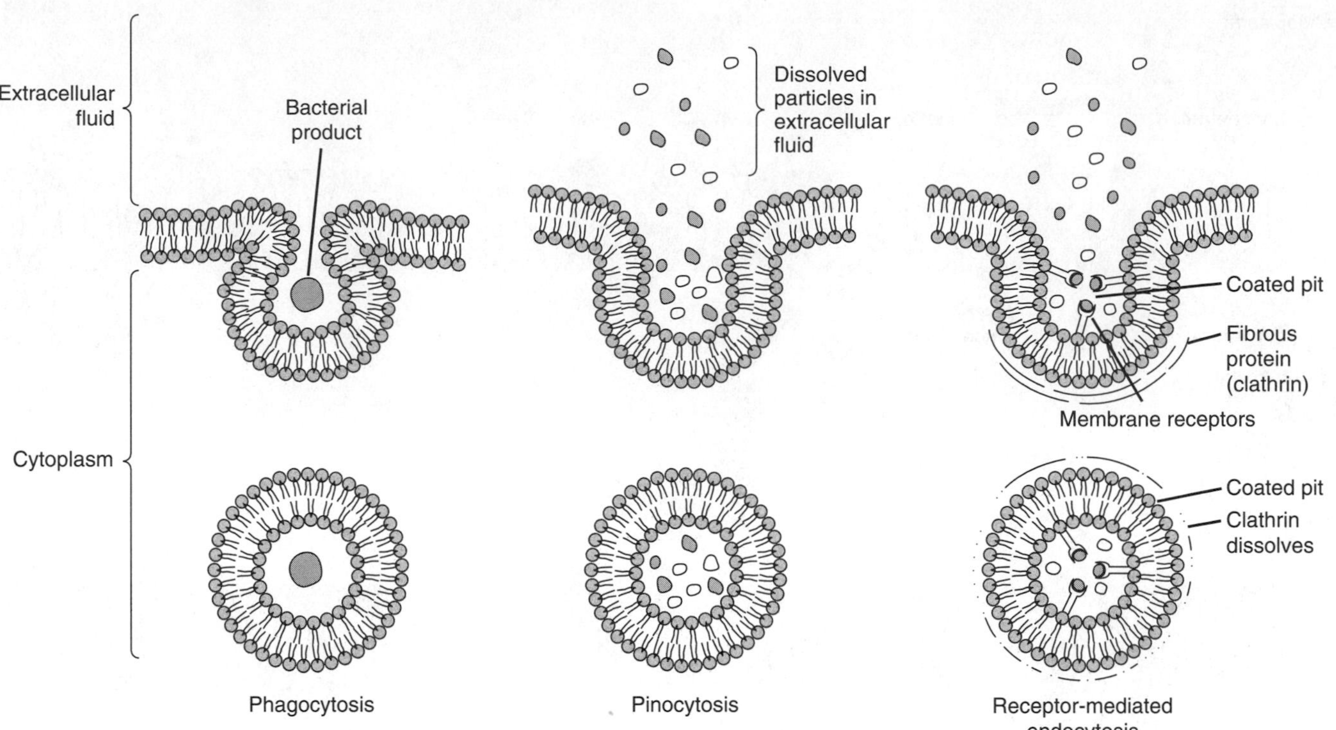

FIGURE 2–11

Three types of endocytosis. Endocytosis is an energy-dependent process. In *phagocytosis,* a white blood cell engulfs bacterial products or cellular debris. Fusion of the engulfed material with lysosomes results in its destruction. In *pinocytosis,* the cell surrounds a small amount of extracellular fluid–containing particles, forming a vesicle, which is taken into the cell. In *receptor-mediated endocytosis,* binding of a specific ligand to a membrane receptor results in the uptake of both ligand and receptor through formation of a specialized vesicle, the coated pit. Lysosomal processing then releases the ligand and recycles membrane components.

Epithelial Transport

Epithelial transport refers to transport across the skin, the intestinal wall, and other biologic membranes composed of adjacent epithelial cells. Different transport processes operate on each side of the cell and between cells (Fig. 2–12). Epithelial cells are said to be *polarized* with respect to transport, and this polarity is critical to the selective permeability of epithelial barriers.

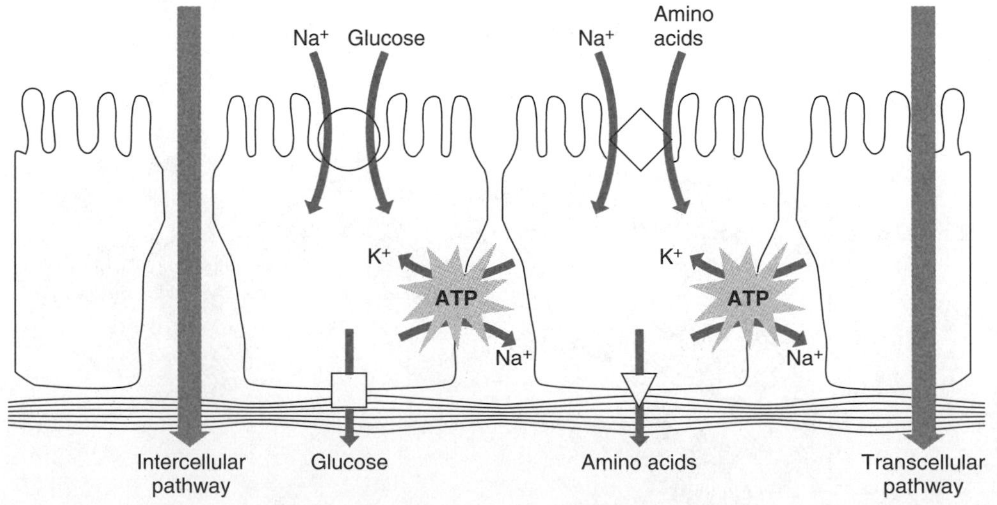

FIGURE 2–12

Epithelial transport. Many biologic membranes are composed of epithelial cells adherent to each other and to a basement membrane. Because different transport processes operate on each side of the cells and between cells, this form of transport is described as *polarized.* Uniports, symports, and antiports transport particles across plasma membranes. Water may move across cells (transcellular pathway) or between cells (intercellular pathway), possibly carrying particles by solvent drag.

Ligand–Receptor Interactions

The final mechanism of intercellular communication is initiated by extracellular signaling molecules, which bind to specific receptors on target cells, inducing a conformational change in the receptor protein that leads to a cellular response. Selectivity of ligand for receptor is variable, but generally a single ligand binds to only one, or very few, receptor types.

Signaling Molecules and Signaling Distances

A wide variety of chemicals serve as signaling molecules. These include endogenous molecules, such as hormones, neurotransmitters, cytokines, lipid mediators, and gases, and exogenous substances, such as drugs, food additives, and other chemicals. Table 2–5 lists examples of common endogenous ligands that act as signaling molecules.

TABLE 2–5
EXAMPLES OF ENDOGENOUS SIGNALING MOLECULES

CATEGORY	EXAMPLES
Hormones	Epinephrine
	Adrenocorticotropic hormone
	Corticotropin-releasing hormone
	Growth hormone
	Prolactin
	Thyroxine
	Insulin
	Cortisol
	Glucagon
	Aldosterone
	Antidiuretic hormone
	Cholecystokinin
	Secretin
	β-Endorphin
Neurotransmitters	Norepinephrine
	Epinephrine
	Acetylcholine
	Dopamine
	Serotonin
	Histamine
	γ-Aminobutyric acid
	Glutamate
Cytokines	Interleukins
	Interferons
	Growth factors
	Colony-stimulating factors
Lipid mediators	Prostaglandins
	Thromboxanes
	Leukotrienes
	Platelet-activating factor
Gases	Nitric oxide

Endocrine signaling occurs when signaling molecules (hormones) travel in the blood to distant target cells, where they bind and exert their effects. In **paracrine** signaling, signaling molecules (neurotransmitters, cytokines, lipid mediators, and gases) bind to target cells located near the releasing cell. In **autocrine** signaling, the target cell is the same cell that released the signaling molecule (typically a growth factor). A given molecule may act simultaneously over more than one signaling distance.

Classification of Receptors

Receptors can be classified on the basis of location, structure, or function. *Transmembrane receptors* are integrated within the plasma membrane, whereas *intracellular receptors* are located within the cytoplasm or nucleus. Transmembrane receptors, also known as *cell surface receptors*, may be classified structurally as group 1 (receptors with a single transmembrane segment), group 2 (receptor–ion channel complexes), or group 3 (receptors with multiple transmembrane segments, linked to **G proteins**).[9] Table 2–6 lists examples of each of these types. Functional classification of receptors may be based on the nature of the ligand (e.g., hormones, neurotransmitters, or cytokines) or on the nature of the signal transduction process that results from receptor binding (see next section).

Signal Transduction

The function of receptors is to recognize and bind specific ligands, which influences conversion of the extracellular signal to an intracellular signal. The processes by which this information is relayed are known collectively as *signal transduction mechanisms*. Transmembrane receptors employ one of three types of signal transduction: (1) opening of ion channels, (2) activation of guanine-nucleotide (G) proteins, or (3) catalytic action of a part of the receptor protein. Intracellular receptors, such as those for steroid and thyroid hormones, transduce signals by a fourth mechanism, in which hormone–receptor complexes bind to DNA in the nucleus and influence gene expression.[10]

Ion Channel Receptors. The fastest and simplest signal transduction occurs when ligand binding to channel-associated receptors opens membrane channels. The resulting ion flux then affects intracellular processes.

G-Protein Transduction. G-protein–associated receptors exist in multiple forms. The most common form is the G-protein–adenylate cyclase system, il-

TABLE 2–6
CLASSIFICATION OF TRANSMEMBRANE RECEPTORS

Receptors	Examples of Ligands
Group 1 (single transmembrane segment)	Insulin Insulin-like growth factor 1 (IGF-1) Epidermal growth factor (EGF) Platelet-derived growth factor (PDGF) Atrial natriuretic hormone (ANH) Low-density lipoprotein (LDL) Nerve growth factor (NGF) Interleukin-2 (IL-2)
Group 2 (receptor–ion channel complexes)	Acetylcholine-nicotinic (Ach_n) γ-Aminobutyric acid (GABA-A) Glycine (GlyR) Glutamate
Group 3 (multiple segments, G-protein linked)	Acetylcholine-muscarinic (ACh_m) Epinephrine Norepinephrine Dopamine Serotonin Adenosine γ-Aminobutyric acid (GABA-B) Glucagon

Data from Haga, T., Haga, K., and Hulme, E.C. (1990). Solubilization, purification, and molecular characterization of receptors: principles and strategy. In: Hulme, E.C. (Ed.). *Receptor Biochemistry: A Practical Approach.* Oxford, UK: IRL Press.

lustrated in Figure 2–13. The receptor is a complex protein that loops back and forth through the membrane, ending in an intracellular "tail." Binding of the ligand first messenger activates an associated G protein on the intracellular surface of the membrane. The activated G protein then exchanges its bound guanosine diphosphate (GDP) for guanosine triphosphate (GTP) on one of its three subunits. This subunit (α) and GTP then activate an intracellular enzyme, adenylate cyclase. Adenylate cyclase catalyzes formation of the second messenger, cyclic adenosine monophosphate (cAMP), from ATP. cAMP then activates the enzyme protein kinase A, which phosphorylates specific intracellular proteins, altering their properties and activities.

In other G-protein systems, the second messenger is not cAMP but rather calcium (Ca^{2+}), inositol 1,4,5,-triphosphate (IP_3), or 1,2-diacylglycerol (DAG). Binding of ligand to the G protein activates an enzyme, phospholipase C, which hydrolyzes a specific membrane phospholipid to form both IP_3 and DAG. IP_3, which is water soluble, binds to a receptor–Ca^{2+} channel on the endoplasmic reticulum, permitting Ca^{2+} flux from the endoplasmic reticulum into the cytosol. DAG, which is lipid soluble, remains associated with the plasma membrane. When cytosolic Ca^{2+} levels rise, an intracellular enzyme, protein kinase C, binds to the plasma membrane and is activated by DAG. Protein kinase C influences cellular activity by phosphorylating intracellular proteins, such as enzymes or transcription factors.

Receptor Tyrosine Kinases. Receptor tyrosine kinase activity best exemplifies signal transduction by the catalytic mechanism. These receptors have ligand-binding sites on the extracellular side of the plasma membrane as well as an intracellular component that is a kinase (phosphorylating) enzyme. Receptor tyrosine kinases bind growth factors or insulin and transduce cellular effects on cell growth and division by a complex signaling pathway that involves activation of a membrane protein, *Ras.* Ligand binding ultimately results in autophosphorylation; that is, the receptor phosphorylates its own intracellular tyrosine segment. The phosphorylated tyrosine then acts as a binding site for intracellular molecules, which dock at the receptor and are then activated by phosphorylation to serve as enzymes or transcription factors.

Intracellular Receptors. Hydrophilic substances, such as steroid and thyroid hormones, easily cross membrane lipids, then bind to receptors inside the cell. Steroid hormones (e.g., androgens, estrogens, cortisol, and aldosterone) and thyroid hormones bind to specific intracellular receptors, causing release of associated inhibitory heat shock proteins (see Chapter 1). The receptor–hormone complex is then able to bind to DNA in the nucleus, influencing transcription of specific segments of the genetic code and subsequent synthesis of regulatory and structural proteins. Genetic mechanisms of regulation are discussed further in Chapter 6.

Cellular Response to Receptor-Mediated Signals

The alteration of intracellular proteins, which is the outcome of signal transduction, may be immediate and short term, or slower onset and long term. Short-term effects usually represent adaptive responses to stressors of various kinds. Examples include the changes in blood vessel caliber, heart rate, and cardiac contractile force mediated by the catecholamines. Epinephrine and norepinephrine are the ligand signals in these cases, and the signals are

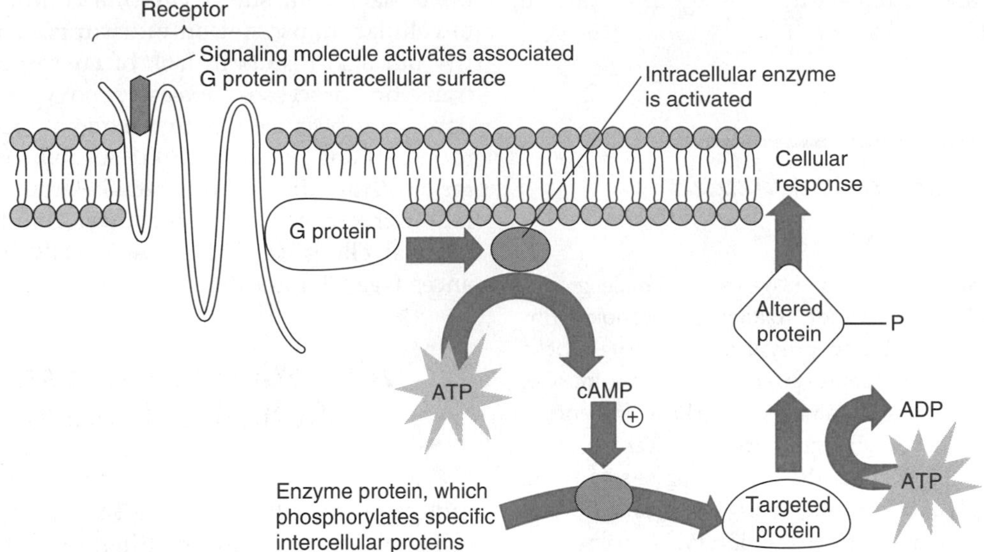

FIGURE 2–13

G-Protein signal transduction. The membrane receptor in this system has multiple segments, ending in a "tail," which is associated with a guanine nucleotide–binding (G) protein. Binding of a signaling molecule first messenger to the receptor causes the G protein to activate an intracellular enzyme, adenylate cyclase, which then catalizes formation of a second messenger, cAMP. cAMP then activates another enzyme protein, protein kinase A, which phosphorylates intracellular target proteins, altering their activity.

transduced by a G-protein–adenylate cyclase system. Phosphorylation of calcium-channel proteins and calcium pumps alters ion flux, which impacts the molecular mechanisms of cardiac conduction and contraction. These mechanisms are detailed in Chapters 4 and 5.

Long-term responses to cellular signals involve alteration of gene expression and protein synthesis. Steroid and thyroid hormone–receptor complexes bind DNA and influence transcription, as has been discussed. Ligands that bind to cell surface receptors may also influence gene expression if the resulting signal transduction phosphorylates intracellular protein transcription factors. These are specific for certain DNA sequences, and binding at these sites influences the expression of the genes encoded there. Defects in these systems have been associated with abnormal or uncontrolled cell growth and differentiation in genetic defects and neoplasia, as discussed in Chapter 7.

Regulation of Receptor-Mediated Functions

Receptor-mediated activity is regulated by negative feedback loops that increase or decrease receptor numbers or alter the affinity of receptor for ligand. Receptor numbers are normally in continuous flux. Up-regulation is mediated by signals that alter the expression of the genes encoding receptor proteins, whereas down-regulation occurs as a result of triggered endocytosis of receptors. Prolonged exposure of receptors to a high concentration of ligand may result in either down-regulation or desensitization (reduced affinity or transduction activity), whereas low levels of ligand may induce opposite effects. Phosphorylation of receptors or transduction pathway components usually results in desensitization, although it may increase the activity of some systems. Removal of phosphate groups reverses this effect.

Certain drugs, such as oral hypoglycemic agents used in the treatment of non–insulin-dependent diabetes mellitus, apparently up-regulate insulin receptors. The affinity of receptor for ligand also varies with alterations in extracellular pH and with binding of other ligands to adjacent receptors. Drugs that are similar in chemical structure to natural ligands may bind to receptors and either induce intracellular activity (act as **agonists**) or block the normal response (act as **antagonists**). Large amounts (nonphysiologic doses) of naturally occurring ligands may be administered as drugs and can induce different effects, referred to as *pharmacologic effects*. For example, the hormone arginine vasopressin does not result in notable vasoconstriction unless given in nonphysiologic doses. Arginine vasopressin may be used as a drug in an effort to control the severe bleeding often associated with end-stage liver failure (see Chapter 26).

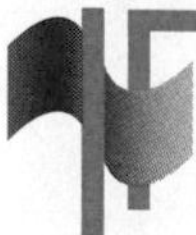

Clinical Scenario

For 6 months, M.J., a 43-year-old female graduate student, has been taking propranolol (Inderal) for high blood pressure. This drug blocks β-adrenergic receptors on cardiac muscle. Binding of catecholamines to these receptors normally causes increased force of cardiac contraction. M.J. reports that "the drug seems to be working," but says she feels light-headed when she "does the stairs" at the library.

1. While taking propranolol, would M.J. exhibit a normal response to stressors?
2. Should the drug be discontinued? What interventions might be considered?

MECHANISMS OF ABNORMAL INTERCELLULAR COMMUNICATION

Alteration of intercellular communication may cause disease or may result from disease. Any pathophysiologic mechanism that impairs membrane integrity, molecular adhesion, gradients, transport processes, or ligand–receptor interaction results in abnormal intercellular communication.

Disruption of Membrane and Cytoskeletal Integrity

Any trauma that disrupts the integrity of the plasma membrane impairs transport processes. For example, in myocardial infarction (heart attack), myocardial cells are damaged by lack of oxygenated blood supply. This results in "spilling" of intracellular enzymes into the blood, where they may be detected with blood testing. Presence of certain enzymes in the blood is indicative of the degree of myocardial damage and thus serves as an important diagnostic tool (see Chapter 16). Similarly, with massive cellular trauma (e.g., crush or burn injuries), the concentration of potassium (predominantly an intracellular ion) rises sharply in the blood and may seriously impair electrolyte balance (see Chapter 9). Hypoxia (lack of tissue oxygen), a common mechanism of cellular injury, not only disrupts membrane integrity but also results in lack of energy to drive active transport processes. Excessive oxygen can also be damaging because reactive oxygen species that bind to membrane lipids or to DNA may form (see Chapter 18). Alteration of the cytoskeleton and extracellular matrix can also result from cellular trauma or from swelling or shrinkage of cells in fluid imbalances (see Chapter 8).

Alteration in Expression of Adhesion Molecules

Congenital and acquired disorders of adhesion molecules may lead to defective tissue defense, disorders of bleeding and clotting, or metastasis of cancer cells. Leukocyte adhesion deficiencies are inherited disorders of integrin expression that result in recurrent infections and possible developmental abnormalities (see Chapter 13). Chronic inflammatory disorders such as asthma and arthritis may involve overproduction of adhesion molecules, and spread of cancer cells may be promoted by their lack of normal cadherin expression (see Focus of Current Research).

Alteration in Gradients

Abnormal gradients may result from excessive or deficient intake or output of water or particles (see Chapters 8 and 9). Many disorders of the cardiovascular, renal, and endocrine systems are characterized by fluid and electrolyte imbalance. An excess of glucose in renal tubules, as occurs in untreated diabetes mellitus, exerts an osmotic force on water, opposing its reabsorption into the blood and causing dehydration. Gradients may be manipulated by drug therapy. For example, mannitol (Osmitrol), a carbohydrate, may be administered to create an osmotic gradient that pulls excess fluid from the interstitium into the blood.

Alteration in Transport Proteins, Pumps, or Channels

Active transport processes are impaired in cardiovascular and respiratory disorders in which oxygenation of tissues is reduced. (As discussed in Chapter 3, energy metabolism is inefficient in oxygen-deficient states.) In conditions such as shock and respiratory failure, cells tend to swell because sodium accumulates intracellularly. Cerebral edema

Focus of Current Research

Study	Objective and Findings
Siitonen, et al. (1996) Reduced E-cadherin expression is associated with invasiveness and unfavorable prognosis in breast cancer.	*Objective:* To examine the relationship between E-cadherin expression and various tumor features *Findings:* Loss of normal E-cadherin expression is an indicator of increased invasiveness and dedifferentiation in breast cancer.
Steinbach, et al. (1996) The influence of cytokines on the adhesion of renal cancer cells to endothelium.	*Objective:* To examine the adherence of renal cell carcinoma lines to endothelium after stimulation with cytokines that induce expression of adhesion molecules *Findings:* Cytokine-induced increases in adhesion of cancer cells to endothelial cells are mediated by vascular cell adhesion molecule 1 and endothelial leukocyte adhesion molecule 1.
Shiota, et al. (1996) Soluble intercellular adhesion molecule 1 (ICAM-1) antigen in sera of bronchial asthmatics	*Objective:* To determine whether bronchial asthma is associated with increased levels of ICAM-1 in serum and to assess the effects of therapy on these levels *Findings:* Active bronchial asthma is associated with increased levels of ICAM-1, and these levels may be modulated with steroid therapy.
Hughes, et al. (1996) Fish oil supplementation inhibits the expression of major histocompatibility complex class II molecules and adhesion molecules on human monocytes.	*Objective:* To test the hypothesis that fish oil can inhibit the expression of functionally associated molecules on the surfaces of monocytes *Findings:* Fish oil can inhibit the expression of surface molecules involved in the function of antigen-presenting cells, potentially suppressing the immune response.
Shing, et al. (1996) Regulation of adhesion molecule expression by human synovial microvascular endothelial cells in vitro	*Objective:* To examine the expression of adhesion molecules in synovial microvascular endothelial cells compared with endothelial cells of neonatal foreskin and umbilical vein *Findings:* Augmented expression of adhesion molecules is present in synovial endothelium, and this may facilitate recruitment of leukocytes to this site in patients with rheumatoid arthritis.

(brain swelling) is a particularly ominous sign in such conditions. Loss of normal transport mechanisms also occurs in renal failure caused by tubular damage and may result in severe fluid, electrolyte, and acid-base imbalances.

The cellular defect in cystic fibrosis is abnormal function of a chloride channel, which leads to accumulation of obstructive secretions in airways and ducts of exocrine glands (see Chapter 18). Pernicious anemia results from lack of intrinsic factor, a glycoprotein that mediates efficient absorption of vitamin B_{12} (see Chapter 12). Uptake of glucose into cells is facilitated by glucose transport proteins, which may be defective in some forms of diabetes mellitus (see Chapter 29).

TABLE 2–7
EXAMPLES OF RECEPTOR DISEASES

DISORDER	RECEPTOR DEFECT
Myasthenia gravis	Autoimmune destruction of acetylcholine receptors at neuromuscular junction
Familial hypercholesterolemia	Deficient numbers of low-density lipoprotein receptors
Type II diabetes mellitus	Defective or deficient numbers of insulin receptors
Cancer (notably breast cancer, some brain tumors)	Expression of increased numbers of growth factor receptors
Vitamin D–resistant rickets	Genetic mutation of vitamin D receptors
Testicular feminization	Defective or deficient numbers of androgen receptors in males

Alteration in Signaling Molecules

Tumors of the endocrine system may result in either overproduction or underproduction of hormones, and tumors arising from nonendocrine tissues may produce hormones ectopically. Tumors may also produce their own growth factors, which signal further tumor development in a positive feedback loop (see Chapter 7). Degenerative disorders of the central nervous system, such as Alzheimer's disease and Parkinson's disease, may alter production of specific neurotransmitters, disrupting the balance among neural signaling pathways (see Chapters 21 and 22).

Dysfunction or Blockade of Receptors

Receptor function may also be affected by hypoxic or physical trauma to cells; however, receptor dysfunction is usually the result of genetic or autoimmune mechanisms or drug therapy. Self-targeted antibodies (autoantibodies) may (1) bind to receptors and destroy them, (2) block receptor-mediated effects, or (3) inappropriately trigger intracellular activity. In myasthenia gravis, a degenerative neurologic condition, autoantibodies destroy the acetylcholine receptors that regulate skeletal muscle contraction in response to nervous stimulation (see Chapter 22). Severe muscle weakness results. Additional examples of receptor diseases are listed in Table 2–7.

Drugs are usually designed to bind to specific receptors and either block or stimulate cellular effects. Narcotic analgesics such as morphine act by binding to central nervous system receptors whose endogenous ligand is β-endorphin (a hormone often associated with exercise-induced euphoria, or "runner's high"). The resultant effect with either the drug or the endogenous ligand is relief of pain and a sense of well-being. Receptor-mediated effects of selected drugs are summarized in Table 2–8.

TABLE 2–8
RECEPTOR-MEDIATED EFFECTS OF SELECTED DRUGS

RECEPTOR*	MECHANISM	DRUG	EFFECT
α_1-Adrenergic	Agonist	Phenylephrine (Neo-Synephrine)	Vasoconstriction
α_2-Adrenergic	Agonist	Clonidine (Catapres)	Decreased heart rate
β_1-Adrenergic	Agonist	Isoproterenol (Isuprel)	Increased cardiac contractility
β_2-Adrenergic	Agonist	Terbutaline (Brethine)	Bronchodilation
α-Adrenergic	Antagonist	Phentolamine (Regitine)	Hypotension
β-Adrenergic	Antagonist	Propranolol (Inderal)	Cardiac depression
Cholinergic (m)	Agonist	Pilocarpine	Miosis
Cholinergic (n)	Agonist	Nicotine (Nicorette)	Selective CNS stimulation or depression
Cholinergic (m)	Antagonist	Atropine	Enhanced cardiac conduction
Histamine (H_1)	Antagonist	Diphenhydramine (Benadryl)	Anti-inflammatory effect
Histamine (H_2)	Antagonist	Cimetidine (Tagamet)	Decreased gastric acid secretion

*These receptor categories are discussed in Chapters 21 and 22.

CLINICAL IMPORTANCE OF INTERCELLULAR COMMUNICATION

For practitioners of the health professions, knowledge of the mechanisms of intercellular communication aids in understanding the etiologic mechanisms of many diseases and permits interpretation of many of the clinical manifestations of disease. On the basis of this understanding, basic researchers are clarifying mechanisms of disease, and clinical researchers are developing new forms of intervention aimed at prevention and treatment of these disorders (see Focus of Current Research). Antibodies against adhesion molecules are being tested in some inflammatory and immune disorders. Nearly all drug development is targeted at manipulation of ligand–receptor interactions. Disruption of microtubular transport of proteins during mitosis provides a means of interrupting division of cancer cells. Gene therapy may permit replacement of genes encoding defective membrane proteins.

As discussed in upcoming chapters in Part One, intercellular communication processes are essential to energy metabolism, action potential formation, and muscle contraction. They are also critical to genetic regulation of cellular function, to embryologic development, and to maintenance of fluid, electrolyte, acid-base, and temperature homeostasis in the extracellular environment. Disruption of intercellular communication is the defining characteristic of cancer cells. Finally, intercellular communication processes are the essence of local regulation in all tissues and of systemic regulation by the neurologic and endocrine systems, which is detailed in Part Two.

Summary of Key Points

- Human cells are bounded by a plasma membrane, with an internal cytoplasm containing a protein cytoskeleton, a nucleus, and functionally specialized organelles. Plasma membrane lipids serve as a lipophilic barrier between the aqueous intracellular and extracellular compartments. Membrane proteins serve as transport channels, transport proteins (transporters and pumps), and receptors. Membrane carbohydrates complexed to proteins or lipids serve as cellular recognition sites that facilitate receptor binding.
- Interaction between protein adhesion molecules and their ligands is the basis for formation of both transient and stable cellular contacts. Transient adhesion mediates cellular interaction during inflammatory and immune responses as well as blood clotting. Stable adhesion involves membrane junction formation, which holds adjacent cells together and fixes them to a basement membrane. Membrane permeability varies on the basis of membrane junction type, presence of membrane channels and transport proteins, and the regulatory processes that govern transport.
- The three types of biologic gradients are derived from differences in concentration, electrical charge, and pressure. Gradient-related transport mechanisms include passive transport along natural gradients and active (energy-consuming) transport in opposition to gradients. Gradient-independent transport mechanisms include the energy-consuming, calcium-mediated processes of endocytosis and exocytosis.
- Endogenous signaling molecules include hormones such as insulin and cortisol, neurotransmitters such as acetylcholine and norepinephrine, cytokines such as interleukins and growth factors, lipid-signaling molecules such as platelet-activating factor, and gases such as nitric oxide. Exogenous signaling molecules include drugs, food additives, and other chemicals.
- Receptors can be classified on the basis of location as transmembrane (cell surface) receptors or intracellular receptors. Three classes of transmembrane receptors can be structurally differentiated, with each having different signal transduction mechanisms. Receptors can also be named and classified on the basis of the ligands they bind.
- The four principal mechanisms of signal transduction are (1) opening of ion channels, (2) activation of G proteins, (3) catalytic action, and (4) regulation of gene transcription.
- Short-term cellular responses to receptor-mediated signals include neuroendocrine adaptive mechanisms such as those induced by the catecholamines. Long-term responses involve alteration of gene expression and protein synthesis.

Summary continued on following page

- Receptor-mediated cellular activity may be regulated by genetic mechanisms (up-regulation and down-regulation of receptor numbers), by alteration of ligand–receptor affinity due to changes in extracellular conditions, or by endogenous or exogenous receptor agonists or antagonists.
- Abnormal intercellular communication may result from disruption of membrane or cytoskeletal integrity; alteration in expression of adhesion molecules; alteration in gradients; alteration in transport proteins, pumps, or channels; alteration in signaling molecules; or receptor dysfunction or blockade.

REFERENCES

1. Singer, S.J., and Nicholson, G.L. (1972). The fluid mosaic model of the structure of the cell membrane. *Science* 175(23), 720–731.
2. Penman, S. (1995). Rethinking cell structure. *Proceedings of the National Academy of Sciences, USA* 92(12), 5251–5257.
3. Pienta, K.J., and Hoover, C.N. (1994). Coupling of cell structure to cell metabolism and function. *Journal of Cellular Biochemistry* 55(1), 16–21.
4. Roskelley, C.D., Srebrow, A., and Bissell, M.J. (1995). A hierarchy of ECM-mediated signalling regulates tissue-specific gene expression. *Current Opinion in Cell Biology* 7(5), 736–747.
5. Frenette, P.S., and Wagner, D.D. (1996). Adhesion molecules —Part I. *The New England Journal of Medicine* 334(23), 1526–1529.
6. Frenette, P.S., and Wagner, D.D. (1996). Adhesion molecules —Part II. *The New England Journal of Medicine* 335(1), 43–45.
7. Haines, T.H. (1994). Water transport across biological membranes. *FEBS Letters* 346(1), 115–122.
8. Burgoyne, R.D., and Morgan, A. (1993). Regulated exocytosis. *Biochemistry Journal* 293 (July 15, Pt. 2), 305–316.
9. Haga, T., Haga, K., and Hulme, E.C. (1990). Solubilization, purification, and molecular characterization of receptors: Principles and strategy. In: Hulme, E.C. (Ed.). *Receptor Biochemistry: A Practical Approach.* Oxford, England: IRL Press. (pp. 1–50).
10. Schwertz, D.W., and Barry, C.P. (1994). Cellular communication through signal transduction: The background. *Journal of Cardiovascular Nursing* 8(3), 1–27.

SELECTED BIBLIOGRAPHY

Albelda, S.M., Smith, C.W., and Ward, P.A. (1994). Adhesion molecules and inflammatory injury. *FASEB Journal* 8(8), 504–512.

Ayala, J.S. (1994). Transport and internal organization of membranes: Vesicles, membrane networks and GTP-binding proteins. *Journal of Cell Science* 107(Apr, Pt. 4), 753–763.

Bajjalieh, S.M., and Scheller, R.H. (1995). The biochemistry of neurotransmitter secretion. *The Journal of Biological Chemistry* 270(5), 1971–1974.

Bevilacqua, M.P., Nelson, R.M., Mannori, G., *et al.* (1994). Endothelial-leukocyte adhesion molecules in human disease. *Annual Review of Medicine* 45(1994), 361–378.

Cooper, D.M.F., Mons, N., and Karpen, J.W. (1995). Adenylyl cyclases and the interaction between calcium and cAMP signalling. *Nature* 374(6521), 421–424.

Cotran, R.S., Kumar, V., and Robbins, S.L. (1994). *Robbins Pathologic Basis of Disease.* (5th Ed.). Philadelphia: W.B. Saunders.

Freifelder, D., and Malcinski, G.M. (1993). *Essentials of Molecular Biology.* (2nd Ed.). Boston: Jones & Bartlett Publishers.

French, A.S. (1992). Mechanotransduction. *Annual Review of Physiology* 54, 135–152.

Gruenberg, J., and Clague, M.J. (1992). Regulation of intracellular membrane transport. *Current Opinion in Cell Biology* 4(4), 593–599.

Hays, R.M., Franki, N., Simon, H., *et al.* (1994). Antidiuretic hormone and exocytosis: Lessons from neurosecretion. *American Journal of Physiology* 267(6 Pt. 1), C1507–C1524.

Hill, C.S., and Treisman, R. (1995). Transcriptional regulation by extracellular signals: Mechanisms and specificity. *Cell* 80(2), 199–211.

Hughes, D.A., Pinder, A.C., Piper, Z., *et al.* (1996). Fish oil supplementation inhibits the expression of major histocompatibility complex class II molecules and adhesion molecules on human monocytes. *American Journal of Clinical Nutrition* 63(2), 267–272.

Janben-Timmen, U., Tomic, I., Specht, E., *et al.* (1994). The arachidonic acid cascade, eicosanoids, and signal transduction. *Annals of the New York Academy of Sciences* 733(Sep 15), 325–334.

Kuhn, M.M. (1991). *Pharmacotherapeutics: A Nursing Process Approach.* (2nd Ed.). Philadelphia: F.A. Davis Co.

Kunkel, E.J., Jung, U., Bullard, D.C., *et al.* (1996). Absence of trauma-induced leukocyte rolling in mice deficient in both P-selectin and intercellular adhesion molecule 1. *Journal of Experimental Medicine* 183(1), 57–65.

LaLonde, J.M., Bernlohr, D.A., and Banaszak, L.J. (1994). The up-and-down beta-barrel proteins. *FASEB Journal* 8(15), 1240–1247.

Lefkowitz, R.J. (1995). G proteins in medicine. *The New England Journal of Medicine* 332(3), 186–187.

Lentze, M.J. (1995). Molecular and cellular aspects of hydrolysis and absorption. *American Journal of Clinical Nutrition* 61(suppl.), 946S–951S.

Liscovitch, M., and Cantley, L.C. (1994). Lipid second messengers. *Cell* 77(3), 329–334.

Lodish, H., Baltimore, D., Berk, A., *et al.* (1995). *Molecular Cell Biology.* (3rd Ed.). New York: Scientific American Books.

Mills, J.W., and Mandel, L.J. (1994). Cytoskeletal regulation of membrane transport events. *FASEB Journal* 8(14), 1161–1165.

Nerum, R.M., Harrison, D.G., Taylor, W.R., *et al.* (1993). Hemodynamics and vascular endothelial biology. *Journal of Cardiovascular Pharmacology* 21(suppl. 1), S6–S10.

Pongs, O. (1992). Structural basis of voltage-gated K+ channel pharmacology. *Trends in Pharmacology Science* 13(9), 359–365.

Saier, M.H. Jr. (1994). Convergence and divergence in the evolution of transport proteins. *BioEssays* 16(1), 23–29.

Shing, S.T., To, P.M., Hyland, V.J., *et al.* (1996). Regulation of adhesion molecule expression by human synovial microvascular endothelial cells in vitro. *Arthritis and Rheumatism* 39(3), 467–477.

Shiota, Y., Wilson, J.G., Marukawa, M., *et al.* (1996). Soluble intercellular adhesion molecule 1 (ICAM-1) antigen in sera of bronchial asthmatics. *Chest* 109(1), 94–99.

Siitonen, S.M., Kononen, J.T., Helin, H.J., *et al.* (1996). Reduced E-cadherin expression is associated with invasiveness and unfavorable prognosis in breast cancer. *American Journal of Clinical Pharmacy* 105(4), 394–402.

Steinbach, F., Tanabe, K., Alexander, J., *et al.* (1996). The influence of cytokines on the adhesion of renal cancer cells to endothelium. *The Journal of Urology* 155(2), 743–748.

Thilo, L. (1994). Endocytosis: Aspects of organellar processing. *Annals of the New York Academy of Sciences* 710 (Mar 9), 209–216.

Tjian, R. (1995). Molecular machines that control genes. *Scientific American* 272(2), 54–61.

Ussing, H.H. (1994). Does active transport exist? *The Journal of Membrane Biology* 137(2), 91–98.

Walsh, D.A., and Van Patten, S.M. (1994). Multiple pathway signal transduction by the cAMP-dependent protein kinase. *FASEB Journal* 8(15), 1227–1236.

Wolfe, S.L. (1993). *Molecular and Cellular Biology*. Belmont, CA: Wadsworth Publishing Co.

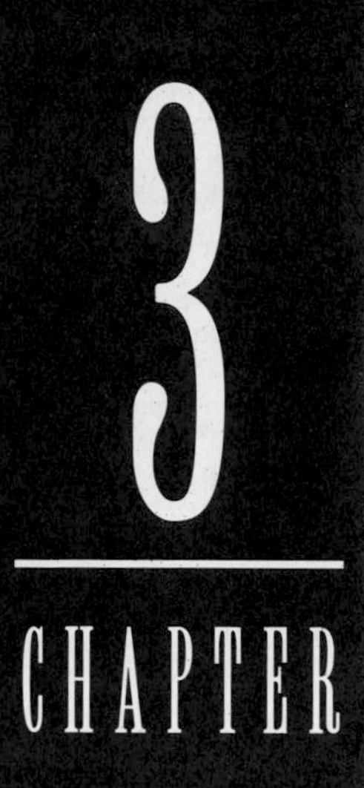

Cellular Nutrition and Energy Metabolism

LEARNING OBJECTIVES

1. Explain the concept of cellular energy balance from a systems perspective.
2. Identify the principal forms of energy input that fuel energy metabolism.
3. Identify the body processes that are energy dependent.
4. List the principal storage forms of energy within the cell.
5. Compare and contrast the cellular locations, fuels, metabolic pathways, and energy outputs of glycolysis, Krebs cycle, and oxidative phosphorylation.
6. Describe the metabolic switching that occurs between the absorptive and postabsorptive states.
7. Discuss mechanisms by which altered energy input can lead to energy imbalance.
8. Discuss conditions in which impaired energy processing promotes energy imbalance.
9. Describe the effects of hypometabolism and hypermetabolism on energy balance.
10. Characterize the relationship between energy imbalance and disease.

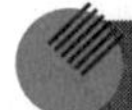

key terms

absorptive state
acetyl CoA
adenosine triphosphate (ATP)
adipose tissue
aerobic metabolism
anabolism
anaerobic metabolism
anorexia
antioxidant
basal metabolic rate (BMR)
β-oxidation
catabolism
Cori cycle
creatine phosphate
fatigue
glucagon
gluconeogenesis
glycogen
glycogenesis
glycogenolysis
glycolysis
guanosine triphosphate (GTP)
hypermetabolic state
hypometabolic state
hypoxia
insulin
keto acid
ketone body
Krebs cycle
lactic acid (lactate)

lipogenesis
lipolysis
malaise
metabolism
negative nitrogen balance
oxidative phosphorylation
oxidative stress
positive nitrogen balance
postabsorptive state
pyruvic acid (pyruvate)
reactive oxygen species
respiratory quotient (RQ)
toxin
trauma

Metabolism refers to the multiple processes by which cells acquire and use energy. Cells must expend energy for active processes, including (1) movement (cell locomotion, intracellular transport, cell division, and muscle contraction), (2) membrane transport (active transport, endocytosis, and exocytosis), and (3) biosynthesis (building of complex molecules from simpler molecules for tissue growth, repair, and remodeling and for regulatory functions). Metabolism couples these energy-consuming processes with energy-producing processes (energy metabolism), metabolic pathways that result in the production of energy from ingested nutrients.

Energy balance requires that energy use and energy metabolism be in equilibrium at all subsystem levels. In this chapter, the major nutrient fuels and metabolic pathways for energy production are discussed along with mechanisms of their regulation. Mechanisms of energy imbalance are introduced, and the relationships of energy imbalance to disease in general and to selected disorders are discussed.

ENERGY BALANCE WITHIN THE CELL

Systems Overview

Systems theory provides a convenient way of conceptualizing cellular energy metabolism. The system, in this case the cell, takes in energy from its environment, processes this energy for its use, and eventually expends energy to the environment as work or heat (Fig. 3–1). Energy homeostasis is governed by the first law of thermodynamics, which requires that energy input into a system must always equal energy output. Energy may be gained by a system and spent by a system, but energy cannot be created or destroyed.

In the human body, nutrition provides energy sources for the cell. Food is ingested, and large molecules are broken down through the mechanical and chemical processes of digestion into simpler forms (see Chapter 25). Carbohydrates are absorbed into the bloodstream primarily as glucose; lipids are absorbed as triglycerides; and proteins are absorbed as amino acids (Fig. 3–2). In the cells, metabolic enzymes continue the breakdown of these nutrient molecules, generating intermediate and end products (metabolites) and free energy. This energy may be stored within cells for future use or may be used almost immediately for cellular work or active processes. In even the most efficient of machines, some energy is unavailable to do work. Instead, it is released into the environment as heat. The body's metabolic machinery is highly efficient, yet 60% of the energy produced by cells is released as heat, generating core body temperature.

Energy Input

Carbohydrates, lipids, and proteins are the fuels that feed the metabolic furnace within body cells. Water and certain vitamins and minerals are essential to energy processing. In most systems, oxygen is also a requirement.

Carbohydrates

Most dietary carbohydrate is derived from plant sources, although a small amount comes from milk (lactose) and even less from the muscle glycogen in meats. Sugars (monosaccharides and disaccharides) and starches (polysaccharides) are ultimately broken down to glucose (a monosaccharide) for use by body cells. The level of glucose in the blood is tightly regulated by the endocrine system because some tissues (i.e., the brain, exercising muscle, and red blood cells) rely almost exclusively on glucose as energy fuel. Glucose levels can be increased by hormonal mechanisms that (1) release glucose from **glycogen** storage, (2) convert lipid or protein metabolites to glucose (**gluconeogenesis**), or (3) preferentially metabolize nonglucose fuels, sparing glucose.

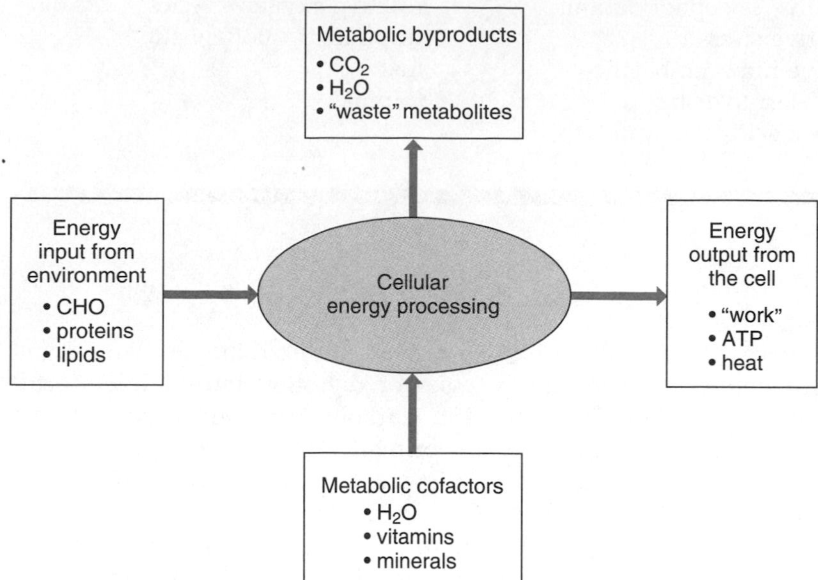

FIGURE 3–1
Systems view of energy balance. Energy is taken into the cell in the form of nutrients. The cell processes these fuels by metabolic pathways and either releases energy as heat or converts it to the chemical "currency" molecule, ATP. ATP is expended in the work of the cell—movement, active transport, or biosynthesis.

Conversely, blood glucose levels can be reduced by glucose uptake into glycogen storage. Glucose homeostasis is briefly discussed later in this chapter, and its regulation is detailed in Chapter 29.

Lipids

Neutral fats (triglycerides) are the most abundant dietary lipids, although some cholesterol and phospholipids are taken in as well. Saturated fats, containing no double carbon–carbon bonds, are found primarily in meats and dairy products. These constitute a major source of cholesterol. Unsaturated fats, containing double bonds, are found in seeds, nuts, and vegetable oils.

Dietary fats are broken down into fatty acids and monoglycerides, then resynthesized into triglycerides for absorption. Triglycerides, phospholipids, and cholesterol are taken up by liver cells for conversion to lipoproteins, in which form they are transported in the bloodstream. Lipids are the major energy fuel used by the heart and by resting skeletal

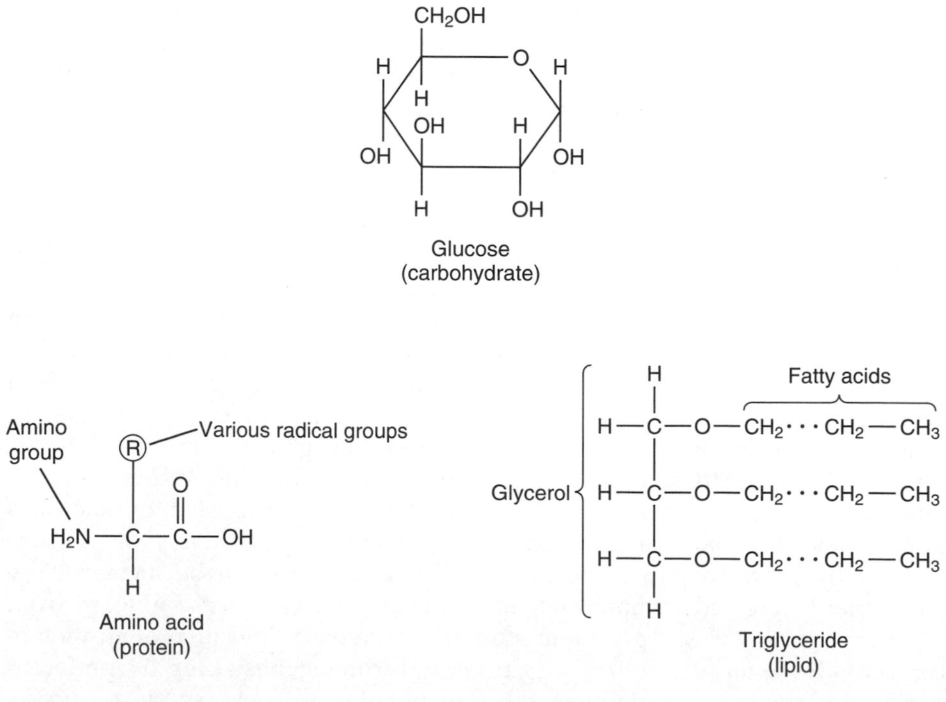

Glucose
(carbohydrate)

Amino group
Various radical groups
Amino acid
(protein)

Glycerol
Fatty acids
Triglyceride
(lipid)

FIGURE 3–2
Principal absorption forms of nutrients. Carbohydrates are absorbed primarily as glucose, although other sugars (e.g., mannose, fructose, and galactose) are absorbed in small amounts. Lipids are absorbed primarily as neutral fats (triglycerides)—three fatty acids attached to a carbohydrate (glycerol) backbone. A small amount of lipid is absorbed as cholesterol or phospholipid. Most proteins are absorbed as single amino acids, characterized by amino (-NH_2) and carboxyl (−COOH) groups. A few proteins are absorbed as peptides (chains of amino acids) or as whole proteins.

muscle; they are used by all cells for synthesis of cell membranes. Lipids are also used by some endocrine cells for the synthesis of steroid hormones (e.g., aldosterone, cortisol, sex hormones). Mediators derived from membrane lipids (e.g., prostaglandins) are also important signaling molecules. Excess lipids are stored in **adipose tissue**, which serves as the body's primary long-term energy reservoir. As discussed in Chapter 25, elevated levels of certain classes of lipoproteins contribute to the development of atherosclerotic lesions in arteries. Atherosclerosis is the pathophysiologic process that underlies coronary artery disease, hypertension, stroke, and peripheral vascular disease (see Chapter 15).

Proteins

Proteins are complex molecules composed of nitrogen-containing amino acids (Fig. 3–2) linked by peptide bonds between their amino (-NH_2) and carboxyl (-COOH) groups. As discussed in Chapter 6, the genetic code directs the synthesis of proteins composed of variable sequences of amino acids. Table 3–1 lists and classifies the 20 amino acids found in proteins. A number of amino acid derivatives are not incorporated into proteins but function as important signaling molecules; these include thyroid hormones, catecholamines, nitric oxide, and γ-aminobutyric acid. Proteins are important structural components of the body and also serve critical functional roles. Enzymes and their precursors are proteins, and cytokines are peptides. Many hormones and neurotransmitters are amino acids, proteins, or peptides. Protein–protein interactions are critical to tissue matrix signaling, molecular adhesion, and signal transduction systems (see Chapter 2). As detailed in other chapters, proteins in the blood (plasma proteins) are integral to fluid balance (e.g., albumin), transport (e.g., albumin, transferrin), blood clotting (e.g., fibrinogen, prothrombin), and immune function (e.g., immunoglobulins).

Amino acids are classified as *essential* if they must be taken in by dietary sources. *Nonessential* amino acids can be synthesized in the body from metabolic precursor molecules. Dietary proteins derived from animal products (eggs, meats, and milk) are *complete proteins*; that is, they contain all of the amino acids required by the body. Vegetables and grains provide *incomplete proteins*, containing some, but not all, essential amino acids. Vegetarian diets must therefore be carefully planned to supply all essential amino acids. Ninety-nine per cent of all protein is absorbed as single amino acids or as peptide bond–linked chains of amino acids (peptides or polypeptides). A few proteins may be absorbed whole; these can also trigger food allergies (see Chapter 13).

Unlike carbohydrate and lipid fuels, excess amino acids are not stored for future use but rather are converted to intermediate products that may enter energy production pathways. Structural and functional body proteins are not used as energy fuel unless glucose and fat are unavailable to tissues. In such states, amino acids derived from the diet, from plasma proteins, or from breakdown of muscle and other tissues can be converted to glucose by liver cells (gluconeogenesis). The condition in which protein is consumed as energy fuel or during biosynthesis at a rate greater than its intake, resulting in breakdown of body proteins, is termed **negative nitrogen balance**. Patients in whom protein intake exceeds protein consumption for energy or biosynthesis are said to be in **positive nitrogen balance**.

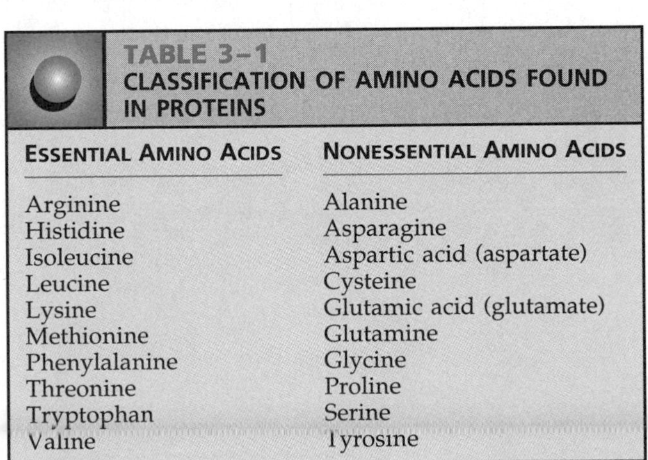

TABLE 3–1
CLASSIFICATION OF AMINO ACIDS FOUND IN PROTEINS

Essential Amino Acids	Nonessential Amino Acids
Arginine	Alanine
Histidine	Asparagine
Isoleucine	Aspartic acid (aspartate)
Leucine	Cysteine
Lysine	Glutamic acid (glutamate)
Methionine	Glutamine
Phenylalanine	Glycine
Threonine	Proline
Tryptophan	Serine
Valine	Tyrosine

Clinical Scenario

C.N., age 3 years, suffered burns over 60% of her body when she turned on the hot-water tap while in the bathtub. (Her mother had left her briefly to answer the telephone.) She is admitted to the Burn Care Unit of a major medical center, where her wounds are cleansed of dead tissue and drainage each day. She is being treated with antibiotics for systemic infection.

1. What factors place C.N. at risk for negative nitrogen balance? Is her age relevant?
2. What clinical manifestations might indicate malnutrition in this case? What interventions might minimize the risk of malnutrition?

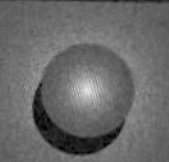

TABLE 3–2
VITAMIN SOURCES, FUNCTIONS, AND MANIFESTATIONS OF EXCESS OR DEFICIT

Vitamin	Sources	Functions	Signs of Excess	Signs of Deficit
Vitamin A (retinol)	Fortified dairy products, eggs, liver, dark green vegetables, deep orange fruits and vegetables	Synthesis of visual pigments, growth and repair of epithelium, immunity, reproduction, antioxidant function	Demineralization of bones and teeth, joint pain, amenorrhea, bleeding tendency, dry skin and hair, nausea and vomiting, enlarged liver and spleen	Stunted growth, joint pain, anemia, night blindness, dry skin and hair, corneal degeneration, hyperkeratosis, diarrhea, immunosuppression
Vitamin D (cholecalciferol)	Sunlight on skin, fortified dairy products, liver, fish	Calcium homeostasis	Hypercalcemia, hyperphosphatemia, kidney stones, calcium deposits	Rickets, osteomalacia, hypocalcemia, hypophosphatemia
Vitamin E (α-tocopherol)	Plant oils, green leafy vegetables, whole grains, liver, egg yolk, nuts, seeds	Antioxidant function, stabilization of cell membranes	Impaired wound healing, hypertension, gastrointestional (GI) discomfort, headache, fatigue, dizziness, visual disturbance	Hemolytic anemia (rare)
Vitamin K	Bacterial synthesis in GI tract, liver, green leafy vegetables, cruciferous vegetables, milk	Synthesis of clotting factors	None	Bleeding tendency
Thiamine (B_1)	Pork, liver, whole grains, legumes, nuts	Coenzyme in energy metabolism	None	Tachycardia, edema, enlarged heart, dysrhythmias, heart failure, muscle weakness, confusion, beriberi
Riboflavin (B_2)	Dairy products, meat, green leafy vegetables	Coenzyme in energy metabolism	None	Glossitis, cheilitis, photophobia, inflammation of cornea, skin rash
Niacin (B_3, nicotinic acid)	Milk, eggs, meat, poultry, fish, whole grains	Coenzyme in energy metabolism, inhibition of cholesterol synthesis	Nausea and vomiting, glossitis, dizziness, flushing, skin rash, excessive sweating, hypotension, abnormal liver function	Diarrhea, anorexia, weakness, dizziness, confusion, skin rash, photosensitivity, pellagra
Vitamin B_6 (pyridoxine)	Green leafy vegetables, meat, fish, poultry, shellfish, legumes, fruits, whole grains	Coenzyme in amino acid metabolism and fatty acid metabolism, glycogenolysis, synthesis of hemoglobin and immunoglobulins	Bloating, depression, fatigue, irritability, headache, numbness, decreased reflexes, gait disturbances	Microcytic anemia, glossitis, cheilitis, abnormal electrocardiogram, muscle twitching, seizures, dermatitis, kidney stones
Folate (folic acid)	Green leafy vegetables, legumes, seeds, liver	Coenzyme in synthesis of amino acids, DNA, and red blood cells	None	Macrocytic anemia, loss of GI villi, constipation, diarrhea, glossitis, embryonic neural tube defects

TABLE 3–2
VITAMIN SOURCES, FUNCTIONS, AND MANIFESTATIONS OF EXCESS OR DEFICIT *Continued*

VITAMIN	SOURCES	FUNCTIONS	SIGNS OF EXCESS	SIGNS OF DEFICIT
Vitamin B_{12} (cyanocobalamin)	Meat, fish, poultry, shellfish, milk, cheese, eggs	Coenzyme in synthesis of GI tract, CNS, and bone marrow cells; synthesis of DNA and amino acids	None	Macrocytic anemia, glossitis, fatigue, peripheral nerve degeneration, skin rash
Biotin	Liver, egg yolk, legumes, nuts, GI bacterial synthesis	Coenzyme in energy metabolism, fat synthesis, amino acid metabolism, and glycogenesis	None	Anorexia, nausea, depression, muscle pain, weakness, fatigue, dry skin, hypercholesterolemia
Pantothenic acid	Liver, egg yolk, legumes, nuts, GI bacterial synthesis	Part of coenzyme A (energy metabolism)	Diarrhea, edema	Vomiting, insomnia, fatigue
Vitamin C (ascorbic acid)	Citrus fruits, cruciferous vegetables, dark green vegetables, melon, strawberries, tomatoes	Synthesis of collagen and thyroxine, antioxidant function, amino acid metabolism, immune function, iron absorption	Hemolysis, nausea, diarrhea, headache, fatigue, hot flashes, skin rash, increased urination, demineralization of bone, kidney stones	Microcytic anemia, atherosclerosis, bleeding tendency, immunosuppression, gingivitis, muscle wasting, depression, bone pain, rough skin, impaired wound healing, scurvy

Vitamins

Vitamins are organic compounds that, although not used for energy themselves, are essential to metabolism of the major nutrients. Most vitamins act as coenzymes in metabolic reactions. As discussed later, the B vitamins riboflavin and niacin are essential to oxidation of glucose for energy.

Vitamins are classified as either fat soluble or water soluble. The fat-soluble vitamins A, D, E, and K are absorbed bound to dietary lipid and may be stored in large amounts in the liver and in adipose tissue (hence the potential for toxicity due to excess amounts of these vitamins). Vitamin D can be synthesized by skin cells exposed to ultraviolet radiation (sunlight), and vitamin K can be synthesized by bacteria within the intestinal tract. Vitamins A and E must be ingested in the diet. In addition, all of the water-soluble vitamins—the B complex and vitamin C—must be ingested on a regular basis. These vitamins are absorbed with water from the gastrointestinal tract, except for vitamin B_{12}, which is absorbed in combination with a glycoprotein, intrinsic factor. Table 3–2 summarizes vitamin sources, functions, and manifestations of excess (toxicity) or deficiency.

Minerals

Minerals are inorganic substancess that, like vitamins, are not used directly for fuel but are in some cases essential to energy metabolism. Iron, for example, is critical to oxidative metabolism in mitochondria. Phosphorus is critical to enzyme activation or inactivation and to the synthesis of molecules used in energy storage and transfer. Table 3–3 summarizes sources, functions, and manifestations of deficiency or excess of the major minerals and several trace elements. The functions of most major minerals (electrolytes) are further detailed in Chapter 9, along with related disorders.

Energy Output

The body consumes energy in muscle contraction, including tension development and movement of skeletal muscles; in constriction of smooth muscle in blood vessels, glandular ducts, and intestinal walls; and in cardiac contraction. Energy is also required for single cell movement, as in transmigration of white blood cells into tissues or movement of cellular appendages such as cilia. Transport of substances

TABLE 3–3
MINERAL SOURCES, FUNCTIONS, AND MANIFESTATIONS OF EXCESS OR DEFICIT

Mineral	Sources	Functions	Signs of Excess	Signs of Deficit
Major Minerals				
Sodium	Table salt, soy sauce, processed foods	Fluid balance, action potential formation	Lethargy, weakness, irritability, twitching, seizures, coma, intracranial bleeding, signs of dehydration	Anorexia, nausea, vomiting, cramping, seizures, lethargy, apathy, confusion, decreased sensation, signs of volume excess
Chloride	Table salt, soy sauce, processed foods	Fluid balance, acid-base balance, gastric HCL synthesis	Same as sodium excess	Same as sodium deficit, alkalosis
Potassium	Meat, milk, fruits, vegetables, grains, legumes	Action potential formation, acid-base balance	Weakness, numbness and tingling, paralysis, dysrhythmias, electrocardiogram changes	Dysrhythmias, weakness, hyporeflexia, paralysis, urinary retention, lethargy, confusion, electrocardiogram changes, alkaline and dilute urine, rhabdomyolysis
Calcium	Dairy products, tofu, green vegetables, legumes, sardines	Synthesis of bones and teeth, muscle contraction, blood clotting, action potential formation, neurotransmitter release	Fatigue, weakness, lethargy, dysrhythmias, urolithiasis, decreased bone density, thirst, anorexia, constipation, encephalopathy, hypercalciuria	Seizures, numbness and tingling, Chvostek's sign, Trousseau's sign, tetany, carpopedal spasm, dysrhythmias, dyspnea, dysphagia, colic, cardiac failure
Phosphorus	All animal tissues	Synthesis of bones and teeth, energy metabolism, DNA and RNA synthesis	Same as calcium deficit	Same as calcium excess
Magnesium	Nuts, legumes, whole grains, dark green vegetables, seafood, chocolate	Synthesis of bones and teeth, enzyme action, action potential formation, enzyme synthesis	Hyporeflexia, nausea, vomiting, weakness, paralysis, hypotension, dysrhythmias	Chvostek's sign, Trousseau's sign, tetany, vertigo, nystagmus, gait disorder, hypokalemia, hypocalcemia, dysrhythmias
Sulfur	All protein foods	Component of protein (S-S bonds), component of vitamins (biotin and thiamine) and of insulin, detoxification reactions	None known	None known
Trace Elements				
Iron	Red meats, fish, eggs, poultry, shellfish, legumes, dried fruits	Component of myoglobin and hemoglobin, energy metabolism	Hemosiderosis	Fatigue, dyspnea, palpitations, angina, tachycardia, hypochromic and microcytic anemia

TABLE 3–3
MINERAL SOURCES, FUNCTIONS, AND MANIFESTATIONS OF EXCESS OR DEFICIT *Continued*

Mineral	Sources	Functions	Signs of Excess	Signs of Deficit
Zinc	Protein foods, grains, vegetables	Part of many enzymes, synthesis of genetic material and proteins, associated with insulin, vitamin A transport, taste perception, wound healing, spermatogenesis, fetal development	Reduced availability of copper, sideroblastic anemia, neutropenia	Skin rash, anergy, growth retardation, impaired taste, impaired immune function, glucose intolerance, alopecia, hypogonadism, depression, diarrhea
Iodine	Iodized salt, seafood, plants in certain regions	Component of thyroid hormones	Iodide myxedema	Cretinism, hypothyroidism
Copper	Meat, drinking water	Absorption and use of iron, myelin synthesis, part of several enzymes	Gastrointestinal problems, hemolysis, liver toxicity	Osteoporosis, bone hematomas, abnormal bone formation, limb edema, neurologic abnormalities, anemia, neutropenia
Manganese	Widely distributed	Facilitates cell processes, with enzymes	Neuropsychiatric symptoms	Hair color change, hypercholesterolemia, prolonged prothrombin time
Fluoride	Drinking water, seafood, tea	Formation of bones and teeth	Loss of appetite, fluorosis	Dental caries
Chromium	Meat, unprocessed foods	Associated with insulin, necessary for release of energy from glucose	None known	Glucose intolerance, insulin resistance, peripheral neuropathy, metabolic encephalopathy, hyperlipidemia
Selenium	Seafood	Antioxidant function	Alopecia, abnormal nails, garlic breath	Myositis, muscle pain, cardiomyopathy, Keshan disease
Molybdenum	Legumes, cereals, organ meats	Facilitates many processes, with enzymes	Gout-like symptoms	None known

across the plasma membrane or across organelle membranes is an energy-dependent process if such movement is against a biologic gradient. Transport of complex molecules by endocytosis or exocytosis also consumes energy (see Chapter 2).

Synthesis of molecules required for growth or tissue building, for regulatory or intercellular signaling, for energy storage, or for alteration of toxic substances into nontoxic or excretable forms also requires the expenditure of energy. Energy released as heat maintains the thermal environment essential to optimal cellular function. Thermoregulation is discussed in Chapter 11.

The **basal metabolic rate (BMR)** is the amount of energy expended during standard resting conditions, typically measured in humans during quiet relaxation after a restful sleep and a 12-hour fast. The BMR is normally about 1.1 kcal/minute but varies depending on lean body mass, hormonal stimulation, and other factors (Table 3–4). (The use of the term *calorie* by nutritionists to quantify dietary energy content actually refers to the kilocalorie. In thermodynamics, the term *joule* is now used in preference to calorie or kilocalorie to refer to a quantity of energy.) There is growing evidence of a genetic basis for variation in BMR as well.[1] Basal metabolism also varies among organ systems. Muscle, even at rest, has a much higher metabolic rate than fat, for example. Proportionately to mass, the brain accounts for the most energy consumption.

TABLE 3–4
FACTORS INFLUENCING BASAL METABOLIC RATE (BMR)

FACTOR	EFFECT
Lean body mass	BMR increases proportionately to lean body mass. Muscle is more actively metabolic than adipose tissue.
Age	BMR decreases as age increases. Increased growth and synthetic activity demand higher metabolism during youth, whereas loss of muscle mass with aging mediates a lower BMR.
Sex	BMR is higher in males. Increased lean body mass and the influence of testosterone account for this.
Climate	BMR increases as ambient temperature increases. Thyroid hormone secretion increases in cool environments to maintain constant body temperature.
Pregnancy	BMR increases by an average of 30% during pregnancy. Metabolism of newly synthesized fetal, placental, and breast tissue accounts for this.

CELLULAR PROCESSING OF ENERGY

Energy Currency and Storage Forms

Within cells, energy is formed and "spent" primarily as **adenosine triphosphate (ATP)**, a nucleic acid derivative thus referred to as the "energy currency" of cells (Fig. 3–3). ATP contains two phosphate bonds that are generated during metabolism of nutrients. When these bonds are cleaved, forming adenosine diphosphate (ADP), energy is liberated for use in movement, transport, or synthesis. Although the phosphate bonds are referred to as *high-energy* bonds, the actual source of free energy is not the bonds themselves but rather the change in structure of the whole molecule when the bonds are cleaved. Several complex physicochemical factors, including fewer repulsive forces between like charges in ADP than in ATP, contribute to the liberation of energy.

Guanosine triphosphate (GTP) is a nucleotide derivative similar to ATP, which is less commonly employed as energy currency. G-protein signal transduction and ribosomal synthesis of proteins are examples of processes that depend on energy from GTP hydrolysis. In muscle, **creatine phosphate** serves as an important energy source in that it can transfer phosphate and energy to ADP, generating ATP (Fig. 3–4).

Longer-term energy storage forms include glycogen stores in liver and muscle and triglycerides in adipose tissue. Under hormonal regulation, these stores may provide glucose and fatty acids that may fuel metabolic pathways for ATP production, discussed later. As has been stated, use of body proteins as fuel occurs only under nonphysiologic conditions, and these proteins are not considered to be energy stores.

Metabolic Pathways for Energy Production

Cells generate ATP from nutrients through three metabolic processes: **glycolysis** (preliminary metabolism, or Embden-Meyerhof pathway), **Krebs cycle** (intermediary metabolism, citric acid cycle, or tricarboxylic acid cycle), and **oxidative phosphorylation** (electron transport chain). These pathways are detailed in the section on carbohydrate metabolism; the potential contributions of lipid and protein derivatives to the pathways are discussed in subsequent sections. Table 3–5 compares the major energy metabolic pathways with respect to their cellular locations, fuel sources, and energy yields.

Chemical Foundations

The metabolic pathways that culminate in energy production consist of sequences of oxidation–reduction (redox) reactions; that is, they involve the removal of pairs of electrons from some molecules (oxidation) and the simultaneous gain of these electrons by other molecules (reduction). Energy is liber-

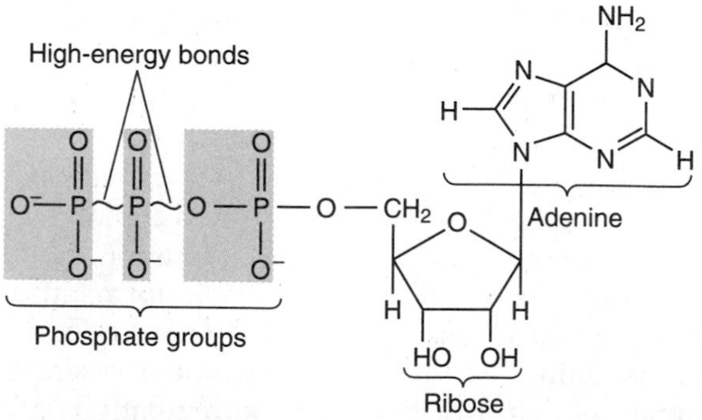

FIGURE 3–3
Adenosine triphosphate. ATP contains two phosphate bonds generated during nutrient metabolism. The energy in ATP is liberated with cleavage of these bonds and may be used to drive active cellular processes.

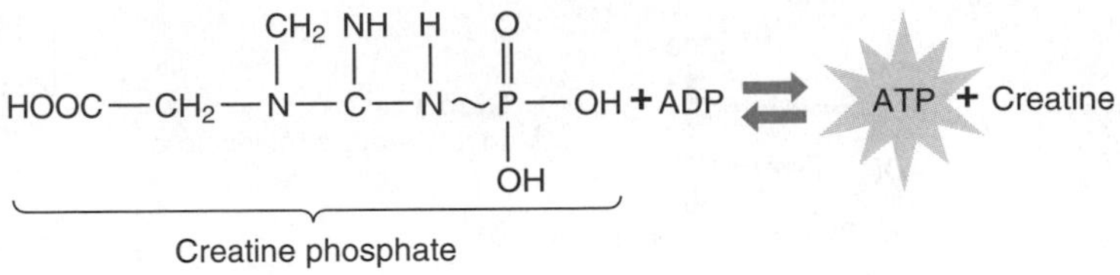

$$HOOC-CH_2-N(CH_2)-C(NH)-N(H)\sim P(=O)(OH)-OH + ADP \rightleftharpoons ATP + \text{Creatine}$$

Creatine phosphate

FIGURE 3–4
Creatine phosphate. In muscle, creatine phosphate serves as an important energy source because cellular ATP is quickly depleted during muscle contraction. Creatine phosphate may then transfer phosphate and energy to ADP, generating ATP for use by the cell. When ATP is again available, creatine phosphate is regenerated.

ated during this exchange because more energy-favorable (or stable) compounds are formed. Oxidation may result from either the gain of oxygen (as in the rusting of iron or the burning of wood) or the loss of hydrogen atoms. Sequential removal of hydrogen atoms (with their electrons) is the mechanism of cellular oxidation of nutrient metabolites for generation of ATP.

The oxidation–reduction reactions of energy metabolism are catalyzed by enzymes (dehydrogenases and oxidases) that require coenzymes (typically B vitamins) for their function. The enzyme catalyzes removal of a hydrogen atom, transferring it temporarily to a hydrogen-accepting coenzyme, thus reducing that coenzyme. The two most important coenzymes in energy metabolism are nicotinamide adenine dinucleotide (NAD), derived from the B vitamin niacin, and flavin adenine dinucleotide (FAD), derived from riboflavin (vitamin B_2).

Carbohydrate Metabolism

Glycolysis. Glycolysis (glucose breakdown) occurs in the cytoplasm of cells (Fig. 3–5) and is the only energy-producing pathway not absolutely dependent on oxygen. Ideally, however, glycolysis occurs in the presence of oxygen (**aerobic metabolism**), in which case glycolysis serves as the first step in complete combustion of glucose by the Krebs cycle and oxidative phosphorylation.

Since glycolysis may proceed in the absence of oxygen (**anaerobic metabolism**), it is a critical energy-producing pathway in situations in which tissues are deprived of oxygen (e.g., strenuous exercise, shock, or respiratory failure). Glycolysis produces little ATP (net gain of two molecules per glucose molecule oxidized) in comparison to the aerobic pathways (38 ATP molecules per glucose molecule). Except for red blood cells, in which glycolysis accounts for all energy metabolism, body cells cannot sustain anaerobic glycolysis for prolonged periods of time. One reason for this is that **lactate** (the dissociated form of **lactic acid**) is produced as an end product of anaerobic glycolysis. Accumulation of lactate results in an increasingly acidic intracellular environment, which may become detrimental to cell function (see Chapter 10). Lactate accumulation and other consequences of cellular **hypoxia**, or lack of oxygen, are discussed later.

As shown in Figure 3–5, glycolysis begins with

TABLE 3–5
COMPARISON OF ENERGY METABOLISM PATHWAYS

PATHWAY	LOCATION	FUELS	OXYGEN REQUIRED	ENERGY OUTPUT
Glycolysis	Cytoplasm	Glucose	No	Net gain of 2 ATP molecules per glucose molecule (plus 2 NADH + H^+ molecules if O_2 present)
Krebs cycle	Mitochondria	Pyruvate, acetyl CoA, keto acids	Yes	1 ATP molecule per turn of the cycle (plus 3 NADH + H^+ and 1 $FADH_2$) 1 NADH + H^+ molecule for each pyruvate converted to acetyl CoA
β-Oxidation	Mitochondria	Fatty acids	Yes	*Consumes* the equivalent of 2 ATP molecules per turn, but produces 1 NADH + H^+ and 1 $FADH_2$, plus 1 acetyl CoA
Oxidative phosphorylation	Mitochondria	Reduced coenzymes (NADH + H^+ and $FADH_2$)	Yes	3 ATP molecules per NADH + H^+; 2 ATP per $FADH_2$

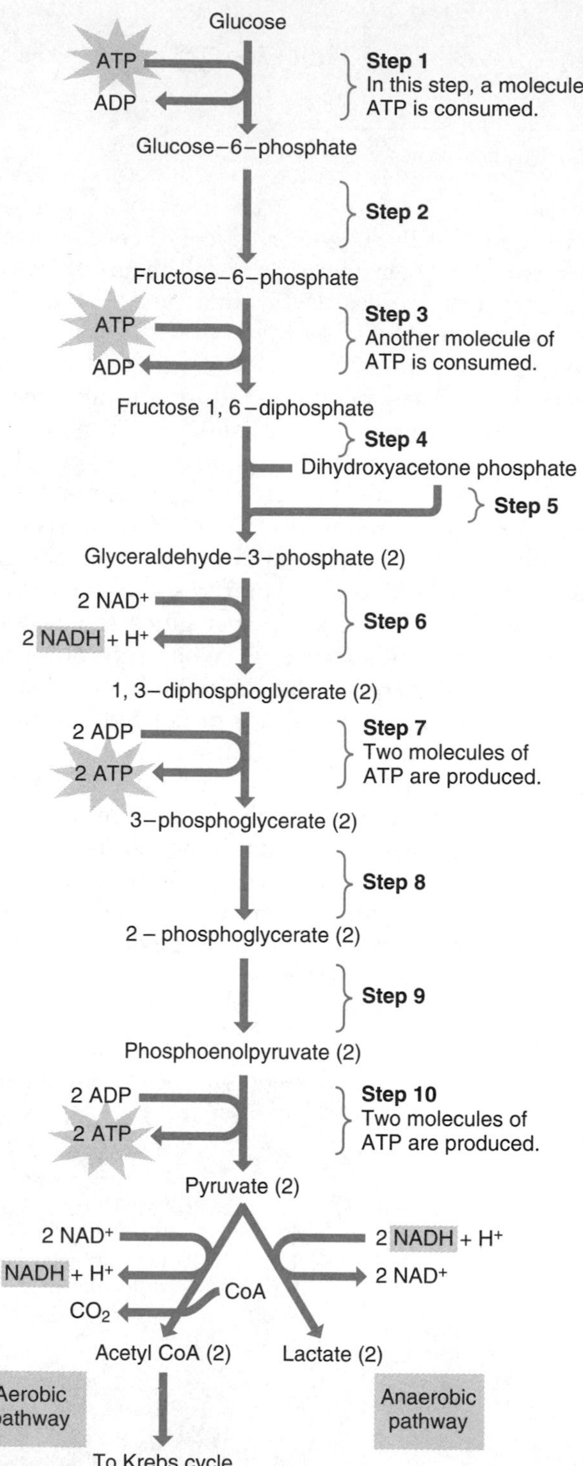

FIGURE 3–5
Glycolysis. Enzymes mediating the glycolytic pathway are located in the cytoplasm. Glycolysis may generate two molecules of ATP per molecule of glucose metabolized in the absence of oxygen. When oxygen is present (aerobic metabolism), reduced coenzymes and pyruvate are also generated, and these may enter the oxidative phosphorylation and the Krebs cycle, respectively, generating additional ATP.

phosphorylation of glucose and conversion to fructose, which is then also phosphorylated. These first steps actually consume two molecules of ATP in activating the pathway. Fructose 1,6-diphosphate is then split into two 3-carbon molecules, which are oxidized, reducing NAD to NADH + H^+. Transfer of phosphate from these metabolic intermediates to ADP, a process referred to as *substrate level phosphorylation*, yields four molecules of ATP (a net gain of two) and two molecules of **pyruvate** (the dissociated form of **pyruvic acid**).

The final steps in glycolysis depend on whether oxygen is present. In the absence of oxygen, NADH + H^+ transfers hydrogen back to pyruvate, reducing it to lactate. Some lactate is transported out of cells to the liver. If oxygen becomes available, this lactate can be (1) converted to pyruvate for use in intermediary metabolism, (2) converted to glucose-6-phosphate for use in hepatic synthesis of glycogen, (3) converted to glucose by an energy-consuming gluconeogenesis pathway known as the **Cori cycle**, or (4) released into the blood, potentially causing acid-base imbalance in body fluids.

The role of lactate in energy metabolism is not completely understood but is certainly not entirely detrimental. Research indicates that significant amounts of lactate are also formed in well-oxygenated tissues.[2] The *lactate shuttle* hypothesis holds that lactate represents an important energy transfer substance because it diffuses easily between tissues. When oxidized to pyruvate, lactate enters intermediary metabolism. When converted to glycogen, it serves as a potential source of glucose, a critical energy substrate.

The outcome of aerobic glycolysis is the delivery of the hydrogen atoms of NADH + H^+ to the enzymes of the electron transport chain for oxidative phosphorylation. NAD is then able to again serve as an electron acceptor, and glycolysis can continue. Pyruvate enters the Krebs cycle for intermediary metabolism.

Krebs Cycle. Although the glycolytic pathway is specific for metabolism of glucose, the Krebs cycle may be fueled by products from carbohydrate, lipid, or protein breakdown. Named for its discoverer, Hans Krebs, this series of reactions occurs in mitochondria. The Krebs cycle is often referred to as *intermediary metabolism* because it uses products from the preliminary metabolism of carbohydrate, lipid, or protein. The Krebs cycle ends when the reduced coenzymes it produces are delivered to the electron transport chain for the final metabolic pathway, oxidative phosphorylation.

The predominant fuel for the Krebs cycle is pyruvate, which enters the mitochondria and is converted to **acetyl CoA** (Fig. 3–6). This conversion is

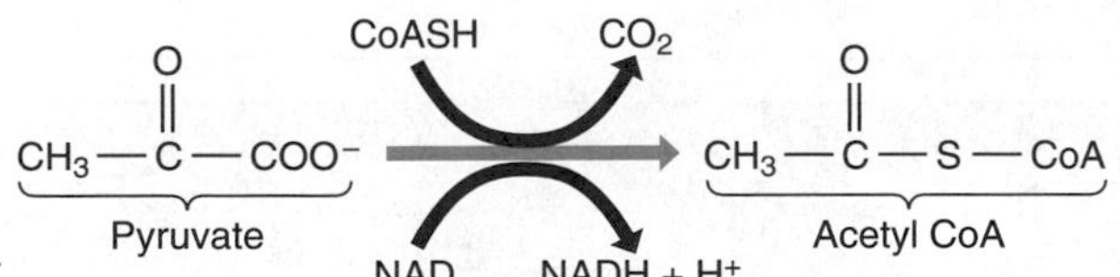

FIGURE 3–6

Conversion of pyruvate to acetyl CoA. Pyruvate (from aerobic glycolysis) must be converted to acetyl CoA before entry into the Krebs cycle. The enzyme pyruvate dehydrogenase catalyzes this reaction, which also generates NADH + H^+ for entry into oxidative phosphorylation.

catalyzed by the enzyme pyruvate dehydrogenase, which reduces NAD to NADH + H^+. Coenzyme A, derived from pantothenic acid (a B vitamin), is added to the resulting acetic acid, producing acetyl coenzyme A (acetyl CoA) and releasing carbon dioxide (CO_2) as a byproduct. Because acetyl CoA can also be synthesized from lipid and protein metabolites, this molecule is often referred to as the *common shuttle*, linking multiple metabolic pathways.

As shown in Figure 3–7, the Krebs cycle begins when acetyl CoA, which contains two carbon atoms, combines with a 4-carbon acid (oxaloacetic acid) to produce citric acid. In eight sequential steps, the six carbons of citric acid are removed or rearranged, producing intermediate products called **keto acids** (acids containing a —C=O group), and eventually regenerating oxaloacetic acid, which can then accept another acetyl CoA. Oxidation generates three NADH + H^+ molecules and one $FADH_2$. Some of the hydrogen atoms are derived from the addition of water during certain steps. Each turn of the Krebs cycle also yields one GTP molecule, which transfers its phosphate to ADP, forming ATP by substrate-level phosphorylation. For the Krebs cycle to continue, the reduced coenzymes must transfer their hydrogen atoms to the electron transport chain for oxidative phosphorylation, the final stage of energy metabolism.

Oxidative Phosphorylation. The electron transport chain is a series of metal-containing enzyme complexes located in the inner mitochondrial membrane (Fig. 3–8). Transfer of electrons down this chain liberates energy, which is used in the phosphorylation of ADP to ATP. Oxygen is the final electron acceptor in the pathway, hence the term oxidative phosphorylation.

The hydrogen atoms delivered to this system by the reduced coenzymes of the Krebs cycle are first

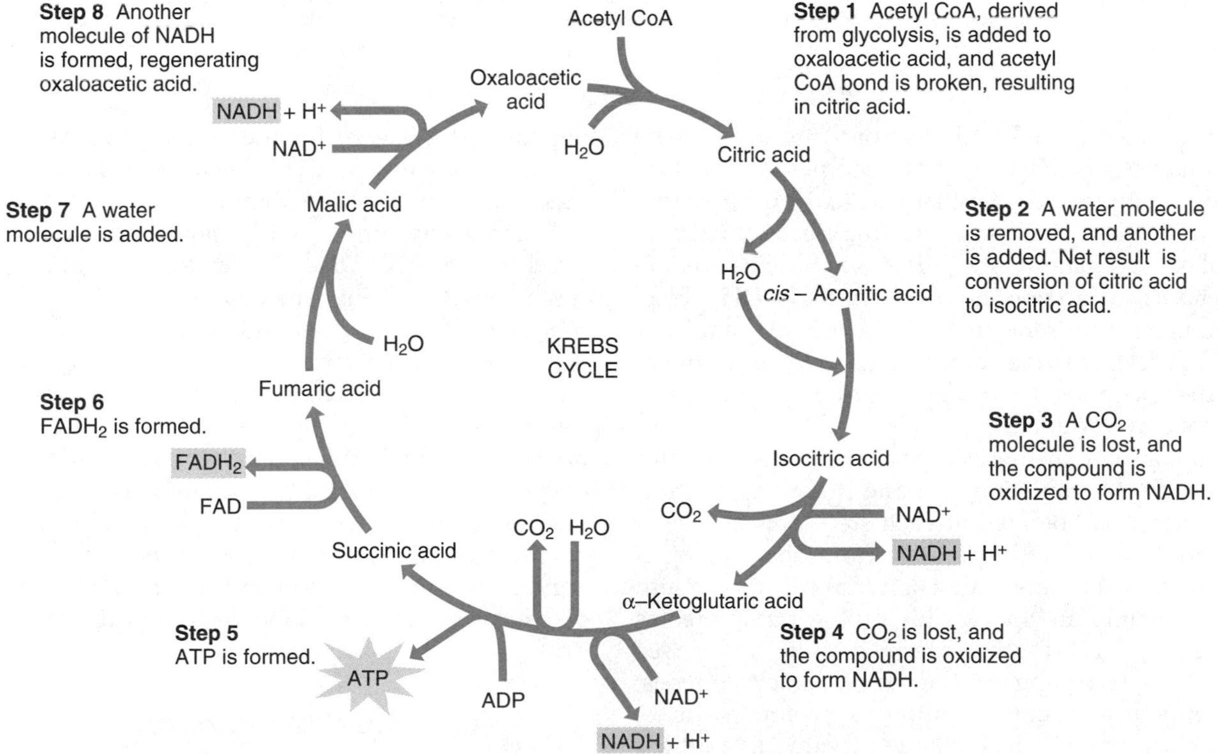

FIGURE 3–7

Krebs cycle. The Krebs cycle, also known as *intermediary metabolism, the citric acid cycle,* or the *tricarboxylic acid* (TCA) *cycle,* is normally fueled by acetyl CoA, which may be derived from pyruvate conversion, β-oxidation of amino acids, metabolism of ketone bodies, or deamination of amino acids. Keto acids (from protein or fatty acid metabolism) may also enter the cycle. Each turn of the cycle produces one ATP molecule and reduced coenzymes for oxidative phosphorylation.

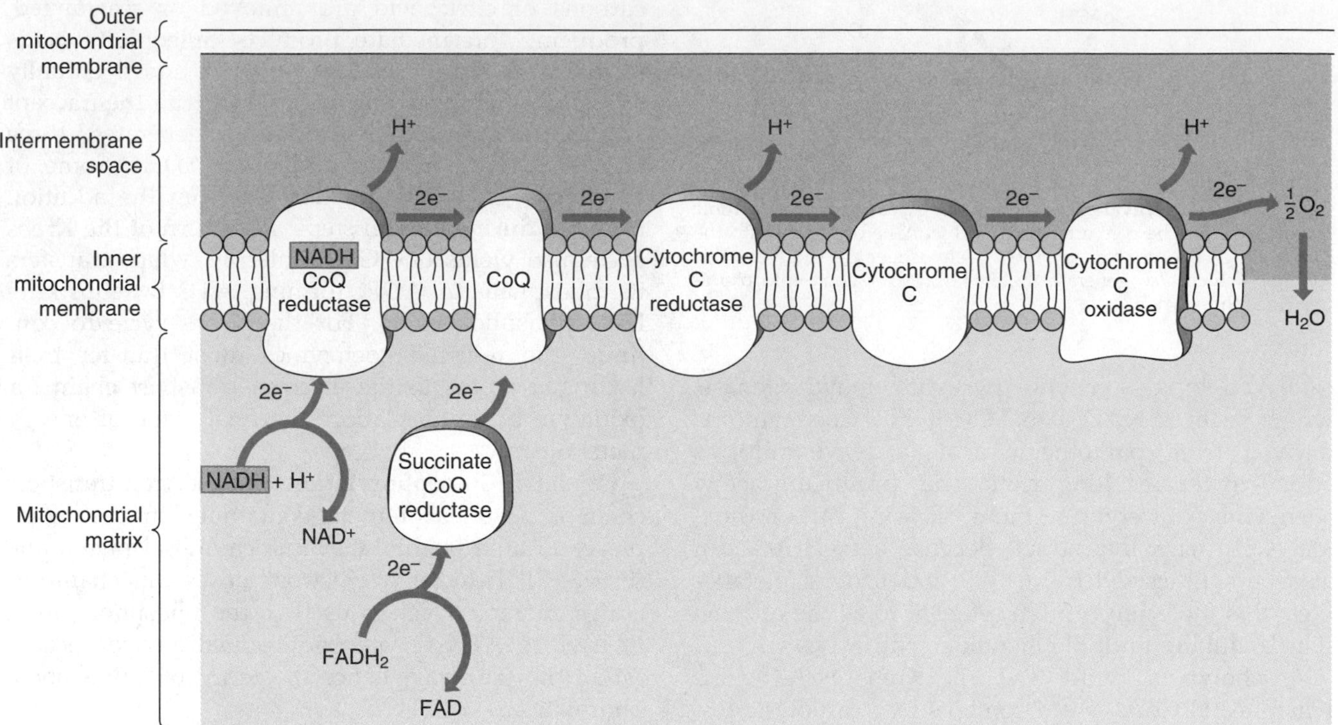

FIGURE 3–8

Electron transport chain. This series of metal-containing enzyme complexes is located in the inner mitochondrial membrane. During the final stage of aerobic metabolism, oxidative phosphorylation, electrons are transferred from reduced coenzymes down this chain of enzyme complexes. Energy is liberated with each transfer as more stable compounds are formed. This energy is coupled to phosphorylation of ADP to ATP by the action of the proton pump.

split into their proton and electron components. The electrons from NADH + H^+ are accepted by the first enzyme complex in the chain, NADH CoQ reductase, and then transferred to the second enzyme complex, succinate–CoQ reductase. Succinate–CoQ reductase also accepts electrons from $FADH_2$. Electron transfer continues down the chain of complexes until the last enzyme, cytochrome *c* oxidase, transfers the electrons to oxygen, forming water as a metabolic by-product.

Each complex in the transport chain has a greater affinity for electrons than the one preceding it; thus, some energy is liberated at each step. This energy is used to transport the protons from the hydrogen atoms across the inner mitochondrial membrane into the intermembrane space. This proton pump creates an excess of H^+ in the intermembrane space (see Fig. 3–8). According to the *chemosmotic hypothesis*, this difference in concentration of proton particles, as well as in electrical charge, creates a gradient (proton-motive force), which favors flow of H^+ back across the membrane (Fig. 3–9). H^+ crosses the membrane through channels in an enzyme complex, ATP synthetase, which uses this energy flow to synthesize ATP from ADP. The proton-motive force also provides energy for the pumping of ADP, inorganic phosphate, pyruvate, and calcium across the inner mitochondrial membrane.

Theoretically, three ATP molecules are synthesized for each NADH + H^+ molecule oxidized, and two for each $FADH_2$. The complete oxidation of one molecule of glucose should yield 38 molecules of ATP. In some analyses, 36 molecules of ATP are generated, apparently because an alternative "shuttle" molecule delivers NADH + H^+ to a site farther down the electron transport chain, liberating less energy for generation of proton-motive force. Direct measurement of energy yield usually indicates lesser amounts of ATP formed, possibly because more energy is consumed in transporting NADH + H^+ from glycolysis between the cytoplasm and the mitochondria.

Lipid Metabolism

Dietary lipids and stored lipids from adipose tissue are important sources of energy. Fatty acids are the preferred energy fuel of resting skeletal muscle, cardiac muscle, and adipose tissue. During periods of fasting or starvation, extended physical exertion,

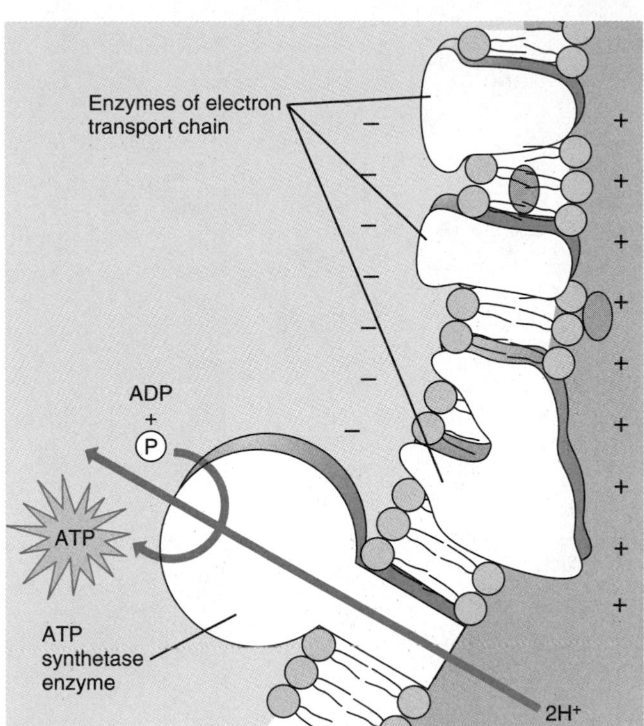

FIGURE 3–9

Proton pump. Energy liberated by the transfer of electrons between the enzyme complexes of the electron transport chain is used to actively transport the protons (H^+) corresponding to those electrons. H^+ is transported from the inner mitochondrial membrane into the intermembrane space (between the double layers of the mitochondrial membrane). The resulting excess of H^+ in this space constitutes concentration and electrical gradients, which then drive H^+ back across the inner mitochondrial membrane. This transport occurs through a channel associated with an enzyme, ATP synthetase, which catalyzes formation of ATP from ADP and inorganic phosphate.

or other forms of stress, many tissues metabolize fats for energy, sparing glucose for the brain and muscle.

Mitochondrial β-Oxidation. Triglycerides are first broken down in the cytoplasm to fatty acids and glycerol. Glycerol is converted to dihydroxyacetone phosphate for entry into glycolysis (see Fig. 3–5, step 5), and fatty acids are converted to acetyl CoA by the process of **β-oxidation**. This cyclic process, shown in Figure 3–10, begins in the cytoplasm and requires the initial consumption of two ATP molecules to synthesize fatty acyl CoA. The fatty acid (acyl) portion of this molecule is then transferred to carnitine, while the CoA is released into the cytosol for reuse. The acyl–carnitine complex is then actively transported into the mitochondrial matrix, where the acyl group is transferred to another CoA. Carnitine is pumped back into the cytosol for reuse.

Within the mitochondria, fatty acyl CoA is oxidized in a sequential process similar to the conversion of succinic acid to oxaloacetic acid within the Krebs cycle. Each turn of the cycle removes two carbons from the original fatty acid and yields one acetyl CoA, one $FADH_2$, and one NADH + H^+. The acetyl CoA enters the Krebs cycle, and the reduced coenzymes enter oxidative phosphorylation. The energy yield depends on the number of carbon atoms in the oxidized fatty acid. An 18-carbon fatty acid, for example, would yield a net of 124 ATP molecules.

Peroxisomal β-Oxidation. Very long chain fatty acids (more than 22 carbons) are first shortened by a similar β-oxidation process in peroxisomes, catalyzed by peroxisomal enzymes. The shorter chains resulting from this process are then transported into the mitochondria for β-oxidation.

Hepatic Ketogenesis. In the liver, a significant portion of the acetyl CoA produced by β-oxidation does not enter the Krebs cycle but instead is converted to **ketone bodies**. These molecules, which are water-soluble equivalents of fatty acids, include acetoacetate, β-hydroxybutyrate, and acetone. (Acetoacetate and β-hydroxybutyrate are also classified structurally as keto acids.) These should not be confused with the α-keto acids, metabolites of some amino acids that may enter the Krebs cycle, as discussed later. Ketone bodies may be converted back to acetyl CoA to serve as metabolic fuel by the liver, skeletal muscle, and other peripheral tissues.

The brain, which normally prefers glucose, may use ketone bodies during starvation. In insulin-dependent diabetes mellitus, impaired glucose uptake results in excessive β-oxidation of lipids for energy. The resulting increase in the formation of ketone bodies produces an acetone odor to the breath and a form of metabolic acidosis known as *diabetic ketoacidosis* (see Chapters 10 and 29).

Protein Metabolism

Proteins are used for energy under two conditions: (1) when dietary protein intake exceeds the rate of tissue **anabolism** (use of protein for growth and repair), and (2) when breakdown of body proteins (**catabolism**) is occurring in states of fasting or starvation and carbohydrate and lipid stores have been depleted.

Deamination. In the cytoplasm, an amino acid is first *deaminated* (NH_2 group removed), with the amino group converted to ammonia (NH_3); or *transaminated* (NH_2 group transferred to an enzyme, which then transfers it to a keto acid acceptor, such as α-ketoglutarate). Ammonia is converted in the liver to urea for excretion in the urine (see Chapter 20). Transamination of α-ketoglutarate yields another amino acid, glutamate, and regenerates the enzyme.

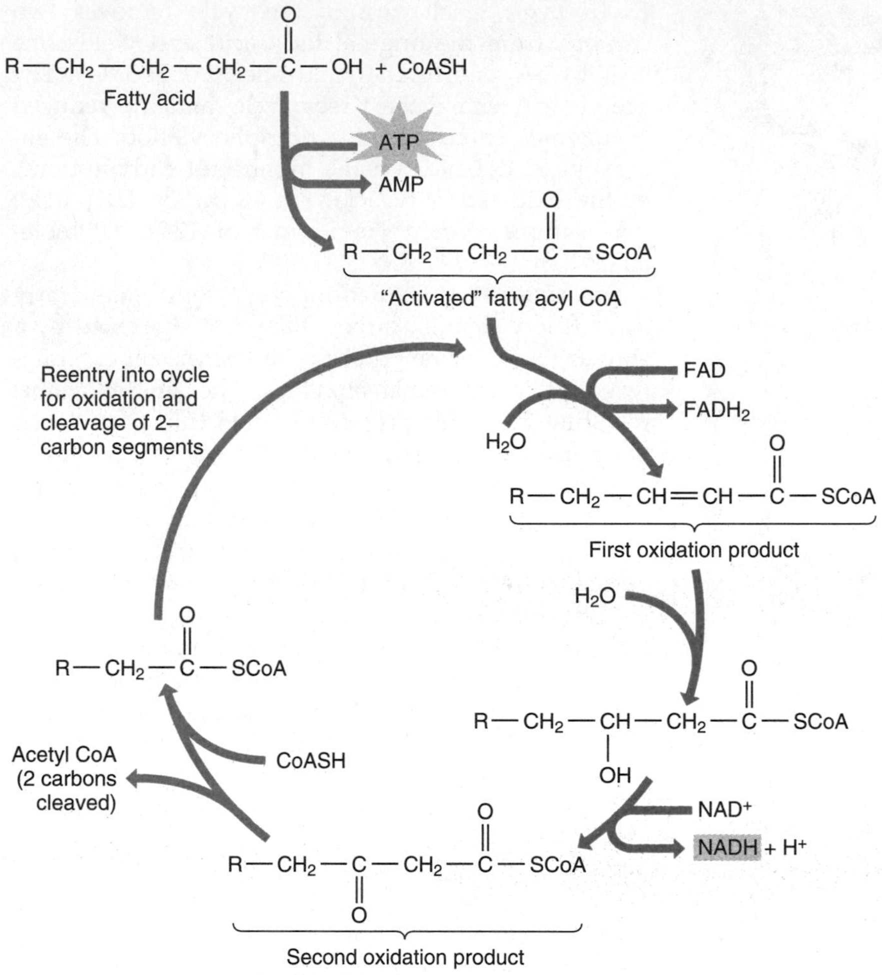

FIGURE 3–10
***β*-Oxidation.** Fatty acids are first activated to fatty acyl CoA in the cytoplasm in an energy-consuming step. After transport into the mitochondrial matrix, sequential oxidation of the fatty acyl CoA yields acetyl CoA for the Krebs cycle and reduced coenzymes for oxidative phosphorylation. (Redrawn from Guyton, A.C., and Hall, J.E. [1995]. *Textbook of Medical Physiology.* [9th ed.]. Philadelphia: W.B. Saunders. [p. 860].)

Metabolism of the Carbon Skeleton. Once its amino group has been removed, the remaining carbon "skeleton" of the amino acid may be converted to pyruvate, acetyl CoA, or ketone bodies; or to one of the intermediate acids of the Krebs cycle (Fig. 3–11). The amount of ATP produced depends on the entry point into the Krebs cycle.

Respiratory Quotient

The amount of CO_2 produced as an end product of metabolism varies depending on the type of metabolic fuel. The ratio of CO_2 produced to O_2 consumed during nutrient metabolism is known as the **respiratory quotient** (RQ). The combustion of carbohydrates (RQ = 1) produces the most CO_2. Proteins, with an RQ averaging 0.8, yield less CO_2, and fat (RQ = 0.7) produces the least CO_2. This concept assumes clinical importance in cases in which nutrition is supplemented. Critically ill patients may receive liquid (tube feeding) diets that are disproportionately high in carbohydrate, producing large amounts of CO_2. The respiratory system normally regulates CO_2 levels, but if this system is compromised, the patient may develop acid-base imbalance as a consequence of increased carbonic acid production as CO_2 combines with water in the blood (see Chapter 10).

Metabolic Regulation and Adaptation

Metabolic processing is differentially regulated depending on the nutrient composition of the diet, with specific enzymes regulating each of the pathways that have been discussed. In addition, metabolic adaptation occurs with regard to the timing of nutrient intake. During the **absorptive state** (during eating and persisting for about 4 hours after a meal), energy is generated from the ingested nutrients, and anabolic processes dominate. Glucose supplies most of the energy, whereas proteins and fats are primarily used in synthesis of new tissues to replace those that have been degraded during normal processes. Excess nutrients are converted in the liver to glycogen (**glycogenesis**) for short-term storage or to fat

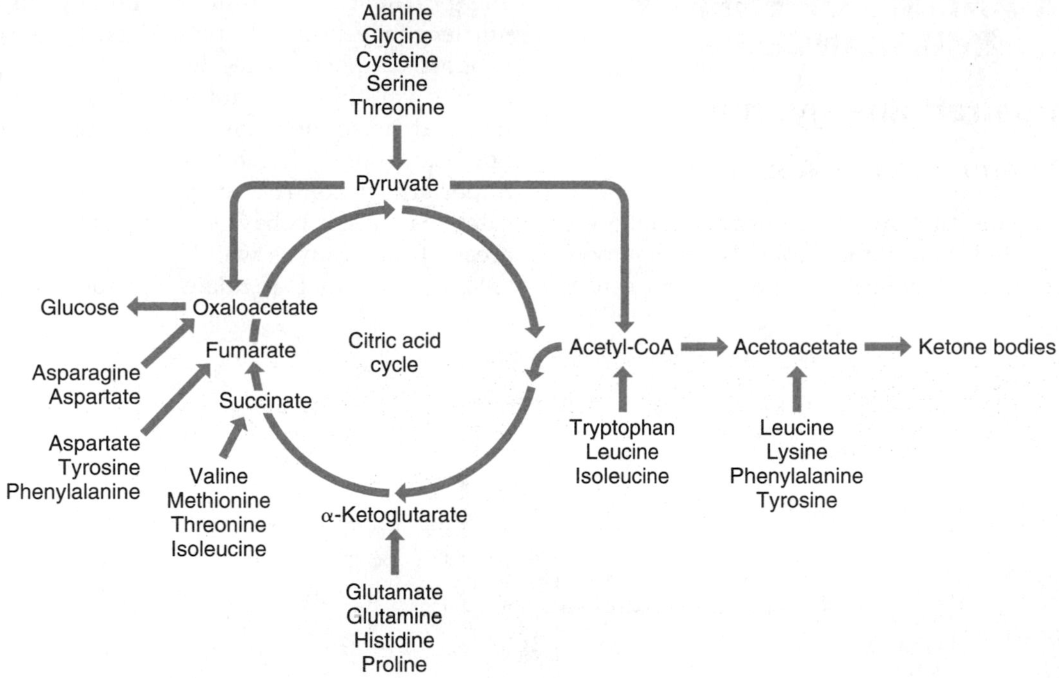

FIGURE 3–11

Entry of amino acid "skeletons" into the Krebs cycle. After deamination, the carbon skeletons of *glucogenic* amino acids are converted to intermediate acids of the Krebs cycle. Skeletons of *ketogenic* amino acids are converted to ketone bodies or to acetyl CoA, which may also enter the cycle. Note that some amino acids are both glucogenic and ketogenic. (Redrawn from Matthews, C.K., and Van Holde K.E. [1996]. *Biochemistry.* [2nd ed.]. Copyright © 1996 by Benjamin Cummings Publishing Company. Reprinted by permission.)

(**lipogenesis**) for long-term storage. The most important regulator of these processes is the pancreatic hormone **insulin** (see Chapter 29).

During the **postabsorptive state**, the gastrointestinal tract is empty, and no nutrients are being absorbed. Because blood glucose levels must be maintained within a narrow range (80 to 120 mg/dL) to supply adequate metabolic fuel to the brain, metabolic adaptations occur that (1) supply glucose from endogenous (internal) sources and (2) spare available glucose for use by the organ systems that need it most.

Four processes may supply blood glucose when none is being taken in. First, liver glycogen is broken down (**glycogenolysis**), releasing glucose into the blood and maintaining normal levels for up to 4 hours. Second, glycogenolysis also begins in skeletal muscle. Muscle glycogen cannot supply glucose to the blood directly; instead, the glucose enters into glycolysis within the muscle cell, producing ATP for use by the cell. Pyruvate and lactate are released into the blood and may be taken up by the liver for reconversion to glucose. The third potential source of glucose is through fat breakdown (**lipolysis**) in liver and adipose cells. This process yields glycerol, which can be converted to glucose by the liver.

Tissue proteins are the fourth endogenous glucose source and are particularly important during prolonged stress (when cortisol influences protein breakdown for energy fuel) or during prolonged fasting or starvation. Most gluconeogenesis from protein occurs in the liver, but the kidneys are also capable of gluconeogenesis. Transport proteins and skeletal muscle proteins are the first to be sacrificed for metabolic fuel. Eventually, if other nutrients are not supplied, vital organ proteins (including cardiac muscle) are cannibalized, resulting in death.

In addition to the processes described to supply glucose from endogenous sources, body organs adapt by switching metabolism to β-oxidation, using fats as their principal energy fuel, and thus sparing glucose for use by the brain. The liver also synthesizes ketone bodies from fats, and these can be used for fuel by other organs, including the brain.

Regulation of events during the postabsorptive state is more complex than regulation during the absorptive state. Although insulin is the only hypoglycemic (glucose-lowering) hormone, several hormones have a hyperglycemic (glucose-elevating) effect. The most important of these is **glucagon**, a pancreatic hormone that opposes the effects of insulin (see Chapter 29).

MECHANISMS OF ENERGY IMBALANCE

Impaired Energy Input

Deregulation of Appetite

The mechanisms that regulate nutrient intake are complex (Fig. 3–12) and incompletely understood. The existence of a set point, or appostat, that senses energy balance and stimulates an appropriate rate of nutrient ingestion is hypothesized because the body weights of most people tend to be relatively stable despite variability in nutrient intake. Specific receptors that sense metabolic rate or nutrient levels have not been found. The hypothalamus is known to be important in control of appetite, but research indicates that eating behavior is regulated in many other areas of the brain as well.[3]

Hormones that regulate metabolism during the

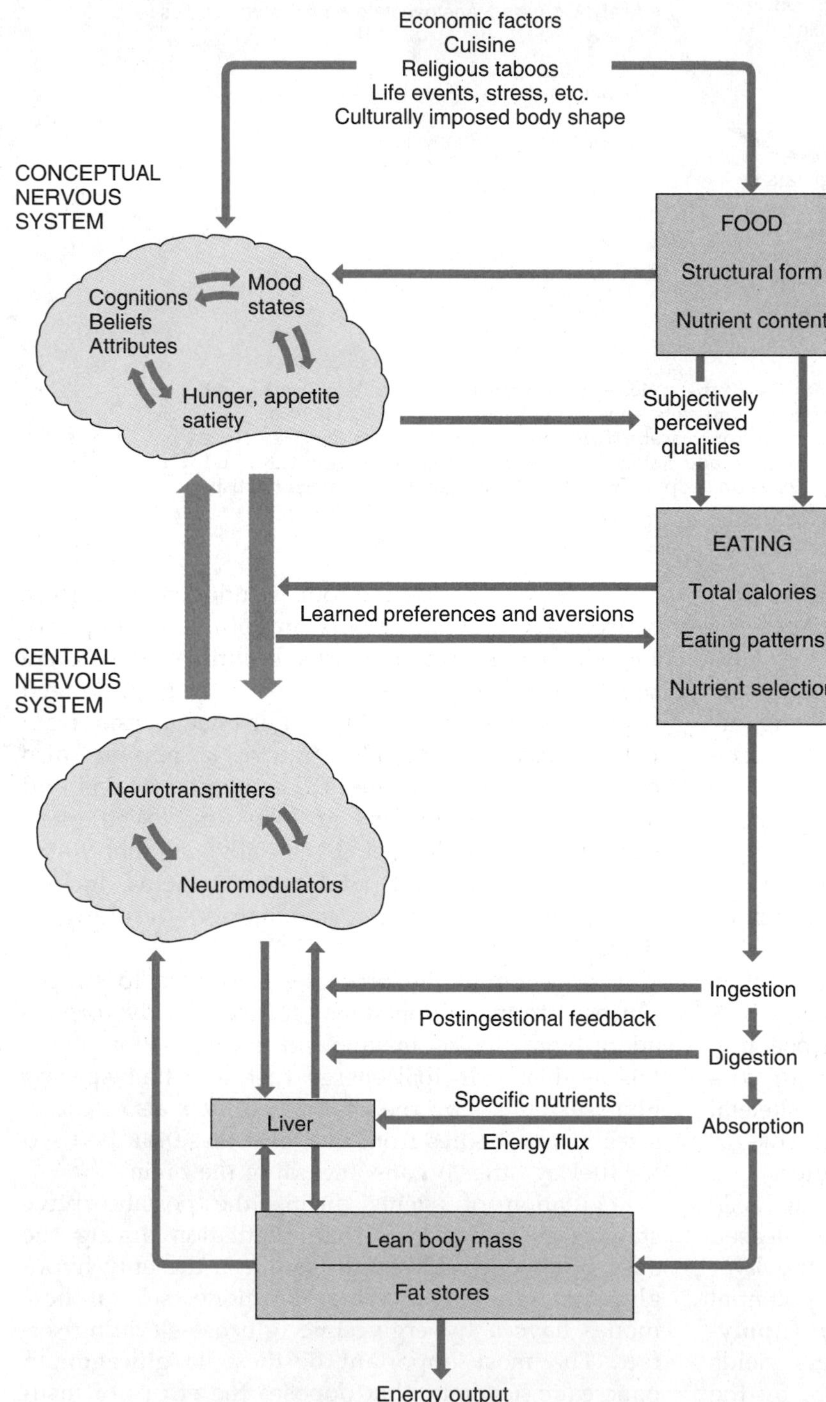

FIGURE 3–12

Factors involved in the regulation of food intake. Regulation is complex and poorly understood. Although the hypothalamus is known to play a central regulatory role, other areas of the brain are also involved. Multiple signaling molecules have been implicated in appetite regulation, including classic hormones, gastrointestinal peptides, and neurotransmitters. Nonphysiologic factors such as availability and palatability of food; psychological factors such as mood and body image; and social contexts also influence food intake. (Redrawn from Blundell, J.E. [1990]. Appetite disturbance and the problems of overweight. *Drugs* 39 [suppl 3], 3. Used with permission.)

absorptive and postabsorptive states may have a direct role in inducing or suppressing appetite. Several hormones secreted by the gastrointestinal tract and several neurotransmitters have been implicated as signaling molecules that may stimulate or inhibit appetite (Table 3–6). Many of these molecules have concurrent effects on the autonomic nervous system. Substances that increase appetite stimulate parasympathetic activity, whereas those that decrease appetite stimulate sympathetic activity. It is uncertain in many cases whether the influence of a signaling molecule on appetite is dependent on the autonomic nervous system or whether its effects are mediated by receptor molecules on target tissues.[4] The possibility of a link between body temperature and appetite has also been proposed, with low temperature signaling increased ingestion, and vice versa.[5] The close anatomic relationship between the appetite centers, thermoregulatory centers, and autonomic integration centers in the hypothalamus lends some support to these theories. Finally, voluntary behavior strongly influences energy balance. Much eating and fasting is not driven by physiologic stimuli but rather occurs independently of or in opposition to body signals. The psychological and social factors that underlie eating and drinking are variable and complex.

Malnutrition

Involuntary starvation (protein-energy malnutrition), in which there is a deficiency of calories from all nutrient sources, is thought to be rare in the United States and other developed countries but continues to be a global problem exacerbated by war and famine.[6] In the United States and other countries, deficiency of selected vitamins and minerals is a common consequence of dietary imbalance. Hospitalized patients, particularly the critically ill, are at high risk for nutritional deficiency due to the **hypermetabolic state** often induced by illness coupled with impaired ability to ingest and absorb an adequate diet.[7] In the United States, psychogenic eating disorders such as anorexia nervosa and bulimia nervosa impose significant risk due to undernutrition, while nutrition in excess of energy demands manifests as obesity (see Chapter 25).

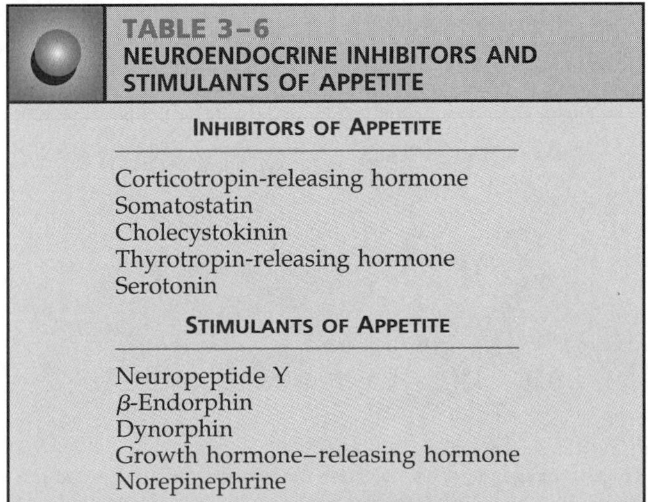

TABLE 3–6
NEUROENDOCRINE INHIBITORS AND STIMULANTS OF APPETITE

Inhibitors of Appetite
Corticotropin-releasing hormone
Somatostatin
Cholecystokinin
Thyrotropin-releasing hormone
Serotonin
Stimulants of Appetite
Neuropeptide Y
β-Endorphin
Dynorphin
Growth hormone–releasing hormone
Norepinephrine

Adapted from Kaiyala, K.J., Woods, S.C., and Schwartz, M.W. (1995). New model for the regulation of energy balance and adiposity by the central nervous system. *American Journal of Clinical Nutrition* 62(suppl.), 1123S–1134S. Copyright © Am J Clin Nutr. American Society for Clinical Nutrition.

Malabsorption

Energy metabolism is also impaired in cases in which, even though nutritional intake is appropriate, nutrients are not absorbed into the blood from the intestinal tract in sufficient amounts. Malabsorption may result from (1) lack of intestinal surface area or blood flow, as in gluten-induced enteropathy or chronic inflammatory syndromes; (2) lack of enzymes or transport proteins necessary for chemical digestion or transport of nutrients; or (3) increased or decreased gastrointestinal motility. Malabsorption syndromes are detailed in Chapter 25.

Impaired Energy Processing

Cellular Hypoxia

Hypoxia is a general term for deficiency of oxygen. Because the most efficient production of energy occurs in the presence of oxygen, any condition that reduces the oxygen content of the blood deprives cells of the capability to efficiently produce large amounts of ATP. Hypoxemia, or decreased oxygen in the blood, results from disorders of the respiratory system such as pneumonia or emphysema (see Chapters 18 and 19), from congenital heart defects in which blood bypasses the oxygenation function of the lungs (see Chapter 16), or from anemias in which the oxygen-carrying capacity of the blood is reduced owing to deficient or defective hemoglobin (see Chapter 12).

In some cases, blood is normally oxygenated by the lungs, but the rate of blood flow to tissues is not sufficient to deliver oxygen in adequate quantities. Such perfusion deficits occur in shock (see Chapter 15), congestive heart failure (see Chapter 16), arterial occlusion by blood clots (see Chapter 14), or vasoconstriction mediated by the sympathetic nervous system (see Chapter 22). Anaerobic energy metabolism predominates in perfusion deficits, producing less energy and increasing tissue acidity due to lactate production. Hypoxic tissue injury (ischemia) and even tissue death (infarction) may occur in severe or prolonged perfusion deficits.

Rarely, the cause of cellular hypoxia is not impaired supply of oxygen but rather the inability of cells to use it. Certain poisons, notably cyanide, block mitochondrial use of oxygen (see section on toxicity).

The cellular mechanism of hypoxia is incompletely understood and undoubtedly complex. As intracellular oxygen tension decreases, oxidative phosphorylation slows, and less ATP is produced. Energy stores (e.g., creatine phosphate, glycogen) are rapidly depleted, and anaerobic glycolysis accelerates, leading to accumulation of lactate and inorganic phosphate. The resulting reduction in intracellular pH leads to clumping of nuclear chromatin and inhibition of certain pH-dependent enzyme systems.

Intracellular accumulation of osmotic particles leads to cellular swelling, which is exacerbated by failure of the Na^+-K^+- ATPase membrane pump. Sodium accumulates intracellularly, while potassium rises extracellularly, preventing normal generation of electrical signals for nerve transmission and muscle contraction. ATP depletion impairs all active transport, and polarity of epithelial cells is lost. Mitochondrial swelling results from impaired pumping of energy metabolites, and ribosomes detach from the rough endoplasmic reticulum.

The plasma membrane may become weakened by detachment from the cytoskeleton due to cellular swelling and phospholipid breakdown. Rising intracellular calcium concentrations (due to impaired pumping) may contribute to activation of enzymes, such as phospholipase A_2, which mediate this breakdown.[8] At some point, cellular injury due to hypoxia is irreversible, and the cell cannot recover even if its oxygen supply is restored. Reoxygenation, or reperfusion of hypoxic tissues, may promote the formation of **reactive oxygen species** (oxygen free radicals), which further damage the cell in a positive feedback loop (discussed later).

Toxicity

A **toxin** is any substance that is harmful to the body, owing either to physical disruption of tissues or to impairment of metabolism. Toxins may be endogenous, arising within the body, such as elevated levels of ammonia in liver disease or accumulation of reactive oxygen species in oxygen toxicity. Exogenous toxins are taken into the human system from the environment and include poisons, environmental pollutants, and, potentially, many drugs.

Carbon monoxide is a toxic gas that impairs energy metabolism by displacing oxygen from hemoglobin, its primary carrier in the blood. As a result, less oxygen is available to cells for energy metabolism. Cyanide is a rapidly acting poison that inactivates cytochrome–enzyme complexes essential to oxidative phosphorylation, instantly asphyxiating cells.

Oxidative stress is a particular form of cellular toxicity related to oxidative phosphorylation within cells. As electrons are transferred from enzyme complexes to oxygen, random errors in oxidation result in the formation of reactive oxygen species instead of the stable water molecule. Reactive oxygen species include atoms or molecules having unpaired electrons in their outer orbits (free radicals) as well as molecules such as hydrogen peroxide or oxygen atoms (singlet oxygen) that readily generate free radicals (Fig. 3–13). The tendency of these species to donate or receive electrons is the source of their toxicity. The combination of free radicals with other molecules may cause a single reaction that does little harm to the cell, or it may trigger chain reactions and branching reactions that generate additional free radicals and continue unimpeded until the cell is destroyed.[9] Free radicals may damage cells by oxidizing membrane lipids (lipid peroxidation), disrupting cell signaling and transport; or they may bind to DNA, inducing breaks that may trigger genetic mutation or programmed cell death.

Because some reactive oxygen species are generated in all cells undergoing oxidative metabolism, cells have **antioxidant** enzyme systems (e.g., superoxide dismutase, catalase, and glutathione peroxidase), which protect against oxidative damage by

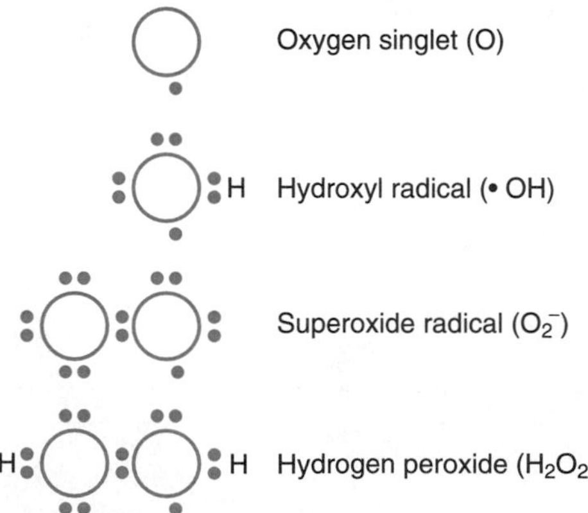

FIGURE 3–13

Reactive oxygen species. Reactive oxygen species are formed randomly during transfer of electrons to oxygen. During normal oxidative phosphorylation, an oxygen molecule accepts four electrons to form the stable water molecule. Acceptance of fewer than four electrons results in the formation of atoms or molecules that have unpaired electrons in their outer orbits (oxygen free radicals) or molecules that can generate these radicals. Free radicals may damage DNA and cell membranes.

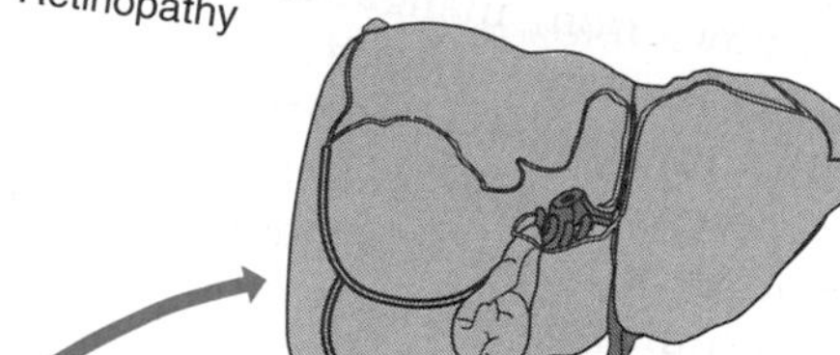

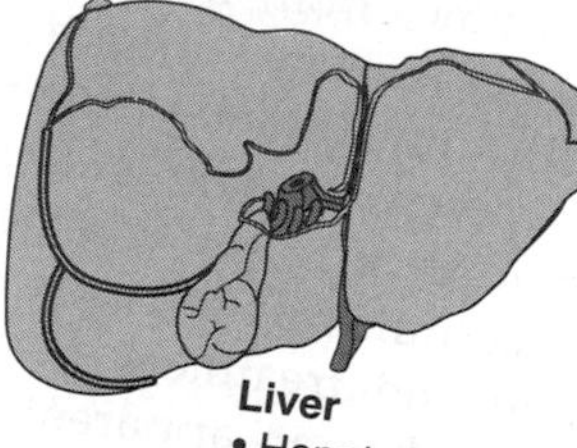

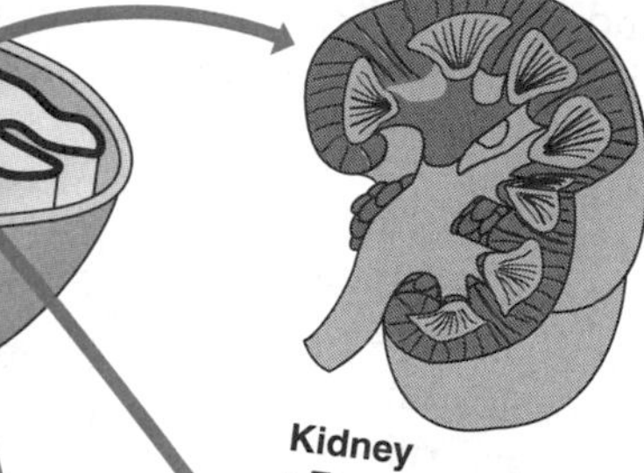

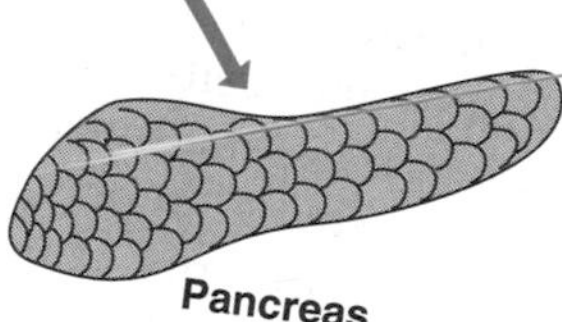

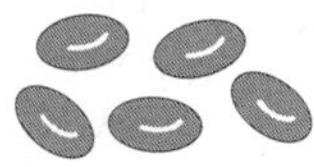

L SYNDROMES

AL MANIFESTATIONS
ysis of eye muscles, nopathy, heart ck, ataxia, hyper- rathyroidism, short ature
oclonus, seizures, taxia, muscle wasting, eafness, dementia
indness in men, movement disorder, encephalomyopathy, abnormal electrocardiogram, retinopathy
Vomiting, lactic acidosis, myopathy, dementia, seizures, deafness, short stature
Infant respiratory distress, weak cry, impaired feeding, impaired vision and hearing, ataxia, weakness, hypotension
r- y- Paralysis of eye muscles, retinopathy, limb myopathy (ragged fibers), CNS dysfunction
le- oci- -
o- o- Seizures, dementia, spasticity, blindness, liver dysfunction, cerebral degeneration

94). The development of mitochondrial *the National Academy of Science, USA* 91(9),

enetic defects in mito-ses, as have defects in phosphorylation affect J. Mitochondrial DNA 1995, Massachusetts

MBALANCE AND DISEASE

both a mechanism of disease e (see Focus of Current Re- for muscle contraction, ac- esis is the common denomi-

in Energy Output or Demand

ometabolic States

rgy output occurs as a consequence apter 6) and is also seen in cases of ty or habitual sedentary lifestyle. In **abolic states**, nutritional intake in ex- owered demands promotes obesity as tion in the serum lipid profile (see

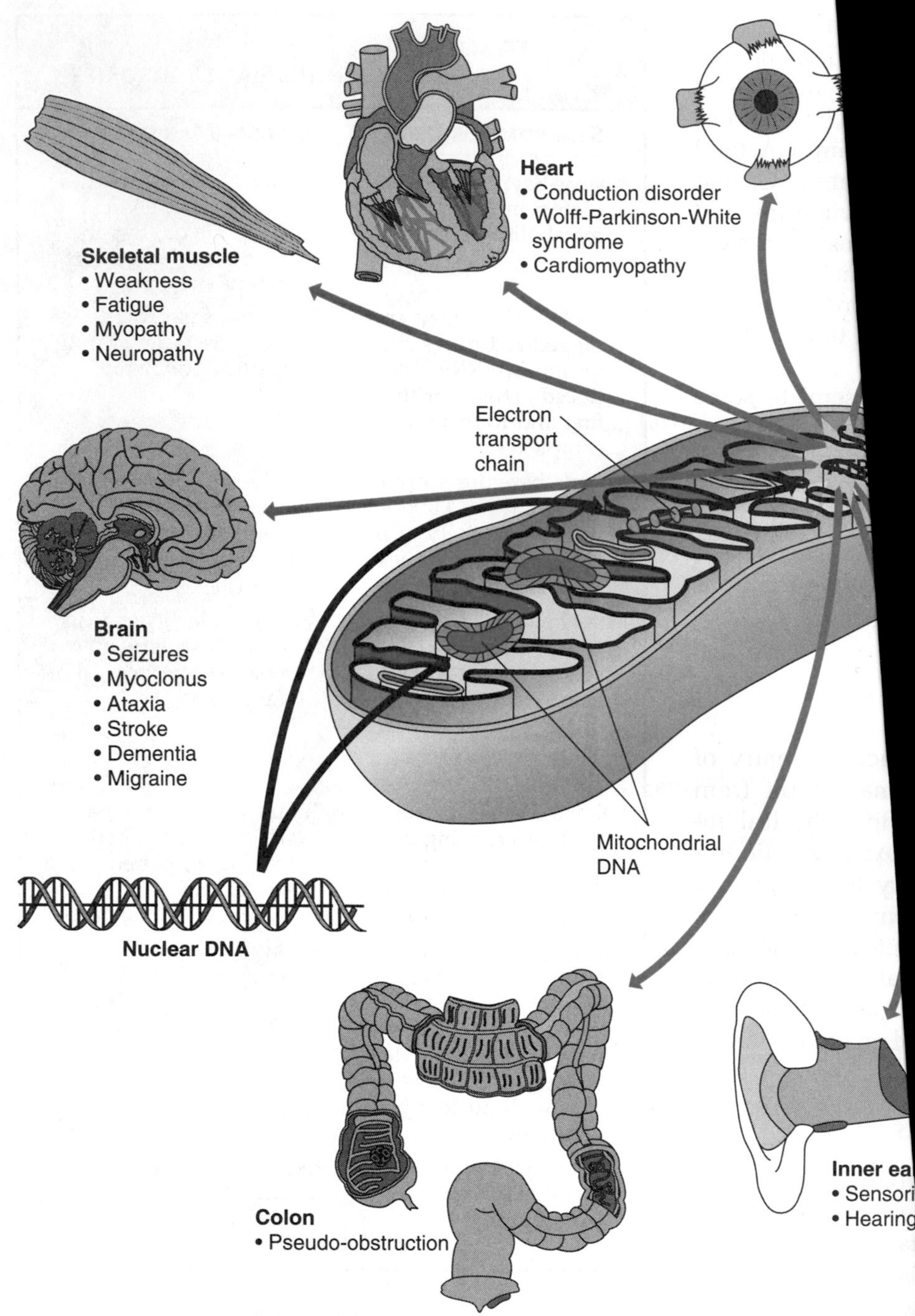

FIGURE 3–14

Systemic disorders associated with defective oxidative phosphorylation. G chondrial DNA (mtDNA) or in nuclear DNA have been implicated in disea signaling between the two types of DNA. These disorders of oxidative virtually all organ systems. (Adapted with permission from Johns, D.R. [1995 and disease. *New England Journal of Medicine* 333 [10], 638–644. Copyrigh Medical Society.)

Hypermetabolic States

Increased energy demands result from stressors such as environmental cold, physical exertion, growth, pregnancy, major trauma, critical illness, and wound healing. These hypermetabolic states manifest as output-derived energy imbalances if input and processing are not also increased.

ENERGY

Energy imbalance and a result of di search). Lack of e tive transport, and

Focus of Current Research

Study	Objective and Findings
Goran, et al. (1994) Determinants of resting energy expenditure in young children.	*Objective:* To examine the effects of body composition, gender, and parental characteristics on variations in resting energy expenditure in children *Findings:* Energy expenditure in children is determined by fat-free mass, gender, and fat mass, similarly to adults. Obesity in children and parents does not negatively influence resting energy expenditure.
Staal-van den Brekel, et al. (1995) Increased resting energy expenditure and weight loss are related to a systemic inflammatory response in lung cancer patients.	*Objective:* To determine whether increased resting energy expenditure and weight loss are related to a systemic inflammatory response in lung cancer patients *Findings:* Hypermetabolism and weight loss are related to an inflammatory response as reflected by increased levels of inflammatory mediators and acute-phase proteins in lung cancer patients.
Hugli, et al. (1996) The daily energy expenditure in stable chronic obstructive pulmonary disease.	*Objective:* To measure the actual 24-hour energy expenditure in patients with stable chronic obstructive pulmonary disease *Findings:* Patients with stable chronic obstructive pulmonary disease have a normal energy expenditure despite an increased basal metabolic rate. They save energy by reducing their level of spontaneous physical activity.
Leibel, et al. (1995) Changes in energy expenditure resulting from altered body weight.	*Objective:* To determine whether changes in body weight lead to metabolic changes in obese versus normal weight subjects *Findings:* Maintenance of body weight at 10% or more below initial weight results in compensatory changes that oppose the maintenance of a body weight that is different from the usual weight. Findings were not related to the degree of adiposity.
Cederholm, et al. (1995) Outcome of protein-energy malnutrition in elderly medical patients.	*Objective:* To assess the impact of malnutrition on mortality and long-term variations in nutritional status *Findings:* The mortality rate was 44% in malnourished patients versus 18% in well-nourished patients during a 9-month period. Malnourished patients with congestive heart failure had an 80% mortality rate.

nator of nonspecific manifestations of disease, such as **fatigue**, **malaise**, and **anorexia**, and specific manifestations of organ system failure, such as heart failure and respiratory failure. Conversely, disease of virtually any organ system potentially impairs energy metabolism. Effective respiratory and gastrointestinal function is essential to intake of nutrients and oxygen, while functional cardiovascular and hematopoietic systems are required for delivery of these substrates to cells. Metabolic adaptation is dependent on normal liver, kidney, and endocrine function. Regulation of these systems requires normal neurologic function, and the nervous system is exquisitely sensitive to any alteration in energy supply.

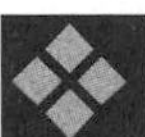

Summary of Key Points

- The first law of thermodynamics requires that energy input (nutrients) equals energy output (work capacity and heat) from the cell.
- The principal forms of cellular energy fuel are carbohydrates, lipids, and proteins. Vitamins, minerals, water, and in most systems, oxygen are required for energy processing.
- Energy-dependent processes include muscle contraction, single cell movement, some forms of membrane transport, synthetic reactions, and maintenance of body temperature.
- Most energy produced by cells is spent in the form of the high-energy molecule adenosine triphosphate (ATP), the "energy currency" of cells. Energy storage forms that can generate ATP include creatine phosphate in muscle, glycogen in liver and muscle, and triglycerides in adipose tissue.
- Carbohydrates may be processed for energy by glycolysis, Krebs cycle, or oxidative phosphorylation. Glycolysis yields a small amount of ATP but may proceed in the absence of oxygen, yielding lactic acid. Krebs cycle and oxidative phosphorylation are oxygen-dependent and yield larger amounts of ATP. Lipids may be metabolized by β-oxidation to yield energy substrates. Lipid and protein metabolites may also enter glycolysis or Krebs cycle.
- Glucose is the preferred metabolic fuel during the absorptive state. Uptake and storage of glucose is mediated by insulin. During the postabsorptive state, glucagon and other hormones mobilize stored glucose, and most body organs switch to β-oxidation of lipid for energy.
- Energy imbalance can result from impaired energy input, as may occur with appetite deregulation, malnutrition, or malabsorption.
- Energy imbalance can result from impaired energy processing, as may occur with hypoxia, toxicity, trauma, or genetic defects.
- Reduced energy demand can result from hypometabolism, as seen with aging and immobility. Hypermetabolism increases energy demand and may occur with environmental cold, exertion, pregnancy, critical illness, wound healing, and other stressors.
- Energy imbalance is both a mechanism of disease and a result of disease.

REFERENCES

1. Bouchard, C., Perusse, L., Deriaz, O., *et al.* (1993). Genetic influences on energy expenditure in humans. *Critical Reviews in Food Science and Nutrition* 33(4/5), 345–350.
2. Brooks, G.A. (1991). Current concepts in lactate exchange. *Medicine and Science in Sports and Exercise* 23(8), 895–906.
3. Read, N., French, S., and Cunningham, C. (1994). The role of the gut in regulating food intake in man. *Nutrition Reviews* 52(1), 1–10.
4. Kaiyala, K.J., Woods, S.C., and Schwartz, M.W. (1995). New model for the regulation of energy balance and adiposity by the central nervous system. *American Journal of Clinical Nutrition* 62 (suppl.), 1123S–1134S.
5. Wilber, J.F. (1991). Neuropeptides, appetite regulation, and human obesity. *Journal of the American Medical Association* 266(2), 257–259.
6. Uvin, P. (1994). The state of world hunger. *Nutrition Reviews* 52(5), 151–161.
7. McMahon, M.M., Farnell, M.B., and Murray, M.J. (1993). Nutritional support of critically ill patients. *Mayo Clinic Proceedings* 68(9), 911–920.
8. Cotran, R.S., Kumar, V., and Robbins, S.L. (1994). *Robbins Pathologic Basis of Disease.* (5th ed.). Philadelphia: W.B. Saunders (pp. 6–11).
9. Kerr, M.E., Bender, C.M., and Monti, E.J. (1996). An introduction to oxygen free radicals. *Heart and Lung* 25(3), 200–209.
10. Barber, D.A., and Harris, S.R. (1994). Oxygen free radicals and antioxidants: a review. *American Pharmacy* NS34(9), 26–35.
11. Luft, R. (1994). The development of mitochondrial medicine. *Proceedings of the National Academy of Science, USA* 91(9), 8731–8738.
12. Vockley, J. (1994). The changing face of disorders of fatty acid oxidation. *Mayo Clinic Proceedings* 69(3), 249–257.

SELECTED BIBLIOGRAPHY

Askew, E.W. (1995). Environmental and physical stress and nutrient requirements. *American Journal of Clinical Nutrition* 61(suppl.), 631S–637S.

Balaban, R.S. (1990). Regulation of oxidative phosphorylation in the mammalian cell. *American Journal of Physiology* 258(3 pt 1), C377–C389.

Baumgartner, T.G. (1993). Trace elements in clinical nutrition. *Nutrition in Clinical Practice* 8(6), 251–263.

Berry, E.M. (1994). Chronic disease: How can nutrition moderate the effects? *Nutrition Reviews* 52(8), S28–S30.

Blundell, J.E. (1990). Appetite disturbance and the problems of overweight. *Drugs* 39(suppl. 3), 1–19.

Blundell, J.E. (1992). Serotonin and the biology of feeding. *American Journal of Clinical Nutrition* 55(1, suppl.), 155S–159S.

Cederholm, T., Jagren, C., and Hellstrom, K. (1995). Outcome of protein-energy malnutrition in elderly medical patients. *The American Journal of Medicine* 98(1), 67–74.

Conway, J.M. (1995). Ethnicity and energy stores. *American Journal of Clinical Nutrition* 62(suppl.), 1067S–1071S.

DuPont, J., and Mathias, M.M. (1994). Future directions for nutrient requirements: Lipids. *Journal of Nutrition* 124(9 suppl.), 1743S–1746S.

Felber, J-P, and Golay, A. (1995). Regulation of nutrient metabolism and energy expenditure. *Metabolism* 44(2, suppl 2), 4–9.

Flatt, J.P. (1995). Body composition, respiratory quotient, and weight maintenance. *American Journal of Clinical Nutrition* 62(suppl.), 1107S–1117S.

Friedman, M.I. (1995). Control of energy intake by energy metabolism. *American Journal of Clinical Nutrition* 62(suppl.), 1096S–1100S.

Goran, M.I., Kaskoun, M., and Johnson, R. (1994). Determinants of resting energy expenditure in young children. *Journal of Pediatrics* 125(3), 362–367.

Guyton, A.C., and Hall, J.E. (1995). *Textbook of Medical Physiology.* (9th ed.). Philadelphia: W.B. Saunders.

Heymsfield, S.B., Darby, P.C., Muhlheim, L.S., *et al.* (1995). The calorie: Myth, measurement, and reality. *American Journal of Clinical Nutrition* 62 (suppl.), 1034S–1041S.

Hotchkiss, R.S., and Karl, I.E. (1992). Reevaluation of the role of cellular hypoxia and bioenergetic failure in sepsis. *Journal of the American Medical Association* 267(11), 1503–1510.

Hugli, O., Schutz, Y., and Fitting, J-W. (1996). The daily energy expenditure in stable chronic obstructive pulmonary disease. *American Journal of Respiratory and Critical Care Medicine* 153, 294–300.

Johns, D.R. (1995). Mitochondrial DNA and disease. (Seminars in Medicine of the Beth Israel Hospital, Boston, J.S. Flier and L.H. Underhill, eds.). *The New England Journal of Medicine* 333(10), 638–644.

King, J.C., Butte, N.F., Bronstein, M.N., *et al.* (1994). Energy metabolism during pregnancy: Influence of maternal energy status. *American Journal of Clinical Nutrition* 59(suppl.), 439S–445S.

Kuczmarski, R.J., Fiegal, K.M., Campbell, S.M., *et al.* (1994). Increasing prevalence of overweight among US adults. *Journal of the American Medical Association* 272(3), 205–211.

LaChance, P., and Langseth, L. (1994). The RDA concept: Time for a change? *Nutrition Reviews* 52(8), 266–270.

Leibel, R.L., Rosenbaum, M., and Hirsch, J. (1995). Changes in energy expenditure resulting from altered body weight. *The New England Journal of Medicine* 332(10), 621–628.

Livesey, G. (1995). Metabolizable energy of macronutrients. *American Journal of Clinical Nutrition* 62(suppl.), 1135S–1142S.

Luke, A., and Schoeller, D.A. (1992). Basal metabolic rate, fat-free mass, and body cell mass during energy restriction. *Metabolism* 41(4), 450–456.

Matthews, C.K., and van Holde, K.E. (1996). *Biochemistry.* (2nd ed.). Menlo Park, CA: Benjamin Cummings Publishing Co.

Misasi, R.S., and Keyes, J.L. (1994). The pathophysiology of hypoxia. *Critical Care Nurse* 14(4), 55–64.

Moe, P.W. (1994). Future directions for energy requirements and food energy values. *Journal of Nutrition* 124(9, suppl.), 1738S–1742S.

Olson, J.A. (1994). Vitamins: The tortuous path from needs to fantasies. *Journal of Nutrition* 124(9, suppl.), 1771S–1776S.

Ravussin, E., and Bogardus, C. (1992). A brief overview of human energy metabolism and its relationship to essential obesity. *American Journal of Clinical Nutrition* 55(1, suppl.), 242S–245S.

Reeds, P.J., and Hutchens, T.W. (1994). Protein requirements: From nitrogen balance to functional impact. *Journal of Nutrition* 124(9, suppl.), 1754S–1764S.

Rosenberg, I.H. (1994). Nutrient requirements for optimal health: What does that mean? *Journal of Nutrition* 124(9, suppl.), 1777S–1779S.

Russel, R.M. (1992). Micronutrient requirements of the elderly. *Nutrition Reviews* 50(12), 463–466.

Saltzman, E., and Roberts, S.B. (1995). The role of energy expenditure in energy regulation: Findings from a decade of research. *Nutrition Reviews* 53(8), 209–220.

Schneeman, B.O. (1994). Carbohydrates: Significance for energy balance and gastrointestinal function. *Journal of Nutrition* 124(9, suppl.), 1747S–1753S.

Schulz, H. (1994). Regulation of fatty acid oxidation in heart. *Journal of Nutrition* 124, 165–171.

Smith, L.C., and Mullen, J.L. (1991). Nutritional assessment and indications for nutritional support. *Surgical Clinics of North America* 71(3), 449–457.

Souba, W.W. (1994). Cytokine control of nutrition and metabolism during critical illness. *Current Problems in Surgery* 31(7), 586–643.

Staal-van den Brekel, A.J., Dentener, M.A., Schols, A.M.W.J., *et al.* (1995). Increased resting energy expenditure and weight loss are related to a systemic inflammatory response in lung cancer patients. *Journal of Clinical Oncology* 13(10), 2600–2605.

Swinburn, B., and Ravussin, E. (1993). Energy balance or fat balance? *American Journal of Clinical Nutrition* 57(suppl.), 766S–771S.

Taylor, D.E., and Piantodosi, C.A. (1995). Oxidative metabolism in sepsis and sepsis syndrome. *Journal of Critical Care* 10(3), 122–136.

Terada, H. (1990). Uncouplers of oxidative phosphorylation. *Environmental Health Perspectives* 87(Jul), 213–218.

Turnlund, J.R. (1994). Future directions for establishing mineral/trace element requirements. *Journal of Nutrition* 124(9, suppl.), 1765S–1770S.

Voet, D., and Voet, J.G. (1995). *Biochemistry.* (2nd ed.). New York: John Wiley & Sons.

Wallace, D.C. (1994). Mitochondrial DNA sequence variation in human evolution and disease. *Proceedings of the National Academy of Science, USA* 91(9), 8739–8746.

Waterlow, J.C. (1994). Where do we go from here? (Alfred E. Harper Symposium on Emerging Aspects of Amino Acid Metabolism.) *Journal of Nutrition* 124(8 suppl.), 1524S–1528S.

Westerterp, K.R. (1993). Food quotient, respiratory quotient, and energy balance. *American Journal of Clinical Nutrition* 57(suppl.), 759S–765S.

Wilson, D.F. (1995). Energy metabolism in muscle approaching maximal rates of oxygen utilization. *Medicine and Science in Sports and Exercise* 27(1), 54–59.

Wilson, D.F. (1991). Factors affecting the rate and energetics of mitochondrial oxidative phosphorylation. *Medicine and Science in Sports and Exercise* 26(1), 37–43.

Young, V.R. (1992). Energy requirements in the elderly. *Nutrition Reviews* 50(4), 95–101.

Young, V.R. (1992). Macronutrient needs in the elderly. *Nutrition Reviews* 50(12), 454–562.

Zawada, E.T. (1996). Malnutrition in the elderly: Is it simply a matter of not eating enough? *Postgraduate Medicine* 100(1), 207–225.

Electrophysiology: Action Potentials and Conduction

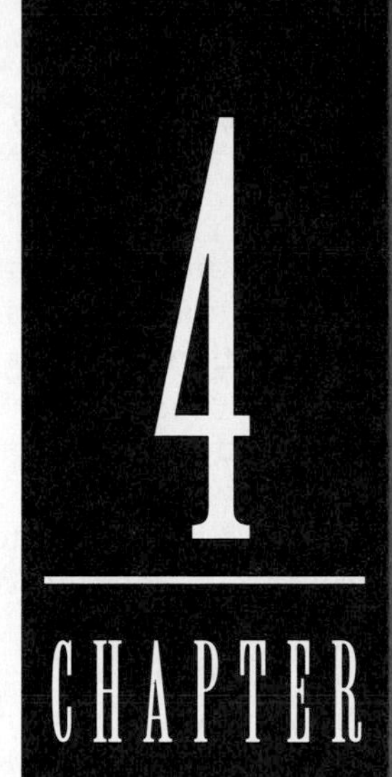

LEARNING OBJECTIVES

1. Comprehend the physiologic processes underlying formation of membrane potentials and action potentials.
2. Identify the significant ion transport that occurs during each phase of the action potential.
3. Discuss the basis and importance of refractoriness in excitable tissues.
4. Differentiate between mechanisms of short-distance and long-distance flow of electrical current in the body.
5. Differentiate among mechanisms of conduction in neurons, cardiac tissue, smooth muscle, and skeletal muscle.
6. Describe the two general mechanisms of altered conduction.
7. Discuss the clinical importance of altered conduction.

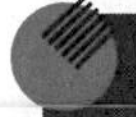

key terms

absolute refractory period
action potential
all-or-none law
anion
automaticity
cation
depolarization
diastolic depolarization
dysrhythmia
electrolyte
electrotonic potential
graded potential
hyperpolarization
ion
membrane potential
myelin
Nernst potential
node of Ranvier
pacemaker cell
plateau
principle of electroneutrality
refractory period
relative refractory period
repolarization
resting membrane potential
rhythmicity
saltatory conduction
supernormal period
threshold

Systems theory holds that the exchange of matter, energy, and information between the human system and the environment is integral to total system function. Information exchange among the excitable tissues of the body (nerve and muscle) is dependent on the generation and transmission of electrical current within these tissues. This means of intercellular signaling regulates neurotransmission, glandular secretion, and the contraction of cardiac, skeletal, and smooth muscle.

The human body is governed by the **principle of electroneutrality**, which requires that total **cations** (positively charged particles) equal total **anions** (negatively charged particles) within the system as a whole. The constant movement of these **ions** within living tissues, however, means that there is inequality in the distribution of charged particles between specific compartments at certain times. Ions flow continuously between the cytoplasm and the extracellular fluid (ECF); this movement is driven by electrical and concentration gradients and by active transport mechanisms. Transport of ions across the plasma membrane results in the generation and conduction of **action potentials**, the mechanisms of electrical communication between excitable cells.

GENERATION OF MEMBRANE POTENTIALS AND ACTION POTENTIALS

Definitions

A **membrane potential** is a difference in electrical charge between the interior and the exterior of a cell. Virtually all body cells display membrane potentials owing to differences in the distribution of charged particles between the two compartments. The term *potential* refers to the potential energy (measurable as voltage, similar to that between the poles of a battery) inherent in the charge separation across the membrane. Because unlike electrical charges attract, a membrane potential represents a potential electrical gradient—a capacity to drive membrane transport. Membrane potentials in excitable cells are called action potentials because the resulting electrical signal produces detectable activity, such as transmission of a nerve impulse or contraction of a muscle cell.

Electrolytes and Ions

Ionization

Generation of action potentials depends on normal permeability and transport functions of plasma membranes and also on gradients derived from normal concentrations of **electrolytes** in intracellular and extracellular fluid. Electrolytes make up the bulk of the solute in body fluids; they consist of particles that dissociate into ions.

Ionization occurs when an atom either loses or gains electrons from its outer orbital shell to achieve a more stable form in water. Sodium, for example, has one electron in its outer shell. By transferring this electron to another particle (such as chlorine), sodium achieves more stability in that its outermost orbital is now complete, containing eight electrons (Fig. 4–1). Because it has lost one negatively charged particle, however, sodium acquires a posi-

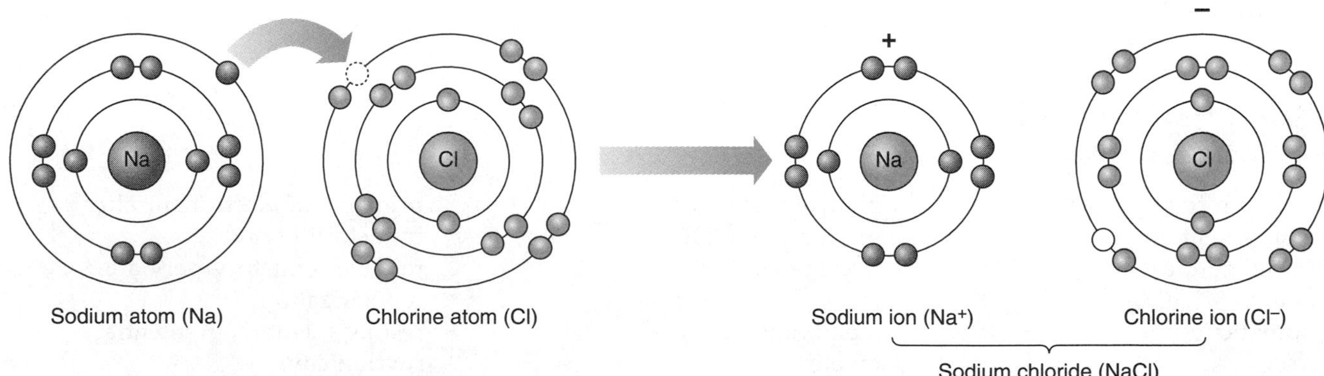

FIGURE 4–1

Chemical basis of ionization. Ionization occurs when an atom gains or loses electrons from its outer orbital shell. Sodium may transfer the single electron from its outer shell to chlorine's, completing its orbit and increasing the stability of both atoms. In the process, sodium acquires a net positive charge and becomes the sodium cation (Na^+). Chlorine acquires a negative charge and becomes the chloride anion (Cl^-). The unlike charges of these ions may result in their forming sodium chloride (NaCl) by ionic bonding.

tive charge and is now the sodium cation (Na^+). Chlorine, on the other hand, has seven electrons in its outer shell, and the acquisition of one electron from sodium completes its orbital and confers stability to it as well. In gaining one electron, chlorine acquires a negative charge and becomes the chloride anion (Cl^-). Their unlike charges cause these ions to attract each other, potentially forming the compound sodium chloride (NaCl) by means of ionic bonding.

Other atoms with one or two electrons in their outer (valence) shells are calcium, potassium, and magnesium. These electrolytes form the cations Ca^{2+}, K^+, and Mg^{2+}. In addition to chlorine, anions are formed from elements—such as iodine, with its seven valence shell electrons—or from compounds such as bicarbonate (HCO_3^-) or phosphate (PO_4^{3-}), which meet similar criteria.

Most ionic compounds exist in a crystalline form in the absence of water (e.g., NaCl as table salt). These crystals dissociate in aqueous body fluids, however, as a result of the polar characteristic of water molecules. The V-shaped structure of the H_2O molecule allows the oxygen to exert a greater pulling force on the electrons it shares with the two hydrogen atoms. A separation of charge (polarity) thus exists; the oxygen end of the molecule is electronegative and the hydrogen region is electropositive. These charges in turn attract ions such as Na^+ and Cl^-. Water molecules surround these ions, causing them to dissociate from their lattice arrangement in the salt form (Fig. 4–2).

Electrolyte Distribution

The electrolyte composition of different body fluids (blood, intestinal juices, sweat, saliva, bile, urine, etc.) is highly variable. Because of their importance in transport functions and in intercellular signaling, electrolyte levels must be tightly regulated. Mechanisms of electrolyte homeostasis and clinical consequences of specific imbalances are detailed in Chapter 9.

Differences between intracellular and extracellular electrolyte concentrations are important to the discussion of action potentials, however. Figure 4–3 illustrates the typical distribution of major electrolytes across the membrane of excitable cells under resting conditions, that is, between action potentials. ECF is high in sodium (Na^+), whereas intracellular fluid is high in potassium (K^+). There is also a major difference in calcium ion (Ca^{2+}) distribution; the extracellular concentration greatly exceeds the intracellular distribution of ionized calcium (a 10,000:1 ratio). (Actually, the concentration of calcium is much greater *intracellularly*, but most of this calcium is in bound form or stored within organelles. In this nonionized form, it is not immediately available for transport.) Chloride (Cl^-) is the major extracellular anion, whereas phosphate (PO_4^{3-}) and negatively charged proteins constitute the main intracellular anions.

As discussed in Chapter 2, charged particles cannot traverse membrane lipids; they must be transported through protein channels in the plasma

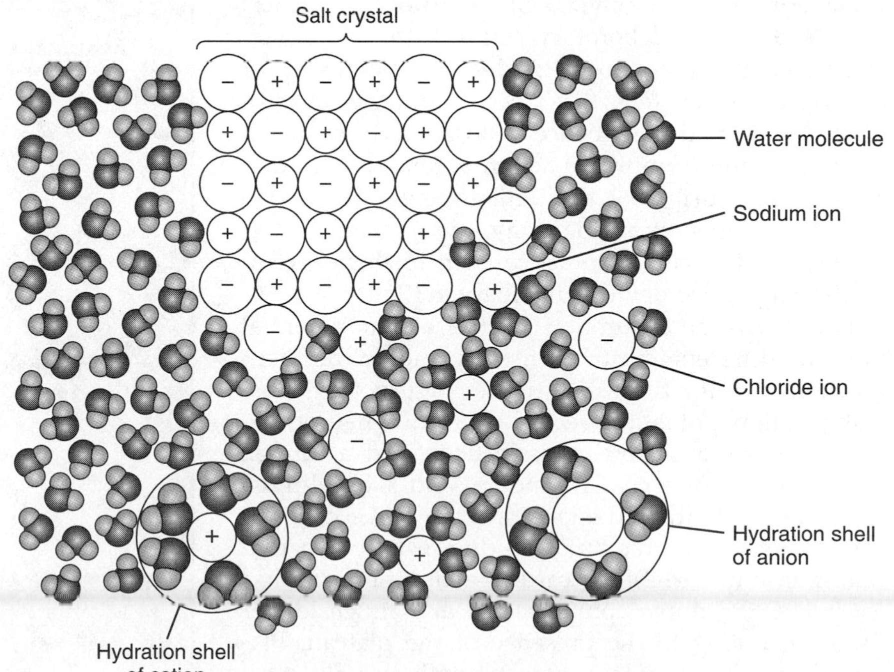

FIGURE 4–2
Dissociation of electrolytes in water. The polarity of the water molecule results in dissociation of electrolytes from crystalline compounds, releasing ions. The negative charge of oxygen in H_2O attracts cations, while the positive charge of hydrogen attracts anions. The resulting hydration shells separate the ions from their crystalline lattice. (Redrawn from Moffett, D.F., Moffett, S.B., and Schauf, C.L. [1993]. *Human Physiology: Foundations and Frontiers*. [2nd ed.]. St. Louis: Mosby–Year Book. [p. 27]. © 1993. Reproduced with permission of the McGraw-Hill Companies.)

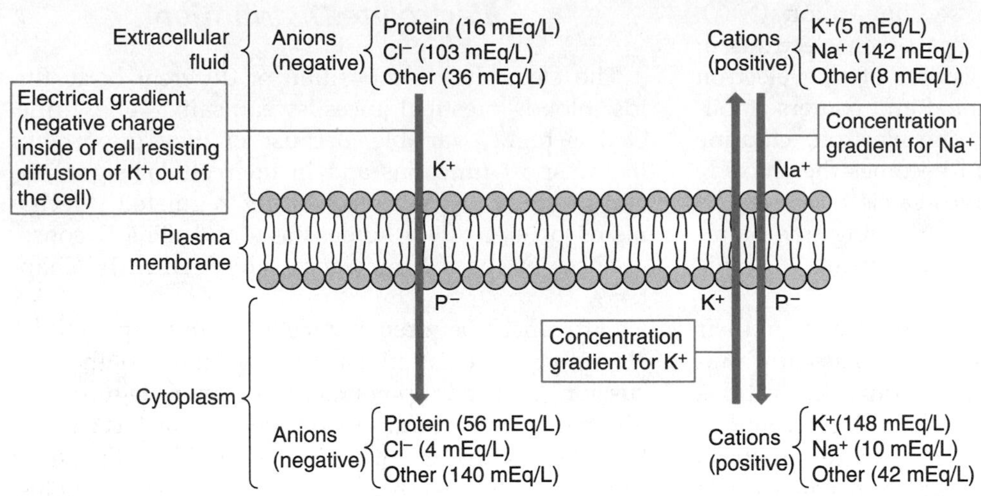

FIGURE 4–3

Distribution of ions in resting cells. The extracellular fluid is high in sodium (Na^+) and chloride (Cl^-), whereas the cytoplasm contains more potassium (K^+) and negatively charged proteins (P^-). Na^+ is attracted inward along electrical and concentration gradients, while K^+ is attracted outward along its concentration gradient and inward along its electrical gradient.

membrane. Ions typically diffuse through specific channels of the appropriate size and charge to accommodate them, and the number of these channels determines permeability of the membrane to specific ions. Most ion channels are gated channels, opening or closing only with appropriate electrical or ligand stimulation; a smaller number are continuously open leak channels, permitting constant passive diffusion.

Phases of the Action Potential

The sequential changes in membrane potential during ion movements may be recorded with microelectrodes (current sensors) placed inside and outside the cell, resulting in a graphic representation of the action potential. Single cell recordings are generally used only in laboratory settings. In clinical settings, the more common modes of monitoring of electrical activity (e.g., electrocardiography, electromyography, and electroencephalography) are based on summation of multiple action potentials recorded at the body surface or through invasive means (Table 4–1). Electrocardiography, in particular, is widely used in clinical practice. Principles of electrocardiography are detailed in Chapter 17.

The shape and duration of the action potential vary in different excitable tissues and in different locations within the same tissue. Figure 4–4 illustrates action potentials recorded from a neuron (α-motoneuron), a skeletal muscle fiber, and a cardiac ventricular muscle cell. The neural and skeletal muscle action potentials demonstrate the spike configuration, with a shorter duration due to lack of a **plateau** phase (phase 2); the cardiac action potential has the spike-and-dome configuration and much longer duration owing to the presence of the plateau. Plateaus are also seen in some smooth muscle cells. These differences relate to functional characteristics of the tissues. Nerve impulse transmission must be rapid for relay of sensory and motor signals (see Chapters 21, 22, and 23), and rapid impulse formation in skeletal muscle permits sustained contraction (tetany) and increased muscle strength (see Chapters 5 and 35). Plateau in cardiac muscle prevents tetany, in which sustained contraction of ventricular walls would prevent adequate filling of the chambers.

The five phases of the cardiac ventricular muscle action potential are labeled in Figure 4–5, for reference during the following discussion of ion trans-

TABLE 4–1
CLINICAL EVALUATION OF ACTION POTENTIALS AND CONDUCTION

EVALUATION MODE	CLINICAL USE
Surface electrocardiography	Diagnosis and monitoring of cardiac dysrhythmias, ischemia and infarction, and effects of drugs and electrolytes
Electrophysiology studies	Evaluation of complex dysrhythmias and abnormal conduction pathways in the heart
Electroencephalography	Evaluation of seizure disorders (epilepsy) and sleep disorders, and determination of brain death
Evoked potentials	Evaluation of blindness, deafness, and brainstem function
Electromyography	Differentiation of neural and muscular effects in neuromuscular disorders

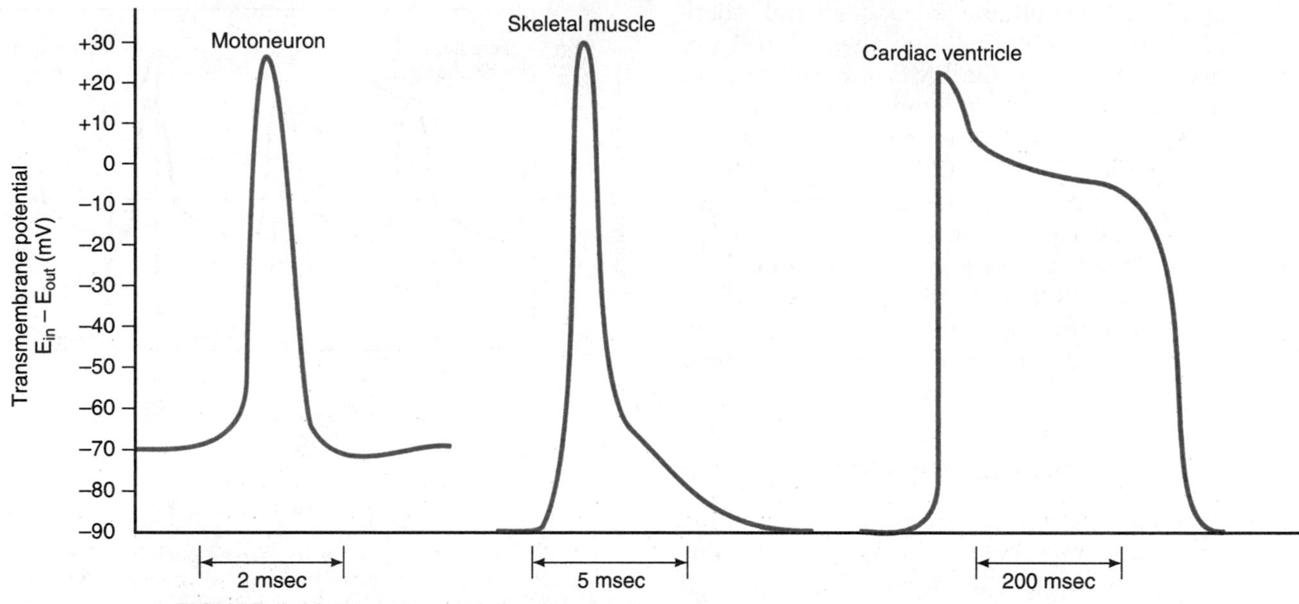

FIGURE 4–4

Action potentials in neuron, skeletal muscle, and cardiac ventricular muscle. The shape and duration of the action potential varies in different excitable tissues because of differences in numbers and types of ion channels. The neural and skeletal muscle action potentials illustrate the spike configuration (without plateau), whereas the cardiac action potential demonstrates the spike and dome, with plateau. (Redrawn from Berne, R.M., and Levy, M.N. [1993]. *Physiology*. [3rd ed.]. St. Louis: Mosby–Year Book. [p. 36]. Used with permission.)

port during each phase. The phase sequence is 4, 0, 1, 2, 3, 4 in action potentials with plateau, and 4, 0, 1, 3, 4 in spike potentials.

Resting Membrane Potential (Phase 4)

In the resting state, the excitable cell is *polarized*: its interior is negative with respect to the exterior. This potential difference is about −70 mV in neurons, −90 mV in skeletal and cardiac muscle, and −50 mV in smooth muscle. This **resting membrane potential (RMP)** is nearly equal to the **Nernst potential** for potassium, which is the point at which the inward electrical gradient and the outward concentration gradient offset. During phase 4, the presence of numerous leak channels for potassium (also called *resting K^+ channels*) permits passive influx and efflux of K^+. Because there is a greater concentration of K^+ inside the cell, a concentration gradient for outward movement (K^+ efflux) exists. At the same time, negatively charged proteins and other anions inside the cell attract K^+ inward. The point at which these two gradients offset each other may be calculated as the equilibrium potential, or Nernst potential.[1]

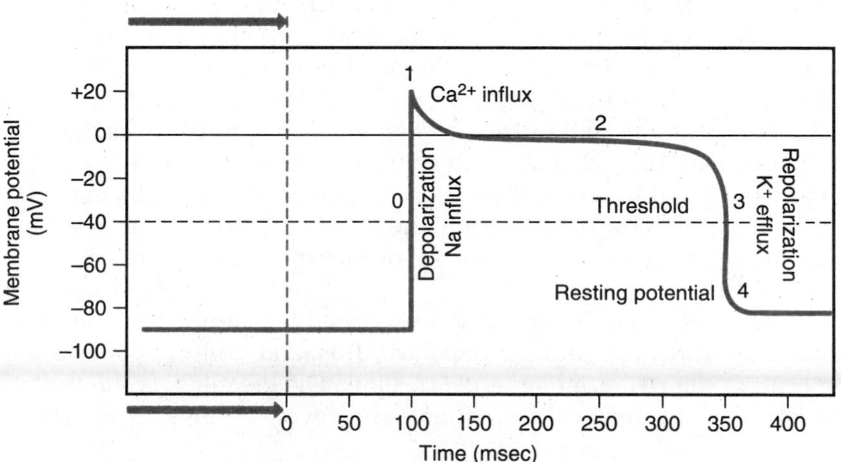

FIGURE 4–5

Phases of the action potential in cardiac muscle. The phase sequence in these cells is 4 (resting membrane potential), 0 (depolarization), 1 (early rapid repolarization), 2 (plateau), and 3 (late rapid repolarization). Spike potentials lack the plateau (phase 2). Principal ion currents during each phase are also shown. *Threshold*, the point where depolarization results in a full action potential, is approximately −40 mV in cardiac muscle cells.

Resting plasma membranes also have leak channels for sodium and chloride, and their Nernst potentials also contribute to the RMP in excitable cells. These ion channels are few in comparison to resting K^+ channels, however, and their contribution is negligible. Some variability in RMP is seen, especially in smooth muscle, and continuous adjustments in the potential occur by passive diffusion of K^+ and Cl^- through leak channels. Voltage-gated sodium channels are *closed but activated* during this phase; that is, their protein subunits are in a conformation in which they are capable of being opened in response to a change in membrane voltage.

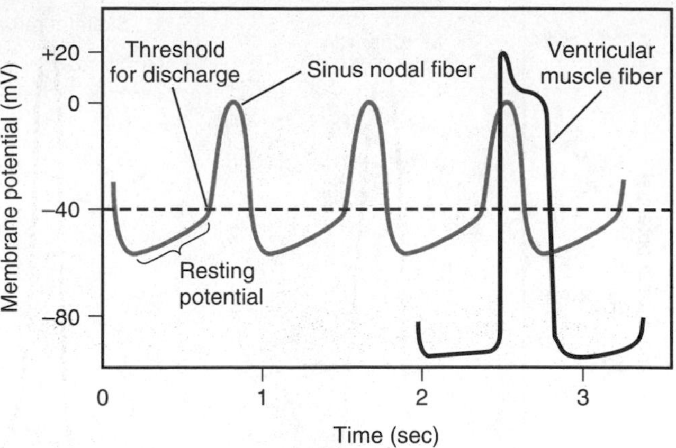

FIGURE 4–6
Action potentials from cardiac pacemaker cells. The *sinus node,* a group of specialized cells in the right atrium, is the normal pacemaker of the heart rate. The action potential from such pacemaker cells has a higher resting membrane potential than that of muscle cells. Resting potential rises gradually owing to Na^+ influx through greater numbers of Na^+ leak channels, resulting in spontaneous triggering of the action potential when threshold is reached. (Redrawn from Guyton, A.C., and Hall, J.E. [1996]. *Textbook of Medical Physiology*. [9th ed.] Philadelphia: W.B. Saunders [p. 122]. Used with permission.)

Depolarization (Phase 0)

During **depolarization** (loss of polarity), the influx of sodium causes membrane potential to become more positive. In most cells, this is due to sudden opening of voltage-gated sodium channels by an electrical stimulus (an action potential or a membrane potential) transmitted from an adjacent cell. The large concentration gradient results in rapid influx of sodium, causing the membrane potential to discharge suddenly, that is, to rise to zero. Passive movement of K^+ (and possibly Cl^-) is still occurring during this phase, but the massive influx of Na^+ overwhelms the effects of these other ion currents.

A specialized category of excitable cells is **pacemaker cells;** these cells have proportionately larger numbers of sodium leak channels in their membranes. In pacemaker cells, depolarization is not sudden but rather occurs gradually owing to slow sodium influx through these channels. Figure 4–6 illustrates an action potential from a pacemaker cell (the sinus node of the heart) in comparison with a cardiac ventricular muscle action potential. Although pacemaker cells may be influenced by electrical stimuli from adjacent cells, they are not dependent on such stimuli. Because of their higher resting membrane potentials and greater numbers of Na^+ leak channels, these cells can spontaneously generate action potentials. Pacemaker cells are found in the sinus node (the normal origin of the heart beat) and in other locations within cardiac tissue (see Chapter 17). Cells of the reticular activating system of the brain stem serve as pacemakers for the rate of impulse transmission to and from the brain, thus determining level of consciousness or alertness (see Chapter 21).

In cardiac muscle cells, voltage-gated calcium channels also open during depolarization and contribute to the rising membrane potential. The greater importance of this calcium influx, however, is in regulation of muscle contraction (see Chapter 5). In smooth muscle cells (e.g., blood vessels, intestinal cells, and glandular ducts), depolarization may also be mediated by both calcium and sodium influx.

As the membrane potential rises during depolarization, it reaches a specified level known as **threshold**. (In cardiac cells, threshold is about −40 to −70 mV.) Consistent with the **all-or-none law**, the excitable cell is committed to a full action potential when the membrane potential rises to this level, whereas depolarizations that fail to reach threshold do not result in action potentials. Subthreshold depolarizations may occur with weak stimuli or when the membrane is hyperpolarized. **Hyperpolarization** is present when the RMP is more negative than normal or when threshold is more positive than normal. Factors influencing the degree of membrane polarization are discussed later in this chapter.

When zero potential is reached, voltage-gated sodium channels begin to undergo a conformational change that renders them *closed and inactive*, that is, incapable of being reopened until RMP is restored. Membrane potential, however, actually "overshoots," or rises above zero, causing the inside of the cell to become briefly positive to the outside. This overshoot is caused by a delay in closure and inactivation of some voltage-gated sodium channels. Depolarization ends as the intracellular sodium concentration approaches, but does not reach, its own equilibrium (Nernst) potential, at about 35 mV.[2]

Early Rapid Repolarization (Phase 1)

Repolarization, the restoration of membrane polarity, begins at the peak of the depolarization upstroke. Voltage-gated Na^+ channels are closed. One type of voltage-gated potassium channel (the A channel) opens at this voltage, and a brief period of unopposed K^+ efflux results in increasingly negative membrane potential. Cl^- influx may also contribute to negativity during this phase.

Plateau (Phase 2)

Plateau, seen in excitable cells in which calcium influx contributes to depolarization, is a steady state of membrane potential caused by the offsetting effects of continued calcium influx while potassium is leaving the cell. Calcium influx continues because these channels are slower to undergo the change in conformation between open and closed forms and because they are responsive to different membrane voltages than are the sodium channels.

Late Rapid Repolarization (Phase 3)

Repolarization ends when RMP is restored. As membrane potential becomes more negative, voltage-gated calcium channels close, and K^+ efflux is unopposed through several types of leak, voltage-gated, and ligand-gated K^+ channels. (In the heart, for example, one type of leak K^+ channel, three types of voltage-gated K^+ channels, and at least five types of ligand-gated K^+ channels have been identified.[3]) The inside of the cell rapidly becomes more negative, approaching RMP, at which point voltage-gated K^+ channels are inactivated. As with depolarization, K^+ efflux overshoots RMP slightly owing to delayed closure of some channels. Small inward potassium currents or outward chloride currents (**diastolic depolarization**) then restore RMP.

Maintenance of Ionic Gradients

During the action potential, the actual number of ions exchanged across the membrane is small relative to the total concentrations in the extracellular and intracellular compartments. The continuous operation of an active transport pump, Na^+-K^+-ATPase, maintains the Na^+ and K^+ gradients near resting level. This antiport simultaneously transports sodium ions out of the cell and potassium ions into the cell in a 3:2 ratio (see Chapter 2). Active transport mechanisms, which probably involve sodium calcium exchange, also maintain the calcium gradient.[4] In the absence of adenosine triphosphate, these ions would diffuse passively across the membrane, equilibrating at their respective Nernst potentials. Membrane potential under these conditions would be zero, and the cell could not be stimulated.

Refractory and Supernormal Periods

Certain time periods during repolarization are of particular importance in the regulation of action potential generation and conduction (Fig. 4–7). The **refractory period** is the period that follows depolarization when the cell usually cannot respond to another stimulus with depolarization because most sodium channels are inactivated over this range of membrane voltage. The **absolute refractory period** is the period immediately following initial depolarization to the point at which the membrane has repolarized to just above threshold. During this time, the cell cannot depolarize again under any circumstances, that is, it is *refractory* to stimulation. Once repolarization has returned the membrane potential to below threshold (although not yet approaching RMP), the cell responds to a greater-than-normal stimulus. This period is known as the **relative refractory period**. There is also a short period late in depolarization when the cell is *more easily depolarized* than normal. During this **supernormal period,** a weaker-than-normal stimulus may trigger an action potential because the cell has activated enough volt-

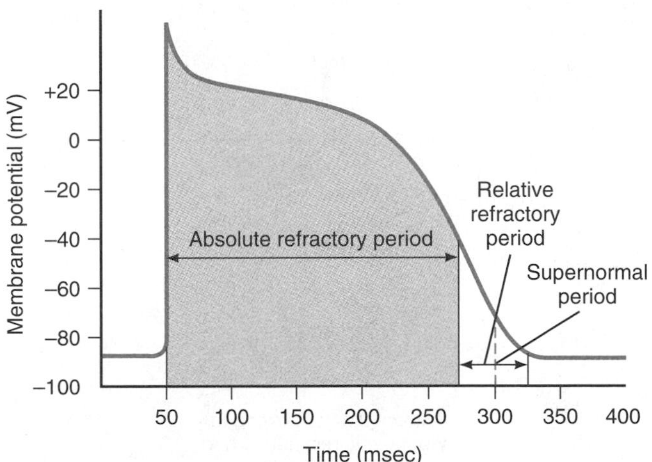

FIGURE 4–7
Refractory and supernormal periods. During the *absolute refractory period,* the cell cannot depolarize again regardless of the strength of the stimulus. During the *relative refractory period,* the cell may depolarize in response to a stronger than normal stimulus. During the *supernormal period,* the cell may depolarize in response to a weaker than normal stimulus.

age-gated sodium channels to depolarize, yet the membrane potential is closer to threshold than the normal RMP. In cardiac cells, stimuli delivered during the supernormal period may result in dangerous rhythm disturbances or **dysrhythmias** (see Chapter 17).

MECHANISMS OF CONDUCTION

Electrical current is conducted in the body as a consequence of ion flow within body fluids. Positively charged particles flow toward more negative areas, and this direction is arbitrarily designated as the direction of current flow. At the same time, negative ions flow toward positively charged areas.

Conduction Over Short Distances

Current flow that is limited to short distances (1 to 2 mm) may result from single action potentials or even subthreshold depolarizations (Fig. 4–8). Such flow is *decremental*, that is, it dies out after a short distance owing to the resistance offered by the

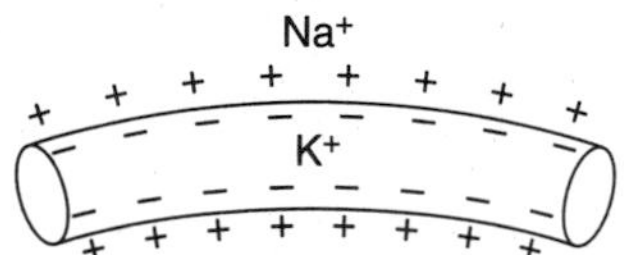

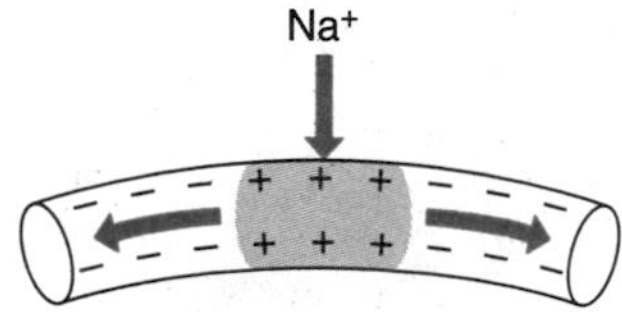

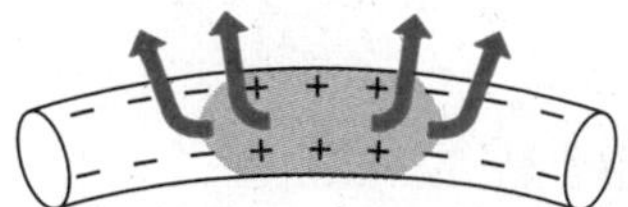

FIGURE 4–8
Conduction over a short distance. The membrane is depolarized in one region by an action potential or a subthreshold membrane potential. In the absence of voltage-gated channels, current is carried only by ion flow in the cytoplasm as entering cations are attracted laterally to anions in adjacent areas. Current dies out after a short distance owing to (1) resistance offered by the cytoplasm and (2) back-leak of positive ions across the membrane.

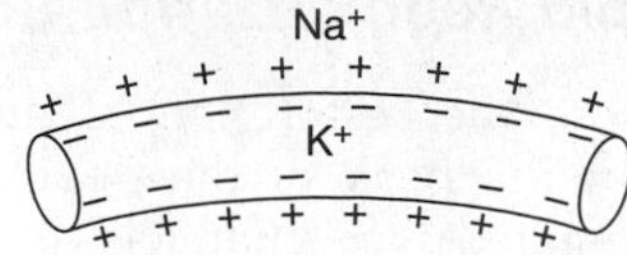

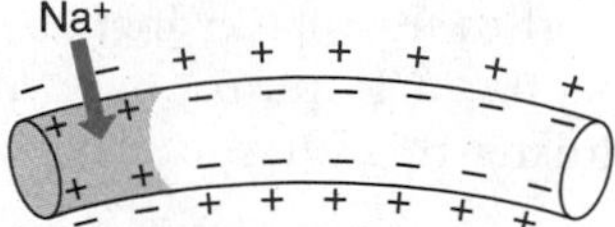

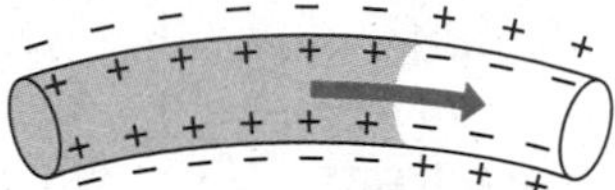

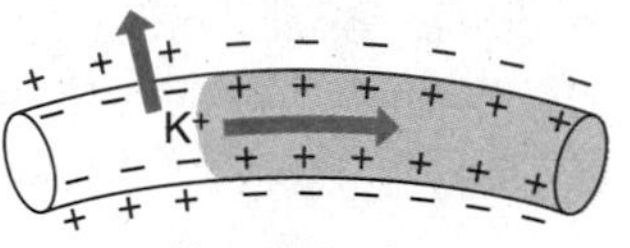

FIGURE 4–9
Conduction over a long distance. An action potential depolarizes an area of the membrane and initiates lateral flow of ions in the cytoplasm. This alteration of the membrane potential opens additional voltage-gated Na^+ (and possibly Ca^{2+}) channels, permitting cation influx and resulting in generation of an action potential in the adjacent membrane areas. This process of action potential propagation continues along the entire length of the membrane. Initially depolarized areas are refractory for a time because of inactivation of the voltage-gated Na^+ channels, resulting in directionality of current flow. At the peak of each action potential, opening of voltage-gated K^+ channels permits K^+ efflux, which repolarizes the membrane.

plasma membrane and by the fluid medium through which the ions flow. In addition, some ions may "escape" across the membrane if channels are open, abolishing the lateral gradient. These short-distance signals are known as **electrotonic potentials** and either serve a local signaling function (such as receptor activation) or initiate the generation of action potentials in adjacent areas. Conduction in dendrites and cell bodies of neurons occurs primarily by this local electrotonic flow.

Subthreshold electrotonic potentials are sometimes referred to as **graded potentials** because the height or amplitude of the depolarization phase depends on the intensity of the stimulus that initiated it.[5] The stimulus, whether electrical, mechanical, or chemical, causes perturbation of the plasma membrane and allows varying degrees of sodium or calcium influx. If threshold is reached, the amplitude of the action potential that results is consistent within tissue types, that is, it is independent of the intensity of the stimulus.

Conduction Over Long Distances

Most nerve circuits are much too long to be traversed by electrotonic potentials. Current flow in these circuits, as well as that between the cells of cardiac and smooth muscle tissues, depends on regeneration, or "propagation," of additional action potentials along the circuit, which depends in turn on the presence of voltage-gated ion channels (Fig. 4–9). Such nondecremental conduction is capable of signaling over distances of 1 meter or more without any loss of signal intensity.

This form of conduction also begins with depolarization in a local area of the membrane, reversing the polarity in that region and causing a lateral flow of positive ions toward adjacent negative areas (electrotonic flow).[6] The rise in membrane potential opens a few voltage-gated Na^+ and Ca^{2+} channels in these areas, resulting in a further rise in voltage, which opens still more channels. If threshold is reached, a full action potential occurs, and the process continues down the membrane.

CONDUCTION IN SPECIFIC EXCITABLE TISSUES

Nervous Tissue

Action potentials in nerves closely resemble those in skeletal muscle and result from the same ionic fluxes (see Fig. 4–4). Multiple subthreshold membrane potentials, generated over the surface of the cell body and dendritic (receiving) fibers, are "added" until threshold is reached. In motor neurons, this results in generation of a full action potential at the axon hillock, the point at which the transmitting nerve fiber leaves the body of the neuron (Fig. 4–10). The action potential can then be propagated down the length of the axon, which is often a considerable distance.

Conduction velocity in axons depends on two factors: (1) the diameter of the axon and (2) whether it is myelinated. Conduction is faster in larger fibers because they offer less resistance to flow of ions in the cytoplasm and because there are more ions present to carry the current. Most larger nerve fibers are surrounded by segments of lipid-derived **myelin,** separated by **nodes of Ranvier**. Myelinated areas are impermeable to ions, whereas nodes of Ranvier are characterized by a high density of voltage-gated channels. Action potentials are generated only at the nodes, and the current thus "skips" between them. This **saltatory conduction** is much faster than in unmyelinated fibers, in which the entire membrane surface must depolarize and repolarize.

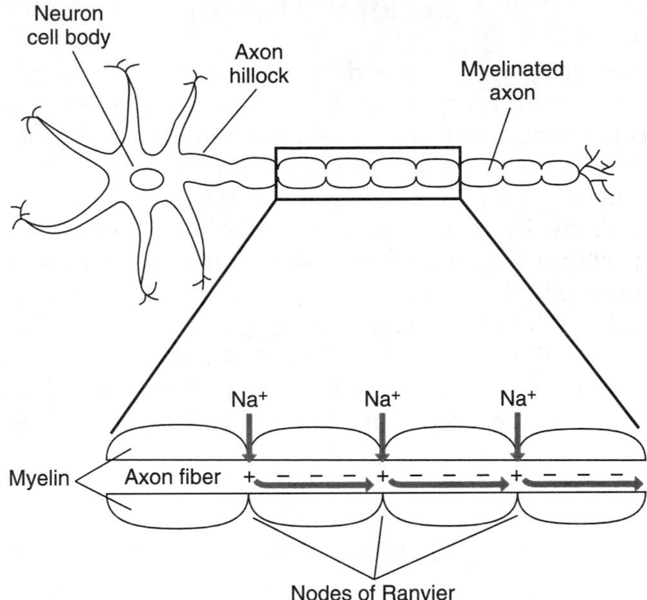

FIGURE 4–10
Current flow in a myelinated axon. The action potential is first generated at the *axon hillock* and is propagated down the length of the myelinated axon. Because the myelinated segments are impermeable to ions, action potentials are generated only at nodes of Ranvier, which have voltage-gated channels. Conduction is fast because the current skips from node to node *(saltatory conduction)*.

Local or electrotonic potentials, similar in configuration but generally lower in amplitude than action potentials, are also important in neurotransmission, serving as signals at contact points (synapses) between nerve cells and at receptors. These specialized aspects of neurotransmission are detailed in Chapters 21, 22, and 23.

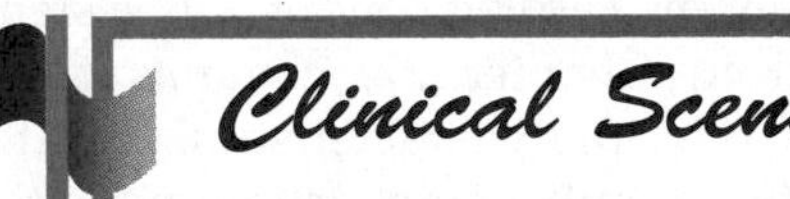

Two months after giving birth to her second child, C.T., age 32 years, began experiencing double vision, muscle weakness, and an unsteady gait. After an extensive clinical work-up, she was diagnosed with multiple sclerosis, a disease characterized by patchy demyelination of motor, sensory, and autonomic nerves.

1. How might C.T.'s clinical manifestations be explained in terms of altered conduction?
2. What additional clinical manifestations might be predicted as the disease progresses to involve additional nerves?

Skeletal Muscle

Skeletal muscle cells do not contract unless stimulated by an action potential from a motor nerve at a connecting point known as the neuromuscular junction. Because current is not conducted from cell to cell in skeletal muscle, each muscle fiber must be individually stimulated (see Chapter 22). As shown in Figure 4–4, the action potential in skeletal muscle has a rapid depolarization phase, which is due to sodium influx through voltage-gated channels. Repolarization due to K^+ efflux is also rapid, without plateau, allowing a high frequency of muscle stimulation, which may result in sustained contraction or spasm.

Cardiac Tissue

The calcium influx that occurs during phase 0 of the ventricular muscle action potential is critical to regulation of contraction of the heart, as discussed in Chapter 5. The presence of plateau lengthens the refractory period of heart muscle, preventing tetanic contraction, as has been discussed. The presence of gap junctions between cardiac cells allows ion flow and electrical current to pass easily from one cell membrane to that of adjacent cells, resulting in coordinated (syncytial) function.

Although the electrical activity of the heart is influenced by signals from the nervous system, it is not dependent on such signals. Transplanted hearts, for example, have neither sympathetic nor parasympathetic innervation but may function for many years.

Embedded within cardiac muscle is a system of specialized noncontractile cells that generates and conducts the electrical signal in a coordinated manner across the heart. This cardiac conduction system, discussed in detail in Chapter 17, contains pacemaker cells that possess the characteristics of **automaticity** (the ability to initiate an action potential without external stimulation) and **rhythmicity** (an intrinsic, regular frequency of action potential generation). Cardiac pacemaker cells have no plateau phase and no significant overshoot (see Fig. 4–6). The automaticity and rhythmicity exhibited by these cells resides in phase 4. The RMP of pacemaker cells is relatively high and is not stable. RMP instead gradually rises until threshold is reached. Phase 0 depolarization is not sudden as in cardiac muscle cells but does cause a steeper rise in membrane potential than that seen during phase 4. The ionic currents that account for this pattern are still uncertain but are believed to involve inward sodium and calcium currents and outward potassium currents.

Smooth Muscle

Smooth muscle is found within the walls of blood vessels and hollow organs. Electrical conduction in smooth muscle is similar to that in cardiac muscle in that this tissue contains some pacemaker cells capable of spontaneously generating action potentials. Although smooth muscle contraction can occur in the absence of any neural stimulation, its rate and force are generally modified by neural signals.

Smooth muscle is variable in its structure, and specific characteristics of action potentials vary among tissues (Fig. 4–11). RMP is highly variable and unstable, often demonstrating an undulating (sine wave) pattern. Superimposed on this baseline are spike potentials, some of which are action potentials and some of which are subthreshold potentials. Pacemaker potentials in smooth muscle resemble

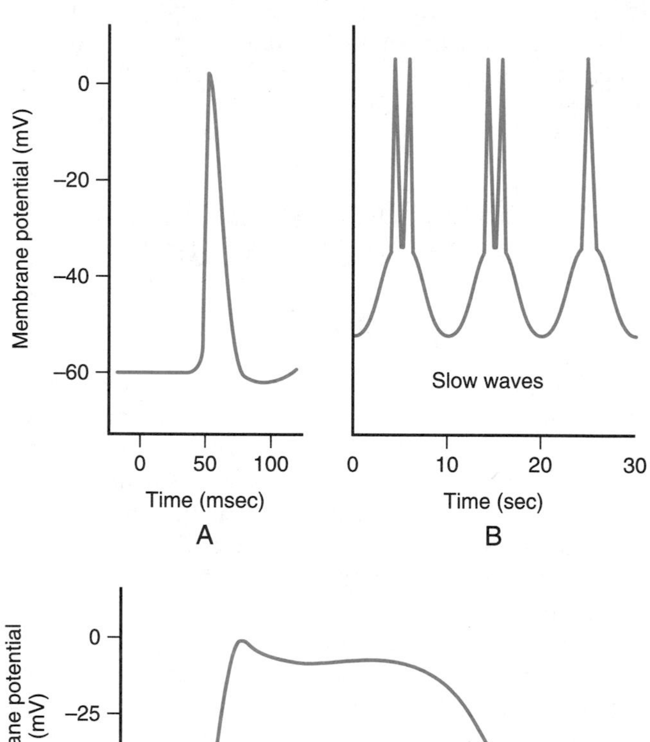

FIGURE 4–11

Action potentials in smooth muscle. Action potential configuration varies in different types of single-unit smooth muscle. *A*, Typical spike potential elicited by an external stimulus. *B*, Spike potentials superimposed on sine wave resting membrane potential (intestinal smooth muscle). *C*, Action potential with plateau (uterine smooth muscle). (Redrawn from Guyton, A.C., and Hall, J.E. [1996]. *Textbook of Medical Physiology*. [9th ed.]. Philadelphia: W.B. Saunders [p. 100]. Used with permission.)

those in cardiac tissue but are not limited to specific locations. In contrast to skeletal and cardiac muscle, the relationship between electrical conduction and subsequent contraction of smooth muscle is uncertain (see Chapter 5). The depolarization phase is the result of influx of calcium, whereas repolarization is due to an outward potassium current.[7]

Most smooth muscle is of the single-unit type, which resembles cardiac tissue in the presence of gap junctions and syncytial function. The less common multiunit type of smooth muscle is more similar in function to skeletal muscle (see Chapter 5).

MECHANISMS OF ALTERED CONDUCTION

Conduction of electrical current within the body depends on normal membrane permeability, transport processes, and ion concentrations. Altered conduction therefore results from abnormality of one or more of these factors.

Altered Membrane Permeability and Transport

As is true of other cells, cardiac, nerve, and muscle cells can be damaged by hypoxia, toxicity, or physical trauma (see Chapter 2). These pathophysiologic processes typically increase the permeability of the plasma membrane and cause instability of the RMP. Cardiac muscle cells, which do not ordinarily generate action potentials spontaneously, may do so under these conditions (see Chapter 17). This increased automaticity, or "irritability," is one mechanism of cardiac dysrhythmia. A similar mechanism may underlie seizure activity (epilepsy or convulsions) seen with trauma or metabolic disturbance of brain tissue (see Chapter 21). Impairment of energy metabolism can directly affect active transport, which is essential for maintenance of ionic gradients in excitable cells. Many drugs that affect conduction do so by virtue of their effects on membrane stability and membrane channel transport, influencing the formation and propagation of action potentials (Table 4–2).

Altered Ionic Concentrations and Gradients

The ion most critical to RMP is potassium; therefore, K^+ is maintained within a narrow range (3.5 to 5 mEq/L) in the blood. In *hyperkalemia* (extracellular potassium excess), RMP is more positive. The cell is slightly depolarized and therefore more irritable, leading to such clinical manifestations as cardiac dysrhythmias, muscle weakness, and intestinal cramping. In extreme cases (e.g., iatrogenic error in K^+ supplementation or lethal injection of KCl as a means of capital punishment), RMP rises to threshold level, preventing the cell from repolarizing and

TABLE 4–2
EXAMPLES OF DRUGS THAT INFLUENCE ACTION POTENTIALS

Drug	Effect	Clinical Use
Potassium chloride	Reduction in negativity of the resting membrane potential	Treatment of hypokalemia
Calcium gluconate (Kalcinate), calcium citrate (Citracal), calcium carbonate (Os-Cal)	Hyperpolarization	Treatment of hypocalcemia or overdose of Mg^{2+} or K^+; prevention of osteoporosis
Magnesium sulfate (Epsom salts, $MgSO_4$)	Hyperpolarization	Treatment of hypomagnesemia, toxemia of pregnancy, preterm labor, or dysrhythmias
Quinidine sulfate (Quinidex), quinidine gluconate (Quinaglute)	Depression of phase 0; prolongation of action potential	Treatment of dysrhythmias
Phenytoin (Dilantin)	Depression of phase 0; shortening of action potential	Treatment of seizures and dysrhythmias
Propranolol (Inderal)	Depression of phase 4	Treatment of heart failure and dysrhythmias
Amiodarone (Cordarone)	Prolongation of phase 3	Treatment of dysrhythmias
Verapamil (Calan)	Prolongation of phases 1 and 2; depression of phase 4	Treatment of dysrhythmias
Halothane (Fluothane)	Prolongation of refractoriness	General anesthesia
Lidocaine (Xylocaine)	Depression of phase 0	Local anesthesia; treatment of dysrhythmias

Focus of Current Research

Study	Objective and Findings
LeGrand, et al. (1995) Alleviation of contractile dysfunction in ischemic hearts by slowly inactivating Na^+ current blockers.	*Objective:* To investigate the role of Na^+ influx in promotion of Ca^{2+} overload seen in cardiac ischemia *Findings:* Na^+ influx through slowly inactivating channels contributes to Ca^{2+} overload. Drugs that block this current may reduce the resulting contractile dysfunction.
Sharma, et al. (1995) Muscular fatigue in Duchenne's muscular dystrophy.	*Objective:* To assess neuromuscular transmission and membrane factors in fatigue in boys with Duchenne's muscular dystrophy (DMD) compared with control subjects *Findings:* Compound muscle potential amplitude was lower in DMD patients, but DMD patients had less central fatigue than did control subjects.
Gallegos & Fry (1994) Alterations to the electrophysiology of isolated human detrusor smooth muscle cells in bladder disease.	*Objective:* To investigate the properties of the inward Ca^{2+} current in human detrusor smooth muscle cells in different pathologic conditions *Findings:* Myocytes from patients with prostatic symptoms had increased membrane surface area and altered Ca^{2+} currents.
Kupersmith, et al. (1994) Marked action potential prolongation as a source of injury current leading to border zone arrhythmogenesis.	*Objective:* To delineate electrophysiologic phenomena in a border zone adjacent to a zone of marked action potential prolongation *Findings:* Action potentials were prolonged and low-amplitude secondary plateaus were frequent in the border zone, owing to an injury current between the two areas.
Stalberg & Sonoo (1994) Assessment of variability in the shape of the motor unit action potential, the "jiggle" at consecutive discharges.	*Objective:* To describe the variability in the motor unit potential recorded during conventional electromyography *Findings:* Variability, or jiggle, was significantly increased in patients with amyotrophic lateral sclerosis.
Wolters, et al. (1994) Ionic currents during action potentials in mammalian skeletal muscle fibers analyzed with loose patch clamp.	*Objective:* To compare membrane currents during extracellularly applied depolarization steps to currents occurring during action potentials *Findings:* Three components were identified in the transmembrane current: a capacitive current, an inward Na^+ current, and an outward K^+ current. Other currents were negligible. The K^+ current was not detectable during extracellularly applied depolarization.

Young, et al. (1993)

T-type and L-type calcium currents in freshly dispersed human uterine smooth muscle cells.

Objective: To characterize the types of voltage-activated calcium currents found in human uterine myocytes and to determine the effects of magnesium and nifedipine on these currents

Findings: Uterine cells exhibit subtypes of calcium currents analogous to those in cardiac muscle. The T-type current may be involved with action potential transmission, while the L-type current increases intracellular free calcium. The differing effects of magnesium and nifedipine explain their potential uses in preterm labor.

responding to another stimulus. This results in cardiac arrest and paralysis. In clinical settings, hyperkalemia is usually the result of renal failure or significant tissue trauma.

Hypokalemia (extracellular potassium deficit) is relatively common, occurring as a result of excessive diuretic therapy, vomiting, or diarrhea. In hypokalemia, the RMP is more negative; that is, the cell is hyperpolarized. Because distance to threshold is greater than normal, the cell is less responsive to stimulation. Clinical manifestations, such as dysrhythmias and decreased muscle tone, are seen. Imbalances of potassium are discussed with those of other electrolytes in Chapter 9.

Calcium imbalances are less common than potassium imbalances, but they also affect action potential formation. Extracellular Ca^{2+} interacts with the negative charges on membrane proteins and phospholipids. This positive ECF charge contributes somewhat to the membrane potential, and when ECF Ca^{2+} is elevated (*hypercalcemia*), the cell is slightly hyperpolarized. Conversely, when ECF Ca^{2+} is low (*hypocalcemia*), the cell is slightly depolarized and therefore more irritable. Conceptually, a rise in calcium increases threshold, whereas a decrease in calcium decreases threshold. As with potassium, ECF calcium levels are tightly regulated. Calcium homeostasis is complex, with multiple hormonal controls and cycling among skeletal calcium stores, bound and unbound forms in the blood, and intestinal absorption (see Chapter 9). The clinical effects of calcium imbalances on action potentials are most apparent as altered contraction of muscle, discussed in Chapter 5.

CLINICAL CONSEQUENCES OF ALTERED CONDUCTION

The human system depends on conduction within excitable tissues for critical functions such as perfusion, mobility, and communication. The cellular processes mediating this type of intercellular signaling in health and disease are still being characterized (see Focus of Current Research). Clinical evaluation of electrical activity is an important aspect of diagnosis and monitoring in disorders of the nervous, cardiovascular, and musculoskeletal systems. Electrical stimulation may be employed as an intervention mode in disorders of excitable tissue. Examples include electrical defibrillation (cardioversion) for dysrhythmias, skeletal muscle stimulation to prevent atrophy, and transcutaneous electrical nerve stimulation for pain reduction. Principles on which such assessment and treatment are based, as well as diseases of altered conduction, are further explored in chapters related to these systems.

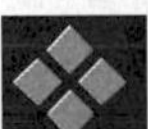

Summary of Key Points

- Generation of membrane potentials and action potentials results from membrane transport processes that produce unequal ion distribution across the plasma membrane. The resulting separation of charge represents an electrical gradient that may be discharged spontaneously in pacemaker cells or in response to electrical, chemical, or mechanical stimulation in other cells.
- Resting membrane potential is determined primarily by the equilibrium (Nernst) potential for potassium. Depolarization is primarily due to inward flux of sodium. Plateau is the result of offsetting inward calcium and outward potassium currents. Repolarization is the result of potassium efflux.
- Refractoriness to repeated stimulation during repolarization is a consequence of insufficient numbers of activated sodium channels

Summary continued on next page

Refractoriness contributes to function (e.g., cardiac filling and muscle recovery) and directionality of current flow.

- Short-distance conduction results from ion flow within body fluids initiated by subthreshold potentials or single action potentials. Long-distance flow requires propagation of action potentials along membranes of cells within the signaling pathway.
- Conduction in cardiac muscle is spontaneously generated but potentially influenced by neural signals. It occurs with least resistance along an anatomic pathway—the cardiac conduction system. Presence of plateau prevents tetany and facilitates ventricular filling. Smooth muscle conduction is similar to cardiac conduction in its pacemaker capacity and syncytial function. Skeletal muscle cells require individual neural stimulation to generate action potentials. Motor neurons are capable of generating full action potentials only at the axon hillock, and they conduct current directionally along nerve fibers. Neural conduction is fastest in larger, myelinated fibers.
- Altered conduction may result from abnormality in membrane permeability or transport or from altered ionic concentrations and gradients.
- Alteration in action potentials may directly contribute to altered muscle contraction and neurotransmission—processes that are essential to the function of all organ systems.

REFERENCES

1. Guyton, A.C., and Hall, J.E. (1996). *Textbook of Medical Physiology*. (9th ed.). Philadelphia: W.B. Saunders. (pp. 49).
2. Ten Eick, R., Whalley, D.W., and Rasmussen, H.H. (1992). Connections: Heart disease, cellular electrophysiology, and ion channels. *Faseb Journal* 6(8), 2568–2580.
3. Ganong, W.F. (1995). *Review of Medical Physiology*. (17th ed.). Norwalk, CT: Appleton & Lange. (pp. 69–70).
4. Noble, D., Noble, S.J., Bett, G.C.L., *et al.* (1991). The role of sodium-calcium exchange during the cardiac action potential. *Annals of the New York Academy of Sciences* 639(1991), 334–353.
5. Moffett, D.F., Moffett, S.B., and Schauf, C.L. (1993). *Human Physiology: Foundations and Frontiers*. (2nd ed.). St. Louis: Mosby-Year Book. (pp. 163–165).
6. Berne, R.M., and Levy, M.N. (1993). *Physiology*. (3rd ed.). St. Louis: Mosby-Year Book. (pp. 49–52).
7. Montgomery, B.S.I., and Fry, C.H. (1992). The action potential and net membrane currents in isolated human detrusor muscle cells. *The Journal of Urology* 147(1), 176–184.

SELECTED BIBLIOGRAPHY

Barchi, R.L. (1993). Ion channels and disorders of excitation in skeletal muscle. *Current Opinion in Neurology and Neurosurgery* 6(1), 40–47.

Bastamante, J. (1994). Nuclear electrophysiology. *Journal of Membrane Biology* 138(2), 105–112.

Franz, M.R. (1994). Bridging the gap between basic and clinical electrophysiology: What can be learned from monophasic action potential recordings? *Journal of Cardiovascular Electrophysiology* 1994(8), 699–710.

Gallegos, C.R.R., and Fry, C.H. (1994). Alterations to the electrophysiology of isolated human detrusor smooth muscle cells in bladder disease. *The Journal of Urology* 151(3), 754–758.

Jayakar, P. (1993). Physiological principles of electrical stimulation. *Advances in Neurology* 63(1993), 17–27.

Kuhn, M.M. (1991). *Pharmacotherapeutics: A Nursing Process Approach*. (2nd ed.). Philadelphia: F.A. Davis.

Kupersmith, J., Li, Z-Y., and Maldonado, C. (1994). Marked action potential prolongation as a source of injury current leading to border zone arrhythmogenesis. *American Heart Journal* 127(6), 1543–1553.

LeGrand, B., Vie, B., Talmant, J.M., *et al.* (1995). Alleviation of contractile dysfunction in ischemic hearts by slowing inactivating Na^+ current blockers. *American Journal of Physiology* 269(2 Pt. 2), H533–H540.

Lesh, M.D. (1993). Interventional electrophysiology: State of the art. *American Heart Journal* 126(3 Pt. 1), 686–698.

Lodish, H., Baltimore, D., Berk, A., *et al.* (1995). *Molecular Cell Biology*. (3rd ed.). New York: Scientific American Books.

Patterson, E., Jackman, W.M., Scherlag, B.J., *et al.* (1991). The monophasic action potential in clinical cardiology. *Clinical Cardiology* 1991(6), 505–510.

Sharma, K.R., Mynhier, M.A., and Miller, R.G. (1995). Muscular fatigue in Duchenne muscular dystrophy. *Neurology* 45(2), 306–310.

Stalberg, E.V., and Sonoo, M. (1994). Assessment of variability in the shape of the motor unit action potential, the "jiggle" at consecutive discharges. *Muscle & Nerve* 17(10), 1135–1144.

Vaughan-Williams, E.M. (1992). The relevance of cellular to clinical electrophysiology in classifying antiarrhythmic action. *Journal of Cardiovascular Pharmacology* 1992(20 suppl. 2), S1–S7.

Weidmann, S. (1993). Cardiac action potentials, membrane currents, and some personal reminiscences. *Annual Review of Physiology* 55(1993), 1–14.

Wolters, H., Wallinga, W., Ypey, D.L., *et al.* (1994). Ionic currents during action potentials in mammalian skeletal muscle fibers analyzed with loose patch clamp. *American Journal of Physiology* 267(6 Pt. 1), C1699–C1706.

Young, R.C., Smith, L.H., and McLaren, M.D. (1993). T-type and L-type calcium currents in freshly dispersed human uterine smooth muscle cells. *American Journal of Obstetrics and Gynecology* 169(4), 785–792.

Yuan, S., Blomstrom-Lundqvist, C., and Olsson, S.B. (1994). Monophasic action potentials: Concepts to practical applications. *Journal of Cardiovascular Electrophysiology* 5(3), 287–308.

Cellular Mechanism of Muscle Contraction

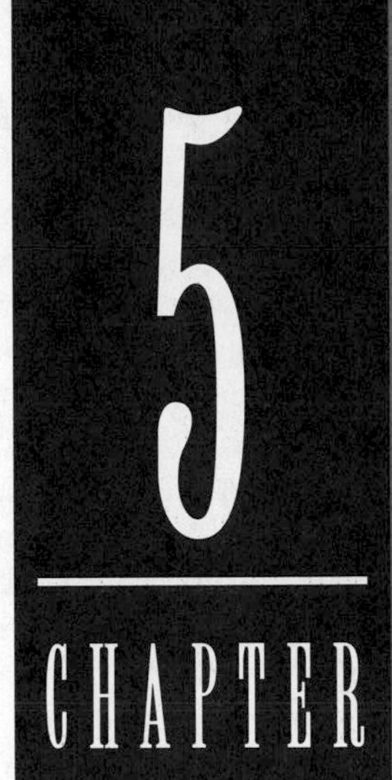

LEARNING OBJECTIVES

1. Identify the major contractile and regulatory proteins found in each type of muscle.
2. Differentiate among skeletal, cardiac, and smooth muscle with regard to striation and T-tubule systems.
3. Describe the stages of the cross-bridge cycle according to the sliding filament model of muscle contraction.
4. Discuss the differences between striated and smooth muscle with regard to the cross-bridge cycle.
5. Differentiate between electromechanical and chemomechanical coupling in regulation of muscle contraction.
6. Identify the principal energy-producing mechanisms in each muscle type.
7. Discuss four general mechanisms that can result in abnormal muscle contraction.
8. Identify clinical manifestations of altered muscle contraction within the major body systems.

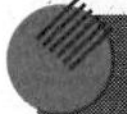

key terms

actin
atrophy
caldesmon
calmodulin
calponin
chemomechanical coupling
connectin (titin)
cross-bridge
dyskinesia
electromechanical coupling
intercalated disk
latch bridge
light chain
myofibrils
myosin
myosin ATPase
myosin light-chain kinase (MLCK)
myosin phosphatase
nebulin
neuromuscular junction
palpitations
paralysis
paresis
peristalsis
rigor mortis
sarcomere
sliding filament theory
spasticity
syncope
tetanus (tetany)
tremor
tropomyosin
troponin
T tubule

Although there are three distinct types of muscle in the body, the topic of muscle contraction typically elicits an image of athletic exertion: the contraction of skeletal muscles during running or weightlifting, for example. Certainly skeletal muscle function in mobility and the performance of work is essential to human function. Contraction of cardiac and smooth muscle is often less apparent, although notable exceptions are the contraction of uterine smooth muscle during labor and childbirth and the forceful contraction of the heart during extreme stress or exertion.

If one includes the smooth muscle of the blood vessels perfusing each system, muscle tissue is found in all organ systems. Nearly half of the total mass of the body is composed of muscle tissue. Table 5–1 summarizes system functions that depend on muscle contraction.

At the cellular level, muscle contraction depends on cellular energy metabolism, transport and receptor functions, and the generation and conduction of action potentials. Energy production and storage in muscle tissue are adapted to the needs of each muscle type (see Chapter 35), and the large quantity of energy released as heat during muscle work is important in maintenance of body temperature (see Chapter 11).

The three types of muscle tissue differ to some extent in their structure and function, but many aspects of the molecular mechanism of muscle contraction are similar in all types. Skeletal muscle is described initially in each section of this chapter, followed by discussion of variations in smooth and cardiac muscle.

MICROANATOMY OF MUSCLE TISSUE

Muscle tissues may be differentiated on the basis of their structural and regulatory proteins. Tissue microstructure also varies among types.

Muscle Proteins

Skeletal Muscle

Muscle tissue contains a number of proteins that serve both structural and regulatory functions. In skeletal muscle, these proteins have a highly regular arrangement.

Actin and Myosin. The essential structural filaments of the contractile apparatus are the proteins **actin** and **myosin**. Actin, the principal component of the *thin filament*, is composed of beaded strands of globular protein subunits, coiled in a double helix configuration (Fig. 5–1). Actin contains binding sites for the *thick filament*, myosin; these sites are cyclically covered and uncovered during the process of contraction.

TABLE 5–1
SYSTEM FUNCTIONS THAT DEPEND ON MUSCLE CONTRACTION

System	Muscle-Dependent Function	Muscle Type
Cardiovascular	Cardiac pumping	Cardiac
	Contraction and dilation of blood vessels (regulation of blood pressure and tissue perfusion)	Smooth
Respiratory	Ventilation (movement of the diaphragm and intercostal muscles)	Skeletal
	Bronchoconstriction and bronchodilation (regulation of airway caliber)	Smooth
Renal and urinary	Ureteral transport and bladder storage and ejection of urine (micturition)	Smooth
	Sphincter control of micturition (urinary continence)	Skeletal
Gastrointestinal	Deglutition (swallowing)	Skeletal Smooth
	Mechanical digestion (chewing; churning movements of the stomach)	Skeletal Smooth
	Bowel motility	Smooth
	Sphincter control of defecation	Skeletal
Hepatobiliary	Bile release and transport	Smooth
Reproductive	Uterine contraction (menstruation; labor and delivery)	Smooth
	Sperm transport through the vas deferens (emission and ejaculation)	Smooth
Musculoskeletal	Antigravity position (contraction of trunk and leg muscles)	Skeletal
	Mobility	Skeletal

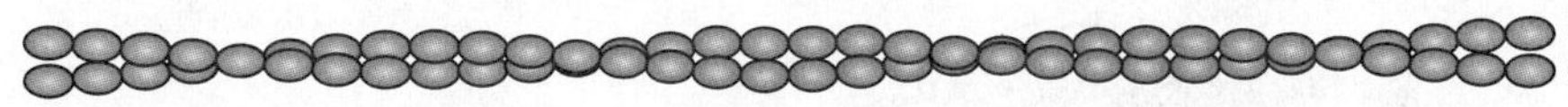

Filamentous actin

FIGURE 5–1

Actin. The major protein of the thin filament of muscle is filamentous actin, which consists of strands of globular subunits, coiled in a double helix.

The type of myosin found in muscle cells differs in structure from that which functions as a motor protein in noncontractile cells (see Chapter 2). The myosin molecule in muscle is composed of two subunits, each of which consists of a fibrous protein "tail" and a globular "head," joined by a "neck" region. About 300 myosin molecules are aggregated parallel to each other to form the thick filament, with the heads projecting laterally 60 degrees apart at opposite ends of the bipolar structure (Fig. 5–2). The head contains binding sites for actin and for adenosine triphosphate (ATP), whereas the neck contains **light chains**, proteins that have regulatory activity. The myosin head also contains a domain that has enzymatic activity. This **myosin ATPase** cleaves ATP to adenosine diphosphate (ADP) and inorganic phosphate during a critical stage of muscle contraction.

When viewed in cross-section, each thick filament associates with six thin filaments in a hexagonal array, and each thin filament associates with three thick filaments (Fig. 5–3). Skeletal muscle is classified as *striated* because of its striped appearance under microscopy. This striation originates in the overlapping bands of thin and thick filaments, arranged in functional units called **sarcomeres** (Fig. 5–4). The sarcomere is bounded at each end by light areas (I bands) with darker middle zones called *Z lines.* Z lines are disk-like protein sheets that serve as the end points for attachment of actin. Dark areas (A bands) result from areas where myosin and actin overlap. The central H zone, a lighter area within the dark A band, is seen only in relaxed muscle when actin and myosin do not overlap in this region. The darker M line, which bisects the H zone, represents the presence of fibers in this region that attach myosin filaments to each other.

Tropomyosin and Troponin. Tropomyosin is a fibrous protein that is coiled with actin in the double helix (Fig. 5–5). Depending on its configuration, it may cover or uncover the binding sites for myosin. **Troponin** is a complex of three protein subunits: troponin T (TN-T), which attaches the complex to actin; troponin C (TN-C), which binds calcium; and troponin-I (TN-I), which induces tropomyosin to cover the binding sites on actin.

Connectin (Titin) and Nebulin. Two large proteins, **connectin** (also known as *titin*) and **nebulin**, are associated with overlapping actin and myosin molecules in muscle cells (Fig. 5–6). The functions of these proteins are still being clarified; however, they are known to be important in maintaining the regular arrangement of thick and thin filaments and in imparting elasticity to the sarcomere. Connectin connects the ends of the myosin thick filaments to the Z disks, and its elastic elements keep the filament centered during contraction.[1] Nebulin is a nonelastic protein that extends from the Z lines adjacent to actin. It apparently acts as a "ruler," regulating the number of actin subunits that make up the length of each thin filament.[2]

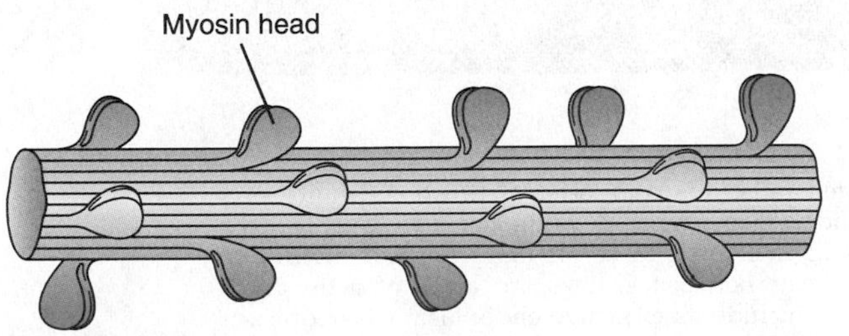

Myosin head

FIGURE 5–2

Structure of the thick filament (myosin). The myosin molecule is composed of two subunits, each with a rod-like "tail" and a globular "head," joined by a "neck" region. About 300 myosin molecules are aggregated parallel to each other to form the thick filament, with the heads projecting 60 degrees apart.

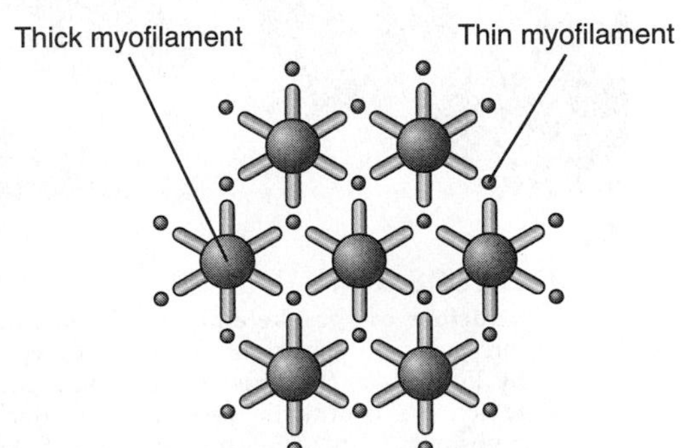

FIGURE 5–3

Hexagonal array of myofilaments. The contractile proteins of skeletal muscle are regularly arranged. As viewed in cross-section, six thin (actin) filaments are associated with each thick (myosin) filament, and each thin filament is associated with three thick filaments.

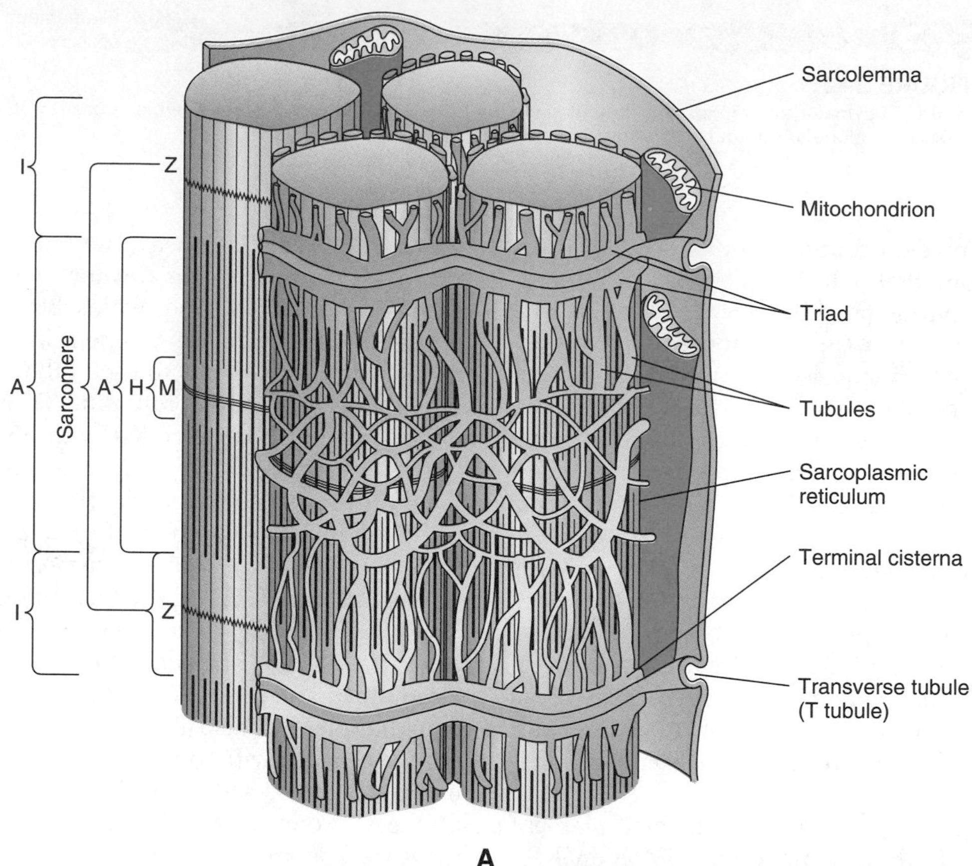

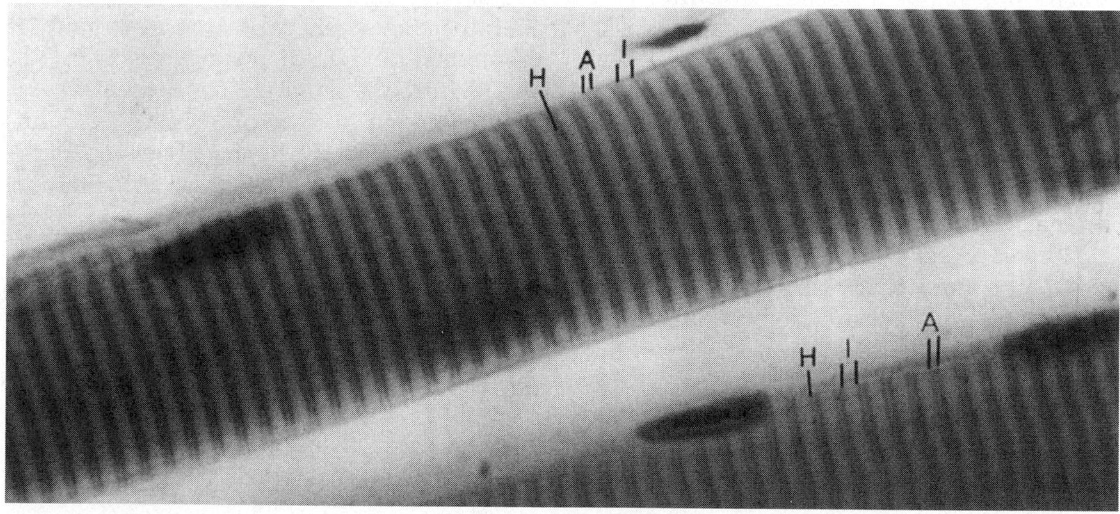

FIGURE 5–4

Structure of the skeletal muscle sarcomere. Striated muscle is composed of functional units, or *sarcomeres. A,* Schematic drawing. *B,* Microscopic slide. The sarcomere's boundaries are established by light areas (I bands) with darker middle zones (Z lines or Z disks). Z disks are end plates to which the contractile proteins are attached. Dark areas between Z lines are areas of actin and myosin overlap. Anatomic features of skeletal muscle include its extensive endoplasmic (sarcoplasmic) reticulum and T-tubule system for regulation of cytosolic calcium levels. The plasma membrane in muscle is known as the *sarcolemma.* (*B* from Leeson, T.S., Leeson, C.R., and Paparo, A.A. [1988]. *Textbook and Atlas of Histology.* Philadelphia: W.B. Saunders. [p. 238].)

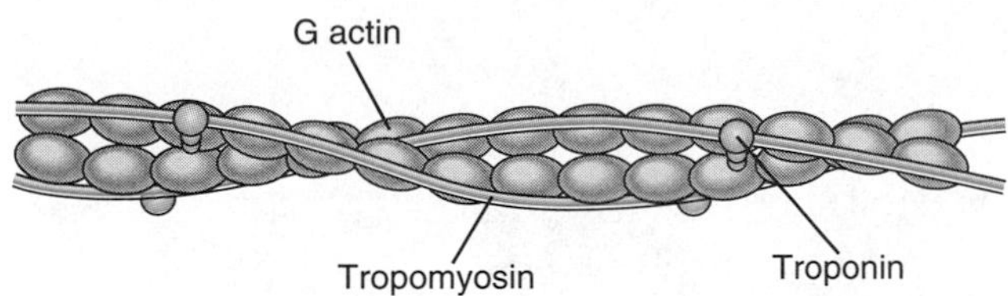

FIGURE 5–5

Tropomyosin and troponin. Tropomyosin is a fibrous protein that is coiled with actin in the thin filament. Seven globular G-actin subunits bind to each molecule of tropomyosin. In striated muscle, the regulatory protein troponin is associated with tropomyosin. Binding of calcium to a troponin subunit initiates a conformational change in tropomyosin, which uncovers myosin-binding sites on actin.

Smooth Muscle

Striation is not apparent on microscopic examination of smooth muscle (Fig. 5–7). Smooth muscle cells contain numerous thin filaments but few thick filaments. Thin filaments are anchored by *dense bodies,* which are much less regularly arranged than are Z lines in skeletal muscle. Thin and thick filaments are aligned along the long axis of the smooth muscle cell but become displaced in several directions when the cell contracts. Smooth muscle also contains noncontractile intermediate filaments, which limit deformation of the cell during contraction (see Chapter 2).

Troponin is not found in smooth muscle. Another protein, **calmodulin,** serves the calcium-binding function. Calmodulin is attached to myosin rather than to actin. The proteins **caldesmon** and **calponin** are associated with actin and, as discussed later, may play an auxiliary role in the mechanism of sustained contraction in smooth muscle.[3] A calcium-dependent enzyme, **myosin light-chain kinase (MLCK),** exposes binding sites for actin on the myosin head in smooth muscle, and **myosin phosphatase** causes dissociation of actin–myosin complexes in smooth muscle.

Cardiac Muscle

Cardiac muscle is similar to skeletal muscle in its striated appearance (Fig. 5–8), although cardiac filaments are not as regular in their array. This lack of precision in fiber arrangement is attributed to the lack of nebulin in cardiac muscle. The other proteins in cardiac muscle are identical to those in skeletal muscle.

Tissue Microstructure

Skeletal Muscle

Skeletal muscle cells have several nuclei and contain large numbers of rod-like **myofibrils,** densely packed together parallel to each other, with organelles such as mitochondria squeezed between them. Because skeletal muscle cells are anatomically separated by tight junctions, each cell must receive its own electrical stimulus (action potential) to contract (see Chapter 4).

Skeletal muscle cells have an extensive endoplasmic reticulum called the *sarcoplasmic reticulum.* The sarcoplasmic reticulum serves the important function of intracellular calcium storage and release. Regulation of intracellular calcium levels is essential to contraction in all muscle tissue, and the sarcoplasmic reticulum stores of Ca^{2+} are particularly important in cardiac and skeletal muscle. In skeletal muscle, an extensive system of transverse tubules (**T tubules**) is a component of the plasma membrane (called the *sarcolemma* in muscle). T tubules penetrate deeply into the cell in the areas where the A and I bands join (Fig. 5–9) and conduct the action potential inward, inducing release of intracellular calcium. Located on each side of the T tubule are terminal cisternae (or calcium reservoirs) of the sarcoplasmic reticulum, forming a functional unit known as a *triad.* Although not anatomically con-

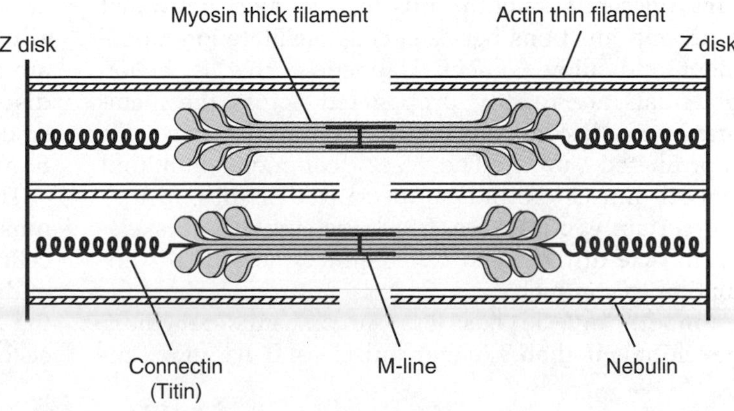

FIGURE 5–6

Connectin and nebulin. Two large proteins associated with actin and myosin contribute to the regularity of the filament arrangement in striated muscle sarcomeres. Connectin (titin) connects myosin to Z disks and also has elastic elements that keep myosin centered and that contribute to muscle tone. Nebulin (in skeletal muscle) extends from the Z lines with actin, apparently acting as a "ruler" that regulates the length of actin strands. (Redrawn from Lodish, H., Baltimore, D., Berk, A. *et al.* [1995]. *Molecular Cell Biology.* [3rd ed.]. © 1995 by Scientific American Books. Used with permission of W.H. Freeman and Company.)

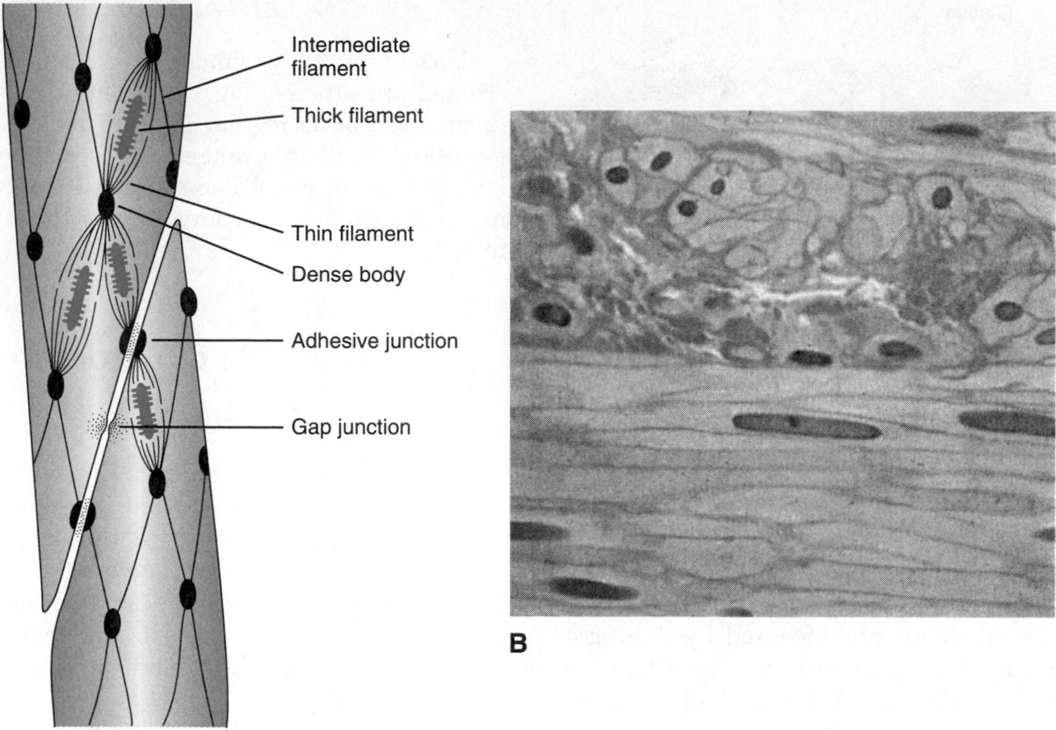

FIGURE 5–7

Structure of smooth muscle. Smooth muscle lacks the regular filament array of striated muscle, containing numerous thin filaments but few thick filaments. *A*, Schematic drawing. *B*, Microscopic slide. Thin filaments are anchored to dense bodies, as are intermediate filaments, which limit cell deformation during contraction. Gap junctions between cells facilitate interstitial function of smooth muscle tissues. Smooth muscle lacks sarcoplasmic reticulum and T-tubule systems. (*B* from Leeson, T.S., Leeson, C.R., and Paparo, A.A. [1988]. *Textbook and Histology.* Philadelphia: W.B. Saunders. [1988].)

nected, the three structures are in close enough proximity to function together in release and reuptake of intracellular calcium, the process that underlies regulation of muscle contraction.

Smooth Muscle

Smooth muscle cells have single nuclei and are much smaller than skeletal muscle cells. In single-unit (visceral) smooth muscle, the most prevalent type, gap junctions between cells facilitate ion movement and allow syncytial function; that is, action potentials are readily propagated across the membranes of adjacent cells, and the tissue functions as a coordinated unit. The less common multiunit smooth muscle, found in specialized tissues, including certain eye muscles, functions similarly to skeletal muscle in that each cell requires individual stimulation to contract.

Smooth muscle has less sarcoplasmic reticulum development than skeletal muscle and has no T tubules. Influx of extracellular fluid (ECF) calcium through membrane channels increases cytoplasmic levels during contraction.

Cardiac Muscle

Cardiac muscle cells are shorter and less regular than skeletal muscle cells, with branches and lateral interconnections between cells in a basketweave-like arrangement. Like smooth muscle, cardiac cells usually contain only one nucleus. Cardiac muscle cells are anatomically separated by **intercalated disks** but display syncytial function similar to single unit smooth muscle because of the presence of gap junctions that allow communication between cells.

The sarcoplasmic reticulum is extensive in cardiac muscle, which depends primarily on release of intracellular calcium to initiate contraction. T tubules are widest and deepest in cardiac muscle, are located at the Z lines, and are associated with a single terminal cisterna, forming a dyad.

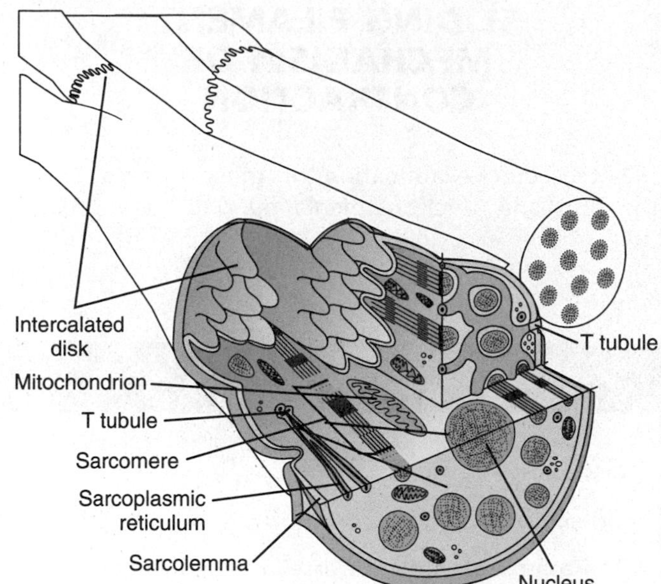

FIGURE 5–8

Structure of cardiac muscle. Cardiac muscle is similar in structure to skeletal muscle, except that cells are shorter, branched, and less regular in their filament arrays. Although cells are anatomically separated by intercalated disks, gap junctions permit syncytial function of cardiac tissue. Extensive sarcoplasmic reticulum and T-tubule systems facilitate regulation of cytosolic calcium levels.

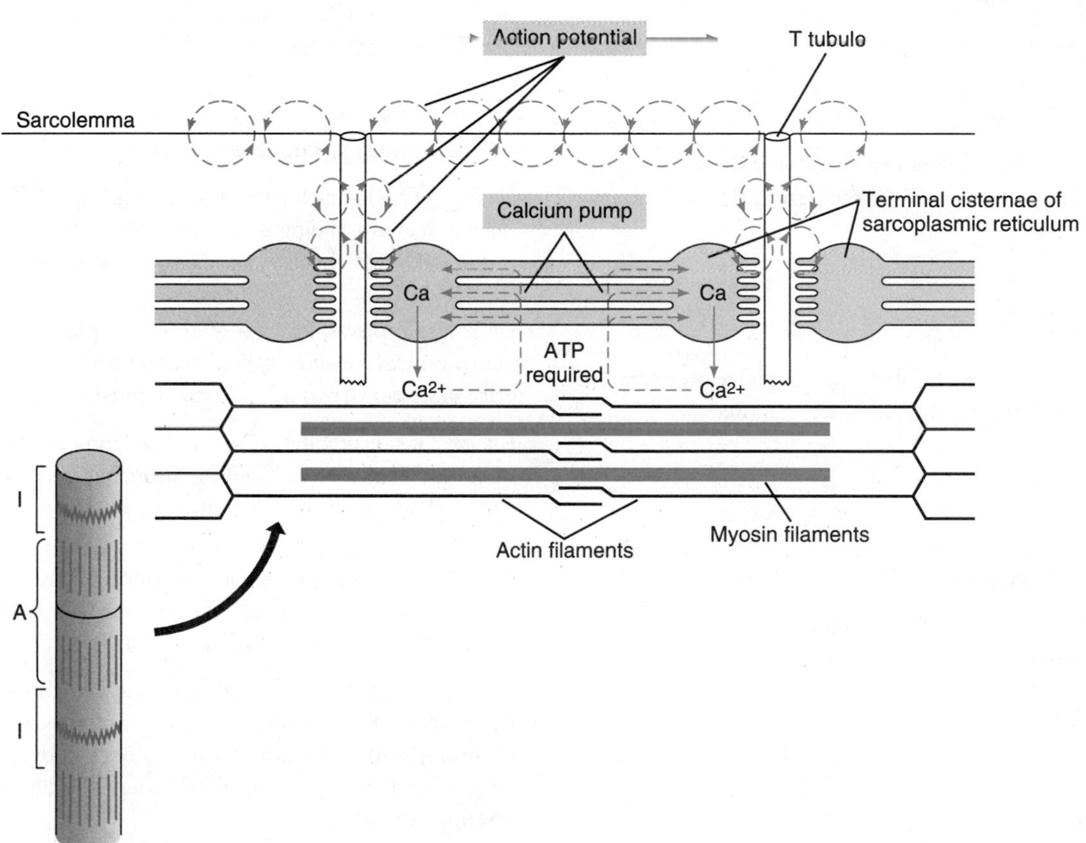

FIGURE 5–9

Calcium-dependent regulation of muscle contraction. In skeletal and cardiac muscle, propagation of action potentials across the sarcolemma and down the T tubule results in opening of voltage-gated calcium channels that permit Ca^{2+} influx from the extracellular fluid and trigger release of Ca^{2+} from the intracellular stores in the sarcoplasmic reticulum. Binding of Ca^{2+} to troponin in the thin filament initiates sliding of actin over myosin, resulting in tension development and shortening of the sarcomere. Pumping of Ca^{2+} out of the cytosol ends actin–myosin interaction. Adenosine triphosphate (ATP) is required for actin–myosin cross-bridge cycling and for active transport of Ca^{2+}. (Modified from Guyton, A.C. [1992]. *Human Physiology and Mechanisms of Disease.* (5th ed.). Philadelphia: W.B. Saunders. [p. 62].)

SLIDING FILAMENT MECHANISM OF CONTRACTION

Microscopic examination of muscle reveals that the thin and thick filaments overlap to a greater extent when muscle is contracted than when it is relaxed. In 1954, Huxley and colleagues[4, 5] proposed the **sliding filament theory** to explain the interactions between actin and myosin that result in filament overlap and development of contractile force. Although subsequent research continues to refine this theory (see Focus of Current Research), the ba-

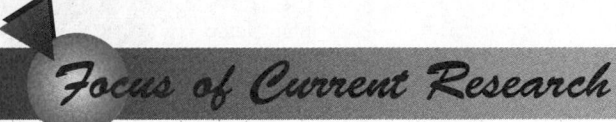

Study	*Objective and Findings*
Cannell, et al. (1995) The control of calcium release in heart muscle.	*Objective:* To examine the control of calcium release from the sarcoplasmic reticulum in cardiac muscle *Findings:* Depolarization resulted in calcium "sparks" through L-type Ca^{2+} channels. These sparks (graded potentials) triggered Ca^{2+} release from the sarcoplasmic reticulum, which was independent of the duration of the spark stimulus.
Irving, et al. (1995) Tilting of the light-chain region of myosin during step length changes and active force generation in skeletal muscle.	*Objective:* To detect changes in the myosin head during contraction using fluorescence polarization *Findings:* The light-chain region of the myosin head tilts during filament sliding and during the subsequent phase, which is thought to signal force generation.
Kahn & Song (1995) Insulin inhibits dog vascular smooth muscle contraction and lowers $Ca^{2+}{}_i$ by inhibiting Ca^{2+} influx.	*Objective:* To examine the effects of a physiologic concentration of insulin on contraction and Ca^{2+} transport in cultured vascular smooth muscle cells *Findings:* Insulin inhibits Ca^{2+} influx from the ECF but does not increase Ca^{2+} efflux and does not inhibit Ca^{2+} release from internal stores.
Higuchi & Goldman (1995) Sliding distance per ATP molecule hydrolyzed by myosin heads during isotonic shortening of skinned muscle fibers.	*Objective:* To measure sliding distance of muscle fibers when known amounts of ATP are made available to the contractile apparatus *Findings:* Distance increases as sliding velocity increases. For each ATPase cycle, a myosin head interacts mechanically with several actin monomers, indicating coupling of hydrolysis of one ATP molecule to more than one movement.
VanBuren, et al. (1994) The essential light chain is required for full force production by skeletal muscle myosin.	*Objective:* To assess how light-chain removal affects cross-bridge cycling *Findings:* Removal of regulatory light chains had little effect on muscle force development, but removal of essential light chains reduced contractile force by more than 50%.

sic mechanism of actin–myosin interaction, or **cross-bridge** formation, is well accepted as the basis of contraction in all types of muscle. The following section describes the mechanism as it occurs in skeletal and cardiac muscle. Differences seen in smooth muscle contraction are discussed subsequently.

Cross-Bridge Cycle in Skeletal and Cardiac Muscle

Stages of the cross-bridge cycle are illustrated in Figure 5–10. In the *relaxed state*, there is no interaction between actin and myosin. Intracellular Ca^{2+} concentration is low, and the TN-I subunit of tropo-

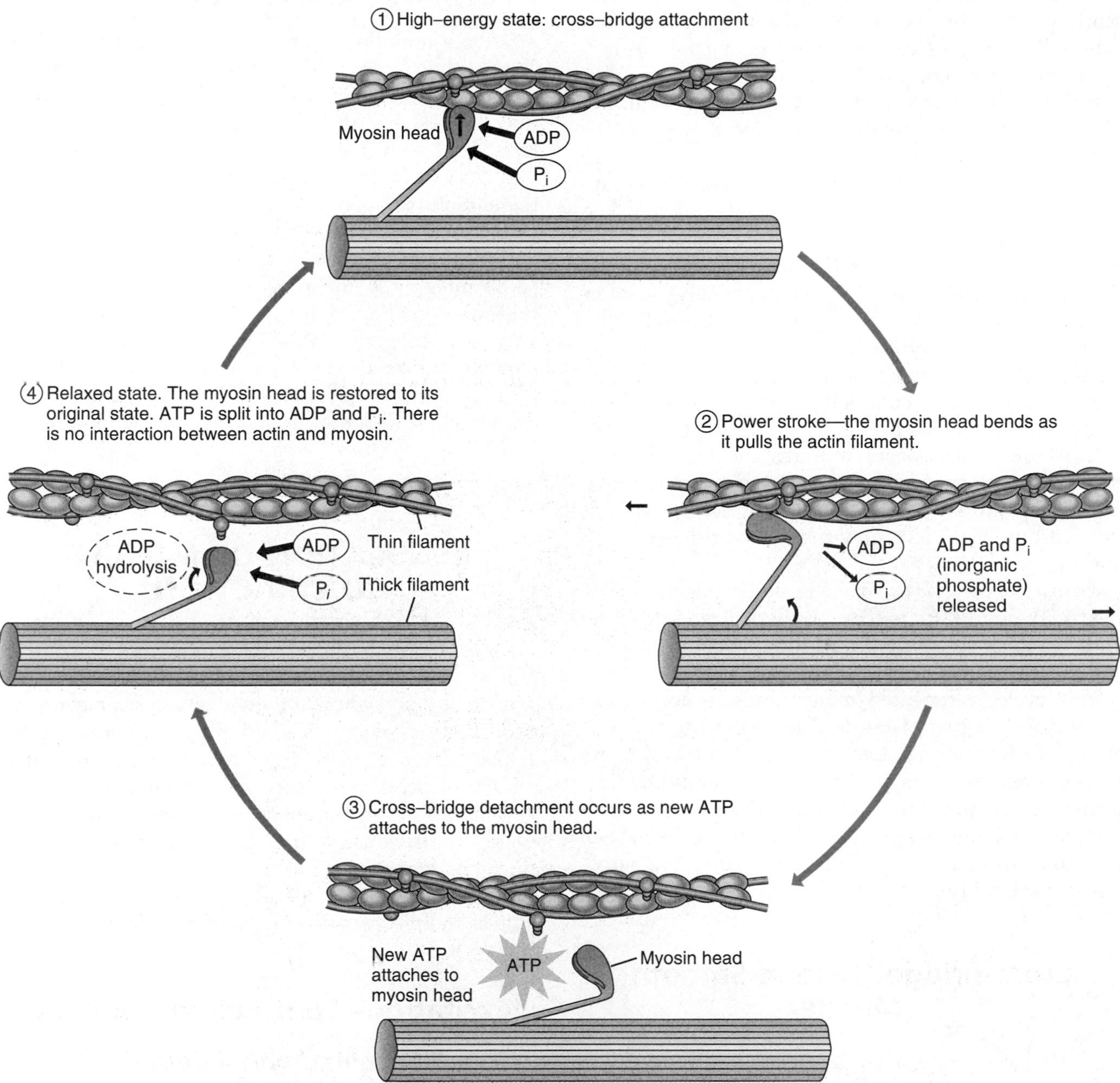

FIGURE 5–10

Cross-bridge cycle in skeletal and cardiac muscle. (1) In the high-energy state, adenosine diphosphate (ADP) and inorganic phosphate (P_i) are bound to a cleft in the myosin head. Affinity of myosin for actin is high, and when calcium binds to troponin, exposing binding sites on actin, cross-bridge attachment occurs. (2) Actin–myosin binding induces release of ADP and P_i from the cleft, and the resulting bending of the myosin head (power stroke) pulls actin over myosin, toward the center of the sarcomere. (3) Binding of adenosine triphosphate (ATP) to the cleft in the myosin head induces a conformational change that detaches myosin from actin. (4) The resting (relaxed) state is restored when ATP is hydrolized to ADP and P_i.

nin causes the binding sites on actin to be covered by tropomyosin. During the previous contraction, myosin ATPase had cleaved ATP to ADP and inorganic phosphate (P_i), both of which remain bound within a cleft in the myosin head. Myosin has high affinity for actin in this configuration, known as the *high-energy state.*

Cross-bridge formation (actin–myosin binding) occurs as a result of a series of events that uncover binding sites on actin. An action potential first causes the entry of calcium into the cytosol, primarily from the sarcoplasmic reticulum but also from the ECF. Ca^{2+} binds to the TN-C subunit of troponin, causing a conformational change that shifts the position of tropomyosin, uncovering binding sites on actin. Due to its high affinity, myosin then rapidly binds to actin.

The *power stroke* occurs when ADP and P_i are released from the cleft on actin–myosin binding, and the myosin head changes to its low-energy conformation. In this state, the myosin head bends in a lever-like action, generating force that pulls the attached actin over the myosin toward the center of the sarcomere, thus contracting the muscle cell. Free energy is released as heat during this stage.

Cross-bridge detachment requires the binding of a new ATP molecule to the myosin head, again inducing conformational change. In this state, myosin has low affinity for actin, and the cross-bridge dissociates.

Return to the relaxed state is accomplished when the ATP bound to myosin is hydrolyzed to ADP and P_i, which remain bound to the myosin head and restore its original conformation.

This cycle is repeated many times to accomplish the desired degree of tension development or shortening of the muscle. Each myosin cross-bridge releases, then attaches at another actin-binding site farther down the thin filament, and so on. Contraction ends when calcium is extruded from the cytosol by active transport into the ECF or into the sarcoplasmic reticulum.

Cross-Bridge Cycle in Smooth Muscle

The precise nature of the cross-bridge cycle in smooth muscle is not well understood and may vary among smooth muscle types. Recall that smooth muscle has tropomyosin but no troponin. The cycle is believed to involve the following steps:

1. Calcium entering the cytoplasm of the smooth muscle cell binds to calmodulin.
2. The calmodulin–Ca^{2+} complex activates MLCK.
3. The MLCK enzyme phosphorylates the myosin head, exposing a binding site for actin. ATP is hydrolyzed in the process, donating the phosphate.
4. Actin and myosin bind, activating myosin ATPase and generating the power stroke.
5. The cross-bridge is dissociated by the action of the enzyme myosin phosphatase, which dephosphorylates the myosin head.

Smooth muscle is unique in its ability to form slow-cycling cross-bridges, known as **latch-bridges**, which allow smooth muscle to maintain tension for long periods with little expenditure of energy. Latch-bridge formation is also calcium-dependent but does not involve increased phosphorylation. Regulation of this phenomenon is still poorly understood. Actin-associated proteins, such as caldesmon and calponin, may be involved but are not believed to be integral to the process.[6] At high Ca^{2+} levels, caldesmon is bound by the calmodulin–Ca^{2+} complex and is inactive. When calcium levels are intermediate, however, caldesmon is inserted between actin and myosin at cross-bridges, preventing them from cycling and thereby halting further hydrolysis of ATP.

REGULATION OF MUSCLE CONTRACTION

As is apparent from discussion of muscle contraction at the molecular level, the final common pathway in its regulation involves changes in cytoplasmic calcium levels. This, in turn, depends on the availability of calcium from extracellular and intracellular sources, the electrical or chemical stimuli that initiate calcium transport, and the availability of energy to drive active transport and cross-bridge cycling. A variety of mechanisms may convert the electrical or chemical energy of an extracellular stimulus to the mechanical energy of muscle contraction.

Excitation–Contraction Coupling

Electromechanical Coupling

Muscle contraction that occurs in response to an electrical stimulus (i.e., an action potential) is known as **electromechanical coupling**.

Skeletal Muscle. In skeletal muscle, the action potential from a motor nerve is propagated across the sarcolemma and down the T tubules. As the impulse passes near the terminal cisternae of the sarcoplasmic reticulum, specialized Ca^{2+} channel proteins in the T-tubule membrane sense the change in membrane voltage and change their conformation. This action opens a second type of gated calcium channel in the sarcoplasmic reticulum, allowing calcium to enter the cytosol from intracellular stores.[7, 8]

The rate of electrical stimulation of skeletal muscle fibers is important in determining the degree of force generated. If the nerve that delivers the electrical stimulus to a skeletal muscle fiber is "firing" (generating action potentials) at a slow rate, each action potential results in a single brief contraction, or twitch, of the muscle. If the frequency of action potentials is high, however, the cytoplasmic calcium level does not return to baseline between twitches but instead continues to rise. Some of the filament overlap generated with previous twitches is retained, and subsequent calcium influx allows additional shortening of the muscle fiber. This process, known as *summation,* is illustrated in Figure 5–11. At high stimulation frequencies, a smooth, continuous (tetanic) contraction is induced. Contraction therefore may last much longer than the time course of a single action potential. **Tetanus** (or tetany) is a continuous contractile state in which maximal force is generated in skeletal muscle.

Smooth Muscle. Smooth muscle is also capable of tetanic contraction, but in many cases action potentials are spontaneously generated by pacemaker cells rather than delivered by nerves. Depolarization of the smooth muscle sarcolemma opens numerous voltage-gated calcium channels, which permit the entry of ECF calcium and support sustained contraction. Indeed, the depolarization stage of the action potential in smooth muscle is entirely due to calcium entry (see Chapter 4).

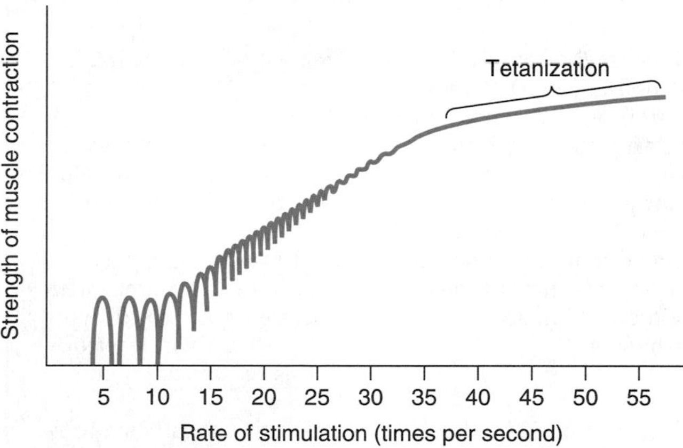

FIGURE 5–11

Summation and tetanus. In skeletal and smooth muscle, lack of plateau in the action potential permits rapid neural stimulation. Under these conditions, cytosolic calcium levels do not return to baseline between contractions but instead continue to rise with each stimulus. The frequency and force of the contraction increase until a state of continuous, forceful contraction (tetanus or tetany) is induced. (Redrawn from Guyton, A.C. [1992]. *Human Physiology and Mechanisms of Disease.* (5th ed.). Philadelphia: W.B. Saunders. [p. 64].)

As has been discussed, smooth muscle has no T tubules and little sarcoplasmic reticulum. Intracellular calcium storage is limited to small vesicles near the sarcolemma. Release of calcium from this pool apparently depends not on a change in membrane potential but rather on activation of a complex second messenger system.

Cardiac Muscle. Cardiac plasma membranes also have voltage-gated calcium channels that open during depolarization. Extracellular calcium enters the cytoplasm, triggering release of calcium from intracellular stores.[8–10] Tetanic contraction does not occur in the heart, owing to the plateau phase of the action potential (see Chapter 4). In cardiac tissue, the sarcomere returns to its original length before the action potential is completed, making summation impossible and preventing sustained contraction, which would adversely affect filling of the ventricles.

Chemomechanical Coupling

Contraction of muscle is also modulated by the actions of various signaling molecules (e.g., cytokines, hormones, neurotransmitters, or drugs) in a process known as **chemomechanical coupling**. These agents ultimately affect calcium levels in the cytosol by blocking voltage-gated calcium channels, by inhibiting membrane pumps that extrude calcium from the cell, or by influencing the release or reuptake of calcium from the sarcoplasmic reticulum by second messenger systems. Enzyme activity and affinity of binding sites on actin and myosin may also be altered. For example, many of the effects of catecholamines seen during the stress response occur as a result of the binding of epinephrine or norepinephrine to receptors on smooth muscle or cardiac muscle. Dilation of bronchial smooth muscle, selective constriction of smooth muscle of arterioles, and increased force of contraction of the heart are examples of such effects (see Chapter 22).

In skeletal muscle, the neurotransmitter acetylcholine (ACh) is released at the connecting point between the motor nerve serving the muscle fiber and the fiber itself, thus serving an important coupling function. (This process of nerve signal transmission at the **neuromuscular junction** is critical to skeletal muscle function and is detailed in Chapter 22.) Many drugs affect muscle contraction either as a desired therapeutic effect (as with muscle relaxant agents) or as toxic or undesirable side effects (as with **dyskinesias** or **tremors**—repetitive movements seen with therapy of many neuropsychiatric disorders). Pharmacologic alteration of muscle contraction is discussed further in Chapter 22. Table 5–2 summarizes effects of selected drugs that influence muscle contraction.

Energy Metabolism in Muscle

Although each muscle type has preferred fuels during resting and active states, all types can metabolize multiple substrates for energy.

Skeletal Muscle

Active skeletal muscle consumes significant amounts of energy in cross-bridge cycling; in operation of the Na^+-K^+-ATPase pumps which maintain ionic gradients for action potential generation; and in pumping calcium out of the cell and into the sarcoplasmic reticulum. Muscle cells store only enough ATP to support a few seconds of activity, however. Muscle also stores energy in the form of creatine phosphate, which can donate its phosphate to ADP, forming ATP and creatine (see Chapter 3). When muscle is at rest, ATP levels rise, driving this reaction in reverse and generating more creatine phosphate. Muscle glycogen also constitutes a short-term energy reserve. Sustained muscle activity depends on the ability of muscle cells to generate ATP by aerobic or anaerobic metabolism of glucose and other nutrient substrates (see Chapter 35).

Skeletal muscle fibers are categorized into three subtypes with respect to energy metabolism: *slow oxidative* (type I slow-twitch fibers), *fast oxidative* (type IIA fast-twitch fibers), and *fast glycolytic* (type IIB fast-twitch fibers). The speed of contraction, or twitch, depends on the degree of myosin ATPase activity in the cell. The more rapidly ATP is cleaved to ADP and P_i, the faster is the cycling of cross-bridges. The functional significance of the different classes of skeletal muscle is discussed in detail in Chapter 35.

Smooth Muscle

Smooth muscle uses ATP for the same purposes as does skeletal muscle. Because of its lower ATP consumption with latch-bridge formation, however, the metabolic demands of this muscle type are relatively low. Smooth muscle employs primarily oxidative phosphorylation to supply energy for contraction, but aerobic glycolysis also occurs in smooth muscle, mainly during the resting state.

Cardiac Muscle

Cardiac muscle relies almost exclusively on aerobic metabolism and has more mitochondria per unit

TABLE 5–2
EFFECTS OF SELECTED DRUGS ON MUSCLE CONTRACTION

Drug	Effect	Mechanism	Clinical Use
Skeletal Muscle			
Pyridostigmine (Mestinon)	Increased contraction	Inhibits breakdown of acetylcholine (ACh) at the neuromuscular junction	Treatment of myasthenia gravis
Succinylcholine (Anectine)	Decreased contraction	Binds and blocks ACh receptors at the neuromuscular junction	Used during anesthesia to facilitate intubation and controlled respiration
Smooth Muscle			
Metoclopramide (Reglan)	Increased contraction	Inhibits dopamine, a neurotransmitter that inhibits ACh effects in some pathways	Used to stimulate gastric motility in patients with slowed gastric emptying due to diabetic gastroparesis or cancer chemotherapy
Atropine	Decreased contraction	Inhibits ACh-mediated contraction	Used with anesthesia to reduce respiratory secretion
Cardiac Muscle			
Digoxin (Lanoxin)	Increased contraction	Inhibits Na^+-K^+-ATPase and promotes intracellular Ca^{2+} accumulation	Treatment of congestive heart failure
Propranolol (Inderal)	Decreased contraction	Blocks β-adrenergic receptors, decreasing sympathetic nervous system–mediated contraction	Treatment of hypertension and angina pectoris

volume than does skeletal muscle. The heart prefers fatty acids as metabolic fuel (see Chapter 16).

MECHANISMS OF ABNORMAL MUSCLE CONTRACTION

Muscle contraction may be altered by abnormality in conduction of nerve impulses to muscle, by alteration in chemical signals, by abnormal calcium gradients or transport, or by impaired energy metabolism.

Alteration in Conduction

Skeletal Muscle

A skeletal muscle fiber will not contract unless stimulated by an action potential from a motor nerve. Severing of the motor nerve prevents the muscle from contracting, and the muscle becomes atonic (without tone) and immobile. *Muscle tone* is the slight resistance to a deforming force felt on palpation of healthy muscle; it results from the elastic recoil of connectin. Atonic muscle is flaccid (floppy) and soon exhibits **atrophy**, or appears wasted, owing to a decrease in the size of the myofibrils with loss of glycogen stores.

Impaired communication between the brain and the spinal cord, such as may occur in spinal cord injury, brain tumor, or stroke, inevitably disturbs electrical stimulation of skeletal muscle. Clinical manifestations can vary from **paresis** (weakness) or **paralysis** to **spasticity** (uncontrollable contraction). Specific effects of such conditions depend on multiple factors, including the location and extent of the lesion. Neuromuscular diseases, such as myasthenia gravis, multiple sclerosis, and amyotrophic lateral sclerosis, affect muscle function secondarily to loss of nerve function (see Chapters 21 and 22). Primary diseases of muscle, such as muscular dystrophy, are discussed in Chapter 35.

Smooth Muscle

In smooth muscle tubes, such as the intestine or the ureter, presence of an obstruction (such as impacted feces in the bowel or a stone in the ureter) triggers neural reflexes that result in increased frequency of action potentials. This causes contractions of high force and frequency, which are intended to assist in propelling the obstruction outward but which are at the same time very painful owing to their intensity. The crampy pain caused by this mechanism is known as *colic.*

Nerve impulses to smooth muscle are important, although not essential, in coordination of contraction. Loss of neural stimulation results in a decrease in the normal rhythmic contractions (**peristalsis**) that propel contents within these organs, and manifestations such as constipation or stagnation of urine may occur. Similarly, interruption of neural stimulation to smooth muscle in some blood vessels causes the vessels to dilate. As discussed in Chapter 15, an increase in vessel diameter decreases resistance to blood flow and causes blood pressure to fall. Conversely, a sudden increase in autonomic stimulation of arterioles may cause a dangerous elevation in blood pressure. This condition, autonomic hyperreflexia, may occur as a complication of spinal cord injury (see Chapter 22).

Cardiac Muscle

Contraction of cardiac muscle (myocardial) cells also follows stimulation by action potentials; thus, cardiac dysrhythmias inevitably result in mechanical dysfunction as well. As discussed in Chapter 16, abnormal cardiac rhythms can cause the heart to fail as a pump, resulting in impaired tissue perfusion, shock, and possibly cardiac arrest. Increased rate and force of cardiac contraction may be subjectively noted by the patient as **palpitations**, whereas a decrease may cause lightheadedness or **syncope** (fainting).

Alteration in Chemical Signaling

Chemical signaling of muscle contraction may be altered by disease or by drugs that affect synthesis, release, receptor binding, signal transduction, or inactivation of signaling molecules.

Skeletal Muscle

Skeletal muscle contraction is dependent on action potentials from motor neurons, which release the neurotransmitter ACh at the neuromuscular junction (see Chapter 22). ACh binds to ligand-gated sodium channels on the muscle fiber, and opening of these channels permits sodium influx, depolarizing the sarcolemma and T-tubule system and releasing calcium ions from the sarcoplasmic reticulum. The enzyme acetylcholinesterase (AChE), also located at the junction, normally inactivates ACh. Alteration of the amount of ACh available at the synapse may result from drug therapy with agonists or antagonists of the ACh receptor (cholinergic or anticholinergic agents) or with agents affecting the AChE enzyme, or from disease of the neuromuscular junction that affects the ACh receptor, AChE enzyme, or synthesis of the signaling molecule (see Chapter 22).

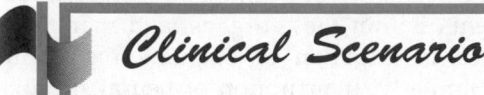

M.M., a 24-year-old construction worker, has myasthenia gravis, a disorder in which some ACh receptors on skeletal muscle cells are blocked or destroyed by an autoimmune process. His symptoms include weakness of upper body and facial muscles, which progressively worsens throughout the day. He reports that his speech becomes slurred and he has trouble keeping his eyes open. His supervisor once confronted him about being "on drugs." M.M. is being treated with edrophonium (Tensilon), a drug that inhibits the activity of AChE.

1. How might M.M.'s sleepy appearance and slurred speech be explained in terms of altered muscle contraction?
2. What is the rationale for M.M.'s drug therapy? What side effects might be anticipated?

Smooth Muscle

Smooth muscle has receptors for numerous hormones, neurotransmitters, cytokines, lipid mediators, and other signaling molecules. The effect of the catecholamines on vascular smooth muscle has been discussed. A number of mediators released by vascular endothelial cells are important in regulation of vessel caliber; and the synthesis, release, and binding of these agents may be altered by disease or pharmacotherapy (see Chapter 15). The smooth muscle of the gastrointestinal tract is responsive to catecholamine hormones as well as to several pancreatic hormones and peptides produced by cells of the stomach and intestine. The effects of alteration of chemical signaling of smooth muscle are complex because the same mediator may cause either contraction or relaxation, depending on the nature of the receptor and the signal transduction system (see Chapter 2). Examples of altered intestinal motility include diarrhea, constipation, and bowel obstruction, discussed in Chapter 24.

Cardiac Muscle

Cardiac muscle also has receptors for a variety of signaling molecules, including the catecholamines and ACh. Contractile force may be altered primarily through manipulation of intracellular calcium levels or may be altered secondary to effects on heart rate, chamber volume, or muscle stretch. Drugs that increase the force of cardiac contraction are known as *positive inotropic agents;* those that decrease contraction are known as *negative inotropic agents* (see Chapter 16).

Alteration in Calcium Gradients or Transport

Calcium Homeostasis

Most calcium in the body is in crystalline form in bones and teeth, whereas only 1% circulates in body fluids. Of the circulating calcium, about half is bound to serum proteins such as albumin, and half is present in ionized form. The ionized fraction is important in muscle contraction. Calcium homeostasis is complex, involving hormonal mechanisms that regulate exchange between the skeletal reserves and the blood, as well as absorption of dietary calcium. These mechanisms, along with causes and consequences of imbalances, are detailed in Chapters 9 and 34.

The fraction of circulating calcium that is ionized varies, depending on the amount of albumin present in the serum and the hydrogen ion concentration. When albumin levels are low, less calcium can be bound, so more exists in ionized form. H^+ displaces calcium from albumin; therefore, in conditions in which H^+ is elevated (i.e., acidosis), more calcium is present in the ionized form. The opposite is true when hydrogen ion concentration is low (i.e., alkalosis).

Hypocalcemia

Hypocalcemia is a decreased concentration of ionized calcium in the blood. This disorder is often seen in children and the elderly due to dietary deficiency. Acute hypocalcemia may be associated with renal failure, metabolic alkalosis, or certain drug therapies that interfere with calcium homeostasis.

Skeletal Muscle. Because low ECF calcium results in lower intracellular calcium, muscle contraction would be expected to decrease owing to lack of calcium to bind to TN-C and initiate the molecular mechanism. In skeletal muscle, however, the threshold-lowering (depolarizing) effect of low ECF Ca^{2+} overrides the effect of lack of calcium on the molecular mechanism (see Chapter 4). The increased frequency of action potentials results in summation and potentially tetany, manifested as severe muscle spasms and possibly seizures. Spasm of laryngeal muscles may close the airway, constituting a medical emergency.

Smooth Muscle. Smooth muscle, lacking sarcoplasmic reticulum for internal storage of Ca^{2+}, depends on influx of ECF calcium for both depolarization and initiation of the cross-bridge cycle. Although hypocalcemia would be expected to manifest consistently as decreased contraction, this is not always the case. Regulation of smooth-muscle contraction is complex, influenced not only by calcium currents but also by numerous local and hormonal mediators and by neural stimulation. In severe hypocalcemia, *increased* contraction of gastrointestinal smooth muscle is manifested because of the threshold-lowering effect. Hyperactive bowel sounds and crampy abdominal pain may occur. *Decreased* contraction is usually seen in vascular smooth muscle, however, for reasons related to endothelial regulation (see Chapter 15). Dietary calcium deficiency has been linked to increased vascular resistance and hypertension in some studies,[11] and use of calcium-channel blocking drugs to treat hypertension results in relaxation of vascular smooth muscle.[12]

Cardiac Muscle. In cardiac muscle, which is incapable of tetanic contraction, the primary manifestation of hypocalcemia is due to decreased influx of ECF calcium, and lack of this triggering current results in release of less Ca^{2+} from sarcoplasmic reticulum stores. The force of cardiac contraction is decreased, potentially contributing to heart failure (see Chapter 16).

Hypercalcemia

Hypercalcemia may be caused by hyperparathyroidism or by bone tumors in which skeletal calcium is liberated into the blood. Clinical manifestations in these situations are the opposite of those seen with hypocalcemia. Elevated ECF Ca^{2+} causes an increase in inward Ca^{2+} flux, which, in cardiac muscle, triggers more Ca^{2+} release from the sarcoplasmic reticulum. Increased force of cardiac contraction results. In skeletal and smooth muscle, however, muscle contraction is weak despite calcium influx because the rise in membrane threshold results in a decrease in the frequency of stimulation by action potentials.

Alteration in Energy Metabolism

Maintenance of calcium gradients is dependent on active transport; thus, any factor that impairs energy metabolism also potentially affects calcium transport, with secondary effects on muscle contraction. Cross-bridge formation and maintenance of gradients for action potentials also consume ATP. As in other tissues, fatigue occurs in muscles when energy consumption exceeds the rate of energy production (see Chapter 3).

When death occurs and no energy is available to the muscle cell, the cross-bridge cycle is arrested after the power stroke. Recall that ATP must bind in order for actin and myosin to dissociate. In the absence of ATP, the cross-bridge persists, and muscle remains contracted. This state of **rigor mortis** is seen for several hours after death, until muscle proteins begin to degenerate.

CLINICAL CONSEQUENCES OF ALTERATION IN MUSCLE CONTRACTION

Because all organ systems contain muscle tissue, at least in their vascular beds, impairment of muscle contraction results in a wide variety of clinical manifestations, many of which have been discussed in this chapter. Table 5–3 summarizes system-specific effects of altered muscle contraction.

In muscle contraction, as in other functions of the human system, interdependence of subsystem functions is apparent. The neurologic and endocrine systems provide electrical and chemical stimuli for con-

TABLE 5–3
CLINICAL MANIFESTATIONS OF ALTERED MUSCLE CONTRACTION

System	Increased Contraction	Decreased Contraction
Cardiac	Palpitations	Cardiac failure
Circulatory	Cool skin; pallor and cyanosis	Warm skin, flushing
Respiratory	Wheezing, dyspnea, hiccoughs	Bronchodilation, hypoventilation
Renal and Urinary	Urinary colic	Urinary stasis
Gastrointestinal	Diarrhea, cramping	Constipation, paralytic ileus
Reproductive	Dysmenorrhea	Uterine atony
Musculoskeletal	Muscle spasms	Paresis or paralysis

traction, whereas the respiratory system provides the oxygen necessary for efficient energy production. The gastrointestinal system delivers nutrients for energy production and for the synthesis of muscle tissue. The cardiovascular system transports oxygen and nutrients to muscle tissue and removes waste products of metabolism.

Disorders that impair function of these and other organ systems adversely affect muscle contraction, which may further impair function of the organ systems. Thus, the potential exists for development of positive feedback loops and continuing decline of function, mandating clinical interventions. Many of the systems disorders discussed in Part Two have impairment of muscle contraction as a pathophysiologic basis.

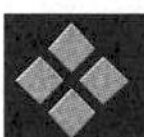

Summary of Key Points

- Actin and myosin are the major contractile proteins in all muscle types, although smooth muscle contains much less myosin. The most important regulatory proteins in skeletal and cardiac muscle are tropomyosin and troponin. Calmodulin is an important calcium-binding protein in smooth muscle.
- Skeletal and cardiac muscle are striated owing to the regular arrangement of thin and thick filaments within the sarcomere. Smooth muscle cells are much smaller and are unstriated owing to their irregular arrangement of actin anchored to dense bodies. Skeletal and cardiac muscle have extensive sarcoplasmic reticulum and T-tubule systems to facilitate regulation of intracellular calcium levels. In smooth muscle, the sarcoplasmic reticulum is less well developed, and there are no T tubules.
- According to the sliding filament theory, muscle contraction occurs as a result of (1) calcium-mediated cross-bridge formation (actin–myosin binding), (2) bending of the myosin head owing to the dissociation of ADP and P_i that occurs with binding, pulling actin centrally over myosin and shortening the sarcomere, (3) cross-bridge detachment as an ATP molecule binds to the myosin head, and (4) return to the relaxed state when ATP is cleaved to ADP and P_i.
- In striated muscle, actin–myosin interaction is regulated by the binding of calcium to troponin, which induces tropomyosin to uncover actin-binding sites. In smooth muscle, calmodulin is the calcium-binding protein. Mechanisms of regulation of smooth muscle contraction are complex and poorly understood.
- Electromechanical coupling is the transduction of an action potential to mechanical activity (muscle contraction) by opening of voltage-gated calcium channels. In chemomechanical coupling, muscle contraction is initiated (in smooth or cardiac muscle) or modulated (in all muscle types) by cytokines, hormones, neurotransmitters, or drugs through various receptor-mediated processes.
- All muscle types may employ both oxidative and anaerobic energy metabolism pathways. The dominant pathway in skeletal muscle depends on fiber type, with glucose preferred as the metabolic fuel. Smooth-muscle contraction normally uses much less energy owing to smooth muscle's ability to form slow-cycling latch-bridges. Oxidative metabolism dominates within cardiac muscle, with fatty acids preferred as the energy fuel.
- The general mechanisms that can result in abnormal muscle contraction are altered conduction, alteration in chemical signaling, abnormal calcium gradients or transport, and alteration in energy metabolism.
- Clinical manifestations of increased muscle contraction include palpitations, wheezing, urinary colic, diarrhea, dysmenorrhea, and muscle spasms. Manifestations of decreased muscle contraction include cardiac failure, hypoventilation, urinary stasis, constipation, uterine atony, and paresis or paralysis.

REFERENCES

1. Ebashi, S. (1991). Excitation-contraction coupling and the mechanism of muscle contraction. *Annual Review of Physiology* 53(1991), 1–16.
2. Lodish, H., Baltimore, D., Berk, A., *et al.* (1995). *Molecular Cell Biology*. (3rd ed.). New York: Scientific American Books.
3. Somlyo, A.P., and Somlyo, A.V. (1994). Signal transduction and regulation in smooth muscle. *Nature* 372(6503), 231–236.
4. Huxley, H.E., and Hanson, J. (1954). Changes in the cross-striations of muscle during contraction and stretch and their structural interpretation. *Nature* 173(4412), 973–976.
5. Huxley, A.F., and Niedergerke, R. (1954). Interference microscopy of living muscle fibres. *Nature* 173(4412), 971–973.
6. Murphy, R.A. (1994). What is special about smooth muscle? The significance of covalent crossbridge regulation. *FASEB Journal* 8(3), 311–318.
7. Ashcroft, F.M. (1991). Ca^{++} channels and excitation-contraction coupling. *Current Opinion in Cell Biology* 3(4), 671–675.
8. Catterall, W.A. (1991). Excitation-contraction coupling in vertebrate skeletal muscle: A tale of two calcium channels. *Cell* 64(5), 871–874.

9. Stern, M.D., and Lakatta, E.G. (1992). Excitation-contraction coupling in the heart: The state of the question. *FASEB Journal* 6(12), 3092–3100.
10. Morgan, J.P., Perreault, C.L., and Morgan, K.G. (1991). The cellular basis of contraction and relaxation in cardiac and vascular smooth muscle. *American Heart Journal* 121(3 Pt. 1), 961–968.
11. Allender, P.S., Cutler, J.A., Follmann, D., *et al.* (1996). Dietary calcium and blood pressure: A meta-analysis of randomized clinical trials. *Annals of Internal Medicine* 124(9), 825–831.
12. Nayler, W.G. (1993). Pharmacological aspects of calcium antagonism: Short term and long term benefits. *Drugs* 46(suppl. 2), 40–47.

SELECTED BIBLIOGRAPHY

Bagshaw, C.R. (1993). *Muscle Contraction*. (2nd ed.). London: Chapman and Hall.

Cannell, M.B., Cheng, H., and Lederer, W.J. (1995). The control of calcium release in heart muscle. *Science* 268, 1045–1049.

D'Angelo, G., and Meininger, G.A. (1994). Transduction mechanisms involved in the regulation of myogenic activity. *Hypertension* 23(6 Pt. 2), 1096–1105.

Farah, C.S., and Beinach, F.C. (1995). The troponin complex and regulation of muscle contraction. *FASEB Journal* 9, 755–767.

Fitts, R.H. (1994). Cellular mechanisms of muscle fatigue. *Physiology Reviews* 74(1), 49–94.

Higuchi, H., and Goldman, Y.E. (1995). Sliding distance per ATP molecule hydrolized by myosin heads during isotonic shortening of skinned muscle fibers. *Biophysical Journal* 69, 1491–1507.

Holmes, K.C. (1995). The actomyosin interaction and its control by tropomyosin. *Biophysical Journal* 68, 2s–7s.

Huxley, H. (1995). The working stroke of myosin crossbridges. *Biophysical Journal* 68, 55s–58s.

Irving, M., Allen, T.S., Sabido-David, C., *et al.* (1995). Tilting of the light-chain region of myosin during step length changes and active force generation in skeletal muscle. *Nature* 375, 688–691.

Jontes, J.J. (1995). Theories of muscle contraction. *Journal of Structural Biology* 115, 119–143.

Kahn, A.M., and Song, T. (1995). Insulin inhibits dog vascular smooth muscle contraction and lowers Ca^{++}_i by inhibiting Ca^{++} influx. *Journal of Nutrition* 125, 1732S–1737S.

Labeit, S., and Kolmerer, B. (1995). Titins: Giant proteins in charge of muscle ultrastructure and elasticity. *Science* 270, 293–296.

Landesberg, A., and Sideman, S. (1994). Mechanical regulation of cardiac muscle by coupling calcium kinetics with cross-bridge cycling: A dynamic model. *Nature* 372(6503), 321–236.

Lowey, S., and Trybus, K.M. (1995). Role of skeletal and smooth muscle myosin light chains. *Biophysical Journal* 68, 120s–127s.

Mombouli, J-V., and Vanhoutte, P.M. (1995). Kinins and endothelial control of vascular smooth muscle. *Annual Review of Pharmacology and Toxicology* 35, 679–705.

Otterson, M.F., and Sarr, M.G. (1993). Normal physiology of small intestinal motility. *Surgical Clinics of North American* 73(6), 1173–1192.

Vale, R.D. (1994). Getting a grip on myosin. *Cell* 78, 733–737.

VanBuren, P., Waller, G.S., Harris, D.E., *et al.* (1994). The essential light chain is required for full force production by skeletal muscle myosin. *Proceedings of the National Academy of Sciences, U.S.A.* 91, 12403–12407.

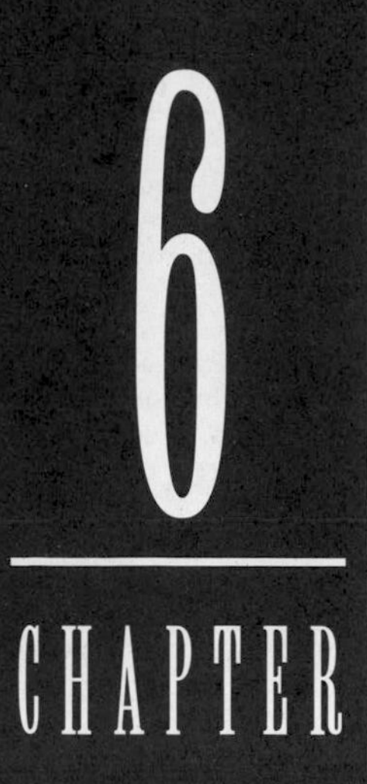

Cellular Development: Genetic Regulation, Embryology, and Aging

LEARNING OBJECTIVES

1. Identify the four cellular developmental processes.
2. Identify the components of the genetic material of the cell.
3. Comprehend the cellular processes of transcription and translation.
4. Describe the phases of the cell cycle and the regulatory processes that determine phase progression.
5. Differentiate among the functions of the four tissue types.
6. Differentiate between necrosis and apoptosis with respect to triggering events, regulation, and process.
7. Briefly describe the major events that occur during the preembryonic, embryonic, and fetal periods of prenatal development.
8. Explain why the first trimester is the most critical period in morphogenesis.
9. Differentiate between primary and secondary aging.
10. Briefly describe the major theories of aging.
11. Identify the typical systemic manifestations of aging.
12. Appreciate the clinical importance of recent major advances in medical genetics.

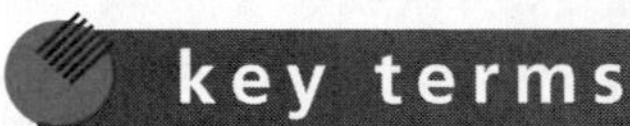

angiogenesis
apoptosis
autosome
carcinogen
cell cycle
chromosome
cleavage
conceptus
congenital
deoxyribonucleic acid (DNA)
differentiation
dysmorphogenesis
ectoderm
embryo
embryonic period
endoderm
fetal period
fetus
gamete
gene
gene therapy
meiosis
mesoderm
mitosis
morphogenesis
mutagen
necrosis
neural tube
neuroectoderm
post-transcriptional processing
post-translational processing
preembryonic period
primary aging
recombinant DNA
ribonucleic acid (RNA)
secondary aging
sex chromosome
telomerase
telomere
teratogen
transcription
transcription factor
translation
zygote

Human development is most broadly defined as the sum of all physiologic and psychological changes occurring from the time of conception until the time of death. Developmental diseases and defects have traditionally been associated with infants and children and have been considered relatively uncommon. Recent advances in molecular genetics have shed new light on this subject. It is now clear that disruption of cellular development underlies not only **congenital** conditions, such as Down syndrome and fetal alcohol syndrome, but also many common diseases that manifest in adults, such as cancer, diabetes mellitus, and coronary heart disease.

Developmental processes at the cellular level include cell division or reproduction, growth, **differentiation**, and programmed cell death (**apoptosis**). These processes are genetically regulated but subject to environmental factors. Environmental agents that may adversely affect cellular development are classified as **mutagens** if they alter cellular genetic material, as **teratogens** if they alter tissues of the developing **embryo** or **fetus**, or as **carcinogens** if they initiate transformation of normally developing cells into cancer cells. Cellular aging is also a developmental process, and the goal of gerontology is the differentiation of normal developmental changes in cell structure and function from changes attributable to disease. The study of cellular development thus integrates the sciences of genetics, embryology, gerontology, and oncology (the study of cancer) and is an important foundation for the study of disease.

In this chapter, the genetic regulation of cellular processes, embryologic development, and aging is discussed. Chapter 7 focuses on abnormal cellular development, specifically congenital defects and neoplasia.

GENETIC REGULATION OF CELLULAR DEVELOPMENT

Genetic Material of the Cell

Nucleic Acids

The "blueprint" for development of the cell is found in its genetic material, the nucleic acids **deoxyribonucleic acid (DNA)** and **ribonucleic acid (RNA)**. DNA is found primarily in the nucleus of the cell, although mitochondria contain DNA as well. Mitochondrial DNA (mtDNA) functions in the regulation of oxidative phosphorylation, discussed in Chapter 3. As illustrated in Figure 6–1, nuclear DNA consists of two linear strands of nucleic acids coiled together in a double helix, which resembles a twisted ladder.

Nucleic acids consist of nucleotide subunits, each of which is composed of a nitrogenous purine or pyrimidine base, a five-carbon sugar (deoxyribose), and a phosphate (P). Nucleotides are linked linearly by phosphodiester bonds, which covalently link the hydroxyl (OH) group in the 3′ position of one deoxyribose to a phosphate in the 5′ position on an

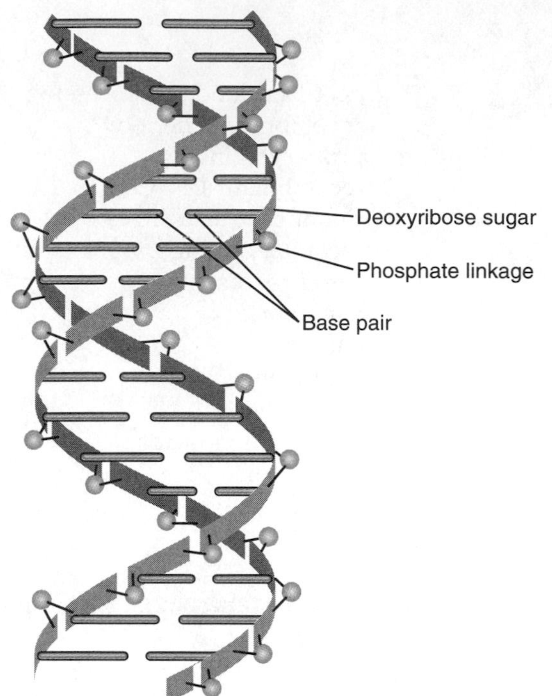

FIGURE 6–1

Structure of DNA. DNA consists of two strands of nucleotides, units composed of deoxyribose, a purine or pyrimidine base, and a phosphate. Nucleotides are linked linearly by phosphodiesterase bonds. Hydrogen bonds between complementary base pairs link the two strands, which are coiled in a double helix.

adjacent deoxyribose. The two DNA strands are joined to each other by hydrogen bonds between complementary bases, forming the "rungs" of the DNA ladder.[1]

DNA contains four different bases: adenine (A), thymine (T), guanine (G), and cytosine (C). Adenine always bonds with thymine, and guanine always bonds with cytosine, permitting one strand to serve as a pattern, or *template*, for the other, for purposes of transcription of the code, DNA repair, or DNA replication before cell division. The two DNA strands are *antiparallel;* that is, the 5′ end of one strand is linked to the 3′ end of the other, and the sugar portion of one strand lies upward, whereas that of the complementary nucleotide lies downward. By convention, base sequences are written in the 5′ to 3′ direction.

RNA differs from DNA in its single-stranded structure, which remains linear in one type (messenger RNA, or mRNA) and is looped back on itself in the two other types, ribosomal RNA (rRNA) and transfer RNA (tRNA). In addition, RNA contains ribose instead of deoxyribose and the base uracil (U), which bonds with adenine, instead of thymine. The function of mRNA is to *transcribe* the genetic code from DNA in the nucleus, then to carry the code into the cytoplasm. There, tRNA and rRNA *translate* the code into proteins. The processes of **transcrip-**

TABLE 6–1
THE GENETIC CODE

Amino Acid	DNA Triplets	RNA Codons
Alanine	CGA CGG CGT CGC	GCU GCC GCA GCG
Arginine	GCA GCG GCT GCC TCC TCT	CGU CGC CGA CGG AGA AGG
Asparagine	TTA TTG	AAU AAC
Aspartic acid	CTA CTG	GAU GAC
Cysteine	ACA ACG	UGU UGC
Glutamic acid	CTT CTC	GAA GAG
Glutamine	GTT GTC	CAA CAG
Glycine	CCA CCG CCT CCC	GGU GGC GGA GGG
Histidine	GTA GTG	CAU CAC
Isoleucine	TAA TAG TAT	AUU AUC AUA
Leucine	AAT AAC GAA GAG GAT GAC	UUA UUG CUU CUC CUA CUG
Lycine	TTT TTC	AAA AAG
Methionine	TAC	AUG
Phenylalanine	AAA AAG	UUU UUC
Proline	GGA GGG GGT GGC	CCU CCC CCA CCG
Serine	AGA AGG AGT AGC TCG TCA	UCU UCC UCA UCG AGC AGU
Threonine	TGA TGG TGT TGC	ACU ACC ACA ACG
Tryptophan	ACC	UGG
Tyrosine	ATA ATG	UAU UAC
Valine	CAA CAG CAT CAC	GUU GUC GUA GUG
START	TAC	AUG
STOP	ATT ATC ACT	UAA UAG UGA

tion and **translation** are detailed later in this chapter.

Genes

Most **genes** consists of a series of three-base units (triplets) necessary to synthesize a specific protein. Contained within each gene are base sequences; some sequences (exons) specify the amino acid sequence of the protein, and others regulate the onset, rate, and termination of protein synthesis. These sequences are not necessarily adjacent to each other; often, they are widely separated by noncoding sequences (introns). It has been estimated that more than 90% of DNA is nonfunctional.[2] This noncoding DNA can be excised without damage to the cell and its progeny, but its insertion into coding sequences causes defects.

Each human cell contains thousands of genes, known collectively as the human *genome* (the precise number is as yet uncertain because of separation, overlapping, and mobility of some gene components). The Human Genome Project, currently in progress under the direction of the National Institutes of Health, has as its goal the construction of a map of the human genome, identifying structural landmarks at 30,000 sites at regular intervals.[3] This map is intended to serve as a consistent reference for localization and isolation of DNA sequences of interest for purposes of research.

Some genes exist not to encode proteins but rather to make the tRNAs and rRNAs essential to protein synthesis. These "housekeeping genes" are frequently repeated throughout the genome because each cell must manufacture these molecules in quantity.

Not all genes are actively directing synthesis at any one time. Protein synthesis by coding genes may be switched on or off by regulatory proteins (**transcription factors**) whose synthesis is directed by other genes.[4] As discussed later in this chapter, most genetic regulation of cell development occurs before transcription.

The four bases found in DNA can be arranged in 64 different triplets, but there are only 20 amino acids. Three of the 64 triplets are termination signals, or "stop signs," which signal the end of a coding sequence. The remaining 61 code for amino acids; thus, certain amino acids are encoded by more than one triplet (Table 6–1).

Chromosomes

Within the cell nucleus, each DNA molecule is tightly wound around a rod-like protein core (histone) to form a **chromosome** (Fig. 6–2). Human body cells normally contain 46 chromosomes (the diploid number), consisting of 22 pairs of homologous **autosomes** and one pair of nonhomologous **sex chromosomes**, designated XX in females and XY in males. Autosomes are common to both sexes, and each member of a homologous pair has an identical arrangement of genes. The site of a particular gene on a chromosome is known as its *locus*, and alternative forms of genes at these loci are known as *alleles*. Human sex cells, or **gametes** (eggs and sperm), contain the haploid number of 23 chromosomes, with 22 autosomes and an X in eggs, and 22 autosomes

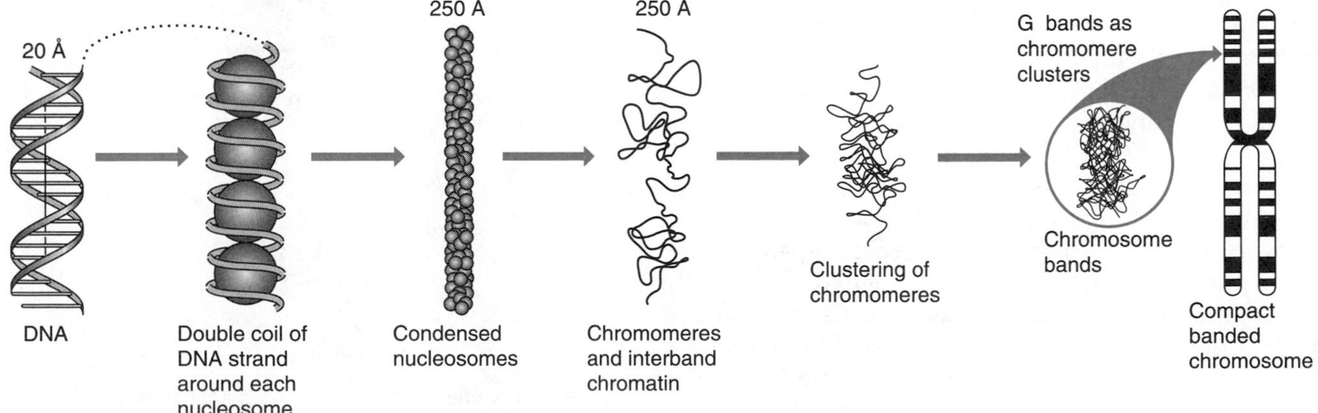

FIGURE 6–2

Chromosome structure. Each chromosome consists of a single DNA molecule tightly wound around a protein core (histone). DNA segments, about 146 base pairs in length, make two turns around histone to form a bead-like nucleosome. Nucleosomes are then condensed into a spiral to form chromomeres, fibers that are further clustered to form chromosomes. Chromosomal regions accept stain differentially, resulting in bands that may serve as landmarks for locating genes.

and either an X or Y in sperm. The union of egg with sperm at fertilization restores the diploid number.

Protein Synthesis by the Cell

The sequential processes by which the genetic instructions on DNA are read and carried out are transcription and translation, illustrated in Figure 6–3 and detailed next.

Transcription

Transcription is the transfer of information from DNA to mRNA in the nucleus. The double-stranded DNA first uncoils, exposing its base sequences. As directed by the enzyme RNA polymerase, binding of appropriate bases of RNA nucleotides to one of these strands results in synthesis of an mRNA strand that is complementary to its DNA template. Each three-base sequence on mRNA is known as a *codon.*

As stated previously, regulation of the onset, rate, and termination of transcription is the primary mechanism of genetic regulation of cell development. This regulation involves binding of transcription factors to regulatory base sequences known as *promoter regions* and *enhancer regions.* Promoters are consistent in their base sequences (usually a thymine-adenine-thymine-adenine, or TATA, box; a cytosine-adenine-adenine-thymine, or CAAT, box; or a guanine-cytosine, or GC, box) and are located within 100 bases upstream (with respect to direction of reading) of the transcription start triplet.[5] The TATA box usually appears immediately before the actual site of initiation of transcription. RNA polymerase, in association with a network of transcription factors, binds at the promoter region, initiating transcription. Enhancers are more variable in structure, location, and effects. Binding of transcription factors to enhancer regions usually increases the rate of transcription but occasionally inhibits it.

The differential expression of genes depends on the response of transcription factor networks to signals originating from the cytoskeletal tissue matrix or from ligands binding to cell surface or intracellular receptors (see Chapter 2). The end result of these signaling pathways is usually the phosphorylation of a transcription factor, which activates it.[6] The structure of the binding site on a particular transcription factor determines its classification as well as the specific DNA sequences to which it may bind. Table 6–2 lists examples of the transcription factors in each classification, or "family," along with some

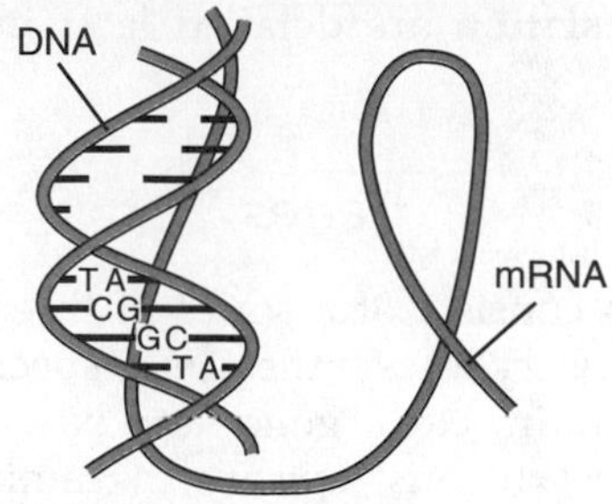

1. mRNA is made in the nucleus (site of transcription) and modified by post–transcriptional processing.

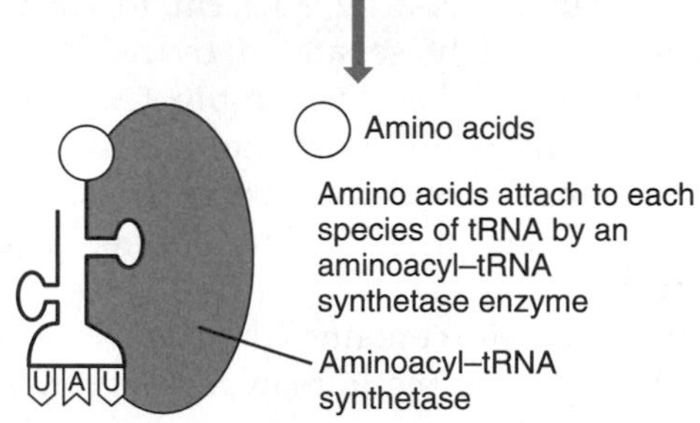

2. mRNA leaves the nucleus and attaches to the ribosome, and translation begins (in the cytoplasm).

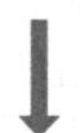

3. Incoming aminoacyl–tRNA hydrogen bonds via its anticodon to complementary mRNA sequence (codon) on the ribosome.

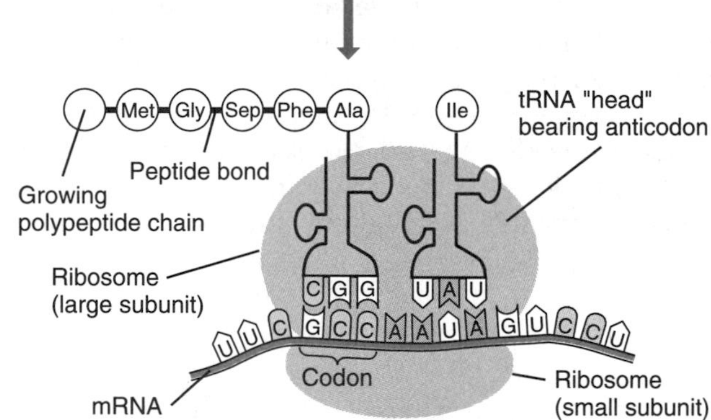

4. A new amino acid is added to the protein chain as the ribosome moves along the mRNA.

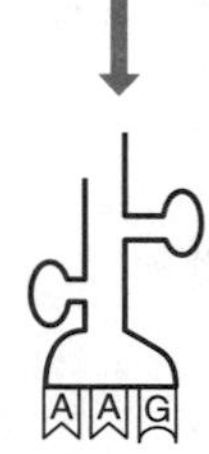

5. Released tRNA reenters the cytoplasmic pool of free tRNA, ready to be bound to a new amino acid.

FIGURE 6–3

Protein synthesis by the cell. The genetic code on DNA is transferred to mRNA in the process of transcription. After modification, the mRNA transcript is transported out of the nucleus to the cytoplasm. On the ribosomes, mRNA directs synthesis of a peptide chain as tRNA links specific amino acids to corresponding codons on mRNA.

TABLE 6–2
TRANSCRIPTION FACTORS

STRUCTURAL FAMILY	EXAMPLES OF TRANSCRIPTION FACTORS	FUNCTIONS
HTH (helix-turn-helix or homeobox)	Pit-1	Differentiation of hematopoietic precursor cells
	Oct-1	Development of childhood leukemias
	Unc-86	Regulation of hormone actions
Zinc finger	Receptors for steroid hormones (glucocorticoids, vitamin D, estrogen)	Regulation of hormone actions Activation of oncogenes in some cancers Tumor suppression
	Thyroid hormone receptor	Differentiation of erythrocytes, megakaryocytes, and mast cells
	Retinoic acid receptor	
	WT-1	Regulation of globin gene expression
	GATA-1	Regulation of gastric proton pump
Leucine zipper	AP-1 (products of *jun* and *fos* proto-oncogenes)	Regulation of cell growth and carcinogenesis Regulation of gluconeogenesis, neurotransmission, circadian rhythms, pituitary growth, opiate tolerance
	CREB	
HLH (helix-loop-helix)	MyoD	Enhancement of synthesis of immunoglobulins
	Muyogenin	Myogenesis
	myc	Growth regulation

Data from Papavassiliou, A.G. (1995). Transcription factors. *New England Journal of Medicine* 332(1), 45–47.

of the physiologic and pathologic effects mediated by these proteins.

Mutations in genes that encode transcription factors have been implicated in genetic defects and neoplasia (see Chapter 7). A number of drugs are known to work by altering the activity of transcription factors. These include the French "abortion pill" RU 486, which suppresses embryologic development and induces abortion, and the immunosuppressants cyclosporine and FK-506, which suppress production of a protein essential to immune cell function.[7]

Transcription proceeds in the 5′ to 3′ direction. The processes by which the action of RNA polymerase is terminated are poorly understood. Some viral proteins (e.g., human immunodeficiency virus [HIV], which causes acquired immunodeficiency syndrome [AIDS]) are able to prevent termination, whereas termination is premature in some cancer cells (e.g., Burkitt's lymphoma).[2]

After initial transcription, the mRNA strand (primary transcript) is modified in several ways. To facilitate later binding to ribosomes, a nucleotide "cap" is added to the upstream end of the mRNA.[1] About 20 bases are trimmed from the downstream end, followed by the addition of a series of adenine bases. This *poly A tail* is believed to stabilize the mRNA molecule. An RNA editing process modifies the base sequence in selected cases. A separate RNA splicing process excises noncoding sequences (introns) from the molecule, leaving uninterrupted coding sequences (exons). At least 100 different proteins have been implicated in the regulation of these modifications.[2]

After this **post-transcriptional processing**, the mRNA carrying the genetic blueprint diffuses into the cytoplasm. Selective transport across the nuclear membrane occurs through nuclear pore complexes, and this transport constitutes another potential site of regulation of protein synthesis.

Translation

Translation, the actual process of protein synthesis, involves all three forms of RNA. The cytoplasm contains many different forms of tRNA, at least one of which is specific for each amino acid, which binds to its helical *acceptor* loop (Fig. 6–4). The opposite loop of the cloverleaf-shaped tRNA contains a three-base sequence (anticodon) complementary to the mRNA codon for that amino acid. Hydrogen bonding of the tRNA anticodon to the mRNA codon thus links mRNA to amino acids.

Assembly of amino acids into polypeptide chains occurs on the ribosomes. First, a specific tRNA recognizes and binds an *initiator* codon on mRNA. Usually, this is the codon for the amino acid methionine. This complex then binds to a ribosome composed of rRNA and protein, with mRNA positioned in a groove between two ribosomal subunits. The ribosome then moves the next mRNA codon into position, and the appropriate amino acid is linked to the ribosome by tRNA. Repetition of this process

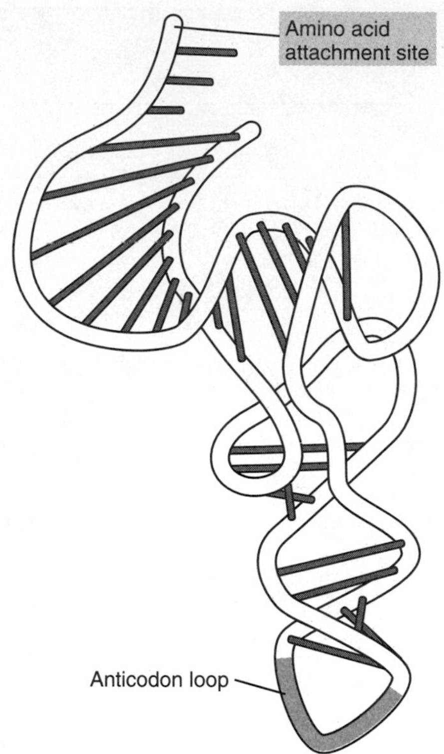

FIGURE 6–4
Structure of tRNA. The cloverleaf-shaped tRNA has a helical acceptor loop that binds a specific amino acid corresponding to an mRNA codon. The anticodon loop of tRNA has a three-base sequence (anticodon) that is complementary to the mRNA codon.

results in a growing peptide chain, with amino acids linked by peptide bonds in the sequence directed by mRNA. As each amino acid is bound in the chain, its tRNA is released into the cytoplasm to pick up another amino acid. As each mRNA codon is read, it is moved off the ribosome.

The translation process continues until a stop codon is read, resulting in release of the newly formed polypeptide from the ribosome. Most polypeptides then undergo further transformation into proteins by a variety of processes known collectively as **post-translational processing**. Chemical attractions between amino acids in the chain determine the folding of proteins into their ultimate shapes, or conformations. Some proteins are modified by the addition of carbohydrates or phosphate groups, and some are cleaved into smaller units. Many hormones, such as insulin and adrenocorticotropic hormone, are cleaved from larger inactive precursors, or *prohormones* (see Chapters 27 and 29).

Most proteins synthesized by the cell are enzymes or other regulatory proteins. Cells that are growing, dividing, and differentiating also synthesize a number of structural proteins.

Processes of Cellular Reproduction

The Cell Cycle

The genetic material of the cell directs the cell division and differentiation that underlie development of the human being from a fertilized ovum. Cells of different tissues, under different regulatory signals, divide at different rates throughout the life span (Table 6–3). Skin cells, for example, divide rapidly throughout life. Dead cells are continuously sloughed from the skin surface, and newly formed cells migrate upward to replace them. Other cells, such as neurons, normally do not divide once the individual reaches maturity.

The sequence of events during which a cell divides is known as the **cell cycle**, illustrated in Figure 6–5. The cell cycle consists of two major phases: interphase and cell division (mitotic, or M, phase). Interphase, the time between cell divisions, is a period of active cell growth and metabolism as well as preparation for division. Interphase consists of three subphases: the first gap phase (G_1), the synthesis phase (S), and the second gap phase (G_2). G_1 is the most variable in length, from hours to years, and is characterized by active protein synthesis. Replication of DNA occurs during the S phase, by a process similar to RNA synthesis. DNA strands uncoil and separate, and complementary free DNA nucleotides

TABLE 6–3
TISSUE VARIATION IN RATE OF CELL DIVISION

Tissue Category	Examples
Postreplicative cells (no physiologic stimulus for division after maturity)	Neuron Skeletal muscle Cardiac muscle Terminally differentiated blood cells
Quiescent cells (usually nondividing but may divide in response to physiologic stimuli, e.g., during wound healing)	Hepatocyte (liver cell) Renal tubular epithelium Connective tissue fibroblast Endothelium
Continuously proliferating cells (stem cells of populations that undergo terminal differentiation and must be constantly renewed)	Hematopoietic stem cells Lining and covering epithelium (e.g., skin, gastrointestinal tract)

Data from Norwood, T.H. (1990). Cellular aging. In: Cassel, C.K., Reisenberg, D.E., Sorenson, L.B., *et al.* (Eds.). *Geriatric Medicine.* (2nd ed.). New York: Springer-Verlag.

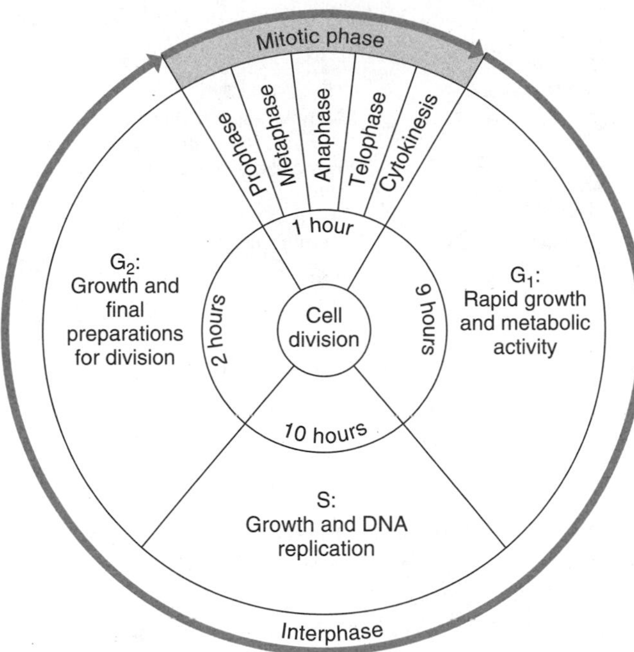

FIGURE 6–5

Cell cycle. The sequence of events during which a cell divides consists of two major phases: mitotic phase (cell division) and interphase (period between divisions). Interphase includes three phases: G_1 (protein synthesis), S (DNA replication), and G_2 (preparation for division). Mitosis includes five phases that culminate in cytokinesis, or cell division (see Fig. 6–6). Time intervals shown are typical, but variation is seen among cell types.

bind to each, forming two new strands identical to the originals. DNA replication takes about 10 to 12 hours to complete. G_2 is a brief phase during which additional protein synthesis occurs and cell constituents are moved into place for cell division.

Phase transition within the cell cycle is regulated by both negative (inhibitory to phase progression) and positive (progression-promoting) mechanisms, which are just beginning to be understood.[8] The most important regulators are transcription factors, which are either activated or inactivated by cyclin-dependent kinase (CDK) enzymes. Regulation of cell cycle phase progression ensures the correct order of events while allowing time for enzymatic repair of any defective or damaged DNA.

DNA Editing and Repair

Enzyme systems encoded by DNA repair genes normally edit newly synthesized DNA, replace any mismatched base pairs (mismatch repair),[9] and excise any defective nucleotide sequences (nucleotide excision repair).[10] The mismatch repair system first distinguishes the newly synthesized strand from the old on the basis of the lesser degree of modification (methylation) of the new strand. In a complex process consisting of at least 10 steps, regulatory proteins recognize and bind the incorrect base and an *endonuclease* enzyme, which induces a strand break on one side of the incorrect sequence. A second enzyme system, including *DNA helicase II* and an *exonuclease,* then binds at the break point and proceeds to the incorrect sequence, excising it.

Nucleotide excision repair is similar but targets damaged bases, that is, bases that have acquired chemical additions (adducts) as a consequence of exposure to ultraviolet radiation or chemical toxins. An *exinuclease* enzyme system hydrolyzes the phosphodiester bonds on both sides of the damaged sequence, excising it. Using the complementary DNA strand as a template, the resulting gap is then filled by synthetic enzymes. Nucleotide excision repair is less specific than mismatch repair and may actually *cause* mutations, owing to excision of key sequences. Optimal function of these DNA repair systems and of systems that edit RNA transcripts consititutes a critical defense against genetic mutations and neoplasia (see Chapter 7).

Mitosis and Meiosis

Two types of cell division (*cytokinesis*) occur in human cells: **mitosis** in body cells and **meiosis** in the formation of gametes or sex cells. Mitotic division of a cell, shown in Figure 6–6, maintains the diploid number of chromosomes and forms two daughter cells that are exact replicas of the original (unless mutation occurs). Mitosis typically takes about 1 to 2 hours. The processes that initiate and regulate mitosis are not completely understood but may involve chemical signals from other cells (e.g., growth factors) or tissue matrix signals triggered by changing cell surface-to-volume relationships (see Chapter 2).

Meiosis, shown in Figure 6–7, consists of two sequential divisions resulting in the formation of four cells, each containing the haploid number of chromosomes. During meiotic division, the genetic material of the original germ cell (reflecting both parents) is recombined, conveying new characteristics to the gametes and potentially contributing to variability of expressed traits in succeeding generations.[11] Regulation of the processes of gamete formation (spermatogenesis and oogenesis) is discussed in Chapters 30 and 31.

Differentiation of Body Cells

Each somatic (body) cell contains the same genetic material. That is, every cell could potentially de-

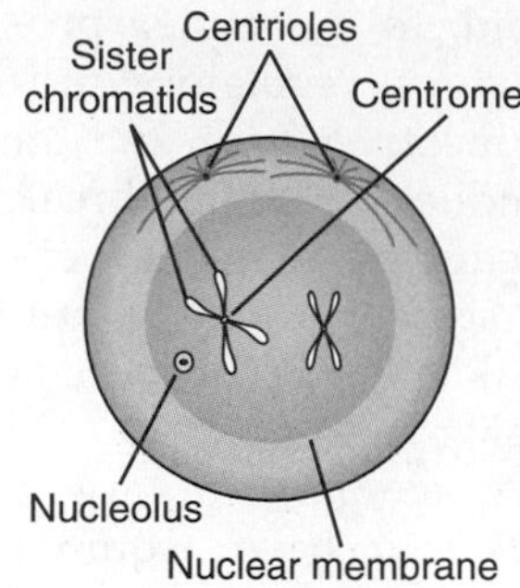

PROPHASE
DNA threads condense into visible chromosomes, each consisting of two sister chromatids joined at the centromere. The nuclear membrane disintegrates, and the centrioles separate and move to opposite sides of the cell. Spindle fibers (microtubules) form.

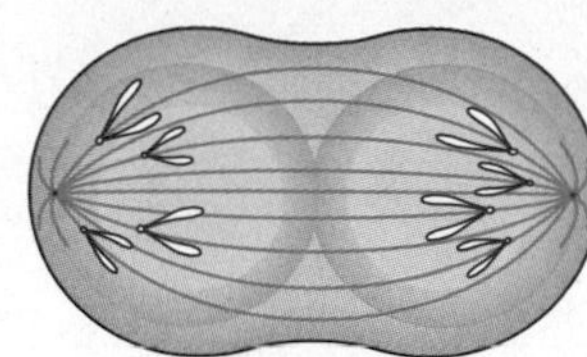

TELOPHASE
At their respective poles, chromosomes uncoil and elongate. The cell constricts along a central plane perpendicular to the spindle fibers, ultimately dividing the cell membrane and creating two cells.

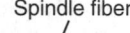

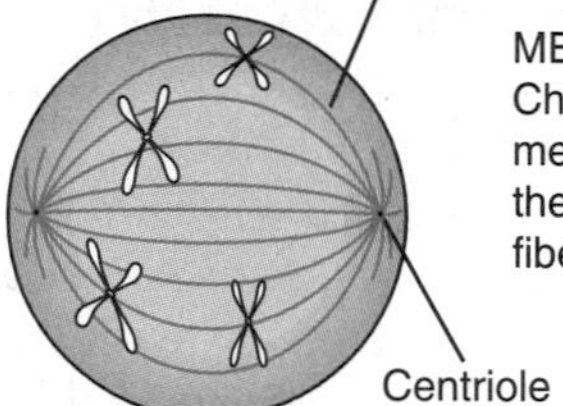

METAPHASE
Chromosomes line up on the metaphase plate at the center of the cell and are attached to spindle fibers at their centromere.

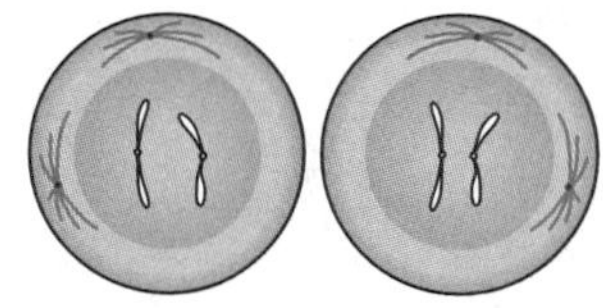

The cell divides, and new daughter cells enter interphase.

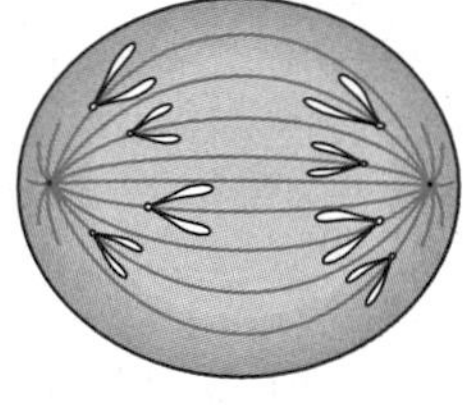

ANAPHASE
Centromeres divide, and single-stranded chromosomes are pulled to opposite sides of the cell.

A

FIGURE 6–6
Mitosis. *A*, Mitosis, the process of cell division in somatic cells, results in formation of two daughter cells, which are replicas of the original, having the diploid number of chromosomes (46).

velop into any of the 200 or so cell varieties found in the human body. The ultimate characteristics of differentiated cells depend on which parts of the genetic code are transcribed and translated into proteins as well as on the timing of these activities. The various types of body cells are organized into four categories of tissues based on their structure and function: epithelial, connective, muscle, and nervous tissues.

Epithelial Tissue

Epithelial tissues consist of two subtypes: covering and lining epithelium, and glandular epithelium. Covering and lining epithelium forms the outer portion of the skin as well as the lining of the gastrointestinal, urinary, and respiratory systems, the blood vessels, and the heart. Glandular epithelium forms glands, or secretory organs. Endocrine glands, such

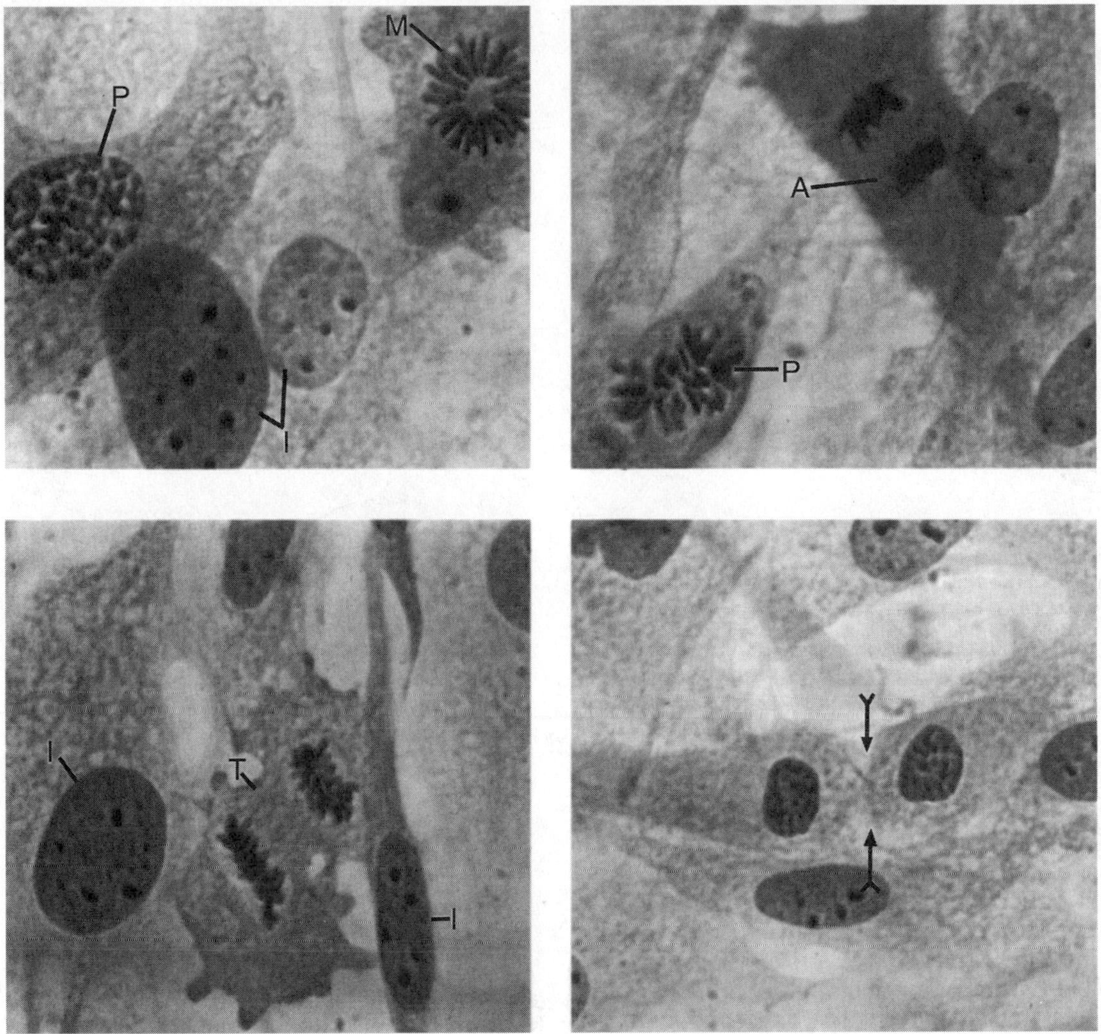

FIGURE 6–6 *continued*

B, Electron micrographs showing the stages of mitosis. *Top left:* interphase (I), one early prophase (P), and metaphase (M). *Top right:* late prophase (P), anaphase (A). *Bottom left:* interphase (I), early telophase (T). *Bottom right:* two daughter cells. (*B* from Leeson, T.S., Leeson, C.R., and Paparo, A.A. [1988]. *Textbook and Atlas of Histology.* [3rd ed.]. Philadelphia: W.B. Saunders [slide 13, p. 88].)

as the pancreas, secrete substances into the blood or lymph, whereas exocrine glands, such as sweat glands, secrete onto the body surface or into body cavities.

Epithelial cells are further classified on the basis of their shape as squamous (flat), cuboidal, or columnar, and on the basis of their arrangement as simple (single layer) or stratified (multilayered). Simple squamous epithelium is found in areas where ease of diffusion is important, such as capillary walls, kidney tubules, and alveoli of the lungs. Simple cuboidal and columnar epithelial cells usually serve a secretory function, as exemplified by mucus-secreting goblet cells of the gastrointestinal and respiratory tracts. Some epithelial cells are ciliated and serve to propel mucus along tracts. Stratified epithelium, such as that found in the epidermis of the skin, is the most prevalent type and serves a protective function.

Epithelial tissue protects underlying structures and is often specialized for cellular transport functions (i.e., absorption, filtration, or secretion). As shown in Table 6–4, epithelial tissue consists primarily of cells, with little extracellular matrix and no blood vessels. Cells are nourished by diffusion of materials from blood vessels in adjacent connective tissue. Epithelial cells secrete a glycoprotein that forms a thin basement membrane, separating the epithelium from underlying connective tissue. Sheets of epithelial cells, adherent to each other and to the

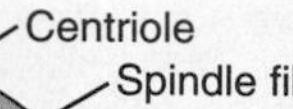

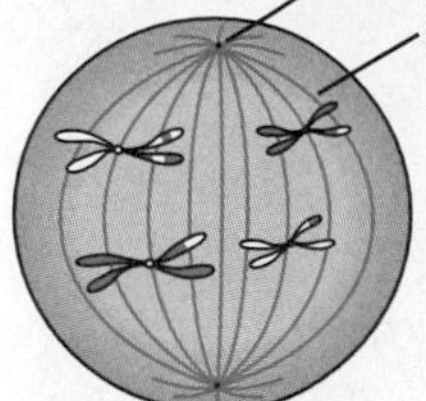

METAPHASE I
Chromosomes line up on the metaphase plate. Homologous chromosomes are paired and attach to spindle fibers at the centromere.

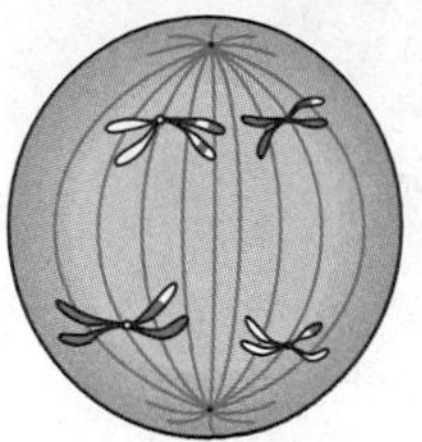

ANAPHASE I
Centromeres are not divided, and the chromatids are pulled to opposite poles. One chromosome of each homologous pair goes to each pole.

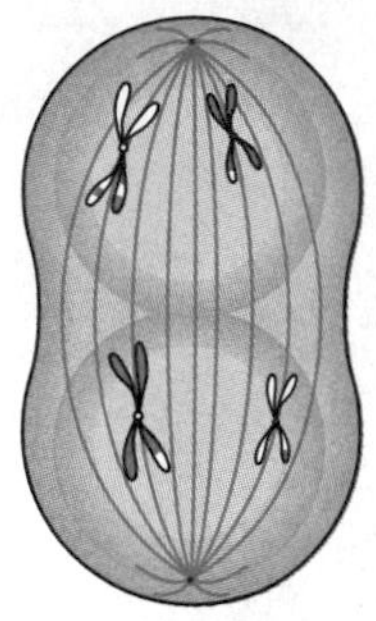

TELOPHASE I
Nuclear membrane reforms, and cell divides, with one duplicated member of each chromosome pair going to each daughter cell.

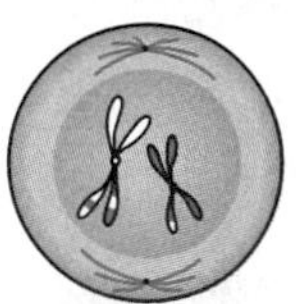

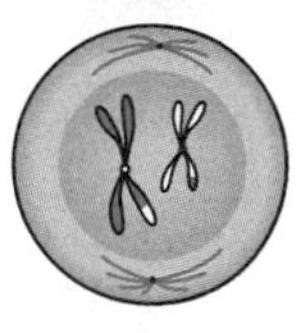

CELL DIVISION
This first division is a reduction division, with each daughter cell containing the haploid number of chromosomes.

A

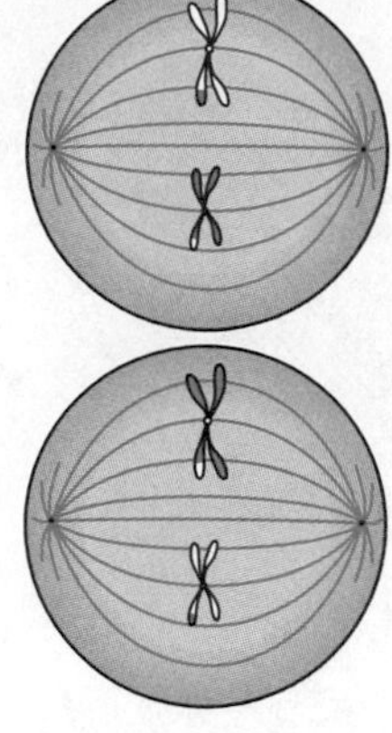

METAPHASE II
Chromosomes line up on the metaphase plate. Centrioles are polarized, and spindle fibers are in place.

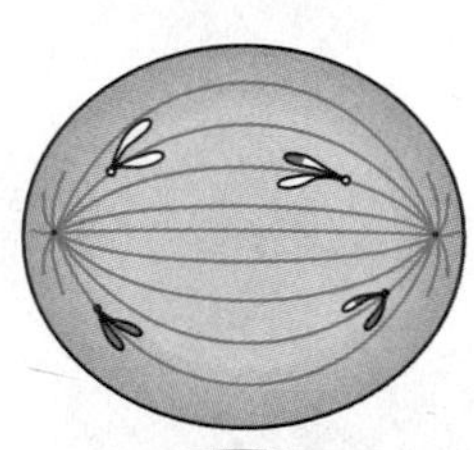

ANAPHASE II
Centromeres divide. Chromatids separate and move to opposite poles.

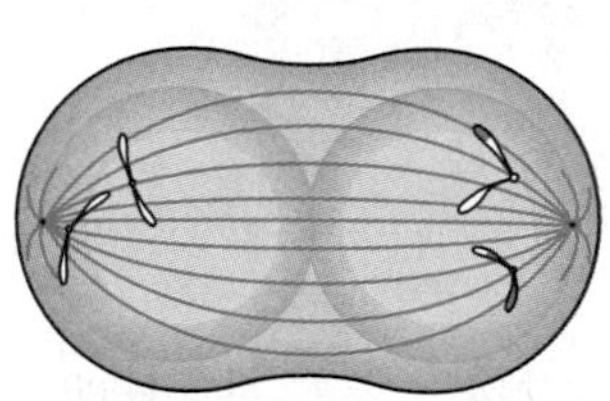

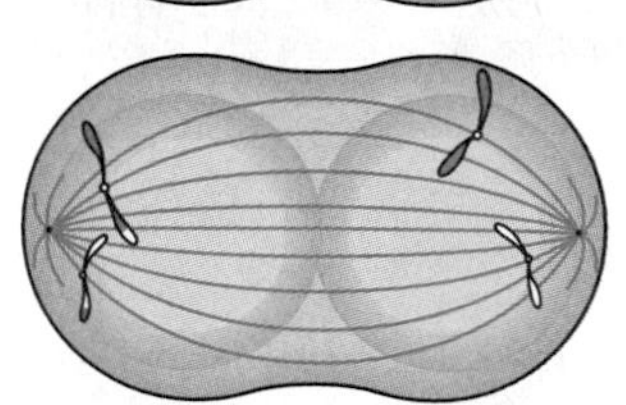

TELOPHASE II
Nuclear membrane reforms, and cell division occurs at end of stage.

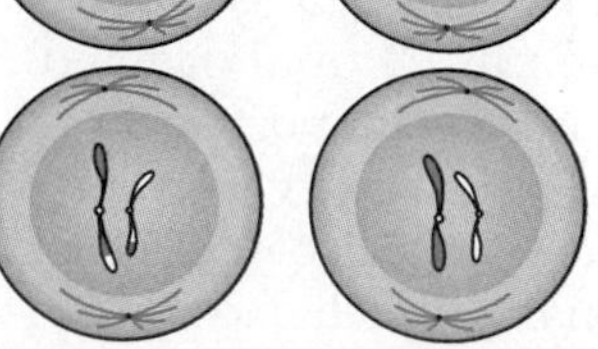

GAMETES
The end result of this equational division is four haploid cells, with one half of each chromosome pair in each cell.

Dark = Maternal origin
Light = Paternal origin

B

FIGURE 6–7 *See legend on opposite page*

basement membrane, constitute many biologic barriers. Movement of molecules across these barriers occurs by polarized transport processes, as discussed in Chapter 2. Epithelial cells divide rapidly and continuously throughout life.

Connective Tissue

Connective tissue, as its name suggests, serves to connect or bind cells together, thus providing support, protection, and insulation for body organs. As discussed in Chapter 2, increasing evidence indicates that connective tissue proteins participate in intercellular communication (tissue matrix signaling). The four subtypes of connective tissue are connective tissue proper, which is widespread throughout the body, and the more specialized cartilage, bone, and blood.

As shown in Table 6–5, most connective tissue has a high ratio of extracellular matrix to cells, and is variable in its vascularity. (The composition of blood is illustrated and discussed in detail in Chapter 12.) The extracellular matrix consists of a ground substance containing water, glycoproteins, and polysaccharides as well as fibrous proteins, such as fibrin, collagen, and elastin. Cell types vary among the subtypes, with connective tissue proper containing primarily fibroblasts (fiber-secreting cells). The *loose* form of connective tissue proper forms the subcutaneous tissue, supporting adipose (fat-storing) cells, blood vessels, and cells that migrate in from the blood, including lymphocytes, mast cells, and macrophages. *Dense* connective tissue proper has a higher proportion of fiber in its matrix and is found in tissues such as fascia, ligaments, tendons, the dermis of the skin, and the vocal cords.

The predominant cell type in cartilage is the chondroblast. Cartilage is more dense than dense connective tissue but less dense than bone. The three types of cartilage are hyaline cartilage, found in many joints, the trachea, the tip of the nose, and the embryonic skeleton; fibrocartilage, found in the knee and in intervertebral disks, and elastic cartilage, found in the ear and the epiglottis.

Bone tissue comprises the skeleton. Its formation is discussed in Chapter 34. Blood is considered a connective tissue because of its composition of cells within an extensive fluid matrix. Blood-forming elements are known collectively as the *hematopoietic system,* discussed in Chapter 12.

Muscle Tissue

The cellular structure and function of muscle tissue, with its skeletal, cardiac, and smooth muscle subtypes, was discussed in Chapter 5. Skeletal muscle function is further detailed in Chapter 35, cardiac muscle in Chapter 16, and smooth muscle in Chapters 15 (vascular smooth muscle), 20 (ureteral and bladder smooth muscle), 24 (intestinal smooth muscle), and 32 (uterine smooth muscle).

Nervous Tissue

The nervous system consists of neurons, which perform its specialized information-processing and transmitting function, and glial cells (neuroglia), which support neuronal function. Some glial cells, the *microglia,* differentiate from hematopoietic cells, which migrate into neural tissue. Neural function is discussed in Chapters 21, 22, and 23.

Programmed Cell Death (Apoptosis)

The same genome that encompasses the blueprint for the life and function of the cell also has the capacity to induce cellular suicide. Apoptosis is an orderly series of events, initiated by an extracellular signal, that culminates in noninflammatory fragmentation of the cell. Specific genes, notably one designated *p53,* are activated during apoptosis, and their protein products serve as enzymes that cleave DNA into fragments. The proteolytic activity of these enzymes, which include interleukin-1B–converting enzyme (ICE), is normally carefully balanced by inhibitors of apoptosis.[12] Imbalance of these factors may contribute to diseases characterized by increased cellular proliferation (e.g., cancer, autoimmune disorders, viral infections) or decreased proliferation (e.g.,

FIGURE 6–7

Meiosis. Meiosis, the process by which gametes (eggs and sperm) are formed from primary germ cells, consists of two sequential divisions resulting in the formation of four cells, each containing the haploid number of chromosomes (23). *A,* The first meiotic division, a reduction division, produces two haploid cells, each containing different alleles. *B,* The second meiotic division, an equational division, produces four haploid cells in which the chromatids of the previous generation are equally distributed.

TABLE 6–4
EPITHELIAL TISSUES

STRUCTURE SUBTYPE	LOCATIONS	FUNCTIONS
Simple squamous 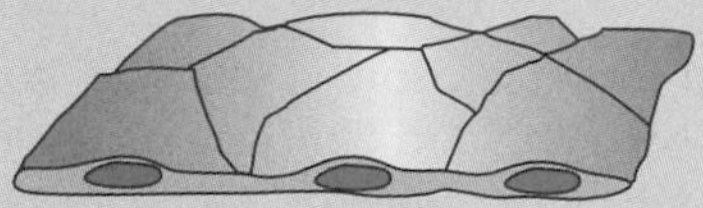 Flat cells in single layer; little extracellular matrix; disk-like central nuclei	Walls of vascular and lymphatic vessels; lining of alveoli of lungs; serosa layer of viscera; lining of Bowman's capsule in kidney	Facilitation of diffusion and filtration
Simple cuboidal Cube-shaped cells with spherical nuclei; may be ciliated	Walls of airways and gastrointestinal tract, renal tubules, ovarian surface	Absorption, secretion, and (if ciliated) propulsion
Simple columnar 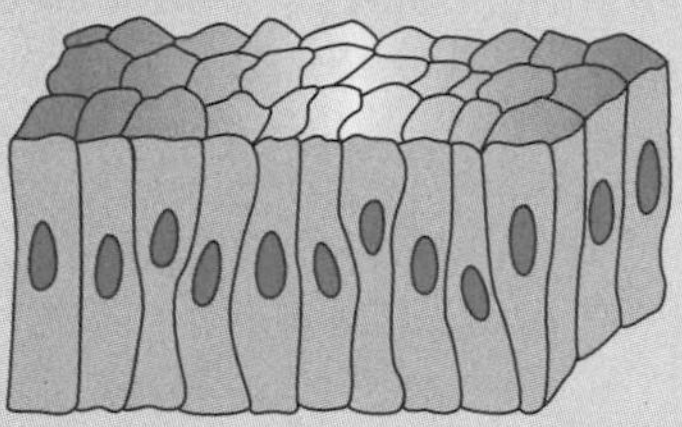 Tall cells with oval nuclei; may be ciliated; may contain mucus-secreting glands (goblet cells)	Walls of airways and gastrointestinal tract, gallbladder and other exocrine glands, uterus and fallopian tubes	Absorption, secretion, and (if ciliated) propulsion)
Stratified squamous 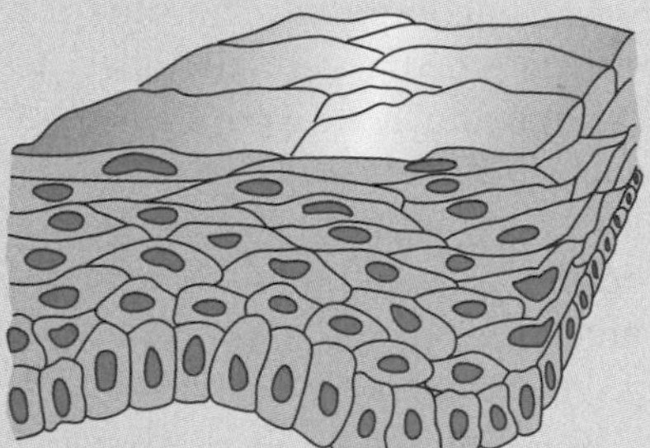 Multilayered with cuboidal base and progressively flatter surface cells	Skin, mucous membranes	Protection
Stratified cuboidal 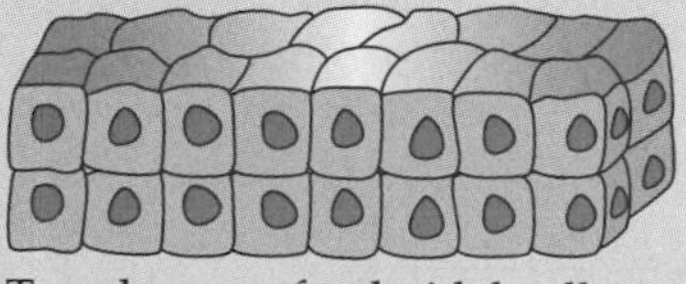 Two layers of cuboidal cells	Ducts of exocrine glands (sweat glands, mammary glands, salivary glands)	Protection

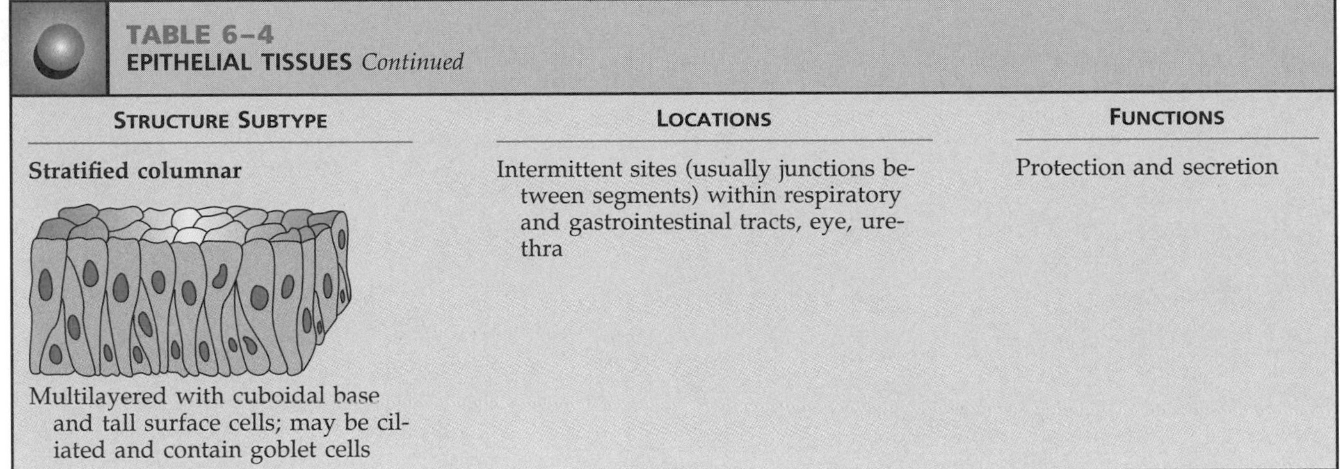

TABLE 6–4
EPITHELIAL TISSUES *Continued*

STRUCTURE SUBTYPE	LOCATIONS	FUNCTIONS
Stratified columnar Multilayered with cuboidal base and tall surface cells; may be ciliated and contain goblet cells	Intermittent sites (usually junctions between segments) within respiratory and gastrointestinal tracts, eye, urethra	Protection and secretion

AIDS, neurodegenerative disorders, ischemic injury, or toxicity).[13]

In contrast to injury-induced inflammatory cell death (**necrosis**), this genetically triggered cell death is critical to many aspects of development. Examples include the selective destruction of cells that shapes organs during embryologic development, the "weeding out" of neurons that fail to connect within signaling pathways, and the destruction of self-sensitized immune cells during maturation in the thymus.

Although the processes by which a single cell differentiates into a complex human being are incompletely understood, the sequence of developmental changes has been precisely observed and documented. Differentiation occurs most rapidly and with the most striking effects during the embryonic and fetal periods.

PRENATAL GROWTH AND DEVELOPMENT

Prenatal development includes all aspects of cellular division, differentiation, and growth that occur between conception and birth. This 40-week period of intrauterine life is traditionally divided into the **preembryonic period**, which includes the first 2 weeks, the **embryonic period**, which includes weeks 3 through 8, and the **fetal period**, which includes the remainder of the period of pregnancy, or gestation. During these prenatal periods, the developing human is referred to as the **conceptus**, the embryo, and the fetus, respectively. By the end of the embryonic period, differentiation has occurred to the extent that the beginnings of all organ systems are apparent, the embryonic membranes are developed, and the placenta is functioning. The fetal period is characterized by some further differentiation but primarily by growth of organ systems and structures. The major stages of prenatal development are illustrated in Figure 6–8.

Preembryonic Development

Fertilization

Fertilization refers to the process by which the ovum of the mother is penetrated by the sperm of the father. Fertilization lasts about 24 hours and occurs within the maternal fallopian tube. The fertilized ovum is called a **zygote**. The sex of the embryo is determined by the father at the time of fertilization. If the sperm carries the X chromosome, the embryo is female; the Y chromosome produces a male. Occasionally, multiple ova are fertilized by sperm, resulting in multizygotic (fraternal, or nonidentical) multiple births.

Cleavage

Mitotic division of the zygote results in formation of the *morula,* a mass of smaller cells within the outer coat of the ovum. This process takes about 3 days, after which the morula leaves the fallopian tube and enters the uterus. In some instances, the zygote splits into identical daughter cells, which undergo separate **cleavage** and development, producing monozygotic (identical) multiple births.

Blastocyst Formation

The blastocyst forms when a fluid-filled cavity separates the cells of the morula into an inner cell mass, which becomes the embryo, and an outer cell layer called the trophoblast, which becomes part of the placenta. The blastocyst floats freely in the

TABLE 6–5
CONNECTIVE TISSUES

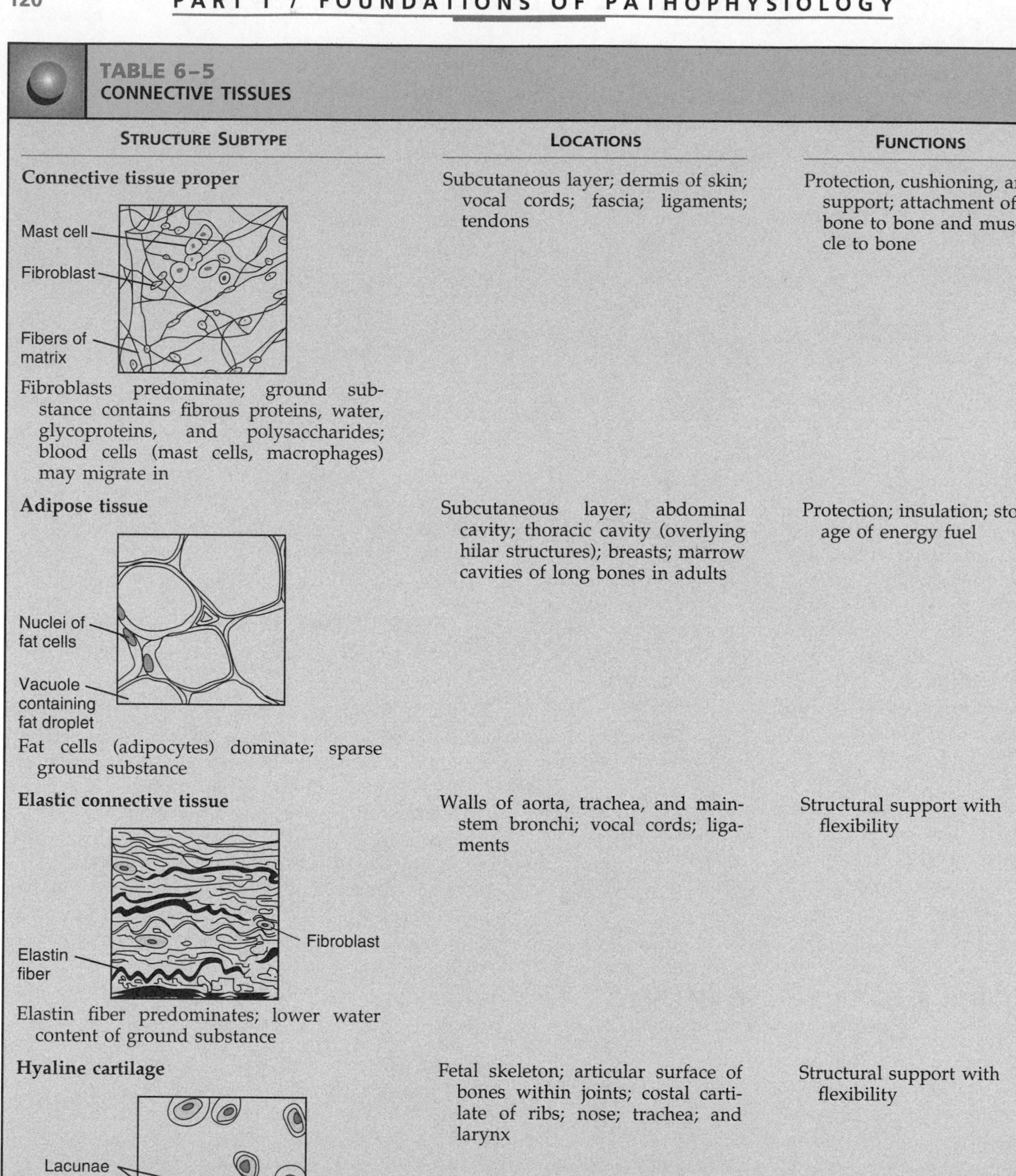

Structure Subtype	Locations	Functions
Connective tissue proper Fibroblasts predominate; ground substance contains fibrous proteins, water, glycoproteins, and polysaccharides; blood cells (mast cells, macrophages) may migrate in	Subcutaneous layer; dermis of skin; vocal cords; fascia; ligaments; tendons	Protection, cushioning, and support; attachment of bone to bone and muscle to bone
Adipose tissue Fat cells (adipocytes) dominate; sparse ground substance	Subcutaneous layer; abdominal cavity; thoracic cavity (overlying hilar structures); breasts; marrow cavities of long bones in adults	Protection; insulation; storage of energy fuel
Elastic connective tissue Elastin fiber predominates; lower water content of ground substance	Walls of aorta, trachea, and mainstem bronchi; vocal cords; ligaments	Structural support with flexibility
Hyaline cartilage Chondroblasts predominate; dense ground substance with collagen fibers; mature chondroblasts (chondrocytes) surrounded by fluid in lacunae	Fetal skeleton; articular surface of bones within joints; costal cartilate of ribs; nose; trachea; and larynx	Structural support with flexibility

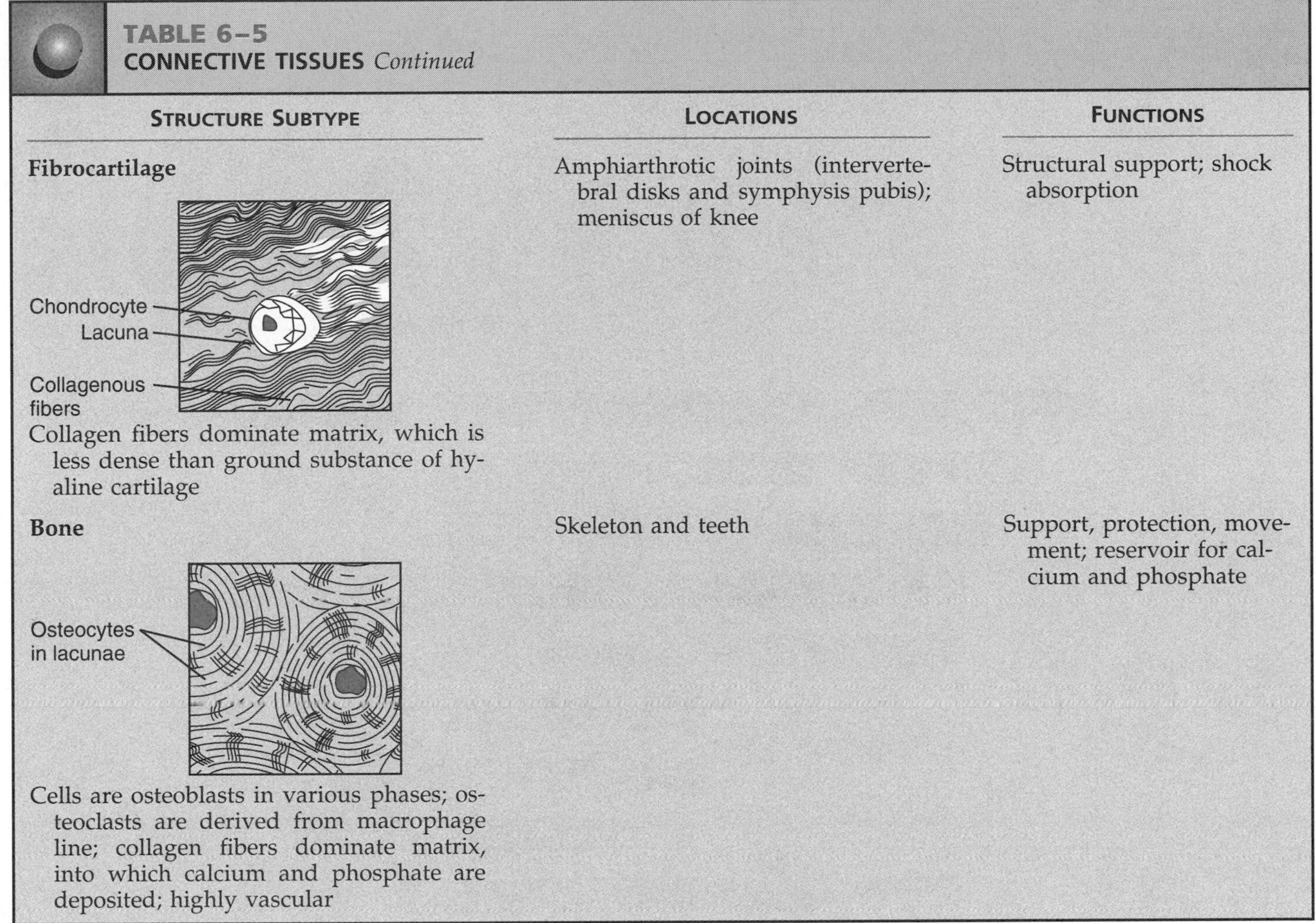

TABLE 6–5
CONNECTIVE TISSUES *Continued*

Structure Subtype	Locations	Functions
Fibrocartilage Chondrocyte Lacuna Collagenous fibers Collagen fibers dominate matrix, which is less dense than ground substance of hyaline cartilage	Amphiarthrotic joints (intervertebral disks and symphysis pubis); meniscus of knee	Structural support; shock absorption
Bone Osteocytes in lacunae Cells are osteoblasts in various phases; osteoclasts are derived from macrophage line; collagen fibers dominate matrix, into which calcium and phosphate are deposited; highly vascular	Skeleton and teeth	Support, protection, movement; reservoir for calcium and phosphate

uterus for about 6 days, obtaining nourishment from uterine fluids.

Implantation

The blastocyst then attaches to the uterine wall, releasing enzymes that erode the uterine lining. Communication with maternal blood is established, and development of the placenta from trophoblast cells and maternal endometrial cells is initiated. Implantation normally occurs in the upper third of the uterus and takes about 2 weeks to complete.

Embryonic Disk Formation

During the process of implantation, additional changes occur within the cell layers of the blastocyst, resulting in formation of a double-layered embryonic disk and in initial formation of the fetal membranes. Trophoblast cells give rise to a primitive membrane known as the *yolk sac,* which serves a nutritive function at this point and later differentiates into tissues of the gut and genitalia. Extraembryonic **mesoderm** then arises from trophoblast cells. Mesodermal tissues ultimately give rise to the connective tissues of the body. Spaces in this mesoderm form a *coelom* (cavity); the coelom later develops into the chorionic sac, which contains the developing embryo with its attached yolk sac and amniotic sac.

The amniotic sac becomes visible as a space between the trophoblast and the inner cell mass, now referred to as the *embryoblast.* The embryoblast differentiates into the bilaminar embryonic disk, with its upper layer (epiblast) associated with the amniotic cavity and its lower layer (hypoblast) adjacent to the blastocyst cavity. The hypoblast develops a thickened area, which becomes the cranial region of the embryo.

Embryonic Development

Gastrulation

Gastrulation is the first stage of embryonic development and consists of the processes by which the bilaminar disk differentiates into the three-layered embryonic disk, or *gastrula.* Gastrulation begins with

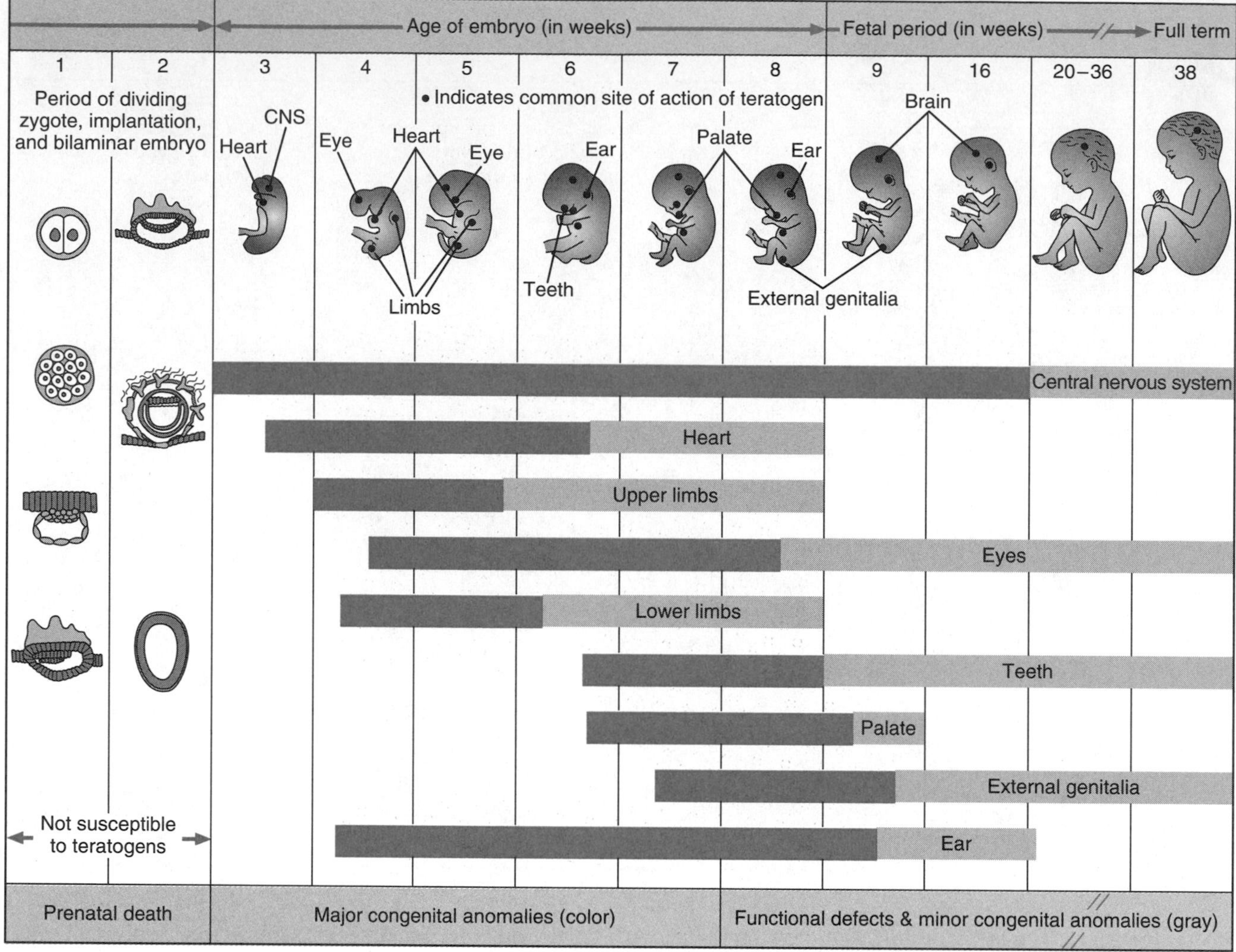

FIGURE 6–8

Stages of prenatal development. The preembryonic period (weeks 1 and 2) begins at fertilization and ends with implantation of the double-layered embryo into the maternal endometrium. The embryonic period (weeks 3 to 8) is characterized by differentiation of all organ systems from three embryonic tissue layers. The fetal period (weeks 9 to 40) is a period of rapid growth and maturation of organ systems. Teratogenic insult during the preembryonic period results in prenatal death. Insult during the embryonic period results in major congenital anomalies, while late insult results in functional defects or minor anomalies. (Modified from Moore, K.L., and Persaud, T.V.N. [1993]. *The Developing Human: Clinically Oriented Embryology.* [5th ed.]. Philadelphia: W.B. Saunders [p. 156]. Used with permission.)

the appearance of the primitive streak, a thickened band of epiblast. Some cells leaving the surface of the primitive streak form a layer of mesoderm, while others displace the hypoblast and form another layer, the **endoderm.** After it begins producing mesoderm by means of the primitive streak, the epiblast becomes known as the **ectoderm**. All of the tissues of the body develop from these three germ layers (Table 6–6).

Notochord Formation

A rod of mesodermal cells forms a central axis within the embryo, giving it some rigidity and separating the ectoderm from the endoderm. This structure canalizes and forms the notochord, around which the vertebral column ultimately develops.

Neural Tube Formation

The developing notochord induces formation of the neural plate, a thickening of the ectoderm in the cranial region. This structure folds inward on itself to form the **neural tube**. The ectoderm of this region becomes further specialized into **neuroectoderm**, which develops into the brain and spinal cord as well as other structures. Cells from the edges of the infolding neural plate, known as *neural crest cells,*

TABLE 6–6
EMBRYONIC ORIGIN OF TISSUES

Endoderm	Mesoderm	Ectoderm
Epithelium of: pharynx trachea bronchi lungs gastrointestinal tract liver pancreas bladder thyroid gland parathyroid gland	Connective tissue: bone blood lymph dermis Gonads Adrenal cortex Cardiovascular system Spleen Serous membranes	Surface ectoderm: epidermis hair nails skin glands mammary glands anterior pituitary gland inner ear lens of eye Neuroectoderm Neural crest cranial and sensory ganglia peripheral nerves adrenal medulla Neural tube central nervous system retina of eye pineal gland posterior pituitary gland

Data from Moore, K.L., and Persaud, T.V.N. (1993). *The Developing Human: Clinically Oriented Embryology.* (5th ed.). Philadelphia: W.B. Saunders Co.

migrate to each side of the neural tube and give rise to ganglia (neuron cell bodies usually located outside the central nervous system), meninges (protective membranes surrounding the brain and cord), Schwann cells (myelin-producing cells for insulation of nerves), the adrenal medulla (a neuroendocrine organ), and some musculoskeletal components of the head.

Somite Development

As the neural tube develops, blocks of mesoderm on each side differentiate and divide into pairs of cube-shaped *somites,* which give rise to the skeleton of the head, neck, and trunk along with the associated muscles and dermis of the skin. Somites are clearly visible in the developing embryo and appear sequentially in pairs in a craniocaudal (head-to-tail) progression. The number of visible somite pairs is a reliable indicator of embryonic age.

Development of the Intraembryonic Coelom

The coelom that first appeared during the preembryonic stage develops into a horseshoe-shaped cavity that divides the mesoderm into two layers: the somatic layer, which is continuous with the amnionic membrane; and the splanchnic layer, which is continuous with the yolk sac membrane. The somatic layer and its overlying ectoderm form the body wall, and the splanchnic layer and its associated endoderm form the wall of the primitive gut. During the second month of gestation, the intraembryonic coelom divides to form the pericardial cavity, enclosing the heart, the pleural cavities, surrounding the lungs, and the peritoneal cavity, containing the abdominal viscera.

Angiogenesis

Angiogenesis, the process of blood vessel development, begins early in the embryonic period and results in formation of the first functional organ system. The cardiovascular system begins pumping blood by the end of the third week, and the heart beat of the embryo is detectable with ultrasonography by the fifth week. Blood vessels are first seen on membranes, then within the embryo. These develop within spaces in the mesoderm, which become lined with endothelial cells, derived from the mesoderm. Primitive vessels unite with each other, forming the circulatory system. The heart begins as paired tubes of endothelial cells that fuse into a single tubular organ in the pericardial cavity. Primitive blood cells are also principally derived from endothelial cells of blood vessels.

Organ System Development

Cell growth and differentiation continue rapidly throughout the embryonic period, resulting in organ system development and sequential changes in the overall form of the embryo. As the trilaminar embryo grows rapidly in length, the tissues at the sides do not grow at the same rate as those in the center. This results in folding of the embryo at the cranial and caudal ends. Buds of limbs appear and develop, and the head becomes more rounded. The tail region eventually disappears.

Organ system development proceeds under genetic control, although specific regulatory mechanisms and signals are uncertain (see Focus of Current Research). Development of organ systems is highly interdependent, however, with adjacent cells communicating during the process by molecular or tissue matrix signals. One structural change often causes or *induces* another, and embryologic development may be viewed as a series of inductions. By the end of the embryonic period, the structure of all of the major organ systems has been substantially developed, although the function of these systems is minimal. Embryologic development of each body system is detailed in Part Two of this textbook.

Fetal Development

From the 9th week of gestation until the time of birth, the developing human, known as the fetus, has a distinctly human appearance. This period is characterized by further differentiation but especially by rapid growth. The head is disproportionately large at the beginning of the fetal period, but more rapid body growth brings structures into proportion. There is little body fat until the later weeks of gestation. Hair appears by the 20th week, and the skin becomes covered with a waxy substance (vernix caseosa). Organ systems continue to develop, with their functional capacity gradually increasing to the

Focus of Current Research

Study	Objective and Findings
Haidet, et al. (1996) Effects of aging per se on arterial stiffness: Systemic and regional compliance in beagles.	*Objective:* To determine whether aging per se results in reduced arterial compliance by using animals that do not develop hypertension and hyperlipidemia and are resistant to atherosclerosis. *Findings:* Systemic arterial compliance is reduced with aging per se.
Lemon & Freedman (1996) Selective effects of ligands on vitamin D_3 receptor- and retinoid X receptor-mediated gene activation in vivo.	*Objective:* To examine the interactions between these receptors and their ligands in inducing effects on target genes. *Findings:* Signals are exchanged between the two hormone systems through the formation of heterodimeric transcription factors.
Tokita, et al. (1994) Genetic influences on type I collagen synthesis and degradation: Further evidence for genetic regulation of bone turnover.	*Objective:* To assess whether genetic effects on bone turnover are detectable with markers of bone collagen turnover. *Findings:* Both synthesis and degradation of type I collagen are genetically determined.
Tamir & Isakov (1994) Cyclic AMP inhibits phosphatidylinositol-coupled and -uncoupled mitogenic signals in T lymphocytes.	*Objective:* To analyze the mechanism by which cAMP inhibits T-cell activation. *Findings:* cAMP alters transcription of the *jun* and *fos* genes.

point at which the fetus is *viable*, or capable of extrauterine life. Fetal physiology and consequences of premature birth are described in Chapter 33.

Development of the Placenta and Fetal Membranes

The developing human is supported during the embryonic and fetal periods by the placenta and fetal membranes, which also develop from the zygote. The placenta functions in the exchange of blood constituents between the embryo and the mother and also secretes hormones that are essential to support and regulation of the pregnancy (see Chapter 32). The fetal membranes include the chorion, amnion, yolk sac, and allantois. These membranes contain fluids and serve to support, protect, and nourish the embryo and fetus at various stages. Beginning at implantation, the chorion develops finger-like projections (chorionic villi) that extend into the maternal endometrium. Blood vessels develop within the villi by the 3rd week, establishing communication with the maternal circulation that continues until the placenta is sufficiently established. The early chorionic cavity, containing the embryo with its attached amniotic and yolk sacs, is obliterated as the embryo grows.

The amnion surrounds the embryo, providing an environment of constant temperature and buoyant support of growth and movement. Amniotic fluid is initially secreted by embryonic cells, then formed from maternal interstitial fluid. Late in gestation, the growing fetus passes urine into the fluid as well. Amniotic fluid is 99% water, which exchanges freely between the cavity and the maternal circulation through placental membranes. The amnion enfolds the point of connection of the embryo to the chorion, forming the umbilical cord.

The yolk sac serves as a nutrient source for the early embryo, while the placenta is being established. It is also the site of early hematopoietic (blood-forming) activity, until the embryonic liver begins to serve this function. Most of the yolk sac atrophies and disappears later in the embryonic period, although parts of it become incorporated into developing tissues of the embryo, including the epithelium of the respiratory and digestive tracts and the germ cells from which eggs or sperm originate.

The allantois is a small pouch-like extension of the yolk sac that also serves in early blood formation. The blood vessels of the allantois develop into the umbilical vein and arteries, which serve as exchange routes between the fetal and maternal circulations. The allantois is continuous with tissues that form the urinary bladder. As the bladder enlarges, the allantois shrinks to form a fibrous chord (the urachus), which extends from the umbilicus to the top of the bladder.

Critical Periods in Morphogenesis

Morphogenesis is the development of human shape and form. **Dysmorphogenesis**, or abnormal physical development, may result from the influence of harmful agents or stimuli (teratogens) from the internal or external environment, resulting in congenital defects. Insults during the preembryonic period usually result in prenatal death and early spontaneous abortion. The most critical period in morphogenesis is the embryonic period. Insults during this time are most likely to result in major anomalies because this is the period of greatest differentiation into organ systems and functional structures. Harmful effects of stimuli during the fetal period generally produce more minor defects because growth predominates over differentiation during this period.

AGING

In studying diseases of various body systems, the impact of age-related structural changes and loss of function is often a primary factor. Even in the healthy elderly, loss of functional reserve or adaptive capacity is of concern, and aging is frequently listed among the risk factors for specific diseases. Aging, per se, is not pathology, however. Aging is a developmental process at the cellular level and at other subsystem levels. A principal focus of gerontologic research is to differentiate the effects of genetically programmed changes in cellular structure and function from potentially preventable outcomes of disease.

Definitions of Aging

Primary aging is defined as the process of physiologic change attributable *only* to advancing age. **Secondary aging** refers to physiologic changes due to diseases that may or may not accompany aging. Some degree of stiffness of arterial walls (arteriosclerosis) is seen in all elderly people and can be considered a primary manifestation of aging. Atherosclerosis (lipid-filled lesions in arteries) often manifests in older people and may account for degenerative effects owing to decreased perfusion of many organ systems. Because not all elderly people develop atherosclerosis, however, this disorder is a secondary manifestation of aging.

Physiologic age must also be differentiated from *chronologic age*. Human bodies age at different rates, regardless of age in years, and the causes of these differences are both genetic and environmental.[14] Many attempts have been made to quantify physiologic age based on norms of clinical assessments, such as blood pressure, body fat, or tests of renal, hepatic, and pulmonary function. Clinical judgment of physiologic age is often noted in medical records with statements such as "patient appears older (or younger) than stated age." Research studies to discover biomarkers of aging are ongoing. The most useful thus far is lipofuscin, a yellow-brown pigment found in aging cells.[15] Such markers show promise as measurable outcomes in studies of factors influencing the rate of physiologic aging in individuals.

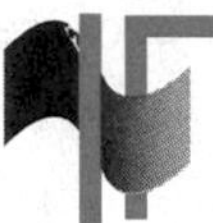

Clinical Scenario

D.F., an 82-year-old widower, lives alone in a high-rise apartment for senior citizens. Despite a history of "heart problems," he claims to be in good health. D.F. cooks his own meals and professes a fondness for "coffee, toast, and a sweet now and then." Most of his days are spent playing cards or checkers with friends, and his evenings are spent watching his favorite television programs. D.F. notes that he has felt "weak" in recent months and has hesitated to walk outdoors because of fear of falling. His legs appear thin, and some atrophy of the muscles of his shoulders and arms is evident.

1. Is loss of muscle mass and bone density inevitable with aging?
2. Are any clinical interventions warranted in D.F.'s case?

Life Expectancy

Since 1900, the average life expectancy in the United States has shown a 30-year gain, which exceeds the gain seen in the time period from 3000 B.C. to 1900.[16] A person born in the United States today can expect to live about 75 years, although race and sex influence this number (Table 6–7). Average life expectancy probably will rise slowly until it approaches 85 years and then level off. This prediction is based on survival curves among various human populations, which have shown a definite change in shape but not in ultimate value over time (Fig. 6–9). A small number of people live significantly longer than 85 years; the maximum documented life span is 122 years.[17] Epidemiologic research has revealed that the major factors influencing increased life expectancy are lowered infant mortality rates and improvement in prevention and treatment of diseases, particularly infectious diseases.[18]

Theories of Aging

Researchers have approached the study of aging from both molecular and organ system perspectives, which has resulted in two bodies of theory: one based on impairment of cellular proliferation due to environmental factors and another focusing on genetically determined changes in functional capacity. Specific theories are summarized in Table 6–8; general categories of theory are discussed in the next sections. In most cases, theories are not mutually exclusive.

Impairment of Cellular Proliferation

Studies of human cell cultures have revealed that all normal body cells, except stem cells, have a finite capacity to reproduce. Only cancer cells are potentially immortal. The best-known theories explaining this phenomenon fall into three categories: genetic

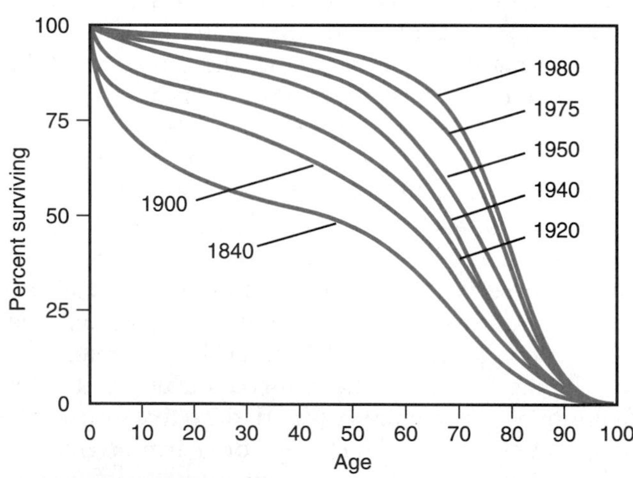

FIGURE 6–9
Survival curves. Life expectancy has risen steadily since the turn of the century. More people are living longer, but the maximal life span has remained constant at about 85 years. (From Cassel, C.K., and Brody, J.A. [1990]. Demography, epidemiology, and aging. In: Cassel, C.K., Reisenberg, D.E., Sorensen, L.B., *et al.* [Eds.]. *Geriatric Medicine.* [2nd ed.]. New York: Springer-Verlag. [p. 17]. Used with permission.)

TABLE 6–7
YEARS OF LIFE EXPECTANCY AT BIRTH BY RACE AND SEX: UNITED STATES

Birth Year	White Female	White Male	Black Female	Black Male	Nonwhite Female	Nonwhite Male
1940	66.6	62.1	—	—	54.9	51.5
1950	72.2	66.5	—	—	62.9	59.1
1960	74.1	67.4	—	—	66.3	61.1
1970	75.6	68.0	68.3	60.0	69.4	61.3
1980	78.1	70.7	72.5	63.8	73.6	65.3
1992	79.8	73.2	73.9	65.0	—	—

Data from National Center for Health Statistics. (1989). Advance report of final mortality statistics, 1987. *Monthly Vital Statistics Report* 38(5 suppl.); and Centers for Disease Control and Prevention. (1992). Mortality patterns: United States 1992. *Morbidity and Mortality Weekly Report* 43(49), 916–920.

mutation theories, oxidative stress theories, and genetic program theories.

Genetic mutation theories hold that age is the result of accumulated mutations in the DNA of body cells, causing progressive impairment of cellular function. Research has focused on the role of **telomerase**, an enzyme expressed in germ cells but not in body cells. **Telomeres**, the ends of chromosomes, have been observed to shorten with each cell cycle in body cells. Telomere shortening has been linked to loss of cell reproductive capacity and ultimately to cell death. Telomerase protects germ cells from this fate by making a DNA copy of its own RNA, then fusing this strand to the chromosomal end, prevent-

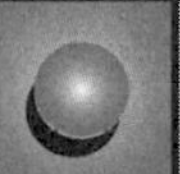

TABLE 6–8
THEORIES OF AGING

Theory	Central Ideas
Cellular senescence	Except for stem cells, human cells have a finite capacity to replicate. Limited replication is an expression of programmed genetic events.
Programmed loss of genetic material (codon restriction)	Loss of redundant DNA sequences with repeated cell divisions results in decreased functional capacity. At a fixed point in life, cells begin to manufacture a substance that inhibits protein synthesis.
Accumulation of random errors (disposable soma)	Random mutations progressively accumulate during transcription or translation. Random errors in protein synthesis ultimately impair cellular function.
Error catastrophe (obligate aging)	Cells develop serious defects in genes that normally repair errors in DNA synthesis or in transcription, resulting in faulty protein synthesis or function.
Free radical oxidative damage (waste product accumulation)	Oxygen free radicals produced during oxidative metabolism or resulting from radiation exposure may result in damage to DNA, particularly mitochondrial DNA.
Telomere shorting	Duplication of DNA during cell division is incomplete in somatic cells, leading to shortening of chromosome ends (telomeres). Length of telomeres is proportionate to remaining replicative capacity. Telomerase protects against shortening in germ and stem cells.
Decreased heat shock response	Heat shock proteins, which mediate the cellular response to various stressors, exhibit reduced expression with aging.
Glycosylation of proteins and nucleic acids (cross-linkage)	Advanced glycosylation end (AGE) products increase with age, cross-linking proteins (e.g., collagen) and nucleic acids and altering their function.
Age-of-onset modifier	Modifier genes, which normally suppress degenerative effects, are inactivated because reproductive potential has been exhausted.
Rate of living	Life span is inversely related to the metabolic rate of the organism.
Endocrine deficiency	The endocrine system acts as a pacemaker for aging.
Neural pacemaker	The central nervous system determines the time of onset of aging and the rate at which it proceeds.
Immune system decline	Decline of immune function results in decreased defense and increased autoantibody formation.

ing shortening. Cancer cells that express telomerase display an unlimited capacity to reproduce.[19] The potential for therapeutic manipulation of telomerase—whether for inhibition of cancer growth or for slowing the aging process—is the subject of intense investigation.[20, 21]

Oxidative stress theories are derived from the knowledge that reactive oxygen species (oxygen free radicals) are generated randomly in any cell with oxidative metabolism (see Chapter 3). These are believed to be potentially damaging to the cell due to their abilities to combine chemically with enzymes and structural proteins and to induce breaks in DNA. Mitochondrial DNA is believed to be particularly vulnerable to this damage because of its proximity to the oxidative metabolism machinery.[14] Antioxidant enzymes, such as superoxide dismutase, normally clear most of these radicals before they damage cells, but activity of these enzyme systems decreases with age. Lipofuscin, the purported biomarker of aging, is thought to be an auto-oxidation product of lipids, proteins, and possibly DNA.

Genetic program theories propose that aging is genetically controlled by regulatory processes that turn off expression of some genes and turn on others. The primary evidence supporting this idea is the observation of extreme variability in maximum life span among mammalian species (a range of 2 to 100 years). In addition, it has been consistently observed that life span is proportional to time span between birth and sexual maturity in all mammalian species, suggesting a developmental basis for longevity. Proponents of these theories frequently study patients with progeria, accelerated aging due to a known genetic defect (Fig. 6–10). Interestingly, progeria patients display pronounced shortening of chromosomal telomeres.[22]

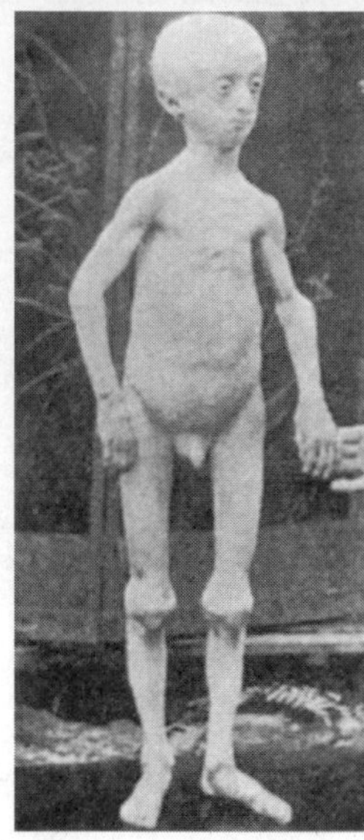

FIGURE 6–10
Child with progeria. This patient is 17 years old.

Genetically Determined Changes in Functional Capacity

It is well accepted that the capacity of cells to divide is finite, and the function of telomeres has been referred to as the "cellular clock." At the systemic level, biologic clocks are believed to reside in the nervous, endocrine, and immune systems.[23]

Research focused on the aging nervous system has established that there are consistent changes in the amounts of the neurotransmitters dopamine, norepinephrine, and serotonin in the basal ganglia, cerebellum, and locus ceruleus. These changes could reasonably account for the tremors, gait disturbances, and sleep disorders that are common among the elderly. It has also been observed that cerebral cortex neurons in the aging brain shrink in volume and that glial cells proliferate. The significance of these findings is uncertain.[24]

Advancing age is also manifested as endocrine system changes, including decreased glucose tolerance and thyroid nodularity.[25] Declining immune function is consistently noted with aging, as evidenced by reduced response to infectious agents and allergens, by increased incidence of immune attacks on one's own tissues (autoimmunity), and possibly by decreased immune surveillance for tumor cells. Degeneration of the thymus gland, in which certain immune cells mature, occurs at puberty and apparently represents genetically programmed apoptosis. The observed decrease in immune function is consistent with the idea that aging is due to a decline in cellular proliferation.

Systemic Manifestations of Aging

Morbidity associated with aging typically displays one of three patterns: (1) progressive illness leading to rapid functional decline (e.g., Alzheimer's disease), (2) a catastrophic event leading to a temporary decline in function, which improves with rehabilitation (e.g., stroke or hip fracture), or (3) "normal" aging, with gradual progressive functional decline.[26]

Table 6–9 summarizes organ-specific changes attributable to primary aging and to secondary age-

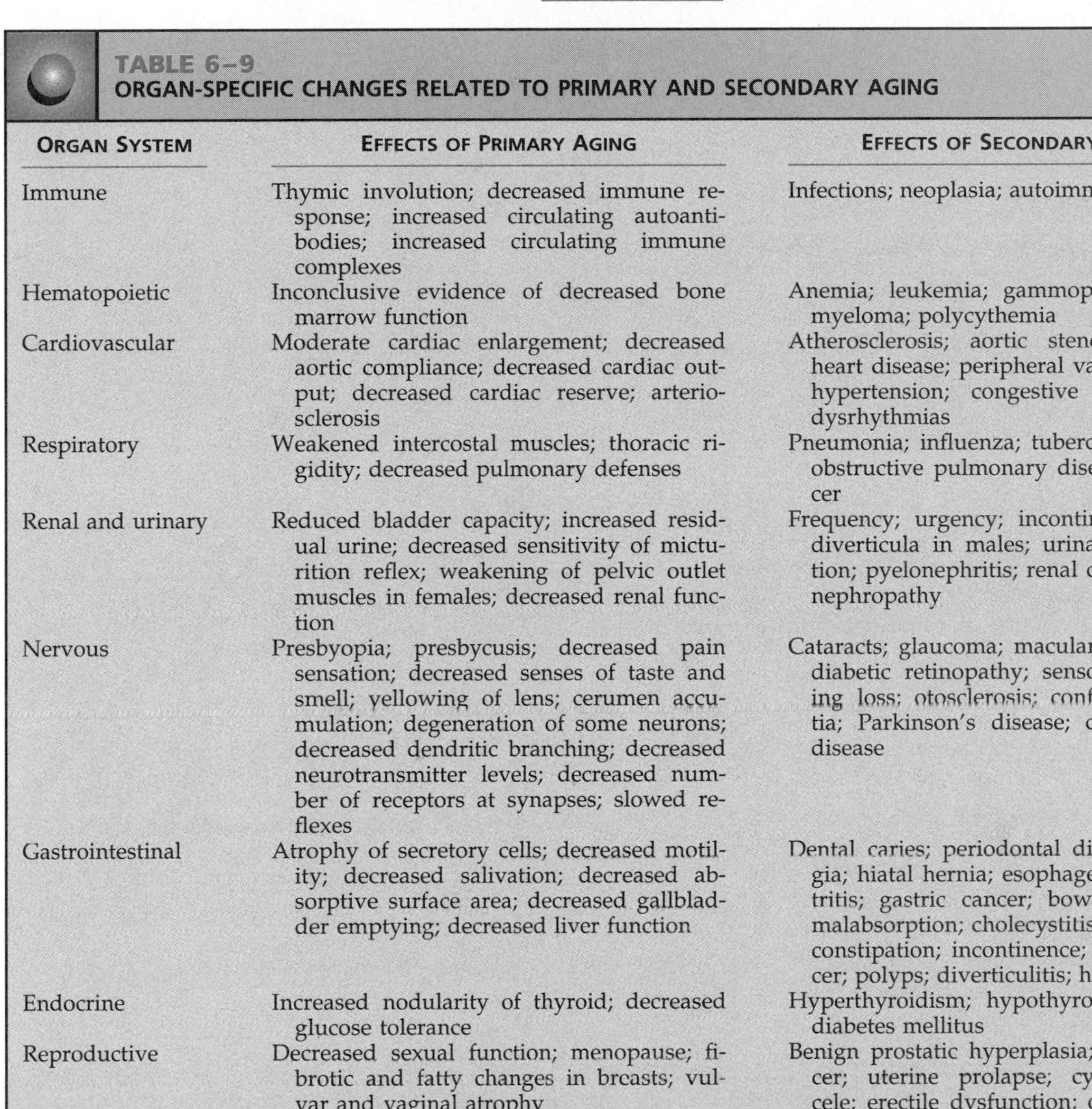

TABLE 6–9
ORGAN-SPECIFIC CHANGES RELATED TO PRIMARY AND SECONDARY AGING

Organ System	Effects of Primary Aging	Effects of Secondary Aging
Immune	Thymic involution; decreased immune response; increased circulating autoantibodies; increased circulating immune complexes	Infections; neoplasia; autoimmune disorders
Hematopoietic	Inconclusive evidence of decreased bone marrow function	Anemia; leukemia; gammopathy; multiple myeloma; polycythemia
Cardiovascular	Moderate cardiac enlargement; decreased aortic compliance; decreased cardiac output; decreased cardiac reserve; arteriosclerosis	Atherosclerosis; aortic stenosis; coronary heart disease; peripheral vascular disease; hypertension; congestive heart failure; dysrhythmias
Respiratory	Weakened intercostal muscles; thoracic rigidity; decreased pulmonary defenses	Pneumonia; influenza; tuberculosis; chronic obstructive pulmonary disease; lung cancer
Renal and urinary	Reduced bladder capacity; increased residual urine; decreased sensitivity of micturition reflex; weakening of pelvic outlet muscles in females; decreased renal function	Frequency; urgency; incontinence; bladder diverticula in males; urinary tract infection; pyelonephritis; renal calculi; diabetic nephropathy
Nervous	Presbyopia; presbycusis; decreased pain sensation; decreased senses of taste and smell; yellowing of lens; cerumen accumulation; degeneration of some neurons; decreased dendritic branching; decreased neurotransmitter levels; decreased number of receptors at synapses; slowed reflexes	Cataracts; glaucoma; macular degeneration; diabetic retinopathy; sensorineural hearing loss; otosclerosis; confusion; dementia; Parkinson's disease; cerebrovascular disease
Gastrointestinal	Atrophy of secretory cells; decreased motility; decreased salivation; decreased absorptive surface area; decreased gallbladder emptying; decreased liver function	Dental caries; periodontal disease; dysphagia; hiatal hernia; esophageal cancer; gastritis; gastric cancer; bowel obstruction; malabsorption; cholecystitis; cholelithiasis; constipation; incontinence; colorectal cancer; polyps; diverticulitis; hemorrhoids
Endocrine	Increased nodularity of thyroid; decreased glucose tolerance	Hyperthyroidism; hypothyroidism; type II diabetes mellitus
Reproductive	Decreased sexual function; menopause; fibrotic and fatty changes in breasts; vulvar and vaginal atrophy	Benign prostatic hyperplasia; prostatic cancer; uterine prolapse; cystocele; rectocele; erectile dysfunction; ovarian cancer; breast cancer
Musculoskeletal	Diminished bone mass; loss of muscle mass; limited joint mobility; stooped posture; shortened stature	Osteoarthritis; rheumatoid arthritis; gout; osteoporosis; falls; fractures; Paget's disease
Integumentary	Uneven pigmentation; dryness and wrinkling; flattening of epidermal junction; hair loss and graying; increased epidermal turnover; decreased immune function of Langerhans cells; decreased dermal vasculature; decreased subcutaneous fat; decreased sweating	Hypothermia; hyperthermia; xerosis; pruritus; skin tumors; pressure sores; herpes zoster virus; photoaging

related disease. It is apparent that many of these are clearly related to decreased cellular proliferation, such as poor wound healing, decreased immune response, muscle atrophy, lens degeneration with cataracts, osteoporosis with loss of bone density, and decreased glucose tolerance due to deficiency of pancreatic β cells. Many other disorders do not fit this model, however, and appear to represent *hyper*proliferation instead. Examples include cancer, benign prostatic hyperplasia, degenerative joint disease, and many skin lesions of aging. It is possible that these represent abnormal responses of cells to signals that, in younger people, induce normal cell division or adaptive apoptosis.

DEVELOPMENTAL FOUNDATIONS OF DISEASE AND INTERVENTION

Medical genetics, the science of biologic variation as it relates to health and disease,[27] has developed its knowledge base during the past 40 years. Technology allows prenatal diagnosis and, in some cases, prenatal treatment of developmental diseases[28] (see Chapter 33). The human genome has been extensively mapped, with more than 800 loci linked to specific disorders.[27] At each of these loci, multiple variants of mutations are being identified. More than 300 different types of mutations are known to be possible at the locus associated with cystic fibrosis, for example.

Recombinant DNA technology, through which virtually unlimited supplies of exact copies of naturally occurring proteins can be generated, has greatly enhanced the treatment of diabetes, thrombosis, hemophilia, and other disorders. This technology was made possible by the identification of *restriction endonuclease* enzymes, which are capable of cleaving double-stranded DNA into fragments.[29] Specific segments encoding the protein of interest may then be inserted into a *vector system*, usually bacterial plasmids (double-stranded circular DNA molecules), which duplicate outside the chromosomes of the bacterial host. Recombinant agents approved by the Food and Drug Administration are listed in Table 6–10 along with the disorders for which they are indicated.

TABLE 6–10
THERAPEUTIC AGENTS DERIVED FROM RECOMBINANT DNA

Agent	Therapeutic Use
Hepatitis B vaccine	Hepatitis B prophylaxis
Insulin	Diabetes mellitus
Tissue plasminogen activator (t-PA)	Coronary thrombosis, pulmonary embolism
Growth hormone	Growth hormone deficiency, constitutional short stature
Erythropoietin	Anemia
Factor VIII	Hemophilia
Interferons	Viral disease, neoplasia
Colony-stimulating factors	Bone marrow depression
Interleukins	Immune deficiency

TABLE 6–11
MODES OF GENE THERAPY

Mode	Description and Use
Ex vivo (outside the living body)	Cells with defective genes are removed from the patient and injected with normal genes before being returned to the body. Primary use has been for treatment of hematopoietic disorders, such as severe combined immunodeficiency (SCID).
In situ (in position)	Carriers bearing corrective genes are introduced directly into the tissue where the genes are needed. Primary use is for localized disorders, such as cystic fibrosis. "Suicide carriers," carrying genes intended to induce apoptosis, have been inserted into tumor cells.
In vivo (inside the living body)	Gene carriers are injected into the bloodstream, from which they target specific cells and transfer their genetic information. This mode is in development but not yet in experimental use.

Data from Anderson, W.F. (1995). Gene therapy. *Scientific American* 272(9), 124–128.

Gene therapy is in its early, experimental stages but shows much promise. Potential applications exist for prevention and treatment of congenital disorders, age-related degenerative disorders, and immune-mediated disease. The three modes of gene therapy being developed are detailed in Table 6–11. Gene therapy of defective body cells affects only the patient being treated and has been most beneficial for disorders of bone marrow stem cells. Gene therapy of germ cell disorders affects the progeny of the patient, raising ethical issues with respect to "designing" the next generation.[30] These concerns notwithstanding, molecular diagnosis and treatment of disease represent the new frontier in health care, holding much promise for the prevention and treatment of the more than 5000 diseases that have been attributed to faulty genetic regulation of cell development.[31]

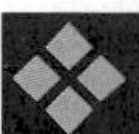

Summary of Key Points

- The primary cellular developmental processes are cell division, growth, differentiation, and apoptosis.
- The genetic material of the cell includes the nucleic acids DNA and RNA. DNA strands in the nucleus are wound around protein cores in the chromosomes, which include 22 pairs of autosomes and one pair of sex chromosomes. The base sequence on DNA determines the genetic code. Messenger RNA transcribes the code and carries it to the cytoplasm, where tRNA and rRNA mediate subsequent protein synthesis.
- Transcription occurs when DNA strands separate, exposing the bases. Regulated by protein transcription factors, RNA polymerase directs synthesis of a complementary mRNA strand from each DNA template. After enzymatic modification, the mRNA strand diffuses into the cytoplasm. Assembly of proteins (translation) occurs on the ribosomes, mediated by tRNA. Transfer RNA links mRNA base codons with appropriate amino acids. Ribosomes, consisting of rRNA and proteins, link the amino acids into peptide chains, thus translating the genetic code into protein.
- The cell cycle begins with phase G_1 (first growth or gap phase) and proceeds to the synthetic phase, S, during which DNA replicates. G_2, the second growth or gap phase, follows, further preparing the cell for division. Actual division (mitosis) occurs during the M phase. Phase transition is promoted or inhibited through the actions of transcription factors. These factors are either activated or inactivated by a family of cyclin-dependent kinase (CDK) enzymes.
- The four tissue types are epithelial, connective, muscle, and nervous tissues. Epithelial tissue forms linings, coverings, and glands. Connective tissue binds and supports other tissues. Muscle contraction is essential to movement, whereas nervous tissue serves an information-processing function.
- Necrosis is injury-induced cell death, mediated by inflammatory cytokines. Apoptosis is initiated by a genetic signal and may be genetically programmed or induced by injury in which DNA is damaged.
- The preembryonic period consists of the first 2 weeks of gestation and includes fertilization, cleavage of the zygote, blastocyst formation, implantation, and formation of the double-layered embryonic disk. The embryonic period follows, during weeks 3 through 8, and includes gastrulation, notochord formation, neural tube formation, somite development, development of the intraembryonic coelom, angiogenesis, and organ system differentiation. Fetal development occurs from the 9th week through term and includes the period of rapid organ system growth.
- The embryonic period is the most critical period of morphogenesis because most organ differentiation is occurring. Teratogenic insults are likely to result in major abnormalities.
- Primary aging is physiologic change attributable only to advancing age, while secondary aging refers to changes due to diseases that may or may not accompany aging.
- The major theories of aging include those related to impairment of cellular proliferation and those related to programmed decline in functional capacity. Cellular proliferation may be impaired by telomere shortening, oxidative damage to DNA, or programmed changes in genetic regulation. Pacemaker theories of aging focus on systemic rather than cellular change and refer to predictable (probably programmed) changes in the function of the body's regulatory systems.
- Common systemic manifestations of aging include those consistent with decreased cellular proliferation, including poor wound healing, decreased immune response, muscle atrophy, cataracts, osteoporosis, and decreased glucose tolerance, as well as those consistent with increased cellular proliferation, including cancer, prostatic hypertrophy, osteoarthritis (degenerative joint disease), and skin lesions.
- Important advances in medical genetics include (1) the capacity to diagnose and treat many genetic disorders prenatally, (2) the technology to produce therapeutic agents using recombinant DNA, and (3) the ability to alter defective genes through gene therapy.

REFERENCES

1. Rosenthal, N. (1994). DNA and the genetic code. *New England Journal of Medicine* 331(1), 39–41.
2. Lodish, H., Baltimore, D., Berk, A., *et al.* (1995). *Molecular Cell Biology.* (3rd ed.). New York: Scientific American Books. (pp. 307, 492, 504).
3. Cox, D.R., Green, E.D., Lander, E.S., *et al.* (1994). Assessing mapping progress in the Human Genome Project. *Science* 265, 2031–2032.
4. Papavassiliou, A.G. (1995). Molecular medicine: Transcription factors. *New England Journal of Medicine* 332(1), 45–47.
5. Rosenthal, N. (1994). Regulation of gene expression. *New England Journal of Medicine* 331(14), 931–933.
6. Hill, C.S., and Treisman, R. (1995). Transcription regulation by extracellular signals: Mechanisms and specificity. *Cell* 80, 199–211.
7. Tijan, R. (1995). Molecular machines that control genes. *Scientific American* 272(2), 54–61.
8. Baringa, M. (1995). A new twist to the cell cycle. *Science* 269, 631–632.
9. Cleaver, J.E. (1994). It was a very good year for DNA repair. *Cell* 76, 1–4.
10. Sancar, A. (1994). Mechanisms of DNA excision repair. *Science* 266, 1954–1956.
11. Sadowski, P.D. (1993). Site-specific genetic recombination: Hops, flips, and flops. *FASEB Journal* 7(9), 760–767.
12. Baringa, M. (1994). Cell suicide: By ICE, not fire. *Science* 263, 754–756.
13. Thompson, C.B. (1995). Apoptosis in the pathogenesis and treatment of disease. *Science* 267, 1456–1462.
14. Martin, G.R., Danner, D.B., and Holbrook, N.J. (1993). Aging: Causes and defenses. *Annual Review of Medicine* 44, 419–429.
15. Davies, I. (1992). Theories and general principles of aging. In: Brocklehurst, J.C., Tallis, R.C., and Fillit, H.M. (Eds.). *Textbook of Geriatric Medicine and Gerontology.* (4th ed.). Edinburgh: Churchill Livingstone. (pp. 26–60).
16. Butler, R.N. (1990). Foreword to the second edition. In: Cassel, C.K., Reisenberg, D.E., Sorensen, L.B., *et al.* (Eds.). *Geriatric Medicine.* (2nd ed.). New York: Springer-Verlag. (pp. vii–ix).
17. Perls, T.T. (1995). The oldest old. *Scientific American* 272(1), 70–75.
18. Fries, J.F. (1980). Aging, natural death, and the compression of morbidity. *New England Journal of Medicine* 303(3), 130–135.
19. Haber, D.A. (1995). Clinical implications of basic research: Telomeres, cancer, and immortality. *New England Journal of Medicine* 332(14), 955–956.
20. Kim, N.W., Piatyszck, M.A., Prowse, K.R., *et al.* Specific association of human telomerase activity with immortal cells and cancer. *Science* 266, 2011–2015.
21. Counter, C.M., Hirte, H.W., Bacchetti, S., *et al.* (1994). Telomerase activity in human ovarian carcinoma. *Proceedings of the National Academy of Sciences, U.S.A.* 91, 2900–2904.
22. Brown, W.T. (1992). Progeria: A human-disease model of accelerated aging. *American Journal of Clinical Nutrition* 55, 1222S–1224S.
23. Butler, R.N. (1994). Cycles, clocks, and power plants. *American Journal of Medicine* 97(suppl. 4A), 35S–39S.
24. Lewis, P.D. (1992). The neuropathology of old age. In: Brocklehurst, J.C., Tallis, R.C., and Fillet, H.M. (Eds.). *Textbook of Geriatric Medicine and Gerontology.* (4th ed.). Edinburgh: Churchill Livingstone. (pp. 258–279).
25. Kart, C.S., Metress, E.K., and Metress, S.P. (1992). *Human Aging and Chronic Disease.* Boston: Jones and Bartlett Publishers. (pp. 237–250).
26. Vellas, B.J., Albarede, J-L., and Garry, P.J. (1992). Diseases and aging. Patterns of morbidity with age: Relationship between aging and age-associated diseases. *American Journal of Clinical Nutrition* 55, 1225S–12230S.
27. McKusick, V.A. (1993). Medical genetics: A 40-year perspective on the evolution of a medical specialty from a basic science. *Journal of the American Medical Association* 270(19), 2351–2356.
28. Jones, S.L. (1994). Genetic-based and assisted reproductive technology of the 21st century. *Journal of Obstetric, Gynecologic, and Neonatal Nursing* 23(2), 160–165.
29. Carroll, W.L. (1993). Introduction to recombinant DNA technology. *American Journal of Clinical Nutrition* 58(suppl.), 249S–258S.
30. Caplan, A. (1995). An improved future? Medical advances challenge thinking on living, dying, and being human. *Scientific American* 272(3), 142–143.
31. Capecchi, M.R. (1994). Targetted gene replacement. *Scientific American* 270(3), 52–59.

SELECTED BIBLIOGRAPHY

Anderson, W.F. (1995). Gene therapy. *Scientific American* 272(9), 124–128.

Artavanis-Tsakonas, S., Matsuno, K., and Fortini, M.E. (1995). Notch signalling. *Science* 268, 225–232.

Blau, H.M., and Springer, M.L. (1995). Gene therapy: A novel form of drug delivery. *New England Journal of Medicine* 333(18), 1204–1207.

Brenner, M.K. (1996). Gene transfer to hematopoietic cells. *New England Journal of Medicine* 335(5), 337–339.

Caskey, C.T. (1993). Molecular medicine: A spin-off from the helix. *Journal of the American Medical Association* 269(15), 1986–1992.

Centers for Disease Control and Prevention. (1994). Mortality patterns: United States, 1992. *Morbidity and Mortality Weekly Report* 43(49), 916–920.

Creditor, M.C. (1993). Hazards of hospitalization of the elderly. *Annals of Internal Medicine* 118, 219–223.

Crystal, R.G. (1995). Transfer of genes to humans: Early lessons and obstacles to success. *Science* 270, 404–410.

Durfy, S.J. (1993). Ethics and the Human Genome Project. *Archives of Pathology and Laboratory Medicine* 117(5), 466–469.

Farabaugh, P.J. (1993). Alternative readings of the genetic code. *Cell* 74, 591–596.

Grody, W.W. (1993). Molecular genetics. *Archives of Pathology and Laboratory Medicine* 117(5), 470–472.

Guyton, A.C., and Hall, J.E. (1995). *Textbook of Medical Physiology.* (9th ed.). Philadelphia: W.B. Saunders Co.

Haidet, G.C., Wennberg, P.W., Finkelstein, S.M., *et al.* (1996). Effects of aging per se on arterial stiffness: Systemic and regional compliance in beagles. *American Heart Journal* 132, 319–327.

Hanawalt, P. (1994). Transcription-coupled repair and human disease. *Science* 266, 1957–1958.

Hannun, Y.A., and Obeid, L.M. (1995). Ceramide: An intracellular signal for apoptosis. *Trends in Biological Science* 20(2), 73–77.

Jazwinski, S.M. (1996). Longevity, genes, and aging. *Science* 273, 54–59.

Jentsch, S. (1996). When proteins receive deadly messages at birth. *Science* 271, 955–956.

Jiminez-Sanchez, A. (1995). On the origin and evolution of the genetic code. *Journal of Molecular Evolution* 41, 712–716.

Joseph, J.A., Cutler, R., and Roth, G.S. (1993). Changes in G protein-mediated signal transduction in aging and Alzheimer's disease. *Annals of the New York Academy of Sciences* 695, 42–45.

Larsen, P.D., and Martin, J.H. (1994). Renal system changes in the elderly. *AORN Journal* 60(2), 298–301.

Latchman, D.S. (1996). Transcription-factor mutations and disease. *New England Journal of Medicine* 334(1), 28–33.

Leigh, J.P., and Fries, J.F. (1994). Education, gender, and the compression of morbidity. *International Journal of Aging and Human Development* 39(3), 233–246.

Lemon, B.D., and Freedman, L.P. (1996). Selective effects of ligands on vitamin D_3 receptor- and retinoid X receptor-mediated gene activation in vivo. *Molecular and Cellular Biology* 16(3), 1006–1016.

Lingner, J., Cooper, J.P., and Cech, T.R. (1995). Telomerase and DNA end replication: No longer a lagging strand problem? *Science* 269, 1533–1534.

Lithgow, G.J., and Kirkwood, T.B.L. (1996). Mechanisms and evolution of aging. *Science* 273, 80.

McConkey, E.H. (1993). *Human Genetics: The Molecular Revolution.* Boston: Jones and Bartlett Publishers.

McKim, K.S., and Hawley, R.S. (1995). Chromosomal control of meiotic cell division. *Science* 270, 1595–1601.

Moore, K.L., and Persaud, T.V.N. (1993). *The Developing Human: Clinically Oriented Embryology.* Philadelphia: W.B. Saunders Co.

Nagata, S., and Goldstein, P. (1995). The *fas* death factor. *Science* 267, 1449–1456.

National Center for Health Statistics. (1989). Advance report of final mortality statistics, 1987. *Monthly Vital Statistics Report* 38(5 suppl.).

Papaconstantinou, J. (1994). Unifying model of the programmed (intrinsic) and stochastic (extrinsic) theories of aging: The stress response genes, signal transduction-redox pathways and aging. *Annals of the New York Academy of Sciences* 719, 195–211.

Pluta, A.F., Mackay, A.M., Ainsztein, A.M., *et al.* (1995). The centromere: Hub of chromosomal activities. *Science* 270, 1591–1594.

Portin, P. (1993). The concept of the gene: Short history and present status. *Quarterly Review of Biology* 68(2), 173–223.

Raff, B.S. (1994). Nursing and genetics for the 21st century. *Journal of Obstetric, Gynecologic, and Neonatal Nursing* 23(6), 477–480.

Rothwell, N.V. (1993). *Understanding Genetics: A Molecular Approach.* New York: Wiley-Liss.

Saks, M.E., Sampson, J.R., and Abelson, J.N. (1994). The transfer RNA identity problem: A search for rules. *Science* 263, 191–197.

Sarkisian, C.A., and Lachs, M.S. (1996). "Failure to thrive" in older adults. *Annals of Internal Medicine* 124, 1072–1078.

Schimmel, P., and de Pouplana, L.R. (1995). Transfer RNA: From minihelix to genetic code. *Cell* 81, 983–986.

Schimmel, P., Giege, R., Moras, D., *et al.* (1993). An operational RNA code for amino acids and possible relationship to genetic code. *Proceedings of the National Academy of Sciences, U.S.A. 90, 8763–8768.*

Schwartz, R.S. (1995). Molecular medicine: Jumping genes. *New England Journal of Medicine* 332(14), 941–944.

Scriver, C.R., Beudeaut, A.L., Sly, W.S., *et al.* (1995). *The Metabolic and Molecular Bases of Inherited Disease.* (7th ed.). New York: McGraw-Hill.

Sohal, R.S., and Weindruch, R. (1996). Oxidative stress, caloric restriction, and aging. *Science* 273, 59–63.

Smith, J.R., and Pereira-Smith, O.M. (1996). Replicative senescence: Implications for in vivo aging and tumor suppression. *Science* 273, 63–67.

Steller, H. (1995). Mechanisms and genes of cellular suicide. *Science* 267, 1445–1449.

Tamir, A., and Isakov, N. (1994). Cyclic AMP inhibits phosphatidylinositol-coupled and -uncoupled mitogenic signals in T lymphocytes. *Journal of Immunology* 152, 3391–3399.

Tokita, A., Kelly, P.J., Nguyen, T.V., *et al.* (1994). Genetic influences on type I collagen synthesis and degradation: Further evidence for genetic regulation of bone turnover. *Journal of Clinical Endocrinology and Metabolism* 78, 1461–1466.

Troncale, J.A. (1996). The aging process: Physiologic changes and pharmacologic implications. *Postgraduate Medicine* 99(5), 111–122.

Vaux, D.L., Haecker, G., and Strasser, A. (1994). An evolutionary perspective on apoptosis. *Cell* 76, 777–779.

Wise, P.M., Krajnak, K.M., and Kashon, M.L. (1996). Menopause: The aging of multiple pacemakers. *Science* 273, 67–70.

Wivel, N.A., and Walters, L. (1993). Germ-line gene modification and disease prevention: Some medical and ethical perspectives. *Science* 262, 533–538.

Zakian, V. (1995). Telomeres: Beginning to understand the end. *Science* 270, 1601–1607.

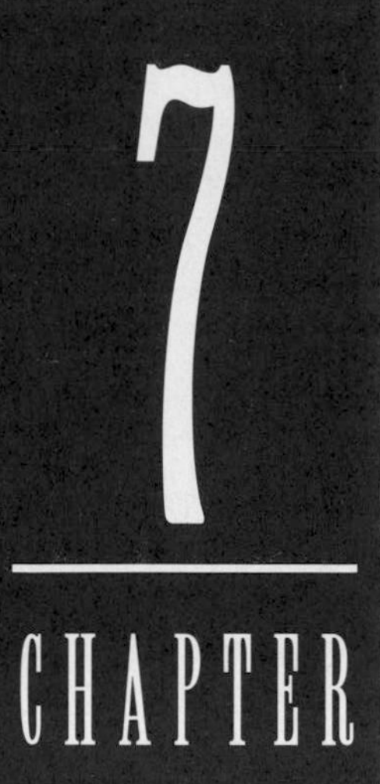

Cellular Development: Congenital Defects and Neoplasia

LEARNING OBJECTIVES

1. Differentiate between physiologic and pathologic forms of atrophy and hypertrophy.
2. Identify the major teratogens and the conditions with which they are associated.
3. Identify the principal mechanisms of single gene mutations.
4. Identify the major mechanisms of chromosomal defects.
5. Comprehend the mendelian principles of inheritance.
6. Differentiate between benign and malignant neoplasms.
7. Identify the major risk factors for cancer.
8. Describe the cellular processes underlying neoplastic transformation.
9. Comprehend the pathophysiologic processes of cancer growth and metastasis.
10. Identify clinical manifestations common to many forms of cancer.
11. Describe the principal modes of cancer prevention and treatment.

key terms

anaphase lag
aneuploid
aplasia
atrophy
autosomal dominant
autosomal recessive
benign
cancer
carcinogen
carcinoma
chromosomal defect
de novo
dysplasia
dystrophy
expressivity
frame shift
genetic polymorphism
genogram
genomic imprinting
genotype
heterozygous
homozygous
hyperplasia
hypertrophy
hypoplasia
karyotype
malignant

mendelian disorder
metastasize
mosaicism
multifactorial inheritance
neoplasia
nondisjunction
neoplasm
oncogene
organomegaly
penetrance
phenotype
point mutation
proto-oncogene
sarcoma
sex-linked
single gene mutation
trisomy
tumor
tumor-associated antigen
tumor suppressor gene
X-linked

Developmental diseases include all disorders of genetic regulation of cellular development, whether apparent at birth or manifesting later in life. These disorders result from irreparable damage to DNA, arising with the affected individual or inherited from one or both parents. The mechanisms of genetic mutation and principles of inheritance described in this chapter are applicable not only to individual humans but also to individual cells and their progeny.

Disorders of cellular growth and development may result from abnormal cell size, number, or differentiation. **Dystrophy** and **dysplasia** are general terms for such conditions. **Neoplasia** (new cell growth) refers to proliferation of abnormal cells and includes both benign and malignant (cancerous) tumors.

Atrophy refers to a decrease in either number or size of cells, with resultant decrease in organ or tissue size. Physiologic atrophy occurs as a result of normally programmed development, as is the case during the embryonic and fetal periods. Pathologic atrophy occurs with poor perfusion of cells, as in starvation or ischemic conditions, or with many idiopathic disorders, such as osteoporosis and some dementias. Disuse atrophy of muscles occurs secondary to immobilization. The terms **hypoplasia** and **aplasia** are also used to describe decreased numbers of cells, particularly with reference to blood cells.

Hypertrophy is an increase in the size of cells, whereas **hyperplasia** refers to an increase in the number of cells. These terms are frequently used interchangeably in clinical settings. True hypertrophy is seen only in muscle, as a response to increased resistance to muscle work. Hyperplasia occurs in many tissue types and usually represents an adaptive response to demands for increased tissue function. In some cases, such as in benign prostatic hyperplasia, the stimulus for increased cell proliferation is unknown. Organ enlargement (**organomegaly**) is frequently due to hyperplasia, although it could also result from engorgement of the organ with fluid, from hypertrophy of muscle tissue within the organ, or from inappropriate new growth of cells (e.g., cancer). Cardiomegaly (heart), splenomegaly (spleen), and hepatomegaly (liver) are common manifestations of clinical disorders.

BPH

The emphasis in this chapter is on genetically induced abnormalities in cell development, specifically defects that manifest at birth and defects that result in the initiation and promotion of cancer.

GENETIC AND CONGENITAL DEFECTS

Congenital defects are present at birth. Frequently, these anomalies arise as a consequence of genetic defects, but this is not always the case. Congenital anomalies may also result when genetically normal fetuses do not receive adequate blood or nutrient supply due to maternal or placental factors, or with complications of labor or delivery (see Chapter 33).

Most congenital defects have a genetic mechanism, with the defect originating within the affected person or inherited from one or both parents. In many cases, however, there is no known exposure to a mutation-inducing agent, nor is there a clear pattern of inheritance.

Teratogenesis

A *teratogen* is any environmental agent that permanently harms the developing fetus.[1] Teratogens can cause congenital structural or functional defects, spontaneous abortion, complications of labor and delivery, or defects that become evident later in development, such as cognitive or behavioral problems or neoplastic transformations. Table 7–1 lists many known teratogens and the conditions with which they are associated.

As discussed in Chapter 6, the timing of exposure to teratogens is important. During the first 2 weeks after conception, significant teratogenic exposure results in loss of the embryo. The embryonic period, when major organ systems are differentiating, is the

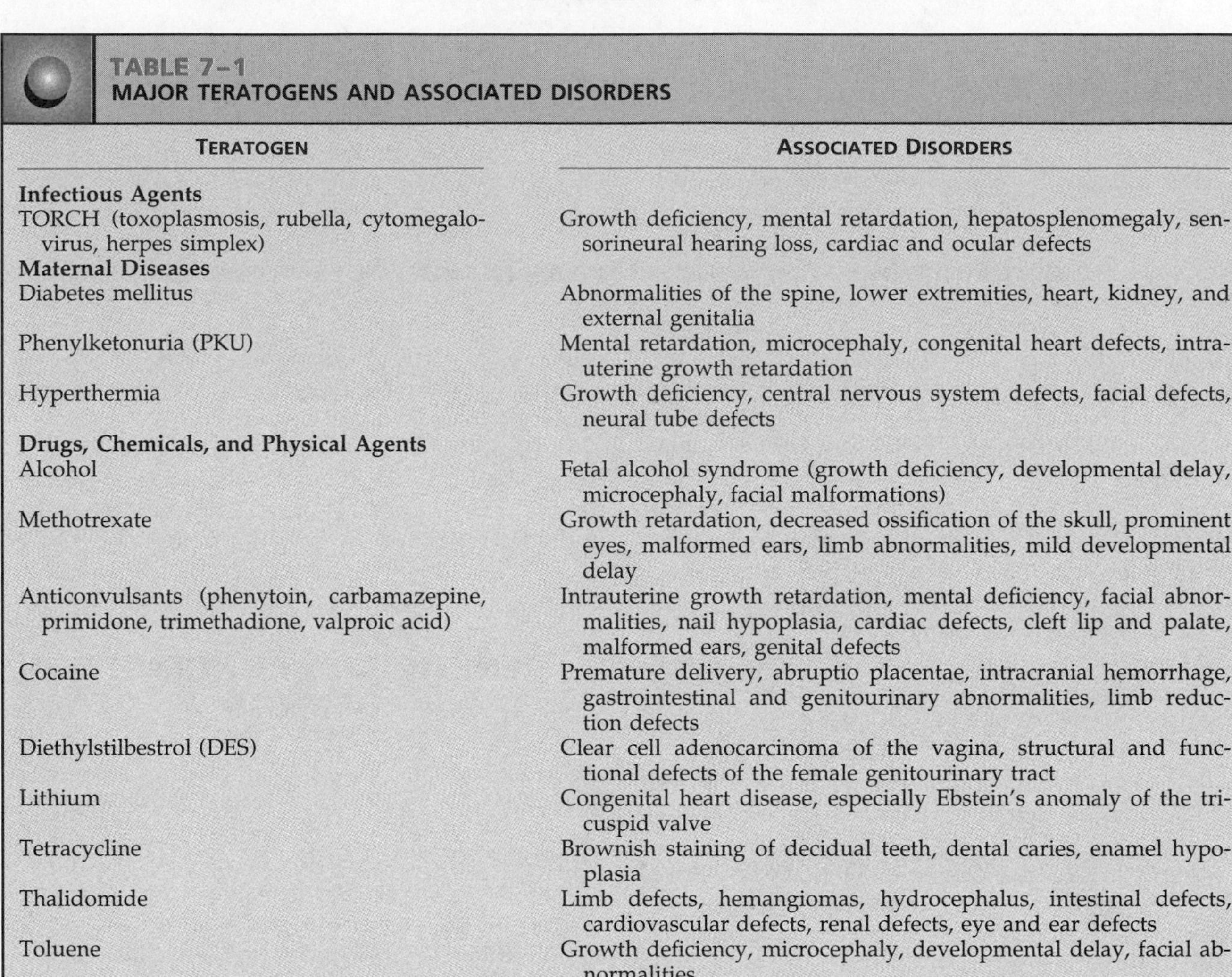

TABLE 7–1
MAJOR TERATOGENS AND ASSOCIATED DISORDERS

Teratogen	Associated Disorders
Infectious Agents	
TORCH (toxoplasmosis, rubella, cytomegalovirus, herpes simplex)	Growth deficiency, mental retardation, hepatosplenomegaly, sensorineural hearing loss, cardiac and ocular defects
Maternal Diseases	
Diabetes mellitus	Abnormalities of the spine, lower extremities, heart, kidney, and external genitalia
Phenylketonuria (PKU)	Mental retardation, microcephaly, congenital heart defects, intrauterine growth retardation
Hyperthermia	Growth deficiency, central nervous system defects, facial defects, neural tube defects
Drugs, Chemicals, and Physical Agents	
Alcohol	Fetal alcohol syndrome (growth deficiency, developmental delay, microcephaly, facial malformations)
Methotrexate	Growth retardation, decreased ossification of the skull, prominent eyes, malformed ears, limb abnormalities, mild developmental delay
Anticonvulsants (phenytoin, carbamazepine, primidone, trimethadione, valproic acid)	Intrauterine growth retardation, mental deficiency, facial abnormalities, nail hypoplasia, cardiac defects, cleft lip and palate, malformed ears, genital defects
Cocaine	Premature delivery, abruptio placentae, intracranial hemorrhage, gastrointestinal and genitourinary abnormalities, limb reduction defects
Diethylstilbestrol (DES)	Clear cell adenocarcinoma of the vagina, structural and functional defects of the female genitourinary tract
Lithium	Congenital heart disease, especially Ebstein's anomaly of the tricuspid valve
Tetracycline	Brownish staining of decidual teeth, dental caries, enamel hypoplasia
Thalidomide	Limb defects, hemangiomas, hydrocephalus, intestinal defects, cardiovascular defects, renal defects, eye and ear defects
Toluene	Growth deficiency, microcephaly, developmental delay, facial abnormalities
Vitamin A derivatives (isotretinoin, etretinate)	Facial defects, cardiac defects, central nervous system defects, thymic defects
Warfarin	Intrauterine growth retardation, mental retardation, seizures, nasal hypoplasia, abnormal calcification of axial skeleton
Radiation	Microcephaly, mental retardation

Data from Seaver, L.H., and Hoyme, H.E. (1992). Teratology in pediatric practice. *Pediatric Clinics of North America* 39(1), 111–134.

most critical period with regard to birth defects. Specific organ systems are more vulnerable when they are actively differentiating (e.g., the heart during weeks 3 to 6, the limbs during weeks 4 to 7, and the palate during weeks 6 to 8). During the fetal period, organ differentiation is complete, but the central nervous system is still maturing. Teratogenic insult during this period usually results in minor structural defects but may cause intrauterine growth retardation or cognitive abnormalities. The major categories of teratogens are infectious agents, maternal systemic diseases, and drugs, chemicals, and physical agents. Although research in this area is problematic because of the many variables involved, teratogenic exposures are believed to represent no more than a 5% to 10% risk of birth defects, as compared with the general population risk of 3% to 5%.[1]

Infectious Agents

One half to one fourth of infants born to women who contract rubella (German measles) in the first trimester of pregnancy exhibit birth defects of tissues arising from mesoderm.[1] These include cataracts, heart defects, and deafness. The widespread use of the measles, mumps, and rubella (MMR) vaccine has decreased the incidence of these conditions in the United States since its introduction in 1963.[2] The most common teratogenic infection is cytomegalovirus, a herpesvirus that may induce microcephaly and microphthalmia (small brain and eyes) or other ectodermal defects in infants of women who are infected in the second or third trimester.[3] Earlier infection usually results in spontaneous abortion. Human immunodeficiency virus (HIV), the virus that causes acquired immunodeficiency syndrome (AIDS), produces immune system and neurologic system defects in infants who contract the disease through maternal blood.

Maternal Diseases

Noninfectious disorders that can induce fetal malformations include: hyperthermia, folic acid deficiency, and obesity, which have been associated with neural tube defects[4]; diabetes mellitus, which is associated with a variety of defects, particularly of the heart; and phenylketonuria (PKU), which can result in microcephaly and heart defects.[5]

Drugs, Chemicals, and Physical Agents

Many drugs have significant teratogenic potential. Alcohol is the most frequently implicated cause of mental retardation in the Western world.[6] Drugs such as cyclophosphamide and vincristine, used in the treatment of cancer, also damage DNA and are thus highly teratogenic. Other notable teratogenic drugs include retinoic acid, used in the treatment of acne, and phenytoin, an anticonvulsant agent.[7]

Ionizing radiation induces DNA breaks in rapidly dividing cells. This is the reason for its use as a therapeutic agent in cancer, but it also potentially affects the cells of the developing embryo. Infants born to women exposed to radiation after the atomic bombing of Hiroshima and Nagasaki during World War II and after the more recent Chernobyl nuclear disaster exhibited many birth defects, particularly microcephaly and skeletal malformations.[8] X-ray exposure during pregnancy is contraindicated because of this risk, and extensive safety measures are indicated for the protection of those who may be exposed to radiation as a consequence of their occupations.

Genetic Variation and Abnormality

Two types of alterations can occur in the genetic material of cells: **single gene mutations** and **chromosomal defects**. Although genetic diseases (birth defects and neoplasia) are emphasized in this chapter, it must be noted that most genetic alterations do not result in disease. In some cases, the resulting protein synthesis is not sufficiently altered to affect the **phenotype**, or manifested expression of the gene; in other cases, the change is consistent with normal variation of traits within a population. Normal variation **(genetic polymorphism)** refers to the presence, within a population, of multiple alleles (gene structures) at specific genetic loci and is believed to apply to at least one third of the human genome.[9]

Single Gene Mutations

A mutation is an alteration in the normal sequence of bases on a region of DNA. Mutations may be **point mutations**, in which one base pair is substituted for another, or **frame shifts**, in which insertion or deletion of a base pair results in misreading of the triplets during transcription and translation (Fig. 7–1). In some cases, entire genes or large parts of genes are deleted or duplicated. Because the ge-

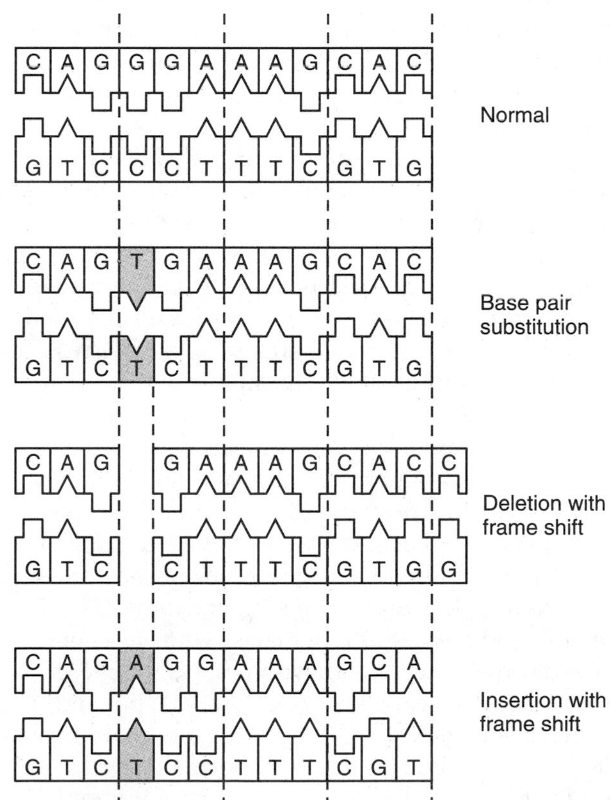

FIGURE 7–1
Single gene defects. Mutations within coding sequences of DNA result in abnormal protein synthesis. Point mutations result when one base pair is substituted for another. Frame shifts, which result in misreading of the sequence during transcription, may be due to insertion or deletion of base pairs.

netic code determines protein synthesis, mutations potentially result in production of abnormal structural elements of cells or in impaired synthesis of regulatory proteins such as enzymes.

Two mechanisms may result in single gene mutations: replication error or induction by a mutation-causing agent, or mutagen. As discussed in Chapter 6, random errors in nucleotide sequence occur during replication of DNA before cell division. Normally, these are repaired by editing and enzymatic repair systems, but when a nonlethal error persists, it is passed on to the cell's progeny when the cell divides. Mutagens may result in chemical alteration of DNA bases or proteins, in formation of DNA adducts (chemical additions to DNA), or in sequence alterations, all of which potentially affect subsequent protein synthesis.

Chromosomal Defects

Chromosomal defects (cytogenetic disorders) are abnormalities of number or structure of chromosomes and can occur in autosomes, sex chromosomes, or both within the same person. These disorders usually result in multiple anomalies because several genes can be affected. Chromosomal abnormalities result from missegregation (unequal separation) or from rearrangement of chromosomal structures during cell division.

Numeric Abnormalities. Abnormalities in the number of chromosomes are the result of missegregation. Mechanisms include **anaphase lag,** in which one chromosome (in meiosis) or one chromatid (in mitosis) lags behind and is left out of the nucleus of the daughter cell or gamete; and **nondisjunction,** the failure of chromatid pairs to separate, resulting in unequal numbers of chromosomes in daughter cells (Fig. 7–2).

Any cell containing neither the diploid nor haploid number of chromosomes is said to be **aneuploid**. Examples of aneuploidy include Down's syndrome, called a **trisomy** because affected individuals have three copies of chromosome 21, an autosome (see Chapter 33); and Turner's syndrome (Fig. 7–3), which produces sterile females with just one sex chromosome (the XO **karyotype**). Klinefelter's syndrome results from the XXY karyotype and produces sterile males with some female characteristics (Fig. 7–4). Cells containing abnormal chromosomes divide if they are capable, resulting in populations of defective cells. In the case of any abnormality occurring *after* fertilization, a normal cell line would be dividing as well, resulting in a mixture of normal and abnormal karyotypes within the same person.

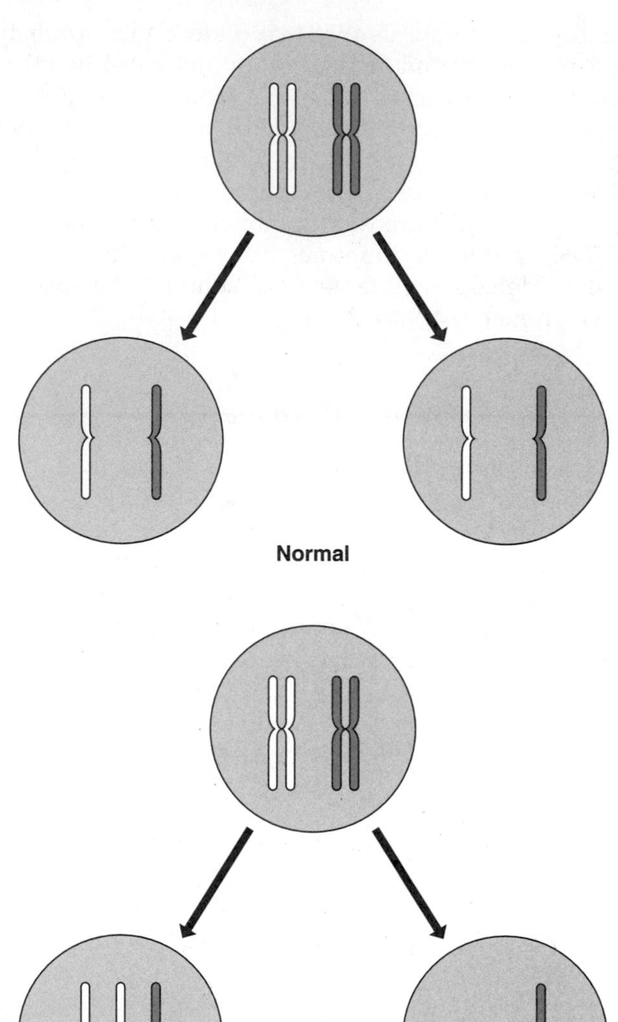

FIGURE 7–2
Nondisjunction. In this mechanism leading to numeric abnormality, chromatid pairs fail to separate during mitosis, leading to unequal numbers in daughter cells. Trisomy, shown on the left, may be compatible with life (*e.g.*, Down's syndrome). Monosomy, shown on the right, is usually lethal.

This state is referred to as **mosaicism**, and the severity of the anomalies depends in part on the ratio of normal to abnormal cells.[10] Table 7–2 summarizes features of the more common chromosomal disorders.

Structural Rearrangements. Figure 7–5 illustrates possible forms of chromosomal rearrangement. *Translocation* occurs when one chromosome breaks during cell division, and part of it becomes attached to another chromosome. If this rearrangement is balanced, that is, if genetic material is evenly ex-

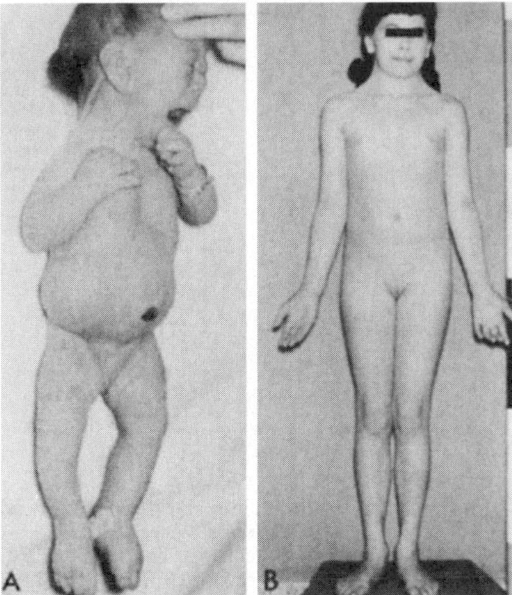

FIGURE 7–3
Turner's syndrome. The 45,XO karyotype produces a syndrome of short stature, webbed neck, and failure of sexual maturation in adult females. (From Moore, K.L. [1966]. *The Sex Chromatin.* Philadelphia: W.B. Saunders.)

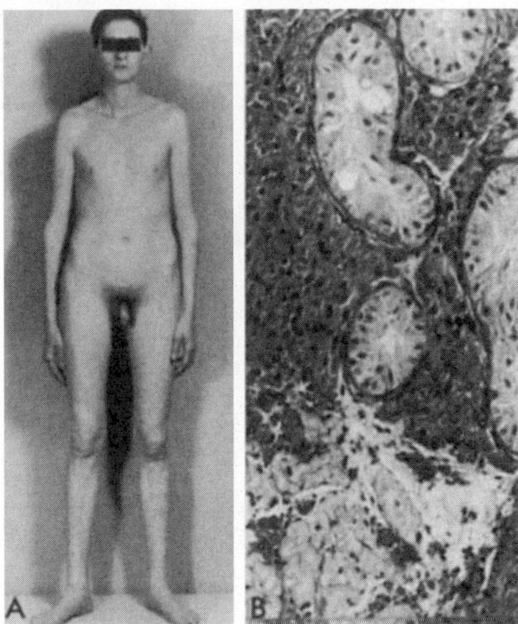

FIGURE 7–4
Klinefelter's syndrome. The 47,XXY karyotype produces a syndrome of tall stature, mental retardation, feminization, and delayed puberty in males. (From Moore, K.L. [1966]. *The Sex Chromatin.* Philadelphia: W.B. Saunders.)

TABLE 7–2
CLINICAL FEATURES OF SELECTED CHROMOSOMAL DISORDERS

Disorder	Incidence	Clinical Features
Trisomy 21 (Down's syndrome)	1 in 800	Mental retardation, characteristic facial features, associated systemic anomalies
Trisomy 18	1 in 8000	Small facial features, cardiac defects, usually death before 3 months
Trisomy 13	1 in 20,000	Mental retardation, hemangiomas, microcephaly, cleft lip and palate, cardiac and urogenital defects, usually death during first year
5p deletion* (cri du chat syndrome)	Rare	Low birthweight, mental retardation, cat-like cry, microcephaly, malformed ears, facial abnormalities
11p deletion* (11p syndrome)	Rare	Mental retardation, growth retardation, absence of the iris, Wilms' tumor, ambiguous genitalia in males
18p* or 18q* deletion	Rare	Variable mental retardation, immunoglobulin A deficiency, whorls on skin of digits
Turner's syndrome (monosomy of short arm of X)	1 in 10,000 live female births	Short stature, abnormal development of sex organs, absence of menstruation, prominent ridges on skin
Klinefelter's syndrome (47,XXY)	1 in 1000 live male births	Infertility, small testes
Poly-X female (three or more X chromosomes)	1 in 1000 live female births	Delayed motor and speech development
Fragile X syndrome (break on long arm of X)	1 in 2000 males; 1 in 1000 females	Mental retardation, enlarged testes
Y-polysomy (more than one Y chromosome)	1 in 1000 males	Aggressive antisocial behavior, tall stature

* p, short arm of chromosome; q, long arm of chromosome.
Data from Behrman, R.E. (Ed.). (1992). *Nelson Textbook of Pediatrics.* (14th ed.). Philadelphia: W.B. Saunders. (pp. 282–295).

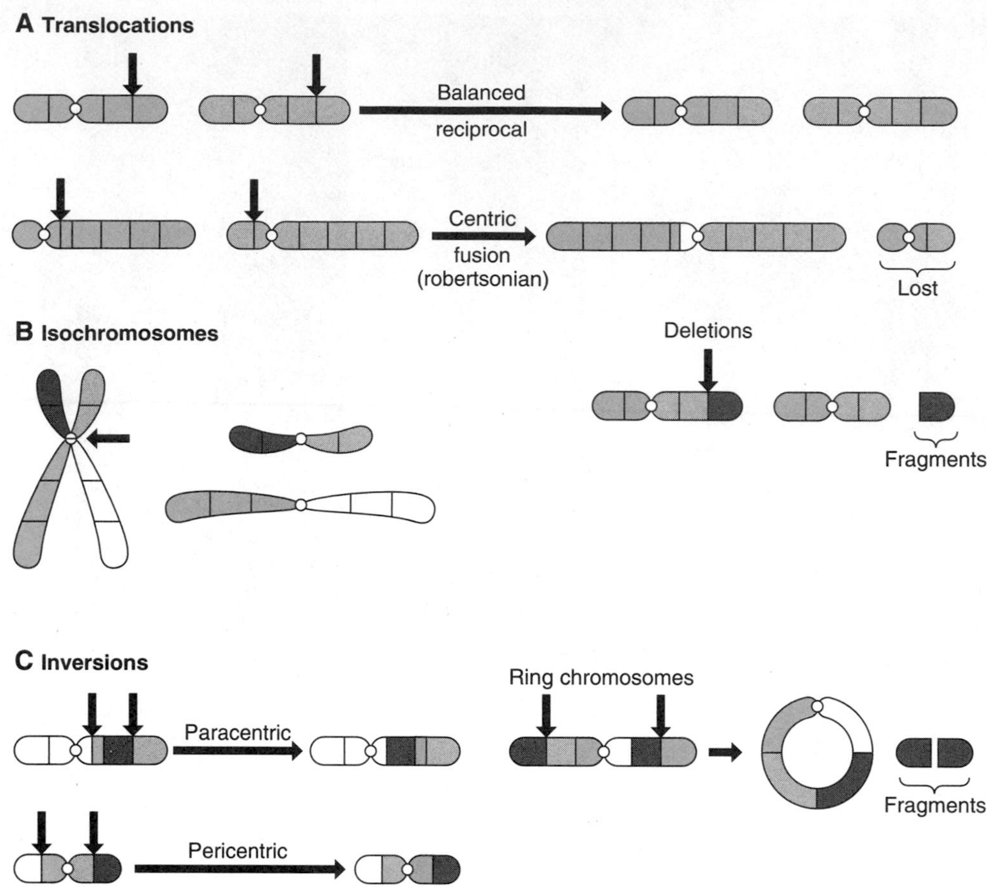

FIGURE 7–5

Forms of chromosomal rearrangement. *A,* Translocation occurs when part of a broken chromosome attaches to another. *B,* Isochromosomes are formed when one arm is lost and the other is duplicated. Deletions occur with fragmentation of chromosomes. *C,* Inversions and ring chromosomes result from abnormal recombination of fragments. (Redrawn from Cotran, R.S., Kumar, V., and Robbins, S.L. [1994]. *Robbins Pathologic Basis of Disease.* [5th ed.]. Philadelphia: W.B. Saunders. [p. 154].)

changed between two chromosomes and the centromere and telomeres are appropriately placed, then the cell may divide normally, and no changes in phenotype would be apparent. If the rearrangement is unbalanced, and chromosomes have deletions or additions in genetic material or have significant structural abnormality, the phenotype is abnormal.

Other forms of structural rearrangements include *deletions* of chromosomal segments, *isochromosomes* formed when one arm is lost and the other is duplicated, *inversions* of chromosomal segments, and *ring chromosomes* formed when a chromosome undergoes two breaks and the ends reunite.

Modes of Inheritance

Genetic defects that first arise in the affected individual are referred to as **de novo** defects, to distinguish them from inherited defects that are passed down from one or both parents. Many inherited defects are governed by the genetic principles first articulated by Gregor Mendel (Table 7–3) and are known as **mendelian disorders**. Inherited disorders originally arise from a de novo defect in a germ cell or gamete. Their effects on offspring are variable, depending on whether the offspring inherit the defect from one or both parents.

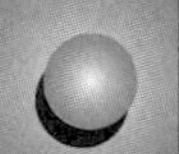

TABLE 7–3
PRINCIPLES OF MENDELIAN INHERITANCE

Principle of dominance: In the competition of two genes at the same locus on paired chromosomes, one gene may mask or conceal the other. The individual manifests the dominant gene's characteristic. The concealed trait is termed recessive.

Principle of segregation: During meiosis, paired chromosomes are separated to form two gametes. Therefore, the genes remain unchanged and are transferred from one generation to the next.

Principle of independent assortment: When displayed traits have alleles at two or more loci, each is distributed within the gametes randomly, independent of each other.

From Blackburn, S.T., and Loper, D.L. (1992). *Maternal, Fetal, and Neonatal Physiology: A Clinical Perspective.* Philadelphia: W.B. Saunders. (p. 8).

Mendelian Inheritance

Dominant Versus Recessive Traits. Mendelian disorders result from abnormality at a single gene locus, affecting a single protein molecule. Three patterns of inheritance are seen: **autosomal dominant, autosomal recessive,** and **X-linked.**[11] Mendelian principles define a recessive trait as a defect that must be inherited from both parents for full expression, that is, for its effects to be fully apparent. A **dominant** trait is expressed when inherited from one parent. **Codominant** traits are equally important in governing expression.

These principles may be illustrated by the ABO blood groups (see also Chapter 13). Three types of genes may be present at blood group alleles: A, B, or O. A and B types are dominant with respect to O, which is recessive, but A and B are codominant with respect to each other. Inheriting one A and one O (AO **genotype**) results in the type A phenotype, while the BO genotype results in the type B phenotype. Inheriting one A and one B produces the AB phenotype. Type O is expressed only when the individual inherits the O gene from both parents. People who inherit identical genes from each parent at a given pair of loci are said to be **homozygous** for the trait governed by those genes, whereas those with different gene forms are **heterozygous**.

Autosomal Versus Sex-Linked Inheritance. Mendelian inheritance patterns are classified as dominant or recessive and are further identified on the basis of location of the defect on an autosome or a sex chromosome. Autosomal dominant disorders include Huntington's chorea, a devastating neurologic disease that becomes apparent in middle adulthood, in which the patient loses motor and intellectual function. Other conditions in this category are summarized in Table 7–4. Autosomal recessive diseases make up the largest category of mendelian disorders. Most of these involve disorders of enzyme function and are referred to as *inborn errors of metabolism.* Well-known examples of autosomal recessive disorders are cystic fibrosis, sickle cell disease, and PKU (Table 7–5).

Sex-linked disorders are caused by defects on the X or Y chromosome. Mutation of genes on the Y chromosome has not been associated with significant functional disorders but may contribute to male infertility (see Chapter 32). It is the X chromosome that is implicated in sex-linked disorders, and the defects are almost always recessive. Expression of these traits is possible in homozygous females, but most are expressed almost exclusively in males, who lack an opposing "normal" gene on an X chromosome. Examples of such X-linked recessive disorders are summarized in Table 7–6 and include hemophilia A and Duchenne's muscular dystrophy. The probability that offspring will express a given trait that obeys Mendel's laws may be calculated using the Punnett square technique, illustrated in Figure 7–6.

Variable Expression and Penetrance. Mendelian inheritance is not an all-or-none phenomenon. Some mendelian disorders display variable **expressivity**, with the degree of expression (or severity of clinical manifestations) dependent on whether the patient is heterozygous or homozygous for the defect, and potentially on environmental factors such as diet or

TABLE 7–4
SELECTED AUTOSOMAL DOMINANT DISORDERS

Disorder	Incidence	Clinical Features
Familial hypercholesterolemia	1 in 500	Defective receptors for low-density lipoprotein uptake leading to early, severe atherosclerosis and coronary artery disease
Adult polycystic kidney disease	1 in 1250	Cystic enlargement of kidneys, manifesting in the teen-age years or later as pain, hematuria, hypertension, and possible renal failure
Huntington's chorea	1 in 10,000	Degeneration of basal ganglia and cortical neurons, manifesting in adulthood as abnormal motor function and progressive dementia
Hereditary spherocytosis	1 in 5000	Spherical abnormality of red blood cells, leading to anemia owing to their increased removal by the spleen
von Willebrand's disease	1 in 8000	Bleeding disorder due to factor VIII defect, which impairs both the clotting cascade and platelet function
Marfan syndrome	1 in 20,000	Abnormal fibrillin (glycoprotein in connective tissue), leading to excessive bone growth, ocular disorders, and cardiac defects
Achondroplasia	1 in 50,000	Dwarfism due to abnormal endochondrial bone formation

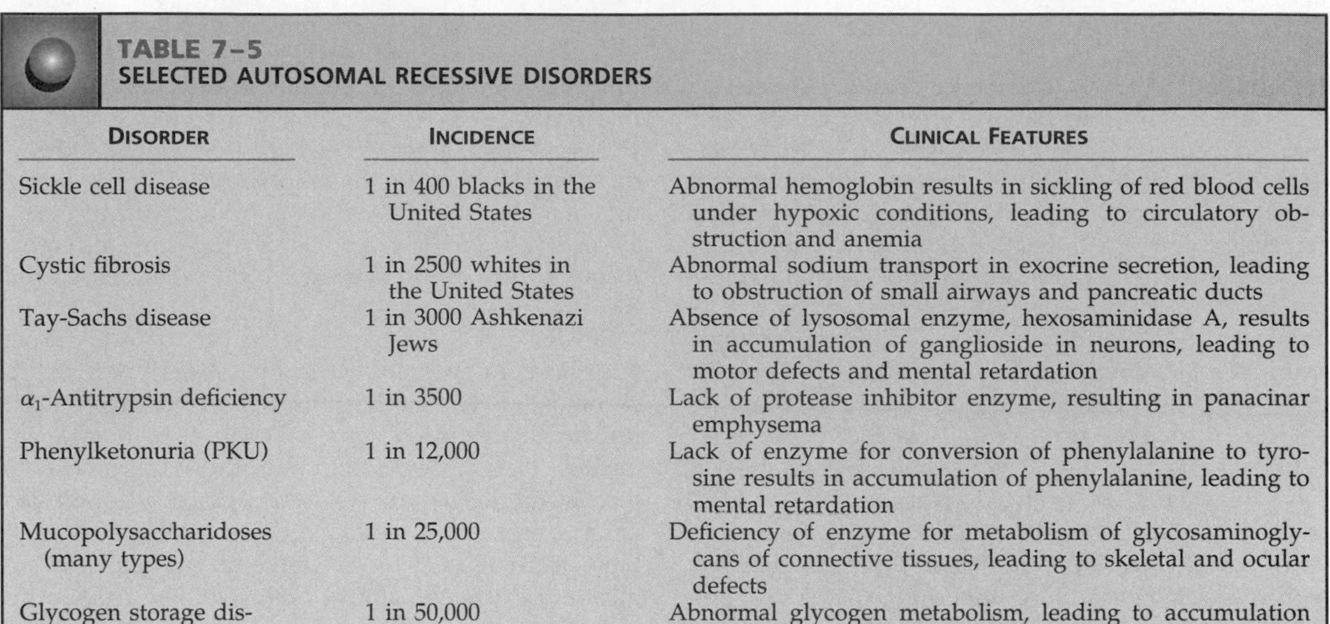

TABLE 7–5
SELECTED AUTOSOMAL RECESSIVE DISORDERS

Disorder	Incidence	Clinical Features
Sickle cell disease	1 in 400 blacks in the United States	Abnormal hemoglobin results in sickling of red blood cells under hypoxic conditions, leading to circulatory obstruction and anemia
Cystic fibrosis	1 in 2500 whites in the United States	Abnormal sodium transport in exocrine secretion, leading to obstruction of small airways and pancreatic ducts
Tay-Sachs disease	1 in 3000 Ashkenazi Jews	Absence of lysosomal enzyme, hexosaminidase A, results in accumulation of ganglioside in neurons, leading to motor defects and mental retardation
α_1-Antitrypsin deficiency	1 in 3500	Lack of protease inhibitor enzyme, resulting in panacinar emphysema
Phenylketonuria (PKU)	1 in 12,000	Lack of enzyme for conversion of phenylalanine to tyrosine results in accumulation of phenylalanine, leading to mental retardation
Mucopolysaccharidoses (many types)	1 in 25,000	Deficiency of enzyme for metabolism of glycosaminoglycans of connective tissues, leading to skeletal and ocular defects
Glycogen storage diseases (many types)	1 in 50,000	Abnormal glycogen metabolism, leading to accumulation of glycogen in various tissues

temperature. In sickle cell anemia, for example, the homozygous patient has the full-blown disease, which results in synthesis of abnormal hemoglobin within red blood cells (see Chapter 12). Such cells assume an elongated sickle shape when they lack oxygen, and in this form they may clump together and occlude blood vessels. They are also removed from the blood by the spleen, leaving the afflicted person severely anemic. The patient who is heterozygous for the trait has less severe disease and does not experience significant sickling of cells unless a state of severe hypoxia is induced. This patient is said to have sickle cell trait and may have a mild degree of anemia at times. Primarily, however, the trait conveys carrier status in that it may be inherited by this person's offspring.

The role of environmental influences in variable expressivity is illustrated by PKU, an inborn error of metabolism of the amino acid phenylalanine. Presence of the amino acid in the diet is essential to full manifestation of the disorder (see Chapter 33).

In X-linked disorders, an additional factor may contribute to variable expression in females. According to the Lyon hypothesis, one of the two X chromosomes in each somatic cell is randomly, irreversibly inactivated (probably by tight coiling of DNA)

TABLE 7–6
SELECTED X-LINKED DISORDERS

Disorder	Incidence	Clinical Features
Duchenne's muscular dystrophy	1 in 3500 males	Progressive fatty degeneration of muscle fibers
Hemophilia A	1 in 5,000 males	Bleeding disorder due to factor VIII deficiency
Fragile X syndrome	1 in 1250 males, 1 in 2000 females	Mental retardation
Lesch-Nyhan syndrome	Rare (males)	Deficiency of enzyme for purine metabolism leads to uric acid accumulation, resulting in poor mental and motor development and often compulsive, self-destructive behavior
Glucose-6-phosphatase deficiency	Rare (blacks)	Lack of enzyme in red blood cells, leading to acute hemolytic anemia when affected patients are given certain drugs (e.g., primaquine or sulfonamide)
Testicular feminization	1 in 64,000 genetic males	Feminine characteristics and ambiguous genitalia due to a defect in receptor-mediated testosterone effects
Color blindness	8% of white males	Defective function of cones for red and green color vision

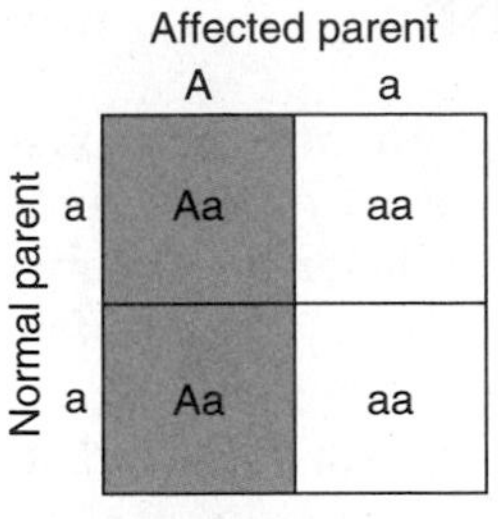

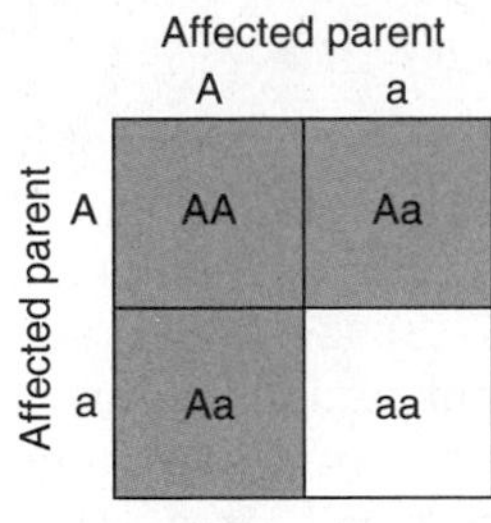

A

PUNNETT SQUARE FOR AUTOSOMAL DOMINANT TRAIT

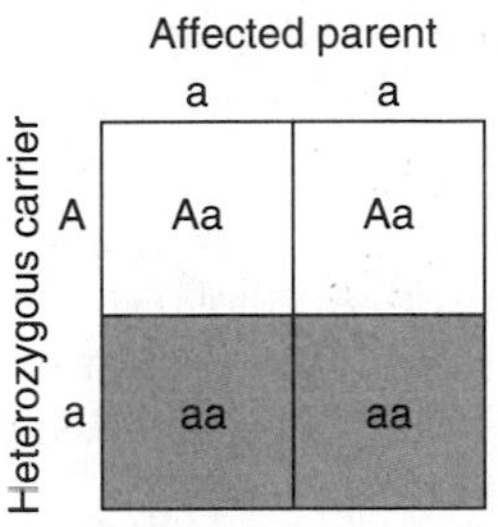

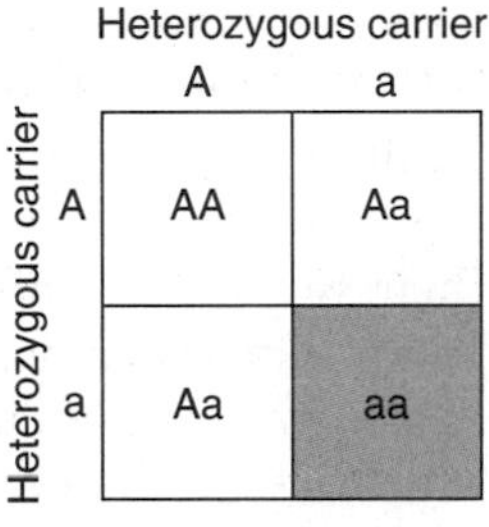

B

PUNNETT SQUARE FOR AUTOSOMAL RECESSIVE TRAIT

FIGURE 7–6

Punnett squares. *A*, For autosomal dominant (A) traits, the probability that the offspring of one normal (aa genotype) parent and one affected (Aa) parent will manifest the trait is 50%. When both parents are affected (both heterozygous, or Aa in this case), the probability is 75%. *B*, For autosomal recessive (a) traits, the probability that offspring of an affected (aa) parent and a carrier (Aa) parent will manifest the trait is 50%. When both parents are heterozygous carriers, 25% of offspring are expected to manifest the trait.

early in embryonic development. Either the maternally derived or the paternally derived X chromosome may be inactivated, with equal probability, and all progeny of this cell line will have this same inactivation. Unless the proportion is disturbed by some factor conferring preferential survival to one cell line, about half of the female's cells will manifest inactivation of the maternal X, and 50% will manifest inactivation of the paternal X. Females thus have the same X-derived "gene dosage" as males, and in X-linked disorders, random inactivation of one X accounts for some variability in expressivity among females.

Genetic defects may also display variable **penetrance**. Penetrance is the degree to which a genetic defect results in abnormality of the protein structure or function governed by that locus. Many autosomal dominant disorders are known to display incomplete penetrance, which limits their impact. **Genomic imprinting**, in which expression of a defect depends on whether it originated from maternal or paternal chromosomes, is an additional variable in some autosomal disorders.[12]

Multifactorial Inheritance

Many common disorders occur with more frequency in certain families but do not follow mendelian patterns. In such cases, defects apparently result from two or more genetic mutations and may involve environmental factors as well. This form of inheritance is termed **multifactorial inheritance**, and disorders in this category are referred to as *complex traits*.[13] A person may be said to have a *genetic predisposition*, that is, to be at higher risk for these disorders, which include cleft lip and palate, congenital heart disease, coronary heart disease, hypertension, gout, diabetes mellitus, pyloric stenosis, and specific types of cancer (Table 7–7).

Construction of **genograms,** or family tree diagrams, may be helpful in analysis of patterns of inheritance. As shown in Figure 7–7, mendelian disorders display a vertical, oblique, or horizontal pattern of inheritance. Multifactorial inheritance manifests more randomly in successive generations.

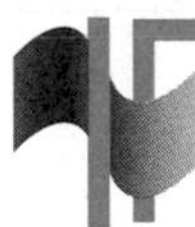

Clinical Scenario

C.K., age 12 years, has Down's syndrome. He has been in generally good health throughout his childhood, although he appears especially prone to fatigue with activity, and his mother says he "catches colds" easily. C.K. has low-normal intelligence and performs well in classes for special needs children at his public elementary school. During a recent physical examination, a heart murmur was heard, and further diagnostic testing revealed a defect in the septum between his cardiac chambers.

1. Is some degree of mosaicism likely in C.K.'s case? What evidence can be cited?
2. Is it probable that C.K.'s cardiac disorder is related to his Down's syndrome? Explain.
3. If C.K. had children of his own, could they inherit his disorder? Explain.

NEOPLASIA

The most significant abnormality of cellular growth and development, by virtue of its prevalence, morbidity, and mortality, is neoplasia. Neoplasia literally means "new growth" and refers to a process of accelerated or uninhibited division and

TABLE 7–7
SELECTED DISORDERS CHARACTERIZED BY MULTIFACTORIAL INHERITANCE

Disorder	Chapter
Alzheimer's disease	21
Atherosclerosis	15
Breast cancer	31
Cleft lip and palate	25
Colon cancer	24
Congenital heart disease	16
Coronary heart disease	16
Diabetes mellitus	29
Gout	34
Hypertension	15
Pyloric stenosis	24
Wilms' tumor	20

growth of genetically abnormal cells. A mass of such cells is referred to as a **neoplasm** or **tumor**, and a malignant tumor is commonly referred to as **cancer.** Cancer is the second leading cause of death in the United States, with lung, breast (in females), and colon cancers accounting for most mortality. Figure 7–8 illustrates recent trends in cancer deaths.

Classification

Classification of a tumor as **malignant** (cancerous) or **benign** has traditionally been based on its microscopic appearance and growth characteristics (Table 7–8). Generally, benign tumors are fairly well differentiated (resemble normal tissue), grow slowly, do not invade adjacent tissues, and remain localized to a small area. Conversely, malignant tumors are more often poorly differentiated, grow rapidly, are invasive, and spread, or **metastasize,** to distant areas of the body through the blood or lymphatic system. This either-or distinction is not always clinically useful, however. Benign tumors within the cranial vault, for example, may be malignant by location in that they damage normal tissues or severely impair their function, owing to their occupation of critical space. On the other hand, some malignant tumors grow so slowly that treatment may not be warranted (e.g., some forms of prostate cancer).

Neoplasms may also be classified on the basis of the cell type from which they originate. Most cancers arise from epithelial cells or connective tissue cells. Malignant tumors of epithelial origin are often referred to as **carcinomas**, whereas connective tissue tumors are commonly called **sarcomas**. Table 7–9

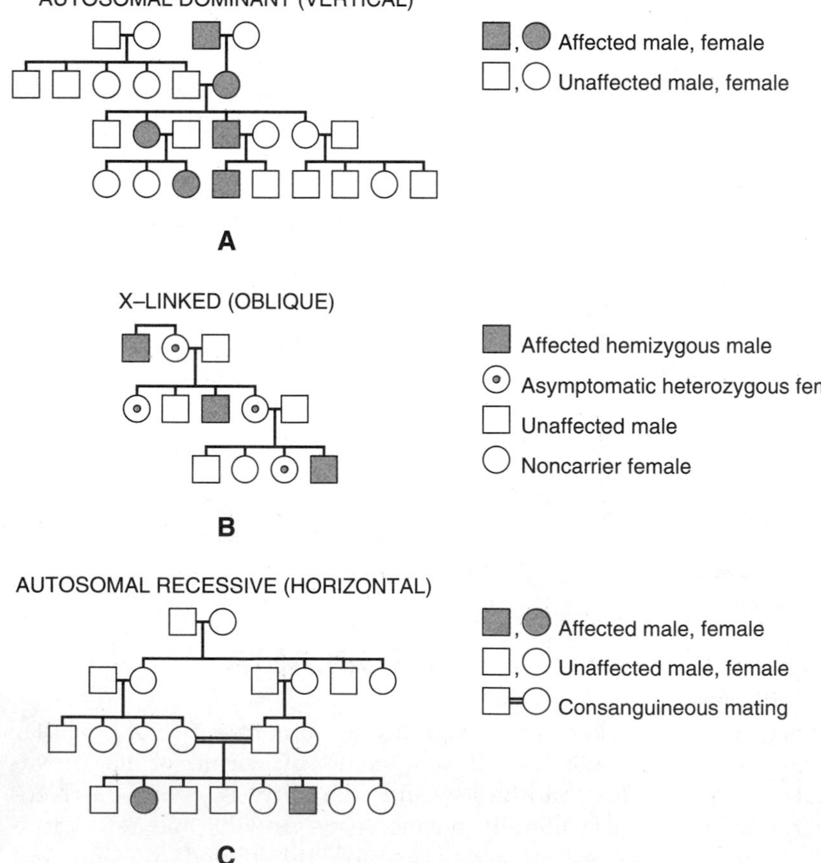

FIGURE 7–7
Genograms showing patterns of inheritance. *A,* Autosomal dominant traits are seen among offspring of both sexes in each generation (vertical pattern). *B,* X-linked disorders manifest only in males in each generation (oblique pattern). *C,* Autosomal recessive disorders manifest in either sex, less commonly than autosomal dominant traits. The initial appearance of two cases among siblings (horizontal pattern) suggests that the defect was inherited from both parents, who were heterozygous carriers. A blood relationship between parents (consanguineous mating) magnifies such risk.

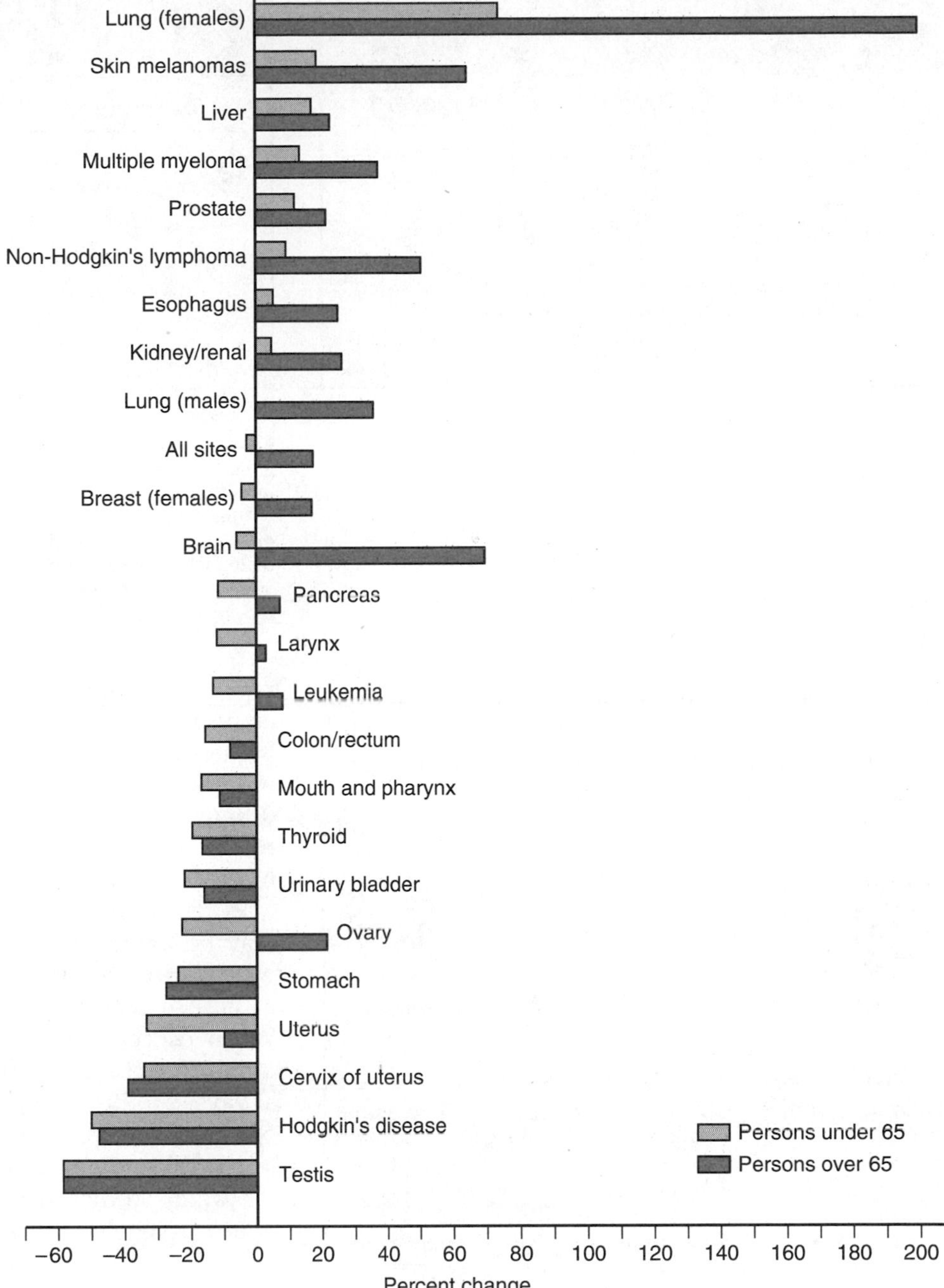

FIGURE 7–8
Changes in cancer death rates in the United States, 1973 to 1990 (age-adjusted). (Data from the National Cancer Institute. [1994]. *Evaluating the national cancer program: An ongoing process.* President's Cancer Panel meeting, September 22, 1993. Bethesda, MD.)

lists common examples of benign and malignant tumors of varying tissue origins.

Malignant tumors may be further classified for purposes of determining prognosis or therapy. As detailed in Table 7–10, the TNM tumor staging system is employed in describing the status of tumors based on degree of tumor mass (T), lymph node involvement (L), and metastasis (M). The tumor grading system (Table 7–11) is based on microscopic examination of cancer cells. Grade I tumors contain well-differentiated cells, whereas grade IV tumor cells are undifferentiated and usually associated with a more unfavorable prognosis.

Epidemiology

With the exception of rare cases of cancers caused by inherited genetic defects (e.g., retinoblastoma) or certain viruses (e.g., Burkitt's lymphoma), the specific cause of cancer is unknown. Several risk factors

TABLE 7–8
TYPICAL CHARACTERISTICS OF BENIGN VERSUS MALIGNANT TUMORS

Characteristic	Benign	Malignant
Differentiation	Well differentiated	Poorly or moderately differentiated
Growth rate	Usually slow	Often rapid
Invasiveness	Noninvasive	Often invasive
Metastasis	Remains localized	Often metastatic
Demarcation	Usually clear margins; may be encapsulated	Often not clearly delimited

have been associated with the development of cancer, however (Table 7–12).

Host Factors

Host factors are intrinsic to the individual patient and include age, sex, genetic factors, psychological factors, immunosuppression, and chronic tissue trauma. A few cancers are found only in children, and these commonly originate from embryonic tissues. In general, however, the incidence of cancer increases with increasing age, giving credence to theories that relate the onset of cancer to faulty genetic regulation or decreased immune surveillance, as discussed later. The overall incidence of cancer is higher in men than in women, although this finding may be due to lifestyle factors rather than biologic differences in susceptibility. Some cancers, such as breast, endometrial, and prostate cancers, are hormonally influenced.

Evidence for a genetic predisposition to cancer may be found in the increased incidence of the disease in people with a known genetic disorder, such as is seen with Down's and Klinefelter's syndromes. When cancer is observed to occur in a number of family members, the pattern of inheritance is nearly always multifactorial, and the possibility then exists of common exposure to environmental agents or of learned lifestyle practices that increase risk.

Several studies have explored potential links between psychological factors such as stress or depres-

TABLE 7–9
NOMENCLATURE OF SELECTED TUMORS

Tissue of Origin	Benign Tumor	Malignant Tumor
Epithelial Tissue		
Glandular epithelium	Adenoma, papilloma	Adenocarcinoma Papillary carcinoma
Squamous epithelium	Papilloma	Squamous cell carcinoma
Melanocyte	Pigmented nevus	Malignant melanoma
Connective Tissue		
Fibrous connective tissue	Fibroma	Fibrosarcoma
Bone	Osteoma	Osteogenic sarcoma
Cartilage	Chondroma	Chondrosarcoma
Meninges	Meningioma	Meningeal sarcoma
Muscle		
Uterine smooth muscle	Leiomyoma	Leiomyosarcoma
Skeletal muscle	Rhabdomyoma	Rhabdomyosarcoma
Nervous Tissue		
Glia (astrocyte)	Astrocytoma (low grade)	Glioblastoma multiforme

TABLE 7–10
TNM CLASSIFICATION SYSTEM FOR CANCER STAGING

Definition	Stage
T: characteristics of primary tumor	T_x: cannot be assessed T_0: no evidence of tumor T_{is}: carcinoma in situ T_{1-4}: increasing size of tumor
N: characteristics of regional lymph nodes	N_x: cannot be assessed N_0: no nodal metastasis N_{1-3}: increasing involvement of regional nodes
M: distant metastasis	M_x: cannot be assessed M_0: no distant metastasis M_1: distant metastasis

Adapted from Groenwald, S.L., *et al.* (Eds.). (1993). *Cancer Nursing: Principles and Practice,* Boston: Jones & Bartlett Publishers. (p. 188). Used with permission of the American Joint Committee on Cancer (AJCC), Chicago, Illinois. The original source for this material is from Beahrs, O.H., *et al.* (1992). *American Joint Committee on Cancer: Manual for Staging of Cancer.* (4th ed.), Philadelphia: Lippincott-Raven Publishers.

TABLE 7–11
TUMOR GRADING SYSTEM

Grade	Interpretation
I	Well differentiated
II	Moderately well differentiated
III	Poorly differentiated
IV	Undifferentiated

Developed by Beahrs, O.H., Hensen, D.E., Hutter, R.V.P., et al. (1992). American Joint Committee on Cancer: *Manual for Staging of Cancer.* (4th ed.). Philadelphia: J.B. Lippincott.
Data from O'Mary, S.S. (1993). Diagnostic evaluation, classification, and staging. In: Groenwald, S.L., Frogge, M.H., Goodman, M., *et al. Cancer Nursing: Principles and Practice.* (3rd ed.). Boston: Jones and Bartlett Publishers. (p. 190).

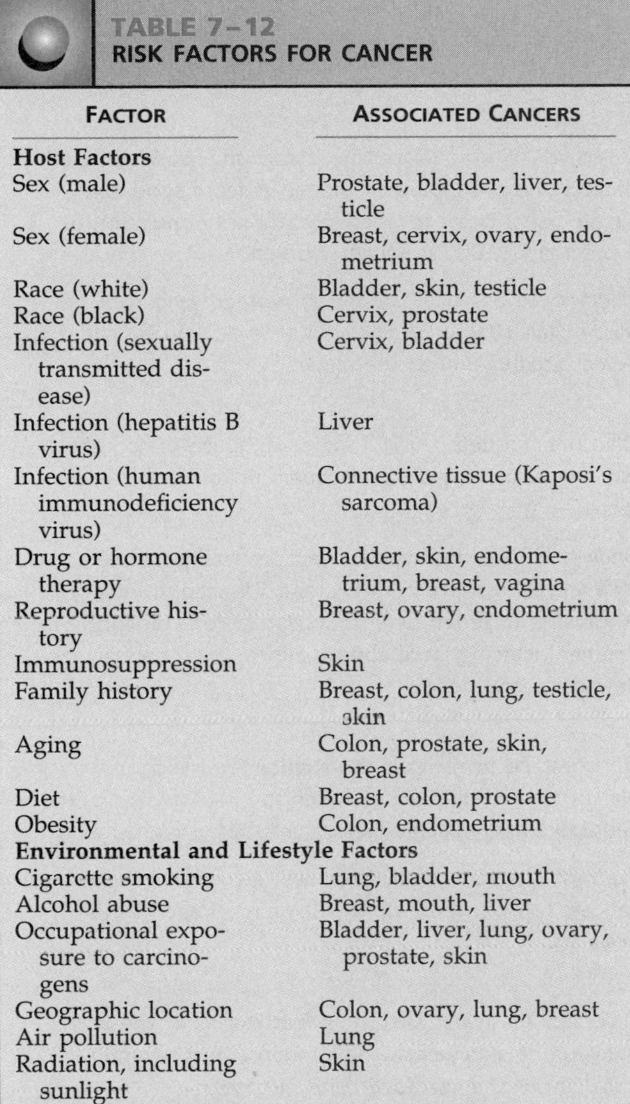

TABLE 7–12
RISK FACTORS FOR CANCER

Factor	Associated Cancers
Host Factors	
Sex (male)	Prostate, bladder, liver, testicle
Sex (female)	Breast, cervix, ovary, endometrium
Race (white)	Bladder, skin, testicle
Race (black)	Cervix, prostate
Infection (sexually transmitted disease)	Cervix, bladder
Infection (hepatitis B virus)	Liver
Infection (human immunodeficiency virus)	Connective tissue (Kaposi's sarcoma)
Drug or hormone therapy	Bladder, skin, endometrium, breast, vagina
Reproductive history	Breast, ovary, endometrium
Immunosuppression	Skin
Family history	Breast, colon, lung, testicle, skin
Aging	Colon, prostate, skin, breast
Diet	Breast, colon, prostate
Obesity	Colon, endometrium
Environmental and Lifestyle Factors	
Cigarette smoking	Lung, bladder, mouth
Alcohol abuse	Breast, mouth, liver
Occupational exposure to carcinogens	Bladder, liver, lung, ovary, prostate, skin
Geographic location	Colon, ovary, lung, breast
Air pollution	Lung
Radiation, including sunlight	Skin
Sedentary lifestyle	Colon

sion and the risk of developing cancer.[14] The mechanisms underlying such risk are unknown, however, and only weak associations have been shown. An increased incidence of cancer has been demonstrated in patients with AIDS and those on immunosuppressive drugs, strongly suggesting a role for immunosuppression in the process of cancer development. Tissues that undergo chronic trauma and healing also demonstrate a slightly increased risk of cancerous transformation, which might be expected owing to the increased cell division inherent in the healing process.

Environmental and Lifestyle Factors

Environmental and lifestyle factors constitute the second category of risk factors for cancer development and include geographic location, nutrition, occupation, and cigarette smoking. Certain cancers are more prevalent in some geographic locations. Breast cancer, for example, is much more common in North America than in Asia.[15] It is often unclear, however, whether such patterns are the result of common exposure to carcinogens, common ancestry, or other factors.

Findings of studies attempting to link nutritional practices with cancer have yielded conflicting results (see Focus of Current Research). The animal models and disproportionately high doses of nutrients often used in such research may limit generalizability of some findings to humans. Preliminary findings suggest possible associations between high fat diet and breast cancer and between low fiber diet and colon cancer. High intake of some foods, such as cruciferous vegetables, high fiber foods, and green tea, may be protective against some forms of cancer (Table 7–13).

TABLE 7–13
NUTRITIONAL FACTORS IN CANCER ETIOLOGY

Organ	Cancer-Promoting Factors	Cancer-Protective Factors
Breast	Fat, protein, sugar	Selenium, low-fat diet
Pancreas	Protein, sugar, ethanol, fried meat, fat	Selenium, low-fat diet, fruits, vegetables
Lung	—	Vitamin A, selenium
Stomach	Salted, pickled, or smoked fish; fava beans; nitrate	Milk, cruciferous vegetables, vitamins C and E
Prostate	Fat, protein	Vitamin A, selenium
Colon, rectum	Fat, protein, selenium(?), fiber(?)	Cruciferous vegetables, milk, selenium(?), pentosans, fiber(?), vitamin A
Larynx	—	Vitamins A and C
Bladder	—	Vitamin A, selenium
Esophagus	Ethanol	Milk, fruits, green and yellow vegetables

Adapted from Guengerich, F.P. (1995). Influence of nutrients and other dietary materials on cytochrome P-450 enzymes. *American Journal of Clinical Nutrition* 61(suppl.), 651S–658S. © Am J Clin Nutr. American Society for Clinical Nutrition.

Focus of Current Research

Study	Objective and Findings
Rothman, et al. (1995) Teratogenicity of high vitamin A intake.	*Objective:* To investigate the relationship between birth defects and the intake of vitamin A from food and supplements in a prospectively studied population of more than 22,000 pregnant women. *Findings:* Among babies born to women who took more than 10,000 IU/day of vitamin A, 1 in 57 had a defect attributable to the intake.
Pearson, et al. (1994) Toluene embryopathy: Delineation of the phenotype and comparison with fetal alcohol syndrome.	*Objective:* To determine if maternal abuse of toluene (sniffing of paint, glue, or lacquer) produces birth defects. *Findings:* 89% of infants exposed prenatally had defects: 39% were born prematurely, and 9% died in infancy. Anomalies included defects similar to fetal alcohol syndrome, including facial abnormalities, microcephaly, and developmental delays.
Bhatia, et al. (1996) Breast cancer and other second neoplasms after childhood Hodgkin's disease.	*Objective:* To investigate the incidence of second neoplasms after treatment of childhood Hodgkin's disease and to identify specific factors associated with the risk. *Findings:* The risk of solid tumors, especially breast cancer, approached 35% by 40 years of age in this population.
Omenn, et al. (1996) (CARET trial) Effects of a combination of beta carotene and vitamin A on lung cancer and cardiovascular disease.	*Objective:* To investigate the effectiveness of the antioxidants beta-carotene and vitamin A in preventing lung cancer and cardiovascular disease. *Findings:* The risk of these disorders was *increased* in the treatment groups, and the trial was stopped 21 months earlier than planned.
Hennekens, et al. (1996) (CARET and ATBC trials) Lack of effect of long-term supplement with beta carotene on the incidence of malignant neoplasms and cardiovascular disease.	*Objective:* To investigate the relationship between use of antioxidant supplements and incidence of neoplasia or cardiovascular disease. *Findings:* Supplementation produced neither benefit nor harm in terms of incidence of malignant neoplasms, cardiovascular disease, or death from all causes.
Bertram & Bortkiewicz (1995) Dietary carotenoids inhibit neoplastic transformation and modulate gene expression in mouse and human cells.	*Objective:* To test the hypothesis that carotenoids, specifically beta-carotene, are protective in an in vitro model system. *Findings:* Carotenoids both with and without provitamin A activity inhibited carcinogen-induced neoplastic transformation and membrane lipid oxidation and caused up-regulation of a gap junction gene.

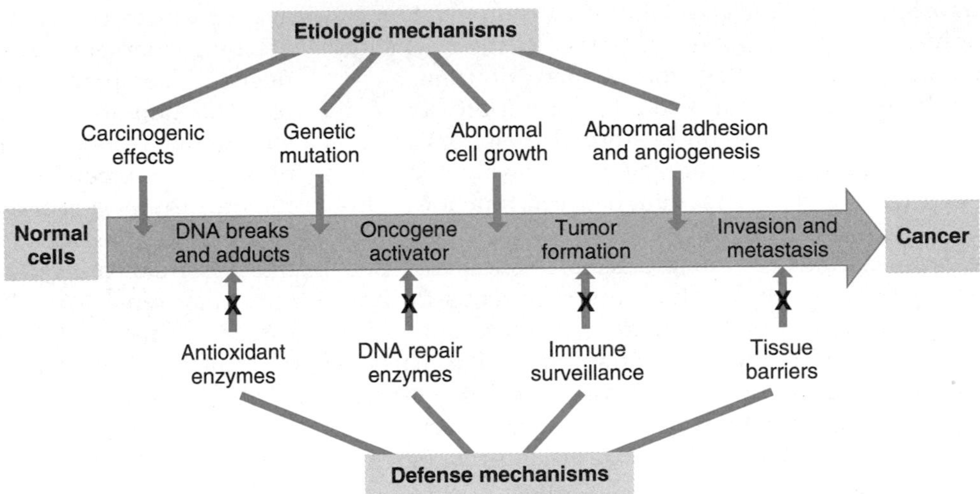

FIGURE 7–9
Etiology of cancer. Cancer develops as a result of initial damaging but sublethal effects of carcinogens on DNA. These effects mark the cell and, if not prevented by cellular antioxidant systems or repaired by DNA editing and repair systems, cause mutation of a gene to an oncogene. The oncogene directs uncontrolled proliferation of the defective cell, resulting in the formation of a neoplasm or tumor. If not detected and destroyed by the immune system, the tumor invades local tissues and may metastasize to distant sites.

Occupational exposure to carcinogens, such as asbestos, pesticides, hydrocarbons, and radiation, has been strongly linked to cancer development. Cigarette smoking has been implicated in 30% of all cancer deaths, particularly those due to lung cancer and colorectal cancer.[16] Because cigarette smoking is also a significant risk factor for cardiovascular diseases, there is little doubt that this habit is the most important preventable cause of disease in the United States.

Etiology

Cancer has no single cause. Its etiology is complex, requiring both DNA damage and inadequate physiologic defense or repair (Fig. 7–9).

Neoplastic Transformation (Initiation of Cancer)

Cancers arise from a single cell that suffers multiple transforming genetic mutations, which may be inherited or acquired.[17] Acquired defects may occur randomly with DNA replication during cell division or may be induced by mutagens, referred to as **carcinogens** in this context. Known carcinogens include chemicals and drugs, toxins, oncogenic viruses, and ionizing radiation (Table 7–14).

Initial DNA damage by carcinogens may convey genetic instability, or cancer predisposition, in that it promotes the accumulation of further damage. Typically, the damage involves genes that normally induce cell proliferation and growth **(proto-oncogenes)** or that inhibit such growth **(tumor suppressor genes)**.[18] Proto-oncogenes may encode growth factor receptors on cells, proteins involved in signal transduction pathways, or positive regulators of the cell cycle. For example, many tumors express the enzyme telomerase, which prevents progressive shortening of telomeres (chromosomal ends). As discussed in Chapter 6, telomere shortening is associated with the limitation of cell division, which is a hallmark of aging in most cells. Presence of telomerase in cancer cells conveys unlimited potential for division. Mutation of a proto-oncogene may convert it to an **oncogene**, capable of inducing malignant

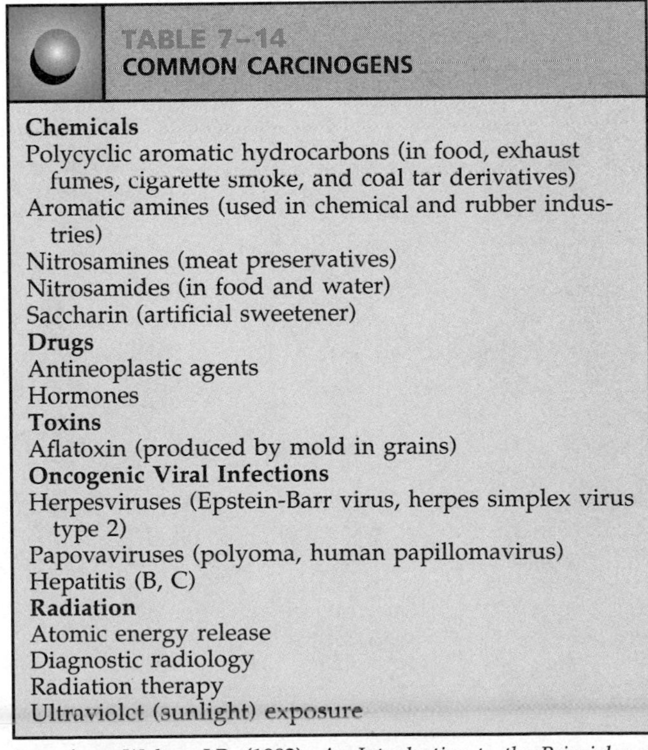
TABLE 7–14
COMMON CARCINOGENS

Chemicals
Polycyclic aromatic hydrocarbons (in food, exhaust fumes, cigarette smoke, and coal tar derivatives)
Aromatic amines (used in chemical and rubber industries)
Nitrosamines (meat preservatives)
Nitrosamides (in food and water)
Saccharin (artificial sweetener)
Drugs
Antineoplastic agents
Hormones
Toxins
Aflatoxin (produced by mold in grains)
Oncogenic Viral Infections
Herpesviruses (Epstein-Barr virus, herpes simplex virus type 2)
Papovaviruses (polyoma, human papillomavirus)
Hepatitis (B, C)
Radiation
Atomic energy release
Diagnostic radiology
Radiation therapy
Ultraviolet (sunlight) exposure

Data from Walter, J.B. (1992). *An Introduction to the Principles of Disease*. (3rd ed.). Philadelphia: W.B. Saunders. (pp. 232–238).

transformation. Such mutations are dominant, with only one defective allele required to transform the daughter cells resulting from the next division.

Alternatively, damage to a tumor suppressor gene may prevent expression of normal inhibitors of cell replication. This type of defect displays a recessive inheritance pattern, and daughter cell function is impaired only if both alleles of the parent cell were defective. Cancers with predictable inheritance patterns occur in people who are homozygous for mutation of tumor suppressor genes. These cancers include retinoblastoma, hereditary neurofibromatosis, and some forms of colon, breast, and lung cancer. People who are heterozygous for such defects have increased predisposition to cancer induced by random mutation or carcinogen exposure.

Promotion of Malignancy

According to the *clonal evolution theory,* cancers become more malignant as mutations accumulate with each generation of transformed cells.[17] Mutations conducive to malignancy would allow neoplastic cells to resist normal growth-inhibiting signals and to escape physical barriers and physiologic defenses.

Because exposure to environmental carcinogens is unavoidable to some extent, the presence of body defenses, such as intact skin and mucous membranes, inflammation, and the immune response, may reduce the risk of acquired damage to DNA. As discussed in Chapter 13, the immune response against cancer cells depends on the cancer cells developing markers (**tumor-associated antigens**) on their cell membranes, which allow them to be recognized as non-normal tissues. These markers initiate an immune response and may be useful in diagnosis or in development of immunotherapy against the tumor. Examples of these are listed in Table 7–15.

Cancer development may also be arrested by intracellular enzyme systems. Antioxidant enzyme systems may repair oxidative damage to DNA, as discussed in Chapter 3. Mismatch repair and nucleotide excision repair systems may correct any defects in DNA before the cell divides, thus preventing transmission to the cell's progeny (see Chapter 6). Regulators of the cell cycle may facilitate this repair by allowing sufficient time in the appropriate phase. Damage that cannot be repaired may trigger cell death by apoptosis, effectively preventing proliferation of defective cells. Impairment of any of these defenses increases the risk, or the pace, of malignant transformation.

TABLE 7–15
TUMOR-ASSOCIATED ANTIGENS*

Category	Description	Examples
Tumor-associated differentiation antigens (TADAs)	Membrane markers on cells transformed by carcinogens	Cluster of differentiation (CD) markers Melanocyte-associated antigen Viral antigen CA-125 Prostate-specific antigen (PSA)
Oncofetal antigens (embryonic antigens)	Membrane markers, normally found only on embryonic cells, which are re-expressed on some tumor cells	α-Fetoprotein (AFP) Carcinoembryonic antigen (CEA)

*Tumor-associated antigens are biologic substances produced by tumors. They can be measured in the blood and are used clinically to detect the presence of tumors and to monitor response to therapy by estimating the quantity of tumor present.

Pathophysiology

Local Growth and Loss of Differentiation

The rate of local tumor growth is dependent on two primary factors: intrinsic cell cycle time (of the cell of origin) and rate of angiogenesis, or development of blood vessels within the tumor. Tumors originating in epithelial tissues, which have shorter cell cycles, typically grow more rapidly than those of connective tissue origin. A tumor cannot enlarge beyond 1 or 2 mm in diameter, however, unless it develops its own blood supply. Angiogenic cytokines that promote vessel growth are apparently secreted by tumor cells as well as by inflammatory cells, such as macrophages, which infiltrate the area.

Initially, the cells within a malignant tumor are monoclonal, or identical daughter cells of the originally mutated cell. By the time such tumors are clinically detectable, however, they have accumulated additional genetic damage. This finding is attributed to the increased risk of random mutation in cells that are dividing rapidly. Each generation of tumor cells thus becomes more poorly differentiated, bearing less resemblance in structure and function to the cell of origin (Fig. 7–10).

Invasion and Metastasis

Cancers typically invade tissues adjacent to the site of origin (primary site) and may metastasize to distant (secondary or metastatic) sites by mechanical

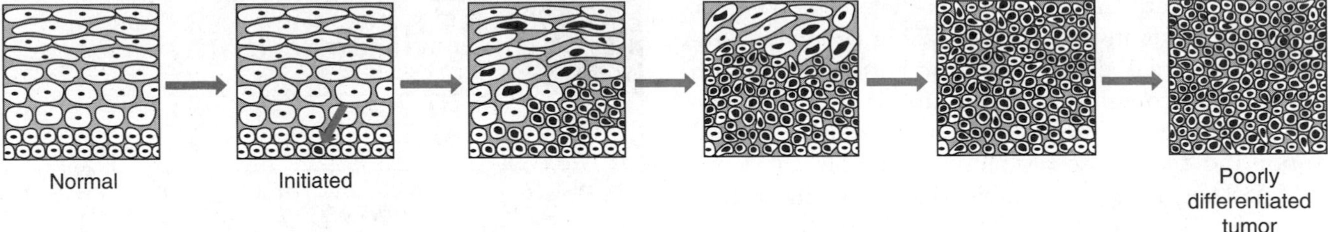

FIGURE 7–10
Progressive loss of differentiation. As cancer progresses, each generation of cells becomes more poorly differentiated, bearing less resemblance in structure and function to the cell of origin.

or gravitational seeding or lymphatic or hematogenous (blood-borne) spread (Fig. 7–11). Tumor cells within a body cavity may fall, by gravity, to lower points, establishing metastatic tumors. During surgery, manipulation of tumors may free some cells within cavities, facilitating spread. More commonly, however, tumor cells travel in the bloodstream or lymphatic system after invasion into these channels.

Cancer cells cannot metastasize unless they first separate from cells at the site of origin, invade a lymphatic or blood vessel, and invade and attach to tissues at distant sites. Physiologic defenses normally oppose each of these processes. As discussed in Chapter 2, cells are held together in tissues by adhesion molecules (cadherins). This adhesion is an important means of intercellular signaling, and cells that become detached are normally destroyed by apoptosis.[19] During the process of neoplastic transformation, cancers cells may lose the ability to express these molecules, promoting detachment; other genetic alterations permit survival in the detached state.

Once detached, cancer cells must breach natural barriers before entering blood or lymphatic vessels. These barriers are the basement membranes of the tissue of origin and the vessel, and the extracellular

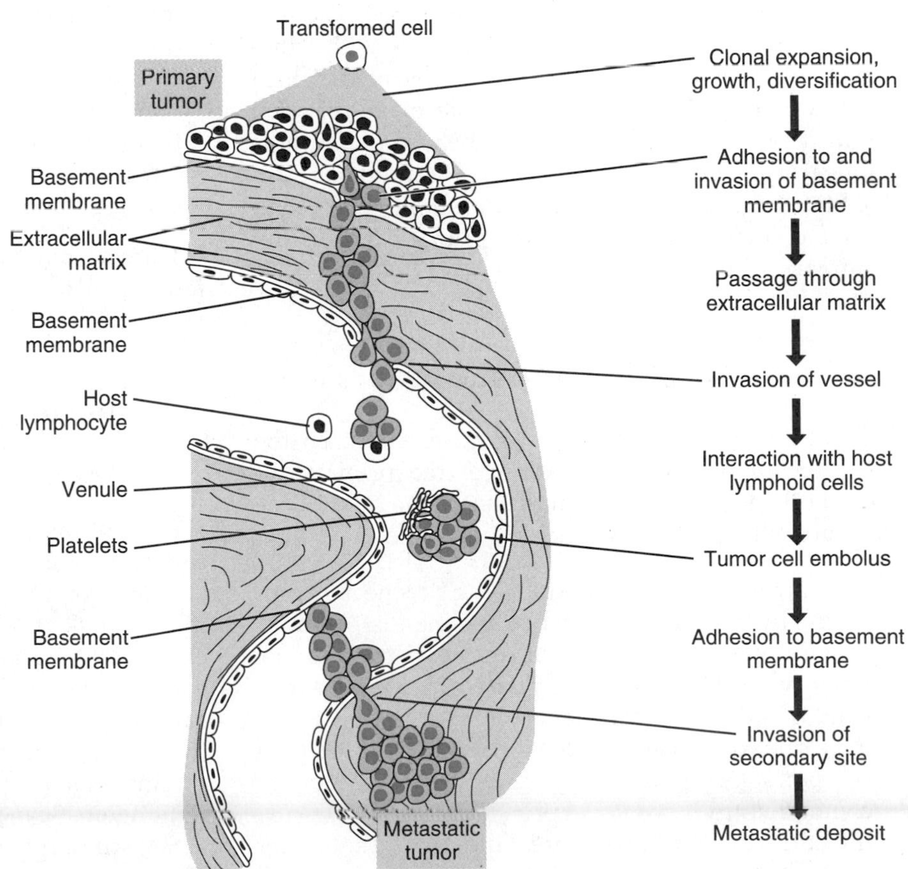

FIGURE 7–11
Hematogenous route of metastasis. Primary tumor cells detach and penetrate the tissue barriers of the extracellular matrix and vascular basement membrane before entering the blood vessel. In the blood, tumor cells are vulnerable to immune attack and platelet adhesion, which may promote their destruction. Tumor cell masses (emboli) that survive may adhere and invade at distal sites, forming secondary (metastatic) tumors. (Redrawn from Cotran, R.S., Kumar, V., and Robbins, S.L. [1994]. *Robbins Pathologic Basis of Disease.* [5th ed.]. Philadelphia: W.B. Saunders. [p. 277].)

matrix between. Cancer cells, like white blood cells, accomplish this invasion by releasing proteolytic enzymes that break down the tissue barriers. Although normal cells contain enzyme-inhibitor systems, these may be overcome, permitting local extension of the tumor and access into the blood or lymph.

Metastasis is not inevitable once the cancer cells are in the blood or lymph, however. In some cases, the cells undergo apoptosis once entering these fluids. Tumor cells may be filtered out of lymph at lymph nodes, or out of blood in the spleen. Immune cells may then destroy the tumor cells at these locations. Metastatic tumors may also form at these sites or within downstream capillaries, where tumor cells become trapped because of the small vessel size.

Attachment and proliferation of cancer cells at metastatic sites depend on several factors. Usually, cancer cells in the blood become trapped within the first capillary bed downstream of their point of entry into the circulation. Blood leaving most organs first enters the capillary beds of the lungs, the most common site of metastasis. Blood from the intestines first encounters the capillary beds of the liver, and this is the second most common metastatic site.[19] Cancer metastasis cannot always be predicted on this basis, however. Some cancers appear to prefer metastatic sites other than those immediately downstream in the blood or lymphatics. Prostate cancer, for example, typically metastasizes to bone. The reason for this selectivity apparently resides with adhesion molecules (integrins) on the cancer cells, which bind preferentially to adhesion molecules (selectins) lining vessels within certain tissues. Secretion of hormones or growth factors by these tissues may also facilitate metastatic growth. Common sites and routes of metastasis for selected primary tumors are summarized in Table 7–16.

TABLE 7–16
COMMON ROUTES AND SITES OF METASTASIS

Primary Site	Metastatic Site	Route
Breast	Brain, adrenals, lung, liver, bone	Blood, lymph
Lung	Brain, adrenals, bone	Blood
Prostate	Bone	Blood
Colon	Liver, lung, bone, brain	Blood, lymph
Kidney	Lung, liver, bone	Blood
Bone	Lung	Blood
Thyroid	Bone, liver, lung	Blood
Pancreas	Liver, lung, adrenals, peritoneal cavity	Blood, lymph, seeding
Stomach	Bone, lung, adrenals, liver, pancreas, peritoneal cavity	Blood, lymph, seeding
Adrenals	Lung, liver	Blood, lymph
Esophagus	Lung, liver, adrenals, bone, brain, kidney	Blood, lymph
Liver	Lungs, bone, adrenals, brain	Blood, lymph

Clinical Manifestations

Effects of cancer depend to a great extent on the cell type of origin, the location of the primary tumor, and the underlying condition of the host. Some common clinical findings include the following:

- Malnutrition due to cytokines (e.g., cachectin) produced by the tumor, metabolic demands of tumor growth, possible obstruction of the gastrointestinal tract, or possible anorexia related to pain, depression, or side effects of therapy
- Pain due to invasion or compression of tissue pain receptors, or nerve injury related to radiation or chemotherapy
- Infection due to barrier breakdown by the cancer or its therapy, or immunosuppression secondary to malnutrition, therapy, or the cancer itself
- Fatigue due to malnutrition, anemia, depression, or the stress of chronic pain
- Bleeding disorders due to vascular invasion, platelet deficiency secondary to therapy, or tumor production of substances that interfere with normal clotting
- Hormonal imbalances due to inappropriate secretion of hormones by tumor cells
- Obstruction of hollow organs by tumor cells occluding lumens or creating external pressure

Clinical manifestations of specific cancers are detailed in Part Two, with discussion of cancers affecting specific body systems.

Prevention and Treatment

Prevention and Early Detection

Prevention of cancer entails assessment of risk factors as well as education and motivation for lifestyle and environmental changes aimed at reducing modifiable risk. Screening examinations, both self-examination and professional evaluation, promote earlier detection and more positive outcomes of cancer. Public information campaigns conducted through the media and warning labels on potential carcinogenic agents such as cigarettes may aid in the fight against cancer.

Several large clinical trials are underway in an effort to establish the efficacy of chemoprevention, the use of micronutrients or drugs to reduce cancer risk. The Breast Cancer Prevention Trial, for example, is evaluating the effectiveness of the antiestrogen drug tamoxifen in prevention of breast cancer in high-risk women.[20] Other studies are evaluating the antioxidant effects and other potentially beneficial effects of vitamins A, C, and E and trace elements such as selenium. Surgical prevention is often employed for removal of precancerous lesions or polyps. In rare cases, healthy tissue may be resected when the risk of malignant transformation is extremely high, as in some forms of hereditary breast and colon cancer.

Treatment

Treatment of cancer may be either palliative or curative. Palliative therapy, designed to relieve symptoms or to retard tumor growth when cure is not possible, may involve surgery, chemotherapy, or radiation therapy to reduce the tumor burden. Analgesics (pain-relieving medications), including anti-inflammatory drugs and opioids, may be administered in doses exceeding normal limits in an effort to ensure comfort of the patient. (Mechanisms of pain relief and related interventions are detailed in Chapter 23.)

Definitive therapy usually involves combinations of methods, with the precise approach depending on the tumor type and its specific stage or grade. Guidelines for therapy may be *investigational*, based on clinical research trial protocols, or *conventional*, based on pooled results of previous trials. Individual preferences and tolerances of therapy are also of primary importance in the choice.

Surgery. Surgical resection of the tumor accounts for the largest number of cures.[21] Removal of the tumor, enclosed by a surrounding layer of normal cells, is indicated in cases in which there is limited direct invasion or metastasis and the location of the tumor is not threatening to vital organs. The outcome of such surgery also must be acceptable to the patient in terms of quality of life issues such as disfigurement or dysfunction.

Radiation Therapy. Radiation therapy, widely used in the treatment of cancer, is the delivery of x-rays or gamma rays to cancerous tissues. The radiation source may be an externally applied beam or internally implanted radioactive pellets. Radiation therapy may be used alone but more often is used in combination with other modes of treatment. Radiation may destroy microscopic metastases missed during surgery or inaccessible to resection.

In target cells, radiation induces sublethal DNA breaks, which are incompletely repaired in radiosensitive cells. Within another cell cycle or two, the damaged cells undergo apoptosis.[22] Many types of cancer cells and some normal cells are highly radiosensitive, particularly epithelial cells of the skin and mucous membranes, bone marrow cells, and germ cells within reproductive organs. During radiation therapy, normal cells are protected to the greatest extent possible with the use of divided doses (fractionation) of radiation, custom-fitted shields for normal tissues, or surgery to temporarily displace reproductive organs from the radiation field.

Chemotherapy. Chemotherapy, or drug therapy of cancer, is a rapidly growing science, with more than 30 antineoplastic agents in common use. The ideal chemotherapeutic agent would preferentially target cancer cells, by virtue of their genetic makeup, increased blood flow, or high oxygen consumption, while sparing normal cells. Unfortunately, few agents have this capability. Most anticancer drugs are *cytotoxic*, that is, they cause DNA damage that can potentially be eliminated by nucleotide excision repair mechanisms. Cancer cells may be deficient in such repair, rendering them vulnerable to apoptosis.[23] Normal cells often have higher thresholds for apoptosis and thus exhibit only cell cycle pauses in response to cytotoxic agents. Nevertheless, normal tissues are nearly always affected to some extent, leading to such adverse effects as sloughing of gastrointestinal epithelial cells, skin lesions, and hair loss. Many chemotherapeutic agents are cell cycle–specific; that is, they attack the cancer cell at a certain stage of the cell cycle. Use of combination therapy targeting different cell cycle stages, as well as different aspects of cell function, maximizes the efficacy of these agents (Table 7–17).

Much research on anticancer drug development is focused on *cytostatic* (growth-arresting), rather than cytotoxic, agents. Cytostatic agents are directed at interruption of genetic and metabolic signal transduction pathways responsible for disordered growth regulation in cancer cells.[23]

Bone Marrow Transplantation. Bone marrow transplantation (BMT) is the treatment of choice for cancers that are responsive to high doses of radiation or chemotherapy, including hematopoietic cancers such as the leukemias and lymphomas and solid tumors such as testicular and breast cancers.[24] In such cases, either the cancer itself or the cancer treatment is toxic to the bone marrow, and BMT is used to "rescue" the patient from this effect. The source of donor marrow may be an immune-matched relative or unrelated donor (*allogenic* transplant) or the patient (*autologous* transplant). In the latter case, some of the patient's own marrow is removed and purged of cancer cells, then reinfused. BMT is discussed further in Chapter 12.

TABLE 7–17
CLASSIFICATION OF CANCER CHEMOTHERAPY (ANTINEOPLASTIC AGENTS)

CLASS	MECHANISM	CELL CYCLE	EXAMPLES
Alkylating agents	Cross-linkage of DNA, preventing transcription and possibly triggering apoptosis	Nonspecific	Busulfan, carboplatin, cisplatin, procarbazine, thiotepa, cyclophosphamide
Antimetabolites	Blockage of enzymes for DNA synthesis or binding to DNA or RNA	S phase	Fluorouracil, mercaptopurine, methotrexate, gemcitabine
Antitumor antibodies	Blockage of enzymes, inhibition of DNA function, alteration of cell membranes	Nonspecific	Bleomycin, doxorubicin, daunorubicin
Plant alkaloids	Blockage of enzymes for DNA replication, inhibition of mitosis	M phase	Etoposide, paclitaxel, vinblastine, vincristine
Topoisomerase inhibitors	Blockage of enzyme which reattaches separated DNA strands after replication	S phase	Doxorubicin, CPT-11

Biologic Response Modifiers. Biologic response modifiers (BRMs) are agents that boost immune system activity or antagonize tumor growth through other biologic effects. These agents may be isolated from human blood, or they may be produced by recombinant DNA technology. BRMs include antibodies and cytokines, such as interferons, interleukins, tumor necrosis factor, and colony-stimulating factors. Although results of early clinical trials of BRMs were often discouraging, recent outcomes have been more favorable.[25]

Gene Therapy. Modes of gene therapy under investigation include the use of synthetic nucleotide strands to bind defective segments of cellular DNA (triplex agents) or mRNA (antisense agents). Such binding prevents production of proteins involved in the molecular mechanisms of neoplastic transformation.[26] Insertion of normal genes into defective cells has been accomplished using viral carriers, resulting in temporary production of normal gene products. Genes that promote apoptosis of cancers cells have also been inserted.[27]

Prognosis and Outcome

Prognosis in cancer varies widely with specific type. Cancer is the second-leading cause of death in the United States, causing more than half a million deaths each year. Between 1975 and 1990, the cancer death rate increased 7%, largely owing to the rising incidence of lung cancer.[28] These mortality statistics, which have been affirmed by the National Cancer Institute of the National Institutes for Health, have been adjusted to remove the effect of population aging.

Cure of cancer is usually clinically defined as 5-year, symptom-free survival. Although some cancers are fatal within a short period, the course of many others is characterized by periods of remission or exacerbation. Most patients with skin cancer and about half of those treated for internal cancers are completely cured. For many patients, cancer is a chronic, rather than acute, disease—one that can be managed, if not cured.

ABNORMAL CELLULAR DEVELOPMENT AND SYSTEMIC DISEASE

Abnormal genetic regulation of cellular development is most closely linked to congenital disorders and neoplasia, further discussed throughout this text in the relevant systems chapters. Disorders of cell growth, division, differentiation, and apoptosis underlie virtually all systemic disorders. Conversely, disorders of anatomic or functional body systems are inevitably expressed at cellular and subcellular levels. Development of rational treatment of disease demands scientific understanding of this subtle, yet most powerful, form of regulation. Along with molecular and cell biology, the sciences of genetics and oncology have had a profound impact on practice within the clinical professions, shifting the focus of pathophysiology to ever more microscopic subsystems.

Summary of Key Points

- Atrophy, a decrease in cell number or cell size within a tissue, may be the result of normally programmed development (physiologic) or pathologic conditions, such as poor tissue perfusion or disuse. Hypertrophy, an increase in cell size, and hyperplasia, an increase in cell numbers, may also be physiologic responses to normal stimuli or pathologic responses, as represented by the cellular proliferation of cancer.
- The major teratogens are infections such as toxoplasmosis, rubella, cytomegalovirus, and herpes simplex (TORCH); maternal diseases such as diabetes mellitus, PKU, and hyperthermia; and drugs, chemicals, and physical agents such as alcohol, methotrexate, anticonvulsants, cocaine, diethylstilbestrol (DES), lithium, radiation, tetracycline, thalidomide, toluene, vitamin A derivatives, and warfarin.
- Single gene mutations are usually base pair substitutions (point mutations) or frame shifts, in which insertion or deletion of a base results in misreading of the genetic code.
- Chromosomal defects are usually due to anaphase lag or nondisjunction, leading to aneuploidy, or to chromosomal breakage, leading to translocation or other structural defects.
- Mendelian principles include the principle of dominance, in which one gene at a locus may mask the expression of the other allele, termed recessive; the principle of segregation, which refers to separation of paired chromosomes in gametes; and the principle of independent assortment, in which traits represented by multiple loci are distributed randomly within the gametes, independent of each other.
- Benign tumors are usually well differentiated, slow growing, noninvasive, localized, clearly demarcated, and encapsulated. Malignant tumors are usually poorly differentiated, rapidly growing, invasive, metastatic, and poorly demarcated.
- Major risk factors for cancer include host factors, such as age, sex, genetic factors, psychologic factors, immunosuppression, and chronic tissue trauma; as well as environmental and lifestyle factors related to geographic location, nutrition, occupation, and cigarette smoking.
- Cancers arise from a single cell that suffers multiple transforming genetic mutations, either inherited or acquired (carcinogen induced). Transformation may activate growth-promoting proto-oncogenes or may inhibit the expression of tumor suppressor genes.
- Local growth and invasion of cancer depend on the intrinsic cell cycle time of the cell of origin and the rate of tumor angiogenesis. Metastatic spread may occur by gravitational seeding or by lymphatic or hematogenous routes.
- Clinical manifestations common to many forms of cancer include malnutrition, pain, infection, fatigue, bleeding disorders, hormonal imbalances, and obstruction of hollow organs.
- Principal modes of cancer prevention include education, screening examination, and chemoprevention. Treatment of cancer may be palliative or definitive. Definitive therapy may include surgical resection, radiation therapy, chemotherapy, BMT, BRMs, or gene therapy.

REFERENCES

1. Conover, E. (1994). Hazardous exposures during pregnancy. *Journal of Obstetric, Gynecologic, and Neonatal Nursing* 23(6), 524–532.
2. Heisler, M.B., and Richmond, J.B. (1994). Lessons from Finland's successful immunization program. *New England Journal of Medicine* 331(21), 1446–1447.
3. Moore, K.L., and Persaud, T.V.N. (1993). *The Developing Human: Clinically Oriented Embryology*. Philadelphia: W.B. Saunders Co. (p. 165).
4. Shaw, G.M., Velie, E.M., and Schaffer, D. (1996). Risk of neural tube defect: Affected pregnancies among obese women. *Journal of the American Medical Association* 275(14), 1093–1096.
5. Behrman, R.E., and Kliegman, R.M., (Eds.). (1992). *Nelson Textbook of Pediatrics*. (14th ed.). Philadelphia: W.B. Saunders Co. (p. 299).
6. West, J.R., Chen, W.A., and Pantazis, N.J. (1994). Fetal alcohol syndrome: The vulnerability of the developing brain and possible mechanisms of damage. *Metabolic Brain Disease* 9(4), 291–321.
7. Seaver, L.H., and Hoyme, H.E. (1992). Teratology in pediatric practice. *Pediatric Clinics of North America* 39(1), 111–134.
8. Walter, J.B. (1992). *An Introduction to the Principles of Disease*. (3rd ed.). Philadelphia: W.B. Saunders Co. (pp. 244–251).
9. Thompson, M.W., McInnes, R.R., and Willard, H.F. (1991). *Thompson & Thompson Genetics in Medicine*. (5th ed.). Philadelphia: W.B. Saunders Co. (p. 120).

10. Bernards, A., and Gusella, J.F. (1994). The importance of genetic mosaicism in human disease. *New England Journal of Medicine* 331(21), 1447–1449.
11. Beaudet, A.L., Scriver, C.R., Sly, W.S., *et al.* (1995). Genetics, biochemistry, and molecular basis of variant human phenotypes. In: Scriver, C.R., Beudet, A.L., Sly, W.S., *et al.* (Eds.). *The Metabolic and Molecular Bases of Inherited Disease.* (7th ed.). Volume 1. New York: McGraw-Hill. (pp. 53–118).
12. Langlis, S. (1994). Genomic imprinting: A new mechanism for disease. *Pediatric Pathology* 14(1), 161–165.
13. Lander, E.S., and Schork, N.J. (1994). Genetic dissection of complex traits. *Science* 265(5181), 2037–2048.
14. Maier, S.F., Watkins, L.R., and Fleshner, M. (1994). Psychoneuroimmunology: The interface between behavior, brain, and immunity. *American Psychologist* 49(12), 1004–1017.
15. Stefanek, M.E. (1990). Counseling women at high risk for breast cancer. *Oncology* 4(1), 27–38.
16. McGinnis, J.M., and Foege, W.H. (1993). Actual causes of death in the United States. *Journal of the American Medical Association* 270(18), 2207–2212.
17. Cavenee, W.K., and While, R.L. (1995). The genetic basis of cancer. *Scientific American* 272(3), 72–79.
18. Marx, J. (1994). How cells cycle toward cancer. *Science* 263, 319–320.
19. Rouslahti, E. (1996). How cancer spreads. *Scientific American* 275(3), 72–77.
20. Greenwald, P. (1996). Chemoprevention of cancer. *Scientific American* 275(3), 96–99.
21. Hellman, S., and Vokes, E.E. (1996). Advancing current treatments for cancer. *Scientific American* 275(3), 118–123.
22. Lichter, A.S., and Lawrence, T.S. (1995). Recent advances in radiation oncology. *New England Journal of Medicine* 332(6), 371–379.
23. Gibbs, J.B., and Oliff, A. (1994). Pharmaceutical research in molecular oncology. *Cell* 79(2), 193–198.
24. Armitage, J.O. (1994). Bone marrow transplantation. *New England Journal of Medicine* 330(12), 827–838.
25. Jassak, P.F. (1993). Biotherapy. In: Groenwald, S.L., Frogge, M.H., Goodman, M., *et al.* (Eds.). *Cancer Nursing: Principles and Practice.* (3rd ed.). Boston: Jones & Bartlett Publishers. (pp. 366–392).
26. Cohen, J.S., and Hogan, M.E. (1994). The new genetic medicines. *Scientific American* 271(6), 76–82.
27. Anderson, W.F. (1995). Gene therapy. *Scientific American* 272(9), 124–128.
28. Beardsley, T. (1994). A war not won. *Scientific American* 270(1), 130–138.

SELECTED BIBLIOGRAPHY

Barker, F.G., and Israel, M.A. (1995). The molecular biology of brain tumors. *Neurologic Clinics* 13(4), 701–714.

Barlow, D.P. (1995). Gametic imprinting in mammals. *Science* 270, 1610–1613.

Bertram, J.S., and Bortkiewicz, H. (1995). Dietary carotenoids inhibit neoplastic transformation and modulate gene expression in mouse and human cells. *American Journal of Clinical Nutrition* 62(suppl.), 1327S–1336S.

Bhatia, S., Robison, L.L., Oberlin, O., *et al.* (1996). Breast cancer and other second neoplasms after childhood Hodgkin's disease. *New England Journal of Medicine* 334(12), 745–751.

Blackburn, S.T., and Loper, D.L. (1992). *Maternal, Fetal, and Neonatal Physiology: A Clinical Perspective.* Philadelphia: W.B. Saunders Co.

Chandley, A.C. (1991). On the parental origin of de novo mutation in man. *Journal of Medical Genetics* 28(4), 217–223.

Cleaver, J.E. (1994). It was a very good year for DNA repair. *Cell* 76(1), 1–4.

Cotran, R.S., Kumar, V., and Robbins, S.L. (1994). *Robbins Pathologic Basis of Disease.* (5th ed.). Philadelphia: W.B. Saunders Co.

Deslypere, J.P. (1995). Obesity and cancer. *Metabolism* 44(9 suppl. 3), 24–27.

Dhami, M.S., and Bona, R.D. (1993). Thrombosis in patients with cancer. *Postgraduate Medicine* 93(8), 131–140.

Fidler, I.J., and Ellis, L.M. (1994). The implications of angiogenesis for biology and therapy of cancer metastasis. *Cell* 79(2), 185–188.

Fisher, D.E. (1994). Apoptosis in cancer therapy: Crossing the threshold. *Cell* 78(4), 539–542.

Greider, C.W., and Blackburn, E.H. (1996). Telomeres, telomerase, and cancer. *Scientific American* 274(2), 92–97.

Guengerich, F.P. (1995). Influence of nutrients and other dietary materials on cytochrome P-450 enzymes. *American Journal of Clinical Nutrition* 61(suppl.), 651S–658S.

Haber, D.A. (1995). Telomeres, cancer, and immortality. *New England Journal of Medicine* 332(14), 955–956.

Hanawalt, P.C. (1994). Transcription-coupled repair and human disease. *Science* 266, 1957–1958.

Hartwell, L.H., and Kastan, M.B. (1994). Cell cycle control and cancer. *Science* 266, 1821–1828.

Hennekens, C.H., Buring, J.E., Manson, J.E., *et al.* (1996). Lack of effect of long-term supplementation with beta carotene on the incidence of malignant neoplasms and cardiovascular disease. *New England Journal of Medicine* 334(18), 1145–1149.

Housman, D. (1995). Human DNA polymorphism. *New England Journal of Medicine* 332(5), 318–320.

Jones, S.L. (1994). Genetic-based and assisted reproductive technology of the 21st century. *Journal of Obstetric, Gynecologic, and Neonatal Nursing* 23(2), 160–165.

Kelley, R.L., and Kuroda, M.I. (1995). Equality for X chromosomes. *Science* 270, 1607–1610.

Kelloff, G.J., Boone, C.W., Steele, V.E., *et al.* (1994). Progress in cancer chemoprevention: Perspectives on agent selection and short-term clinical intervention trials. *Cancer Research* 54(suppl.), 2015s–2024s.

Korf, B. (1995). Molecular medicine: Molecular diagnosis. *New England Journal of Medicine* 332(18 Pt. 1), 1218–1220.

Korf, B. (1995). Molecular medicine: Molecular diagnosis. *New England Journal of Medicine* 332(22 Pt. 2), 1499–1502.

Krontiris, T.G. (1995). Molecular medicine: Oncogenes. *New England Journal of Medicine* 333(5), 303–306.

Latchman, D.S. (1996). Transcription factor mutations and disease. *New England Journal of Medicine* 334(1), 28–33.

Lokich, J., and Anderson, N. (1995). Infusional cancer chemotherapy: Historical evolution and future development at the cancer center of Boston. *Cancer Investigation* 13(2), 202–226.

Modrich, P. (1994). Mismatch repair, genetic stability, and cancer. *Science* 266, 1959–1960.

Naber, S.P. (1994). Molecular medicine. Molecular pathology: Detection of neoplasia. *New England Journal of Medicine* 331(22), 1508–1510.

Nussbaum, R.H., and Kohnlein, W. (1994). Inconsistencies and open questions regarding low-dose health effects of ionizing radiation. *Environmental Health Perspectives* 102(8), 656–667.

Omenn, G.S., Goodman, G.E., Thornquist, M.D., *et al.* (1996). Effects of a combination of beta carotene and vitamin A on lung cancer and cardiovascular disease. *New England Journal of Medicine* 334(18), 1150–1155.

Pathmanathan, R., Prasad, U., Sadler, R., *et al.* (1995). Clonal proliferation of cells infected with Epstein-Barr virus in preinvasive lesions related to nasopharyngeal carcinoma. *New England Journal of Medicine* 333(11), 693–698.

Pearson, M.A., Hoyme, H.E., Seaver, L.H., *et al.* (1994). Toluene embryopathy: Delineation of the phenotype and comparison with fetal alcohol syndrome. *Pediatrics* 93(2), 211–215.

Perera, F.P. (1996). Uncovering new clues to cancer risk. *Scientific American* 274(5), 54–62.

Rabbitts, T.H. (1994). Chromosomal translocations in human cancer. *Nature* 372, 143–149.

Rader, P.M. (1995). Developing brain as a target of toxicity. *Environmental Health Perspectives* 103(suppl. 6), 73–76.

Raff, B.S. (1994). Nursing and genetics for the 21st century. *Journal of Obstetric, Gynecologic, and Neonatal Nursing* 23(6), 477–480.

Rothman, K.J., Moore, L.L., Singer, M.R., *et al.* (1995). Teratogenicity of high vitamin A intake. *New England Journal of Medicine* 333(21), 1369–1373.

Sadowski, P.D. (1993). Site-specific genetic recombination: Hops, flips, and flops. *FASEB Journal* 7, 760–767.

Salvatore, J.R. (1996). Low-frequency magnetic fields and cancer. *Postgraduate Medicine* 100(2), 183–190.

Sancar, A. (1994). Mechanisms of DNA excision repair. *Science* 266, 1954–1956.

Schutte, D. (1995). Genetic illness in the adult ICU: Implications for nursing practice. *Critical Care Nurse* 15(3), 49–56.

Schwartz, R.S. (1995). Jumping genes. *New England Journal of Medicine* 332(14), 941–944.

Sidransky, D. (1996). Advances in cancer detection. *Scientific American* 275(3), 104–107.

Smith, J.R., and Pereira-Smith, O.M. (1996). Replicative senescence: Implications for in vivo aging and tumor suppression. *Science* 273, 63–67.

Steinbach, F., Tanabe, K., Alexander, J., *et al.* (1996). The influence of cytokines on the adhesion of renal cancer cells to endothelium. *Journal of Urology* 155, 743–749.

Studzinski, G.P., and Moore, D.C. (1995). Sunlight: Can it prevent as well as cause cancer? *Cancer Research* 55, 4014–4022.

Trichopoulos, D., Li, F.P., and Hunter, D.J. (1996). What causes cancer? *Scientific American* 275(3), 80–87.

Weinberg, R.A. (1996). How cancer arises. *Scientific American* 275(3), 62–70.

Wertz, D.C., Fanos, J.H., and Reilly, P.R. (1994). Genetic testing for children and adolescents: Who decides? *Journal of the American Medical Association* 272(11), 875–881.

West, J.R., Chen, W-J.A., and Pantazis, N.J. (1994). Fetal alcohol syndrome: The vulnerability of the developing brain and possible mechanisms of damage. *Metabolic Brain Disease* 9(4), 291–321.

Willett, W.C., Colditz, G.A., and Mueller, N.E. (1996). Strategies for minimizing cancer risk. *Scientific American* 275(3), 88–95.

Unit III

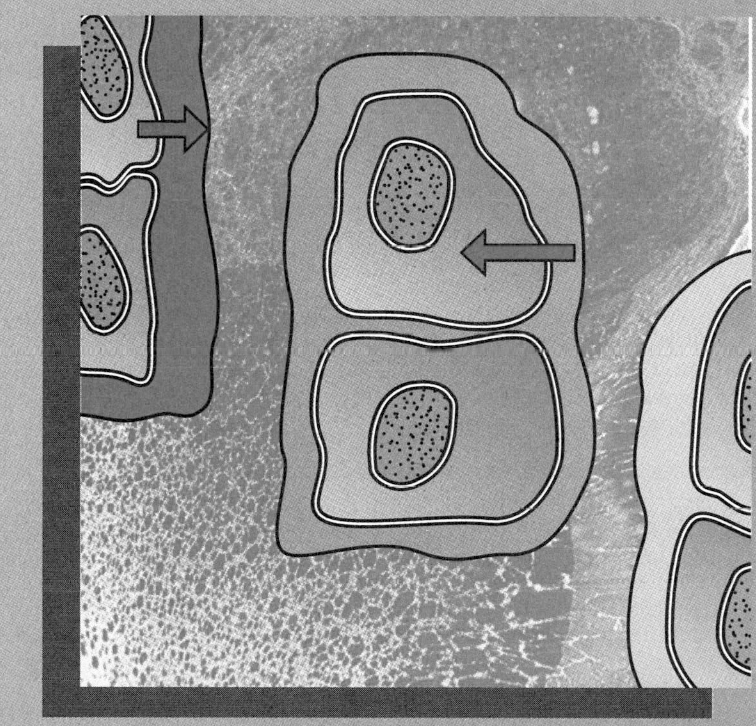

Chapter 8
Fluid Balance

Chapter 9
Electrolyte Balance

Chapter 10
Acid-Base Balance

Chapter 11
Thermoregulation

THE CELLULAR ENVIRONMENT

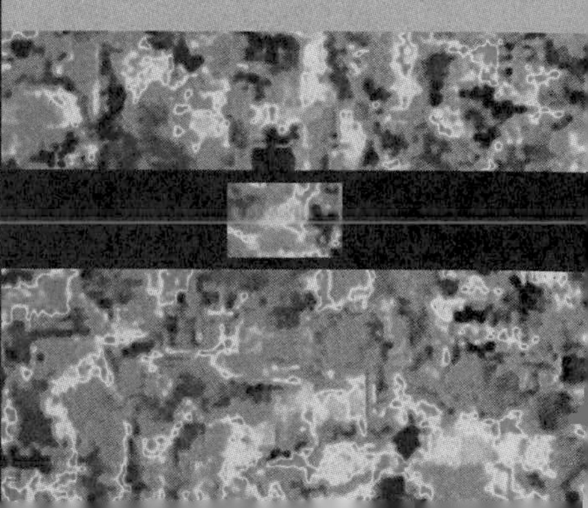

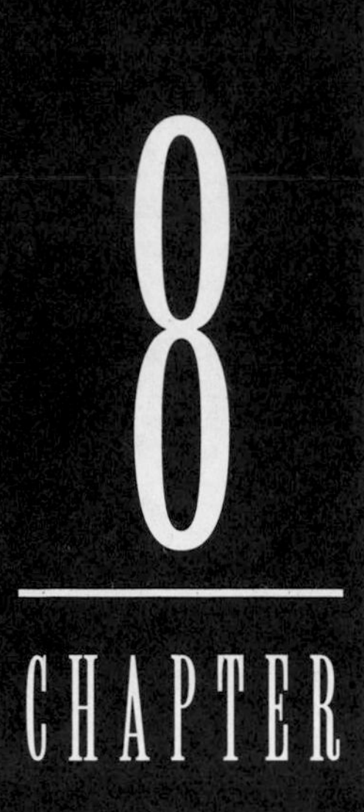

Fluid Balance

LEARNING OBJECTIVES

1. Differentiate among the body fluid compartments in terms of location and contribution to total body water.
2. Identify the principal sources of fluid intake and routes of fluid output.
3. Describe the physical and hormonal mechanisms that regulate systemic fluid balance.
4. Describe the effects of osmotic pressure gradients on fluid exchange between the intracellular and interstitial spaces.
5. Discuss the dynamics of capillary fluid exchange within the context of Starling's law of the capillary.
6. Discuss the clinical significance of fluid shift from the plasma to the interstitial space or from the interstitial space to the plasma.
7. Contrast the clinical features of hypovolemia and hypervolemia.
8. Contrast the clinical features of hypo-osmolar and hyperosmolar imbalances.
9. Identify developmental variables that influence fluid balance.

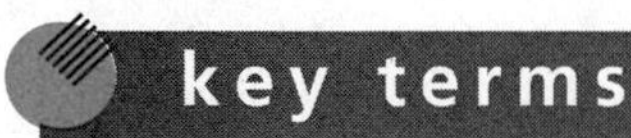

key terms

aldosterone
angioedema
angiotensin-converting enzyme
angiotensin I
angiotensin II
angiotensinogen
antidiuretic hormone (ADH)
arginine vasopressin
atrial natriuretic peptide (ANP)
capillary hydrostatic pressure (CHP)
colloid
diuresis
Donnan effect
edema
effusion
extracellular fluid (ECF)
exudate
filtration
glomerular filtration rate
hyperosmolar imbalance
hypertonic
hypervolemia
hypo-osmolar imbalance

hypotonic
hypovolemia
interstitial fluid
intracellular fluid (ICF)
intravascular fluid
isotonic
lymphedema
oliguria
organic osmolyte
osmolality
osmolarity
osmoreceptor
plasma colloid osmotic pressure
polydipsia
reabsorption
renin
renin–angiotensin–aldosterone system (RAAS)
specific gravity
third spacing
tissue hydrostatic pressure
tissue osmotic pressure
transcellular fluid
transudate
turgor

Water is the medium within which the human system and all its subsystems function. Water surrounds cells and is contained within them. *Fluid balance* refers to processes that establish and maintain equilibrium in the exchange of water among the internal fluid compartments of the body and between the body and the external environment. Fluid balance depends on mechanisms that regulate fluid volume and the proportions of water and particles, quantified as **osmolality** or **osmolarity**. (Osmolality is expressed as osmoles of solute per *kilogram* of solvent, while osmolarity is expressed as osmoles per *liter* of solvent.) Conditions that disrupt fluid balance are common in clinical practice, involving every organ system.

DISTRIBUTION OF BODY FLUIDS

In adults, about 60% of total body weight is derived from water, although considerable variation exists depending on the proportion of lean body mass to adipose tissue. Total body water volume (in liters) can be estimated by dividing the body weight in pounds by 4, then adjusting the result by adding 10% for more muscle mass (typical in men) or by subtracting 10% for less muscle or more fat (because adipose tissue excludes water).[1] Accordingly, obese people, women, infants, and the elderly are at greater risk for dehydration in clinical conditions that cause fluid loss.

Water is found within two major compartments in the body: **intracellular fluid (ICF)** and **extracellular fluid (ECF)** (Fig. 8–1). ICF comprises about two thirds of fluid volume, and ECF constitutes about one third. ECF may be subdivided into three compartments: **intravascular fluid**, the plasma of the blood as well as the fluid inside blood cells; **interstitial fluid**, the fluid found in the interstices (extracellular matrix) between cells, in connective tissues, and in the lymphatic capillaries; and **transcellular fluid**, consisting of fluids other than blood that are exchanged within the body, such as saliva, pleural fluid, peritoneal fluid, intraocular fluids, synovial fluids, and cerebrospinal fluid.

Because fluids in the intracellular and interstitial compartments are normally inaccessible for clinical analysis, their status is usually evaluated indirectly, on the basis of testing of blood or transcellular fluids. Fluids in each compartment differ in their composition of electrolytes and other solutes. Transport between compartments is the basis of action potential formation and other forms of intercellular communication (see Chapter 2). Furthermore, because evaporation of water from the surface of the body is the body's most important cooling mechanism, fluid balance also affects temperature regulation (see Chapter 11).

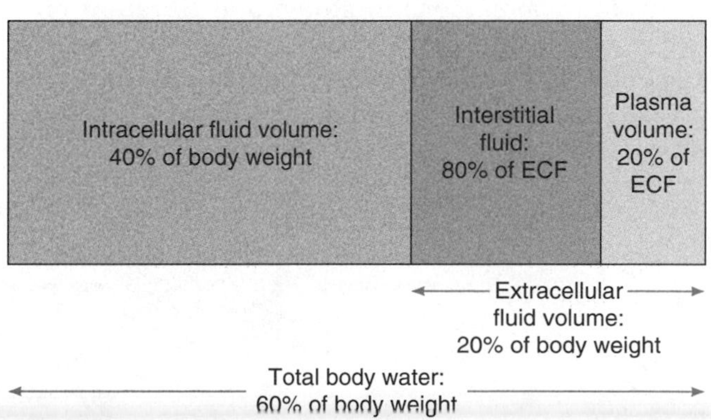

FIGURE 8–1
Distribution of body water.

SYSTEMIC FLUID BALANCE: INTAKE AND OUTPUT

Normal sources of fluid intake and routes of output are illustrated in Figure 8-2.

Sources of Fluid Intake

The body's primary source of fluid intake is dietary; the typical adult consumes about 2200 mL/day of water. Water is also gained as a by-product of metabolic reactions within the body. This water of metabolism has been estimated at 200 to 300 mL/day and is not considered clinically significant.

Water is lost to the external environment through the urine (about 1500 mL/day) and stool (100 mL/day). These amounts may be altered considerably with disorders of renal or gastrointestinal function. *Insensible* water loss (about 900 mL/day) occurs through evaporation from the skin or respiratory tract. This loss is not usually detectable and is not clinically significant in most cases. An exception to this occurs in the case of severe burns, when large volumes of fluid may be lost as water vapor from the surface of the burn wounds. Water loss through sweating is detectable and therefore distinct from insensible loss through the skin. The volume of sweat is normally low (100 mL/day or less) but may approach 5000 mL with heavy exertion in a hot, dry environment.

Regulation of Systemic Fluid Balance

Fluid volume and osmolarity are maintained within normal limits by the hypothalamic thirst mechanism, which governs the amount of water taken in; by alterations in **glomerular filtration rate,** which influences urine output; and by several hormones, notably **aldosterone, antidiuretic hormone (ADH)**, and **atrial natriuretic peptide (ANP)**, which act on the kidney to regulate urine volume and osmolality. A number of researchers are attempting to clarify cellular and molecular mechanisms of this regulation (see Focus of Current Research).

Thirst Mechanism

The role of the hypothalamus in coordination of the stress response is discussed in Chapter 1. Physiologic regulation of thirst is another of the many regulatory functions of this neuroendocrine organ (Fig. 8-3). Specialized receptor cells in the hypothalamus sense alterations in the fluid surrounding them. These **osmoreceptors** shrink when interstitial fluid is more concentrated than the ICF because ICF leaves the cells along the osmotic gradient. Alterations in the cell membranes of these receptors trigger nerve impulses along sensory pathways to areas of the brain that interpret the sensation as thirst, subsequently motivating the person to drink. Dry mouth due to decreased salivation may also be a triggering factor. Intake of fluid increases the volume and lowers the osmolarity of the ECF, completing a negative feedback loop.

Glomerular Filtration Rate

The most direct mechanism by which the kidney regulates fluid volume is by altering its rate of removal of fluid from the blood through specialized capillaries (glomeruli). The greater the blood volume, the greater is the hydrostatic pressure driving fluid out of glomerular capillaries into the renal tubules. Fluid entering the tubules is excreted as urine unless it is later reabsorbed into the blood under the influence of the hormones aldosterone and ADH. Glomerular filtration and tubular transport mechanisms of the kidney are detailed in Chapter 20.

Aldosterone and the Renin–Angiotensin–Aldosterone System

Aldosterone is a steroid hormone released from the adrenal cortex when ECF volume is low or when the serum sodium concentration [Na^+] is elevated, that is, when serum osmolarity is high. Regulation occurs by a complex negative feedback loop

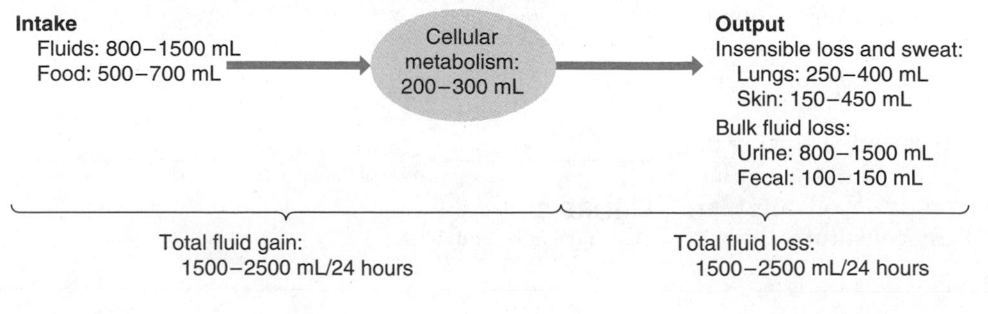

FIGURE 8-2
Systemic fluid balance. Daily fluid gain from dietary sources and from metabolism must balance daily fluid loss.

Focus of Current Research

Study	*Objective and Findings*
Goldman, et al. (1996) The influence of polydipsia on water excretion in hyponatremic, polydipsic, schizophrenic patients	*Objective:* To determine whether polydipsia is responsible for altered water excretion in schizophrenic patients who exhibit excessive water intake *Findings:* Hyponatremia occurs in some patients because the relationship between free water excretion and plasma osmolality is shifted to the left; that is, water clearance is decreased at lower osmolalities.
Folkesson, et al. (1996) Transepithelial water permeability in microperfused distal airways	*Objective:* To investigate the mechanism of water movement across the airway epithelium *Findings:* Water is transported through specific channels and is generally driven by osmotic gradients produced by active ion transport.
Zhang, et al. (1995) Identification and activation of autocrine renin-angiotensin system in adult ventricular myocytes	*Objective:* To determine whether components of the renin–angiotensin system were present in cardiac muscle cells *Findings:* Expression of genes for renin, angiotensinogen, angiotensin-converting enzyme, and angiotensin II receptors was detected.
Sone, et al. (1995) Restoration of urine concentrating ability and accumulation of medullary osmolytes after chronic diuresis	*Objective:* To investigate the cellular processes responsible for restoration of osmolarity within the medullary interstitium of the nephron after chronic diuresis. *Findings:* After diuresis, accumulation of organic osmolytes and restoration of urine osmolality proceed in parallel.
Takamata, et al. (1995) Body temperature modification of osmotically induced vasopressin secretion and thirst in humans	*Objective:* To investigate the effect of increased body temperature on secretion of vasopressin (antidiuretic hormone). *Findings:* Increased body temperature increases vasopressin secretion in a P_{osm}-dependent manner.
Kraly, et al. (1995) Drinking after intragastric NaCl without increase in systemic plasma osmolality in rats	*Objective:* To determine whether increased plasma osmolality always accompanies initiation of drinking *Findings:* Administration of a hypertonic solution into the stomach elicited a drinking response even though P_{osm} was unchanged, supporting the hypothesis of a neural osmosensitive mechanism regulating this behavior.

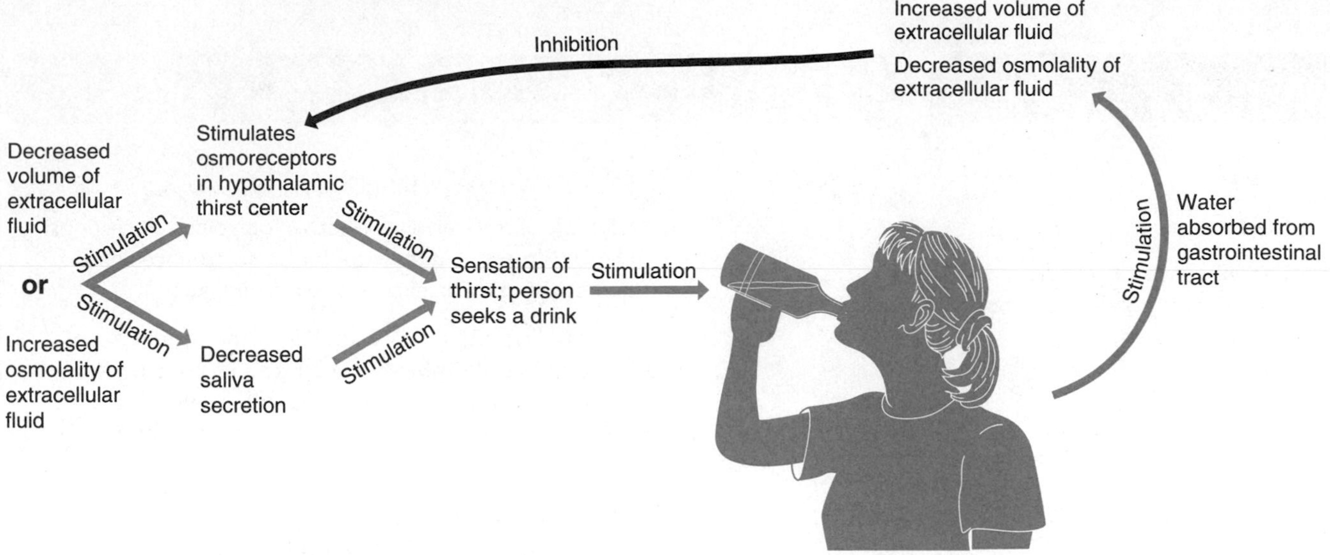

FIGURE 8–3

Regulation of thirst. Osmoreceptors in the hypothalamus trigger the thirst sensation when extracellular fluid volume is low or osmolality is high. Decreased saliva and dry mouth may also stimulate thirst.

known as the **renin–angiotensin–aldosterone system (RAAS)**, shown in Figure 8–4. Two types of receptor cells, osmoreceptors and baroreceptors, trigger this mechanism in the kidney.

The juxtaglomerular cells, located in the walls of the blood vessels leading into the kidney, are examples of baroreceptors in that they sense the degree of pressure within these vessels. This pressure is proportional to the volume of blood entering the kidney, which in turn depends on vascular volume in the system as a whole. When blood volume is low, juxtaglomerular cells stimulate the release of the hormone **renin** from renal cells. Renin enters the blood and converts a precursor protein, **angiotensinogen**, to **angiotensin I**. AGT I is then activated to **angiotensin II** by **angiotensin-converting enzyme**, produced primarily by lung cells. Angiotensin II stimulates the synthesis and release of aldosterone from the adrenal cortex. Aldosterone induces active **reabsorption** of sodium from kidney tubules, that is, the transport of sodium from the tubular fluid back into the blood. Sodium reabsorption creates an osmotic gradient for more water to be retained, and blood volume rises, completing the loop.

The RAAS cycle may also be triggered by low serum osmolality, sensed by the osmoreceptor macula densa cells of the distal tubules of the kidney. These cells stimulate renin release in response to low sodium chloride (NaCl) concentration in the distal tubular fluid. Although lack of tubular sodium has long been believed to be the primary stimulus, more recent research indicates that chloride might be the more important initiator of RAAS by this mechanism.[2] The RAAS results in sodium retention, restoring osmolality in a negative feedback effect.

A number of other stimuli influence the RAAS, including sympathetic nervous system stimulation of juxtaglomerular cells, which initiates renin release in low-volume states; adrenocorticotropic hormone, which promotes aldosterone release to a minor extent by the hypothalamic–pituitary endocrine axis (Chapter 27); increased serum potassium, which directly stimulates aldosterone release (Chapter 9); and a number of locally released signaling molecules, including prostaglandins, kinins, and adenosine, which are involved in autoregulation of renal blood flow.

In addition to the circulating RAAS system all components of the system, including angiotensinogen, angiotensin-converting enzyme, and angiotensin II, have been found in several tissues, including the arterial wall, kidney, adrenal cortex, heart, pituitary, gonads, and brain.[3] This suggests that angiotensin II plays an important role in local regulation as well.

Antidiuretic Hormone

Diuresis is an increase in the volume of urine output. As its name suggests, ADH has an *anti*diuretic action; that is, it results in retention of water in the blood and in decreased urine output (Fig. 8–5). ADH is synthesized by the hypothalamus and

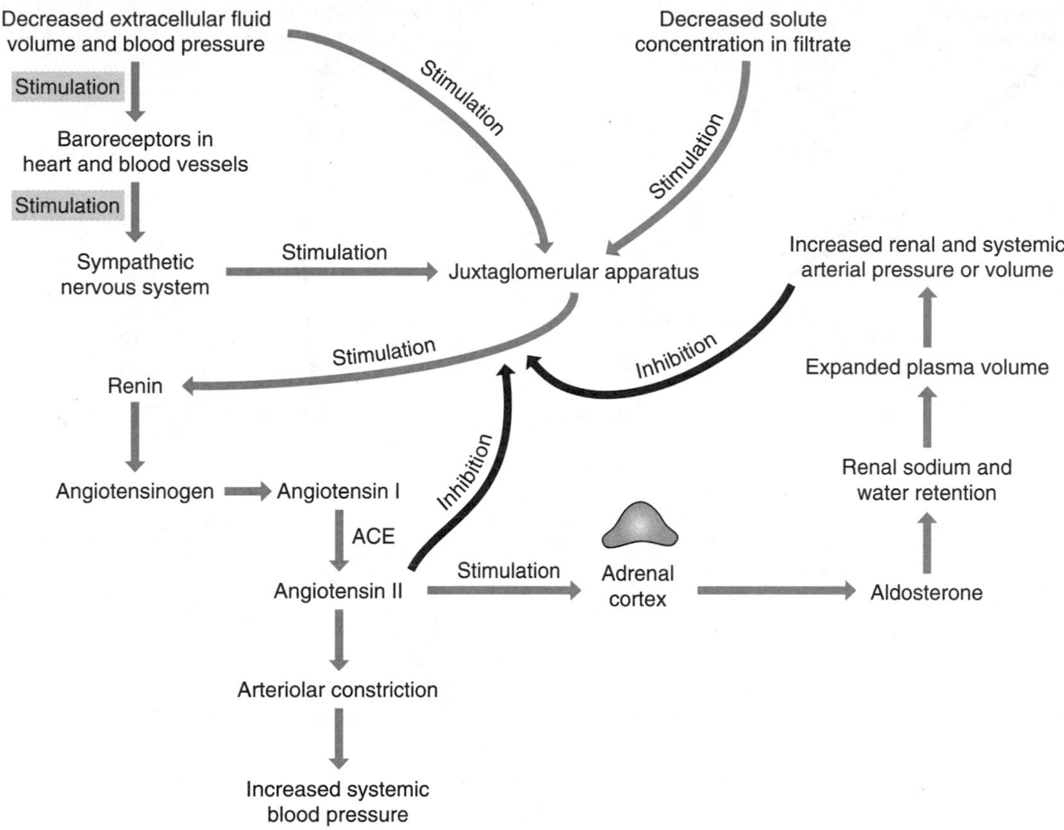

FIGURE 8–4

Renin–angiotensin–aldosterone system. This system is a complex endocrine response that may be initiated by decreased blood volume or pressure, decreased tubular solute, or sympathetic nervous system stimulation. A sequence of hormonal actions results in activation of angiotensin II, a potent vasoconstrictor, which also stimulates release of aldosterone from the adrenal cortex. Aldosterone stimulates the reabsorption of sodium, which establishes an osmotic gradient for reabsorption of water (ACE, angiotensin-converting enzyme).

released from the posterior pituitary gland. ADH release is stimulated when the hypothalamus is signaled in either of two ways: by hypothalamic osmoreceptors, probably distinct from those mediating thirst, when ECF osmolarity is high; and by baroreceptors in large blood vessels, which signal the hypothalamus when blood volume is low. The primary stimulus for ADH release is high osmolarity. If ECF osmolarity is elevated, ADH is released regardless of volume status. As discussed later with fluid imbalances, a number of other stimuli may also initiate ADH release, often detrimentally.

ADH initiates expression of water channels in the distal convoluted tubule and collecting duct of the nephron, rendering them permeable to water. Water can only be reabsorbed into the blood from the tubules if ADH is present. In summary, high ECF osmolarity (or low volume) stimulates release of ADH from the posterior pituitary. ADH permits reabsorption of water from tubular fluid into the blood, lowering osmolarity and increasing volume, completing the negative feedback loop.

ADH is also known as **arginine vasopressin**, a term that reflects its ability to mediate vasoconstriction. ADH is occasionally used pharmacologically for this purpose and may be replaced therapeutically in ADH-deficient states such as diabetes insipidus (see Chapter 27).

Atrial Natriuretic Peptide

Atrial natriuretic peptide is generally considered to be a cardiac hormone because it is primarily released from cells of the atrial myocardium in response to volume-induced atrial stretch. ANP is also found in several locations in the brain and has multiple forms and functions.[4] In regulation of fluid balance, ANP functions as a relatively weak antagonist of RAAS and ADH, protecting the body against fluid overload.[5] ANP is of particular importance in regulation of serum sodium, blood pressure, and cardiac output and is discussed further in chapters relevant to these functions (see Chapters 9, 15, and 16).

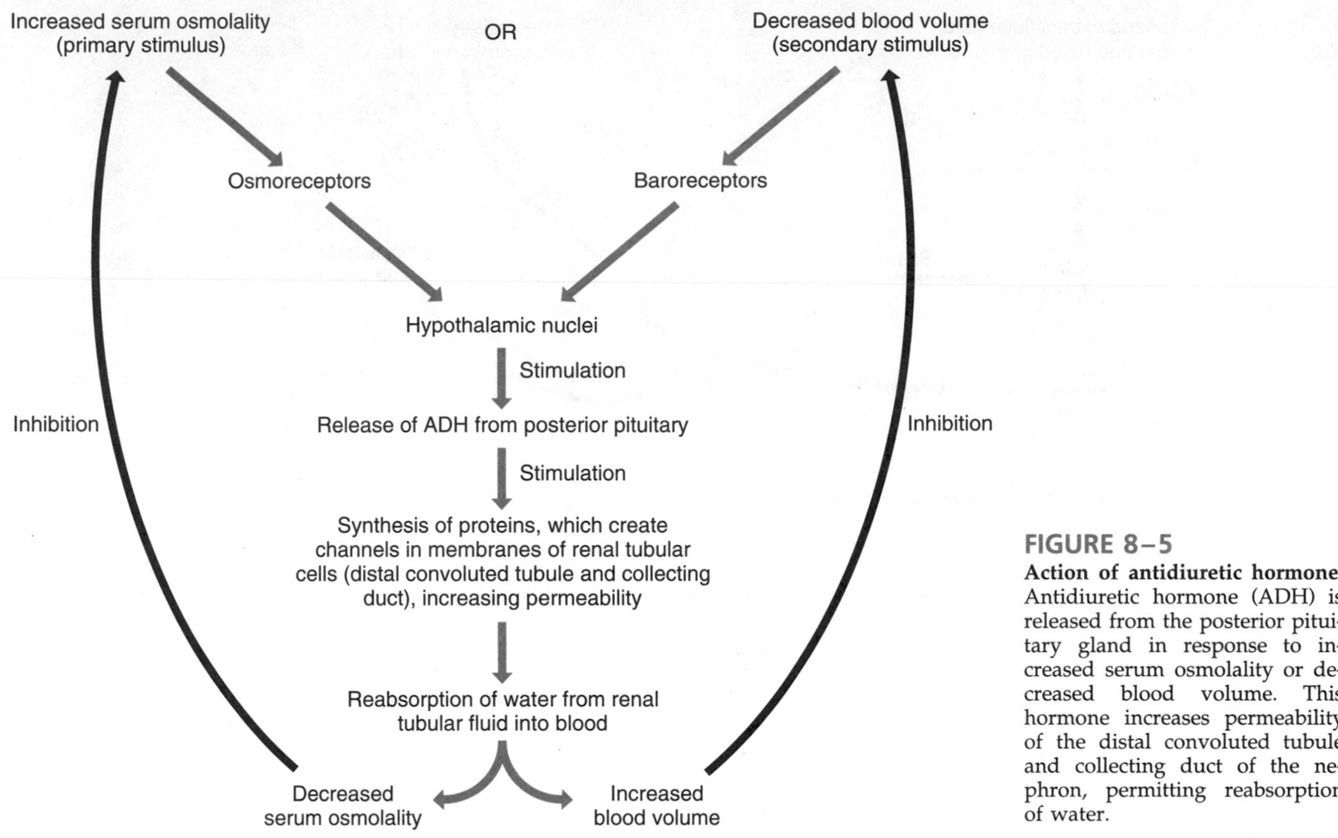

FIGURE 8–5
Action of antidiuretic hormone. Antidiuretic hormone (ADH) is released from the posterior pituitary gland in response to increased serum osmolality or decreased blood volume. This hormone increases permeability of the distal convoluted tubule and collecting duct of the nephron, permitting reabsorption of water.

COMPARTMENTAL FLUID BALANCE: PRESSURE GRADIENTS AND CAPILLARY EXCHANGE

Internal fluid balance involves exchange of water between the ICF and the ECF and among ECF compartments. Exchange of fluid between the cytoplasm and the interstitial space is driven by osmotic gradients created by the active and passive transport of particles. Exchange between the interstitial and vascular spaces involves transport across the capillary membrane along both osmotic and hydrostatic pressure gradients. The emphasis in this chapter is on general mechanisms of compartmental fluid balance—those affecting all body systems. Mechanisms regulating balance between transcellular fluid systems and the blood are highly specialized and are discussed in the appropriate systems chapters.

Osmotic Pressure

As discussed in Chapter 2, osmosis is movement of water from an area of lesser concentration of particles to an area of greater concentration of particles. This pulling force on water depends on a compartmental membrane that is more permeable to water than to solute. In clinical situations, plasma osmolality (P_{osm}) may be measured directly or may be estimated by the following formula[2]:

$$P_{osm} = 2 \times \text{plasma } [Na^+] + [glucose]/18 + BUN/2.8$$

As is apparent from the formula, sodium, glucose, and urea (BUN refers to blood urea nitrogen) are the principal solutes contributing to plasma osmolality. Glucose and BUN values are divided by 18 and 2.8, respectively, to correct for differences in measurement units. Because plasma membranes are highly permeable to urea, however, this solute is not effective in attracting or holding water in the extracellular space. The *effective* P_{osm} can thus be calculated without including the BUN term. The normal P_{osm} range is 275 to 290 mOsm/kg, whereas the range for effective P_{osm} is 270 to 285 mOsm/kg.[2] Urine osmolality is also measured in clinical settings because it reflects the plasma solute load as well as renal tubular function and the renal response to ADH and aldosterone. The solute concentration of the urine may also be assessed by measurement of

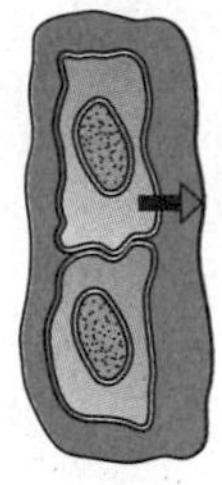
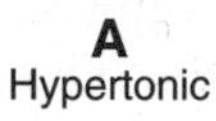
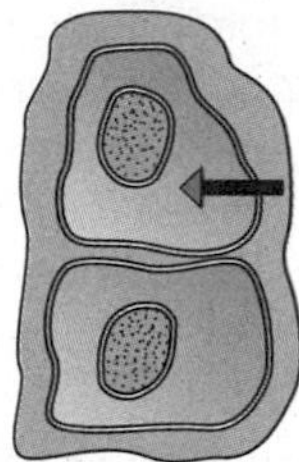
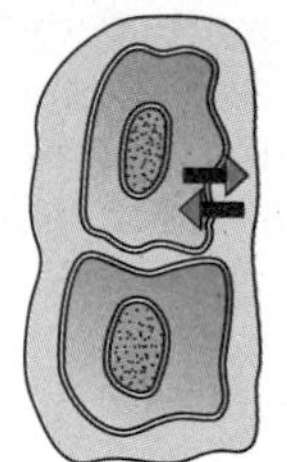

FIGURE 8–6

Cellular response to altered osmolality of the extracellular fluid (ECF). *A,* Cells placed in hypertonic ECF shrink as water leaves along the osmotic gradient. *B,* Cells placed in hypotonic ECF swell as water enters. *C,* With isotonic fluid imbalances, there is no osmotic effect on cells.

the **specific gravity**, the weight of the urine compared with that of an equal volume of distilled water. The specific gravity of water is 1.000, whereas the urine value rises about 0.001 unit for each 30 to 35 mOsm/kg of solute.[2]

Solutions containing unequal concentrations of particles may be described in terms of their *relative* osmolarity. **Isotonic** solutions are similar in concentration to body fluids such as cytoplasm and plasma. **Hypertonic** solutions are more concentrated than plasma, and **hypotonic** solutions are more dilute than plasma.

When body cells are surrounded by hypertonic ECF, the cells shrink because intracellular water leaves to restore osmotic equilibrium across the membrane (Fig. 8–6). Conversely, cells exposed to a hypotonic environment swell as extracellular water enters the cell along the osmotic gradient.

Osmolar imbalances trigger the thirst mechanism, the RAAS, and ADH secretion, as has been discussed. An additional mechanism, the cellular uptake or release of **organic osmolytes**, protects cells from extreme volume disturbances secondary to osmolar imbalances. Organic osmolytes are small organic molecules present in all cells. These solutes contribute to osmotic gradients but, unlike electrolytes, do not disrupt action potentials, acid-base balance, or other metabolic processes.[6] Organic osmolytes include carbohydrates such as sorbitol, amino acid derivatives, and methylamines. Cell swelling induces adaptive loss of organic osmolytes owing to passive diffusion through a swelling-induced membrane channel. Furthermore, swelling inhibits transcription of the genes encoding the synthesis of these molecules as well as the transport proteins involved in their uptake. Cell shrinkage induces opposite effects.

Osmolar imbalances that cannot be alleviated by normal regulation result in detrimental effects on body cells. Cells of the central nervous system are especially sensitive to osmolar imbalance. Swelling or shrinkage of these cells may result in clinical manifestations such as headache, apathy, confusion, stupor, seizures, or coma.

Hydrostatic Pressure

The second force governing the transport of fluid is hydrostatic pressure. As discussed in Chapter 2, hydrostatic pressure originates from two sources: the force of gravity and hemodynamic pumping forces. The gravitational pressure exerted on a column of fluid causes the fluid to flow to the most dependent (lowest) position. This force explains why excess fluid in the interstitial space (**edema**) accumulates first in the lowermost areas of the body (i.e., the ankles and feet). The greater the mass of the blood, the greater is the gravitational pressure on it. Hemodynamic pumping forces originate primarily from the contraction of the heart and secondarily from accessory pumps, such as smooth muscle contraction and elastic recoil in blood vessels and contraction of skeletal muscles surrounding blood vessels (see Chapter 15).

Capillary Dynamics

Hydrostatic pressure and osmotic pressure are the forces that determine transport of fluid in and out of capillaries. As shown in Figure 8–7, a typical capillary wall consists of a single layer of endothelial cells curved in a tubular shape and arranged end to end. In an example of epithelial transport, water may move through the two sides of the cell membrane or through spaces between cells. Most tissues

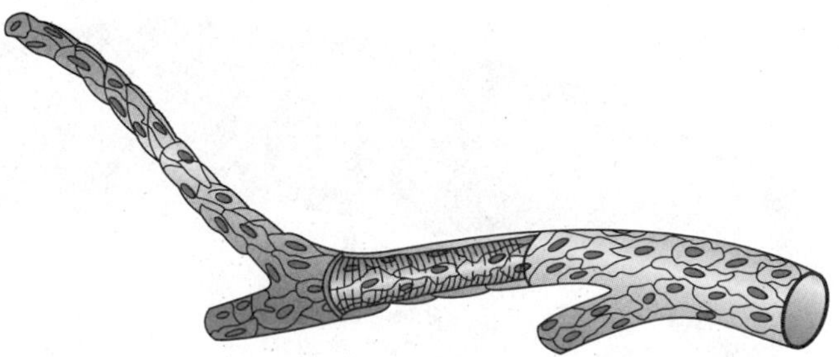

FIGURE 8–7

Capillary structure. The typical capillary wall consists of a single layer of epithelial cells. Water may be transported across the plasma membrane or through spaces between cells.

TABLE 8–1
VARIATION IN TISSUE CAPILLARY PERMEABILITY*

TISSUE TYPE	PERMEABILITY
Renal glomeruli	High
Hepatic sinusoids	High
Skin	Moderate
Muscle	Moderate
Brain	Low

*All capillaries are freely permeable to water. Permeability to proteins is low in all tissue capillaries. Permeability to other solutes, such as glucose and electrolytes, is variable.

of the body contain both vascular capillaries and lymphatic capillaries. The lymphatic system is a one-way fluid transport system, serving to remove excess fluid and larger particles from the interstitial space. Lymphatic channels contain filters (lymph nodes) and immune system cells, which remove and destroy some bacteria and other proteins originating from the tissues (see Chapter 13).

Capillaries of different organs display variable permeability to solutes because of anatomic differences (Table 8–1). All capillaries are highly permeable to water. Normal function of all organs and tissues of the body depends on the balanced movement of fluid (containing nutrients and oxygen) out of capillaries, into the interstitial fluid, and then into body cells. Similarly, fluid containing cellular wastes and carbon dioxide must move from cells to the interstitial fluid, and then into capillaries.

Starling's law of the capillary holds that net forces driving fluid movement into capillaries must equal net forces favoring outward movement to maintain compartmental fluid balance. (In actuality, there is a slight disequilibrium favoring outward fluid movement, but this extra fluid in the interstitial space is removed by lymphatic capillaries.) As shown in Figure 8–8, the most important forces driving outward fluid movement (**filtration**) are **capillary hydrostatic pressure (CHP)** and interstitial fluid osmotic pressure. The major force favoring inward movement of fluid is **plasma colloid osmotic pressure (PCOP)**, although interstitial fluid hydrostatic pressure may be a factor in certain pathologies.

Capillary hydrostatic pressure is derived from the blood pressure, which in turn depends on blood volume; blood vessel resistance, including autoregulation of capillary blood flow; and the pumping force of the heart (see Chapters 15 and 16). CHP is a positive pressure, or pushing force, that drives fluid out of capillaries into the interstitial space. **Tissue osmotic** (or oncotic) **pressure** is normally a slight negative pressure, or pulling force, exerted by small amounts of protein in the interstitial space. It has been proposed that lymphatic pumping also contributes to this slight negative pressure. Tissue osmotic pressure is clinically insignificant unless large amounts of protein leak into the interstitial space (as in capillary damage due to burns) or lymphatics become obstructed (as in lymphatic cancers). In these conditions, water is pulled into the interstitium, and **tissue hydrostatic pressure** rises rapidly to oppose CHP.

Plasma colloid osmotic pressure favors inward movement of fluid (reabsorption). This force originates from an osmotic gradient created mainly by the presence of **colloids** (albumin and other plasma proteins), which are too large to leave the plasma under normal conditions. Because plasma proteins have several negative surface charges, they exert an attractive force on cations referred to as the **Donnan effect**. The free exchange of sodium and other cations is impeded to some extent, and these cations also contribute to the osmotic force that holds or draws water into the blood.

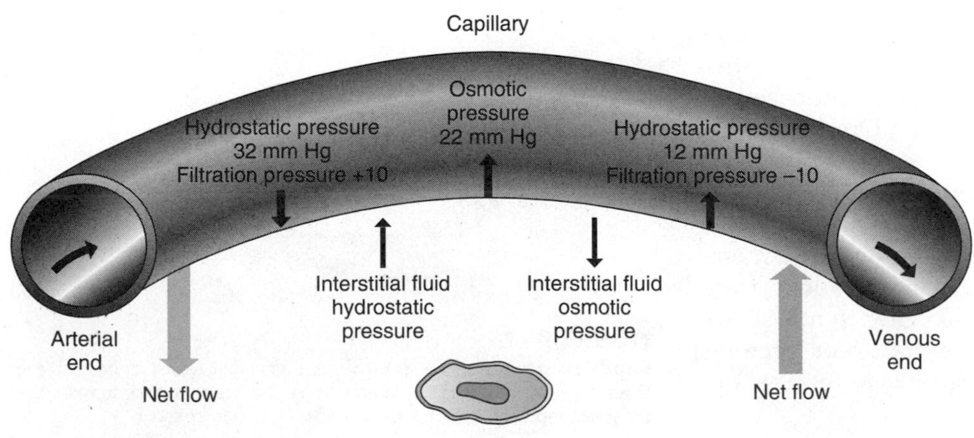

FIGURE 8–8
Starling's law of the capillary. Compartmental fluid balance depends on maintenance of an equilibrium between forces favoring outward and inward movement of water from the capillary. Capillary hydrostatic pressure and interstitial fluid osmotic pressure are the major forces favoring outward movement (filtration), whereas plasma colloid osmotic pressure favors inward movement (reabsorption). Interstitial fluid hydrostatic pressure may also promote reabsorption if it is elevated.

DISORDERS OF FLUID BALANCE

Fluid imbalance is present when regulatory mechanisms are insufficient to compensate for abnormal intake or output of fluid. Disorders of fluid volume or osmolarity result. Many clinical conditions also affect capillary exchange, resulting in *fluid shifts,* or abnormalities in distribution of fluid among internal compartments.

Fluid Shifts

Third Spacing (Plasma-to-Interstitial Shift)

Definition. Third spacing refers to the presence of excess fluid in the interstices and connective tissues between cells (edema) or in potential fluid spaces of the body (**effusion**). Potential fluid spaces are body cavities that normally contain small amounts of fluid but have the capacity for much more. Examples include the peritoneal cavity containing the abdominal organs, the pericardial sac covering the heart, synovial cavities of joints, alveoli of the lungs, and the intrapleural spaces surrounding the lungs.

Epidemiology. Although the precise incidence is unknown, third spacing of fluid is common. Risk factors are the underlying conditions with which it is associated, including major trauma, heart and kidney failure, and lymphatic cancers.

Etiology. Third spacing occurs when capillary dynamics are altered to favor filtration in excess, or when reabsorption of interstitial fluid is impaired.

Pathophysiology. Third spacing is a consequence of increased CHP, decreased PCOP, or both. In the case of lymphatic obstruction, the normal slight excess of tissue fluid is not removed. Edema due to lymphatic obstruction is referred to as **lymphedema**, whereas that caused by altered capillary forces is called **angioedema**. Potential fluid spaces provide convenient reservoirs for excess filtered fluid.

Mechanisms producing third spacing and edema include *inflammation,* in which local tissue factors mediate vasodilation and increased permeability (see Chapter 13); *increased blood volume,* as occurs in fluid overload, congestive heart failure, and renal failure; *venous obstruction,* in which high pressure at the venous end of the capillary prevents CHP from being dissipated as filtration occurs; and *decreased serum albumin,* as occurs with malnutrition, burns, liver disease, and kidney disease.

Third-spaced fluid that contains protein is called **exudate**. Exudation not only removes protein from the vascular space, decreasing PCOP, but also increases tissue PCOP. Both of these mechanisms favor excessive filtration. Exudation occurs with inflammation, in which capillary permeability is increased such that even large protein molecules may be filtered (see Chapter 13). Third-spaced fluid not containing protein is called **transudate**. Transudation is associated with noninflammatory or hemodynamic causes of fluid shift.

Clinical Manifestations. Figure 8–9 illustrates *pitting edema* of the lower leg, so called because compression of the edematous tissue leaves an indentation that persists for several seconds after the pressure is removed. This represents a severe degree of edema, although even more fluid accumulation is possible, resulting in visible water efflux from pores in the skin, referred to as *weeping edema. Dependent edema* is the presence of visible and palpable interstitial fluid in lowermost body tissues. In the upright person, ankle edema is usually most apparent. In a bedridden person, edema fluid may accumulate in the lower back, or in the scrotal sac of the male. Dependent edema is a common manifestation of mild or moderate congestive heart failure. *Generalized edema* occurs with severe heart failure, major burns, and end-stage liver or kidney disease.

Pulmonary edema, the accumulation of fluid in the interstitial spaces of the lungs, may occur as a result

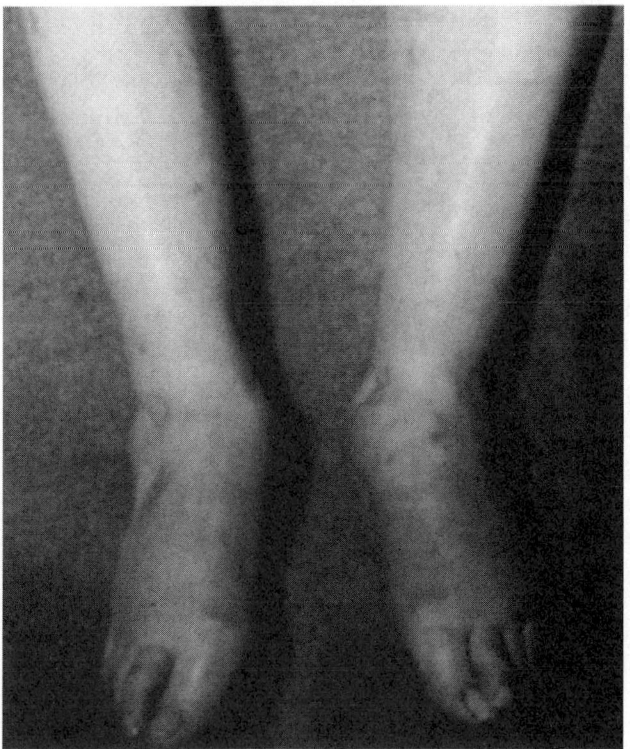

FIGURE 8–9

Pitting edema. (From Cotran, R.S., Kumar, V., and Robbins, S.L. [1994]. *Robbins Pathologic Basis of Disease.* [5th ed.]. Philadelphia: W.B. Saunders.)

of inflammatory lung disease or, more commonly, in congestive heart failure, with increased CHP resulting from increased pulmonary venous pressure behind a weakened left ventricle (see Chapter 16). Pulmonary edema may be detected as abnormal lung sounds, difficult breathing (dyspnea), or opacity on chest radiograph. This form of third spacing can be life-threatening because it increases the diffusion distance for exchange of oxygen between alveoli and the blood (see Chapter 19).

Prevention and Treatment. Prevention and treatment are ideally focused on the underlying cause. Surgical drainage of third-spaced exudate is controversial because it results in protein loss, but it may be necessary if organ function is impaired. For example, paracentesis (removal of fluid from the peritoneal cavity) and thoracentesis (removal of fluid from the intrapleural space) may be necessary to facilitate ventilation, while pericardiocentesis may facilitate ventricular filling during diastole.

Prognosis and Outcome. Outcome is variable depending on the nature of the underlying cause.

Interstitial-to-Plasma Shift

Definition. Interstitial-to-plasma shift refers to movement of fluid from the interstitial space to the vascular space along a hydrostatic gradient. (A fluid shift in this direction also occurs along an osmotic gradient in hyperosmolar imbalance, as discussed later in this chapter.)

Epidemiology. Interstitial-to-plasma shift is less common than third spacing, occurring primarily in patients with hypovolemic shock and burns. Risk factors are those associated with these underlying conditions (see Chapters 15 and 36).

Etiology. Shift of fluid from the interstitium to the vascular space is a short-term adaptive response to a sudden decrease in plasma volume or to high interstitial volume.

Pathophysiology. When blood volume is suddenly decreased, as in acute hemorrhage, plasma CHP is low. Under these conditions, some interstitial fluid may shift into the vascular space. This process apparently takes several hours and may represent normal equilibration among compartments rather than an active compensatory process (see Chapter 15). Major burn injury directly damages capillaries, causing increased permeability to fluid and to protein. Extensive edema occurs early; however, as capillaries heal, edema fluid begins to remobilize back into the vascular compartment. This shift is apparently mediated by cytokines (see Chapter 36).

Clinical Manifestations. Augmentation of intravascular volume may be reflected as stabilization of hemodynamic variables, such as blood pressure and heart rate in patients with **hypovolemia**. Urine output may also remain stable for a time. In patients with burns, remobilization of edema fluid may result in manifestations of **hypervolemia** (isotonic volume excess), discussed later in this chapter.

Prevention and Treatment. Intervention is directed toward the underlying cause.

Prognosis and Outcome. Outcome is determined by the severity of the underlying disorder.

Volume Imbalances

Volume imbalance is present when there is an excess or a deficit of total body water. When volume imbalance is not accompanied by osmolar abnormality, a state of isotonic imbalance is said to exist.

Hypovolemia (Isotonic Volume Deficit)

Definition. Hypovolemia is a decrease in ECF volume (intravascular and interstitial fluid volume).

Epidemiology. Isotonic volume deficit may result from inadequate intake of isotonic fluids, excessive vomiting or diarrhea, hemorrhage, or excessive urine output due to overtreatment with diuretic drugs. These conditions are commonly encountered in clinical settings. Risk factors relate to the underlying causes of the disorder.

Etiology. Hypovolemia is the result of disorders in which there is inadequate intake or excessive loss of isotonic fluids.

Pathophysiology. Volume deficit results in decreased CHP and decreased filtration. Cells are thus deprived of normal substrates for energy metabolism and other intracellular functions. Because there is no osmolar imbalance, there is no swelling or shrinkage of cells. Decreased renal blood flow triggers the RAAS, resulting in an adaptive increase in sodium and water reabsorption.

Clinical Manifestations. Clinical manifestations are those of tissue dehydration (loss of skin **turgor**, possible temperature elevation), and decreased blood volume and tissue perfusion (low blood pressure, rapid heart rate, decreased urine output). In severe deficit, hypovolemic shock syndrome is present (Chapter 15).

Prevention and Treatment. Prevention is directed at the underlying cause. Patients at risk should be closely monitored to ensure adequate hydration. Treatment of isotonic volume deficit consists of replacement of isotonic fluid by oral intake or intravenous infusion. Table 8–2 lists examples of intravenous fluid solutions of varying osmolarities.

TABLE 8–2
COMPOSITION OF SELECTED INTRAVENOUS FLUIDS

SOLUTION	GLUCOSE (g/dL)	Na^{2+}	K^+	Ca^{2+} (mEq/L)	Cl^-	LACTATE	OSMOLARITY (mOsm/L)
5% Dextrose in H_2O	5.0	—	—	—	—	—	Isotonic* (278)
10% Dextrose in H_2O	10.0	—	—	—	—	—	Hypertonic (556)
5% Dextrose in 0.9% saline	5.0	154	—	—	—	154	Hypertonic (586)
5% Dextrose in 0.45% saline	5.0	77	—	—	—	77	Hypertonic (432)
5% Dextrose in 0.225% saline	5.0	38.5	—	—	—	38.5	Hypertonic (355)
Half-strength saline (0.45%)	—	77	—	—	77	—	Hypotonic (154)
Normal saline (0.9%)		154	—	—	154	—	Isotonic (308)
Lactated Ringer's solution		130	4	3	109	28	Isotonic (274)

*5% Dextrose in water is an isotonic solution; however, because its glucose is metabolized immediately, administration of this solution contributes to hypotonicity of the extracellular fluid.

Prognosis and Outcome. Outcome depends on the severity of the underlying disorder and the adequacy of fluid resuscitation.

Hypervolemia (Isotonic Volume Excess)

Definition. Hypervolemia without osmolar imbalance is an excess of isotonic fluid in the intravascular and interstitial spaces.

Epidemiology. Because it is associated with common disorders, hypervolemia is frequently encountered in clinical settings. Risk factors are those related to the underlying disorders, as discussed next.

Etiology. Isotonic volume excess is usually caused by **oliguria** associated with renal failure, in which the kidneys are not excreting sufficient urine. Rarely, hyperaldosteronism, the excessive secretion of aldosterone, results in inappropriate reabsorption of sodium and water (see Chapter 29). Administration of excessive intravenous fluids is also a common iatrogenic cause of hypervolemia.

Pathophysiology. Excess blood volume results in elevated CHP and third spacing. Congestive heart failure may also occur owing to the increased workload imposed on the heart (see Chapter 16).

Clinical Manifestations. Clinical manifestations include edema, high blood pressure, bounding pulse, and high urine output (if the kidneys are functional).

Prevention and Treatment. Iatrogenic fluid overload is preventable with appropriate monitoring of therapy. Optimal management of underlying cardiac or renal disorders is also warranted. Treatment consists of diuretics to stimulate urine output from functional kidneys, or dialysis in cases of renal failure (see Chapter 20). Sodium may be restricted to decrease PCOP and increase glomerular filtration rate.

Prognosis and Outcome. Outcome depends on the severity of the underlying disorder.

Osmolar Imbalances

Hypo-osmolar Imbalance

Definition. Hypo-osmolar imbalance is present when a disproportionate amount of free water is retained in the extracellular compartment. ECF volume is normal in pure hypo-osmolar imbalance.

Epidemiology. Hypo-osmolar imbalance is common in critical care settings. Risk factors are those pertaining to the underlying disorders, discussed next.

Etiology. Retention or increased reabsorption of free water may occur in end-stage renal failure or in the syndrome of inappropriate ADH secretion. This syndrome is present when ADH is secreted in excess, in response to various stimuli such as extreme pain, nausea, stress, or certain drugs, including morphine and some cancer chemotherapeutic agents.

Pathophysiology. In hypo-osmolar imbalance, cells swell as water enters them along the osmotic gradient. Swelling initiates the efflux of organic osmoles, which may modulate cellular effects to some degree.

Clinical Manifestations. Laboratory evidence of hypo-osmolarity of the ECF includes a decrease in serum osmolality (below 275 mOsm/kg) and a decrease in the hematocrit owing to hemodilution. A low serum sodium level (below 135 mEq/L) is usually apparent, owing to actual sodium deficit or to dilution. (see discussion of hyponatremia in Chapter 9). Urine specific gravity is usually low (below 1.010), but impairment of renal function can affect this parameter. Because central nervous system cells are most sensitive to volume changes, clinical manifestations of headache, confusion, or other alteration of consciousness are most apparent.

Prevention and Treatment. Prevention and treatment are directed at the underlying cause. Free water intake is restricted in an effort to normalize serum osmolarity. Administration of hypertonic fluids is used only in extreme imbalances because overcorrection of the imbalance may lead to cellular dehydration and increased cardiac workload.

Prognosis and Outcome. Outcome depends on the severity of the underlying disorder.

Hyperosmolar Imbalance

Definition. Hyperosmolar imbalance is a disorder in which ECF is more concentrated than normal.

Epidemiology. In clinical situations, the risk of this form of dehydration is highest among patients who are receiving a hypertonic liquid diet through an enteric feeding tube or who are severely hyperglycemic, as in diabetic ketoacidosis or hyperglycemic, hyperosmolar nonketotic state (see Chapter 29). Patients with diabetes insipidus, who excrete large volumes of dilute urine owing to lack of ADH secretion or lack of response to ADH, are at risk for hyperosmolar imbalance if their intake of free water is not adequate to replace losses (see Chapter 27).

Etiology. The cause of this imbalance is insufficient intake or increased loss of free water, or accumulation of excess solute (e.g., sodium or glucose) in the serum.

Pathophysiology. Cells shrink in their hypertonic ECF environment, and uptake of organic osmolytes is initiated to modulate the osmotic gradient. ADH release is initiated by osmoreceptors, triggering a compensatory increase in reabsorption of water from renal tubules. The thirst mechanism is also triggered.

Clinical Manifestations. Serum osmolality is elevated, as are serum sodium or glucose levels. As in hypo-osmolar imbalance, central nervous system manifestations are most apparent. Tissue dehydration may manifest as decreased skin turgor. Increased thirst and compensatory water intake (**polydipsia**) are evident.

Prevention and Treatment. Preventive measures are directed at the underlying cause. Care must be taken to ensure adequate free water intake in situations in which impairment of consciousness may alter the patient's thirst mechanism or ability to access water. Treatment consists of replacement of free water and definitive therapy of the underlying cause (see discussions of hypernatremia, Chapter 9, and diabetes mellitus, Chapter 29).

Prognosis and Outcome. Outcome depends on the severity of the underlying disorder.

Combined Imbalances

In clinical practice, most fluid imbalances represent abnormality of *both* volume and osmolarity. Although four combinations are possible, only two occur commonly with pathology. *Hypovolemic, hyperosmolar* imbalance usually results from excessive sweating (as in heat exhaustion, discussed in Chapter 11) or from loss of hypotonic gastrointestinal fluids with severe vomiting or diarrhea (see Chapter 24). *Hypervolemic, hypo-osmolar* imbalance may be seen in end-stage renal failure (see Chapter 20). The other two combined imbalances are uncommon and are usually iatrogenically induced. *Hypovolemic, hypo-osmolar* imbalance may occur if isotonic fluid loss is replaced with free water or with hypotonic intravenous solutions. Balanced electrolyte solutions, such as Ringer's lactate (see Table 8–2), are appropriately used in treatment of such imbalances. *Hypervolemic, hyperosmolar* imbalance may result from too-rapid administration of hypertonic intravenous solutions, such as total parenteral nutrition (TPN) preparations.

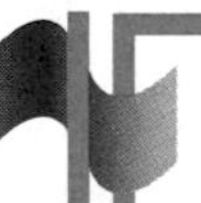

Clinical Scenario

R.S., a 56-year-old father of two, is admitted to the intensive care unit following renal transplantation. For 13 years, he had suffered from chronic renal failure and congestive heart failure, both secondary to hypertension. Before surgery, R.S. was undergoing hemodialysis four times per week. His weight after surgery is 40 pounds above his ideal body weight.

1. What factors place R.S. at risk for a postoperative fluid imbalance? How might this risk be minimized?
2. Could R.S.'s excess body weight be due, at least in part, to a fluid imbalance? Explain.

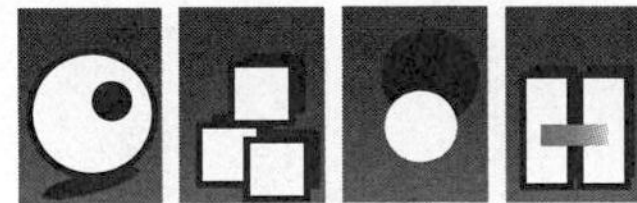

Developmental Perspective

Embryonic and Fetal Periods

The fetal kidneys begin to produce urine at the end of the first trimester, contributing to the formation of amniotic fluid. Intrauterine fluid balance is primarily reflective of maternal mechanisms, however. Excessive amniotic fluid production (*polyhydramnios*) is associated with fetal abnormality.

Infancy and Childhood

Nephron formation is complete at term birth, and renal function increases gradually over several months. Infants, especially if premature, are at increased risk of fluid imbalance owing to immature renal mechanisms. Infants have an increased body water–to–body mass ratio, with water comprising 70% to 80% of body weight. Premature infants, with their decreased body fat, demonstrate the upper end of this range. Manifestations of dehydration due to gastrointestinal water loss or fever are often more severe in infants. During childhood growth, body water gradually declines to 60% of body weight, the adult norm.

Adolescence and Young Adulthood

Pregnancy, muscle mass, and obesity constitute variables influencing fluid balance. The hormones of pregnancy mediate significant increases in total blood volume and circulatory capacity, and the gravid uterus may impede venous return, promoting third spacing. Muscle tissue incorporates water, while adipose tissue excludes it. Dietary, genetic, and conditioning factors may thus contribute to variation in total body water.

Middle and Older Adulthood

Degeneration of muscle tissue accompanies aging, and the relative proportion of adipose tissue to lean mass typically increases, decreasing total body water and increasing the risk of dehydration. Declines in cardiac and renal function are typical, although not universal, with aging, and contribute to risk of fluid imbalances. Insulin resistance may contribute to hyperglycemia, which promotes hyperosmolar imbalance.

CLINICAL IMPORTANCE OF FLUID IMBALANCES

Disturbances of fluid volume and osmolarity are common in clinical situations. Risk of imbalance must be anticipated in situations in which intake may be impaired owing to decreased level of consciousness, immobility, or lack of access to fluids. Impaired output of fluids occurs with renal disease or gastrointestinal disorders, and blood loss may result in acute hypovolemia. Abnormal regulation of fluid balance occurs with renal failure or with endocrine disorders such as hyperaldosteronism and diabetes insipidus. Fluid shifts, such as edema and effusion, accompany fluid imbalances and circulatory disorders. Certain types of therapy, such as diuretics, parenteral nutrition, and liquid diets, increase the risk of fluid imbalance. Humans in each stage of development face risks of particular types of imbalance originating from developmental changes in anatomy, organ function, regulatory processes, disorders common to developmental stage, or therapy associated with these disorders (see Developmental Perspective).

Fluid imbalances and shifts may be detected and evaluated through monitoring of fluid intake and output and by clinical symptoms such as thirst, headache, and confusion. Objective signs of fluid imbalance include weight fluctuations and alterations in mucous membranes and skin turgor. Laboratory analysis of serum electrolyte concentrations, albumin, hematocrit, and osmolality allows evaluation of fluid balance, as does measurement of the specific gravity of urine.

The fluid environment in which cells exist must be precisely regulated as a basis for normal cellular function and for the communication between cells that underlies all organ system function. Fluid balance depends on regulation of solutes such as electrolytes, acids, and bases (pH regulation) and on cooling of the body (thermoregulation). These concepts are discussed in the remaining three chapters of Unit III.

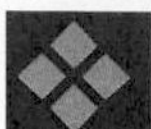

Summary of Key Points

- The two major body fluid compartments are the ICF, constituting two thirds of body water, and the ECF, constituting one third of body water. ECF may be subdivided into three compartments: intravascular fluid (plasma and fluid inside blood cells), interstitial fluid (fluid in cellular interstices, connective tissues, and lymphatics), and transcellular fluid (fluids other than blood that are exchanged within the body).
- The principal source of fluid intake is dietary. Water is lost to the environment through the urine and stool, and as insensible water loss through the skin and respiratory tracts.
- Systemic fluid balance (intake and output) depends on regulation by the hypothalamic thirst mechanism, glomerular filtration, and hormonal mechanisms. Thirst sensation is initiated by an increase in serum osmolality, sensed by osmoreceptors. The glomerular filtration rate increases proportionately to fluid volume increases. The RAAS is a hormonal cascade culminating in increased reabsorption of sodium and water from the distal kidney. ADH, secreted in response to increased osmolality or decreased volume of ECF, permits water reabsorption from the distal kidney. Atrial natriuretic peptide weakly antagonizes the effects of the RAAS and ADH.
- Body cells shrink in hypertonic ECF because water leaves along the osmotic gradient. Conversely, cells swell in hypotonic ECF. Cells of the central nervous system are most sensitive to this effect.
- Starling's law of the capillary holds that forces favoring outward movement of water (filtration) must equal inward forces (reabsorption). Forces favoring filtration include CHP and negative tissue osmotic pressure. Forces favoring reabsorption include PCOP and, in edematous states, positive tissue hydrostatic pressure.
- Third spacing, fluid shift from the plasma to the interstitium, occurs when capillary dynamics are altered to favor excess filtration. Third spacing is a clinical consequence of inflammation, hypervolemia, venous obstruction, lymphatic obstruction, or decreased serum albumin. Interstitial-to-plasma fluid shift is seen adaptively in hypovolemic shock and in major burns, owing to the effects of local cytokines.
- Hypovolemia manifests as tissue dehydration, decreased tissue perfusion, and possible temperature elevation or shock. Hypervolemia manifests as edema, hypertension, increased cardiac workload, and diuresis (except in renal failure). If osmolality is normal, there is no swelling or shrinkage of cells.
- Hypo-osmolar imbalances result in swelling of cells, and hyperosmolar imbalances result in shrinkage of cells along abnormal osmotic gradients. Because central nervous system cells are most sensitive to these effects, manifestations of these imbalances are headache, confusion, and other alterations of consciousness.
- Developmental variables influencing fluid balance include body water–to–body mass ratio, relative proportions of lean body mass to adipose tissue, alterations in renal function due to immaturity or age-related degeneration, or alterations in cardiovascular function due to age-related degeneration or pregnancy.

REFERENCES

1. Oh, M.S., and Carroll, H.J. (1985). Regulation of extra- and intracellular fluid composition and content. In: Arieff, A.I., and DeFronzo, R.A. (Eds.). *Fluid-Electrolyte and Acid-Base Disorders.* Volume 1. New York: Churchill Livingstone (pp. 1–38).
2. Rose, B.D. (1994). *Clinical Physiology of Acid-Base and Electrolyte Disorders.* (4th ed.). New York: McGraw-Hill. (pp. 32, 385, 641–642).
3. Aguilera, G., Kiss, A., Luo, X., *et al.* (1995). The renin angiotensin system and the stress response. *Annals of the New York Academy of Sciences* 771, 173–186.
4. Thrasher, T.N., and Ramsay, D.J. (1993). Interactions between vasopressin and atrial natriuretic peptides. *Annals of the New York Academy of Sciences* 689, 426–437.
5. Tan, A.C., Russel, F.G., Thien, T., *et al.* (1993). Atrial natriuretic peptide: An overview of clinical pharmacology and pharmacokinetics. *Clinical Pharmacokinetics* 24(1), 28–45.
6. McManus, M.L., Churchwell, K.B., and Strange, K. (1995). Regulation of cell volume in health and disease. *New England Journal of Medicine* 333(19), 1260–1266.

SELECTED BIBLIOGRAPHY

Black, J.M., and Matassarin-Jacobs, E. (1993). *Luckmann and Sorensen's Medical Surgical Nursing: A Psychophysiologic Approach.* (4th ed.). Philadelphia: W.B. Saunders Co.

Brown, R.G. (1993). Disorders of water and sodium balance. *Postgraduate Medicine* 93(4), 227–246.

Chernoff, R. (1994). Nutritional requirements and physiological changes in aging: Thirst and fluid requirements. *Nutrition Reviews* 52(8), S3–S5.

Fallo, F. (1993). Renin-angiotensin-aldosterone system and physical exercise. *Journal of Sports Medicine and Physical Fitness* 33(3), 306–312.

Folkesson, H.G., Matthay, M.A., Frigeri, A., *et al.* (1996). Transepithelial water permeability in microperfused distal airways. *Journal of Clinical Investigation* 97(3), 664–671.

Funder, J.W. (1993). Aldosterone action. *Annual Review of Physiology* 1993(53), 115–130.

Goldman, M.B., Robertson, G.L., Luchins, D.J., *et al.* (1996). The influence of polydipsia on water excretion in hyponatremic, polydipsic, schizophrenic patients. *Journal of Clinical Endocrinology and Metabolism* 81(4), 1456–1470.

Gregoire, J.R. (1994). Adjustment of the osmostat in primary aldosteronism. *Mayo Clinic Proceedings* 69(11), 1108–1110.

Hays, R.M., Franki, N., Simon, H., *et al.* (1994). Antidiuretic hormone and exocytosis: Lessons from neurosecretion. *American Journal of Physiology* 267, C1507–C1524.

Hill, L.L. (1990). Body composition, normal electrolyte concentrations, and the maintenance of normal volume, tonicity, and acid-base metabolism. *Pediatric Clinics of North America* 37(2), 241–256.

Inagami, T. (1994). Atrial natriuretic factor as a volume regulator. *Journal of Clinical Pharmacology* 34(5), 424–426.

Johnston, C.I., Fabris, B., and Yoshida, K. (1993). The cardiac renin-angiotensin system in heart failure. *American Heart Journal* 126(3 Pt. 2), 756–760.

King, J.A., Lush, D.J., and Fray, J.C. (1993). Regulation of renin processing and secretion: Chemiosmotic control and novel secretory pathway. *American Journal of Physiology* 265(2 Pt. 1), C305–C320.

Kraly, F.S., Kim, Y-M., Dunham, L.M., *et al.* (1995). Drinking after intragastric NaCl without increase in systemic plasma osmolality in rats. *American Journal of Physiology* 269, R1085–R1092.

Schrier, R.W. (1990). Body fluid volume regulation in health and disease: A unifying hypothesis. *Annals of Internal Medicine* 113(2), 155–159.

Sone, M., Ohno, A., Albrecht, G.J., *et al.* (1995). Restoration of urine concentrating ability and accumulation of medullary osmolytes after chronic diuresis. *American Journal of Physiology* 269, F480–F490.

Takamata, A., Mack, G.W., Stachenfeld, N.S., *et al.* (1995). Body temperature modification of osmotically induced vasopressin secretion and thirst in humans. *American Journal of Physiology* 269, R874–R880.

Trachtman, H. (1995). Sodium and water homeostasis. *Pediatric Clinics of North America* 42(6), 1343–1363.

Wagner, B.K., and D'Amelio, L.F. (1993). Pharmacologic and clinical considerations in selecting crystalloid, colloidal, and oxygen-carrying resuscitation fluids. *Clinical Pharmacy* 12(5 Pt. 1), 335–346.

Weinberg, A.D., Minaker, K.L., and the Council on Scientific Affairs, American Medical Association. (1995). Dehydration: Evaluation and management in older adults. *Journal of the American Medical Association* 274(19), 1552–1556.

White, P.C. (1994). Disorders of aldosterone biosynthesis and action. *New England Journal of Medicine* 331(4), 250–258.

Zhang, X., Dostal, D.E., Reiss, K., *et al.* (1995). Identification and activation of autocrine renin-angiotensin system in adult ventricular myocytes. *American Journal of Physiology* 269, H1791–H1802.

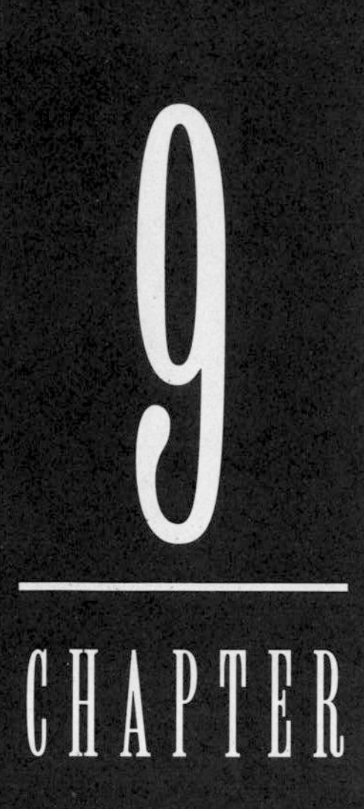

Chapter 9 Electrolyte Balance

LEARNING OBJECTIVES

1. Identify the general functions of electrolytes in body system homeostasis.
2. Differentiate among electrolyte concentrations in intracellular versus extracellular fluids.
3. Comprehend the regulatory roles of aldosterone, atrial natriuretic peptide, and parathyroid hormone in regulation of electrolyte balance.
4. Discuss the principal effects of sodium excess or deficit in body fluids.
5. Discuss the principal effects of potassium excess or deficit in body fluids.
6. Discuss the principal effects of calcium excess or deficit in body fluids.
7. Discuss the principal effects of magnesium excess or deficit in body fluids.
8. Identify developmental variables influencing electrolyte homeostasis.

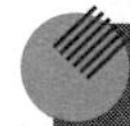

key terms

aldosterone
anion
ascites
atrial natriuretic peptide (ANP)
bicarbonate (HCO_3^-)
calcitonin
calcium (Ca^{2+})
cation
chloride (Cl^-)
Chvostek's sign
electrolyte
hemolysis
hydrogen (H^+)
hyperaldosteronism
hypercalcemia
hyperchloremia
hyperglycemia
hyperkalemia
hypermagnesemia
hypernatremia
hyperparathyroidism
hyperphosphatemia
hyperreflexia
hypoaldosteronism
hypocalcemia
hypochloremia
hypokalemia
hypomagnesemia
hyponatremia
hypophosphatemia
magnesium (Mg^{2+})
natriuresis
osmotic demyelination syndrome
parathyroid hormone (PTH)

paresthesia
phosphate (PO_4^{3-})
potassium (K^+)
pseudohyponatremia
sodium (Na^+)
syndrome of inappropriate antidiuretic hormone secretion (SIADH)
tetany
Trousseau's sign
urolithiasis
vitamin D

Electrolytes are a critical component of the extracellular fluid (ECF) and intracellular fluid (ICF) environments. These charge-carrying particles make up 95% of the solute in body fluids. The importance of the **cations sodium (Na^+), potassium (K^+),** and **calcium (Ca^{2+})** in action potential formation and conduction is detailed in Chapter 4. The pivotal role of calcium ions in the molecular mechanism of muscle contraction is discussed in Chapter 5, and the importance of sodium in establishing and maintaining osmotic gradients for fluid balance is discussed in Chapter 8. **Hydrogen (H^+)** and **bicarbonate (HCO_3^-)** are electrolytes, and their regulation is interdependent with that of other ions. Their principal importance, however, is in regulation of the pH of body fluids, so these electrolytes are discussed separately in Chapter 10. In this chapter, regulation of the composition of major electrolytes within body compartments is discussed, along with the causes and clinical consequences of electrolyte imbalances.

Table 9–1 illustrates the composition of specific electrolytes in plasma and intracellular fluid. The electrolytes calcium, **magnesium (Mg^{2+}),** and **phosphate (PO_4^{3-})** are also found in significant amounts in the nonfluid reservoirs of the bones, teeth, and soft tissues. Regulation of electrolyte concentrations within these compartments depends on a balance between adequate intake of food and drink containing electrolytes and output of electrolytes in urine, feces, and sweat. Transport of electrolytes between the ECF and ICF compartments is also essential to electrolyte balance and is hormonally regulated.

TABLE 9–1
ELECTROLYTE COMPOSITION OF BODY FLUIDS

Electrolyte	Compartmental Concentration (mEq/L)	
	Intracellular	Extracellular
Sodium (Na^+)	10	142
Potassium (K^+)	140	4
Calcium (Ca^{2+})	0.0001	2.4
Magnesium (Mg^{2+})	58	1.2
Chloride (Cl^-)	4	103
Bicarbonate (HCO_3^-)	10	28
Phosphate (PO_4^{3-})	75	4
Protein (Pr^-)	40	5

Data from Guyton, A.C., and Hall, J.E. (1996). *Textbook of Medical Physiology.* (9th ed.). Philadelphia: W.B. Saunders.

ELECTROLYTE BALANCE MECHANISMS

Dietary Intake of Electrolytes

Principal dietary sources of the major electrolytes are listed in Chapter 3. Intake of food is driven by appetite, which is regulated by complex hormonal signals, integrated in the hypothalamus and other centers of the brain, as well as by access and social factors (see Chapter 3). It is evident that humans have a specific salt appetite, although its precise regulation is not understood. Under normal circumstances, humans ingest electrolytes well in excess of their daily needs.

Regulation of Electrolyte Output

Rate-Dependent Output

To a significant extent, the quantity of electrolytes excreted in urine, feces, and sweat depends on the rates of fluid production and flow within the renal tubules, gastrointestinal tract, and sweat glands, respectively. These depend on fluid intake as well as hormonal regulation (see Chapter 8). At higher flow rates, a smaller fraction of secreted or filtered electrolytes is reabsorbed from the fluid, and more are lost from the body.

Direct Hormonal Regulation

The hormones of greatest importance in regulation of the electrolyte concentrations in plasma are **aldosterone, atrial natriuretic peptide (ANP), parathyroid hormone (PTH), vitamin D,** and **calcitonin.** The importance of aldosterone and the renin–angiotensin–

aldosterone system (RAAS) in fluid balance is detailed in Chapter 8. Aldosterone, a steroid hormone produced by the adrenal cortex, acts on the distal kidney tubules to promote increased reabsorption of sodium, which in turn causes increased water reabsorption by osmosis. The tubular "pump" that actively reabsorbs sodium from the tubular fluid is a countertransport mechanism that simultaneously secretes potassium (or hydrogen, when it is present in excess) into the tubules for potential excretion in the urine. Similar pumps are found in intestinal wall cells and in salivary ducts. These, too, are influenced by aldosterone and result in sodium reabsorption and potassium secretion into the intestinal juices or saliva. The RAAS is triggered by several stimuli, including decreased renal blood flow, sympathetic nervous system stimulation, and decreased renal tubular solute concentrations.

Apart from its role in the RAAS, aldosterone is also released by a *direct* effect of potassium on the adrenal cortex. When serum potassium is high, aldosterone release is stimulated, resulting in increased secretion of K^+ and its subsequent removal from the body, primarily by the kidneys (see Chapter 20). Aldosterone directly affects sodium and potassium concentrations in the blood, creating gradients that influence fluid volume and levels of **anions,** such as **chloride (Cl^-)** and bicarbonate.

The recently discovered hormone ANP opposes the effects of the RAAS on sodium and fluid balance. Elevation of serum sodium increases fluid volume, stretching atrial walls (Fig. 9–1). Atrial baroreceptors sense this stimulus, and this primary factor and other secondary factors (norepinephrine, angiotensin II) trigger release of ANP into the blood. ANP suppresses aldosterone-mediated effects on the kidney, resulting in decreased reabsorption of sodium. Increased urinary output of sodium (**natriuresis**) and water then occurs, completing the negative feedback loop.

PTH (also called parathormone) and vitamin D (1,25-dihydroxycholecalciferol) are essential to calcium and phosphate balance. PTH is produced by the parathyroid glands, four small endocrine glands attached to the posterior surface of the thyroid (see Chapter 28). PTH secretion is stimulated by a low serum calcium concentration, and acts to increase Ca^{2+} by (1) causing calcium release from bone (bone resorption), (2) increasing renal reabsorption of calcium while decreasing phosphate reabsorption, and (3) increasing the rate of activation of vitamin D. Vitamin D is ingested in inactive form in the diet or synthesized by the liver from cholesterol. Chemical transformation of vitamin D to its active hormonal form involves ultraviolet irradiation of the skin (sunlight exposure), further processing by the liver, and finally activation in the kidney. Vitamin D stimulates increased calcium and phosphate absorption from the intestine. Calcium homeostasis is depicted in Figure 9–2.

Ionized calcium and phosphate exist in a reciprocal relationship in the blood: when calcium is high, phosphate is low, and vice versa. As phosphate levels rise, calcium and phosphate bind, reducing the concentration of free or ionized calcium. The fact that PTH increases renal output of phosphate is therefore an important aspect of calcium balance.

Calcitonin, produced by the thyroid gland, has effects that weakly oppose those of PTH. Although important in animals, calcitonin is believed to play a

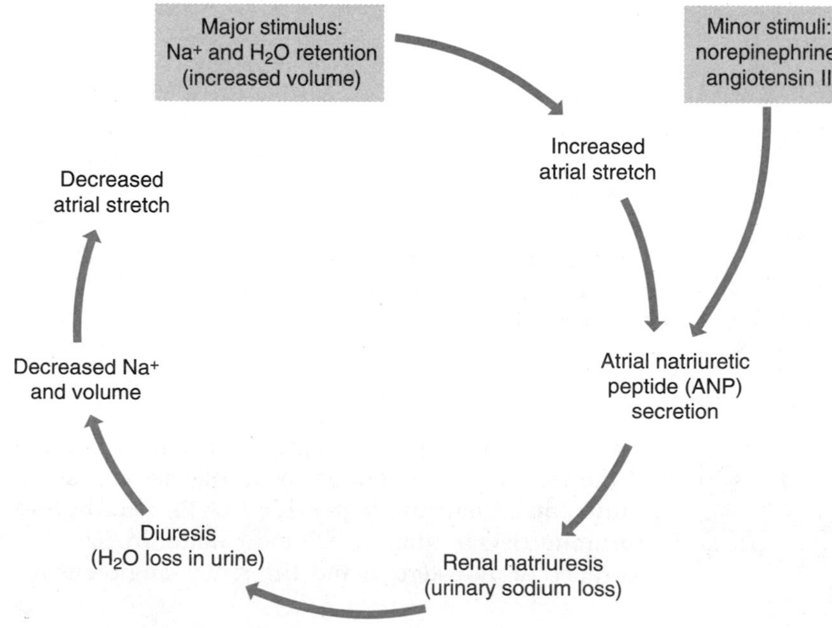

FIGURE 9–1

Actions of atrial natriuretic peptide (ANP). Baroreceptors in atrial walls sense an increase in stretch due to an increase in volume within the chambers. This stretch is the primary stimulus for ANP release, although hormones such as norepinephrine and angiotensin II may serve as weak stimuli. ANP opposes the actions of the Na^+-K^+-ATPase in the distal nephron, resulting in urinary loss of sodium (natriuresis).

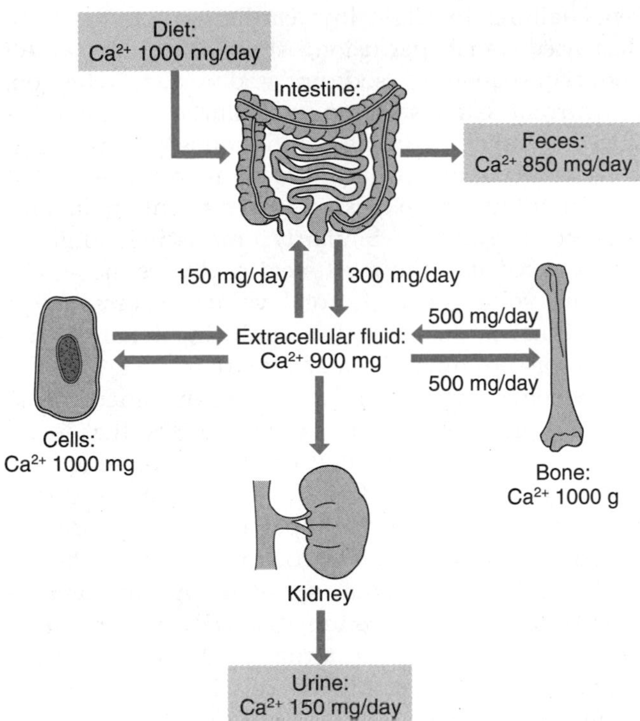

FIGURE 9–2

Calcium homeostasis. Most body calcium is in crystalline form in the bones and teeth, which serve as a reservoir for serum Ca^{2+} by an exchangeable pool of mobile calcium. Dietary intake is normally offset by Ca^{2+} losses in the urine and feces as well as by uptake into bone for structural purposes and body cells for metabolic purposes.

limited role in calcium and phosphate regulation in humans. When calcitonin is secreted in excess, as in the case of a calcitonin-secreting tumor, it can cause a significant deficiency of serum calcium owing to decreased bone resorption.

Indirect Hormonal Influences

Because electrolyte balance mechanisms are interdependent with fluid balance and metabolic regulation, other hormones influence electrolyte balance secondarily. Antidiuretic hormone (ADH), for example, regulates serum volume and osmolarity and affects urinary output (see Chapter 8). Retention of water in the blood dilutes electrolyte concentrations, and increased urinary output "washes out" some electrolytes in the urine. Insulin, a pancreatic hormone, is required by most cells for uptake of glucose from the blood (see Chapter 29). Membrane transport of glucose is linked to that of sodium and potassium, and insulin also stimulates transport of potassium from the ECF to the ICF of liver and muscle cells, independently of its effects on glucose. The stress hormone epinephrine also promotes cellular uptake of potassium. Hormones such as cholecystokinin, gastrin, and secretin influence the rate of secretion of enzymes (primarily) and electrolytes (secondarily) into the gut (see Chapter 24). Normal levels of the sex hormones estrogen and testosterone are necessary for the maintenance of bone mass and thus secondarily affect calcium and phosphate balance. Weight-bearing and the pull of muscle on bone with activity also influence bone density.

SPECIFIC ELECTROLYTES: FUNCTIONS AND IMBALANCES

Sodium

Sodium is the most abundant cation, found predominantly in the ECF (normal range, 135 to 148 mEq/L). Its primary clinical importance is in regulation of osmolarity and volume of body fluids, as discussed in Chapter 8. In conjunction with potassium and calcium, sodium is essential to the establishment and maintenance of gradients for action potentials. Because most membrane transport is linked to sodium in some way, sodium balance influences virtually all cellular functions.

Hyponatremia

Definition. Hyponatremia is defined as a serum sodium concentration of less than 135 mEq/L. *True* hyponatremia must initially be differentiated from **pseudohyponatremia**, in which the measured serum sodium is low, but serum osmolality is normal.[1] In pseudohyponatremia, excessive amounts of other particles, such as proteins or lipids, reduce the proportion of water in which sodium may dissolve, yielding artifactually low sodium concentrations.

Epidemiology. Hyponatremia is the most common electrolyte imbalance encountered in clinical settings, occurring in an estimated 2.5% of hospitalized patients.[2] Risk factors are related to the specific etiology.

Etiology. As shown in Table 9–2, hyponatremia may be caused by a deficit of sodium (pure sodium deficit), an excess of water in the ECF (dilutional hyponatremia), or a combination of both.

Pure sodium deficits may result from inadequate dietary intake, but this is rare because of the innate salt appetite and the availability of dietary sources. Hyponatremia may occur by this mechanism in patients who are on sodium-restricted diets *and* diuretic therapy, typically patients being treated for congestive heart failure (CHF) or hypertension.

Hyponatremia may be associated with hypovolemia, hypervolemia, or normal volume (*euvolemic*)

TABLE 9–2
CLINICAL FEATURES OF HYPONATREMIA

Mechanism	Examples
Etiologies	
Deficient sodium intake	Sodium-restricted diet (usually coupled with diuretic therapy)
Renal sodium loss in excess of water	Diuretic therapy Hypoaldosteronism Hyperglycemia
Water and sodium gain (water in excess of sodium)*	CHF Cirrhosis with ascites Nephrotic syndrome Renal failure
Free water gain	Hypothyroidism SIADH Water intoxication Exogenous ADH administration Replacement of hypotonic fluid losses (vomiting, diarrhea, sweating) with free water
Clinical Manifestations	
Osmotic swelling of cells	Anorexia Nausea, vomiting Muscle cramps Seizures Lethargy Apathy, confusion Decreased sensation

*Signs and symptoms of volume excess also are apparent.

states. The imbalance occurs in hypovolemic patients when deficits in total body sodium and water exist, but the sodium deficit is proportionately greater. This is the case in loss of fluids from the gastrointestinal tract (e.g., vomiting or diarrhea), followed by volume replacement with free water. Excessive sweating replaced only by free water can also cause coexistent hyponatremia and hypovolemia. Excessive renal losses of sodium and water due to **hypoaldosteronism** can produce hyponatremia, as can overdiuresis coupled with volume replacement with hypotonic fluids. Diuresis can be induced by an excess of osmotically active solutes in the serum, most notably glucose. **Hyperglycemia** in poorly controlled diabetes mellitus increases tubular flow rates and may promote renal sodium loss in excess of water.

Hyponatremia with hypervolemia occurs in conditions in which both water and sodium are retained, with water excess proportionately greater than sodium excess. Examples of such conditions include CHF, liver disease with **ascites**, and, rarely, chronic renal failure. In CHF, low cardiac output leads to decreased renal perfusion, stimulating the RAAS and, consequently, sodium and water retention. Concurrent salt restriction and diuretic therapy, reduced tubular flow rates, and nonosmotically triggered ADH secretion are among many factors that can contribute to excessive water retention in proportion to sodium. Similarly, in ascites, fluid is third-spaced into the peritoneal cavity, reducing circulating volume despite total volume excess. As in CHF, renal perfusion is low, inducing renal mechanisms for sodium and water retention.

Euvolemic hyponatremia is seen in patients who have no physical signs of volume excess, that is, no edema. These patients often have an increase in total body water, but total body sodium remains stable, producing a dilutional hyponatremia. Conditions producing hyponatremia secondary to free water retention include the **syndrome of inappropriate antidiuretic hormone secretion (SIADH)**, water intoxication, and a number of iatrogenic causes. SIADH is defined by increased ADH levels in the absence of osmotic or volume-related stimuli for its release and may result from inappropriate hypothalamic stimulation or lack of renal responsiveness to ADH (see Chapter 27).

Water intoxication is a rare cause of hyponatremia but may occur with voluntary ingestion of very large fluid volumes, especially in patients who have some deficiency in renal mechanisms for dilution of urine. The usual setting of water intoxication is mental illness in which water ingestion is an uncontrollable compulsion.

Pathophysiology. Hyponatremia induces a shift of water from the ECF to the ICF because of alteration of normal osmotic gradients. Cells swell, and, as discussed in Chapter 8, tissues of the central nervous system are most sensitive to this effect. The brain protects itself from edema to some extent by decreasing the number of other osmotically active particles (e.g., potassium and organic osmolytes) within cells, but this mechanism occurs over a period of days.[3] Some cerebral edema occurs nevertheless, resulting in adaptive decreases in thirst and ADH secretion.

Clinical Manifestations. Nausea and vomiting may be present if edema affects receptors in the brain or the vomiting center of the brain stem (see Table 9–2). Decreased cellular excitability produces effects related to altered neurotransmission; these range from lethargy and confusion to seizures and coma, depending on the degree of hyponatremia. Effects on muscle include weakness and spasm. Additional clinical signs of hyponatremia vary depending on whether the condition is associated with volume imbalance.

Prevention and Treatment. Prevention entails reduction of risk related to underlying causes. Treatment of pure sodium deficits consists of cautious replacement of sodium. Mild hyponatremia may respond to increased dietary intake of sodium, whereas intravenous replacement with hypertonic saline is used for more severe imbalance. Too rapid correction of hyponatremia has been shown to cause **osmotic demyelination syndrome**, in which osmotic injury to myelinated nerve fibers (white matter) may result in paralysis or death.[4] Patients who have a concurrent deficiency of potassium may be at higher risk for this iatrogenic syndrome. In dilutional hyponatremia, restriction of free water is the treatment of choice. The underlying cause of the imbalance must also be corrected, if possible.

Prognosis and Outcome. Hyponatremia is normally responsive to treatment. Outcome is variable depending on the degree and duration of hyponatremia and the potential for correction of the underlying cause.

Hypernatremia

Definition. Hypernatremia, a relative excess of sodium in the ECF, is present if Na^+ exceeds 147 mEq/L.

Epidemiology. Hypernatremia is a common electrolyte imbalance. Risk factors relate to the specific etiology.

Etiology. Hypernatremia may be caused by either a gain of sodium or a loss of free water (Table 9–3). Sodium gain is an infrequent cause of hypernatremia because increased dietary intake of sodium is normally offset by increased renal excretion. Hypernatremia may be induced iatrogenically with overtreatment of acidosis (hydrogen ion excess) with sodium bicarbonate (see Chapter 10). Rare causes of hypernatremia due to sodium gain in excess of water include **hyperaldosteronism** (see Chapter 29) and near-drowning in salt water (see Chapter 19).

Deficit of free water is the usual cause of hypernatremia and may occur with inadequate intake owing to immobility, confusion, dependent status (e.g., in infants), or damage to the hypothalamic thirst center (e.g., by tumor or stroke). More commonly, however, hypernatremia is the result of excessive loss of free water. This may occur with increased insensible loss due to fever or respiratory infection, with profuse sweating, or with watery diarrhea. Renal loss of water in excess of sodium may result from osmotic diuresis due to proteinuria or therapy with osmotic diuretics such as mannitol. Diabetes insipidus, in which the hypothalamus produces too little ADH or the kidneys fail to respond to ADH, results in excessive output of hypotonic urine (see Chapter 27).

TABLE 9–3
CLINICAL FEATURES OF HYPERNATREMIA

ETIOLOGIES

Mechanism	Examples
Increased sodium intake	High sodium diet (especially accompanied by renal dysfunction) Iatrogenic excess of sodium bicarbonate administration
Sodium gain in excess of water	Hyperaldosteronism Near-drowning in salt water Iatrogenic administration of hypertonic saline
Unreplaced loss of free water or hypotonic fluids*	Sweating Burns Respiratory infection Diabetes insipidus Diarrhea Osmotic diuresis Injury to hypothalamic thirst center Inability to respond to thirst stimulus

CLINICAL MANIFESTATIONS

Mechanism	Examples
Altered cellular metabolism Osmotic shrinkage of cells	Lethargy Weakness Irritability Twitching Seizures Coma Intracranial bleeding

*Signs and symptoms of dehydration (hypovolemia) also are present.

Pathophysiology. Hypernatremia results in cellular dehydration due to a shift of water from the ICF to the ECF along the altered osmotic gradient. The central nervous system is most sensitive to this effect and protects itself by retaining other solutes, such as potassium, magnesium, and organic osmolytes.

Clinical Manifestations. When adaptive mechanisms are overcome, or in cases of acute hypernatremia, brain cells shrink and capillaries swell, increasing the risk of hemorrhage and clotting. Signs of hyperirritability include restlessness, muscle twitching, and seizures, although lethargy, coma, and muscle weakness are seen as well owing to altered cellular metabolism. The patient may have a low-grade fever due to altered thermoregulation (see Chapter 11). The fluid shift also may manifest as increased thirst, dry mucous membranes, and pulmonary edema, depending on overall fluid balance.

Prevention and Treatment. The significant number of cases that are iatrogenic are preventable with appropriate monitoring of fluid and electrolyte therapy. Hypernatremia is usually corrected with removal of the precipitating cause or treatment of the underlying condition. In severe cases, slow administration of salt-free isotonic fluids, such as 5% dextrose in water (D_5W), may be used to dilute serum sodium. Diuretic therapy and dialysis may also be used to restore sodium and water balance (see Chapter 20).

Prognosis and Outcome. The mortality rate associated with hypernatremia has been estimated at 42% to 60%.[5]

Potassium

Potassium has a narrow normal range of 3.5 to 5 mEq/L in the ECF. It is the major ICF electrolyte, exerting an osmotic pressure that maintains cell volume. K^+ is important in carbohydrate metabolism in that it is needed for glycogen deposition in liver and skeletal muscle. Exchange of K^+ for H^+ at renal and cellular levels occurs in compensation for acid-base imbalances, as discussed in Chapter 10.

The most critical function of potassium, however, is in action potential formation. As discussed in Chapter 4, the resting membrane potential (RMP) of excitable cells is determined by the Nernst potential for potassium, that is, the point at which the concentration and electrical gradients for ICF–ECF potassium flux offset each other. Although sodium, calcium, and magnesium are also involved in action potentials, electrolyte-induced alterations of neurotransmission and muscle contraction are most commonly due to potassium imbalances.

Hypokalemia

Definition. Hypokalemia is defined as a serum potassium level below 3.5 mEq/L. Most body potassium, however, is *inside* cells. Only 2% is in the serum, readily accessible for measurement, and in cases in which hypokalemia is due to an ECF-to-ICF shift in K^+, serum levels do not reflect true potassium status.

Epidemiology. Hypokalemia is common in clinical situations as a consequence of the narrow homeostatic range of K^+ as well as the high prevalence of its associated disorders and iatrogenic causes.

Etiology. As shown in Table 9–4, hypokalemia may be caused by decreased K^+ intake, shift of extracellular potassium into cells, or increased loss of K^+ from the urinary or gastrointestinal tracts. Dietary deficiency of K^+ is unusual but may occur in cases of very poor nutrition, as in some elderly patients, in alcoholic patients, or in patients with eating disorders (see Chapter 25). Shift of K^+ into cells occurs with increased cell division and maturation, such as occurs with the healing of major trauma or the adaptive increase in hematopoiesis that follows blood loss. Alkalosis (hydrogen ion deficit) also induces hypokalemia as K^+ moves into cells to compensate for the cation deficit.

Increased loss of potassium is the usual cause of hypokalemia. Loss of intestinal fluids through vomiting, diarrhea, or drainage causes direct loss of small amounts of potassium, but the primary mechanism of hypokalemia in these conditions is stimula-

TABLE 9–4
CLINICAL FEATURES OF HYPOKALEMIA

Mechanism	Examples
ETIOLOGIES	
Decreased potassium intake	Poor diet associated with poverty, aging, eating disorders, or alcoholism Liquid protein diets
Shift of potassium from ECF to ICF	Alkalosis Insulin excess Increased sympathetic nervous system activity Anabolic states
Increased potassium loss	Vomiting, diarrhea Intestinal drainage Sweating Diuretic therapy (loop and thiazide diuretics) Dialysis Hypovolemia Hypomagnesemia
CLINICAL MANIFESTATIONS	
Altered action potentials (decreased resting membrane potential)	Cardiac dysrhythmias Muscle weakness Decreased reflexes Paralysis Paralytic ileus Urinary retention Lethargy Confusion
Delayed repolarization of cardiac cells	Electrocardiographic changes (flat or inverted T wave, prominent U wave, peaked P wave, widened QRS complex, prolonged QT interval)
Renal exchange of hydrogen for potassium	Increased urinary pH

tion of the RAAS by volume depletion. Aldosterone release causes renal reabsorption of sodium and simultaneous secretion of potassium, which is lost in urine. Hyperaldosteronism due to an adrenocortical tumor or other cause also depletes serum potassium. Magnesium deficit is associated with hypokalemia and is thought to involve renal regulation, although the exact mechanism by which K^+ loss occurs is unknown. Increased tubular flow rates enhance urinary loss of potassium; thus, therapy with "loop" diuretics (e.g., furosemide) or osmotic diuretics (e.g., mannitol) is a risk factor for hypokalemia (see Chapter 20). Potassium-sparing diuretics, such as spironolactone, inhibit sodium reabsorption and potassium secretion in the distal renal tubule and thus do not contribute to hypokalemia. A rare genetic disorder, *periodic hypokalemia*, causes intermittent attacks of weakness associated with hypokalemia.[6]

Pathophysiology. The most serious clinical effects of hypokalemia are those due to alteration of RMP in excitable cells. As illustrated in Figure 9–3, hypokalemia lowers RMP, thus hyperpolarizing these cells. Cells are less excitable, and ventricular repolarization is delayed, resulting in cardiac dysrhythmias and muscle weakness. With prolonged or chronic hypokalemia, carbohydrate metabolism is altered, with decreased insulin secretion and glycogen synthesis. The ability of the kidneys to concentrate urine may be impaired owing to lack of potassium for countertransport with sodium.

Clinical Manifestations. Cardiac dysrhythmias include sinus bradycardia, atrioventricular blocks, premature ventricular contractions, and paroxysmal supraventricular tachycardia (see Chapter 17). The electrocardiogram typically reveals decreased T wave amplitude or T wave inversion, increased U wave amplitude, ST segment depression, and, in severe cases, peaked P waves and prolongation of the QRS complex. Patients being treated with digitalis for CHF are at increased risk for toxicity because the drug effects are similar to those induced by the hypokalemic state.

Alteration of the RMP also affects skeletal and smooth muscle. Skeletal muscle effects range from weakness to paralysis, with possible diaphragmatic involvement and respiratory arrest. Smooth muscle effects include constipation, urinary retention, and possible paralysis of the bowel (paralytic ileus).

Prevention and Treatment. Serum K^+ must be closely monitored in patients at risk. Treatment of hypokalemia consists of cautious replacement of K^+, preferably by oral dietary sources, although slow intravenous K^+ replacement is commonly employed in clinical settings. Correction of acid-base imbalance may be warranted and further K^+ loss should be prevented with removal of the underlying cause if possible.

Prognosis and Outcome. Hypokalemia may result in fatal dysrhythmia if untreated. Replacement therapy relieves the imbalance, but ultimate outcome depends on the underlying disorder.

Hyperkalemia

Definition. Hyperkalemia is an elevation of serum K^+ concentration above 5.5 mEq/L.

Epidemiology. Hyperkalemia is much less common than hypokalemia because renal excretion and

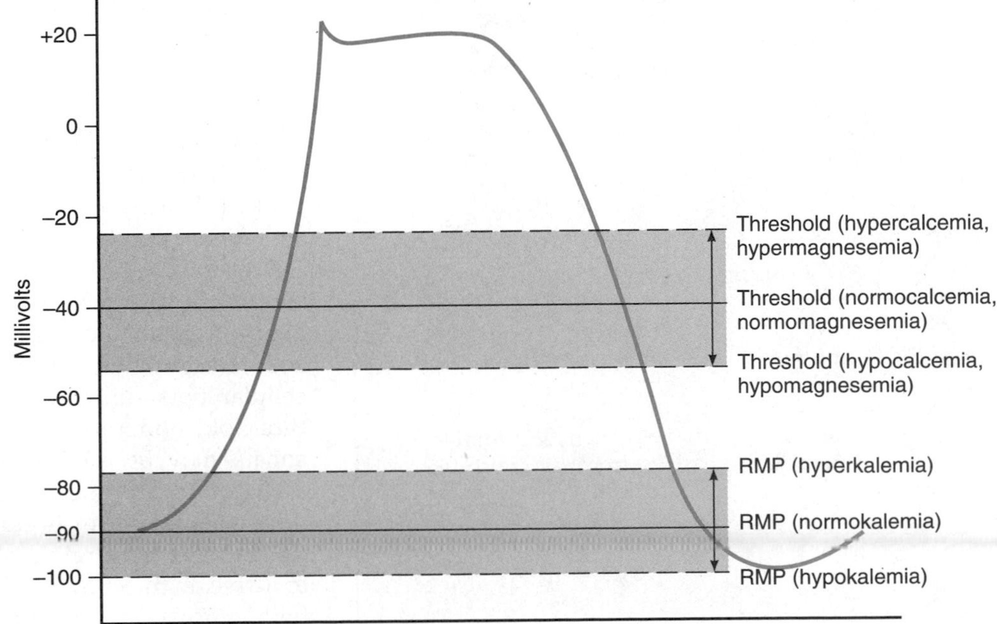

FIGURE 9–3
Effects of potassium and calcium imbalances on the cardiac action potential. Resting membrane potential (RMP) rises (becomes less negative) as extracellular fluid (ECF) K^+ rises, and it falls as K^+ falls. Threshold rises as Ca^{2+} rises and falls as Ca^{2+} falls. Magnesium imbalances also affect threshold. Any disorder that increases the distance between RMP and threshold hyperpolarizes the cell, rendering it less excitable. Conversely, any disorder that decreases this distance results in increased excitability.

ECF-to-ICF shifting usually prevent K^+ accumulation in the plasma. Risk factors are associated with the underlying causes.

Etiology. Causes of hyperkalemia are summarized in Table 9–5. Hyperkalemia due to increased intake of K^+ is infrequent but can occur iatrogenically with transfusion of large quantities of stored whole blood (K^+ leaves red blood cells during storage), with excessive or rapid administration of potassium-containing antibiotics such as penicillin G, or with too rapid intravenous administration of K^+ in treatment of hypokalemia. Patients may accidentally ingest excessive amounts of potassium-based salt substitutes, although this is rarely harmful except in those with renal failure.

Shift of potassium from the ICF to the ECF occurs with mechanical disruption of cell membrane integrity due to trauma or ischemia. Patients suffering severe burns or crush injuries or those undergoing major surgery are at risk of hyperkalemia by this mechanism. **Hemolysis** (red blood cell breakdown) may cause hyperkalemia in disorders such as sickle cell crisis or transfusion incompatibility. Because K^+ is actively transported into excitable cells to maintain baseline gradients during the action potential, hypoxic conditions (which reduce available adenosine triphosphate [ATP]) result in equilibration of K^+ at higher ECF levels. Serum K^+ levels rise during strenuous exercise, probably by this mechanism. Acidosis is accompanied by hyperkalemia because of the interdependence of H^+ and K^+ secretion by the distal kidney. When H^+ is present in excess, the kidney secretes it instead of K^+, causing secondary hyperkalemia. In addition, entry of H^+ into cells causes an ICF-to-ECF shift in K^+, contributing to an apparent hyperkalemia in acidosis.

The most common cause of hyperkalemia is renal failure in which renal excretion of K^+ is insufficient. Conditions in which the Na^+-K^+-ATPase in the distal kidney is inhibited lead to a decrease in sodium reabsorption and potassium secretion and, if severe, can cause hyperkalemia. These conditions include hypoaldosteronism, digitalis overdose, and overuse of potassium-sparing diuretics. A genetic disorder producing *periodic hyperkalemia* has also been demonstrated; however, like its counterpart, which produces hypokalemia, the mechanism is unknown.

Pathophysiology. The effects of hyperkalemia depend on the degree of imbalance and the rate of its development. With mild or moderate elevation of K^+, RMP is less negative than normal, and the cell is slightly depolarized, or more excitable (see Fig. 9–3). When K^+ is elevated above 8 mEq/L, however, RMP may reach threshold, and the cell cannot repolarize.

Clinical Manifestations. Typical clinical manifestations include restlessness, intestinal cramping, and diarrhea. Decreased neurotransmission may cause muscle weakness and decreased sensation. At very high levels, hyperkalemia may cause death due to respiratory and cardiac arrest. Electrocardiographic signs of dangerously high serum K^+ levels include peaked T waves, shortened QT interval, depressed ST segment, and widened QRS complex (Fig. 9–4).

Prevention and Treatment. Careful monitoring of serum K^+ is warranted in patients at risk. Emergency treatment of acute hyperkalemia is aimed at counteracting the cardiac effects and shifting extracellular potassium into cells. Because calcium raises threshold and prolongs repolarization, calcium gluconate may be administered to decrease irritability of cardiac cells (see Chapter 4). Intravenous solutions of glucose (in nondiabetic patients) or of insulin (in hyperglycemic diabetic patients) may be used to drive extracellular K^+ into cells. In some cases, both glucose and insulin are administered for this

TABLE 9–5
CLINICAL FEATURES OF HYPERKALEMIA

Mechanism	Examples
ETIOLOGIES	
Increased potassium intake	Iatrogenic excess of KCl or potassium penicillin Transfusion with stored whole blood Overuse of potassium-containing salt substitutes
Shift of potassium from ICF to ECF	Acidosis Uncontrolled diabetes mellitus Catabolic states Use of β-blockers Hypoxia Hemolysis Strenuous exercise
Decreased renal potassium excretion	Renal failure Hypoaldosteronism Overuse of potassium-sparing diuretics Digitalis toxicity
CLINICAL MANIFESTATIONS	
Inactivation of membrane sodium channels Hypopolarization Alteration in repolarization	Muscle weakness Paralysis Paresthesias Cardiac dysrhythmias Electrocardiographic changes (peaked T waves, shortened QT interval, depressed ST segment, widened QRS complex)

purpose. β-Adrenergic agonists, such as albuterol (Proventil, Ventolin), tend to drive K^+ into cells by increasing the activity of the Na^+-K^+-ATPase pump.

Serum levels of potassium may also be lowered with dialysis or by the oral or rectal administration of cation exchange resins such as sodium polystyrene sulfonate (Kayexalate), which exchange sodium for potassium in the bowel. Na^+ is reabsorbed, whereas K^+ is excreted in the feces. Once potassium levels are reduced to the point at which they are not life-threatening, treatment is aimed at correction of acidosis and removal of the underlying cause.

Prognosis and Outcome. Hyperkalemia is normally responsive to treatment. Mortality with unrecognized hyperkalemia is high as a consequence of lethal dysrhythmia.

Calcium

Ninety-nine per cent of body calcium is contained within the bones and teeth, whereas just 1% is found in body fluids. The small amount in body fluids (normal range, 8.8 to 10 mg/dL) is of critical importance, however. Calcium is essential to action potentials and to muscle contraction. Because it is a cofactor in many enzyme systems, it is critical to metabolism. Calcium is required for synaptic release of neurotransmitters and is therefore essential to both electrical and chemical aspects of neurotransmission (see Chapter 21). As discussed in Chapter 14, calcium is a clotting factor and as such is essential to prevention of major bleeding from minor trauma. Recent research indicates a possible link between lack of dietary calcium and essential hypertension, although the precise role of calcium in blood pressure regulation remains speculative (see Focus of Current Research).

Most of the calcium in body fluids is in bound form within cells. It is the unbound (ionized) form that participates in metabolic functions. The ECF-to-ICF ratio of Ca^{2+} is about 10,000:1; thus, a large concentration gradient exists for movement of calcium into cells when calcium channels are open.

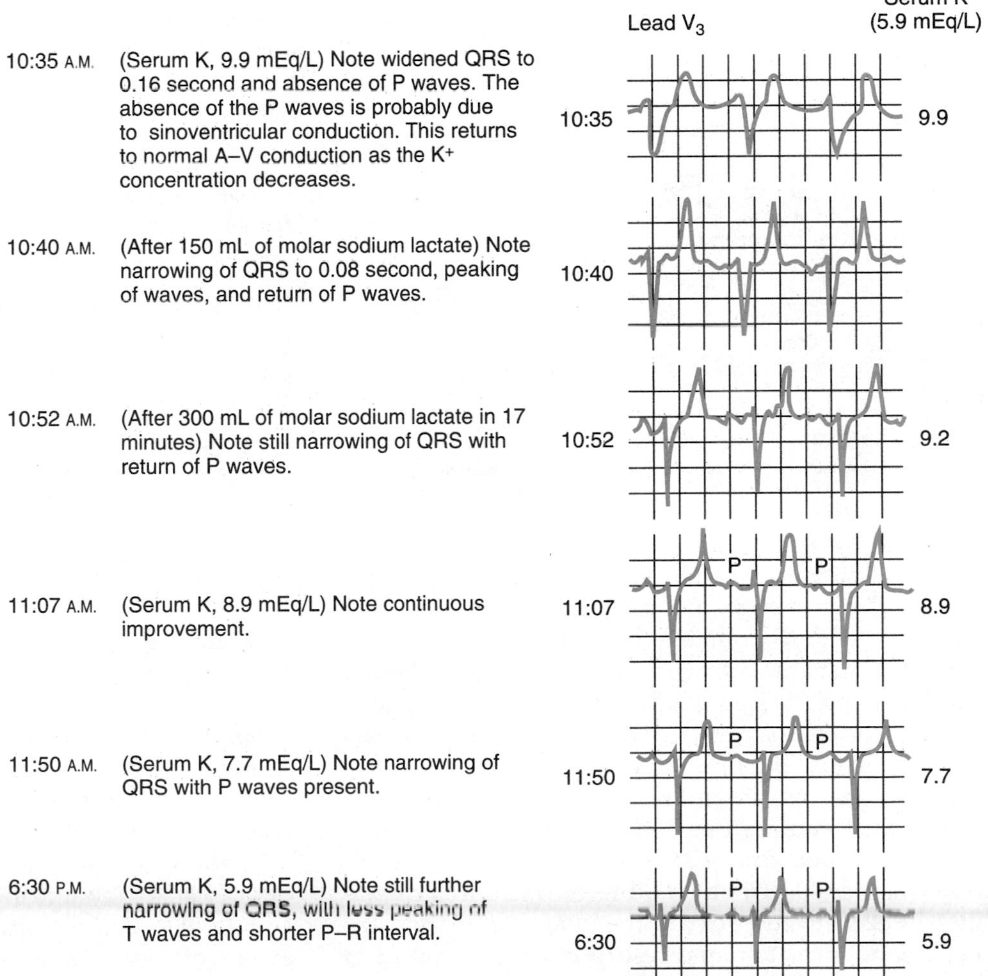

Lead V_3
Serum K (5.9 mEq/L)
10:35 A.M. (Serum K, 9.9 mEq/L) Note widened QRS to 0.16 second and absence of P waves. The absence of the P waves is probably due to sinoventricular conduction. This returns to normal A–V conduction as the K^+ concentration decreases.
10:35
9.9
10:40 A.M. (After 150 mL of molar sodium lactate) Note narrowing of QRS to 0.08 second, peaking of waves, and return of P waves.
10:40
10:52 A.M. (After 300 mL of molar sodium lactate in 17 minutes) Note still narrowing of QRS with return of P waves.
10:52
9.2
11:07 A.M. (Serum K, 8.9 mEq/L) Note continuous improvement.
11:07
8.9
P
P
11:50 A.M. (Serum K, 7.7 mEq/L) Note narrowing of QRS with P waves present.
11:50
7.7
P
P
6:30 P.M. (Serum K, 5.9 mEq/L) Note still further narrowing of QRS, with less peaking of T waves and shorter P–R interval.
6:30
5.9
P
P

FIGURE 9–4
Electrocardiographic effects of hyperkalemia. An alkalinizing agent (sodium lactate) was used in this patient to drive K^+ into cells, lowering ECF K^+. (Redrawn from Bellet, S., and Wasserman, F. [1957]. *Archives of Internal Medicine* 100, 565. Copyright 1957, American Medical Association.)

Focus of Current Research

Study	Objective and Findings
Bucher, et al. (1996) Effects of dietary calcium supplementation on blood pressure	*Objective:* To review the effect of supplemental calcium on blood pressure *Findings:* Calcium supplementation may lead to a small reduction in systolic but not diastolic blood pressure.
Allender, et al. (1996) Dietary calcium and blood pressure: A meta-analysis of randomized clinical trials	*Objective:* To assess the effect of dietary calcium supplementation on blood pressure *Findings:* A statistically significant decrease in systolic blood pressure was shown with calcium supplementation, but the effect was too small to support the use of calcium for preventing or treating hypertension.
Thiagarajan, et al. (1996) Hyponatremia caused by a reset osmostat in a neonate with cleft lip and palate and panhypopituitarism	*Objective:* To report a case of persistent hyponatremia caused by a reset osmostat *Findings:* The diagnosis was confirmed by inappropriate elevation of plasma ADH relative to the plasma osmolality accompanied by increased urine osmolality. ADH could be suppressed with a reduction in serum osmolality, excluding a diagnosis of SIADH.
Fogh-Andersen, et al. (1995) Composition of interstitial fluid	*Objective:* To calculate the composition of the interstitial fluid from changes in hematocrit and plasma composition in 20 subjects before and after lying down *Findings:* The concentrations of protein-bound calcium and magnesium were lower in interstitial fluid than in plasma. The activity of free cations was also lower. There was no escape of leukocytes or platelets from the plasma.

This gradient is maintained by active transport pumps that transport ICF calcium into organelles or extrude calcium from the cell. Within the plasma, calcium exists in an equilibrium: half is unbound Ca^{2+}, and half is bound to plasma proteins such as albumin or complexed to anions such as bicarbonate or phosphate. Because H^+ and Ca^{2+} compete for binding sites on albumin, alterations in serum pH affect this equilibrium, with alkalosis promoting lower Ca^{2+} and acidosis causing higher Ca^{2+} levels (see Chapter 10.) About 500 mg of calcium is continuously exchanged between the bone surface and the ECF. Bone formation and resorption are discussed in Chapter 34.

Hypocalcemia

Definition. Hypocalcemia is defined as a total serum calcium (bound and ionized) of less than 8.5 mg/dL.

Epidemiology. Chronic, stable hypocalcemia is relatively common, whereas severe hypocalcemic emergencies are rare.[7] Risk factors are related to the underlying causes.

Etiology. As shown in Table 9–6, hypocalcemia can be caused by nutritional deficiency of calcium or vitamin D. Cancers involving bone may result in excess of either bone formation or resorption. For example, in "hungry tumor" syndrome, seen in pa-

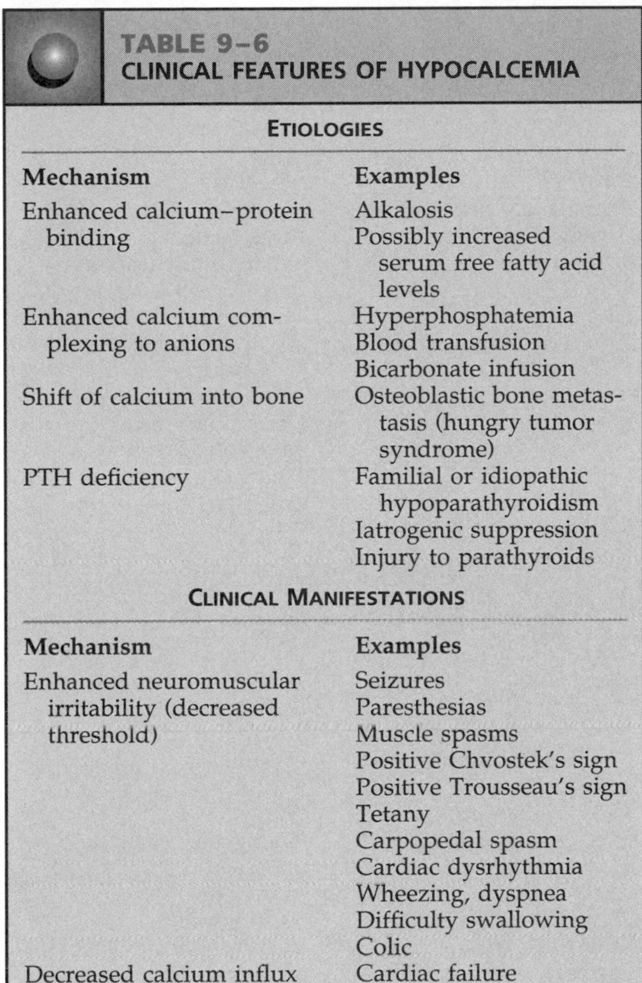

TABLE 9–6
CLINICAL FEATURES OF HYPOCALCEMIA

ETIOLOGIES	
Mechanism	**Examples**
Enhanced calcium–protein binding	Alkalosis Possibly increased serum free fatty acid levels
Enhanced calcium complexing to anions	Hyperphosphatemia Blood transfusion Bicarbonate infusion
Shift of calcium into bone	Osteoblastic bone metastasis (hungry tumor syndrome)
PTH deficiency	Familial or idiopathic hypoparathyroidism Iatrogenic suppression Injury to parathyroids
CLINICAL MANIFESTATIONS	
Mechanism	**Examples**
Enhanced neuromuscular irritability (decreased threshold)	Seizures Paresthesias Muscle spasms Positive Chvostek's sign Positive Trousseau's sign Tetany Carpopedal spasm Cardiac dysrhythmia Wheezing, dyspnea Difficulty swallowing Colic
Decreased calcium influx	Cardiac failure

tients with metastatic prostate cancer, treatment with estrogen enhances bone formation, depleting ECF calcium.[7] Alkalosis causes clinical manifestations of hypocalcemia due to a decrease in the ionized fraction of ECF calcium. Less common causes of hypocalcemia include anion binding (*chelation*) secondary to hyperphosphatemia or exogenous bicarbonate administration (because binding reduces ionized calcium) and massive blood transfusion (because citrate used to prevent clotting binds calcium). Inadvertent removal or injury of the parathyroid glands during thyroidectomy is a common iatrogenic cause of PTH deficiency and resulting hypocalcemia.

Pathophysiology. Hypocalcemia manifests as altered neurotransmission and increased irritability of muscle cells. Calcium deficit lowers the threshold for depolarization and shortens repolarization in cardiac cells (see Chapter 4).

Clinical Manifestations. Symptoms of confusion and **paresthesias** ("pins and needles" sensation) are common. Cramping and diarrhea may result from increased motility and secretion of the gastrointestinal system. Cardiac dysrhythmias may occur. In severe hypocalcemia, seizures and **hyperreflexia** with muscle spasm (**tetany**) are seen. Classic indications of impending tetany are **Chvostek's sign**, in which twitching of facial muscles is elicited by tapping over the facial nerve, and **Trousseau's sign**, in which carpopedal spasm is stimulated with inflation of a blood pressure cuff (Fig. 9–5).

Prevention and Treatment. Serum calcium must be closely monitored in patients at risk. Treatment of hypocalcemia consists of replacement of calcium and vitamin D in cases of nutritional deficiency. Intravenous calcium administration may be used in acute cases, although never in combination with bicarbonate, which could result in crystal formation and precipitation.[7] Attention is also given to the underlying cause.

Prognosis and Outcome. Hypocalcemia is usually responsive to calcium replacement. Outcome is de-

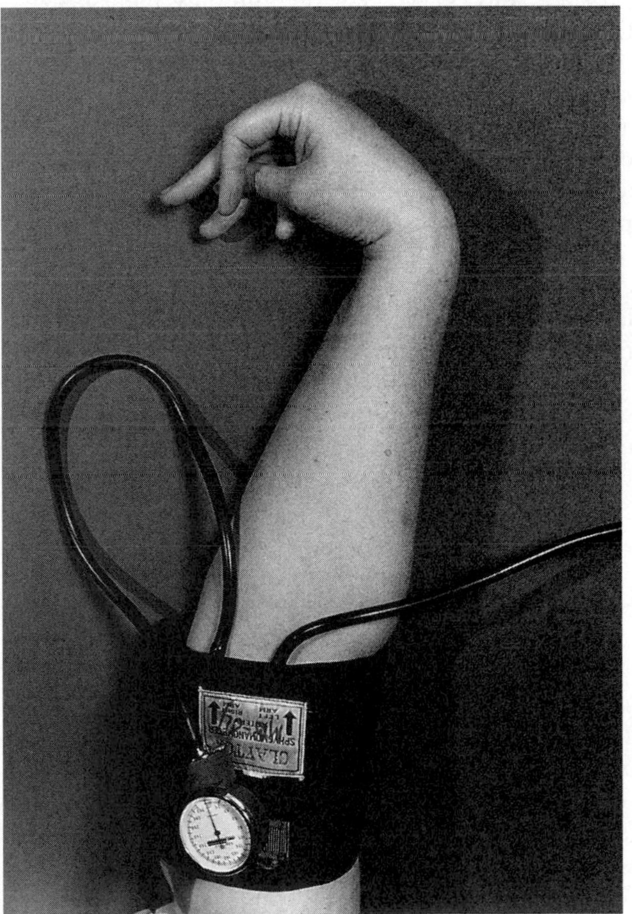

FIGURE 9–5
Carpopedal spasm. Compression of the upper arm with a blood pressure cuff elicits spasm at the wrist (Trousseau's sign), typical of hypocalcemia and impending tetany. (From Ignatavicious, D.D., Workman, M.L., Mishler, M.A. [1995]. *Medical–Surgical Nursing: A Nursing Process Approach.* [2nd ed.]. Philadelphia: W.B. Saunders.)

termined primarily by the severity of the underlying disorder.

Hypercalcemia

Definition. Hypercalcemia is present when serum Ca^{2+} exceeds 10.5 mg/dL.

Epidemiology. On routine laboratory testing, hypercalcemia has been found in 1.5% of healthy patients.[8] Risk factors are related to the primary causes.

Etiology. More than 90% of cases of hypercalcemia are due to either primary **hyperparathyroidism** or malignancy.[8] Hyperparathyroidism is usually caused by a PTH-secreting tumor (parathyroid adenoma) but may also occur with noncancerous parathyroid hyperplasia. Hypercalcemia of malignancy occurs as a result of resorptive bone metastasis, in which a primary tumor produces parathyroid hormone-related protein or other cytokines that are structurally similar to PTH.[9] Cancers of the breast, prostate, and cervix, which commonly metastasize to the bone, and multiple myeloma, which locally invades bone, are examples of cancers in which bone resorption is common. Prolonged immobilization is also associated with bone resorption and hypercalcemia. Rarely, excessive ingestion of calcium antacids is a contributing cause. Clinical features of hypercalcemia are summarized in Table 9–7.

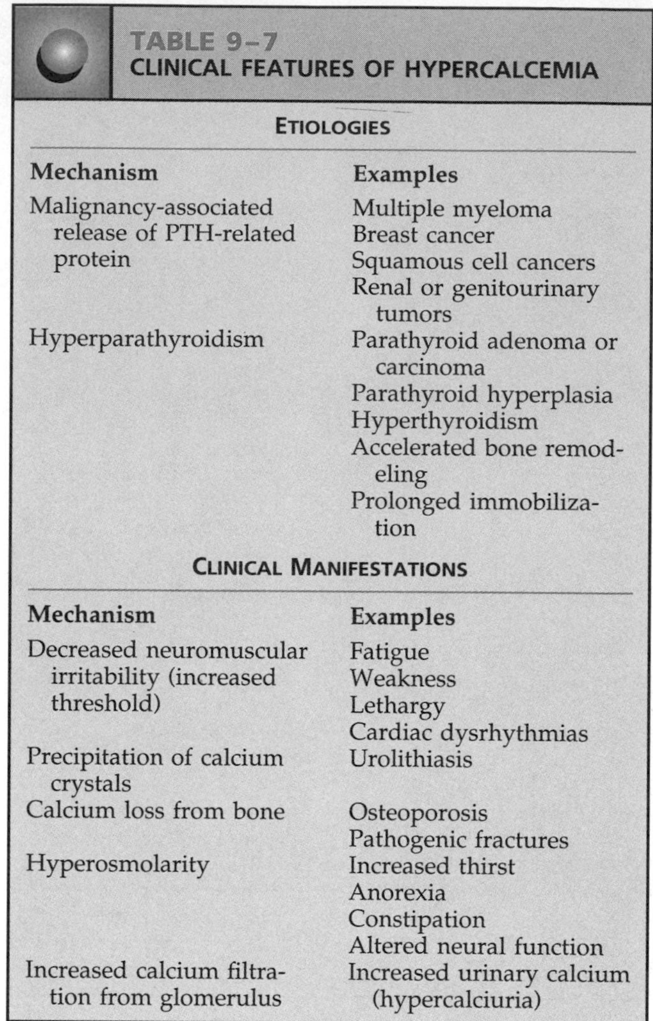

TABLE 9–7
CLINICAL FEATURES OF HYPERCALCEMIA

Mechanism	Examples
ETIOLOGIES	
Malignancy-associated release of PTH-related protein	Multiple myeloma Breast cancer Squamous cell cancers Renal or genitourinary tumors
Hyperparathyroidism	Parathyroid adenoma or carcinoma Parathyroid hyperplasia Hyperthyroidism Accelerated bone remodeling Prolonged immobilization
CLINICAL MANIFESTATIONS	
Decreased neuromuscular irritability (increased threshold)	Fatigue Weakness Lethargy Cardiac dysrhythmias
Precipitation of calcium crystals	Urolithiasis
Calcium loss from bone	Osteoporosis Pathogenic fractures
Hyperosmolarity	Increased thirst Anorexia Constipation Altered neural function
Increased calcium filtration from glomerulus	Increased urinary calcium (hypercalciuria)

Pathophysiology. Hypercalcemia results in decreased neuromuscular irritability and, if serum Ca^{2+} levels reach a critical point, calcium precipitation from body fluids into tissues.

Clinical Manifestations. Early signs are often vague and may include fatigue, weakness, lethargy, nausea and vomiting, and constipation. In more severe hypercalcemia, cardiac dysrhythmias may occur. Precipitation of calcium may result in **urolithiasis** (kidney stones), discussed in Chapter 20. If bone resorption is the underlying cause, bone pain may be present, and pathologic fractures may occur due to bone weakness.

Prevention and Treatment. Serum Ca^{2+} levels should be closely monitored in patients at risk. Treatment of hypercalcemia is directed at the underlying cause. Primary hyperparathyroidism is usually treated with surgical removal of the glands (see Chapter 28). Malignancies are optimally treated with surgery, radiation, or chemotherapy (see Chapter 7).

To normalize serum calcium levels in acute hypercalcemia, fluids and diuretics may be administered to dilute serum calcium and enhance its excretion. Calcium-chelating agents such as plicamycin (Mithracin) may be used to decrease ionized calcium, and dialysis may be employed in hypercalcemic emergencies. In metastatic cancers, drugs such as calcitonin (Calcimar, Miacalcin) and biphosphonates such as etidronate disodium (Didronel) may be given to inhibit bone resorption.

Prognosis and Outcome. Hypercalcemia is usually successfully managed with definitive therapy. Ninety per cent of patients with hyperparathyroidism are surgically cured.[8]

Magnesium

Magnesium is the second most abundant ICF cation after potassium. Mg^{2+} levels are not routinely monitored in clinical situations because serum levels (normal range, 1.5 to 2.5 mEq/L) do not correlate well with total body magnesium. The functions of magnesium overlap those of potassium and calcium, however, and when clinical manifestations cannot be attributed to imbalance of those cations, magnesium balance is assessed.

Like calcium, much of the body's magnesium (40% to 60%) is stored in bone. Additional magnesium is found in soft tissues and in muscle cells. One third of ECF magnesium is bound to plasma proteins. Regulation of magnesium levels is poorly understood, with no single factor or hormone identified as being of primary importance in either absorption or excretion of magnesium.[10] Magnesium is conserved by the kidneys when serum Mg^{2+} levels are low and is excreted when levels are high. Regulation of calcium, potassium, and magnesium homeostasis is apparently interrelated. Magnesium and potassium levels often increase or decrease together in a direct linear relationship. Increased secretion of PTH causes increased renal excretion of magnesium, and magnesium deficiency promotes hypocalcemia, possibly owing to increased resistance of bone to the actions of PTH.

The effects of magnesium on action potentials are similar to those of calcium, raising or lowering threshold (see Chapter 4). Mg^{2+} influences bone metabolism and serves as a cofactor in hundreds of intracellular reactions, including the conversion of ATP to cyclic adenosine monophosphate in second messenger systems.

Hypomagnesemia

Definition. Hypomagnesemia is defined by a serum Mg^{2+} level less than 1.5 mEq/L.

Epidemiology. A 6.9% incidence of hypomagnesemia was found on routine serum evaluation in one study.[11] In intensive care units, the incidence is about 20%.[12] Risk factors are related to the underlying causes.

Etiology. As detailed in Table 9–8, hypomagnesemia may result from decreased intake or absorption (e.g., malabsorption syndromes or malnutrition, often associated with chronic alcohol abuse), increased demand (e.g., pregnancy), or increased loss of magnesium (e.g., renal tubular dysfunction or use of thiazide diuretics).

Pathophysiology. Hypomagnesemia nearly always coexists with hypokalemia and hypocalcemia. Hypokalemic patients have a 42% incidence of hypomagnesemia.[11] Hypomagnesemia may cause decreased release of PTH or decreased target organ response to PTH, promoting hypocalcemia. Separation of the pathophysiologic effects of magnesium deficiency is therefore difficult, but increased irritability of excitable cells is usually apparent. Epidemiologic studies indicate a possible relationship between Mg^{2+} deficiency and atherosclerosis (see Chapter 15).

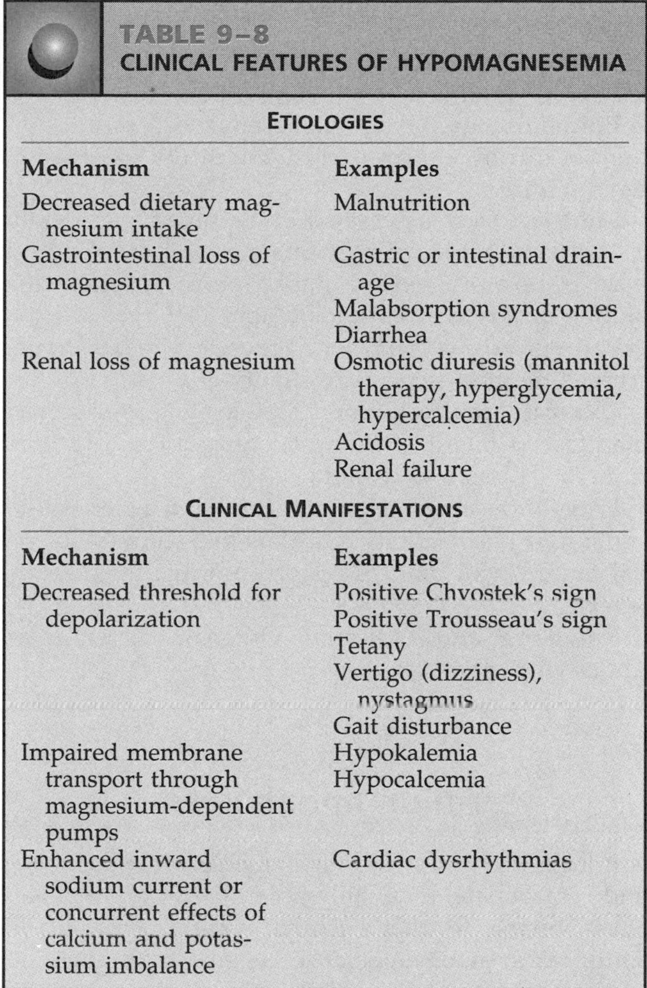

TABLE 9–8
CLINICAL FEATURES OF HYPOMAGNESEMIA

Mechanism	Examples
ETIOLOGIES	
Decreased dietary magnesium intake	Malnutrition
Gastrointestinal loss of magnesium	Gastric or intestinal drainage Malabsorption syndromes Diarrhea
Renal loss of magnesium	Osmotic diuresis (mannitol therapy, hyperglycemia, hypercalcemia) Acidosis Renal failure
CLINICAL MANIFESTATIONS	
Decreased threshold for depolarization	Positive Chvostek's sign Positive Trousseau's sign Tetany Vertigo (dizziness), nystagmus Gait disturbance
Impaired membrane transport through magnesium-dependent pumps	Hypokalemia Hypocalcemia
Enhanced inward sodium current or concurrent effects of calcium and potassium imbalance	Cardiac dysrhythmias

Clinical Manifestations. Although there are no clinical signs and symptoms specific for hypomagnesemia, signs of increased neuromuscular irritability reflect a general disturbance in electrolyte homeostasis. These clinical findings include behavioral disturbances, hyperreflexia, muscle spasms with possible tetany, seizures, nystagmus, and cardiac dysrhythmias.

Prevention and Treatment. Risk factors for hypomagnesemia should be minimized, and serum Mg^{2+} levels should be monitored in those at risk. The condition is treated with administration of magnesium, either orally (in magnesium-containing antacids such as Maalox or Mylanta) or as intravenous magnesium sulfate.

Prognosis and Outcome. Outcome depends on the degree of Mg^{2+} deficiency and on the severity of the underlying disorder. Both hypomagnesemia and hypermagnesemia have been correlated with increased risk of sudden death in patients with CHF.[11]

Hypermagnesemia

Definition. Hypermagnesemia is present when the serum level of Mg^{2+} is greater than 2.5 mEq/L.

Epidemiology. Hypermagnesemia is a rare condition, occurring almost exclusively in the presence of renal failure.

Etiology. Decreased renal excretion of magnesium is the usual cause of hypermagnesemia, although it may be exacerbated by intake of magnesium-containing laxatives or antacids (Table 9–9).

Pathophysiology. Hypermagnesemia results in decreased neuromuscular excitability.

Clinical Manifestations. Magnesium excess may manifest as muscle weakness, bradycardia, hypotension, or nausea and vomiting.

Prevention and Treatment. Intake of magnesium-containing medications is curtailed. Treatment of renal failure with dialysis restores normal magnesium levels.

Prognosis and Outcome. Outcome depends on underlying renal status.

Anion Imbalances

Imbalances of anions, such as chloride, phosphate, and bicarbonate, invariably accompany cation imbalances owing to the electroneutrality principle. In some cases, anion imbalance is the initiating condition. Imbalance of one anion often causes a compensatory imbalance in another. Bicarbonate imbalances are discussed in conjunction with acid-base homeostasis in Chapter 10.

TABLE 9–9
CLINICAL FEATURES OF HYPERMAGNESEMIA

Mechanism	Examples
ETIOLOGIES	
Decreased renal magnesium excretion	Renal failure Adrenal insufficiency
Excess magnesium intake (in patients with renal impairment)	Iatrogenic excess of $MgSO_4$ therapy of eclampsia Overuse of magnesium-containing antacids
CLINICAL MANIFESTATIONS	
Mechanism	**Examples**
Increased threshold for depolarization	Decreased relfexes Nausea, vomiting Muscle weakness Paralysis Hypotension
Decreased inward sodium current	Cardiac dysrhythmias

Chloride

Chloride and bicarbonate are the major extracellular anions, whereas phosphate is primarily intracellular. **Hypochloremia** (serum Cl^- below 95 mEq/L) commonly accompanies hyponatremia. It may also result from loss of gastric hydrochloric acid with severe vomiting. A compensatory decrease in chloride is seen in acid-base disorders in which bicarbonate is increased, such as metabolic alkalosis. **Hyperchloremia** (serum Cl^- greater than 103 mEq/L) accompanies hypernatremia and one form of metabolic acidosis. Clinical manifestations of chloride imbalance are attributable to sodium or acid-base disturbance, and treatment is directed at the underlying disorder.

Phosphate

Phosphate is stored with calcium in bones and teeth as well as in other cells. Like calcium, some phosphate is continuously exchanged between the skeleton and the ECF. The major transportable ICF anion, phosphate is a component of ATP, membrane phospholipids, DNA, and RNA. It is also essential for glycolysis and many other intracellular reactions.

Hypophosphatemia is defined as a serum level below 2.7 mg/dL. It may occur as a result of vitamin D deficiency or hyperparathyroidism, or may be caused iatrogenically with the use of aluminum-containing antacids, such as Amphojel, which bind phosphate. Impairment of metabolism and bone formation results in clinical manifestations of confusion, numbness, weakness, seizures, and possibly coma. Chronic hypophosphatemia can cause bone deformities such as rickets and osteomalacia (see Chapter 34). Treatment is directed at the underlying cause. Phosphate replacement (dietary supplements or intravenous administration of phosphate salts) may be indicated in some cases. Replacement is generally contraindicated in hypophosphatemia associated with hypercalcemia or renal failure because the likelihood of calcium precipitation is increased with such therapy.

Hyperphosphatemia, serum phosphate level above 4.5 mg/dL, is common in renal failure. It may also result from cellular hypoxia or trauma in which intracellular constituents "spill" into the plasma, or from overuse of enemas or laxatives containing phosphate (e.g., Fleet phosphate enema). Clinical manifestations of neuromuscular irritability are due to increased $Ca-PO_4$ binding, which results in hypocalcemia. Treatment of the underlying cause is central, and aluminum-based antacids may be used to bind phosphate, thus reducing serum levels of the ionized form.

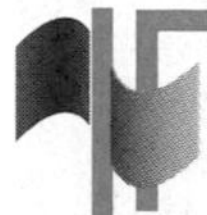

Clinical Scenario

A.G., a 68-year-old retired teacher, is being treated on an outpatient basis for multiple myeloma. She also suffers from chronic hypertension, for which she takes a thiazide diuretic and restricts her sodium intake. Recently, A.G. has been bothered by frequent "heartburn," which she has been self-treating with Tums (calcium carbonate).

1. What factors in A.G.'s history predispose her to electrolyte imbalance?
2. For what specific imbalances is she at highest risk? Why?
3. What preventive measures are indicated?

CLINICAL SIGNIFICANCE OF ELECTROLYTE IMBALANCES

Electrolyte imbalances are common, occurring with disorders of many organ systems and in patients at all developmental stages (see Developmental Perspective). Serum levels may or may not reflect total body levels of electrolytes owing to shifts between the ECF and ICF, alterations in protein binding, and hormonal mechanisms influencing electrolyte storage in bone or other tissues.

Because of the many functions served by electrolytes, clinical manifestations of imbalance are extensive. Acute imbalances of potassium, calcium, and magnesium may lead to fatal cardiac dysrhythmias or to respiratory arrest. Prevention of imbalances depends on identifying patients at risk, ensuring optimal nutritional intake, and treating renal or gastrointestinal conditions that may impair regulation or excretion of electrolytes.

Electrolyte balance affects, and is affected by, fluid balance, discussed in Chapter 8, and acid-base balance, discussed in Chapter 10. Regulation of electrolyte levels in the cellular environment underlies nor-

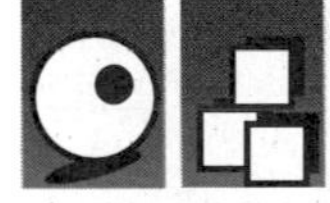
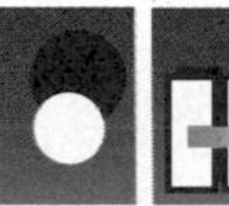

Developmental Perspective

Embryonic and Fetal Periods

Cells of the embryo and fetus incorporate the ICF electrolytes, which are essential to normal development. Maternal requirements for potassium, magnesium, and calcium are thus increased.

Infancy and Childhood

Immaturity of renal and endocrine mechanisms for fluid and electrolyte balance imposes increased risk of imbalances. The greater proportion of body water to body mass also constitutes risk. Because the rate of fluid intake and output is high during infancy, any disruption of this homeostasis may quickly lead to rate-dependent imbalances. The inability of infants to ask for water in response to thirst may contribute to dehydration risk. Childhood growth imposes increased mineral needs, predisposing to deficiencies if dietary intake is marginal.

Adolescence and Young Adulthood

Growth spurts during adolescence are accompanied by increased demand for calcium, potassium, magnesium, and phosphate.

Middle and Older Adulthood

Age-related declines in renal function, cardiac function, and ability to sweat may predispose to electrolyte imbalances, particularly hyponatremia and hypokalemia. Hypercalcemia of malignancy is chiefly a problem of older adults, owing to their increased incidence of cancer. Calcium homeostasis may also be disrupted by estrogen removal at menopause and by the reduced mobility that often accompanies aging. Impaired mental or physical capacity may result in dependence on caregivers, with increased risk of imbalances associated with negligence. Treatment of multiple illnesses may impose risk of iatrogenic imbalances secondary to diuretics or electrolyte replacement therapy.

mal function of all organ systems, and diseases of all systems can produce electrolyte imbalances, as discussed in Part Two.

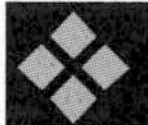

Summary of Key Points

- Electrolytes are essential to action potential formation, which underlies neurotransmission, cardiac function, and muscle contraction. Maintenance of osmotic gradients and pH balance also involves electrolyte-dependent processes.
- The predominant ICF electrolytes are potassium, magnesium, phosphate, and protein, whereas sodium and chloride are the major ECF electrolytes.
- Aldosterone promotes sodium reabsorption and potassium excretion in the distal nephron. ANP induces renal sodium excretion, protecting against hypervolemia. PTH induces elevation of serum calcium through effects on renal excretion and bone resorption of calcium, and indirectly through activation of vitamin D.
- Sodium deficit (hyponatremia) results in swelling of cells due to water influx along an abnormal osmotic gradient, manifesting primarily as central nervous system dysfunction. Similar manifestations are seen in hypernatremia, owing to shrinkage of cells.
- The most significant effects of potassium imbalance result from alteration of RMP in excitable cells, with hypokalemia lowering and hyperkalemia raising this potential. Excitability is decreased in hypokalemia and increased in hyperkalemia, leading to altered neuromuscular function and cardiac dysrhythmias.
- Calcium imbalance affects threshold of action potentials and the molecular mechanisms of muscle contraction and secretion. Hypocalcemia lowers threshold in skeletal and smooth muscle, increasing contraction and neurotransmission. Decreased force of cardiac contraction results from reduction of the ECF–ICF calcium gradient. Hypercalcemia has opposite effects, and, in addition, calcium deposition into urinary structures and soft tissues may occur.
- The effects of magnesium imbalance are similar to those of calcium imbalance and result from raising of threshold (with hypermagnesemia) and lowering of threshold (with hypomagnesemia). Alteration of many enzymatic reactions is also apparent. Manifestations of hypomagnesemia include hyperreflexia, seizures, and cardiac dysrhythmias. Hypermagnesemia is rare but may manifest as muscle weakness and bradycardia.
- Developmental variables influencing electrolyte balance originate primarily from differences in fluid compartments, renal function, mineral needs during growth, and capacity to acquire water in response to thirst.

REFERENCES

1. Mulloy, A.L., and Caruana, R.J. (1995). Hyponatremic emergencies. *Medical Clinics of North America* 79(1), 155–168.
2. Anderson, R.J., Chung, H.M., Kluge, R., *et al.* (1985). Hyponatremia: A prospective analysis of its epidemiology and the pathogenic role of vasopressin. *Annals of Internal Medicine* 102(2), 164–168.
3. Rose, B.D. (1994). *Clinical Physiology of Acid-Base and Electrolyte Disorders.* (4th ed.). New York: McGraw-Hill (pp. 651–694).
4. Lohr, J.W. (1994). Osmotic demyelination syndrome following correction of hyponatremia: Association with hypokalemia. *American Journal of Medicine* 96(5), 408–413.
5. Palevsky, P.M., Bhagrath, R., and Greenberg, A. (1996). Hypernatremia in hospitalized patients. *Annals of Internal Medicine* 124(2), 197–203.
6. Saggar-Malik, A.K., and Cappuccio, F.P. (1993). Potassium supplements and potassium-sparing diuretics: A review and guide to appropriate use. *Drugs* 46(6), 986–1008.
7. Reber, P.M., and Heath, H. (1995). Hypocalcemic emergencies. *Medical Clinics of North America* 79(1), 93–106.
8. Kaye, T.B. (1995). Hypercalcemia: How to pinpoint the cause and customize treatment. *Postgraduate Medicine* 97(1), 153–160.
9. Hall, T.C., and Schaiff, R.A.B. (1993). Update on the medical treatment of hypercalcemia of malignancy. *Clinical Pharmacy* 12(2), 117–125.
10. Rude, R.K. (1993). Magnesium metabolism and deficiency. *Endocrinology and Metabolism Clinics of North America* 22(2), 377–395.
11. Whang, R., Hampton, E.M., and Whang, D.D. (1994). Magnesium homeostasis and clinical disorders of magnesium deficiency. *Annals of Pharmacotherapy* 28(2), 220–226.
12. Wong, E.T., Rude, R.K., Singer, R.F., *et al.* (1983). A high prevalence of hypomagnesemia and hypermagnesemia in hospitalized patients. *American Journal of Clinical Pathology* 79, 348–352.

SELECTED BIBLIOGRAPHY

Allender, P.S., Cutler, J.A., Follman, D., *et al.* (1996). Dietary calcium and blood pressure: A meta-analysis of randomized clinical trials. *Annals of Internal Medicine* 124(9), 825–831.

Bilezikian, J.P. (1993). Management of hypercalcemia. *Journal of Clinical Endocrinology and Metabolism* 77(6), 1445–1449.

Brown, G.R., and Greenwood, J.K. (1994). Drug- and nutrition-induced hypophosphatemia: Mechanisms and relevance in the critically ill. *Annals of Pharmacotherapy* 28(5), 626–632.

Brown, R.G. (1993). Disorders of water and sodium balance. *Postgraduate Medicine* 93(4), 227–246.

Bucher, H.C., Cook, R.J., Guyatt, G.H., *et al.* (1996). Effects of dietary calcium supplementation of blood pressure. *Journal of the American Medical Association* 275(13), 1016–1022.

Edelson, G.W., and Kleerekoper, M. (1995). Hypercalcemic crises. *Medical Clinics of North America* 79(1), 79–92.

Fogh-Andersen, N., Altura, B.M., Altura, B.T., *et al.* (1995). Composition of interstitial fluid. *Clinical Chemistry* 41(10), 1522–1525.

Guyton, A.C., and Hall, J.E. (1995). *Textbook of Medical Physiology.* (9th ed.). Philadelphia: W.B. Saunders Co.

Kamel, K.S., Quaggin, S., Scheich, A., *et al.* (1994). Disorders of potassium homeostasis: An approach based on pathophysiology. *American Journal of Kidney Diseases* 24(4), 597–613.

Lier, C.V., Dei Cas, L., and Metra, M. (1994). Clinical relevance and management of the major electrolyte abnormalities in congestive heart failure: Hyponatremia, hypokalemia, and hypomagnesemia. *American Heart Journal* 128(3), 564–574.

McDonald, R.A. (1995). Disorders of potassium balance. *Pediatric Annals* 24(1), 31–37.

McLean, R.M. (1994). Magnesium and its therapeutic uses: A review. *American Journal of Medicine* 96(1), 63–75.

Metheny, N.M. (1992). *Fluid and Electrolyte Balance: Nursing Considerations.* (2nd ed.). Philadelphia: J.B. Lippincott Co.

Narins, R.G. (Ed.). *Maxwell & Kleeman's Clinical Disorders of Fluid and Electrolyte Metabolism.* (5th ed.). New York: McGraw-Hill.

Orlov, S.N., Dam, T-V., Tremblay, J., *et al.* (1996). Apoptosis in vascular smooth muscle cells: Role of cell shrinkage. *Biochemical and Biophysical Research Communications* 221, 708–715.

Thiagarajan, R., La Gamma, E., Dey, S., *et al.* (1996). Hyponatremia caused by a reset osmostat in a neonate with cleft lip and palate and panhypopituitarism. *Journal of Pediatrics* 128(4), 561–563.

White, J.R., and Campbell, R.K. (1993). Magnesium and diabetes: A review. *Annals of Pharmacotherapy* 27(6), 775–780.

Wysolmerski, J.J., and Broadus, A.E. (1994). Hypercalcemia of malignancy: The central role of parathyroid hormone-related protein. *Annual Review of Medicine* 45, 189–200.

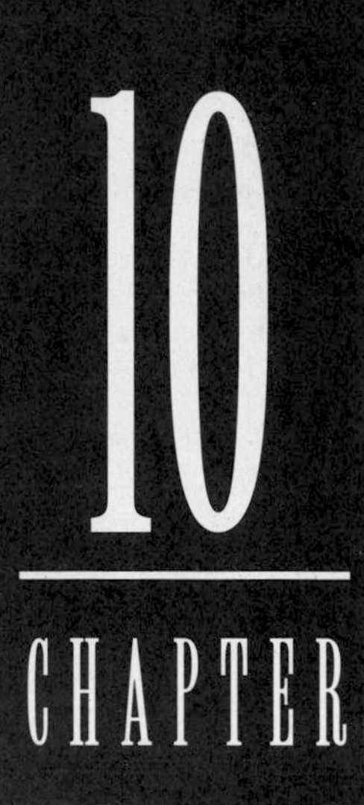

Acid-Base Balance

LEARNING OBJECTIVES

1. Appreciate the importance of maintaining the pH of body fluids within a narrow range.
2. Comprehend respiratory mechanisms for regulation of volatile acid excretion.
3. Describe the process by which the kidney may reclaim filtered bicarbonate from the tubule.
4. Compare and contrast the three principal buffer systems that permit secretion of H^+ into the urine while minimizing changes in urinary pH.
5. Discuss the mutual effects of acid-base imbalance and imbalance of other electrolytes.
6. Explain the importance of the carbonic acid–bicarbonate buffer system in the extracellular fluid.
7. Identify the relationships among serum pH, carbonic acid, and bicarbonate with reference to the Henderson-Hasselbalch equation.
8. Compare and contrast clinical features of the four principal acid-base imbalances: respiratory acidosis, respiratory alkalosis, metabolic acidosis, and metabolic alkalosis.
9. Identify clinical settings in which more than one acid-base disorder may coexist in the same patient.
10. Differentiate between compensation and correction of acid-base imbalances.

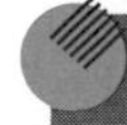

key terms

acid
acidemia
acidosis
alkalemia
alkalosis
anion gap (A^-)
arterial blood gases (ABGs)
base
bicarbonate (HCO_3^-)
bicarbonate reclamation
bicarbonate regeneration
buffer
carbamino compound
carbonic acid (H_2CO_3)
carbonic acid–bicarbonate buffer system
carbonic anhydrase (CA)
chloride (Cl^-)
chloride shift
Henderson-Hasselbalch equation
hydrogen ion (H^+)
hydrolysis
ketoacidosis
Kussmaul's respiration
lactic acidosis
metabolic acidosis

metabolic alkalosis
mixed acid-base imbalance
pH
pKa
renal tubular acidosis
respiratory acidosis
respiratory alkalosis
titratable acid
uremic acidosis
urinary buffer
ventilation

Regulation of the extracellular fluid (ECF) environment is reflected in the volume, composition, and temperature of body fluids. An important aspect of this regulation involves the ratio of **acids** to **bases**, measured clinically as **pH**. pH, the negative logarithm of the **hydrogen ion** (H^+) concentration, is proportional to the reciprocal of the concentration ($1/[H^+]$). This means that lower pH values represent greater acidity, and higher pH indicates alkalinity, or an excess of base.

Normal serum pH ranges from 7.35 to 7.45, with lower values demonstrating **acidemia** (relative excess of acid in the blood) and higher values demonstrating **alkalemia** (relative excess of base in the blood). These serum findings suggest, but are not synonymous with, conditions producing relative acid excess (**acidosis**) or base excess (**alkalosis**) within the body as a whole. pH values for other body fluids vary more widely, from the extremely acidic gastric juice (pH 1.0) to the very alkaline pancreatic juice (pH 7.6 to 8.2). Urine pH averages 6.0 but varies depending on the acid load that the kidneys are required to excrete from the body.

Serious impairment of cellular function occurs when serum pH falls outside the 7.2 to 7.55 range. pH values below 6.8 or above 7.8 may be incompatible with life. Because the body's mechanisms for regulation of pH are time dependent, the impact of pH changes on the human system depends not only on the degree of change but also on the rapidity of the change, with gradual changes being better tolerated. Acid-base imbalances are common in clinical settings and involve virtually all body systems.

MECHANISMS OF ACID-BASE BALANCE

Intake and Output of Acids and Bases

Acid-base homeostasis and maintenance of normal serum pH require that the addition of acid or base to body fluids is counterbalanced by equivalent losses. Meats in the diet are the principal sources of acid intake. The average daily intake of acid associated with a typical Western diet has been estimated at 1 mEq per kilogram of body weight per day.[1] This amount may vary considerably, however. Those on vegetarian diets may ingest a net excess of base.

Output of acid or base occurs through three primary routes: the respiratory system, the renal system, and the gastrointestinal system. Exhalation of variable amounts of carbon dioxide (CO_2) gas by the lungs removes substrate for carbonic acid production in the blood. The kidneys may excrete acid and base in proportion, or either in excess. Except in cases of gastrointestinal pathology, loss of acid and base in the feces remains relatively constant. Isolated losses of acid-rich gastric fluids (through vomiting or nasogastric drainage) or bicarbonate-rich intestinal fluids (through diarrhea or intestinal drainage) may lead to acid-base imbalance (see Chapter 24). The gastrointestinal system does not alter the secretion of acid or base in response to changes in serum pH, however. The respiratory and renal systems do respond to such changes and are of primary importance in regulation of the pH of body fluids, as detailed subsequently.

Metabolic Production of Acids

Acid-base balance must account for acids produced as a consequence of energy metabolism. As discussed in Chapter 3, the complete metabolism of glucose for energy yields CO_2 and water as end products, along with adenosine triphosphate. Excessive metabolic production of CO_2 is unusual but may occur in patients in whom nearly all caloric intake is derived from carbohydrate. Lactic acid is a product of glycolysis, with increased amounts produced during anaerobic metabolism. Ketoacids may be produced as byproducts of lipid and protein metabolism. In states in which glucose is not available (e.g., starvation) or cannot be taken into cells (e.g., diabetes mellitus), ketoacids may be produced in excess. In states characterized by increased protein catabolism for energy, acid production is also increased. Acid-base imbalance occurs if these acid gains cannot be offset by increased acid output or adaptive retention of base.

Principles of Buffering

The respiratory and renal systems, along with a number of **buffer** systems in the intracellular fluid (ICF) and ECF, interact to regulate serum pH. A buffer system consists of a weak acid (one that does not readily dissociate, or release free H^+) and a corresponding base (e.g., $NaHCO_3$). Examples of buffering reactions are shown in Figure 10–1. When a strong acid (one that readily dissociates) is added to a solution containing this buffer, it combines with the buffer pair to form a weaker acid. When a strong base is added, a weaker base is formed. Because only free H^+ contributes to pH, formation of weaker acids minimizes changes in pH.

Table 10–1 lists the most important ICF and ECF buffer systems. As detailed later in this chapter, buffers constitute an immediate defense against fluctuations in pH but do not actually eliminate acid or base from the body. Such elimination, as well as maintenance of normal concentrations of buffer system components, is dependent on respiratory and renal mechanisms.

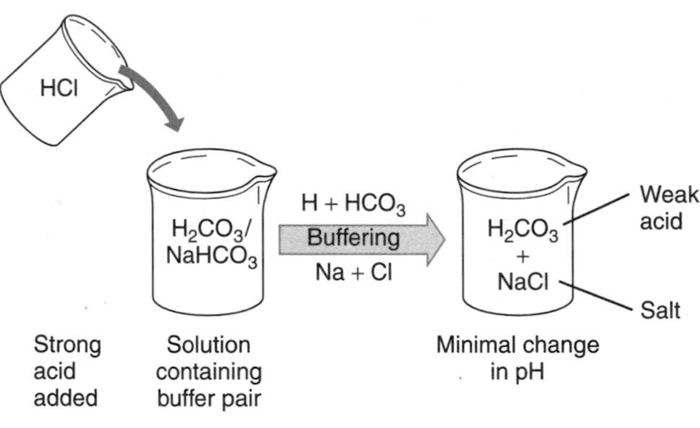

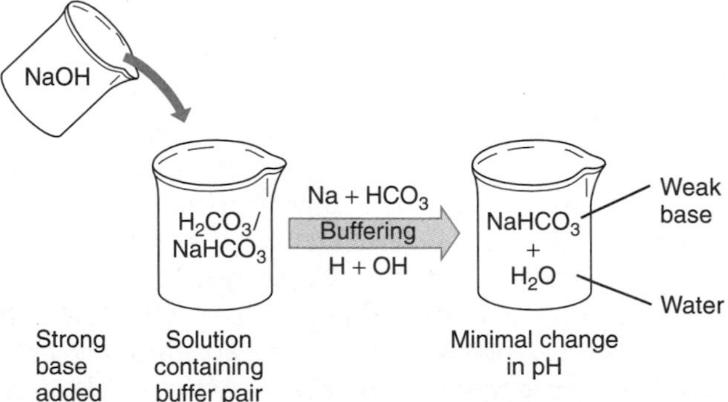

FIGURE 10–1
Principles of buffering. When a strong acid is added to a solution containing a buffer system, it combines with the buffer pair to form a weaker acid. When a strong base is added, a weaker base is formed. Because only free H^+ contributes to pH, formation of weaker compounds (which do not readily dissociate into ions) minimizes changes in pH.

TABLE 10–1
EXTRACELLULAR FLUID (PLASMA) AND INTRACELLULAR FLUID BUFFER SYSTEMS

Buffer System	Location
Carbonic acid–bicarbonate ($H^+ + HCO_3^- \rightleftarrows H_2CO_3 \rightleftarrows CO_2 + H_2O$)	ECF > ICF
Phosphate ($2H^+ + PO_4^{2-} \rightleftarrows H_2PO_4$)	ICF > ECF
Sulfate ($2H^+ + SO_4^{2-} \rightleftarrows H_2SO_4$)	ICF > ECF
Protein ($H^+ + Pr^- \rightleftarrows HPr$)	ICF > ECF
Hemoglobin ($H^+ + HB^- \rightleftarrows HHb$)	ICF (RBCs)
Ammonium ($H^+ + NH_3 \rightleftarrows NH_4^+$)	ECF (renal tubules)

Respiratory Mechanisms of pH Regulation

Hydrolysis of Carbon Dioxide

The lungs exhale large amounts of potential acid in the form of CO_2 gas. A product of energy metabolism, CO_2 diffuses from cells into the plasma, where it reacts with water to form **carbonic acid (H_2CO_3)**. Carbonic acid then dissociates, releasing hydrogen ions into the blood and causing a decrease in pH. This reversible **hydrolysis** reaction is shown in Figure 10–2. As CO_2 is eliminated from the body by the lungs, less carbonic acid is formed, and pH rises.

Regulation of Carbon Dioxide Elimination

The rate at which the lungs eliminate CO_2 depends on the rate and depth of **ventilation**, that is, the amount of air moved into and out of the alveoli during a given time period. The regulation of ventilation, discussed in detail in Chapter 18, involves neural signals coordinated in the respiratory centers of the brain stem. Chemoreceptor cells in the brain and in large blood vessels sense the degree of acidity of the blood or cerebrospinal fluid and initiate signals that result in alteration of ventilation. When ventilation increases, pH rises because less acid is formed through hydrolysis. When ventilation decreases, more CO_2 is retained in the blood, more carbonic acid is formed, and pH decreases.

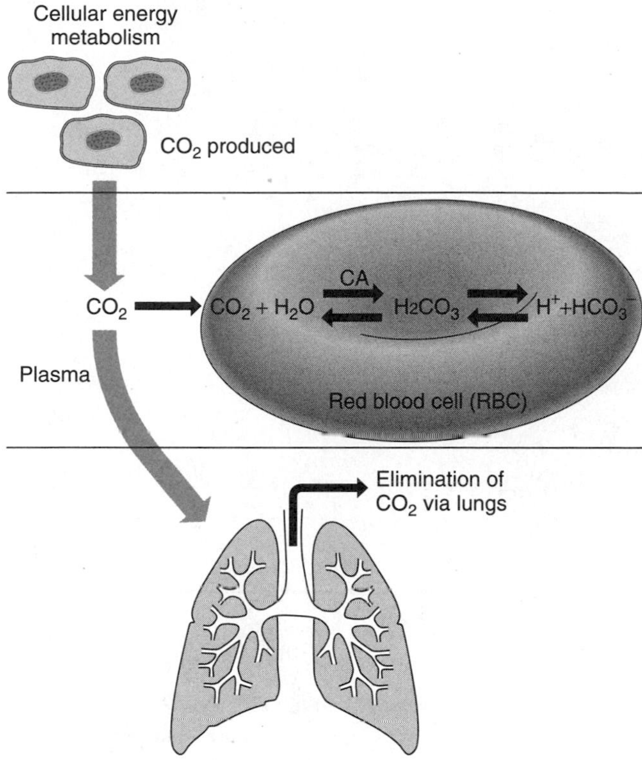

FIGURE 10–2
Production of acid from CO_2. Carbon dioxide gas (CO_2) is formed continuously as a product of cellular energy metabolism. CO_2 diffuses easily into plasma, then into red blood cells, where it reacts with water to form carbonic acid (H_2CO_3). This acid immediately dissociates, releasing H^+ into the blood and decreasing pH. This *hydrolysis* reaction occurs most rapidly in the presence of the enzyme carbonic anhydrase (CA). At the lungs, exhalation of CO_2 eliminates this source of acid and drives the hydrolysis reaction in the reverse direction (dehydration).

Bicarbonate Transport and the Chloride Shift

The hydrolysis reaction demonstrates that some of the CO_2 entering the blood ultimately forms the base **bicarbonate (HCO_3^-)**. Most hydrolysis occurs, not in the plasma, but rather in erythrocytes (red blood cells [RBCs]), which contain the enzyme **carbonic anhydrase (CA).** Hydrolysis occurs much more slowly in the plasma owing to absence of this catalyst, and it is also slowed by accumulation of the end products H^+ and HCO_3^-. These end products do not accumulate inside RBCs; instead, in an example of intracellular buffering, H^+ combines with hemoglobin, and HCO_3^- diffuses out of the cell into the plasma. Removal of the end products allows the hydrolysis reaction to continue unimpeded in the forward direction.

Seventy per cent of the CO_2 in the body is transported in the serum as HCO_3^-; 23% forms **carbamino compounds** by combining with hemoglobin in RBCs; and 7% circulates as dissolved CO_2 gas.[2] The amount of carbonic acid in the blood is negligible because it dissociates immediately.

The diffusion of bicarbonate from the RBC to the plasma must be offset by the inward diffusion of another negatively charged ion to maintain electroneutrality. The **chloride (Cl^-)** anion serves this purpose, and the exchange of anions across the RBC membrane is known as the **chloride shift**. As blood circulates through the lungs, the chloride shift occurs in the opposite direction. Removal of CO_2 by exhalation drives the hydrolysis reaction in the reverse direction (dehydration). HCO_3^- reenters the RBC and recombines with H^+ to form CO_2 and H_2O. CO_2 diffuses from the RBC into the plasma, then into the alveoli of the lungs for elimination by ventilation. Bicarbonate is consumed in this reaction, and removal of the anion from the plasma allows chloride to reenter. This sets the stage for another chloride shift as cellular metabolism produces more CO_2 for excretion (Fig. 10–3).

Renal Mechanisms of pH Regulation

Acids that cannot be converted to gaseous form (nonvolatile, or fixed, acids) must be eliminated in the urine. These acids include the inorganic sulfuric and phosphoric acids produced by protein metabolism as well as lactic acid, ketoacids, creatinine, uric acid, and other intermediate products of metabolism. The kidney filters both H^+ and HCO_3^- from the blood into the tubular fluid (see Chapter 20). As stated earlier, an excess of acid is produced under normal dietary and metabolic conditions. This means that all, or nearly all, the filtered bicarbonate is consumed in buffering H^+. The usual task of the kidney in acid-base balance is to replenish this HCO_3^- while excreting the excess H^+.

Bicarbonate Reclamation in the Proximal Convoluted Tubule

As a relatively large, charged molecule, HCO_3^- cannot be directly reabsorbed from the tubular lumen into tubular cells. Instead, the bicarbonate is reclaimed through a specialized process. **Bicarbonate reclamation** occurs primarily in the proximal tubule of the renal nephron (Fig. 10–4). The combination of filtered and secreted H^+ with HCO_3^- in the tubule first generates CO_2 in a reversal of the hydrolysis reaction. CO_2 easily diffuses from the fluid into the tubular cell, where its hydrolysis produces

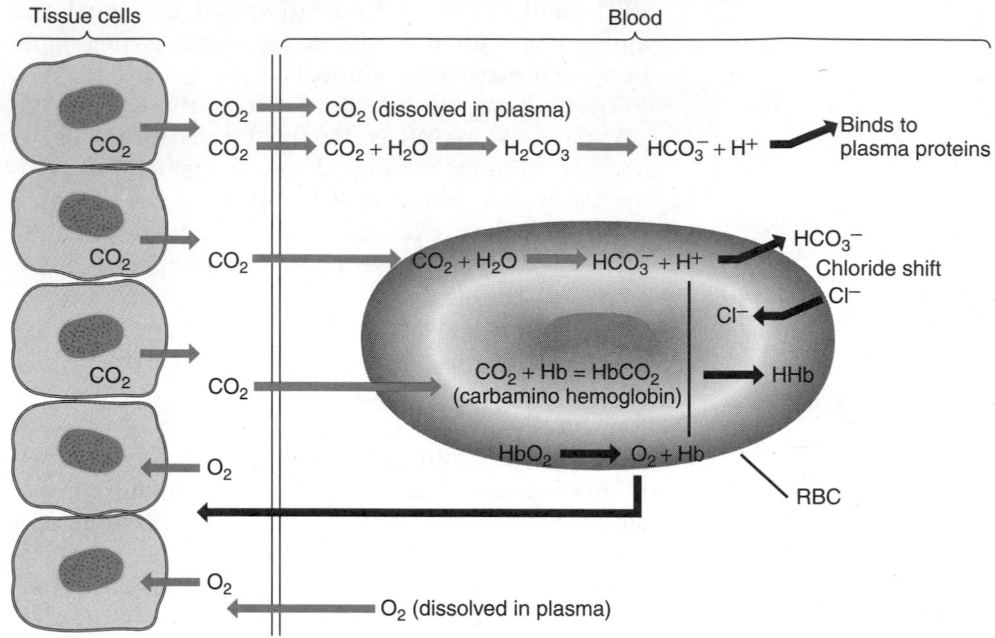

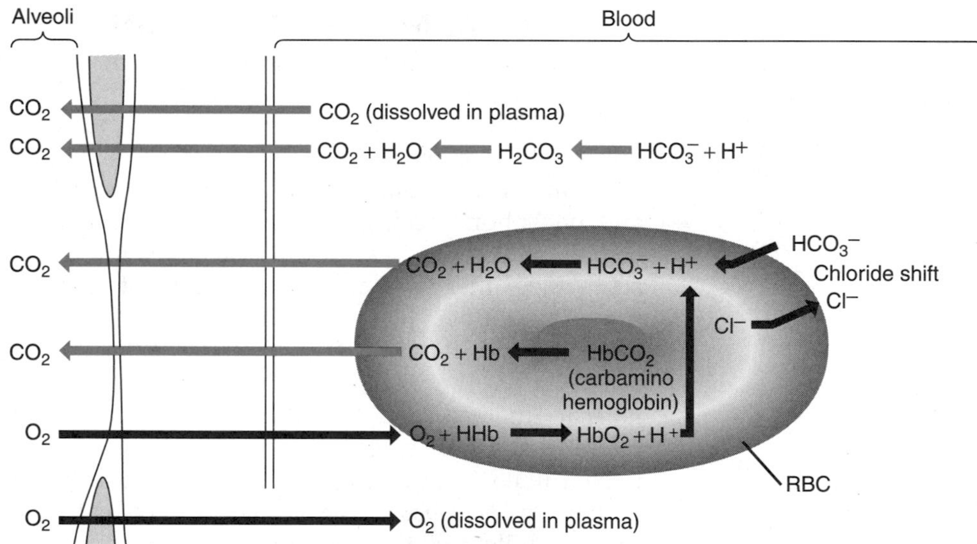

FIGURE 10–3

Bicarbonate transport and the chloride shift. Hydrolysis of CO_2 inside red blood cells (RBCs) produces hydrogen ions (H^+) and bicarbonate ions (HCO_3^-). H^+ is buffered by hemoglobin, and HCO_3^- diffuses out of the RBC in exchange for chloride (Cl^-). This *chloride shift* maintains electroneutrality of the intracellular and extracellular fluid compartments. Bicarbonate is transported in the plasma to the lungs, where exhalation of CO_2 drives the hydrolysis reaction in the reverse direction within RBCs. Oxygenation induces the release of H^+ from hemoglobin. Consumption of HCO_3^- in this reaction creates a gradient for bicarbonate to enter the RBC from the plasma, and chloride exits the RBC in a reversal of the chloride shift.

$H^+ + HCO_3^-$. HCO_3^- is then actively reabsorbed, with Na^+, into the blood, and H^+ is secreted into the tubular fluid. Normally, more than 90% of filtered HCO_3^- is replenished by this mechanism.

In acidosis, bicarbonate reclamation normally replenishes the base component of the most important buffer system in blood, the **carbonic acid–bicarbonate buffer system** (discussed later). In alkalosis, more bicarbonate ions are filtered into the tubule than hydrogen ions. Because bicarbonate reclamation is linked to hydrogen ion secretion, the excess HCO_3^- ions remain in the tubule for excretion in the urine.

Acid Secretion by the Distal Nephron

When excess H^+ is present in the plasma, the acid load is handled by the distal parts of the nephron as well as the proximal tubule. Unfiltered H^+ is actively secreted by distal convoluted tubule and collecting duct cells into the tubular fluid, increasing its acidity. This transport system operates only until tubular fluid pH falls to about 4.5 because, at lower pH values, the tubular epithelium permits significant back-leak of H^+ from the lumen into the blood. Therefore, for this system to be effective, **urinary**

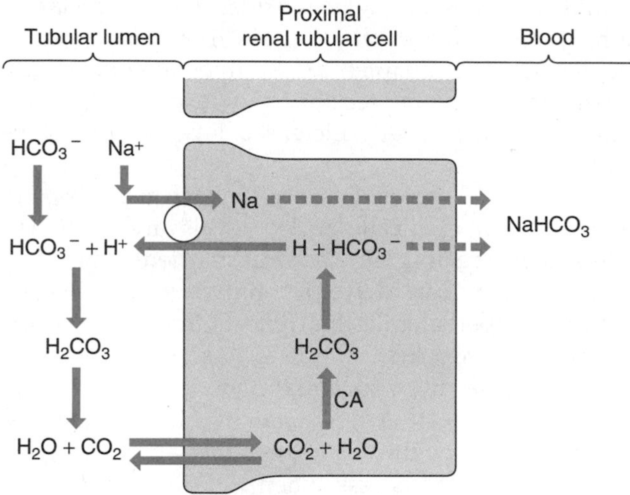

FIGURE 10–4

Bicarbonate reclamation in the proximal tubule. Bicarbonate (HCO_3^-) is filtered or secreted from the blood into the proximal convoluted tubule of the renal nephron. It is too large to be reabsorbed easily but must instead be reclaimed through the generation of CO_2 in the tubule. The combination of HCO_3^- with filtered or secreted H^+ in the tubule produces H_2O and CO_2, both of which are easily reabsorbed into tubular cells. There, the hydrolysis reaction yields HCO_3^-, which may be actively reabsorbed into the blood with sodium (Na^+). The H^+ is actively secreted into the tubule in the exchange for Na^+. For every H^+ secreted into the tubule, one molecule of HCO_3^- reenters the blood. (CA, carbonic anhydrase.)

buffers in the tubular fluid must operate to permit the acceptance of large quantities of H^+ with minimal changes in urine pH.

The most important urinary buffers are bicarbonate and **titratable acids** (primarily ammonium and phosphate). Because of their dissociation characteristics, titratable acids can serve as buffers of stronger acids. These systems all begin in the renal tubular cell, where the hydrolysis reaction occurs at rapid rates owing to the presence of carbonic anhydrase.

Bicarbonate Urinary Buffer. In the bicarbonate system, the buffer pair consists of carbonic acid and sodium bicarbonate. As illustrated in Figure 10–5, H^+ ions are secreted into the urine in exchange for Na^+. In the tubule, addition of H^+ drives the hydrolysis reaction in reverse. H^+ combines with HCO_3^- to form carbonic acid (H_2CO_3), which then forms CO_2 and H_2O. CO_2 is reabsorbed into the tubular cell, then into the blood, for excretion by the lungs. H_2O remains in the tubule for excretion in the urine. The sodium that was initially exchanged for hydrogen is reabsorbed into the blood, carrying HCO_3^- with it along the electrical gradient. For every H^+ ion excreted, one HCO_3^- ion is reabsorbed from the tubular cell into the blood. This buffering process, often referred to as **bicarbonate regeneration**, is identical to bicarbonate reclamation in the proximal tubule, except that the H^+ is excreted in the urine.

Ammonium Urinary Buffer. Tubular buffering by ammonium begins when tubular cells synthesize ammonia (NH_3) from amino acids such as glutamine. NH_3 gas diffuses into the tubular fluid where it may combine with secreted H^+ ions to form ammonium (NH_4^+), a particle prevented from reabsorption into the tubular cell by its size and charge (Fig. 10–6). Ammonium is thus trapped in the tubular fluid, where it combines with Cl^- (from NaCl) and is excreted in the urine. Na^+ is reabsorbed, carrying HCO_3^- with it.

Phosphate Urinary Buffer. In this system, sodium phosphate salt in the tubule combines with secreted H^+ ions to form H_2PO_4, a weak acid excreted in the urine (Fig. 10–7). Na^+ and HCO_3^- enter the blood, as with the other urinary buffer systems.

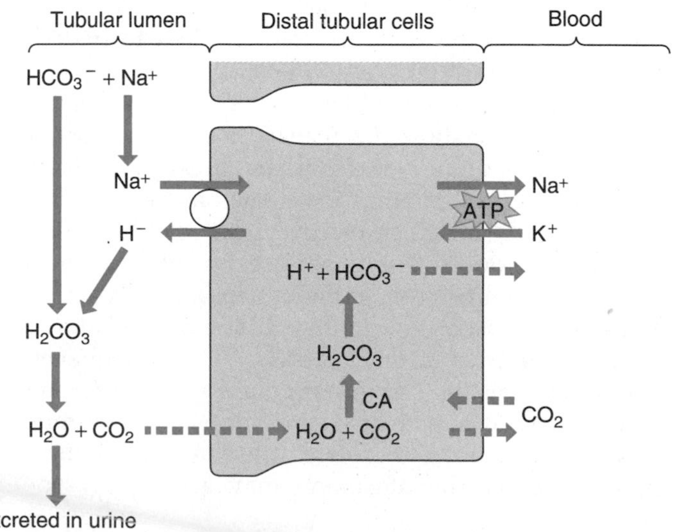

FIGURE 10–5

Bicarbonate urinary buffer (bicarbonate regeneration). H^+ secreted into the distal tubule drives the hydrolysis reaction in reverse, combining with bicarbonate (HCO_3^-) to form carbonic acid (H_2CO_3), then H_2O and CO_2. The CO_2 may be reabsorbed into the blood for ventilatory excretion or may be reabsorbed into the tubular cell, driving regeneration of bicarbonate for reabsorption with sodium (Na^+). The H_2O is excreted in the urine. Note that sodium reabsorption in the distal tubule is linked to potassium transport into the tubular cell. (CA, carbonic anhydrase.)

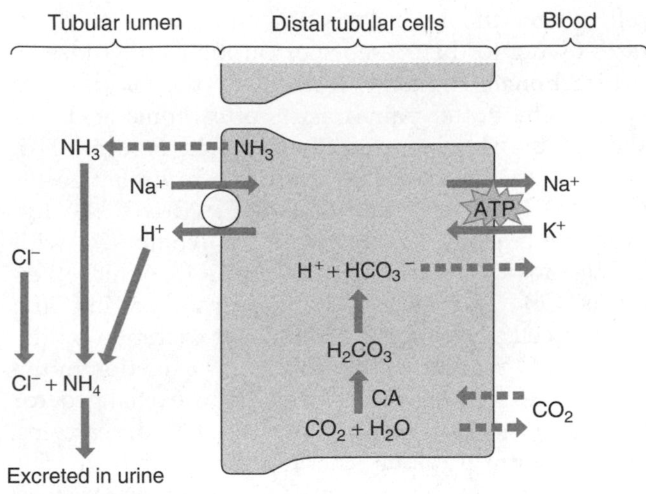

FIGURE 10–6

Ammonium urinary buffer. Ammonia (NH_3), synthesized in tubular cells from amino acids such as glutamine, diffuses into the tubular lumen. Secreted H^+ combines with NH_3 to form ammonium (NH_4^+), which cannot be reabsorbed because of its large size and positive charge. The secreted H^+ is thus trapped in the tubule, and NH_4^+ is excreted in the urine in combination with an anion such as chloride. (CA, carbonic anhydrase.)

Bicarbonate Secretion by the Distal Tubule

In less common conditions in which an alkaline load must be excreted, the distal tubule secretes bicarbonate instead of hydrogen ions through an antiport linked to chloride reabsorption. The collecting duct may also secrete bicarbonate by a similar mechanism.

Effects on Renal Transport of Other Electrolytes

Because H^+ is a cation and HCO_3^- is an anion, acid-base regulation inevitably has secondary effects on renal handling of other electrolytes.

Sodium. Sodium reabsorption is linked to hydrogen ion secretion into the tubule and to reabsorption of bicarbonate, as illustrated by the processes of bicarbonate reclamation and urinary buffering. Plasma and tubular sodium concentrations directly influence fluid balance and tubular flow rates as well as the concentrations of other electrolytes, notably potassium and chloride. Bicarbonate reabsorption is particularly dependent on volume status, and volume status may contribute to both acidosis and alkalosis, as discussed later in this chapter. As a consequence of hypovolemia, the renin–angiotensin–aldosterone system (RAAS) is activated, and aldosterone stimulates sodium reabsorption from the renal tubule (see Chapter 8). Bicarbonate anion may accompany sodium. H^+ secretion, which drives HCO_3^- reclamation, is stimulated by angiotensin II, a component of the RAAS (see Chapter 8). In hypovolemic states, bicarbonate may be reclaimed in excess as a consequence of chronically increased levels of angiotensin II.[1]

Potassium. Hyperkalemia often accompanies H^+ excess. When extracellular H^+ levels are high, H^+ enters cells, creating an electrical gradient. This electrical gradient can drive K^+ outward, causing an apparent hyperkalemia that reflects the shift in compartments rather than a true K^+ excess. Over time, however, true hyperkalemia may develop as the kidney secretes H^+ while retaining K^+ for electroneutrality. The degree of hyperkalemia occurring by these mechanisms is less when H^+ excess is due to retention of organic acids (e.g., lactic acid, ketoacids) because organic acids may enter cells in undissociated form.[1]

Hypokalemia is associated with volume-depleted states and with alkalemia. Stimulation of the RAAS in volume-depleted or sodium-depleted states results in potassium excretion through the Na^+-K^+-ATPase pump in the distal tubule (see Chapter 9). Typically, the kidney sacrifices acid-base balance in defense of volume. Hypokalemia stimulates ammonia production and increases the capacity of the distal nephron to secrete acid, promoting alkalemia.[1]

Chloride. Chloride, the most abundant anion in ECF, is secreted into the distal tubular lumen when bicarbonate is reabsorbed. In chloride depletion (hypochloremia), less Cl^- is available for reabsorption

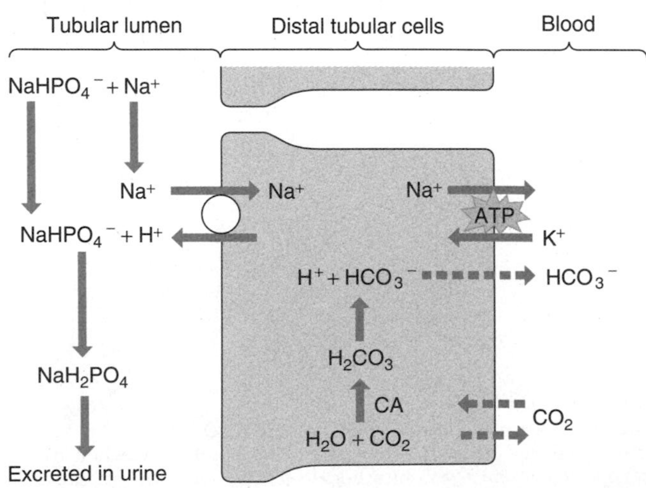

FIGURE 10–7

Phosphate urinary buffer. Sodium phosphate salt ($NaHPO_4^-$), present in the tubule, combines with secreted H^+ to form H_2PO_4, a weak acid that is excreted in the urine in combination with sodium. (CA, carbonic anhydrase.)

by the proximal tubule, resulting in reduced proximal reabsorption of sodium. More sodium is then delivered to the distal tubule and collecting duct, stimulating increased Na^+ reabsorption in exchange for increased H^+ and K^+ secretion. Lack of Cl^- in distal tubular fluid impairs secretion of bicarbonate by the $Cl-HCO_3$ antiport. Hypochloremia thus promotes alkalosis and hypokalemia.[3]

Plasma and Intracellular Buffer Systems

As shown in Table 10–1, several buffer systems are present in ECF or ICF, and many are present in both compartments. Urinary buffers were discussed previously. The most important buffers in the plasma and ICF are detailed next.

Focus of Current Research

Study	Objective and Findings
Cinnella, et al. (1996) Effects of assisted ventilation on the work of breathing: Volume-controlled versus pressure-controlled ventilation	*Objective:* To compare the effects of two forms of assisted ventilation on respiratory work *Findings:* At high tidal volumes, all patients exhibited respiratory alkalosis. At moderate tidal volumes, normal pH was achieved.
Gerhardt, et al. (1995) Acid dialysate correction of metabolic alkalosis in renal failure	*Objective:* To describe a case in which acid dialysate was used in an effort to correct severe metabolic alkalosis in a patient with chronic renal failure *Findings:* Rapid correction of the metabolic alkalosis was achieved.
Chang, et al. (1995) Pulmonary vascular resistance in infants after cardiac surgery: Role of carbon dioxide and hydrogen ion	*Objective:* To describe the effects of altering $PaCO_2$ and pH on pulmonary vascular resistance in infants after cardiopulmonary bypass for cardiac surgery *Findings:* Increasing pH with bicarbonate administration lowers pulmonary arterial pressure and decreases pulmonary vascular resistance. These changes were independent of alteration in $PaCO_2$.
Stacpoole, et al. (1994) Natural history and course of acquired lactic acidosis in adults	*Objective:* To determine the course of lactic acidosis in adults receiving standard medical care *Findings:* Nearly all cases had both hemodynamic and nonhemodynamic causes, most of which did not respond to standard care.
Giovambattista, et al. (1994) Bicarbonate transport along the loop of Henle	*Objective:* To assess the role of the loop of Henle in modulating bicarbonate transport *Findings:* The loop of Henle reabsorbs about 15% of filtered HCO_3^-.

Plasma Buffer Systems

Carbonic Acid–Bicarbonate Buffer. Although not the most abundant blood buffer, the plasma carbonic acid–bicarbonate buffer is the system that is most accessible for clinical monitoring. Because all buffers operate interdependently, status of this system reflects all others. The acid component of this system is carbonic acid (H_2CO_3), and the base is sodium bicarbonate ($NaHCO_3$).

The carbonic acid–bicarbonate buffer is of physiologic importance for two reasons. First, it is an *open* buffer system. That is, the end products of acid buffering (CO_2 and water) can be continuously eliminated from the body by the lungs and kidneys, allowing the reaction to continue indefinitely. When bases must be buffered, the CO_2 consumed in carbonic acid formation can be readily replenished by normal metabolism.

The second reason underlying the importance of the carbonic acid–bicarbonate buffer system is that it has an optimal dissociation constant **(pKa)**. The pKa of a buffer system is the pH at which half of its components are in acid form and half are in base form. At normal serum pH, the carbonic acid–bicarbonate system has about 10% of its constituents in acid form and 90% in base form. This proportion is ideal when metabolism produces a net acid load, which is the usual case.[4] The plasma carbonic acid–bicarbonate system buffers more than half of all acids or bases added to the ECF.

Plasma Proteins. Serum proteins, such as albumin and other globulins, play a minor role in the regulation of acid-base balance (see Focus of Current Research).[5] The weakly acidic and weakly basic amino acids within these proteins may participate in buffering, but when serum albumin levels are normal, this buffer is apparently of little clinical importance. In cases of hyperproteinemia or hypoproteinemia, however, the determination of total anions may be complicated by the unmeasured anions provided by negatively charged proteins (see later discussion of anion gap in acidosis).

Intracellular Buffers

Although not directly monitored in clinical practice, intracellular buffers, including bicarbonate, carbonate, phosphate, and proteins, bind large quantities of hydrogen ions. Buffering of H^+ by hemoglobin in RBCs is critical to respiratory mechanisms of pH balance, as has been discussed. Skeletal anions are also of primary importance in buffering acid loads. Acidosis directly stimulates the release of calcium and the anions carbonate and bicarbonate from bone. The anions buffer acid, and the kidneys excrete more calcium in the urine.[1] Parathyroid hormone, also released in response to acidosis, may partially mediate this resorption of bone minerals into the blood. Cellular buffers respond within 2 to 4 hours of addition of an acid load.[2]

Compartmental Shifting of Acids and Bases

Shifting of added acid from the ECF to the ICF may prevent wide fluctuations in serum pH, and this transport is an important component of buffering of acid loads. The hydrogen ions dissociated from inorganic (mineral) acids such HCl, H_2SO_4, and HNO_3 are exchanged almost immediately by membrane pumps for intracellular sodium or potassium, and the associated anions are exchanged for intracellular bicarbonate.[1] This mechanism may buffer up to half of a mineral acid load but is of minimal importance in buffering of organic acids.

Shifting in the opposite direction can provide buffering of an alkaline load. Intracellular acids may shift into the ECF, accompanied by intracellular transport of bicarbonate in exchange for chloride.

Interaction of Acid-Base Regulatory Systems

Henderson-Hasselbalch Equation

The relationship between the mechanisms that regulate acid-base balance is characterized by the **Henderson-Hasselbalch equation**:

$$pH = pKc + \log [base]/[acid]$$

TABLE 10–2
NORMAL VALUES OF ARTERIAL BLOOD GAS PARAMETERS

CONSTITUENT (MEASURED OR CALCULATED)	NORMAL RANGE
Partial pressure of oxygen (PaO_2)	75–100 mm Hg
Partial pressure of carbon dioxide ($PaCO_2$)	35–45 mm Hg
pH	7.35–7.45
Bicarbonate ion concentration [HCO_3^-]	22–26 mEq/L
Base excess (BE)	−2 to +2
Oxygen content (O_2CT)	15%–23%
Oxygen saturation of hemoglobin (O_2Sat)	94%–100%

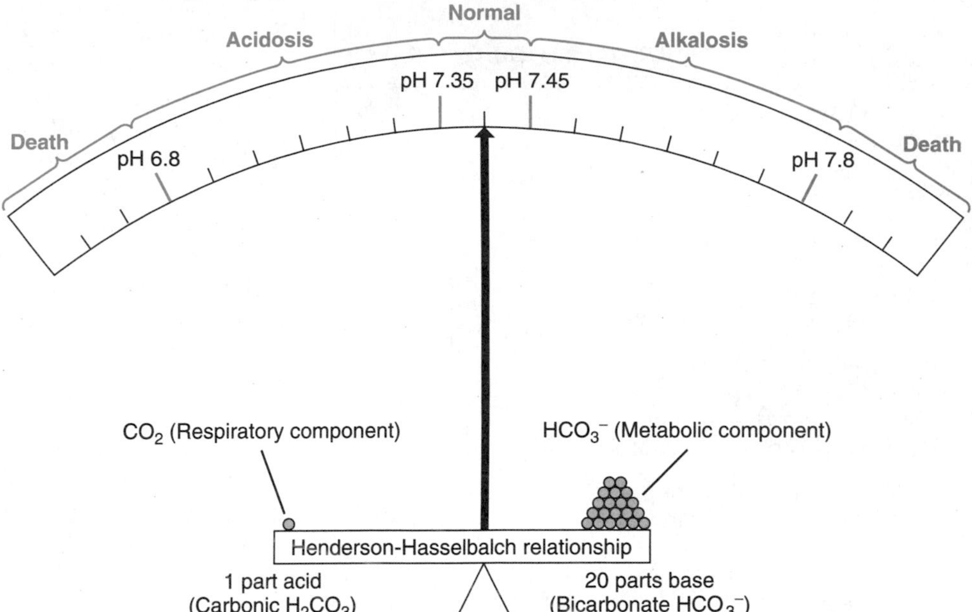

FIGURE 10–8
Interaction of pH regulatory systems. The Henderson-Hasselbalch relationship demonstrates that maintenance of normal serum pH (7.4). requires a ratio of 20 parts base to 1 part acid in plasma and intracellular fluid. Alteration of either the base or acid component by disease may result in acid-base imbalances, which may be incompatible with life outside the pH range of 6.8 to 7.8. The physiologic systems that regulate acid-base balance may alter the absolute amounts of acid or base in a compartment to maintain the ratio, that is, to compensate for imbalances.

In this equation, pKc is a constant value, 6.1, the pKa of the carbonic acid–bicarbonate buffer system. The base concentration is represented by serum HCO_3^-, and the acid by H_2CO_3. Because the concentration of H_2CO_3 in body fluids is negligible, however, the dissolved CO_2 concentration (which is proportional to carbonic acid concentration) is substituted. This value is calculated from the clinically measured pressure of CO_2 in arterial blood ($Paco_2$), by multiplying the $Paco_2$ by a unit conversion factor of 0.03. Substituting normal values for these parameters (Table 10–2), the equation becomes:

$$7.4 = 6.1 + \log 24/1.2$$

It is then apparent that a ratio of 20 parts base to 1 part acid must be present to yield a normal pH. An increase in the numerator (base) tends to increase blood pH, whereas a decrease tends to decrease pH. An increase in the denominator (acid) lowers pH, whereas a decrease causes a rise in pH (Fig. 10–8).

Compensation Versus Correction of Acid-Base Imbalance

When primary disease processes alter either the base or acid component of the 20:1 ratio, the lungs or the kidneys (whichever is unaffected by pathology) act to restore the ratio and normalize pH. This compensation is evidenced by abnormality of both the lung ($Paco_2$) and kidney (HCO_3^-) parameters *in the same direction*, whereas pH is near normal. When kidney disease impairs excretion of acid, for example, the respiratory system can increase ventilation to "blow off" excess acid as CO_2. The kidneys may compensate for retention of acid (CO_2) in hypoventilation by reclaiming HCO_3^- and excreting H^+.

In most cases, compensation does not fully restore normal pH (Table 10–3). For example, compensa-

TABLE 10–3
PREDICTED COMPENSATORY RESPONSES

PRIMARY DISORDER	MAXIMAL COMPENSATION
Respiratory acidosis	Increase in HCO_3^- of 1 mEq/L (in acute) to 4 mEq/L (in chronic) for each 10 mm Hg increase in $Paco_2$
Respiratory alkalosis	Decrease in HCO_3^- of 2 mEq/L (in acute) to 5 mEq/L (in chronic) for each 10 mm Hg decrease in $Paco_2$
Metabolic acidosis	Decrease in $Paco_2$ equal to 1.3 times the decrease in HCO_3^-
Metabolic alkalosis	Increase in $Paco_2$ equal to 0.6 times the increase in HCO_3^-

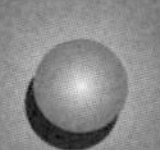

TABLE 10–4
ANALYSIS OF ARTERIAL BLOOD GASES

STEP 1: CLASSIFY THE pH
Normal: 7.35–7.45
Acidemia: <7.35
Alkalemia: >7.45

STEP 2: ASSESS $PaCO_2$
Normal: 35–45 mm Hg
Respiratory acidosis: >45 mm Hg
Respiratory alkalosis: <35 mm Hg

STEP 3: ASSESS HCO_3^-*
Normal: 22–26 mEq/L
Metabolic acidosis: <22 mEq/L
Metabolic alkalosis: >26 mEq/L

STEP 4: DETERMINE PRESENCE OF COMPENSATION
Compensation present: $PaCO_2$ and HCO_3^- are abnormal (or nearly so) in the same direction, e.g., both increased or both decreased.†
Compensation absent: One component ($PaCO_2$ or HCO_3^-) is abnormal, the other normal.

STEP 5: IDENTIFY PRIMARY DISORDER, IF POSSIBLE
If pH is clearly abnormal: The acid-base component most consistent with pH is the primary disorder.
If pH is normal or near-normal: The more deviant component is probably primary.‡ To verify, note whether pH is on acidotic or alkalotic side of 7.4. The more deviant value should be consistent with this pH.

STEP 6: CLASSIFY DEGREE OF COMPENSATION, IF PRESENT
Limits of Complete Compensation
Metabolic acidosis: The decrease in $PaCO_2$ is equal to 1.3 times the decrease in HCO_3^-.
Metabolic alkalosis: The increase in $PaCO_2$ is equal to 0.6 times the increase in HCO_3^-.
Respiratory acidosis: For every 10-mm Hg increase in $PaCO_2$, the HCO_3^- is increased by 1 mEq/L (in acute acidosis) or 4 mEq/L (in chronic acidosis).
Respiratory alkalosis: For every 10-mm Hg decrease in $PaCO_2$, the HCO_3^- is decreased by 2 mEq/L (in acute alkalosis) or 5 mEq/L (in chronic alkalosis).

"Compensation" beyond these limits suggests the presence of a mixed disorder.

*Base excess (BE) is also reported with ABGs and is a second index of metabolic status. Normal BE is −2 to +2. Because fluctuation in BE exactly parallels that of bicarbonate, it is not necessary to classify both.
†It is possible, but less likely, that two or more primary imbalances (i.e., a mixed disorder) are present, which results in the *appearance* of compensation. The detection of mixed disorders is facilitated by the use of acid-base maps or nomograms and by the formulas in step 6, but a mixed disorder cannot always be differentiated from compensation.
‡It is unlikely that the more deviant value represents compensation because the body does not overcompensate for imbalance. When pH approaches the normal range, compensatory mechanisms are no longer triggered.
Adapted from Hansen, M. (1997). Acid-base disorders. In: Black, J.M., and Matassarin-Jacobs, E. (Eds.). *Medical-Surgical Nursing: Clinical Management for Continuity of Care.* (5th Ed.). Philadelphia: W.B. Saunders, 1997. (p. 338).

tory hypoventilation in response to alkalosis caused by renal acid losses is limited by the hypoxemia that develops. Because hypoxemia is a respiratory stimulant, ventilation then increases. Similarly, renal compensation for ventilatory disorders is potentially limited by many factors, including renal blood flow, tubular flow rates, and saturability of tubular transport mechanisms.

The plasma and intracellular buffer systems act instantaneously to modulate pH changes. The lungs respond to changes in pH within minutes, but maximal compensation takes up to 24 hours. The kidneys may require up to 72 hours to achieve maximal compensation. Although compensation may nearly restore the 20:1 *ratio* of base to acid, the actual *amounts* of base or acid are still abnormal. Absolute quantities of acid or base are returned to normal only with correction of the underlying disease process.

Clinical Evaluation of Acid-Base Balance

Acid-base balance is monitored clinically through the serial measurement of **arterial blood gases (ABGs)**. A typical ABG report includes values for pH, $PaCO_2$, and HCO_3^- as determined from a sample of arterial blood. From these parameters, the presence of acid-base imbalance, as well as the degree of compensation, can be determined (Table 10–4). ABGs, however, only provide evidence of the blood picture (acidemia or alkalemia). Evaluation of acidosis and alkalosis requires consideration of the total clinical picture, including patient history, signs, symptoms, and laboratory values indicative of fluid and electrolyte balance, function of critical regulatory systems, and tissue response to acidemia or alkalemia.

ACID-BASE IMBALANCES

Four primary acid-base imbalances are described: **respiratory acidosis, respiratory alkalosis, metabolic acidosis,** and **metabolic alkalosis.** Respiratory acid-base imbalances are the result of impaired ventilation. Metabolic acid-base imbalances are due to a variety of renal or other, nonrespiratory, conditions. Table 10–5 compares the ABG parameters typical of each of these disorders.

Mixed acid-base imbalances consist of a combina-

TABLE 10–5
ARTERIAL BLOOD GAS VALUES IN PRIMARY ACID-BASE IMBALANCES

DISORDER	pH	$PaCO_2$	HCO_3^-
Respiratory acidosis	↓	↑	Normal or ↑ if compensation
Respiratory alkalosis	↑	↓	Normal or ↓ if compensation
Metabolic acidosis	↓	Normal or ↓ if compensation	↓
Metabolic alkalosis	↑	Normal or ↑ if compensation	↑

tion of two or three primary imbalances. Because hyperventilation and hypoventilation cannot occur simultaneously, respiratory acidosis and respiratory alkalosis cannot coexist, but all other combinations are possible. Acid-base imbalances are common in clinical settings, with respiratory alkalosis being most common, followed in frequency by respiratory acidosis, metabolic alkalosis, metabolic acidosis, and mixed disorders.[6]

Respiratory Acidosis

Definition. Respiratory acidosis is a relative excess of acid in body fluids resulting from carbon dioxide retention.

Epidemiology. Respiratory acidosis is common in disorders associated with hypoventilation (see later). Rarely, the imbalance is associated with increased metabolic production of CO_2.

Etiology. Respiratory acidosis is nearly always due to hypoventilation, which is seen in many clinical disorders (Table 10–6; see Chapter 18). Chronic obstructive pulmonary disease, also known as chronic airflow limitation, includes such disorders as emphysema, chronic bronchitis, asthma, and cystic fibrosis. Hypoventilation, due to airway obstruction, and disturbances of ventilation–perfusion relationships in the lungs characterize these disorders. Hypoventilation may also result from neuromuscular disorders such as spinal cord injury, amyotrophic lateral sclerosis, or Guillain-Barré syndrome, in which diaphragmatic movement is impaired. Head injury, stroke, or overdose of central nervous system depressant drugs can inhibit the respiratory center in the medulla, causing hypoventilation secondary to loss of the central drive or neural signal that initiates ventilation. Iatrogenic causes of respiratory acidosis include inadequate mechanical ventilation or suppression of the hypoxic stimulus for ventilation with excessive administration of oxygen to patients with chronic CO_2 retention. Increased metabolic production of CO_2 may occur iatrogenically with high-carbohydrate tube feedings or parenteral nutrition, but this is usually not significant unless the patient also has severely compromised ventilation.

Pathophysiology. CO_2 is easily able to diffuse across biologic membranes, permitting the distribution of the acid load to all body compartments. During *acute respiratory acidosis* (first 3 days of increased CO_2, or hypercapnea), buffering occurs within both plasma and ICF. The addition of CO_2 to body fluids drives the synthesis of carbonic acid by the hydrolysis reaction, and buffering occurs by nonbicarbonate buffers. Renal excretion of acid is accompanied by increased bicarbonate reclamation in the proximal tubule and increased bicarbonate regeneration in the distal tubule and collecting duct.

Hypercapnea persisting longer than 3 days is termed *chronic respiratory acidosis* and involves further renal compensation by an adaptive increase (up-regulation) in the number of membrane transport proteins for secretion of H^+ and reabsorption of HCO_3^-.[1] Renal ammonia production also increases, enhancing the function of the ammonium urinary buffer in the excretion of acid.

Clinical Manifestations. Respiratory acidosis is indicated on ABG analysis by a low pH, signifying acidosis, and a high $PaCO_2$, indicating retention of

TABLE 10–6
CAUSES OF RESPIRATORY ACIDOSIS

MECHANISM	EXAMPLES
Hypoventilation	Chronic obstructive pulmonary disease Obstructive sleep apnea Neuromuscular disorders Depression of medullary respiratory center Errors in mechanical ventilation Excess oxygen therapy in hypercapnea Chest wall trauma or congenital defect
Excess metabolic production of CO_2	Enteral or parenteral feedings high in carbohydrate Hypermetabolism

CO_2 in the blood. HCO_3^- values are normal or, if renal compensation is occurring, elevated. Compensatory elevation of HCO_3^- occurs to a greater degree in chronic acidosis than in acute acidosis (see Table 10–3). Clinical manifestations of acidosis are present to varying degrees (Table 10–7). Acute hypercapnea induces vasodilation as a local response of vascular smooth muscle (see Chapter 15). Cardiac dysrhythmias may also occur.[7]

Prevention and Treatment. Patients at risk should be carefully monitored for development of hypoxia and acidosis. Treatment is aimed at the underlying disorder, and ventilatory support is a major component. Administration of exogenous base (e.g., sodium bicarbonate) is *not* warranted because the acidosis is normally well compensated by physiologic mechanisms.[1] In patients with chronic respiratory acidosis, such treatment may induce posthypercapneic metabolic alkalosis after correction of the respiratory disorder (see later). Furthermore, the lower pH in respiratory acidosis may stimulate ventilation (see Chapter 18).

Prognosis and Outcome. The most critical problem for patients with respiratory acidosis is not the acidosis itself but rather the hypoxia that also results from ventilatory failure. The clinical outcome thus depends primarily on the degree and duration of tissue hypoxia and the responsiveness of the underlying disorder to treatment.

TABLE 10–7
CLINICAL MANIFESTATIONS OF ACIDOSIS

Affected System and Effects	Manifestations
Cardiovascular	Arterial vasodilation
Decreased vascular tone	Venoconstriction
Blunted response to catecholamines (EPI and NE)	Decreased cardiac output
Decreased myocardial contractility	Dysrhythmias
Disruption of conduction	
Central nervous system	Tremors
Depression of neurotransmission	Seizures
Increased cerebral blood flow	Lethargy
	Stupor
	Papilledema
Respiratory system	Hypoventilation in respiratory acidosis
Altered ventilation	Hyperventilation in metabolic acidosis
Rightward shift in oxyhemoglobin dissociation curve	Enhanced unloading of oxygen from hemoglobin
Electrolyte balance	Increased serum Ca^{2+}, K^+, and possibly Cl^-
Altered renal regulation	
Cellular ion shifts	

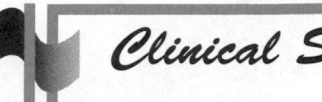

J.S., a 76-year-old retired mechanic, has advanced chronic obstructive lung disease associated with a long history of cigarette smoking. He sees his physician in the clinic, complaining of a "cold" that "just keeps hanging on." ABGs drawn during the visit reveal a pH of 7.34, $PaCO_2$ of 65 mm Hg, and HCO_3^- of 34 mEq/L.

1. What acid-base disorder is represented?
2. What additional information would be helpful in planning J.S.'s care?

Respiratory Alkalosis

Definition. Respiratory alkalosis is a relative excess of base in body fluids secondary to increased ventilatory elimination of CO_2.

Epidemiology. Respiratory alkalosis is the most common of the acid-base imbalances. Risk factors are those associated with hyperventilation (see later).

Etiology. The most common cause of respiratory alkalosis is hypoxemia, apparent on ABGs, as a PaO_2 (pressure of oxygen in arterial blood) lower than normal. As discussed in Chapter 18, low levels of oxygen in the blood are sensed by receptors, which feed back this information to the respiratory center in the brain stem. Rate and depth of ventilation increase in an attempt to improve oxygenation of the blood, but excess CO_2 may be lost concurrently. As detailed in Table 10–8, respiratory alkalosis commonly occurs with respiratory diseases such as pneumonia, pulmonary fibrosis, or adult respiratory distress syndrome. It is also seen in low blood flow states such as shock, owing to increased oxygen extraction by tissues, and in severe anemia, in which lack of hemoglobin reduces the oxygen-carrying capacity of the blood (see Chapter 12). The respiratory center may also trigger increased ventilation in response to other stimuli, including extreme emotional stress and severe pain. Certain drugs, including caffeine and theophylline, stimulate respiration. Hypermetabolic states induced by fever or strenuous exercise may produce hypoxemia due to increased oxygen consumption, resulting in increased stimulation of the respiratory center.

TABLE 10–8
CAUSES OF RESPIRATORY ALKALOSIS

MECHANISM	EXAMPLES
Hyperventilation	
Hypoxemia	Pneumonia Pulmonary embolism Asthma Pulmonary edema High altitude
Psychogenic	Extreme anxiety
Drugs (respiratory stimulants)	Theophylline Catecholamines Salicylates Progesterone Doxapram
Central nervous system disease	Stroke Cheyne-Stokes respirations
Hypermetabolism	Fever Sepsis Pregnancy
Iatrogenic	Mechanical ventilation error

Pathophysiology. Respiratory alkalosis of less than 24 hours' duration is considered to be acute, whereas that lasting longer than 24 hours is chronic. The acute buffering response is due to shifting of acid from the ICF to the blood and by movement of bicarbonate into cells in exchange for chloride. Alkalemia also triggers an adaptive increase in lactic acid production, secondary to stimulation of the glycolytic enzyme phosphofructokinase (see Chapter 3). Renal compensation in acute respiratory alkalosis involves decreased acid secretion by the distal tubule and collecting duct (thereby decreasing HCO_3^- regeneration) as well as excretion of excess filtered and secreted bicarbonate in the urine. In chronic respiratory alkalosis, further compensation results from down-regulation of tubular transport proteins for acid secretion.

Clinical Manifestations. ABG signs of respiratory alkalosis are elevated pH, $PaCO_2$ lower than normal, and HCO_3^- normal or low owing to compensation. The degree of renal compensation is greater in chronic respiratory alkalosis (see Table 10–3). Serum lactate levels are elevated. Clinical manifestations of alkalosis are summarized in Table 10–9. Central nervous system dysfunction is predominant, with lightheadedness, confusion, and possibly seizures occurring as a consequence of decreased cerebral blood flow.[7]

Prevention and Treatment. Patients at risk should be closely monitored for development of the disorder. Treatment is aimed at the underlying disorder and often involves the administration of oxygen to correct hypoxia. In some cases, rebreathing of CO_2 may be beneficial.

Prognosis and Outcome. Outcome depends on the severity of the underlying disorder and the response to treatment. Compensation for respiratory alkalosis depletes the bicarbonate buffer, placing the patient at risk if subsequently exposed to an increased acid load.

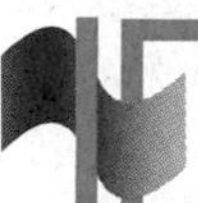

Clinical Scenario

M.A., a 19-year-old college student, is brought to the emergency department at 4:30 A.M. by her friends. She had been studying for final exams and had grown increasingly anxious during this "cram session." She repeatedly voiced doubts about passing a particularly difficult science course. M.A.'s breathing became labored, and she seemed dazed and confused. She said her "face felt numb." Two years ago, M.A. had been diagnosed with bleeding duodenal ulcers. ABGs drawn in the emergency department reveal a pH of 7.58, $PaCO_2$ of 21 mm Hg, and HCO_3^- of 20 mEq/L.

1. What acid-base imbalance is represented?
2. What interventions might prevent future episodes?

TABLE 10–9
CLINICAL MANIFESTATIONS OF ALKALOSIS

AFFECTED SYSTEM AND EFFECTS	MANIFESTATIONS
Cardiovascular Increased myocardial irritability	Dysrhythmias
Central nervous system Decreased seizure threshold Reduced cerebral blood flow	Seizures Lightheadedness Confusion
Respiratory system Altered ventilation	Hyperventilation in respiratory alkalosis Hypoventilation in metabolic alkalosis
Electrolyte balance Altered renal regulation Cellular ion shifts	Decreased serum Ca^{2+}, K^+

Metabolic Acidosis

Definition. Metabolic acidosis is the clinical syndrome resulting from loss of bicarbonate or gain of nonvolatile acid.

Epidemiology. Metabolic acidosis is common in clinical settings. Risk factors are those associated with conditions in which there is increased ingestion or metabolic production of nonvolatile acid, or increased loss or decreased production of base (see below).

Etiology. Metabolic acidosis is classified as *high-anion gap acidosis* if due to excess of organic acids (e.g., **lactic acidosis**, **ketoacidosis**, or **uremic acidosis**). Metabolic acidosis due to excess of inorganic acid (mineral acids such as HCl) or increased loss of base is classified as *non-anion gap acidosis*. Table 10-10 lists causes of both forms of metabolic acidosis.

The **anion gap (A^-)** is the difference obtained when the sum of the major ECF anions, HCO_3^- and Cl^-, is subtracted from the major cation, Na^+:

$$A^- = [Na^+] - ([HCO_3^-] + [Cl^-]) = 12 \pm 4 \text{ mEq/L}$$

TABLE 10-10
CAUSES OF METABOLIC ACIDOSIS

Mechanisms	Examples
Non-Anion Gap Acidosis	
Renal loss of bicarbonate	Proximal renal tubular acidosis
	End-stage renal failure with chloride retention
Gastrointestinal loss of bicarbonate	Diarrhea
	Pancreatic fistula
	Intestinal drainage
Gain of mineral acid	Parenteral nutrition
	Overtreatment of alkalosis
High-Anion Gap Acidosis	
Excess endogenous production of organic acids	Ketoacidosis
	Diabetes mellitus
	Starvation
	Alcoholism
	Lactic acidosis
	Anaerobic metabolism
	Hypermetabolism
	Cirrhosis
	Diabetes mellitus
	Cancer
	Salicylate poisoning
	Abuse of methanol or ethylene glycol
Decreased renal H^+ secretion	Uremic acidosis
	End-stage renal failure
	Distal renal tubular acidosis

The gap represents anionic proteins and other anions that are not routinely measured in clinical settings.

Non-Anion Gap Acidosis. In cases of $NaHCO_3$ loss (e.g., diarrhea), the kidneys retain NaCl to restore sodium and water balance. Cl^- thus rises, offsetting HCO_3^- loss and maintaining a normal anion gap. In mineral acid ingestion, such as may occur iatrogenically with parenteral nutrition, chloride anion is ingested with the acid, and bicarbonate is excreted proportionately. In some forms of **renal tubular acidosis,** failure of renal reclamation or regeneration of bicarbonate results in proportional retention of chloride. In end-stage renal failure, mechanisms for restoration of the bicarbonate component of the principal buffer may also fail, and acid may be retained as a consequence of a decline in ammonia production. Chloride retention offsets low serum levels of bicarbonate, and the gap remains normal. Because of the associated chloride retention, non-anion gap metabolic acidosis is often referred to as *hyperchloremic metabolic acidosis*.

High-Anion Gap Metabolic Acidosis. Ketoacidosis results from a shift in metabolism from glucose to nonglucose sources (primarily fatty acids) for energy fuel. The usual setting is diabetes mellitus, in which relative or absolute lack of insulin inhibits uptake of glucose into cells (see Chapter 29). In starvation states, lack of nutrient intake and rapid depletion of glycogen stores lead to use of adipose stores of fatty acids for fuel. Alcoholic patients are prone to ketoacidosis when they limit their caloric intake *and* their alcohol intake (e.g., owing to vomiting). In these cases, starvation induces ketoacid formation, and lack of alcohol, which normally suppresses ketoacid formation, permits development of acidosis. Ketoacids are produced as metabolic byproducts in these states and manifest as acidosis if renal function is not adequate to clear them from the circulation.

Lactic acidosis occurs as a consequence of either increased production of lactate with anaerobic metabolism or failure of the liver and kidneys to convert lactate to pyruvate or bicarbonate (see Chapter 3). The former results from tissue hypoxia, and the latter results from primary disease of the liver or kidneys. Diabetes may promote lactic acidosis by a combination of these mechanisms.

Uremic acidosis occurs in a small percentage of patients with end-stage renal disease. (Most develop non-anion gap acidosis, discussed earlier.) Lack of ammonium buffering reduces acid excretion, and retention of unmeasured anions may induce an anion gap.

Salicylate poisoning (typically due to aspirin overdose) induces high–anion gap acidosis by inhibiting oxidative phosphorylation in mitochondria (see Chapter 3). This promotes lactic acidosis and ketoacidosis, as alternate forms of energy metabolism are employed. Although rare causes of metabolic acidosis, ingestion of methanol (wood alcohol) and ethylene glycol (antifreeze) induce high–anion gap acidosis by the production of formic acid and lactic acid, respectively.[1]

Recent research has called the validity of anion gap assessment into question.[8] Many cases of metabolic acidosis originate from retention of *both* organic and inorganic acids. Absolute correlation between high–anion gap acidosis and organic acidosis is seen only with an A^- of 30 or greater, and, in lactic acidosis, A^- often does not rise proportionately to lactate accumulation. Calculation of the anion gap is still important in clinical practice, but this assessment is gradually being replaced by more specific tests, such as measurement of serum lactate and ketone levels and evaluation of renal function.

Pathophysiology. Unless there is a coexisting respiratory disorder, metabolic acidosis is accompanied by a compensatory increase in ventilation. Hyperkalemia also accompanies metabolic acidosis, owing to shifting of acid into ICF with corresponding shift of K^+ extracellularly or to renal retention of K^+ in exchange for H^+. In diabetic patients, insulin deficiency may also promote hyperkalemia because insulin normally promotes cellular uptake of K^+ along with glucose.

Clinical Manifestations. Metabolic acidosis is revealed by blood gases showing a decreased pH, decreased HCO_3-, and a $PaCO_2$ that is normal or decreased owing to compensation. Clinical manifestations of acidosis are detailed in Table 10–7. Respiratory compensation in severe metabolic acidosis is evident as hyperventilation or **Kussmaul's respirations** and is particularly effective (see Table 10–3). Local vasodilation is common, and the oxyhemoglobin dissociation curve shifts to the right, inducing an adaptive increase in tissue oxygenation (see Chapter 19). Acidosis and hyperkalemia are both associated with cardiac dysrhythmias and central nervous system dysfunction.

Prevention and Treatment. Careful monitoring is warranted in patients who have underlying disorders that place them at risk for metabolic acidosis. Treatment is aimed at the underlying disorder. Administration of sodium bicarbonate is limited to severe metabolic acidosis, that is, HCO_3^- less than 5 mEq/L or pH less than 7.10.[7,9]

Prognosis and Outcome. Outcome depends on the severity and response to treatment of the underlying disorder.

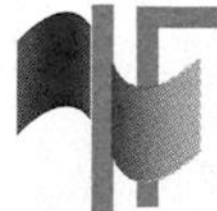

Clinical Scenario

S.R., a 65-year-old widow, has a long history of non–insulin-dependent diabetes mellitus. She was a heavy smoker for 40 years but has not smoked in the past 5 years. She is admitted to the general medical unit because of a 1-week history of diarrhea, attributed to "food poisoning." She appears to be in respiratory distress. Her admission ABGs are pH of 7.26, $PaCO_2$ of 13 mm Hg, and HCO_3^- of 5 mEq/L.

1. What acid-base imbalance is represented?
2. Other than ABGs, what laboratory parameters should be closely monitored in this case? Why?

Metabolic Alkalosis

Definition. Metabolic alkalosis is the clinical syndrome that results from accumulation of bicarbonate or loss of nonvolatile acid from the body.

Epidemiology. Metabolic alkalosis is commonly encountered in clinical settings. The usual risk factors are those associated with hypovolemia. Less commonly, risk factors for primary excess of aldosterone or iatrogenic excess of base administration are implicated (see later).

Etiology. This imbalance is caused by either loss of nonvolatile acid or accumulation of base, in a two-stage process. *Generation* of alkalosis involves a triggering event in which there is acid loss or base gain. Under normal circumstances, however, renal excretion of HCO_3^- quickly restores homeostasis. *Maintenance* of metabolic alkalosis requires the additional presence of renal impairment in HCO_3^- elimination, which may be induced by hypovolemia or, less commonly, hyperaldosteronism. Table 10–11 lists common causes of metabolic alkalosis in hypovolemic states (*contraction alkalosis*) versus normovolemic states.

Metabolic alkalosis due to acid loss may occur with prolonged vomiting, which causes loss of gastric HCl. Base may be gained as a consequence of loss, through diarrhea or drainage, of intestinal fluids containing more chloride than bicarbonate. The hypovolemia that also results from these fluid losses

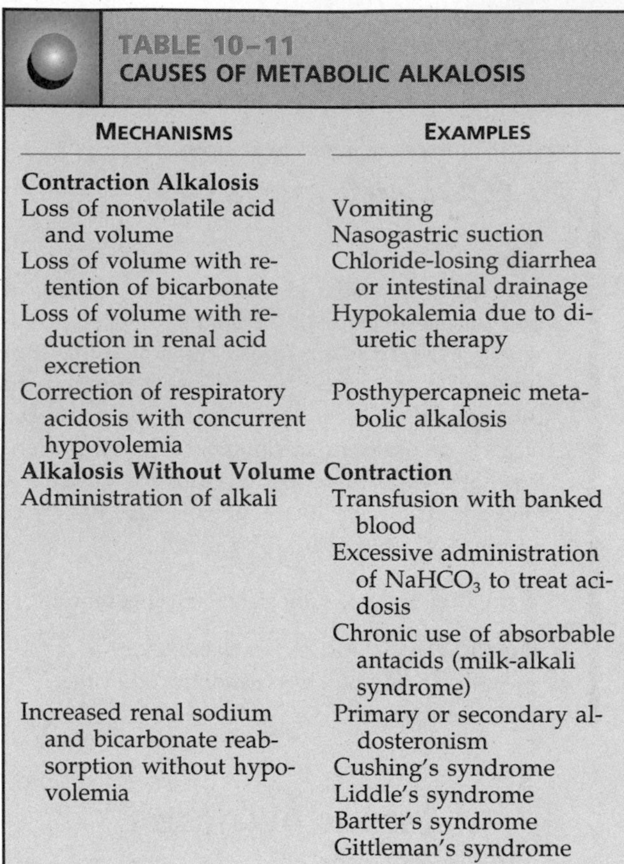

TABLE 10–11
CAUSES OF METABOLIC ALKALOSIS

MECHANISMS	EXAMPLES
Contraction Alkalosis	
Loss of nonvolatile acid and volume	Vomiting Nasogastric suction
Loss of volume with retention of bicarbonate	Chloride-losing diarrhea or intestinal drainage
Loss of volume with reduction in renal acid excretion	Hypokalemia due to diuretic therapy
Correction of respiratory acidosis with concurrent hypovolemia	Posthypercapneic metabolic alkalosis
Alkalosis Without Volume Contraction	
Administration of alkali	Transfusion with banked blood Excessive administration of $NaHCO_3$ to treat acidosis Chronic use of absorbable antacids (milk-alkali syndrome)
Increased renal sodium and bicarbonate reabsorption without hypovolemia	Primary or secondary aldosteronism Cushing's syndrome Liddle's syndrome Bartter's syndrome Gittleman's syndrome

then perpetuates the imbalance. The RAAS is activated (see Chapter 8), and increased Na^+ reabsorption by the distal kidney is accompanied by increased H^+ secretion and HCO_3^- regeneration.

A number of iatrogenic mechanisms may produce metabolic alkalosis. Diuretic therapy may contribute to hypovolemia and hypokalemia (see Chapters 8 and 9). In an effort to protect serum K^+ levels, the kidney retains K^+ and secretes H^+, thereby regenerating additional bicarbonate. Exchange of K^+ for H^+ across cell membranes also occurs in hypokalemia, contributing to alkalosis. Less commonly, alkalosis results from alkali administration, as with overcorrection of acidosis with administration of sodium bicarbonate or massive transfusion of whole blood. Alkalosis occurs in the latter case because citrate, used as an anticoagulant in banked blood, is converted to bicarbonate in the body. Another iatrogenic cause of metabolic alkalosis is the rapid correction of respiratory acidosis in which renal compensation had generated increased amounts of HCO_3^-. After treatment restores normal ventilation, adequate fluid volume must be available to deliver Cl^- to the distal tubule for exchange with HCO_3^-. If the patient is hypovolemic, the elevated bicarbonate persists as a primary metabolic alkalosis (posthypercapneic metabolic alkalosis).

An unusual cause of metabolic alkalosis, unrelated to hypovolemia, is a hormonal imbalance in which there is a primary or secondary excess of aldosterone or other mineralocorticoid (see Chapter 29). In this case, aldosterone inappropriately stimulates distal sodium reabsorption, with concurrent secretion of H^+ and regeneration of HCO_3^-, as described earlier.

Pathophysiology. The mechanisms that buffer metabolic alkalosis are much weaker than those that buffer an acid load, and most buffering occurs in the ECF.[1] Respiratory compensation is limited, but some hypoventilation does occur (see Table 10–3). Metabolic alkalosis is associated with hypokalemia and hypochloremia, as described earlier.

Clinical Manifestations. Metabolic alkalosis is manifested on ABGs by an elevated pH, elevated HCO_3^-, and normal or elevated (with compensation) $PaCO_2$. Table 10–9 summarizes clinical manifestations of alkalosis. Adaptive hypoventilation may induce some degree of hypoxia. Signs of volume deficit are associated with the underlying cause in many cases (see Chapter 8). Hypokalemia may manifest as cardiac dysrhythmias (see Chapter 9). Central nervous system manifestations may result from alkalosis, hypoxia, hypovolemia, or electrolyte imbalance. These include lethargy, confusion, muscle twitching, and possibly seizures.

Prevention and Treatment. Patients at risk should be closely monitored for development of alkalosis. Overcorrection of acidosis with sodium bicarbonate administration and too rapid correction of hypoventilation in respiratory acidosis should be avoided. Treatment of metabolic alkalosis centers on identification and removal of the underlying cause, if possible. In contraction alkalosis, restoration of fluid volume and chloride levels (usually with intravenous normal saline) permits the kidney to excrete the excess bicarbonate over a few days. Potassium replacement is often necessary as well. Intravenous administration of acetazolamide (Diamox), a carbonic anhydrase inhibitor, may be used in severe alkalosis to enhance renal bicarbonate excretion.[9] Cautious administration of exogenous acid in the form of hydrochloric acid or HCl precursors (e.g., ammonium chloride or arginine monohydrochloride) may be warranted for severe metabolic alkalosis. These agents are corrosive, however, and can promote dangerous hyperkalemia.[7]

Prognosis and Outcome. Uncorrected metabolic alkalosis may carry significant risk of mortality due to dysrhythmia and poor tissue perfusion. Outcome is primarily associated with the severity of the underlying disorder.

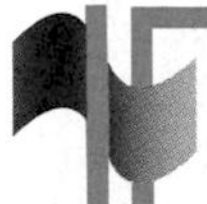

Clinical Scenario

R.G. is a 60-year-old woman whose chronic renal failure has been treated at home with peritoneal dialysis for 3 years. She is admitted to the medical intensive care unit in a near coma. Her husband reports that for several days, she had complained of abdominal pain and had experienced frequent episodes of nausea and vomiting. Her abdomen is grossly distended, and she is diagnosed with peritonitis and bowel obstruction. Her ABGs on admission show a pH of 7.47, $PaCO_2$ of 67 mm Hg, and HCO_3^- of 49 mEq/L.

1. What acid-base disorder is represented?
2. What factors in R.G.'s history account for the development of this imbalance? Explain.

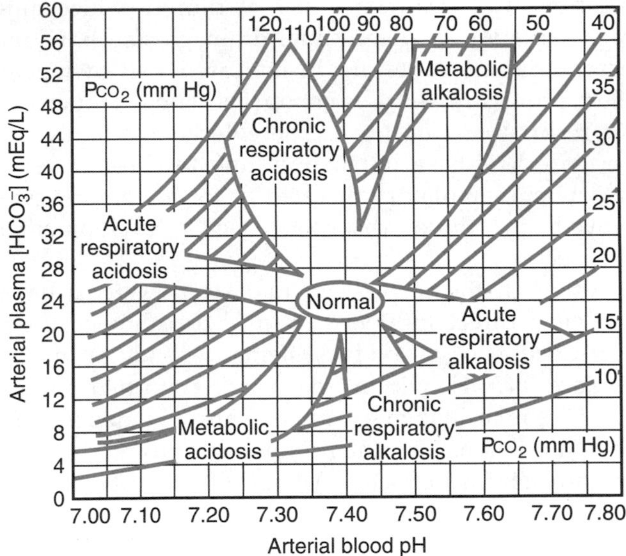

FIGURE 10–9

Acid-base nomogram. This nomogram, or map, is derived from predicted arterial blood gas (ABG) values for specific primary acid-base imbalances. HCO_3^- is plotted on the vertical axis, arterial pH on the horizontal axis, and $PaCO_2$ on the isobars. If plotted ABG values converge at a point outside the usual range for any of the primary imbalances, a mixed disorder is suspected. (Adapted from Brenner, B.M. [Ed.]. [1986]. *Brenner & Rector's The Kidney*. Philadelphia: W.B. Saunders.)

TABLE 10–12
EXAMPLES OF MIXED ACID-BASE IMBALANCES

MIXED DISORDERS	ETIOLOGY
Metabolic and respiratory acidosis	Acute pulmonary edema and cardiac arrest Poisons that depress ventilation and yield acid metabolites
Metabolic and respiratory alkalosis	Hepatorenal failure with hypoventilation due to ascites and volume depletion secondary to diuretic therapy Heart failure and diuretic therapy
Metabolic alkalosis and respiratory acidosis	Chronic obstructive pulmonary disease and diuretic therapy Respiratory failure and gastric drainage
Metabolic acidosis and respiratory alkalosis	Chronic renal failure and hyperventilation Septic shock and lactic acidosis Salicylate overdose
Metabolic acidosis and metabolic alkalosis	Chronic renal failure and vomiting
Respiratory acidosis, metabolic acidosis, and metabolic alkalosis	Methanol ingestion, vomiting, and respiratory arrest
Respiratory alkalosis, metabolic acidosis, and metabolic alkalosis	Heart failure, pneumonia, and diuretic therapy

Mixed Acid-Base Imbalances

Two or three primary acid-base disorders may coexist in mixed imbalances (Table 10–12). Because hypoventilation and hyperventilation are mutually exclusive conditions, only one primary respiratory imbalance may be present. Metabolic acidosis and alkalosis may occur simultaneously, however, due to different etiologies. On ABG analysis, a mixed imbalance is suspected when $PaCO_2$ and HCO_3^- levels do not correlate with pH, or when evidence of compensation exceeds predicted levels (see Table 10–3). Acid-base nomograms are also useful in clinical evaluation of mixed imbalances (Fig. 10–9). If plotted ABG values converge at a point outside the usual range for a primary imbalance, a mixed disorder is likely.

CLINICAL SIGNIFICANCE OF ACID-BASE IMBALANCES

Health care professionals must identify and monitor the many patients at risk for acid-base disorders. Respiratory and renal diseases commonly cause imbalances, and treatments such as diuretics, mechanical ventilation, and intestinal drainage also have inherent risks. Infants are at increased risk owing to their immature renal function and their propensity for respiratory infections. The elderly commonly experience acid-base imbalances due to chronic respiratory and circulatory diseases or to the therapy employed in these disorders (see Developmental Perspective).

Although the respiratory and renal systems have the most direct influence on acid-base homeostasis, the function of all body systems depends on maintenance of pH within the narrow normal range. Most cellular enzyme systems are pH dependent, and alterations in their function produce widespread clinical effects. Alterations in pH induce local adaptive responses in tissue perfusion, including that of critical systems (e.g., coronary and cerebral circulations). Because H^+ and HCO_3^- are electrolytes, acid-base abnormalities are inevitably associated with imbalance of potassium, chloride, and other electrolytes. Fluid balance influences and is influenced by renal handling of acids and bases.

Although homeostatic mechanisms may compensate for acid-base imbalances to a significant degree, *correction* of acid-base disorders only occurs when absolute amounts of acids and bases are returned to normal. This requires resolution of the underlying cause. Specific disorders associated with acid-base imbalances are detailed in the relevant systems chapters in Part Two.

Developmental Perspective

Embryonic and Fetal Periods

Processes that affect maternal respiration, uterine blood flow, placental gas exchange, and fetal cardiovascular function may affect fetal acid-base balance. Fetal lactate levels are increased with maternal smoking and alcohol use and with rapid administration of intravenous glucose during labor and delivery. Maternal respiratory acidosis and alkalosis may be manifested by the fetus and can occur with hypoventilation (i.e., with use of analgesic drugs) or hyperventilation (i.e., with anxiety, pain, or improper breathing techniques) during labor.

Infancy and Childhood

Because residual lung volume is low in infants, any alteration in ventilation rapidly affects $PaCO_2$. The higher metabolic rate of infants and young children produces increased acid end products that, when coupled with immaturity of the kidneys, increases the risk of acidosis. Many disorders of infancy and childhood may contribute to acid-base imbalance, including infant respiratory distress syndrome, asthma, diabetes mellitus, and accidental aspirin ingestion. Voluntary hypoventilation, or breath-holding, is also common in young children and can contribute to transient, benign respiratory acidosis.

Adolescence and Young Adulthood

Patients in this age group are at highest risk for acid-base disorders caused by the respiratory and renal effects of chronic drug use or of acute overdose. Spinal cord injury and head injury have their highest incidence in this group and can result in paralysis of ventilatory muscles or alteration in the brain-stem respiratory control centers. Mild respiratory alkalosis is common during pregnancy because uterine displacement of the diaphragm induces a more rapid, shallow type of ventilation.

Middle and Older Adulthood

Age-associated declines in homeostatic systems (i.e., reduced ventilatory capacity and renal function) enhance the rate with which acid-base disorders may develop. Diseases that can underlie severe acid-base imbalance, such as congestive heart failure, renal failure, respiratory failure, and diabetes mellitus, occur with greatest frequency in the elderly.

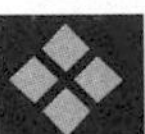

Summary of Key Points

- Most of the body's metabolic processes are pH dependent; thus, the pH of body fluids must be tightly regulated. pH outside the range of 6.8 to 7.8 may be incompatible with life.
- The lungs regulate the excretion of CO_2 by alteration of the rate and depth of ventilation. Because hydrolysis of CO_2 yields carbonic acid, CO_2 exhalation constitutes excretion of potential acid.
- The bicarbonate filtered into the renal tubular fluid undergoes dehydration to generate CO_2, which diffuses into the tubular cell. CO_2 is hydrolyzed to bicarbonate in the cell and is then actively reabsorbed into the blood.
- H^+ secreted into the renal tubular fluid may combine with bicarbonate, with ammonia, or with other anions such as phosphate. Binding of H^+ limits changes in urinary pH. With bicarbonate buffering, CO_2 and H_2O are formed, and bicarbonate is regenerated. With ammonia buffering, H^+ combines with NH_3 to form NH_4, which is too large to be reabsorbed. Instead, it is excreted with Cl^- or another anion. Phosphate buffering results in the formation of a weak acid, which is excreted.
- Because H^+ and HCO_3^- are electrolytes, acid-base imbalances influence the regulation of other electrolytes. Hyperkalemia may develop in H^+ excess due to transcellular H^+–K^+ shifts. Also, the kidney may excrete excess H^+ while retaining K^+ for electroneutrality. Na^+ reabsorption is accompanied by HCO_3^-. Chloride may be retained or excreted in compensation for HCO_3^- excess or deficit.
- The importance of the carbonic acid–bicarbonate buffer system lies in its ECF location, which facilitates monitoring; in its pKa, which is ideal for buffering a predominantly acid load; and in the fact that it is an *open* system, the components of which are readily regenerated or excreted.
- The Henderson-Hasselbalch equation illustrates that maintenance of a normal pH requires a 20:1 ratio of base to acid in body fluids.
- Respiratory acidosis results from CO_2 retention secondary to hypoventilation. Respiratory alkalosis results from CO_2 deficit due to hyperventilation, which is often induced by hypoxemia. Metabolic acidosis may be caused by retention or ingestion of fixed acid or by loss of base. Metabolic alkalosis results from base ingestion or loss of fixed acid.
- Mixed acid-base disorders are common in settings in which both respiratory function and metabolic function are compromised, such as cardiac arrest, liver disease with ascites, coexisting respiratory and renal disease, and coexisting respiratory and cardiac disease. Drug therapy of these conditions may also contribute.
- In acid-base compensation, the unaffected system (lungs or kidneys) retains or excretes acid, or, in the case of the kidneys, reclaims base to restore the 20:1 ratio of base to acid, normalizing pH. Actual amounts of acid and base remain abnormal until the condition is corrected with resolution of the underlying disorder.

REFERENCES

1. Laski, M.E., and Kurtzman, N.A. (1996). Acid-base disorders in medicine. *Disease-A-Month* 42(2), 59–125.
2. Guyton, A.C., and Hall, J.E. (1996). *Textbook of Medical Physiology*. (9th ed.). Philadelphia: W.B. Saunders Co. (p. 520).
3. Koch, S.M., and Taylor, R.W. (1992). Chloride ion in intensive care medicine. *Critical Care Medicine* 20(2), 227–240.
4. Preisig, P. (1994). Renal acidification. *ANNA Journal* 21(5),251–259.
5. Figge, J., Rossing, T.H., and Fencl, V. (1991). The role of serum proteins in acid-base equilibria. *Journal of Laboratory and Clinical Medicine* 117, 453–467.
6. Palange, P., Carlone, S., Galassetti, P., *et al.* (1990). Incidence of acid-base and electrolyte disturbances in a general hospital: A study of 110 consecutive admissions. *Recenti Progressi in Medicine (Roma)* 81(12), 788–791.
7. McLaughlin, M.L., and Kassirer, J.P. (1990). Rational treatment of acid-base disorders. *Drugs* 399(6), 841–855.
8. Badrick, T., and Hickman, P.E. (1992). The anion gap: A reappraisal. *American Journal of Clinical Pathology* 98(2), 249–252.
9. Toto, R.D. (1991). Acid-base balance in the CCU patient. *Hospital Medicine* 27(8), 103–117.

SELECTED BIBLIOGRAPHY

Chang, A.C., Zucker, H.A., Hickey, P.R., *et al.* (1995). Pulmonary vascular resistance in infants after cardiac surgery: Role of carbon dioxide and hydrogen ion. *Critical Care Medicine* 23, 568–574.

Cinnella, G., Conti, G., Lofaso, F., *et al.* (1996). Effects of assisted ventilation on the work of breathing: Volume-controlled versus pressure-controlled ventilation. *American Journal of Respiratory Critical Care Medicine* 153, 1025–1033.

D'Addesio, J. (1992). Metabolic and respiratory acidosis. *Topics in Emergency Medicine* 14(1), 51–55.

Dirks, J.L. (1995). Innovations in technology: Continuous intra-arterial blood gas monitoring. *Critical Care Nurse* 15(2), 1995, 19–27.

Gerhardt, R.E., Koethe, J.D., Glickman, G.D., *et al.* (1995). Acid dialysate correction of metabolic alkalosis in renal failure. *American Journal of Kidney Diseases* 25(2), 343–345.

Gilbert, H.C., and Vender, J.S. (1995). Arterial blood gas monitoring. *Critical Care Clinics* 11(1), 233–248.

Gilfix, B.M., Bique, M., and Magder, S. (1993). A physical chemical approach to the analysis of acid-base balance in the clinical setting. *Journal of Critical Care* 8(4), 187–197.

Giovambattista, C., Unwin, R., Ciani, F., *et al.* (1994). Bicarbonate transport along the loop of Henle. II. Effects of acid-base, dietary, and neurohumoral determinants. *Journal of Clinical Investigations* 94, 830–838.

Grillo, J.A., and Gonzalez, E.R. (1993). Changes in the pharmacotherapy of CPR. *Heart and Lung* 22(6), 548–553.

Hanna, J.D., Scheinman, J.I., and Chan, J.C.M. (1995). The kidney in acid-base balance. *Pediatric Clinics of North America* 42(6), 1365–1395.

Hansen, M. (1997). Acid-base disorders. In: Black, J.M., and Matassarin-Jacobs, E. (Eds.). *Medical-Surgical Nursing: Clinical Management for Continuity of Care.* (5th ed.). Philadelphia: W.B. Saunders Co. (pp. 328–341).

Levine, R.L. (1993). Ischemia: From acidosis to oxidation. *FASEB Journal* 7, 1242–1246.

Marik, P.E., Kussman, B.D., Lipman, J., *et al.* (1991). Acetazolamide in the treatment of metabolic alkalosis in critically ill patients. *Heart and Lung* 20(5 Pt. 1), 455–459.

Mays, D. (1995). Turn ABGs into child's play. *RN* 58(1), 36–39.

Mitch, W.E., Price, S.R., May, R.C., *et al.* (1994). Metabolic consequence of uremia: Extending the concept of adaptive responses to protein metabolism. *American Journal of Kidney Diseases* 23(2), 224–228.

Narins, R. (Ed.). (1994). *Maxwell & Kleeman's Clinical Disorders of Fluid and Electrolyte Metabolism.* (5th ed.). New York: McGraw-Hill.

Preuss, H.G. (1993). Fundamentals of clinical acid-base evaluation. *Clinics in Laboratory Medicine* 13(1), 103–116.

Rose, B. (1994). *Clinical Physiology of Acid-Base and Electrolyte Disorders.* (4th ed.). New York: McGraw-Hill.

Russell, J.M. (1991). Successful methods for arterial blood gas interpretation. *Critical Care Nurse* 11(1), 14–19.

Sica, D.A. (1994). Renal disease, electrolyte abnormalities, and acid-base imbalance in the elderly. *Clinics in Geriatric Medicine* 10(1), 197–211.

Stacpoole, P.W., Wright, E.C., Baumgartner, T.G., *et al.* (1994). Natural history and course of acquired lactic acidosis in adults. *American Journal of Medicine* 97, 47–53.

Stringfield, Y.N. (1993). Back to basics: Acidosis, alkalosis, and ABGs. *American Journal of Nursing* 93(11), 43–44.

Tasota, F.J., and Wesmiller, S.W. (1994). Assessing ABGs: Maintaining the delicate balance. *Nursing 94* 24(5), 34–44.

Williamson, J.C. (1995). Acid-base disorders: Classification and management strategies. *American Family Physician* 52(2), 584–590.

Yancey, M.K., and Harlass, F.E. (1993). Extraneous factors and their influences on fetal acid-base status. *Clinical Obstetrics and Gynecology* 36(1), 60–72.

Thermoregulation

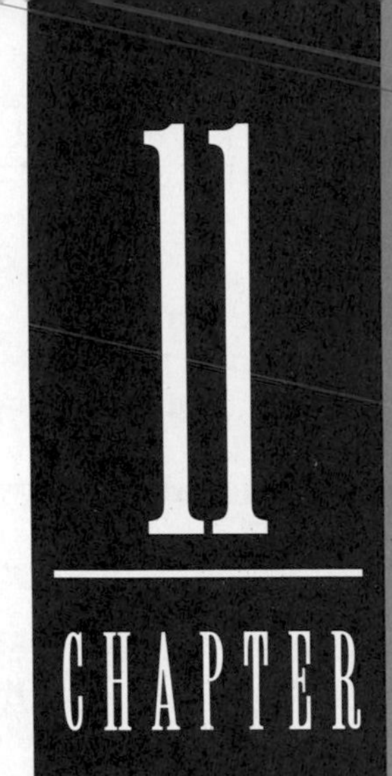

LEARNING OBJECTIVES

1. Identify the four major mechanisms by which the body can generate heat.
2. Identify the four mechanisms by which the body can lose heat to the environment.
3. Identify the four mechanisms by which the body can conserve heat.
4. Describe the components of the thermoregulatory system and their specific functions.
5. Differentiate among mechanisms of pyrogenic hyperthermia (fever) and other forms of hyperthermia.
6. Relate the four stages of fever to the underlying thermoregulatory responses.
7. Differentiate among the clinical features of the mild and major forms of environmental hyperthermia.
8. Discuss modes of clinical intervention in hyperthermia.
9. Describe the pathophysiologic mechanisms that underlie the clinical manifestations of hypothermia.

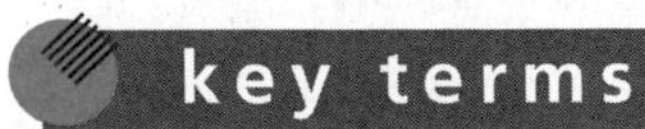

acclimation
afterdrop
antipyretic
brown fat
conduction
convection
cryogen
defervescence
environmental hyperthermia
evaporation
febrile seizures
fever
fever of unknown origin
heat exhaustion
heatstroke

hyperthermia
hypothermia
malignant hyperthermia
neurogenic hyperthermia
neuroleptic malignant syndrome
nonshivering thermogenesis
piloerection
pyrogen
pyrogenic hyperthermia
radiation
shivering thermogenesis
thermogenesis
thermoreceptor
thermoregulation

Regulation of the temperature of the extracellular environment, or **thermoregulation,** requires a precise balance of the body's mechanisms for heat production, heat conservation, and heat loss. Normal body temperature is generally considered to be 98.6°F (37°C), although temperature varies among people of different ages (Table 11–1) and among specific organ systems, depending on metabolic activity. The time of temperature measurement and method of measurement must also be considered in temperature evaluation. Body temperature displays a circadian pattern, being highest in the early evening (Fig. 11–1), as well as a monthly cycle in women, corresponding to the menstrual cycle. In clinical settings, pulmonary arterial temperatures most closely approximate core temperature, and rectal temperature measurement yields slightly higher readings than oral, tympanic, axillary, or skin surface methods (Fig. 11–2).

Cellular function is altered when body temperature is too high (**hyperthermia**) or too low (**hypothermia**); although in many cases, this alteration is adaptive rather than pathologic. Elevated body temperature that accompanies infection, for example, may be adaptive in that it promotes the activity of some immune functions and creates an unfavorable environment for proliferation of microorganisms.[1] Hypothermia may be employed therapeutically during surgery or in cases of shock or trauma to reduce metabolic demands for oxygen and thereby minimize harmful effects of tissue hypoxia.[2] It has also been proposed that the hypothermia that often accompanies severe trauma is a protective response.[3] These views are controversial, however, and recent research has indicated that the hypothermia traditionally induced during major surgeries is associated with worse outcomes (see Focus of Current Research).[4]

Each organ system has an optimal thermal environment for its function, and this function is ultimately impaired in states of thermal imbalance. For example, production of spermatozoa by the male testis requires a scrotal temperature that is 2 to 3 degrees cooler than intra-abdominal temperature. Spermatogenesis is impaired in cryptorchidism, or undescended testicle, because the testis is too warm in its ectopic abdominal environment (see Chapter 30).

TABLE 11–1
VARIATION IN BODY TEMPERATURE WITH AGE

Age	Temperature (Degrees)	
	Fahrenheit	Centigrade
Newborn	98.6–99.8	37–37.7
3 years	98.5–99.5	36.9–37.5
10 years	97.5–98.6	36.4–37
16 years	97.6–98.8	36.4–37.1
Adult	96.8–99.5	36–37.5
Older adult	96.5–97.5	35.8–36.4

Adapted from Morton, P.G. (1993). *Health Assessment in Nursing.* (2nd ed.) (p. 95). Philadelphia: F.A. Davis.

MECHANISMS OF HEAT PRODUCTION (THERMOGENESIS)

In the unusual circumstance in which ambient temperature is warmer than body temperature, the body gains heat from the environment. The usual state, however, requires the body to *generate* heat to maintain normal temperature; this process is called **thermogenesis**. The body produces heat as a byproduct of basal metabolism, voluntary muscle activity, involuntary muscle movements, and, in infants, metabolism of **brown fat**.

Energy Metabolism

As discussed in Chapter 3, a significant fraction of the energy produced during cellular metabolism is released in the form of heat. The metabolic rate is highest in core organs such as the liver, heart, and brain. Metabolic rates vary depending on energy demands, and each 7% increase in metabolic rate is accompanied by a 1°F increase in temperature. When heat production mechanisms are accelerated,

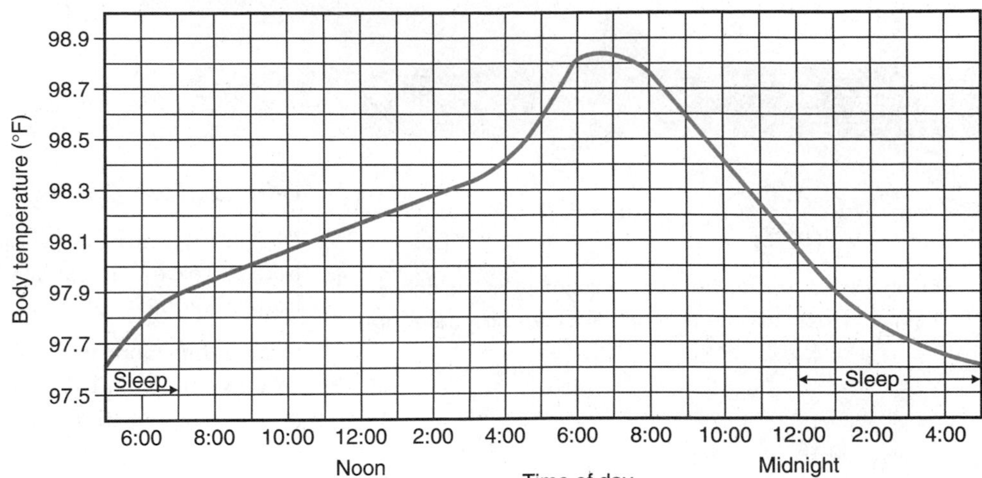

FIGURE 11–1
Circadian variation in body temperature. Body temperature displays a predictable pattern during the 24-hour cycle, with the highest readings obtained in the early evening and the lowest during sleep.

such as during the prodrome stage of **fever**, the fraction of energy released as heat increases, and adenosine triphosphate production decreases. This is the basis of such associated symptoms as weakness and fatigue.

Voluntary Muscle Activity

During muscle work and exercise, about one fourth of energy expenditure is in the form of work, and three fourths is released as heat. Although heat production with basal metabolism is normally stable, heat production due to skeletal muscle activity varies widely depending on the nature and duration of the physical activity. The potential for production of heat by this mechanism is high, although limitations are eventually imposed by the energy demands of the exercising muscle.

Involuntary Muscle Movements

Shivering and teeth chattering are the result of rapid, fine muscle movements in which nearly all of the energy expended is in the form of heat. This activity (**shivering thermogenesis**), which is initiated by the hypothalamus, may increase heat production to three to five times the normal level.

Brown Fat Metabolism

Heat production by basal metabolism and brown fat metabolism is categorized as **nonshivering thermogenesis**. Brown fat metabolism is important in infants, who lose heat easily owing to their high surface area–to–body mass ratios. Because brown fat develops late in gestation, lack of this tissue in premature infants predisposes them to hypothermia.

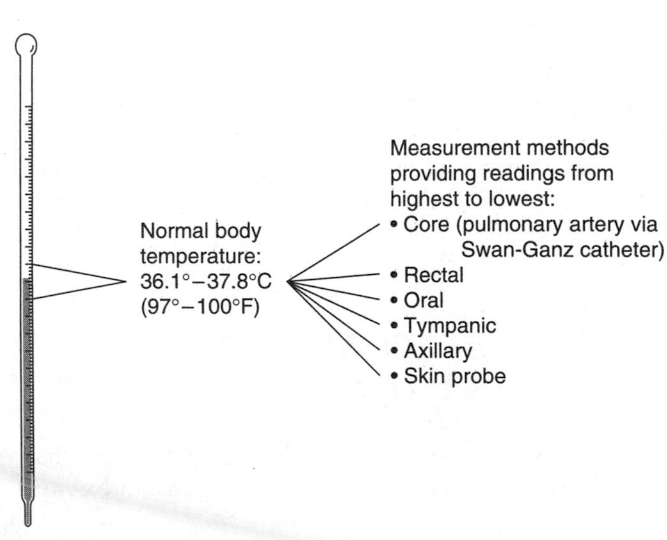

FIGURE 11–2
Temperature variation with method of measurement. Body temperature measurements vary depending on the proximity of the thermometer probe to core organs. Readings obtained from the thermistor on pulmonary artery catheters most closely approximate core temperature, whereas those obtained from more distal sites yield lower values.

Focus of Current Research

Study	Objective and Findings
Kurz, et al. (1996) Perioperative normothermia to reduce the incidence of surgical-wound infection and shorten hospitalization	*Objective:* To test the hypothesis that hypothermia both increases susceptibility to infection and lengthens hospitalization *Findings:* Infections were more frequent (19% compared with 6%) in hypothermic versus normothermic patients, and length of stay was prolonged by 2.6 days in hypothermic patients.
Miller, et al. (1996) Prolonged fevers of unknown origin in children: Patterns of presentation and outcome	*Objective:* To review the presentation, clinical characteristics, and outcome of children with fevers of unknown origin *Findings:* Fever of unknown origin usually has a benign outcome, but 29% of children were later found to have neurologic problems.
Semenza, et al. (1996) Heat-related deaths during the July 1995 heat wave in Chicago	*Objective:* To determine who was at greatest risk for heat-related death *Findings:* Those at greatest risk were people with medical illnesses who were socially isolated and did not have access to air-conditioning.
Dicker, et al. (1995) Halothane selectively inhibits nonshivering thermogenesis	*Objective:* To explain the susceptibility of infants to hypothermia during halothane anesthesia *Findings:* A much diminished or abolished thermogenic response to injected norepinephrine was demonstrated in anesthetized hamsters.

Brown fat is highly vascular and contains large numbers of mitochondria, both of which account for its color and differentiate it from other adipose tissue. Metabolism of brown fat produces significant amounts of heat during the first 4 weeks of life, after which this tissue gradually atrophies.

MECHANISMS OF HEAT LOSS

Heat may be lost from the body by four mechanisms: **radiation, conduction, convection,** and **evaporation** (Fig. 11–3).

Radiation

Heat is lost by radiation when a gradient exists for transfer of electromagnetic "heat waves" from a warm object to cooler surrounding (ambient) air. Because the human body is usually warmer than the ambient environment, heat radiates from the skin surface. Heat loss is enhanced by vasodilation of surface vessels, which shunts more blood from the warm core to the cooler peripheral tissues and causes the person to appear flushed (Fig. 11–4). Maintenance of tissue perfusion during this vasodilation requires increased cardiac output, placing demands on the heart that may be detrimental in people with underlying cardiac disease.

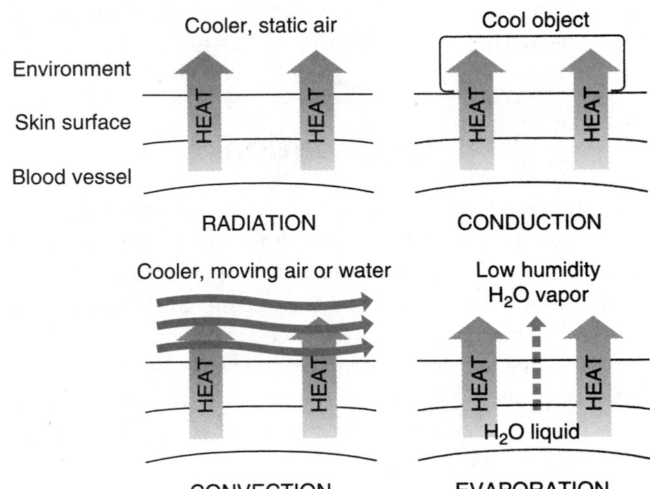

FIGURE 11–3
Mechanisms of heat loss. Heat may be lost from the body by four mechanisms. *Radiation* occurs when electromagnetic heat waves are transferred from the warm body to cooler ambient air. *Conduction* transfers heat from the warm body to a cooler object. *Convection* enhances radiant or conductive loss of heat by means of currents that carry transferred heat away from the body, maintaining the thermal gradient. *Evaporation* of water from the body surface consumes heat in the change of state (from liquid to gas). Evaporation is the only means of heat loss when ambient temperature is warmer than body temperature.

Conduction

Conduction refers to heat transfer between two objects or media that have different temperatures. The warm body may lose heat to cool water, ice application, or cold surfaces such as x-ray film cassettes or examination tables.

Convection

Heat loss due to conduction may be enhanced if convection currents are present that continuously carry transferred heat away from the warm object, thus maintaining the gradient. These currents, created by wind, fans, or moving water, accelerate heat

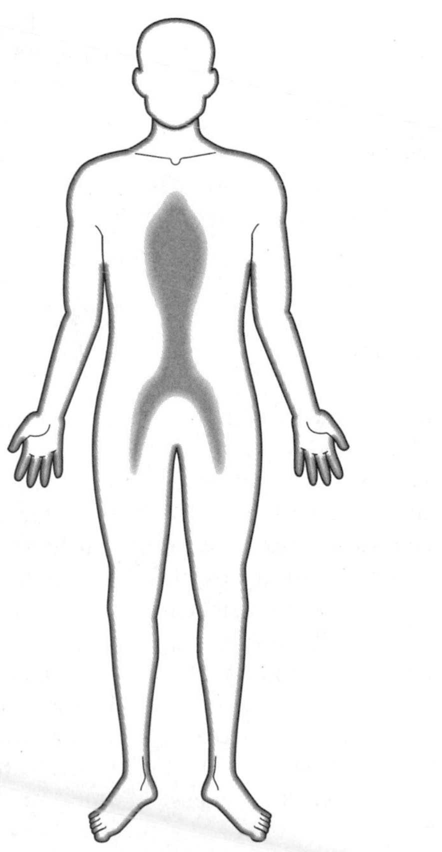

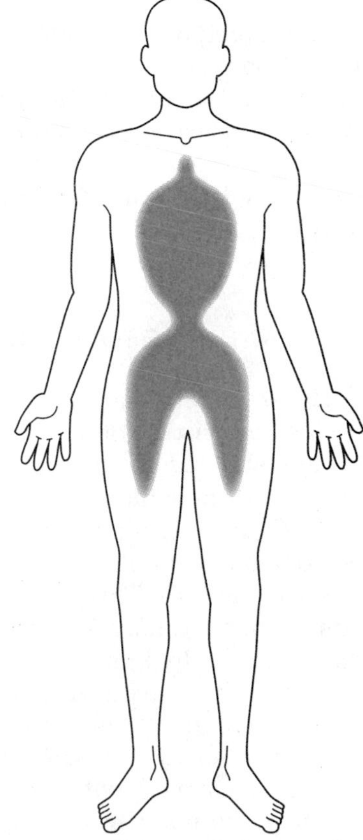

FIGURE 11–4
Vascular response to environmental temperature. In a warm environment, vasodilation of surface vessels enhances radiant heat loss. In a cold environment, surface blood vessels constrict, shunting most blood flow to the warmer core and inhibiting radiant heat loss from the surface.

loss detrimentally (as in wind chill) or therapeutically (as with fans or cooling blankets).

Evaporation

Conversion of a liquid to a gaseous state during evaporation consumes heat and cools the surface from which the evaporation occurs. Because loss of water from the body by sweating and insensible losses is the *only* means of cooling when ambient temperature exceeds body temperature, people who have impaired ability to sweat (e.g., the elderly, or those being treated with drugs affecting the autonomic nervous system) are at increased risk of hyperthermia. Sweat must *evaporate* from the body, not merely drip from the skin, to effect maximal heat loss. The degree of evaporative cooling possible is affected not only by the temperature gradient but also by the humidity gradient. Thus, dry heat is generally better tolerated than an environment that is warm *and* humid. For each 1 g of water lost due to evaporation, 0.5 calorie of heat is dissipated.

MECHANISMS OF HEAT CONSERVATION

Thermoregulation is also influenced by the ability of the body to retain the heat it produces, that is, to oppose loss of heat by radiation to a cooler environment. Heat conservation is facilitated by four mechanisms: vasoconstriction, **piloerection**, adipose tissue insulation, and positioning to decrease surface area.

Vasoconstriction

The most important mechanism of heat conservation is constriction of superficial vessels. More blood is thus shunted to the warm core of the body (see Fig. 11–4), and the skin appears pale or even cyanotic (blue), owing to enhanced deoxygenation of hemoglobin with slowed blood flow in skin vessels (see Chapter 15). This mechanism of heat conservation is often diminished in the elderly, increasing their risk of hypothermia. Vasoconstriction is also impaired by excessive consumption of alcohol, which increases the subjective sensation of warmth while producing vasodilation and flushing. Heat loss is accelerated without the person's awareness, and hypothermia risk is increased.

Piloerection

Contraction of superficial piloerector muscles causes "goose bumps" in response to environmental cold. This response is believed to decrease surface area for radiant heat loss.

Adipose Insulation

Layers of adipose tissue overlying normal muscle mass in obese people enhance heat conservation because this tissue is much less vascular than lean subcutaneous tissue. Adipose tissue differs from muscle tissue and brown fat, however, in its lack of mitochondria for oxidative metabolism. Although adipose tissue insulates against heat loss, it does not *produce* much heat. Adipose tissue commonly constitutes a greater proportion of body mass in the elderly; nevertheless, their simultaneous loss of muscle mass may place them at risk of hypothermia.

Positioning to Decrease Surface Area

In a cold environment, people instinctively assume positions that minimize exposed surface area. Ambulatory people may huddle, or bend over, wrapping their arms around their bodies. People lying down commonly flex into a fetal position, slowing the rate of radiant loss of heat.

REGULATION OF THE THERMAL ENVIRONMENT

Timely and appropriate activation of heat gain, loss, or conservation measures is mediated by both neural and hormonal mechanisms and is regulated primarily by a neuroendocrine organ—the hypothalamus. The hypothalamus, discussed in detail in Chapter 27, serves many regulatory functions and is particularly important in integration of autonomic nervous system reflexes (e.g., the stress response) and in initiation of hormone secretion.

The neural axis of the thermoregulatory system consists of (1) temperature sensors (**thermoreceptors**) in the skin, abdominal organs, spinal cord, and hypothalamus; (2) sensory nerves, which carry the impulse to the neurons of the *preoptic nucleus* ("thermostat") in the anterior hypothalamus; (3) autonomic nerves, which mediate vasoconstriction or vasodila-

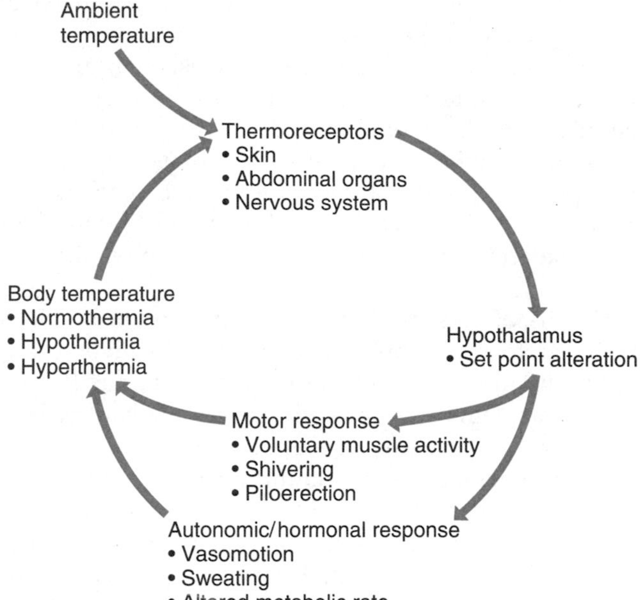

FIGURE 11–5
Thermoregulatory responses. Changes in body temperature as a result of metabolic or environmental factors are detected by thermoreceptors, which signal the preoptic nucleus of the hypothalamus. In this physiologic thermostat, incoming signals permit comparison of actual body temperature with the set point. If body temperature is lower than the set point, heat gain mechanisms are activated. If body temperature is higher, heat loss mechanisms are activated.

tion, sweating, piloerection, and short-term increases in basal metabolic rate; and (4) motor nerves, which initiate voluntary and involuntary muscle movement (Fig. 11–5). It is unknown whether there are separate thermoreceptors for hot and cold sensations or whether these receptors are activated *only* by thermal stimuli. The temperature sensed by these receptors is compared with a physiologic set point in the hypothalamic thermostat. If body temperature is lower than the set point, heat gain and conservation mechanisms are activated; if body temperature exceeds that of the set point, heat loss mechanisms are initiated.

Long-term adaptation to changes in body temperature or environmental temperature (**acclimation**) requires at least 10 to 14 days of exposure and is regulated by hormonal mechanisms through activation of the hypothalamic–pituitary axis. As discussed in Chapter 27, the hypothalamus synthesizes releasing hormones, which it secretes into the blood on appropriate neural stimulation. These releasing hormones trigger the hypothalamic–pituitary axis, a chain reaction of hormonal mechanisms that culminates in release of hormones from target endocrine organs. With respect to thermoregulation, the most important effect is on the thyroid gland, which increases its output of thyroxine (T_4). Thyroxine has two effects that increase body temperature: (1) it acts on the adrenal medulla to stimulate epinephrine output, thus mobilizing energy stores; and (2) it increases the basal metabolic rate of most body tissues (see Chapter 28).

THERMAL IMBALANCES

Hyperthermia

Hyperthermia is present when body temperature rises above 100°F (37.8°C). Disorders characterized by hyperthermia include **pyrogenic hyperthermia**, **environmental hyperthermia, neurogenic hyperthermia**, and **malignant hyperthermia**. Hyperthermia may also result from extremely high output of thyroid hormone ("thyroid storm") as discussed in Chapter 28.

Pyrogenic Hyperthermia (Fever)

Definition. Pyrogenic hyperthermia, also known as fever, is an elevation in body temperature induced by a **pyrogen**.

Epidemiology. Fever is a common occurrence with infections and is seen in people of all ages. Particular risk factors for infection are detailed in Chapter 13. Fever may also be associated with the inflammatory responses of malignancy and rheumatic diseases.

Etiology. Fever is most commonly the result of pyrogens, or fever-producing agents. Pyrogens can be exogenous or endogenous. Exogenous pyrogens include bacterial toxins and cell wall components, and endogenous pyrogens include many of the cytokines produced during an inflammatory response. As detailed in Chapter 13, inflammation is a local adaptive response to tissue injury or invasion. Macrophages and other cells activated as part of this response release pyrogenic cytokines, including interleukin-1, interleukin-6, and others. These agents circulate in the blood to the circumventricular organs, areas where absence of the blood–brain barrier permits access of pyrogens to receptors in the hypothalamus. Receptor binding then "resets" the hypothalamic thermostat to an abnormally high set point.

Details of this mechanism are unknown, but it is believed to be highly regulated and to involve another inflammatory mediator, prostaglandin E. The pyrogenic signal is modulated somewhat by the presence of **cryogens**, agents such as arginine vasopressin, melanocyte-stimulating hormone, glucocorticoids, and possibly tumor necrosis factor.[5] The hypothalamus activates heat gain mechanisms until the new set point is reached. Fever due to this mechanism rarely exceeds 105.8°F (41°C). When pyrogen is removed with resolution of inflammation, the thermostat is reset to normal, and heat loss mechanisms are activated.

Fever of unknown origin is defined as a temperature elevation of 101°F (38.3°C) or higher for 3 weeks or longer, the cause of which is not diagnosed after 1 week of intensive investigation.[6] In most cases, these fevers are due to undiagnosed infections, but they may also result from malignancy or autoimmune disorders.

Pathophysiology. Figure 11–6 illustrates the four stages of fever: (1) the *prodrome,* during which the patient usually feels cold and during which heat activation mechanisms predominate; (2) *chills,* during which heat activation mechanisms are even more pronounced and shivering is present; (3) *flushing,* when vasodilation occurs to enhance heat loss due to removal of the pyrogenic stimulus; and (4) **defervescence,** or "breaking" of the fever, when heat loss is accelerated by evaporative cooling due to sweating. Infants and children may suffer **febrile seizures** during stages 1 and 2 owing to the heightened sensitivity of their central nervous system cells to the altered thermal environment.

Clinical Manifestations. Clinical manifestations of hyperthermia are summarized in Table 11–2. Fever is evidenced by increased body temperature, which typically reaches a maximum of 105°F (39.1°C) but which may be higher in some patients. Signs and symptoms parallel the four stages, with a subjective feeling of cold early, then shivering and teeth chattering as temperature is rising. Flushing and sweating are evident later as the temperature falls to normal. Fatigue and malaise are associated with increased energy expenditure during the early heat-gain stages.

Prevention and Treatment. Intervention is ideally aimed at the underlying cause (e.g., antibiotic therapy in known bacterial infection). Reduction of fever is not warranted in cases in which the condition induces only minor discomfort because the temperature elevation is believed to be adaptive. Higher fevers with systemic manifestations may be treated with **antipyretic** drugs, such as aspirin and acetaminophen, which block prostaglandin synthesis and prevent upward resetting of the hypothalamic ther-

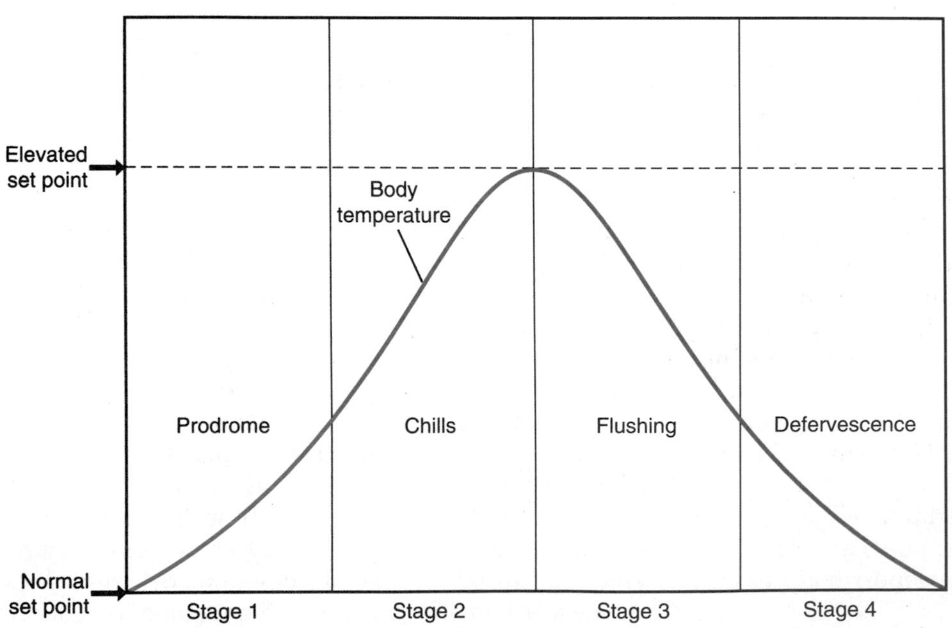

FIGURE 11–6
Stages of fever. Body temperature rises during stage 1 (prodome), in which the set point is elevated and heat gain mechanisms are activated. The patient feels cold. Temperature continues to rise during stage 2 (chills), as shivering and teeth chattering generate more heat. Stage 3 (flushing) is evidenced when the removal of the pyrogen resets the set point to normal, activating heat loss mechanisms including vasodilation. Heat loss is accelerated during stage 4 (defervescence) by evaporative cooling owing to sweating, and body temperature returns to normal.

TABLE 11–2
CLINICAL MANIFESTATIONS OF HYPERTHERMIA

SYSTEM	EFFECTS
Cardiovascular	Heart rate may increase by 8.5 beats/minute for each 1°C rise in temperature during fever, and up to 25 beats/minute in other forms of hyperthermia.
	Decreased perfusion and high metabolic rate promote metabolic acidosis.
Nervous	Febrile seizures occur in 2%–4% of young children with high temperatures.
	Hypoxia and decreased perfusion result in sleepiness and confusion in lower-grade fevers and in delirium, stupor, or coma in extreme hyperthermia.
Respiratory	Increased metabolic rate and activation of heat loss mechanisms induces hypoxia and respiratory alkalosis.
Renal	Increased metabolic rate and dehydration promote electrolyte imbalances and accumulation of metabolic wastes in the blood (azotemia). Thermal injury to muscle may cause rhabdomyolysis (release of myoglobin), which obstructs renal tubules.
Hematologic	Dehydration results in hemoconcentration. Disseminated intravascular coagulation can occur secondary to tissue injury.

mostat. Use of these agents may provide the additional benefit of reducing inflammation and pain associated with the underlying disorder, but they carry some associated risks. Aspirin, for example, has been associated with the development of Reye's syndrome when given to young children with influenza or varicella (measles) (see Chapter 26).[1] Sponging with tepid water probably provides little additional benefit when used in combination with antipyretic drugs. Other physical measures, such as air-conditioning, fans, and cooling blankets, may also be used, but care must be taken to prevent induction of shivering and vasoconstriction with these rapid-cooling measures.

Prognosis and Outcome. In most patients, fever is of short duration.

Environmental Hyperthermia

Definition. Environmental hyperthermia is an elevated temperature resulting from inability of the thermoregulatory system to offset heat gains from the environment. This category includes the specific disorders of **heat exhaustion** and **heat stroke** as well as several minor manifestations of exposure to high ambient temperatures.

Epidemiology. Environmental hyperthermia is common and can be life-threatening. During 1979 to 1988, more than 4500 deaths in the United States were attributed to heat exposure.[7] In 1980 alone, 1700 deaths occurred during a severe heat wave. Risk factors for environmental hyperthermia include age (the very young and the very old), lower socioeconomic status, habitual exertion in hot environments (work or recreational activity), and use of certain drugs that can affect thermoregulation (Table 11–3).

Etiology. In environmental hyperthermia, the set point is normal, but the body's cooling mechanisms are inadequate to offset heat gain by radiation from the warmer environment. Factors such as heart disease, dehydration, obesity, and impaired cognition or mobility may contribute to the etiology in these situations.

Heat exhaustion results from volume depletion associated with excessive sweating. **Heatstroke,** the most dangerous form of environmental hyperthermia, is present when there is heat-associated permanent damage to body tissues. Neurologic impairment must be present to establish this diagnosis. Heatstroke is further classified according to its etiology as *exertional* or *classic.* Patients suffering exertional heatstroke overload their thermoregulatory systems in that the large amount of heat generated through muscle activity is superimposed on the environmental heat gain. Classic heat stroke usually occurs in elderly people, commonly those with heart disease or on diuretic therapy, who become progressively dehydrated during prolonged heat waves. Lack of circulating blood volume, cardiac reserve, and capacity to sweat contribute to inadequate cooling.

Pathophysiology. With the initial increase in sweating, the patient may replace hypotonic losses of sweat with water only, leading to depletion of electrolytes. With heat exhaustion, hypovolemia limits cooling to the extent that body temperature rises to a range of 100.4° to 104°F (38°–40°C). Lack of neurologic impairment differentiates heat exhaustion from heatstroke, in which core temperature exceeds 104°F (40°C).

Clinical Manifestations. At first, body temperature may be normal, but manifestations arise from fluid and electrolyte imbalance. Muscle cramps (heat cramps) are common in these cases and are attributed primarily to hyponatremia. People who sit

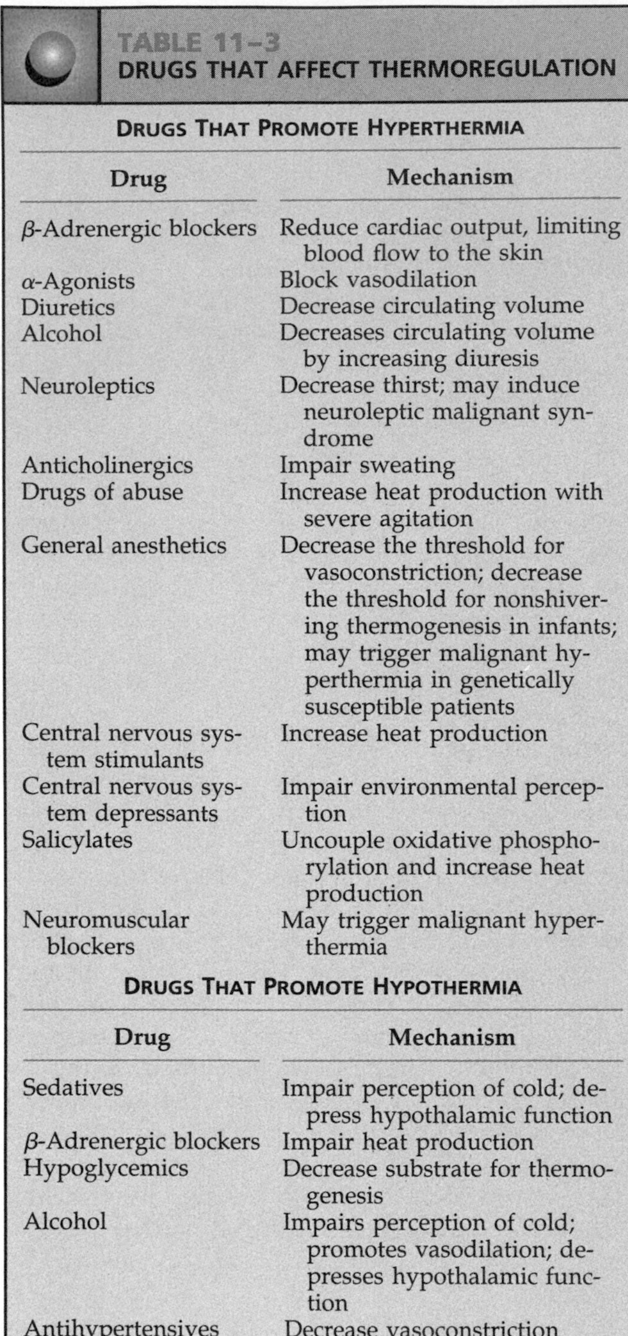

TABLE 11-3
DRUGS THAT AFFECT THERMOREGULATION

DRUGS THAT PROMOTE HYPERTHERMIA

Drug	Mechanism
β-Adrenergic blockers	Reduce cardiac output, limiting blood flow to the skin
α-Agonists	Block vasodilation
Diuretics	Decrease circulating volume
Alcohol	Decreases circulating volume by increasing diuresis
Neuroleptics	Decrease thirst; may induce neuroleptic malignant syndrome
Anticholinergics	Impair sweating
Drugs of abuse	Increase heat production with severe agitation
General anesthetics	Decrease the threshold for vasoconstriction; decrease the threshold for nonshivering thermogenesis in infants; may trigger malignant hyperthermia in genetically susceptible patients
Central nervous system stimulants	Increase heat production
Central nervous system depressants	Impair environmental perception
Salicylates	Uncouple oxidative phosphorylation and increase heat production
Neuromuscular blockers	May trigger malignant hyperthermia

DRUGS THAT PROMOTE HYPOTHERMIA

Drug	Mechanism
Sedatives	Impair perception of cold; depress hypothalamic function
β-Adrenergic blockers	Impair heat production
Hypoglycemics	Decrease substrate for thermogenesis
Alcohol	Impairs perception of cold; promotes vasodilation; depresses hypothalamic function
Antihypertensives	Decrease vasoconstriction

or stand for long periods of time in the heat may develop dependent edema (heat edema), which results from peripheral vasodilation and hydrostatic pooling of blood.[8] In some cases, vasodilation and venous pooling cause hypotension (low blood pressure) and even fainting (heat syncope). Manifestations of hypovolemia in heat exhaustion include malaise, weakness, headache, anorexia, nausea, vomiting, tachycardia, and hypotension.

In exertional heatstroke, the patient is still sweating early in the condition. In both exertional and classic types, however, the skin eventually becomes very hot and dry. Early symptoms of heatstroke are nonspecific and may include tachycardia, dyspnea, nausea, and vomiting. Soon after, muscle swelling and pain, delirium, and seizures are manifested.

Prevention and Treatment. The first priority in prevention of environmental hyperthermia is education of people at risk. When air temperature and humidity are high, they should seek cooler environments if at all possible (e.g., air-conditioned libraries, malls, and theaters). Light clothing should be worn, and physical activity should be limited. Dietary salt may be increased, and fluid intake should be increased to 2 to 3 L/day (unless contraindicated by cardiac or renal disease). Misting the skin with lukewarm water and drying it in front of a fan can facilitate cooling if air-conditioning is not available.

Heat cramps are effectively treated with replacement of sodium and fluids. When heat exhaustion or heatstroke are suspected, the patient should be removed from the warm environment immediately, and medical assistance should be sought. Cooling with water mist and fans may be instituted during transport. Treatment of heat exhaustion consists of replacement of fluids and electrolytes, usually with isotonic intravenous fluids. Treatment of heatstroke centers on cooling the patient with physical measures, such as ice packs, tepid sponge baths, fans, and cooling blankets. Fluid and electrolyte status is normalized, and manifestations of specific organ damage, such as cardiac or renal failure, are addressed.

Prognosis and Outcome. Heat exhaustion and minor heat-related ailments respond well to fluid and electrolyte replacement, with no permanent damage. Prognosis in heatstroke depends on the duration of coma. The mortality rate is high with classic heatstroke, approaching 10%.[9] Decreased heat tolerance may persist for up to 1 year in surviving patients.[10]

Neurogenic Hyperthermia

Definition. Neurogenic hyperthermia is present in primary neurologic diseases in which temperature elevation is a presenting sign. These disorders may include neurotrauma (head injury or spinal cord injury), seizure disorders, stroke, heatstroke, infections of the central nervous system, and rare genetic disorders such as **neuroleptic malignant syndrome**.

Epidemiology. Incidence of neuroleptic malignant

syndrome is rare. It usually occurs in young and middle-aged adults and has been estimated to occur in 0.2% of patients who receive neuroleptic drugs, used in the treatment of psychological disorders.[11] Epidemiology of head injury, stroke, meningitis, and seizure disorders is discussed in Chapter 21, and spinal cord injury is detailed in Chapter 22.

Etiology. Direct injury to the hypothalamus may result in altered thermoregulation, manifesting as either hypothermia or hyperthermia. Neuroleptic malignant syndrome results from an abnormal reaction to drugs that block dopamine receptors in the basal ganglia deep within the cerebral cortex, resulting in (1) spastic contraction of skeletal muscles, which generates excessive heat; and (2) autonomic dysfunction, which prevents normal heat loss mechanisms from being triggered.[9]

Pathophysiology. A vicious circle may be generated in patients suffering head injury or stroke, in which hyperthermia, with the patient's temperature approaching 108°F (43.3°C), can result in further damage to the hypothalamus. Neuroleptic malignant syndrome may also produce permanent damage to tissues, but this disorder is usually anticipated in psychiatric treatment settings and is interrupted by intervention before extensive tissue injury occurs.

Clinical Manifestations. Temperature in excess of 104°F (40°C) is usual. Central nervous system manifestations include altered consciousness (confusion or coma) and muscle rigidity, and autonomic nervous system dysfunction may manifest as wide fluctuations in blood pressure and pulse.

Prevention and Treatment. Awareness of this complication of drug therapy mandates careful monitoring of patients, and neuroleptic drugs must be discontinued immediately in patients exhibiting signs of the disorder. Like environmental hyperthermia, neurogenic hyperthermia does not respond to antipyretic drugs but must instead be treated with measures such as sponging with tepid water to accelerate evaporative cooling, or application of cooling pads or blankets, which circulate cool water to enhance conductive loss of heat. Care must be taken not to cool the body to the extent that shivering occurs because this results in heat gain and increased oxygen consumption. Dantrolene (Dantrium), a muscle relaxant more commonly used in treatment of malignant hyperthermia (see later), has also been used experimentally.[9]

Prognosis and Outcome. Tolerance of neurogenic hyperthermia varies widely; most people can withstand temperatures as high as 107°F (41.8°C) for several hours with little or no organ damage.[12] In others, the metabolic stress associated with the high temperature may precipitate heart failure or renal failure. The mortality rate is still about 20% despite optimal therapy.[9]

Malignant Hyperthermia

Definition. Malignant hyperthermia is a hypermetabolic disorder of skeletal muscle in which muscular rigidity induced by anesthesia results in significant temperature elevation.

Epidemiology. This disorder is more common in males and has been estimated to occur in 1 in 15,000 children and 1 in 50,000 to 100,000 adults undergoing anesthesia.[13]

Etiology. Malignant hypothermia is caused by an inherited enzyme defect, usually an autosomal dominant but occasionally a multifactorial disorder.[14] The most common triggering agents are halogenated inhalation anesthetics and depolarizing muscle relaxants (e.g., halothane, isoflurane, trichloroethylene, succinylcholine, enflurane, methoxyflurane, ketamine).

Pathophysiology. Massive release of intracellular calcium from the sarcoplasmic reticulum of muscle cells occurs within minutes to hours after induction of anesthesia. Calcium initiates sustained, uncontrolled muscle contraction, which rapidly produces heat. Acidosis results, and muscle breakdown with myoglobin release (rhabdomyolysis) may precipitate renal failure. Increased metabolic demands may also result in cardiac failure, especially in compromised patients.

Clinical Manifestations. Muscle rigidity is severe. The hypermetabolic state first manifests as increased carbon dioxide concentration in arterial blood ($Paco_2$) and venous blood (CO_2 content). A mixed respiratory and metabolic acidosis is present (see Chapter 10). Rapid heart rate (tachycardia) and rapid breathing (tachypnea) are seen. Blood pressure is elevated and cardiac dysrhythmias are common. Late complications include seizures and bleeding due to disseminated intravascular coagulation (see Chapter 14).[13] Temperature elevation occurs in about one third of patients; temperature may rise as high as 113°F (45°C).[9]

Prevention and Treatment. There are no reliable screening tests for malignant hyperthermia. A detailed family history before anesthesia can reveal risk for the disorder, but such history is absent in half of cases.[12] The patient may have had previous anesthesia without incident.[13] Malignant hyperthermia is treated with dantrolene, a drug that decreases the muscle rigidity by preventing further calcium release.

Prognosis and Outcome. With increasing awareness and prompt treatment of the disorder, mortality in malignant hyperthermia has decreased to 7%.[12]

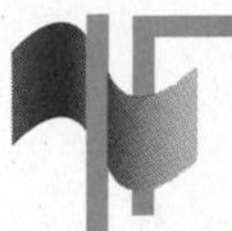

Clinical Scenario

H.H., a 10-week-old girl weighing 6.4 kg, is admitted to the pediatric ward. She had been seen in the clinic 2 days earlier and was thought to have a viral infection. Earlier today, she began gasping for breath, and her mother called 911. Her mother now reports that H.H. has had a fever of 102° to 103° F for 3 days, and "won't take her bottle." The baby's vital signs on admission are temperature of 101.3°F, pulse of 164, and respirations of 60.

1. What is the mechanism of hyperthermia in this case?
2. Should the baby's fever be treated? Why or why not?
3. What developmental characteristics of infants must be considered in such cases?

Hypothermia

Definition. Hypothermia is defined as a decline in core body temperature below 94°F (34.4°C). Unintentional hypothermia, which excludes therapeutic hypothermia, is classified as *primary accidental hypothermia* if it occurs in an otherwise healthy person subjected to exposure to environmental cold stress, or *secondary accidental hypothermia* if it occurs despite mild environmental conditions and is due to injury- or illness-induced alterations in thermoregulation.[3]

Epidemiology. The annual incidence of accidental hypothermia has been estimated at between 0.6% and 15%.[8] Accidental exposure to cold most commonly occurs with boating accidents or falls through ice-covered bodies of water, in children and confused elderly people who become lost in cold weather, in the poor or homeless who live in inadequately heated conditions, or in people whose vehicles become stranded in blizzards. Risk factors relate to these causes. Consumption of alcohol is associated with up to 80% of hypothermia cases. Presence of hypothyroidism, hypoglycemia, malnutrition, or neuromuscular disease may also predispose to hypothermia owing to impaired thermoregulation. Developmental factors may also relate, with the very young and the very old at highest risk (see Developmental Perspective).

Etiology. Prolonged exposure to environmental cold is the most frequent direct cause of hypothermia, although developmental or disease factors may contribute. The most common disease process associated with hypothermia is hypothyroidism, in which basal metabolic rate is lower than normal (see Chapter 28). Hypoglycemia, which most commonly results from excess insulin administration in diabetics, may lead to hypothermia owing to lack of metabolic fuel. Hypoxic conditions, such as acute respiratory failure, impair energy production by oxidative metabolism. Disorders that can cause hypothermia due to direct affects on the hypothalamus include stroke, head injury, and brain tumors. Drugs may impair thermoregulation by depression of hypothalamic function, reduction of metabolic rate, or inhibition of muscle contraction or vasoconstriction (see Table 11–2).

Hypothermia may be deliberately induced to reduce metabolic demands of compromised tissues. During cardiac surgery, for example, the ambient environment is kept cool, and cold solutions (cardioplegics) are used to stop cardiac contraction. Blood temperature may be cooled as a component of the cardiopulmonary bypass procedure. Hypothermia has also been used in treatment of spinal cord injury and increased intracranial pressure.

Pathophysiology. The cold environment initially lowers metabolic demands and delays the onset of hypoxic tissue damage. (Survival in near-drowning victims is greater with cold water submersion than warm for this reason.) Heat-production mechanisms are soon initiated, however, which increases metabolic demands and oxygen consumption. Proteins of tissues become denatured (altered in shape and function) by cold, resulting in peripheral tissue damage. Denaturation of serum proteins increases blood viscosity and inhibits platelet function and blood clotting. Increased viscosity and vasoconstriction result in poor perfusion of tissues. Ultimately, organ damage occurs.

Clinical Manifestations. Clinical consequences of hypothermia are summarized in Table 11–4. Initially, as body temperature falls below the set point, heat production mechanisms are evidenced as tachycardia, shivering, and cool skin. Poor perfusion becomes increasingly evident as confusion, fatigue, and slurred speech. As tissue damage progresses, heart rate and respiratory rate decrease, blood pressure drops, and diuresis occurs. Coma ensues, and electrocardiographic changes and cardiac dysrhythmias are common. When temperature falls below 87.8°F (31°C), a characteristic electrocardiographic sign, the Osborne wave (J wave) is frequently seen (Fig. 11–7).[15] The electroencephalogram may be flat, indicating no brain activity. If body temperature

TABLE 11–4
CLINICAL MANIFESTATIONS OF HYPOTHERMIA

SYSTEM	EFFECTS
Cardiovascular	Decreased perfusion results from increased blood viscosity and denaturation of serum proteins. Vasoconstriction further decreases peripheral perfusion, promoting injury of peripheral tissues with freezing (frostbite). Lactic acidosis develops. First tachycardia then bradycardia is the typical cardiac rhythm. Decreased cardiac perfusion produces electrocardiographic changes, including Osborne (J) waves following the QRS complex, and lengthening of the PR, QRS, and QT intervals. Blood pressure drops. Atrial and ventricular dysrhythmias are induced by myocardial hypoxia. Asystole occurs at temperatures below 82.4°F (28°C).
Nervous	Hypothalamic heat gain mechanisms are activated early, including vasoconstriction, shivering, and increased metabolic rate. Shivering stops with moderate hypothermia as muscles stiffen. Stupor and coma occur with reduced cerebral perfusion. Pupils become nonreactive, and reflexes disappear. Response to pain decreases. Electroencephalogram may be flat with severe hypothermia.
Respiratory	Respiratory rate is initially increased but soon decreases as oxygen consumption declines. Arterial blood gas values obtained from hypothermic patients are unreliable. A 50% decrease in CO_2 production occurs with a decrease of 8°C in temperature. Bronchorrhea and cough suppression are apparent at first, followed by pulmonary edema. Hypothermia shifts the oxyhemoglobin dissociation curve to the left, decreasing oxygen delivery to tissues.
Renal	Cold-induced diuresis occurs. Renal acid excretion is impaired. Glycosuria and electrolyte imbalances develop.
Hematologic	Hematocrit increases 2% for each 1°C decline in temperature, contributing to hypercoagulability. Cold directly inhibits the clotting cascade. Production of thromboxane B_2 by platelets declines, and thrombocytopenia results from bone marrow suppression and hepatic sequestration.

falls below 82.4°F (28°C), death is likely, owing to lethal dysrhythmia (ventricular fibrillation; see Chapter 17).

Prevention and Treatment. Prevention of accidental hypothermia involves reduction of controllable risk, including application of cold-weather precautions, such as appropriate clothing, use of winter survival kits, and implementation of appropriate behavior if stranded in a cold environment. Young children and the confused elderly must be adequately supervised.

Accidental hypothermia may be treated with any

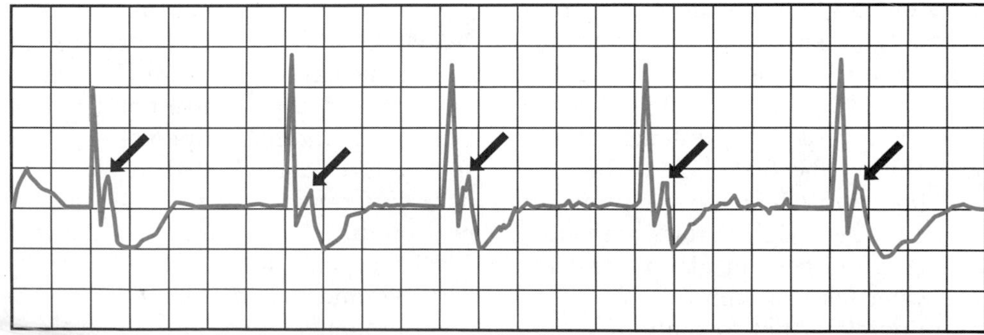

FIGURE 11–7

Osborne (J) waves of hypothermia. Cardiac conduction is altered in hypothermia, leading to dysrhythmias and the appearance of Osborne, or J, waves on the electrocardiogram. These waves are common when temperature is below 91.4°F (33°C) and are nearly always seen at temperatures below 77°F (25°C). (Modified from Carrier-Kohlman, V., Lindsey, A.M., and West, C.M. [1993]. *Pathophysiologic Phenomena in Nursing: Human Responses to Illness.* [2nd ed.]. Philadelphia: W.B. Saunders. [p. 161].)

of three rewarming techniques: (1) passive external rewarming, (2) active external rewarming, and (3) active core rewarming. Passive external rewarming consists of placing the patient in a warm environment and covering the head and body to retain heat while the body's heat production mechanisms raise body temperature. This mode is used for patients who are still shivering and whose body temperature is above 86°F (30°C).[8] Active external rewarming involves use of warm water baths, heating pads, blankets, or radiant warmers. This rewarming mode raises temperature more rapidly but may impose risk of burns when devices are applied to vasoconstricted skin. Another concern is that of potential **afterdrop,** in which peripheral vasodilation permits cold blood to return to the core organs, decreasing core temperature and inducing acidosis and potential dysrhythmias.[8] In extreme cases, internal rewarming measures may be employed. These methods include the administration of warmed intravenous fluids, lavage of the pleural or peritoneal cavities with warmed solution, dialysis with warmed dialysate, and cardiopulmonary bypass. In the course of rewarming the hypothermic patient, care must be taken not to induce hypovolemia due to increased insensible fluid loss as body temperature approaches the normal range.

Prognosis and Outcome. In patients with hypothermia due to exposure, the mortality rate is about 21% when core temperature decreases to 82.4° to 89.6°F (28° to 32°C). In trauma victims with hypothermia, the mortality rate approaches 100%.[3] The mortality rate in elderly people with severe hypothermia approaches 90%.[8] Patients (usually children)

Developmental Perspective

Embryonic and Fetal Periods

Maternal hyperthermia has been shown to be teratogenic in animal studies, but its risk in humans is as yet unproved. Brown fat is deposited around core organs late in gestation to protect against hypothermia.

Infancy and Childhood

Newborns are hypothermic for several hours after birth because of heat loss due to exposure in the delivery room and possibly because of hypoglycemia during the first few days of life. Hypoglycemia (low blood glucose level) results from removal of maternal glucose as an energy source while the infant's insulin level is still high. Brown fat is rapidly metabolized by the infant to offset the lack of glucose for energy fuel, and infants are fed glucose and water during the first days of life. Infants (particularly premature infants) are prone to hypothermia owing to their high surface area–to–body mass ratio, lack of adipose insulation, and increased insensible water loss through thin skin. Use of aspirin as an antipyretic agent is contraindicated in children because of the risk of triggering Reye's syndrome, characterized by cerebral edema and liver failure.

Adolescence and Young Adulthood

Adolescents and young adults are more likely to engage in outdoor activities during temperature extremes, predisposing them to environmental hyperthermia and hypothermia. Alcohol use in conjunction with such activities exacerbates risk because of associated dehydration and impaired judgment. Body temperature measurement may be used to track female ovulatory cycles as a means of contraception (natural family planning) or of enhancing fertility.

Middle and Older Adulthood

The elderly are at risk for hypothermia because of their decreased sensitivity to environmental temperature changes as well as their more limited ability to respond to alterations in ambient temperature. Peripheral vasoconstriction in response to cold is blunted in older people, and they have less capacity to increase basal metabolism for heat production. The elderly are less likely to have a febrile response to inflammation and, paradoxically, may become hypothermic in the presence of infection. Prolonged exposure to heat may precipitate cardiac failure in elderly people with limited reserve because vasodilation demands increased cardiac output to maintain tissue perfusion.

with temperatures as low as 60.8°F have been successfully resuscitated.

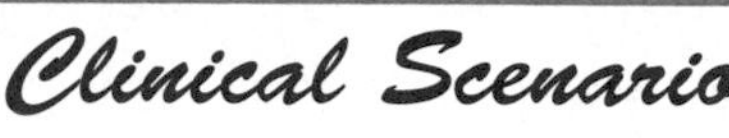

Clinical Scenario

An elderly man is brought by ambulance to the emergency department after being found in an alley behind a homeless shelter. Overnight temperatures have averaged 15° to 20°F during the past 2 days. When found, the man was unresponsive, with a weak carotid pulse and barely perceptible respirations. Ambulance personnel had been unable to obtain a blood pressure. Oxygen and intravenous normal saline were started en route to the hospital. In the emergency room, his systolic blood pressure is 40 mm Hg by palpation, and his respiratory rate is 4 breaths/minute. A special thermometer registers his rectal temperature at 86°F (30°C).

1. What systemic responses to hypothermia are revealed by the clinical findings?
2. For what complications is this patient at risk? How might these be minimized?
3. What are the priorities for treatment in this case?

CLINICAL SIGNIFICANCE OF ALTERED THERMOREGULATION

Measurement of body temperature is perhaps the most basic of clinical assessments. Alterations in body temperature may signify systemic disease or inadequacy of thermoregulatory mechanisms in the face of environmental extremes. People of all ages are subject to thermal imbalance, although infants and the elderly may be at higher risk (see Developmental Perspective).

Maintenance of thermal homeostasis is clearly dependent on cellular mechanisms of energy metabolism and fluid balance. In hypothermic or hyperthermic states, cellular function is altered, and this alteration may be either harmful or beneficial, depending on the clinical situation. Clinical trials of therapeutic hypothermia and hyperthermia are ongoing. Specific disorders manifested by alterations in thermoregulation are detailed in upcoming systems chapters.

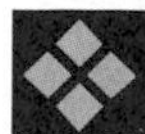

Summary of Key Points

- When the environmental temperature is cooler than body temperature, the body must generate heat by four mechanisms: energy metabolism, voluntary muscle activity, involuntary muscle movements (shivering thermogenesis), and, in neonates, brown fat metabolism (nonshivering thermogenesis).
- Heat may be lost from the body to a cooler environment by radiation, conduction, and convection. Heat can be lost from the body to a warmer environment only by evaporation.
- The body conserves heat through vasoconstriction, piloerection, adipose insulation, and positioning to decrease surface area.
- The thermoregulatory system consists of thermoreceptors in the skin and core organs; sensory nerves carrying impulses to the preoptic nucleus of the hypothalamus; autonomic nerves mediating vasomotion, sweating, piloerection, and short-term increases in basal metabolic rate; and motor nerves that initiate muscle movement, generating heat. Long-term thermoregulation (acclimation) depends on hormonal mechanisms mediated through the hypothalamic–pituitary axis.
- In pyrogenic hyperthermia (fever), the body's heat gain mechanisms are activated in response to an abnormally high set point induced by pyrogens. In other forms of hyperthermia, the set point is normal, but heat loss mechanisms are inadequate to overcome hyperthermia induced by environmental gain, hypothalamic injury or malfunction, or abnormal muscle contraction.
- During the first stage of fever (prodrome), the patient feels cold, and heat activation mechanisms are activated. Chills are evident when shivering thermogenesis begins in an effort to attain the abnormally high set point. When the set point returns to normal, heat loss mechanisms are initiated, as manifested by flushing due to vasodilation and

Continued on next page

sweating (defervescence) to effect evaporative cooling.

- Mild forms of environmental hyperthermia include (1) heat cramps due to hyponatremia induced by replacement of hypotonic fluid losses (sweat) with free water, (2) heat edema due to vasodilation and venous pooling, and (3) heat syncope, resulting from decreased cerebral perfusion, which is also due to vasodilation and venous pooling. Major forms of environmental hyperthermia are heat exhaustion, in which hypovolemia induces shock-like symptoms, and heatstroke, in which neurologic impairment is evident and permanent thermal injury to tissues occurs.

- Cooling measures that may be instituted in hyperthermia include antipyretic drugs for fever, lukewarm water misting and fans, cooling blankets, and sponging with tepid water.

- In hypothermia, activation of heat production mechanisms increases metabolic demands and oxygen consumption. Proteins of tissues become denatured by cold, resulting in peripheral tissue damage. Protein denaturation increases blood viscosity and inhibits blood clotting and tissue perfusion.

REFERENCES

1. Klein, N.C., and Cunha, B.A. (1996). Treatment of fever. *Infectious Disease Clinics of North America* 10(1), 211–216.
2. Marion, D.W., Leonov, Y., Ginsberg, M., *et al.* (1996). Resuscitative hypothermia. *Critical Care Medicine* 24(2 suppl.), S81–S89.
3. Gentillelo, L.M. (1995). Advances in the management of hypothermia. *Surgical Clinics of North America* 75(2), 243–256.
4. Kurz, A., Sessler, D.I., and Lenhardt, R. (1996). Perioperative normothermia to reduce the incidence of surgical-wound infection and shorten hospitalization. *New England Journal of Medicine* 334(19), 1209–1215.
5. Kluger, M.J., Kozak, W., Conn, C.A., *et al.* (1996). The adaptive value of fever. *Infectious Disease Clinics of North America* 10(1), 1–20.
6. Cunha, B.A. (1996). Fever of unknown origin. *Infectious Disease Clinics of North America* 10(1), 111–127.
7. Centers for Disease Control and Prevention. (1993). Heat-related deaths: United States, 1993. *Journal of the American Medical Association* 270(7), 810. (Excerpted from *Morbidity and Mortality Weekly Report* 42, 558–560.)
8. Brody, G.M. (1994). Hyperthermia and hypothermia in the elderly. *Clinics in Geriatric Medicine* 10(1), 213–229.
9. Simon, H.B. (1993). Hyperthermia. *New England Journal of Medicine* 329(7), 483–487.
10. Tom, P.A., Garmel, G.M., and Auerbach, P.S. (1994). Environment-dependent sports emergencies. *Medical Clinics of North America* 78(2), 305–325.
11. Caroff, S.N., and Mann, S.C. (1993). Neuroleptic malignant syndrome. *Medical Clinics of North America* 77(1), 185–202.
12. Powers, J.H., and Scheld, W.M. (1996). Fever in neurologic diseases. *Infectious Disease Clinics of North America* 10(1), 45–66.
13. Heiman-Patterson, T.D. (1993). Neuroleptic malignant syndrome and malignant hyperthermia. *Medical Clinics of North America* 77(2), 477–492.
14. Donnelly, A.J. (1994). Malignant hyperthermia. *AORN Journal* 59(2), 393–405.
15. Lee-Chiong, T.L., and Stitt, J.T. (1996). Accidental hypothermia: When thermoregulation is overwhelmed. *Postgraduate Medicine* 99(1), 77–88.

SELECTED BIBLIOGRAPHY

Benarroch, E.E. (1993). The central autonomic network: Functional organization, dysfunction, and perspective. *Mayo Clinic Proceedings* 68(10), 988–1001.

Berg, A.T. (1993). Are febrile seizures provoked by a rapid rise in temperature? *American Journal of Diseases in Children* 147(10), 1101–1103.

Bross, M.H., Nash, B.T., and Carlton, F.B. (1994). Heat emergencies. *American Family Physician* 50(2), 389–396.

Cabanac, M. (1993). Selective brain cooling in humans: "Fancy" or fact? *FASEB Journal* 7(12), 1143–1147.

Cunha, B.A. (1996). The clinical significance of fever patterns. *Infectious Disease Clinics of North America* 10(1), 33–44.

Danzl, D.F., and Pozos, R.S. (1994). Accidental hypothermia. *New England Journal of Medicine* 331(26), 1756–1760.

Delaney, K.A. (1992). Heatstroke: Underlying processes and lifesaving management. *Postgraduate Medicine* 91(4), 379–388.

Dicker, A., Ohlson, K.B.E., Johnson, L., *et al.* (1995). Halothane selectively inhibits nonshivering thermogenesis. *Anesthesiology* 82(2), 495–501.

Drake, D.K., and Nettina, S.M. (1994). Recognition and management of heat-related illness. *Nurse Practitioner* 19(8), 43–47.

Guyton, A.C., and Hall, J.E. (1996). *Textbook of Medical Physiology.* (9th ed.). Philadelphia: W.B. Saunders Co. (pp. 911–922).

Harchelroad, F. (1993). Acute thermoregulatory disorders. *Clinics in Geriatric Medicine* 9(3), 621–639.

Kaus, S.J., and Rockoff, M.A. (1994). Malignant hyperthermia. *Pediatric Clinics of North America* 41(1), 221–237.

Lee-Chiong, T.L., and Stitt, J.T. (1995). Heatstroke and other heat-related illnesses: The maladies of summer. *Postgraduate Medicine* 98(1), 26–36.

Miller, L.C., Sission, B.A., Tucker, L.B., *et al.* (1996). Prolonged fevers of unknown origin in children: Patterns of presentation and outcome. *Journal of Pediatrics* 129(3), 419–423.

Norman, D.C., and Yoshikawa, T.T. (1996). Fever in the elderly. *Infectious Disease Clinics of North America* 10(1), 93–99.

Perlstein, P.H. (1995). Thermoregulation. *Pediatric Annals* 25(10), 531–537.

Phillips, R. (1993). Hypothermia. In: Carrieri-Kohlman, V., Lindsey, A.M., and West, C.M. *Pathophysiological Phenomena in Nursing: Human Responses to Illness.* (2nd ed.). Philadelphia: W.B. Saunders Co. (pp. 153–173).

Rescorl, D. (1995). Environmental emergencies. *Critical Care Nursing Clinics of North America* 7(3), 445–456.

Semenza, J.C., Rubin, C.H., Falter, K.H., *et al.* (1996). Heat-related deaths during the July 1995 heat wave in Chicago. *New England Journal of Medicine* 335(2), 84–90.

Sessler, D.I. (1993). Perianesthetic thermoregulation and heat balance in humans. *FASEB Journal* 7(8), 638–644.

Weinberg, A.D. (1993). Hypothermia. *Annals of Emergency Medicine* 22(2 Pt. 2), 370–377.

Wilson, D. (1995). Assessing and managing the febrile child. *Nurse Practitioner* 20(11), 59–74.

PART TWO

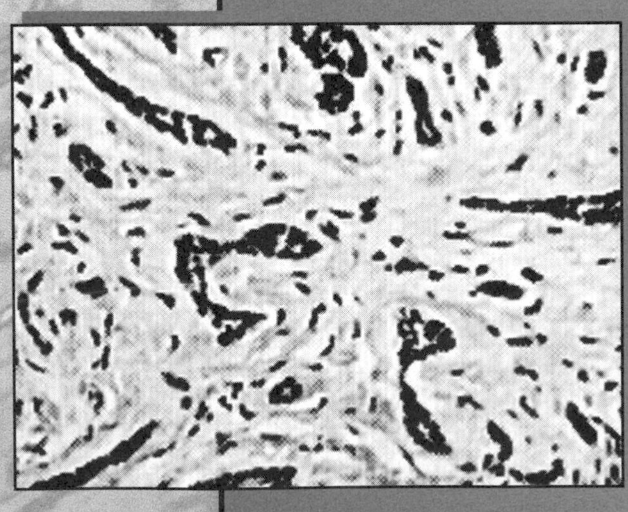

PATHOPHYSIOLOGY OF ORGAN SYSTEMS

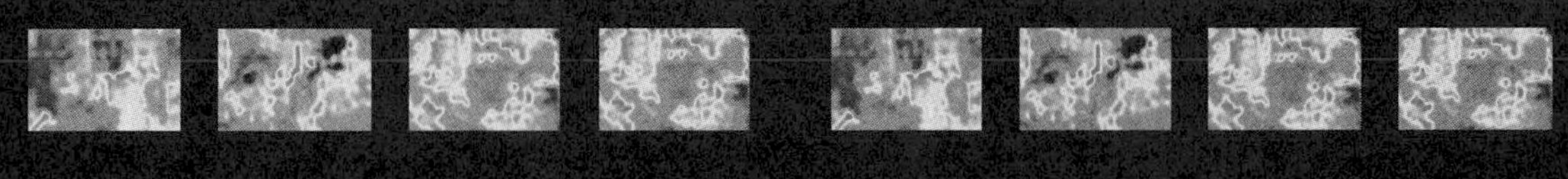

UNIT IV
Hematologic System

Unit IV

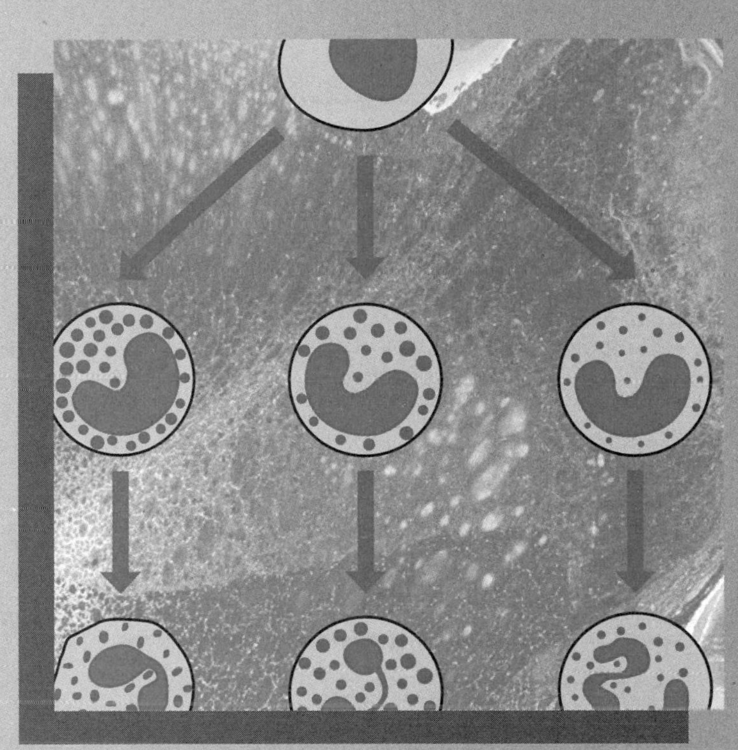

HEMATOLOGIC SYSTEM

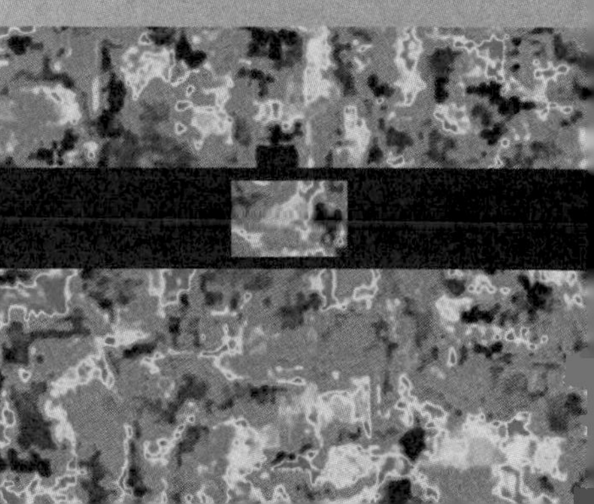

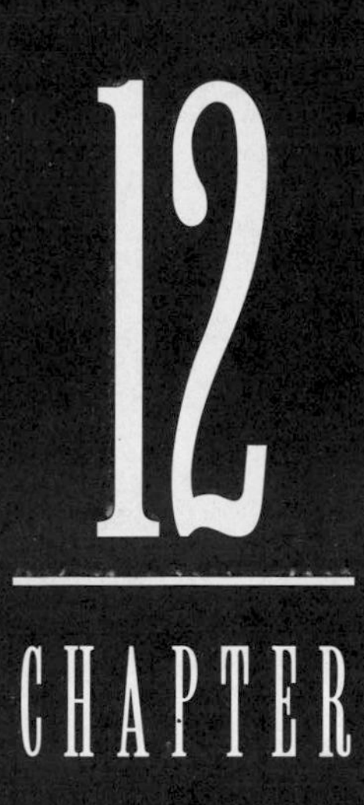

Hematopoiesis and Related Disorders

LEARNING OBJECTIVES

1. Identify the general functions of each of the fluid and cellular components of the blood.
2. Describe the processes by which erythrocytes, leukocytes, and thrombocytes develop from the pluripotent stem cell in the bone marrow.
3. Compare and contrast the mechanisms that may result in excess or deficiency of hematopoietic cells of different lineages.
4. Discuss the clinical consequences of excess or deficit of each type of hematopoietic cell.
5. Explain the rationale for the principal modes of clinical intervention in hematopoietic disorders.
6. Appreciate the clinical significance of disorders of hematopoiesis.

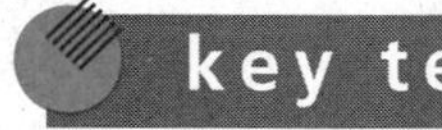

key terms

acute lymphoblastic leukemia
acute myeloid leukemia
anemia
basophil
bone marrow transplantation
chronic lymphocytic leukemia
chronic myeloid leukemia
eosinophil
erythrocyte
erythropoiesis
erythropoietin
essential thrombocythemia
exchange transfusion
granulocyte
hairy-cell leukemia
hematocrit
hematology
hematopoiesis
heme
hemochromatosis
hemoglobin
hemoglobinopathy
hemolysis
hereditary spherocytosis
iron-deficiency anemia
leukemia
leukocyte
leukocytosis
leukopenia
leukopoiesis

lymphocyte
megakaryopoiesis
monocyte-macrophage
neutrophil
pernicious anemia
platelet
polycythemia vera
porphyria
reactive thrombocytosis
red blood cell indices
reticulocyte
sickle cell disease
thrombocyte
thrombocytopenia

The discipline of **hematology** is concerned with the composition and function of the blood, a specialized connective tissue with both fluid and formed (cellular) elements. The blood is the essential transport medium within the body, facilitating communication between cells and serving to nourish them while carrying away their waste products. **Hematopoiesis** (or *hemopoiesis*) refers to the differentiation and proliferation of blood cells from a single type of stem cell in the bone marrow. Mature blood cells have short life spans, and must be constantly replenished by the hematopoietic system. The hematopoietic processes regulating the synthesis and degradation of each cell type must be precisely controlled to maintain optimal quantities of functional blood cells. Rapid cell turnover mandates significant rates of DNA replication and cell division, increasing the risk of genetic mutation and neoplastic transformation.

This chapter provides an overview of the composition and general functions of the blood, and details the processes of red blood cell (RBC) formation (**erythropoiesis**), white blood cell (WBC) formation (**leukopoiesis**), and **platelet** formation (**megakaryopoiesis**). Selected disorders related to each of these processes are discussed, including the **anemias**, **polycythemia vera**, the **porphyrias**, **hemochromatosis**, the **leukemias**, **thrombocytopenia**, and **essential thrombocythemia**. Additional hematologic disorders associated with inflammation and immune function are detailed in Chapter 13; Chapter 14 addresses disorders manifesting primarily as altered hemostasis (blood clotting).

COMPONENTS OF THE BLOOD

Plasma (Serum)

More than half of the blood, by volume, is composed of fluid, or *plasma*. In clinical settings, the term *serum* is used to describe characteristics of blood constituents, such as serum sodium and serum osmolality. Serum is plasma from which protein clotting factors have been removed.

Ninety per cent of the plasma is composed of water, underlying the fundamental purpose of the blood as a transport medium. Dissolved and suspended particles comprise the remaining 10% of the plasma. These include proteins, inorganic particles, and organic substances (Table 12–1). The plasma

TABLE 12–1
COMPOSITION OF BLOOD

Component	Functions
Plasma	
Water	Transport medium Solvent Suspending medium Thermoregulation
Plasma proteins	
Albumin	Osmotic pressure Binding and transport of drugs, hormones, ions
Globulins	Immune response
Fibrinogen	Hemostasis Inflammation Wound healing
Nitrogenous metabolites (urea, uric acid, creatinine)	Metabolic wastes Osmotic pressure Establishment of renal medullary gradient (urea)
Nutrients	Substrate for energy metabolism
Enzymes, hormones, neurotransmitters	Regulation
Blood gases	Respiration Acid-base balance
Electrolytes and other minerals	Neurotransmission Muscle contraction Metabolism
Formed Elements	
Erythrocytes (RBCs)	Blood gas transport Acid-base balance
Leukocytes (WBCs)	
Neutrophils	Phagocytosis
Eosinophils	Immune response to parasites and allergens
Basophils	Vasoactive effect in inflammation
Monocytes	Phagocytosis (as macrophage) Immune response (as macrophage)
Lymphocytes	Immune response
Platelets (thrombocytes)	Hemostasis

proteins include albumin (53%), which exerts colloid osmotic pressure to maintain normal compartmental distribution of body fluids (see Chapter 8). Albumin also serves as a binding and transport medium for many hormones and drugs. The globulin fraction (43%) of plasma proteins includes antibodies (a component of the immune response), complement and kinin system proteins important in inflammation, and clotting factors. The fibrinogen fraction constitutes the final 4% of plasma protein and is important in inflammation, wound healing, and hemostasis.

Blood Cells

Three types of cells are suspended in plasma: RBCs (**erythrocytes**), WBCs (**leukocytes**), and platelets (**thrombocytes**) (Color Fig. 12–1). RBCs are critical to the transport of oxygen to tissues (see Chapter 19), and as such supply essential energy substrate for all active processes. Platelets are an essential component of the hemostatic system, and WBCs are of primary importance in the inflammatory and immune responses.

HEMATOPOIESIS

Organs and Tissues of the Hematopoietic System

Although the embryonic yolk sac and the fetal liver and spleen are involved in early blood cell formation, the principal site of hematopoiesis in children and adults is the bone marrow (see Developmental Perspective). Blood cells may continue to differentiate and mature in other tissues, such as the spleen, liver, and other lymphatic tissues.

Blood cells form in the red (hematopoietic) marrow of flat bones, such as the sternum (breastbone) and ilia (hip bones), and, to a lesser extent, in the proximal ends (epiphyses) of the long bones. In infancy, the central marrow cavities of long bones, such as the humerus of the arm and the femur of the leg, also contain red marrow, but this is gradually replaced by yellow (fatty) marrow. Yellow marrow ordinarily has limited hematopoietic activity. Although the distribution of hematopoietic marrow differs, the total amount is the same in adults and children.[1] In addition to its hematopoietic function, bone marrow is also the site of origin of osteoblasts and osteoclasts, the cells that mediate bone formation and remodeling (see Chapter 34).

Red bone marrow resembles thick blood owing to the concentration of cellular elements within it. It is liquid enough to be removed by needle aspiration and can be reinfused by intravenous administration. As discussed later in this chapter, **bone marrow transplantation** is employed in the treatment of a number of hematopoietic and neoplastic disorders.

Hematopoietic Cascade

Figure 12–1 illustrates development of the three principal cell types and their subtypes. Activation of a single precursor cell, the pluripotent stem cell, may give rise to any of the blood cell types in a stepwise activation sequence, or cascade. Stem cells, which make up only 0.1% of all marrow cells, are unique in their ability to self-replicate by asymmetric mitosis.[2] When activated by molecular signals, the stem cell divides into two daughter cells, one of which enters into a differentiation sequence that gives rise to a particular blood cell type, and the other of which remains in reserve as part of the stem cell pool. The total number of stem cells thus remains constant while functional cells of all lineages are regenerated.

In response to regulatory signals, the differentiating stem cell is committed to form either a lymphoid or a myeloid progenitor or stem cell. Committed lymphoid progenitor cells undergo further differentiation into B **lymphocytes**, T lymphocytes, or natural killer (NK) cells. Committed myeloid progenitor cells give rise to other lineage-specific progenitor cells, from which all remaining cell lines differentiate, resulting in the formation of thrombocytes, **granulocytes** (nonlymphocytic WBCs), and erythrocytes. Mature hematopoietic cells are terminally differentiated; that is, they are unable to divide and proliferate further.

Small numbers of pluripotent stem cells and lineage-specific progenitor cells leave the bone marrow and circulate in peripheral blood. As an alternative or adjunct to bone marrow transplantation, these peripheral blood progenitor cells may be isolated from blood, induced to proliferate, and infused to stimulate hematopoiesis in patients with bone marrow failure due to disease or therapy.[3]

Regulation of Hematopoiesis

Hematopoiesis is controlled by the combined effects of (1) local signaling molecules (hematopoietic growth factors), which promote cellular growth and proliferation; and (2) transcription factors, which activate the specific genes that direct differentiation of

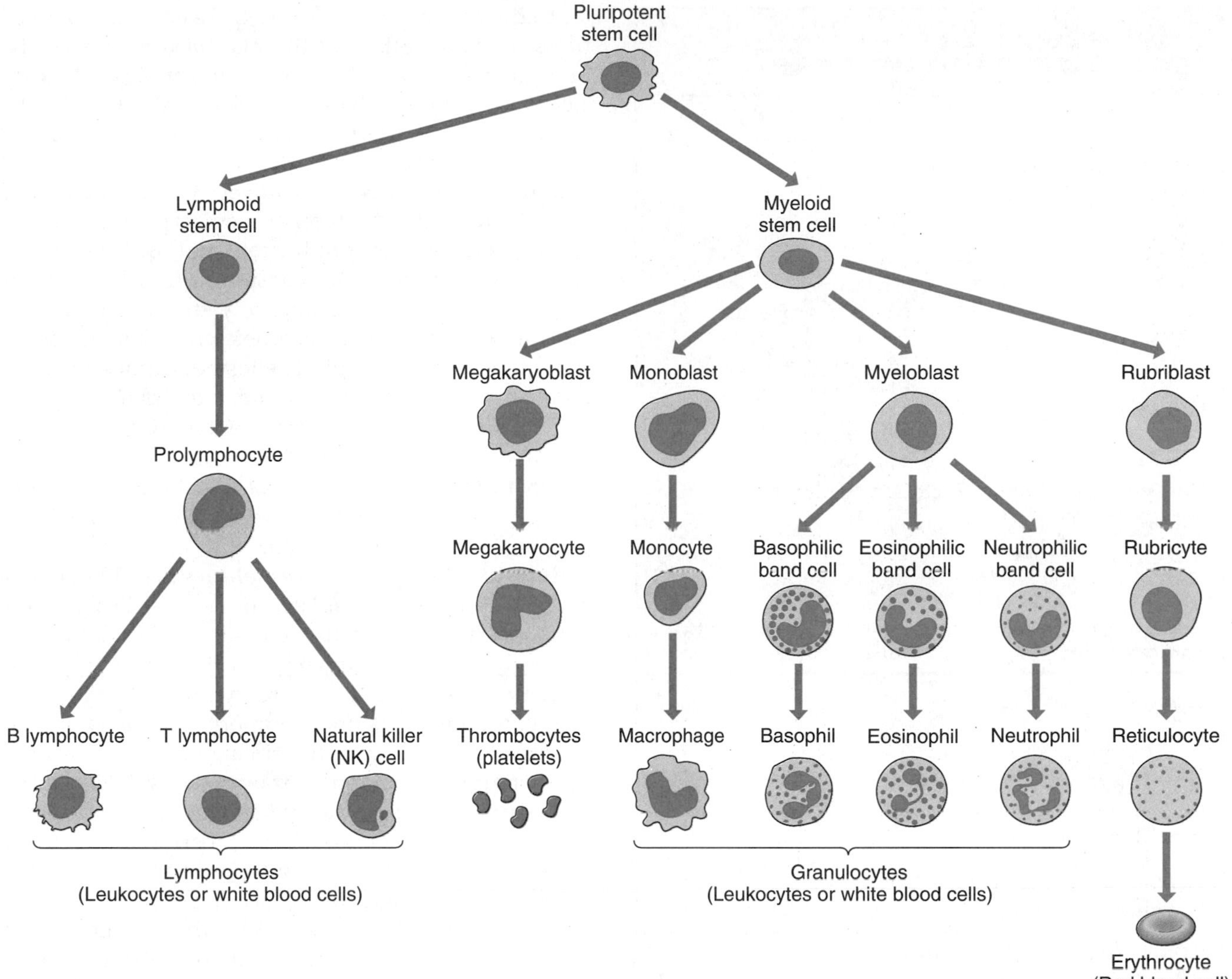

FIGURE 12–1
Hematopoietic cascade. Activation of the pluripotent stem cell may give rise to any of the blood cell types in a stepwise activation sequence mediated by hematopoietic growth factors and transcription factors.

pluripotent stem cells and committed progenitor cells (see Chapter 6). Table 12–2 lists examples of hematopoietic growth factors and transcription factors known to be important in the regulation of hematopoiesis.

The production of RBCs is increased in the presence of **erythropoietin** (EPO), a hematopoietic growth factor that acts as a hormone. Ninety per cent of the circulating EPO originates from the kidney, whereas 10% is from extrarenal sources. Fetal EPO production occurs in the liver. The cellular source of renal EPO is believed to be a type of peritubular interstitial cell located in the inner cortex and outer medulla, whereas hepatic EPO is apparently synthesized in both hepatocytes and Kupffer cells.[4] Erythropoietin is secreted in response to tissue hypoxia, resulting in an increase in the rate of bone marrow release and maturation of erythrocytes for oxygen transport (see Chapter 19).

Both pluripotent stem cells and lineage-specific progenitors contain receptors for specific hematopoietic growth factors. Abnormalities in these receptors may be linked to a number of congenital hematopoietic diseases (Table 12–3).[5]

Development of Specific Cell Types

Erythropoiesis

Stages in Red Blood Cell Development. Erythrocytes develop from committed erythroid progenitors (rubriblasts) through a series of stages in which they

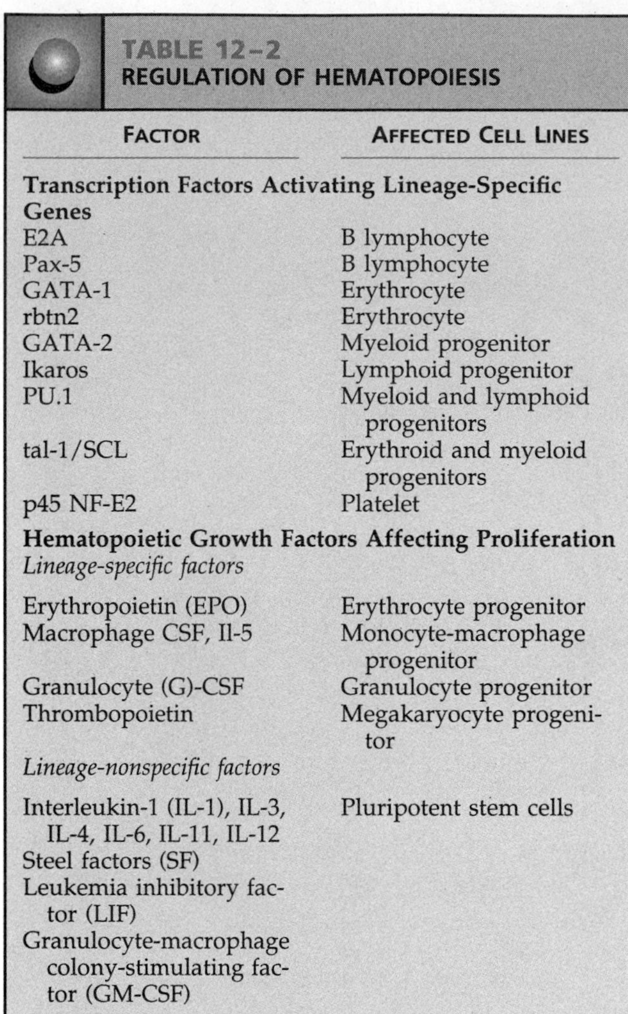

TABLE 12–2
REGULATION OF HEMATOPOIESIS

Factor	Affected Cell Lines
Transcription Factors Activating Lineage-Specific Genes	
E2A	B lymphocyte
Pax-5	B lymphocyte
GATA-1	Erythrocyte
rbtn2	Erythrocyte
GATA-2	Myeloid progenitor
Ikaros	Lymphoid progenitor
PU.1	Myeloid and lymphoid progenitors
tal-1/SCL	Erythroid and myeloid progenitors
p45 NF-E2	Platelet
Hematopoietic Growth Factors Affecting Proliferation	
Lineage-specific factors	
Erythropoietin (EPO)	Erythrocyte progenitor
Macrophage CSF, Il-5	Monocyte-macrophage progenitor
Granulocyte (G)-CSF	Granulocyte progenitor
Thrombopoietin	Megakaryocyte progenitor
Lineage-nonspecific factors	
Interleukin-1 (IL-1), IL-3, IL-4, IL-6, IL-11, IL-12	Pluripotent stem cells
Steel factors (SF)	
Leukemia inhibitory factor (LIF)	
Granulocyte-macrophage colony-stimulating factor (GM-CSF)	

Data from Orkin, S.H. (1995). Transcription factors and hematopoietic development. *Journal of Biological Chemistry* 270(10), 4955–4958; and Ogawa, M. (1994). Hematopoiesis. *Journal of Allergy and Clinical Immunology* 94(3 Pt. 2), 645–650.

accumulate **hemoglobin**, lose their RNA and their mitochondria, and extrude their nuclei. This differentiation process normally takes about 3 to 5 days, beginning in the bone marrow and concluding in the plasma. **Reticulocytes** are newly released RBCs that still contain some RNA. Increased numbers of these immature RBCs in the plasma (reticulocytosis) indicate a state of accelerated erythropoiesis. Mature RBCs are compact, biconcave disks (see Fig. 12–1). Hemoglobin normally constitutes about 33% of the weight of mature RBCs.

Rate of Erythrocyte Turnover. Under regulation by erythropoietin and other hematopoietic growth factors, the rate of production and maturation of erythrocytes is normally constant, offsetting normal RBC destruction. RBCs normally degenerate within 120 days because their anaerobic energy metabolism cannot produce enough adenosine triphosphate to maintain cellular processes and membrane integrity beyond this time. Aged (senescent) RBCs, as well as any abnormal or damaged cells, are destroyed by either intravascular or extravascular **hemolysis**. Normally, most aged erythrocytes are destroyed by phagocytic cells of the spleen.

Role of the Spleen. The spleen (Fig. 12–2) is a highly vascular, encapsulated organ that lies just under the diaphragm in the left side of the abdominal cavity, between the stomach and the left kidney. The spleen serves as a site of RBC synthesis during fetal life. After birth, its most important role is in the clearance of RBCs from the circulation.

Arterial blood enters through the splenic artery and empties through the splenic vein into the portal venous circulation, which then perfuses the liver. Blood vessels entering the spleen are surrounded for much of their length by a sheath of lymphoid cells known as the *white pulp*. These arteries then enter the *red pulp*, a region of vascular tubes (sinuses) and net-like connective tissue (cords) containing phagocytic tissue macrophages. Some blood enters sinuses directly, whereas other blood first flows through the cords, where aged or defective RBCs are selectively lysed and phagocytized.

Although the spleen is important in immune function as well as in RBC clearance, it is not considered to be an essential organ. Because of its vascularity

TABLE 12–3
DISORDERS ASSOCIATED WITH DEFECTS IN CYTOKINE RECEPTORS ON HEMATOPOIETIC CELLS

Receptor Type	Affected Cell	Disease of Overproduction	Disease of Underproduction
Erythropoietin	Erythrocyte progenitor	Familial erythrocytosis	—
Granulocyte colony-stimulating factor	Granulocyte	—	Kostmann's syndrome
Growth hormone	Lymphocyte	—	Laron dwarfism
Interleukin-2	T lymphocyte	—	X-linked severe combined immunodeficiency

Adapted from D'Andrea, A.D. (1994). Cytokine receptors in congenital hematopoietic disease. *New England Journal of Medicine* 330(12), 841.

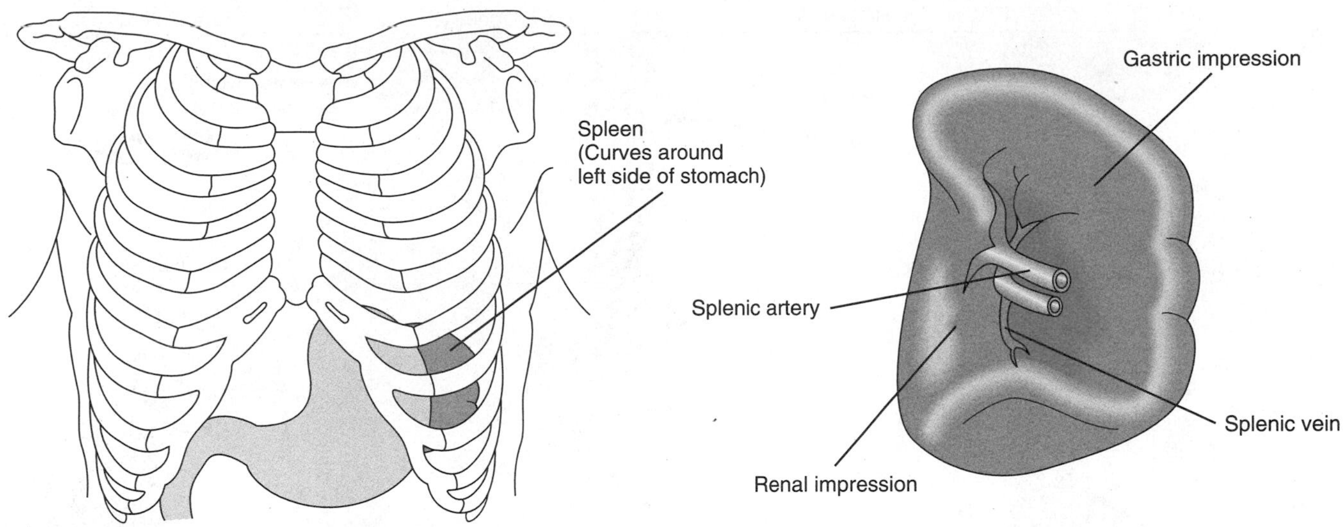

FIGURE 12-2
Spleen. The spleen, a highly vascular organ lying in the left upper quadrant of the abdomen, serves as a site of hematopoiesis during fetal life. After birth, its most important role is in the clearance of senescent or defective red blood cells from the circulation.

and proximity to the ribs, the spleen is vulnerable to hemorrhage with trauma. It may also be a site of infiltration of neoplastic cells. Splenic enlargement (splenomegaly) may occur with such infiltration, with lymphocyte proliferation within the spleen, or with engorgement by increased numbers of RBCs or platelets. When the spleen must be surgically removed (splenectomy), its functions are served by the liver and other tissue macrophage systems.

Red Blood Cell Synthesis. Adequate amounts of protein, iron, folic acid, and vitamin B_{12} are essential to DNA synthesis and cell division in the process of erythropoiesis. Activation of more than two dozen genes on chromosomes 11 and 16 directs the synthesis of hemoglobin within developing erythrocytes. The most prevalent adult hemoglobin (hemoglobin A) consists of four protein (globin) chains, two α and two β, complexed to four molecules of **heme** (Fig. 12-3). Heme consists of a protoporphyrin ring into which an iron atom has inserted. Protoporphyrin is a basic substance that may accumulate to toxic levels when heme biosynthesis is abnormal, resulting in one of a group of disorders known as the porphyrias (discussed later). Heme is contained not only in hemoglobin but also in the myoglobin of skeletal muscle, in the cytochrome oxidase enzyme complexes of the mitochondrial electron transport chain, and in the cytochrome P-450 oxidase system of liver cells. Heme thus functions not only in oxygen transport but also in energy metabolism and hepatic biotransformation of drugs and hormones.

Iron Homeostasis. Iron availability for hemoglobin synthesis is normally stable despite fluctuations in dietary intake, rate of erythropoiesis, and iron losses in urine, feces, sweat, and menstrual flow (Fig. 12-4). The reason for this is tight control of the rate of iron absorption by intestinal epithelial cells. When body iron stores are low, the rate of iron absorption is increased, probably by active transport. Absorbed iron binds loosely to the serum protein *transferrin;* it then circulates to the bone mar row for use in erythropoiesis and to cells of the liver, spleen, and skeletal muscle for storage. When total body iron is sufficient and the rate of erythropoiesis is normal, dietary iron is absorbed passively into intestinal epithelial cells, where it binds to the protein *ferritin.* This iron is gradually lost in

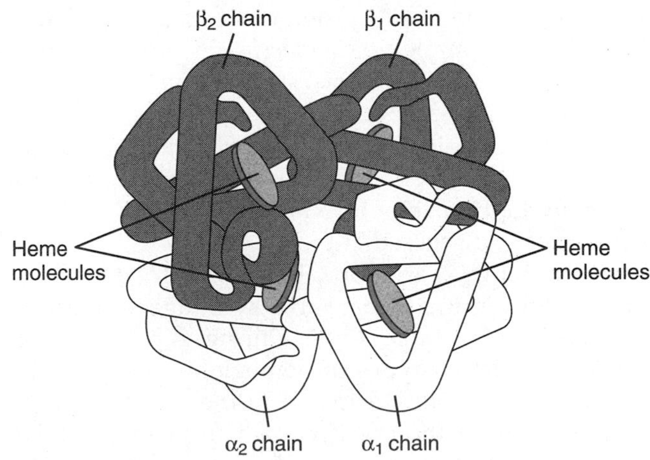

FIGURE 12-3
Hemoglobin A. Adult hemoglobin consists of four protein chains, two of the α family and two of the β structural family of globins. One molecule of heme is complexed to each protein chain. Heme consists of a protoporphyrin ring into which an iron atom has inserted.

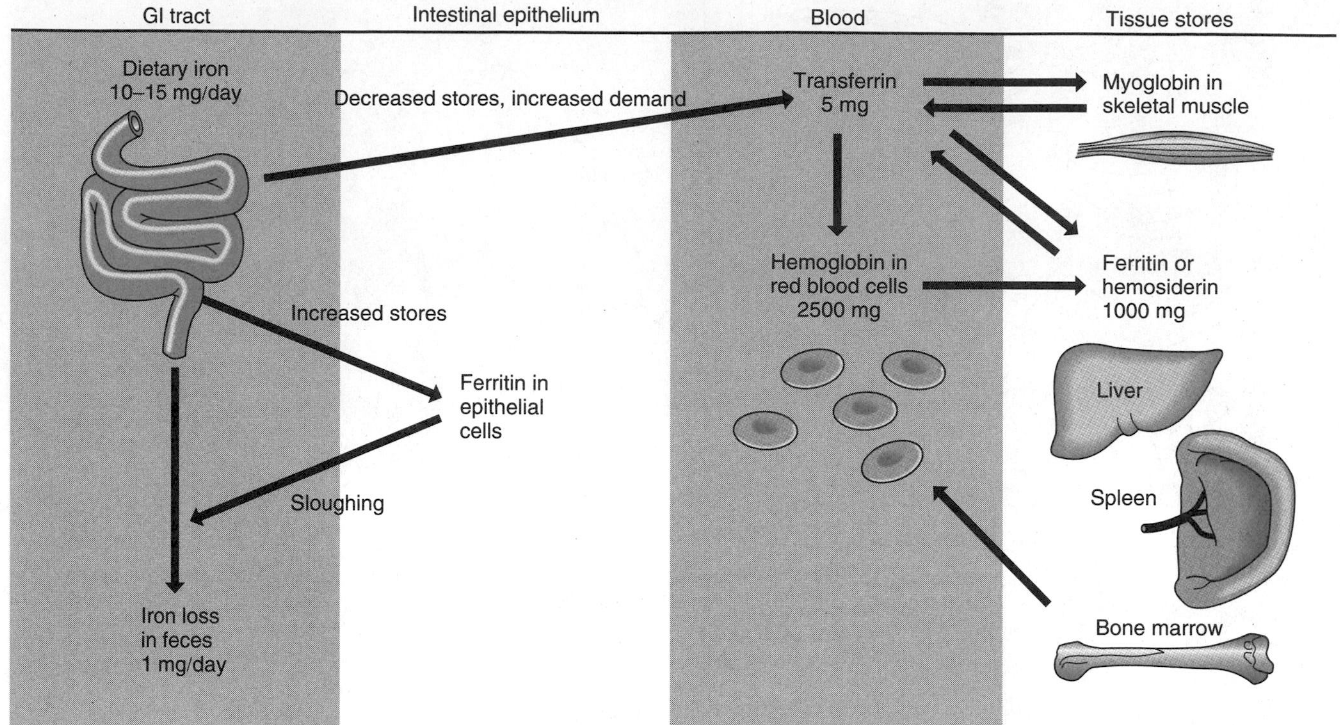

FIGURE 12–4

Iron homeostasis. Regulation of the rate of iron absorption by intestinal epithelial cells normally offsets iron losses to maintain stable tissue iron stores. When iron stores are low or demand is increased, the rate of active iron absorption is increased. Absorbed iron binds to the plasma protein transferrin and circulates to the bone marrow for use in hemoglobin synthesis. Iron not needed for erythropoiesis is complexed to ferritin or hemosiderin for tissue storage or is used for myoglobin synthesis in skeletal muscle. When iron availability is sufficient, dietary iron is absorbed passively by intestinal epithelial cells and is lost in the feces with normal sloughing of these cells.

the feces with normal turnover of these epithelial cells.

Because free iron is toxic, it must exist in the body in complex with other substances. About 65% of body iron is found in the hemoglobin of RBCs; the remainder is bound to protein as ferritin or another iron-protein complex, *hemosiderin,* in the bone marrow, liver, or spleen. This stored iron, along with that in the myoglobin of muscle, serves as a reservoir from which additional iron can be drawn during periods of accelerated erythropoiesis. Abnormally high rates of iron absorption lead to hemochromatosis, discussed later.

Hemoglobin Variation. The normal quantity of hemoglobin in the blood varies with age and sex, as summarized in Table 12–4. During a person's lifetime, six different types of hemoglobin are normally produced. Variability arises from the structure of the globin chains, although two each from the α and β families are always present. Three of these hemoglobins are found only during embryonic life. Production of a fourth type, hemoglobin F (fetal hemoglobin) begins at about 6 weeks' gestation. As discussed in Chapter 33, hemoglobin F displays higher affinity for oxygen than does hemoglobin A (adult hemoglobin) promoting fetal oxygen uptake from maternal blood during placental exchange. Hemoglobin A, the fifth type, replaces hemoglobin F by about 6 months of age. Hemoglobin A_2, the sixth type, appears at birth and gradually increases throughout adulthood. It never exceeds 1% of the total hemoglobin, however, and is believed to be clinically insignificant.[1]

Genetic defects in synthesis of the globin chains of hemoglobin give rise to a group of disorders known as **hemoglobinopathies**. The most prevalent of these, **sickle cell disease**, is detailed later in this chapter; other, less common hemoglobinopathies are summarized in Table 12–5.

Clearance of Plasma Hemoglobin. Although some free hemoglobin is released into the plasma as a result of extravascular hemolysis, most hemoglobin is first degraded to iron, amino acids, and the yellow pigment, *bilirubin* (discussed later). Rupture of RBCs due to mechanical stress within the circulation (intravascular hemolysis) releases their hemoglobin into the blood. Normally, hemoglobin is rapidly cleared from the plasma by *haptoglobin,* a

TABLE 12–4
HEMOGLOBIN VARIATION WITH SEX AND AGE

Age and Sex	Hemoglobin (g/dL)
28 weeks' gestation	14.5
34 weeks' gestation	15.0
Neonatal day 1	18.4
2 weeks	16.8
2 months	9.0–14.0
6–12 years	11.5–15.5
12–18 years; male	13.0–16.0
12–18 years; female	12.0–16.0
18–49 years; male	13.5–17.5
18–49 years; female	12.0–16.0
65–74 years; male	14.9
65–74 years; female	13.8

Data from Blackburn, S.T., and Loper, D.L. (1992). *Maternal, Fetal, and Neonatal Physiology: A Clinical Perspective.* Philadelphia: W.B. Saunders Co.; Foster, R.L.R., Hunsberger, M.M., and Anderson, J.J.T. (1989). *Family-Centered Nursing Care of Children.* Philadelphia: W.B. Saunders Co.; and Johnson, M.A., Fischer, J.G., Bowman, B.A., *et al.* (1994). Iron nutriture in elderly individuals. *FASEB Journal* 8(9), 609–621.

plasma protein that binds free hemoglobin and transports it to the liver for degradation. The amount of circulating haptoglobin is limited, however, and when the capacity of this mechanism is exceeded, renal and plasma clearance mechanisms are activated. Some hemoglobin is filtered by the glomerulus into renal tubules, where it is then taken up by tubular cells for degradation. The released iron is stored within these cells. When tubular cell capacity is exceeded, hemoglobin is lost in the urine (hemoglobinuria). Alternatively, the hemoglobin iron is oxidized within the circulation, forming *methemoglobin*. The ferric (Fe^{3+}) heme then dissociates from this compound, binds to albumin and other transport proteins, and is carried to the liver for degradation. Excessive methemoglobin accumulation in the blood, due to either hereditary or acquired etiologies, leads to tissue hypoxia because of the inability of this form of hemoglobin to bind oxygen (see Chapter 19).

Anemia and Polycythemia. The anemias are disorders characterized by a reduction in either numbers of functional erythrocytes or amount of functional hemoglobin. Anemia is commonly encountered in clinical practice, and the more prevalent types are detailed later. Polycythemia, an excess of erythrocytes, may occur as a primary condition (polycythemia vera) or, more commonly, secondary to disorders characterized by chronic tissue hypoxia and increased erythropoietin production. Secondary polycythemia is discussed in Chapter 19. Polycythemia vera is discussed later in this chapter.

Leukopoiesis

Five distinct types of leukocytes are recognized: lymphocytes, **monocyte-macrophages, neutrophils, eosinophils,** and **basophils**. Their development from the lymphoid and myeloid progenitor cells is regulated by hematopoietic growth factors and transcription factors, as previously discussed. In addition, numerous cytokines and lipid mediators released during the immune and inflammatory responses may stimulate leukopoiesis (see Chapter 13).

Lymphocytes. Lymphocytes originate from the lymphoid progenitor cell (see Fig. 12–1). Lymphocyte differentiation into T lymphocytes, B lymphocytes, and NK cells represents sequential changes in activation and function rather than distinct structural stages. Most lymphocytes differentiate outside the bone marrow, in lymphatic tissues such as the thymus gland, lymph nodes, and spleen. Specific processes of lymphocyte maturation and activation are detailed in Chapter 13.

Granulocytes. Neutrophils, eosinophils, and basophils are collectively known as granulocytes because of their irregularly shaped nuclei and cytoplasmic granules. They are sometimes referred to as *polymorphonuclear leukocytes* because their nuclei are segmented into multiple lobes. (Monocytes, in contrast, are agranular and mononuclear.) These leukocyte classes develop exclusively in the bone marrow, from the myeloid progenitor cell.

Neutrophils. Neutrophils are phagocytic cells that comprise more than half of the WBCs in the peripheral circulation.[6] Neutrophil development within the bone marrow normally takes about 1 week. Once released, neutrophils circulate for 6 to 12 hours before irreversibly entering sites of inflammation in tissues (see Chapter 13). Their life cycles are then completed within 24 hours.[7] Each mature neutrophil is capable of inactivating 5 to 20 bacteria. Presence of an increased fraction of band cells (immature neutrophils) in the blood indicates increased leukopoiesis. This "shift to the left" generally signifies the presence of infection. An increase in the fraction of hypermature segmented neutrophils ("shift to the right") may be seen in conditions in which nuclear segmentation is impaired, as in liver disease and some anemias.

Eosinophils. Eosinophils are phagocytic cells that target foreign (antigenic) proteins and antigen–antibody complexes. These cells are often increased in number in cases of allergy or parasitic infection (see Chapter 13).

Basophils. Basophils are the circulating equivalent of tissue mast cells and are identical to these in function but fewer in number. As detailed in Chapter 13, basophils and mast cells synthesize and re-

TABLE 12–5
CONGENITAL HEMOGLOBINOPATHIES*

Disease	Defect	Clinical Features
Sickle cell disease	Hemoglobin S, resulting from substitution of valine for glutamic acid in the β chain of the globin protein	Severity of anemia depends on genotype. Disease occurs almost exclusively in blacks. Deoxygenation promotes RBC sickling, hemolysis, and infarction.
Thalassemias	Group of disorders of the rate of synthesis of the α or β chains (decreased or absent synthesis)	Disease occurs in those of Mediterranean, African, or Asian ancestry. Severity of anemia varies with specific defect and heterozygous versus homozygous state.
Hereditary persistence of fetal hemoglobin (Hb F)	Group of disorders in which Hb F production continues in adult life.	Hb F is present in all RBCs in pancellular type. Homozygous patients have 100% Hb F, a disorder seen in blacks. Heterozygotes have 30% Hb F.
Unstable hemoglobins Hb Koln Hb Gun Hill Hb Hammersmith Hb M Hb C Hb Kansas Hb Chesapeake Hb C-Harlem Hb J-Singapore Hb H Hb Bart's Hb Lepore Hb Cranston Hb Constant Spring Hb Seattle Hb Ranier Hb Hiroshima Hb San Francisco Hb G	Many autosomal dominant disorders	Homozygous state usually is incompatible with life. Variable effects of heterozygous state include hemolysis, increased or decreased affinity, compensatory erythrocytosis, and decreased solubility.

* Clinically important disorders are listed; more than 300 variants have been identified.
Data from Moya, C.E., Shah, S., and Sodeman, T.M. (1985). The erythrocyte. In: Sodeman, W.A., and Sodeman, T.M. (Eds.). *Sodeman's Pathologic Physiology: Mechanisms of Disease.* (7th ed.). Philadelphia: W.B. Saunders. [pp. 648–703].

lease histamine and other mediators of inflammation.

Monocyte-Macrophages. Monocyte-macrophages are mononuclear phagocytic cells that function similarly to neutrophils in inflammation except that their development within the bone marrow is more rapid (3 to 4 days) and their circulation time is longer (24 hours) before entry into tissues.[1] Monocytes are the inactive, circulating precursors, while macrophages represent the mature, active, phagocytic form. In comparison to neutrophils, macrophages are present for a longer period at sites of inflammation. These cells are important not only in phagocytosis of microorganisms and cellular debris but also in preparation of the area for healing and in processing and presentation of antigen for the cellular immune response (see Chapter 13).

Leukopenia and Leukocytosis. Leukopenia, a reduction in the number of circulating leukocytes, may be present in a variety of disorders (Table 12–6). Logically, these disorders are manifested by a high risk of infection. **Leukocytosis**, an elevation in circulating leukocytes, may represent either a normal proliferation of phagocytic cells in response to infection or allergy, or a hematopoietic malignancy. One type of malignancy, leukemia, is detailed in this chapter. Reactive leukocytosis is discussed in Chapter 13.

Megakaryopoiesis

Platelet (Thrombocyte) Formation. Megakaryocytes, the precursor cells that disintegrate to form platelets, are large cells with variably shaped nuclei. Like granulocytes and monocytes, they originate from the myeloid line. The megakaryocyte grows rapidly within the bone marrow, acquiring cytoplasmic granules and the ability to secrete von Willebrand factor, a substance critical to platelet aggregation in blood clotting (see Chapter 14). The cytokine thrombopoietin has been characterized as a principal regulator of megakaryocyte production, but a number of other hematopoietic growth factors also affect this process (see Table 12–2). After two to five cycles of DNA replication, the megakaryocyte fragments into individual platelets, and its nucleus is phagocytized by macrophages. Platelet formation from committed stem cells takes about 5 days.[1] New platelets circulate for about 10 days before being removed by the spleen.

TABLE 12–6
CONDITIONS ASSOCIATED WITH LEUKOPENIA

White Blood Cell Deficiency	Associated Conditions

Neutropenia (granulocytopenia; referred to as *agranulocytosis* if severe)	Aplastic anemia
	Megaloblastic anemias
	Some leukemias and lymphomas
	Myelosuppressive drug therapy
	  Cancer chemotherapy (antimetabolites and alkylating agents)
	  Idiosyncratic reaction to chloramphenicol, sulfonamides, phenylbutazone, or other drugs
	CD8+ lymphocytosis
	Felty's syndrome
	Hypersplenism
	Overwhelming sepsis
	Chronic benign neutropenia of childhood (CBN)
	Kostmann's syndrome (congenital agranulocytosis)
	Cyclic neutropenia
	Shwachman's syndrome
	Chédiak-Higashi syndrome
	Reticular dysgenesis
	Glycogenosis type Ib

Lymphopenia	Congenital immunodeficiency
	  DiGeorge's syndrome
	  Severe combined immunodeficiency disease (SCID)
	  Wiskott-Aldrich syndrome
	Acquired immunodeficiency syndrome (AIDS)
	Hodgkin's disease
	Nonlymphocytic leukemias
	Corticosteroid therapy

Data from Bernini, J.C. (1996). Diagnosis and management of chronic neutropenia during childhood. *Pediatric Clinics of North America* 43(3), 773–792; and Cotran, R.S., Kumar, V., and Robbins, S.L. (Eds.). (1994). *Robbins Pathologic Basis of Disease*. (5th ed.). Philadelphia: W.B. Saunders. (pp. 216–231, 630–631).

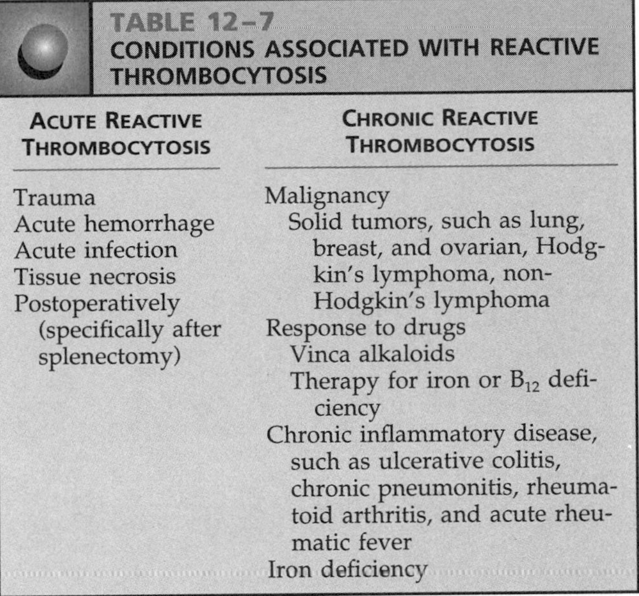

TABLE 12–7
CONDITIONS ASSOCIATED WITH REACTIVE THROMBOCYTOSIS

Acute Reactive Thrombocytosis	Chronic Reactive Thrombocytosis

Trauma
Acute hemorrhage
Acute infection
Tissue necrosis
Postoperatively (specifically after splenectomy)
	Malignancy
	  Solid tumors, such as lung, breast, and ovarian, Hodgkin's lymphoma, non-Hodgkin's lymphoma
	Response to drugs
	  Vinca alkaloids
	  Therapy for iron or B_{12} deficiency
	Chronic inflammatory disease, such as ulcerative colitis, chronic pneumonitis, rheumatoid arthritis, and acute rheumatic fever
	Iron deficiency

From Shucy, K.M. (1996). Platelet-associated bleeding disorders. *Seminars in Oncology Nursing* 12(1), 16.

Thrombocytopenia and Thrombocytosis. Deficiency of circulating platelets (thrombocytopenia), which may result from a number of congenital and acquired disorders, is detailed later in this chapter. **Reactive thrombocytosis**, an increase in platelets resulting from increased production of plasma platelet-stimulating factor, may occur as a response to anemia, hemorrhage, malignancy, inflammation, or iron deficiency (Table 12–7).[8] Essential thrombocythemia, an increase in platelets due to abnormal proliferation of the myeloid stem cell, is discussed later in this chapter. Mechanisms of platelet activation, adhesion, and aggregation in hemostasis are examined in Chapter 14.

HEMATOPOIETIC DISORDERS

Anemias

Transport of oxygen is impaired in the anemias, a variety of conditions characterized by deficiency or functional abnormality of RBCs. Table 12–8 summarizes clinical features of the anemias, which may result from blood loss, excessive RBC destruction (hemolysis), nutritional deficiency (dietary deficiency or malabsorption), or hereditary defects in RBC synthesis. Anemias are classified on the basis of the size of RBCs as *normocytic*, *microcytic* (small), or *macrocytic* (large), and on the basis of their color (reflective of hemoglobin concentration) as *normochromic* or *hypochromic* (pale). **Iron-deficiency anemia, perni-**

TABLE 12–8
CLINICAL FEATURES OF THE ANEMIAS

Anemia	Etiology	RBC Characteristics
Hemorrhagic	Acute blood loss	Normocytic, normochromic, reticulocytosis
Iron-deficiency	Chronic, slow blood loss; insufficient intake relative to demands	Microcytic, hypochromic
Hemolytic	Hereditary defect of RBCs; immune, infectious, mechanical, or traumatic injury of RBCs; hypersplenism	Variable morphology in hereditary forms (e.g., sickle or spherical shape); normocytic, normochromic in other etiologies
Sickle cell disease		
Hereditary spherocytosis		
Prosthetic heart valves		
Autoimmune		
Transfusion mismatch		
Hemoglobinopathies		
Glucose-6-phosphate dehydrogenase deficiency		
Aplastic or hypoplastic	Hereditary or nutritional deficiency of substrate for erythropoiesis; bone marrow depression; chronic disease	Macrocytic (megalobastic) in substrate deficiency; normocytic, normochromic in bone marrow depression; microcytic, hypochromic in chronic disease
Idiopathic		
Drug induced		
Radiation induced		
Pure red cell aplasia (PRCA)		
Anemia of chronic disease		
Alcoholism		
Pernicious anemia		
Folate deficiency		

cious anemia, sickle cell disease, and **hereditary spherocytosis** are discussed in detail next.

Iron-Deficiency Anemia

Definition. Iron-deficiency anemia is a disorder of oxygen transport due to deficiency of hemoglobin synthesis.

Epidemiology. With its 11% prevalence worldwide, iron-deficiency anemia is the most common type of anemia, usually resulting from slow blood loss, possibly combined with deficient dietary intake of iron.[9] Women of childbearing age are at highest risk because of menstrual blood losses and the increased iron demands of the growing fetus during pregnancy. Other risk factors for slow blood loss include presence of gastrointestinal irritation (often induced by alcohol abuse or excessive intake of aspirin), ulceration, diverticula, or malignancy (see Chapter 24). Gastrointestinal conditions may also result in malabsorption of iron and other nutrients.

Inadequate dietary intake of iron is less common in the United States than in developing countries. Those at particular risk include vegetarians, pregnant women, infants and young children, and the elderly. Dietary sources of iron are listed in Table 12–9.

Etiology. Iron-deficiency anemia is caused by negative iron balance due to insufficient intake, impaired absorption, excessive iron demand, or chronic blood loss.

Pathophysiology. Iron stores are gradually depleted, sparing hemoglobin at first. Circulating iron is also decreased, and finally hemoglobin and myoglobin synthesis are impaired. Oxygen-carrying capacity is reduced, and tissues become hypoxic. Erythropoietin release stimulates erythropoiesis, but RBC production is limited by lack of substrate.

Because iron is critical to the function of mitochondrial and hepatic enzymes, the metabolism of

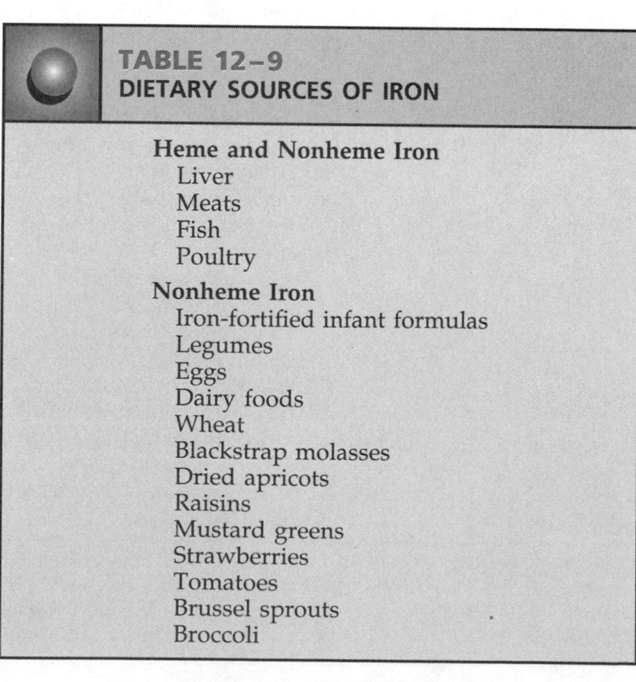

TABLE 12–9
DIETARY SOURCES OF IRON

Heme and Nonheme Iron
- Liver
- Meats
- Fish
- Poultry

Nonheme Iron
- Iron-fortified infant formulas
- Legumes
- Eggs
- Dairy foods
- Wheat
- Blackstrap molasses
- Dried apricots
- Raisins
- Mustard greens
- Strawberries
- Tomatoes
- Brussel sprouts
- Broccoli

all tissues is affected. Iron deficiency is known to be particularly detrimental to brain development in infancy and childhood and may alter central nervous system metabolism later in life as well.[10]

Clinical Manifestations. Microscopic study of a peripheral blood smear reveals several abnormalities, as does analysis of the complete blood count (Table 12–10). Hemoglobin and **hematocrit** (the percentage of blood volume composed of RBCs) are reduced. RBCs have a microcytic, hypochromic appearance due to lack of hemoglobin, expressed quantitatively as low mean corpuscular volume and mean corpuscular hemoglobin concentration (Color Fig. 12–2). Serum iron is low, and total iron-binding capacity is high because the greater fraction of transferrin is not bound to iron.

TABLE 12–10
HEMATOLOGY STUDIES

Test	Clinical Significance
Red Blood Cell Tests	
RBC count	Variable with age; increased in polycythemia or hemoconcentration; decreased in anemia
RBC morphology	Abnormal RBCs may vary in size (anisocytosis), color (anisochromia), or shape (poikilocytosis)
Hematocrit	Percentage by volume of packed RBCs in whole blood; decreased in anemia, or hemodilution; increased in polycythemia, or hemoconcentration
RBC indices	Includes mean corpuscular volume (MCV), hemoglobin (MCH), and hemoglobin concentration (MCHC); indicates whether RBCs are microcytic, macrocytic, or normocytic; normochromic or hypochromic; aids in classifications of anemias
Erythrocyte sedimentation rate (ESR)	Degree of RBC settling during a specified time period; increased if fibrinogen and globulin are present in excess (during inflammation)
Reticulocyte count	Immature RBC forms present in blood for 24–48 hours after release from bone marrow; index of bone marrow activity
Osmotic fragility	Degree of resistance of RBCs to hemolysis when exposed to hypotonic solutions; supplements RBC morphology data in classifying hemolytic anemias
Hemoglobin Tests	
Total hemoglobin	Supplies data for calculation of RBC indices; useful for monitoring severity of anemia or response to therapy
Hemoglobin electrophoresis	Separates forms of hemoglobin for detection of abnormal forms
Sickle cell test	Presence of spontaneous sickling of RBCs on a peripheral blood smear indicates sickle cell disease; induction of sickling with addition of a reducing agent indicates sickle cell trait or another hemoglobinopathy
Serum iron	Measures amount of iron bound to transferrin; decreased in iron-deficiency anemia or chronic inflammation; increased in iron overload (hemochromatosis)
Total iron-binding capacity (TIBC)	Measures amount of iron that would be present in plasma if all transferrin were saturated; dividing serum Fe by TIBC reveals percentage of saturation and evaluates capacity to store iron
Serum ferritin	Proportional to total body iron stores
White Blood Cell Tests	
WBC count	Variable with stress, exercise, and digestion (within 2000/μL); elevated with inflammation or leukemia; decreased with bone marrow depression
WBC differential	Classifies WBCs into five types: neutrophils, eosinophils, basophils, lymphocytes, and monocytes; identifies abnormal forms; indicates inflammation, allergy, pancytopenia, leukemia, lymphoma
Platelet Tests	
Platelet count	Used in screening for platelet function in hemostasis (assessment of risk of bleeding); increased in reactive thrombocytosis or essential thrombocythemia; decreased in thrombocytopenia due to primary disease or in response to radiation therapy or chemotherapy

Skin and mucous membranes appear pale owing to lack of the red color of oxyhemoglobin. Although the patient may lack symptoms, fatigue and muscle weakness are often present owing to impairment of oxidative metabolism. Shortness of breath, palpitations, and chest pain may occur with exertion. Relatively uncommon signs of severe and prolonged iron deficiency include an appetite for dirt or other unusual substances (pica), and atrophic changes in epithelial cells, resulting in inflammation of the lips or tongue (cheilitis or glossitis), formation of web-like membranes in the esophagus, or spoon-like deformation of the nails (koilonychia).

Prevention and Treatment. Prevention requires early identification and treatment of any source of chronic blood loss as well as assurance of adequate dietary intake of iron. Treatment consists of replacement of iron, usually as oral ferrous sulfate. Patients who have impaired iron absorption may require administration of iron by deep injection into muscle.

Prognosis and Outcome. A positive response to therapy is usually seen within 10 days, as evidenced by increased numbers of immature RBCs (reticulocytosis) and improvement in the **red blood cell indices** (see Table 12–10). Up to 6 months of therapy may be necessary to fully replenish iron stores.

Pernicious Anemia

Definition. Pernicious anemia is a deficiency of vitamin B_{12} (cobalamin), resulting in impaired erythropoiesis and oxygen transport and in demyelination of peripheral nerves.

Epidemiology. The annual incidence of new cases is 100 per 1 million population.[11] Dietary deficiency of B_{12} is extremely rare, although strict vegetarians may be at increased risk. Surgical resection of a portion of the stomach or small intestine predisposes to pernicious anemia because of lack of absorption of B_{12}. Patients with autoimmune disorders such as type I diabetes, Addison's disease, or Hashimoto's thyroiditis are at increased risk of pernicious anemia, which, in most cases, has an autoimmune etiology. The incidence of pernicious anemia is increased after the age of 50 years.[12] Although the disorder was once believed to be more prevalent in fair-skinned people of northern European descent, it is now known to affect all ethnic groups. A familial predisposition is evident.

Etiology. Cobalamin release from its dietary protein-bound state depends on the acidic gastric environment. Achlorhydria, a reduction in gastric HCl secretion, may contribute to lack of cobalamin absorption. In nearly all cases, however, pernicious anemia is caused by lack of *intrinsic factor (IF)*, a glycoprotein secreted by the parietal cells of the stomach lining. Factors causing gastric atrophy disrupt the secretion of both HCl and IF.

Vitamin B_{12}, once freed from dietary protein, is not absorbed efficiently unless it is first complexed to IF (Fig. 12–5). Loss of parietal cells owing to surgical resection or chronic inflammatory disease results in lack of IF. An autoimmune mechanism is believed to underlie most cases of chronic gastritis, which precedes the pernicious anemia found in older people. Autoantibodies may be directed at parietal cells or at intestinal receptors for the B_{12}–IF complex (see Chapter 13). Rarely, pernicious anemia is caused by a genetic defect in IF production, in which case it manifests in children younger than 2 years of age.

Pathophysiology. Lack of vitamin B_{12} impairs DNA synthesis and cell division, with significant effects on erythropoiesis and myelination of nerves. RBC precursors do not divide normally; instead, they form large, poorly functional cells known as *megaloblasts*. Myelin is an insulating substance surrounding larger nerves. As discussed in Chapter 21, loss of myelin interferes with impulse transmission, leading to abnormality of sensation or movement in affected tissues. Abnormal erythropoiesis is believed to be secondary to impairment of folic acid metabolism induced by lack of vitamin B_{12}, whereas demyelination is apparently a direct effect of vitamin B_{12} deficiency.

Clinical Manifestations. Erythrocytes are reduced in number, and cells are macrocytic and irregularly shaped (Color Fig. 12–3). Manifestations of gastrointestinal inflammation, such as diarrhea and abdominal pain, may be present. Weakness and fatigue are proportionate to the degree of anemia. Neurologic manifestations include numbness and paresthesias and, in severe cases, loss of reflexes, gait disturbance, and decreased mental function.

Prevention and Treatment. Early detection is important in patients at risk. The Schilling test, in which radioactive vitamin B_{12} is administered and its urinary excretion measured, may be used to evaluate vitamin B_{12} absorption. The widespread use of vitamin B_{12} supplements as "tonics" for anyone complaining of fatigue or poor appetite is unwarranted. Because a small fraction (1% to 3%) of cobalamin is absorbed without IF, high-dose replacement therapy with an oral form of the vitamin may be used. This form of therapy is common in Europe. In the United States, however, documented vitamin B_{12} deficiency is usually treated with monthly intramuscular injection of vitamin B_{12} throughout the lifetime of the patient.

Prognosis and Outcome. If not treated, pernicious anemia is fatal. The patient succumbs to heart failure as the heart attempts to meet the demands of

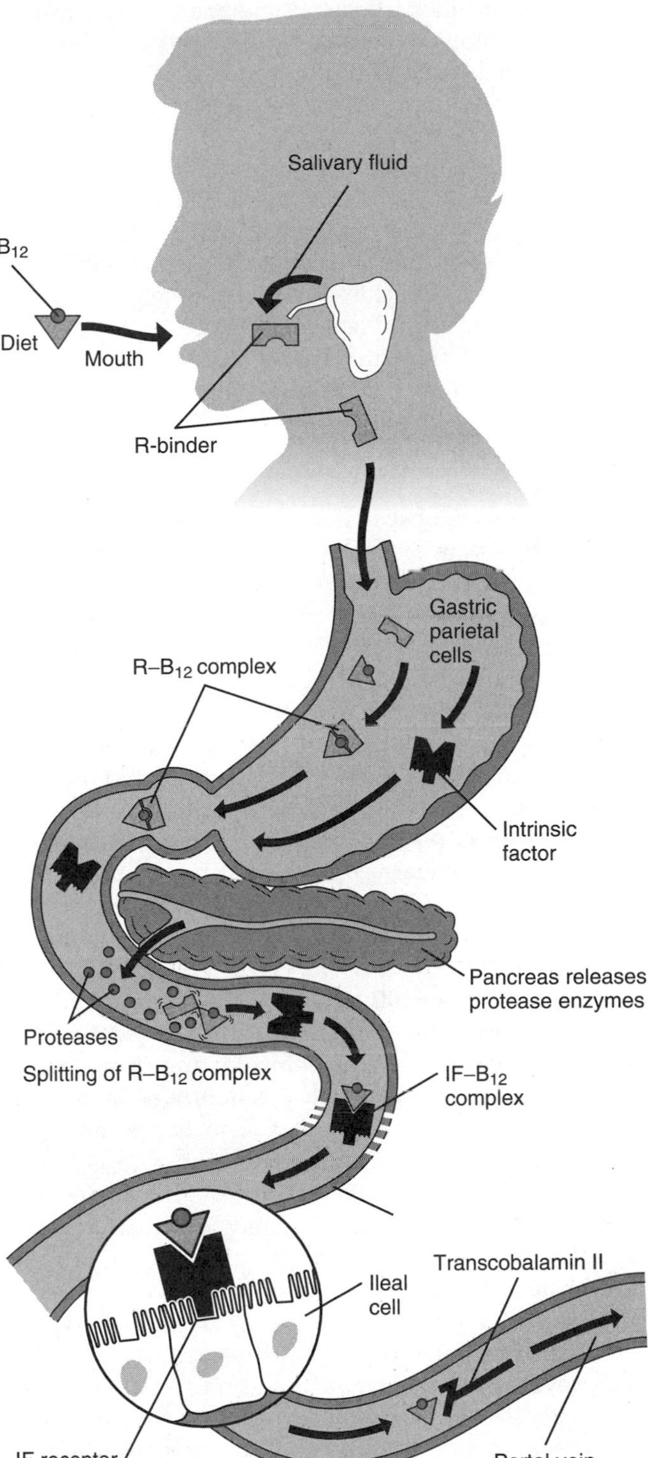

FIGURE 12–5
Absorption of vitamin B_{12}. Vitamin B_{12} is first released from its protein-bound form in ingested food by the proteolytic enzyme pepsin, secreted by the stomach. The vitamin then binds primarily to salivary binding proteins, with a smaller amount binding to intrinsic factor (IF). IF is a glycoprotein secreted by the gastric parietal cells. In the small intestine, pancreatic protease enzymes release more vitamin B_{12} from the salivary binding proteins, and the released vitamin then binds to IF. In the ileum, the IF–B_{12} complex binds to IF receptors, and the vitamin is taken into ileal cells. It is then bound to a plasma protein, transcobalamin II, for transport in the blood to the liver and bone marrow. (R, rapidly-mobile salivary vitamin B_{12}-binding proteins.) (Redrawn from Cotran, R.S., Kumar V., and Robbins, S.L. [Eds.], [1994]. *Robbins Pathologic Basis of Disease.* [5th ed.]. Philadelphia: W.B. Saunders. [p. 606].)

hypoxic tissues. With treatment, manifestations of anemia subside, but some neurologic deficits may be permanent.

Sickle Cell Disease

Definition. Sickle cell disease is an inherited disorder of hemoglobin synthesis resulting in tissue hypoxia and circulatory obstruction due to abnormal erythropoiesis.

Epidemiology. Sickle cell disease occurs almost exclusively in blacks. In the United States, about 1 in 400 blacks is homozygous for the defect and has sickle cell anemia, whereas 1 in 12 is heterozygous and has sickle cell trait, a milder form of the disease. Worldwide, sickle cell disease is the most common form of inherited hemolytic anemia. The trait is prevalent among blacks in Africa, possibly because the abnormal hemoglobin (Hb S) is more resistant to the parasite that causes the malaria endemic to the area.

Etiology. The genetic defect results in substitution of the amino acid valine for glutamine on one of the globin chains of the hemoglobin molecule. This Hb S is less soluble than normal adult hemoglobin (Hb A) and assumes a sickle or crescent shape when it is deoxygenated. The defect is inherited as an autosomal recessive trait with variable expressivity.

Pathophysiology. Deoxygenation of Hb S produces a conformational change in the globin protein, resulting in flattening and elongation of the RBC. Blood viscosity is increased, and sickled cells may clump together, obstructing the microcirculation and leading to tissue ischemia. Anemia results from removal of sickled RBCs by phagocytic cells of the spleen, which further exacerbates tissue hypoxia. The course of the disease is characterized by periods of remission and exacerbation (sickling crises).[13]

Clinical Manifestations. Infants younger than 6 months of age do not usually have any clinical signs because fetal hemoglobin (Hb F) persists in sufficient amounts to allow normal gas transport. After this period, Hb S is predominant, and clinical manifestations are seen, usually precipitated by respiratory or gastrointestinal infections toward the latter part of the first year of life.[13] Sickled cells are apparent in the peripheral blood (Color Fig. 12–4). Anemia is usually severe, resulting in weakness, fatigue, and growth impairment. The spleen is enlarged early in the disease but usually atrophies owing to infarction by the time the child reaches school age (a process referred to as *autosplenectomy*). The hands and feet may become swollen and painful owing to ischemic effects resulting from obstruction of the microcirculation. Vascular obstructions may eventually cause ischemic damage to the lungs, kidneys, heart, and central nervous system.

Acute exacerbations (crises) may be caused by respiratory infections or other stressors that reduce PaO_2 levels below normal. Five types of crises may be seen: (1) *vaso-occlusive* or *pain crisis*, in which there is pain originating from the area of vascular occlusion, with no change in hematology findings; (2) *aplastic crisis*, in which there may be some pain, but the predominant sign is bone marrow hypoplasia with decreased hemoglobin and reticulocytes; (3) *hemolytic* or *hyperhemolytic crisis*, in which there is fever and increased RBC destruction; (4) *sequestration crisis*, in which there is sudden and massive RBC trapping by the visceral organs, especially the spleen; and (5) *mixed crisis*, in which manifestations of more than one crisis type are seen.[14]

Prevention and Treatment. Premarital genetic screening for the sickle cell defect is routine within the black population, and genetic counseling is available. In people with sickle cell trait or anemia, the risk of hypoxia is minimized with immunization against pneumonia and influenza, and prompt treatment of upper respiratory infections or other illnesses. Manifestations of the disorder are treated supportively with analgesics for pain, fluids to decrease blood viscosity, and oxygen therapy. Blood transfusions are indicated when the patient's hemoglobin level drops more than 2 g/dL below normal, and **exchange transfusion** is used to remove sickled cells in cases of severe occlusive crisis. Care must be taken not to overuse transfusion therapy because blood-borne infections, such as hepatitis, and toxicity due to iron overload and increased hemosiderin deposition (hemosiderosis) may result.[14]

Prognosis and Outcome. Half of patients with sickle cell anemia survive beyond the fifth decade (see Focus of Current Research).[15] Morbidity and mortality depend on the frequency and severity of sickling crises. High levels of Hb F in children with sickle cell anemia are associated with improved survival. Early death is usually due to myocardial infarction, renal failure, chronic infections, or stroke.

Hereditary Spherocytosis

Definition. Hereditary spherocytosis is an inherited defect of the RBC membrane, resulting in abnormal erythrocyte shape and anemia due to an increased rate of RBC hemolysis by the spleen.

Epidemiology. Hereditary spherocytosis occurs in about 1 in 5000 people.[9] It is the most common inherited disorder of the RBC membrane.

Etiology. The disorder is inherited as an autosomal dominant trait in about 75% of cases.[16] Autosomal recessive inheritance confers a milder form of the disease.

Pathophysiology. The genetic defect results in abnormally low levels of spectrin, a structural protein that is a component of the cytoskeleton supporting the RBC membrane. The membrane is more rigid than normal, and it fragments more readily owing to shear stress during circulation. Cells assume a spherical shape rather than the normal biconcave disk shape, and these abnormally shaped cells are filtered, stored, and ultimately phagocytized in the spleen. Spherocyte membranes are also abnormally permeable to sodium. The inward Na^+ leak results in increased active transport of sodium out of the cell, and the energy demands of this process mandate increased demands for glucose and other energy substrates. When these demands cannot be met, the cell is destroyed.[1] Hemoglobin synthesis is

Focus of Current Research

Study	Objective and Findings
Lozoff, et al. (1996) Iron-deficiency anemia and infant development: Effects of extended oral iron therapy.	*Objective:* To determine whether oral iron therapy corrects lower developmental test scores in infants with iron-deficiency anemia *Findings:* Lower mental test scores persisted despite extended iron therapy and an excellent hematologic response.
Wurapa, et al. (1996) Primary iron overload in African Americans.	*Objectives:* To report on African Americans with primary iron overload diagnosed during life and to study iron stores in those undergoing autopsy *Findings:* Living patients had elevated iron stores and one or more of the following: liver enlargement, cirrhosis, cardiomyopathy, diabetes, and impotence. Four of 326 patients had elevated iron stores at autopsy.
Kurtzberg, et al. (1996) Placental blood as a source of hematopoietic stem cells for transplantation into unrelated recipients.	*Objective:* To examine results of transplantation using partially HLA-mismatched placental blood from unrelated donors *Findings:* HLA-mismatched placental blood is an acceptable alternative to bone marrow transplantation.
Ravindranath, et al. (1996) Autologous bone marrow transplantation versus intensive consolidation chemotherapy for acute myeloid leukemia in childhood.	*Objective:* To compare the efficacy and safety of the two modes of intervention in AML *Findings:* Treatment of children with AML in first remission with either mode of therapy prolongs event-free survival equally.
Mele, et al. (1996) Risk factors for essential thrombocythemia: A case-control study.	*Objective:* To determine possible risk factors for essential thrombocythemia *Findings:* In 39 patients in Italy, risk factors included use of hair dye, selected occupations, and residence in houses composed of radiation-emitting materials.
Gruppo Italiano Studio Policitemia (1995) Polycythemia vera: The natural history of 1213 patients followed for 20 years.	*Objective:* To obtain estimates of incidence of thrombosis and survival in polycythemia vera *Findings:* Cytoreduction favorably effects the incidence of thrombosis but may be associated with increased risk for neoplasia.

Box continued on following page

Box continued from previous page

Rapaport, et al. (1995) Relationship of growth hormone deficiency and leukemia.	*Objective:* To investigate the risk of leukemia associated with growth hormone deficiency *Findings:* An increased risk may exist and is unrelated to use of exogenous growth hormone replacement.
Platt, et al. (1994) Mortality in sickle cell disease: Life expectancy and risk factors for early death.	*Objective:* To determine life expectancy and risk factors for early death among patients with sickle cell disease *Findings:* Half of patients survive beyond the fifth decade. A large number of those who died had an acute episode of pain, chest syndrome, or stroke. A high level of fetal hemoglobin was associated with increased life expectancy.

normal, and intact spherocytes transport oxygen normally.

Clinical Manifestations. Hemolysis results in manifestations of anemia that are proportional to the degree of RBC destruction. Increased release of hemoglobin and iron from lysed cells may result in jaundice and hemosiderosis, and gallstones are common later in life if the spleen is not removed (see Chapter 26). Hereditary spherocytosis, like sickle cell disease, is characterized by self-limited hemolytic crises triggered by infections or other stressors. Less frequently, aplastic crises occur, in which the synthesis of all types of bone marrow cells ceases.

Prevention and Treatment. Genetic counseling may be indicated in cases of known inheritance. The child with hereditary spherocytosis is treated supportively with transfusions (for anemia) or phototherapy (for jaundice) until the age of 5 or 6 years, when splenectomy is done.

Prognosis and Outcome. Splenectomy cures the anemia.

Polycythemia Vera

Definition. Polycythemia vera ("true" polycythemia) is a chronic disorder characterized by excessive bone marrow production of erythrocytes, leukocytes, and platelets due to excessive activation of pluripotent stem cells.

Epidemiology. Polycythemia vera is rare, with an estimated annual incidence of 4.5 to 16 new cases per 1 million people.[17] It is slightly more prevalent in men. The typical age at diagnosis is 55 to 60 years. Secondary polycythemia, due to chronic tissue hypoxia, does *not* progress to polycythemia vera.

Etiology. The precise etiology of polycythemia vera is unknown, but the disorder is believed to be associated with increased responsiveness to hematopoietic growth factors, such as interleukin-3 or insulin-like growth factor. Because it often precedes the development of leukemia, polycythemia vera may represent a precancerous genetic transformation. One form of polycythemia displays familial inheritance.

Pathophysiology. The volume and viscosity of the blood are increased, resulting in engorgement of vessels and sludging of blood flow. Tissue perfusion is decreased, and blood is hypercoagulable owing to slowed flow. The color of increased amounts of hemoglobin (whether oxygenated or not) is visible below the surface of the skin and mucous membranes.

Clinical Manifestations. Clinical manifestations are primarily due to the increased mass of erythrocytes in the blood (Color Fig. 12–5). In contrast to secondary polycythemia, erythropoietin levels are *decreased* in polycythemia vera. Vessel engorgement results in headache, hypertension, distention of superficial veins, hepatomegaly, and splenomegaly. Pruritus (itching) is also common, although the causative mechanism is unclear. The skin and mucous membranes have a characteristic reddish-blue color known as *plethora*. Erythromyalgia, a syndrome demonstrated by burning pain, redness, and warmth of the fingers and toes, is seen in many cases. Deep vein thrombosis and other manifestations of inappropriate clotting are common. Hemorrhagic complications may also occur if platelet function is impaired.

Prevention and Treatment. Polycythemia vera is treated with phlebotomy (periodic removal of blood) to maintain a hematocrit near 45%.[17] Bone marrow suppression with radiation or chemotherapy may be used in combination with occasional phlebotomy in patients who do not respond to phlebotomy alone. α-Interferon and platelet inhibitors have been used experimentally. Splenomegaly may necessitate splenectomy in some cases.

Prognosis and Outcome. Polycythemia vera demonstrates an overall mortality rate of 2.9% per year.[18] Patients with severe polycythemia vera are at high risk for developing **acute myeloid leukemia**. Bone marrow suppression decreases the risk of thrombosis but increases the risk of neoplasia.

Porphyrias

Definition. The porphyrias are a group of inherited enzyme disorders that affect the synthesis of heme and result in the accumulation of porphyrins. This accumulation may primarily affect the skin, the nervous system, or both.

Epidemiology. The incidence of the different types of porphyria is variable. *Porphyria cutanea tarda* is the most common porphyria, but its precise incidence is unknown. It is seen worldwide but is especially prevalent among the Bantus of South Africa because of their high incidence of hemosiderosis.[19] High alcohol intake and estrogen supplementation also increase the risk of this type. Prevalence of a second type, *acute intermittent porphyria,* has been estimated at 5 to 10 per 100,000 population in the United States.[20] Attacks of acute intermittent porphyria are more frequent in women than men, and onset of symptoms is usually in the third or fourth decade of life. Use of certain drugs, including barbiturates, sulfonamides, and estrogens, as well as infection and reduced-calorie diet, are associated with exacerbation of attacks. *Plumboporphyria* is similar to acute intermittent porphyria but results in milder disease. A fourth type, *hereditary coporphyria,* is less common than acute intermittent porphyria. In Denmark, its incidence has been estimated at 2 per 1 million population.[19] *Variegate porphyria* is similar in its epidemiology to porphyria cutanea tarda, with highest incidence in South Africa. Other types of porphyria have been identified, but these are extremely rare.

Etiology. The porphyrias are caused by defects in one or more enzymes within the heme biosynthetic pathway. Heme, consisting of iron within a protoporphyrin ring, is synthesized in erythropoietic tissues and in the liver through a multistage pathway involving eight enzymatically mediated reactions. The enzyme defects are usually inherited through an autosomal dominant mechanism, although a few are autosomal recessive. Penetrance is low, however, and most affected people have the genetic trait but do not express the disease.[21] Symptomatic attacks are usually precipitated by factors that induce heme synthesis for the production of cytochrome enzymes.

Pathophysiology. Heme synthesis is decreased, and porphyrin precursors accumulate in tissues and are excreted in the urine and feces. The specific enzyme defect determines whether the porphyria affects neural tissue, dermatologic tissue, or both. If the enzyme acts early in the synthetic pathway, neural tissues are most affected by porphyrin accumulation. If the enzyme acts later in the pathway, the skin is most affected. Enzyme defects affecting both early and late stages produce effects in both types of tissues. Porphyrin intermediates in the first half of the pathway are water soluble and are excreted primarily in the urine. Those in the last half are fat soluble and are excreted primarily in the feces through the bile.

Clinical Manifestations. Cutaneous porphyrias, such as porphyria cutanea tarda, result in dermatologic manifestations such as photosensitivity (skin irritation with exposure to sunlight), blistering, edema, facial hyperpigmentation, and facial hirsutism (hairiness). Neuroporphyrias, such as acute intermittent porphyria and plumboporphyria, may manifest as attacks of abdominal pain, vomiting, constipation, rapid heart rate, and high blood pressure due to autonomic nerve dysfunction. Psychiatric manifestations are also seen, along with fever, leukocytosis, numbness and tingling, and possibly the syndrome of inappropriate antidiuretic hormone secretion (SIADH). Neurocutaneous porphyrias, such as hereditary coporphyria and variegate porphyria, result in both types of manifestations.

Attacks are transient but usually persist for several days. Urine containing porphyrin precursors turns dark on standing, whereas that containing porphyrins is red. Increased levels of porphyrin precursors may also be assayed in the blood, urine, and feces.

Prevention and Treatment. Family members of patients with porphyria should be genetically screened and counseled regarding their risk of transmitting the defect. Patients should avoid factors that may precipitate acute attacks, such as certain drugs, alcohol, and restrictive diets. Acute attacks are treated with removal of the triggering agent, if possible. Symptoms such as pain, agitation, and SIADH are treated supportively. Hematin (Panhematin), a heme derivative, has been used to decrease the synthesis of heme precursors but has not been consistently effective in clinical studies.[22] Tin protoporphyrin, an inhibitor of heme degradation, has been shown to prolong remissions but not to affect the course of the disease.

Prognosis and Outcome. Outcome is variable depending on the specific type of porphyria. Some patients remain asymptomatic, whereas others have only two or three attacks in a lifetime. Others may experience transient exacerbations two or three times per year, with each episode lasting days to months. Among Finnish patients with acute intermittent porphyria, the porphyria was reported to be the cause of death in 32%.[23]

Hemochromatosis

Definition. Hemochromatosis is a disorder characterized by the accumulation of excess iron in many organs, leading to cell damage and functional insufficiency.[24]

Epidemiology. Hereditary hemochromatosis is the most common autosomal recessive disorder among whites, with a prevalence of 4 cases per 1000 among those of northern European descent.[24] One in eight whites is a carrier of the disorder. Clinically evident disease is five times more common in men than women, probably because of normal blood losses to menstruation and pregnancy in women. Clinical disease usually has its onset between the ages of 30 and 50 years. Family history and northern European heritage constitute risk factors for the disease. Research has demonstrated that primary iron overload also occurs in African Americans, but the prevalence and mechanisms are uncertain.[25] Excessive iron intake imposes risk of a secondary hemochromatosis in some people.

Etiology. Seventy per cent of patients with hereditary hemochromatosis have a particular HLA subtype (HLA-A3), which is believed to be located near the hemochromatosis gene on the short arm of chromosome 6.[26] (HLA antigens are markers for native, or self, cells, as discussed in Chapter 13.) Although the precise location of the hemochromatosis gene is uncertain, the two genes are said to be *linked* in that their traits are often transmitted together. Hemochromatosis is inherited as an autosomal recessive trait. Secondary hemochromatosis may result from excessive intake of iron as a result of iron supplementation or repeated blood transfusions.

Pathophysiology. In hereditary hemochromatosis, iron absorption by the intestinal mucosal cells is inappropriately high, although the precise nature of the defect is unknown.[27] Iron thus accumulates in the tissues. The liver is predominantly involved because of its normal role in iron storage, and cirrhosis may develop as a result of iron toxicity (see Chapter 26). Pancreatic iron loading may induce damage that results in diabetes mellitus (see Chapter 29). Deposition of iron in the heart may cause cardiomyopathy (see Chapter 16). Deposition of iron into the skin causes increased production of the pigment melanin.

Clinical Manifestations. The classic description of manifestations of hemochromatosis, "bronze diabetes," is present only in a minority of patients.[28] More often, iron overload is discovered through routine laboratory testing or after evaluation of abdominal pain, joint pain, fatigue, or weakness. The liver is usually enlarged, and the serum levels of the hepatic aminotransferase enzymes may be elevated. Serum iron, transferrin, ferritin, and transferrin saturation are increased. Liver biopsy reveals greatly increased iron storage. In severe disease, hepatic fibrosis and cirrhosis, congestive heart failure, and hypogonadism may be seen.

Prevention and Treatment. Secondary hemochromatosis is preventable with normalization of iron intake. First- and second-degree relatives of patients with hereditary hemochromatosis should be screened for the disorder. Phlebotomy is the treatment of choice. Removal of one unit (500 mL) of blood removes 250 mg of excess iron. Phlebotomy is done once or twice a week at first, until iron stores are depleted, then less frequently to maintain desired iron levels. Patients who are too anemic to tolerate frequent phlebotomy may be treated with a chelating agent, deferoxamine (Desferal), which binds and detoxifies iron.[28]

Prognosis and Outcome. Prognosis depends on the severity of associated cirrhosis and diabetes. Overall survival rates are 76% at 10 years and 49% at 20 years.[27] Patients with cirrhosis have a high risk of death due to hepatocellular carcinoma (see Chapter 26).

Leukemias

Leukemias are traditionally classified on the basis of their onset and course as acute or chronic, and on the basis of their cell of origin as lymphoid or myeloid, with subclasses within each of these cell lines (Fig. 12–6). Leukemias often defy precise classification in that acute conditions may become chronic, and chronic conditions may undergo acute transformation (blast crisis). Classification based on cell type is also problematic in that neoplastic cells of either line may be further transformed during the course of the illness. In some cases, the leukemic cells are

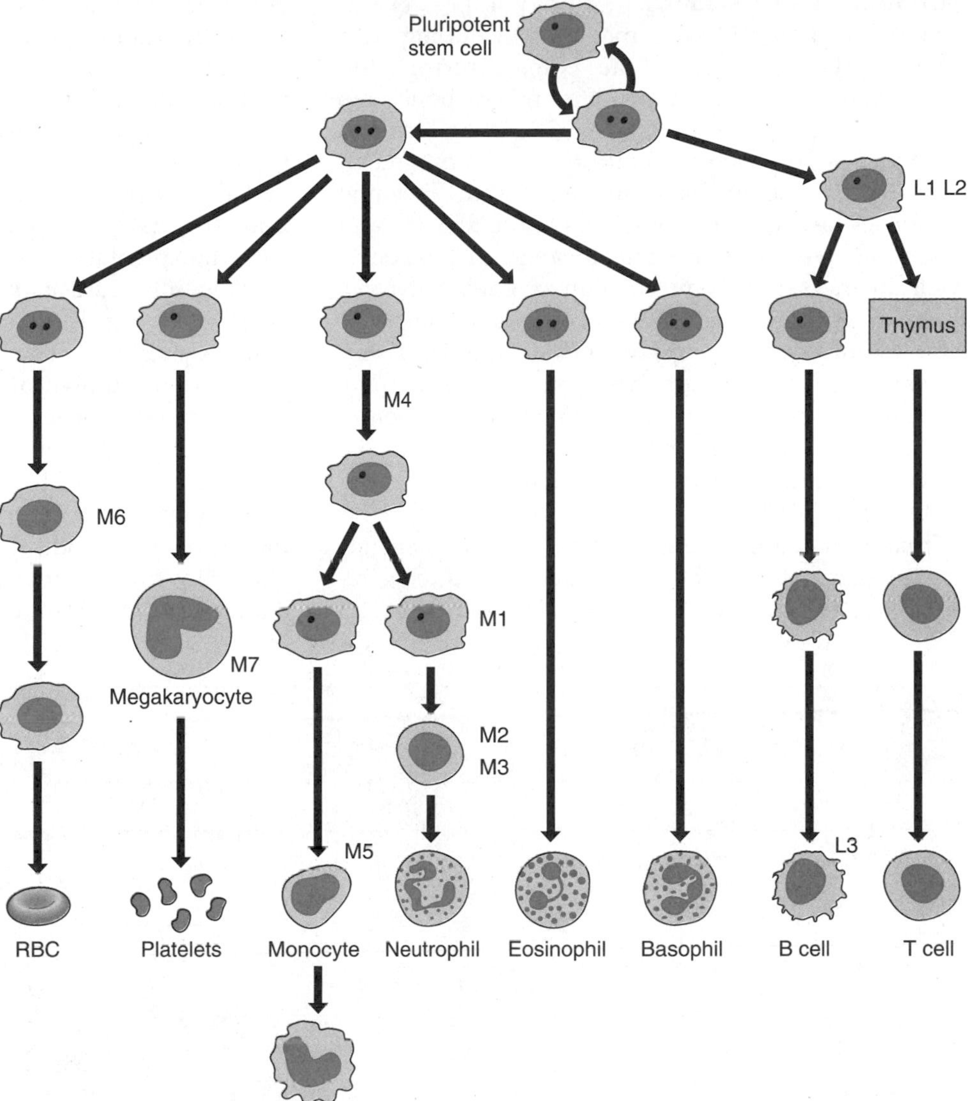

FIGURE 12–6
Morphologic classification of leukemias. According to the French-American-British classification, leukemias may be classified according to the degree of differentiation of the transformed cell. The L subtypes represent the lymphoid line, whereas the M subtypes originate within the myeloid line (see Table 12–13). The higher numbers are more highly differentiated cells, generally associated with a more favorable prognosis. (Redrawn from Groenwald, S.L., Frogge, M.H., Goodman, M., *et al.* [1993]. *Cancer Nursing: Principles and Practice.* [3rd ed.]. © Boston: Jones and Bartlett Publishers. [p. 1152]. Reprinted with permission.)

so primitive that they most closely resemble pluripotent stem cells. Leukemias affect all age groups, with certain types being more prevalent in children and one chronic form occurring exclusively in older adults.

Acute Lymphoblastic Leukemia

Definition. Acute lymphoblastic leukemia (ALL) is a malignant neoplasm of lymphocyte precursors that originates in the bone marrow. The transformed cell is usually a B lymphocyte.

Epidemiology. ALL is primarily a disease of children, although it also occurs in adults. About 2000 children in the United States are afflicted with ALL each year (3 per 100,000 children younger than 15 years), representing 80% of all childhood leukemias.[29] White children are at higher risk than blacks, and boys are at slightly higher risk than girls. Viral infection and exposure to radiation have been implicated as risk factors in the development of ALL.

Etiology. The etiology of ALL, like that of most cancers, is unknown. Mechanisms of neoplastic transformation are reviewed in Chapter 7.

Pathophysiology. Rapid proliferation of neoplastic cells (immature lymphocytes or lymphoblasts) occurs within the bone marrow, consuming energy and substrates and crowding out functional WBCs, RBCs and platelets. Nonfunctional, leukemic cells enter the blood and lymph, eventually infiltrating bone and other organs.

Clinical Manifestations. ALL typically begins with pallor and profound malaise developing over several days or weeks. Bone pain, bruising, and lymph node enlargement are often noted. Bone pain results from infiltration of bone with leukemic cells. Bleeding is typically manifested as ecchymosis (bruising), but hemorrhage may also occur. Bleeding tendencies are due to deficiency of platelets, and pallor and weakness are due to anemia. Leukocyte levels in the serum may be high or low, but functional lymphocytes are lacking, predisposing the child to infections by opportunistic organisms. Enlargement of the spleen, liver, and the testes may occur with infiltration by leukemic cells. The meninges covering the brain and spinal cord may also be infiltrated, and the resulting inflammation may cause severe headaches and vomiting.

Treatment. ALL is treated with early, intensive, multiple-agent chemotherapy aimed at inducing remission of the disease (Table 12–11). Destruction of abnormal cells allows normal hematopoiesis to resume. Immunosuppression resulting from the disease and its therapy renders the patient susceptible to infection, and in clinical settings, protective isolation (neutropenic precautions) may be employed (Table 12–12).

Radiation may be used in ALL to destroy leukemic cells that have infiltrated organs, and bone marrow transplantation has been accepted as standard therapy for acute leukemias in which remission is short-lived (Fig. 12–7).[30] Both allogenic grafts (donor marrow or stem cells from peripheral blood, placental blood, or umbilical cord blood) and autologous grafts (marrow or stem cells harvested from the patient and purged of tumor cells before reinfusion) have been used with variable efficacy. Purging may be accomplished with in vitro chemotherapy or monoclonal antibody treatment (immunotherapy). In allogenic transplants, the patient's residual bone marrow is irradiated or destroyed with chemother-

TABLE 12–11
CHEMOTHERAPY OF LEUKEMIAS

LEUKEMIA TYPE	THERAPEUTIC PURPOSE	AGENTS
Acute lymphoblastic leukemia (ALL)	Remission induction	Prednisolone Vincristine Asparaginase Cytosine arabinoside Daunorubicin Cyclophosphamide
	Consolidation and intensification (elimination of minimal residual disease)	Methotrexate Cyclophosphamide Asparaginase Cytosine arabinoside Etoposide 6-Mercaptopurine
	Prevention of central nervous system relapse (agents injected intrathecally)	Methotrexate Hydrocortisone Cytosine arabinoside
	Continuation and maintenance	6-Mercaptopurine Methotrexate Vincristine
Acute myeloid leukemia (AML)	Remission induction	Cytosine arabinoside Daunorubicin *Trans*-retinoic acid
	Consolidation	Induction drugs in very high doses
	Intensification	Mitoxantrone
Chronic lymphocytic leukemia (CLL)	Remission induction (initial therapy)	Chlorambucil Prednisone
	Remission induction (if no response to initial therapy)	Fludarabine Cladribine
Chronic myeloid leukemia (CML)	Chronic-phase therapy	Busulfan Hydroxyurea
	Terminal-phase therapy	α-Interferon
Hairy-cell leukemia	Remission induction	2′-Deoxycoformycin Cladribine α-Interferon

TABLE 12–12
PROTECTIVE ISOLATION MEASURES (NEUTROPENIC PRECAUTIONS)

MEASURE	PROCEDURE
Cutaneous and gastrointestinal decontamination	Nonabsorbable antibiotics are applied to the patient's skin and also ingested to destroy the normal flora before the patient enters the room.
Laminar air-flow room	Room air is filtered and circulated unidirectionally to reduce air turbulence and the risk of microbial precipitation.
Decontamination of food and objects	Raw foods are excluded. Water and objects coming in contact with the patient are sterilized.
Protective barriers	People coming in contact with the patient are masked, gowned, and gloved.

apy to minimize risk of graft-versus-host disease and rejection (see Chapter 13).

It is hoped that gene therapy will soon be available as an adjunct to bone marrow transplantation for those patients whose leukemia does not respond to standard therapies (see Chapter 7). The genetic defect within harvested leukemic cells could be repaired and normal hematopoiesis stimulated with reinfusion of the patient's cells after this repair.[31] ALL is unique among the leukemias in that maintenance of remission requires prolonged chemotherapy (up to 3 years) to ensure eradication of all leukemic cells.

Prognosis and Outcome. With improved treatment protocols, the prognosis in ALL is increasingly favorable. Ninety-nine per cent of children with lower-risk cell types and lower numbers of leukemic cells achieve complete remission with chemotherapy, and 80% achieve cure.[31] These survivors are at higher risk of developing other cancers, however, and their risk of developing brain tumors is 22 times that of the general population.[30] Surviving children are also more likely to have decreased educational attainment.[32] In adults, cure rates range from 20% to 35%.[33]

Acute Myeloid Leukemia

Definition. Acute myeloid leukemia (AML) is a malignant neoplasm of immature hematopoietic cells of the myeloid line. Originating in the bone marrow, AML has many subtypes (Table 12–13) and may also be referred to as *acute granulocytic leukemia* or *acute nonlymphoblastic leukemia*. The transformed cell may be any of several in the myeloid line, and stem cell leukemia is also classified with these.

Epidemiology. AML accounts for 80% of acute leukemias in adults and occurs primarily in young adults, 15 to 39 years of age.[16] AML is diagnosed in about 500 children each year in the United States.[30]

Etiology, Pathophysiology, Clinical Manifestations, and Treatment. The clinical features of AML are similar to those of ALL, discussed previously.

Prognosis and Outcome. AML has a less favorable prognosis than ALL. Nearly all patients relapse after initial remission. Median 1-year survival is 50%, although there have been some long-term survivors after bone marrow transplantation.[34]

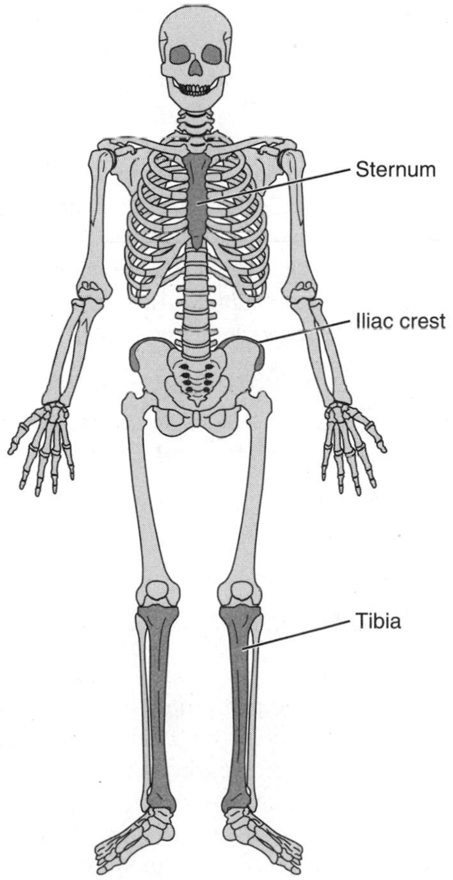

FIGURE 12–7
Sites of bone marrow aspiration. Hematopoeitic marrow for transplantation is usually aspirated from the posterior iliac crests, but the anterior iliac crests and sternum may also be used in adults. In infants, the proximal end of the tibia is the preferred site for aspiration of marrow for diagnostic examination (biopsy).

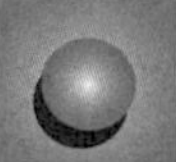

TABLE 12–13
MORPHOLOGIC CLASSIFICATION OF ACUTE MYELOID LEUKEMIAS (FRENCH-AMERICAN-BRITISH SYSTEM)

Classification		Morphology of Transformed Cell
M0	Minimally differentiated AML	Minimal myeloid differentiation
M1	AML without differentiation	Poorly differentiated myeloblasts; very immature cells
M2	AML with maturation	Myeloblastic with differentiation; fully mature granulocytes
M3	Acute promyelocytic leukemia	Promyelocytic; hypergranular cells
M4	Acute myelomonocytic leukemia	Myeloblastic and monoblastic
M5	Acute monocytic leukemia	Monoblastic and promonoblastic
M6	Acute erythroleukemia	Erythroleukemic (abnormnal erythroblasts)
M7	Acute megakaryocytic leukemia	Megakaryoblastic (abnormal platelet precursors)

Adapted from Cotran, R.S., Kumar, V., and Robbins, S.L. (Eds.). (1994). *Robbins Pathologic Basis of Disease.* (5th ed.). Philadelphia: W.B. Saunders. (p. 653).

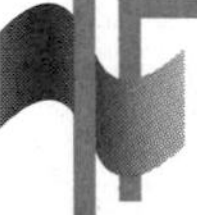

Clinical Scenario

D.Y., a 57-year-old machinist, underwent a bone marrow biopsy 2 weeks ago because of severe weakness. He was diagnosed with acute myeloid leukemia, M-5 type. He is now admitted to the oncology unit because of a frequent cough and a fever of 102.8°F. During the past year, D.Y. has lost 10 pounds unintentionally. He has been a lifelong pipe smoker and continues to smoke. He also has a history of peptic ulcer disease and herniated lumbar disk. Hematology studies reveal a low WBC count and a hemoglobin of 6.9. Three different antibiotics are ordered for D.Y., and he is scheduled for remission induction chemotherapy.

1. Could D.Y.'s leukemia account for his weakness, fever, and cough? Explain.
2. Why were antibiotics ordered? What additional interventions might be warranted?

Chronic Lymphocytic Leukemia

Definition. Chronic lymphocytic leukemia (CLL) is a slowly progressive malignant neoplasm of bone marrow origin in which the transformed cell is a mature B lymphocyte expressing the CD5 antigen.[35]

Epidemiology. CLL is the most common form of leukemia in Western countries. Median onset is at age 65 years, and more men than women are diagnosed.[36]

Etiology. The etiology of CLL is unknown.

Pathophysiology. Gradual acceleration of production of leukemic lymphocytes occurs within the marrow, crowding out normal cells, and infiltration of other organs with these cells eventually occurs, as in the acute leukemias. The leukemic B cells are greatly increased in number, but they are small cells that do not function normally in the humoral immune response (Color Fig. 12–6). If they do produce antibodies, these are inappropriately targeted to the patient's own RBCs.

Clinical Manifestations. CLL begins with the insidious onset of fatigue due to anemia. Increased numbers of lysed RBCs are filtered by the spleen, contributing to splenomegaly, and lymph node enlargement and hepatomegaly are also common. Deficiency in humoral immunity results in increased susceptibility to infections, and platelet deficiency causes bleeding tendencies.

Treatment. The disease is usually treated with chemotherapy (see Table 12–11).

Prognosis and Outcome. The clinical course of CLL is variable; some patients have normal life spans, whereas others die within 5 years of diagnosis. Median survival is 9 years.[36] Several staging systems have been identified as determinants of prognosis in CLL (Table 12–14).

Chronic Myeloid Leukemia

Definition. Chronic myeloid leukemia (CML) is a malignant neoplasm of bone marrow origin in which the transformed cell is the committed progenitor cell of the myeloid line.

Epidemiology. CML accounts for 15% to 20% of all leukemias and occurs primarily in middle-aged adults.[16] The prevalence of CML has been estimated at 1 to 1.5 cases per 100,000 population. Slightly more men than women are affected.[37] Exposure to ionizing radiation may confer increased risk.

Etiology. The etiology of CML is unknown. There does not appear to be a hereditary basis.

Pathophysiology. The genetic defect in the transformed cells is often a specific chromosomal translocation abnormality known as the *Philadelphia chromosome.* All cells originating from this precursor are

TABLE 12–14
STAGING SYSTEMS FOR CHRONIC LYMPHOCYTIC LEUKEMIAS

Stage	Risk	Clinical Features	Median Survival (mo)
Rai Staging System			
0	Low	Lymphocytosis alone	>150
I	Intermediate	Lymphocytosis; lymphadenopathy	101
II	Intermediate	Lymphocytosis; spleen or liver enlargement	>71
III	High	Lymphocytosis; anemia	19
IV	High	Lymphocytosis; thrombocytopenia	19
Binet Staging System			
A		No anemia; no thrombocytopenia; less than three lymphoid areas enlarged	>84
B		No anemia; no thrombocytopenia; three or more lymphoid areas enlarged	<60
C		Anemia or thrombocytopenia	<24

Adapted from Kipps, T.J. (1995). In: Beutler, E., Lichtmann, M.A., Coller, B.S., *et al.* (Eds.). *Williams Hematology.* (5th ed.). New York: McGraw-Hill. (pp. 1027–1028). Reproduced with permission of the McGraw-Hill Companies.

affected, resulting in rapid, disordered proliferation of the myeloid line. Because these cells, although abnormal, are usually functional, CML is often classified as a myeloproliferative disorder, along with polycythemia vera and essential thrombocythemia.

The disease progresses in two, or sometimes three, phases, beginning with a chronic phase in which leukocytes are elevated but manifestations are relatively moderate. An accelerated phase follows and may serve as a transition to a highly symptomatic, blastic phase. About half of patients with CML experience blast crisis, a sudden onset of accelerated proliferation of bone marrow cells, including pluripotent stem cells. Cells are immature and nonfunctional and include both myeloid cells and lymphoid cells.

Clinical Manifestations. Clinical manifestations of CML are due to the hypermetabolic state induced by rapid proliferation of myeloid cells. There is gradual onset of fatigue, weakness, and weight loss. Splenomegaly occurs due to increased RBC numbers and may cause obstructive abdominal symptoms. Large numbers of neutrophils, basophils, eosinophils, T lymphocytes, and possibly platelets are present in the blood. Neutrophil function is usually normal, and patients do not have an increased risk of infection during the chronic phase. Some patients have thrombocytopenia and anemia. During blast crisis, the clinical picture resembles acute leukemia with severe anemia, bleeding disorder, and immunodeficiency.

Prevention and Treatment. Exposure to ionizing radiation should be minimized, as discussed in Chapter 7. Chemotherapy with busulfan or hydroxyurea is beneficial in controlling cellular proliferation but has not significantly improved outcomes. More recently, α-interferon therapy has been associated with improved survival.[38] Allogenic bone marrow transplantation has resulted in long-term survival rates of 50% to 80%.[38]

Prognosis and Outcome. Median survival after diagnosis of CML depends on the phase of the disease. For those in the chronic phase, the long-term survival rate is 50% to 60%. This rate falls to 15% to 40% for those in the accelerated phase, and to less than 15% for those in the blastic phase.[38]

Hairy-Cell Leukemia

Definition. Hairy-cell leukemia (HCL) is a variant of the chronic leukemias in which the transformed cell is probably an immunoglobulin-bearing B cell. The term *hairy* refers to the prominent cytoplasmic projections on these cells.

Epidemiology. Risk factors and incidence groups are similar to those for CLL. HCL represents about 2% of all leukemias, with about 600 cases diagnosed each year in the United States.[38] Weak associations have been shown between HCL and prior exposure to organic chemicals or employment in woodworking or farming. The disease is four times more common in men. Onset is usually at about 50 years of age.

Etiology. The etiology is unknown. A genetic basis has been suggested by the finding of a familial pattern in some cases, with affected patients having the same HLA subtype (see Chapter 13).

Pathophysiology. The course of HCL is similar to that of CLL.

Clinical Manifestations. Massive splenomegaly is characteristic of HCL, and most patients also have pancytopenia with symptomatic anemia, bleeding, and infection.

Prevention and Treatment. Environmental and occupational risk factors should be minimized. Patients with HCL are closely monitored for the development of a reduction in all bone marrow cell lines (pancytopenia), which is treated with splenectomy, chemotherapy with nucleoside analogs (e.g., deoxycoformycin and chlorodeoxyadenosine), and α-interferon.

Prognosis and Outcome. Chemotherapy is palliative for all patients and curative for some. Without treatment, survival is about 4 years.[38]

Thrombocytopenias

Definition. Thrombocytopenia is a reduction (below 100,000/μL of blood) in the number of circulating platelets due to diminished production, altered distribution, or increased destruction of these cells.[39] True thrombocytopenia must be differentiated from pseudothrombocytopenia, in which the low platelet count is an artifact of laboratory procedures in which an anticoagulant (usually EDTA) used to preserve the specimen for analysis causes clumping of the platelets. Dilutional thrombocytopenia, which may result from rapid administration of large quantities of packed RBCs (platelet-poor blood) in treatment of hemorrhage, must also be differentiated from the true thrombocytopenias.[40]

Epidemiology. Thrombocytopenia may be congenital or acquired. Congenital forms are rare, whereas acquired thrombocytopenias, as a whole, are relatively common. Risk factors relate to the specific etiology.

Etiology. Three etiologic mechanisms may produce thrombocytopenia: decreased production or function, abnormal distribution, and increased destruction of platelets. Table 12–15 lists specific disorders associated with thrombocytopenia. Rare hereditary forms of thrombocytopenia include thrombocytopenia–absent radius (TAR) syndrome, Wiskott-Aldrich syndrome, May-Hegglin anomaly, Fanconi's anemia, and Alport's syndrome. In some of these conditions, platelets alone are reduced; in others, platelet reduction precedes reduction in other bone marrow cell lines. Acquired thrombocytopenia is much more common, and decreased platelet production or function may be associated with infection, nutritional deficiency, or bone marrow suppression secondary to toxins, neoplasia, radiation, and drugs such as antineoplastics, alcohol, or cocaine. Mechanisms resulting in acquired thrombocytopenia include impaired synthesis or damage to megakaryocytes and immune-mediated platelet destruction.

Thrombocytopenia secondary to altered distribution of platelets occurs with *hypersplenism,* a syndrome of splenic enlargement and reduction of circulating blood cells despite bone marrow hyperactivity. Although the total body platelet pool is normal, platelets are differentially trapped within the spleen, reducing their circulating numbers. Platelets are also sequestered in the liver and spleen during hypothermia.

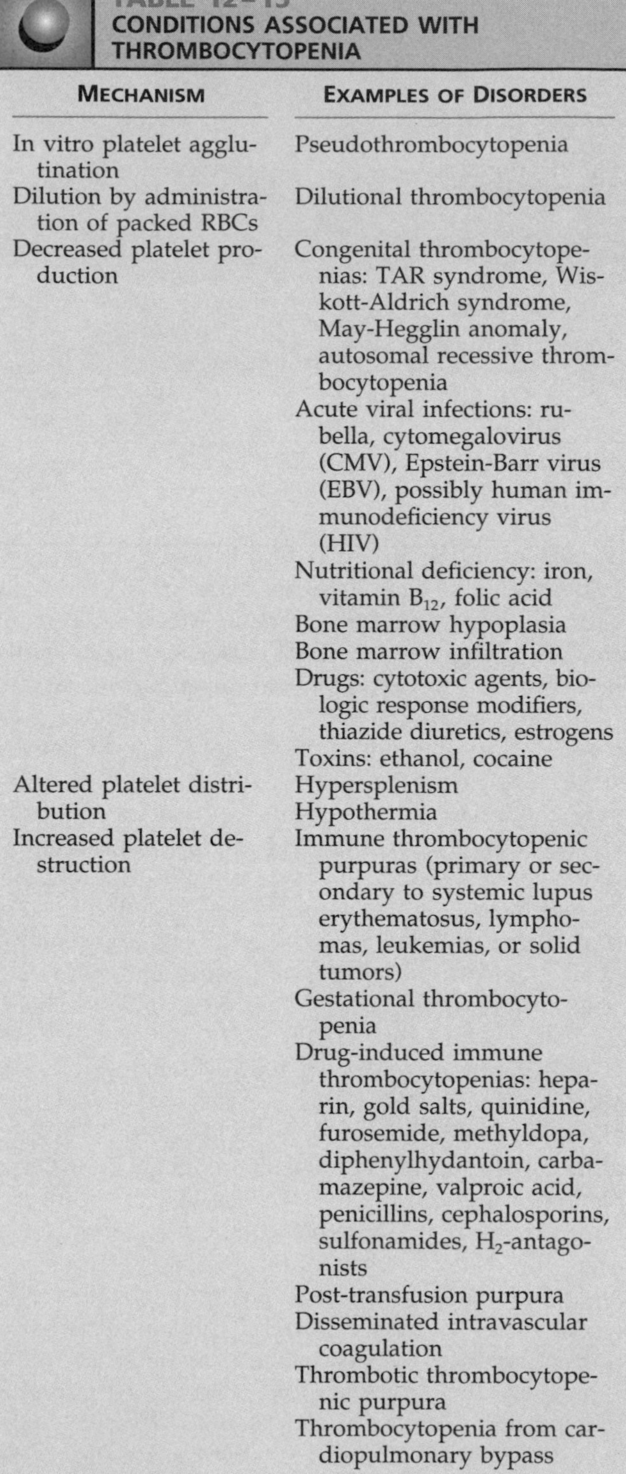

TABLE 12–15
CONDITIONS ASSOCIATED WITH THROMBOCYTOPENIA

Mechanism	Examples of Disorders
In vitro platelet agglutination	Pseudothrombocytopenia
Dilution by administration of packed RBCs	Dilutional thrombocytopenia
Decreased platelet production	Congenital thrombocytopenias: TAR syndrome, Wiskott-Aldrich syndrome, May-Hegglin anomaly, autosomal recessive thrombocytopenia
	Acute viral infections: rubella, cytomegalovirus (CMV), Epstein-Barr virus (EBV), possibly human immunodeficiency virus (HIV)
	Nutritional deficiency: iron, vitamin B_{12}, folic acid
	Bone marrow hypoplasia
	Bone marrow infiltration
	Drugs: cytotoxic agents, biologic response modifiers, thiazide diuretics, estrogens
	Toxins: ethanol, cocaine
Altered platelet distribution	Hypersplenism
	Hypothermia
Increased platelet destruction	Immune thrombocytopenic purpuras (primary or secondary to systemic lupus erythematosus, lymphomas, leukemias, or solid tumors)
	Gestational thrombocytopenia
	Drug-induced immune thrombocytopenias: heparin, gold salts, quinidine, furosemide, methyldopa, diphenylhydantoin, carbamazepine, valproic acid, penicillins, cephalosporins, sulfonamides, H_2-antagonists
	Post-transfusion purpura
	Disseminated intravascular coagulation
	Thrombotic thrombocytopenic purpura
	Thrombocytopenia from cardiopulmonary bypass

Data from Rutherford, C.J., and Frenkel, E.P. (1994). Thrombocytopenia: Issues in diagnosis and therapy. *Medical Clinics of North America* 78(3), 555–575.

Increased platelet destruction results in thrombocytopenia when the capacity of the bone marrow to increase megakaryocyte production, which is normally about three-fold, is exceeded. Three conditions are associated with thrombocytopenia by this mechanism: immune thrombocytopenic purpura, disseminated intravascular coagulation, and thrombotic thrombocytopenic purpura. The latter two are detailed in Chapter 14.

Immune thrombocytopenic purpura includes several disorders in which antibodies or immune complexes bound to the platelet membrane cause removal of these cells from the circulation. Primary autoimmune thrombocytopenic purpura, formerly known as idiopathic thrombocytopenic purpura, is common in adults, particularly in young women. Secondary immune thrombocytopenic purpura is seen in association with other autoimmune disorders, including systemic lupus erythematosus, with human immunodeficiency virus infection, and with neoplasias, particularly leukemias and lymphomas. About 8% of pregnant women have a mild thrombocytopenia that subsides after delivery. The cause of this gestational thrombocytopenia is unknown but is not believed to be immune mediated.[40]

Many drugs are known to induce thrombocyte destruction by an immune mechanism. As discussed in Chapter 13, drugs may act as partial antigens (haptens) that initiate antibody production, or may bind circulating antibody and create immune complexes that initiate an inflammatory response. The platelet membrane may be a target of these processes. Destruction of platelets may also be caused by increased consumption during thrombosis in disseminated intravascular coagulation and thrombotic thrombocytopenic purpura, as discussed in Chapter 14. Finally, platelets may be depleted as a consequence of their adhesion to artificial surfaces, as during cardiopulmonary bypass.

Pathophysiology. Deficiency of platelets impairs the platelet phase of the hemostatic response (see Chapter 14), predisposing the patient to bleeding.

Clinical Manifestations. At platelet counts below 100,000/μL, laboratory coagulation studies are abnormal, with progressively prolonged bleeding times (see Chapter 14). When counts fall below 50,000, excessive bleeding is apparent with trauma or surgery. Spontaneous bleeding is not usually seen until platelets fall below 15,000/μL.[40]

Prevention and Treatment. Frequent monitoring of platelet counts is warranted in patients at risk due to disease or therapy, as is clinical assessment for signs of bleeding (see Chapter 14). Offending drugs are discontinued if possible. The treatment of choice for thrombocytopenias due to decreased production or function is transfusion of platelets. Antifibrinolytic drugs, such as aminocaproic acid (Amicar), may also be used to decrease bleeding in relatively mild thrombocytopenias. Thrombocytopenia due to hypersplenism usually does not require intervention because platelets may be mobilized from the spleen during stress. Rewarming of hypothermic patients reverses platelet sequestration in these cases. Immune-mediated thrombocytopenias may be treated with corticosteroids, splenectomy, or cytotoxic drugs, such as cyclosporin A, cyclophosphamide, and azathioprine.

Prognosis and Outcome. Many mild thrombocytopenias are self-limited. Severity and outcome are variable with immune-mediated thrombocytopenias and hereditary disorders. Although some hereditary thrombocytopenias (e.g., Fanconi's anemia and TAR syndrome) lead to early death, most of these syndromes run a chronic course, and life-threatening bleeding episodes are uncommon.

Essential Thrombocythemia

Definition. Essential, or primary, thrombocythemia is a myeloproliferative disorder resulting from proliferation of the myeloid stem cell.[41]

Epidemiology. Essential thrombocythemia was once considered rare but is now known to be increasing in incidence in younger patients, probably as a consequence of improved screening of platelet counts. Most patients are between the ages of 50 and 70 years, with men and women equally affected. Known risk factors include use of dark hair dyes, exposure to organic solvents or radon, and employment as an electrical worker.[41] Rarely, a familial pattern is seen.

Etiology. The precise etiology is unknown.

Pathophysiology. The fraction of megakaryocytes in the bone marrow is increased, possibly due to abnormal responsiveness of this line to hematopoietic growth factors. The reason for the preferential proliferation of megakaryocytes rather than other myeloid lines is unknown.[42]

Clinical Manifestations. The serum platelet count is greater than 600,000/μL. Mild splenomegaly is present in 40% of patients and may be the only physical sign.[42] Others may have thickening of the aortic and mitral valves. The incidence of bleeding or clotting abnormalities is highly variable among patients with essential thrombocythemia. If abnormal clotting occurs, it is more often arterial than venous.

Prevention and Treatment. Asymptomatic patients may not require therapy, but they should be closely monitored for bleeding or clotting complications. Bleeding may result from adsorption of von Willebrand factor (which promotes platelet clumping in early blood clotting) by the large numbers of platelets.[43] Inappropriate clotting (thrombosis) is more

Developmental Perspective

Embryonic and Fetal Periods

Fetal uptake of oxygen is favored by the 50% greater hemoglobin concentration in fetal versus maternal blood, and by the higher affinity of fetal hemoglobin, hemoglobin F. Erythropoiesis begins in the "blood islands" of the yolk sac at about 14 days' gestation. At 6 to 8 weeks' gestation, erythropoiesis begins in the fetal liver and spleen, under the influence of erythropoietin. The embryonic hemoglobins, Gower 1, Gower 2, and Portland, are produced during erythropoiesis in the yolk sac. Production of hemoglobin F begins in the liver and at term constitutes up to 95% of hemoglobin. Hemoglobin A synthesis begins in the fetal marrow and may constitute up to 45% of hemoglobin at term. Genetic defects in hemoglobin synthesis (hemoglobinopathies) may occur. At term, bone marrow erythropoiesis is fully established. Leukopoiesis begins with granulocyte production in the fetal liver by the 7th week of gestation and in the bone marrow by the 10th week. Lymphocyte production is observed in fetal lymphatic tissues at 9 to 11 weeks. Megakaryocytes are present in the yolk sac and liver by 6 weeks of gestation, in the spleen by 10 weeks, and in the bone marrow by 13 weeks. Maternal use of drugs, such as diazoxide and thiazide diuretics, may induce thrombocytopenia.

Infancy and Childhood

Normally, the term infant is somewhat polycythemic, with an increase in the number of reticulocytes reflecting the rapid rate of erythropoiesis. Premature infants are prone to anemia, which may be iatrogenic, physiologic, or nonphysiologic. Iatrogenic anemia is due to frequent drawing of blood samples for testing. Physiologic anemia is due to the normal hemolysis of fetal RBCs, which have a life span two thirds as long as that of adult RBCs. Also, increased tissue oxygenation results in decreased erythropoietin stimulation of erythropoiesis. Nonphysiologic anemia of prematurity is due to an idiopathic reduction in erythropoietin. Growing children have increased requirements for iron, vitamin B_{12}, and folic acid and are thus at increased risk of nutritional anemias. Neutrophil counts are lower in preterm infants than in term infants, with a higher proportion of immature forms (bands). Infants and young children are at higher risk of morbidity and mortality due to infection than are older children and adults. Newborn platelet counts are similar to adult values in healthy term and preterm infants, but thrombocytopenia is common in those with respiratory distress, sepsis, intrauterine growth retardation, and congenital anomalies.

Adolescence and Young Adulthood

Young women are prone to iron-deficiency anemia related to menstrual blood loss or to the increased demands of pregnancy. Deficiency of folic acid during pregnancy results in megaloblastic anemia in the mother and increases the risk of neural tube defects in the fetus. Adherence to a strict vegetarian diet is also more common in this age group and may predispose to nutritional anemia. Many leukemias have their onset during this period, and thrombotic thrombocytopenic purpura has its highest incidence in this age group.

Middle and Older Adulthood

Anemia is never the result of old age, per se. Although iron stores are increased in the elderly, iron-deficiency anemia is common and is usually caused by slow blood loss secondary to gastrointestinal disorders, such as polyps, peptic ulcer disease, hiatal hernia, diverticulitis, gastritis, or colon cancer. The cellularity of the bone marrow decreases in old age, possibly related to a reduction in the volume of cancellous bone due to osteoporosis. This constitutes a reduction in marrow reserve capacity rather than a primary deficiency syndrome. Neutrophil counts do not decrease with age. The lymphocyte count is usually stable as well, but the immune response is diminished. Although the platelet count does not change with age, platelets are more reactive to mediators of clotting.

likely. Treatment in those at high risk may include cytoreductive drugs such as hydroxyurea, anagrelide, or α-interferon. Removal of platelets from the serum (pheresis) has also been used, but the reduction in platelets is transient and may induce a rebound increase in bone marrow production.[8]

Prognosis and Outcome. Most patients with essential thrombocythemia have a normal life expectancy.[43] About one third of patients experience thrombotic complications.

CLINICAL SIGNIFICANCE OF ALTERED HEMATOPOIESIS

Clinical examination of the blood is not limited to disorders of the hematopoietic system; indeed, it is routine in the diagnosis and monitoring of disorders of *all* body systems. Blood is easily accessed for study, and hematologic research is rapidly clarifying the mechanisms underlying altered hematopoiesis in many disease states (see Focus of Current Research). Hematologic disorders may affect the developing fetus as well as patients of all ages (see Developmental Perspective). Normal function of hematopoietic cells underlies the critical processes of tissue oxygenation, tissue defense against invasion, wound healing, and maintenance of the integrity of the circulation. These processes are further examined in Chapters 13 and 14.

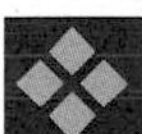

Summary of Key Points

- Blood is composed of a fluid component (plasma) and a cellular component, which consists of RBCs (erythrocytes), WBCs (leukocytes), and platelets (thrombocytes). Plasma serves as a transport medium for water and for suspended particles and cells. Erythrocytes are critical to the transport of oxygen within the blood. Leukocyte function underlies the inflammatory and immune responses, and thrombocytes are essential to hemostasis.
- All blood cells originate from a single type of bone marrow cell: the pluripotent stem cell. Under the selective regulation of hematopoietic growth factors and transcription factors, these stem cells differentiate and proliferate in a cascade mechanism that culminates in the formation of lineage specific cells. Because hematopoietic stem cells also have the unique ability to self-replicate by asymmetric mitosis, a constant supply of stem cells is maintained within the bone marrow.
- An excess of RBCs (polycythemia) may result from a primary idiopathic process or, more commonly, may occur secondary to hypoxia-induced excess of the growth factor erythropoietin. Increased numbers of WBCs (leukocytosis) may occur with neoplasia (e.g., leukemia) or in response to mediators of inflammation or immune responses. Thrombocyte excess (thrombocytosis) may result from inappropriate stimulation of megakaryopoiesis (as in essential thrombocythemia) or may be a reaction to a number of disorders in which release of platelet-stimulating factor is increased. Deficiencies of any or all three cell types may result from decreased production of cells, increased consumption or sequestration of cells, or increased destruction of cells.
- Erythrocyte excess (polycythemia) manifests as engorgement of blood vessels due to the increased blood volume and viscosity, which slow tissue perfusion. Anemia generally manifests as hypoxia due to deficient oxygen-carrying capacity of the blood. Leukocyte excess (leukocytosis) may be adaptive, manifesting as enhanced inflammatory and immune responses. If WBCs are nonfunctional, however, the excess cells may infiltrate tissues and consume substrates that would otherwise be available to normal hematopoiesis. Leukocyte deficiency (leukopenia) confers increased risk of infection and neoplasia owing to diminished immune capacity. Excess or deficit of thrombocytes manifests as a disorder of bleeding or inappropriate blood clotting.
- Clinical intervention in hematopoietic disorders may include transplantation of bone marrow or peripheral blood stem cells to compensate for bone marrow failure due to primary disease or therapy. Excess numbers of cells may be removed by plasmapheresis or exchange transfusion, with subsequent infusion of normal blood or plasma. Hematopoietic processes may be enhanced or suppressed with drugs that facilitate or inhibit the hematopoietic cascade. When the substrate for erythrocyte synthesis is deficient, supplementation (e.g., of iron, folic acid, or vitamin B_{12}) is indicated.
- The importance of hematopoietic disorders is evident in the critical nature of the functions

Summary continued on following page

served by blood cells: delivery of oxygen to tissues, defense against tissue invasion and neoplasia, healing of tissue injuries, and maintenance of the integrity of the circulation.

REFERENCES

1. Babior, B.M., and Stossel, T.P. (1990). *Hematology: A Pathophysiologic Approach.* (2nd ed.). New York: Churchill-Livingstone. (pp. 5, 106, 132, 205, 278).
2. Sahai, J., and Louie, S.G. (1993). Overview of the immune and hematopoietic systems. *American Journal of Hospital Pharmacy* 50(suppl. 3), S4–S9.
3. Champlin, R.E. (1996). Peripheral blood progenitor cells: A replacement for marrow transplantation? *Seminars in Oncology* 23(2 suppl. 4), 15–21.
4. Porter, D.L., and Goldberg, M.A. (1994). Physiology of erythropoietin production. *Seminars in Hematology* 31(2), 112–121.
5. D'Andrea, A.D. (1994). Cytokine receptors in congenital hematopoietic disease. *New England Journal of Medicine* 330(12), 839–846.
6. Loeb, S. (Ed.), *et al.* (1994). *Illustrated Guide to Diagnostic Tests.* (Student Version). Springhouse, PA: Springhouse Corporation. (p. 9).
7. Bernini, J.C. (1996). Diagnosis and management of chronic neutropenia during childhood. *Pediatric Clinics of North America* 43(2), 773–792.
8. Shuey, K.M. (1996). Platelet-associated bleeding disorders. *Seminars in Oncology Nursing* 12(1), 15–27.
9. Erickson, J.M. (1996). Anemia. *Seminars in Oncology Nursing* 12(1), 2–14.
10. Beard, J. (1995). One person's view of iron deficiency, development, and cognitive function. *American Journal of Clinical Nutrition* 62(4), 709–710.
11. Karnad, A.B., and Krozser-Hamati, A. (1992). Pernicious anemia: Early identification to prevent permanent sequelae. *Postgraduate Medicine* 91(2), 231–237.
12. Pruthi, R.K., and Tefferi, A. (1994). Pernicious anemia revisited. *Mayo Clinic Proceedings* 69(2), 144–150.
13. Samuels-Reid, J.H. (1994). Common problems in sickle cell disease. *American Family Physician* 49(6), 1477–1486.
14. Burdick, E. (1994). Sickle cell disease: Still a management challenge. *Postgraduate Medicine* 96(8), 107–115.
15. Platt, O.S., Brambilla, D.J., Rosse, W.F., *et al.* (1994). Mortality in sickle cell disease: Life expectancy and risk factors for early death. *New England Journal of Medicine* 330(23), 1639–1644.
16. Cotran, R.S., Kumar, V., and Robbins, S.L. (1994). *Robbins Pathologic Basis of Disease* (5th ed.). Philadelphia: W.B. Saunders Co. (pp. 589, 606, 651, 654).
17. Knoop, T. (1996). Polycythemia vera. *Seminars in Oncology Nursing* 12(1), 70–77.
18. Gruppo Italiano Studio Policitemia. (1995). Polycythemia vera: The natural history of 1213 patients followed for 20 years. *Annals of Internal Medicine* 123(9), 656–664.
19. Sassa, S. (1995). The porphyrias. In: Beutler, E., Lichtman, M.A., Coller, B.S., *et al.* (Eds.). *Williams Hematology.* (5th ed.). New York: McGraw-Hill. (pp. 726–750).
20. Resor, S.S., and Beare, P.G. (1995). Acute intermittent porphyria: A nursing case study. *Critical Care Nurse* 15(6), 35–43.
21. Tefferi, A., Solberg, L.A. Jr., and Ellefson, R.D. (1994). Porphyrias: Clinical evaluation and interpretation of laboratory tests. *Mayo Clinic Proceedings* 69(3), 289–290.
22. Tefferi, A., Colgan, J.P., and Solberg, L.A. Jr., (1994). Acute porphyrias: Diagnosis and management. *Mayo Clinic Proceedings* 69(10), 991–995.
23. Kauppinen, R., and Mustajoki, P. (1992). Prognosis of acute porphyria: Occurrence of acute attacks, precipitating factors, and associated diseases. *Medicine* 71(1), 1–13.
24. Tavel, A.S., and Bacon, B.R. (1990). Hemochromatosis: Iron metabolism and the iron overload syndromes. In: Zakim, D., and Boyer, T.D. (Eds). *Hepatology: A Textbook of Liver Disease.* Philadelphia: W.B. Saunders Co. (pp. 1273–1294).
25. Wurapa, R.K., Gordeuk, V.R., Brittenham, G.M., *et al.* (1996). Primary iron overload in African Americans. *American Journal of Medicine* 1996(101), 9–18.
26. Edwards, C.Q., and Kushner, J.P. (1993). Screening for hemochromatosis. *New England Journal of Medicine* 328(220), 1616–1620.
27. Olynyk, J.K., and Bacon, B.R. (1994). Hereditary hemochromatosis: Detecting and correcting iron overload. *Postgraduate Medicine* 96(5), 151–165.
28. Little, D.R. (1996). Hemochromatosis: Diagnosis and management. *American Family Physician* 53(8), 2623–2528.
29. Pui, C-H., and Crist, W.M. (1994). Biology and treatment of acute lymphoblastic leukemia. *Journal of Pediatrics* 124(4), 491–503.
30. Pui, C-H. (1995). Childhood leukemias. *New England Journal of Medicine* 332(24), 1618–1630.
31. Cline, M.J. (1994). The molecular basis of leukemia. *New England Journal of Medicine* 330(5), 328–336.
32. Haupt, R., Fears, T.R., Robison, L.L., *et al.* (1994). Educational attainment in long-term survivors of childhood acute lymphoblastic leukemia. *Journal of the American Medical Association* 272(18), 1427–1432.
33. Kantarjian, H.M. (1994). Adult acute lymphocytic leukemia: Critical review of current knowledge. *American Journal of Medicine* 1994(97), 176–183.
34. Wujcik, D. (1993). Leukemia. In: Groenwald, S.L., Frogge, M.H., Goodman, M., *et al.* (Eds.). *Cancer Nursing: Principles and Practice.* (3rd ed.). Boston: Jones & Bartlett. (p. 1151).
35. Foon, K.A., Thiruvengadam, R., Saven, A., *et al.* (1993). Genetic relatedness of lymphoid malignancies: Transformation of chronic lymphocytic leukemia as a model. *Annals of Internal Medicine* 119(1), 63–73.
36. Rozman, C., and Montserrat, E. (1995). Chronic lymphocytic leukemia. *New England Journal of Medicine* 333(16), 1052–1057.
37. Cortes, J.E., Talpaz, M., and Kantarjian, H. (1996). Chronic myelogenous leukemia: A review. *American Journal of Medicine* 1996(100), 555–570.
38. Kipps, T.J., and Robbins, B.A. (1995). Hairy-cell leukemia. In: Beutler, E., Lichtman, M.A., Coller, B.S., *et al.* (Eds.). *Williams Hematology.* (5th ed.). New York: McGraw-Hill. (pp. 1040–1047).
39. Homans, A. (1996). Thrombocytopenia in the neonate. *Pediatric Clinics of North America* 43(3), 737–756.
40. Rutherford, C.J., and Frenkel, E.P. (1994). Thrombocytopenia: Issues in diagnosis and therapy. *Medical Clinics of North America* 78(3), 555–575.
41. Mele, A., Visani, G., Pulsoni, A., *et al.* (1996). Risk factors for essential thrombocythemia: A case-control study. *Cancer* 77(10), 2157–2161.
42. Schafer, A.J. (1995). Essential (primary) thrombocythemia. In: Beutler, E., Lichtman, M.A., Coller, B.S., *et al. Williams Hematology.* (5th ed.). New York: McGraw-Hill. (pp. 340–345).
43. Tefferi, A., and Hoagland, H.C. (1994). Issues in the diagnosis and management of essential thrombocythemia. *Mayo Clinic Proceedings* 69(7), 651–655.

SELECTED BIBLIOGRAPHY

Abshire, T.C. (1996). The anemia of inflammation: A common cause of childhood anemia. *Pediatric Clinics of North America* 43(3), 623–637.

Adamson, J.W. (1996). Regulation of red blood cell production. *American Journal of Medicine* 101(suppl. 2A), 4S–6S.

Aoki, R.Y., and Saad, S.T.O. (1995). Enalapril reduces the albuminuria of patients with sickle cell disease. *American Journal of Medicine* 1995(98), 432–435.

Armitage, J.O. (1994). Bone marrow transplantation. *New England Journal of Medicine* 330(12), 827–838.

Blackburn, S.T., and Loper, D.L. (1992). *Maternal, Fetal, and Neonatal Physiology: A Clinical Perspective*. Philadelphia: W.B. Saunders Co.

Brenner, M.K. (1996). Gene transfer to hematopoietic cells. *New England Journal of Medicine* 335(5), 337–339.

Craig, W.J. (1994). Iron status of vegetarians. *American Journal of Clinical Nutrition* 59(suppl.), 1233S–1237S.

Davenport, J. (1996). Macrocytic anemia. *American Family Physician* 53(1), 155–162.

Foster, R.L.R., Hunsberger, M.M., and Anderson, J.J.T. (1989). *Family-Centered Nursing Care of Children*. Philadelphia: W.B. Saunders Co.

Fraser, J.K., Lill, M.C.C., and Figlin, R.A. (1996). The biology of the cytokine sequence cascade. *Seminars in Oncology* 23(2 suppl. 4), 2–8.

George, J.N., El-Harake, M.A., and Raskob, G.E. (1994). Chronic idiopathic thrombocytopenic purpura. *New England Journal of Medicine* 331(18), 1207–1211.

Goldstein, K.H., and Abramson, N. (1996). Efficient diagnosis of thrombocytopenia. *American Family Physician* 53(3), 915–920.

Greenburg, A.G. (1996). Pathophysiology of anemia. *American Journal of Medicine* 1996(101 suppl. 2A), 7S–11S.

Johnson, M.A., Fischer, J.G., Bowman, B.A., *et al.* (1994). Iron nutriture in elderly individuals. *FASEB Journal* 8(9), 609–621.

Klein, H.G. (1996). New insights into the management of anemia in the surgical patient. *American Journal of Medicine* 1996(101 suppl. 2A), 12S–15S.

Kurtzberg, J., Laughlin, M., Graham, M.L., *et al.* (1996). Placental blood as a source of hematopoietic stem cells for transplantation into unrelated recipients. *New England Journal of Medicine* 335(3), 157–166.

Lane, P.A. (1996). Sickle cell disease. *Pediatric Clinics of North America* 43(3), 639–664.

Laporte, J-P., Gorin, N-C., Rubinstein, P., *et al.* (1996). Cord-blood transplantation from an unrelated donor in an adult with chronic myelogenous leukemia. *New England Journal of Medicine* 335(3), 167–170.

Louie, S.G., and Jung, B. (1993). Clinical effects of biological response modifiers. *American Journal of Hospital Pharmacy* 50(suppl. 3), S10–S18.

Lozoff, B., Wolf, A.W., and Jiminez, E. (1996). Iron-deficiency anemia and infant development: Effects of extended oral iron therapy. *Journal of Pediatrics* 129(3), 382–389.

Medeiros, D., and Buchanan, G.R. (1996). Current controversies in the management of idiopathic thrombocytopenic purpura during childhood. *Pediatric Clinics of North America* 43(3), 757–772.

Montserrat, E., and Rozman, C. (1994). Current approaches to the treatment and management of chronic lymphocytic leukemia. *Drugs* 47(suppl. 6), 1–9.

Moore, D.F., and Sears, D.A. (1994). Pica, iron deficiency, and the medical history. *American Journal of Medicine* 1994(97), 390–393.

Moses, P.L., and Smith, R.E. (1995). Endoscopic evaluation of iron deficiency anemia: A guide to diagnostic strategy in older patients. *Postgraduate Medicine* 98(2), 213–226.

Ogawa, M. (1994). Hematopoiesis. *Journal of Allergy and Clinical Immunology* 94(3 Pt. 2), 645–650.

Orkin, S.H. (1995). Transcription factors and hematopoietic development. *Journal of Biological Chemistry* 270(10), 4955–4958.

Rapaport, R., Oberfield, S.E., Robison, L., *et al.* (1995). Relationship of growth hormone deficiency and leukemia. *Journal of Pediatrics* 126(5 Pt. 1), 759–761.

Ravindranath, Y., Yeager, A.M., Chang, M.N., *et al.* (1996). Autologous bone marrow transplantation versus intensive consolidation chemotherapy for acute myeloid leukemia in childhood. *New England Journal of Medicine* 334(22), 1428–1434.

Rowe, J.M., Ciobanu, N., Ascensao, J., *et al.* (1994). Recommended guidelines for the management of autologous and allogenic bone marrow transplantation. *Annals of Internal Medicine* 120(2), 143–158.

Sanders, T.A.B. (1995). Vegetarian diets and children. *Pediatric Clinics of North America* 42(2), 955–965.

Shpall, E.J., Gee, A.P., Hogan, C., *et al.* (1996). Bone marrow metastasis. *Hematology/Oncology Clinics of North America* 10(2), 321–343.

Sodeman, W.A. Jr., and Sodeman, T.M. (1985). *Sodeman's Pathologic Physiology: Mechanisms of Disease*. (7th ed.). Philadelphia: W.B. Saunders Co.

Spivak, J.L. (1993). Recombinant erythropoietin. *Annual Review of Medicine* 44, 243–253.

Stasi, R., Stipa, E., Masi, M., *et al.* (1995). Long-term observation of 208 adults with chronic idiopathic thrombocytopenic purpura. *American Journal of Medicine* 1995(98), 436–442.

United States Public Health Service. (1995). Adult screening for anemia and hemoglobinopathies. *Nurse Practitioner* 20(12), 48–51.

Walters, M.C., and Abelson, H.T. (1996). Interpretation of the complete blood count. *Pediatric Clinics of North America* 43(3), 599–622.

CHAPTER 13

Inflammation, Immunity, and Related Disorders

LEARNING OBJECTIVES

1. Define inflammation and immunity within the context of tissue defense.
2. Describe the roles of plasma constituents, blood cells, the hematopoietic system, the tissue macrophage system, mast cells, endothelial cells, and epithelial cells in the inflammatory and immune responses.
3. Discuss the possible ways in which the inflammatory and immune responses may be initiated.
4. Explain the physiologic basis of the local and systemic clinical manifestations of inflammation.
5. Differentiate among the usual outcomes of inflammation: healing, chronic inflammation, and granuloma formation.
6. Discuss the variables that may affect the process of wound healing.
7. Describe the nature of antigens and the process of antigen challenge in initiation of the immune response.
8. Discuss the principal elements of the humoral and cell-mediated immune responses.
9. Differentiate among the four categories of immunopathology.
10. Comprehend the pathophysiologic processes that predict clinical manifestations and rationalize clinical interventions in selected disorders of tissue defense.

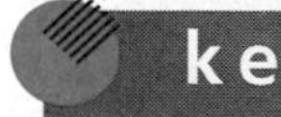

key terms

ABO incompatibility
acquired immunodeficiency syndrome
allergen
allergy
anaphylactoid reaction
anaphylaxis
antibody
antigen
arachidonic acid
autoantibody
autoantigen
autoimmunity
cell-mediated immunity
chemotaxis

complement
epitope
exudation
fibrin
graft rejection
graft-versus-host disease
hapten
Hodgkin's disease
human leukocyte antigen
humoral immunity
hyperemia
hypersensitivity
immunity
immunization
immunodeficiency
immunoglobulin
infection
infectious mononucleosis
inflammation
isoimmunity
lymphoma
lymphoproliferative disorder
non-Hodgkin's lymphoma
regeneration
repair
resolution
Rh incompatibility
sepsis
superantigen
systemic inflammatory response syndrome
transfusion reaction

Cells can be injured by many different agents and mechanisms, and cellular injury is the common denominator in all disease. The human system has three lines of defense against injury and invasion. The physical and chemical barriers of the intact skin and mucous membranes constitute the first line of defense (Table 13–1). When these barriers are breached, **inflammation** and nonspecific mechanisms of **immunity** form the second line of defense. These responses are essentially the same regardless of the nature of the injuring or invading agent. The third line of defense consists of the *specific* immune responses mounted by antibodies and activated cells that target invading microorganisms (**infection**) or neoplastic cells. These lines of defense are interdependent.

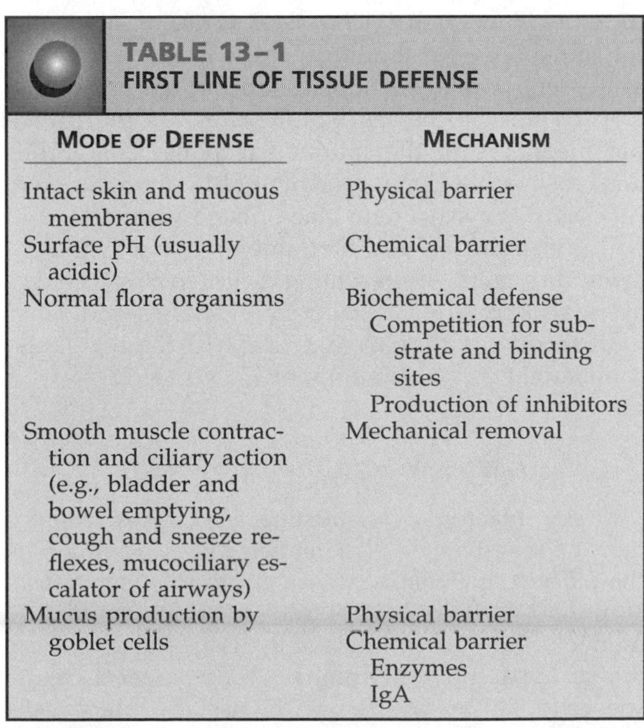

TABLE 13–1
FIRST LINE OF TISSUE DEFENSE

Mode of Defense	Mechanism
Intact skin and mucous membranes	Physical barrier
Surface pH (usually acidic)	Chemical barrier
Normal flora organisms	Biochemical defense Competition for substrate and binding sites Production of inhibitors
Smooth muscle contraction and ciliary action (e.g., bladder and bowel emptying, cough and sneeze reflexes, mucociliary escalator of airways)	Mechanical removal
Mucus production by goblet cells	Physical barrier Chemical barrier Enzymes IgA

Inflammation is a critical homeostatic process that is activated by cellular injury regardless of the mechanism of that injury. Inflammation is essentially local in nature, although cellular mediators released during inflammation may initiate systemic responses as well. **Systemic inflammatory response syndrome** is the most extreme form of inflammatory response and may be life-threatening in critically ill patients. This syndrome nearly always occurs in the setting of systemic infection and is termed **sepsis** in such cases.

The immune system is a functional network of cells and tissues that constitutes the most powerful line of tissue defense. This system defends against injury to body cells by foreign, or nonself, proteins (**antigens**), including microorganisms and genetically altered self antigens such as those produced by cancer cells. The cells that mount immune responses are derived primarily from bone marrow stem cells. Lymphocyte function is central to the immune response, although monocyte-macrophages are as important to immunity as to inflammation.

Immunologic mechanisms often trigger inflammation and the complement cascade as a means of destroying invading agents. Immune responses may also destroy or inactivate invading agents without inflammation, however, and the hallmark of the immune response is the development of specific proteins (**antibodies** or **immunoglobulins**) and activated lymphocytes (cytotoxic T lymphocytes) directed against these agents.

Immune responses differ from inflammation not only in their specificity but also in the time course of the reactions. The local inflammatory response begins instantaneously with cell injury, and clinical manifestations are apparent within 1 to 2 hours. Systemic manifestations of inflammation (the acute phase response) occur within 8 to 12 hours.[1] Specific immune responses are generated more slowly, often requiring days to weeks to establish an adequate serum level of antibodies or an adequate population of activated cytotoxic T lymphocytes.

Inflammatory processes are defensive or adaptive by design; however, they may contribute to distressing clinical manifestations of disease at the same time they are helping to eradicate it. In some cases, such as when inflammation is excessive or when it occurs in enclosed spaces (e.g., joints, cranium), inflammation may contribute to additional cellular injury. In systemic inflammatory response syndrome, a hypermetabolic response often results in multiple organ failure. Sepsis is the 13th leading cause of death in the United States.[2]

Like inflammation, immune responses evolved for an adaptive purpose; but when dysfunctional, immune responses may constitute mechanisms of disease. Adaptive immune responses require the system to (1) differentiate self from nonself antigens and (2) destroy nonself antigens. Direct cellular communication, the complexity of which is increasingly appreciated, is essential to achieve the specificity in target selection and response that defines adaptive immunity.

In this chapter, the phases, components, and regulation of the inflammatory and immune responses are detailed. Both adaptive and pathologic forms of inflammation and immunity are discussed. Specific disorders characterized by inflammation and immune responses are found throughout subsequent systems chapters; however, selected disorders influencing multiple systems are included here as examples of alterations in tissue defense. These include the **lymphomas, infectious mononucleosis,** and **acquired immunodeficiency syndrome (AIDS).**

INFLAMMATION AND HEALING

Overview of the Inflammatory Response

The sequence of events in inflammation may be summarized as follows: (1) cellular injury; (2) local vasodilation, increased capillary permeability, cellular adhesion, and exudation to bring inflammatory cells and chemical mediators to the injured area; (3) destruction of injurious agents by phagocytes; (4) clearing away of cellular debris; and (5) deposition of a protein framework for tissue healing. During the course of inflammation, cellular mediators are released, and in the plasma, chain reaction (cascade) responses activate other protein mediators. These reactions result in formation of substances that augment the inflammatory response and produce systemic signs and symptoms. The ideal outcome of inflammation is complete removal of the injurious agent and return of tissues to their preinjury state. Numerous factors, including the nature and extent of the injury, the type of tissue injured, and the ability of the body's systems to deliver adequate nutrients and oxygen, influence the potential for tissue healing.

Components of the Inflammatory Response System

The components of the inflammatory response system are found in connective tissues of the body, primarily in the blood, blood vessels, and tissues adjacent to vessels.

Plasma Constituents

Antibodies are found in the globulin fraction of plasma proteins. This fraction also contains the **complement** and kinin system proteins, which are important in inflammation. Another protein, fibrinogen, forms a physical barrier around the site of inflammation and lays down a meshwork scaffold for the healing process.

Blood Cells

As discussed in Chapter 12, the primary functions of white blood cells (WBCs; leukocytes) relate to the inflammatory and immune responses. Neutrophils are essential phagocytic cells during the inflammatory response, whereas lymphocytes are the principal mediators of the immune responses. Basophils and eosinophils have a similar, but more limited, role, as discussed later. Macrophages are critical to both inflammation and immunity, serving as phagocytes and antigen-presenting cells (APCs). Leukocytes also secrete a number of cytokines and other local mediators that are important in the regulation of inflammation and immunity (Table 13–2).

Tissue Macrophage System

Tissue macrophages (histiocytes) are a component of a system of phagocytic cells also known as the *reticuloendothelial system* or *lymphoreticular system.* Some of these cells are derived from circulating monocytes, which migrate into tissues and mature; others apparently differentiate from connective tissue cells within the tissues themselves. These cells

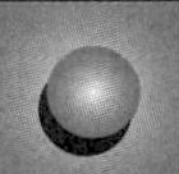

TABLE 13–2
CELLULAR MEDIATORS OF INFLAMMATION

Mediator	Source	Effect
Cytokines		
Interleukins		
IL-1	Macrophages, lymphocytes, neutrophils, epithelial cells, fibroblasts	Regulation of hematopoiesis Pyrogenic activity Tissue catabolism Stimulation of prostaglandin and adhesion molecule synthesis Activation of neutrophils
IL-3	T lymphocytes, monocytes	Colony-stimulating factor
IL-4	T lymphocytes	Colony-stimulating factor
IL-5	T lymphocytes	Eosinophil differentiation Monocyte-macrophage differentiation
IL-6	Monocytes, endothelial cells, fibroblasts, T lymphocytes	Colony-stimulating factor Antiviral effects
IL-8	Monocytes, neutrophils, endothelial cells, virally infected fibroblasts	Activation of neutrophils Chemotactic factor
IL-9	T lymphocytes	Colony-stimulating factor Mast cell stimulation
IL-10	Lymphocytes	Immune response regulation Mast cell stimulation
IL-13	T lymphocytes	Inhibition of proinflammatory interleukins
Tumor necrosis factor	T lymphocytes, endotoxin-stimulated macrophages	Pyrogenic factor Phagocyte activation
Transforming growth factor	Macrophages	Hematopoietic regulation Stimulation of endothelial and fibroblast growth
Transforming growth factor-β	Platelets	Tissue remodeling during wound healing Limitation of inflammatory response
Platelet-derived growth factor	Platelets, macrophages, endothelial cells	Stimulation of wound healing
Basic fibroblast growth factor	Endothelial cells and others	Stimulation of blood vessel growth Stimulation of mitosis
Interferons	Leukocytes, fibroblasts, activated T lymphocytes	Antiviral effects Phagocyte activation
Colony-stimulating factors	Monocyte-macrophages, endothelial cells, fibroblasts	Activation of neutrophils, monocyte-macrophages, eosinophils, basophils Hematopoietic growth and differentiation
Lipid Mediators		
Platelet-activating factor	Neutrophils, monocytes, platelets	Increase in capillary permeability Neutrophil activation Neutrophil chemotaxis
Arachidonic acid products	Most cell types	Regulation of vasomotor tone (prostaglandins and leukotrienes) Capillary permeability Neutrophil activation Pyrogenic factor (prostaglandins)
Other		
Reactive oxygen species	Leukocytes	Destruction of pathogens
Nitric oxide	Endothelial cells	Vasodilation Mediation of pain Regulation of adhesion
Proteases	Leukocytes	Tissue remodeling during healing

"lie in wait" for foreign proteins to enter their domain, ingesting and destroying them. Examples of tissue macrophages include the Kupffer cells of the liver and the alveolar macrophages (type I cells) of the lungs.

Mast Cells

Mast cells are a migratory population of cells found primarily at mucosal surfaces and in connective tissues surrounding blood vessels. They are believed to be of bone marrow origin, but their precise lineage is uncertain. The secretion of vasoactive amines, such as histamine and serotonin, by mast cells is of primary importance in immune-mediated inflammation.

Endothelial Cells

The past decade has brought growing recognition of the importance of the vascular endothelium in the regulation of many physiologic functions. Endothelial cells line the blood vessels, serving as a critical interface between the blood and the body tissues. These cells sense physical (hemodynamic) and chemical (vasoactive mediators) stimuli and respond by synthesizing and secreting a variety of small molecules, lipids, and proteins (Table 13–3). These endothelium-derived relaxing factors and endothelium-derived contracting factors regulate vascular tone and platelet function and may constitute a chemical barrier against the toxic effects of reactive oxygen species[3] (see Chapter 3). These functions are important not only to the inflammatory response but also to circulatory regulation and to the potential development of atherosclerosis (see Chapter 15). During inflammation, the expression of adhesion molecules on the endothelial surface facilitates leukocyte adherence and exudation (see Chapter 2).

TABLE 13–3
ENDOTHELIUM-DERIVED MEDIATORS

ENDOTHELIUM-DERIVED RELAXING FACTORS (VASODILATORS)
Lipids
Prostacyclin (PgI_2)
Other Small Molecules
Histamine
Nitric oxide (endothelium-derived relaxing factor)
Endothelium-derived hyperpolarizing factor
ENDOTHELIUM-DERIVED CONTRACTING FACTORS (VASOCONSTRICTORS)
Proteins
Endothelin
Angiotensin II
Lipids
Endoperoxide (PgH_2)
Thromboxane A_2
Other Small Molecules
Reactive oxygen species
OTHER ENDOTHELIUM-DERIVED MEDIATORS
Proteins
Growth factors
Matrix proteins
Coagulation factors
Anticoagulation factors
Fibrinolytic factors
Antigens
Enzymes
Receptors
Other Small Molecules
Adhesion molecules

Epithelial Cells

As linings and coverings, epithelial cells function as a physical barrier in the first line of tissue defense. Epithelial cells also respond to injury or infection with cytokine secretion, and many of these mediators are involved in regulation of inflammation, immune responses, hemostatic responses, and wound healing.[4]

Initiation of the Inflammatory Response

Cellular Injury

Cells can be damaged by many agents in many ways, and the mechanisms of cellular injury are logically consistent with the mechanisms of disease (see Chapter 1). Trauma, toxicity, and hypoxia, discussed in Chapter 3 within the context of impairment of energy metabolism, are common triggers of inflammation secondary to cellular injury.

Immune Mechanisms

Immune mechanisms initiate the inflammatory response in two ways. First, an immune attack against a specific antigen results in activation of macrophages, and these secrete cytokines, which mediate an inflammatory response even in the absence of specific cellular damage. Second, immune complexes (antigen–antibody combinations) may precipitate into tissues, causing toxic cellular injury. These mechanisms are detailed later in this chapter.

Infection

Infection is a common trigger of inflammation. Infectious agents include bacteria, viruses, fungi, and parasites. Table 13–4 summarizes mechanisms by which specific infectious agents induce inflammation, which may include physical disruption of cell membranes, competition for nutrients, and production of destructive enzymes or secretions (endotoxins). Viruses damage cells by replicating within

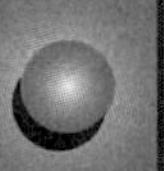

TABLE 13–4
MECHANISMS OF CELLULAR INJURY BY INFECTIOUS AGENTS

Agent	Mechanisms of Injury	Examples	
Bacteria	Secretion of exotoxins Endotoxin-induced injury (inner cell wall lipopolysaccharide of gram-negative bacteria) Release of proteolytic enzymes Immune response	**Bacterium**	**Disorder**
		Clostridium sp	Tetanus Botulism Soft tissue infections
		Bacillus sp	Anthrax Food poisoning
		Corynebacterium diphtheriae	Diphtheria
		Vibrio cholerae	Cholera
		Bordetella pertussis	Pertussis
		Staphylococcus aureus	Skin infections Soft tissue infections Toxic shock syndrome
		Staphylococcus epidermidis	Infections associated with indwelling catheters in blood vessels
		Streptococcus sp	Pharyngitis Periodontal disease Endocarditis Pneumonia Neonatal meningitis
		Gram-negative rods (*Escherichia coli, Pseudomonas* sp, *Proteus* sp)	Urinary tract infections Pneumonia Systemic inflammatory response syndrome Central nervous system infections
		Haemophilus influenzae	Bronchitis Pneumonia Septicemia
		Neisseria sp	Gonorrhea Meningitis
		Klebsiella pneumoniae	Opportunistic infections Pneumonia
		Bacteroides fragilis	Septicemia secondary to tissue necrosis or trauma
		Salmonella sp	Food poisoning Typhoid fever Septicemia
		Legionella sp	Sepsis
		Listeria monocytogenes	Sepsis Meningitis Neonatal infections
		Mycobacterium sp	Tuberculosis Hansen's disease (leprosy)
		Treponema sp	Syphilis Lyme disease
		Helicobacter pylori	Peptic ulcer disease
Viruses	Direct cytopathic effects (parasitic effect on intracellular substrate; replication with possible cell lysis) Immune response	**Virus**	**Disorder**
		Influenza viruses	Influenza
		Respiratory syncytial virus	Upper respiratory infection in adults Bronchiolitis and pneumonia in children
		Measles virus	Measles Atypical severe disease
		Hepatitis viruses	Hepatitis
		Herpesviruses	Chicken pox (varicella) Shingles (herpes zoster) Genital herpes Coldsores Infectious mononucleosis

Table continued on following page

TABLE 13–4
MECHANISMS OF CELLULAR INJURY BY INFECTIOUS AGENTS *(Continued)*

Agent	Mechanisms of Injury	Examples	
		Virus	**Disorder**
		Papillomaviruses	Common warts (verrucae) Genital warts
		Human immunodeficiency virus	AIDS
Fungi	Invasive injury (including blood vessel injury producing tissue infarction) Immune response	**Fungus**	**Disorder**
		Epidermophyton sp	Dermatophytosis (skin infection)
		Blastomyces dermatitidis	Blastomycosis (systemic infection)
		Coccidioides immitis	Coccidioidomycosis (systemic infection)
		Histoplasma capsulatum	Histoplasmosis (systemic infection)
		Candida albicans	Candidiasis (opportunistic infection of skin, mucous membranes, with possible systemic spread)
		Pneumocystis carinii	Pneumocystosis (interstitial pneumonia, often opportunistic)
Parasites	Invasion and cellular lysis Immune response	**Parasite**	**Disorder**
		Plasmodium sp (protozoan)	Malaria
		Toxoplasma sp (protozoan)	Toxoplasmosis
		Schistosoma sp (helminth)	Schistosomiasis Swimmer's itch
		Ancylostoma duodenale (nematode)	Hookworms
		Trichinella spiralis (nematode)	Trichinosis
		Ascaris sp (nematode)	Roundworm

them, using the host cell's genetic machinery for nucleotide synthesis. As viral DNA (or, less commonly, RNA) accumulates, the host cell ruptures, and viruses are released to infect other cells. The immune response to viral infection may induce further cellular injury.

The presence of microorganisms (colonization) does not result in an inflammatory response unless cell injury occurs. Indeed, normal flora microorganisms are continuously present on the skin, in the gastrointestinal tract, in the upper respiratory tract, and in the lower genitourinary tracts. Because they compete with potentially pathogenic organisms, they are actually a component of first-line defense. The terms *infection* and *sepsis* connote an inflammatory response to an organism. The casual interchangeable use of the terms *infection* and *inflammation* is common in clinical settings but should be avoided. Infection is but one trigger of inflammation.

Phases of the Inflammatory Response

Vasomotor Responses

The immediate response to cellular injury is a brief spasm of arterioles in the injured area (Fig. 13–1). This vasoconstriction is mediated by endothelial factors and is believed to be a protective reflex designed to minimize bleeding or to limit the extent of the injury. The dominant vascular response in inflammation is not vasoconstriction, however, but vasodilation, with resulting increased blood flow (**hyperemia**). Arterioles in the injured area dilate, and thoroughfare channels in capillary beds close. Because these channels bypass many exchange vessels, their closure causes increased blood flow to the injured tissues (Fig. 13–2). The hyperemic response serves three important purposes: (1) to bring WBCs (primarily neutrophils and monocytes) to the area, (2) to supply nutrients and oxygen because inflammation is an energy-consuming process, and (3) to dilute any toxins present, minimizing their damaging effects.

Adhesion and Chemotaxis

Under the activating stimulus of several cellular mediators, circulating neutrophils are attracted by **chemotaxis** to the area of injury, where their motility is slowed within postcapillary venules. Neutrophils first roll along the surface of the endothelium in a process mediated by selectins, adhesion molecules that are expressed by endothelial cells and that bind reversibly to sites on the leukocyte membrane.

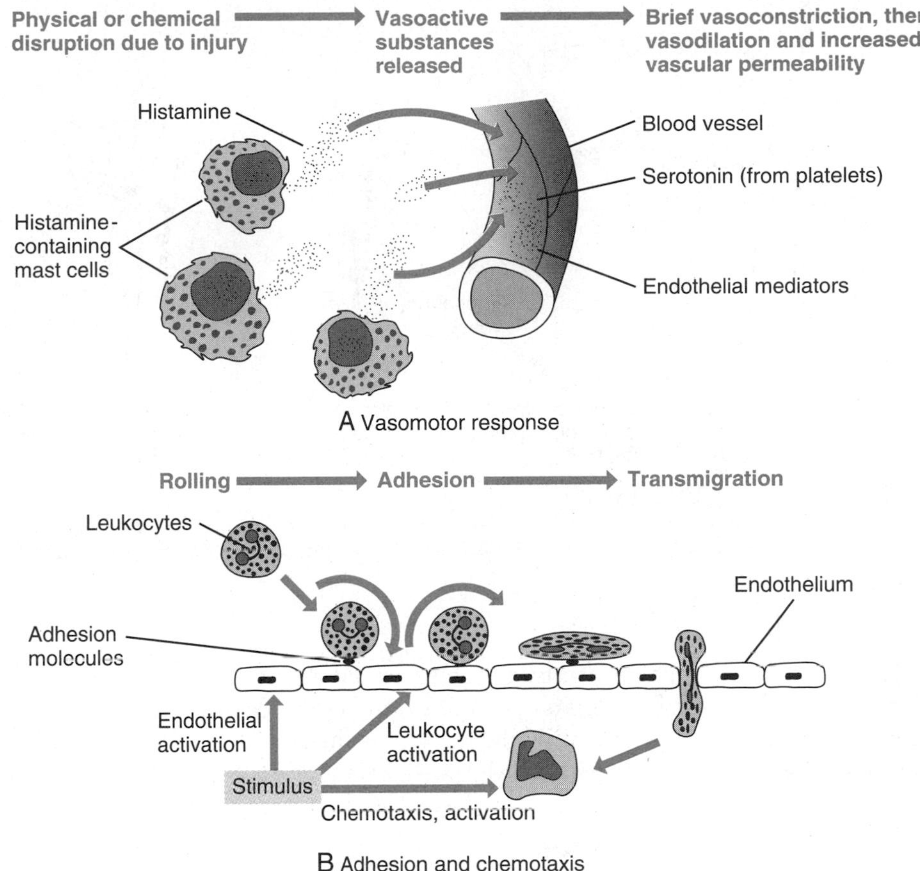

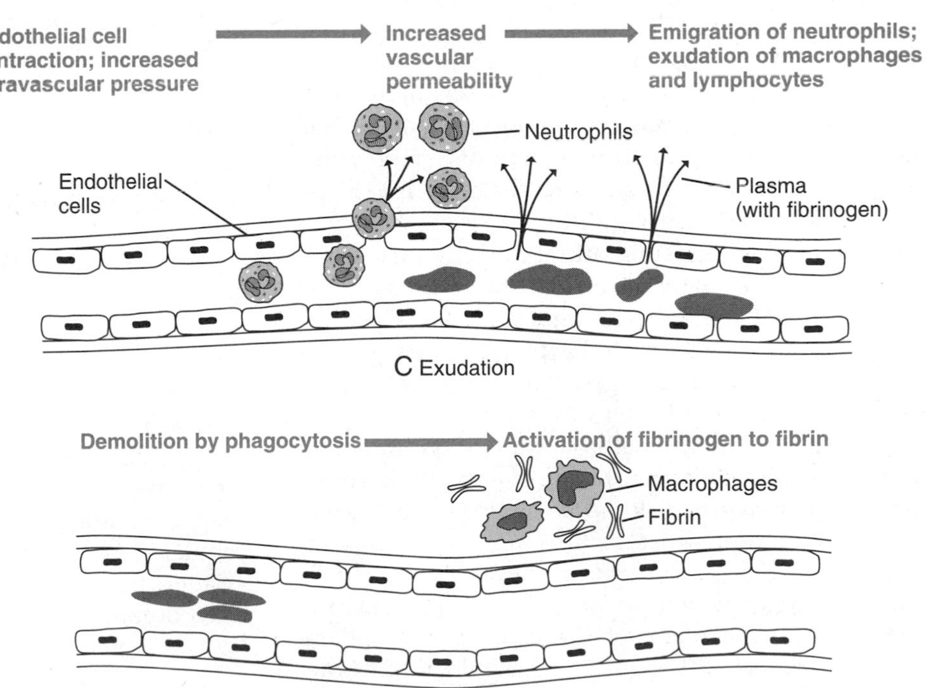

FIGURE 13–1

Phases of inflammation. *A*, Cellular injury triggers a brief vasospasm, followed by vasodilation and increased capillary permeability in the area of injury. *B*, Local mediators attract leukocytes (neutrophils) to the area by chemotaxis. Adhesion molecules expressed on neutrophils and endothelial cells slow the neutrophils, inducing rolling and adhesion of these cells to the endothelium. *C*, Neutrophils, and later macrophages, exude into the injured tissues, where they engulf and digest injurious agents. Lymphocytes may also mediate a specific immune attack against these agents. *D*, Phagocytosis clears the area in preparation for wound healing. Fibrinogen exudes into the area and is activated to fibrin. Fibrin forms a barrier around the area of injury as well as a matrix for deposition of new tissue during wound healing.

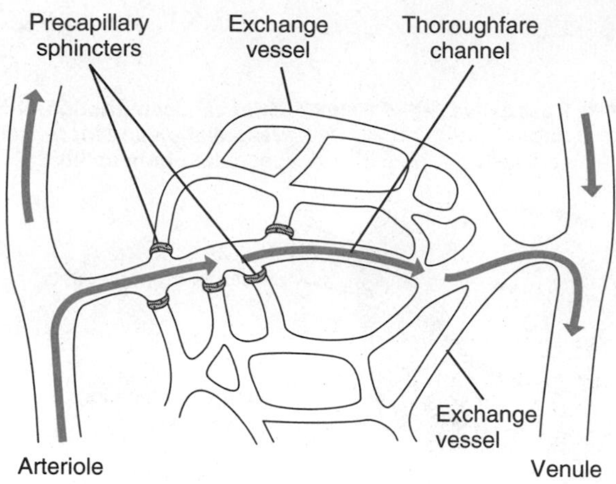

A Normal capillary bed circulation. Most blood flows through thoroughfare channel, bypassing exchange vessels ("true" capillaries).

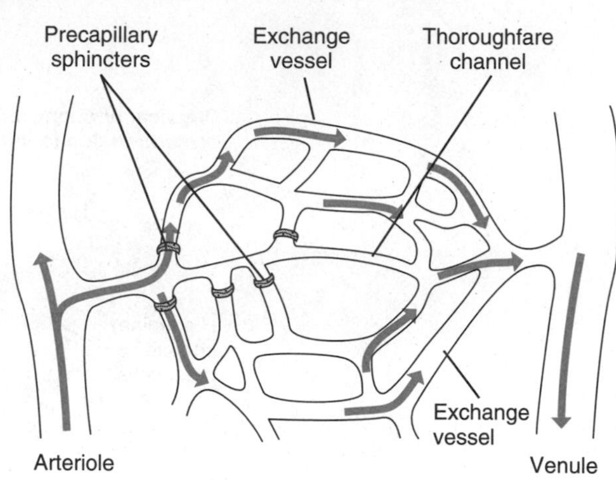

B Hyperemia. Arteriole dilates, and thoroughfare channel closes, routing more blood through exchange vessels.

FIGURE 13–2

Hyperemia. Arteriolar dilation and closure of thoroughfare channels in capillary beds occurs in response to inflammatory mediators, bringing phagocytic cells, oxygen, and nutrients to the area of injury.

Later, neutrophils become firmly adherent to the endothelium by binding of leukocyte adhesion molecules (integrins) to endothelial ligands, such as intercellular adhesion molecule-1 (I-CAM-1).

Exudation

The dilated vessels in the injured area become more permeable because increased pressure within them widens the spaces between the endothelial cells forming the vessel walls. These changes result in **exudation** of plasma, containing fibrinogen, into the interstitial space. Rearrangement of action within WBCs enables them to squeeze through spaces between cells in the vessel wall by a process known as *diapedesis*. WBC transmigration into the tissues is also mediated by chemotactic factors and by platelet–endothelial cell adhesion molecule-1 (P-CAM-1).[5] Within the interstitium of the injured area, phagocytic WBCs engulf and digest bacteria or other injurious agents and dead cells.

At first, the inflammatory exudate is thin and clear, resembling plasma, but it eventually becomes thicker and white or colored as cellular debris accumulates. In the presence of infection, the exudate is referred to as *pus* or *purulent exudate* and may be foul smelling. The nature of the exudate may provide a cue to the phase or the cause of the inflammatory response (Table 13–5). The fluid that exudes into the interstitium during inflammation may drain from the wound surface or may be cleared by the lymphatic system (see Chapter 15).

Fibrin Barrier Formation

During inflammation, the plasma protein fibrinogen also exudes into the interstitium, where it becomes activated to **fibrin**, a thread-like protein. Fibrin serves three functions in inflammation: (1) to wall off the injured area, limiting the spread of microorganisms or toxins, (2) to form a mesh-like framework for new tissue formation during healing, and (3) to participate in hemostasis (blood clotting) in the case of damage to local blood vessels (see Chapter 14).

Regulation of Inflammation

Because inflammation is essentially a local response, its regulation is primarily locally mediated by the autocrine and paracrine stimulation of cytokines and other cell products. Ordinarily, the influence of neural and endocrine regulation is minimal, although the anti-inflammatory effect of the adrenocortical hormone cortisol may be amplified when a stress response is superimposed (see Chapter 1). Cellular mediators of inflammation may originate from cellular components of the inflammatory response system, from injured tissue cells, or from invading microorganisms (see Table 13–2).

Cytokines

Many of the physiologic effects of inflammation are mediated by the *proinflammatory* cytokines tumor

TABLE 13–5
CHARACTERISTICS OF INFLAMMATORY EXUDATE IN COMMON DISEASES

Type of Exudate	Characteristics	Clinical Significance
Serous	Watery and copious Low protein content	Typical of mild or early inflammation
Fibrinous	Thick and sticky High protein (fibrinogen) content	Typical of more severe inflammation with greater degree of capillary permeability
Mucinous	High mucus content Contains sloughed epithelial cells	Typical of inflammation of mucous membranes, e.g., common cold, hay fever
Membranous	Incorporation of necrotic cells into mucous membranes, forming a thick coat	Typical of diphtheria, moniliasis, pseudomembranous colitis
Purulent	High content of liquified leukocytes, tissue debris, and protein May be foul smelling Color may suggest specific causative agent Also known as suppurative exudate or pus	Typical of infection with pyogenic (pus-producing) bacteria and within cysts or abscesses
Hemorrhagic	Significant erythrocyte content	Indicates involvement of blood vessels due to injury or necrosis
Serosanguinous	Contains both serous and hemorrhagic components	Indicates involvement of blood vessels due to injury or necrosis

necrosis factor (TNF), interleukin-1 (IL-1), and IL-8.[6] TNF and IL-1 act together to mediate neutrophil activation, lower pain threshold and blood pressure, and stimulate release of lipid mediators. IL-8 is an important chemotactic factor and also stimulates the release of enzymes and reactive oxygen species from neutrophils, leading to tissue damage and increased capillary permeability. Each of these cytokines promotes the synthesis and release of other factors in a positive feedback loop. Positive feedback is adaptive in this case because it is limited by the inhibitory effects of the *anti-inflammatory* cytokines IL-4, IL-10, and transforming growth factor-β.

Monocyte-macrophages and other cells secrete colony-stimulating factors (CSFs), which stimulate production of more WBCs from the bone marrow during inflammation. During the immune response, lymphocytes secrete cytokines (lymphokines), which stimulate macrophage activity. Lymphocytes and macrophages produce a variety of other interleukins, which may act as CSFs, mediate fever, promote wound healing, or activate immune system cells (see Table 13–2).

Platelets secrete the vasoactive amine serotonin as well as cytokines that promote wound healing, known generally as *tissue growth factors*. The primary role of the platelet products, however, is in mediation of hemostasis (see Chapter 14).

Mast cells synthesize and store histamine within cytoplasmic granules. During inflammation, mast cell degranulation occurs as histamine is released by exocytosis. Histamine then binds to receptors in vessel walls to mediate vasodilation and increased permeability. Mast cells also release chemotactic factors and serotonin, which has effects similar to those of histamine.

Eosinophils secrete a chemical that damages the surface membrane of parasites but that also opposes the effects of histamine slightly (possibly a fine-tuning mechanism). Eosinophil levels tend to be elevated in immune-mediated inflammation rather than in infection. Basophils, a type of circulating granulocyte, function similarly to mast cells.

Arachidonic Acid Derivatives

Among the most important of the lipid mediators of inflammation and other biologic processes are the products of the degradation of **arachidonic acid**, a fatty acid derived from membrane lipids (Fig. 13–3). The enzymes mediating this biochemical pathway are found within many types of cells, including mast cells. The products of the pathway, known collectively as *eicosanoids* because of their fatty acid structure, include prostaglandins, thromboxanes, and leukotrienes. Leukotrienes cause vasodilation and increased permeability, similarly to histamine, but the effects of leukotrienes begin more gradually and are more prolonged. Prostaglandins also have histamine-like effects and are involved in fever and in transmission of pain impulses. Thromboxanes are particularly important in the platelet response to blood vessel injury, as discussed in Chapter 14. As detailed later in this chapter, drugs such as cortisone and aspirin suppress inflammation through blockade of enzymes within the arachidonic acid pathway.

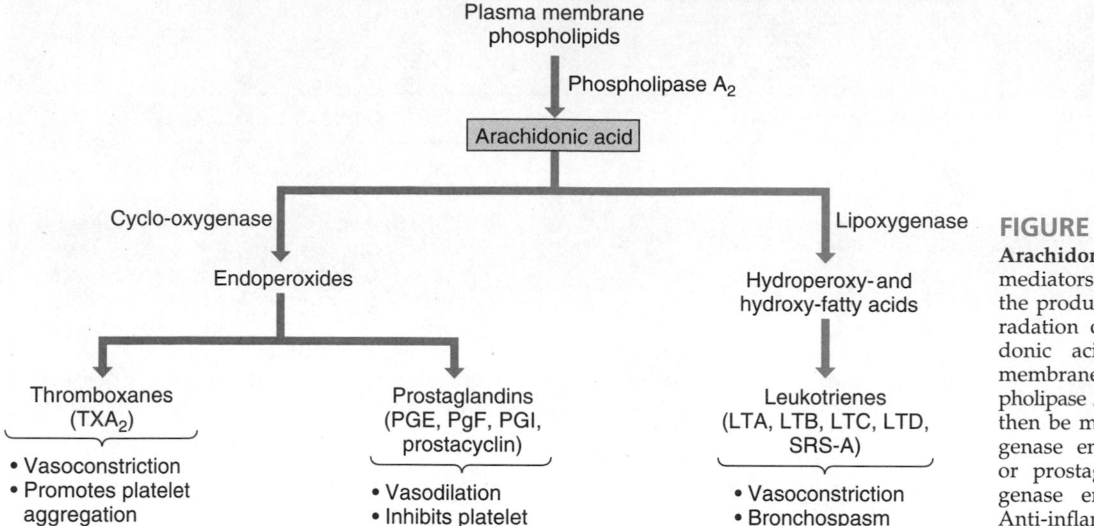

FIGURE 13–3
Arachidonic acid pathway. Lipid mediators of inflammation include the products of the metabolic degradation of the fatty acid arachidonic acid, released from cell membranes by the enzyme phospholipase A_2. Arachidonic acid may then be metabolized by cyclo-oxygenase enzyme to thromboxanes or prostaglandins, or by lipoxygenase enzyme to leukotrienes. Anti-inflammatory drugs may inhibit these enzymes, suppressing the inflammatory response.

Other Small Molecules

Small molecules such as nitric oxide and reactive oxygen species mediate vasodilation and tissue damage in inflammation.

Plasma Protein Systems

Three interrelated cascade systems are associated with inflammation: the complement system, the hemostatic–fibrinolytic system (clotting cascade), and the kinin system.

Complement System. As illustrated in Figure 13–4, the complement system is a series of about 30 enzymes. These plasma proteins are labeled C1 through C9; some have several subunits designated with lower-case letters. Complement proteins circulate in inactive (proenzyme) form. Activation of one protein during inflammation or an immune response results in stepwise activation of the others. The two

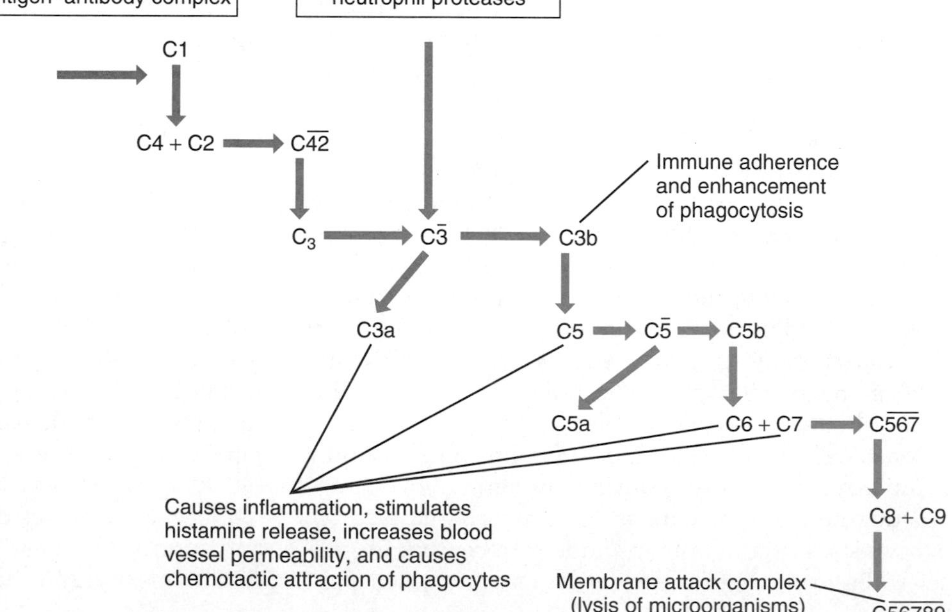

FIGURE 13–4
The complement cascade. Complement proteins circulate in inactive form until activation by either an antigen–antibody complex (classic pathway) or microorganisms (alternate pathway). Activation of one protein causes sequential activation of others, enhancing the inflammatory response and leading to formation of a membrane attack complex. This complex destroys invading microorganisms by perforating their walls.

mechanisms of complement activation are the classic pathway, in which an antigen–antibody complex activates the system, and the alternative pathway, in which chemicals produced by leukocytes or invading bacteria activate the cascade. The complement system thus plays a role in both inflammatory and immune defenses.

Regardless of the mechanism of activation, the last steps of the complement cascade are identical. Proteins C_1 through C_5 *opsonize* bacteria (roughen their surfaces and clump them together to facilitate phagocytosis), are chemotactic for WBCs, and act as *anaphylatoxins,* which enhance mast cell secretion and the immune response. C_6 through C_9 form circular membrane attack complexes, which tunnel through bacterial cell walls, causing lysis of the cells.

Hemostatic–Fibrinolytic System. As illustrated and discussed in detail in Chapter 14, the clotting cascade is a series of reactions designed to form a fibrin clot in a damaged vessel while that vessel heals. In the latter portion of the cascade, the fibrinolytic system is activated to break down the clot and restore patency of the vessel. This system is interactive with the inflammatory response in that fibrin is activated for walling off the injured area and for deposition of a matrix for new tissue formation. Intermediate products of the clotting cascade also enhance vascular permeability and are chemotactic for neutrophils. Because most tissue injury involves vascular damage, the concurrent activation of both systems is a logical homeostatic collaboration.

Kinin System. The kinin system begins with activation of a plasma protein known as the *Hageman factor,* which is also a component of the clotting cascade. As shown in Figure 13–5, in the presence of circulating high-molecular-weight kininogen, activated Hageman factor converts plasma prekallikrein to the enzyme kallikrein, which in turn releases small peptides (kinins). The most important of these is bradykinin, which mediates vasodilation and increased vascular permeability as well as pain sensation. These effects duplicate those of the mast cell products but are of slower onset and are more prolonged.

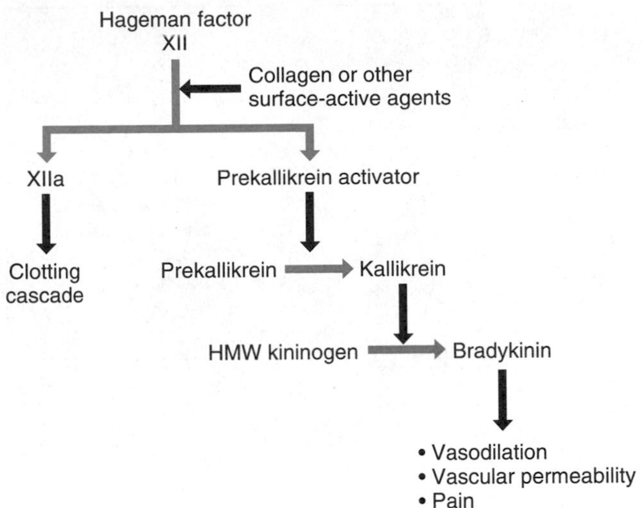

FIGURE 13–5

The kinin cascade. Activation of a plasma protein, Hageman factor (clotting factor XII), results in activation of the enzyme kallikrein. Kallikrein releases kinins (e.g., bradykinin), which mediate vasodilation, increased capillary permeability, and pain sensation during the inflammatory response. HMW, high molecular weight.

Clinical Manifestations of Inflammation

Cardinal Signs and Symptoms

The five local effects of inflammation were first described centuries ago and still retain their Latin names: *rubor* (redness), *tumor* (swelling or edema), *calor* (heat), *dolor* (pain), and *functiolaesa* (loss of function). Redness and heat result from hyperemia, and swelling occurs as a result of exudation. Pain is typical in inflammation due to mechanical disruption or chemical irritation of pain receptors in the injured area, and the transmission of pain impulses to the brain is believed to be facilitated by local chemicals, including prostaglandins (see Chapter 23). Loss of function of the inflamed part is secondary to pain and swelling.

Systemic Effects

Within the systems perspective, it is not surprising that, although inflammation is essentially a local phenomenon, it also has systemic effects. These include malaise and fatigue, fever, leukocytosis, increased erythrocyte sedimentation rate, and alterations in serum levels of several proteins (acute phase reactants) synthesized primarily by the liver (Table 13–6).

Much energy is consumed during inflammation, fever, and tissue repair, and the afflicted person may feel sick and tired. As detailed in Chapter 11, fever may be present, owing to release of pyrogenic cytokines from microorganisms or WBCs. Fever is believed to be an adaptive response in that it creates an unfavorable environment for growth of bacteria. Leukocytosis, an elevation in serum WBCs, is evidence that the bone marrow is responding appropriately to stimuli, making more WBCs available for the inflammatory response. Typically, neutrophils are elevated to the greatest extent, and increased numbers of immature cells (bands) are seen. The

TABLE 13–6
ACUTE PHASE REACTANTS

Reactant	Significance
C-reactive protein	Binds to bacterial proteins, initiating complement activation by the alternative pathway
Fibrinogen	Involved in barrier formation, clotting, and tissue preparation for healing
Complement proteins	Components of complement cascade that augments inflammatory response
α_1-Antitrypsin	Inhibits tissue breakdown by protease enzymes
α_2-Macroglobulin	Inhibits tissue breakdown by protease enzymes
Fibronectin	Involved in cellular attachment
	Chemotactic factor (attracts neutrophils)
Ceruloplasmin	Inhibits reactive oxygen species
Haptoglobin	Accelerates wound healing

latter response is sometimes referred to as a *shift to the left*. (Leukocytosis is further described in Chapter 12).

The rate at which red blood cells (RBCs) precipitate out of serum is increased during inflammation because increased fibrinogen levels cause RBCs to become sticky and stack together in particles of increased mass. Fibrinogen is among the acute phase reactants elevated in inflammation. Leukocytosis, increased erythrocyte sedimentation rate, and presence of acute phase reactants are commonly used nonspecific markers for the presence of inflammation.

Patients with systemic inflammatory response syndrome manifest systemic signs of inflammation along with hypermetabolism, hypotension, and possibly septic shock (see Chapter 15).

Outcomes of Inflammation

The optimal outcome of an acute inflammatory response is tissue healing, either by **resolution** (recovery of cells sustaining nonlethal damage), **regeneration** (replacement of dead cells with functional duplicates), or **repair** (replacement of dead cells with nonfunctional scar tissue). Wound healing is discussed later in this chapter.

When the exudative phase of inflammation lasts longer than 2 weeks, chronic inflammation is said to be present. Inflammation may persist indefinitely, owing to the virulence of the invading organism, the severity of trauma, or the inadequacy of the patient's inflammatory or immune response system. The severe, prolonged inflammatory response of systemic inflammatory response syndrome is characterized by a superimposed acute stress response, hypermetabolism, and potential multiple organ dysfunction, including cardiac, respiratory, and renal failure.[7]

In some instances of infection, the outcome of the inflammatory response is not healing but rather granuloma formation. In such cases (e.g., tuberculosis), the inflamed area is walled off, but the organism is not destroyed. A lesion is formed that at first has a grainy center and may later become necrotic or calcified. Granulomas may persist for the life of the patient without causing any problems, but if the person becomes vulnerable (immunosuppressed, highly stressed, or afflicted with another illness), the initial organism could again cause an acute inflammatory response.

Wound Healing

Process and Regulation

When cell injury is nonlethal, inflammation serves to clear debris (dead microorganisms or cells), facilitating restoration of normal cellular structure and function. When tissue is lost as a result of injury, creating a wound, inflammation serves not only to clear the area but also to set up a fibrin framework for wound healing by regeneration or repair. Wound healing, like inflammation, is locally regulated by tissue growth factors released by a variety of cells, including macrophages, platelets, and the injured cells themselves. At the genetic level, transcription factors mediate a process that resembles embryologic mechanisms of tissue formation, including cell migration, proliferation, and differentiation[8] (see Chapter 6).

After inflammation and the deposition of the fibrin mesh, reconstruction of the area of tissue deficit occurs by division of adjacent normal cells (in tissues capable of cell division) or by inward migration of other epithelial or connective tissue cells, forming granulation tissue. Named for its grainy appearance, this tissue contains cells that secrete fibrous, collagen-like proteins and contractile proteins. Under the influence of specific growth factors, adjacent blood vessels, lymphatic vessels, and nerve fibers also grow into the wound, and the dense network of blood vessels gives the wound a pink appearance. If exposed, the surface of the granulation tissue eventually dries, forming a scab.

Healing by Regeneration Versus Repair

In tissues capable of mitosis (see Chapter 6), wound healing occurs by regeneration, or replacement of lost tissue with tissue that is structurally and functionally identical to that which was lost, and there is no permanent scar, or cicatrix. Regenerative capacity varies among tissues, but generally the more specialized the tissue, the less capable it is of regeneration. Under optimal conditions of wound size, nutrition, and oxygenation, tissues of the skin, epithelium of gastrointestinal and genitourinary tracts, and bone marrow are highly regenerative. Muscle, bone, liver, kidney, and lung tissues are moderately regenerative; whereas heart muscle (myocardium) and neuron cell bodies are generally incapable of mitosis in adults. In the case of nervous tissue, axons (long fibrous projections of nerve cells) may regenerate if the cell body is intact. Scarring occurs even in highly regenerative tissues if the wound is large or complicated by infection, malnutrition, or poor tissue perfusion.

When regeneration is not possible, lost tissue is repaired with fibrous connective tissue. Although not functional, the scar serves to restore the structural integrity of the damaged tissue. Wound healing by repair is more prolonged than healing by regeneration and is highly dependent on adequate nutrition and oxygenation of the area to supply substrates and energy for new tissue synthesis. Epithelial cells from the wound edges divide and grow inward, displacing the scab. The fibrous component of the granulation tissue also continues to grow, and the contractile proteins eventually squeeze out excess blood vessels, causing the scar to become less red, smaller in size, and stronger. This process of maturation of scar tissue may take several weeks.

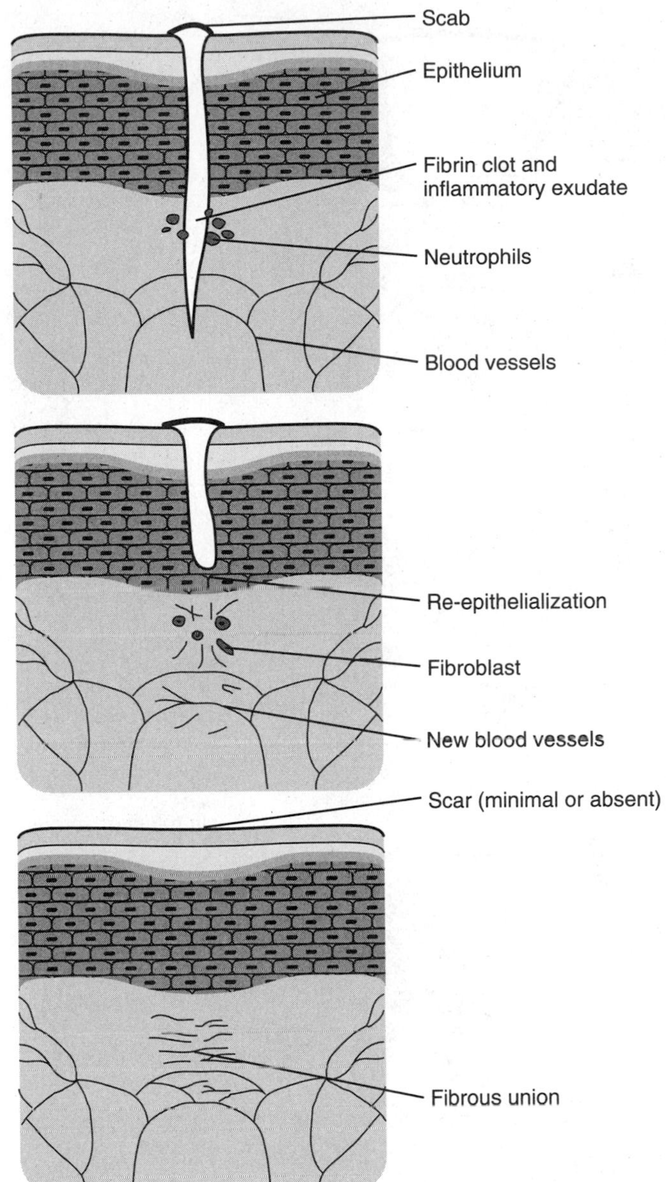

FIGURE 13–6
Healing by primary intention. When wound edges are well approximated and tissue loss is minimal, healing occurs from the edges in, with little or no scarring.

Healing by Primary Versus Secondary Intention

Healing by *primary intention* occurs when tissue loss is minimal, wound edges are close together (well approximated), and there is no wound infection. These wounds, which include clean cuts and sutured surgical incisions, heal from the edges inward, with little or no scarring (Fig. 13–6). Healing by *secondary intention* occurs with deep or large wounds, such as draining ulcers. Healing proceeds from the bottom upward, and scarring is more extensive (Fig. 13–7). The term *tertiary intention* is sometimes used in reference to intentional delay of wound closure or intentional reopening of a previously sutured wound. This approach is employed for infected wounds, or for wounds at high risk of infection, to ensure that the area is free of debris and that the deeper recesses of the wound are well granulated before primary closure of more superficial tissues takes place.[9]

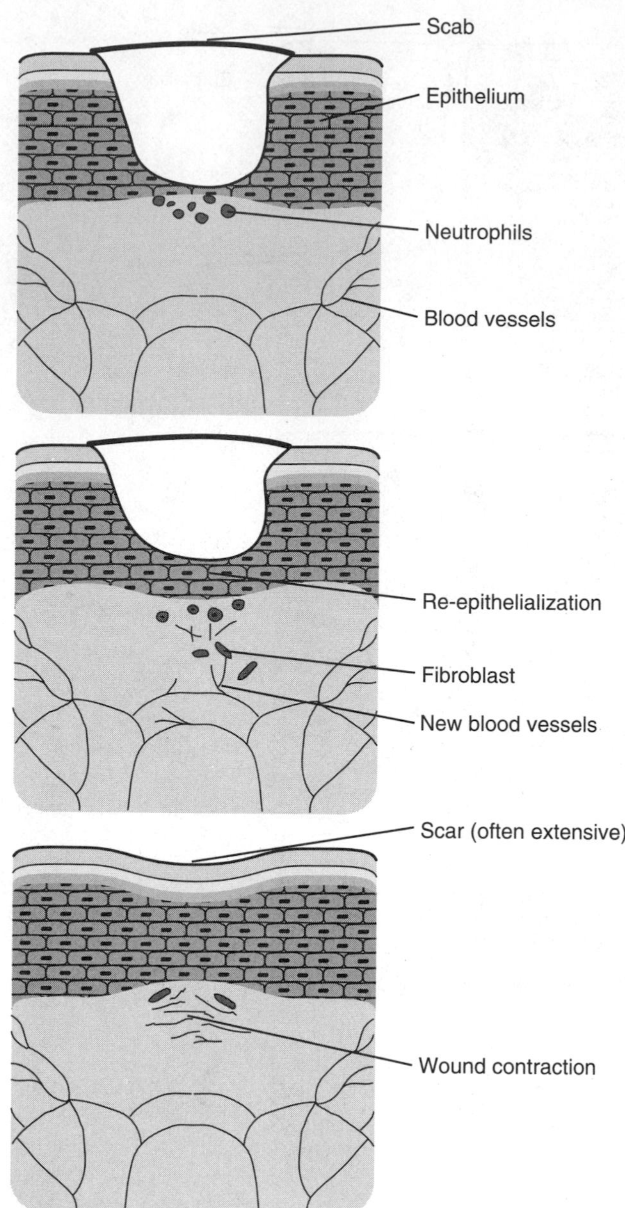

FIGURE 13–7
Healing by secondary intention. In the case of larger or deeper wounds, healing proceeds from the bottom upward, leading to more extensive scarring.

Maladaptive Inflammation and Healing

Insufficient Inflammatory Response

Because inflammation and healing depend on the adequacy of hematopoiesis and the availability of sufficient energy and nutrients, conditions in which any of these is compromised may result in an insufficient inflammatory response or delayed wound healing. Patients who are malnourished or immunosuppressed may be unable to mount an adequate defense. Those who have compromised perfusion (e.g., diabetes mellitus, cardiac or respiratory failure) may also be at risk.

Excessive or Inappropriate Inflammatory Response

Excessive or inappropriately triggered inflammation may result from abnormal expression of adhesion molecules or from immunopathology (hypersensitivity or allergy), as discussed later in this chapter. As has been mentioned, appropriately triggered inflammation may be harmful if it occurs within enclosed spaces. The morbidity and mortality due to head injury, spinal cord injury, and stroke, for example, are more often attributable to the pressure of edema associated with inflammation rather than to the original lesion.

Ineffective Wound Healing

Inadequacy of tissue healing may predispose wound edges to separate when subjected to mechanical stress or pressure. The same factors that contribute to an insufficient inflammatory response also result in ineffective wound healing. Obesity, excessive activity or violent coughing without sufficient wound support, and inadequate suture technique or materials further promote wound dehiscence (separation of the wound edges). Dehiscence may be complicated by hemorrhage, evisceration, and infection.

Scar tissue formation may pose problems, owing to the location of the injury. Burns involving joints may heal with scars that "freeze" the joints in nonfunctional positions (contractures) as the scar tissue contracts with maturation (Fig. 13–8). Scar tissue

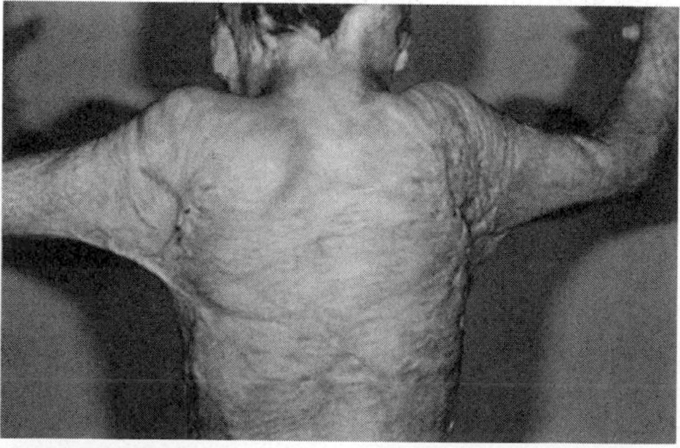

FIGURE 13–8
Contracture. Scar tissue involving joints may restrict mobility as scar tissue contracts during maturation. Here, axillary contractures limit movement of the shoulders and arms. (From McCarthy, J.G., May, J.W., Jr., and Littler, J.W. [1990]. *Plastic Surgery.* Volume 8. Part 2. Philadelphia: W.B. Saunders [p. 5475].)

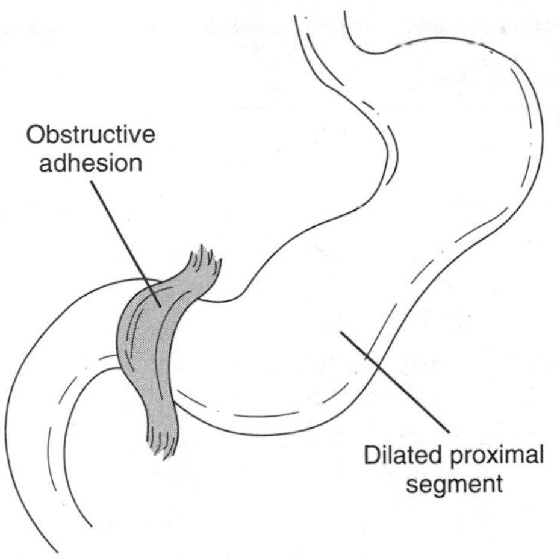

FIGURE 13–9
Adhesion. Inflammation and healing within body cavities may produce bands of fibrous scar tissue, which obstruct hollow organs.

within body cavities may fuse membranous structures or form obstructive bands or adhesions (Fig. 13–9). Adhesions are a common complication of abdominal surgery. Some patients are prone to excessive scar tissue formation, possibly owing to genetic variation. These excessive scars (keloids) may be disfiguring and are most likely to occur with burns, with upper body wounds, and in adolescents (Color Fig. 13–1).

Developmental Variables

Developmental variables also influence inflammation and healing, as a consequence of variable probability of exposure to triggers of inflammation or variable efficacy of the inflammatory response (see Developmental Perspective).

Clinical Management of Inflammation

Common sense dictates that an adaptive inflammatory response should be allowed to continue unimpeded. Many patients, however, find the clinical manifestations distressing, or at least inconvenient, and seek to suppress inflammation. Other clinical interventions may be employed to support or enhance an adaptive inflammatory response. Maladaptive inflammation and healing require clinical intervention specific to the cause. Manifestations of hypermetabolism and organ failure secondary to systemic inflammatory response syndrome mandate nutritional support as well as support of critical systems.

Local Application of Heat or Cold

In localized inflammation, application of cold (e.g., ice packs) causes vasoconstriction and may be helpful in limiting fluid exudation and edema when joints are injured. The cold sensation also occupies pain transmission pathways and decreases discomfort. Compression and elevation may also be employed to inhibit swelling. Warm soaks or pads promote vasodilation and enhance the hyperemic response. They may also reduce pain by reducing muscle tension in areas surrounding the injury.

Wound Drainage and Débridement

Removal of pus and debris (drainage and débridement) supports the demolition phase of inflammation when injury is extensive, as in severe burns or deep ulcers. Wound drainage may be collected on dressings or may be routed to an external receptacle through drains or tubes inserted into the wound. Débridement involves manual removal of nonviable tissue from the healing wound so that healthy granulation tissue is uppermost.

Drug Therapy

Anti-inflammatory drugs in common use are summarized in Table 13–7. These include steroids, such as cortisone, which interrupts the formation of arachidonic acid from membrane phospholipids, suppressing production of prostaglandins and leukotrienes. Steroids (glucocorticoids) relieve the pain and swelling of inflammation but introduce the risk of further damage and significant metabolic side effects. Steroids are similar to the adrenocortical hormone cortisol, which has widespread metabolic effects (see Chapter 29). Many nonsteroidal anti-inflammatory drugs are available in both prescription and nonprescription strengths. These agents, which include aspirin, ibuprofen, and naproxen, suppress inflammation primarily by interrupting prostaglandin synthesis by the arachidonic acid pathway. Nonsteroidal anti-inflammatory drugs have fewer side effects than cortisol but may also have less capacity to relieve symptoms. Agents such as gold salts may be used in an effort to induce remission in chronic inflammatory conditions such as arthritis. Cytotoxic agents such as methotrexate have been employed in some disorders. When inflamma-

Developmental Perspective

Embryonic and Fetal Periods

A number of maternal infections are known to be teratogenic. Intrauterine infection is one mode of vertical transmission of the HIV virus. Fetal surgery is being performed in prenatal repair of certain congenital disorders, and owing to enhanced tissue proliferation and differentiation, fetal wounds heal without scarring. The first precursors of immune cells appear about 9 weeks after conception. The thymus gland differentiates during the sixth week of embryonic development. The thymus does not have the capability of mounting an immune response in utero because it is protected from exposure to antigen by epithelial membranes surrounding its blood vessels. Its role instead is to provide the environment for differentiation and maturation of T cells. Fetal immunity is derived passively from maternal transfer of immunoglobulins across the placenta. Impaired development of the fetal thymus results in congenital immunodeficiency. Erythroblastosis fetalis may develop in the Rh-positive fetus if anti-Rh antibodies develop during pregnancy in the Rh-negative mother.

Infancy and Childhood

The barrier function of the skin in infants is not established until about 4 months of age. Fragility and lack of bacteriostatic chemical properties thus predispose newborns (especially premature infants) to infection. Neonates also are deficient in the normal mucous layer of membranes of the respiratory, gastrointestinal, and genitourinary tracts. Neonates have immature neutrophils and decreased complement levels, limiting their phagocytic responses. Neutrophil diapedesis is impaired, and release of CSFs and interleukins is diminished. Immaturity of thermoregulatory systems typically results in higher fevers with inflammation in infants and young children than are seen in adults. The causative organism in many bacterial infections often can be predicted based on the child's age. Neonates are most often infected with group B streptococci, enterococci, and *Listeria* and *Pseudomonas* spp. Older children may also be susceptible to these, and in addition may be infected by *Haemophilus influenzae, Streptococcus pneumoniae,* and *Neisseria meningitidis.* Children have more viral infections than adults, owing to more frequent exposures and less development of acquired immunity.

The immune response is not fully developed until about 5 years of age. Childhood immunization against a number of communicable diseases is mandated by school immunization laws. Breast-fed infants receive antibodies that are highly targeted against pathogens in the infant's immediate environment because these antigens stimulate maternal development of the antibodies. Secretory IgA in breast milk protects the infant's mucous membranes and, unlike most other antibodies, may destroy pathogens without causing inflammation—a beneficial effect, considering the delicacy of membranes in young children. The first breast secretion, colostrum, is particularly high in interferon, which has antiviral activity. Breast milk also contains lymphocytes (20% B cells and 80% T cells), which produce cytokines promoting the infant's own immune response. Children are vulnerable to vertically transmitted AIDS and to some forms of leukemia and lymphoma, disorders that result in immunodeficiency. Many allergies, particularly bronchial asthma, are more common in childhood.

Adolescence and Young Adulthood

Healthy adolescence and young adulthood is normally a period of decreased incidence of inflammatory disease, with the exception of an inflammatory skin disorder, acne vulgaris. Unprotected sexual activity may increase the risk of sexually transmitted diseases during this period (see Chapter 30). Use of illicit drugs is highest in this group and may contribute to blood-borne infections such as AIDS and hepatitis B. The thymus gland continues to grow until puberty, after which it normally begins to atrophy. Some lymphomas, notably Hodgkin's disease, target this age group. A number of autoimmune disorders may have their onset during this period, including systemic lupus erythematosus, myasthenia gravis, Addison's disease, multiple sclerosis, and rheumatoid arthritis.

Middle and Older Adulthood

Although it is widely believed that the elderly are at higher risk for maladaptive inflammation and healing, there is no evidence that age, per se, is a risk factor. Rather, the risk is associated with poor nutrition or with poor tissue oxygenation secondary to chronic illnesses to which the elderly are more prone. The elderly also have thinner, more friable skin and mucous membranes, with decreased Langerhans cell function. The oral flora of elderly people may include gram-negative bacteria. Mucociliary transport and cough efficacy are decreased, predisposing to respiratory infection. Decreased gastric acidity may predispose some elderly people to overgrowth of gastric bacteria, which may be aspirated. Diabetes mellitus, which predisposes to infection by several mechanisms, is most frequent among middle-aged and older adults. The systemic response to inflammation is often atypical among the elderly, manifesting as a change in mental status, weakness, confusion, anorexia, drowsiness, hyperglycemia or hypoglycemia, acidosis, or altered hemostasis. Lack of fever is usual. Older people are clearly more susceptible than younger adults to a number of infectious diseases, to autoimmune disorders, and to cancer, suggesting a decline in immune function with aging. Reduction in the proportions of CD4+ and CD8+ T cells is seen with aging, with a slightly greater reduction in CD4+ (helper T) cells. T cells do not respond as well to antigenic challenge, owing to impairment of intercellular signaling and gene expression. A decrease in the activity of NK cells is seen, although macrophage function is normal. Total immunoglobulin levels are unchanged, although the proportions of IgA and IgG are increased. An increase in circulating autoantibodies is seen. Antibody response to a number of antigens is decreased, probably owing to defective T-cell–mediated regulation.

tion is initiated by an immune mechanism, immunosuppressive agents or antihistamines may be used.

When inflammation is caused by infection, antibiotic therapy may be indicated. Table 13–8 lists examples of several categories of antibiotics. These agents kill or weaken microorganisms by a variety of mechanisms, thus supporting the inflammatory response. The Age of Antibiotics, which began in the early 1950s, has eradicated many of the infectious diseases that at one time were the leading causes of morbidity and mortality in the world. The efficacy of anti*viral* drugs, however, is still limited. Of growing concern is the development of mutant forms of microorganisms that are resistant to many (in some cases *all*) antibiotics.[10] Indiscriminate use of antibiotics for mild infections, use of multiple antibiotics to defend against all possible organisms, and inappropriate use of antibacterial agents for viral infections, such as the common cold, have undoubtedly contributed to this multiple resistance. With antibiotic "pressure," a natural selection process is set up whereby the stronger, more resistant organisms survive and reproduce. Subsequent exposure to the same drug is then less effective or ineffective.

Standard Precautions

Limitation of spread of the infectious agent is critical in many cases and may involve isolation of the infected patient or special handling of the patient's blood, body fluids, or excrement (see Focus of Current Research). Since the advent of the AIDS epidemic, the Centers for Disease Control and Prevention have mandated implementation of the Standard Precautions to control transmission of the human immunodeficiency virus (HIV) and other infections in health care settings[11] (Table 13–9).

TABLE 13–7
ANTI-INFLAMMATORY DRUGS IN COMMON USE

Anti-Inflammatory Class	Examples	Actions
Group I agents: salicylates and nonsteroidal anti-inflammatory drugs	Aspirin Ibuprofen Naproxen	Inhibition of cyclo-oxygenase enzyme of arachidonic acid pathway, decreasing prostaglandin synthesis
Group II agents; remission-inducing drugs	Gold salts Penicillamine Hydroxychloroquine	Unknown mechanism, inhibition of phagocytosis, inhibition of lysosomal enzymes, decrease in immunoglobulins
Group III agents: glucocorticoids	Cortisol Cortisone Hydrocortisone Prednisone	Inhibition of arachidonic acid formation from membrane lipids
Group IV agents: cytotoxic agents	Cyclophosphamide Methotrexate	Inhibition of lymphocyte activity

TABLE 13–8
ANTIBIOTICS IN COMMON USE

ANTIBIOTIC CLASS	EXAMPLES	MECHANISMS OF ACTION
β-Lactams	Penicillins Cephalosporins Monobactams Carbapenems	Bind enzymes that regulate bacterial cell wall synthesis
Aminoglycosides	Amikacin Gentamicin Kanamycin Tobramycin Streptomycin	Inhibit bacterial protein synthesis by irreversibly binding to the 30S ribosomal subunit
Sulfonamides	Sulfadiazine Sulfadoxine Sulfamethoxazole Trimethoprim-sulfamethoxazole	Inhibit bacterial conversion of para-aminobenzoic acid to folate, impairing DNA synthesis
Tetracyclines	Chlortetracycline Oxytetracycline Tetracycline HCl Demeclocycline	Inhibit bacterial protein synthesis by binding irreversibly to the 30S ribosomal subunit
Urinary tract anti-infectives	Methenamine Nitrofurantoin	Decompose in acid urine to form formaldehyde, which is toxic to gram-negative bacteria
Quinolones	Ciprofloxacin Norfloxacin	Inhibit bacterial DNA gyrase enzyme
Antituberculins	Isoniazid	Interferes with synthesis of mycolic acid and other essential metabolites within the bacillus
	Rifampin	Inhibits RNA polymerase
	Ethambutol	Unknown
	Streptomycin	Aminoglycoside (see earlier)
Miscellaneous	Erythromycins Clindamycin Chloramphenicol Vancomycin Metronidazole	Inhibit bacterial protein synthesis by binding irreversibly to the 50S ribosomal subunit
Antifungals	Amphotericin B	Binds fungal cell membrane sterols, inducing leakage
	Miconazole	Inhibits fungal cell membrane synthesis
	Nystatin	Inhibits fungal cell membrane synthesis
	Flucytosine	Disrupts fungal protein synthesis
	Griseofulvin	Impairs fungal DNA replication
Antivirals	Acyclovir	Inhibits viral DNA polymerase
	Vidarabine	Unknown
	Zidovudine	Inhibits viral reverse transcriptase in retroviruses
	Amantadine	Prevents viral uncoating after attachment to hose cell; slightly inhibits penetration of influenza A virus
	Idoxuridine	Inhibits DNA polymerase
	Ribavirin	Inhibits RNA polymerase, processing of mRNA; reduces guanosine triphosphate concentration
Antiparasitics	Pentamidine	Impairs energy metabolism and nucleic acid synthesis of protozoans
	Mebendazole	Direct toxic action on worms
	Chloroquine	Interacts with DNA of the malaria parasite

Biologic Response Modifiers

The newest form of therapy in inflammation involves the use of CSFs, tissue growth factors, and other biologic response modifiers that have been duplicated with recombinant DNA technology.[12] Cytokine antagonists, such as α-melanocyte-stimulating hormone (which influences communication between the neuroendocrine and immune systems), IL-1 receptor antagonist, and soluble TNF receptor, are being investigated as modulators of the inflammatory response.[13]

Focus of Current Research

Study	Objectives and Findings
Chiu, et al. (1996) Diet and risk of non-Hodgkin's lymphoma in older women.	*Objective:* To test whether high dietary intake of fat, protein, and milk is associated with the development of non-Hodgkin's lymphoma in older women *Findings:* A high-meat diet and a high intake of animal fat are associated with increased risk.
Karon, et al. (1996) Prevalence of HIV infection in the United States, 1984–1992.	*Objective:* To estimate the number of people infected with HIV living in the United States and the change in HIV prevalence since 1984 *Findings:* As of 1992, 650,000 to 900,000 people were infected. The proportion infected was higher among non-Hispanic blacks and Hispanics than among non-Hispanic whites.
Landesman, et al. (1996) Obstetrical factors and the transmission of human immunodeficiency virus type 1 from mother to child.	*Objective:* To evaluate the relationship of obstetrical factors to vertical transmission of HIV *Findings:* Risk of transmission increases when the fetal membranes rupture more than 4 hours before delivery.
Schacker, et al. (1996) Clinical and epidemiologic features of primary HIV infection.	*Objective:* To describe the presentation of the primary HIV infection *Findings:* Primary HIV infection causes a recognizable clinical syndrome characterized by fever, sore throat, fatigue, weight loss, and myalgia.
Slaughter, et al. (1996) A comparison of the effect of universal use of gloves and gowns with that of glove use alone on acquisition of vancomycin-resistant enterococci in a medical intensive care unit.	*Objective:* To compare the efficacy of two methods in the prevention of nosocomial transmission of vancomycin-resistant enterococci *Findings:* There was no difference between the two methods.
Cao, et al. (1995) Virologic and immunologic characterization of long-term survivors of human immunodeficiency virus type 1 infection.	*Objective:* To describe common characteristics of people who remain healthy and immunologically normal for 12 to 15 years after HIV infection *Findings:* These people have low levels of the virus and a combination of strong virus-specific immune responses with some degree of attenuation of the virus.

Continued on following page

Continued

Macallan, et al. (1995) Energy expenditure and wasting in human immunodeficiency virus infection.	*Objective:* To determine the contribution of total energy expenditure to weight changes in people with HIV-associated wasting *Findings:* Reduced energy intake, not elevated energy expenditure, is the prime determinant of weight loss.
Heddle, et al. (1994) The role of the plasma from platelet concentrates in transfusion reactions.	*Objective:* To determine whether substances in the plasma or the cells in the blood product cause reactions to transfused platelets *Findings:* Bioreactive substances in the plasma cause most febrile reactions associated with platelet transfusions. Removal of the plasma before transfusion can minimize or prevent these reactions.

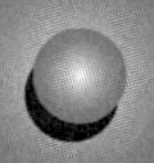

TABLE 13–9
STANDARD PRECAUTIONS*

HANDWASHING

Hands and other skin surfaces are washed immediately and thoroughly if contaminated with blood or other body fluids, whether or not gloves are worn. Hands are washed between patient contacts. Plain soap is sufficient for routine handwashing. An antibacterial agent may be appropriate in specific circumstances.

GLOVES

Clean, nonsterile gloves are worn when touching blood and body fluids, mucous membranes, or nonintact skin of all patients and when handling items or surfaces soiled with blood or body fluids.

MASK, EYE PROTECTION, FACE SHIELD

To prevent exposure of mucous membranes of the mouth, nose, and eyes, masks and protective eyewear or face shields are worn during procedures that are likely to generate droplets of blood or other body fluids.

GOWN

Gowns are worn during procedures that are likely to generate splashes of blood or other body fluids.

PATIENT CARE EQUIPMENT

Disposable articles contaminated with body substances are bagged and discarded according to local and state regulations. Reusable equipment is appropriately cleaned and reprocessed between patients.

ENVIRONMENTAL CONTROL

Adequate procedures for cleaning and disinfection of environmental surfaces and equipment are implemented.

LINEN

Used linen is handled in a manner that prevents contamination of the skin and mucous membranes of linen handlers and other patients.

OCCUPATIONAL HEALTH AND BLOOD-BORNE PATHOGENS

Care is taken to prevent injuries when using sharp instruments. Used needles are not recapped unless a one-handed scoop technique or mechanical device is used. Used needles and other sharp items are placed in a designated puncture-resistant container as close as possible to the point of use. Mouthpieces, resuscitation bags, or other ventilation devices are used as an alternative to mouth-to-mouth resuscitation methods in areas where the need for their use is predictable.

PATIENT PLACEMENT

Patients who impose risk of environmental contamination are placed in private rooms, if available, or in acceptable alternative environments for minimization of transmission risk.

*These guidelines apply to the care of all hospitalized patients, regardless of their diagnosis or presumed infectious status. An additional tier of guidelines applies to those who may be colonized or infected with epidemiologically important pathogens that can be transmitted by airborne or droplet transmission or by contact with dry skin or contaminated surfaces.

Data from Garner, J.D. (1996). Hospital Infection Control Practices Advisory Committee. *Guidelines for Isolation Precautions in Hospitals.* Public Health Service, U.S. Department of Health and Human Services, Centers for Disease Control and Prevention, Atlanta, Georgia.

Supportive Care

The oldest form of therapy for inflammatory conditions is supportive care: rest (to conserve energy), fluids (to replace those lost to exudation and to facilitate thermoregulation), and optimal nutrition (to supply energy fuel and substrate for wound healing). These measures are without risk and are sufficient intervention in most cases of adaptive inflammation.

IMMUNE RESPONSES

As has been stated, both inflammatory and immune responses are induced in most forms of cell injury, and the two processes intersect at several points. Immune responses differ from inflammation in that they are initiated by, and targeted against, specific antigens.

Classification of Immune Responses

Natural Versus Acquired Immunity

Natural immunity is inborn and is derived from nonspecific aspects of tissue defense. Certain species or races have evolved a genetic resistance to some invading agents, and although the mechanisms of this resistance are usually uncertain, natural immunity is believed to depend primarily on the actions of physical and chemical barriers, local mediators such as interferons and the proinflammatory cytokines, and cellular defense by natural killer (NK) cells and phagocytes. Whatever the mechanism, physiologic characteristics of the organism and the host are incompatible, to the benefit of the host. During the great epidemics of history, a few individuals invariably displayed this innate resistance. It is also readily apparent that many disorders of animals do not occur in humans, and vice versa, as a consequence of natural immunity.

Acquired immunity develops after birth, as immune cells proliferate and differentiate within lymphoid tissues. Immunity is acquired as a result of contact with (1) autoantigens initiating selective developmental processes and (2) foreign antigens initiating defensive immunity.

Acquired immunity develops *actively* in most cases, as when the patient develops an immune response to a microorganism with which he or she has been colonized or infected. This type of immunity usually persists for many years, possibly for life. The organism may have been communicated from other infected people, or it may have been purposively administered to initiate the immune response. **Immunization** involves the injection or oral administration of *vaccine*, which usually consists of a small amount of killed or attenuated (weakened) organism or its toxin. Table 13–10 summarizes recommendations for active immunization.

Short-term immunity may be acquired *passively* if antibodies or activated T cells are developed outside the body and transferred to the person. Passive immunity occurs by transfer of antibodies from mother to fetus across the placenta, or from mother to infant during breastfeeding. Injection of immune sera containing antibodies or other immune agents also confers passive immunity. Such agents have been used after known exposure to infectious antigens such as hepatitis B virus and in treatment of certain cancers. These substances may be developed in other people or animals, or by recombinant DNA technology (Table 13–11).

Humoral Versus Cell-Mediated Immunity

Active immune responses have long been classified as either **humoral immunity**, which is mediated by antibodies and occurs mainly in the blood and other body fluids, or **cell-mediated immunity**, which involves cytotoxic T cells and occurs mainly within cells. This distinction is becoming less clear, however, because research focusing on molecular mechanisms of immune function and on regulation of immune responses has revealed critical interactions between these two mechanisms. As discussed later, each system is involved in activation and regulation of the other, and each is active both within body fluids and within cells.

Components of the Immune System

Lymphoid Organs and Tissues

The immune system is not a specific anatomic system; rather, it is a functional system made up of organs that serve many purposes other than generation of immune responses (Fig. 13–10). *Primary* organs of the immune system are those in which lymphocytes and other immune system cells form and mature; these include the bone marrow, the thymus gland, and the liver. *Secondary* organs and tissues contain mature immune cells and are capable of generation of immune responses directed against circulating antigen or antigen that is trapped in cells. These include lymph nodes throughout the body,

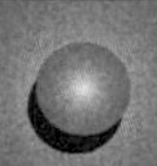

TABLE 13-10
RECOMMENDED IMMUNIZATIONS FOR CHILDREN AND ADULTS

ROUTINE IMMUNIZATIONS

Age	Recommended Immunizations
Birth	Hepatitis B (HBV)
2 months	Hepatitis B (HBV) Poliomyelitis (OPV) Diphtheria, tetanus, pertussis (DTP) *Haemophilus influenzae*, type B (HbCV)
4 months	Poliomyelitis (OPV) Diphtheria, tetanus, pertussis (DTP) *Haemophilus influenzae*, type B (HbCV)
6 months	Hepatitis B (HBV) Diphtheria, tetanus, pertussis (DTP)
12 months	*Haemophilus influenzae*, type B (HbCV)
15 months	Diphtheria, tetanus, pertussis (DTP) Poliomyelitis (OPV) Measles, mumps, rubella (MMR) *Haemophilus influenzae* booster
4–6 years	Diphtheria, tetanus, pertussis (DTP) Poliomyelitis (OPV)
14–16 years	Tetanus and diphtheria toxoids (Td)
Adult	Td every 10 years

IMMUNIZATIONS FOR THOSE AT RISK

Typhoid (ViCPS) if traveling to and from countries in which typhoid is endemic

Hepatitis A (HAVRIX) for (1) military personnel and others traveling to areas in which HAV is endemic, (2) homosexual men, (3) illicit drug users, (4) people with chronic liver disease, (5) those at occupational risk

Varicella (VARIVAX) for (1) infants and children, (2) health care workers, (3) susceptible household contacts of infected people, (4) day care center and school workers, (5) young adults in closed populations, e.g., college students, military, (5) nonpregnant women of childbearing age, (6) international travelers, (7) other susceptible adolescents and adults.

Pneumococcal pneumonia (Pneumovax 23, Pnu-Imune 23) for children with congenital and chronic illness and for susceptible adults older than 50 years

Influenza (Fluogen, Fluzone, Flu-Shield) annually for (1) adults older than 65 years, (2) chronically ill residents of long-term care facilities, and (3) adults and children with chronic pulmonary, cardiovascular, or metabolic disorders, including asthma, renal failure, hemoglobinopathies, and immunosuppression

Meningitis (Menomune-A/C/Y/W-135) for (1) high-risk children older than 2 years, (2) people with complement deficiency or asplenia, (3) close contacts of people with meningitis due to serotype B *Neisseria meningitidis*.

Data from Gardner, P., Eickhoff, T., Poland, G.A., *et al.* (1996). Adult immunizations. *Annals of Internal Medicine* 12(1 Pt. 1), 35–40; Vetter, R.T., and Johnson, G.M. (1995). Vaccination update: Diphtheria, tetanus, pertussis, mumps, rubella, measles. *Postgraduate Medicine* 98(4), 133–148; Vetter, R.T., and Johnson, G.M. (1995). Vaccination update: Hib, hepatitis, polio, varicella, influenza, pneumococcal and meningococcal disease. *Postgraduate Medicine* 98(5), 141–150.

Peyer's patches in the intestines, the appendix, the tonsils and adenoids, and the spleen.

The thymus gland, an endocrine organ, is located in the chest behind the sternum. This gland grows rapidly during childhood and reaches maximum size during puberty. The thymus then normally shrinks and becomes essentially nonfunctional, although in some adults, it persists. Overfunction of the thymus in adults has been implicated in some cases of inappropriate immune function, notably the neuromuscular disease myasthenia gravis (see Chapter 22).

The position and tissue structure of secondary immune organs facilitates the capture of antigens and also brings immunocompetent cells in contact with each other and with antigen. The tonsils and adenoids of the oropharynx are well placed to attack antigen entering through the mouth and nose, whereas immune cells in the Peyer's patches and appendix attack intestinal antigens.

The lymph nodes and spleen act as specialized filters that harbor immune cells and promote destruction of antigens in the lymph and blood, respectively. The structure and function of the spleen was discussed in Chapter 12. Figure 13–11 illustrates a typical lymph node, with its four distinct compartments: the subcapsular sinus, the diffuse cortex, the paracortical regions, and the B-cell follicles. The subcapsular sinus is lined with macrophages, typically the first immune cells to encounter antigen. The diffuse cortex of lymph nodes consists of dense networks of reticular fibers, which slow the movement of circulating cells, increasing the probability that specific antigens and their counterpart immune cells or products will contact each other as

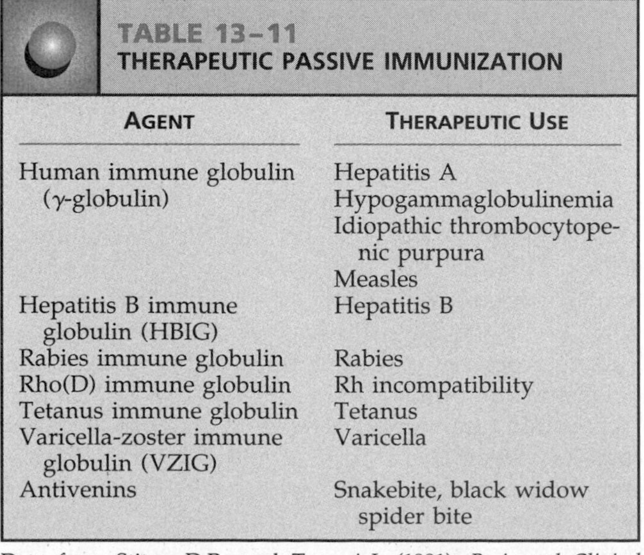

TABLE 13-11
THERAPEUTIC PASSIVE IMMUNIZATION

AGENT	THERAPEUTIC USE
Human immune globulin (γ-globulin)	Hepatitis A Hypogammaglobulinemia Idiopathic thrombocytopenic purpura Measles
Hepatitis B immune globulin (HBIG)	Hepatitis B
Rabies immune globulin	Rabies
Rho(D) immune globulin	Rh incompatibility
Tetanus immune globulin	Tetanus
Varicella-zoster immune globulin (VZIG)	Varicella
Antivenins	Snakebite, black widow spider bite

Data from Stites, D.P., and Terr, A.I. (1991). *Basic and Clinical Immunology*. (7th ed.). Norwalk, CT: Appleton & Lange.

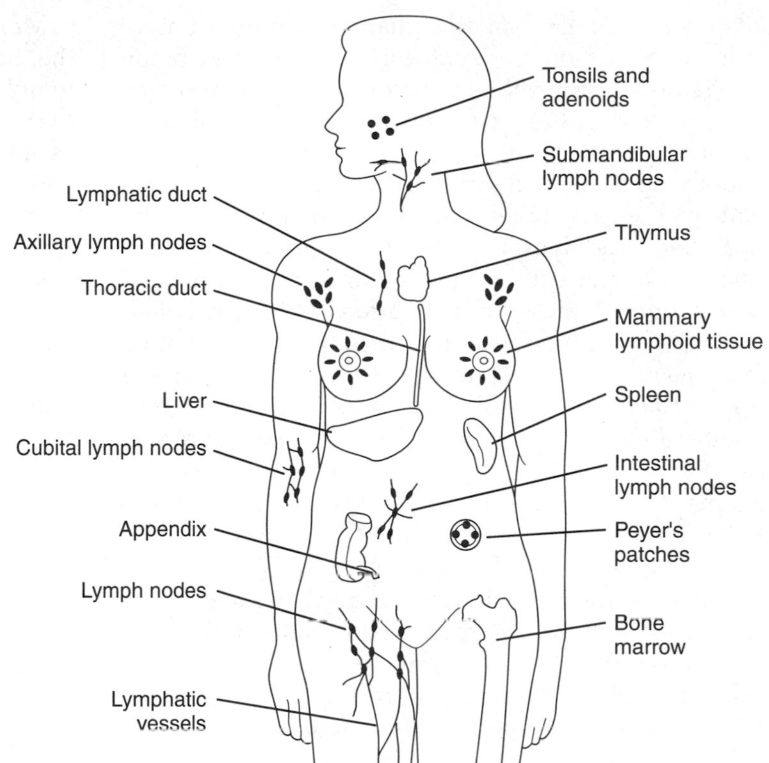

FIGURE 13–10

Immune system. The immune system is a functional system that includes primary organs (those in which immune cells form and mature) and secondary organs (those containing mature immune cells). Primary organs of the immune system include the bone marrow, thymus, and liver. Secondary organs are the lymph nodes, Peyer's patches of the intestines, the appendix, the tonsils and adenoids, and the spleen.

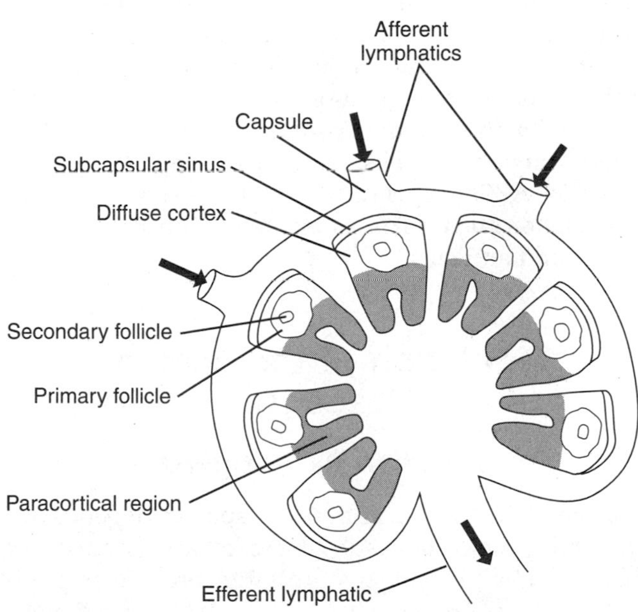

FIGURE 13–11

Lymph node structure. Lymph nodes act as filters within the lymphatic circulation, a one-way accessory circulation that carries excess fluid and particles (lymph) from the interstitium to the venous blood. Lymph fluid enters nodes through afferent lymphatic vessels and exits through efferent lymphatics. The typical lymph node has four compartments: (1) the subcapsular sinus, which is lined with macrophages; (2) the diffuse cortex, composed of net-like fibers that slow the movement of cells circulating through the node; (3) the paracortical regions, which are rich in T lymphocytes; and (4) the primary and secondary follicles, which are sites of active B-lymphocyte differentiation.

they "percolate" through the node. The paracortical regions are rich in T lymphocytes, and the B-cell follicles are sites of active B-lymphocyte differentiation.

Under neural and hormonal influences, blood flow into the lymph node is increased, promoting lymphocyte delivery, and constriction of the efferent lymphatic vessel occurs, decreasing lymphocyte outflow during an active immune response. The enlargement of lymph nodes (lymphadenopathy) that characterizes an active immune response results from these vascular responses as well as from immune-mediated inflammatory responses within nodes. Because the lymphatic system joins the venous system at the thoracic duct in the chest (see Chapter 15), antigens in either circulatory system are vulnerable to immune challenge within the lymph nodes and spleen.

Immunocompetent Cells

Lymphocytes are the critical cells of the immune response because they alone are capable of recognizing and responding to specific antigens. Lymphocytes circulate freely between lymphoid tissues and body fluids. The development of immunocompetence by these cells refers to their ability to distinguish self from nonself proteins and to generate a response specifically directed against nonself antigens. As discussed further later in this chapter, immunocompetence depends on the synthesis of specific cytokine mediators and on the expression of specific receptor proteins and adhesion molecules on the membranes of these lymphocytes.

B Lymphocytes. B lymphocytes, or B cells, originate in the fetal bone marrow, then migrate to the fetal liver and lymphoid tissues to mature. (The *B* refers to bursal equivalent; the bursa is the organ of maturation of these cells in birds.) When activated during the immune response, these cells differentiate into plasma cells and memory cells (clones of the original activated B cell). Plasma cells secrete immunoglobulins, whereas memory cells (sensitized B cells) are kept in reserve for later immune responses against the same agent. About 10% to 20% of circulating lymphocytes are B cells.

T Lymphocytes. T lymphocytes, or T cells, also originate in the bone marrow and are identical to B-cell precursors before their maturation in the thymus (*T* refers to thymus derived). Under the regulation of thymic hormones, T cells differentiate into three subclasses: helper T cells, cytotoxic T cells, and suppressor T cells. Like B cells, T cells display primary responses on initial contact with antigen and more rapid responses on subsequent contact, mediated by previously sensitized cytotoxic T lymphocytes in a memory response. On activation, helper T cells secrete cytokines that regulate the immune response. Cytotoxic T cells bind to infected or neoplastic cells, lysing them. Suppressor T cells temper the immune response by preventing inappropriate recognition of self antigens as foreign and by opposing the activation of B and T cells, thus preserving native tissues and limiting the immune response. T cells constitute about 60% to 70% of circulating lymphocytes.

Natural Killer Cells. NK cells are lymphocytes that originate and differentiate in the bone marrow but that are neither T nor B cells. NK cells do not require activation against specific antigen but are innately able to destroy some tumor cells, virally infected cells, and normal cells. These cells thus act similarly to T cells but are less specific. Additionally, NK cells are able to destroy cells that have been coated with immunoglobulin G (IgG), thereby augmenting the B-cell immune response. NK cells also secrete the cytokine γ-interferon, which promotes cell-mediated immunity. The effect of NK cells on selected normal cells is believed to be genetically programmed and to serve in embryologic tissue development and normal tissue remodeling during growth and repair. This programmed cell death (apoptosis) may also underlie cellular aging and the developmental processes that normally suppress proliferation of T cells, which could attack self tissues.

Monocyte-Macrophages. Monocytes develop in the bone marrow and circulate in the blood and lymph, with some entering and maturing in tissues. Mature monocytes, known as macrophages, function as phagocytes and in regulation of inflammation and healing. Their additional importance in the immune response is evident during the initial encounter with antigen. Macrophages line the subcapsular sinus of lymph nodes, near the afferent lymphatic vessels. In their role as the principal antigen-presenting cells (APCs) of the cellular immune response, macrophages bind and engulf antigen, breaking it into pieces and expressing some of these pieces on the macrophage surface. Binding of the antigen-containing macrophage and a helper T cell results in activation of the helper T cell and initiates secretion of T-cell cytokines for regulation of the specific immune response. Monocytes also secrete cytokines, which have many functions, including promotion of maturation of T and B cells (Table 13–12).

Dendritic and Langerhans Cells. These cells are distinguished by their cytoplasmic processes or extensions (dendritic processes). Like monocyte-macrophages, they serve as APCs; but unlike macrophages, they are not phagocytic. Langerhans cells are located in the epidermis of the skin (see Chapter 36). There are two subclasses of dendritic cells: one is bone marrow derived, and the other originates within the follicles of lymph nodes. In addition to its antigen-presenting role, the follicular dendritic cell functions in regulation of B-lymphocyte function. The ability of monocyte-macrophages, dendritic cells, Langerhans cells, and also some B cells to serve as APCs depends on their expression of self antigens on their surfaces as well as on their capacity to bind antigens.

Regulation of the Immune Response

Initiation by Antigens

Generation of the immune response depends on the ability of certain substances to act as antigens. Usually, foreign antigens are large protein or polysaccharide molecules such as those associated with microorganisms or their toxins, venoms, foods, and protein-based drugs, such as streptokinase. Regions on the membranes of neoplastic cells may also be antigenic (tumor antigens), and the body's own cell membranes have sites (often receptors for hormones or neurotransmitters) that may serve as self antigens.

Haptens, or incomplete antigens, are low-molecular-weight molecules that are too small to elicit an

TABLE 13–12
CELLULAR MEDIATORS OF IMMUNITY

MEDIATOR	FUNCTION
Cytokines	
Interleukin-2 (IL-2), IL-4, IL-5, IL-12	Promotion of lymphocyte growth, activation, and differentiation
IL-10, transforming growth factor-β	Inhibition of immune response
Colony-stimulating factors	Stimulation of hematopoiesis
Secreted immunoglobulins	Direct and indirect effects that lyse antigen-bearing cells
Recognition Molecules	
T-cell receptors	Enabling of T cell to recognize specific antigen and major histocompatibility complex and to become activated
Membrane-bound immunoglobulin	Antigen receptor on B cells
CD receptors and ligands	Membrane markers that function in recognition of specific types of immune cells and as binding sites mediating intercellular signaling
Major histocompatibility complex gene products	Recognition markers for self proteins on immune cells and nucleated body cells
Adhesion Molecules	
LFA, ICAM, CD2	Enhancement of affinity for cell–cell interaction

immune response by themselves but may do so if they first combine with a larger molecule. Most drug allergies are elicited by haptens, as are immune responses to pollens, dusts, and animal dander. Agents that cause **allergy** (an excessive or inappropriate immune response) are often referred to as **allergens**.

Antigens induce the immune response when they breach membrane barriers and nonspecific defenses and bind to APCs, such as macrophages, or in some cases, directly to B cells. The binding regions on antigens are referred to as antigenic determinants, or **epitopes**, and a single antigen may have many different epitopes on its surface membrane. Antigens do not induce the formation of specific epitope receptors on B and T cells; rather, they determine which pre-existing antigen-specific cells will be selected for activation during the immune response.

Some antigens, known as **superantigens**, bind to T-cell regions other than those associated with specific epitope. The result is nonspecific activation of more than one subpopulation of T cells, triggering an excessive immune response. An example of superantigen-initiated immunopathology is toxic shock syndrome, associated with *Staphylococcus aureus* toxin.[14]

Intercellular Recognition and Binding

The multiple cellular interactions of the immune response require that appropriate cells recognize each other at appropriate times so that appropriate binding occurs. Two recognition systems within the immune system are of clinical importance: the CD (cluster of differentiation) membrane proteins and the major histocompatibility complex (MHC) gene products. The CD system differentiates between cell types based on consistent groups of molecules expressed on cell membranes. The many CD groups are seen in varying combinations on immune system cells, but the ones of particular importance are CD4, found on some helper T cells, and CD8, present on some cytotoxic T cells. Recognition of CD sites *and* MHC antigens is essential to binding of antigen by these T cells.

The MHC genes direct the synthesis of membrane surface proteins, which serve as self antigens. The most important of these genes, clustered on chromosome 6, code for antigens that are sometimes referred to as **human leukocyte antigens** (HLA). First identified on leukocytes, HLA have since been found on all cells except neurons and RBCs. Each of the HLA genes exists in at least 50 different forms, and HLA patterns are inherited. The particular HLA subtype of a person is thus a combination of the gene forms originating from each parent, giving rise to a wide variability in HLA patterns among the general population. HLA tissue typing is one basis of tissue matching to enhance the success of organ transplantation.

Two classes of MHC gene products have been described. Class I antigens are present on nearly all nucleated body cells and on platelets. Class II antigens are found mainly on the APCs, on B cells, and on some activated T cells. Under certain conditions, one form of the cytokine interferon can induce expression of class II antigen on other cells, including fibroblasts, endothelial cells of blood vessels, and renal tubular epithelium.

Intercellular Signaling

Direct communication between immunocompetent cells has been likened to the physical and chemical connections (synapses) that exist between nerve cells in that it is local, specific, and directional. Unlike neurotransmission, however, the immunologic synapse does not depend on an electrical stimulus but instead depends on interactive effects of membrane receptors and the molecules that bind to them. The soluble mediators of immunity include a large number of cytokines (see Table 13–12).

The secreted immunoglobulins produced by B cells are also cytokines, while membrane-bound immunoglobulin proteins serve as receptors, binding to specific surface proteins on other cells. Two types of T-cell receptors have been identified: the $\alpha\beta$ type on T cells in the blood and in lymphoid tissues, and the $\gamma\delta$ type in epithelial tissues. T-cell receptors recognize epitope presented within the cleft of MHC molecules on the surfaces of APCs. Adhesion molecules expressed on cell membranes during the immune response may attract circulating inactive lymphocytes to lymph nodes or may attract activated T and B lymphocytes to areas of tissue inflammation.[15]

Hormonal Regulation

During childhood, the thymus gland produces thymic hormones that regulate the proliferation, differentiation, and maturation of T lymphocytes within the gland. As each T cell matures, it develops membrane receptors specific for a single type of antigen. Those T cells acquiring receptors for self antigens are normally weeded out by apoptosis during this maturation process.

The role of the anterior pituitary hormones in immune function has been studied extensively. Although much of the evidence is still indirect, it appears that prolactin stimulates proliferation of lymphocytes in a concentration-dependent manner.[16] If prolactin levels are too high or too low, lymphocyte reproduction is inhibited. Prolactin levels are often abnormal in patients with autoimmune diseases, such as rheumatoid arthritis and systemic lupus erythematosus (see Chapter 34) and multiple sclerosis (see Chapter 22). Both B and T cells have receptors for prolactin and also secrete prolactin-like cytokines, which may regulate immune function.

The stress hormones, specifically the glucocorticoid hormone cortisol and the catecholamines epinephrine and norepinephrine, are known to mediate effects on the immune response through receptors on T and B cells. The generalization that stress suppresses immunity cannot be supported on the basis of current research, however. Different stressors produce different effects on immunity in different people. Research in the growing field of psychoneuroimmunology aims to clarify the subtle, complex relationships between the body's major regulatory systems.[1, 17]

Neural Influences

The sympathetic nervous system innervates the thymus, bone marrow, spleen, and lymph nodes and may have direct synaptic contacts on some lymphocytes.[18] Lymphocytes, macrophages, and other immune cells have receptors for norepinephrine, the sympathetic nervous system neurotransmitter. As previously discussed, the flow of blood and lymph into nodes is differentially mediated by sympathetic stimulation to enhance the antigen-trapping and lymphocyte accumulation functions of the nodes. In laboratory studies, sympathetic agonists have been shown to modulate all aspects of the immune response, altering cytokine production, lymphocyte proliferation, and antibody secretion.[18] The progressive decline in neural stimulation of lymphoid organs with aging may underlie some of the decrease in immunoresponsiveness that also occurs.

Phases of the Immune Response

Antigen Challenge

When antigen invades the body, it is usually intercepted initially by a macrophage or other APC, which processes it so that epitope is readily accessible. Usually, but not always, the first encounter of invading antigen with a specific immunocompetent cell occurs in a lymph node or in the spleen. If the immune cell is a B cell, the humoral response is initiated; if a T cell is encountered, the cell-mediated response begins. Often, both are initiated simultaneously.

Humoral (Antibody-Mediated) Immune Response

Phases of the humoral immune response are illustrated in Figure 13–12.

Activation of B Lymphocytes. Inactive B cells circulate in the blood and migrate across specialized vascular areas into sites of trapped antigen in lymphoid organs. B cells enter the T-cell–rich paracortical areas of lymph nodes, where they bind to trapped antigen. B cells with the highest affinity for the antigen are selected for proliferation, and others undergo apoptosis. Each dividing B cell produces two daughter cell lines: plasma cells and memory cells. Some of the immunoglobulin produced by plasma cells remains attached to the B-cell membrane, where it serves as a receptor for antigen; but most is secreted into the blood or other body fluids, where it mediates the humoral response.

The production of antibodies on first exposure to a specific antigen is known as the *primary immune*

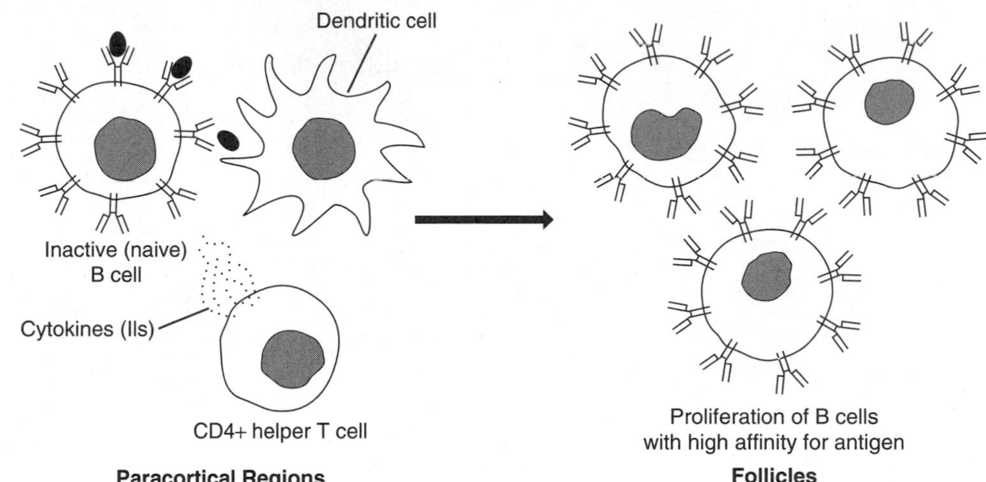

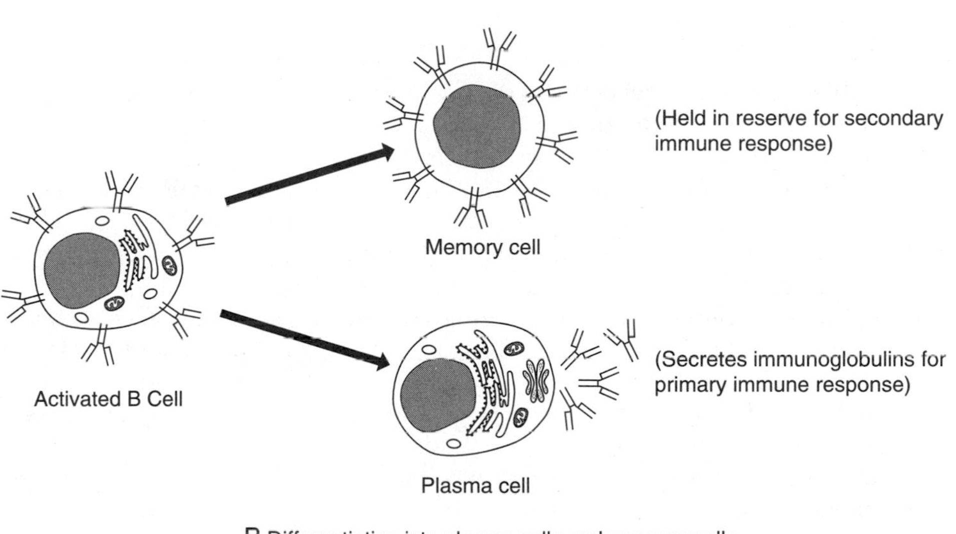

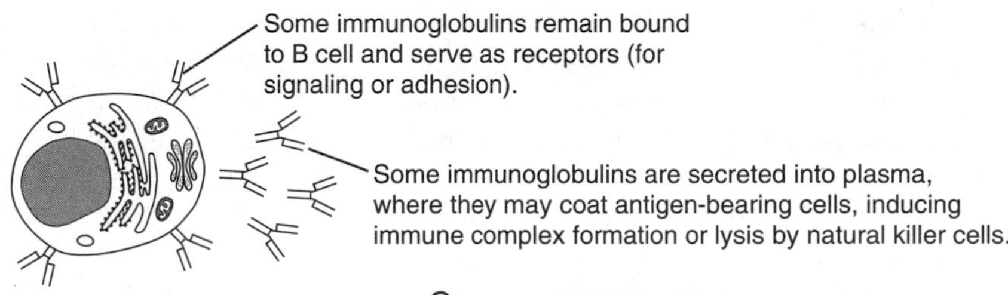

FIGURE 13–12
Humoral immune response. *A,* Circulating inactive B lymphocytes enter the paracortical regions of lymph nodes, where they bind to trapped antigen. B cells that have the highest affinity for the antigen are selected for proliferation and activated. *B,* Each dividing B cell produces two daughter cell lines: plasma cells, which secrete immunoglobulins on the first encounter with antigen (primary immune response), and memory cells, which are held in reserve. Memory cells, which are clones of the original activated B cell, are able to mount a more rapid and potent response in the case of a subsequent encounter with the antigen (secondary immune response). *C,* Immunoglobulins may remain attached to the B-cell membrane, serving as receptors for regulation of the immune response, or may be secreted into the blood for direct or indirect actions against antigen-bearing cells.

response. Memory cells lie dormant until a second or subsequent encounter with the same antigen, when their increased numbers facilitate a more rapid and potent humoral response (*secondary immune response,* or memory response).

Immunoglobulin Structure. B cells synthesize five classes of immunoglobulins, all of which are composed of the same basic Y-shaped structural unit consisting of two heavy and two light polypeptide chains (Fig. 13–13). The classes are differentiated by the amino acid sequences in their constant (Fc) regions, which bind the immunoglobulin to cell surfaces or to complement. Immunoglobulin molecules also contain variable or antigen-binding (Fab) regions that have at least two binding sites for specific epitope. The five classes of immunoglobulins, IgA, IgD, IgE, IgG, and IgM, are depicted in Table 13–13, which also summarizes their characteristics and functions.

Actions of Immunoglobulins. Binding of anti-

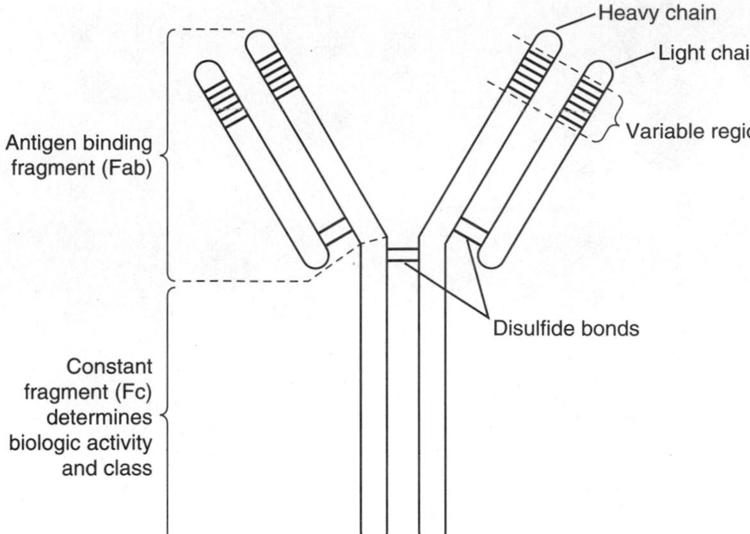

FIGURE 13–13
Immunoglobulin structure. Five classes of immunoglobulins are synthesized by B lymphocytes. All classes are derived from a basic structural unit consisting of two heavy-chain and two light-chain peptides linked by disulfide bonds in a Y shape. The amino acid sequence of the constant fragment (Fc) segment determines the immunoglobulin class. The Fc region serves to bind the immunoglobulin to cell surfaces or to complement proteins. The antigen-binding segment (Fab) has at least two binding sites for antigen.

body to antigen results in several direct and indirect effects aimed at destruction of the antigen. Direct effects include complement fixation, precipitation, agglutination, and neutralization (Fig. 13–14). If the antigen is a cell, such as a bacterium, binding induces a change in the shape of the immunoglobulin, which exposes binding sites for complement and attaches, or fixes, complement to the antigen–antibody complex, eventually destroying the cell. If two or more antigen-bearing particles are bound to the immunoglobulin, the complex may be large enough to precipitate out of solution in body fluids. This may be effective in destroying the antigen, but the precipitated immune complexes may also trigger inappropriate or excessive inflammation, as discussed later in this chapter. Agglutination (clumping) of antigen-bearing particles occurs by the same mechanism and may inactivate antigen or make it more accessible to phagocytic cells. Immunoglobulins may also neutralize bacterial toxins by preventing their secretion or binding.

Indirect effects of the humoral response include facilitation of inflammation through activation of the complement cascade by the classic pathway. In addition, coating of antigen-bearing cells with immunoglobulin facilitates inflammation by attracting phagocytic neutrophils. Antibody-coated cells are also more susceptible to destruction by NK cells. B cells, which express class II MHC on their membranes, may also act as APCs for the cell-mediated immune response.

Cell-Mediated Immune Response

Encounter of an antigen with a specific immunocompetent T cell sets off a chain of events that is regulated and amplified by several cytokines released during the process. Antigen cannot initiate the cell-mediated response unless it is first processed by an APC.

Activation of Helper T Cells. The cell-mediated response typically begins with presentation of antigen by a macrophage expressing epitope on its surface (Fig. 13–15). A small number of helper T cells possessing CD4 receptors (which recognize *both* the epitope and the class II MHC self antigen on the macrophage) bind the antigen. This binding causes the macrophage to secrete IL-1, which in turn binds to an IL-1 receptor on the helper T cell, activating it. Once activated, the helper T cell secretes regulatory cytokines, the most important of which is probably IL-2. IL-2 is involved in B-cell activation and is essential to the activation of cytotoxic T cells (discussed later). On the basis of differential cytokine secretion, two subclasses of helper T cells have been identified.[19, 20] The first subclass of helper T cells, Th1 cells, promotes differentiation of activated B cells that secrete IgM, IgG2a, and IgG3 and that also induce the activity of macrophages. The second subclass, Th2 cells, promotes proliferation of inactive B cells and differentiation of active B cells into IgM-, IgG1-, and IgG3-secreting cells. Th1-mediated activities tend to enhance cell-mediated immunity, whereas Th2-mediated responses may inhibit the tissue-damaging effects of Th1 responses to some extent. Depending on the pattern of cytokines produced, helper T cells may develop into either active cells or memory cells.

Activation of Cytotoxic T Cells. Cytotoxic T cells are activated when they encounter specific epitope presented within the groove of the class I MHC protein complex on body cell membranes (Fig. 13–16). Cytotoxic T cells with α β T-cell receptors that recognize both the epitope and the class I MHC

TABLE 13–13
CHARACTERISTICS AND FUNCTIONS OF THE IMMUNOGLOBULIN CLASSES

IMMUNOGLOBULIN	CHARACTERISTICS	FUNCTIONS
IgA (IgA1, IgA2) J chain IgA	15% of serum Ig Primary Ig in secretions and breast milk	Barrier to mucosal invasion Antiviral defense
IgD IgD	0.2% of serum Ig Most on B-cell surface Initial Ig expressed (with IgM)	May be involved in attack against certain antigens Primary role is probably in intercellular signaling
IgE IgE	0.004% of serum Ig	Defense against parasitic infection Mediates immediate hypersensitivity ("true" allergy)
IgG (IgG1, IgG2, IgG3, IgG4) IgG	75% of serum Ig Able to cross placenta	Mediates secondary immune response Complement fixation Binds to macrophages, activating them
IgM J chain IgM	10% of serum Ig Initial Ig expressed (with IgD) 10 binding sites	Mediates primary immune response Complement fixation Mediates some blood transfusion reactions Agglutination

(designated CD8+) bind to the epitope. Specific recognition and binding is regulated by five additional membrane proteins associated with the T-cell receptor, and the cytotoxic T cell is induced to express receptors for IL-2 on its surface. Binding of IL-2 (from activated helper T cells) then induces rapid proliferation of clones of activated, antigen-specific cytotoxic T cells.

Actions of Cytotoxic T Cells

In a process known as *immune surveillance*, activated cytotoxic T cells circulate throughout the blood, lymph, and lymphoid tissues in search of specific cellular antigen (typically on cells infected with viruses or other intracellular pathogens such as *mycoplasmas* or *chlamydiae*, or on neoplastic cells). When such antigen is bound by a T cell, the epitope-containing cell is destroyed by one of three effector mechanisms: (1) proteolytic enzymes contained within T-cell granules; (2) release of cytokines known as *perforins*, which create pores in the cell membrane of the target cell (similar to the effects of the membrane attack complex of complement); and (3) by a pathway mediated by a T-cell surface molecule, Fas (APO-1), which triggers apoptosis.[21] After inflicting its cytotoxic injury, the T cell then detaches and continues its surveillance. Activated cytotoxic T

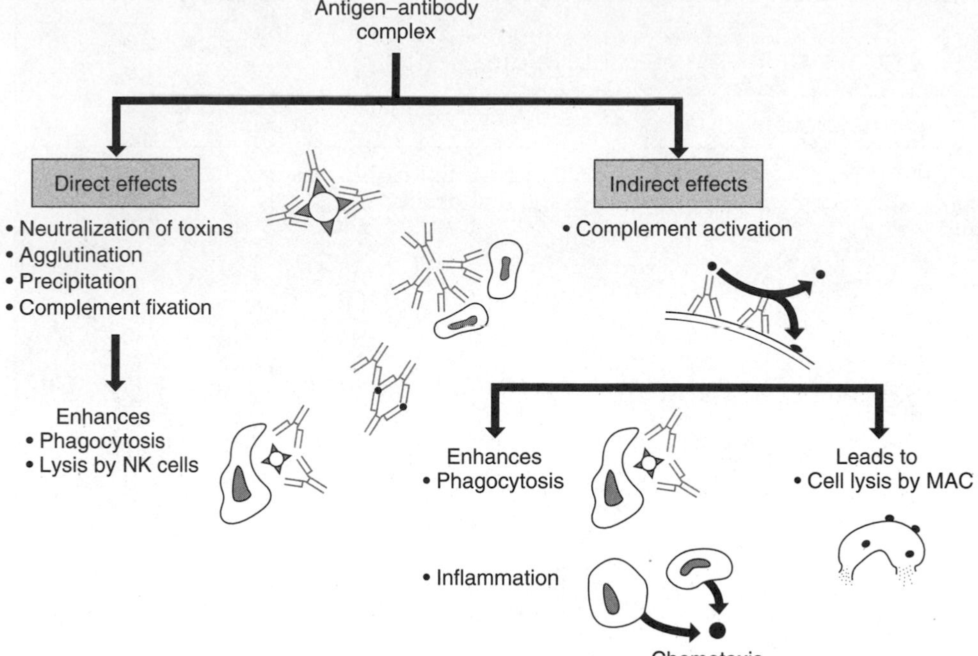

FIGURE 13–14
Actions of immunoglobulins. Binding of antigen to immunoglobulin (antibody) initiates multiple effects designed to destroy the antigen-bearing cell. Fixation (binding) of complement to the antigen–antibody complex attracts phagocytic cells, enhances the inflammatory response, and leads to lysis of the antigen-bearing cell through the membrane attack complex (MAC) of complement. Coating of antigen-bearing cells with immunoglobulin may (1) neutralize bacterial toxins, and (2) agglutinate (clump) cells so that they precipitate out of solution or are more accessible to phagocytes or natural killer (NK) cells.

cells also secrete a wide variety of cytokines, including interferons and regulators of macrophage activity. As with B cells and helper T cells, some activated cytotoxic T cells differentiate into memory cells, which may effect a more rapid response than that mediated by "naive" cells, which require activation.

Mechanisms of Immunopathology

As is also the case with inflammation, the immune response may cause or contribute to disease if it is excessive, inappropriately triggered, or deficient. Four broad categories of immunopathology

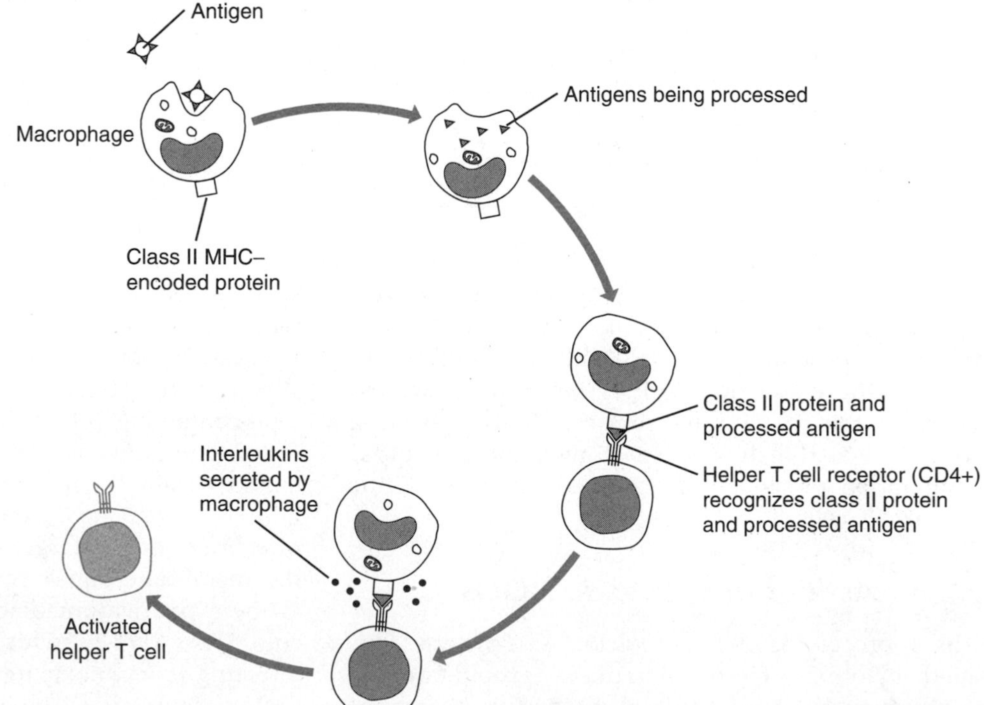

FIGURE 13–15
Activation of helper T cells. Antigens are processed and presented by an antigen-presenting cell, typically a macrophage. Certain CD4+ helper T cells, which recognize the specific antigen *and* major histocompatibility complex (MHC) class II self-antigen on the macrophage, bind the antigen. Binding induces the secretion of interleukin-1 by the macrophage, and interleukin-1 binds to its receptor on the helper T cell, activating it and inducing it to secrete interleukin-2.

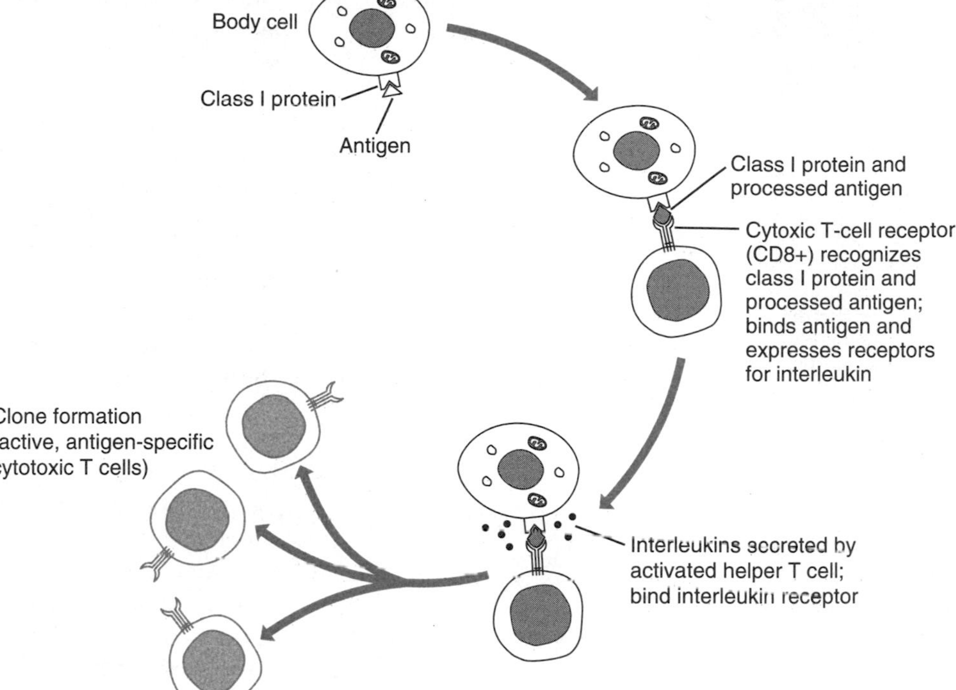

FIGURE 13–16

Activation of cytotoxic T cells. Certain CD8+ cytotoxic T cells, which recognize the specific antigen and major histocompatibility complex class I (on the body cell bearing the antigen) bind to the antigen. Binding induces the T cell to express receptors for interleukin-2 on its membrane. Binding of interleukin-2 (from activated helper T cells) induces rapid proliferation of clones of the activated cytotoxic T cell.

are recognized: **hypersensitivity, autoimmunity, isoimmunity,** and **immunodeficiency**.

Hypersensitivity

Hypersensitivity refers to an excessively intense immune response that may cause tissue damage or possibly even death of the host. Two major forms of hypersensitivity are defined based on the time course of the response: *immediate hypersensitivity* results in clinical manifestations within about 30 minutes, and *delayed hypersensitivity* may take several days to develop.

Immediate Hypersensitivity. Clinical features of allergy, **anaphylaxis**, and **anaphylactoid reactions**, the three types of immediate hypersensitivity, are summarized in Table 13–14. These syndromes all result from mast cell degranulation. In the cases of allergy and anaphylaxis, mast cell degranulation is mediated by IgE through the cross-linking mechanism illustrated in Figure 13–17. Two adjacent IgE molecules bound to mast cells or basophils are

TABLE 13–14
CLINICAL SYNDROMES OF IMMEDIATE HYPERSENSITIVITY

Syndrome	Mechanism	Clinical Manifestations	Examples
Allergy	Mast cell degranulation by cross-linking of IgE, releasing inflammatory mediators	Vasodilation Edema Inflammatory exudation Smooth muscle spasm Increased vascular permeability	Asthma Seasonal allergic rhinitis Eczema Urticaria
Anaphylaxis	Same as allergy, except on a massive scale	Bronchospasm Vomiting Laryngeal edema Vascular collapse or shock	Response to insect venoms, drugs, foods
Anaphylactoid reaction	Mast cell degranulation by a non-IgE mechanism	Similar to anaphylaxis, but usually milder	Response to drugs, IV contrast media

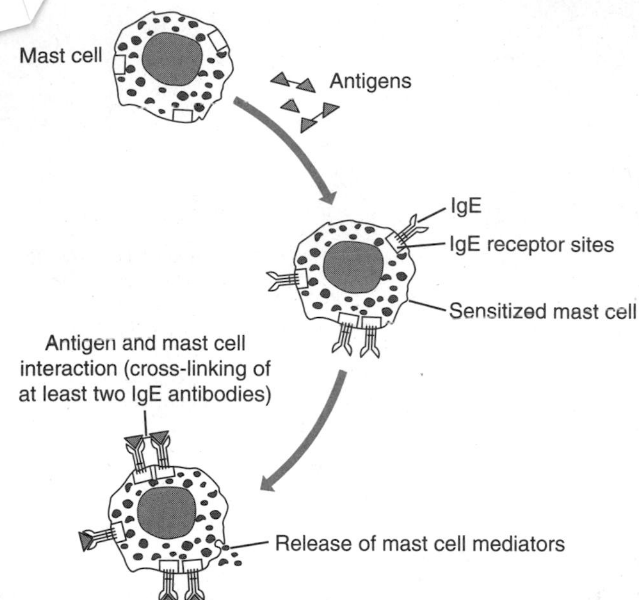

FIGURE 13–17

Mechanism of mast cell degranulation. Immediate hypersensitivity reactions result from the release of mast cell mediators of inflammation by antigen cross-linking of immunoglobulin E (IgE) molecules bound to the mast cell surface.

simultaneously bound by antigen, resulting in secretion of histamine, prostaglandins, and other inflammatory mediators.

The adaptive function of IgE-mediated humoral immunity is to protect against infection of parasites entering through the skin, lungs, or gastrointestinal tract, and IgE-secreting B cells are abundant in these tissues. In allergy, IgE is overproduced or inappropriately produced in response to common environmental allergens. True allergy is always mediated by IgE, but the term allergy is often used inappropriately in reference to any abnormal or unpleasant response to an agent, such as a food or drug. Allergy generally refers to a local or more limited reaction, whereas anaphylaxis refers to a generalized or systemic response. Both are more likely to occur in atopic people, who have a genetic predisposition to type I hypersensitivity. Atopy is familial; but usually, no consistent pattern of inheritance is seen. More than 20% of the U.S. population suffers from one or more forms of allergy, and its prevalence appears to be increasing rapidly.[22]

Examples of conditions caused by true allergy are the respiratory conditions allergic (intrinsic) asthma and seasonal allergic rhinitis (hay fever) (see Chapter 18) and the dermatologic disorders atopic dermatitis (eczema) and urticaria (hives) (see Chapter 36). Local inflammation results in edema and fluid exudation as well as other manifestations specific to the tissues involved. Anaphylaxis, usually triggered by insect venoms or injected drugs, is a life-threatening state of systemic circulatory collapse (anaphylactic shock), with airway obstruction due to laryngeal edema and bronchial constriction (see Chapter 15).

Allergic responses are ideally prevented by identifying and avoiding contact with specific allergens. Often, this is not possible or desirable, however, and hyposensitization therapy is instituted in an effort to prevent or decrease the intensity of the immune response. Hyposensitization therapy consists of the regular administration of small but increasing amounts of allergen ("allergy shots") in an effort to increase the patient's tolerance of the agent. This therapy is successful in many people, although the mechanisms by which tolerance is established are uncertain.[23] In most cases, IgE levels are not altered, but increased levels of IgG-class antibody directed against the allergen are usually seen. IgG may attack the allergen, rendering it less able to trigger the IgE-mediated response. Basophils also release much less histamine in hyposensitized people.

Antihistamines (which block histamine binding to target cells), mast cell stabilizers (which inhibit histamine release), and steroids (which block formation of prostaglandin and leukotriene mediators of inflammation) are commonly used, nonspecific drugs that may temper the allergic response (see Chapter 18).

Anaphylactoid reactions are often classified with the immediate hypersensitivity reactions because they also involve mast cell degranulation. Although clinical manifestations are similar, IgE is *not* involved. The mechanism that induces release of inflammatory mediators is unknown. Agents commonly causing anaphylactoid reactions are contrast media (used in diagnostic radiographs), drugs, and foods. Anaphylactoid reactions are less intense than anaphylactic responses and are usually immediately reversible with administration of antihistamines.

Delayed Hypersensitivity. Delayed hypersensitivity is a T-cell–mediated response that is usually initiated by a skin irritant such as those found in some plant secretions (e.g., poison ivy or poison oak), detergents, lotions, cosmetics, adhesive tape, jewelry, clothing, and linens. Sunburn is also considered by many to be a delayed hypersensitivity response to ultraviolet light rather than a true burn injury (see Chapter 36). Delayed hypersensitivity may also play a role in rejection of transplanted tissues, as discussed later. The effects of cytotoxic T lymphocytes, activated tissue macrophages, NK cells, and interferons account for the damage to surrounding normal tissue as well as to the irritating agent. Clinical manifestations of inflammation appear in response to the tissue injury within 3 days and are mediated by T-cell lymphokines rather than mast cell mediators.

Delayed hypersensitivity reactions are usually localized to the area of contact. Clinical manifestations are more severe on second or subsequent contact with the agent because the proliferation of specific memory T cells (sensitization) has been stimulated by the prior contact. It is this sensitization that is the basis of tuberculin skin testing (Mantoux or PPD), in which TB antigen is injected between the layers of the skin. Redness and induration (hardness due to edema) of the area occurs if the person has been previously sensitized to the organism (see Chapter 19).

Autoimmunity

Autoimmune responses are inappropriately directed at self antigens (**autoantigens**) and may involve either humoral or cell-mediated immune mechanisms, or both. Many diseases are now known to be caused, entirely or partly, by autoimmunity (Table 13–15). These disorders are discussed in the systems chapters relevant to the affected tissues and organs. The mechanisms of autoimmunity are incompletely understood, but their common denominator is loss of self-tolerance.

Self-tolerance is essential to the immune system's ability to differentiate self from nonself antigens and to spare native cells from immune attack. Immune cells develop self-tolerance during their maturation, as clones of lymphocytes that develop receptors for self proteins are selectively destroyed by apoptosis. This process is thought to be more important in cell-mediated immune tolerance than in the humoral response because self-reactive B cells and immunoglobulins (**autoantibodies**) are commonly seen in body fluids and lymphoid tissues. These antibodies may function normally in the removal of aged or defective cells.

TABLE 13–15
AUTOIMMUNE DISEASES

SYSTEM	DISEASES	CHAPTER
Cardiovascular	Thrombocytopenic purpura	14
	Henoch-Schönlein purpura	14
	Rheumatic fever	16
Renal	Glomerulonephritis	20
Nervous	Myasthenia gravis	22
	Amyotrophic lateral sclerosis	22
	Multiple sclerosis	22
Gastrointestinal	Ulcerative colitis	24
Endocrine	Hashimoto's thyroiditis	28
	Diabetes mellitus	29
Musculoskeletal	Rheumatoid arthritis	34
	Systemic lupus erythematosus	34

Self-reactive immune cells are rendered functionally inactive by a variety of mechanisms. Antigen binding to immature immune cells may prevent expression of receptors, recognition of MHC antigen on APCs, or immunoglobulin secretion. These cells are then unable to respond to a subsequent challenge by antigen. Finally, it is believed that suppressor T cells play a role in limiting autoimmune responses, but the mechanisms of this suppression are unknown.

The loss of self-tolerance, which is the hallmark of autoimmune disorders, may result from the single or combined effects of processes that alter either the antigenic determinants on body cells or the function of immunocompetent cells. Native tissue cells that were previously tolerated may become antigenic if their cell membranes are structurally altered by injury, disease, or age-related degeneration. Genetic mutations may result in expression of antigenic epitopes in tissues that have high mitotic rates, a tendency that increases with aging (see Chapter 6).

Infection may induce the activation of clones of immune cells against epitopes that are similar enough to native antigens to allow cross-reaction with both the invading organism and some normal cells. Microorganisms may also produce toxins that stimulate proliferation of several clones of immunocompetent cells, inducing an increased risk of autoimmune attack.

Inherited variations in class II MHC gene products have been associated with autoimmune diseases, notably type I diabetes mellitus. During T-cell maturation in the thymus, deletion of self-reactive clones depends on recognition of self antigens on cells presented by class II APCs. When this presentation is defective, some self-reactive T cells may not be deleted, predisposing the patient to autoimmune disorders.

Finally, the ratio of T-cell subclasses appears to be important in autoimmunity. Decreases in suppressor T cells and increases in cytotoxic T cells or helper T cells may increase the risk of autoimmune responses. Such alterations can be seen with aging or with immunodeficiency disorders such as AIDS (discussed later).

Isoimmunity

Isoimmunity is immune attack against tissues originating from another human being. Specifically, isoimmunity includes rejection of infused or surgically implanted tissues from a human donor, or attack of the maternal immune system against fetal tissues. Examples of the former include **transfusion reactions** against whole blood or its components (Table 13–16), **ABO incompatibility, Rh incompatibility, graft rejection,** and **graft-versus-host disease (GVHD),** associated with organ transplantation. The antigens in each case are genetically derived and include the blood group antigens and the HLA antigens.

ABO Incompatibility. There are many antigens in the blood, but the two that are most important clinically are found on the erythrocyte membrane: the ABO system and the Rh system. The ABO group consists of genetically determined combinations of A or B antigens on the RBC membrane and anti-A or anti-B antibodies in the serum. Four ABO types are possible: type A, with A antigen and anti-B antibody; type B, with B antigen and anti-A antibody; type AB, with both antigens and neither antibody; and type O, with neither antigen and both antibodies (Fig. 13–18). If a type A patient were infused with type B blood, the anti-A antibodies in the donor blood (usually a minimal amount) would attack the recipient's erythrocytes, and the recipient's anti-B antibodies would destroy the donor erythrocytes, a much more detrimental effect.

Clinical manifestations result from agglutination and lysis of RBCs and from the inflammatory response to tissue injury.[24, 25] Inflammatory mediators are released, resulting in vascular spasm followed by dilation, fever, hypotension, pain and redness at the infusion site, flushing of the skin, headache, and possibly bronchoconstriction. Low back pain and renal failure may occur if renal blood flow is compromised by vascular spasm, hypotension, or intravascular clots. Hemolytic anemia is apparent from hematology studies, and hemoglobin is evident in the urine. Severity of the transfusion reaction is proportional to the amount of incompatible blood transfused.

Type O blood is often referred to as the universal donor if transfused in small amounts. Because it contains neither antigen, the antibodies of the recipient will not attack the donor cells. The antibodies contained in the donor serum will attack recipient cells; but with limited volumes transfused, this effect is minimal. Type AB patients, with neither antibody, are universal recipients in that they may receive any type of blood in small amounts.

The possibility of transfusion reaction is minimized in clinical settings with careful blood typing and cross-matching (checking for incompatibility before infusion). Volumes of blood transfused are kept to a minimum, and whenever possible packed RBCs are infused rather than whole blood, thus eliminating the effects of serum antibodies in the donor units. When blood losses are anticipated before surgery, autotransfusion of the patient's own blood is often done. Patients may bank their own blood in

TABLE 13–16
TRANSFUSION REACTIONS

Reaction	Mechanism	Clinical Manifestations
Acute hemolysis	Lysis of donor RBCs by antibodies in host plasma (ABO incompatibility)	Fever, chills, back pain, flushing, nausea, lightheadedness, hemoglobinuria, dyspnea, hypotension, shock, renal failure
Delayed hemolysis	Extravascular clearance of IgG-coated RBCs by the tissue macrophage system (donor RBCs have antigens to which host has previously been sensitized)	Fever, jaundice, anemia, hemoglobinuria (usually 7–14 days after transfusion)
Anaphylactoid reaction	IgA-deficient host develops antibodies against IgA in donor serum, resulting in immune complex–induced inflammation	Hypotension, flushing, chills, laryngeal edema, bronchospasm, GI distress, urticaria
Fever without hemolysis	Immunoglobulins in recipient plasma react against antigens on donor WBCs or platelets	Fever
Transfusion-associated lung injury	Altered permeability of pulmonary capillary beds due to histamine or complement	Pulmonary edema, dyspnea, chills, fever, cyanosis, hypotension

Data from Gloe, D. (1991). Common reactions to transfusions. *Heart and Lung* 20(5 Pt. 1), 506–512; Sloop, G.D., and Friedberg, R.C. (1995). Complications of blood transfusion: How to recognize and respond to noninfectious reactions. *Postgraduate Medicine* 98(1), 159–172.

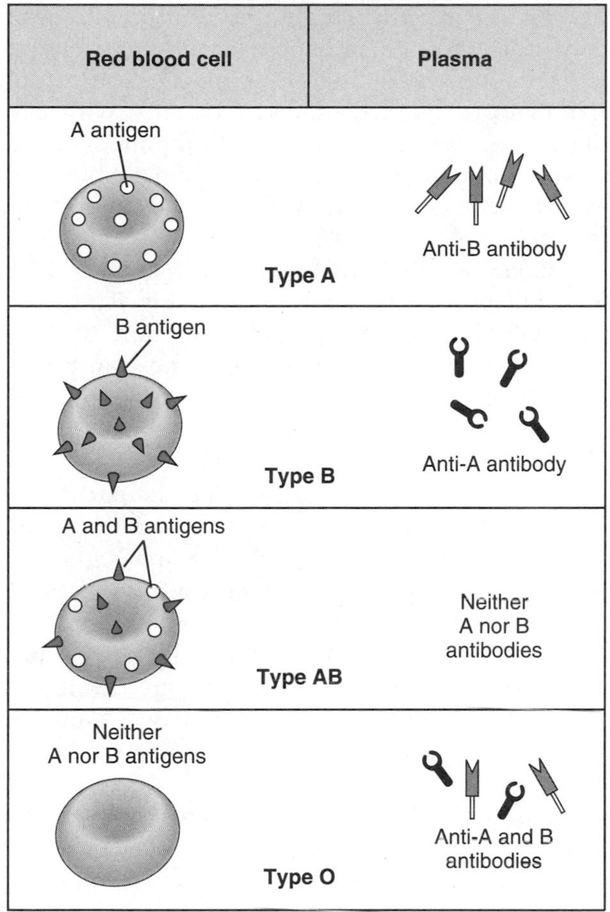

FIGURE 13–18
ABO blood group system. Type A blood has A antigen on the red blood cell surface and anti-B antibody in the plasma. Type B blood has B antigen and anti-A antibody. Type AB has both antigens and neither antibody, whereas type O has neither antigen and both antibodies.

advance of procedures, and blood lost intraoperatively or with postoperative wound drainage may be collected, processed, and reinfused. Research aimed at development of artificial blood and blood products is ongoing.

Rh Incompatibility. Typing for Rh antigen is routinely done and is of particular importance in obstetrics. Rh antigen, named for the initial research done with rhesus monkeys, is present on the erythrocytes of about 85% of whites and virtually 100% of blacks in the United States. There are more than 30 antigens in the Rh group, but those of the D group are usually the ones involved in Rh incompatibility.[26] For this reason, Rh incompatibility is sometimes referred to as Rho(D) isoimmunization.

People who have Rh antigen on RBCs are designated Rh positive, whereas those lacking the antigen are Rh negative. Rh-negative people develop anti-Rh antibodies if exposed to Rh-positive blood, as a result of either incompatible transfusion or, in the case of childbearing women, exposure to the blood cells of an Rh-positive fetus.

Usually, the first Rh-positive infant born to an Rh-negative mother is not affected because the placenta effectively separates fetal RBCs from maternal plasma, preventing formation of anti-Rh antibodies during the pregnancy. In some conditions, such as pregnancy-induced hypertension or other obstetrical complications, sensitization may occur during pregnancy. In most cases, however, sensitizing contact occurs only during delivery, inducing development of maternal anti-Rh antibodies that, with subsequent pregnancies in which the fetus is Rh-positive, cross the placenta and lyse fetal RBCs. The resultant condition, erythroblastosis fetalis (hemolytic disease of the newborn), has potentially devastating effects on the infant. Destruction of fetal RBCs leaves the infant severely anemic, resulting in poor tissue oxygenation and possible organ failure (see Chapter 12). Bilirubin released from lysed RBCs may lead to kernicterus, or toxicity of the brain (see Chapter 26). The most severe form (hydrops fetalis) is characterized by enlargement of the liver and spleen due to the large numbers of lysed RBCs, bleeding tendencies due to diversion of bone marrow stem cells to erythrocyte production at the expense of platelets, and third spacing of fluid secondary to cardiac failure.

Hemolytic disease of the newborn is preventable with prenatal monitoring and maternal injection of anti-Rh antibody (RhoGAM or RhIG) at the time of delivery of the first infant, or after any potentially sensitizing event (e.g., abortion, ectopic pregnancy). These anti-Rh antibodies lyse any fetal Rh-positive RBCs shortly after they enter the maternal circulation, preventing development of large amounts of anti-Rh antibody. If erythroblastosis fetalis does develop, the condition may be treated with exchange transfusion (replacement of the infant's blood with antibody-free blood). Intrauterine transfusion (into the umbilical cord) may also be done when fetal effects of Rh incompatibility are detected during pregnancy.

Organ Transplantation. Tissues transplanted from one human being to another are known as *allografts*, and tissues (usually skin or bone marrow) transplanted from one area of the body to another within the same person are known as *autografts*. An *isograft* is a tissue transplant from a genetically identical donor (e.g., an identical twin), whereas a *xenograft* is a transplant from another species. Xenografts are temporary, as exemplified by the use of pigskin grafts for short-term coverage of burn wounds.

Allografts, because they are foreign tissues, inevitably induce an immune response in the recipient or ost. Rejection of the graft occurs unless the immune response is minimized through careful tissue typing before transplantation and, often, therapeutic suppression of the host immune response with radiation or chemotherapy. Organs commonly transplanted include skin, bone marrow, bone, cornea, kidney, liver, heart, and lung.

Tissue typing for compatibility is based on laboratory identification of the blood group antigens and MHC gene products produced by both potential donor and recipient. The closer the tissue match, the higher the probability of a successful graft. Ideally, a close relative (often a sibling) is the living donor for bone marrow or kidney transplantation. Cadaver donors also provide kidneys and other tissues. Unrelated living donors may provide bone marrow if there is a sufficient match of critical blood group and HLA antigens. Computerized national registries are used to facilitate identification of potentially compatible donors.

Graft Rejection. Both humoral and cell-mediated immune responses may be involved in rejection of grafts. Cell-mediated delayed hypersensitivity is the classic form of rejection. Clinical manifestations are apparent within 10 to 14 days (acute rejection) if the host is not immunosuppressed, or may appear months later (chronic rejection) in others, typically when immunosuppressive therapy is discontinued. In this reaction, lymphoid cells containing both class I and class II MHC (most likely dendritic cells) in the grafted tissue provide the antigens. Because these cells have class II MHC, they are able to activate CD4+ helper T cells of the host. Simultaneously, specific CD8+ cytotoxic T cells (which recognize class I MHC) become activated, and an immune attack is directed against the graft. Cytokines released during this process appear to further activate macrophages and B cells, although the precise mechanisms of cell-mediated rejection are as yet unknown. Clinical manifestations result from local and systemic effects of inflammatory mediators, failure of the transplanted organ, and renal failure resulting from vascular spasm and occlusion by products of cell lysis.

Hyperacute or immediate rejection of the grafted tissue becomes apparent within minutes to hours after organ transplantation. This form of rejection is antibody mediated and occurs only if the host has been presensitized against donor tissues by previous transplantation or, less commonly, by blood transfusion or maternal–fetal transfer. Clinical manifestations include widespread inflammation, occlusion of blood vessels, and necrosis of tissues (including the graft) served by those vessels.

Immunosuppressive measures are nearly always employed to enhance the success of transplantation. These measures reduce the numbers of immunocompetent cells through radiation of the bone marrow and other lymphoid tissues, administration of anti-inflammatory steroids, or chemotherapy with cytotoxic agents. This induced state of immunodeficiency places the patient at risk for opportunistic infections and neoplasms, however, as discussed later in this chapter.

Graft-Versus-Host Disease. GVHD may occur when transplanted tissue contains viable T cells, typically with bone marrow transplantation or blood transfusions (which are actually tissue transplants). These T cells recognize the host tissue antigens as foreign and mount an immune response against them.[27] Acute GVHD usually occurs within 3 months of the transplantation and is particularly damaging to cells of the skin (rash or desquamation), liver (venous occlusion), gastrointestinal tract (necrosis), and immune system (opportunistic infection). Chronic GVHD occurs more than 100 days after transplantation and usually affects multiple organs.[28] Acute GVHD occurs in 20% to 80% of patients undergoing bone marrow transplantation, despite prior host immunosuppression. Removal of T cells from the graft decreases the risk of GVHD but also increases the risk of graft failure.

Immunodeficiency

Disorders in which the immune response is absent or insufficient may be primary (congenital), secondary (acquired), or iatrogenic. Clinical features of the congenital immunodeficiencies, which are relatively rare, are summarized in Table 13–17. Secondary immunodeficiencies are commonly encountered in clinical practice, as a consequence of neoplasia of the immune system or infections directed at immune cells (e.g., AIDS). Iatrogenic destruction of immune cells may occur during treatment of neoplasia with radiation, steroids, or cytotoxic agents, or with intentional immunosuppression to promote successful organ transplantation or suppress chronic inflammation.

Because hematopoietic cells are highly mitotic, they are at increased risk for developing genetic mutations that may transform them into neoplastic cells. The leukemias, a group of malignant disorders that arise within the bone marrow, may affect both the lymphoid and myeloid cell lines (see Chapter 12). Multiple myeloma, a neoplasm originating from plasma cells, primarily manifests as direct invasion of bone (see Chapter 34). Lymphomas, including Hodgkin's disease and non-Hodgkin's lymphomas, are detailed later, along with two infec-

TABLE 13-17
CLINICAL FEATURES OF PRIMARY IMMUNODEFICIENCY

Disorder	Etiology or Pathophysiology	Manifestations
X-linked agamma-globulinemia	X-linked recessive deficiency of IgG and absence of IgM and IgA; normal cell-mediated immunity	Recurrent pyogenic infections in affected males
Hyper-IgM syndrome	X-linked recessive elevation of IgM, but no IgA and very low levels of IgG; normal cell-mediated immunity	Recurrent pyogenic and opportunistic infections, autoimmune disorders
Common variable immunodeficiency	Inherited deficiency of B-cell activation with low serum IgG, IgA, and IgM, presenting in the second or third decade	Recurrent sinus and lung infections, 50-fold risk of gastric carcinoma, autoimmune disorders common
Severe combined immunodeficiency (SCID)	Inherited (usually X-linked) deficiency of both humoral and cell-mediated immunity	Fatal infection in infancy unless isolated or treated with bone marrow transplantation or gene therapy
Wiskott-Aldrich syndrome	X-linked recessive disorder in which patient cannot make antibodies against CHO antigens and has a poor response to protein antigens	Recurrent bloody diarrhea, thrombocytopenia, eczema, pyogenic infections, risk of neoplasia

Data from Rosen, F.S., Cooper, M.D., and Wedgwood, R.J.P. (1995). The primary immunodeficiencies. *New England Journal of Medicine* 333(7), 431–440.

tious disorders that influence inflammatory and immune responses: infectious mononucleosis and AIDS.

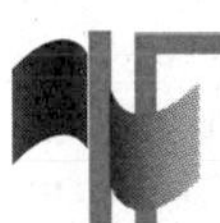

Clinical Scenario

B.H., aged 3 months, is examined in the pediatric clinic because of the development of skin lesions. The lesions are determined to be due to infection with herpesvirus and *Candida* sp. The infant also has a low-grade fever and cough, and a chest radiograph reveals pneumonia. No lymph node enlargement is noted. Her serum immunoglobulin levels are found to be greatly reduced, and no T cells are evident. B.H. was born after a normal pregnancy, and her birth weight and neonatal course were normal. Recently, however, she stopped gaining weight. Her condition is diagnosed as severe combined immunodeficiency syndrome.

1. What clinical manifestations of immunosuppression are evident?
2. What are the priorities of clinical intervention for B.H. at this time?
3. Is definitive treatment available for B.H.? Explain.

SELECTED DISORDERS OF TISSUE DEFENSE

Lymphomas

Hodgkin's Disease

Definition. Hodgkin's disease is a malignant neoplasm originating in secondary lymphoid tissues (lymph nodes or spleen), in which the transformed cell is a Reed-Sternberg (RS) cell. The RS cell is a large, multinucleated cell of uncertain origin. It apparently arises from B cells in some cases and T cells in others.

Epidemiology. Hodgkin's disease typically occurs in people of two age groups: 20 to 24 years, and 60 to 65 years.[29] Incidence in men is slightly higher. Hodgkin's disease in young adults has been associated with higher social class, advanced education, and small family size.

Etiology. The onset of Hodgkin's disease has been correlated with infection by the Epstein-Barr virus (EBV) in some studies, and a familial basis has been proposed. Hodgkin's disease is also seen as an opportunistic cancer in patients with AIDS.

Pathophysiology. Under the influence of a transforming stimulus, RS cells grow and proliferate in lymphoid tissues. Painless enlargement of a single lymph node is usually the first clinical sign of the disease, with spread of the disease along lymphatic channels to other nodes and to the spleen. Organs outside the lymphatic system are eventually infiltrated as well.

Clinical Manifestations. Lymphatic spread and progression of clinical manifestations from local to systemic constitute the basis for staging of the disease (Table 13–18). Weight loss, fever, and night sweats result from the hypermetabolic state, in which energy is consumed and heat is produced as a by-product of rapid cellular proliferation.

Treatment. Choice of treatment mode depends on the clinical stage of the disease (Table 13–19). Standard therapy is based on radiation and chemotherapy, alone or in combination.

Prognosis and Outcome. In patients with stage I or II disease, standard therapy achieves cure in 85%.[29] Patients who relapse, or those with more advanced disease, have demonstrated increased survival with the use of combination chemotherapy or autologous or allogenic bone marrow transplantation, or both.

TABLE 13–19
TREATMENT OF HODGKIN'S DISEASE

STAGES	TREATMENT
I, IIA	Radiation therapy to involved lymph nodes and adjacent lymphatic regions
IIB, III, IV	Combination chemotherapy with one of the following regimens: MOPP (mechlorethamine, Oncovin [vincristine] procarbazine, prednisone) ABVD (Adriamycin [doxorubicin], bleomycin, vinblastine, dacarbazine) ChlVPP (chlorambucil, vinblastine, procarbazine, prednisone) MOPP-ABVD in alternating monthly cycles MOPP-ABV hybrid (mechlorethamine, vincristine, procarbazine, prednisone, doxorubicin, bleomycin, vinblastine)

Non-Hodgkin's Lymphoma

Definition. Non-Hodgkin's lymphomas are malignant neoplasms of secondary lymphoid tissue origin, in which the transformed cell is not an RS cell. Non-Hodgkin's lymphoma originates from a variety of lymphoid cell types, of which most are B cells. These lymphomas are classified on the basis of cell type and malignant potential (low, intermediate, or high grade), and this classification determines choice of treatment (Table 13–20).

Epidemiology. Non-Hodgkin's lymphoma occurs in people of all ages and both sexes, although specific subclasses are more restricted in their incidence groups. Of great concern, yet still unexplained, is the 73% increase in incidence of this disease between 1973 and 1991.[30] Non-Hodgkin's lymphoma is diagnosed in 43,000 people in the United States each year. Immunodeficiency is a known risk factor for this disease. Other proposed risk factors include exposure to pesticides, use of hair dyes, prior blood transfusion, and higher dietary intake of meat and animal fats.

TABLE 13–18
CLINICAL STAGES OF HODGKIN'S DISEASE (ANN ARBOR SYSTEM)

STAGE*	DEFINING FEATURES
I	Involvement of a single lymph node region (I) or a single extralymphatic organ or site (I_E)
II	Involvement of two or more lymph node regions on the same side of the diaphragm (II), or one or more lymph node regions with an extralymphatic site (II_E)
III	Involvement of lymph node regions on both sides of the diaphragm (III), possibly with an extralymphatic organ or site (III_E), the spleen (III_S), or both (III_{SE})
IV	Diffuse or disseminated involvement of one or more extralymphatic organs (identified by symbols), with or without associated lymph node involvement

* All stages are futher classified as A (asymptomatic) or B (fever, sweats, and loss of more than 10% of body weight).

Etiology. With the exception of Burkitt's lymphoma, the etiology of non-Hodgkin's lymphoma is unknown. Burkitt's lymphoma, caused and transmitted by EBV, is endemic in some regions of Africa and South America. Failure of T-cell–mediated immune surveillance has been implicated in immunosuppressed patients.[31]

Pathophysiology and Clinical Manifestations. There is considerable variation among the non-Hodgkin's lymphoma subclasses, but clinical manifestations of this disease are usually caused by mechanical obstruction resulting from enlarged lymph nodes or lymphocytic infiltration of tissues within the abdomen or oropharynx. Abdominal pain, peptic ulcer, and constipation are frequently seen, whereas systemic signs such as fever are unusual. The central nervous system may be infiltrated in advanced disease.

Treatment and Prognosis. Table 13–20 summarizes specific treatment of the more common subclasses. Low-grade non-Hodgkin's lymphoma is curable with radiation alone in 90% of cases; combination chemotherapy and radiation are used for more advanced disease, with a 50% remission rate. Clinical trials evaluating the efficacy of bone marrow transplantation in patients with non-Hodgkin's lymphoma are under way.[32]

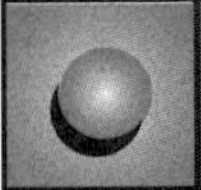

TABLE 13–20
CLASSIFICATION AND TREATMENT OF NON-HODGKIN'S LYMPHOMA

CLASSIFICATION*	TREATMENT
Low Grade	
Small lymphocytic Follicular, small cleaved Follicular, mixed small cleaved and large cell	Localized radiation for early stages Palliative radiation or chemotherapy for advanced stages
Intermediate Grade	
Follicular, large cell Diffuse, small cleaved Diffuse, mixed small and large cell Diffuse, large cell	Combination chemotherapy† with localized radiation for early stages Combination chemotherapy for advanced stages
High Grade	
Immunoblastic, large cell Lymphoblastic	Combination chemotherapy with localized radiation for early stages
Small, noncleaved Burkitt's lymphoma	Combination chemotherapy for advanced stages

* According to the Working Formulation of the National Cancer Institute.
† Combination chemotherapy with ProMACE/MOPP protocol: prednisone, methotrexate, doxorubicin, cyclophosphamide, etoposide, followed by mechlorethamine, vincristine, procarbazine, and prednisone after maximal response.

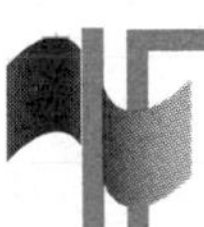

Clinical Scenario

D.V., a 72-year-old man, is admitted with intractable pain in his right leg. D.V. is 5 feet, 7 inches tall and weighs 192 pounds. Eight months earlier, his condition was diagnosed as stage I, high-grade non-Hodgkin's lymphoma. He was treated with induction chemotherapy with the CHOP protocol (cyclophosphamide, hydroxydaunomycin [doxorubicin], Oncovin [vincristine], and prednisone) and received radiation to lymph nodes on the left side of his neck. The pain in his leg is found to be due to extension of the lymphoma to his lower abdomen, causing compression of the sacral nerve roots.

1. What was the rationale for treatment of D.V.'s lymphoma with both radiation and chemotherapy?
2. What is the priority for intervention at this time?
3. What prognosis is suggested by the stage of D.V.'s disease at the time of diagnosis?

Infectious Mononucleosis

Definition. Infectious mononucleosis is a self-limited disorder characterized by proliferation of T lymphocytes in lymphoid tissues and non-neoplastic abnormality of circulating lymphocytes. It is the most common of the benign **lymphoproliferative disorders**. (Other examples of benign and malignant disorders characterized by excessive production of lymphocytes or their products are listed in Table 13–21.)

Epidemiology. Infectious mononucleosis has its highest incidence in the 15- to 25-year-old age group.[33] Approximately 1% to 3% of all college students are affected each year. The disease may also occur in young children and older adults but is uncommon after 40 years of age. Immunosuppressed patients are at higher risk for complications of the disorder.

Etiology. The usual cause is infection with EBV, a herpesvirus. EBV is usually transmitted in saliva from person to person by hand contact or kissing.

Pathophysiology. The incubation period between infection and the appearance of clinical signs of disease is 4 to 6 weeks.[34] The virus first enters and replicates within epithelial cells of the oropharynx and B lymphocytes of tonsillar tissue. Instead of lysing infected cells as viruses commonly do, EBV initiates alteration of the shape and function of the infected cells. Infected B cells produce proteins that activate cell-mediated immunity, with proliferation

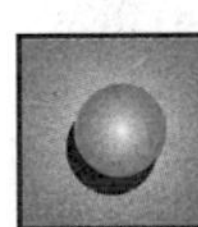

TABLE 13–21
LYMPHOPROLIFERATIVE DISORDERS

ETIOLOGIC MECHANISM	DISORDERS
Infection	Cat-scratch fever Infectious mononucleosis AIDS Toxoplasmosis Histoplasmosis Other local and systemic infections
Autoimmunity	Rheumatoid arthritis Systemic lupus erythematosus
Malignancy	Hodgkin's disease Non-Hodgkin's lymphoma Leukemias Lymph node metastasis Multiple myeloma
Iatrogenic	Serum sickness Drug hypersensitivity
Idiopathic	Sarcoidosis Kawasaki disease Lysosomal storage diseases Hyperthyroidism Waldenström's macroglobulinemia

of abnormal cytotoxic T lymphocytes in lymphoid tissues and in the circulation. Lymphoproliferation stops when cytotoxic T lymphocytes are able to destroy the population of infected B lymphocytes.

Clinical Manifestations. Although some patients (particularly young children) may not have symptoms, most patients develop an acute viral illness over 1 to 2 weeks, with fever, lymphadenopathy, and sore throat. The posterior cervical chain of lymph nodes in the neck is most often involved, and these nodes are enlarged and tender. Inflammatory exudate may be visible in the throat and may be grayish green or white.[33] There may be pinpoint red spots (petechiae) on the soft palate. The spleen and, less commonly, the liver may be enlarged. The patient usually manifests extreme fatigue, malaise, headache and body aches, and anorexia.

Hepatic enzymes (liver function tests) are usually elevated (see Chapter 26). Lymphocytosis is seen on hematology testing and on the peripheral blood smear, with atypical lymphocytes composing up to 30% of the total WBC count. The heterophile antibody rapid slide test (Monospot test), which detects anti-EBV antibodies, is positive in 50% of cases by the first week and in 90% of cases by the fourth week.[33] This test often remains negative in infected children, however.

Prevention and Treatment. Prevention involves avoidance of contact with infected people. Immunosuppressed patients must be especially vigilant. Treatment is symptomatic and supportive, with antibiotic therapy used only if secondary bacterial infection is present. Aspirin use should be avoided because this drug appears to promote further lymphoproliferation and may trigger Reye's syndrome in young children (see Chapter 26). Acetaminophen may be used to relieve fever and discomfort. To reduce the risk of splenic rupture, those with splenomegaly should be cautioned against use of motor vehicles or participation in contact sports.

Prognosis and Outcome. Most patients recover fully from infectious mononucleosis within 1 to several weeks. Complications are rare but may include splenic rupture, pericarditis, Guillain-Barré syndrome, pneumonia, meningitis, liver failure, pancreatitis, and bone marrow suppression.[34] Affected patients may continue to shed the virus for a year or more after infection, and 15% to 20% become long-term carriers. Infection confers a high degree of immunity to the virus.

Acquired Immunodeficiency Syndrome

Definition. AIDS is defined as documented infection with HIV in an adolescent or adult, together with a CD4+ T-lymphocyte count of less than 200/mm^3 or a percentage of these lymphocytes of less than 14% of the total.[35] This definition, which originated in 1993 from the Centers for Disease Control and Prevention, represents a broadened case definition from prior definitions, which specified the presence of certain clinical diseases as well.

Epidemiology. HIV infection is pandemic, affecting nearly all of the world. HIV is well accepted as the most significant emerging pathogen of the century. More than half a million cases have been reported in the United States, with 99% of these occurring in adults or adolescents.[35] The median age at diagnosis is 30 to 34 years.

TABLE 13–22
MODES OF TRANSMISSION OF HUMAN IMMUNODEFICIENCY VIRUS IN THE UNITED STATES

Mode and High-Risk Group	Percentage of Cases
Adults	
Bidirectional venereal transmission	
Homosexual or bisexual males	60
Heterosexual contacts of HIV-infected people	6
Parenteral transmission	
Intravenous drug abusers	23
Hemophiliac patients (before 1985)	1
Nonhemophiliac recipients of blood or blood components (before 1985)	2
Other and unknown transmissions	6
Children	
Vertical transmission from infected mothers	89
Parenteral transmission	10
Other or unknown transmissions	<1

Data from Cotran, R.S., Kumar, V, and Robbins, S.L. (Eds.). (1994). *Robbins Pathologic Basis of Disease* (5th ed.). Philadelphia: W.B. Saunders; Chadwick, E.G., and Yogev, R. (1995). Pediatric AIDS. *Pediatric Clinics of North America* 42(4), 969–992.

HIV is transmitted by contact with blood and other body fluids. Specific modes of transmission are listed in Table 13–22, with the most important routes being sexual contact, contact with contaminated blood, and perinatal transmission. In about 3% of cases, the route of transmission is unknown.

Before 1985, HIV was communicable by transfusion of blood or blood products, and AIDS frequently occurred among hemophiliac patients (see Chapter 14). Blood is now screened for anti-HIV antibody, but a small risk of transmission, estimated at 3.3 per 1 million transfusions, remains if recently infected people (who have not yet developed detectable levels of antibody to HIV) donate blood.[36]

Etiology. AIDS is caused by infection with HIV. There are two major types of the virus: HIV-1 and HIV-2. HIV-1 is predominant in most areas of the world, whereas HIV-2 is found primarily in West Africa. HIV-1 is further subclassified on the basis of viral genotype into group M (types A through I) and group O. The distribution of these subtypes varies geographically and may reflect different modes of transmission. HIV-1 subtype B is most prevalent in the United States. HIV subtypes may also vary in their capacity to inflict clinical disease. HIV-2 demonstrates slower progression and a lesser degree of resulting immunosuppression than does HIV-1.

Pathophysiology. HIV is a retrovirus, containing RNA and an enzyme, reverse transcriptase, which allows the viral RNA to be transcribed to DNA within the host cell. Other enzymes, including protease, and regulatory proteins are also involved in viral replication. HIV initially targets CD4+ cells, which are either helper T cells or macrophages. A surface glycoprotein, gp120, on HIV binds to the CD4+ region of the target cell, permitting entry of the virus. At least two other receptors on target cells are also required during this process. The viral DNA is integrated into the host cell's genome, where it directs activities of the cell. When immune resistance is overcome, viral replication lyses the cell. Loss of helper T cells produces immunodeficiency, particularly of the cell-mediated response.

Clinical Manifestations. The typical course of HIV-1 infection occurs in three phases: (1) an acute viral illness, which may be mild or severe; (2) a period of latency, or absence of clinical manifestations; and (3) clinical disease, resulting from viral infiltration, opportunistic infections, or neoplasms. Antibody to HIV-1 may be detectable in the blood after a variable window period. A positive enzyme immunoassay for antibody is followed by the more sensitive Western blot test to confirm the infection. Viral assays are also available but are not in wide clinical use.[37] Lymphocyte reduction ultimately is evident.

Symptoms characteristic of acute viral infection are first seen; malaise, fever, rash, diarrhea, and lymphadenopathy are commonly reported and last about 2 weeks. Children with HIV infection also display delayed development. After the immediate immune response curtails replication of the virus in the blood, symptoms may subside, and presence of the virus is then detectable only with blood testing. During this period, HIV-1 is bound to follicular dendritic cells and coated with antibody, but it continues to replicate within CD4+ cells in lymphoid tissues. As infected cells are lysed, new cells are produced to replace them. The new CD4+ cells are then infected, and a period of rapid turnover of CD4+ cells persists throughout the latent period. As the disease progresses, production of new cells by the immune system cannot keep pace, and defi-

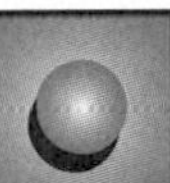

TABLE 13–23
ACQUIRED IMMUNODEFICIENCY DISEASE–ASSOCIATED DISORDERS

Opportunistic Infections Due to Immunosuppression
Candidiasis of bronchi, trachea, or lungs
Candidiasis, esophageal
Coccidioidomycosis, disseminated or extrapulmonary
Cryptococcosis, extrapulmonary
Cryptosporidiosis, chronic intestinal
Cytomegalovirus disease (other than liver, spleen, or nodes)
Cytomegalovirus retinitis (with loss of vision)
Herpes simplex: chronic ulcers, bronchitis, pneumonitis, or esophagitis
Histoplasmosis, disseminated or extrapulmonary
Isosporiasis, chronic intestinal
Mycobacterium avium complex or *Mycobacterium kansasii*, disseminated or extrapulmonary
Mycobacterium tuberculosis
Mycobacterium (other species)
Pneumocystis carinii pneumonia
Pneumonia, recurrent
Salmonella sp septicemia, recurrent
Toxoplasmosis of brain
Opportunistic Neoplasms Due to Immunosuppression
Cervical cancer, invasive
Kaposi's sarcoma
Lymphoma, Burkitt's
Lymphoma, immunoblastic
Lymphoma, primary, of brain
Disorders Due to HIV Infiltration
Encephalopathy, HIV related
Progressive multifocal leukoencephalopathy
Wasting syndrome due to HIV

Data from Centers for Disease Control. (1992). 1993 revised classification system for HIV infection and expanded surveillance case definition for AIDS among adolescents and adults. *Morbidity and Mortality Weekly Report* 41, 1–19.

ciency of lymphocytes is manifested. Immunosuppression predisposes the patient to the third phase, marked by a wasting syndrome, central nervous system involvement, and complications of opportunistic infections and neoplasms such as Kaposi's sarcoma (Color Fig. 13–2). These AIDS-defining illnesses are listed in Table 13–23.

Prevention and Treatment. The greatest hope for eradicating the AIDS epidemic currently lies in educational programs aimed at reduction of high-risk sexual practices and intravenous drug abuse. In clinical settings, Standard Precautions are implemented to reduce the risk of transmission among patients and health care personnel (see Table 13–9). There is no definitive therapy for AIDS, but in recent years, combination drug therapy with reverse transcriptase inhibitors and protease inhibitors (the "AIDS cocktail") has been successful in reducing the viral load and slowing the progression of the disease in many patients (Table 13–24). Prophylaxis against opportunistic disorders such as tuberculosis, influenza, and pneumonia may be warranted in many. Attempts to develop a vaccine against HIV have been unsuccessful thus far, owing in part to the rate of mutation of the virus and the difficulty of accessing the virus within cells.

Prognosis and Outcome. Although AIDS is ultimately a fatal disease, the rate of progression is variable, depending on multiple factors, such as the virulence of the infecting HIV subtype, adequacy of drug therapy, and resistance of the host. Eighty per cent of those infected with HIV develop third-phase complications leading to death within 10 years. Ten to 15% progress within 2 to 3 years, and 5% to 10% remain symptom free after 7 to 10 years.[38] The latter group, termed nonprogressors or long-term survivors, is the subject of intense study to determine the factors that may account for their positive course.

TABLE 13–24
DRUG THERAPY FOR ACQUIRED IMMUNODEFICIENCY DISEASE

CATEGORY AND MECHANISM	EXAMPLES
Reverse transcriptase inhibitors	
Nucleosides: become incorporated into the growing viral DNA strand and cause premature termination of translation	Zidovudine (AZT, ZDV) Didanosine (ddI) Zalcitabine (ddC) Stavudine (D4T) Lamivudine (3TC)
Nonnucleosides: bind directly to reverse transcriptase enzyme, inhibiting its function	Nevirapine Delavirdine Thiobenzimidazolines
Protease inhibitors: inhibit the viral proteinase enzyme that is essential to cleavage of the provirus to functional viral particles, thereby inhibiting replication of infected cells and inhibiting cell–cell spread of HIV	Saquinavir Ritonavir Indinavir

Data from Threlkeld, S.C., and Hirsch, M.S. (1996). Antiretroviral therapy. *Medical Clinics of North America* 80(6), 1263–1282.

CLINICAL SIGNIFICANCE OF INFLAMMATORY AND IMMUNE DISEASES

Because it may be initiated by any form of cellular injury, inflammation is among the most common mechanisms of disease. Although inflammation is inherently adaptive, its mediators and effects may contribute to the clinical manifestations of disease. In a significant number of cases, inflammation is maladaptive as a consequence of either disease or host factors.

The importance of the immune system and its functions in health and disease is being increasingly appreciated in clinical practice. Because many of its components and mechanisms are still poorly understood, the immune system is considered to be a frontier of biomedical science. It is likely that the immune system is as important as the endocrine and neurologic systems in regulating function of the total human system, and interactions between these regulatory systems are becoming increasingly clear. The immune system also affects, and is affected by, genetic control systems within cells. It has been called the "pacemaker of aging," and mediates programmed cell death (see Chapter 6). As further detailed in subsequent systems chapters, the pathophysiology of many disorders involves altered immune function, and prevention or cure of these disorders may require manipulation of the immune response.

Summary of Key Points

- Inflammation is the body's second line of defense (after intact physical and chemical barriers) to any form of tissue injury. It is a nonspecific response aimed at limitation of extent of injury, destruction of the injurious agent, and preparation of the injured tissue for healing.
- Immunity, the third line of defense, is a response that differentiates self from nonself

antigens, then mounts an attack against nonself antigens. Nonself antigens include invading microorganisms and proteins on neoplastic cells.

- The plasma complement and kinin cascades are activated during inflammation and serve to augment the destructive effects of the cytokine mediators on injurious agents. Products of the hemostatic–fibrinolysic system are important to repair of vascular injury and also participate in walling off the inflamed area. WBCs (macrophages and neutrophils) are phagocytic and also release regulatory mediators. Mast cell mediators are of greatest importance in immune-mediated inflammation. The vascular endothelium affects the vasomotor responses of inflammation. The cellular products of the inflammatory and immune response system components are the principal regulators of inflammation and immunity.
- Many aspects of immunity intersect with the nonspecific inflammatory response. Immunologic mechanisms often trigger inflammation and the complement cascade as a means of destroying invading agents. Macrophages, which are phagocytic during inflammation, act as APCs during immune responses. Antibody-coated cells are more susceptible to lysis by NK lymphocytes.
- The inflammatory response may be initiated by any form of cellular injury, including trauma, toxicity, hypoxia, immune mechanisms, or infection. The immune response is normally triggered by the contact of an immune cell with antigen.
- The local manifestations (cardinal signs) of inflammation are rubor (redness) and calor (heat), which result from hyperemia; tumor (swelling), caused by exudation; dolor (pain), due to physical and chemical stimulation of pain receptors and transmission mediated by prostaglandins and other cellular mediators; and functiolaesa (loss of function), which is secondary to the other manifestations. Systemic effects result from increased synthesis of acute phase proteins, increased hematopoietic activity, pyrogenic cytokines or toxins, and increased energy demands of the inflammatory process.
- The usual outcomes of inflammation are tissue healing (by resolution, regeneration, or repair), chronic inflammation, or granuloma formation. Resolution is the recovery of cells sustaining nonlethal damage. Regeneration is healing by replacement of dead cells with functional duplicates. Repair is the replacement of dead cells with nonfunctional scar tissue. Chronic inflammation is the persistence of the exudative phase of inflammation longer than 2 weeks. In granuloma formation, the invading organism is walled off but not destroyed.
- Wound healing may be affected by the extent of injury, regenerative potential of the injured tissue, presence of infection, adequacy of nutrition and perfusion, and developmental factors. Maladaptive inflammation and healing may manifest as either an insufficient or an excessive response. Insufficient inflammation and delayed wound healing may result from inadequate hematopoiesis or lack of sufficient energy and nutrients. Inflammation may be excessive and inappropriately triggered in allergy and other forms of hypersensitivity. A normal inflammatory response occurring in an enclosed space may also result in pressure-induced tissue injury. Scar tissue formation may impede the function of joints and may be excessive and disfiguring. Scar tissue may also obstruct hollow organs.
- Antigens are usually proteins or large carbohydrate molecules. Antigen that breaches the surface and mucosal defenses is usually intercepted in the blood or in lymphoid tissues by a macrophage or other APC, which processes it so that its specific recognition region (epitope) is readily accessible. Presentation of epitope to B cells initiates the humoral response, whereas presentation to T cells initiates cell-mediated immunity.
- The humoral response begins with binding of an inactive B cell to antigen, usually within a lymph node. Activation and division of these B cells produces two cell lines: plasma cells, which secrete antibody and mount the primary response; and memory cells, clones of the activated B cell. Memory cells lie dormant until a second challenge with the antigen, when they mount a more rapid and intense secondary immune response (memory response). Antigen–antibody binding initiates complement fixation, precipitation, aggluti-

Continued on following page

nation, and neutralization of antigen. The complement cascade is activated by the classic pathway, and cell lysis by NK cells is facilitated by antibody coating of antigen-bearing cells. The cell-mediated response begins with macrophage presentation of antigen to a CD4+ helper T cell. Secretion of IL-1 by the macrophage results in activation of the CD4+ cell, which then induces proliferation of antigen-specific cytotoxic T cells. Cytotoxic T cells destroy the antigen-containing cell by the effects of proteolytic enzymes, membrane-perforating proteins, and initiation of apoptosis.

- Four broad categories of immunopathology are recognized: hypersensitivity, autoimmunity, isoimmunity, and immunodeficiency. Hypersensitivity is an excessively intense immune response, such as allergy or anaphylaxis. Autoimmunity is an immune attack against native tissues, as occurs in disorders such as rheumatoid arthritis. Isoimmunity is immune attack against tissues originating from another human being, such as incompatible blood transfusion and organ transplantation. Immunodeficiency is an insufficient immune response, which may be primary (congenital) or secondary (acquired).
- Hodgkin's disease is a malignant neoplasm originating in secondary lymphoid tissues, in which the transformed cell is the RS cell. Non-Hodgkin's lymphomas also originate in secondary lymphoid tissues, but from a number of cell types other than the RS cell. Intervention in these lymphomas is designed to inhibit neoplastic proliferation. Infectious mononucleosis is the most common type of benign lymphoproliferative disorder. It is a self-limited disorder, generally requiring only supportive care. AIDS results from destruction of helper T cells by the HIV virus. Immunodeficiency is profound and renders the patient vulnerable to opportunistic infections and cancers, which are ultimately fatal. Intervention aims to reduce the viral burden and prevent opportunistic diseases, thus slowing the progression of AIDS.

REFERENCES

1. Maier, S.F., Watkins, L.R., and Fleshner, M. (1994). Psychoneuroimmunology: The interface between behavior, brain, and immunity. *American Psychologist* 49(12), 1004–1017.
2. Mehra, I.V., Gottlieb, J.E., and Nash, D.B. (1993). Monoclonal antibody therapy for gram-negative sepsis: Principles, applications, and controversies. *Pharmacotherapy* 13(2), 128–134.
3. Rubanyi, G.M. (1993). The role of endothelium in cardiovascular homeostasis and diseases. *Journal of Cardiovascular Pharmacology* 22(suppl. 4), S1–S14.
4. Stadnyk, A.W. (1994). Cytokine production by epithelial cells. *FASEB Journal* 8(13), 1041–1047.
5. Albelda, S.M., Smith, C.W., and Ward, P.A. (1994). Adhesion molecules and inflammatory injury. *FASEB Journal* 8(8), 504–512.
6. Dinarello, C.A., Gelfand, J.A., and Wolff, S.M. (1993). Anticytokine strategies in the treatment of the systemic inflammatory response syndrome. *Journal of the American Medical Association* 269(14), 1829–1835.
7. Beal, A.L., and Cerra, F.B. (1994). Multiple organ failure syndrome in the 1990s. *Journal of the American Medical Association* 271(3), 226–233.
8. Raghow, R. (1994). The role of extracellular matrix in postinflammatory wound healing and fibrosis. *FASEB Journal* 8(11), 823–831.
9. Black, J.M., and Matassarin-Jacobs, E. (1993). *Luckmann and Sorensen's Medical Surgical Nursing: A Psychophysiologic Approach*. (4th ed.). Philadelphia: W.B. Saunders. (p. 382).
10. Tomasz, A. (1994). Multiple antibiotic-resistant pathogenic bacteria: A report on the Rockefeller University Workshop. *New England Journal of Medicine* 330(17), 1247–1251.
11. Centers for Disease Control and Prevention. (1987). Recommendations for prevention of HIV transmission in health-care settings. *Morbidity and Mortality Weekly Report* 36(2S), 3–17.
12. Louie, S.G., and Jung, B. (1993). Clinical effects of biologic response modifiers. *American Journal of Hospital Pharmacy* 50(7 suppl. 3), S10–S18.
13. Catania, A., Manfredi, G., Airaghi, L., *et al.* (1994). Cytokine antagonists in infectious and inflammatory disorders. *Annals of the New York Academy of Sciences* 741(Nov 25), 149–161.
14. Moffett, D.F., Moffett, S.B., and Schauf, C.L. (1993). *Human Physiology: Foundations and Frontiers*. St. Louis: Mosby-Year Book. (p. 771).
15. Weissman, I.L. (1994). Developmental switches in the immune system. *Cell* 78(2), 207–218.
16. Reber, P. M. (1993). Prolactin and immunomodulation. *American Journal of Medicine* 1993(95), 637–643.
17. Ader, R., and Cohen, N. (1993). Psychoneuroimmunology: Conditioning and stress. *Annual Review of Psychology* 1993(44), 53–85.
18. Madden, K.S., Sanders, V.M., and Felten, D.L. (1995). Catecholamine influences and sympathetic neural modulation of immune responsiveness. *Annual Review of Pharmacology and Toxicology* 1995(35), 417–448.
19. Paul, W.E., and Seder, R.A. (1994). Lymphocyte responses and cytokines. Cell 76(2), 241–251.
20. Labro, M.T. (1994). *Host Defense and Infection*. New York: Marcel Dekker.
21. Doherty, P.C. (1993). Cell-mediated cytotoxicity. *Cell* 75(4), 607–612.
22. Sutton, B.J., and Gould, H.J. (1993). The human IgE network. *Nature* 366(6454), 421–428.
23. Terr, A.I. (1991). Allergy desensitization. In: Stites, D.P., and Terr, A.I. (Eds.). *Basic and Clinical Immunology* (7th ed.). Norwalk, CT: Appleton & Lange.
24. Gloe, D. (1991). Common reactions to transfusions. *Heart & Lung* 20(5), 506–512.
25. Sloop, G.D., and Friedberg, R.C. (1995). Complications of blood transfusion. *Postgraduate Medicine* 98(1), 159–172.
26. Blackburn, S.T., and Loper, D.L. (1992). *Maternal, Fetal, and Neonatal Physiology: A Clinical Perspective*. Philadelphia: W.B. Saunders. (pp. 459–464).
27. Schwinghammer, T.L., and Bloom, E.J. (1993). Pharmacologic prophylaxis of acute graft-versus-host disease after allogenic marrow transplantation. *Clinical Pharmacy* 12(10), 736–761.
28. Rowe, J.M., Ciobanu, N., Ascensao, J., *et al.* (1994). Recommended guidelines for the management of autologous and allogeneic bone marrow transplantation: A report from the Eastern Cooperative Oncology Group (ECOG). *Annals of Internal Medicine* 1994(120), 143–158.
29. Erickson, J.M. (1994). Update on Hodgkin's disease. *Nurse Practitioner* 19(11), 63–68.

30. Chiu, B.C.-H., Cerhan, J.R., Folsom, A.R., *et al.* (1996). Diet and risk of non-Hodgkin lymphoma in older women. *Journal of the American Medical Association* 275(17), 1315–1321.
31. Sandlund, J.T., Downing, J.R., and Crist, W.M. (1996). Non-Hodgkin's lymphoma in childhood. *New England Journal of Medicine* 334(19), 1238–1248.
32. Armitage, J.O. (1993). Treatment of non-Hodgkin's lymphoma. *New England Journal of Medicine* 328(14), 1023–1030.
33. Cozad, J. (1996). Infectious mononucleosis. *Nurse Practitioner* 21(3), 15–28.
34. Schaffer, S. (1996). Benign lymphoproliferative disorders. *Seminars in Oncology Nursing* 12(1), 28–37.
35. Gourevitch, M.N. (1996). The epidemiology of HIV and AIDS. *Medical Clinics of North America* 80(6), 1223–1236.
36. Carson, J.L., Russell, L.B., Taragin, M.I., *et al.* (1992). The risks of blood transfusion: The relative influence of acquired immunodeficiency syndrome and non-A, non-B hepatitis. *American Journal of Medicine* 1992(92), 45–52.
37. Gold, J.W.M. (1996). The diagnosis and management of HIV infection. *Medical Clinics of North America* 80(6), 1283–1307.
38. Hardy, W.D., Jr. (1996). The human immunodeficiency virus. *Medical Clinics of North America* 80(6), 1239–1261.

SELECTED BIBLIOGRAPHY

Ackerman, M.H., Evans, N.J., and Ecklund, M.M. (1994). Systemic inflammatory response syndrome, sepsis, and nutritional support. *Critical Care Nursing Clinics of North America* 6(2), 321–340.

Alteration in circulating intercellular adhesion molecule-1 and L-selectin: Further evidence for chronic inflammation in ischemic heart disease. *American Heart Journal* 132(1 Pt. 1), 1–8.

Armitage, J.O. (1994). Bone marrow transplantation. *New England Journal of Medicine* 330(12), 827–838.

Baumert, P.W. (1995). Acute inflammation after injury. *Postgraduate Medicine* 97(2), 35–49.

Beeson, P.B. (1994). Age and sex associations of 40 autoimmune diseases. *American Journal of Medicine* 1994(96), 457–462.

Bevilacqua, M.P., Nelson, R.M., Mannori, G., *et al.* (1994). Endothelial-leukocyte adhesion molecules in human disease. *Annual Review of Medicine* 45(1994), 361–378.

Blumberg, N., and Heal, J.M. (1996). Immunomodulation by blood transfusion: An evolving scientific and clinical challenge. *American Journal of Medicine* 101, 299–308.

Bone, R.C. (1996). Immunologic dissonance: A continuing evolution in our understanding of the systemic inflammatory response syndrome (SIRS) and the multiple organ dysfunction syndrome (MODS). *Annals of Internal Medicine* 125(8), 680–687.

Border, W.A., and Noble, N.A. (1994). Transforming growth factor beta in tissue fibrosis. *New England Journal of Medicine* 331(19), 1286–1292.

Brandtzaeg, P. (1992). Humoral immune response patterns of human mucosae: Induction and relation to bacterial respiratory tract infections. *Journal of Infectious Diseases* 1992(165 suppl. 1), S167–S176.

Bryan, R.T., Pinner, R.W., and Berkelman, R.L. (1994). Emerging infectious diseases in the United States: Improved surveillance, a requisite for prevention. *Annals of the New York Academy of Sciences* 740(Dec 15), 346–361.

Cao, Y., Qin, L, Zhang, L., *et al.* (1995). Virologic and immunologic characterization of long-term survivors of human immunodeficiency virus type I infection. *New England Journal of Medicine* 332(4), 201–208.

Carpenter, C.C.J., Fischi, M.A., Hammer, S.M., *et al.* (1996). Antiretroviral therapy for HIV infection in 1996: Recommendations of an international panel. *Journal of the American Medical Association* 276(2), 146–154.

Centers for Disease Control. (1992). 1993 Revised classification system for HIV infection and expanded surveillance case definition for AIDS among adolescents and adults. *Morbidity and Mortality Weekly Report* 41, 1–19.

Chandra, R.K., and Kumari, S. (1994). Nutrition and immunity: An overview. *Journal of Nutrition* 124(suppl. 8), 1433S–1435S.

Chrousos, G.P. (1995). The hypothalamic-pituitary adrenal axis and immune-mediated inflammation. *New England Journal of Medicine* 332(20), 1351–1362.

Church, M.K., Okayama, Y., and Bradding, R. (1994). The role of the mast cell in acute and chronic allergic inflammation. *Annals of the New York Academy of Sciences* 725(May 28), 13–21.

Cohen, M.S. (1995). HIV and sexually transmitted diseases: The physician's role in prevention. *Postgraduate Medicine* 98(3), 52–64.

Corley, M.D., and Sneed, G. (1994). Criteria in the selection of organ transplant recipients. *Heart & Lung* 23(6), 446–457.

Cotran, R.S., Kumar, V., and Robbins, S.L. (1994). *Robbins Pathologic Basis of Disease.* (5th ed.). Philadelphia: W.B. Saunders.

D'Aquila, R.T., Hughes, M.D., Johnson, V.A., *et al.* (1996). Nevirapine, zidovudine, and didanosine compared with zidovudine and didanosine in patients with HIV-1 infection. *Annals of Internal Medicine* 124(12), 1019–1030.

Davis, S.F., Byers, R.H., Lindegren, M.L., *et al.* (1995). Prevalence and incidence of vertically acquired HIV infection in the United States. *Journal of the American Medical Association* 274(12), 952–955.

DeVita, V.T., and Hubbard, S.M. (1993). Hodgkin's disease. *New England Journal of Medicine* 328(8), 560–565.

Dinarello, C.A., and Wolff, S.M. (1993). The role of interleukin-1 in disease. *New England Journal of Medicine* 328(2), 106–113.

Ellis, R.W., and Douglas, R.G. (1994). New vaccine technologies. *Journal of the American Medical Association* 271(12), 929–931.

Fauci, A.S. (Moderator). (1996). Immunopathologic mechanisms of HIV infection (NIH Conference). *Journal of the American Medical Association* 124(7), 654–663.

Gailit, J., and Clark, R.A.F. (1994). Wound repair in the context of extracellular matrix. *Current Opinion in Cell Biology* 6(5), 717–725.

Gardner, P., Eickhoff, T., Poland, G.A., *et al.* (1996). Adult immunizations. *Annals of Internal Medicine* 12(1 Pt. 1), 35–40.

Gershon, R.R.M., Karkashian, C., and Felknor, S. (1994). Universal precautions: An update. *Heart & Lung* 23(4), 352–358.

Gilsdorf, J.R. (1994). Vaccines: Moving into the molecular era. *Journal of Pediatrics* 125(3), 339–344.

Gold, H.S., and Moellering, R.C. (1996). Antimicrobial drug resistance. *New England Journal of Medicine* 335(19), 1445–1453.

Goldmann, D.A., Weinstein, R.A., Wenzel, R.P., *et al.* (1996). Strategies to prevent and control the emergence and spread of antimicrobial-resistant microorganisms in hospitals: A challenge to hospital leadership. *Journal of the American Medical Association* 275(3), 234–240.

Graham, B.S., and Wright, P.F. (1995). Candidate AIDS vaccines. 333(20), 1331–1339.

Groenwald, S.L., Frogge, M.H., Goodman, M., *et al.* (1993). *Cancer Nursing: Principles and Practice.* (3rd ed.). Boston: Jones & Bartlett.

Haas, D.W., and Des Prez, R.M. (1994). Tuberculosis and acquired immunodeficiency syndrome: A historical perspective on recent developments. *American Journal of Medicine* 1994(96), 439–449.

Hazinski, M.F. (1994). Mediator-specific therapies for the systemic inflammatory response syndrome, sepsis, severe sepsis, and septic shock: Present and future approaches. *Critical Care Nursing Clinics of North America* 6(2), 309–319.

Heddle, N.M., Klama, L., Singer, J., *et al.* (1994). The role of the plasma from platelet concentrates in transfusion reactions. *New England Journal of Medicine* 331(10), 625–628.

Henderson, W.R. (1994). The role of leukotrienes in inflammation. *Annals of Internal Medicine* 121(9), 684–697.

Hirschtick, R.E., Glassroth, J., Jordan, M.C., *et al.* (1995). Bacterial pneumonia in persons infected with the human immunodeficiency virus. *New England Journal of Medicine* 333(13), 845–851.

Hoffman-Goetz, L., and Pedersen, B.K. (1994). Exercise and the immune system: A model of the stress response? *Immunology Today* 15(8), 382–387.

Hu, D.J., Dondero, T.J., Rayfield, M.A., *et al.* (1996). The emerging genetic diversity of HIV: The importance of global surveillance for diagnostics, research, and prevention. *Journal of the American Medical Association* 275(3), 210–216.

Institute for Clinical Systems Integration, Minneapolis. (1996). Pediatric immunization. *Postgraduate Medicine* 100(5), 213–225.

Johnson, H.M., Bazer, F.W., Szente, B.E., *et al.* (1994). How interferons fight disease. *Scientific American* 270(5), 68–75.

Just, J.J., Abrams, E., Louie, L.G., *et al.* (1995). Influence of host genotype on progression to acquired immunodeficiency syndrome among children with human immunodeficiency virus type 1. *Journal of Pediatrics* 127(4), 544–549.

Karon, J.M., Rosenberg, P.S., McQuillan, G., *et al.* (1996). Prevalence of HIV infection in the United States, 1984–1992. *Journal of the American Medical Association* 276(2), 126–131.

Kliks, S.C., Wara, D.W., Landers, D.V., *et al.* (1994) Features of HIV-1 that could influence maternal-child transmission. *Journal of the American Medical Association* 272(6), 467–473.

Kyle, R.A. (1994). The monoclonal gammopathies. *Clinical Chemistry* 40(11B), 2154–2161.

Labro, M.T. (1994). *Host Defense and Infection.* New York: Marcel Dekker.

Landesman, S.H., Kalish, L.A., Burns, D.N., *et al.* (1996). Obstetrical factors and the transmission of human immunodeficiency virus type 1 from mother to child. *New England Journal of Medicine* 334(25), 1617–1623.

Lawler, D.A. (1994). Hormonal response in sepsis. *Critical Care Nursing Clinics of North America* 6(2), 265–274.

Lehne, R.A. (1994). *Pharmacology for Nursing Care.* (2nd ed.). Philadelphia: W.B. Saunders.

Levy, J.A. (1996). Infection by human immunodeficiency virus: CD4 is not enough. *New England Journal of Medicine* 335(20), 1528–1530.

Lipton, J.M., Ceriani, G., Macaluso, A., *et al.* (1994). Antiinflammatory effects of the neuropeptide alpha-MSH in acute, chronic, and systemic inflammation. *Annals of the New York Academy of Sciences* 741(Nov 25), 137–148.

Lipton, S.A., and Gendelman, H.E. (1995). Dementia associated with the acquired immunodeficiency syndrome. *New England Journal of Medicine* 332(14), 934–940.

Liu, C.-C., Young, L.H.Y., and Young, J.D.-D. (1996). Lymphocyte-mediated cytolysis and disease. *New England Journal of Medicine* 335(22), 1651–1659.

Lober, B. (1996). Are all diseases infectious? *Annals of Internal Medicine* 125(10), 844–851.

Lotan, M., and Schwartz, M. (1994). Cross talk between the immune system and the nervous system in response to injury: Implications for regeneration. *FASEB Journal* 8(13), 1026–1033.

Macallan, D.C., Noble, C., Baldwin, C., *et al.* (1995). Energy expenditure and wasting in human immunodeficiency virus infection. *New England Journal of Medicine* 333(2), 83–88.

Manno, C.S. (1996). What's new in transfusion medicine? *Pediatric Clinics of North America* 43(3), 793–808.

Marchalonis, J.J., and Schluter, S.F. (1994). Development of an immune system. *Annals of the New York Academy of Sciences* 712, 1–12.

Marrack, P., and Kappler, J. (1994). Subversion of the immune system by pathogens. *Cell* 75, 323–332.

Miller, R.A. (1996). The aging immune system: Primer and prospectus. *Science* 273, 70–74.

Montserrat, E., and Rozman, C. (1994). Current approaches to the treatment and management of chronic lymphocytic leukemia. *Drugs* 47(suppl. 6), 1–9.

Moore, F.D. (1994). Therapeutic regulation of the complement system in acute injury states. *Advances in Immunology* 56(1994), 267–299.

Moqbel, R. (1994). Eosinophils, cytokines, and allergic inflammation. *Annals of the New York Academy of Sciences* 725(May 28), 223–233.

Naber, S.P. (1994). Molecular pathology: Diagnosis of infectious disease. *New England Journal of Medicine* 331(18), 1212–1215.

Newman, J. (1995). How breast milk protects newborns. *Scientific American* 273(6), 76–79.

Nowak, M.A., and McMichael, A.J. (1995). How HIV defeats the immune system. *Scientific American* 273(2), 58–65.

Paul, W.E. (1995). Can the immune response control HIV infection? *Cell* 82(2), 177–182.

Peckham, C., and Gibb, D. (1995). Mother-to-child transmission of the human immunodeficiency virus. *New England Journal of Medicine* 333(5), 298–302.

Peggs, J.F., Shimp, L.A., and Opdycke, R.C. (1995). Antihistamines: Old and new. *American Family Physician* 52(2), 593–600.

Pellacani, A., Brunner, H.R., and Nussberger, J. (1992). Antagonizing and measurement: Approaches to understanding of hemodynamic effects of kinins. *Journal of Cardiovascular Pharmacology* 20(suppl. 9), S28–S34.

Pinner, R.W., Teutsch, S.M., Simonsen, L., *et al.* (1996). Trends in infectious diseases mortality in the United States. *Journal of the American Medical Association* 275(3), 189–193.

Pirofsky, B., and Kinzey, D.M. (1992). Intravenous immune globulins: A review of their uses in selected immunodeficiency and autoimmune diseases. *Drugs* 43(1), 6–14.

Playfair, J.H. (1992). *Immunology at a Glance.* (5th ed.). Oxford: Blackwell Scientific Publications.

Raud, J., Thorlacius, J., Xie, X., *et al.* (1994). Interactions between histamine and leukotrienes in the microcirculation: Aspects of relevance to acute allergic inflammation. *Annals of the New York Academy of Sciences* 744(Nov 15), 191–198.

Reiser, H., and Stadecker, M.J. (1996). Costimulatory B7 molecules in the pathogenesis of infectious and autoimmune diseases. *New England Journal of Medicine* 335(18), 1369–1377.

Rett, K., Wicklmayr, M., and Dietze, G.J. (1990). Metabolic effects of kinins: Historical and recent developments. *Journal of Cardiovascular Pharmacology* 15(suppl. 6), S57–S59.

Rosen, F.S., Cooper, M.D., and Wedgwood, R.J.P. (1995). The primary immunodeficiencies. *New England Journal of Medicine* 333(7), 431–440.

Ross, R. (1994). The role of T lymphocytes in inflammation. *Proceedings of the National Academy of Sciences, U.S.A.* 91(8), 2879.

Saez-Llorens, X., and McCracken, G.H. (1993). Sepsis syndrome and septic shock in pediatrics: Current concepts of terminology, pathophysiology, and management. *Journal of Pediatrics* 123(4), 497–508.

Saksela, K., Stevens, C.E., Rubinstein, P., *et al.* (1995). HIV-1 messenger RNA in peripheral blood mononuclear cells as an early marker of risk for progression to AIDS. *Annals of Internal Medicine* 123(9), 641–648.

Sanford, G.G. (1994). The stress response to trauma and critical illness. *Critical Care Nursing Clinics of North America* 6(4), 693–702.

Schacker, T., Collier, A.C., Hughes, J., *et al.* (1996). Clinical and epidemiologic features of primary HIV infection. *Annals of Internal Medicine* 125(4), 257–264.

Schoenwetter, W.F. (1996). Safe allergen immunotherapy: The correct allergen, the appropriate patient, the adequate dose. *Postgraduate Medicine* 100(2), 123–135.

Schreiber, G.B., Busch, M.P., Kleinman, S.H., *et al.* (1996). The risk of transfusion-transmitted viral infections. *New England Journal of Medicine* 334(26), 1685–1690.

Secor, V.H. (1994). The inflammatory/immune response in critical illness. *Critical Care Nursing Clinics of North America* 6(2), 251–264.

Siminoff, L.A., Arnold, R.M., Caplan, A.L., *et al.* (1995). Public policy governing organ and tissue procurement in the United States: Results from the National Organ and Tissue Procurement Study. *Annals of Internal Medicine* 1995(123), 10–17.

Slaughter, S., Hayden, M.K., Nathan, C., *et al.* (1996). A comparison of the effect of universal use of gloves and gowns with that of glove use alone on acquisition of vancomycin-resistant enterococci in a medical intensive care unit. *Annals of Internal Medicine* 125(6), 448–456.

Snow, E.C., and Noelle, R.J. (1993). The role of direct cellular communication during the development of a humoral immune response. *Advances in Cancer Research* 1993(62), 241–266.
Sperling, R.S., Shapiro, D.E., Coombs, R.W., *et al.* (1996). Maternal viral load, zidovudine treatment, and the risk of transmission of human immunodeficiency virus type 1 from mother to infant. *New England Journal of Medicine* 335(22), 1621–1629.
Stallone, D.D. (1994). The influence of obesity and its treatment on the immune system. *Nutrition Reviews* 52(2), 37–50.
Stengle, J., and Dries, D. (1994). Sepsis in the elderly. *Critical Care Nursing Clinics of North America* 6(2), 421–427.
Stites, D.P., and Terr, A.I. (Eds.). (1991). *Basic and Clinical Immunology.* (7th ed.). Norwalk, CT: Appleton & Lange.
Streit, W.J., and Kincaid-Colton, C.A. (1995). The brain's immune system. *Scientific American* 273(5), 54–61.

Tenover, F.C., and Hughes, J.M. (1996). The challenge of emerging infectious diseases: Development and spread of multiply-resistant bacterial pathogens. *Journal of the American Medical Association* 275(4), 300–304.
Threlkeld, S.C., and Hirsch, M.S. (1996). Antiretroviral therapy. *Medical Clinics of North America* 80(6), 1263–1282.

Vetter, R.T., and Johnson, G.M. (1995). Vaccination update: Diphtheria, tetanus, pertussis, mumps, rubella, measles. *Postgraduate Medicine* 98(4), 133–148.
Vetter, R.T., and Johnson, G.M. (1995). Vaccination update: Hib, hepatitis, polio, varicella, influenza, pneumococcal and meningococcal disease. *Postgraduate Medicine* 98(5), 141–150.

Wang, C., Brodland, G., and Su, W.P.D. (1995). Skin cancers associated with acquired immunodeficiency syndrome. *Mayo Clinic Proceedings* 1995(70), 766–772.
Wang, C., Schroeter, A.L., and Su, W.P.D. (1995). Acquired immunodeficiency syndrome-related Kaposi's sarcoma. *Mayo Clinic Proceedings* 1995(70), 869–879.
Wang, C., Snow, J.L., and Su, W.P.D. (1995). Lymphoma associated with human immunodeficiency virus infection. *Mayo Clinic Proceedings* 1995(70), 665–672.
Weissman, I.L., and Cooper, M.D. (1993). How the immune system develops. *Scientific American* 269(3), 65–71.
Witek-Janusek, L., and Cusack, C. (1994). Neonatal sepsis. *Critical Care Nursing Clinics of North America* 6(2), 405–419.
Wyatt, R. (1996). Anaphylaxis: How to recognize, treat, and prevent potentially fatal attacks. *Postgraduate Medicine* 100(2), 87–99.

Yocum, M.W., and Khan, D.A. (1994). Assessment of patients who have experienced anaphylaxis: A 3-year survey. *Mayo Clinic Proceedings* 1994(69), 16–23.
Yoshikawa, T.T., and Norman, D.C. (1995). Treatment of infections in elderly patients. *Medical Clinics of North America* 79(3), 651–661.

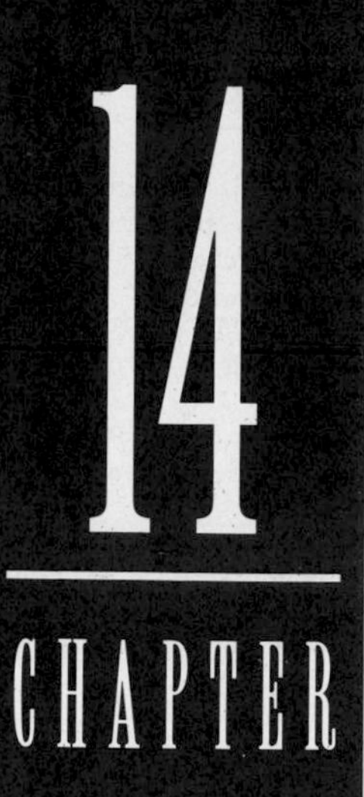

Disorders of Hemostasis and Fibrinolysis

LEARNING OBJECTIVES

1. Comprehend the physiologic purpose and potential activators of the hemostatic system.
2. Discuss the phases of hemostasis, including tissue components and regulation.
3. Identify the stages of fibrinolysis.
4. Compare and contrast factors promoting hypocoagulable versus hypercoagulable states.
5. Describe the process of embolization of blood clots.
6. Discuss the pathophysiology underlying the clinical manifestations and rationalizing the treatment of selected disorders of hemostasis and fibrinolysis.
7. Discuss the general clinical significance of altered hemostasis.

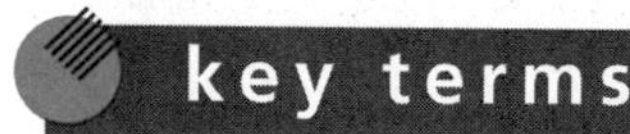

key terms

acrocyanosis
α_2-antiplasmin
anticoagulant
antithrombin III
clotting cascade
clotting factor
disseminated intravascular coagulation
deep vein thrombosis
ecchymosis
embolus
fibrin
fibrinogen
fibrinolysis
gangrene
hemophilia
hemostasis
heparan sulfate
heparin
hypercoagulability
hypocoagulability
mottling
petechiae
plasmin
plasminogen
platelet-activating factor
postphlebitic syndrome
procoagulant
protein C
protein S
prothrombin
purpura
stasis ulcer
streptokinase
thrombin
thromboembolism

thrombomodulin
thrombophlebitis
thrombotic thrombocytopenic purpura
thrombus
tissue factor pathway inhibitor
tissue plasminogen activator
urokinase
venous stasis
von Willebrand's disease
von Willebrand factor (vWF)

Hemostasis (literally, "blood stoppage") is a complex process that defends against uncontrolled hemorrhage in the event of damage to blood vessels. Components of this defense system include the vessel endothelium, platelets (thrombocytes), and serum protein **clotting factors** along with a number of regulatory cytokines and adhesion molecules. The hemostatic mechanism can be activated by vessel injury, tissue injury, or presence of a foreign body in the bloodstream. Mechanisms of hemostasis include spasm of the injured vessels to restrict blood flow, formation of a short-term platelet plug to seal minor vessel defects, and formation of a strong fibrin clot or **thrombus** in the event of more significant vessel damage. Thrombus formation effectively prevents blood loss but also occludes the injured vessel for a time, inhibiting blood flow to organs and tissues served by the vessel. For hemostasis to be adaptive, the thrombus must be degraded as soon as the injured vessel has healed, restoring tissue perfusion. Dissolution of the clot (**fibrinolysis**) is the normal conclusion of hemostasis.

Adaptive hemostasis depends on maintenance of a balance of **procoagulant** and **anticoagulant** factors within the bloodstream and surrounding tissues. Normally, the balance is tipped slightly in favor of anticoagulation, preventing inappropriate clotting in response to the tiny vessel tears that frequently occur with normal vasomotion and circulation. This state of **hypocoagulability**, along with the positive charges on the surfaces of the intact vessel endothelium and the circulating blood cells, normally keeps blood flowing smoothly in vessels.

Like the inflammatory and immune responses, hemostasis is a locally regulated process (see Chapter 13). Many of the mediators that regulate inflammation are also active in hemostasis. And, like the other tissue defenses, the hemostatic–fibrinolytic system may be a source of disease if it is deficient or inappropriately activated. If hemostasis is ineffective, excessive bleeding occurs with minor trauma or even normal "wear and tear" of vessels. If hemostasis is inappropriate or excessive, clotting may occlude vessels and cause tissue ischemia; or portions of clots may break free in the bloodstream, forming **emboli** that can lodge in distal tissues. Thromboembolitic disorders commonly affect the lungs (pulmonary embolism), the heart (myocardial infarction), and the brain (stroke), all with potentially devastating consequences. These conditions are detailed in relevant chapters on the affected systems.

In this chapter, mechanisms of hemostasis and fibrinolysis are detailed, along with disorders that involve excessive bleeding (**hemophilia** and **von Willebrand's disease**) or inappropriate clotting (**deep vein thrombosis** [DVT]). **Disseminated intravascular coagulation** (DIC) and **thrombotic thrombocytopenic purpura** (TTP), conditions characterized by *both* inappropriate clotting and bleeding, are also discussed.

PHASES OF HEMOSTASIS

Figure 14–1 illustrates the four principal phases of the hemostatic mechanism: vasospasm, formation of the platelet plug, formation of the fibrin thrombus, and fibrinolysis.

Vasospasm

Acute injury to a blood vessel causes an immediate constriction of the vessel, which may persist for 20 to 30 minutes. This response serves to limit blood flow and subsequent blood loss, and the slowing of blood flow is believed to cause a local accumulation of procoagulant factors, favoring later clot formation. This reaction is probably due in part to a sympathetic nervous system reflex in response to local pain stimuli; however, it is primarily mediated by locally released molecules such as thromboxane A_2 (TXA_2), a product of the arachidonic acid pathway in platelets, and endothelin, a cytokine produced by endothelial cells lining the vessel (see Chapter 13).

Formation of the Platelet Plug

Platelet Activation

Platelets may become activated by any of several physiologic or pathologic activators released or ex-

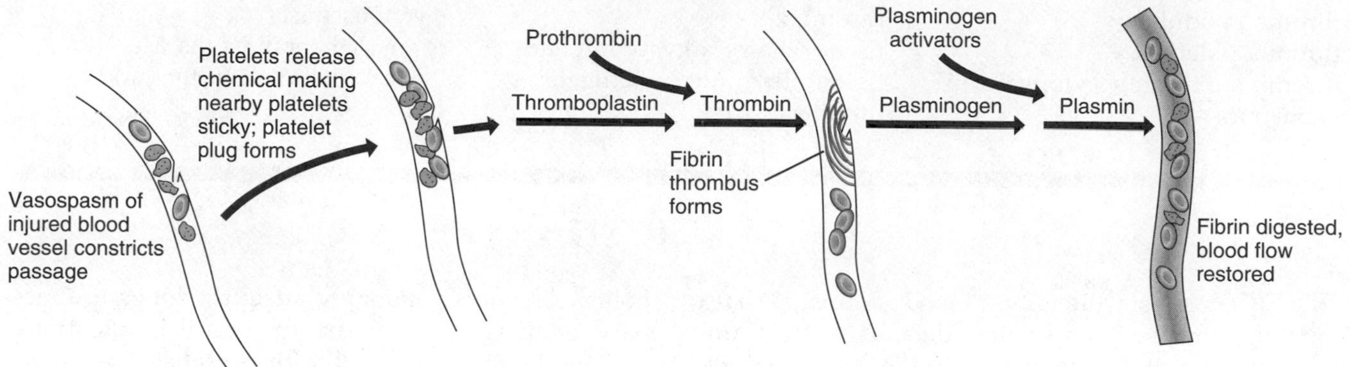

FIGURE 14–1

Phases of hemostasis. Acute vessel injury results in a brief period of vasospasm, which limits blood loss. Exposure of the vessel endothelium initiates the release of local mediators, which activate platelets. The vessel defect is initially sealed with a temporary plug composed of aggregated platelets. A strong clot forms by a cascade mechanism that culminates in activation of thrombin, an enzyme that converts fibrinogen to fibrin. Fibrin threads incorporate platelets and red blood cells within the clot, and clot retraction further strengthens the clot and may permit some blood flow past the clot. When the vessel defect is healed, the fibrinolytic process ensues. Plasminogen is activated to plasmin, a proteolytic enzyme that digests fibrin, restoring blood flow within the vessel.

posed at the site of injury. These activators include collagen, thrombin, adenosine diphosphate (ADP), TXA_2, epinephrine, serotonin, arginine vasopressin (AVP or ADH), and **platelet-activating factor** (PAF). Platelet activators are counterbalanced by the presence of several inhibitors of activation, including flowing blood and the endothelial products prostacyclin (PgI_2) and nitric oxide.[1]

Platelet Adhesion

Injury (or disease) of the vessel endothelium exposes a number of adhesive subendothelial proteins, including **von Willebrand factor** (vWF), collagen, and fibronectin. Platelets also express vWF. The platelet membrane contains glycoprotein receptors for many of these proteins, and binding of platelet to platelet, and platelet to endothelium, promotes formation of a platelet plug.[2] A single layer of platelets first binds to the exposed endothelium.

Platelet Aggregation

Platelet aggregation follows adhesion as additional platelets stick to the first layer, forming a loose plug that initially seals the defect. Platelet aggregation is mediated by a limited positive feedback loop in which ADP, serotonin, and other mediators released by the adherent platelets, endothelial cells, or possibly endotoxins cause the platelets to become more rounded and to develop extensions, facilitating clumping of the cells. ADP also causes platelets to produce more TXA_2, which causes the aggregating platelets to become sticky.

Formation of the Fibrin Thrombus

Cascade Mechanism

The process that culminates in formation and dissolution of the fibrin clot is extremely complex, involving a stepwise series of reactions known as the **clotting cascade** (Fig. 14–2). Each reaction activates a precursor, which is usually a plasma protein clotting factor. As shown in Table 14–1, the clotting factors are labeled with the roman numerals I through XIII. (Note that there is no factor VI because it was ultimately found to duplicate factor V.) Protein clotting factors are synthesized primarily by the liver but also by endothelial cells.

Clotting factors normally circulate in inactive form in the plasma as part of the procoagulant fraction. Some of these proteins, when activated, serve as critical enzymes in activation of others in the cascade, whereas others (factors V and VIII) are necessary cofactors in the reactions. Still other factors catalyze the formation of the components of the fibrin clot. Vitamin K is essential to the synthesis of prothrombin (factor II), and calcium (factor IV) is a required cofactor for several steps of the clotting cascade.

The clotting cascade may begin in two different ways, known as the *intrinsic* and *extrinsic* pathways. These pathways coincide at the point of formation of activated factor X (factor Xa), and the remaining steps constitute the *common* pathway. An additional link between the two pathways occurs at an earlier step of the extrinsic pathway, at the point of forma-

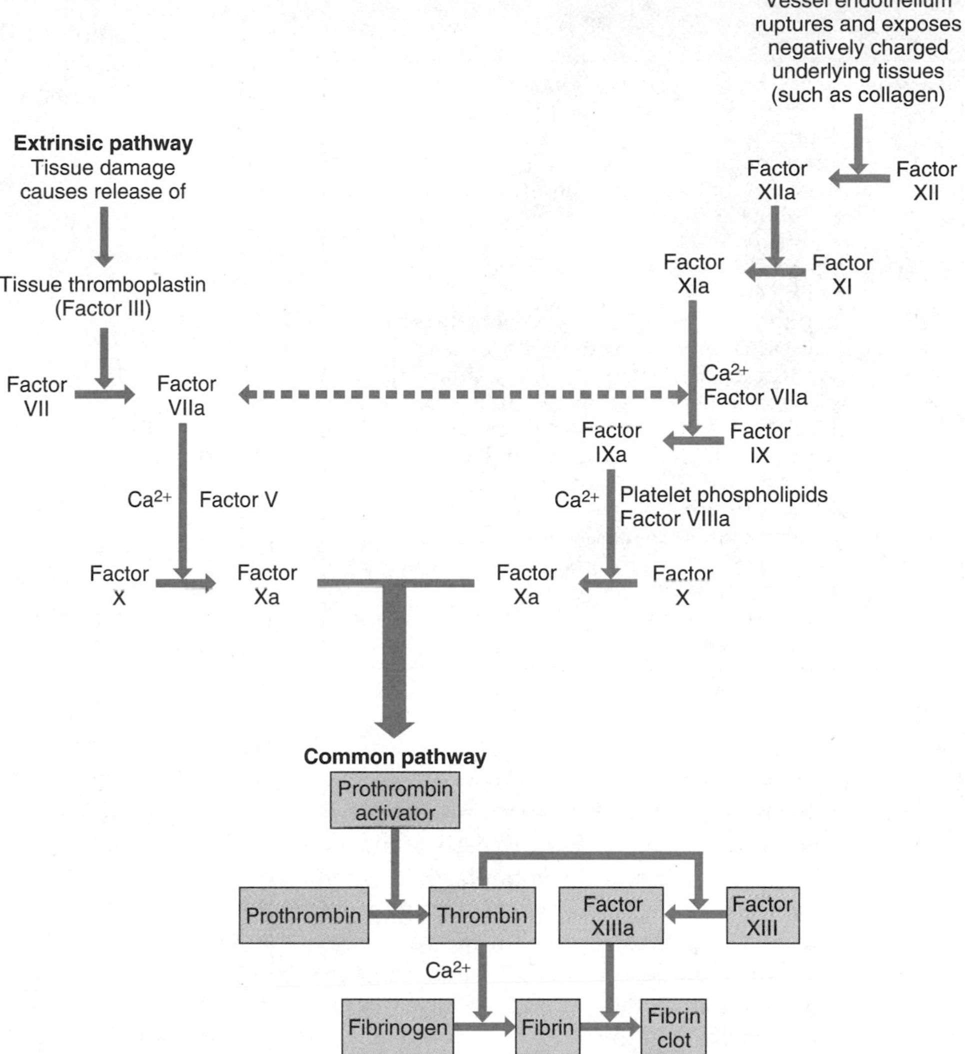

FIGURE 14–2
The clotting cascade. Sequential activation of clotting factors culminates in formation of the fibrin clot. The coagulation system may be activated in either of two ways. The more rapid, extrinsic pathway begins with release of tissue thromboplastin by injured cells. The slower, more complex intrinsic pathway is initiated by contact of the blood with the injured vessel endothelium. Both pathways converge at the point of activation of factor X.

tion of the thromboplastin–factor VIIa complex, which may directly activate factor IX of the intrinsic pathway. Most mechanisms of vessel injury ultimately activate both pathways. A large number of locally produced substances promote the reactions of the clotting cascade, including proteins of the kinin system, such as Hageman factor, HMW kininogen, and prekallikrein (see Chapter 13). Much of this local regulation is still incompletely understood.

Intrinsic Pathway

All of the components of the intrinsic pathway are contained within the blood. The intrinsic pathway, which is slower and more complex than the extrinsic pathway, is initiated by contact of the blood with negatively charged surfaces. In the body, this contact is with exposed collagen of the injured or diseased (e.g., atherosclerotic) vessel lining. Blood in a test tube or on a laboratory slide also clots by this mechanism.

Contact of serum with exposed collagen results in activation of factor XII and also causes platelets to release phospholipids. Factor XIIa then activates factor XI; factor XIa, with a calcium cofactor, activates factor IX. Prior activation of factor VIII (antihemophilic factor), also critical to this pathway, results from separation of factor VIII from its circulating complex with vWF during the hemostatic process. Factor IXa, calcium, platelet phospholipids, and factor VIIIa then bond together on the surface of platelets, forming a complex that activates factor X and leads to the common pathway.

Extrinsic Pathway

The extrinsic pathway relies on factors outside the bloodstream for its activation. Because it involves

TABLE 14–1
CLOTTING FACTORS

FACTOR	COMMON NAMES
I	Fibrinogen
II	Prothrombin
III	Tissue thromboplastin, thromboplastin, thrombokinase
IV	Calcium
V	Proaccelerin, labile factor, accelerator-globulin (AcG)
VII	Serum prothrombin conversion accelerator (SPCA), proconvertin, stable factor
VIII	Antihemophilic factor (AHF), antihemophilic globulin (AHG), antihemophilic factor A
IX	Plasma thromboplastin component (PTC), Christmas factor, antihemophilic factor B
X	Stuart factor, Stuart-Prower factor
XI	Plasma thromboplastin antecedent (PTA), antihemophilic factor C
XII	Hageman factor, contact factor, antihemophilic factor D
XIII	Fibrin-stabilizing factor (FSF), fibrinase, plasma transglutaminase

fewer steps, this is the more rapid pathway, resulting in the beginning of clot formation within 15 seconds. This pathway begins with release of an intracellular lipoprotein, tissue thromboplastin (factor III), by injured cells outside the vessel. In the presence of calcium, tissue thromboplastin activates factor VII. The thromboplastin–factor VIIa complex then activates factor X of the common pathway and factor IX of the intrinsic pathway.

Common Pathway

The common pathway requires the presence of the activated cofactor proaccelerin (factor V), which may be derived from platelets, vascular endothelial cells, or plasma sources. Factor Xa combines with factor Va, platelet phospholipids, and calcium to form a prothrombin activator complex, which activates **prothrombin** (factor II) to **thrombin**, an enzyme that has several important roles in coagulation. The primary role of thrombin is to convert circulating **fibrinogen** (factor I) molecules into long strands of **fibrin**. Thrombin also activates factor XIII (fibrin-stabilizing factor). Factor XIIIa and calcium then cross-link the fibrin strands, forming an insoluble meshwork that is incorporated into the platelet plug, forming a stable clot. Other roles of thrombin in hemostasis include acceleration of the activation of factors IX, X, XI, and XII, and activation of an enzyme, **protein C**, which inactivates factors Va and VIIIa, slowing the coagulation process.

Clot Retraction

After formation of the fibrin mesh, the clot is further stabilized by contraction of proteins within the entrapped platelets. Clot retraction squeezes out serum from the clot, compressing it for increased strength, and pulls the edges of the vessel wound together, promoting healing. Clot retraction may also permit blood to flow past the clot, augmenting tissue perfusion.

Inhibition of Excessive or Inappropriate Clotting

The fibrinolytic system normally limits the clotting cascade (see later). In addition, inappropriate activation of the clotting cascade is normally prevented by characteristics of the intact endothelium as well as by a number of circulating inhibitors of coagulation.

Circulating Anticoagulants. When activated by thrombin, **protein C**, a vitamin K–dependent protein synthesized by the liver, inactivates factors V and VIII. Another vitamin K–dependent factor, **protein S**, enhances protein C activity. **Antithrombin III** (AT III), synthesized by liver and endothelial cells, binds and inactivates any activated thrombin outside the clot. **Heparin**, a polysaccharide continuously produced by mast cells and basophils, combines with AT III to enhance its anticoagulant activity. **Tissue factor pathway inhibitor** forms a complex with factors Xa and VIIa and tissue thromboplastin in the presence of calcium, suppressing the extrinsic pathway.[3]

Endothelial Mechanisms. The intact endothelium normally prevents thrombus formation by serving as the site of several procoagulant–anticoagulant interactions. Endothelial cells express a protein, **thrombomodulin**, which induces thrombin to activate protein C. These cells also express proteoglycans containing **heparan sulfate**, which enhances the anticoagulant function of AT III on the endothelial surface. Endothelial cell products are also involved in the generation of **tissue plasminogen activator (TPA)** during fibrinolysis, as discussed later.[4]

Fibrinolysis

When the vessel defect has healed and the clot is no longer needed, the fibrinolytic pathway is activated to dissolve the clot. As shown in Figure 14–3, an anticoagulant protein, **plasminogen**, continuously circulates in the plasma in inactive form. As the clot forms, plasminogen is deposited into it. Plasminogen may be activated to the proteolytic enzyme **plasmin** by a number of agents, including TPA,

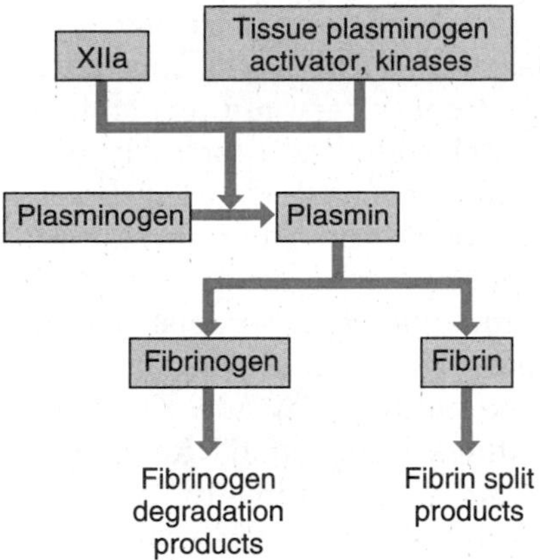

FIGURE 14–3

Fibrinolysis. The fibrinolytic pathway is activated to dissolve the clot, restoring vessel patency. The anticoagulant protein plasminogen circulates in inactive form and is deposited into the growing clot. A number of agents, including tissue plasminogen activator (tPA), may activate plasminogen to plasmin, a proteolytic enzyme that digests fibrin as well as any fibrinogen in the area. The serum level of fibrin split products serves as an indicator of the degree of fibrinolytic activity. Fibrinogen degradation products bind fibrin strands, preventing further clot formation.

released by vascular endothelial cells in the presence of thrombin and fibrin, and **urokinase**, a similar substance released by renal cells. The release of tPA is stimulated not only by clotting but also by exercise and stress. If streptococcal infection is present, **streptokinase**, a toxin produced by these bacteria, may also induce plasminogen activation as a pathologic mechanism. The presence of Hageman factor (factor XIIa) accelerates plasmin activation. Several enzyme systems exist to prevent inappropriate activation of tPA (e.g., α_2-plasmin inhibitor, α_2-macroglobulin, and C1 inactivator).[4] Any plasmin outside the clot is inactivated by a circulating anticoagulant enzyme, **α_2-antiplasmin.**

Within the clot, plasmin digests fibrin, producing *fibrin split products*, which may be monitored clinically as an indicator of fibrinolytic activity. Plasmin also breaks down fibrinogen, and the resulting *fibrinogen degradation products* serve as anticoagulants in that they bind to fibrin strands, preventing further clot formation.

Laboratory Evaluation of Hemostasis and Fibrinolysis

Monitoring of serum indicators of the different phases of hemostasis and fibrinolysis is routine in most clinical settings, either for diagnostic purposes or for assessment of the outcomes of anticoagulant or procoagulant interventions. Examples of these laboratory tests are listed in Table 14–2.

MECHANISMS OF MALADAPTIVE BLEEDING AND CLOTTING

Hypocoagulability

Excessive bleeding may be caused by deficiency or abnormal function of clotting factors, deficiency of platelets (thrombocytopenia), or conditions in which blood vessels are abnormally fragile. Examples of conditions that may induce hypocoagulability are summarized in Table 14–3. A hypocoagulable state may also be induced therapeutically with drug therapy (Table 14–4). Antiplatelet agents, such as aspirin and dipyridamole, have been shown to

TABLE 14–2
LABORATORY EVALUATION OF HEMOSTATIC FUNCTION

TEST	CLINICAL USE
Prothrombin time (PT)	Identification of deficiencies in activity of fibrinogen, prothrombin, and factors V, VII, and X Monitoring of oral anticoagulant therapy
Activated partial thromboplastin time (aPTT)	Identification of deficiencies or inhibitors of factors VIII, IX, and XI Monitoring of heparin therapy Screening for lupus anticoagulants (antiphospholipid antibodies)
Fibrinogen assay	Identification of deficiencies due to consumption, hereditary disorders, liver disease, or thrombolytic therapy Screening for excess, a risk factor for cardiovascular disease
Specific factor assays	Identification of deficiencies due to hereditary or acquired coagulation disorders
Factor VIII inhibitor assay	Detection of presence of inhibitors, which may impede replacement therapy
Euglobin clot lysis time	Assessment of overall efficacy of fibrinolytic system
Fibrin(ogen) degradation products (FDPs)	Identification of excess, suggesting disseminated intravascular coagulation or hyperfibrinolysis
Bleeding time	Screening for platelet disorder or von Willebrand's disease
Coagulation time	Assessment of overall efficacy of hemostatic system Monitoring of heparin therapy

TABLE 14–3
CONDITIONS ASSOCIATED WITH HYPOCOAGULABILITY

Causative Mechanism	Examples
Platelet Abnormaltiy	
Decreased platelet production	Hereditary thrombocytopenias Aplastic anemia Bone marrow neoplasia Radiation Immunosuppressive drugs Viral infection Nutritional deficiency
Increased platelet destruction or sequestration	Thrombocytopenic purpuras Pregnancy Hypersplenism Hypothermia
Abormal platelet function	Inherited glycoprotein abnormalities Defects in arachidonic acid metabolism Uremia Antiplatelet drugs Liver disease Disseminated intravascular coagulation
Vascular Disorders	
Increased vascular pressure	Valsalva Coughing Vomiting Childbirth Weight-lifting
Increased fragility of the microcirculation and connective tissue support	Aging Glucocorticoid excess Hormonal effects in females
Vessel trauma	Physical injuries or abuse Radiation Emboli Neoplastic infiltration Toxicity
Vasculitis	Henoch-Schönlein purpura Collagen vascular diseases
Disorders of the Clotting Cascade	
Congenital deficiency of clotting factor activity	Hemophilia A Factor XI deficiency von Willebrand's disease Factor V deficiency
Acquired deficiency of clotting factor activity	Vitamin K deficiency Liver disease Amyloidosis Nephrotic syndrome Disseminated intravascular coagulation

Data from Williams, W.J. (1995). Classification and clinical manifestations of disorders of hemostasis. In: Beutler, E., Lichtman, M.A., Coller, B.S., *et al* (Eds.). *Williams Hematology* (5th ed.). New York: McGraw-Hill.

reduce the risk of myocardial infarction and stroke, and the plasminogen activator substances tPA, urokinase, and streptokinase are available as thrombolytic agents ("clot busters") for early intervention in these conditions as well as in pulmonary emboli. Heparin has long been used to restore hemostatic balance in patients who are prone to clotting (e.g., owing to immobility and sluggish blood flow), and anticoagulants such as warfarin inhibit specific phases of the clotting cascade. Developmental factors also influence hemostatic function; infants and the elderly are more prone to excessive bleeding, and the elderly are at higher risk for inappropriate clotting (see Developmental Perspective).

Hypercoagulability

During a state of **hypercoagulability**, clots may form inappropriately in either arteries or veins.

Venous Thrombosis

Venous thrombi usually form in undamaged vessels owing to the combined effects of sluggish blood

TABLE 14–4
ANTICOAGULANT DRUGS

Category	Examples of Actions
Antiplatelet agents	Aspirin and other nonsteroidal anti-inflammatory drugs: inhibit cyclooxygenase enzyme within arachidonic acid pathway, decreasing production of thromboxane A_2 Dipyridamole (Persantine): inhibits release of adenosine diphosphate from platelets
Clotting factor antagonists	Heparin: decreases stickiness of platelets; has antithromboplastin, antiprothrombin, and antithrombin effects; combines with antithrombin III to inhibit fibrin formation Coumarin derivatives (warfarin sodium, dicumarol, anisindione): interfere with hepatic synthesis of vitamin K–dependent clotting factors II, VII, IX, and X
Thrombolytics	Streptokinase, urokinase, recombinant tissue plasminogen activator: activate the endogenous fibrinolytic system

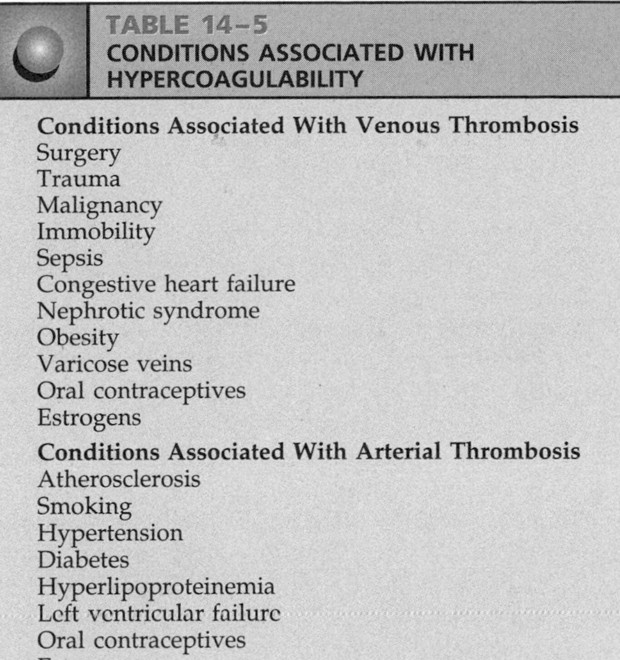

TABLE 14–5
CONDITIONS ASSOCIATED WITH HYPERCOAGULABILITY

Conditions Associated With Venous Thrombosis
Surgery
Trauma
Malignancy
Immobility
Sepsis
Congestive heart failure
Nephrotic syndrome
Obesity
Varicose veins
Oral contraceptives
Estrogens

Conditions Associated With Arterial Thrombosis
Atherosclerosis
Smoking
Hypertension
Diabetes
Hyperlipoproteinemia
Left ventricular failure
Oral contraceptives
Estrogens
Polycythemia

Data from Bick, R.L. (1994). Hypercoagulability and thrombosis. *Medical Clinics of North America* 78(3), 635–665.

flow (stasis) and inappropriate activation of clotting factors. Venous stasis apparently increases the likelihood of clotting by reducing clearance of activated clotting factors by the liver and by facilitating concentration of clotting factors in areas of particularly slowed circulation. (This mechanism provides the rationale for the traditional first aid measure of applying direct pressure to bleeding wounds.) Venous clots are often referred to as *red thrombi* because they consist primarily of red blood cells enmeshed in fibrin.[5]

Inherited or acquired disorders may contribute to hypercoagulability (Table 14–5). Increased estrogen levels, as in pregnancy, result in increased coagulability by an unknown mechanism, probably as a defense against blood loss with delivery. This hypercoagulability, along with slowed venous return from the legs due to occlusion of the iliac veins by the enlarged uterus, makes pregnancy a high-risk state for inappropriate clotting.

Arterial Thrombosis

Conditions such as hypertension and atherosclerosis are associated with chronic injury of the vascular endothelium, promoting inappropriate clotting by the intrinsic pathway. Exposure of the blood to foreign bodies, such as intravenous needles and catheters, artificial heart valves, and tubing for dialysis or extracorporeal circulation (heart–lung bypass), may also induce clotting by the intrinsic system. Arterial injury tends to increase the velocity of blood flow, promoting further endothelial trauma by *shear stress* (frictional forces). In contrast to venous thrombi, arterial clots often consist primarily of platelets and may be referred to as *white clots*.[5] These differences are not absolute, however, and both the platelet responses and clotting cascade mechanisms are activated in either case.

Embolization

An embolus is an aggregate of solid, liquid, or gaseous material that travels freely within the bloodstream from its site of origin to a downstream site, where it lodges[6] (Fig. 14–4). Emboli arise from thrombi in nearly all cases (**thromboembolism**), but in rare cases may consist of fragments of bone (with

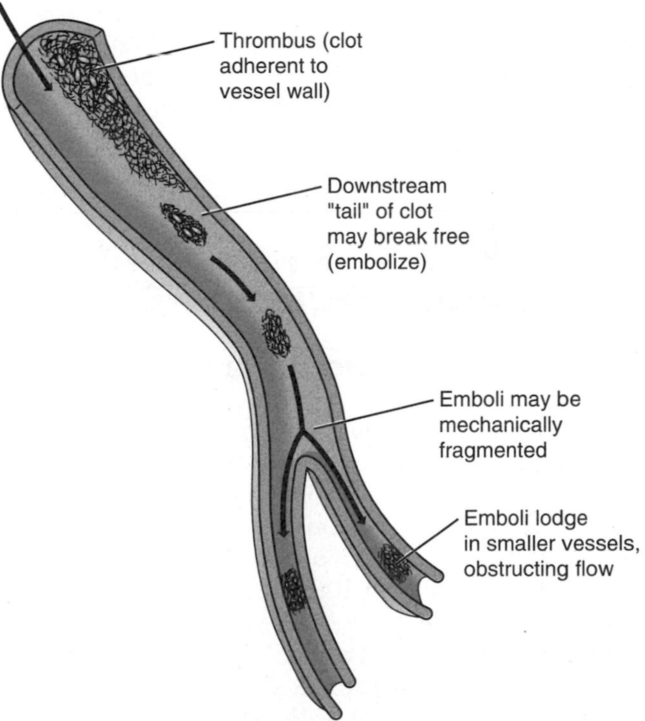
Thrombus (clot adherent to vessel wall)
Downstream "tail" of clot may break free (embolize)
Emboli may be mechanically fragmented
Emboli lodge in smaller vessels, obstructing flow

FIGURE 14–4
Embolization. A portion of a thrombus, typically the downstream "tail," may break free and travel within the bloodstream. Embolization probably occurs during the early phases of hemostasis, before the clot has fully incorporated fibrin and retracted. Emboli may be mechanically fragmented to smaller particles as a result of vasomotion, impact at vessel bifurcations, cardiac contraction, or valve closure. Ultimately, emboli lodge in distal sites, impeding blood flow.

fractures), atherosclerotic plaque, tumors, droplets of fat (from yellow bone marrow), amniotic fluid, foreign bodies (e.g., parts of intravenous needles or catheters), or air bubbles. The risk of thromboembolization is highest during the earlier phases of hemostasis, before the clot becomes well organized with cross-linked fibrin strands (i.e., during the first 7 to 10 days after vessel injury).

Most thromboemboli originate from clots within the deep veins of the legs and pelvis, lodging within the pulmonary arterial system. DVT is discussed later in this chapter, and pulmonary embolism is detailed in Chapter 19. Arterial emboli usually arise from mural thrombi (clots forming on the walls of the heart) or from areas of aneurysm or atherosclerotic plaque (see Chapter 15). Rarely, a venous clot may access the arterial circulation through a structural defect in the heart. Emboli arising from the right side of the heart normally lodge in the pulmonary circulation, whereas other arterial emboli lodge in the systemic circulation.

Systemic emboli result in tissue hypoxia (ischemia) and possible tissue death (infarction), such as occurs in stroke, myocardial infarction, or acute arterial occlusion. The clinical manifestations of embolization depend on the size of the embolus, where it lodges, and the impact of the resulting loss of tissue perfusion. The precise incidence of embolization is uncertain because many cases are believed to be asymptomatic.

DISORDERS OF HEMOSTASIS AND FIBRINOLYSIS

Hemophilia

Definition. Hemophilia is a congenital bleeding disorder that results from deficiency or abnormal function of one or more components of the clotting cascade. The most common types are hemophilia A (classic hemophilia), manifesting as factor VIII deficiency, and hemophilia B (Christmas disease), manifesting as factor IX deficiency.

Epidemiology. Hemophilia A is the most common hemophilia, with an estimated incidence of 20 per 100,000 males.[7] It occurs with equal frequency in all races and geographic locations. The incidence of hemophilia B is one fourth to one sixth that of hemophilia A.[8] In most cases, the defect is inherited from the patient's mother, an asymptomatic carrier; although in as many as 30% of cases, the defect apparently arises from a de novo mutation.[9]

Etiology. The defect of hemophilia A occurs in a specific gene on the X chromosome that codes for factor VIII synthesis. An inversion at intron 22 accounts for 40% to 50% of abnormalities. The factor IX gene is also located on the X chromosome, and more than 300 different base pair substitutions have been associated with hemophilia B.[8] There is no linkage between the inheritance of factor VIII and factor IX defects. Variability in the nature of the genetic defect produces variability in factor VIII and IX levels as well as in degrees of severity of bleeding tendencies.

Pathophysiology. Factors VIII and IX are components of the intrinsic pathway. Factor IX is essential, and factor VIII is a critical cofactor that accelerates the rate of factor X activation by several thousandfold. When these factors are reduced by more than 75%, the clotting cascade is significantly inhibited, resulting in excessive bleeding. Patients with no detectable factor VIII or IX activity have severe hemophilia; those with 1% to 4% activity have moderate hemophilia; and those with 5% to 25% of normal activity have mild hemophilia.

Clinical Manifestations. Laboratory findings and clinical manifestations related to each degree of hemophilia are summarized in Table 14–6. Clinical terms related to bleeding are listed and defined in Table 14–7. Patients with mild hemophilia often do not have symptoms unless subjected to major surgery or trauma, which results in prolonged bleeding from wounds or incisions. Their disease is often undiagnosed until they are adults. In moderate or severe hemophilia, the disease usually becomes apparent during the first year of life. Excessive bleeding may be evident during circumcision. Later, when the boy begins to walk, bleeding into joints (hemarthrosis) is usually seen, often involving the knees, elbows, ankles, shoulders, and hips. This bleeding triggers an inflammatory response, which causes pain and swelling and may initiate a cycle of further joint damage and still more bleeding. If untreated, joint damage can result in permanent disability. Bleeding into the skin causes **ecchymosis**, and muscle hemorrhages result in pain and loss of function. Intracranial bleeding is uncommon but can result in death.

Prevention and Treatment. Genetic counseling, detection of female carrier status, and prenatal diagnosis are preventive options available to those in whom hemophilia is hereditary. Patient and family education regarding lifestyle and activity modification is warranted to reduce the risk of bleeding. Patients with mild hemophilia may be treated prophylactically before dental procedures or minor surgery with a vasopressin analogue, desmopressin (DDAVP), to release stored vWF and factor VIII.[9] The mainstay of treatment of more severe hemophilia is factor replacement with plasma-derived

TABLE 14–6
CLINICAL MANIFESTATIONS OF HEMOPHILIA

Factor VIII/IX Activity Level			
Normal (0.5–1.5 U/mL)	Severe (<0.01 U/mL)	Moderate (0.01–0.05 U/mL)	Mild (>0.05 U/mL)
% of all hemophilia A	70%	15%	15%
% of all hemophilia B	50%	30%	20%
Bleeding Manifestations			
Age of onset	≤1 year	1–2 years	2 years–adult
Neonatal symptoms	PCB: usually ICH: occasionally	PCB: usually ICH: uncommonly	None Rare
Muscle/joint hemorrhage	"Spontaneous" requires no trauma	Requires minor trauma	Requires major trauma
CNS hemorrhage	High risk (2%–8%)	Moderate risk	Rare
Postsurgical hemorrhage (without prophylaxis)	Frank bleeding, severe	Wound bleeding common	Wound bleeding with factor <0.3 U/mL
Oral hemorrhage following trauma, tooth extraction	Usual	Common	Often

PCB, postcircumcisional bleeding; ICH, intracranial hemorrhage.
From DiMichele, D. (1996). Hemophilia 1996: New approach to an old disease. *Pediatric Clinics of North America* 43(3), 711.

TABLE 14–7
CLINICAL TERMINOLOGY RELATED TO BLEEDING

TERM	DEFINITION
Ecchymosis	Bruise; nonelevated blue or purplish patch due to hemorrhage into the skin
Hemarthrosis	Blood in joint spaces
Hematemesis	Bloody vomitus
Hematochezia	Blood surrounding or coating fecal material
Hematoma	Localized collection of blood in tissues
Hematuria	Bloody urine
Hemoperitoneum	Blood in the peritoneal cavity
Hemoptysis	Production of blood with coughing
Hemorrhage	Overt bleeding from wounds, incisions, membrane surfaces, body cavities or orifices
Hemothorax	Blood in the pleural space
Melena	Mahogany or black stools, indicating presence of digested blood
Occult blood	Presence of blood in stool or vomitus indicated only by laboratory testing, e.g., guaiac, Hemoccult, Hematest
Petechiae	Minute, pinpoint, nonelevated, round, purplish red spots caused by hemorrhage into the skin or submucosa
Purpura	Collective term for hemorrhage into the skin or mucous membranes, producing spontaneous ecchymoses or petechiae

products or products manufactured by recombinant DNA technology (see Chapter 6).

Plasma-derived factor VIII and factor IX products of varying purity are available, and all are similarly effective in restoring clotting function. The risk of viral transmission is reduced by pasteurization or solvent detergent treatment, except in cases in which a single, screened plasma donor is used. Factor replacement is commonly administered intravenously in the home, by the patient or his parents, and has been effective in preventing bleeding episodes. Tragically, before 1985, blood products were not screened for human immunodeficiency virus (HIV), and many hemophiliac patients developed acquired immunodeficiency syndrome (AIDS) as a result of factor replacement (see Chapter 13).

Factor IX products of low purity contain significant amounts of activated factors VII and X and prothrombin. Frequent and prolonged use of this form of replacement therapy imposes risk of thrombosis or DIC[8] (see later discussion). A recombinant form of factor IX is not yet available for clinical use.

Recombinant factor VIII has been approved for use since 1993. This product carries no risk of virus transmission but is much more expensive than plasma-derived factor VIII. Both forms of factor replacement may stimulate production of antifactor antibodies (factor inhibitors) in some patients.[10] In patients who have no native factor, this protein is a foreign antigen and may stimulate antibody production, reducing the effectiveness of the treatment. Inhibitors develop in an estimated 20% to 33% of patients with hemophilia A and in 1% to 4% of those with hemophilia B.[8] It is expected that gene therapy, in which hemophilia can be cured with repair of specific gene defects, will soon be available.[11]

Prognosis and Outcome. Before 1964, moderate to severe hemophilia inevitably caused death at an early age. With the advent of replacement therapy, life expectancy increased to 68 years by 1980. Between 1981 and 1990, however, life expectancy dropped sharply as a consequence of the AIDS epidemic. When deaths due to HIV infection are excluded, life expectancy for patients with hemophilia A is now similar to that of the general male population.[12]

von Willebrand's Disease

Definition. von Willebrand's disease is a family of bleeding disorders caused by an abnormality of vWF.

Epidemiology. von Willebrand's disease is the most common congenital bleeding disorder, affecting an estimated 1% of the population.[13] The gene encoding vWF synthesis is located on chromosome 12. Gene defects range from complete deletion to amino acid sequence abnormalities. More than 20 subtypes have been identified, which give rise to variable severity in bleeding manifestations.

Etiology. von Willebrand's disease is inherited as an autosomal dominant defect or acquired in association with other disorders, including hypothyroidism, malignancies, congenital heart disease, systemic lupus erythematosus, and thalassemia.[13] The etiologic mechanism of acquired von Willebrand's disease is unknown, and it is possible that its occurrence with other disease states is coincidental.

Pathophysiology. vWF, released from endothelial cells and platelets, is essential to both the platelet aggregation and coagulation phases of hemostasis. In binding to glycoprotein receptors, vWF serves as a cofactor for platelet adhesion. vWF also functions as a carrier protein for factor VIII, protecting it from degradation in the plasma by activated protein C. When vWF is reduced, factor VIII levels are also reduced, owing to increased clearance from the plasma. vWF deficiency thus results in defects in both platelet plug formation and thrombus formation, predisposing to bleeding.

Clinical Manifestations. von Willebrand's disease usually manifests as mucosal bleeding, recurrent epistaxis (nosebleed), menorrhagia (excessive menstrual bleeding), ecchymosis, and excessive bleeding after surgery, childbirth, or trauma. Deep tissue bleeding similar to that in hemophilia may occur in the more severe types. Laboratory analysis reveals prolonged bleeding times, reduced vWF protein, and reduced platelet aggregation in response to the antibiotic ristocetin (i.e., reduced vWF activity).

Prevention and Treatment. Patient and family education regarding accident prevention is warranted, as for hemophilia. Ethanol and medications such as aspirin with antiplatelet effects should be avoided (see Table 14–3). Patients with mild von Willebrand's disease are treated with desmopressin, which causes a two- to five-fold increase in plasma vWF and factor VIII in responsive patients.[13] Because desmopressin is an analog of antidiuretic hormone, care must be taken to prevent the development of fluid overload and hyponatremia with this therapy (see Chapters 8 and 9). Low-purity, plasma-derived factor VIII contains vWF and has been used for patients who do not respond to desmopressin. Anti-vWF antibodies may develop, reducing the effectiveness of this therapy in some. Platelet transfusion and antifibrinolytic drugs, such as aminocaproic acid (Amicar), may be used in treatment of severe bleeding episodes.

Prognosis and Outcome. Most patients with von Willebrand's disease respond well to desmopressin therapy, and most have markedly reduced clinical manifestations by the second or third decade of life. Fatal bleeding episodes are rare.

Deep Vein Thrombosis

Definition. DVT is a state of excessive or inappropriate clotting in one or more deep veins, typically of the legs or pelvis. DVT may or may not be associated with chronic venous insufficiency, in which clotting may occur in superficial varicose veins (see Chapter 15).

Epidemiology. DVT is common, with yearly incidence in the United States estimated at between 5 million and 20 million cases.[14] Any of the factors known to induce a hypercoagulable state (see Table 14–4) may constitute risk factors for DVT. Bed rest, obesity, pregnancy, and occupations requiring prolonged sitting or standing are commonly implicated. Trauma to leg vessels secondary to fractures, infection, surgery, or other invasive procedures is also associated with DVT. A single point mutation in the factor V gene has been reported to be the most common hereditary cause of venous thrombosis.[15] This defect results in resistance to activated protein C.

DVT has been found at autopsy in 65% of fatally injured trauma patients, with older patients being

Focus of Current Research

Study	Objective and Findings
Triemstra, et al. (1996) Mortality in patients with hemophilia.	*Objective:* To determine causes of death and mortality rates in patients with hemophilia during a 20-year period *Findings:* Acquired immunodeficiency syndrome and hepatitis strongly influence mortality in hemophilia. In the absence of viral infections, life expectancy in hemophilia would nearly equal that of the general population.
den Heijer, et al. (1996) Hyperhomocysteinemia as a risk factor for deep-vein thrombosis.	*Objective:* To assess the risk of venous thrombosis associated with elevated plasma levels of homocysteine, a metabolite of the amino acid methionine *Findings:* High homocysteine levels are a risk factor for deep vein thrombosis, possibly owing to a toxic effect on the vascular endothelium.
Siragusa, et al. (1996) Low-molecular weight heparins and unfractionated heparin in the treatment of patients with acute venous thromboembolism: Results of a meta-analysis.	*Objective:* To estimate the efficacy and safety of low-molecular weight heparins and unfractionated heparins in the treatment of venous thromboembolism *Findings:* Low-molecular-weight heparins are more effective in preventing recurrent venous thromboembolism.
Prandoni, et al. (1996) The long-term clinical course of acute deep venous thrombosis.	*Objective:* To determine the clinical course of patients during the 8 years following their first episode of symptomatic deep vein thrombosis *Findings:* These patients have a high risk of recurrence that persists for many years. One third have post-thrombotic syndrome.
Geerts, et al. (1994) A prospective study of venous thromboembolism after major trauma.	*Objective:* To determine the frequency and associated risk factors for deep vein thrombosis after major trauma *Findings:* Deep vein thrombosis was found in the lower extremities of 58% of 349 patients, and proximal vein thrombosis was found in 18%. Three patients died of massive pulmonary embolism.

particularly susceptible[16] (see Focus of Current Research). Thirty per cent of surgical patients would be expected to develop DVT postoperatively if prophylactic anticoagulation and other antithrombotic measures were not employed.[17] Clinical incidence of DVT in cancer patients has been reported to be as high as 50%, particularly in those with pancreatic and lung cancers.[18] Further evidence of the link between cancer and DVT is the finding that patients with DVT have a one in six chance of having a malignancy diagnosed within 2 years.[14] The etiologic mechanism of hypercoagulability in malignancy is uncertain and probably multifactorial.

Etiology. Virchow's triad of **venous stasis** (slow venous flow, hypercoagulability, and inflammation of the vessel wall) describes the underlying etiology of all DVT. Venous stasis permits local concentration of procoagulant factors and acts as a platelet-activating factor. Hypercoagulable states tip the balance in favor of clotting, as has been discussed. Vessel wall inflammation may expose collagen and induce the expression of mediators promoting hemostasis.

Pathophysiology. Venous clotting obstructs return of blood to the heart. At the capillary level, high pressure at the venous end causes elevation of capillary hydrostatic pressure and a shift of fluid from the vascular to the interstitial space (see Chapter 8). Tissue edema results in poor perfusion of cells and tissue injury. An inflammatory response (**thrombophlebitis**) ensues, causing more edema and more fibrin deposition in the clot, inhibiting its breakdown and trapping blood cells within it. Venous flow is slowed even more by the growing clot, promoting further extension or "propagation" of the clot. Portions of the clot, particularly the downstream "tail" of the thrombus, may embolize within the venous system (see Fig. 14–4). Clots most commonly form in the veins of the calves, but these do not usually embolize unless they are propagated above the knee. Clots in the thigh or pelvic areas are at high risk to embolize to the lungs.

Clinical Manifestations. Only 25% of cases of DVT can be detected on the basis of clinical findings.[14] Edema may occur in the area of the clot owing to venous obstruction and inflammation, but this is usually too deep to be palpable. Discrepancy in limb size is suggestive of DVT, but most venous thrombi are nonobstructing and produce little swelling. Calf pain on dorsiflexion of the foot (Homans' sign) is a classic sign of calf thrombi but is present in fewer than one third of patients with DVT.[17] Often, DVT can only be confirmed with Doppler measurement of blood flow, ultrasound imaging, or venography. In chronic DVT, tissue ulceration (**stasis ulcer**) may occur due to ischemia (Color Fig. 14–1). Pulmonary emboli may result in chest pain and heart failure (see Chapter 19).

Prevention and Treatment. Reduction of risk factors is critical to prevention of DVT. Patients on bed rest are ambulated as soon as possible to promote venous flow. Compression stockings are used to support the walls of veins, limiting venous pooling. In patients on bed rest, sequential compression devices (inflatable wraps) are used to simulate the rhythmic pressure of skeletal muscles on veins, which occurs normally during ambulation. Oral contraceptives and hormone replacement therapies that are high in estrogen are avoided, if possible, as is use of leg veins for intravenous therapy. In patients with recurrent DVT and history of embolism, the vena cava may be divided surgically, or screening devices may be implanted to filter out emboli before they reach the heart or lungs (Fig. 14–5).

Infected stasis ulcers are treated with débridement, drainage, and antibiotic therapy. Anticoagulant drugs, such as heparin and warfarin, may be used to prevent further clotting. Thrombolytic agents (e.g., tPA) or surgical embolectomy are the treatments of choice in patients in whom pulmonary embolization occurs (see Chapter 19).

Prognosis and Outcome. Treatment of DVT without embolization is effective, but the rate of recurrence is high if risk factors are not removed. More than half of DVT patients develop chronic deep venous insufficiency (**postphlebitic syndrome**), suffering chronic pain, inflammation (cellulitis), and stasis ulceration (see Chapter 15). An estimated 40% of DVT patients develop pulmonary embolism, which has a high rate of morbidity and mortality.[14]

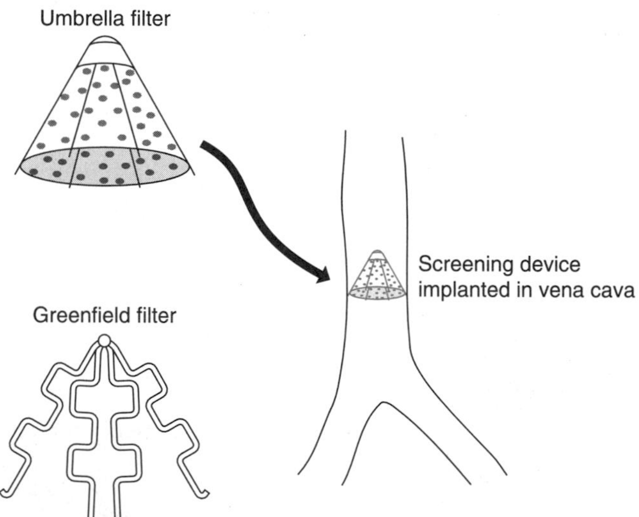

FIGURE 14–5

Antiembolic devices. Patients with recurrent thromboembolism may benefit from the insertion of screening devices within the vena cava. These devices, which are placed using a catheter inserted into the femoral vein, entrap larger venous emboli before they reach the pulmonary vasculature. The clots then dissolve as a consequence of fibrinolysis and the shearing forces of the rapid blood flow in the vena cava. (Adapted from Black, J.M., and Matassarin-Jacobs, E. [1993]. *Luckman and Sorensen's Medical-Surgical Nursing: A Psychophysiologic Approach* [4th ed.]. Philadelphia: W.B. Saunders. [p. 1083].)

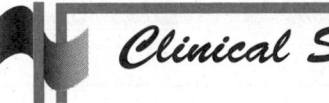

H.F., a 73-year-old man with a history of diabetes and hypertension, is admitted because of severe leg pain after falling down a flight of stairs in his home. His lower right leg is swollen, red, and extremely sensitive to touch. Noninvasive imaging studies reveal the presence of DVT. Intravenous infusion of heparin is begun. Four days after admission, H.F. develops petechiae, ecchymosis, epistaxis, and gastrointestinal bleeding.

1. Is it likely that H.F.'s medical history contributed to the development of DVT? Explain.

2. What is the probable cause of the bleeding that H.F. experienced? What measures might be taken to minimize the occurrence of such complications?

Disseminated Intravascular Coagulation

Definition. DIC is a systemic thrombohemorrhagic disorder seen in association with well-defined situations and laboratory evidence of: (1) procoagulant activation, (2) fibrinolytic activation, (3) inhibitor consumption, and (4) biochemical evidence of end-organ damage or failure.[19]

Epidemiology. The incidence of DIC in major medical centers is 12 to 49 patients per year.[20] The reported incidence of DIC in septic patients ranges from 16% to 73%.[2] Risk factors are those related to the underlying disorders (see later discussion).

Etiology. Two separate mechanisms may initiate DIC. Massive tissue damage due to trauma, burns, intravascular hemolysis, or shock (particularly septic shock) may cause large amounts of tissue thromboplastin to be released into the blood, triggering the clotting cascade on a massive scale. In cardiovascular diseases, cancer, obstetrical complications such as amniotic fluid embolus (see Chapter 32), or milder infections, a more benign form of DIC may be triggered by a substance (e.g., a tumor cell cytokine, an amniotic fluid protein, or a bacterial toxin) that is structurally similar to the prothrombin activator complex.

Pathophysiology. Large-scale clotting occurs in smaller blood vessels where flow is slowest. This causes tissue ischemia and release of more tissue thromboplastin, which triggers more clotting. Circulating clotting factors and platelets are depleted during this process, and large quantities of fibrinogen degradation products are produced during fibrinolysis. Two fibrinogen degradation product fragments (D and E) have a high affinity for platelet membranes and induce significant platelet dysfunction. The stage is then set for bleeding from larger, unclotted vessels. Circulating plasmin may activate the complement cascade, leading to increased vascular permeability and contributing to hypotension and shock. Generation of factor XIIa activates the kinin cascade, also promoting increased permeability, hypotension, and shock.

Clinical Manifestations. Clinical manifestations depend on which part of the coagulation–fibrinolysis cycle predominates. Some patients demonstrate excessive clotting; in others, uncontrolled bleeding is more apparent. Many have both simultaneously. Profuse bleeding from surgical incisions, wounds, or invasive lines and tubes may be evident. Vascular lesions (**petechiae**, **purpura**, ecchymosis, hemorrhagic bullae) due to bleeding into the skin are common (Color Figs. 14–2 and 14–3). Signs of tissue ischemia include coolness and **mottling** of the skin, **acrocyanosis**, and possibly **gangrene**. Gastrointestinal bleeding may manifest as nausea, vomiting of blood (hematemesis), abdominal pain, or rectal bleeding. Hypovolemic shock results in worsening of tissue ischemia, causing absence of peripheral pulses, hypotension, and tachycardia (see Chapter 15). Organ failure eventually results owing to decreased perfusion; adult respiratory distress syndrome is especially common with DIC (see Chapter 19).

Prevention and Treatment. Patients who are at risk for DIC should be closely monitored for evidence of bleeding. Efforts should be made to minimize invasive procedures that can result in bleeding. Treatment of DIC is aimed at the underlying disorder, for example, antibiotic therapy of sepsis or delivery of the infant in obstetrical emergencies. Replacement of platelets and protein clotting factors may be necessary in patients in whom bleeding predominates. If blood transfusion is necessary, washed packed red blood cells are used to avoid concurrent administration of anticoagulant substances. The use of heparin is controversial, but this anticoagulant may be used in patients in whom inappropriate thrombosis predominates, as evidenced by acute renal shutdown or skin necrosis.[21]

Prognosis and Outcome. Multiple organ failure is common, and, when superimposed on underlying critical illness, DIC is fatal in 50% to 80% of cases.[21]

Developmental Perspective

Embryonic and Fetal Periods

Maternal aspirin use may impair fetal platelet aggregation. Warfarin, an anticoagulant, crosses the placenta. This agent not only depresses fetal clotting factors but also is teratogenic. Administration of heparin during pregnancy appears safe because this drug does not cross the placenta. Antiepileptic agents (e.g., phenytoin sodium [Dilantin], phenobarbital) and antituberculin drugs (e.g., isoniazid, rifampin) may also reduce fetal clotting factors.

Infancy and Childhood

The increased bleeding tendency in infants is normally due to capillary fragility rather than coagulation disorder. Newborns commonly have petechiae associated with the trauma of vaginal delivery, but these usually disappear within a few days. Congenital bleeding disorders, including hemophilia, usually present during childhood. Bleeding is also common with childhood leukemias. Arterial and venous thrombosis are more frequent in newborns than in other childhood age groups, although the precise reasons for this are unknown.

Adolescence and Young Adulthood

Females of childbearing age experience changes in coagulability with the menstrual cycle, owing to the effects of estrogen and progesterone on blood vessels. Many leukemias and lymphomas have their onset during this period, and these are often associated with bleeding. Trauma, the leading cause of death in adolescents and young adults, is associated with maladaptive bleeding and clotting. TTP has its highest incidence in this age group.

Middle and Older Adulthood

An increased tendency toward maladaptive bleeding and clotting has been noted in the elderly. Although the platelet count does not change with age, platelets are more reactive to mediators of aggregation. Clotting cascade activity is also increased. Immobility, atherosclerosis, and congestive heart failure, more prevalent in the elderly, may also contribute to a hypercoagulable state. Bleeding tendencies in the elderly may stem from capillary fragility, liver disease, or increased responsiveness to anticoagulant therapy.

Thrombotic Thrombocytopenic Purpura

Definition. TTP is a syndrome of target organ dysfunction caused by marked platelet aggregation in the microcirculation.[21]

Epidemiology. TTP is rare, occurring in 1 in 50,000 hospital admissions.[22] It affects women slightly more often than men (3:2), and its usual onset is between the ages of 10 and 50 years. In most patients, there are no obvious risk factors or precipitating conditions, although associations with infections (including HIV), pregnancy, cancer, autoimmune disorders, drug allergies, and environmental influences have been reported.

Etiology. The specific stimuli for the formation of microthrombi in TTP are unknown. One theory proposes that deficiency of a depolymerase enzyme leaves TPP patients unable to cleave polymers of coagulation factors, leading to the formation of large molecules of vWF and factor VIII that predispose to platelet aggregation.[23] Deficiency of substances that mediate fibrinolysis, inhibit platelet aggregation, or decrease prostacyclin release has also been postulated as a cause of TTP, as has presence of a substance that promotes platelet aggregation.[21]

Pathophysiology. White microthrombi composed principally of platelets form in capillaries and arterioles throughout the body, resulting in vessel injury, consumption of platelets, and intravascular hemolysis as erythrocytes attempt to pass through the partially occluded vessels. Tissue ischemia leads to end-organ failure, for example, renal failure, infarction of the intestinal tract or pancreas, myocardial infarction, and neurologic dysfunction.

Clinical Manifestations. The typical signs of TTP are thrombocytopenia, anemia, purpura or other signs of bleeding, fever, renal failure, and neurologic abnormalities such as headache, confusion, paresis, and dysphasia. Diabetes mellitus may occur secondary to pancreatic microthrombi, and dysrhythmias or myocardial infarction may result from cardiac microthrombi.[22]

Treatment. Treatment of TPP is empiric and may include plasma infusion to provide potential inhibitors of platelet aggregation and plasmapheresis to remove triggering substances. Other treatments shown to increase survival, although their rationale is unclear, are splenectomy, steroids, dextran, antiplatelet agents, and cytotoxic agents.[21, 22]

Prognosis and Outcome. The mortality rate in TTP is 90% without therapy.[21] Initial treatment is successful in about 70% of patients.[22]

CLINICAL SIGNIFICANCE OF ALTERED HEMOSTASIS

Either extreme of inappropriate bleeding or clotting may be incompatible with life. In clinical settings, immobilization, invasive procedures, and iatrogenic manipulation of the hemostatic system are common, imposing risks in addition to those inherent in specific illnesses. For these reasons, clinical monitoring of the hemostatic system is routine. Bleeding and clotting are manifestations of a wide variety of disorders, discussed in forthcoming systems chapters.

Summary of Key Points

- The hemostatic system defends against uncontrolled hemorrhage in the event of damage to blood vessels. The hemostatic mechanism may be activated by vessel injury, tissue injury, or presence of a foreign body in the bloodstream.
- Vessel injury first induces reflex vasospasm to limit blood loss. This reflex may be mediated by the sympathetic nervous system but also involves local mediators such as TXA_2 and endothelin. Formation of a platelet plug follows, by the processes of platelet activation, platelet adhesion, and platelet aggregation. Platelet plug formation is regulated locally by a number of cytokines and endothelial adhesive molecules. Formation of a stronger fibrin clot is the result of a series of enzymatic activations, which may begin with either surface contact or tissue injury. Regulation of the clotting cascade depends on a balance of procoagulant and anticoagulant factors. The fibrin clot then retracts, compressing it for strength and permitting some blood flow past the clot.
- The fibrinolytic pathway dissolves the clot when the vessel injury has healed. Plasminogen, deposited into the clot during its formation, is activated to plasmin by a number of agents. Within the clot, plasmin digests fibrin, lysing the clot. Plasmin also degrades fibrinogen, preventing its activation to fibrin, and producing degradation products, which serve an anticoagulant function.
- Factors that promote a hypocoagulable state include hormones, genetic and developmental factors, bleeding disorders, liver disease, and anticoagulant therapy. A hypercoagulable state may be induced by sluggish blood flow, hormones, endothelial injury or disease, and exposure of the blood to foreign surfaces.
- Embolization occurs when a portion of a thrombus breaks free and travels in the bloodstream to a distal site, where it lodges. The risk of embolization is highest during the early phases of hemostasis, before the clot becomes well organized and cross-linked with fibrin. Arterial emboli may lodge in the brain, the coronary arteries, or peripheral arteries, resulting in ischemia and infarction. Venous emboli usually lodge in the pulmonary arterial system, potentially impairing gas exchange and promoting heart failure.
- Both hemophilia and von Willebrand's disease promote a bleeding tendency, although hemophilia is due to deficiency of factor VIII activity and von Willebrand's disease is due to deficiency of vWF. Both disorders result from genetic defects, although an acquired form of von Willebrand's disease has been described. DVT results from venous stasis, hypercoagulability, or vessel inflammation. Clinical manifestations of edema, stasis ulceration, and pain may occur due to venous obstruction, and venous clots may embolize to the lungs. DIC and TTP are disorders that manifest as tissue ischemia and end-organ damage due to the formation of microthrombi. Sequentially or simultaneously, bleeding occurs as a result of consumption of coagulation factors during this process. In

Continued on following page

DIC, fibrinolytic activity follows clotting, leading to bleeding from wound sites and mucosal surfaces. In TTP, the clots are composed primarily of platelets, leading to thrombocytopenic purpura.

- Either extreme of inappropriate bleeding or clotting may be incompatible with life. Because bleeding and clotting are manifestations of a wide variety of disorders, clinical monitoring of hemostasis is routine.

REFERENCES

1. Ware, J.A., and Coller, B.S. (1995). Platelet morphology, biochemistry, and function. In: Beutler, E., Lichtman, M.A., Coller, B.S., *et al.* (Eds.). *Williams Hematology.* (5th ed.). New York: McGraw-Hill. (pp. 1161–1201).
2. Shelton, B.K. (1994). Disorders of hemostasis in sepsis. *Critical Care Nursing Clinics of North America* 6(2), 373–387.
3. Brose, G.J. (1995). Tissue factor pathway inhibitor and the revised theory of coagulation. *Annual Review of Medicine* 46, 103–112.
4. Nachman, R.L., and Silverstein, R. (1993). Hypercoagulable states. *Annals of Internal Medicine* 119(8), 819–827.
5. Schafer, A.I. (1996). Antiplatelet therapy. *American Journal of Medicine* 101, 199–209.
6. Cotran, R.S., Kumar, V., and Robbins, S.L. (1994). *Robbins Pathologic Basis of Disease.* (5th ed.). Philadelphia: W.B. Saunders. (pp. 111–114).
7. Hoyer, L.W. (1994). Hemophilia A. *New England Journal of Medicine* 330(1), 38–47.
8. DiMichele, D. (1996). Hemophilia 1996: New Approach to an Old Disease. *Pediatric Clinics of North America* 43(3), 709–736.
9. Cohen, A.C., and Kessler, C.M. (1995). Treatment of inherited coagulation disorders. *American Journal of Medicine* 99, 675–682.
10. Peterson, C.W. (1994). Treating hemophilia. *American Pharmacy* NS34(8), 57–69.
11. Lozier, J.N., and Brinkhous, K.M. (1994). Gene therapy and the hemophilias. *Journal of the American Medical Association* 271(1), 47–51.
12. Triemstra, M., Rosendaal, F.R., Smit, C., *et al.* (1995). Mortality in patients with hemophilia. *Annals of Internal Medicine* 123, 823–827.
13. Werner, E.J. (1996). von Willebrand disease in children and adolescents. *Pediatric Clinics of North America* 43(3), 683–707.
14. Stephen, J.M., and Feied, C.F. (1995). Venous thrombosis: Lifting the clouds of misunderstanding. *Postgraduate Medicine* 97(1), 36–47.
15. Bertina, R.M., Koeleman, B.P.C., and Koster, T., *et al.* (1994). Mutation in blood coagulation factor V associated with resistance to activated protein C. *Nature* 369, 64–67.
16. Geerts, W.H., Code, K.I., Jay, R.M., *et al.* (1994). A prospective study of venous thromboembolism after major trauma. *New England Journal of Medicine* 331(24), 1601–1606.
17. Weinmann, E.E., and Salzman, E.W. (1994). Deep-vein thrombosis. *New England Journal of Medicine* 331(24), 1630–1641.
18. Dhami, M.S., and Bona, R.D. (1993). Thrombosis in patients with cancer. *Postgraduate Medicine* 93(8), 131–140.
19. Bick, R.L. (1994). Disseminated intravascular coagulation: Objective criteria for diagnosis and management. *Medical Clinics of North America* 78(3), 511–543.
20. Seligsohn, U. (1995). Disseminated intravascular coagulation. In: Beutler, E., Lichtman, M.A., Coller, B.S., *et al.* (Eds.). *Williams Hematology.* (5th ed.). New York: McGraw-Hill. (pp. 1497–1516).
21. Dabrow, M.B., and Wilkins, J.C. (1993). Hematologic emergencies: Management of hyperleukemic syndrome, DIC, and thrombotic thrombocytopenic purpura. *Postgraduate Medicine* 93(5), 193–202.
22. Kajs-Wyllie, M. (1995). Thrombotic thrombocytopenic purpura: Pathophysiology, treatment, and related nursing care. *Critical Care Nurse* 15(16), 44–52.
23. Kuter, D.J., Ellman, L., and McCluskey, R.T. (1991). An 85-year old woman with renal failure, neurologic deterioration, and seizures. *New England Journal of Medicine* 325(4), 265–273.

SELECTED BIBLIOGRAPHY

Beutler, E., Lichtman, M.A., Coller, B.S., *et al.* (Eds.). (1995). *Williams Hematology.* (5th ed.). New York: McGraw-Hill.

Bick, R.L. (1994). Hypercoagulability and thrombosis. *Medical Clinics of North America* 78(3), 635–665.

den Heijer, M., Koster, T., Blom, H.J., *et al.* (1996). Hyperhomocysteinemia as a risk factor for deep-vein thrombosis. *New England Journal of Medicine* 334(12), 759–762.

Fareed, M., Hoppensteadt, D., Walenga, J.M., *et al.* (1994). Current trends in the development of anticoagulant and antithrombotic drugs. *Medical Clinics of North America* 78(3), 713–731.

George, J.N., El-Harake, M.A., and Raskob, G.E. (1994). Chronic idiopathic thrombocytopenic purpura. *New England Journal of Medicine* 331(18), 1207–1211.

Goldstein, K.H., and Abramson, N. (1996). Efficient diagnosis of thrombocytopenia. *American Family Physician* 53(3), 915–920.

Ibrahim, S., MacPherson, D.R., and Goldhaber, S.Z. (1996). Chronic venous insufficiency: Mechanisms and management. *American Heart Journal* 132(4), 856–860.

Landefeld, C.S., and Beyth, R.J. (1993). Anticoagulant-associated bleeding: Clinical epidemiology, prediction, and prevention. *American Journal of Medicine* 95, 315–328.

Levi, M., ten Cate, H., van der Poll, T., *et al.* (1993). Pathogenesis of disseminated intravascular coagulation in sepsis. *Journal of the American Medical Association* 270(8), 975–979.

Litin, S.C., and Gastineau, D.A. (1995). Current concepts in anticoagulant therapy. *Mayo Clinic Proceedings* 70, 266–272.

Lusher, J.M. (1996). Screening and diagnosis of coagulation disorders. *American Journal of Obstetrics and Gynecology* 175(3 Pt. 2), 778–783.

Lusher, J.M., Arkin, S., Abildgaard, C.F., *et al.* (1993). Recombinant factor VIII for the treatment of previously untreated patients with hemophilia A: Safety, efficacy, and development of inhibitors. *New England Journal of Medicine* 328(7), 453–459.

Mammen, E.F. (1994). Coagulation defects in liver disease. *Medical Clinics of North America* 78(3), 545–554.

Moser, D.M., Fedullo, P.F., Littejohn, J.K., *et al.* (1994). Frequent asymptomatic pulmonary embolism in patients with deep venous thrombosis. *Journal of the American Medical Association* 271(3), 223–225.

Patrono, C. (1994). Aspirin as an antiplatelet drug. *New England Journal of Medicine* 330(18), 1287–1294.

Phillips, D.E., Payne, D.K., and Mills, G.M. (1994). Heparin-induced thrombotic thrombocytopenia. *Annals of Pharmacotherapy* 28, 43–46.

Prandoni, P., Lensing, A.W.A., Cogo, A., *et al.* (1996). The long-term course of acute deep venous thrombosis. *Annals of Internal Medicine* 125(1), 1–7.

Rutherford, C.J., and Frenkel, E.P. (1994). Thrombocytopenia: Issues in diagnosis and therapy. *Medical Clinics of North America* 78(3), 555–575.

Sbarouni, E., Bradshaw, A., Andreotti, F., *et al.* Relationship between hemostatic abnormalities and neuroendocrine activity in heart failure. *American Heart Journal* 127(3), 607–612.

Schafer, A.I. (1995). Effects of nonsteroidal antiinflammatory drugs on platelet function and systemic hemostasis. *Journal of Clinical Pharmacy* 35, 209–219.

Seremetis, S.V., and Aledort, L.M. (1993). Congenital bleeding disorders: Rational treatment options. *Drugs* 45(4), 541–547.

Shuey, K.M. (1996). Platelet-associated bleeding disorders. *Seminars in Oncology Nursing* 12(1), 15–27.

Siragusa, S., Cosmi, B., Piovella, F., *et al.* (1996). Low-molecular weight heparins and unfractionated heparin in the treatment of patients with acute venous thromboembolism: Results of a meta-analysis. *American Journal of Medicine* 100, 269–277.

Stasi, R., Stipa, E., Masi, M., *et al.* (1995). Long-term observation of 208 adults with chronic idiopathic thrombocytopenic purpura. *American Journal of Medicine* 98, 436–442.

Toglia, M.R., and Weig, J.G. (1996). Venous thromboembolism during pregnancy. *New England Journal of Medicine* 335(2), 108–114.

Unit V

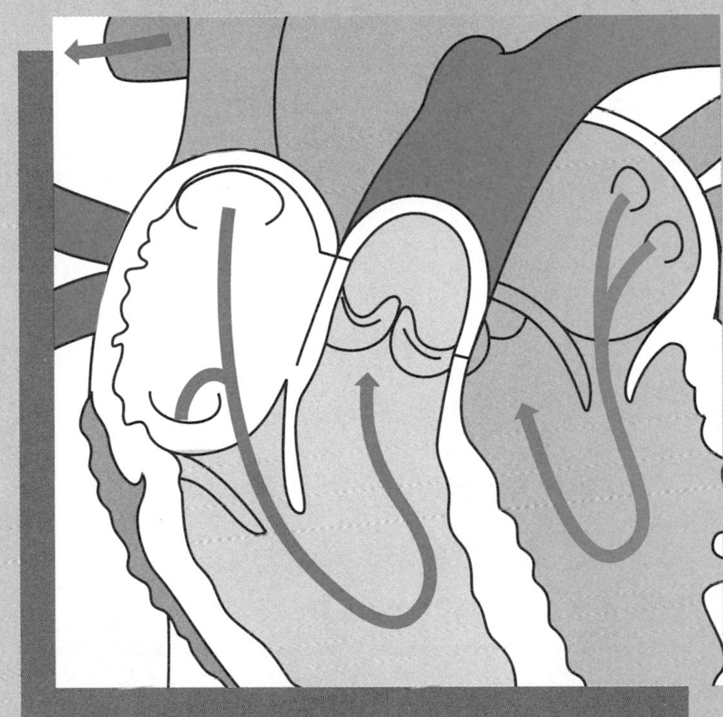

Chapter 15
Disorders of the Circulation

Chapter 16
Cardiac Failure

Chapter 17
Cardiac Dysrhythmias

CARDIOVASCULAR SYSTEM

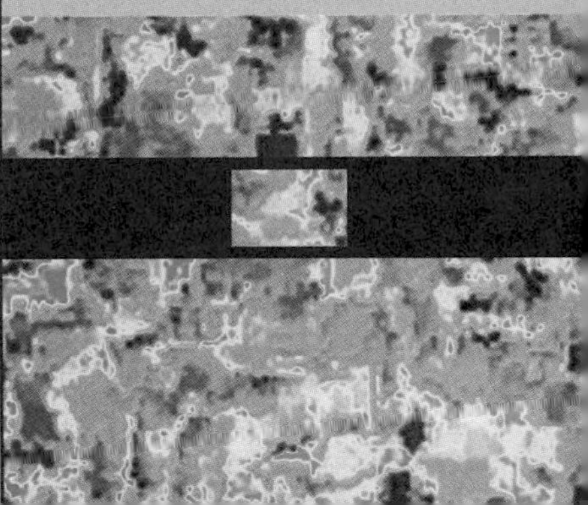

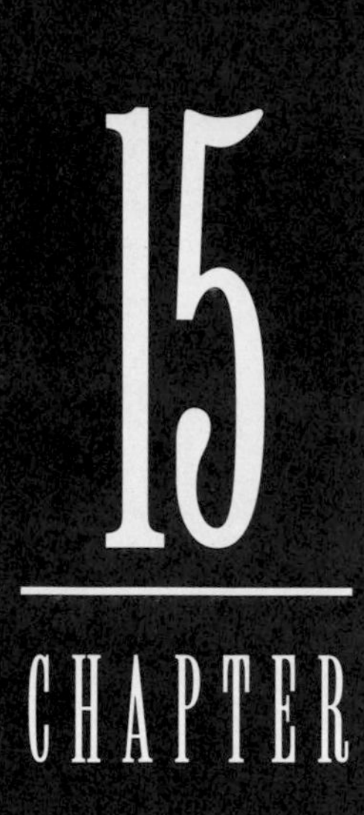

15 CHAPTER Disorders of the Circulation

LEARNING OBJECTIVES

1. Differentiate between functions of the systemic and pulmonary circulations.
2. Describe the primary and secondary pumps of the circulatory system.
3. Identify the principal functions of each type of vascular and lymphatic vessel.
4. Discuss the relationships among the hemodynamic factors influencing blood flow.
5. Differentiate among the neuroendocrine and endothelial mechanisms of circulatory regulation.
6. Discuss the epidemiology and etiologic mechanisms of atherosclerosis.
7. Discuss the epidemiology and etiologic theories underlying the development of hypertension.
8. Differentiate among the three general categories of shock.
9. Identify the pathophysiologic mechanisms that predict clinical manifestations and rationalize treatment of selected disorders of peripheral circulation.

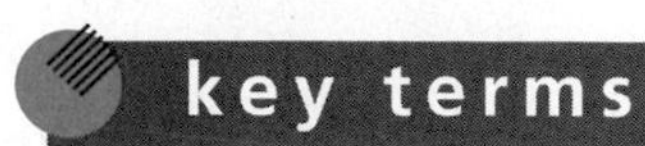

key terms

abdominal aortic aneurysm
anaphylactic shock
aneurysm
arteriosclerosis
arteriosclerosis obliterans (ASO)
atherosclerosis
baroreceptor reflex
burn shock
cardiac output
cardiogenic shock
central nervous system (CNS) ischemic response
central venous pressure (CVP)
chronic venous insufficiency
dissecting aneurysm
distributive shock
essential hypertension
general resistance equation
hemodynamics
hemorrhagic shock
hypertension
hypotension
hypovolemic shock
intermittent claudication
isolated systolic hypertension
Kawasaki disease
lipodermatosclerosis
mean arterial pressure (MAP)
neurogenic shock
orthostatic (postural) hypotension

perfusion
peripheral vascular disease (PVD)
pulse pressure
Raynaud's syndrome
septic shock
shock
spinal shock
systemic vascular resistance (SVR)
varicose veins
vascular remodeling
vasculitis
vasogenic shock
vasomotor center
vasovagal syncope
venous stasis ulcer

The cardiovascular system serves the general function of **perfusion** of body cells with blood containing oxygen, nutrients, hormones, and other elements essential to homeostasis. Circulating blood also carries waste products of cellular metabolism away from cells for processing by other systems. Normal perfusion of tissues depends on (1) establishment of the normal volume and constituents of the blood, and (2) movement of blood through vessels, which requires maintenance of normal patency and resistance of vessels as well as an adequate driving force to generate blood pressure and flow.

Despite significant improvement in outcomes, disease of the cardiovascular system, including the "pump" (heart) and "pipes" (blood vessels), is still the leading cause of death in the United States and other industrialized nations. During the 15-year period from 1973 to 1987, cardiovascular mortality rates decreased by 42% for people younger than 54 years and by 33% for those between 55 and 84 years of age.[1] (Fig. 15–1). More recent data indicate that this trend is continuing, with much of the decline due to risk reduction and improved treatment of coronary heart disease (associated with myocardial infarction) and cerebrovascular disease (associated with stroke).[2] In contrast to this overall positive trend, deaths due to congestive heart failure have increased since 1980.

Coronary heart disease and congestive heart failure are discussed in detail in Chapter 16, and cerebrovascular disease is reviewed in Chapter 21. Function and disorders of the hematopoietic system are discussed in Chapter 12. Emphasis in this chapter is on function and disorders of the blood vessels.

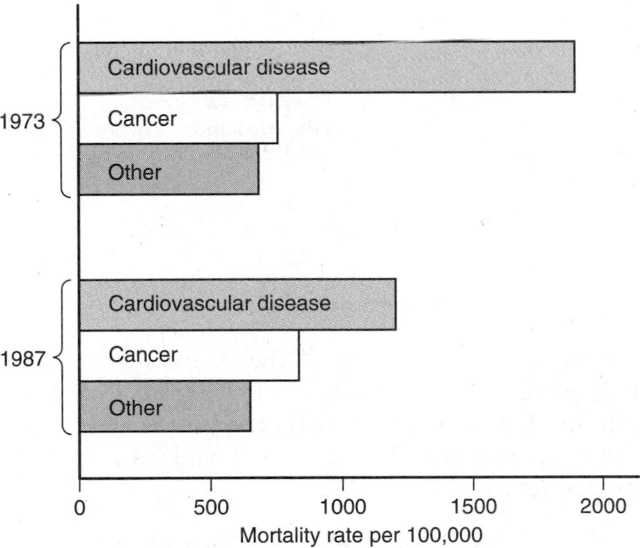

FIGURE 15–1

Trends in mortality due to cardiovascular diseases. During the 15-year period illustrated, deaths due to cardiovascular diseases declined by nearly 40% among whites. In contrast, deaths due to cancer increased slightly. (Data from The Centers for Disease Control and Prevention. Reported in Davis, D.L., Dinse, G.E., and Hoel, D.G. [1994]. Decreasing cardiovascular disease and increasing cancer among whites in the United States from 1973 through 1987: Good news and bad news. *Journal of the American Medical Association* 271[6], 431–437.)

FUNCTIONAL ANATOMY OF THE CIRCULATION

Major Divisions

Figure 15–2 illustrates the two major divisions of the circulation: the larger *systemic circulation,* in which blood leaves the left ventricle of the heart, perfuses all organ systems except the lungs, and returns to the right atrium of the heart; and the *pulmonary circulation,* in which blood leaves the right ventricle of the heart, circulates through the lungs, and returns to the left atrium of the heart.

The perfusion pressure within the systemic circulation, called the **mean arterial pressure (MAP),** is five to seven times that of the pulmonary system perfusion pressure because of the greater resistance to blood flow within the systemic circulation. Factors contributing to vessel resistance, pressure, and blood flow, collectively known as **hemodynamics,** are discussed later in this chapter. The systemic circulation is the focus of this chapter; the pulmonary circulation is detailed in Chapter 19, in the context of respiratory function.

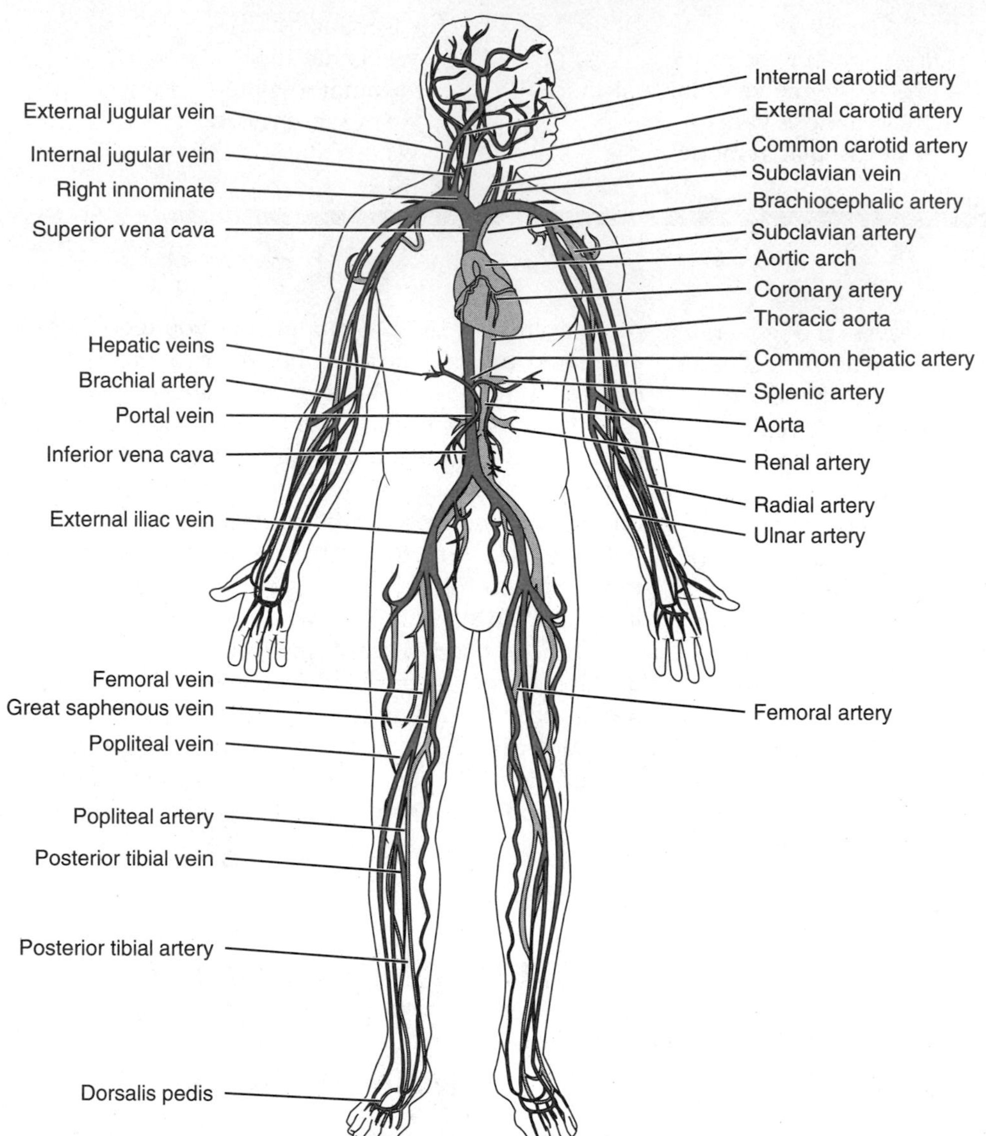

FIGURE 15–2
The circulation. Principal arteries and veins are illustrated.

Pumps

The heart serves as the primary pump within the circulation. Contraction of cardiac muscle (myocardium) pushes blood into the vessels in a cyclic or pulsatile manner (see Chapter 16). The left and right ventricles of the heart serve as separate pumps for the systemic and pulmonary circulations, respectively. Although the heart is by far the most important pumping force, it is not the *only* force that moves blood within the system. Secondary pumping forces are derived from the Windkessel effect, the skeletal muscle pump, the diaphragmatic pump, and the intrinsic vasomotion of the vessels themselves.

Windkessel Effect

With each contraction of the heart, the expelled volume stretches elastic fibers in the walls of larger arteries. Recoil of these fibers (the Windkessel effect) smoothes out the flow of blood and assists in its propulsion.

Skeletal Muscle Pump

The external pressure of skeletal muscle contraction on thin-walled, one-way vessels (i.e., veins and lymphatics) assists with flow in these vessels. Loss of this skeletal muscle pump with immobilization contributes to slowed venous flow and deep vein thrombosis (see Chapter 14).

TABLE 15–1
ANATOMIC AND FUNCTIONAL CHARACTERISTICS OF VESSELS

VESSEL	DIAMETER	WALL THICKNESS	CHARACTERISTICS
Aorta	25 mm	2 mm	Increased compliance due to elastic tissue
Artery	4 mm	1 mm	More muscular, less compliant
Arteriole	30 μm	6 μm	Prominent circular smooth muscle
Capillary	8 μm	0.5 μm	Single layer of endothelium surrounded by basement membrane
Venule	20 μm	1 μm	Nonmuscular, fixed diameter
Vein	5 mm	0.5 mm	Muscular and compliant owing to elastin; larger veins have semilunar valves
Vena cava	30 mm	1.5 mm	Muscular, compliant, and tough owing to fibrous tissue

Diaphragmatic Pump

During respiration, contraction and relaxation of the diaphragm cause cyclic pressure changes in the thoracic and abdominal cavities, which alternately impede and promote flow through vessels in these cavities. Intrathoracic pressure changes also influence ejection of blood from the ventricles of the heart, as discussed in Chapter 16.

Vasomotion

Many blood vessels also contribute directly to propulsion of blood within them through vasomotion, or cyclic contraction and relaxation of their smooth muscle and elastic elements. Vasomotion is influenced by signals from the autonomic nervous system but is primarily regulated by endothelial mediators, as discussed later.

Conduits

The conduits, or pipes, of the circulatory system are the blood vessels (vascular circulation). The lymphatic vessels comprise a one-way accessory circulation. The vascular circulation consists of the arteries, arterioles, capillaries, venules, and veins. The arterioles, capillary beds, and venules are often collectively referred to as the *microcirculation.*

Anatomic and functional characteristics of each vessel type are summarized in Table 15–1.

Arteries

The arteries serve primarily as conductance vessels. As shown in Figure 15–3, arteries have a three-layered structure consisting of the inner intima (endothelium and smooth muscle), the media (smooth muscle), and the outer adventitia (fibroblasts and smooth muscle). The muscular structure of arteries allows them to withstand the pressure load derived from their proximity to the major pump, and their large diameters allow for rapid conductance of blood from the heart to the arterioles of the tissues.

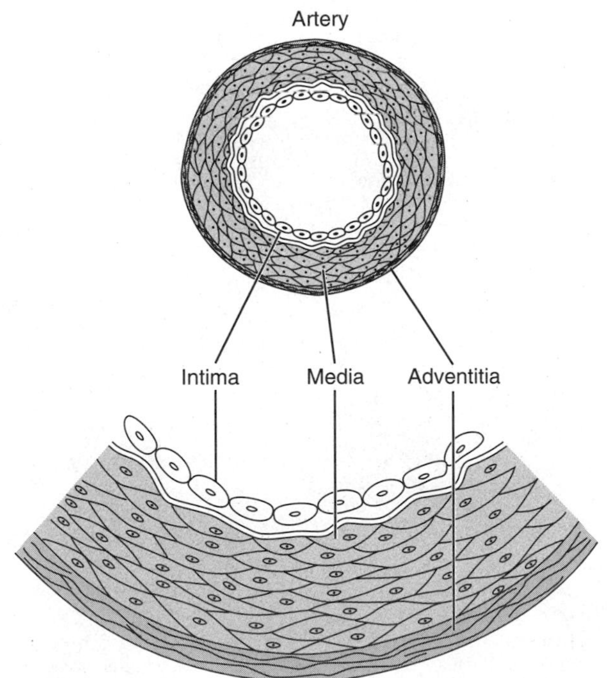

FIGURE 15–3
The arterial wall. The three layers of the arterial wall are the inner intima (endothelium), the media (smooth muscle layer), and the outer adventitia (fibrous layer). Some smooth muscle is found in all three layers.

Arterioles

The arterioles serve as the major *resistance* vessels because of their variable diameters and their thick walls of smooth muscle. Arterioles may provide increased or decreased resistance to flow in response to either autonomic nervous system stimulation or to local mediators secreted by endothelial cells. Because arterioles are positioned between larger arteries and capillary beds, variation in their diameter affects both blood pressure and capillary hydrostatic pressure (CHP), as discussed subsequently.

Capillary Beds

The smallest vessels, the capillaries, serve as *exchange* vessels, transporting substances between the blood and the interstitial fluid surrounding cells. As discussed in detail in Chapter 8, capillary walls are composed of single endothelial cells. The capillary lumen is just large enough for red blood cells to squeeze through. Although variability exists among tissues, capillaries are usually highly permeable to water and to the dissolved constituents in plasma.

As illustrated in Figure 15–4, capillaries are arranged in networks, or "beds," within tissues. In addition to exchange vessels (true capillaries), these beds contain thoroughfare channels, which, when open, allow blood to pass through without participating in the exchange process. They also contain metarterioles, vessels that have a structure midway between that of arteriole and capillary. Some capillaries are encircled by smooth muscle bands (precapillary sphincters).

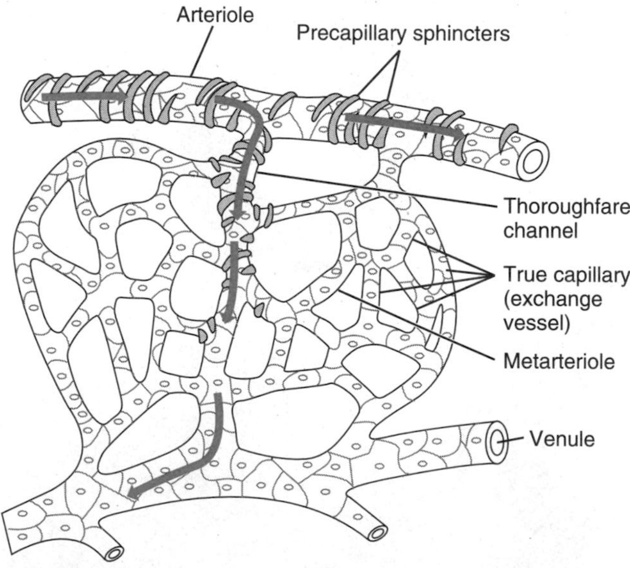

FIGURE 15–4
Structures of the capillary bed. Capillary beds are composed of (1) true capillaries, which exchange fluid and dissolved substances between the blood and the interstitium; (2) thoroughfare channels, which shunt blood through capillaries with little or no exchange when open; (3) metarterioles, which constrict to direct flow within the capillary bed; and (4) precapillary sphincters, which constrict or relax to regulate flow from the arteriole into the capillary bed.

As a result of contraction of their smooth muscle, metarterioles and precapillary sphincters regulate CHP within true capillaries while simultaneously influencing systemic resistance and blood pressure. As discussed later, metarterioles and precapillary sphincters are believed to be the principal sites of autoregulation of tissue perfusion, whereby tissues locally regulate their own blood supply. Much of the driving pressure in the arterial system is normally dissipated in the capillaries as fluid leaves the vessels along the CHP gradient and enters the interstitium (see Starling's Law of the Capillary, Chapter 8).

Venules

Capillary beds exit into the venules, the smallest vessels of the venous system. The immediate postcapillary venules have fixed diameters; but because of their small size, they provide some resistance to blood flow, contributing to venous pressure. Larger venules are able to stretch passively when blood volume is high, thus serving a *capacitance,* or *reservoir,* function. These vessels also have smooth muscle in their walls and are innervated by the autonomic nervous system. When blood volume is low, a neural signal causes contraction of venules and shifts pooled blood into the central circulation.

Veins

Veins, the largest vessels in the body, serve both conductance and capacitance functions. Veins of the systemic circulation conduct blood from the tissues back to the heart, often in opposition to gravity. This *venous return* is facilitated by the presence of one-way valves, which normally prevent backflow, and by the skeletal muscle pump (Fig. 15–5).

Lymphatic Circulation

The lymphatic system is a one-way circulation that parallels the venous system both anatomically

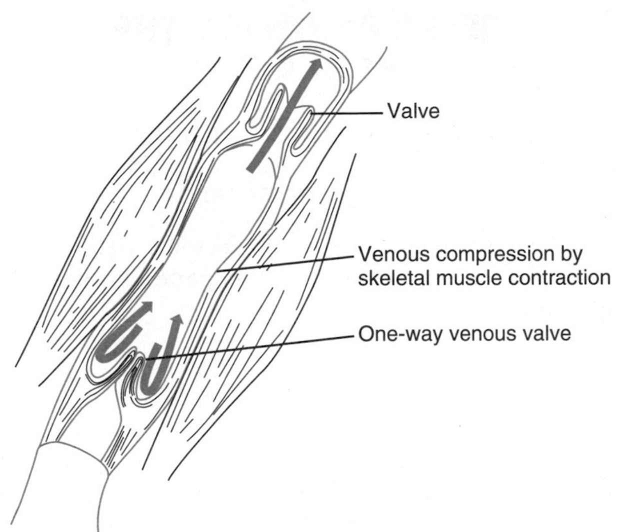

FIGURE 15–5
Skeletal muscle pump. One-way flow of blood in veins is facilitated by external compression with skeletal muscle contraction. Semilunar valves in veins prevent backflow.

and functionally (see Chapter 13). Blind-ended lymphatic capillaries are present near vascular capillary beds in most tissues (Fig. 15–6). These vessels receive excess interstitial fluid and large particles, such as proteins, cellular debris, or bacterial products associated with inflammation or infection. Lymphatic capillaries converge into lymphatic vessels, which are filtered by lymph nodes, where immunologic attack may be mounted against foreign antigens. The lymphatic system ultimately joins the venous system at the thoracic duct.

Reservoirs

The capacity of the vascular system to pool or store excess blood when volume is high is an important aspect of regulation of perfusion. The systemic venous system, with its larger, thin-walled vessels, is an important blood reservoir. The pulmonary vessels are an additional vascular reservoir, as are two distensible organs—the liver and spleen. Clinical enlargement of these organs is frequently due to high blood volume or backup of volume and pressure due to cardiac failure (see Chapter 16). In low-volume states (e.g., **hypovolemic shock**), reflex contraction of vascular and organ reservoirs occurs as an adaptive response, shunting more blood into the central circulation.

Circuits

Many clinical manifestations of cardiovascular disorders reflect the specific sequences or pathways of blood flow within the system. Classification of vascular circuits as *series* or *parallel* circuits is based on concepts derived from the study of electrical circuits. With respect to the circulation of blood, two circuits aligned in series receive the *same* blood supply, sequentially. As shown schematically in Figure 15–7, the pulmonary and systemic circulations are in series with each other, as are the intestinal tract and liver circulations. That is, virtually all of the blood flowing through the pulmonary circulation then flows through the systemic circulation; and the blood leaving the intestines flows through the liver before re-entering the main venous circulation. Series circuitry is functionally essential in both cases. Blood is first oxygenated and cleared of carbon dioxide in its circuit through the lungs. This blood then enters the systemic circulation to perfuse tissues, supplying them with oxygen and removing carbon dioxide. Blood leaving the intestine contains absorbed nutrients and dietary bacteria. Nutrients must be processed by liver cells (hepatocytes) and bacteria cleared by fixed macrophages (Kupffer cells) in the liver before blood re-enters the general circulation.

The other organ systems of the body are arranged in parallel with respect to each other. The blood supplied by the systemic circulation is divided

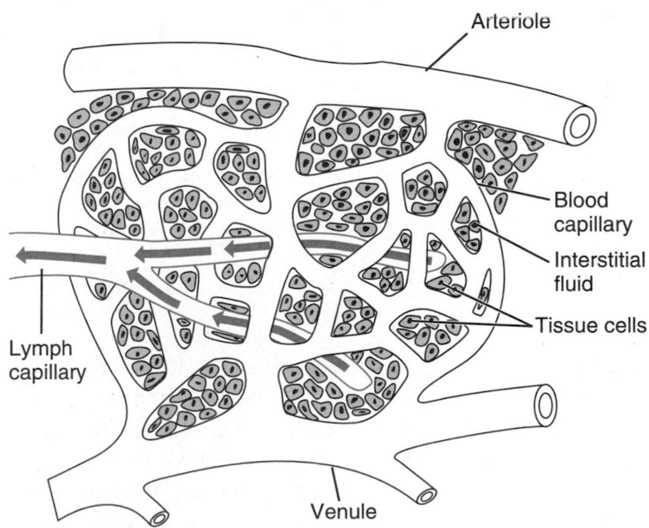

FIGURE 15–6
Lymphatic capillaries. Most vascular capillary beds are associated with lymphatic capillaries. These blind-ended vessels transport excess interstitial fluid and larger particles from the tissues to the venous system through the lymph.

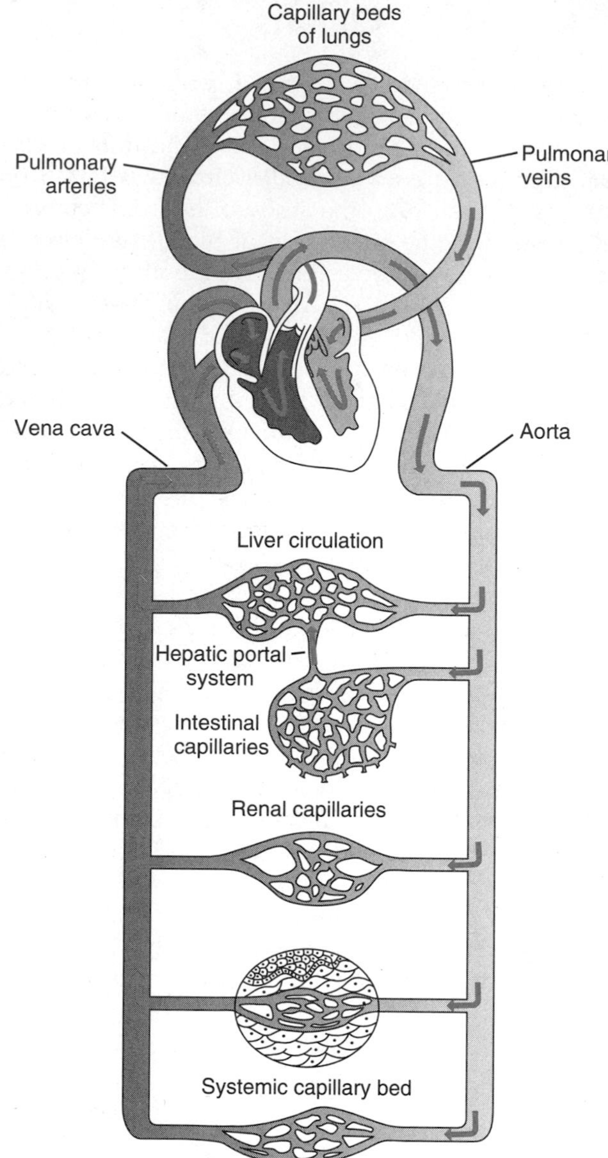

FIGURE 15–7

Series and parallel circuits. The pulmonary and systemic circulations are aligned in series in that each receives the same blood sequentially. The intestinal and liver circulations are also connected in series. Other organ systems are perfused by parallel circuitry, with each receiving a fraction of the systemic circulation.

among them, with each receiving a fraction that varies according to its metabolic needs during an unstressed state (Table 15–2). During stress, however, the sympathetic nervous system (SNS) is activated, resulting in selective vasoconstriction, which redistributes blood flow to the most essential organ systems (see Chapter 1). A similar response occurs in **shock** states, as discussed later. This adaptive redistribution of blood would be impossible if not for the parallel circuitry of these systems.

REGULATION OF THE CIRCULATION

Hemodynamic Principles

Flow Determinants

The relationship between factors determining blood flow is expressed by the **general resistance equation:**

$$F = (P_a - P_v)/R$$

Blood flow (F) is expressed as a volume per unit time, for example, milliliters per minute or liters per minute. The general resistance equation holds that blood flow is directly related to the pressure gradient within the circuit ($P_a - P_v$) and inversely related to the resistance (R) within the circuit. In the systemic circulation, the pressure gradient is the difference in pressure between the beginning of the circuit (P_a, quantified as mean arterial pressure [MAP]) and the end of the circuit (P_v, quantified as **central venous pressure [CVP]**).

Factors Influencing the Pressure Gradient

The general resistance equation illustrates that any factor that decreases the arterial pressure or increases the venous pressure would decrease the pressure gradient within the system. Arterial pressure is generated within the heart on the basis of blood volume, heart rate, and contractile force (see Chapter 16). If resistance is held constant, alteration of any of these three parameters would be *directly* reflected as a change in MAP. A change in resistance *indirectly* influences MAP because the pressure gradient is altered adaptively to maintain constant

TABLE 15–2
DISTRIBUTION OF BLOOD AMONG ORGAN SYSTEMS

ORGAN SYSTEM	CARDIAC OUTPUT (%)
Gastrointestinal	24
Musculoskeletal	21
Renal-urinary	19
Cerebrovascular	13
Integumentary	9
Coronary circulation	4
All other organ systems	10

flow. MAP is calculated from the measured blood pressure as follows:

$$MAP = (\text{systolic BP} + 2 \text{ diastolic BP})/3$$

Blood pressure (BP) is most often measured clinically by the noninvasive auscultatory method (Fig. 15–8) and documented as a fraction with systolic pressure over diastolic pressure. Systolic pressure primarily results from the pumping force of the heart during contraction and emptying (*systole*), whereas diastolic pressure is maintained by the resistance of the vessels while the heart is refilling (*diastole*). Because the heart is typically in diastole twice as long as it is in systole, the calculation of MAP is weighted accordingly.

Central venous pressure must be measured invasively, which is often done by introducing a catheter into the vena cava just outside the right atrium, or into the right atrium itself (Fig. 15–9). Because almost all of the pressure within the arterial system is dissipated in the capillaries, pressure at the end of the systemic circuit normally approaches zero. CVP may be elevated in conditions of volume overload or in cardiac failure.

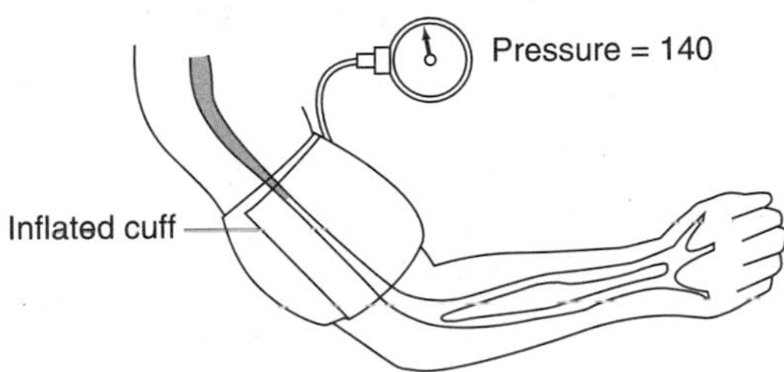

A The artery is occluded by the pressure of the cuff. No sound is audible with a stethescope over the brachial artery.

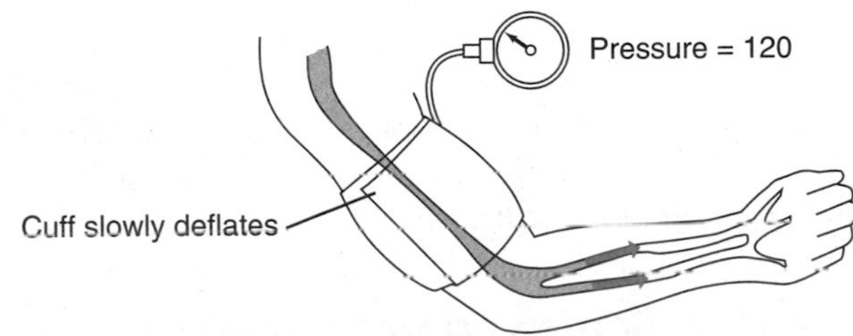

B Eddy currents distal to the compressed vessel produce vibrations that cause noise (Korotkoff's sounds) as the cuff is slowly deflated. The first sound is the systolic pressure.

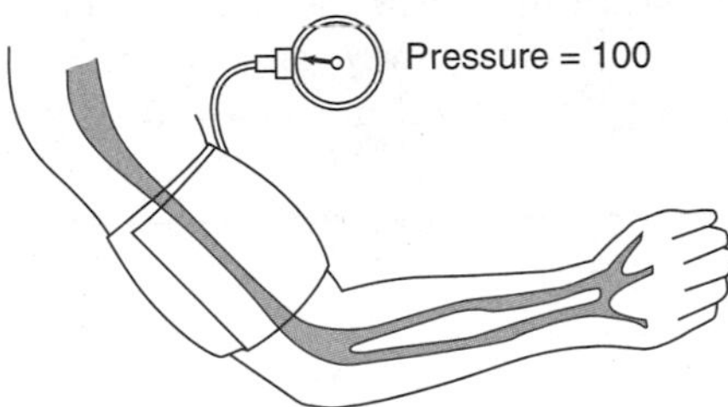

C Sounds that are produced change in character as more blood flows.

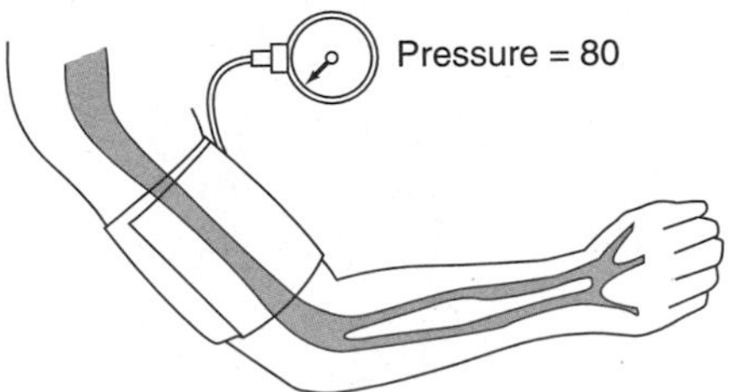

D At the diastolic pressure, the vessel is fully open. No eddy currents are produced, and Korotkoff's sounds disappear. Pressure is recorded as 120/80.

FIGURE 15–8

Auscultatory method of blood pressure measurement.

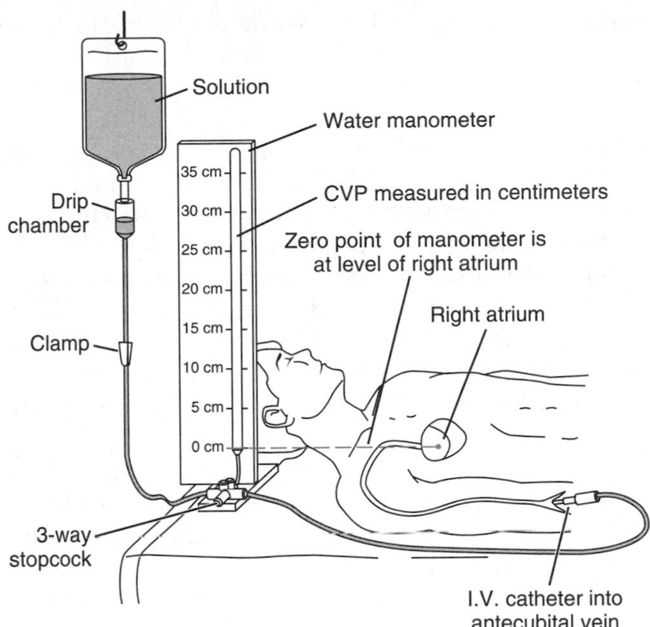

FIGURE 15–9

Measurement of central venous pressure (CVP). A water manometer connected to a catheter introduced into the vena cava or right atrium provides an estimate of the pressure at the end of the systemic circuit. Such catheters (CVP lines) may be connected to electronic pressure transducers in critical care settings. (Redrawn from Long, B.C., Phipps, W.J., and Cassmeyer, V.L. [1993]. *Medical-Surgical Nursing: A Nursing Process Approach.* St. Louis: Mosby-Year Book. [p. 147].)

Factors Affecting Resistance

Factors that increase resistance decrease flow, and vice versa. These factors include alterations in (1) vessel radius, (2) blood viscosity (thickness or stickiness), (3) directional flow characteristics, and (4) vascular distensibility, or compliance.

Vessel Radius. Because of its physiologic variability, vessel radius is the most important factor determining resistance. Resistance varies inversely in proportion to the fourth power of the radius. For example, a decrease in vessel radius from 2 mm to 1 mm would result in a 16-fold increase in resistance to flow within that vessel. Vessel caliber varies anatomically as well as in response to neural, hormonal, and local regulatory stimuli. Occlusion of vessels by atherosclerotic plaque or clots also decreases lumen size and increases resistance.

Blood Viscosity. Blood viscosity refers to the fluidity of the blood, that is, the degree of friction generated through contacts among its constituents. The more viscous the blood, the greater are the frictional forces and resistance to flow. Blood viscosity depends primarily on the proportion of blood volume composed of red blood cells, measured clinically as the *hematocrit* (see Chapter 12). Hyperosmolarity (as in hyperglycemia) also increases blood viscosity and resistance to flow.

Laminar Versus Turbulent Flow. Blood flow within smooth, straight vessels is normally laminar, and clinically silent. As shown in Figure 15–10, blood flows in a single direction in concentric layers, with little resistance. Turbulent blood flow occurs in areas of vessel branching, damage, or partial occlusion. Turbulent flow generates eddy currents in which blood flows in several directions at once, creating a high-resistance state. Turbulent flow may result in vibratory sounds (bruits), which are audible with a stethoscope.

Vessel Compliance. *Compliance* refers to the degree of distensibility of a vessel or hollow organ. Compliant tissues typically have more elastic connective tissue and less fibrous tissue. The more compliant a tissue, the more easily it increases its volume or length in response to a pressure load. Compliance and resistance are reciprocals: the more compliant a vessel, the less resistance it offers. Veins normally offer little resistance to flow, whereas arteries offer more resistance, maintaining higher pressures per unit volume within them. Arteries stiffened by **atherosclerosis** offer even higher resistance.

Clinical Assessment of Resistance. Resistance cannot be directly measured in clinical settings but may be calculated from the measurable parameters of MAP, CVP, and **cardiac output** using the general resistance equation (see earlier). Cardiac output, the volume of blood ejected from the heart per minute, represents flow (F) in this assessment, and may be measured by various means, discussed in Chapter 16. Resistance within the systemic circulation **(systemic vascular resistance [SVR]**) is often used as a monitoring parameter to determine the efficacy of vasoactive medications in the critically ill. In other clinical situations, resistance is evaluated indirectly on the basis of blood pressure measurements and signs and symptoms reflective of perfusion of specific organs.

Neural Regulation

Physiologic regulation of blood flow involves short-term and long-term mechanisms affecting both the pressure gradient and resistance. The short-term mechanisms are neural reflexes, of which the **baroreceptor reflex** is most important.

Baroreceptor Systems

Baroreceptors are specialized sensory nerve endings located in the carotid sinuses, aortic arch, great veins, right atrium, and both ventricles of the heart (Fig. 15–11). Baroreceptors alter their rate of transmission of neural impulses in response to the degree of pressure or stretch within the tissues. Action potentials are conducted along sensory nerves to the

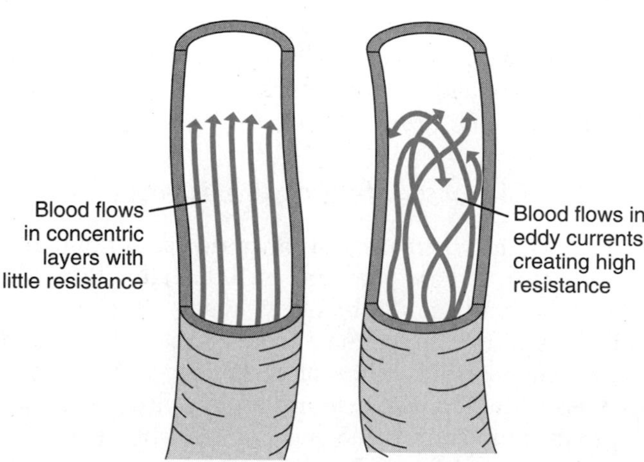
Blood flows in concentric layers with little resistance
Blood flows in eddy currents, creating high resistance
Laminar flow
Turbulent flow

FIGURE 15–10

Laminar versus turbulent flow. In smooth, straight vessels, blood flows in concentric layers with little resistance. In branched, damaged, or partially occluded vessels, blood flow generates eddy currents and increased resistance.

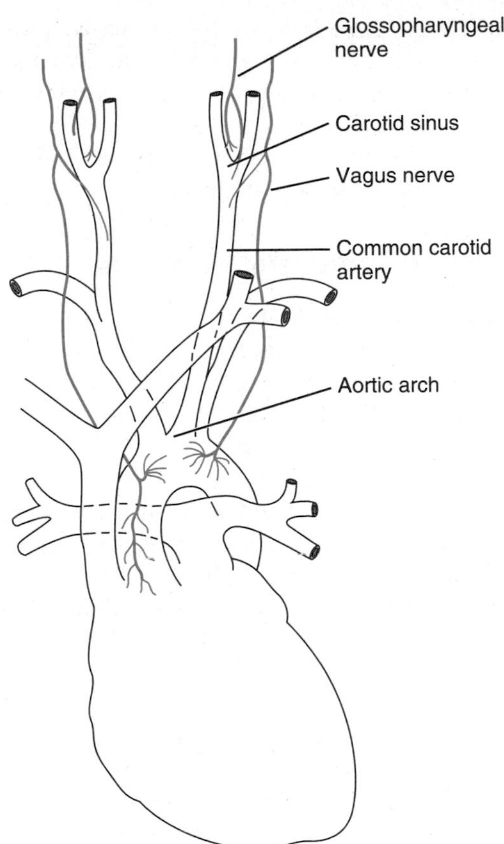

FIGURE 15–11
Baroreceptor reflex. Baroreceptors in the carotid sinuses and aortic arch initiate neural signals in response to the degree of pressure or stretch in these vessels. Heart rate and contractility are altered to restore baseline blood pressure.

vasomotor center in the medulla of the brain stem and are then relayed to the hypothalamus for processing. Output signals travel from the hypothalamus back to the vasomotor center, then along autonomic (sympathetic and parasympathetic) nerves to the heart and blood vessels. The arterial baroreceptors mediate the *high-pressure baroreflex*, responding to increases in blood pressure; whereas the cardiopulmonary baroreceptors mediate the *low-pressure baroreflex*, responding to altered tissue stretch due to changes in blood volume.

If blood pressure or volume is decreased (e.g., in hypovolemic shock), sympathetic output dominates, resulting in increased heart rate and contractile force as well as selective vasoconstriction, primarily at the arteriolar level. Blood pressure rises to maintain consistent flow under conditions of increased resistance. The rate of baroreceptor firing then returns to the baseline state, completing the negative feedback loop.

The baroreceptor reflex may be impaired with aging, hypovolemia, or antihypertensive drug therapy, resulting in a condition known as **orthostatic (postural) hypotension**, a sudden drop in blood pressure with symptoms of cerebral hypoperfusion when a person changes positions from lying or sitting to standing. Orthostatic hypotension is often objectively defined as a decline in systolic blood pressure of more than 20 mm Hg or a reduction in diastolic blood pressure of more than 10 mm Hg.[3] The change in position causes a gravitational shift in blood volume, with more blood pooling in the veins of the legs. Venous return is suddenly lower, and cardiac output falls. Normally, the baroreceptor reflex is triggered, and blood pressure is immediately restored by increased heart rate and contractility. In orthostatic hypotension, however, there is a delayed or insufficient response. Tissue perfusion to the brain is compromised, and the person may become dizzy or lose consciousness.

Regulatory systems such as the baroreceptor system, which are not dependent on conscious input from higher centers of the brain, are known as *reflex arcs.* As detailed in Chapter 22, these are automatic or stereotyped motor responses to sensory inputs. Although reflex arcs do not require input from higher centers, they may be influenced by such input. The cerebral cortex can over-ride the hypothalamus in certain instances. Blood vessels may be dilated in anticipation of exercise, for example, or with extreme emotional stress. In the latter case, the person may lose consciousness (faint or swoon) owing to inappropriate parasympathetic stimulation, which results in low blood flow to areas of the brain governing consciousness. This condition is known as **vasovagal syncope**.

Chemoreceptor Systems

Chemoreceptors initiate reflex arcs in response to chemical alterations in the fluids surrounding them. *Peripheral chemoreceptors* in the carotid and aortic bodies sense changes in blood gases (oxygen and carbon dioxide) and pH. These receptors are more important in regulation of respiration than of circulation, and are discussed in detail in Chapter 18. They do have some cardiac effect, however, resulting in circulatory changes. Decreased pH, increased P_{CO_2}, or decreased P_{O_2} causes parasympathetic stimulation, slowing the heart rate and causing decreased contractile force.

Cardiopulmonary chemoreceptors in the walls of the heart and large airways of the lungs detect chemicals released owing to ischemia, resulting in a similar reflex. The chemoreceptor reflexes result in *decreased* systemic blood flow in states of poor tissue perfusion, the adaptive purpose of which apparently is to protect the heart (by minimizing oxygen demands). This protection occurs at the expense of peripheral tissues.

Central Nervous System Ischemic Response

Like the chemoreceptor systems, the **central nervous system (CNS) ischemic response** is designed to protect a critical organ, the brain in this case, in low-perfusion states (e.g., end-stage shock). When MAP falls to very low levels, neurons of the vasomotor center are directly stimulated, causing a short burst of tachycardia (heart rate of about 200 beats/minute). In addition, vasoconstriction virtually shuts down all blood flow to the kidneys, abdominal organs, skin, and muscles. This response is a final effort to preserve cerebral function in extreme shock, but unfortunately, it often leads to a downward spiral that ends in death.

Endocrine Regulation

Longer-term regulation of circulation is mediated by the mechanisms governing fluid volume. Hormones regulating these mechanisms, discussed in detail in Chapter 8, include the renin–angiotensin–aldosterone system (RAAS), antidiuretic hormone (ADH), and atrial natriuretic peptide. Volume-dependent alterations in glomerular filtration rate are also relevant to regulation of the circulation.

Renin–Angiotensin–Aldosterone System

Unlike the immediate-acting neural reflexes, the renal-hormonal mechanisms influencing circulation take days or weeks to act. In low-perfusion states, decreased flow to the kidneys triggers the system, which culminates in release of the hormone aldosterone from the adrenal cortex (see Chapter 8). Aldosterone then acts on the kidney to increase reabsorption of sodium, causing a secondary reabsorption of water by osmosis. Increased fluid volume results in increased cardiac output and an increased pressure gradient for blood flow within the circulation.

The RAAS also influences vessel resistance through its intermediate product, angiotensin II, which is a potent vasoconstrictor. Recently, the existence of RAAS components in other tissues, including the heart and vascular wall, has been demonstrated. These tissue systems function independently of the hormonal RAAS, in the local tonic control of tissue function and vascular resistence.[4] Use of angiotensin-converting enzyme (ACE) inhibitors is one pharmacologic approach to treatment of hypertension. These drugs prevent the activation of the inactive precursor, angiotensin I, to the active angiotensin II. In addition, ACE inhibition potentiates the action of kinins in normalizing endothelial regulation of blood flow, as discussed later.

Antidiuretic Hormone

The importance of ADH in regulation of circulation relates primarily to its role in regulation of fluid volume and osmolarity, discussed in Chapter 8. Volume influences the pressure gradient, whereas osmolarity affects resistance to a minor degree. ADH, also known as arginine vasopressin, is a significant vasoconstrictor only if used as a drug, in nonphysiologic doses. As a local cytokine, ADH is known to have a growth-promoting effect on the vascular endothelium and to induce the release of vasoconstrictor substances from the endothelium, as discussed later.

Atrial Natriuretic Peptide

Atrial natriuretic peptide, released from cardiac cells in response to increased blood volume, inhibits the aldosterone-dependent Na^+-K^+-ATPase pump in the distal nephron (see Chapter 8). Sodium and water reabsorption are decreased in response to atrial natriuretic peptide, resulting in decreased blood volume and completing the negative feedback loop.

Glomerular Filtration Rate

The most basic means by which the body regulates fluid volume is by varying the rate of volume filtered by renal glomerular capillaries (see Chapter 20). As blood volume increases, renal plasma flow is also increased, promoting glomerular filtration in response to higher CHP. Neural and hormonal inputs may influence the filtration fraction by selective constriction of the arterioles on either side of the glomerular capillary tuft. Glomerular filtration is directly responsive to blood flow, and renal mechanisms are critical to regulation of blood volume. The coexistence of renal failure and circulatory disorders is common in clinical settings, as discussed later with regard to **hypertension** and shock.

Endothelial Regulation

Tissue perfusion is locally regulated by several endothelial cell products that affect contraction of vascular smooth muscle, hemostasis, cellular proliferation for vascular growth and remodeling, and inflammatory and immune responses within the vessel wall.[5] Although the precise mechanisms are incompletely understood, the importance of this autoregulation is clear. Within limits, autoregulation maintains constant flow to specific tissues despite fluctuations in MAP. Excessive flow with high blood pressure would otherwise cause pressure damage (barotrauma) to tissues; and with low blood pressure, tissue ischemia would quickly develop. During unstressed states, autoregulation "fine-tunes" perfusion of tissues, optimally matching tissue demand and supply.

The endothelium responds to stretch, shear stress (frictional force resulting from flow), and numerous chemical mediators with the production of signaling molecules.[6] These may promote vasodilation, vasoconstriction, or proliferation of endothelial or smooth muscle cells. Through the differential release of relaxing or constricting factors, the endothelium functions as the regulator of local tissue perfusion and hemostasis.

Endothelial-Derived Relaxing Factors

Endothelial-derived relaxing factors, which promote vasodilation, include prostacyclin, nitric oxide, and endothelial-derived hyperpolarizing factor. Endothelial derived relaxing factors are released owing to endothelial stimulation by thrombin, ADH, and bradykinin as well as due to shear stress and vascular wall tension.

Prostacyclin, a product of arachidonic acid metabolism, relaxes vascular smooth muscle and inhibits platelet aggregation by increasing the cellular level of cyclic adenosine monophosphate (see Chapters 13 and 14). Nitric oxide, derived from the metabolism of the amino acid L-arginine, causes vasodilation and inhibits platelet activation by elevating cellular levels of cyclic guanosine monophosphate. Nitric oxide also inhibits proliferation of vascular cells. Reactive oxygen species produced with tissue injury and inflammation inactivate nitric oxide, promoting local hemostasis and enhancing vascular permeability. Endothelial-derived hyperpolarizing factor opens membrane K^+ channels, hyperpolarizing the membrane and relaxing smooth muscle.

Endothelial-Derived Contracting Factors

Under stimulation by local substances (e.g., acetylcholine, arachidonic acid, norepinephrine, thrombin, antidiuretic hormone, angiotensin II, low-density lipoprotein [LDL] cholesterol), tissue hypoxia, stretch, or pressure, the endothelium may release *endothelial-derived contracting factors,* which cause vasoconstriction. Endothelial-derived contracting factors include the arachidonic acid metabolites endoperoxide and thromboxane A_2, and endothelin.

Endothelin is the most potent vasoconstrictor substance known to be produced by the body.[7] Endothelin influences gene expression by vascular smooth muscle cells and causes an increase in the intracellular pH. Increased pH enhances the sensitivity of the smooth muscle myofilaments to calcium, augmenting contraction.

Short-Term Versus Long-Term Autoregulation

In the short term, autoregulatory mechanisms respond to an increased demand for tissue perfusion with closure of thoroughfare channels in capillary beds to route flow through exchange vessels, and with opening of metarterioles and precapillary sphincters, leading into exchange vessels. If the need for increased perfusion is sustained, **vascular remodeling** occurs under the regulation of growth-promoting cytokines (angiogenic factors), vasoactive substances, and hemodynamic stimuli. Vascular remodeling is an active process of structural alteration that involves changes in cell growth, cell death (apoptosis), cell migration, and alteration of the extracellular matrix.[8] In response to chronically increased pressure, the vessel wall thickens as a result of an increase in smooth muscle mass or rearrangement of the extracellular matrix. A sustained increase in blood flow results in an increase in lumen size, with little change in wall thickness, effected by reconstruction of the vessel wall components. Sustained decreases in flow result in reduction of lumen caliber.

Growth of new blood vessels (angiogenesis) occurs adaptively in the case of increased tissue demands during normal growth and development as well as during wound healing. Angiogenesis is also a critical factor in the growth of most tumors. When blood vessels serving a tissue become chronically occluded (as with atherosclerosis), *collateral circulation* may develop over time, owing to the growth of new vessels and enlargement of others to bypass the blocked area. This important long-term mechanism may sustain organ function in atherosclerotic conditions such as coronary heart disease and cerebrovascular disease.

CIRCULATORY DISORDERS

Function of the circulation is compromised by pump failure or pipe failure, that is, any syndrome

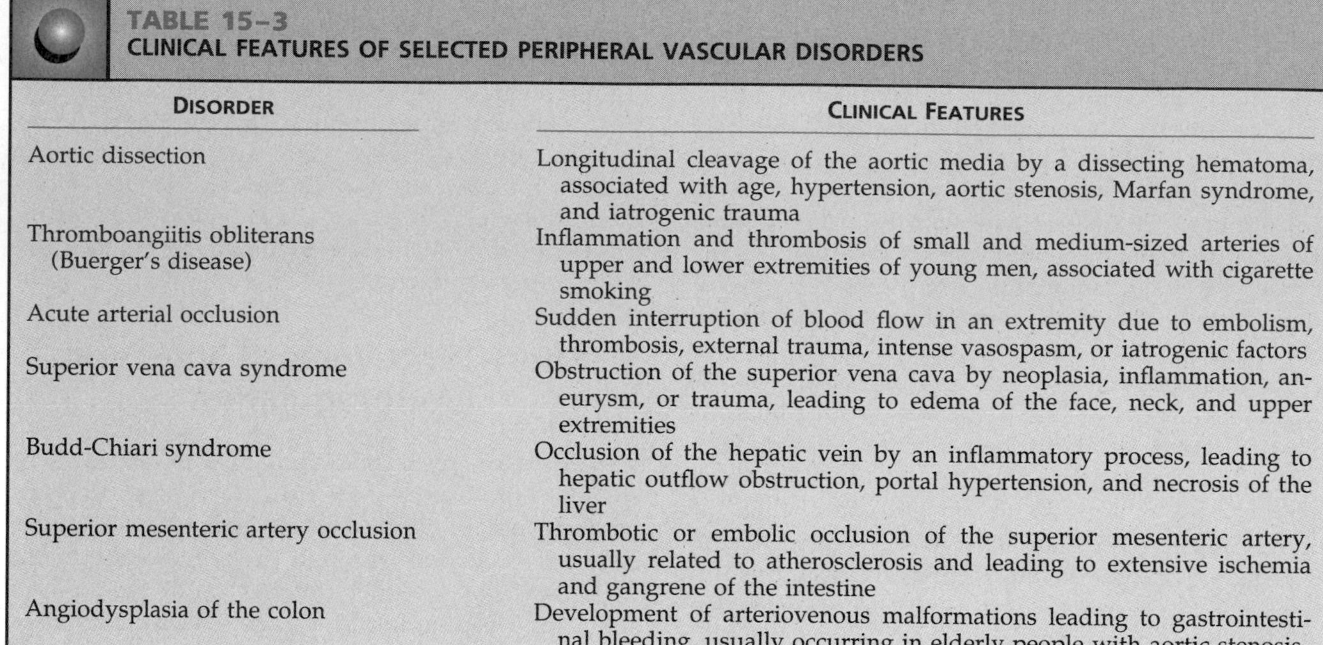

TABLE 15–3
CLINICAL FEATURES OF SELECTED PERIPHERAL VASCULAR DISORDERS

Disorder	Clinical Features
Aortic dissection	Longitudinal cleavage of the aortic media by a dissecting hematoma, associated with age, hypertension, aortic stenosis, Marfan syndrome, and iatrogenic trauma
Thromboangiitis obliterans (Buerger's disease)	Inflammation and thrombosis of small and medium-sized arteries of upper and lower extremities of young men, associated with cigarette smoking
Acute arterial occlusion	Sudden interruption of blood flow in an extremity due to embolism, thrombosis, external trauma, intense vasospasm, or iatrogenic factors
Superior vena cava syndrome	Obstruction of the superior vena cava by neoplasia, inflammation, aneurysm, or trauma, leading to edema of the face, neck, and upper extremities
Budd-Chiari syndrome	Occlusion of the hepatic vein by an inflammatory process, leading to hepatic outflow obstruction, portal hypertension, and necrosis of the liver
Superior mesenteric artery occlusion	Thrombotic or embolic occlusion of the superior mesenteric artery, usually related to atherosclerosis and leading to extensive ischemia and gangrene of the intestine
Angiodysplasia of the colon	Development of arteriovenous malformations leading to gastrointestinal bleeding, usually occurring in elderly people with aortic stenosis

or disease affecting the pressure gradient or resistance. Because dysfunction of one component stimulates adaptive effects within the other, most cardiovascular disorders reflect both aspects of the system. Cardiac failure is further detailed in Chapter 16, whereas vascular disorders are the focus here.

Three major circulatory syndromes are discussed: atherosclerosis, hypertension, and shock. These syndromes are integral to the pathophysiology of many diseases. **Peripheral vascular disease (PVD)** encompasses disorders of the veins, arteries, and lymphatics. The two most commonly occurring venous disorders are deep vein thrombosis, discussed in Chapter 14, and **chronic venous insufficiency**, discussed in this chapter; features of other forms of PVD are summarized in Table 15–3. The two disorders that most commonly affect peripheral arteries, **arteriosclerosis obliterans (ASO)** and **aneurysms**, are discussed in this chapter, as are the most prevalent form of **vasculitis, Kawasaki disease,** and **Raynaud's syndrome**, a vasospastic disorder. Lymphatic system disorders include lymphedema (discussed in Chapter 8) and several uncommon conditions, which are summarized in Table 15–4.

Atherosclerosis

Definition. Atherosclerosis is a pathologic process of arterial wall damage and luminal occlusion associated with infiltration of lipids and formation of a characteristic lesion (plaque).

TABLE 15–4
DISORDERS OF THE LYMPHATIC SYSTEM

Disorder	Clinical Features
Lymphedema	Abnormal accumulation of lymph in the extremities due to infection, thrombosis, congenital arrest of lymphatic growth, traumatic injury to lymphatics, essential lymphedema (Milroy's disease), allergy, or obstruction secondary to venous insufficiency or neoplasia
Lymphangitis	Infection spreading into lymphatic channels (usually group A β-hemolytic streptococcus) and resulting in painful red streaks along the lymphatics and enlargement of regional lymph nodes
Lymphadenopathy	Lymph node enlargement secondary to one of several primary disorders, including infections, immunologic disorders, neoplasms, hyperthyroidism, lipid storage diseases (Gaucher's disease, Niemann-Pick disease), sarcoidosis, amyloidosis, and Kawasaki disease

Epidemiology. About 45% of the population of the Western world will die from atherosclerotic diseases, particularly coronary heart disease and stroke.[9] Risk factors for the development of atherosclerosis are summarized in Table 15–5. Atherosclerosis increases with age, possibly owing to genetic factors or cumulative effects of long-term exposure to risk, and is more prevalent in men. Higher estrogen levels appear to protect the vessels of premenopausal women, possibly because they are associated with higher levels of high-density lipoprotein (HDL). HDL ("good" cholesterol) assists with removal of LDL ("bad" cholesterol) from the body (see Chapter 25). After menopause, atherosclerosis risk in women approaches that of men. Elevation of serum LDL cholesterol due to diet, hereditary factors, or both is strongly correlated with atherosclerosis.

Atherosclerosis is accelerated in hypertension and diabetes mellitus, two disorders that are also strongly correlated with each other. In hypertension, it is believed that mechanisms other than chronic vessel barotrauma are involved. Impairment of the endothelial balance between relaxing and contracting factors, as well as inappropriate stimulation of factors promoting vascular smooth muscle proliferation and vessel remodeling, may play a role in atherogenesis.[10] Accelerated atherosclerosis in diabetic patients is probably a result of insulin resistance rather than hyperglycemia.[11] Most people with insulin resistance have high serum levels of insulin. Insulin is a potent growth factor that stimulates proliferation of arterial smooth muscle cells, enhances cholesterol synthesis in the arterial wall, and increases the number of endothelial LDL receptors. Hyperinsulinemia induces abnormalities in circulating serum lipids, increasing LDL cholesterol and triglycerides, and decreasing HDL cholesterol.

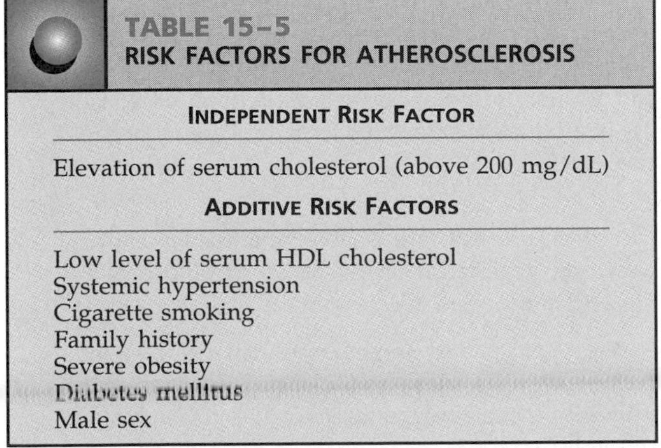

TABLE 15–5
RISK FACTORS FOR ATHEROSCLEROSIS

Independent Risk Factor
Elevation of serum cholesterol (above 200 mg/dL)
Additive Risk Factors
Low level of serum HDL cholesterol
Systemic hypertension
Cigarette smoking
Family history
Severe obesity
Diabetes mellitus
Male sex

Data from Roberts, W.C. (1995). Preventing and arresting coronary atherosclerosis. *American Heart Journal* 130(3 Pt 1), 580–600.

Obese people are often at higher risk for atherosclerosis owing to associated conditions, such as high fat diet, diabetes mellitus, hyperinsulinemia, hypertension, or lack of exercise. Aerobic exercise is considered to be an antirisk factor for atherosclerosis because it increases levels of HDL. Moderate alcohol intake (1 to 3 drinks per day) has also been associated with increased HDL levels and lower risk, whereas heavy alcohol use (more than 5 drinks per day) has been shown to increase the risk of cardiovascular disease.[12]

Another significant risk factor for atherosclerosis is abuse of tobacco, whether smoked or chewed. In 1990, 179,820 deaths due to cardiovascular disease (myocardial infarction and stroke) were attributed to cigarette smoking.[13] Components of tobacco damage the vascular endothelium, promote vascular spasm, and increase platelet aggregation, blood viscosity, and fibrinogen levels. Tobacco use adversely affects serum lipids, causing increased LDL and decreased HDL levels. Smoking also results in increased production of carbon monoxide, promoting ischemic damage of the endothelium (see Chapter 19).

Of all the factors associated with development of atherosclerosis, only one is *essential* to atherogenesis. That factor is serum lipid abnormality.[9] An elevated serum total cholesterol or LDL cholesterol, a low HDL cholesterol, or both constitute independent risk for atherosclerosis. The other factors discussed serve to accelerate the process, but only when lipid abnormality is also present.

Etiology. The precise mechanisms that account for the development of atherosclerosis are uncertain. The endothelial dysfunction and smooth muscle replication that underlie plaque development probably reflect a multifactorial etiology, and research in the field is consequently diverse (see Focus of Current Research).

The best-accepted mechanism of atherogenesis is the lipid infiltration hypothesis, which presupposes a high circulating level of LDL cholesterol. As shown in Figure 15–12, oxidation of LDL by enzymes from monocytes, platelets, and endothelial cells stimulates the expression of leukocyte adhesion molecules and the release of cytokines. Among these are monocyte chemoattractant protein-1 and monocyte colony-stimulating factor, which mediate the adhesion of monocytes to the endothelial wall as well as their eventual migration into the subintimal tissue.[14]

Within subintimal tissue, the monocytes are activated to macrophages, which are able to ingest LDL through scavenger receptors and to further stimulate monocyte activation and oxidation of LDL. The macrophages take up increasing amounts of oxidized LDL, forming foam cells, which eventually coalesce,

Focus of Current Research

Study	Objective and Findings
Lampert, et al. (1996) The concept of Raynaud's phenomenon of the lung revisited.	*Objective:* To examine two groups of patients suffering from primary and secondary Raynaud's phenomenon *Findings:* Raynaud's phenomenon in the lung is due to vasodilation rather than vasoconstriction of the pulmonary artery.
Boushey, et al. (1995) A quantitative assessment of plasma homocysteine as a risk factor for vascular disease.	*Objective:* To determine the risk of elevated plasma homocysteine with respect to vascular disease *Findings:* Elevated homocysteine is associated with increased risk of vascular disease.
Brun-Buisson, et al. (1995) Incidence, risk factors, and outcome of severe sepsis and septic shock in adults.	*Objective:* To examine the incidence, risk factors, and outcome of severe sepsis in intensive care unit patients *Findings:* Only three of four patients with severe sepsis have documented infection. Risk factors are similar for septic shock with or without documented infection, and all patients are at high risk of death.
Rosenfeld, et al. (1995) Kawasaki disease in infants less than one year of age.	*Objective:* To identify risk factors for severe sequelae, analyze disease characteristics, and assess efficacy of immune globulin therapy in infants with Kawasaki disease *Findings:* Patients younger than 6 months of age are at high risk for developing coronary artery aneurysms. Immune globulin therapy reduces this risk.
Petrakis (1995) Earlobe crease in women: Evaluation of reproductive factors, alcohol use, and Quetelet Index and relation to atherosclerotic disease.	*Objective:* To investigate the relationship of diagonal earlobe crease to factors associated with atherosclerosis *Findings:* Age and Quetelet index (body mass-to-height ratio) were positively associated with earlobe crease, and alcohol use was negatively associated. Diagonal earlobe crease is associated with increased atherosclerosis.
Caulfield, et al. (1994) Linkage of the angiotensinogen gene to essential hypertension.	*Objective:* To investigate whether there is linkage between the angiotensinogen gene on chromosome 1q42-43 and essential hypertension *Findings:* Linkage between essential hypertension and regions within or close to the angiotensinogen gene exists. Precisely how mutations in this region may result in hypertension remains to be determined.

box continued on following page

Davis, et al. (1994) Decreasing cardiovascular disease and increasing cancer among whites in the United States from 1973 through 1987: Good news and bad news.	*Objective:* To assess trends in cancer mortality and cardiovascular mortality *Findings:* Incidence of cardiovascular mortality decreased between 1973 and 1987 (42% for ages 0–54 and 33% for ages 55–84 years).
Terres, et al. (1994) Changes in cardiovascular risk profile during the cessation of smoking.	*Objective:* To evaluate the intraindividual changes in serum lipids, blood pressure, adrenergic stimulation, and platelet reactivity in chronic smokers undergoing controlled smoking cessation *Findings:* Cessation of smoking results in favorable serum lipid changes, increase in diastolic blood pressure, and reduced platelet aggregation.
Markovitz, et al. (1993) Psychological predictors of hypertension in the Framingham Study.	*Objective:* To test the hypothesis that heightened anxiety, anger, and suppression of anger increase the risk of hypertension *Findings:* Among middle-aged men, but not women, anxiety levels are predictive of later incidence of hypertension.

forming fatty streaks beneath the intima. Activated macrophages release a number of cytokines, including interleukin-1, which stimulate smooth muscle cells to release growth factors. These growth factors regulate both proliferation and migration of smooth muscle cells. In addition, oxidized LDL is directly cytotoxic to endothelial and smooth muscle cells, contributing to vascular injury, which may trigger inflammatory, immune, and hemostatic responses.

Factors that promote the oxidation of LDL include inherited variation in the size and density of LDL cholesterol particles; low serum HDL levels; elevated serum triglycerides; cigarette smoking; diabetes mellitus; hypertension; low levels of vitamins E and C, β-carotene, and selenium; and high levels of serum iron and copper.[15] Research evaluation of the use of antioxidant vitamins (A, C, and E) in prevention of atherosclerosis has yielded conflicting results.[16]

Pathophysiology. The atheromatous lesions that result from these processes range from soft, fatty plaques to hard, calcified plaques. The early, soft lesions contain mainly foam cells and extracellular lipid deposits, with some platelets and a few smooth muscle cells.[14] Local vasospasm and platelet aggregation may reduce flow rates in the vessel episodically. As the lesion progresses, smooth muscle cells and extracellular matrices proliferate. The plaque may contain areas of necrosis into which calcium may deposit along with areas of thrombus formation. Areas of plaque may develop fissures and rupture, triggering hemorrhage into the plaque and further thrombosis. Such events may result in rapid progression of a nonsignificant lesion into a significant vessel stenosis.

Plaque progression is not inevitable, however. Lesions may regress as a consequence of fibrinolytic processes, removal of cholesterol by HDL, or vascular remodeling. Risk of plaque rupture and thrombosis is also variable. Higher-risk lesions are associated with higher LDL levels and typically have larger lipid cores and more fragile fibrous caps.[17]

Clinical Manifestations. Atherosclerosis often occludes one or more of the major arteries serving the heart muscle, resulting in coronary heart disease, which may present as angina pectoris or myocardial infarction (see Chapter 16). Atherosclerosis within the peripheral arterial circulation is manifested as ASO, discussed later in this chapter. Atherosclerosis affecting the carotid arteries and other arteries serving the brain (cerebrovascular disease) is discussed in Chapter 21. Atherosclerosis within the systemic circulation is the most prevalent mechanism associated with hypertension and aneurysms and is discussed later in this chapter.

Prevention and Treatment. Many of the risk factors for development of atherosclerosis are removable or modifiable with lifestyle alterations. Cessation of tobacco use, adoption of a diet lower in fat, and regular, moderately strenuous aerobic exercise have been shown to slow the progression of athero-

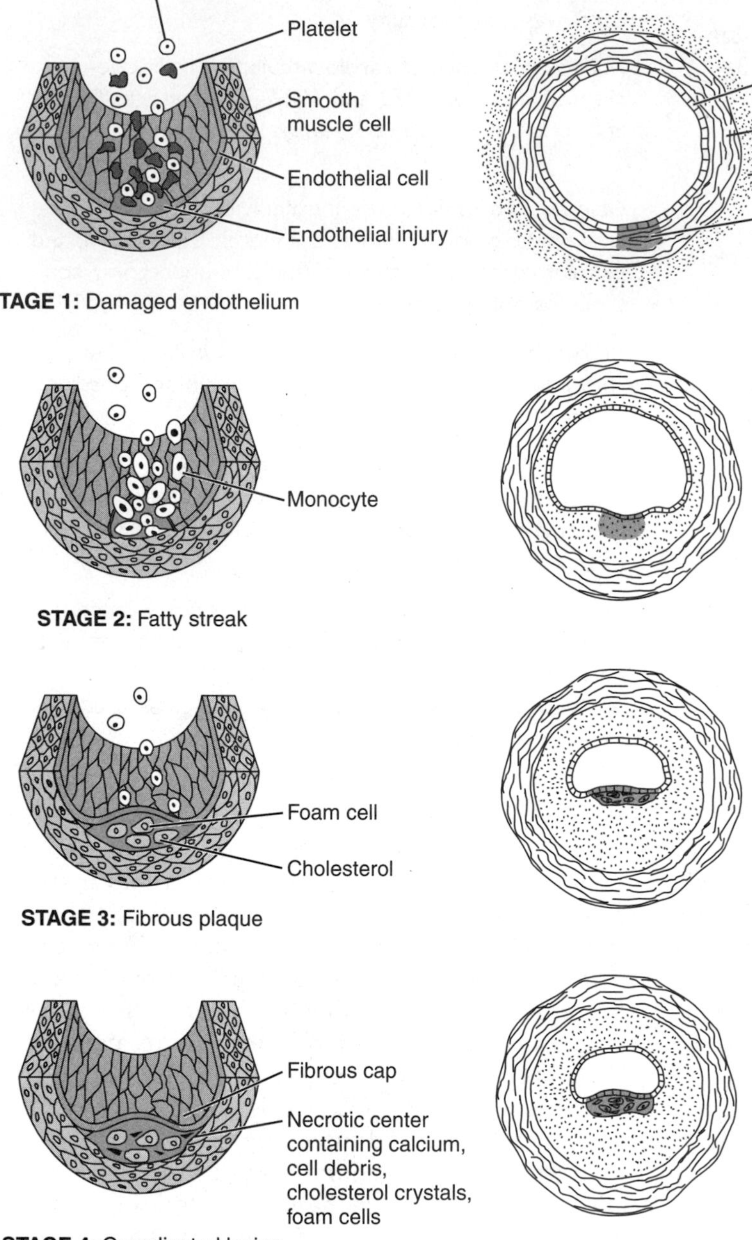

FIGURE 15–12

Formation of atherosclerotic plaque. 1. Low-density lipoprotein (LDL) cholesterol is first oxidized by endothelial and blood cell enzymes, stimulating the release of local mediators that cause monocytes to adhere and migrate into the vessel wall. 2. Monocytes are activated to macrophages, which ingest oxidized LDL. LDL-filled macrophages become foam cells, which coalesce to form fatty streaks beneath the injured or intact intima. 3. A fibrous cap of variable thickness forms over the cholesterol core of the lesion. 4. Calcium may be deposited into the growing plaque, and the lesion may undergo necrosis, leading to rupture and possible thrombus formation.

sclerosis significantly, and even to reverse the process of plaque formation in some instances. When serum lipid abnormality does not respond adequately to dietary and other lifestyle modifications, lipid-lowering drugs may be employed (see Chapter 25). Weight reduction in the obese, control of serum glucose and hyperinsulinemia in diabetic patients, and treatment of hypertension are also beneficial. The use of antioxidant agents such as probucol (Lorelco) and vitamin E in the treatment of atherosclerosis remains controversial.[18]

Invasive approaches to the removal of atherosclerotic plaque include endarterectomy, in which a surgical incision is made in an affected vessel and plaque is scraped free. Surgical bypass of vessels occluded by plaque is among the most common of surgical procedures and involves use of grafts (vein or artery segments or synthetic materials) to create a route for blood flow around the occluded segment. Balloon angioplasty involves insertion of a balloon-tipped catheter into an occluded area (Fig. 15–13). Inflation of the balloon compresses plaque against the walls of the vessel, restoring blood flow. Newer angioplastic procedures employ lasers or other cutting devices to pulverize or remove plaque by this less invasive approach (atherectomy). The effective-

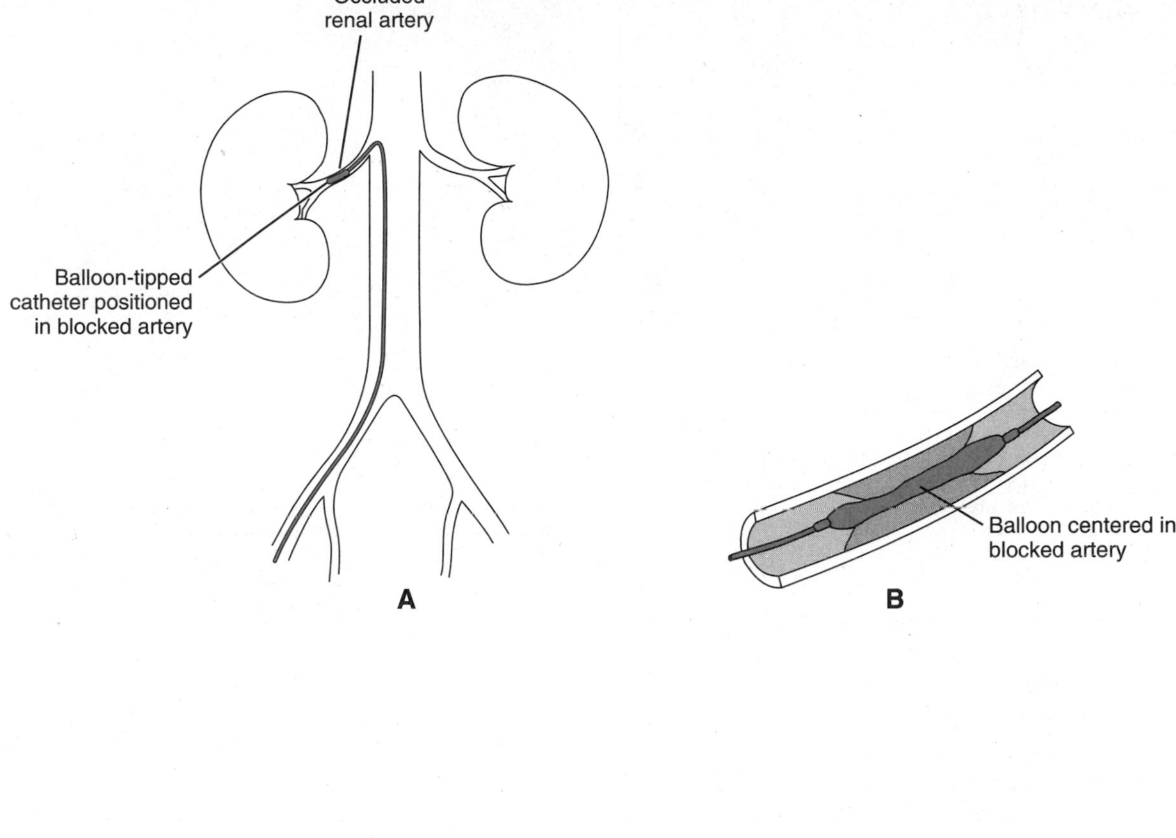

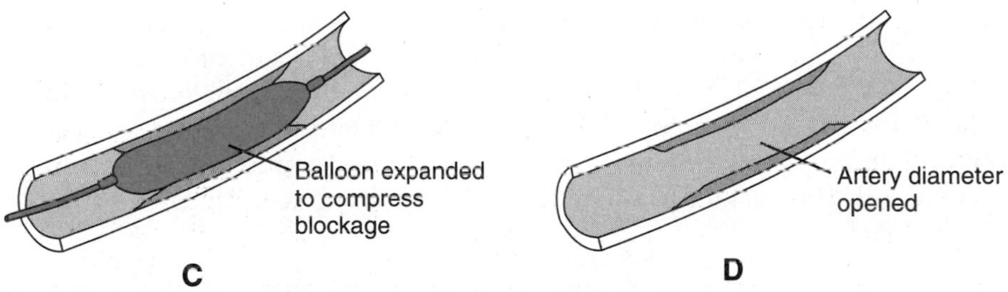

FIGURE 15–13

Balloon angioplasty. A balloon-tipped catheter is introduced into an area of occlusion due to atherosclerotic plaque. Inflation of the balloon compresses plaque against vessel walls, restoring blood flow.

ness of angioplasty has been limited by a frequent rate of early reocclusion, although the use of tubular endovascular stents to support vessel walls in the damaged area has improved outcomes.[19]

Prognosis and Outcome. Mortality due to atherosclerotic disorders has been steadily declining, as has been stated. The absolute prevalence of atherosclerosis is increasing, however, as a consequence of the aging population.[15]

Hypertension

Definition. Hypertension is usually defined as a consistent elevation of blood pressure greater than 140 mm Hg systolic or 90 mm Hg diastolic in adults.[20] Staging of hypertension according to severity is based on either the systolic or diastolic pressures, whichever is higher (Table 15–6). Specific norms vary with age, with lower pressures at birth

TABLE 15–6
CLASSIFICATION OF SEVERITY OF HYPERTENSION

Stage	Systolic (mm Hg)	Diastolic (mm Hg)
None	<130	<85
None or very mild	130–139	85–89
Mild	140–159	90–99
Moderate	160–179	100–109
Severe	180–209	110–119
Very severe	210 or greater	≥120

Highest level of either systolic or diastolic blood pressure is used for staging.

From the Joint National Committee on Detection, Evaluation, and Treatment of High Blood Pressure. (1993). The Fifth Report of the Joint National Committee on Detection, Evaluation, and Treatment of High Blood Pressure (JNC V). *Archives of Internal Medicine* 153(2), 154–183.

TABLE 15–7
AGE-SPECIFIC NORMS FOR BLOOD PRESSURE

Age	Mean Blood Pressure (mm Hg)
1 mo	80/50
6 mo	90/60
2 y	99/64
5 y	100/60
12 y	113/59
15 y	115/70
20 y	126/74
30 y	122/76
40 y	128/80
50 y	134/80
60 y	142/82
70 y	148/80
80 y	148/80
90 y	145/78

Data from Marlow, D.R., and Redding, B.A. (1988). *Textbook of Pediatric Nursing*. Philadelphia: W.B. Saunders; and Jarvis, C. (1996). *Physical Examination and Health Assessment* (2nd ed.). Philadelphia: W.B. Saunders.

gradually rising to adult levels (Table 15–7). Hypertension is classified according to etiology as *primary* or **essential hypertension**, in which the cause is unknown; or *secondary* to a specific disorder, such as renal disease, neoplasia, or pregnancy. Ninety-five per cent of cases of hypertension are essential hypertension, the focus of this discussion. Disorders associated with secondary hypertension are summarized in Table 15–8 and detailed in relevant systems chapters.

Epidemiology. The overall prevalence of hypertension in the United States is about 20%, and the rate of newly diagnosed hypertensive patients is about 3% per year.[21] The incidence of pediatric hypertension has been estimated at 1% to 3%.[22] Table 15–9 lists known risk factors for the development of essential hypertension. Many of these are also implicated in atherosclerosis, including increasing age, obesity, hyperinsulinemia, hyperlipidemia, and alcohol abuse. Presence of hypertension accelerates development of atherosclerosis, as has been discussed, and atherosclerosis contributes to hypertension by increasing resistance secondary to loss of compliance and laminar flow. The relationship of alcohol use to hypertension is the same as that in atherosclerosis:

TABLE 15–8
DISORDERS ASSOCIATED WITH SECONDARY HYPERTENSION

Disorder	Clinical Features
Renal artery stenosis	Renal artery obstruction by stricture or atherosclerosis leads to chronic stimulation of the RAAS
Renal disease (e.g., acute glomerulonephritis, polycystic kidney disease)	Hypervolemia
Wilms' tumor	Paraneoplastic renin secretion
Primary aldosteronism	Aldosterone stimulation of sodium and fluid retention
Cushing's syndrome	Glucocorticoid excess mimics aldosterone effects
Pheochromocytoma	Catecholamine-secreting tumor induces increased resistance
Polycythemia	Increased hematocrit results in increased resistance due to blood viscosity
Coarctation of the aorta	Blood pressure rises upstream to congenital aortic stricture
Autonomic hyper-reflexia	Uncontrolled sympathetic nervous system stimulation produces high resistance
Pregnancy-induced hypertension (preeclampsia, eclampsia)	Hypertension and possible seizures; mechanisms uncertain but possibly related to lipid mediators
Sleep apnea syndrome	Highly associated with hypertension; mechanisms uncertain.
Drug therapy (e.g., sympathetic nervous system agonists, estrogens, electrolytes, cortisone)	Impact regulation of blood pressure by multiple mechanisms

TABLE 15–9
RISK FACTORS FOR ESSENTIAL HYPERTENSION

FACTOR	COMMENTS
Age	Highest incidence among middle-aged and older
Sex	By middle age, women have higher systolic pressures
Genetic factors	Familial tendency apparent, probably reflecting both genetic and environmental factors; gene locus for essential hypertension is near the locus that codes for angiotensinogen
Race	Blacks in the United States have more severely elevated blood pressures and more end-organ damage than whites
Sodium intake	Blood pressure correlates to a minor degree with sodium intake; higher correlation in salt-sensitive people
Potassium intake	Higher levels of K^+ intake may correlate with lower blood pressure
Calcium intake	Higher levels of Ca^{2+} intake may correlate with lower blood pressure
Alcohol intake	Moderate alcohol intake has no harmful effect, and possibly a slight beneficial effect, on blood pressure. Intake of more than three to five drinks per day increases blood pressure.
Weight	Weight gain increases blood pressure, and weight loss decreases blood pressure.
Diabetes mellitus	Hypertension is secondary to diabetic nephropathy and microvascular changes in type 1 diabetes. In type 2 diabetes, hypertension may be due to insulin resistance. High insulin levels may lead to sympathetic nervous system stimulation and endothelial effects.
Atherosclerosis	Increased vessel stiffness increases vascular resistance.

moderate levels appear to be protective, but heavy drinking increases the incidence of hypertension.

Age is a significant risk factor for hypertension. More than 60% of women older than 60 years are hypertensive.[20] Women are at slightly higher risk than men, and blacks are three times as likely to have severe hypertension as whites.[23] Cigarette smoking has not been established as an independent risk factor in the development of hypertension. Tobacco use does contribute to atherosclerosis, however, and vasoconstriction due to nicotine causes an immediate, short-term increase in resistance, which may exacerbate an existing hypertensive condition. Several drugs may contribute to hypertension. These are summarized in Table 15–10.

Hypertension displays a multifactorial inheritance pattern. This familial tendency is most likely due to both genetic and environmental factors.

Etiology. The specific mechanisms of essential hypertension are unknown, but the condition is generally attributed to failure of regulatory mechanisms governing cardiac output, vessel resistance, or both. It is likely that environmental factors contribute to development of essential hypertension, especially when superimposed on a genetic predisposition.

The *hemodynamic hypothesis* holds that a primary increase in cardiac output is the cause. Persistent hypervolemia develops because of failure of sodium excretion and volume regulation by the RAAS, ADH, or glomerular filtration rate. Increased volume causes increased flow to tissues, triggering autoregulation, which, in turn, increases resistance.

The *vasoconstrictor hypothesis* proposes a mechanism by which increased vessel resistance is due to dysfunction at the level of tissue autoregulation. Imbalance of neural, hormonal, or endothelial regulation leads to increased intracellular calcium levels and increased contraction of vascular smooth muscle. Research has linked essential hypertension to genetic regions within or close to the gene that encodes angiotensinogen, the precursor of the vasoconstricting hormone, angiotensin II.[24] Most patients with hypertension are not hypervolemic, however,

TABLE 15–10
DRUGS ASSOCIATED WITH DEVELOPMENT OF HYPERTENSION

MECHANISM	DRUGS
Sympathetic agonism: vasoconstriction and increased cardiac contractility	Epinephrine Norepinephrine Dopamine Caffeine Nicotine Cocaine
Prevention of reuptake of catecholamines at synapses	Amphetamines Tricyclic antidepressants
Prevention of enzymatic degradation of catecholamines	Monoamine oxidase inhibitors
Sodium and water retention	Adrenocorticotropin (adrenocorticotrophic hormone) Corticosteroids
Increase in hepatic synthesis of angiotensinogen	Estrogens

nor do they have elevated serum levels of sodium, calcium, or hormones associated with activation of the SNS or RAAS. An imbalance of endothelial mediators is likely in such cases.

Pathophysiology. Hypertension causes three major circulatory abnormalities: increased arteriolar resistance, increased large artery stiffness, and early or premature reflection of arterial pulse waves.[25] Increased resistance and vessel stiffness in younger hypertensive patients result from structural changes, including thinning and fracturing of elastin, increased collagen deposition, and increased wall thickness. These changes manifest primarily as a greater rise in systolic than diastolic pressure. In the elderly, increased arterial stiffness is the greater factor and may contribute to **isolated systolic hypertension**, in which systolic pressure is elevated but diastolic pressure is normal or low (increased **pulse pressure**). Patients with isolated systolic hypertension are at substantially increased risk for stroke, coronary heart disease, and congestive heart failure.[26] *Pulse wave reflection* refers to the backward rebound of some of the cardiac output as it encounters the resistance of the arteries. When arteries are normally compliant, this reflected flow occurs during diastole and assists with filling of the coronary arteries. In hypertension, however, reflection occurs prematurely, during systole, contributing to vascular overload in the aortic arch and in the coronary, carotid, and renal arteries.

Clinical Manifestations. Virtually every organ system of the body is affected by high pressure within its circulation. Usually, there are no signs and symptoms until significant organ damage has occurred, although some patients may experience headaches, nosebleeds (epistaxis), or orthostatic hypotension. Organs that are particular targets of hypertensive injury include the heart, brain, kidneys, and retinas.

Hypertensive heart disease culminates in cardiac failure due to acceleration of atherosclerosis within coronary arteries, which decreases myocardial blood supply. At the same time, the heart must pump against the increased resistance offered by the hypertensive systemic circulation, resulting in left ventricular hypertrophy and dilation. Ultimately, left ventricular failure ensues, with an increased tendency toward ventricular dysrhythmias and sudden cardiac death.[27] High blood pressure is a significant risk factor for stroke (see Chapter 21). Cerebral blood flow is impeded by atherosclerotic vessels, and high pressure within them may contribute to aneurysm formation and hemorrhage. Peripheral vascular disease is associated with hypertension in the same manner. In the kidneys, hypertension leads to pressure necrosis of renal cells (hypertensive nephropathy), producing renal failure, which may lead to a positive feedback loop of fluid overload and worsening hypertension (see Chapter 20). Similarly, pressure trauma in retinal vessels of the eyes may lead to hypertensive retinopathy, characterized by retinal hemorrhage and potentially leading to blindness (see Chapter 23).

Prevention and Treatment. Modification of risk factors is warranted, as discussed with atherosclerosis. Because of the absence of early clinical manifestations, routine monitoring of blood pressure is important to detect the condition as early as possible. Individual risk factors and stage of hypertension determine the approach to treatment. As a consequence of recent research, the traditional stepped-care approach, in which nonpharmacologic measures (e.g., weight loss, sodium restriction, exercise) are employed before drug therapy, has been replaced by early pharmacologic intervention *in addition to* nonpharmacologic measures.[28] Antihypertensive drugs include diuretics, to treat or prevent hypervolemia; vasodilators (e.g., calcium antagonists, β-blockers, α-blockers) to decrease peripheral resistance, and ACE inhibitors to interrupt the RAAS, inhibiting fluid retention and reducing circulating levels of the vasoconstrictor angiotensin II (Table 15–11).

Prognosis and Outcome. Treatment of hypertension significantly reduces the occurrence of strokes.[29] Presence of hypertension with left ventricular hypertrophy has been shown to increase overall mortality rates 5.6 times in men and 5.4 times in women and to increase the risk of sudden death 6.9 times in men and 3.5 times in women.[27]

TABLE 15–11
ANTIHYPERTENSIVE DRUGS

CLASSIFICATION	EXAMPLES
Diuretics	Furosemide (Lasix) Hydrochlorothiazide (Dyazide) Spironolactone (Aldactone)
β-Adrenergic blockers	Metoprolol (Lopressor) Propranolol (Inderal)
α-Adrenergic blocker	Prazosin (Minipress)
α- and β-blocker	Labetalol (Normodyne)
Centrally acting sympathetic nervous system antagonists	Clonidine (Catapres) Methyldopa (Aldomet)
Angiotensin-converting enzyme inhibitors	Captopril (Capoten) Enalapril (Vasotec)
Calcium-channel blockers	Diltiazem (Cardizem) Nicardipine (Cardene) Nifedipine (Procardia) Verapamil (Calan)

Clinical Scenario

C.R. is a 47-year-old obese man with a 10–year history of essential hypertension. Despite therapy with furosemide, clonidine, and enalapril, his blood pressure is still uncontrolled at 160/110 mm Hg. His compliance with the medication plan has been good, with prescriptions refilled consistently. C.R. has been unable to maintain weight loss achieved with a number of programs, and his exercise capacity is limited by shortness of breath and occasionally by chest pain. He has recently been diagnosed with type 2 diabetes mellitus, which is being treated with an oral hypoglycemic agent.

1. What risk factors for hypertension are present in C.R.'s case?
2. Why is he being treated with this combination of drugs?
3. What further intervention might be warranted?

Shock

Definition. Shock is a state of severe, generalized deficit in tissue perfusion. Shock states can be categorized according to etiologic mechanisms as **hypovolemic shock** (due to an absolute reduction in circulating blood volume), **distributive shock** (also known as **vasogenic shock**, due to a maldistribution of circulating blood volume secondary to loss of vascular tone), and **cardiogenic shock** (due to cardiac pump failure).

Epidemiology

Hypovolemic Shock. Hypovolemic shock is common in the setting of major trauma, major surgery, and burns. Hypovolemic shock due to acute blood loss is termed **hemorrhagic shock,** whereas that due to fluid water vapor loss and third spacing in major burns is termed **burn shock**. Risk factors for hemorrhage include hypocoagulable states (see Chapter 14) as well as factors that increase the risk for trauma or the necessity of surgery. Risk factors for burn injury are discussed in Chapter 36.

Distributive Shock. **Septic shock**, resulting from systemic vasodilation due to massive release of inflammatory mediators, is the leading cause of death in critical care units and the 13th most common cause of death in the United States.[30] Two hundred thousand cases are estimated to occur annually. Risk factors for infection are detailed in Chapter 13 and include those related to the presence and virulence of the causative organism as well as those related to vulnerability of the host. Other forms of distributive shock include **neurogenic shock**, associated with head injury (see Chapter 21); **spinal shock**, seen in spinal cord injury (see Chapter 22); and **anaphylactic shock**, resulting from a severe hypersensitivity reaction to an allergen (see Chapter 13).

Cardiogenic Shock. The incidence of cardiogenic shock among survivors of myocardial infarction has been estimated at 6% to 20%.[31] Cardiogenic shock is synonymous with end-stage cardiac failure. Coronary heart disease constitutes the major risk factor for cardiogenic shock. Conditions associated with acute cardiac failure include not only myocardial infarction but also cardiomyopathy, pericarditis (cardiac tamponade), cardiac valve disease (see Chapter 16), and cardiac dysrhythmias (see Chapter 17).

Etiology

Hypovolemic Shock. Hypovolemic shock may develop due to decreased blood volume secondary to external or internal hemorrhage, third spacing of fluid (e.g., hepatic cirrhosis or peritonitis), excessive gastrointestinal losses (e.g., diarrhea, vomiting, or drainage), excessive sweating (e.g., heat exhaustion or heatstroke), or excessive renal losses (e.g., diuretic phase of acute renal failure or iatrogenic excess of diuretic therapy).

Distributive Shock. In response to inflammatory mediators induced by infection or allergy (in septic shock or anaphylactic shock), peripheral vessels produce massive amounts of endothelial-derived relaxing factors, including nitric oxide and prostaglandin I_2, which overwhelm the effects of the SNS in maintaining vascular tone.

Decreased vascular tone (vasodilation) initially results in increased volume at the tissue level, but the resulting decrease in venous return soon compromises cardiac output and effective circulation (*movement* of blood) is decreased. Vasodilation also reduces SVR and induces a maldistribution in the microcirculation. Intraorgan shunts develop, reducing perfusion in some tissues. Inflammatory mediators also induce increased capillary permeability, promoting third spacing, which further reduces circulating blood volume. Injury and increased permeability of pulmonary capillary beds may result in adult respiratory distress syndrome (see Chapter 19). Endothelial injury resulting from inflammatory mediators and ischemia may lead to microvascular occlusion, which promotes further ischemia and may precipitate disseminated intravascular coagulation (DIC) (see Chapter 14).

In neurogenic and spinal shock, vasodilation is a

consequence of autonomic nervous system failure rather than inflammatory mediators. Unless autonomic reflex arcs are directly injured by spinal trauma, shock is a transient state in this condition. Autonomic function and vascular tone return after a period of weeks; however, higher-level regulation is absent or abnormal, conferring risk of vasospasm and hypertensive crisis (see Autonomic Hyper-reflexia, Chapter 22).

Cardiogenic Shock. Cardiac muscle is destroyed in myocardial infarction and in cardiomyopathy, weakening the primary circulatory pump and decreasing the pressure gradient for perfusion. In constrictive pericarditis, the heart is prevented from filling adequately by the fibrous pericardium; and in cardiac tamponade, the rapid accumulation of fluid between the pericardial sac and the heart also impedes ventricular filling. Valve disorders disrupt the efficiency or directly obstruct ventricular filling and ejection. These disorders are detailed in Chapter 16.

Pathophysiology. Although there are some mechanisms unique to each etiology, the shock syndrome typically proceeds through three stages (Table 15–12).

Initial (Compensatory) Stage. During the initial stage of shock, adaptive mechanisms (e.g., the baroreceptor system and fluid balance mechanisms) are triggered by the decreased flow. At the capillary level, an interstitial-to-plasma fluid shift occurs, and the blood reservoirs constrict. Sympathetic stimulation triggered by baroreceptors mediates increased cardiac output and selective vasoconstriction, which shunts most flow to the heart, lungs, and brain. These measures are effective in restoring essential tissue perfusion for a time.

Intermediate (Progressive) Stage. The intermediate stage of shock begins when adaptive mechanisms fail. Positive feedback loops develop as a consequence of increased cardiac workload and prolonged vasoconstriction. Tissue perfusion is compromised to the point at which ischemia occurs due to lack of oxygenated blood. Anaerobic metabolism dominates (see Chapter 3), producing metabolic acidosis (see Chapter 10). Tissue hypoxia causes release of endothelial mediators, resulting in vasodilation and endothelial imbalance. Fluid leaks from the plasma to the interstitium, worsening the hypovolemic state, if present. Slowed blood flow due to cardiac failure and vasodilation results in damage to specific organs and sets the stage for development of DIC, which further compromises perfusion.

Irreversible (Refractory) Stage. The irreversible stage of shock begins at the point at which cellular damage within vital organs is so extensive that the patient cannot recover, even if positive feedback loops are interrupted with treatment and hemodynamic balance is restored.

Clinical Manifestations. In hypovolemic shock, the clinical findings may be used to estimate the degree of blood loss (Table 15–13). In critical care

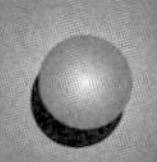

TABLE 15–12
CLINICAL STAGES OF SHOCK

Pathophysiology	Clinical Manifestations
Initial (Compensatory) Stage Decreased perfusion triggers baroreceptor reflexes and fluid regulation mechanisms.	Anxiety Tachycardia Bounding pulse Cool, clammy skin (except in sepsis) Narrowed pulse pressure (except in distributive shock) Decreased urine output Hyperventilation
Intermediate (Progressive) Stage Adaptive mechanisms fail and positive feedback loops develop owing to increased cardiac workload and tissue hypoxia.	Mental confusion, restlessness Skin cyanotic or mottled Hypotension Little or no urine output Lactic acidosis Respiratory distress Possible disseminated intravascular coagulation or adult respiratory distress syndrome Myocardial depression
Irreversible (Refractory) Stage Ischemic damage to vital organs is so extensive that patient cannot recover even if hemodynamic paremeters are restored.	Apathy or coma Undetectable blood pressure Anuria Severe metabolic acidosis Multiple-system organ failure

TABLE 15–13
CLINICAL CLASSIFICATION OF HYPOVOLEMIC SHOCK

Class	Blood Volume Lost	Clinical Findings
I	<15% (<750 mL)	Pulse <100 beats/minute; normal blood pressure, respirations, and urine output; slightly anxious
II	15%–30% (750–1500 mL)	Pulse ≥100 beats/minute; normal systolic blood pressure but decreased pulse pressure; delayed capillary refill; respirations 20–30 per minute; urine output 20–30 mL/h; anxious
III	>30%–40% (1500–2000 mL)	Pulse >120 beats/minute; decreased blood pressure (both systolic and diastolic); decreased pulse pressure; respirations 30–40 per minute; urine output 5–15 mL/h; confused
IV	>40% (>2000 mL)	Pulse >140 beats/minute; respirations ≥35; minimal urine output; confused and lethargic

Data from Guthrie, D. (Ed.). (1989). *Advanced Trauma Life Support Course for Physicians.* (Revised ed.). Chicago: American College of Surgeons. (pp. 57–88).

settings, invasive monitoring of CVP, cardiac output, and SVR permits differentiation of the etiologies (Table 15–14). Methods of hemodynamic monitoring are detailed in Chapter 16.

Clinical manifestations reflecting SNS stimulation due to reduced circulating volume in early shock include restlessness, tachycardia, bounding pulse, and cool, clammy skin. Vasoconstriction causes the diastolic blood pressure to rise, whereas the systolic pressure usually remains stable. This clinical hallmark of early shock is known as a *narrowed pulse pressure*. The baroreceptor response, however, is impaired in distributive shock owing to altered autonomic pathways or the presence of vasodilator substances, and these signs will be absent or altered. Furthermore, if cardiac reserve is limited (as in cardiogenic shock), or if hypovolemia is severe, cardiac output remains low despite SNS stimulation, and bounding pulse is not seen.

SNS-mediated vasoconstriction in hypovolemic and cardiogenic shock deprives the skin to maintain perfusion to critical systems. The skin is thus cool, pale, or mottled owing to lack of perfusion. In early septic shock, however, vasoconstriction is absent, and infection induces fever with warm, flushed skin. SNS stimulation results in clamminess or diaphoresis (sweating), except in neurogenic shock, in which sympathetic pathways are interrupted as a consequence of the primary cause of the shock state. Glomerular filtration is decreased, resulting in little or no urine output. Eventually, necrosis of renal tubular cells occurs, leading to renal failure, which worsens acidosis and fluid imbalance (see Chapter 20). Decreased blood flow to the gastrointestinal tract leads to bowel ischemia, which may allow bacterial translocation from the gut lumen to the blood, producing bacteremia. Consequently, hypovolemic or cardiogenic shock may be complicated by septic shock at this stage. Liver failure ("shock liver") leads to abnormalities in hemostasis and loss of Kupffer cell function, contributing to DIC and sepsis. Cells of the ischemic pancreas release myocardial depressant factor, which inhibits cardiac contraction. Sluggish circulation and extensive tissue damage may trigger DIC, with further impairment of perfusion.

TABLE 15–14
HEMODYNAMIC PARAMETERS IN SHOCK

Type of Shock	Central Venous Pressure	Cardiac Output	Systemic Vascular Resistance*
Hypovolemic	Low	Low	High
Cardiogenic	High	Low	High
Distributive	Low or normal	Low or normal	Low

* Reflecting vasoconstriction.

Although the CNS is protected as long as possible by autoregulation and adaptive mechanisms, including the CNS ischemic response, cerebral edema and anoxia eventually occur. Microvascular damage, microthrombi, and cardiac failure may result in critical injury to the lungs, kidneys, and liver (multiple-system organ failure). At this irreversible stage, the patient cannot recover, even if treatment restores normal blood pressure and tissue perfusion.

Prevention and Treatment. Prevention of shock involves anticipation of risk in patients with associated etiologies. Clinical monitoring of the skin and sensorium is important in early detection of decreased perfusion. Blood pressure and urine output are monitored in most inpatient settings, and cardiac output and SVR may be monitored in critical care units.

General aspects of treatment of shock include administration of oxygen to enhance delivery to poorly perfused tissues. The patient is kept cool (but not to the point of shivering) to minimize metabolic demands. The patient's legs may be elevated to shift any pooled venous blood to central organs, but the head-down (Trendelenburg) position, long used as an emergency intervention in shock, is no longer advocated because of detrimental effects on diaphragmatic movement and cerebral circulation.

In hypovolemia, volume is replaced with crystalloid intravenous fluids (electrolyte and glucose solutions), colloids such as albumin or dextran, whole blood, or plasma. In cardiogenic shock, cardiac contractility is supported with inotropic drugs, such as dopamine, or with circulatory assist devices (see Chapter 16). If fluid volume is adequate, vasodilators such as nitrates (e.g., nitroglycerin or nitroprusside) or ACE inhibitors (e.g., enalapril) may be administered to improve perfusion.

Vasoconstrictors such as epinephrine and norepinephrine have been used to augment the SNS response in shock, but this is usually considered to be a last resort owing to the detrimental effects on tissue perfusion in most organs. In emergency settings or in the field (at accident or injury sites), external pressure applied by inflatable trousers (military antishock trousers) may be useful in increasing resistance in the legs, maintaining higher perfusion pressure in vital organs. Treatment of the underlying condition is instituted as soon as the patient is hemodynamically stable and may include surgery for hemorrhage or trauma, antibiotic therapy for sepsis, or steroids for anaphylactic shock.

Prognosis and Outcome. In hypovolemic shock occurring secondary to trauma in otherwise healthy people, the prognosis is favorable if volume replacement is appropriate and the underlying cause is treatable. The mortality rate in septic shock ranges from 20% to 80%,[30] and mortality rate in cardiogenic shock ranges from 30% to 90%.[31] Multiple-system organ failure occurs in 15% of patients with shock.[32]

Chronic Venous Insufficiency

Definition. Chronic venous insufficiency includes a spectrum of disorders resulting from elevated venous pressure in the legs. Chronic venous insufficiency ranges in severity from **varicose veins**, which are dilated and twisted superficial veins that are of only cosmetic significance, to induration and fibrosis of the skin (**lipodermatosclerosis**) and chronic **venous stasis ulcers.**

Epidemiology. Varicosities of the superficial veins of the legs are common, occurring in an estimated 10% to 20% of the U.S. population.[33] About 6 million Americans have the skin changes of lipodermatosclerosis, and almost half a million have chronic stasis ulcers.[34] A familial tendency is apparent, and incidence increases with age over 50 years, female gender, obesity, sedentary lifestyle, and pregnancy. In men, cigarette smoking confers increased risk.

Etiology. Varicose veins usually occur as a primary condition, associated with a genetic weakness of superficial, communicating, or perforating vein walls that results in incompetence of the vein valves. Secondary varicose veins are associated with recurrent deep vein thrombosis as a component of the postphlebitic syndrome (see Chapter 14). In such cases, occlusion, pooling, and valve damage in the deeper venous system lead to increased pressure in superficial veins, which serve as collateral channels for venous return. Lipodermatosclerosis and leg ulcers are usually associated with secondary varicosities.

Pathophysiology. In primary varicose veins of the legs, genetic weakness of the vein wall results in dilation and distortion of superficial veins by venous pressure. It is believed that all veins are afflicted with this weakness, but effects are seen in superficial veins that are not supported by skeletal muscle. Vessel trauma may induce inflammatory and hemostatic responses. Venous damage may be exacerbated by (in primary varicosities) or caused by (in secondary varicosities) abnormally high venous pressure.

The precise mechanism by which high venous pressure leads to skin changes and ulcers is uncertain. The fibrin cuff hypothesis holds that increased venous pressure leads to leakage of plasma proteins and fibrinogen, forming a cuff around capillaries that restricts perfusion of skin tissues.[34] The white cell–trapping hypothesis proposes that white blood cells are trapped in capillaries as a result of sluggish blood flow. Release of proteolytic enzymes, reactive oxygen species, and lipid mediators from these white blood cells damages the capillary endothelium. Leakage of fibrinogen leads to formation of the fibrin cuff.

Clinical Manifestations. Small clusters of visible leg veins become increasingly apparent over time. Signs and symptoms of inflammation (e.g., edema, itching, aching) are variable but usually mild. Superficial thrombophlebitis may occur but imposes minimal risk of embolization. Legs may ache or feel heavy. If the condition worsens, red or brown discoloration of the skin occurs due to hemosiderin deposition. Dermatitis develops and may lead to lipodermatosclerosis (Fig. 15–14). Mild trauma may result in ulceration, commonly in the area of the medial malleolus.

Prevention and Treatment. Prevention of deep vein thrombosis is relevant to secondary varicosities and is discussed in Chapter 14. Leg elevation is warranted to reduce venous pressure. Vascular compression measures, such as elastic wraps or pressure stockings, may support vein walls and provide an upward pressure gradient that inhibits venous pooling and fibrin cuff formation. Topical ointments may be used to facilitate ulcer healing.

Small varicose veins may be treated with laser coagulation or with sclerotherapy, which consists of injection of irritating agents that close the veins with scar tissue. Larger varicosities may be treated surgically with ligation and stripping. In such cases, after ascertaining the patency of the deep venous system and collateral vessels, the affected vein is accessed with small incisions, tied off and removed. Surgical reconstruction of vein valves may be beneficial in deep venous insufficiency, and transplantation of valves from upper to lower extremities is under investigation.[34]

Prognosis and Outcome. Treatment of primary varicosities usually achieves a satisfactory cosmetic outcome. Complications of the condition or its surgical treatment, such as infection, bleeding, or thromboembolism, are rare. Varicosities frequently reappear after several years, however, and further treatment may be required.[35]

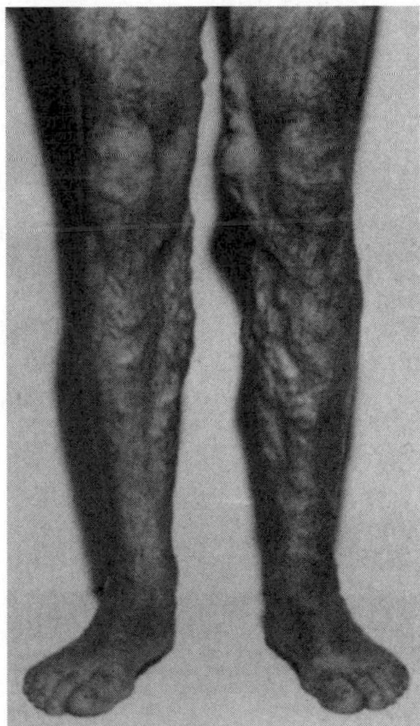

FIGURE 15–14

Chronic venous insufficiency. Severe varicose veins and lipodermatosclerosis are illustrated here. (From Lofgren, K.A. [1976]. Varicose veins. In: Wilson, S., et al. [Eds.]. *Vascular Surgery: Principles and Techniques*. New York: McGraw-Hill. [pp. 799–811]. Copyright 1976. Reproduced with permission of The McGraw-Hill Companies.)

Arteriosclerosis Obliterans

Definition. ASO is a peripheral vascular disorder characterized by chronic, progressive hardening and occlusion of arteries due to lesions consisting primarily of atherosclerotic plaque. **Arteriosclerosis** is a general term referring to hardening of arteries.

Epidemiology. The prevalence of ASO has been estimated at up to 14% of American men and women older than 65 years. Women generally demonstrate a lower prevalence than men.[36] Risk factors include increasing age, cigarette smoking, high systolic blood pressure, obesity, diabetes mellitus, and elevation of serum levels of lipids, fibrinogen, or leukocytes.

Etiology. ASO is almost always a manifestation of atherosclerosis, in which vessel hardening is due to lipid deposition, intimal proliferation, and calcification of plaque. Nonatherosclerotic mechanisms may also contribute to arteriosclerosis, however. These include degeneration of smooth muscle cells and connective tissue proliferation (hyalinization).

Pathophysiology. Progressive atherosclerotic occlusion of middle-sized arteries occurs over a period of 20 to 40 years. Although there is much variation in the sites of occlusion, areas of bifurcation (branching) in the pelvis and lower extremities are most commonly affected (Fig. 15–15). Increased resistance in these areas reduces perfusion of tissues served by these vessels, producing manifestations of ischemia in a syndrome referred to as *arterial insufficiency*. Collateral circulation develops to offset ischemic effects for a limited time. Slowed flow may induce thrombosis, and weakening of the vessel wall in these areas may cause aneurysm.

Clinical Manifestations. The most specific sign of ASO is crampy pain in the lower extremities occurring with exercise. This ischemic pain, known as **intermittent claudication**, is analogous to the angina pectoris of coronary heart disease (see Chapter 16). Exercise (e.g., walking) triggers pain because it increases the deficit between tissue oxygen supply and demand, worsening the ischemic state and accelerating anaerobic metabolism. The location of the pain depends on the level of the occlusion, but the muscles of the buttocks, thighs, and calves are most frequently involved. Intermittent claudication disappears with rest as the products of anaerobic metabolism are cleared from the muscle. As arterial insufficiency worsens, however, exercise tolerance declines, and pain may also be present at rest. Tissues of the legs are chronically deprived of oxygen, leading to

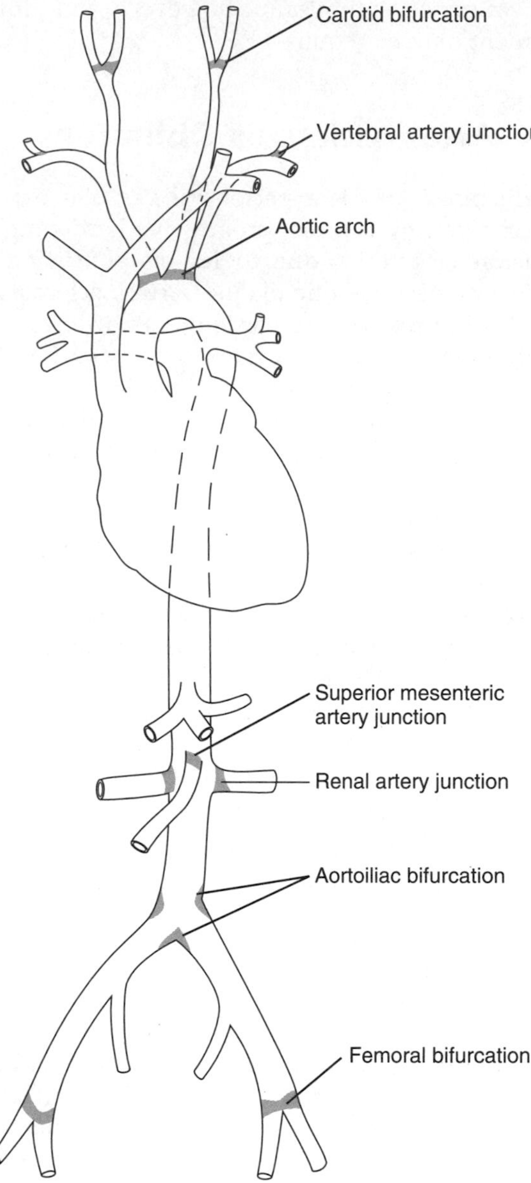

FIGURE 15–15
Sites of obstruction in arteriosclerosis obliterans. Occlusion of peripheral arteries by atherosclerotic plaque usually occurs in areas of branching. Middle-sized arteries of the pelvis and legs are most commonly affected.

loss of hair, pallor, coolness, and degenerative changes of the nails. Peripheral pulses distal to the occlusion are absent or diminished. Paresthesias may occur as peripheral nerves are deprived of oxygen. End-stage ASO manifests as tissue atrophy, necrosis, ulceration, and gangrene.

Prevention and Treatment. Reduction of risk factors associated with atherosclerosis is warranted. Lipid-lowering measures, such as a low fat diet and drug therapy, may be indicated (see Chapter 25). Cigarette smoking should be discontinued, and hypertension and diabetes should be appropriately managed. In early ASO, the patient may benefit from an exercise program in which walking distances are gradually increased. Exercise tolerance may be improved with such programs, possibly owing to acceleration of the development of collateral circulation. Sympathectomy (surgical interruption of sympathetic vasoconstrictor nerves to the affected vessels) may prevent claudication in early disease. Vasodilator drugs such as pentoxifylline (Trental) have been used in the treatment of ASO, but the benefits of such therapy are as yet unproved.[35]

Angioplasty, atherectomy, and surgical bypass (aortoiliac, aortofemoral, and femoropopliteal) are employed in treatment of advanced ASO (Fig. 15–16). When tissue necrosis is extensive, amputation may be necessary to arrest gangrene and prevent bacteremia.

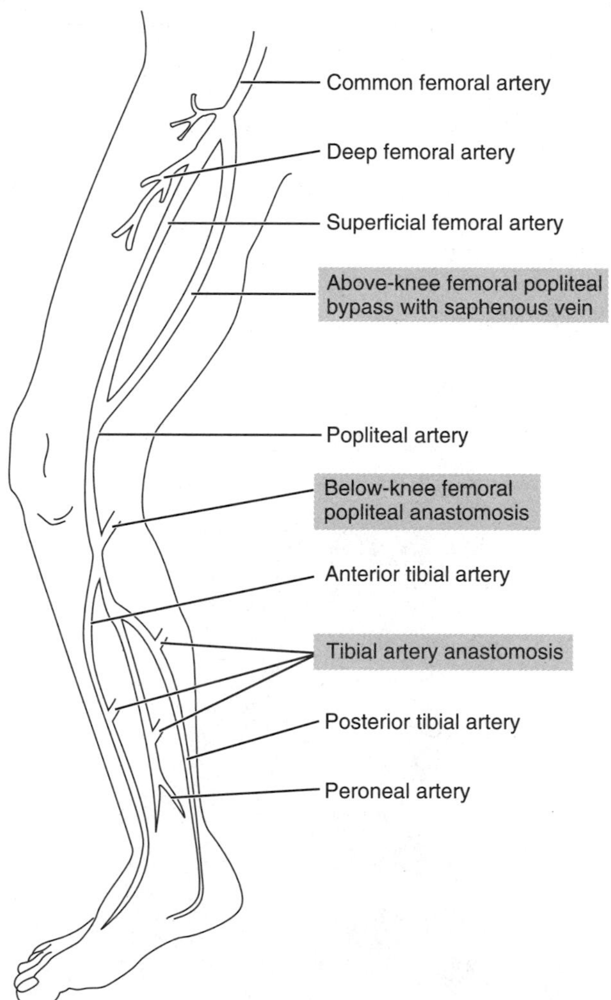

FIGURE 15–16
Surgical treatment of arteriosclerosis obliterans. Grafts composed of reversed veins may be used to bypass areas of occlusion. Reconstruction of the arterial system may involve anastomosis of artery branches to sites distal to occluded areas. (Redrawn from *Critical Care Nursing Quarterly* 8[2], 43. © 1985 Aspen Publishers, Inc.)

Prognosis and Outcome. Typically, patients with ASO also have more life-threatening manifestations of atherosclerosis, including coronary heart disease and cerebrovascular disease. Morbidity and mortality due to ASO are uncertain owing to the association of ASO with these significant disorders.

Aortic Aneurysms

Definition. An aortic aneurysm is a focal dilation (ballooning) of the aorta involving an increase in diameter of at least 50%.[37]

Epidemiology. Ninety-eight per cent of aneurysms are located in the lower aorta **(abdominal aortic aneurysm).** Abdominal aortic aneurysm is increasing in prevalence, with one study demonstrating a rise from 12.2 per 100,000 to 36.2 per 100,000 population during the three decades from 1951 to 1980.[38] This trend most likely reflects the increasing age of the population. Aneurysm is diagnosed more frequently in men than women, and most patients are older than 55 years. Risk factors for atherosclerosis, including age, are applicable to aortic aneurysm development.

Etiology. Aneurysms are most often due to vessel weakening associated with atherosclerosis, especially when hypertension is also present. Rarely, aneurysms are due to congenital defects of the arterial wall, direct trauma to arteries, or infection.

Pathophysiology. Aneurysms are most likely to form at bifurcations (due to reflective pulse waves), in areas where the artery is not well-supported by muscle, or where the artery is subjected to frequent bending with physical activity. In response to intraluminal pressure, the weakened vessel may balloon out on one side (saccular aneurysm) or may enlarge circumferentially in a spindle shape (fusiform aneurysm). If weakening creates a defect in the intima, blood may be forced between the arterial layers, separating them **(dissecting aneurysm).** The different types of aneurysms are illustrated in Figure 15–17. The growing aneurysm is a space-occupying mass, causing pressure on adjacent structures. Rupture of the vessel is possible, with consequences depending on the location of the aneurysm.

Clinical Manifestations. The intact aneurysm is asymptomatic until it becomes large enough to be detectable as a pulsating mass or to create pressure on surrounding organs. Vascular obstruction may occur, resulting in renal failure, and bowel obstruction may result in peritonitis. Blood supply to nerves may be compromised, resulting in pain, numbness, and in rare cases, paralysis. Acute dissection is acutely painful, and because it often occurs in the aortic arch, the chest pain may simulate the pain of myocardial infarction. Rupture of peripheral aneurysms results in hemorrhage and shock. Fortunately, most abdominal aortic aneurysms rupture posteriorly into the retroperitoneal space, surrounding the kidneys. The pressure of the blood accumulating in this small space quickly rises to oppose further bleeding.

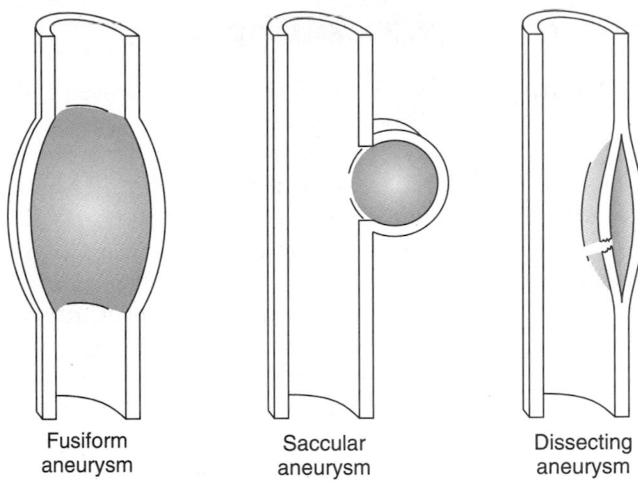

FIGURE 15–17

Types of aneurysm. Fusiform aneurysms develop when the vessel wall is weakened circumferentially. Weakness on one side results in saccular aneurysm formation. A defect in the intima may force blood between arterial wall layers, separating them and resulting in dissection.

Prevention and Treatment. Reduction of risk factors for atherosclerosis is indicated. Because many aneurysms are asymptomatic, routine physical examination is essential in detecting aneurysms in their early development. Aneurysms that are dissecting or that have ruptured retroperitoneally may be repaired with emergency surgery. Depending on their shape and extent, aneurysms may be clamped off (clipped), or the diseased segment removed and the artery repaired with a tubular or patch graft of a synthetic elastic material. Lower-risk aneurysms (generally those less than 5 cm in diameter) may be treated with elective surgery if the benefits of such treatment outweigh the risks. Smaller aortic dissections involving the descending aorta may be managed medically with antihypertensive medications to lower vessel wall stress.

Prognosis and Outcome. The mortality rate associated with elective surgery for intact aneurysms is 6%. The overall mortality rate due to rupture of aneurysms has been estimated at 90%. About 50% of those who reach the hospital alive survive.[37]

Kawasaki Disease

Definition. Kawasaki disease, also known as mucocutaneous lymph node syndrome, is an acute febrile illness of children that is the most common form of vasculitis. Vasculitis is an inflammatory, destructive process affecting arteries, veins, or capillaries.[39] Table 15–15 summarizes clinical features of other vasculitis syndromes.

Epidemiology. Kawasaki disease is most prevalent in Japan, where the annual incidence is 67 per 100,000 children younger than 5 years. In the United States, 2126 cases were reported to the Centers for Disease Control and Prevention between 1976 and 1985. Kawasaki disease is the leading cause of acquired heart disease in children.[40]

Etiology. The specific cause of Kawasaki disease is unknown. Several factors have been implicated, including microorganisms (*Rickettsia* sp., *Propionibacterium acnes*, Epstein-Barr virus, retroviruses) as well as exposure to environmental toxins, such as rug-cleaning solutions or mercury. None of these has been shown with certainty to trigger the disease, however.[41]

Pathophysiology. Vasculitis results in a systemic inflammatory response as well as local inflammatory changes within blood vessels. Vascular inflammation may compromise the vessel lumen, leading to ischemia of tissues, as well as the integrity of the vascular wall, leading to hemorrhage, thrombosis, or aneurysm. Antibody specific to vascular endothelial cells may contribute to the inflammatory pathology.

In Kawasaki disease, vasculitis primarily affects small- and medium-sized muscular arteries, often including the coronary arteries. Coronary artery aneurysms may develop, some of which resolve during the disease, and others that may become obstructive.

The vasculitis syndrome of Kawasaki disease progresses in three phases. The *acute febrile phase* begins at the onset of fever and lasts from 10 to 14 days. The *subacute febrile phase* extends from days 10 to 14 through days 21 to 25 and is characterized by resolution of acute signs of systemic inflammation and appearance of signs of cardiac involvement and desquamation (skin sloughing). The *convalescent phase* begins at day 25 or earlier, and during this period, systemic function returns to normal unless cardiac complications ensue.[41]

Clinical Manifestations. During the acute febrile phase, patients have spiking temperatures that sometimes exceed 104°F. Other signs of systemic inflammation include elevated acute-phase proteins, conjunctivitis (inflammation of the eyes); erythema (redness) of the oral mucosa and tongue; dry, cracked lips; erythema, edema, and desquamation of the palms of the hands and soles of the feet; diffuse skin rash; and cervical lymphadenopathy. Less commonly, signs of arthritis, liver disease, or meningitis

TABLE 15–15
VASCULITIS SYNDROMES

Syndrome	Clinical Features
Kawasaki disease	Inflammatory process affecting small and medium-sized arteries, veins, and capillaries; produces acute febrile illness in children; may be complicated by coronary artery aneurysm (see text)
Henoch-Schönlein purpura (HSP)	Leukocytoclastic vasculitis of small vessels, producing palpable purpura, polyarthritis, abdominal pain, and nephritis
Hypersensitivity vasculitis (HSV)	Morbilliform or urticarial rash on the fingers, palms, and soles of the feet; possible arthritis, nephritis, carditis, and neuropathy
Polyarteritis nodosa (PAN)	Involvement of vessels of the kidney, central nervous system, skeletal muscle, heart, and viscera
Systemic necrotizing vasculitis (SNV)	Intense inflammation of small and medium-sized arteries, resulting in vascular obstruction, ischemia, and infarction (e.g., bowel perforation, renal failure, neuritis, stroke)
Allergic angiitis and granulomatosis (AAG)	Intense, destructive inflammation and fibrinoid necrosis of small and medium-sized muscular arteries, preceded by a long history of allergic asthma
Wegener's granulomatosis (WG)	Clinical triad of granulomatous vasculitis of the respiratory tract, glomerulonephritis, and small vessel vasculitis
Giant cell vasculitis (GCV) (temporal arteritis)	Generalized vasculitis affecting large and medium-sized arteries with an elastic lamina (usually above the neck)
Takayasu's arteritis	Similar to GCV but affecting primarily young females, 15–20 years of age

Data from Athreya, B.H. (1995). Vasculitis in children. *Pediatric Clinics of North America* 42(5), 1239–1261; and Ledford, D.K. (1992). Immunologic aspects of cardiovascular disease. *Journal of the American Medical Association* 268(20), 2923–2929.

are present. Cardiac involvement may take the form of myocarditis, cardiac ischemia, myocardial infarction, or sudden cardiac death.

Treatment. Standard therapy of Kawasaki disease consists of high-dose aspirin to decrease coronary artery inflammation and prevent thrombosis. A single infusion of γ-globulin may be used in an empiric effort to modulate the level of immune activation.[41]

Prognosis and Outcome. Most patients recover completely. The mortality rate ranges from 0.08% to 2%, with death due to cardiac complications.[42]

Raynaud's Syndrome

Definition. Raynaud's syndrome is a condition characterized by digital vasospasm, that is, inappropriate or excessive vasoconstriction in the fingers or, less commonly, the toes, in response to cold, vibration, or stress. *Raynaud's phenomenon* is Raynaud's syndrome occurring secondary to an underlying systemic disease (see later). Raynaud's syndrome occurring as a benign primary disorder is termed *Raynaud's disease.*

Epidemiology. Raynaud's disease is most common among young women between the ages of 20 and 49 years, and there is an apparent familial predisposition. Raynaud's phenomenon may occur in either sex and usually develops after the age of 30.[43] Disorders associated with Raynaud's phenomenon are listed in Table 15–16. Risk factors for acute attacks include exposure to cold, vibration, and stress. Because of their concurrent vasoconstrictor effects, tobacco abuse and excessive caffeine intake exacerbate this risk.

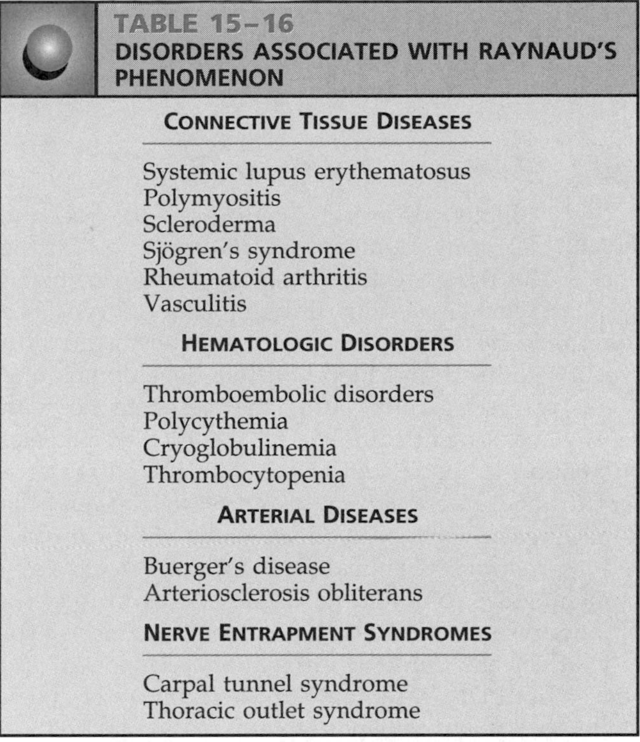

TABLE 15–16
DISORDERS ASSOCIATED WITH RAYNAUD'S PHENOMENON

CONNECTIVE TISSUE DISEASES
Systemic lupus erythematosus
Polymyositis
Scleroderma
Sjögren's syndrome
Rheumatoid arthritis
Vasculitis
HEMATOLOGIC DISORDERS
Thromboembolic disorders
Polycythemia
Cryoglobulinemia
Thrombocytopenia
ARTERIAL DISEASES
Buerger's disease
Arteriosclerosis obliterans
NERVE ENTRAPMENT SYNDROMES
Carpal tunnel syndrome
Thoracic outlet syndrome

Adapted with permission from Davis, E. (1993). The diagnostic puzzle and management challenge of Raynaud's syndrome. *Nurse Practitioner* 18(3), 21.

Etiology. The precise etiologic mechanism of Raynaud's syndrome is unknown. Postulated mechanisms include local hypersensitivity within sympathetic reflex arcs and inappropriate release or response to serotonin.

Pathophysiology. Local vasospasm results in ischemia of the fingers or toes. Relief of spasm then produces a hyperemic response (see Chapter 13).

Clinical Manifestations. The classic sign of Raynaud's phenomenon or disease is the triphasic response, in which the affected digit turns white, then blue, then red. The white response (pallor) dominates and is due to decreased blood flow resulting from vasospasm. The blue response (cyanosis) develops as oxygen is extracted in greater quantities owing to the sluggish blood flow. (Deoxygenated hemoglobin is blue.) When the spasm releases, blood rushes through the digital arterioles, and this hyperemia leads to redness. Other clinical manifestations also relate to the sequential vascular changes. Ischemia may be accompanied by pain or numbness and a cold sensation. With frequent recurrence of attacks, the skin and nails may become thickened. Prolonged ischemia during a single attack may cause ulceration or even gangrene of the tips of the fingers or toes, but this is rare. Hyperemia may manifest as throbbing pain or paresthesias. Attacks of vasospasm are bilateral and symmetric.

Prevention and Treatment. Stress management, cessation of smoking, reduction of caffeine intake, and measures to ensure warmth of the digits may reduce the frequency of attacks. Some patients are able to interrupt an attack at its onset by swinging their arms in a circular motion, which increases arterial flow to the hands by means of centrifugal force. Vasodilators, such as calcium-channel blockers (e.g., nifedipine) are beneficial to most patients with chronic disease. Sympathectomy, the surgical interruption of sympathetic nerves to the vessels, may be used in the treatment of Raynaud's syndrome affecting the toes. Rarely, amputation is necessitated by gangrene. Associated systemic disorders should be optimally managed in Raynaud's phenomenon.

Prognosis and Outcome. Raynaud's syndrome is usually responsive to preventive measures and treatment.

Developmental Perspective

Embryonic and Fetal Periods

Initially, diffusion is sufficient to meet the perfusion demands of the embryo. By the end of the third week of gestation, however, blood can be seen circulating through the embryo. The lymphatic system begins to develop during the fifth week. The heart and blood vessels develop simultaneously, but separately, from the mesenchyme, with most development complete by the 10th week. Fetal circulation is specialized to facilitate placental transfer of blood gases, nutrients, and wastes because the fetal lungs are collapsed and hepatic and renal function is minimal. Congenital abnormalities of vessel branching are common but usually benign. Congenital aneurysms and arteriovenous malformations usually affect the cerebral circulation. Congenital absence of LDL receptors or deficiency of HDL cholesterol may predispose to atherosclerosis.

Infancy and Childhood

Atherosclerotic plaque formation may begin in childhood. Obesity, type 1 diabetes, and hypertension may have their onset during childhood and are associated with earlier development of atherosclerosis. Some vasculitis syndromes, including Kawasaki disease, affect children. Tumors of blood vessels often present during childhood, particularly the benign hemangiomas.

Adolescence and Young Adulthood

Cigarette smoking commonly begins during this period, and habitual smoking constitutes a major risk for development of atherosclerosis. In those with familial hypercholesterolemia, atherosclerosis may be severe, precipitating myocardial infarction or stroke as early as the teens or 20s. Many young adults engage in aerobic exercise regimens or athletic activities, which increase HDL cholesterol, protecting against development of atherosclerosis.

Middle and Older Adulthood

Aging is a risk factor for atherosclerosis and hypertension, two syndromes that underlie the major cardiovascular disorders. The arterial wall demonstrates a progressive increase in stiffness with age, owing to loss of elasticity and increased connective tissue. There is also a diminished vasomotor response to catecholamines and decreased sensitivity of the baroreceptor reflex.

CLINICAL SIGNIFICANCE OF CIRCULATORY DISORDERS

Circulatory disorders affect people of all ages, but have their greatest impact on the elderly (see Developmental Perspective). Risk factors for atherosclerosis, however, may be evident even in childhood, warranting early screening of blood pressure and serum lipid levels. Establishment of healthy dietary and exercise habits ideally begins early in life. Cardiovascular disorders constitute the leading cause of death in the United States, and the impact of these conditions on quality of life is inestimable. Because many cardiovascular conditions are preventable to a significant degree, risk reduction measures may reduce not only morbidity and mortality but also the staggering costs associated with treatment of these disorders.

The impact of circulatory disorders justifies the extensive research being done in the area. Epidemiologic research is focused on clarification of factors associated with positive mortality and morbidity trends because such trends are not uniform across age, sex, and race. The role of psychological characteristics, such as personality type, anxiety, hostility, and depression, in determining cardiovascular risk continues to be explored. Basic research into the mechanisms of essential hypertension continues to be a high priority. Much research now centers on genetic factors regulating vascular function in health and disease and on the role of endothelial mediators in autoregulation. Several large clinical trials are in progress in an effort to determine the most effective modes of prevention and treatment of circulatory disorders.

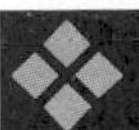

Summary of Key Points

- The major divisions of the circulation are the larger systemic circulation, in which oxygenated blood leaves the left ventricle of the heart, perfuses (by arteries) all organ systems except the lungs, and returns (by veins) to the right atrium of the heart; and the pulmonary circulation, in which unoxygenated blood leaves the right ventricle, circulates through the lungs where it is oxygenated, and returns to the left atrium of the heart.
- The heart serves as the primary pump within the circulation, assisted by the secondary pumps derived from the Windkessel effect; contraction of skeletal muscle, including the diaphragm; and the intrinsic vasomotion of the vessels.
- The principal function of the arteries is conductance, and the arterioles serve as the major resistance vessels. Capillaries serve as exchange vessels between the blood and the interstitial fluid surrounding cells. The smallest veins, the venules, serve as resistance vessels because of their fixed diameters, and the large veins serve as blood reservoirs. Lymphatic vessels collect and transport excess fluid and cellular debris from interstitial space to the venous system.
- Blood flow is directly proportional to the circulatory pressure gradient and inversely proportional to the systemic resistance.
- Neural mechanisms mediating short-term regulation of the blood pressure gradient and systemic resistance include the baroreceptor reflexes, chemoreceptor systems, and the CNS ischemic response. Endocrine mechanisms include the regulatory systems for fluid volume regulation, namely the RAAS, ADH, atrial natriuretic peptide, and glomerular filtration. Endothelial regulation of blood flow depends on the balance of local mediators influencing vasoconstriction and vasodilation.
- About 45% of the population of the Western world will die of atherosclerotic diseases, particularly coronary artery disease and stroke. Elevation of serum LDL cholesterol is the definitive risk factor for atherosclerosis, although other factors, including aging, menopause in women, diabetes, hypertension, tobacco abuse, sedentary lifestyle, and obesity, exacerbate the development of plaques. The best-accepted mechanism of atherogenesis is the lipid infiltration hypothesis, which proposes that LDL cholesterol is oxidized and taken up by macrophages, which penetrate the intact arterial wall.
- The overall prevalence of hypertension in the United States is 20%. Ninety-five per cent of cases of hypertension are essential hypertension, in which the precise cause is unknown. Theoretical mechanisms include the hemodynamic hypothesis, which holds that persistent hypervolemia due to defective sodium excretion and volume regulation is the cause; and the vasoconstrictor hypothesis, which proposes that increased vessel resistance is due to dysfunction at the level of local endothelial regulation.
- The three categories of shock are hypovolemic shock, due to volume deficit secondary to hemorrhage or third spacing; cardiogenic shock, due to inadequate cardiac pumping secondary to myocardial infarction or cardiomyopathy; and distributive shock, due to loss of vascular tone secondary to endothelial mediators or autonomic dysfunction.
- Kawasaki disease is the most common form of vasculitis in children and may be associated with the development of coronary artery aneurysms. Arteriosclerosis obliterans results from atherosclerosis in peripheral arteries, producing intermittent claudication and potential gangrene secondary to ischemia. Aortic aneurysms are dilations in weak areas of the aortic wall, which may be congenital or traumatic but more often are the result of atherosclerosis. Raynaud's syndrome is a vasospastic disorder of the fingers and toes, which may be primary (benign) or secondary to a systemic disorder.

REFERENCES

1. Davis, D.L., Dinse, G.E., and Hoel, D.G. (1994). Decreasing cardiovascular disease and increasing cancer among whites in the United States from 1973 through 1987: Good news and bad news. *Journal of the American Medical Association* 271(6), 431–437.
2. Centers for Disease Control and Prevention. (1994). Mortality from congestive heart failure—United States, 1980–1990. *Journal of the American Medical Association* 271(11), 813–814.
3. Stumpf, J.L., and Mitrzyk, B. (1994). Management of orthostatic hypotension. *American Journal of Hospital Pharmacy* 51(5), 640–698
4. Falkenhahn, M., Gohlke, P., Paul, M., *et al.* (1994). The renin-angiotensin system in the heart and vascular wall: New therapeutic aspects. *Journal of Cardiovascular Pharmacology* 24(suppl. 2), S6–S13.

5. Rubanyi, G.M. (1993). The role of endothelium in cardiovascular homeostasis and diseases. *Journal of Cardiovascular Pharmacology* 22(4 suppl.), S1–S14.
6. Loscalzo, J. (1995). Nitric oxide and vascular disease. *New England Journal of Medicine* (Editorial). 333(4), 251–253.
7. Tamirisa, P., Frishman, W.H., and Kumar, A. (1995). Endothelin and endothelin antagonism: Roles in cardiovascular health and disease. *American Heart Journal* 130(3 Pt.1), 601–610.
8. Gibbons, G.H., and Dzau, V.J. (1994). The emerging concept of vascular remodeling. *New England Journal of Medicine* 330(20), 1431–1438.
9. Roberts, W.C. (1995). Preventing and arresting coronary atherosclerosis. *American Heart Journal* 130(3 Pt. 1), 580–600.
10. Rossi, G.P., Pavan, E., and Pessina, A.C. (1994). Role of genetic, humoral, and endothelial factors in hypertension-induced atherosclerosis. *Journal of Cardiovascular Pharmacology* 23(suppl. 5), S75–S84.
11. Arrants, J. (1994). Hypertension and cardiovascular risk. *Heart & Lung* 23(2), 118–124.
12. Fuchs, C.S., Stampfer, M.J., Colditz, G.A., *et al.* (1995). Alcohol consumption and mortality among women. *New England Journal of Medicine* 332(19), 1245–1250.
13. Bartecchi, C.E., MacKenzie, T.D., and Schrier, R.W. (1994). The human costs of tobacco use. (Pt. 1). *New England Journal of Medicine* 330(13), 907–912.
14. Dzau, V.J. (1994). Pathobiology of atherosclerosis and plaque complications. *American Heart Journal* 128(6 Pt. 2), 1300–1304.
15. Mehra, M.R., Lavie, C.J., Ventura, H.O., *et al.* (1995). Prevention of atherosclerosis. *Postgraduate Medicine* 98(1), 175–184.
16. Meyers, D.G., and Maloley, P.A. (1993). The antioxidant vitamins: Impact on atherosclerosis. *Pharmacotherapy* 13(6), 574–582.
17. O'Brien, K.D., and Chait, A. (1994). The biology of the artery wall in atherogenesis. *Medical Clinics of North America* 78(1), 41–67.
18. Jha, P., Flather, M., Lonn, E., *et al.* (1995). The antioxidant vitamins and cardiovascular disease: A critical review of epidemiologic and clinical trial data. *Annals of Internal Medicine* 123(11), 860–872.
19. Kimura, T., Yokoi, H., Nakagawa, Y., *et al.* (1996). Three-year follow-up after implantation of metallic coronary-artery stents. *New England Journal of Medicine* 334(9), 561–566.
20. Black, H.R. (1996). Blood pressure control. *American Journal of Medicine* 101(suppl. 4A), 50S–55S.
21. Fletcher, E.C. (1995). The relationship between systemic hypertension and obstructive sleep apnea: Facts and theory. *American Journal of Medicine* 98(2), 118–128.
22. Lieberman, E. (1994). Pediatric hypertension: Clinical perspective. *Mayo Clinic Proceedings* 69(11), 1098–1107.
23. Sollek, M.V., and Lee, K.A. (1989). High blood pressure. In: Underhill, S.L., Woods, S.L., Froelicher, E.S.S., *et al.* (Eds.). *Cardiac Nursing*. (2nd ed.). Philadelphia: J.B. Lippincott. (pp. 814–857).
24. Caulfield, M., Lavender, P., Farrall, M., *et al.* (1994). Linkage of the angiotensinogen gene to essential hypertension. *New England Journal of Medicine* 330(23), 1629–1633.
25. Franklin, S.S., and Weber, M.A. (1994). Measuring hypertensive cardiovascular risk: The vascular overload concept. *American Heart Journal* 128(4), 793–803.
26. Sagie, A., Larson, M.G., and Levy, D. (1993). The natural history of borderline isolated systolic hypertension. *New England Journal of Medicine* 329(26), 1912–1917.
27. Prisant, L.M., Houghton, J.L., Bottini, P.B., *et al.* (1994). Hypertensive heart disease: How does blood pressure affect left ventricular mass? *Postgraduate Medicine* 95(6), 59–76.
28. Opie, L.H. (1993). Individualised selection of antihypertensive therapy. *Drugs* 46(suppl. 2), 142–148.
29. Littenberg, B. (1995). A practice guideline revisited: Screening for hypertension. *Annals of Internal Medicine* 122(12), 937–939.
30. Parillo, J.E. (1993). Pathogenic mechanisms of septic shock. *New England Journal of Medicine* 328(20), 1471–1477.
31. Califf, R.M., and Bengtson, J.R. (1994). Cardiogenic shock. *New England Journal of Medicine* 330(24), 1724–1730.
32. McMahon, K. (1995). Multiple organ failure: The final complication of critical illness. *Critical Care Nurse* 15(6), 20–28.
33. Schoen, F.J. (1994). Blood vessels. In: Cotran, R.S., Kumar, V., and Robbins, S.L. (Eds.). *Robbins Pathologic Basis of Disease.* (5th ed.). Philadelphia: W.B. Saunders. (pp. 467–516).
34. Ibrahim, S., MacPherson, D.R., and Goldhaber, S.Z. (1996). Chronic venous insufficiency: Mechanisms and management. *American Heart Journal* 132(4), 856–860.
35. Krikorian, R.K., and Vacek, J.L. (1995). Peripheral arterial disease: When to consider percutaneous revascularization. *Postgraduate Medicine* 97(6), 109–119.
36. Balkau, B., Vray, M., and Eschwege, E. (1994). Epidemiology of peripheral arterial disease. *Journal of Cardiovascular Pharmacology* 23(suppl. 3), S8–S16.
37. Ernst, C.B. (1993). Abdominal aortic aneurysm. *New England Journal of Medicine* 328(16), 1167–1172.
38. Smith, R.B., and Perdue, G.D. (1990). Diseases of the peripheral arteries and veins. In: Hurst, J.W., Schlant, R.C., Rackley, C.E., *et al.* (Eds.). *The Heart, Arteries, and Veins.* (7th ed.). New York: McGraw-Hill Information Services Company, Health Professions Division. (pp. 1423–1445).
39. Athreya, B.H. (1995). Vasculitis in children. *Pediatric Clinics of North America* 42(5), 1239–1261.
40. Ledford, D.K. (1992). Immunologic aspects of cardiovascular disease. *Journal of the American Medical Association* 268(20), 2923–2929.
41. Applegate, B.L. (1995). Kawasaki syndrome: An important consideration in the febrile child. *Postgraduate Medicine* 97(2), 121–126.
42. Rosenfeld, E.A., Corydon, K.E., and Shulman, S.T. (1995). Kawasaki disease in infants less than one year of age. *Journal of Pediatrics* 126(4), 524–529.
43. Davis, E. (1993). The diagnostic puzzle and management challenge of Raynaud's syndrome. *Nurse Practitioner* 18(3), 18–25.

SELECTED BIBLIOGRAPHY

Alyn, I.B., and Baker, L.K. (1992). Cardiovascular anatomy and physiology of the fetus, neonate, infant, child, and adolescent. *Journal of Cardiovascular Nursing* 6(3), 1–11.

Amsterdam, E.A., Hyson, D., and Kappagoda, C.T. (1994). Nonpharmacologic therapy for coronary artery atherosclerosis: Results of primary and secondary prevention trials. *American Heart Journal* 128(6 Pt. 2), 1344–1352.

Barron, R.L. (1993). Pathophysiology of septic shock and implications for therapy. *Clinical Pharmacy* 12(11), 829–845.

Blackburn, S.T., and Loper, D.L. (1992). *Maternal, Fetal, and Neonatal Physiology: A Clinical Perspective.* Philadelphia: W.B. Saunders.

Bonner, G. (1994). Hyperinsulinemia, insulin resistance, and hypertension. *Journal of Cardiovascular Pharmacology* 24(suppl. 2), S39–S49.

Boushey, C.J., Beresford, S.A.A., Omenn, G.S., *et al.* (1995). A quantitative assessment of plasma homocysteine as a risk factor for vascular disease. *Journal of the American Medical Association* 274(13), 1049–1057.

Brun-Buisson, C., Doyon, F., Carlet, J., *et al.* (1995). Incidence, risk factors, and outcome of severe sepsis and septic shock in adults: A multicenter prospective study in intensive care units. *Journal of the American Medical Association* 274(12), 968–974.

Carr, A.A., Prisant, L.M., and Bottini, P.B. (1994). Hypertension: Not solely a blood pressure problem. *Postgraduate Medicine* 95(6), 79–86.

Cotran, R.S., Kumar, V., and Robbins, S.L. (Eds.). (1994). *Robbins Pathologic Basis of Disease.* (5th ed.). Philadelphia: W.B. Saunders.

Erstad, B.L. (1994). Oxygen transport goals in the resuscitation of critically ill patients. *Annals of Pharmacotherapy* 28(11), 1273–1284.

Freis, E.D. (1995). The efficacy and safety of diuretics in treating hypertension. *Annals of Internal Medicine* 122(3), 223–226.

Guthrie, D. (Ed.). (1989). *Advanced Trauma Life Support Course for Physicians*. (Revised ed.). Chicago: American College of Surgeons. (pp. 57–88).

Hazinski, M.F. (1994). Mediator-specific therapies for the systemic inflammatory response syndrome, sepsis, severe sepsis, and septic shock: Present and future approaches. *Critical Care Nursing Clinics of North America* 6(2), 309–319.

Hennekens, C.H. (1994). Platelet inhibitors and antioxidant vitamins in cardiovascular disease. *American Heart Journal* 128(6 Pt. 2), 1333–1336.

Hodis, H.N., Mack, W.J., LaBree, L., *et al.* (1995). Serial coronary angiographic evidence that antioxidant vitamin intake reduces progression of coronary artery atherosclerosis. *Journal of the American Medical Association* 273(23), 1849–1854.

Hunder, G. (1996). Vasculitis: Diagnosis and therapy. *American Journal of Medicine* 100(suppl. 2A), 37S–45S.

Hurst, J.W., Schlant, R.C., Rackley, C.E., *et al.* (1990). *The Heart, Arteries, and Veins*. (7th ed.). New York: McGraw-Hill Information Services Company, Health Professions Division.

Jarvis, C. (1996). *Physical Examination and Health Assessment*. (2nd ed.). Philadelphia: W.B. Saunders.

Joint National Committee. (1993). The fifth report of the Joint National Committee on Detection, Evaluation, and Treatment of High Blood Pressure (JNC V). *Archives of Internal Medicine* 153(2), 154–183.

Kaplan, J.R., and Manuck, S.B. (1994). Antiatherogenic effects of β-adrenergic blocking agents: Theoretical, experimental, and epidemiologic considerations. *American Heart Journal* 128(6 Pt. 2), 1316–1328.

Kasiske, B.L., Ma, J.Z., Kalil, R.S.N., *et al.* (1995). Effects of antihypertensive therapy on serum lipids. *Annals of Internal Medicine* 122(2), 133–141.

Lampert, E., Charloux, A., Lonsdorfer, J., *et al.* (1996). The concept of Raynaud's phenomenon of the lung revisited. *American Journal of Medicine* 101, 468–471.

Landsberg, L. (1994). Pathophysiology of obesity-related hypertension: Role of insulin and the sympathetic nervous system. *Journal of Cardiovascular Pharmacology* 23(suppl. 1), S1–S8.

Lehne, R.A. (1994). *Pharmacology for Nursing Care*. (2nd ed.). Philadelphia: W.B. Saunders.

Levin, E.R. (1995). Endothelins. *New England Journal of Medicine* 333(6), 356–363.

Levine, G.N., Keaney, J.F., and Vita, J.A. (1995). Cholesterol reduction in cardiovascular disease. *New England Journal of Medicine* 332(8), 512–521.

Markovitz, J.H., Matthews, K.A., Kannel, W.B., *et al.* (1993). Psychological predictors of hypertension in the Framingham Study: Is there tension in hypertension? *Journal of the American Medical Association* 270(20), 2439–2443.

Marlow, D.R., and Redding, B.A. (1988). *Textbook of Pediatric Nursing*. Philadelphia: W.B. Saunders.

Mazzonim M.C., Warnke, K.C., Arfors, K.E., *et al.* (1994). Capillary hemodynamics in hemorrhagic shock and reperfusion: In vivo and model analysis. *American Journal of Physiology* 267(5 Pt. 2), H1928–H1935.

Mombouli, J.V., and Vanhoutte, P.M. (1995). Kinins and endothelial control of vascular smooth muscle. *Annual Review of Pharmacology and Toxicology* 35, 679–705.

Moncada, S., and Higgs, A. (1993). The L-arginine-nitric oxide pathway. *New England Journal of Medicine* 329(27), 2002–2012.

Nayler, W.G. (1993). Pharmacological aspects of calcium antagonism: Short term and long term benefits. *Drugs* 46(suppl. 2), 40–47.

Ohno, T., Gordon, D., San, H., *et al.* (1994). Gene therapy for vascular smooth muscle cell proliferation after arterial injury. *Science* 265(5173), 781–784.

Petrakis, N.L. (1995). Earlobe crease in women: Evaluation of reproductive factors, alcohol use, and Quetelet Index and relation to atherosclerotic disease. *American Journal of Medicine* 99, 356–361.

Phillips, G.R., Kauder, D.R., and Schwab, C.W. (1994). Massive blood loss in trauma patients: The benefits and dangers of transfusion therapy. *Postgraduate Medicine* 95(4), 61–72.

Pitt, B. (1994). Angiotensin-converting enzyme inhibitors in patients with coronary atherosclerosis. *American Heart Journal* 128(6 Pt. 2), 1328–1332.

Saez-Llorens, X., and McCracken, G.H. (1993). Sepsis syndrome and septic shock in pediatrics: Current concepts of terminology, pathophysiology, and management. *Journal of Pediatrics* 123(4), 497–508.

Schaefer, E.J., Lichtenstein, A.H., Lamon-Fava, S., *et al.* (1995). Lipoproteins, nutrition, aging, and atherosclerosis. *American Journal of Clinical Nutrition* 61(3 Suppl.), 726S–740S.

Schmidt, E.B., and Dyerberg, J. (1994). Omega-3 fatty acids: Current status in cardiovascular medicine. *Drugs* 47(3), 405–424.

Schmieder, R.E. (1992). Hypertensive heart disease: Significance of left ventricular hypertrophy. *Journal of Cardiovascular Pharmacology* 20(suppl. 6), S50–S55.

Schwartz, S.M., deBlois, D., and O'Brien, E.R.M. (1995). The intima: Soil for atherosclerosis and restenosis. *Circulation Research* 77(3), 445–465.

Smith, J.J., Porth, C.J., and Erickson, M. (1994). Hemodynamic response to the upright posture. *Journal of Clinical Pharmacology* 34(5), 375–386.

Stein, P.P., and Black, H.R. (1993). The role of diet in the genesis and treatment of hypertension. *Medical Clinics of North America* 77(4), 831–847.

Stone, N.J. (1996). The clinical and economic significance of atherosclerosis. *American Journal of Medicine* 101(suppl. 4A), 6S–9S.

Strausbaugh, L.J. (1993). Toxic shock syndrome: Are you recognizing its changing presentations? *Postgraduate Medicine* 94(6), 107–118.

Taylor, A.A. (1994). Autonomic control of cardiovascular function: Clinical evaluation in health and disease. *Journal of Clinical Pharmacology* 34(5), 363–374.

Teba, L., Banks, D.E., and Balaan, M.R. (1992). Understanding circulatory shock: Is it hypovolemic, cardiogenic, or vasogenic? *Postgraduate Medicine* 91(7), 121–129.

Terres, W., Becker, R., and Rosenberg, A. (1994). Changes in cardiovascular risk profile during the cessation of smoking. 97(3), 242–249.

Underhill, S.L., Woods, S.L., Froelicher, E.S.S., *et al. Cardiac Nursing*. (2nd ed.). Philadelphia: J.B. Lippincott.

Waters, D., and Lesperance, J. (1994). Calcium channel blockers and coronary atherosclerosis: From the rabbit to the real world. *American Heart Journal* 128(6 Pt. 2), 1309–1316.

Weidmann, P., Boehlen, L.M., and de Courten, M. (1993). Pathogenesis and treatment of hypertension associated with diabetes mellitus. *American Heart Journal* 125(5 Pt. 2), 1498–1513.

Wiessner, W.H., Casey, L.C., and Zbilut, J.P. (1995). Treatment of sepsis and septic shock: A review. *Heart and Lung* 24(5), 380–392.

Wolfe, T.A., and Dasta, J.F. (1995). Use of nitric oxide synthase inhibitors as a novel treatment for septic shock. *Annals of Pharmacotherapy* 29(1) 36–46.

Zhu, B., and Parmley, W.W. (1995). Hemodynamic and vascular effects of active and passive smoking. *American Heart Journal* 130(6), 1270–1275.

16 CHAPTER

Cardiac Failure

LEARNING OBJECTIVES

1. Describe the structure and function of the three cardiac layers.
2. Identify the local and neuroendocrine mechanisms by which cardiac contraction is regulated.
3. Discuss the phases and events of the cardiac cycle.
4. Discuss the factors that determine cardiac output.
5. Discuss the principles on which cardiac failure may be classified.
6. Describe the clinical features of the syndrome of congestive heart failure.
7. Differentiate among the following disorders, all of which may culminate in congestive heart failure: coronary heart disease, cardiomyopathy, inflammatory heart disorders, cardiac valve disease, and congenital heart defects.
8. Discuss the clinical significance of disorders of cardiac contraction.

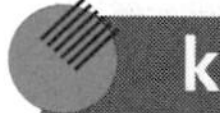

key terms

afterload
angina pectoris
aortic insufficiency
aortic stenosis
atrial septal defect
cardiac cycle
cardiac failure
cardiac index
cardiac output
cardiac reserve
cardiac tamponade
cardiomyopathy
coarctation of the aorta
congenital heart defect
congestive heart failure (CHF)
constrictive pericarditis
coronary heart disease (CHD)
coronary steal syndrome
diastole
ejection fraction
Frank-Starling mechanism
gallop rhythm
hypertrophic cardiomyopathy
idiopathic dilated cardiomyopathy (IDC)
infective endocarditis
intrinsic contractility
mitral insufficiency
mitral stenosis
mitral valve prolapse
murmur
myocardial infarction
myocarditis
no-reflow phenomenon
patent ductus arteriosus

pericarditis
persistent truncus arteriosus
preload
pulmonary edema
pulmonic stenosis
restrictive cardiomyopathy
stroke volume
systole
tetralogy of Fallot
transposition of the great vessels
ventricular septal defect (VSD)

The ability of the cardiovascular system to perfuse tissues with blood depends not only on the integrity of the vessels but also on the contraction of the major pump, the heart. **Cardiac failure** is the inability of the heart to contract with sufficient rate and force to satisfy the metabolic demands of tissues. Quantitatively, cardiac failure is usually defined by abnormally low **cardiac output**, the volume of blood pumped by the left ventricle per minute. The clinical syndrome most closely associated with cardiac failure is **congestive heart failure (CHF)**, discussed in detail later in this chapter. Despite declining death rates for cardiac disease in general, mortality due to CHF is increasing. Because more than 90% of CHF deaths occur in people older than 65 years, the aging of the population is a possible contributing factor to this trend.[1]

Cardiac failure may occur as a result of impairment of the heart by congenital or acquired disease. Diseases of other organs may impose excessive volume loads or metabolic demands that could precipitate failure of the compromised heart. Less commonly, extreme metabolic demands, such as those imposed by iatrogenic fluid overload, thyroid crisis, or high temperature, may precipitate failure of normal hearts. Cardiac failure in the latter case is referred to as *high-output failure*, in contrast to the low cardiac output that is the hallmark of CHF.

Function of the heart as a pump may be impaired owing to anatomic abnormality or impaired regulation of heart rate and contractility. The cellular basis of contractility is cardiac muscle contraction, which depends on energy metabolism, action potential formation, and calcium flux (see Chapters 3, 4, and 5). Because cardiac muscle cells normally contract in response to an electrical signal, disorders of conduction of electrical impulses within the heart (dysrhythmias) represent an important mechanism of cardiac failure. These disorders are discussed in detail in Chapter 17. This chapter focuses on the mechanisms of failure that involve congenital defects in cardiac anatomy or acquired diseases affecting the tissue layers of the heart wall.

CARDIAC ANATOMY

The heart is positioned behind the sternum or breastbone, tipped toward the left side, with its uppermost border (paradoxically referred to as the *base*) at the level of the second rib and its lowermost tip or *apex* at the level of the fifth or sixth rib (Fig. 16–1). Its normal size may be approximated by the closed fist. The heart, esophagus, and trachea are contained within the mediastinal space, which lies between the two pleural spaces enclosing the lungs.

The heart wall consists of three layers: the inner *endocardium* or lining, which includes the valves separating chambers and major vessels; the middle *myocardium*, the muscle layer; and the outer *pericardium*, a protective sac containing a small amount of lubricating fluid that facilitates the contraction and relaxation of the myocardium. Figure 16–2 illustrates the interior anatomy of the heart, with its four chambers, valves, and major vessels.

The myocardium is perfused by three arteries that

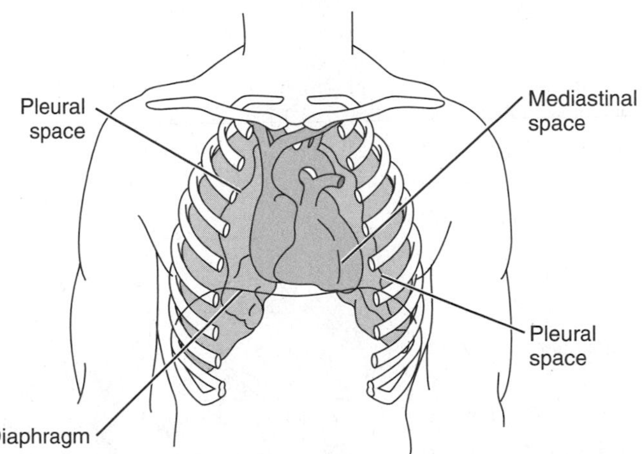

Figure 16–1
Position of the heart in the thoracic cavity. The heart is positioned behind the sternum in the mediastinal space. Its upper border (base) is at the level of the second rib, and its lower tip (apex) is at the level of the fifth rib. The mediastinal space is bordered by the left and right pleural spaces, containing the lungs. The diaphragm separates the thoracic and abdominal cavities.

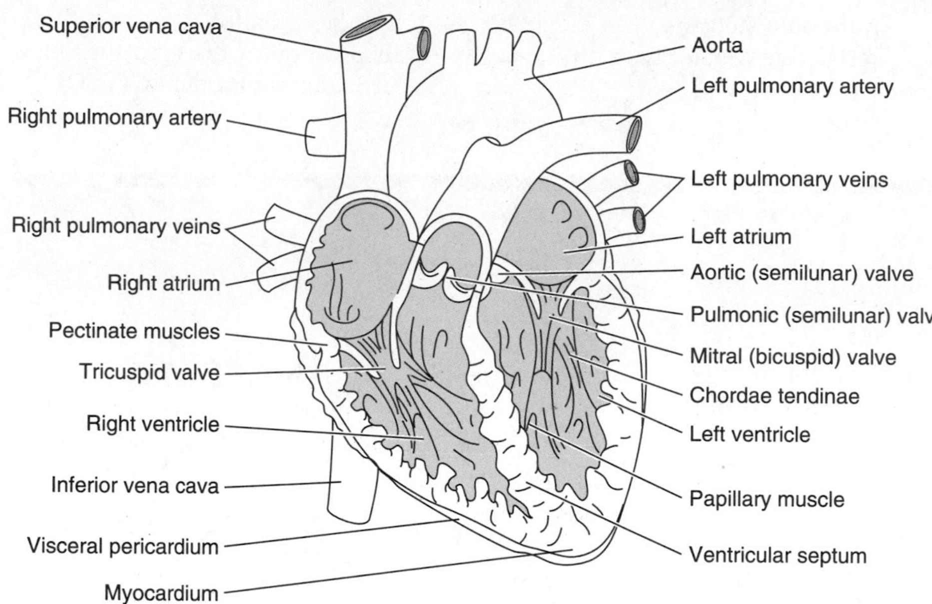

Figure 16–2
Interior structures of the heart. The four cardiac chambers are separated by the septum and by valves that facilitate directional flow of blood. The right atrium is separated from the right ventricle by the tricuspid valve. The pulmonic valve separates the right ventricle from the pulmonary artery. The mitral valve separates the left atrium from the left ventricle, and the aortic valve separates the left ventricle from the aorta.

branch off the aorta just beyond the aortic valve: the *right coronary artery*, and the two principal branches of the left main coronary artery, the *left anterior descending artery* and the *circumflex artery* (Figs. 16–3 and 16–4). The right coronary artery supplies the right atrium, right ventricle, and the posterior and inferior (lower) portions of the left ventricle. The left anterior descending artery supplies parts of the left ventricle and most of the septum (wall) between the right and left sides. The circumflex branch supplies the left atrium and parts of the left ventricle.

Variations in coronary artery anatomy are common, with the most important variation determined by the vessel that supplies blood to the atrioventricular nodal artery and the posterior descending artery. In 85% of hearts, the right coronary artery supplies these vessels, and the person is said to be *right dominant.*[2] In 8%, the circumflex artery supplies these arteries, and the person is then *left dominant.* The remaining 7% are *codominant.* Atherosclerotic occlusion of one or more of the coronary arteries or their branches constitutes **coronary heart disease (CHD),** discussed later in this chapter.

Although the bulk of the blood supply to the myocardium is provided by the coronary arteries and their branches, some of the subendocardial fibers are

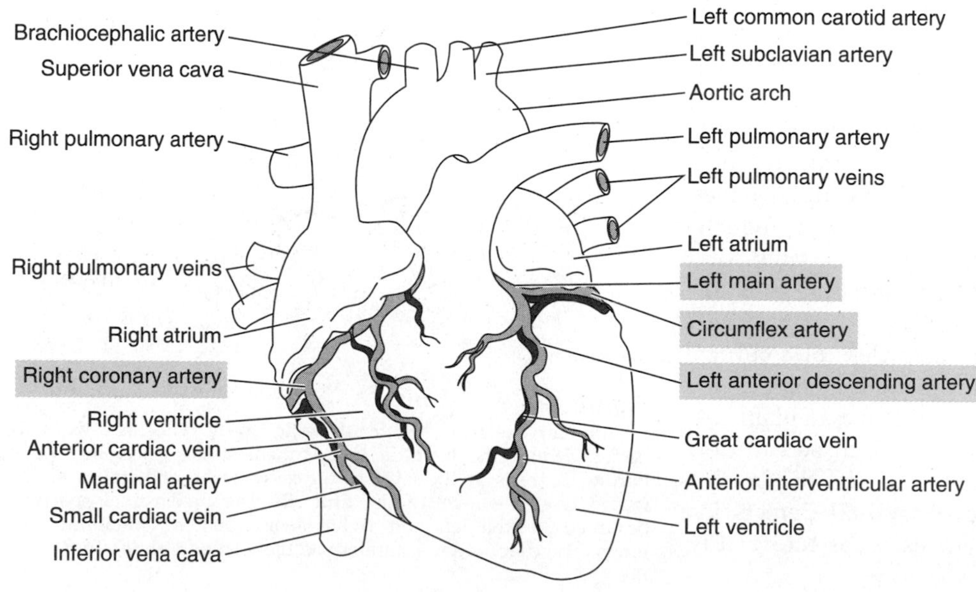

Figure 16–3
Coronary circulation (anterior view). The principal coronary arteries are the right coronary artery and the left main coronary artery, which divides into the left anterior descending and circumflex branches.

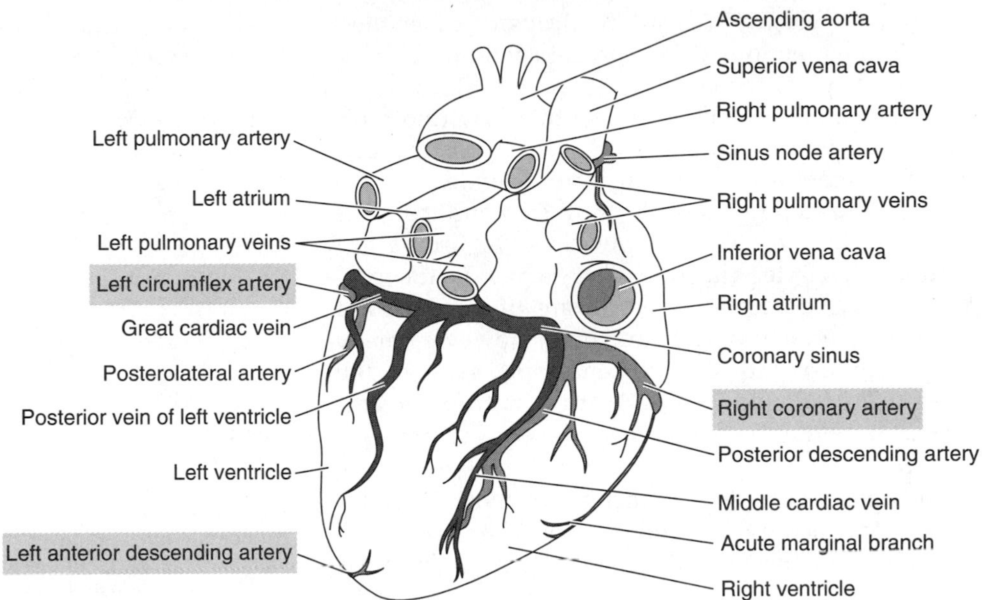

Figure 16–4
Coronary circulation (posterior view). The posterior myocardium is perfused primarily by the right coronary artery and the circumflex branch of the left coronary artery.

perfused directly from the ventricle by small channels known as the *thebesian veins*. Venous drainage of the heart is into the right atrium, and lymphatics empty into the superior vena cava leading into the right atrium. Venous and lymphatic drainage are not usually impaired by diseases of the heart.

CARDIAC CONTRACTION

Regulation of Contraction

Like most other physiologic processes, contraction of cardiac muscle displays both local autoregulation and neuroendocrine control.

Autoregulatory Mechanisms

The **Frank-Starling mechanism**, illustrated in Figure 16–5, describes the relationship between the degree of tension generated within myocardial fibers and the contractile force generated during their subsequent contraction. *Up to a maximal point*, the greater the myocardial fiber stretch or tension (i.e., the greater the volume contained within the chamber), the greater is the force of contraction that ejects that volume (and the greater the cardiac output). The physiologic basis of the Frank-Starling mechanism is uncertain, but the most prevalent theory is that at certain fiber lengths, overlap of the contractile proteins actin and myosin is optimal (see Chapter 5). As the Frank-Starling curve indicates, filling of the cardiac chambers beyond a maximal point does not result in further enhancement of contractility; that is, the curve levels off. The Frank-Starling mechanism is impaired in conditions such as hypertensive heart disease and chronic CHF, in which the cardiac muscle is less compliant (stiffer) than normal

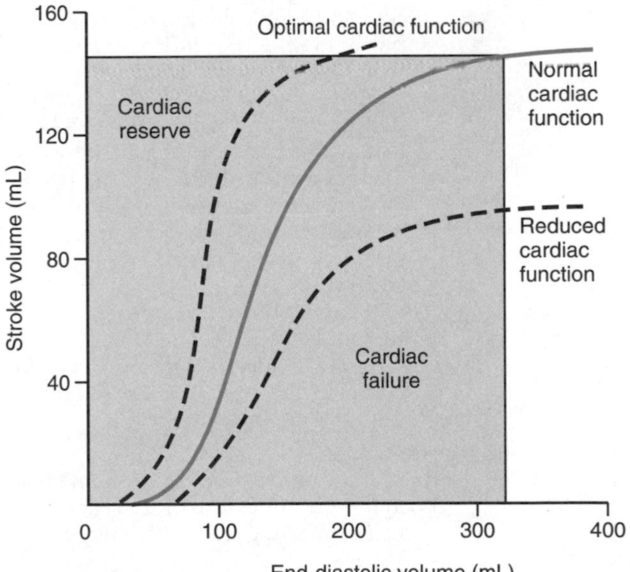

Figure 16–5
Frank-Starling curve. Up to a maximal point, an increase in end-diastolic volume (preload) results in an increase in the contractile force that ejects that volume. In cardiac failure, a rightward shift (more limited increase in stroke volume with increased preload) is evident. The slope of the curve may be altered in the leftward direction by cardiac reserve mechanisms.

owing to hypertrophy. Diuretic drugs or other therapeutic interventions that alter fluid volume also affect the shape of the curve.

Autoregulation of **intrinsic contractility** (inotropic state) involves alteration of the velocity of myocardial fiber contraction, which is independent of the effects of volume or stretch. Intrinsic contractility is based on the *rate* of actin–myosin cross-bridge formation: the faster the rate, the greater is the contractile force generated. Mechanisms of regulation of intrinsic contractility are unknown; however, many drugs are used to alter the inotropic state of the myocardium (Table 16–1). Positive inotropic agents increase contractility (but increase myocardial oxygen demand as a result), whereas negative inotropic agents decrease contractility. Alterations in intrinsic contractility are reflected as changes in the *slope*, but not the maximal point, of the Frank-Starling curve.

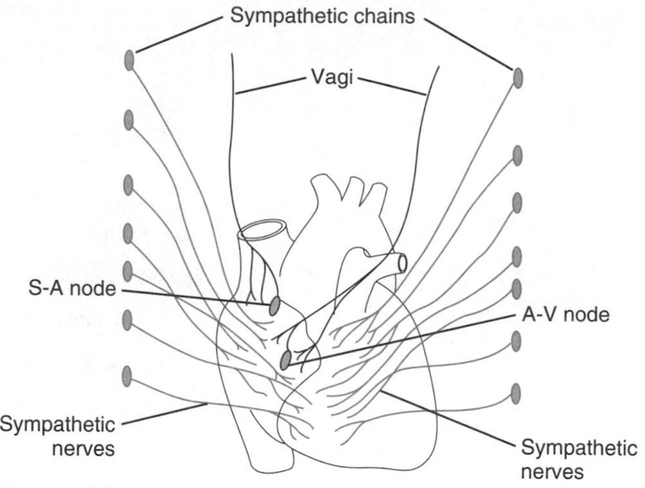

Figure 16–6

Autonomic innervation of the myocardium. Sympathetic nerves innervate the atrial and ventricular myocardium as well as the cardiac conduction system (S-A and A-V nodes). Sympathetic nervous system stimulation increases the rate and force of myocardial contraction. Parasympathetic fibers also innervate the conduction system, with parasympathetic nervous system (PNS) stimulation slowing the heart rate. PNS fibers also innervate the atrial myocardium, but the decrease in contractility resulting from vagal stimulation is primarily due to the effect of slowed rate. (Modified from Guyton, A.C. [1992]. *Human Physiology and Mechanisms of Disease.* [5th ed.]. Philadelphia: W.B. Saunders. [p. 86].)

TABLE 16–1
DRUGS USED TO ALTER CARDIAC CONTRACTILITY

Drug	Mechanism of Action
Positive Inotropic Agents	
Digoxin (Lanoxin)	Inhibition of Na^+-K^+-ATPase activity, causing sodium accumulation in the cell. Na^+ is exchanged for extracellular fluid calcium by the T tubules, with Ca^{2+} influx mediating more forceful contraction.
Amrinone (Inocor)	Inhibition of cyclic adenosine monophosphate (cAMP) phosphodiesterase, leading to an increase in intracellular cAMP, which mediates intrinsic contractility. Calcium movement into the cell, and Ca^{2+} storage within the cell, are also increased.
Dobutamine (Dobutrex)	Direct stimulation of β_1-adrenergic receptors in the myocardium, increasing intracellular cAMP and increasing contractility without inducing vasoconstriction.
Negative Inotropic Agents	
Propranolol (Inderal)	Inhibition of release of norepinephrine and antagonism of catecholamine binding to β-adrenergic receptors.
Verapamil (Calan)	Blocks entry of extracellular fluid calcium into the myocardial cell.
Alcohol	Inhibition of Ca^{2+} binding and reuptake by the sarcoplasmic reticulum; inhibition of mitochondrial function; inhibition of myosin ATPase activity, decreasing actin–myosin cross-bridge cycling.

Neuroendocrine Regulation of Contractility

Autonomic innervation of the myocardium is illustrated in Figure 16–6. As discussed in Chapter 15, neural control of cardiovascular function is primarily automatic or reflex. The most important reflex arc begins with stimulation of baroreceptors in the carotid sinus and aortic arch by pressure or stretch within the walls of these vessels. Baroreceptors signal the vasomotor center in the medulla, and the signal is relayed upward to the hypothalamus for integration with other reflexes. If arterial pressure is high, descending signals along parasympathetic nerves cause a decrease in the rate and force of cardiac contraction; if pressure is low, a sympathetic nervous system (SNS) signal initiates an increased rate and force of cardiac contraction. Higher centers in the central nervous system (e.g., cerebral cortex, limbic system) may influence this reflex regulation, as exemplified by the response to emotional stress (see Chapter 1).

Myocardial fibers contain receptors for norepinephrine, which is the neurotransmitter at sympathetic nerve endings and which is released as a hormone after sympathetic stimulation of the adrenal medulla. Binding of norepinephrine (and also epinephrine from the adrenal medulla) to these β_1-adrenergic receptors results in an increased rate and force of contraction, that is, a positive inotropic effect. Coronary arteries have β_2-adrenergic receptors to which epinephrine binds, resulting in dilation, which facilitates myocardial perfusion and energy metabolism. Sympathetic nervous system stimulation thus accounts for the familiar cardiac manifestations of stress, with the person often aware of a racing, pounding heart.

Parasympathetic fibers (primarily vagus nerve) also innervate the myocardium, and vagal stimulation decreases contractility by cholinergic receptors. Because most parasympathetic fibers are found in the atria rather than in the primary pumps—the ventricles—vagal stimulation is more important in slowing heart rate than in directly influencing contraction (see Chapter 17). Conduction, however, reflected in heart rate and rhythm, significantly influences contraction. Anatomy and physiology of the autonomic nervous system are detailed in Chapter 22.

Cardiac Cycle

The **cardiac cycle** is the series of events occurring during one complete heart beat, or contraction–relaxation sequence.

Sequence of Blood Flow Through the Heart

Figure 16–7 illustrates the normal sequence of blood flow through the heart, beginning arbitrarily at the point at which systemic venous blood returns to the right atrium through the superior and inferior vena cavae. Blood then flows through the tricuspid valve, into the right ventricle, through the pulmonic valve, and into the pulmonary arterial circulation, where it is oxygenated. Pulmonary veins empty into the left atrium, and this blood then flows through the mitral valve into the left ventricle. The left ventricular volume is ejected through the aortic valve into the aorta, leading into the systemic circulation.

Systole and Diastole

Systole (contraction and ejection) and **diastole** (relaxation and filling), the two physiologic components of each cardiac cycle, are generally described with reference to the ventricles. As shown in Figure 16–8, the ventricles are full at the end of diastole. In response to an electrical stimulus, systole begins with *isovolumetric ventricular contraction*, an increase in myocardial tension that closes the tricuspid and mitral valves. As contraction continues, ventricular chamber pressure rises until it exceeds pressure in the aortic and pulmonic valves, causing them to open (*ventricular ejection*). Ejection of a portion of the ventricular volume (normally, 50% to 70%, known as the **ejection fraction**) then occurs, with the right ventricle pumping into the pulmonary artery and the left ventricle pumping into the aorta. As the volume is depleted during ejection, ventricular chamber pressure falls.

Ventricular diastole begins when ventricular chamber pressure falls below pressure in the pulmonary artery and the aorta, causing the pulmonic and aortic valves to close. The myocardium relaxes (*isovolumetric ventricular relaxation*), and ventricular

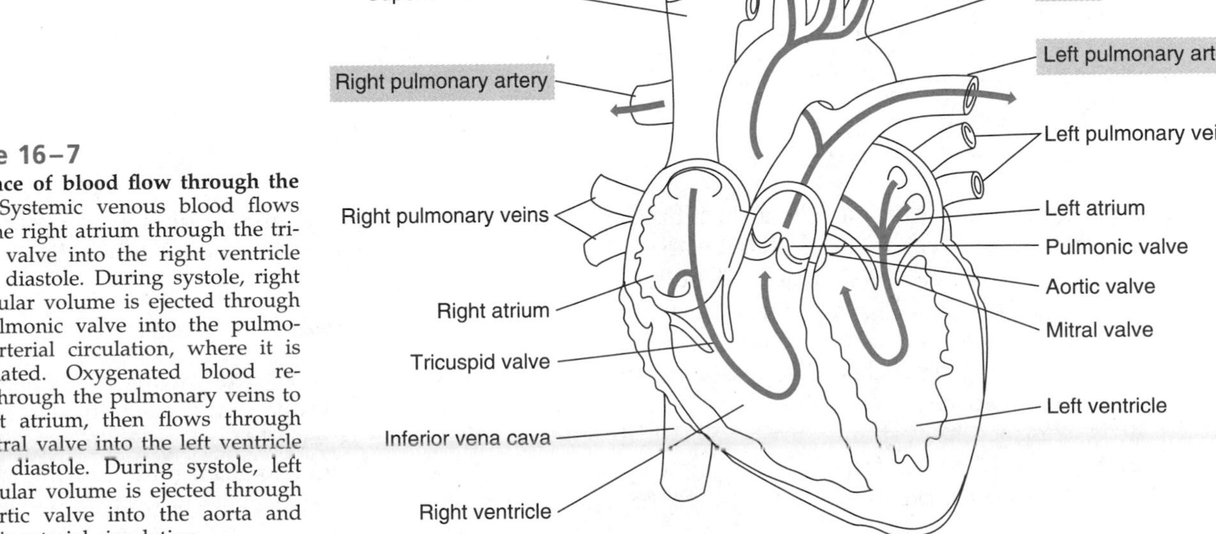

Figure 16–7
Sequence of blood flow through the heart. Systemic venous blood flows from the right atrium through the tricuspid valve into the right ventricle during diastole. During systole, right ventricular volume is ejected through the pulmonic valve into the pulmonary arterial circulation, where it is oxygenated. Oxygenated blood returns through the pulmonary veins to the left atrium, then flows through the mitral valve into the left ventricle during diastole. During systole, left ventricular volume is ejected through the aortic valve into the aorta and systemic arterial circulation.

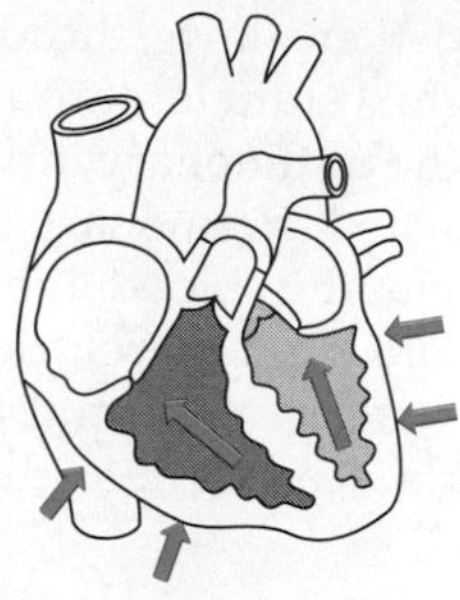

1. Isovolumetric ventricular contraction
Electrical stimulation of the ventricular muscle causes a rise in myocardial wall tension, closing the tricuspid and mitral valves.

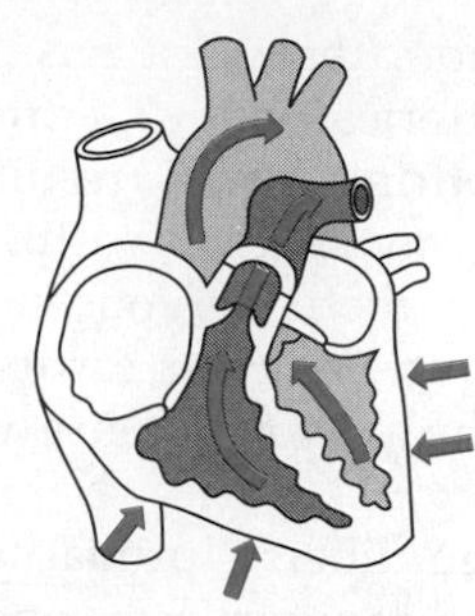

2. Ventricular ejection
Wall tension continues to rise, increasing ventricular chamber pressure, which opens the aortic and pulmonic valves and ejects the ventricular volume.

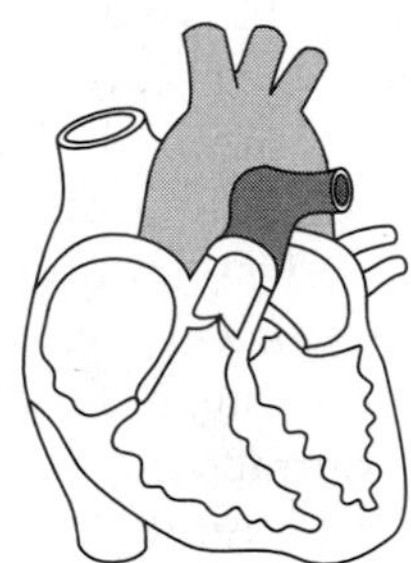

3. Isovolumetric ventricular relaxation
The electrical stimulus ends, and myocardial tension falls.

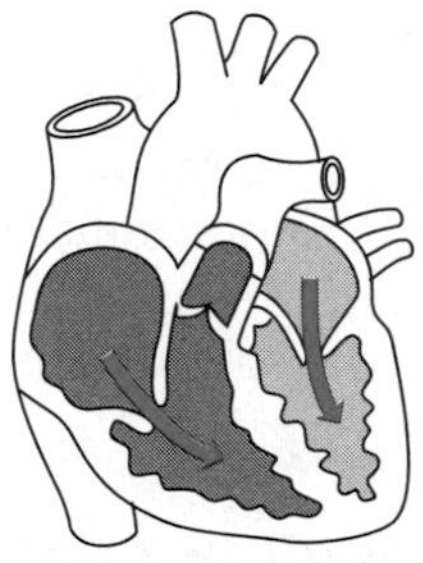

4. Late diastole
The atria, then the ventricles, begin to fill passively because venous pressure exceeds chamber pressure.

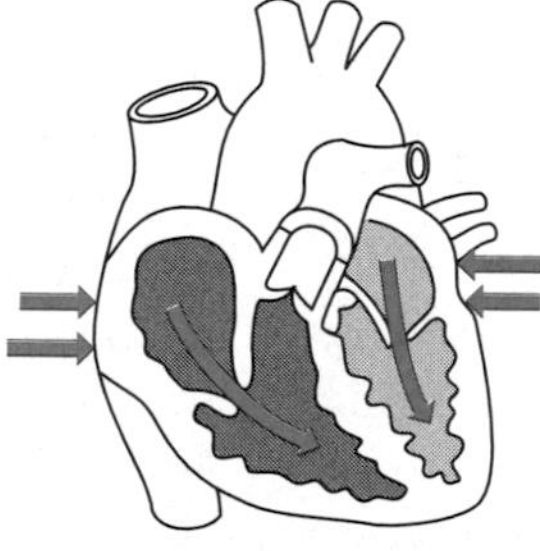

5. Atrial systole
Electrical stimulation of the atria causes atrial contraction, which pumps the final 25% of atrial volume into the ventricles.

Figure 16–8

Phases of the cardiac cycle. The cardiac cycle (systole and diastole) is illustrated, beginning arbitrarily at the point where the ventricles are full (at end-diastole), and the electrical stimulus is received by the ventricular myocardium.

chamber pressure continues to fall. The atria fill passively during this time because atrial chamber pressure is less than that in the vena cavae and pulmonary veins. During *late diastole,* when atrial pressure exceeds ventricular pressure, the atrioventricular valves open, and the ventricles fill passively to about 75% of their capacity. Near the end of diastole, the atria contract in response to an electrical stimulus, and this *atrial systole* (atrial "kick") actively pumps the final 25% of atrial blood into the ventricles. When the electrical stimulus is conducted to the ventricles, ventricular systole begins again.

Heart Sounds

Normal Heart Sounds. The cardiac cycle produces sounds that are audible with a stethoscope, and these heart sounds provide an important noninvasive method of diagnosing and monitoring abnormalities of the cardiac cycle. The normal cycle produces two primary sounds, S_1 (the first heart sound) and S_2 (the second heart sound), often characterized as "lub dub." The relationship of the normal heart sounds to the cardiac cycle is diagrammed in Figure 16–9. The heart sounds are generated from the *closure* of valve pairs during the cycle (valve opening is normally silent). S_1 is produced by closure of the tricuspid and mitral valves at the beginning of systole. S_2 is produced by closure of the aortic and pulmonic valves at the beginning of diastole. At normal heart rates, diastole is longer than systole, and the sounds are perceived as coupled, with a brief pause between each cycle. At more rapid heart rates, the pause may not be discernible.

Adventitious Sounds. Adventitious sounds (added sounds) may be superimposed on the normal sounds. Although these sounds may be normal variants in some cases, they often signify abnormality of the cardiac cycle. A **gallop rhythm** (so called because it mimics the sound of the hoofbeats of a galloping horse) is present when a third heart sound (S_3) is heard in early diastole, or when a fourth heart sound (S_4) is heard late in diastole (see Fig. 16–9). In some cases, both S_3 and S_4 are heard, and the condition is referred to as a *summation gallop*. S_3 is believed to be an echo caused by very rapid filling of a noncompliant ventricle, whereas S_4 is produced by abnormally forceful atrial contraction. Both of these conditions are typical of CHF.

Other adventitious sounds may originate from splitting of a normal heart sound into two components, due to asynchronous closure of the valve pairs. In some cases, this may be a normal variant due to slight differences in left-sided and right-sided pressures, which are enhanced during respiration. In other cases, splitting indicates pathology of a valve. Valve opening may become audible in valve disease or when artificial valves have been implanted, producing opening sounds such as clicks and snaps.

Murmurs are vibratory (blowing or rushing) sounds produced by increased turbulence of blood flow during the cycle. Murmurs may be normal variants ("innocent" or functional murmurs) in children and young adults if they are low grade (barely audible) and if they occur during systole. Transient murmurs may be present during acute cardiac failure with very rapid flow through the heart. Higher-grade murmurs or those occurring during diastole or throughout the cycle always signify congenital or acquired defects of the heart wall, major vessels, or valves (Table 16–2). Low-grade murmurs *may* also indicate advanced valve disease because severe narrowing of a valve opening would permit little flow.

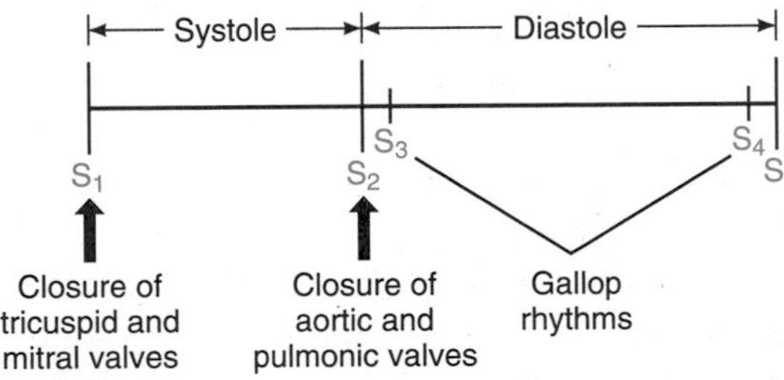

Figure 16–9

Heart sounds. The normal heart sounds are S_1, the first heart sound, and S_2, the second heart sound. These "lub dub" sounds are produced by closure of the atrioventricular (tricuspid and mitral) valves at the beginning of systole, and by the closure of the semilunar (aortic and pulmonic) valves at the beginning of diastole. The third and fourth heart sounds (S_3 and S_4) are added sounds that are usually abnormal. S_3, heard early in diastole, signifies rapid filling of a noncompliant ventricle; whereas S_4 indicates increased force of atrial contraction. These *gallop rhythms* are often present in cardiac failure.

Cardiac Output

Calculation and Measurement

Cardiac output (CO), the volume of blood pumped by the left ventricle in 1 minute, is calculated from the following formula:

$$CO = HR \times SV$$

Cardiac output is determined by heart rate (HR) and **stroke volume** (SV). Stroke volume is the volume of blood ejected by the left ventricle during each systole. Normal cardiac output ranges from 4 to 8 liters/minute, a range so wide that it is not useful as a diagnostic parameter. Serial measurements of cardiac output are commonly employed in critical care units to monitor trends, however. **Cardiac index** is calculated by dividing cardiac output by the body surface area of the person, thus adjusting for body size and making cardiac index a more useful normative reference. Normal cardiac index is 2.4 to 3.8 liters/minute.

In clinical settings, cardiac output may be measured by the thermodilution method using a pulmonary artery (Swan-Ganz) catheter (Fig. 16–10). This catheter, which has a thermal sensor near its tip, is inserted into a central vein, threaded into the right side of the heart, and floated into the pulmonary artery. To measure cardiac output, a cool or room-temperature bolus of fluid (usually 5% dextrose in water) is injected into the right atrium through an opening in the catheter. This induces cooling of the blood flowing past the sensor in the pulmonary artery, and cardiac output is then calculated by com-

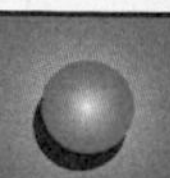

TABLE 16-2
CLASSIFICATION OF CARDIAC MURMURS

CLASSIFICATION PARAMETERS

Timing
Systolic
Diastolic
Continuous

Intensity (Grade)
For systolic murmurs:
- Grade 1 (barely audible)
- Grade 2 (faint, but immediately audible)
- Grade 3 (easily heard)
- Grade 4 (easily heard and associated with a palpable vibration [thrill] over the precordium)
- Grade 5 (very loud; heard with stethoscope lightly on chest)
- Grade 6 (audible without the stethoscope directly on chest wall)

For diastolic murmurs:
- Grade 1 (barely audible)
- Grade 2 (faint, but immediately audible)
- Grade 3 (easily heard)
- Grade 4 (very loud)

Location
Aortic area
Pulmonic area
Tricuspid area
Mitral area

Shape
- Crescendo–decrescendo or diamond-shaped (murmur increases, then decreases in intensity throughout cardiac cycle)
- Crescendo (murmur increases in intensity)
- Decrescendo (murmur decreases in intensity)
- Uniform or pansystolic (murmur is constant in intensity)

CLASSIFICATION OF COMMON MURMURS

Aortic stenosis—systolic murmur, crescendo–decrescendo
Mitral insufficiency—systolic murmur, pansystolic
Ventricular septal defect—systolic murmur, pansystolic
Aortic insufficiency—diastolic, decrescendo
Mitral stenosis—diastolic, decrescendo
Atrial septal defect—late diastolic, decrescendo
Patent ductus arteriosus—continuous, crescendo–decrescendo

Data from Lilly, L.S. (Ed.) (1993). *Pathophysiology of Heart Disease.* Philadelphia: Lea & Febiger. (pp. 24–28).

puter as proportional to the rate and degree of this temperature change.

Determinants of Cardiac Output

As indicated by the formula, any factor altering heart rate, stroke volume, or both affects cardiac output. A significant decline in cardiac output defines most cardiac failure. Heart rate is regulated by the baroreceptor reflex as well as by intrinsic pacemaker mechanisms within the cardiac conduction

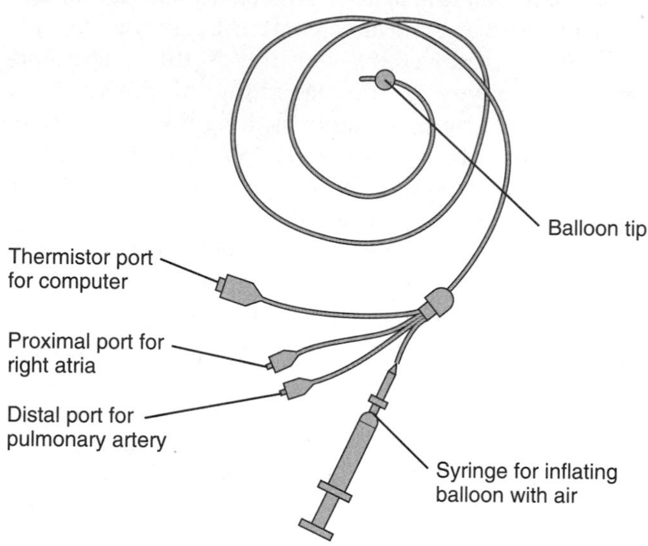

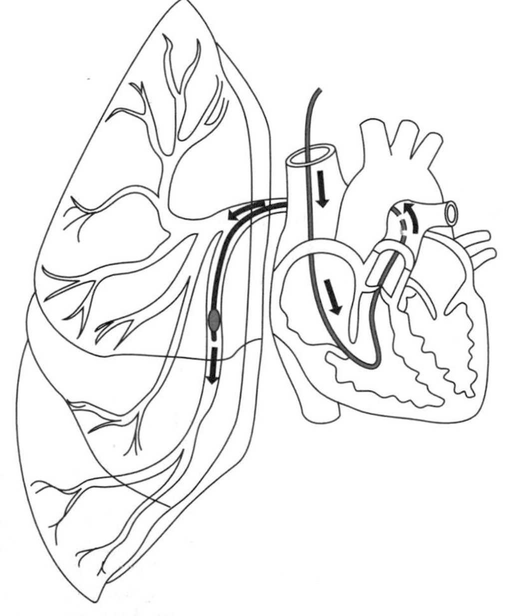

Figure 16–10
Pulmonary artery catheter. Hemodynamic monitoring in critical care settings involves the use of a flow-directed catheter inserted through the right side of the heart into the pulmonary artery. Cardiac output may be calculated as proportional to the rate and degree of temperature change, sensed by a thermistor at the catheter tip, when a bolus of cool solution is injected into the right atrium. Right atrial pressure (RAP), pulmonary artery pressure (PAP), and pulmonary artery wedge pressure (PAWP) may also be measured with this device. RAP evaluates right-sided preload, and PAP indicates right ventricular afterload. PAWP (in which a balloon is briefly inflated to wedge the catheter in a pulmonary artery branch) indicates left-sided pressure.

system, discussed in Chapter 17. If stroke volume is held constant, a decrease in heart rate results in a decrease in cardiac output and could possibly precipitate cardiac failure.

Stroke volume is influenced by four factors: **preload, afterload,** intrinsic contractility, and heart rate. Preload is the amount of stretch or tension of the ventricular myocardium just prior to contraction. Preload is derived from venous return (which reflects circulating volume) and is often quantified as the pressure or volume of a ventricle at the end of diastole, or left ventricular end-diastolic volume. Central venous pressure and right atrial pressure are clinical indicators of right ventricular preload; whereas pulmonary artery wedge pressure is a measure of left ventricular preload. Pulmonary artery wedge pressure and right atrial pressure measurements may be obtained from the Swan-Ganz catheter (see Fig. 16–10). Increasing left ventricular preload (e.g., with fluid administration) results in increased stroke volume, up to the maximum point indicated by the Frank-Starling curve. Beyond this point, increasing preload may precipitate failure due to increased wall stress and pericardial restraint of ventricular filling.

Afterload is the force *opposing* ventricular ejection, originating primarily from pressure or resistance in the systemic circulation for the left ventricle and the pulmonary circulation for the right ventricle. Increasing afterload (e.g., with vasoconstriction due to hormone effects or to drug therapy) decreases stroke volume except in cases in which vasodilation is present as a baseline state. In these cases (e.g., septic shock), vasoconstriction shunts pooled venous blood back to the heart, temporarily increasing preload and cardiac output.

Increasing contractility results in increased stroke volume up to the point at which increased myocardial oxygen consumption becomes a limiting factor. In addition to its independent effect on cardiac output, heart rate affects stroke volume. With rapid heart rates (*tachycardias*), diastole is shortened, potentially decreasing ventricular filling time and reducing stroke volume. Up to a point, however, the summation phenomenon compensates for decreased filling time by increasing the force of contraction proportionately to the increase in heart rate (see Chapter 5). This compensation is limited, however. Very rapid rates result in a decrease in cardiac output not only because of lack of filling time but also because of reduced coronary artery perfusion. The coronary arteries are unique in that they fill during diastole as aortic blood rebounds against the closed aortic valve. Furthermore, tachycardia causes an increase in myocardial oxygen consumption; thus, increased metabolic demand may offset increased cardiac output.

Concept of Cardiac Reserve

Cardiac reserve is the degree to which the heart can increase cardiac output in response to increased metabolic demands (e.g., physical exertion or psychological stress). Normally, cardiac reserve allows for about a three-fold increase by mechanisms that increase heart rate, stroke volume, or both. Heart rate may increase as a result of autonomic reflexes, but this compensation is limited owing to decreases in filling time and coronary perfusion. Dilation of cardiac chambers may allow increased preload up to the Frank-Starling maximum. Hypertrophy of the ventricular myocardium occurs in response to increased afterload, increasing contractile force and ejection fraction to a point. The hypertrophied ventricle becomes less compliant as it thickens, however, and may eventually impinge on the coronary arteries embedded within it. Compensatory mechanisms, such as tachycardia, hypertrophy, and dilation, thus compensate for increased demands to the extent of the person's cardiac reserve. Cardiac failure occurs when these mechanisms are insufficient, and this is the basis for use of the term *cardiac decompensation* as a synonym for failure.

Patients with chronic cardiac failure usually rely on their cardiac reserve to fulfill their activities of daily living, leaving no additional reserve for unusual demands. The elderly have diminished cardiac reserve, even in the absence of cardiac disease. Aerobically conditioned athletes have increased cardiac reserve owing to increased efficiency of cardiac and skeletal muscle in both extraction and use of oxygen (see Chapter 35).

Classification of Cardiac Failure

Cardiac failure may be classified not only on the basis of cardiac output as high-output or low-output failure, discussed earlier, but also with regard to its onset and course. Failure may be acute or chronic; left-sided, right-sided, or biventricular; systolic or diastolic. Acute failure may develop suddenly with severe **myocardial infarction** if destruction of heart muscle is extensive, or with certain dysrhythmias. Chronic failure is more usual, however, and is often associated with gradual worsening of coronary heart disease or hypertension.

Left-sided versus right-sided failure refers to clinical manifestations associated with disease of a specific ventricle. Failure of the left ventricle is associated with decreased cardiac output and pulmonary congestion, whereas failure of the right ventricle results in increased central venous pressure and hepatomegaly. As discussed later in this chapter, functional interdependence of the ventricles ultimately results in failure of both ventricles in nearly all cases, regardless of the site of the initial failure.

Recently, the terms *systolic* and *diastolic* have been used to differentiate the pathophysiologic mechanism of cardiac failure. Systolic heart failure is present when the heart's ability to contract during systole is decreased (as in myocardial infarction or other ischemic heart disease), and diastolic heart failure refers to the heart's inability to relax during diastole (as in ventricular hypertrophy or hypertensive heart disease). Systolic failure results in decreased cardiac output, whereas diastolic failure produces pulmonary or systemic vascular congestion. Often, both forms are present simultaneously.

DISORDERS OF CARDIAC CONTRACTION

The clinical syndrome of CHF is discussed next, followed by selected disorders that may culminate in CHF.

Congestive Heart Failure

Definition. CHF is a syndrome in which cardiac output is not adequate to meet tissue metabolic demands, usually accompanied by rising pressure and volume in the pulmonary or systemic venous systems. Because increased filling pressures and venous congestion are not always present, the recent practice guideline issued by the U.S. Department of Health and Human Services Agency for Health Care Policy and Research has recommended that the term *congestive* no longer be used as broadly as in the past.[3]

Epidemiology. The prevalence of CHF has been estimated at up to 3 million in the United States, with about 400,000 new cases diagnosed each year.[4] Aging is an independent risk factor for development of CHF, owing to degenerative changes in cardiac tissues. As discussed in Chapter 33, premature birth also carries increased risk owing to persistence of fetal structures (see Developmental Perspective). A number of disorders of the heart and other organs may result in abnormal preload, afterload, contractility, or metabolic demands, thus constituting risk factors for CHF.

Etiology. CHF may be caused by increased preload, decreased preload, increased afterload, or less commonly, greatly increased metabolic demands (Table 16–3).

Increased Preload. Fluid overload, whether iatrogenic or pathologic (e.g., due to renal failure), results in increased venous return, potentially overwhelming the capacity of the heart to eject blood at the same rate. Pressure and volume rise behind the failing ventricle, creating congestion. Structural heart defects (e.g., valve disorders or septal defects) in which a divided flow state is created increase preload in that some of the blood is inefficiently recycled through the heart or lungs rather than being pumped into the systemic circulation.

Decreased Preload. Decreased venous return or limitation of ventricular filling reduces stroke volume, resulting in inadequate cardiac output. Venous

TABLE 16–3
MECHANISMS OF CONGESTIVE HEART FAILURE WITH ASSOCIATED DISORDERS

MECHANISM	EXAMPLES OF DISORDERS
Increased preload	Iatrogenic fluid overload Renal failure Hyperaldosteronism Mitral insufficiency Left-to-right intracardiac shunting
Decreased preload, limitation of ventricular filling	Hemorrhagic shock Dehydration Overdiuresis Constrictive pericarditis Cardiac tamponade Tachyarrhythmias Ventricular hypertrophy
Increased afterload	Hypertension Aortic stenosis Aortic outflow tract obstruction Coarctation of the aorta Hypoxic pulmonary vasoconstriction
Decreased contractility	Myocardial infarction Myocardial ischemia Ventricular hypertrophy Ventricular dilation Ventricular aneurysm Myocardial depression in shock Cardiomyopathies Negative inotropic drugs Primary neuromuscular disorders Starvation Dysrhythmias
Greatly increased metabolic demands	Pregnancy Thyroid storm Malignant hyperthermia Sepsis Status asthmaticus Status epilepticus Profound anemias

return is decreased in hypovolemia (e.g., hemorrhagic shock), third spacing (e.g., ascites), or systemic vasodilation (e.g., septic shock). Reduced filling may result from decreased compliance of the ventricle, as with aging or with myocardial hypertrophy. Ventricular filling may be impaired by the pericardium if it is noncompliant due to **constrictive pericarditis**, or if myocardial dilation exceeds the elastic limits of the pericardium (*pericardial restraint*). Rarely, **cardiac tamponade**, in which the pericardial sac or mediastinal space fills with blood or exudate, impedes ventricular filling and leads to acute heart failure.

Increased Afterload. High pulmonary vascular resistance (e.g., **pulmonary edema**) and systemic vascular resistance (e.g., hypertension and some **congenital heart defects**) oppose ventricular ejection, limiting stroke volume and inducing ventricular remodeling (hypertrophy and, ultimately, dilation), which may eventually compromise myocardial perfusion and contractility.

Decreased Contractility. Intrinsic contractility may be compromised by poor myocardial perfusion secondary to coronary atherosclerosis, by primary disease of the myocardium (e.g., **myocarditis** or **cardiomyopathy**), by degenerative changes with aging, or by necrosis of myocardium secondary to myocardial infarction. A number of drugs also have negative inotropic effects.

Increased Metabolic Demands. Metabolic demands that exceed cardiac reserve may also precipitate failure, especially in hearts compromised by structural disorder.

Pathophysiology. Although isolated right-sided or left-sided cardiac failure is possible, preload–afterload relationships nearly always cause both ventricles to fail eventually, regardless of the site of the original defect. Failure of the left ventricle (e.g., with myocardial infarction) leads to increased pressure in the pulmonary system. This congestion creates increased afterload against which the right ventricle must pump, causing it to fail as well. If the right ventricle fails first (as in *cor pulmonale* due to high pulmonary resistance), less volume is pumped into the pulmonary system and left atrium. Left ventricular preload is thus decreased, causing left ventricular failure by this mechanism.

Similarly, either systolic or diastolic failure may be present, and many patients have aspects of both. In systolic failure, inadequate cardiac contractility results in "forward" effects of CHF, represented by a rightward shift in the Frank-Starling curve. Decreased cardiac output leads to decreased tissue perfusion (ischemia) as well as to an increase in the volume remaining in the ventricle at the end of systole. Anaerobic metabolism predominates in ischemic tissues, resulting in lactic acidosis. Cardiogenic shock syndrome may ensue if the perfusion deficit is severe (see Chapter 15).

"Backward" effects of CHF are those due to increased end-systolic volume as congestion develops behind (i.e., upstream to) the failing chamber. Retention of volume in the left ventricle generates pressure, which is projected backward into pulmonary vessels; whereas increased right ventricular pressure is projected into the systemic venous system. Compensatory fluid retention or associated diastolic failure may also contribute to congestion.

Decreased circulating blood volume and tissue perfusion trigger compensatory neuroendocrine responses, including (1) vasoconstriction and increased contractility mediated by the SNS, (2) fluid retention and vasoconstriction mediated by antidiuretic hormone, and (3) sodium and water retention and vasoconstriction mediated by the renin–angiotensin–aldosterone system (RAAS). Increased end-systolic volume results in (1) increased secretion of atrial natriuretic peptide, which offsets the effects of RAAS stimulation at first (see Chapter 8); and (2) ventricular remodeling (hypertrophy and dilation), presumably mediated by local cytokines released in response to altered ventricular wall stress. Unless precipitating factors are removed, these initially compensatory responses culminate in a positive feedback loop. Continued fluid retention increases preload, vasoconstriction increases afterload, and increased contractility magnifies the oxygen demand of the failing myocardium.

Up to 40% of patients with CHF have isolated diastolic failure, in which ventricular contractility is normal or even enhanced, but one or both ventricles are too stiff to fill adequately at normal (low) diastolic pressures, leading to decreased stroke volume and decreased cardiac output.[5]

In diastolic failure, increased stiffness (decreased compliance) shifts the Frank-Starling curve to the left, indicating that a higher filling pressure is required to produce a given end-diastolic volume. Under these conditions, passive ventricular filling during diastole is limited, and the contribution of atrial systole becomes more important. A rise in atrial pressure reflects the rise in ventricular pressure, and atrial wall stress leads to hypertrophy and dilation. The proportion of ventricular filling attributed to atrial systole may rise as high as 40%.[6]

Clinical Manifestations. Clinical manifestations of CHF are categorized in Table 16–4. The cardiovascular system manifests signs of adaptation or compensation for decreased cardiac output, namely poor exercise tolerance, weakness and fatigue, increased heart rate (tachycardia), cardiomegaly due to dilation and hypertrophy, gallop rhythm, and possibly

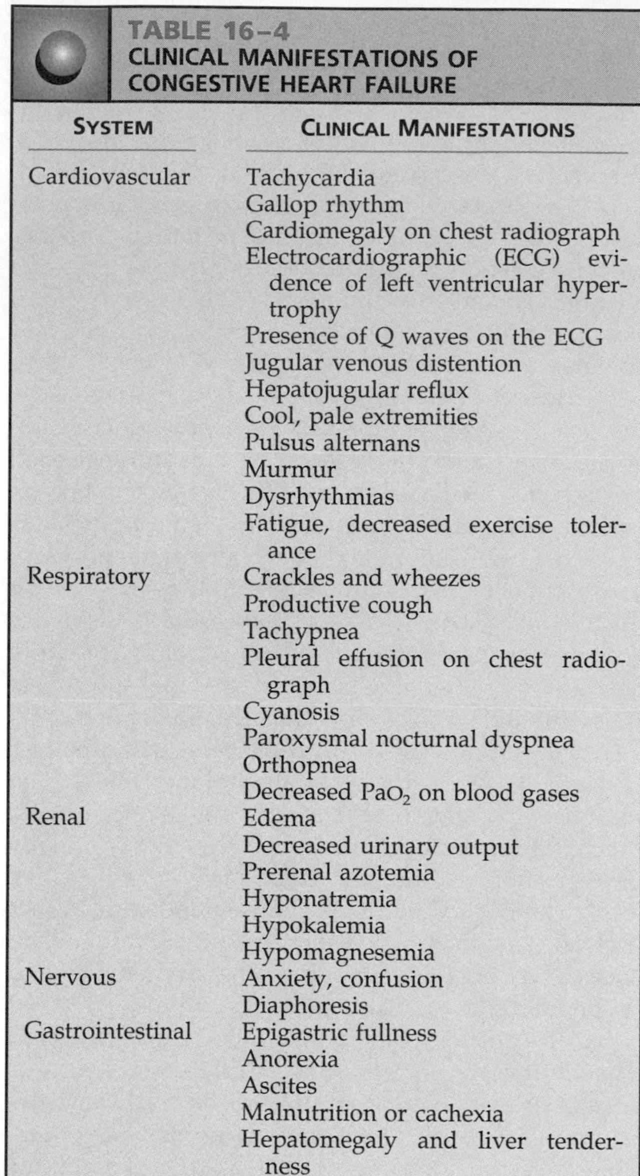

TABLE 16–4
CLINICAL MANIFESTATIONS OF CONGESTIVE HEART FAILURE

System	Clinical Manifestations
Cardiovascular	Tachycardia Gallop rhythm Cardiomegaly on chest radiograph Electrocardiographic (ECG) evidence of left ventricular hypertrophy Presence of Q waves on the ECG Jugular venous distention Hepatojugular reflux Cool, pale extremities Pulsus alternans Murmur Dysrhythmias Fatigue, decreased exercise tolerance
Respiratory	Crackles and wheezes Productive cough Tachypnea Pleural effusion on chest radiograph Cyanosis Paroxysmal nocturnal dyspnea Orthopnea Decreased PaO_2 on blood gases
Renal	Edema Decreased urinary output Prerenal azotemia Hyponatremia Hypokalemia Hypomagnesemia
Nervous	Anxiety, confusion Diaphoresis
Gastrointestinal	Epigastric fullness Anorexia Ascites Malnutrition or cachexia Hepatomegaly and liver tenderness

cardiogenic shock. Congestion of blood behind the failing right ventricle results in jugular venous distention. Dilation and ischemia may disrupt cardiac conduction, leading to dysrhythmias, and sudden cardiac death is possible (see Chapter 17). Slowed blood flow and possibly neuroendocrine factors lead to a hypercoagulable state, increasing the risk for myocardial infarction, stroke, and deep vein thrombosis. The New York Heart Association criteria are often used to grade the severity of CHF on the basis of fatigue and dyspnea (Table 16–5).

When the left ventricle fails, congestion of the pulmonary venous system occurs, resulting in difficulty breathing (dyspnea), orthopnea (the need to sit upright to breathe), pallor, or cyanosis. When pulmonary venous pressure rises greatly, fluid exudes from pulmonary capillaries into the interstitium, and possibly into the alveoli, obstructing airways and compromising gas exchange. This condition, pulmonary edema, is discussed in Chapter 19. Fluid may also accumulate in the potential fluid space between the pleural membranes, creating pleural effusion and compromising ventilation, as discussed in Chapter 18.

Hepatomegaly (liver enlargement) occurs because of venous congestion behind the failing right ventricle. Gentle pressure over the liver may produce hepatojugular reflux, a sustained rise in the level of jugular venous pulsation due to increased venous return with this maneuver. Gastrointestinal veins also become engorged with blood, leading to a feeling of fullness and anorexia, and third spacing into the peritoneal cavity (ascites) may occur. In chronic CHF, the patient may become markedly malnourished (cardiac cachexia). Renal function is compromised in CHF, with fluid retention resulting in weight gain and dependent edema. Decreased renal perfusion in severe CHF may lead to acute renal failure (see Chapter 20). Electrolyte imbalances are common owing to the disease and its therapy, with hyponatremia, hypokalemia, and hypomagnesemia most frequently seen[7] (see Chapter 9).

Prevention and Treatment. Prevention of CHF involves reduction of risk factors for atherosclerosis and hypertension (see Chapter 15) as well as monitoring and treatment of the specific disorders associated with CHF syndrome. For some patients, cardiac reserve may be increased with rehabilitative exercise programs. General treatment of CHF is aimed at reduction of metabolic demands with rest and oxygen therapy and at augmentation of cardiac function with drug therapy, mechanical assist devices, or in selected cases, cardiac transplantation (Table 16–6).

Drug therapy of CHF may include diuretics to reduce preload, positive inotropic agents to enhance contractility, β-blocking agents to prevent inappropriate down-regulation of β-adrenergic receptors, in-

TABLE 16–5
NEW YORK HEART ASSOCIATION (NYHA) CLASSIFICATION OF HEART FAILURE

Class	Defining Criteria
NYHA I	No dyspnea or fatigue
NYHA II	Dyspnea or fatigue with ordinary activity
NYHA III	Dyspnea or fatigue with less than ordinary activity
NYHA IV	Dyspnea or fatigue at rest

Adapted from Lilly, L.S. (Ed.). (1993). *Pathophysiology of Heart Disease*. Philadelphia: Lea & Febiger. (p. 160).

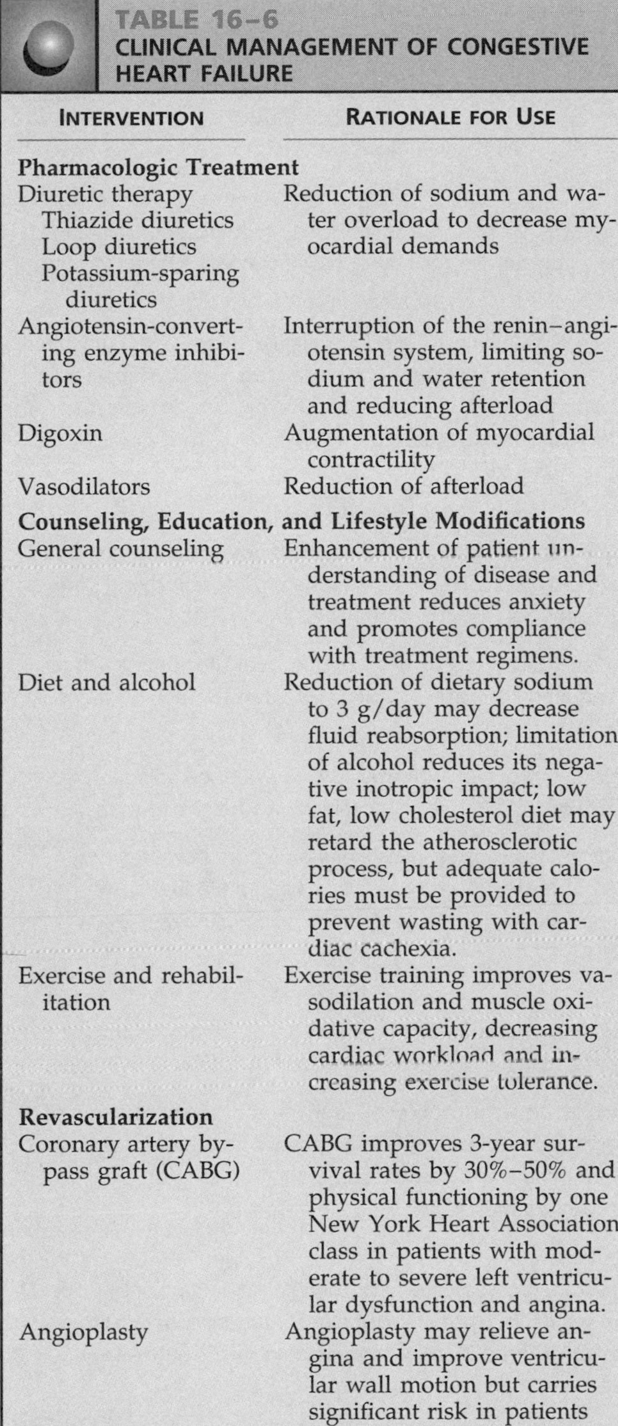

TABLE 16–6
CLINICAL MANAGEMENT OF CONGESTIVE HEART FAILURE

INTERVENTION	RATIONALE FOR USE
Pharmacologic Treatment	
Diuretic therapy Thiazide diuretics Loop diuretics Potassium-sparing diuretics	Reduction of sodium and water overload to decrease myocardial demands
Angiotensin-converting enzyme inhibitors	Interruption of the renin–angiotensin system, limiting sodium and water retention and reducing afterload
Digoxin	Augmentation of myocardial contractility
Vasodilators	Reduction of afterload
Counseling, Education, and Lifestyle Modifications	
General counseling	Enhancement of patient understanding of disease and treatment reduces anxiety and promotes compliance with treatment regimens.
Diet and alcohol	Reduction of dietary sodium to 3 g/day may decrease fluid reabsorption; limitation of alcohol reduces its negative inotropic impact; low fat, low cholesterol diet may retard the atherosclerotic process, but adequate calories must be provided to prevent wasting with cardiac cachexia.
Exercise and rehabilitation	Exercise training improves vasodilation and muscle oxidative capacity, decreasing cardiac workload and increasing exercise tolerance.
Revascularization	
Coronary artery bypass graft (CABG)	CABG improves 3-year survival rates by 30%–50% and physical functioning by one New York Heart Association class in patients with moderate to severe left ventricular dysfunction and angina.
Angioplasty	Angioplasty may relieve angina and improve ventricular wall motion but carries significant risk in patients with ejection fractions below 40%.

Data from Baker, D.W., Konstam, M.A., Bottorff, M., *et al.* (1994). Management of heart failure. I. Pharmacologic treatment. *Journal of the American Medical Association* 272(17), 1361–1366; Dracup, K., Baker, D.W., Dunbar, S.B., *et al.* (1994). Management of heart failure. II. Counseling, education, and lifestyle modifications. *Journal of the American Medical Association* 272(18), 1442–1446; and Baker, D.W., Jones, R., Hodges, J., *et al.* (1994). Management of heart failure. III. The role of revascularization in the treatment of patients with moderate or severe left ventricular systolic dysfunction. *Journal of the American Medical Association* 272(19), 1528–1534.

hibitors of the RAAS to decrease fluid and water retention and vasoconstriction, and vasodilators to decrease afterload and improve coronary perfusion. The most significant advance in the treatment of CHF in the last decade has been the introduction of angiotensin-converting enzyme (ACE) inhibitors as first-line treatment.[8] Total mortality and hospitalization for CHF have been shown to be significantly reduced in a broad range of patients treated with these drugs (see Focus of Current Research). ACE inhibitors interrupt the detrimental effects of the RAAS (fluid retention and vasoconstriction). Nonpeptide angiotensin II receptor blockers have recently been introduced and may serve to augment the effects of ACE inhibitors.[9]

The use of other drugs in the treatment of CHF is traditional but less well documented in terms of efficacy and toxicity. Diuretics reduce preload but may limit the atrial natriuretic peptide response and may predispose to renal failure and electrolyte imbalances. Digoxin, a positive inotropic agent, has been used in the treatment of heart failure for more than 200 years. It has been shown to be of benefit in reducing symptoms in patients with left ventricular systolic failure, but its impact on mortality is unknown.[9] In critical care settings, intravenous dopamine and dobutamine are commonly used to enhance contractility. Direct-acting vasodilators, such as hydralazine and isosorbide dinitrate, may be used to reduce afterload if ACE inhibitors are not well tolerated. Intravenous nitroprusside may be used for this purpose in critical care settings. Calcium-channel blockers are generally contraindicated as vasodilators in CHF because of their negative inotropic effect.[10] β-blockers reduce myocardial oxygen demands but must be used judiciously because their negative effects on heart rate and contractility could worsen failure.[11]

When drug therapy is insufficient, cardiac assist devices may be used on a short-term basis to augment cardiac output. Figure 16–11 illustrates the intra-aortic balloon pump, a cylindrical balloon that is inserted into the aorta and inflated during diastole. This inflation propels blood ahead of the balloon into the systemic circulation and behind it into the coronary circulation. During systole, the balloon is deflated so as not to obstruct ventricular ejection. A number of ventricular assist devices (implantable pumps) have also been used to assist patients awaiting cardiac transplantation. A new surgical technique, dynamic cardiomyoplasty, is under investigation as a bridge to transplantation or for patients who are not candidates for transplantation. This procedure involves wrapping the heart with the patient's latissimus dorsi muscle, then stimulating the muscle to contract using a pacemaker current.[12]

Focus of Current Research

Study	Objective and Findings
Multiple Risk Factor Intervention Trial Research Group (1997) Multiple Risk Factor Intervention trial: Risk factor changes and mortality results.	*Objective:* To test the effect of a multifactor intervention program on mortality from coronary heart disease (CHD) *Findings:* Measures to reduce cigarette smoking and to lower cholesterol may have reduced CHD mortality in certain subgroups. There may have been an unfavorable response to antihypertensive drug therapy in some hypertensive subjects.
The Digitalis Investigation Group (1997) The effect of digoxin on mortality and morbidity in patients with heart failure.	*Objective:* To study the effect of digoxin on mortality and hospitalization in a randomized, double-blind clinical trial *Findings:* Digoxin did not reduce overall mortality, but it reduced the rate of hospitalization for heart failure.
Nwasokawa, et al. (1997) Higher prevalence and greater severity of coronary disease in short versus tall men referred for coronary arteriography.	*Objective:* To test whether the prevalence and severity of coronary disease is variable with height in men *Findings:* Short men had a higher frequency of greater than 50% diameter stenosis, a higher frequency of three-vessel disease, and more total coronary occlusions.
Blair, et al. (1996) Influences of cardiorespiratory fitness and other precursors on cardiovascular disease and all-cause mortality in men and women.	*Objective:* To quantify the relation of cardiorespiratory fitness to cardiovascular disease mortality *Findings:* Low fitness level is an important precursor of mortality. Moderate fitness appears to protect against other predictors of mortality, such as smoking, elevated cholesterol, and hypertension.
The Bypass Angioplasty Revascularization Investigation (BARI) Investigators (1996) Comparison of coronary bypass surgery with angioplasty in patients with multivessel disease.	*Objective:* To test the hypothesis that angioplasty does not result in a poorer outcome than coronary artery bypass grafting in selected patients with multivessel disease *Findings:* As compared with grafting, an initial strategy of angioplasty did not compromise 5-year survival, although subsequent revascularization was required more often. For diabetic patients, 5-year survival was better after bypass.

box continued on following page

Spielberg, et al. (1996). Circadian, day-of-week, and seasonal variability in myocardial infarction: Comparison between working and retired patients.	*Objective:* To analyze the relationships between working status and variability in acute myocardial infarction *Findings:* Infarction occurred more frequently on Monday mornings and during winter months. Working patients demonstrated a second peak at about 4 PM and an additional seasonal peak in September.
Jiang, et al. (1996) Mental stress-induced myocardial ischemia and cardiac events.	*Objective:* To assess the significance of mental stress–induced myocardial ischemia in patients with coronary heart disease *Findings:* Mental stress–induced ischemia is associated with higher rates of fatal and nonfatal cardiac events.
Morrison, et al. (1996) Serum folate and risk of fatal coronary heart disease.	*Objective:* To assess the relationship between serum folate levels and the risk of fatal coronary heart disease *Findings:* Low serum folate levels are associated with an increased risk of fatal coronary heart disease.

For some patients in whom degeneration of myocardium is extensive, cardiac transplantation is the only effective option. Candidates for transplantation generally have an ejection fraction below 25% and are unstable despite medical therapy.[13]

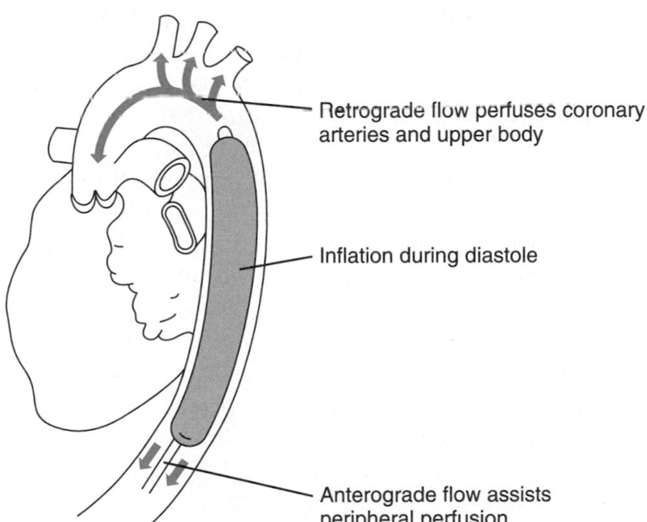
Retrograde flow perfuses coronary arteries and upper body
Inflation during diastole
Anterograde flow assists peripheral perfusion

Figure 16–11
Intra-aortic balloon pump. The failing heart may be assisted by a cylindrical balloon inserted into the descending aorta through the femoral artery. Inflation and deflation of the balloon are synchronized with the cardiac cycle by an arterial pressure or electrocardiogram monitor. Deflation during systole permits flow past the balloon. Inflation during diastole assists in the forward propulsion of blood into the descending aorta and also propels blood backward toward the closed aortic valve. This retrograde flow perfuses the coronary arteries and upper body.

Prognosis and Outcome. The annual mortality rate in CHF patients whose ejection fractions are above 35% has been estimated at 10%. For those with ejection fractions below 20%, the annual mortality rate is 20% to 30%.[14]

Coronary Heart Disease

Definition. Coronary heart disease (CHD) is a condition of decreased perfusion of the myocardium due to occlusion of one or more coronary arteries by atherosclerosis, thrombosis, or spasm. CHD is also known as coronary artery disease, ischemic heart disease, and atherosclerotic cardiovascular disease.

Epidemiology. Despite a continuing decline in mortality over the past several decades, CHD is still the leading cause of death in the United States. About 1.5 million Americans have an acute myocardial infarction each year, and about one third of those people die from sudden cardiac death.[15] The rate of decline in the incidence of CHD is only half as great in women as in men. Although CHD onset is typically later in women, nearly half of all deaths due to myocardial infarction are among women.[16] Risk factors for CHD are essentially the same as those for atherosclerosis, discussed in Chapter 15. Some of these factors, such as age, male sex, and family history, are not amenable to clinical intervention. *Modifiable* coronary risk factors are summarized in Table 16–7 along with interventions designed to reduce risk.

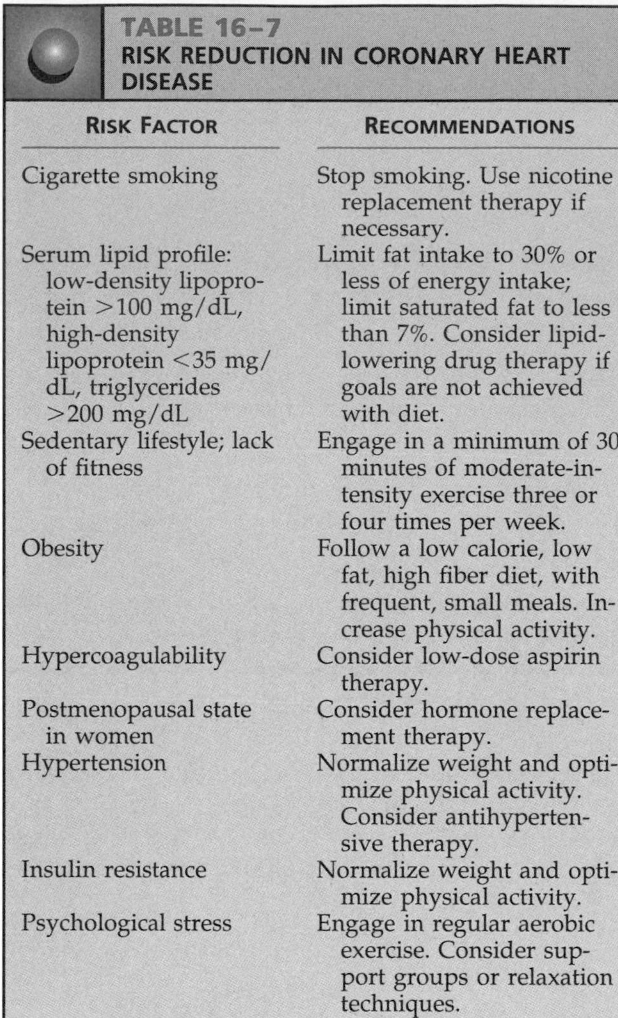
TABLE 16–7
RISK REDUCTION IN CORONARY HEART DISEASE

RISK FACTOR	RECOMMENDATIONS
Cigarette smoking	Stop smoking. Use nicotine replacement therapy if necessary.
Serum lipid profile: low-density lipoprotein >100 mg/dL, high-density lipoprotein <35 mg/dL, triglycerides >200 mg/dL	Limit fat intake to 30% or less of energy intake; limit saturated fat to less than 7%. Consider lipid-lowering drug therapy if goals are not achieved with diet.
Sedentary lifestyle; lack of fitness	Engage in a minimum of 30 minutes of moderate-intensity exercise three or four times per week.
Obesity	Follow a low calorie, low fat, high fiber diet, with frequent, small meals. Increase physical activity.
Hypercoagulability	Consider low-dose aspirin therapy.
Postmenopausal state in women	Consider hormone replacement therapy.
Hypertension	Normalize weight and optimize physical activity. Consider antihypertensive therapy.
Insulin resistance	Normalize weight and optimize physical activity.
Psychological stress	Engage in regular aerobic exercise. Consider support groups or relaxation techniques.

Etiology

Coronary Atherosclerosis. Atherosclerosis underlies nearly all CHD. Gradual occlusion of the coronary artery lumen occurs owing to growing plaque and infiltration by intimal smooth muscle, as discussed in Chapter 15. In response to the action of local plaque-associated cytokines or to the shear stress of blood flow (possibly increased by physical exertion or circadian variation in SNS stimulation), plaque may rupture or develop fissures, exposing the vascular endothelium. Along with slowed flow due to the presence of plaque, endothelial and inflammatory cell mediators trigger inappropriate thrombosis, which may totally occlude the vessel.

The likelihood that plaque will rupture depends on its mechanical properties rather than its size. The core of the plaque (foam cell contents), the composition of the fibrous cap, and the relationship of the plaque to the adjacent arterial wall are apparently key factors.[17] The degree of luminal occlusion with plaque does not correlate directly with acute coronary events, such as thrombosis and infarction. In fact, recent research has revealed that smaller, angiographically insignificant plaques are more likely to rupture. This finding has called into question the practice of routine coronary angiography (cardiac catheterization) to quantify the degree of occlusion.[17] Cardiac catheterization involves insertion of a wire-guided catheter, with injection of x-ray contrast media into coronary arteries and heart chambers.

Coronary Artery Spasm. Coronary spasm is a poorly understood phenomenon that is frequently observed in areas of mild-to-moderate plaque deposition but that may also occur in nonatherosclerotic coronary arteries. Spasm may slow blood flow through the vessel, promoting thrombosis. In rare instances, prolonged spasm totally occludes the vessel, resulting in myocardial infarction. Many factors have been shown to provoke spasm, including the vasoactive amines epinephrine, norepinephrine, and histamine; exposure to cold; and coronary instrumentation (such as catheter insertion during diagnostic coronary angiography).

Pathophysiology. Occlusion of one or more coronary arteries or their branches results in decreased perfusion of the areas of myocardium served by those vessels. When perfusion is insufficient to meet metabolic demands, myocardial ischemia occurs, with accumulation of lactic acid (see Chapter 3). Toxic injury and impaired membrane transport result in pain and impairment of electrical conduction and muscle contraction. Prolonged ischemia results in myocardial infarction, death of myocardial cells.

The extent of myocardial damage depends on the degree and duration of occlusion. Because coronary arteries penetrate the myocardium at 90-degree angles to the surface, the smallest vessels are found deep in the muscle, next to the endocardium. Tissues served by these vessels are first deprived, leading to less extensive *subendocardial* infarction. With more significant occlusion, myocardial damage may extend through the entire thickness of the myocardium in the affected area (*transmural* infarction).

Ischemic damage to cells triggers an inflammatory response, and necrosis of myocardial cells releases intracellular enzymes into the blood. By definition, myocardial infarction results in lethal ischemic injury to a central zone of myocardium. Surrounding the infarcted area is a region of "stunned" myocardial cells, which are damaged but still viable. These cells are dysfunctional for a time but recover if perfusion is restored and drug therapy is instituted to stimulate their contraction.[18] Myocardial damage may become complete and irreversible within 3 or 4 hours or less, unless the infarct zone is adequately perfused by collateral circulation or the occluded artery is opened by medical or surgical intervention.[19]

The injured area of the ventricle expands as cardiac muscle cells slide apart, and the noninfarcted area dilates adaptively. This ventricular remodeling leads to an increased risk of heart failure and dysrhythmias.

Clinical Manifestations. The hallmark of coronary heart disease is ischemic chest pain, known as **angina pectoris** ("strangling in the chest"). Angina may be subclassified as *stable* (occurring predictably with effort or exertion and relieved with rest), *unstable* (occurring unpredictably), or *variant* (having atypical characteristics). Angina is commonly described as severe pressure over the precordium (chest wall overlying the heart), with possible radiation of this pain down one or both arms (often the left arm) or up to the shoulders, neck, or jaw. Episodes of angina pectoris, which signify myocardial ischemia but not necessarily infarction, usually last less than 10 minutes, and the pain rarely changes in either location or quality in a given person.[20] Angina may, however, vary in intensity and radiation. Extreme fatigue with minimal exertion is also typical and, together with angina, forms the basis of the most common system of classification of CHD severity (Table 16–8).

The precise manifestations of myocardial infarction depend on the location and extent of infarction, which depend in turn on the affected coronary arteries and the patient's individual coronary anatomy (Table 16–9). Myocardial infarction may result in chest pain similar to angina, but the pain is usually more severe and prolonged and is not relieved by rest or the patient's usual drug therapy (e.g., nitroglycerin). In about 25% of patients, however, myocardial infarction is "silent," causing no pain.[15] These patients are often elderly or diabetic, with diminished capacity to perceive pain.

Electrical conduction is impaired in the infarcted area, resulting in characteristic abnormalities of the electrocardiogram that reveal the location of the damage (see Chapter 17). Enzymes from damaged or dead myocardial cells are released into the blood in a characteristic pattern that is diagnostic of myocardial infarction, and the degree of elevation of

TABLE 16–8
CANADIAN CARDIOVASCULAR SOCIETY (CCS) CLASSIFICATION OF ANGINA

Class	Defining Criteria
CCS 1	No angina with ordinary activity such as walking and stair-climbing; angina is present with strenuous, rapid, or prolonged activity.
CCS 2	Slight limitation of ordinary activity; walking more than two blocks on the level or climbing more than one flight of stairs induces angina.
CCS 3	Marked limitation of ordinary activity; walking one to two blocks on the level and climbing one flight of stairs induces angina.
CCS 4	Inability to carry on any physical activity without discomfort; anginal symptoms may be present at rest.

Modified from Campeau, L. (1976). Letter to the editor. *Circulation* 54, p. 522, as cited in Hurst, J.W., Schlant, R.C., Rackley, C.E., *et al.* (Eds.). (1990). *The Heart, Arteries, and Veins.* (7th ed.). New York: McGraw-Hill, p. 120.

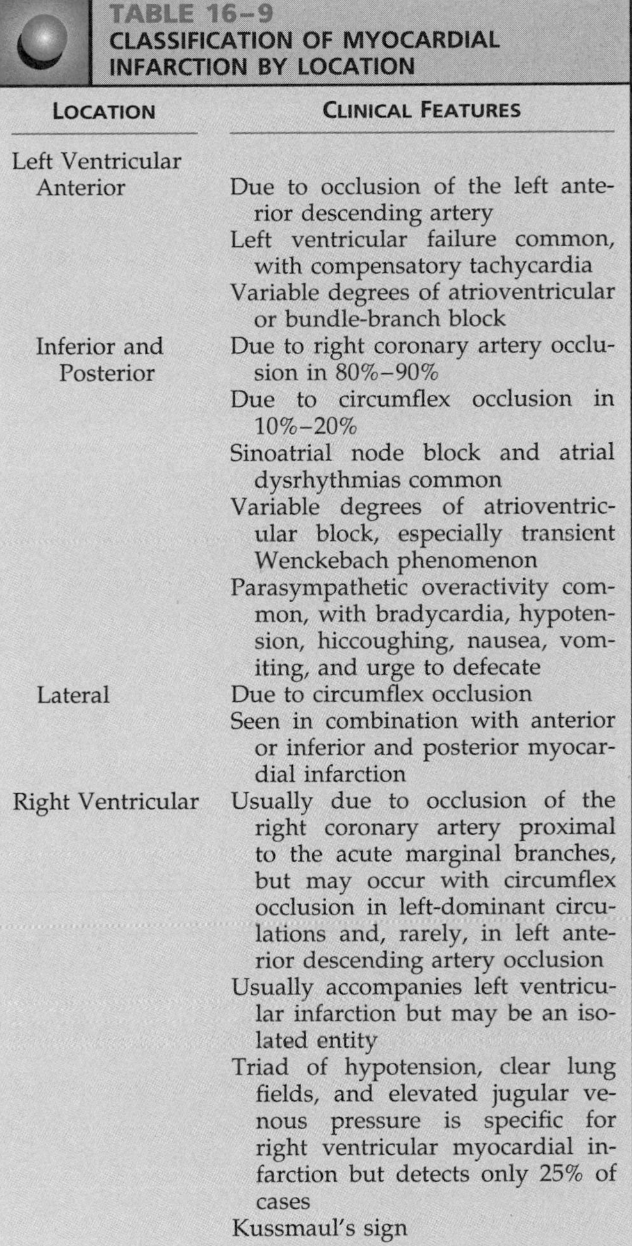

TABLE 16–9
CLASSIFICATION OF MYOCARDIAL INFARCTION BY LOCATION

Location	Clinical Features
Left Ventricular	
Anterior	Due to occlusion of the left anterior descending artery Left ventricular failure common, with compensatory tachycardia Variable degrees of atrioventricular or bundle-branch block
Inferior and Posterior	Due to right coronary artery occlusion in 80%–90% Due to circumflex occlusion in 10%–20% Sinoatrial node block and atrial dysrhythmias common Variable degrees of atrioventricular block, especially transient Wenckebach phenomenon Parasympathetic overactivity common, with bradycardia, hypotension, hiccoughing, nausea, vomiting, and urge to defecate
Lateral	Due to circumflex occlusion Seen in combination with anterior or inferior and posterior myocardial infarction
Right Ventricular	Usually due to occlusion of the right coronary artery proximal to the acute marginal branches, but may occur with circumflex occlusion in left-dominant circulations and, rarely, in left anterior descending artery occlusion Usually accompanies left ventricular infarction but may be an isolated entity Triad of hypotension, clear lung fields, and elevated jugular venous pressure is specific for right ventricular myocardial infarction but detects only 25% of cases Kussmaul's sign

Data from Woods, S.L., and Underhill, S.L. (1989). Myocardial ischemia and infarction. In: Underhill, S.L., Woods, S.L. Froelicher, E.S.S., *et al. Cardiac Nursing.* (2nd ed.). Philadelphia: J.B. Lippincott. (pp. 488–508); and Kinch, J.W., and Ryan, T.J. (1994). Right ventricular infarction. *New England Journal of Medicine* 330(17), 1211–1217.

three "cardiac enzymes" has long been used to estimate the extent of myocardial damage (Fig. 16–12). More recently, assay of serum levels of cardiac troponins T and I have been used to stratify risk after acute myocardial infarction.[21, 22] These enzymes, critical to regulation of cardial muscle contraction, are even more specific for cardiac injury than the classic cardiac enzymes. Coronary angiography may reveal areas of coronary occlusion or areas of the myocardial wall that are contracting poorly. A decreased ejection fraction might be detected with angiography or with noninvasive imaging techniques, such as radionucleotide scans or echocardiography.

A significant number of patients suffering myocardial infarction develop acute CHF, which manifests as cardiogenic shock in those with extensive muscle damage (see Chapter 15). Dysrhythmias are common owing to impaired conduction with ischemia and may also occur when treatment restores patency of the blocked coronary artery. Reperfusion dysrhythmias are discussed in Chapter 17. Reperfusion (restored coronary arterial flow) may induce a paradoxical *decrease* in blood flow to the microvasculature of the myocardium. This **no-reflow phenomenon** may be due to impaired endothelial function or to mechanical plugging of capillaries by neutrophils and red blood cells.[23] Dysrhythmias may be lethal (see Sudden Cardiac Death, Chapter 17).

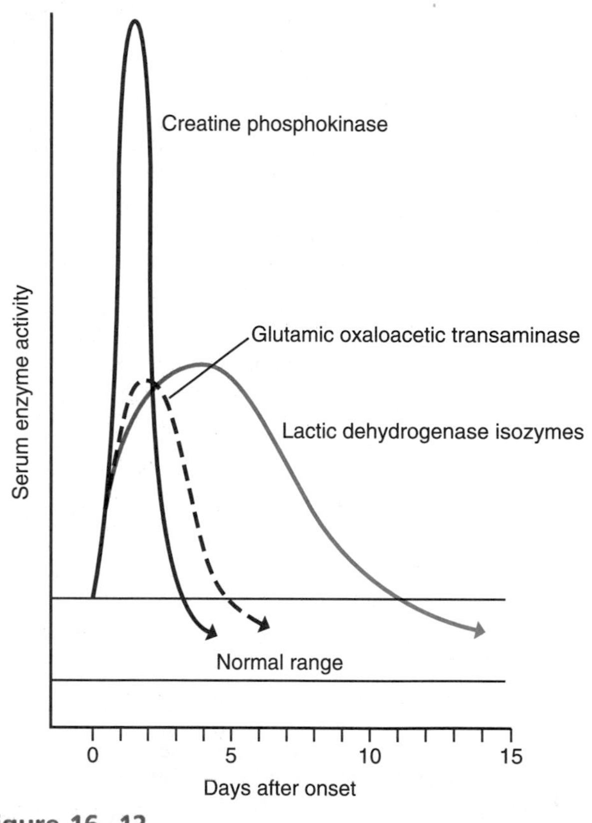

Figure 16–12

Cardiac enzymes. Myocardial ischemia disrupts the integrity of cell membranes, releasing intracellular enzymes into the blood. Serum creatine phosphokinase (CPK, also known as creatine kinase or CK) rises first, followed by glutamic oxaloacetic transaminase (also known as aspartate transaminase or AST), then lactic dehydrogenase (LDH). Certain forms of these enzymes *(isoenzymes)* are more specific to cardiac tissue. The degree of elevation of the MB band of creatine phosphokinase, for example, correlates with the degree of myocardial damage. A rise in LDH(2) greater than LDH(1) also indicates necrosis of myocardial cells. (From Braunwald, E., Alpert, J.S., and Ross, R.S. [1980]. *Harrison's Principles of Internal Medicine.* [9th ed.]. New York: McGraw-Hill. Copyright 1980. Reproduced with permission of the McGraw-Hill Companies.)

Less common clinical manifestations that may complicate myocardial infarction include mural thrombosis, papillary muscle dysfunction, **pericarditis**, and ventricular aneurysm. A mural thrombus is a blood clot that forms on the infarcted area of the myocardial wall. This inappropriate clotting may be triggered by local blood pooling due to impaired contraction or physical defect (e.g., aneurysm). Mural thrombi may embolize into the cerebral circulation, resulting in stroke (see Chapter 21).

Ischemic dysfunction of the papillary muscle, which closes the mitral valve leaflets during systole, may lead to acute mitral regurgitation and heart failure. If severe, this condition may be fatal unless surgical mitral valve replacement is done on an emergency basis.

Pericarditis, inflammation of the pericardial sac, may complicate a transmural infarction if the inflammatory response to myocardial damage extends to the pericardium. During the acute phase of pericarditis, inflammatory exudate may accumulate within the pericardial sac or mediastinal space and impose external pressure on the heart. This cardiac tamponade impedes ventricular filling, reducing preload and precipitating or worsening failure. Later, contraction of pericardial scar tissue may restrict ventricular filling. This late complication is known as *Dressler's syndrome.*

Ventricular aneurysm, a ballooning dilation of the area of infarction, may occur with extensive transmural damage. These aneurysms impede effective contraction and may contribute to mural thrombosis, as discussed earlier. Rupture of a ventricular aneurysm is a potentially lethal complication of myocardial infarction.

Prevention and Treatment. Modifiable risk factors for atherosclerosis should be reduced insofar as possible, including reduction of dietary lipids, maintenance of regular physical activity, and cessation of smoking (see Table 16–7). Underlying conditions, such as obesity, hypertension, and diabetes, should be managed. The preventive use of antiplatelet agents, such as aspirin and ticlopidine (Ticlid), is still a matter of some controversy, but several large studies have indicated a significant reduction in risk of myocardial infarction in patients taking daily low-dose aspirin.[24] Use of drugs to lower lipid levels may be indicated in cases in which hyperlipidemia does not respond to dietary measures (see Chapter 25). Because estrogen apparently exerts a protective effect on the endothelium and on blood lipids, hormone replacement therapy may be indicated for postmenopausal women at high cardiovascular risk[25] (see Chapter 31). Moderate alcohol consumption may also decrease the risk of heart disease, possibly by increasing endothelial production of an endogenous tissue plasminogen activator that inhibits coronary thrombosis.[26]

Medical therapy in coronary heart disease may include a variety of agents, depending on severity of ischemia and presence of dysrhythmia or CHF (Table 16–10). Patients suffering from angina pectoris are appropriately treated with antiplatelet agents and coronary dilators (nitrates, calcium-channel blockers, or β-blockers). In patients with stable angina, this therapy is highly effective in suppressing symptoms.[27] Hemostatic balance is altered therapeutically to favor clot breakdown, as discussed in Chapter 14.

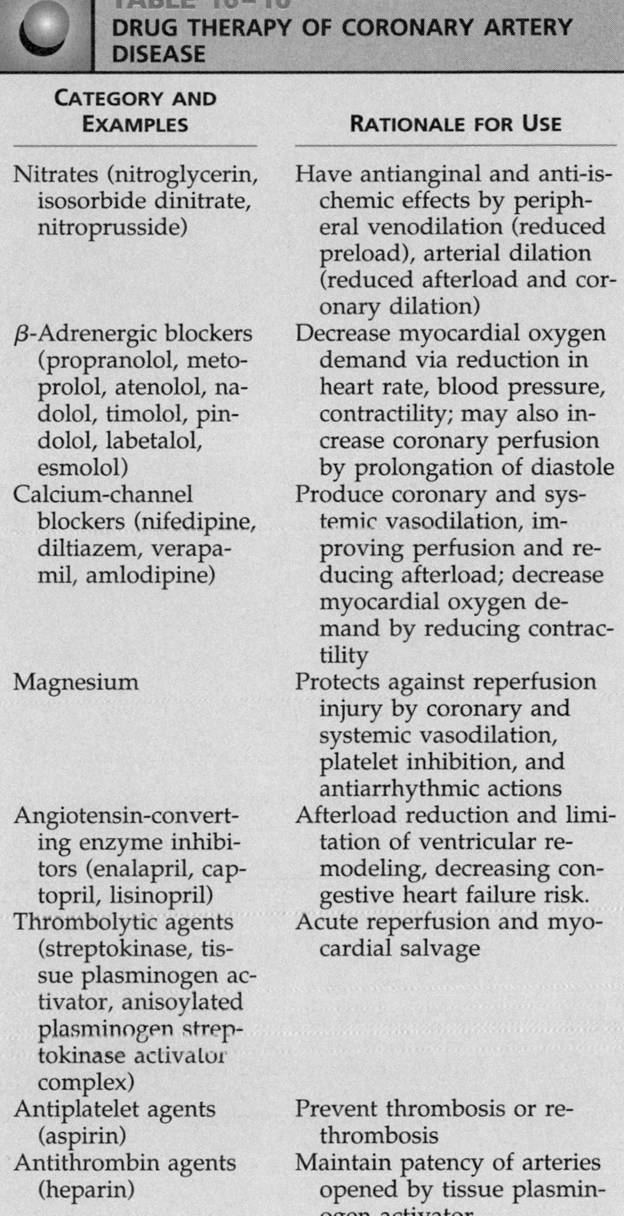

TABLE 16–10
DRUG THERAPY OF CORONARY ARTERY DISEASE

Category and Examples	Rationale for Use
Nitrates (nitroglycerin, isosorbide dinitrate, nitroprusside)	Have antianginal and anti-ischemic effects by peripheral venodilation (reduced preload), arterial dilation (reduced afterload and coronary dilation)
β-Adrenergic blockers (propranolol, metoprolol, atenolol, nadolol, timolol, pindolol, labetalol, esmolol)	Decrease myocardial oxygen demand via reduction in heart rate, blood pressure, contractility; may also increase coronary perfusion by prolongation of diastole
Calcium-channel blockers (nifedipine, diltiazem, verapamil, amlodipine)	Produce coronary and systemic vasodilation, improving perfusion and reducing afterload; decrease myocardial oxygen demand by reducing contractility
Magnesium	Protects against reperfusion injury by coronary and systemic vasodilation, platelet inhibition, and antiarrhythmic actions
Angiotensin-converting enzyme inhibitors (enalapril, captopril, lisinopril)	Afterload reduction and limitation of ventricular remodeling, decreasing congestive heart failure risk.
Thrombolytic agents (streptokinase, tissue plasminogen activator, anisoylated plasminogen streptokinase activator complex)	Acute reperfusion and myocardial salvage
Antiplatelet agents (aspirin)	Prevent thrombosis or rethrombosis
Antithrombin agents (heparin)	Maintain patency of arteries opened by tissue plasminogen activator

Acute reperfusion of ischemic myocardium in early myocardial infarction may be attempted with intracoronary or intravenous administration of a thrombolytic agent, immediate coronary angioplasty, or emergent coronary artery bypass surgery. Three thrombolytic agents are approved for use in acute myocardial infarction: streptokinase, anistreplase (anisoylated plasminogen streptokinase activator complex), and alteplase (recombinant tissue plasminogen activator).[19] Third-generation thrombolytic agents are under active investigation. Follow-up therapy may include administration of heparin or other anticoagulants.

Percutaneous transluminal coronary angioplasty has been used since 1977, either emergently during early myocardial infarction or for relief of angina and manifestations of cardiac failure not manageable by medical therapy (see Fig. 15–13 in Chapter 15). More than 300,000 of these procedures were performed in the United States in 1990.[28] Inflation of a catheter-induced balloon within the atherosclerotic lesion compresses and fractures the plaque and also stretches the underlying media and adventitia, inducing an aneurysm-like dilation. *Directional coronary atherectomy* is a newer nonballoon catheter approach that resects plaque using a rotational cutting device at the catheter tip.[17]

Surgical treatment of coronary artery disease involves bypassing occluded vessels with grafts composed of reversed saphenous veins harvested from the patient's legs, or with myocardial implantation of the distal ends of small thoracic arteries such as the internal mammary artery (Fig. 16–13). Coronary artery bypass graft, a common surgical procedure, is most often done electively for class III or IV coronary artery disease, but may also be done emergently for evolving myocardial infarction that does not respond to thrombolytic agents or angioplasty. Vein grafts are prone to atherosclerotic reocclusion after several years, necessitating reoperation or other reperfusion measures. Arterial grafts do not develop atherosclerotic plaque; however, **coronary steal syndrome** may develop in a small number of patients with atherosclerotic stenosis of the left subclavian artery proximal to the origin of the graft.[29] In this situation, pressure gradients induce retrograde flow through the graft (from the myocardium to the sub-

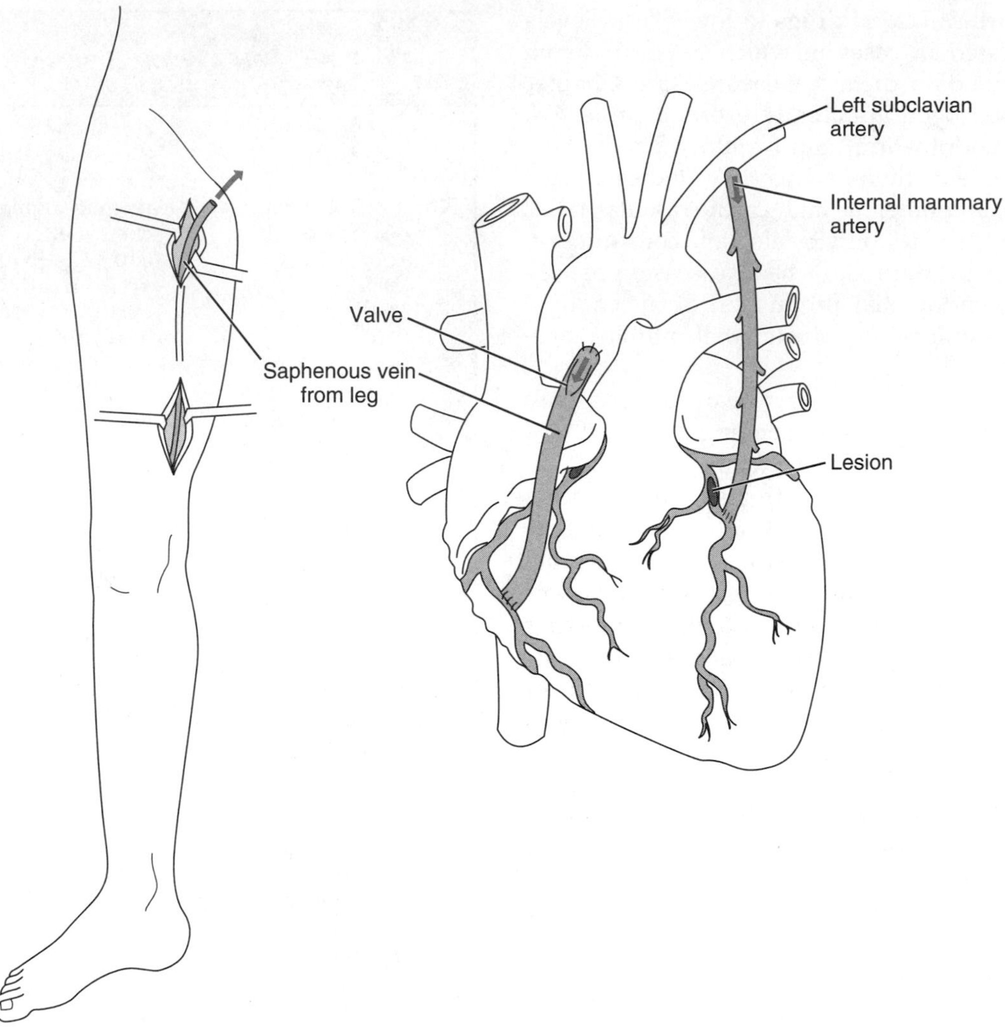

Figure 16–13

Coronary artery bypass graft surgery. Areas of occlusion in coronary arteries may be bypassed with grafts composed of reversed veins (typically saphenous veins, harvested from the legs) or with implantation of the distal end of the internal mammary artery. These procedures route aortic blood around the plaque-filled area to revascularize the myocardium.

clavian artery), "stealing" myocardial perfusion and inducing ischemia.

Prognosis and Outcome. Survival statistics indicate no significant difference between medical and surgical therapy of coronary artery disease, although greater improvement in functional capacity and quality of life have been reported with surgical treatment.[30, 31] In those who die of myocardial infarction, 60% expire during the first hour from lethal arrhythmia. Severe cardiac failure and cardiogenic shock account for other deaths occurring within 3 or 4 days. Surgical mortality with coronary artery bypass surgery is about 5%. The long-term prognosis is highly variable, depending on the nature of the atherosclerotic plaque, degree of coronary occlusion, amount of collateral circulation, and presence of dysrhythmias or CHF. Most infarct-related deaths occur within 3 months. Of those patients whose initial hospital stays are uneventful, one third have a future cardiac event (unstable angina, recurrent infarction, or death) within 3 years.[32]

Clinical Scenario

J.H., a 74-year-old man, is admitted to a small community hospital with chest pain radiating to the jaw and left arm, unrelieved by three sublingual nitroglycerin tablets. Four months earlier, he had suffered an inferior myocardial infarction. Coronary angiography performed at that time revealed atherosclerotic lesions in the right coronary artery and the diagonal branch of the left anterior descending artery. J.H. underwent angioplasty, which was successful in restoring flow through these occlusions.

During the present admission, J.H. is started on intravenous heparin, intravenous fluids, and dopamine to stabilize his low blood pressure, but he continues to experience chest pain throughout the day. He is transferred to a major medical center, where coronary angiography reveals that restenosis of his previous lesions has occurred.

1. Is J.H.'s chest pain more typical of angina pectoris or myocardial infarction? Explain.

2. What portions of J.H.'s myocardium are likely to be affected? What clinical consequences might be expected in this case?

Cardiomyopathies

Definition. Cardiomyopathy usually refers to impairment of cardiac contraction due to primary disease of myocardium, unrelated to the effects of hypertension or CHD. In some cases, however, the term *secondary cardiomyopathy* is used to refer to the syndrome of hypertrophy or dilation resulting from adaptation to CHD or hypertension.

Epidemiology. The annual incidence of the most common type of cardiomyopathy, **idiopathic dilated cardiomyopathy (IDC)**, has been estimated at 5 to 8 per 100,000 in the United States, accounting for 10,000 deaths.[33] It is believed that these figures underestimate the true incidence, however, because many cases are asymptomatic. The risk of cardiomyopathy is greater in men and in blacks. Alcohol consumption, pregnancy, hypertension, and use of β-adrenergic agonists are also associated with increased risk. Some forms of cardiomyopathy display familial inheritance.

Etiology. In a minority of cases, cardiomyopathy is caused by infection (myocarditis). An autoimmune mechanism may be involved in these cases. Altered metabolism in alcoholism or pregnancy may produce substances that are toxic to the myocardium. In most cases, the precise etiology is unknown. In those with familial inheritance, autosomal dominant, autosomal recessive, and X-linked recessive patterns have all been seen. In a very few cases, the disorder is linked to a specific defect in mitochondrial DNA, influencing some aspect of myocardial energy metabolism. Cardiomyopathy is commonly seen along with skeletal muscle disease in muscular dystrophy (see Chapter 35).

Pathophysiology. The pathophysiologic mechanisms of cardiomyopathy are unclear, but the disease displays one of three characteristic patterns (Fig. 16–14). In dilated cardiomyopathy, which may be idiopathic or associated with alcoholism, pregnancy, and viral infection, both ventricles dilate. CHF occurs when the Frank-Starling maximum is exceeded. In **hypertrophic cardiomyopathy**, associated with familial inheritance, the walls of both ventricles become greatly hypertrophied, with small chamber sizes. Hypertrophy of the septum obstructs aortic outflow. CHF occurs due to decreased compliance, decreased coronary artery perfusion, decreased preload, and increased left ventricular afterload. In **restrictive cardiomyopathy**, the least common type, the myocardium becomes fibrous and noncompliant, although not hypertrophied. Restrictive cardiopathy may result from amyloidosis (deposition of immunoglobulin or other protein, common in the elderly), from scarring secondary to radiation or drug toxicity, or from a number of rare disorders.[34] Restrictive cardiomyopathy is often idiopathic. CHF occurs owing to decreased preload and decreased contractility.

Clinical Manifestations. Except for the small number of patients who do not have symptoms, the clinical manifestations of cardiomyopathy are those of CHF (see Table 16–4). Onset and course of the disease are highly variable, but heart failure is usually first noted between the ages of 20 and 50 years.[33] In cases in which the disease progresses slowly, ejection fraction may fall to single-digit levels.

Prevention and Treatment. Primary prevention of cardiomyopathy is limited. Intervention in alcohol abuse is warranted, and genetic counseling may be beneficial in those rare patients in whom the inheritance pattern is clear. Treatment of the disorder is founded on treatment of CHF, as previously discussed. Transplantation is employed much more frequently in cardiomyopathy than in other causes of CHF.

Prognosis and Outcome. The average 5-year mortality rate in IDC is 20%. Most deaths occur within 3 years of onset of symptoms.[33]

Myocarditis

Definition. Myocarditis is defined as inflammation and injury of the myocardium in the absence of ischemia.

Epidemiology. The true incidence of myocarditis is uncertain because it may be transient and asymptomatic. Among patients with IDC, the incidence of myocarditis at biopsy has ranged from 1% to 17% in

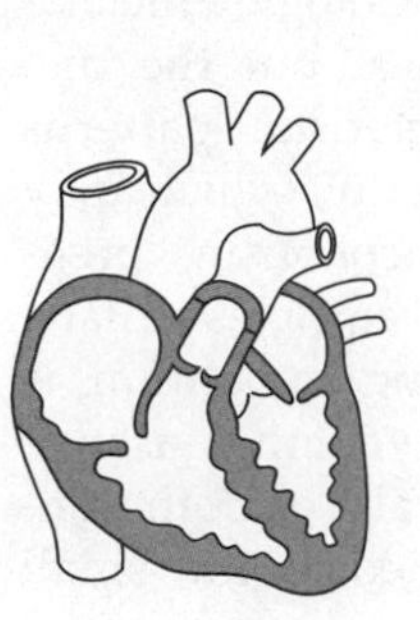

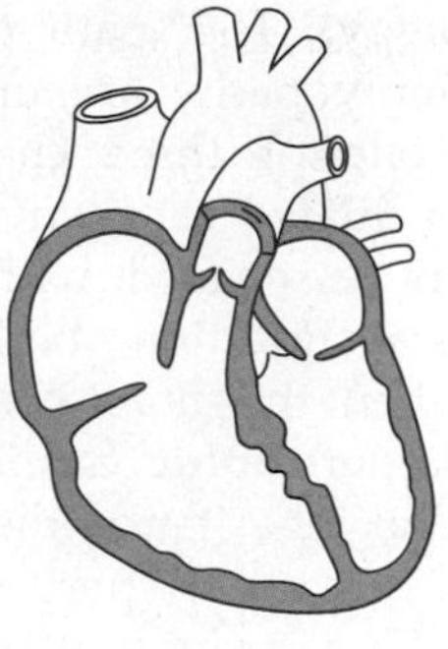

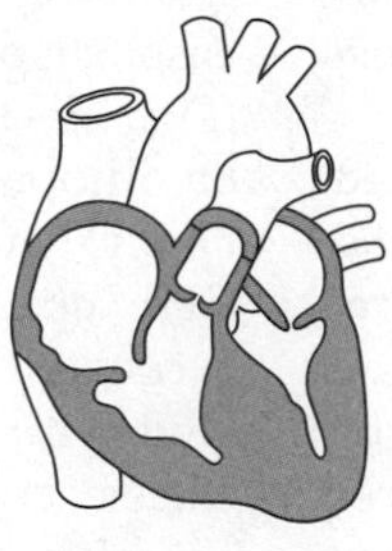

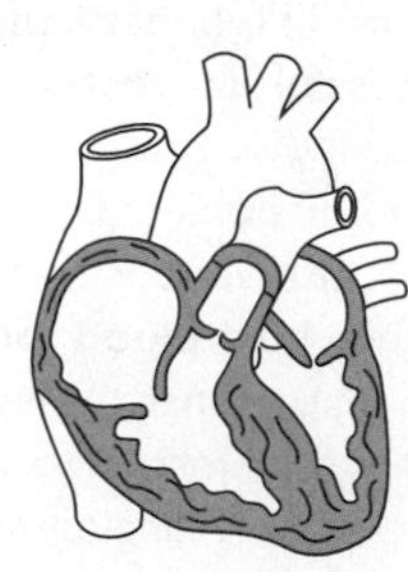

Figure 16–14
Types of cardiomyopathy. The normal heart is illustrated for comparison. *Dilated cardiomyopathy* is characterized by enlargement of both ventricular chambers. *Hypertrophic cardiomyopathy* demonstrates greatly thickened myocardial walls, with reduced chamber sizes. *Restrictive cardiomyopathy* results from myocardial fibrosis, which greatly reduces ventricular compliance, although hypertrophy and dilation are absent.

different studies.[33] Specific risk factors are the same as those for IDC.

Etiology. Myocarditis is believed to be caused in most cases by an infection that triggers an autoimmune attack on myocardial cells.[35] Causative agents include viruses (coxsackievirus B, echovirus, influenza, hepatitis B, human immunodeficiency virus, Epstein-Barr virus, cytomegalovirus), bacteria (*Corynebacterium diphtheriae, Salmonella* sp., *Chlamydia* sp., *Mycobacterium tuberculosis,* β-hemolytic streptococci, Lyme disease), and fungi (aspergillosis, candidiasis, histoplasmosis).

Pathophysiology. The initial infection triggers an autoimmune, cellular, and possibly humoral response, leading to myocardial inflammation and necrosis.[35] This process usually leads to IDC and heart failure.

Clinical Manifestations. An influenza-like syndrome may be present during the initial infection. The disease may be clinically silent for a variable period. Overt heart failure, with symptoms of fatigue, dyspnea, palpitations, and chest pain, is usually evident late in the disease, and the clinical syndrome is that of IDC. A small number of patients suffer sudden cardiac death.

Prevention and Treatment. Preventive measures involve reduction of risk of IDC. Treatment involves management of heart failure, as discussed earlier. Corticosteroids have been used in the treatment of myocarditis, but their benefit is unproved.[35]

Prognosis and Outcome. Mortality rates are the same as those for IDC. Patients undergoing cardiac transplantation for active myocarditis with IDC have a poorer 1-year survival rate (52% versus 82%) than those transplanted for other reasons and have double the usual rejection rate.[35]

Infective Endocarditis

Definition. Infective endocarditis is infection of the endocardial surface of the heart, including the valves.

Epidemiology. The annual incidence of infective endocarditis is thought to be about 1 per 1000 hospital admissions, or 4 per 100,000 population.[36] Although some people with infective endocarditis have no apparent risk factors, most patients have underlying structural heart disease, such as valve disease or congenital heart disease, or an autoimmune systemic illness, such as rheumatic heart disease or systemic lupus erythematosus. Procedures associated with introduction of causative organisms into the bloodstream include dental work, bladder catheterization, gastrointestinal intubation or surgery, and vaginal delivery. Those who abuse intravenous drugs are also at increased risk.

Etiology. Conditions that must be present for infective endocarditis to occur include: (1) endocardial surface injury, (2) thrombus formation at the site of injury, (3) bacterial entry into the circulation, and (4) bacterial adherence to the injured endocardial surface.[2] Endocardial damage usually results from high-velocity turbulent blood flow induced by structural abnormality, although immune complex deposition has been implicated in patients with autoimmune disorders. Injury triggers endothelial hemostatic mechanisms, resulting in formation of a sterile thrombus (nonbacterial thrombotic endocarditis) at the site. Bacteria, if present, may then adhere to this thrombus and produce the bacterial vegetations (fern-like deposits) that are characteristic of endocarditis. Procedure-associated bacteremia is transient, often peaking 30 minutes after the procedure, but this is thought to be sufficient to cause endocarditis in susceptible patients.

Pathophysiology. Inflammatory and immune responses may further damage the endocardial structures, leading to worsening of valve lesions and potentially precipitating CHF. Local extension of inflammation may cause myocardial abscesses, pericarditis, or dysrhythmia. Bacterial vegetations may break off and embolize to the coronary arteries, causing myocardial infarction. Septic emboli may also serve as foci for infectious processes elsewhere in the circulation, inducing vascular injury (mycotic aneurysm) or other focal infections.

Clinical Manifestations. Signs of systemic infection are common, including fever, sweats, chills, anorexia, fatigue, weight loss, joint pain, back pain, and muscle pain. Cardiovascular signs may include heart murmur due to valve dysfunction and signs of CHF. Septic emboli may cause manifestations of arthritis, osteomyelitis, pericarditis, brain abscess, or meningitis.

Prevention and Treatment. Although no study has proved its efficacy, prophylactic antibiotic therapy before dental work and other invasive procedures is routine in those who have structural heart disease.[37] Treatment of endocarditis involves appropriate antibiotic therapy and, if necessary, surgical replacement of defective cardiac valves.

Prognosis and Outcome. Endocarditis is fatal in 10% to 20% of those infected.[36]

Pericarditis

Definition. Pericarditis is inflammation of the pericardial layers—the visceral pericardium overlying the myocardium, and the fibrous parietal pericardium overlying the visceral layer.

Epidemiology. Infectious pericarditis is believed to be uncommon but may occur as a component of trauma or viral or neoplastic illness, or as an extension of transmural myocardial infarction (Dressler's syndrome). Patients with chronic renal failure are at increased risk for unknown reasons. Most pericarditis risk is associated with procedures, including radiation therapy, drugs, or surgical entry into the pericardial sac during open heart surgery (postcardiotomy syndrome).

Etiology. Pericarditis may be infectious, neoplastic, autoimmune, allergic, traumatic, or iatrogenic (Table 16–11).

TABLE 16–11
ETIOLOGY OF PERICARDITIS

CATEGORY	EXAMPLES
Trauma	Blow to chest Surgical incision of pericardium Radiation
Infection	Viruses: coxsackievirus, echovirus, influenza, varicella, human immunodeficiency virus, Epstein-Barr virus Bacteria: staphylococcus, meningococcus, pneumococcus, tuberculosis, *Haemophilus influenzae* Extension of myocarditis or infective endocarditis
Neoplasm	Primary: mesothelioma Metastatic: leukemia, lymphoma, melanoma, breast cancer, lung cancer
Autoimmune disease	Rheumatic fever, systemic lupus erythematosus, rheumatoid arthritis, vasculitis, scleroderma, dermatomyositis, myxedema
Ischemic extension	Dressler's syndrome after myocardial infarction
Drug toxicity	Heparin, warfarin, procainamide, cromolyn sodium, hydralazine, dantrolene, methysergide, penicillin, isoniazid, phenytoin, minoxidil, phenylbutazone
Idiopathic	Renal disease

Pathophysiology. Pericardial inflammation in acute pericarditis may result in local inflammation that does not significantly affect cardiac function. More extensive inflammation may cause third spacing of exudate into the potential space between pericardial layers (*pericardial effusion*). When this fluid volume exceeds a critical point, restriction of diastolic filling (cardiac tamponade) occurs. Rarely, and usually associated with chronic or recurrent pericarditis, scarring of the pericardial layers may cause them to fuse and thicken, and this constrictive pericarditis may lead to CHF due to restricted diastolic filling.

Clinical Manifestations. Signs of inflammation, including fever, are often present. Chest pain may be sharp and severe and is differentiated from ischemic pain by its aggravation by deep inspiration or coughing. A scratchy sound (pericardial friction rub) may be heard on auscultation and is produced by the rubbing of the inflamed pericardial layers against each other. Inflammation extending to the myocardium may manifest as an electrocardiogram abnormality consistent with ischemia (see Chapter 17). Pericardial effusion may be apparent on chest radiograph. Signs of diastolic heart failure may be present if filling is impeded; jugular venous distention is especially prominent. A classic sign of cardiac tamponade is *pulsus paradoxus*, in which the systolic blood pressure is significantly decreased during each inspiration. This cyclic pattern results from the additional reduction of left ventricular filling due to increased intrathoracic pressure. Constrictive pericarditis is usually manifested by *Kussmaul's sign*, a cyclic increase in jugular venous distention due to restriction of right-sided filling during inspiration.

Prevention and Treatment. Reduction of risk factors may be possible in some cases, but there is no specific prevention for pericarditis. Treatment of uncomplicated viral pericarditis is supportive, consisting of rest and anti-inflammatory drugs. Appropriate antibiotic therapy is indicated for bacterial infections, such as *M. tuberculosis*. Treatment of pericardial effusion is aimed at the underlying cause, if possible. Surgical drainage of exudate (pericardiocentesis) may be necessary in cases of tamponade. Constrictive pericarditis is treated with surgical excision of the pericardium (pericardiectomy).

Prognosis and Outcome. Prognosis is highly variable, depending on the underlying cause and severity of pericarditis. Uncomplicated viral pericarditis is self-limiting, running its course in 1 to 3 weeks. The surgical mortality rate in constrictive pericarditis is 5% to 15%.[38] In infectious pericarditis with purulent exudation, the mortality rate is as high as 70% to 80%.[2]

Cardiac Valve Disease

Definition. Cardiac valve disease is a congenital or acquired disorder in which a cardiac valve is unable to open or close effectively, resulting in disruption of the cardiac cycle. The term *stenosis* refers to incomplete valve opening, whereas *insufficiency* denotes incomplete closure. Stenosis and insufficiency may coexist if a valve is fused in a partially open state. *Regurgitation* is the backward flow of blood through an insufficient valve.

Epidemiology. Valve defects are present in association with a number of congenital heart disorders, including **aortic stenosis** (6%) and **pulmonic stenosis** (8%).[2] Risk factors include teratogenic infections such as rubella, maternal use of alcohol, and maternal use of antiepileptic drugs such as phenytoin (Dilantin). Infants of diabetic mothers are at increased risk, as are infants with other anomalies such as Down syndrome (see Chapter 33).

Acquired valve disease is still relatively common, although its epidemiologic patterns are changing. Almost 3% of all people 75 to 86 years old have critical aortic stenosis, and 13% have moderate to severe **aortic insufficiency**.[39] As the population ages, degenerative valvular changes with calcium deposition are seen with greater frequency, although these do not impair function in most cases. The elderly are at increased risk for acquired valve disease as a result of having acquired rheumatic fever in early adulthood, coupled with the degenerative changes of aging. After a long period of declining incidence due to eradication of rheumatic fever in the United States, acquired disease of the aortic and mitral valves is again occurring with more frequency in younger people. Most of these people are immigrants from Mexico, Vietnam, India, and eastern Mediterranean countries, where rheumatic fever is still prevalent. The inflammatory response to this form of infective endocarditis may damage valves owing to scar tissue formation.

One fourth of patients with rheumatic heart disease have **mitral stenosis**, and 40% have combined stenosis and **mitral insufficiency.**[40] Two thirds of these patients are women, and pregnancy may precipitate symptoms of CHF. Mitral insufficiency also commonly results from papillary muscle dysfunction secondary to myocardial infarction, and from severe left ventricular hypertrophy and dilation, which physically pulls valve leaflets apart.

The most common form of valvular heart disease in the United States is **mitral valve prolapse**, with a reported prevalence of 6% to 17% in women and 2% to 4% in men.[41] Mitral prolapse may be a primary condition, associated with autosomal dominant inheritance, or secondary to a number of other disorders, including Marfan syndrome, muscular dystrophy, rheumatic fever, systemic lupus erythematosus, and athletic cardiac enlargement.

Etiology. Specific genetic defects accounting for congenital valve disorders are usually unknown. The most common cause of acquired valvular disease is rheumatic fever, an inflammatory disorder affecting the heart, joints, and skin, caused by group A streptococcus. During the acute phase of infection, there is little or no hemodynamic disturbance, but scarring of heart valves occurs during the healing process. The left-sided mitral and aortic valves are most vulnerable, apparently because they are subjected to higher pressures during the cardiac cycle. Left ventricular pressure exceeds right ventricular pressure because of the differences in afterload against which these muscles must pump.

Pathophysiology

Aortic Stenosis. As shown in Figure 16–15, aortic stenosis results in left ventricular hypertrophy and, later, dilation due to increased left ventricular afterload. Atrial kick also increases adaptively, and loss of effective atrial contraction due to a dysrhythmia such as atrial fibrillation may precipitate CHF acutely. Usually, CHF is of gradual onset as adaptive mechanisms are overcome by increasing left ventricular afterload. Ventricular hypertrophy and dilation increase dysrhythmia risk, increase myocardial oxygen demands, and reduce coronary artery flow because of high pressure during diastole.

Aortic Insufficiency. In aortic insufficiency, shown in Figure 16–16, CHF may develop due to increased left ventricular preload because this chamber must pump both the volume entering from the left atrium and the volume that regurgitates backward from the aorta during diastole. Effective cardiac output is decreased, leading to compensatory mechanisms (hypertrophy and dilation), which further increase the workload of the heart. Chronic aortic insufficiency

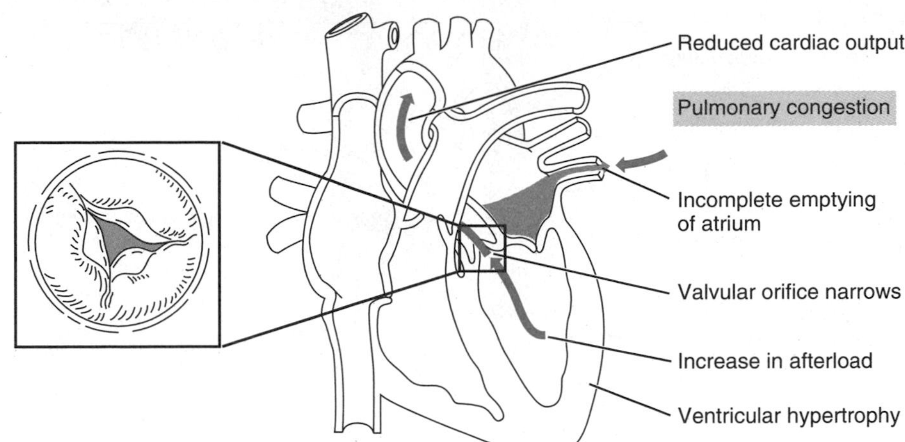

Figure 16–15
Aortic stenosis. Narrowing of the aortic valve orifice results in left ventricular hypertrophy secondary to increased afterload. Left ventricular failure may result, with decreased cardiac output and pulmonary congestion. (Modified from Black, J.M., and Matassarin-Jacobs, E. [1997]. *Medical-Surgical Nursing: Clinical Management for Continuity of Care.* [5th ed.]. Philadelphia: W.B. Saunders. [p. 1345].)

may cause the heart to become larger than in any other form of chronic heart disease.[39]

Mitral Stenosis. Mitral stenosis impairs left ventricular filling during diastole and causes a rise in left atrial pressure and pulmonary hypertension. CHF may result from increased left atrial afterload and decreased left ventricular preload (Fig. 16–17).

Mitral Insufficiency. In mitral insufficiency (Fig. 16–18), failure of the insufficient valve to close completely during systole permits regurgitation of left ventricular blood back into the left atrium, dividing the cardiac output into forward and backward components. Cardiac output falls, and adaptive mechanisms result in increased heart rate and volume retention (increased preload). CHF results from the increased cardiac workload required to generate adequate cardiac output in this inefficient condition of divided flow.

Mitral Prolapse. Mitral prolapse, illustrated in Figure 16–19, is an abnormal enlargement of the mitral valve leaflets. During systole, the large valve leaflets project (prolapse) into the left atrium. Mitral valve prolapse usually does not significantly impair valvular function, but these patients are at higher risk for developing infective endocarditis. In some cases, the prolapsed mitral valve is also insufficient. The degree of mitral insufficiency correlates with the risk of complications, such as CHF, atrial fibrillation, and embolization.[42]

Clinical Manifestations. Signs and symptoms of CHF may be seen with both stenosis and insufficiency (see Table 16–4). Hypertrophy of chambers affected by increased afterload or preload may be detected with radiography, electrocardiography, or echocardiography. Murmur is apparent owing to turbulent flow through damaged valves. Mitral valve prolapse is usually asymptomatic; however, some patients experience benign dysrhythmias or chest pain that is atypical of ischemia. Manifestations of anxiety are also common.

Prevention and Treatment. Antibiotic therapy has resulted in a decline in the incidence of rheumatic fever in the United States, although rheumatic heart disease is still prevalent in other countries. Antibiotic therapy may be used preventively in people

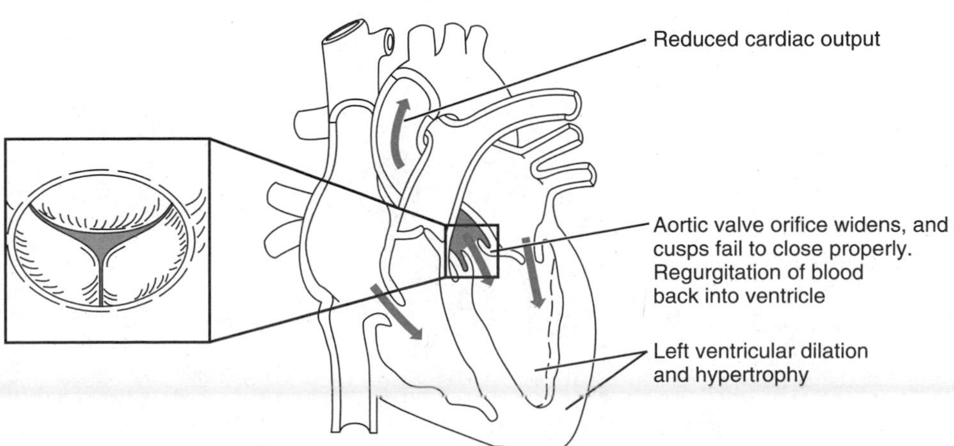

Figure 16–16
Aortic insufficiency. Failure of aortic valve cusps to close completely during diastole permits regurgitation of aortic blood back into the left ventricle, increasing the workload of this chamber. Divided flow also reduces cardiac output. (Modified from Black, J.M., and Matassarin-Jacobs, E. [1997]. *Medical-Surgical Nursing: Clinical Management for Continuity of Care.* [5th ed.]. Philadelphia: W.B. Saunders. [p. 1345].)

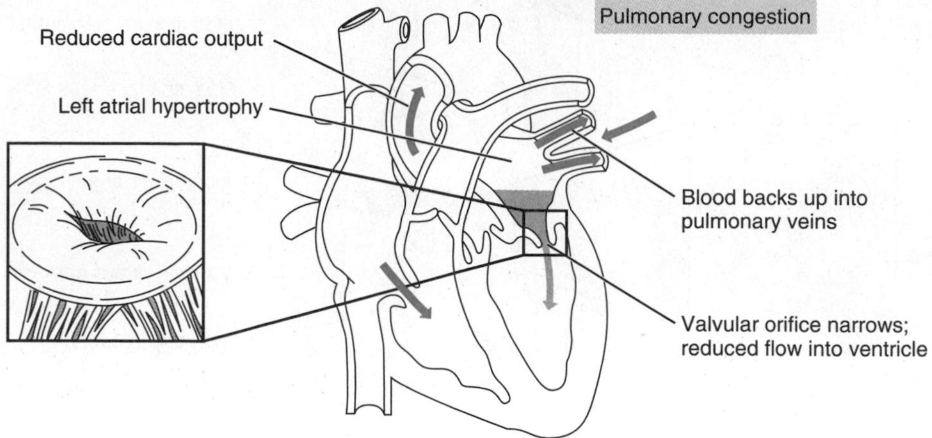

Figure 16–17
Mitral stenosis. Narrowing of the mitral valve orifice impedes flow of blood from the left atrium during diastole. Left atrial hypertrophy and pulmonary congestion develop in response to the increased afterload, and cardiac output falls as a consequence of reduced left ventricular preload. (Modified from Black, J.M., and Matassarin-Jacobs, E. [1997]. *Medical-Surgical Nursing: Clinical Management for Continuity of Care.* [5th ed.]. Philadelphia: W.B. Saunders. [p. 1345].)

with defective or diseased hearts, to reduce the risk of infective endocarditis.

CHF is treated medically insofar as possible (see Table 16–6). Balloon valvuloplasty has been employed in the treatment of stenosis. This procedure is similar to angioplasty in that a balloon-tipped catheter is threaded into the stenosed valve. Inflation of the balloon compresses scar tissue, relieving stenosis to some degree. Surgical repair or replacement is indicated when CHF due to valve disease does not respond to these therapies. Stenosed valves may be opened surgically, and incompetent valve leaflets may be repaired. Damaged valves may be removed and replaced with artificial (prosthetic) valves or porcine grafts (Figure 16–20).

Prognosis and Outcome. Prognosis in valve disease is variable depending on type, severity, and patient age. Patients may be symptom free for 10 to 20 years after rheumatic fever before onset of CHF symptoms. The operative mortality rate ranges between 2% and 10%. The 10-year mortality rate for those with New York Heart Association class IV CHF due to valve disease approaches 70% to 100%.[43]

Congenital Heart Defects

Definition. Congenital heart defects are structural disorders of the heart that are present at birth.

Epidemiology. The prevalence of congenital heart defects has been estimated at 2 to 10 cases per 1000 live births.[44] The actual prevalence is probably much higher because many spontaneously aborted fetuses display heart defects, and many defects may go undetected if they do not significantly impair function. There are many types of congenital heart defects, with **ventricular septal defects (VSD)** being the most common (Table 16–12).

The risk of congenital heart disease is increased with exposure to the common teratogens, as discussed in Chapter 7. Fetal alcohol syndrome and first-trimester maternal rubella are associated with congenital heart defects, but in most cases, there is no known exposure to teratogens. Prematurity is a risk factor owing to incomplete development and persistence of fetal structures, especially if complicated by infant respiratory distress syndrome with high pulmonary pressures (see Chapter 33). Further-

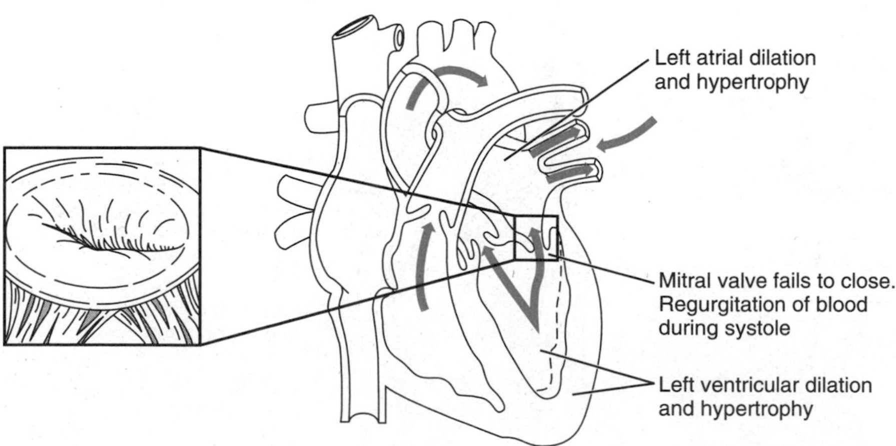

Figure 16–18
Mitral insufficiency. Failure of the mitral valve to close completely during systole permits regurgitation of blood from the left ventricle back into the left atrium. The workload of both chambers is increased, resulting in hypertrophy and dilation. Cardiac output falls due to divided flow. (Modified from Black, J.M., and Matassarin-Jacobs, E. [1997]. *Medical-Surgical Nursing: Clinical Management for Continuity of Care.* [5th ed.]. Philadelphia: W.B. Saunders. [p. 1345].)

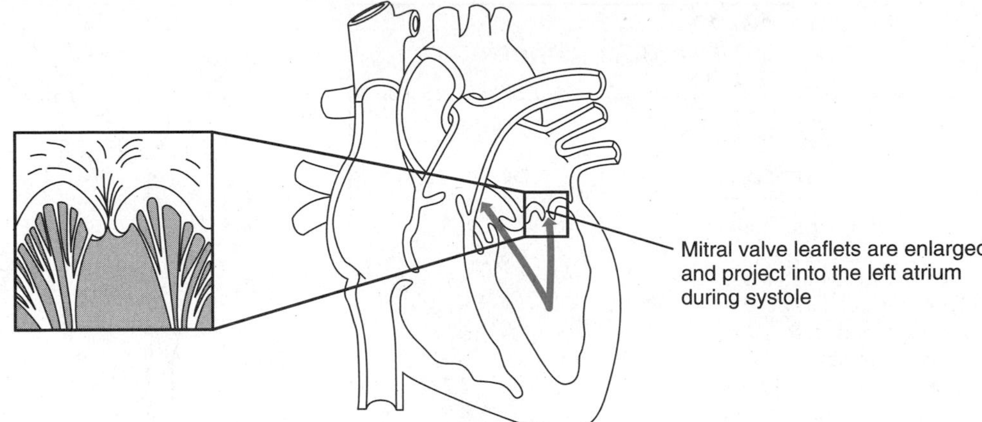
Mitral valve leaflets are enlarged and project into the left atrium during systole

Figure 16–19
Mitral prolapse. Abnormally enlarged valve leaflets project back into the left atrium during systole. Mitral prolapse does not significantly affect cardiac output unless mitral insufficiency is also present.

more, infants with genetic defects, including heart defects, are often born prematurely.

Etiology. Congenital heart defects are usually caused by de novo genetic abnormalities occurring early in the embryonic period and resulting in defective synthesis of structural proteins of the heart. Some defects display multifactorial inheritance, but the relative contribution of genetic versus environmental factors is uncertain. Prematurity is highly associated with a specific defect, **patent ductus arteriosus**, in which the fetal channel between the pulmonary artery and the aorta fails to close soon after birth.

Pathophysiology. Congenital heart defects result in impairment of blood flow through the heart or lungs to varying degrees. Defects are classified as *acyanotic* if they do not impair oxygenation of blood in the lungs, or *cyanotic* if oxygenation is compromised. Cyanosis is a clinical manifestation resulting from accumulation of deoxygenated hemoglobin (which is blue in color), due either to poor initial oxygenation of hemoglobin by the lungs (central cyanosis) or to increased extraction of oxygen from hemoglobin in cases of slowed blood flow through tissues (peripheral cyanosis). Cyanosis is evidenced by a blue tinge to the skin, nailbeds, or mucous membranes of the lips and mouth.

Two mechanisms may result in cyanosis with congenital heart defects: right-to-left shunt and admixture. Right-to-left shunt refers to flow from the right side of the heart directly to the left through an abnormal opening, bypassing the lungs. Admixture occurs with mixing of oxygenated and unoxygenated blood in a common vessel or chamber before its ejection into the systemic circulation.

CHF is a common outcome of congenital heart defects, due to a variety of mechanisms that impair cardiac output and tissue perfusion (Table 16–13).

Acyanotic Heart Defects. In **coarctation of the aorta** (Fig. 16–21), CHF may occur as a result of increased left ventricular afterload caused by stricture of the aorta. Aortic pressure is elevated behind the stricture and may be manifested as high pressure in the arteries of the head and neck as well as the left ventricle. Perfusion distal to the coarctation is decreased. Because blood flow through the lungs is normal and there is no admixture, coarctation is

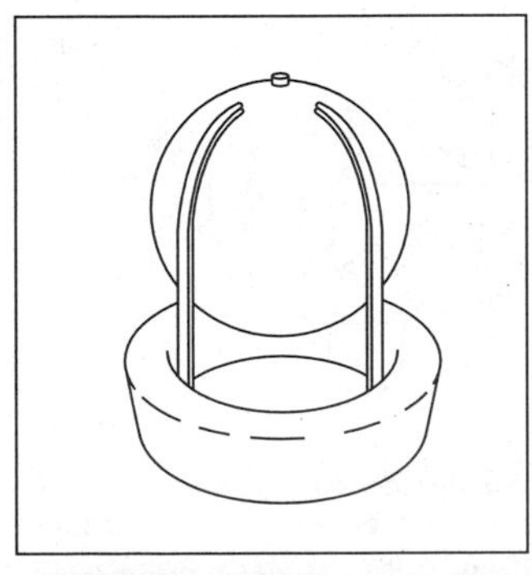
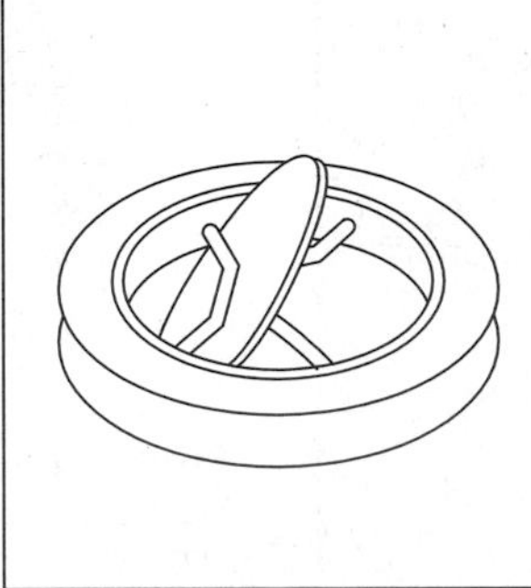
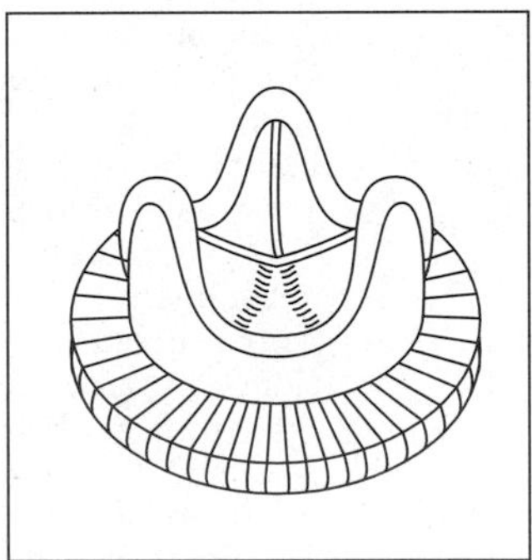

A Caged-ball valve **B** Tilting-disk valve **C** Porcine tissue valve

Figure 16–20
Prosthetic heart valves. Diseased valves may be surgically replaced with synthetic or porcine tissue valves.

TABLE 16–12
INCIDENCE OF SELECTED CONGENITAL HEART DEFECTS

Defect	Congenital Heart Defects (%)
Ventricular septal defect	28.3
Pulmonic stenosis	9.5
Patent ductus arteriosus	8.7
Tetralogy of Fallot	6.8
Atrial septal defect	6.7
Aortic stenosis	4.4
Coarctation of the aorta	4.2
Atrioventricular canal	3.5
Transposition of the great vessels	3.4
Aortic atresia	2.4
Truncus arteriosus	1.6
Tricuspid atresia	1.2
Total anomalous pulmonary venous return	1.1
Double-outlet right ventricle	0.8
Pulmonary atresia	0.3

Adapted with permission from Nugent, E.W., Plauth, W.H., Jr., Edwards, J.E., (1990). The pathology, abnormal physiology, clinical recognition, and medical and surgical treatment of congenital heart disease. In: Hurst, J.W. (Ed.). *The Heart, Arteries, and Veins.* New York: McGraw-Hill Information Services. (p. 657). Copyright 1990. Reproduced with permission of The McGraw-Hill Companies.

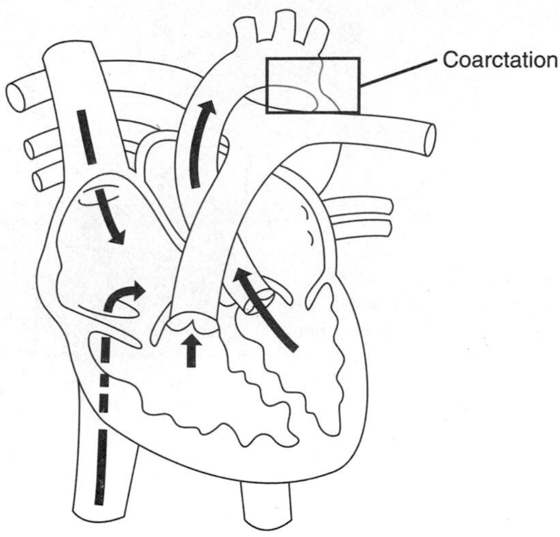

Figure 16–21
Coarctation of the aorta. A stricture in the aorta increases left ventricular afterload and results in elevated pressure in the head and upper extremities while pressure in the lower extremities is reduced. (Modified and used with permission of Ross Products Division, Abbott Laboratories, Columbus, OH 43216. © 1997 Ross Products Division, Abbott Laboratories.)

an acyanotic defect. If the child experiences cardiac failure, however, congestion in the lungs could impair oxygenation and result in cyanosis.

Defects such as VSD (Fig. 16–22), **atrial septal defect** (Fig. 16–23), and patent ductus arteriosus (Fig. 16–24) are classified as acyanotic because they are associated with left-to-right shunting of blood. That is, although oxygenated blood is inappropriately and inefficiently directed back to the right side of the heart, there is no impairment of oxygenation in the lungs. The direction of the shunt in these defects is determined by the normally higher pressure of the left side, due to higher resistance in the

TABLE 16–13
MECHANISMS OF CONGESTIVE HEART FAILURE IN CONGENITAL HEART DISEASE

Mechanism	Examples of Defects
Increased preload	Valve regurgitation
	Ventricular septal defect
	Transposition of the great vessels
	Complete atrioventricular canal
	Patent ductus arteriosus
	Truncus arteriosus
	Total anomalous pulmonary venous return
Increased afterload	Aortic atresia
	Coarctation of the aorta
	Interruption of the aortic arch
	Aortic stenosis
	Tetralogy of Fallot
	Pulmonic stenosis
Decreased filling	Mitral stenosis
	Tricuspid atresia
Decreased contractility	Endocardial fibroelastosis

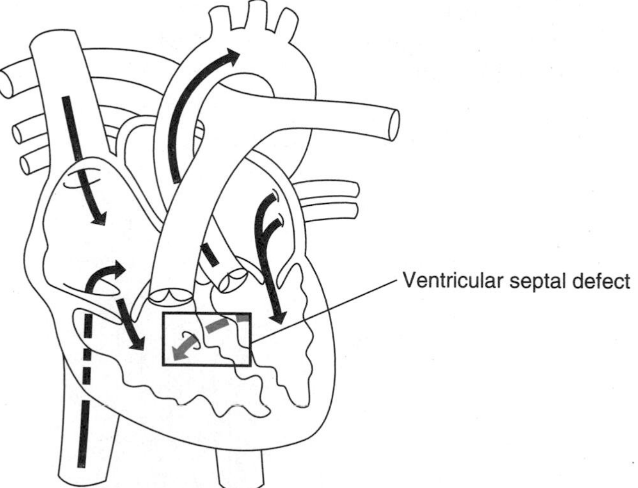

Figure 16–22
Ventricular septal defect. An opening in the septum between the ventricles permits flow between the chambers. The direction of the shunt is normally left to right because pressure is higher in the left side of the heart. Oxygenation of blood is not impaired, but cardiac workload is increased. (Modified and used with permission of Ross Products Division, Abbott Laboratories, Columbus, OH 43216. © 1997 Ross Products Division, Abbott Laboratories.)

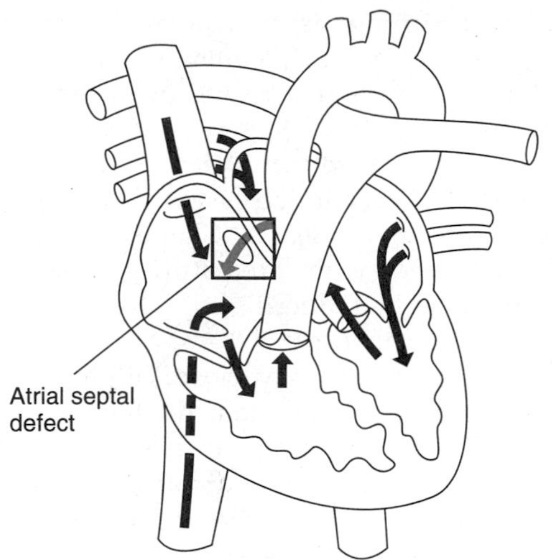

Figure 16–23

Atrial septal defect. An opening in the septum between the atria permits flow between the chambers. The direction of the shunt is normally left to right because pressure is higher in the left side of the heart. Oxygenation of blood is not impaired, but cardiac workload is increased. (Modified and used with permission of Ross Products Division, Abbott Laboratories, Columbus, OH 43216. © 1997 Ross Products Division, Abbott Laboratories.)

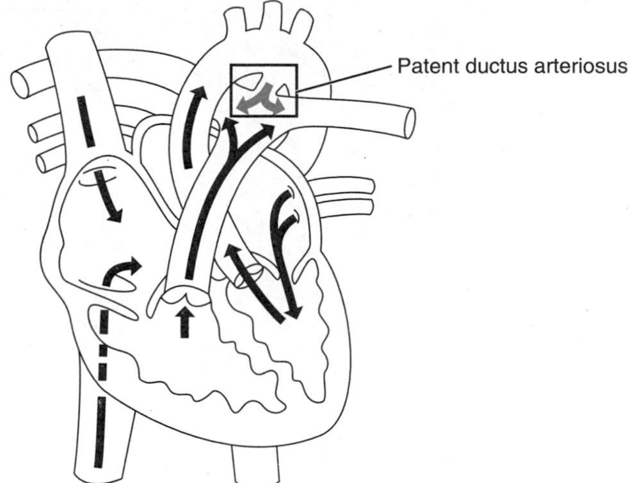

Figure 16–24

Patent ductus arteriosus. The ductus arteriosus, which permits most of the pulmonary arterial blood to bypass the collapsed fetal lungs in utero, normally closes soon after birth. High pulmonary vascular resistance or other factors may cause this fetal channel to remain open, resulting in shunting of some aortic blood back into the pulmonary artery. This left-to-right shunt does not impair oxygenation of the blood; however, cardiac workload is increased and cardiac output is reduced by the divided flow. (Modified and used with permission of Ross Products Division, Abbott Laboratories, Columbus, OH 43216. © 1997 Ross Products Division, Abbott Laboratories.)

systemic as opposed to the pulmonary circulation (see Chapter 15). CHF may develop in these defects owing to the divided flow (forward, into the systemic circulation, and backward, through the defect). Cardiac output is decreased, and the heart must contract more frequently to eject the increased preload originating from venous return and regurgitated volume. Children with these defects may become cyanotic if they develop respiratory infections, which increase right-sided congestion and pressure, reversing the direction of the shunt.

Cyanotic Heart Defects. Cyanosis due to right-to-left shunting is seen in **tetralogy of Fallot** (Fig. 16–25). Tetralogy of Fallot is a combination of four defects: pulmonic stenosis, VSD, abnormal position of the aorta such that it overrides the VSD, and right ventricular hypertrophy (which develops due to the afterload imposed by the pulmonic stenosis). Right-sided pressure is high because of the pulmonic stenosis and right ventricular hypertrophy, resulting in right-to-left shunting through the VSD. A portion of the right ventricular output thus bypasses the lungs, and oxygenation of the blood is impaired. Cardiac output is decreased and workload increased by the divided flow. Right ventricular failure results in systemic venous congestion and leads to a decrease in left ventricular preload, culminating in biventricular failure.

Admixture defects include **transposition of the great vessels** (Fig. 16–26), and **persistent truncus arteriosus** (Fig. 16–27). In transposition, the pulmonary artery and aorta are transposed, with the pulmonary artery arising from the left ventricle and the aorta arising from the right, creating separate pulmonary and systemic circulations. Because systemic blood would have no source of oxygen, this condi-

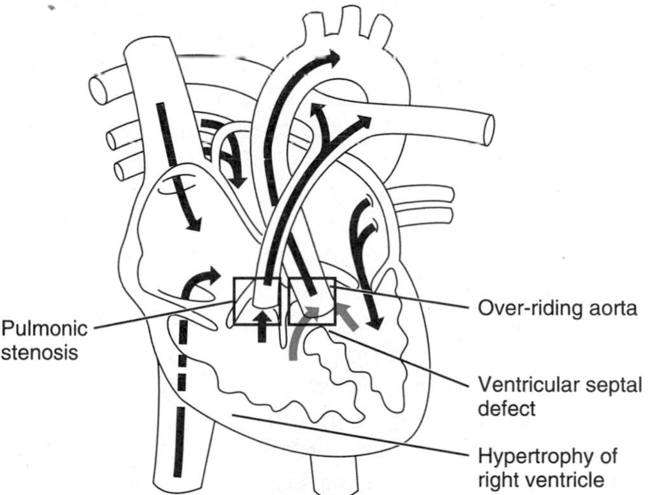

Figure 16–25

Tetralogy of Fallot. Tetralogy of Fallot is a combination of four anomalies: (1) pulmonic stenosis, (2) ventricular septal defect (VSD), (3) abnormal position of the aorta (over-riding the VSD), and (4) compensatory right ventricular hypertrophy. Blood is shunted from right to left through the VSD because of high right-sided pressure, which develops in response to the increased afterload imposed by pulmonic stenosis. Oxygenation of the blood is impaired, resulting in cyanosis. (Modified and used with permission of Ross Products Division, Abbott Laboratories, Columbus, OH 43216. © 1997 Ross Products Division, Abbott Laboratories.)

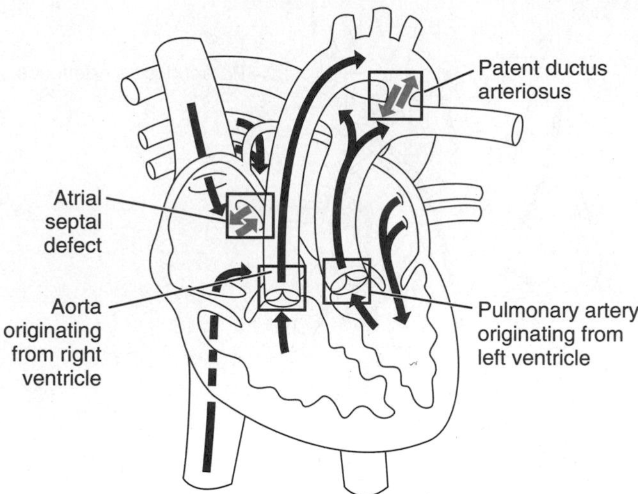

Figure 16–26

Transposition of the great vessels. The pulmonary artery and aorta arise from the left ventricle and the right ventricle, respectively. This anatomy results in separate pulmonary and systemic circulations, a condition that is incompatible with life unless an abnormal communication permits mixing of blood between the two systems. In this example, a patent ductus arteriosus and an atrial septal defect permit admixture, resulting in cyanosis due to perfusion of both systems with poorly oxygenated blood. (Modified and used with permission of Ross Products Division, Abbott Laboratories, Columbus, OH 43216. © 1997 Ross Products Division, Abbott Laboratories.)

tion is incompatible with life unless an abnormal communication, such as a septal defect or patent ductus arteriosus, allows mixing of blood between the two circulations.

Truncus arteriosus is an uncommon defect in which the embryologic common vessel fails to separate at its origin into the pulmonary artery and aorta. This common vessel, or truncus, usually arises centrally from a VSD, creating a common ventricular chamber, and divides distally into pulmonary and aortic vessels leading into the respective circulations. In some cases, pulmonary vessels are small or entirely absent; the lungs are then perfused by bronchial arteries arising from the aorta. Cyanosis arises from admixture of oxygenated and deoxygenated blood in the ventricles and common truncus.

Clinical Manifestations. Cyanosis is present to varying degrees in cyanotic defects and may be precipitated by respiratory infection or CHF in others. Chronic tissue hypoxia may result in clubbing of the extremities and secondary polycythemia, as discussed in Chapter 19. CHF is common with significant defects and manifests with both forward and backward effects, as detailed previously in Table 16–4. In children, chronically deficient tissue perfusion results in abnormal growth and development (see Developmental Perspective). Pulmonary congestion imposes increased risk of respiratory infection, and structural heart defects predispose to infective endocarditis. Murmur is present in defects such as atrial septal defect, VSD, patent ductus arteriosus, and valvular stenosis due to turbulent flow through abnormal openings.

Prevention and Treatment. Risk reduction in congenital heart defects involves avoidance of teratogenic exposure, discussed in Chapter 7. Modifiable factors associated with prematurity, discussed in Chapter 33, may be reduced with appropriate prenatal care and screening.

Small septal defects may close without intervention as the child grows. Patent ductus arteriosus in the premature infant may close spontaneously if lung disease is prevented or managed. Administration of a prostaglandin inhibitor, such as indomethacin, may result in closure of the ductus in some cases. The rationale for this therapy is that local mediators, such as prostaglandins, are believed to play a role in maintaining ductal patency during fetal life. Acyanotic defects may not require treatment if they do not significantly impair activity, growth, or development. If incidence of CHF is rare, the condition may be treated medically.

Surgical repair is indicated for congenital defects that significantly impair cardiac function. Whether surgery is done emergently, soon after birth, or later depends on the nature and severity of the defect. Early repair is the usual approach and may involve ligation of vessels or abnormal channels, relief of

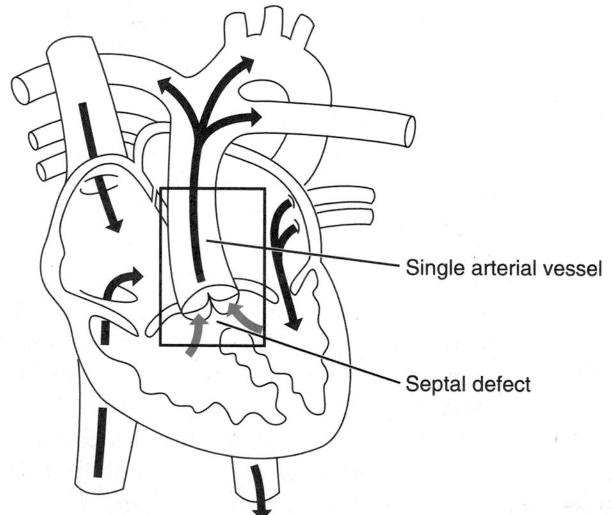

Figure 16–27

Persistent truncus arteriosus. The pulmonary artery and aorta fail to separate during embryologic development and are instead fused into a common vessel, the truncus arteriosus. The truncus usually arises from a ventricular septal defect and divides distally, leading into separate pulmonary and systemic circulations. Admixture of oxygenated and unoxygenated blood in the ventricles and truncus results in cyanosis. (Modified and used with permission of Ross Products Division, Abbott Laboratories, Columbus, OH 43216. © 1997 Ross Products Division, Abbott Laboratories.)

Developmental Perspective

Embryonic and Fetal Periods

The cardiovascular system develops from the mesenchyme and begins to function by the end of the third week of gestation, necessitated by the metabolic demands of the rapidly growing embryo. This system is therefore vulnerable to early teratogenic insults, and congenital anomalies are relatively common. Congenital heart defects may also result from single-gene or chromosomal mechanisms, such as Down syndrome. Because oxygenation of the blood occurs by placental exchange, specialized fetal structures, the foramen ovale between the atria and the ductus arteriosus between the pulmonary artery and the aorta, permit bypass of the collapsed fetal lungs. These structures may give rise to congenital heart defects (atrial septal defect and patent ductus arteriosus) in premature infants or in those with high pulmonary pressures due to infant respiratory distress syndrome.

Infancy and Childhood

Most congenital heart defects manifest at birth or during early childhood with signs of CHF. Growth and development impose increased metabolic demands during this period and may be impaired owing to lack of critical organ perfusion. Because neonates have little cardiac reserve, CHF may have a sudden onset. As the child grows, the adult left-to-right pressure gradient develops, and myocardial cells become longer and thicker. Ventricular size and compliance increase, and by adolescence, cardiac function is similar to that of adults. Evidence of the dyslipidemia that contributes to coronary artery disease may be present during early childhood, especially in those with an inherited lipid disorder or familial predisposition.

Adolescence and Young Adulthood

Although it is unusual, CHD may manifest in young adults as myocardial infarction in those with familial dyslipidemia. Cardiomyopathies are common in young adults and may also have a familial basis. Young immigrants from countries where rheumatic fever is still prevalent may manifest signs of cardiac valve disease. Young people with congenital heart defects are particularly prone to infective endocarditis and subsequent development of valve disease. The metabolic demands of pregnancy or athletic activities may uncover congenital defects in this age group. The term *athletic heart syndrome* is used to describe the electrocardiographic alterations and increase in ventricular mass that result from intense physical training. The eating disorder anorexia nervosa is particularly prevalent during this developmental period and may result in heart failure if cardiac muscle is cannibalized during this self-imposed starvation.

Middle and Older Adulthood

CHF occurs with greatest frequency in this age group, owing to the cumulative effects of coronary atherosclerosis, hypertension, diabetes, sedentary lifestyle, and obesity. Degenerative changes with aging include accumulation of lipofuscin, amyloid, and collagen as well as calcification of cardiac valves. These changes decrease cardiac reserve and increase the risk of failure when stressors are imposed. Elderly people may manifest valve disease owing to the combined effects of rheumatic fever suffered in young adulthood and the degenerative changes of aging.

constrictions, or use of synthetic patches or grafts. Cardiac transplantation has been employed in a small number of infants.[45]

Prognosis and Outcome. Mortality due to congenital heart disease during the first year of life is 71.2 deaths per 100,000 live births.[44] Defects amenable to early surgical repair are associated with increasingly favorable prognoses, although survival rates are still lower than those in the general population.[46]

CLINICAL SIGNIFICANCE OF DISORDERS OF CARDIAC CONTRACTION

The prevalence of cardiac disorders, particularly CHF and CHD, establishes their clinical importance, as does the availability of effective clinical interventions for risk reduction and treatment of these conditions. Cardiovascular disorders are the leading cause of mortality in the United States. Furthermore, these diseases significantly limit independence, capacity to work, and quality of life for many. Cardiovascular disorders consume the bulk of the nation's health care resources.

As summarized in the Focus of Current Research, many aspects of cardiac disease and its treatment are being actively investigated. The impact of traditional risk reduction measures, such as low fat diet and exercise programs, has yet to be determined with precision. Women have been poorly represented as subjects of cardiovascular research, but large studies such as the Nurses' Health Study are being undertaken to provide information on differential risk and treatment. The importance of estrogen replacement therapy in reducing risk of cardiovascular disease in postmenopausal women is under particular scrutiny because this treatment may impose increased risk of breast or endometrial cancers (see Chapter 31). The roles of sudden physical exertion and other factors in the precipitation of acute myocardial infarction in people with CHD is also being evaluated. The mechanisms of coronary occlusion in myocardial infarction are still incompletely understood, particularly with regard to the contributions of plaque rupture, intimal proliferation, and spasm. A number of large clinical trials are ongoing for the purpose of establishing the relative efficacy of treatment measures in these conditions.

Summary of Key Points

- The heart wall consists of three layers: the inner endocardium, which includes the valves mediating directional flow; the middle myocardium, the muscle layer; and the outer pericardium, a protective sac containing a small amount of lubricating fluid that facilitates the contraction and relaxation of the myocardium.

- Cardiac contraction is regulated locally by the Frank-Starling mechanism and intrinsic contractility (inotropic state). The Frank-Starling mechanism results in increased force of contraction as end-diastolic volume increases, up to a maximal point, and is presumably derived from optimal actin–myosin overlap for cross-bridge formation. Intrinsic contractility is derived from the rate of cross-bridge formation, which is influenced by autonomic innervation and by local factors that are poorly understood. The neuroendocrine regulation of contractility involves autonomic reflexes triggered by baroreceptors and chemoreceptors. Circulating catecholamines exert similar effects.

- The cardiac cycle is the series of events occurring during one complete contraction (systole) and relaxation (diastole) sequence. Synchronous opening and closing of valve pairs facilitates appropriate directional flow through the heart and into the pulmonary and systemic circulations.

- Cardiac output is determined by heart rate and stroke volume. Heart rate varies on the basis of autonomic stimulation and intrinsic pacemaker mechanisms. Increased rate increases cardiac output up to the point at which decreased filling time becomes a limiting factor. Stroke volume depends on preload, afterload, intrinsic contractility, and heart rate. Preload depends primarily on volume through the Frank-Starling mechanism, and afterload depends primarily on the resistance in the circulation. The neuroendocrine factors mediating these states thus indirectly influence cardiac output. Intrinsic contractility may be influenced by numerous factors but is limited by its concurrent effect on myocardial oxygen consumption. Increased heart rate results in increased force of contraction due to summation.

- Cardiac failure, the inability of the heart to pump sufficient blood to meet metabolic demands, may be classified on several physiologic bases: low (usual) versus high output; acute versus chronic; left-sided, right-sided, or biventricular; and systolic, diastolic, or both.

- CHF may result from primary cardiac disease or may occur secondarily when increased stress places demands on a compromised heart. Etiologic mechanisms include increased preload, increased afterload, decreased contractility, and impaired ventricular filling. Decreased tissue perfusion results in the forward effects of failure, which include sodium and water retention, lactic acidosis, and possible cardiogenic shock with multiple-system organ failure. The congestive effects of failure are not always seen but include pulmonary hypertension with possible pulmonary edema and effusion, jugular venous hypertension, hepatomegaly, ascites, and dependent edema.

- Many clinical disorders can culminate in CHF. CHD and cardiomyopathy result in CHF due to decreased myocardial contractility. CHD results from decreased myocardial perfusion secondary to coronary atherosclerosis, whereas cardiomyopathy results from nonischemic myocardial disease. Inflammatory heart disorders include infective endocarditis, myocarditis, and pericarditis. Infective endocarditis may precipitate CHF if it results in cardiac valve disease. Myocarditis precedes some forms of cardiomyopathy. Pericarditis may cause CHF if pericardial effusion is severe enough to limit ventricular filling (cardiac tamponade), or if pericardial scarring imposes external restraint on ventricular filling. Valve disease may increase afterload in the case of stenosis, or preload in the case of insufficiency. Congenital heart defects may trigger CHF by a variety of mechanisms, depending on the specific structural abnormality.

- Cardiovascular disorders are the leading cause of mortality in the United States. These diseases significantly limit independence, capacity to work, and quality of life for many, and they consume the bulk of the nation's health care resources.

REFERENCES

1. Centers for Disease Control and Prevention. (1994). Mortality from congestive heart failure: United States, 1980–1990. *Journal of the American Medical Association* 271(11), 813–814.
2. Lilly, L.S. (Ed.). (1993). *Pathophysiology of Heart Disease.* Philadelphia: Lea & Febiger. (p. 8, 130–146).
3. Dracup, K., Dunbar, S.B., and Baker, D.W. (1995). Rethinking heart failure. *American Journal of Nursing* 95(7), 22–27.
4. Young, J.B. (1995). Contemporary management of patients with heart failure. *Medical Clinics of North America* 79(5), 1171–1190.
5. Miller, M.M. (1994). Current trends in the primary care management of chronic congestive heart failure. *Nurse Practitioner* 19(5), 64–70.
6. Goldsmith, S.R., and Dick, C. (1993). Differentiating systolic from diastolic heart failure: Pathophysiologic and therapeutic considerations. *American Journal of Medicine* 95(12), 645–655.
7. Leier, C.V., and Metra, M. (1994). Clinical relevance and management of the major electrolyte abnormalities in congestive heart failure: Hyponatremia, hypokalemia, and hypomagnesemia. *American Heart Journal* 128(3), 564–574.
8. Baker, D.W., Konstam, M.A., Bottorff, M., *et al.* (1994). Management of heart failure. I. Pharmacologic treatment. *Journal of the American Medical Association* 272(17), 1361–1366.
9. Weber, K.T. (1993). Role of aldosterone in congestive heart failure. *Postgraduate Medicine* 93(5), 203–221.
10. Piepho, R.W. (1995). Calcium antagonist use in congestive heart failure: Still a bridge too far? *Journal of Clinical Pharmacology* 35(5), 443–453.
11. Hjalmarson, A., and Waagstein, F. (1994). The role of β-blockers in the treatment of cardiomyopathy and ischaemic heart failure. *Drugs* 47(suppl. 4), 31–40.
12. Bove, L.A., Mancini, M.G., Duris, L., *et al.* (1995). Nursing care of patients undergoing dynamic cardiomyoplasty. *Critical Care Nurse* 15(3), 96–104.
13. Stevenson, L.W. (1993). Advanced congestive heart failure. *Postgraduate Medicine* 94(5), 97–116.
14. Rector, T.S. (1994). Prognosis in congestive heart failure. *Annual Review of Medicine* 45, 341–350.
15. Creel, C.A. (1994). Silent myocardial ischemia and nursing implications. *Heart and Lung* 23(3), 218–227.
16. Cochrane, B.L. (1992). Acute myocardial infarction in women. *Critical Care Nursing Clinics of North America* 4(2), 279–289.
17. Rosenschein, U., and Topol, E.J. (1996). Uncoupling clinical outcomes and coronary angiography: A review and perspective of recent trials in coronary artery disease. *American Heart Journal* 132(4), 910–920.
18. Walton, J., and Westrope, P. (1996). Stunned myocardium: Theoretical mechanisms of injury. *Critical Care Nurse* 16(2), 23–28.
19. Rogers, W.J. (1995). Contemporary management of acute myocardial infarction. *American Journal of Medicine* 99(8), 195–206.
20. Seager, L.H. (1995). Diagnosis of chest pain: Pluses and minuses of stress tests. *Postgraduate Medicine* 97(2), 131–145.
21. Ohman, E.M., Armstrong, P.W., Christenson, R.H., *et al.* (1996). Cardiac troponin T levels for risk stratification in acute myocardial ischemia. *New England Journal of Medicine* 335(18), 1333–1341.
22. Antman, E.M., Tanasijevic, M.J., Thompson, B., *et al.* (1996). Cardiac-specific troponin I levels to predict the risk of mortality in patients with acute coronary syndromes. *New England Journal of Medicine* 335(18), 1342–1349.
23. Velasco, C.E., Turner, M., Inagami, T., *et al.* (1994). Reperfusion enhances the local release of endothelin after regional myocardial ischemia. *American Heart Journal* 128(3), 441–451.
24. Fitch, L.F., Buchwald, H., Matts, J.P., *et al.* (1995). Effect of aspirin use on death and recurrent myocardial infarction in current and former cigarette smokers. *American Heart Journal* 129(4), 656–662.
25. Manson, J.E. (1994). Postmenopausal hormone therapy and atherosclerotic disease. *American Heart Journal* 128(6 Pt. 2), 1337–1343.
26. Ridker, P.M., Vaughan, D.E., Stampfer, M.J., *et al.* (1994). Association of moderate alcohol consumption and plasma concentration of endogenous tissue-type plasminogen activator. *Journal of the American Medical Association* 272(12), 929–933.
27. Carbajal, E.V., and Deedwania, P.C. (1995). Contemporary approaches in medical management of patients with stable coronary artery disease. *Medical Clinics of North America* 79(5), 1063–1084.
28. Landau, C., Lange, R.A., and Hillis, L.D. (1994). Percutaneous transluminal coronary angioplasty. *New England Journal of Medicine* 330(14), 981–993.
29. Cosgrove, L.E. (1995). Coronary-subclavian steal after CABG surgery. *Critical Care Nurse* 15(3), 19–22.
30. Hamm, C.W., Reimers, J., Ischinger, T., *et al.* (1994). A randomized study of coronary angioplasty compared with bypass surgery in patients with symptomatic multivessel coronary disease. *New England Journal of Medicine* 331(16), 1037–1043.
31. King, S.B., Lembo, N.J., Weintraub, W.S., *et al.* (1994). A randomized trial comparing coronary angioplasty with coronary bypass surgery. *New England Journal of Medicine* 331(16), 1044–1050.
32. Fowles, R.E. (1995). Myocardial infarction in the 1990s: Complications, prognosis, and changing patterns of management. *Postgraduate Medicine* 97(6), 155–168.
33. Dec, G.W., and Fuster, V. (1994). Idiopathic dilated cardiomyopathy. *New England Journal of Medicine* 331(23), 1564–1575.
34. Kushwaha, S.S., Fallon, J.T., and Fuster, V. (1997). Restrictive cardiomyopathy. *New England Journal of Medicine* 336(4), 267–276.
35. Brown, C.A., and O'Connell, J.B. (1995). Myocarditis and idiopathic dilated cardiomyopathy. *American Journal of Medicine* 99(9), 309–314.
36. Nunley, D.L., and Perlman, P.E. (1993). Endocarditis: Chang-

ing trends in epidemiology, clinical and microbiologic spectrum. *Postgraduate Medicine* 93(5), 235–247.
37. Durak, D.T. (1995). Prevention of infective endocarditis. *New England Journal of Medicine* 332(1), 38–44.
38. Pauker, S.G., Kopelman, R.I., and Lechan, R.M. (1995). Diverted by the chief complaint. *New England Journal of Medicine* 333(1), 45–48.
39. Mangion, J.R., and Tighe, D.A. (1995). Aortic valvular disease in adults: A potentially lethal clinical problem. *Postgraduate Medicine* 98(1), 127–140.
40. Feldman, T. (1993). Rheumatic mitral stenosis: On the rise again. *Postgraduate Medicine* 93(6), 93–104.
41. Alpert, M.A., Mukerji, V., Sabeti, M., *et al.* (1991). Mitral valve prolapse, panic disorder, and chest pain. *Medical Clinics of North America* 75(5), 1119–1133.
42. Kim, S., Kuroda, T., Nishinaga, M., *et al.* (1996). Relation between severity of mitral regurgitation and prognosis of mitral valve prolapse: Echocardiographic follow-up study. *American Heart Journal* 132(2 Pt. 1), 348–355.
43. Underhill, S.L., and McGregor, M.S. (1989). Acquired valvular heart disease. In: Underhill, S.L., Woods, S.L., Froelicher, E.S.S., *et al. Cardiac Nursing*. (2nd ed.). Philadelphia: J.B. Lippincott.
44. Gillum, R.F. (1994). Epidemiology of congenital heart disease in the United States. *American Heart Journal* 127(4 Pt. 1), 919–927.
45. Zales, V.R., and Stapleton, P.L. (1993). Neonatal and infant heart transplantation. *Pediatric Clinics of North America* 40(5), 1023–1046.
46. Higgins, S.S., and Reid, A. (1994). Common congenital heart defects: Long-term follow-up. *Nursing Clinics of North America* 29(2), 233–248.

SELECTED BIBLIOGRAPHY

Amsterdam, E.A., Hyson, D., and Kappagoda, C.T. (1994). Nonpharmacologic therapy for coronary artery atherosclerosis: Results of primary and secondary prevention trials. *American Heart Journal* 128(6 Pt. 2), 1344–1352.

Ascherio, A., and Willett, W.C. (1995). New directions in dietary studies of coronary heart disease. *Journal of Nutrition* 125(3 Suppl), 647S–655S.

Ayanian, J.Z., Guadagnoli, E., and Cleary, P.D. (1995). Physical and psychosocial functioning of women and men after coronary artery bypass surgery. *Journal of the American Medical Association* 274(22), 1767–1770.

Baker, D.W., Jones, R., Hodges, J., *et al.* (1994). Management of heart failure. III. The role of revascularization in the treatment of patients with moderate or severe left ventricular systolic dysfunction. *Journal of the American Medical Association* 272(19), 1528–1534.

Baker, D.W., and Wright, R.F. (1994). Management of heart failure. IV. Anticoagulation for patients with heart failure due to left ventricular systolic dysfunction. *Journal of the American Medical Association* 272(20), 1614–1618.

Barrett-Connor, E. (1993). Estrogen and estrogen-progestogen replacement: Therapy and cardiovascular diseases. *American Journal of Medicine* 95(suppl. 5A), 40S–43S.

Beery, T.A. (1995). Gender bias in the diagnosis and treatment of coronary artery disease. *Heart and Lung* 24(6), 427–435.

Bernadet, P. (1995). Benefits of physical activity in the prevention of cardiovascular diseases. *Journal of Cardiovascular Pharmacology* 25(suppl. 1), S3–S8.

Blair, S.N., Kampert, J.B., Kohl III, H.W., *et al.* (1996). Influences of cardiorespiratory fitness and other precursors on cardiovascular disease and all-cause mortality in men and women. *Journal of the American Medical Association* 276(3), 205–210.

The Bypass Angioplasty Revascularization Investigation (BARI) Investigators. (1996). Comparison of coronary bypass surgery with angioplasty in patients with multivessel disease. *New England Journal of Medicine* 335(4), 217–225.

Cameron, A., Davis, K.B., Green, G., *et al.* (1996). Coronary bypass surgery with internal-thoracic-artery grafts: Effects on survival over a 15-year period. *New England Journal of Medicine* 334(4), 216–219.

Carroll, J.D., and Feldman, T. (1993). Percutaneous mitral balloon valvotomy and the new demographics of mitral stenosis. *Journal of the American Medical Association* 270(14), 1731–1736.

Chang, A.C., Hanley, F.L., Lock, J.E., *et al.* (1994). Management and outcome of low birth weight neonates with congenital heart disease. *Journal of Pediatrics* 124(3), 461–466.

Chu, E., and Cheitlin, M.D. (1993). Diagnostic considerations in patients with suspected coronary artery anomalies. *American Heart Journal* 126(12), 1427–1438.

Conti, J.B., and Curtis, A.B. (1993). Antiarrhythmic therapy in patients with congestive heart failure. *Postgraduate Medicine* 94(5), 121–137.

Davis, J.S., and Small, B.M. (1995). Advances in treatment of aortic stenosis across the lifespan. *Nursing Clinics of North America* 30(2), 317–332.

The Digitalis Investigation Group. (1997). The effect of digoxin on mortality and morbidity in patients with heart failure. *New England Journal of Medicine* 336(8), 525–533.

Dracup, K., Baker, D.W., Dunbar, S.B., *et al.* (1994). Management of heart failure. II. Counseling, education, and lifestyle modifications. *Journal of the American Medical Association* 272(18), 1442–1446.

Elliott, W.J. (1994). Cardiovascular risk factors: Which ones can and should be remedied? *Postgraduate Medicine* 96(3), 49–61.

Gagnon, D.R., Zhang, T., Brand, F.N., *et al.* (1994). Hematocrit and the risk of cardiovascular disease. The Framingham Study: A 34-year follow-up. *American Heart Journal* 127(3), 674–682.

Garg, R., and Yusuf, S. (1995). Overview of randomized trials of angiotensin-converting enzyme inhibitors on mortality and morbidity in patients with heart failure. *Journal of the American Medical Association* 273(18), 1450–1456.

Gaziano, J.M., Buring, J.E., Breslow, J.L., *et al.* (1993). Moderate alcohol intake, increased levels of high-density lipoprotein and its subfractions, and decreased risk of myocardial infarction. *New England Journal of Medicine* 329(25), 1829–1834.

Gheorghiade, M., Ruzumna, P, Borzak, S., *et al.* (1996). Decline in the rate of hospital mortality from acute myocardial infarction: Impact of changing management strategies. *American Heart Journal* 131(2), 250–256.

The GUSTO Angiographic Investigators. (1993). The effects of tissue plasminogen activator, streptokinase, or both on coronary-artery patency, ventricular function, and survival after acute myocardial infarction. *New England Journal of Medicine* 329(22), 1615–1622.

Handlin, L.R., and Vacek, J.L. (1994). Angioplasty versus thrombolysis for acute myocardial infarction. *Postgraduate Medicine* 95(4), 87–92.

Hilleman, D.E. (1993). Assessing the treatment of congestive heart failure: Inotropic agents and calcium channel blockers. *Pharmacotherapy* 13(5 Pt. 2), 88S–93S.

Hurst, J.W. (Ed.). (1990). *The Heart, Arteries, and Veins*. New York: McGraw-Hill Information Services.

Jiang, W., Babyak, M., Krantz, D.S., *et al.* (1996). Mental stress-induced myocardial ischemia and cardiac events. *Journal of the American Medical Association* 275(21), 1651–1656.

Johnson, C.M. (1993). Adherence events in the pathogenesis of infective endocarditis. *Infectious Disease Clinics of North America* 7(1), 21–36.

Karlson, B.W., Herlitz, J., and Hartford, M. (1994). Prognosis in myocardial infarction in relation to gender. *American Heart Journal* 128(3), 477–482.

Katz, N.M. (1995). Current surgical treatment of valvular heart disease. *American Family Physician* 52(2), 559–568.
Kelly, D.P., and Strauss, A.W. (1994). Inherited cardiomyopathies. *New England Journal of Medicine* 330(13), 913–919.
Kinch, J.W., and Ryan, T.J. (1994). Right ventricular infarction. *New England Journal of Medicine* 330(17), 1211–1217.
Kiowski, W., and Osswald, S. (1993). Circadian variation of ischemic cardiac events. *Journal of Cardiovascular Pharmacology* 21(suppl. 2), S45–S48.
Kohr, L.M., and O'Brien, P. (1995). Current management of congestive heart failure in infants and children. *Nursing Clinics of North America* 30(2), 261–290.
Koster, N.K. (1994). Physical activity and congenital heart disease. *Nursing Clinics of North America* 29(2), 345–356.
Krumholz, H.M., Seeman, T.E., Merrill, S.S., *et al.* (1994). Lack of association between cholesterol and coronary heart disease mortality and morbidity and all-cause mortality in persons older than 70 years. *Journal of the American Medical Association* 272(17), 1335–1340.

Lange, L.G., and Schreiner, G.F. (1994). Immune mechanisms of cardiac disease. *New England Journal of Medicine* 330(16), 1129–1134.
Lenihan, D.J., Gerson, M.C., Hoit, B.D., *et al.* (1995). Mechanisms, diagnosis, and treatment of diastolic heart failure. *American Heart Journal* 130(1), 153–166.
Liuzzo, G., Biasucci, L.M., Gallimore, J.R., *et al.* (1994). The prognostic value of C-reactive protein and serum amyloid A protein in severe unstable angina. *New England Journal of Medicine* 331(7), 418–424.

Maseri, A. (1992). Abnormal coronary vasomotion in ischemic heart disease. *Journal of Cardiovascular Pharmacology* 20(suppl. 7), S30–S31.
Mattioni, T.A. (1992). Long-term prognosis after myocardial infarction. *Postgraduate Medicine* 92(8), 107–114.
McClellan, M., McNeil, B.J., and Newhouse, J.P. (1994). Does more intensive treatment of acute myocardial infarction in the elderly reduce mortality? Analysis using instrumental variables. *Journal of the American Medical Association* 272(11), 859–866.
Miner, P.D. (1994). Infective endocarditis: Implications for care of the adult with congenital heart disease. *Nursing Clinics of North America* 29(2), 269–283.
Miner, P.D., and Canobbio, M.M. (1994). Care of the adult with cyanotic congenital heart disease. *Nursing Clinics of North America* 29(2), 249–267.
Mittleman, M.A., Maclure, M., Tofler, G.H., *et al.* (1993). Triggering of acute myocardial infarction by heavy physical exertion. *New England Journal of Medicine* 329(23), 1677–1683.
Moliterno, D.J., Willard, J.E., Lange, R.A., *et al.* (1994). Coronary-artery vasoconstriction induced by cocaine, cigarette smoking, or both. *New England Journal of Medicine* 330(7), 454–459.
Morris, D.L., Kritchevsky, S.B., and Davis, C.E. (1994). Serum carotenoids and coronary heart disease: The Lipid Research Clinics Coronary Primary Prevention Trial and Follow-Up Study. *Journal of the American Medical Association* 272(18), 1439–1441.
Morrison, H.I., Schaubel, D., Desmeules, M., *et al.* (1996). Serum folate and risk of fatal coronary heart disease. *Journal of the American Medical Association* 275(24), 1893–1896.
Multiple Risk Factor Intervention Trial Research Group. (1997). Multiple Risk Factor Intervention Trial: Risk factor changes and mortality results. *Journal of the American Medical Association* 277(7), 582–594.
Muscari, A., Bozzoli, C., Puddu, G.M., *et al.* (1995). Association of serum C3 levels with the risk of myocardial infarction. *American Journal of Medicine* 98(4), 357–364.

Nayler, W.G. (1993). Pharmacological aspects of calcium antagonism: Short term and long term benefits. *Drugs* 46(suppl. e), 40–47.
Norris, S.L., deGuzman, M., Sobel, E., *et al.* (1993). Risk factors and mortality among black, Caucasian, and Latina women with acute myocardial infarction. *American Heart Journal* 126(6), 1312–1318.
Nwasokwa, O.N. (1995). Coronary artery bypass graft disease. *Annals of Internal Medicine* 123(xx), 528–545.
Nwasokwa, O.N., Weiss, M., and Bodenheimer, M.M. (1997). Higher prevalence and greater severity of coronary disease in short versus tall men referred for coronary arteriography. *American Heart Journal* 133(2), 147–152.
Nygard, O., Vollset, E., Refsum H., *et al.* (1995). Total plasma homocysteine and cardiovascular risk profile: The Hordaland Homocysteine Study. *Journal of the American Medical Association* 274(19), 1526–1533.

Patterson, J.H., and Adams, K.F. (1993). Pathophysiology of heart failure. *Pharmacotherapy* 13(5 Pt. 2), 73S–81S.
Petrakis, N.L. (1995). Earlobe crease in women: Evaluation of reproductive factors, alcohol use, and Quetelet index and relation to atherosclerotic disease. *American Journal of Medicine* 99(10), 356–361.
Piano, M.R., and Schwertz, D.W. (1994). Alcoholic heart disease: A review. *Heart and Lung* 23(1), 3–17.
Price, V.A., Friedman, M., Ghandour, G., *et al.* (1995). Relation between insecurity and type A behavior. *American Heart Journal* 129(3), 488–491.

Rabah, M.M., Gangadharan, V., Brodsky, M., *et al.* (1996). Unstable coronary ischemic syndromes caused by coronary-subclavian steal. *American Heart Journal* 131(2), 374–378.
Ramsey, J.D. (1995). Use of ventricular stroke work index and ventricular function curves in assessing myocardial contractility. *Critical Care Nurse* 15(1), 61–67.
Resnekov, L. (1993). Aortic valve stenosis: Management in children and adults. *Postgraduate Medicine* 93(6), 107–122.
Rich-Edwards, J.W., Manson, J.E., Hennekens, C.H., *et al.* (1995). The primary prevention of coronary heart disease in women. *New England Journal of Medicine* 332(26), 1758–1766.
Rickenbacher, P.R., Rizeq, M.N., Hunt, S.A., *et al.* (1994). Long-term outcome after heart transplantation for peripartum cardiomyopathy. *American Heart Journal* 127(5), 1318–1323.
Riley, D.J., Weir, M., and Bakris, G.L. (1994). Renal adaptation to the failing heart. *Postgraduate Medicine* 95(8), 141–156.
Roberts, W.C., Kragel, A.H., Gertz, S.D., *et al.* (1994). Coronary arteries in unstable angina pectoris, acute myocardial infarction, and sudden coronary death. *American Heart Journal* 127(6), 1588–1593.

Sbarouni, E., Bradshaw, A., Andreotti, F., *et al.* (1994). Relationship between hemostatic abnormalities and neuroendocrine activity in heart failure. *American Heart Journal* 127(3), 607–612.
Schaefer, E.J. (1994). Familial lipoprotein disorders and premature coronary artery disease. Medical Clinics of North America 78(1), 21–39.
Schulz, H. (1994). Regulation of fatty acid oxidation in heart. *Journal of Nutrition* 124(2), 165–171.
Seed, M. (1994). Postmenopausal hormone replacement therapy: Coronary heart disease and plasma lipoproteins. *Drugs* 47(suppl. e), 25–34.
Sempos, C.T., Looker, A.C., Gillum, R.F., *et al.* (1994). Body iron stores and the risk of coronary heart disease. *New England Journal of Medicine* 330(16), 1119–1124.
Sharkey, A.M., and Clark, B.J. (1991). Common complaints with cardiac implications in children. *Pediatric Clinics of North America* 38(3), 657–666.
Sigurdsson, E., Thorgeirsson, G., Sigvaldason, H., *et al.* (1995). Unrecognized myocardial infarction: Epidemiology, clinical characteristics, and the prognostic role of angina pectoris. *Annals of Internal Medicine* 122(2), 96–102.
Sparacino, P.S. (1994). Adult congenital heart disease: An emerging population. *Nursing Clinics of North America* 29(2), 213–219.
Spielberg, C., Falkenhahn, D., Willich, S.N., *et al.* (1996). Circadian, day-of-week, and seasonal variability in myocardial infarction: Comparison between working and retired patients. *American Heart Journal* 132(3), 579–585.
Spyer, K.M. (1994). Central nervous mechanism contributing to cardiovascular control. *Journal of Physiology* 474(1), 1–19.

Steckelberg, J.M., and Wilson, W.R. (1993). Risk factors for infective endocarditis. *Infectious Disease Clinics of North America* 7(1), 9–19.

Subramaniam, P.M. (1994). Complications of acute myocardial infarction. *Postgraduate Medicine* 95(2), 143–148.

Sudhir, K., Mullen, W.L., Hausmann, D., *et al.* (1995). Contribution of endothelium-derived nitric oxide to coronary artery distensibility: An in vivo two-dimensional intravascular ultrasound study. *American Heart Journal* 129(4), 726–732.

Tashiro, H., Shimokawa, H., Yamamoto, K., *et al.* (1995). Monocyte-related cytokines in acute myocardial infarction. *American Heart Journal* 130(3 Pt. 1), 446–452.

Thompson, S.G., Kienast, J., Pyke, S.D.M., *et al.* (1995). Hemostatic factors and the risk of myocardial infarction or sudden death in patients with angina pectoris. *New England Journal of Medicine* 332(10), 635–641.

Underhill, S.L., Woods, S.L., Froelicher, E.S.S., *et al.* (Eds.). (1989). *Cardiac Nursing* (2nd ed.). Philadelphia: J.B. Lippincott.

Van de Werf, F., Topol, E.J., Lee, K.L., *et al.* (1995). Variations in patient management and outcomes for acute myocardial infarction in the United States and other countries: Results from the GUSTO trial. *Journal of the American Medical Association* 273(20), 1586–1591.

Verschuren, W.M.M., Jacobs, D.R., and Bloemberg, B.P.M. (1995). Serum total cholesterol and long-term coronary heart disease mortality in different cultures. *Journal of the American Medical Association* 274(2), 131–136.

Werns, S.W., Rote, W.E., Davis, J.H., *et al.* (1994). Nitroglycerin inhibits experimental thrombosis and reocclusion after thrombolysis. *American Heart Journal* 127(4 Pt. 1), 727–737.

Willett, W.C.K., Manson, J.E., Stampfer, M.J., *et al.* (1995). Weight, weight change, and coronary heart disease in women: Risk within the "normal" weight range. *Journal of the American Medical Association* 273(6), 461–465.

Willich, S.N., Lewis, M., Lowel, H., *et al.* (1993). Physical exertion as a trigger of acute myocardial infarction. *New England Journal of Medicine* 329(23), 1684–1690.

Woo, K.S., and White, H.D. (1994). Factors affecting outcome after recovery from myocardial infarction. *Annual Review of Medicine* 45, 325–339.

Zhu, B., Sievers, R.E., Sun, Y., *et al.* (1994). Is the reduction of myocardial infarct size by dietary fish oil the result of altered platelet function? *American Heart Journal* 127(4 Pt. 1), 744–755.

Cardiac Dysrhythmias

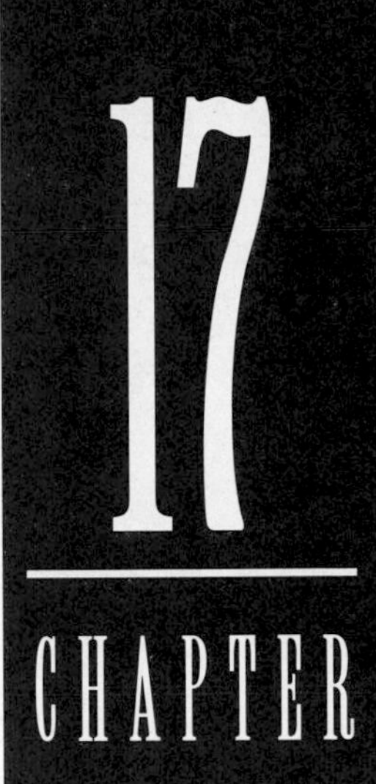

LEARNING OBJECTIVES

1. Describe the normal anatomy of the cardiac conduction system.
2. Discuss the normal physiology of cardiac conduction, including pacemaker function (automaticity), neural regulation, and variation in the cardiac axis.
3. Differentiate between normal and abnormal configurations of the PQRST complex on the basis of electrocardiographic principles, cellular pathophysiology, and the cardiac action potential.
4. Identify the steps in systematic evaluation of the cardiac axis, PQRST complex, and cardiac rhythm.
5. Describe the clinical features of the more common cardiac dysrhythmias in each of five categories: tachycardias, flutter and fibrillation, bradycardias, premature contractions, and conduction disturbances.

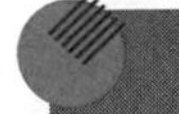

key terms

asystole
atrial fibrillation
atrial flutter
atrial tachycardia
atrioventricular (AV) block
automaticity
axis deviation
bradycardia
bundle branch block
cardiac axis
cardiopulmonary resuscitation (CPR)
conduction disturbance
dysrhythmia
ectopic pacemaker
electrocardiogram (ECG)
first-degree AV block
idioventricular rhythm
junctional rhythm
normal sinus rhythm (NSR)
pacemaker
paroxysmal supraventricular tachycardia (PSVT)
premature atrial contraction (PAC)
premature junctional contraction (PJC)
premature ventricular contraction (PVC)
pulseless electrical activity

reentry
second-degree AV block
sick sinus syndrome
sinus arrest
sinus arrhythmia
sinus bradycardia
sinus exit block
sinus pause
sinus tachycardia
sudden cardiac death (SCD)
supraventricular tachycardia
tachycardia
third-degree AV block
triggered activity
ventricular fibrillation (VF)
ventricular flutter
ventricular tachycardia (VT)
wandering atrial pacemaker
Wenckebach phenomenon
Wolff-Parkinson-White (WPW) syndrome

Cardiac muscle is an excitable tissue. Its contraction is stimulated by electrical signals (action potentials) that are self-generated within cardiac **pacemaker** cells. This signal flows directionally through the cardiac conduction system, initiating a wavefront of current that spreads across the membranes of myocardial cells. As detailed in Chapter 4, generation and propagation of action potentials are based on appropriate membrane transport of electrolytes, which is in turn dependent on normal energy metabolism and electrolyte balance mechanisms. Action potentials result in altered membrane voltage, with opening and closing of voltage-gated membrane channels for sodium, potassium, and calcium. Because calcium is essential to actin–myosin cross-bridge cycling, calcium transport links conduction and muscle contraction (see Chapter 5).

Cardiac **dysrhythmia** (or arrhythmia) refers to abnormal origin, rate, or direction of conduction of the electrical impulse, which may result in impairment of cardiac contraction. Dysrhythmias may be detected indirectly by manifestations of cardiac failure or myocardial ischemia (see Chapter 16), and some dysrhythmias result in **sudden cardiac death (SCD)** if not immediately terminated.

Dysrhythmias may be evaluated directly with electrocardiography, in the form of the **electrocardiogram (ECG)**, by bedside or ambulatory monitoring, or by invasive electrophysiology studies. Analysis of electrocardiographic data may reveal the origin and mechanism of dysrhythmia, sites of ischemia or infarction, effects of drug therapy or electrolyte imbalances, and direction of current flow within the heart. Initial clinical evaluation of the cardiac rhythm is based on graphic recording of summed action potentials by electrodes placed on the body surface.

This chapter discusses the anatomy and function of the cardiac conduction system, principles of surface electrocardiography, methods for analysis of electrocardiographic data, and mechanisms of dysrhythmia. The electrocardiographic characteristics, mechanisms, clinical manifestations, and treatment of the more common dysrhythmias are detailed.

ANATOMY OF THE CARDIAC CONDUCTION SYSTEM

The cardiac conduction system, illustrated in Figure 17–1, is a network of noncontractile cells that serves to originate and conduct action potentials at the appropriate rate and in the appropriate sequence from the atria to the ventricles. The normal pacemaker, or origin of the electrical impulse, is the sinoatrial (SA) node. Also referred to as the *sinus node,* the normal pacemaker consists of a group of cells located in the wall of the right atrium, near the point of entry of the superior vena cava. From the SA node, current is conducted across the atrial myocardium in a radiating pattern, causing atrial systole, and also downward more quickly through the internodal pathways of the conduction system to the atrioventricular (AV) junction.

The AV junction, located near the septum, is normally the only route through which atrial current may be conducted to the ventricles. It is composed of three zones: the high (atrionodal) zone, located in the lower atria; the middle zone or AV node, located in the septum between the atria and ventricles; and the low (nodal–His) zone, in or adjacent to the *bundle of His* in the ventricles. Because the AV node consists of small fibers with few gap junctions, it provides increased resistance to current flow, slowing the impulse long enough for atrial conduction and contraction to be completed before current reaches the ventricles.

In the ventricular septum, the common bundle of His divides into the right and left bundle branches, and the left bundle branch further divides into the anterior and posterior fascicles. The bundle branches terminate in finely branched Purkinje fibers, which are embedded in the ventricular myocardium. Rapid conduction of the impulse across the ventricles results in ventricular systole.

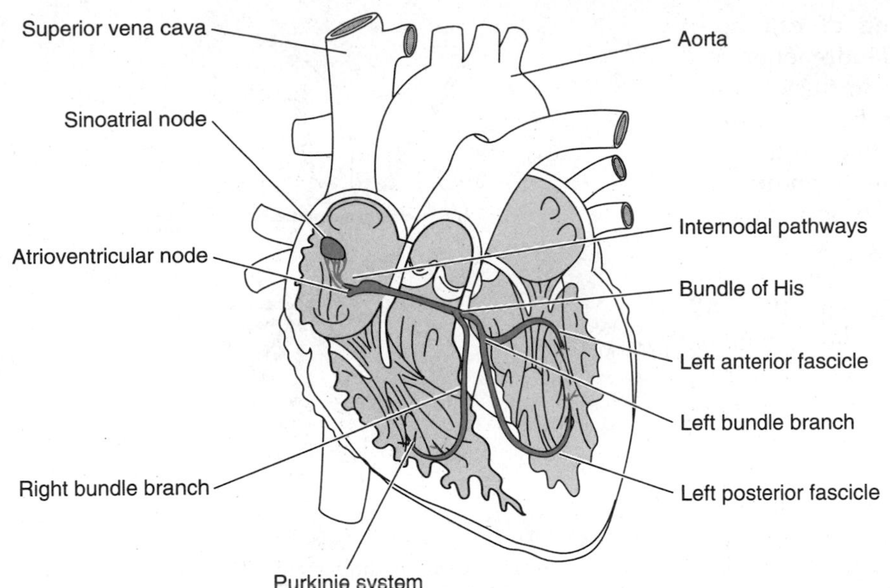

FIGURE 17–1
Cardiac conduction system. The cardiac impulse normally originates with the pacemaker cells of the sinoatrial node and is conducted sequentially across the internodal pathways, atrial myocardium, atrioventricular node, bundles of His, bundle branches, Purkinje system, and ventricular myocardium.

CARDIAC CONDUCTION

Pacemaker Function (Automaticity)

The ability of selected cells to serve as pacemakers depends on their membrane characteristics, which endow them with the quality of **automaticity**, the ability to self-generate an action potential. As discussed in Chapter 4, potential pacemakers have sufficient "leak" channels to allow a slow phase 4 (diastolic) depolarization. These continuously open channels permit a slow influx of sodium or calcium even in the absence of a stimulus to open voltage-gated "fast" sodium channels. Membrane potential becomes more positive as sodium cations enter the cell; and when threshold is reached, the membrane is depolarized. The action potential thus generated is then propagated across gap junctions to adjacent cardiac muscle cells or along the fibers of the conduction system. The intrinsic rate of spontaneous depolarization appears to depend on the number of open slow calcium channels present in the membrane.

Within the cardiac conduction system, there are numerous potential, or latent, pacemakers other than the SA node, each with a different intrinsic rate. Cells of the AV node may pace the heart at 40 to 60 beats/minute, whereas ventricular pacemakers have a slow intrinsic rate of 30 to 40 beats/minute. The SA node is the normal pacemaker of the heart because its intrinsic rate is 60 to 100 beats/minute. This faster rate normally results in depolarization of the pacemaker cells in the AV junction and ventricles by the conducted SA nodal impulse *before* these cells reach threshold on their own, a process known as *overdrive suppression*. The existence of latent pacemakers is important in cases of SA node disease or damage, or blockage of the atrial impulse at the AV node. A latent pacemaker may initiate an "escape" rhythm in such cases, preventing cardiac failure or arrest.

Myocardial cells that do not normally serve as pacemakers may acquire automaticity if their membranes are damaged by ischemia (as in coronary heart disease) or deformed by dilation or hypertrophy (as in congestive heart failure). If the intrinsic rate of these cells exceeds the normal SA nodal rate, a state of myocardial irritability exists in which these cells may act as **ectopic pacemakers** for abnormal beats or rhythms.

Neural Regulation of Conduction

The intrinsic rate of generation and conduction of action potentials may be influenced by autonomic nervous system reflexes, particularly the baroreceptor reflex (see Chapter 15). Reflex regulation of heart rate is controlled by the vasomotor center of the brain stem, integrated with other reflexes in the hypothalamus, and potentially modified by input from higher centers, such as the limbic system and cerebral cortex (see Chapter 21). Sympathetic fibers innervate the SA and AV nodes as well as the atrial and ventricular myocardium. Binding of catecholamines, particularly epinephrine, to β_1-adrenergic receptors results in an increase in the intrinsic pacemaker rate of these cells, probably by increasing permeability to sodium and calcium through ligand-gated channels. Increased heart rate and conduction through the AV node results, as is typical in enhanced sympathetic activity during exercise or stress.

Parasympathetic (vagal) fibers innervate the SA and AV nodes and the atrial myocardium, where binding of acetylcholine to cholinergic receptors results in decreased heart rate, probably by opening ligand-gated potassium channels. This increased permeability to potassium lowers resting membrane potential, hyperpolarizing the cell. The cell is thus less automatic or irritable. Indeed, very strong vagal stimuli can cause cardiac arrest by slowing SA nodal impulse generation or blocking conduction through the AV node. Vagal stimuli may be initiated inappropriately with extreme emotional stress (see *vasovagal syncope*, Chapter 15) or with abdominal muscle contraction during vomiting, straining to defecate, lifting heavy objects, or performing isometric exercise while holding the breath. In clinical settings, vagal stimuli may be initiated therapeutically for treatment of rapid heart rates. The patient may be instructed in the Valsalva maneuver, which involves diaphragmatic and abdominal contraction in an attempt to forcibly exhale against a closed glottis (like trying to blow up a stiff balloon that resists inflation.) Massage of the carotid sinus area or application of manual pressure over the eyeballs also provokes vagal impulses.

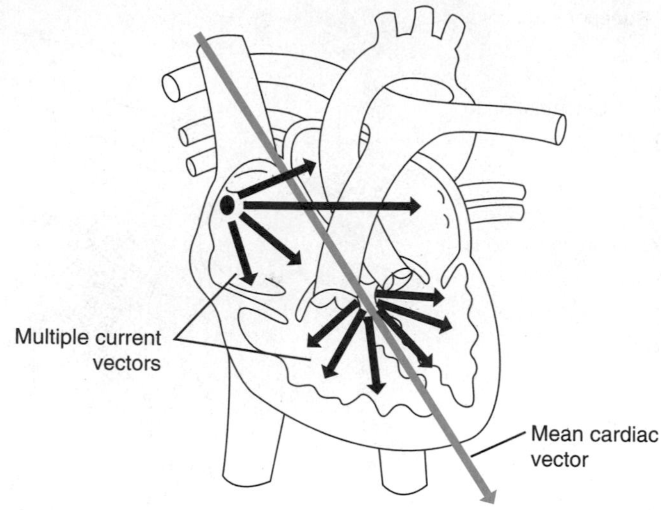

FIGURE 17–2
Cardiac vectors and mean cardiac axis. The multiple vectors of current flowing through the myocardium can be averaged geometrically to determine the mean direction (mean cardiac axis) during systole.

Cardiac Axis

The **cardiac axis** is defined as the mean direction or vector of current flow within the contracting heart, that is, the geometric average of the multiple current vectors present in the heart during systole (Fig. 17–2). In clinical settings, axis is usually approximated on the basis of electrocardiographic data, as discussed later in this chapter. The normal range of the cardiac axis is between −30 and +120 degrees, as illustrated on the *hexaxial figure* (Fig. 17–3), or along an imaginary line from the right shoulder to the left hip. Most current flow is in this direction when the heart is positioned normally and when the impulse is conducted through a normal conduction system and healthy myocardium.

Abnormal axis is referred to as left or right **axis deviation.** Left axis deviation may result from a more horizontal position of the heart in the chest, as occurs normally in many short people. Left axis deviation is also seen normally during pregnancy because the gravid uterus pushes the diaphragm and apex of the heart upward. Very tall people often have more vertically positioned hearts, with normal right axis deviation. Axis may also be altered with cardiomegaly secondary to athletic conditioning. A rare congenital condition, dextrocardia, causes right axis deviation because the heart is tipped toward

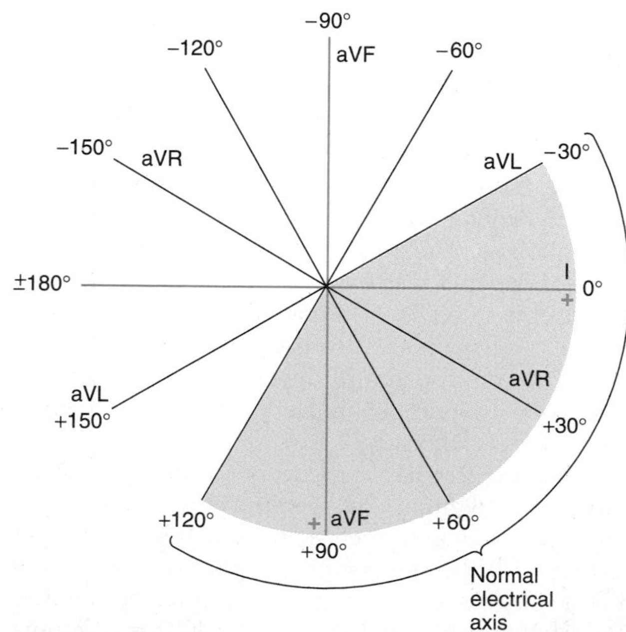

FIGURE 17–3
Range of normal cardiac axis. A cardiac axis outside the normal range (axis deviation) may be due to abnormal position of the heart within the thorax but is more often due to altered myocardial current flow.

the right side of the chest. Other internal organs are also reversed, in a mirror image of the normal; however, organ function is not impaired.

Except for these normal variations, axis deviation indicates pathology. Current vectors may be altered by areas of ischemia or infarction, in which current flow is abnormal or absent. Cardiomegaly secondary to congestive heart failure may cause deviation of the axis. Hypertrophy of one ventricle, as may be seen in congenital heart disease, pulmonary disease, or hypertensive heart disease, may extend the duration of current flow in the enlarged area. Dysrhythmias alter cardiac axis if the rhythm originates in an abnormal site, altering the direction of individual current vectors. In some cases, determination of axis is helpful in identifying the dysrhythmia. Clinical evaluation of axis and dysrhythmias requires an understanding of the principles and procedures of electrocardiography.

ELECTROCARDIOGRAM

PQRST Complex

The graphic representation of one cardiac cycle is illustrated in Figure 17–4. The vertical axis of the graph represents *amplitude* of current, in which 10 mm (two large squares) equal 1 mV for standardized ECGs. The horizontal axis represents *time*, with 1 mm (one small square) equal to 0.04 second (1 large square then equals 0.20 seconds).

Each PQRST complex represents the flow of electrical current through the heart during one cardiac cycle, as detected by surface electrodes. Normal characteristics of each component of the complex are summarized in Table 17–1. Depolarization of the SA node does not generate enough current flow to be detected at the surface; thus, the tracing remains at the baseline (i.e., is *isoelectric*) while the normal pacemaker fires. Atrial depolarization produces the first visible deflection, the P wave. The tracing is again isoelectric while current flows through the AV junction. The time period including the P wave and the isoelectric line that follows is known as the *PR interval* (PRI).

The *QRS complex* represents depolarization of the

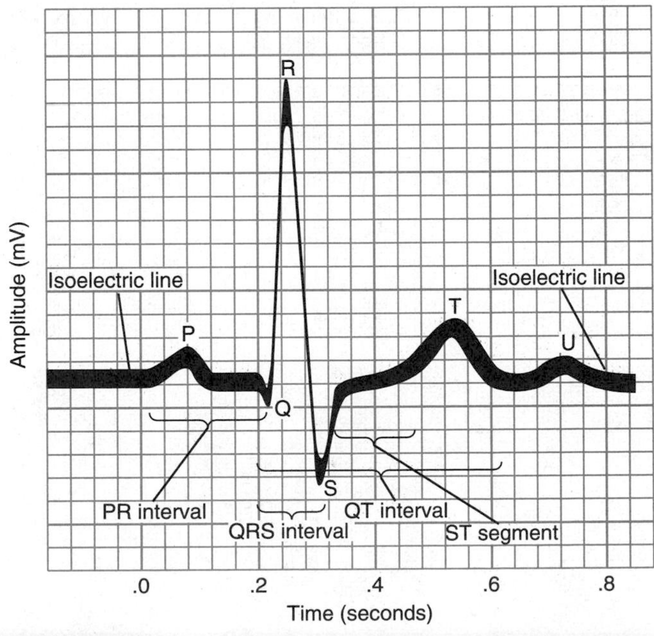

FIGURE 17–4

ECG graph and PQRST complex. Each PQRST complex represents the flow of current through the heart during one cardiac cycle.

TABLE 17–1
NORMAL CHARACTERISTICS OF THE PQRST COMPLEX

ECG COMPONENT	NORMAL PARAMETERS
P wave	Present, uniformly shaped, no notching or peaking Preceding QRS complex Maximum 0.11 second in duration Maximum 3 mm in height Positive deflection in leads I, II, aVF, and V_4–V_6, and inverted in aVR. Variable deflection in other leads.
PR interval	0.12–0.2 second in duration
QRS complex	0.05–0.10 second in duration Configuration may be qRs, QS, Rs, qR, or rSR′ (R waves are positive, large Q or small q waves are negative and precede the R; large S or small s waves are negative and follow the R)
ST segment	May be slightly elevated (1 mm or less in leads I, II, and III; 2 mm or less in some V leads) Should not be depressed more than 0.5 mm in any lead Curves slightly upward into the T wave
QT interval	Should not exceed 0.5 second Should not be variable in length
T wave	Same polarity as the QRS complex Rounded and asymmetric Notching is normal in children Maximum height of 5 mm in leads I, II, and III; 10 mm in V leads
U wave	Low voltage Same polarity as T wave

* Data from Conover, M.B. (1988). *Understanding Electrocardiography: Arrhythmias and the 12-lead ECG.* (5th ed.). St. Louis: C.V. Mosby.

His-Purkinje system and ventricles. An isoelectric interval, the *ST segment*, represents the plateau phase of ventricular repolarization, during which there is little net current flow. The T wave that follows is produced by current flow during rapid repolarization of the ventricles. (NOTE: Atrial repolarization occurs during the QRS complex but is not detectable as an event separate from the greater current flow caused by ventricular depolarization. Atrial repolarization is thus referred to as being "buried" in the QRS complex.) In some cases, a detectable U wave follows the T wave. Although the significance of the U wave is uncertain, one theory is that it represents repolarization of the His-Purkinje system, usually not seen owing to very low voltage.

Principles of Electrocardiography

The standard ECG is often referred to as a 12-lead ECG. A *lead* is an imaginary straight line (axis) between two *electrodes*, or current sensors. Each lead has one electrode designated as positive and another that is either a negative electrode or a zero-voltage reference point. The current flowing through the heart between these electrodes is recorded on the ECG. Because each of the 12 leads offers a different perspective or "camera angle" on the same electrical events, the amplitude and direction of the waveforms vary in each lead (Fig. 17–5).

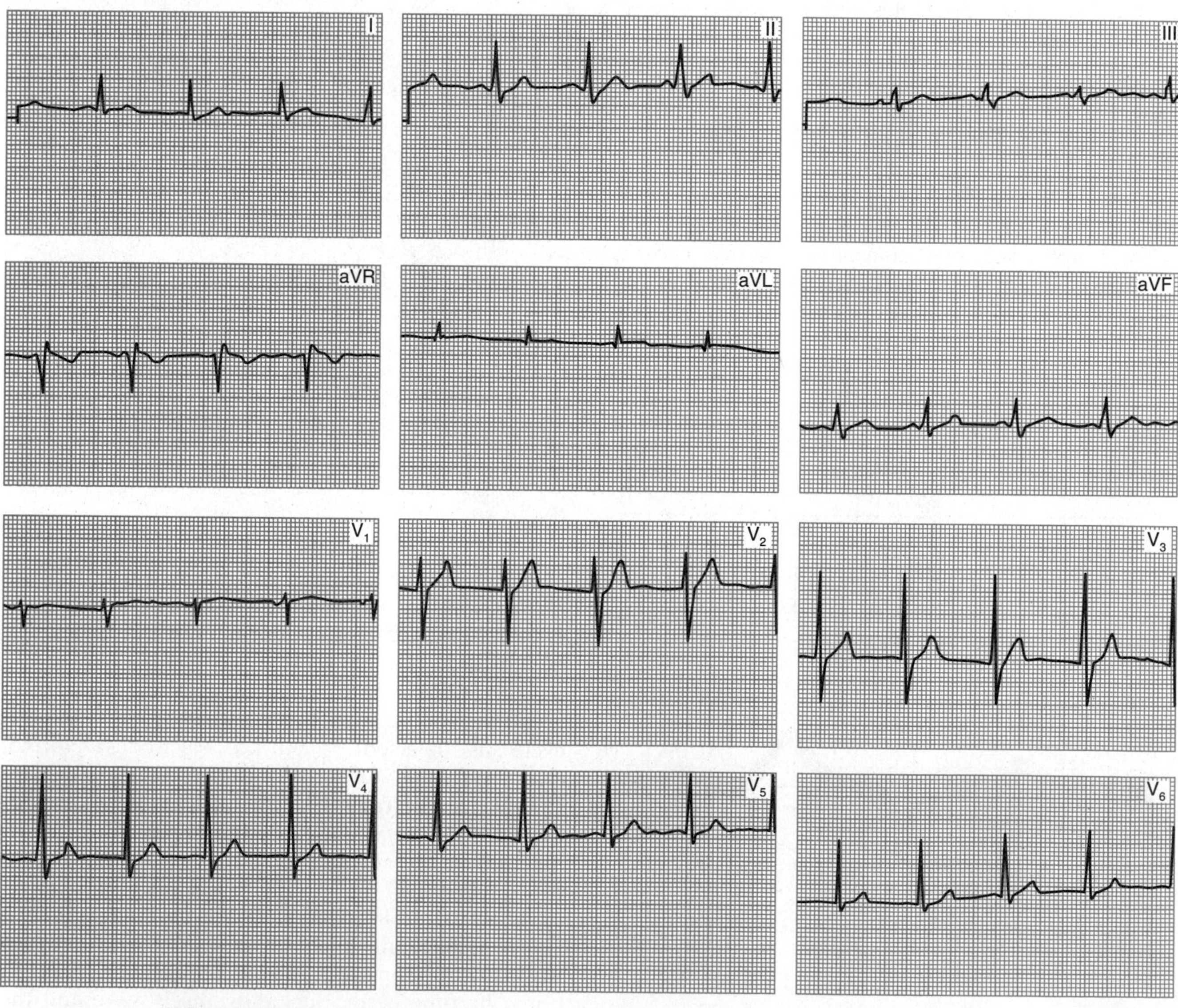

FIGURE 17–5

Normal 12-lead ECG. Each lead represents a different perspective of the same electrical events. (Courtesy of M. Martha Vorvick, MS, RNC, Assistant Professor. Moorhead, MN: Tri-College University Nursing Program.)

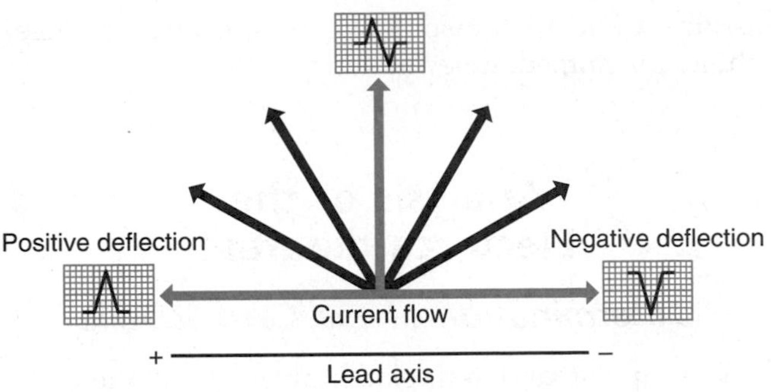

FIGURE 17–6
Relationship of ECG waveform to lead axis. Current flowing toward the positive electrode of a lead produces a positive deflection in that lead, whereas current flowing away from the positive electrode produces a negative deflection. If current flow is perpendicular to the lead axis, an equiphasic deflection results.

As shown in Figure 17–6, current flowing toward the positive electrode of a lead produces an upward (positive) deflection in that lead, whereas current flowing away from the positive electrode produces a downward or negative deflection. Current flowing parallel to the axis of the lead creates the greatest amplitude. If current flow is perpendicular to the lead axis, an *equiphasic* deflection (half up, half down) results.

Three types of leads are used to obtain the standard ECG: bipolar limb leads, unipolar limb leads, and unipolar chest leads. The three bipolar limb leads, I, II, and III, form the classic Einthoven's triangle, shown in Figure 17–7. In lead I, the positive electrode is placed on the left arm, and the negative on the right arm. In lead II, the positive electrode is on the left leg, and the negative on the right arm. Lead III is formed from placement of the positive electrode on the left leg and the negative on the left arm. Of the limb leads, lead II is closest to the normal cardiac axis.

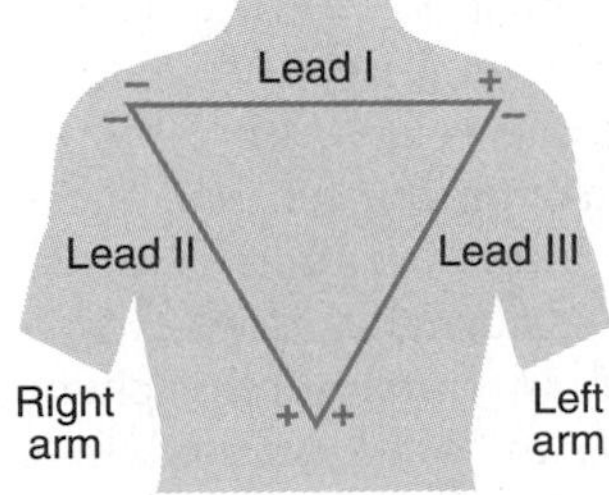

FIGURE 17–7
Einthoven's triangle (the bipolar limb leads). Lead I is obtained by placing the positive electrode on the left arm and the negative electrode on the right arm. Lead II is obtained by placing the positive electrode on the left leg and the negative on the right arm. In lead III, the positive electrode is on the left leg and the negative is on the left arm. Bipolar limb leads are used to assess current flow in the frontal plane.

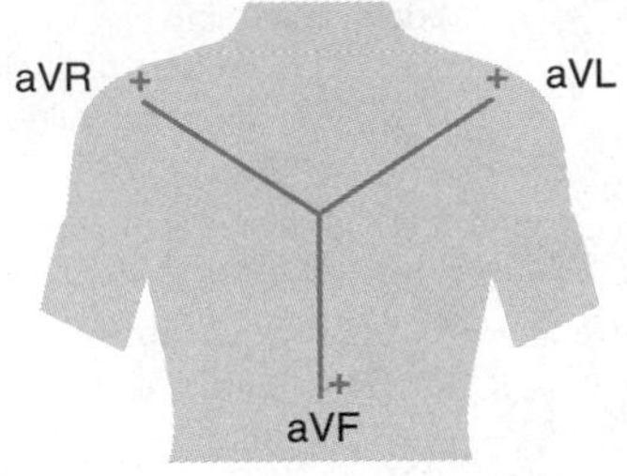

FIGURE 17–8
Augmented limb leads. Leads aVR, aVL, and aVF are obtained with positive electrodes on the right arm, left arm, and left leg, respectively, and a zero reference point at midchest. Augmented leads are located between the bipolar limb leads; they also detect current flow in the frontal plane.

The unipolar (augmented) limb leads are three additional leads, each perpendicular to a bipolar limb lead. As shown in Figure 17–8, the unipolar leads consist of one positive electrode and a zero reference point at midchest, produced by summing the voltages of leads I, II, and III. Lead aVR has its positive electrode on the right arm, lead aVL on the left arm, and lead aVF on the left leg. The axes of the bipolar and augmented limb leads may be "collapsed," or drawn through a common point at midchest, forming the hexaxial figure (Fig. 17–9). Leads are 30 degrees apart on this reference figure, with the positive electrode of lead I representing zero degrees.

The remaining six leads of the standard ECG are the unipolar chest leads, also known as *precordial* or *V leads* (Fig. 17–10). These leads consist of a positive electrode and a zero reference point. Placement of

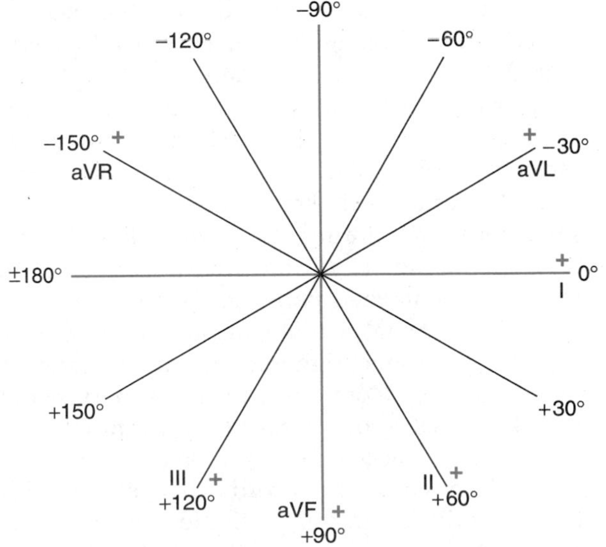

FIGURE 17–9
Hexaxial reference figure. This figure is formed when the axes of the bipolar and augmented limb leads are drawn through a common point at midchest.

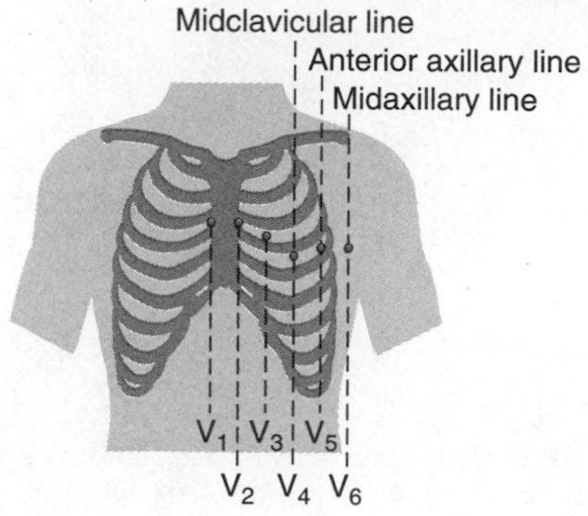

FIGURE 17–10
Precordial leads. These V leads consist of a positive electrode in each of six positions: V_1—fourth intercostal space (ICS) at the right sternal border; V_2—fourth ICS at the left sternal border; V_3—midway between V_2 and V_4; V_4—fifth ICS at the midclavicular line; V_5—fifth ICS at the anterior axillary line; and V_6—fifth ICS at the midaxillary line. A zero reference point at midchest serves as the negative pole of each lead. Precordial leads detect current flow in the horizontal plane.

the positive electrode in six positions over and around the heart is particularly useful in detection of current flow in the horizontal plane, as opposed to the limb leads, which primarily detect current flow in the frontal plane.

Clinical Applications of Electrocardiography

The standard 12-lead ECG is adequate for routine screening and diagnosis of many conditions, including axis deviation, myocardial ischemia, and myocardial infarction affecting the left ventricle. If pathology affecting the right side of the heart is suspected, additional right-sided chest leads may be evaluated. For evaluation of complex dysrhythmias, other specialized leads may be obtained with esophageal lead placement or with electrophysiology studies, which involve placement of electrodes within the heart by cardiac catheterization.

Continuous monitoring for evaluation of dysrhythmias or ischemic episodes may be done at the bedside for hospitalized patients. Oscilloscopes visually display electrical activity in one or more leads, with paper printouts triggered by any abnormality in rate or rhythm. Monitoring during supervised exercise is the basis of the stress ECG, commonly used in evaluation of chest pain. Ambulatory monitoring (e.g., Holter monitoring) records the patient's ECG continuously during normal activities during a specified time period. A tape of the electrical activity may be evaluated at a later time. Some event monitoring systems permit the patient to place a recorder over the chest during palpitations, chest pain, or dizziness and to transmit the rhythm over the telephone for immediate evaluation.

Analysis of the Electrocardiogram

Determination of the Cardiac Axis

The bipolar and unipolar limb leads of the standard ECG allow determination of the cardiac axis. Although there are several methods, the following approach illustrates electrocardiographic principles (Fig. 17–11):

Step 1: Identify the lead with the most equiphasic QRS complex. Most current flow in the heart is perpendicular to the axis of this lead.

Step 2: Examine the lead that is perpendicular to the one identified in step 1. (This lead is parallel to the cardiac axis and provides the shaft of the axis arrow.) If the QRS complex is upright in this lead, current is toward the positive end of the lead; if the QRS complex is downward, current is toward the negative end. The direction of the QRS deflection provides the arrowhead, and the cardiac axis may be estimated in degrees using the hexaxial figure.

Analysis of the PQRST Complex

Inspection of components of the PQRST complex in different leads may provide evidence of ischemia, infarction, cardiomegaly, electrolyte imbalance, or drug effect.

Ischemia. Electrocardiography is useful in determining whether incidents of chest pain are due to myocardial ischemia (angina pectoris) or to noncardiac causes, such as skeletal muscle strains or gastrointestinal conditions. During an episode of myocardial ischemia, lack of oxygen deprives the myocardial cell of the energy required for active Na^+ and K^+ transport during repolarization. Calcium pumping is also decreased, and calcium accumulates within the cell. Resting membrane potential rises, hypopolarizing the cell and increasing its automaticity. Early repolarization is represented by the ST segment. The normally isoelectric ST segment becomes elevated in transmural ischemia or in coronary artery spasm, or depressed in subendocardial ischemia[1] (Fig. 17–12). The T wave, which represents phase 3 repolarization, becomes flattened or inverted owing to delayed repolarization of ischemic tissue.

Myocardial Infarction. The presence and progression of myocardial infarction can usually be determined through analysis of the ECG (Fig. 17–13).

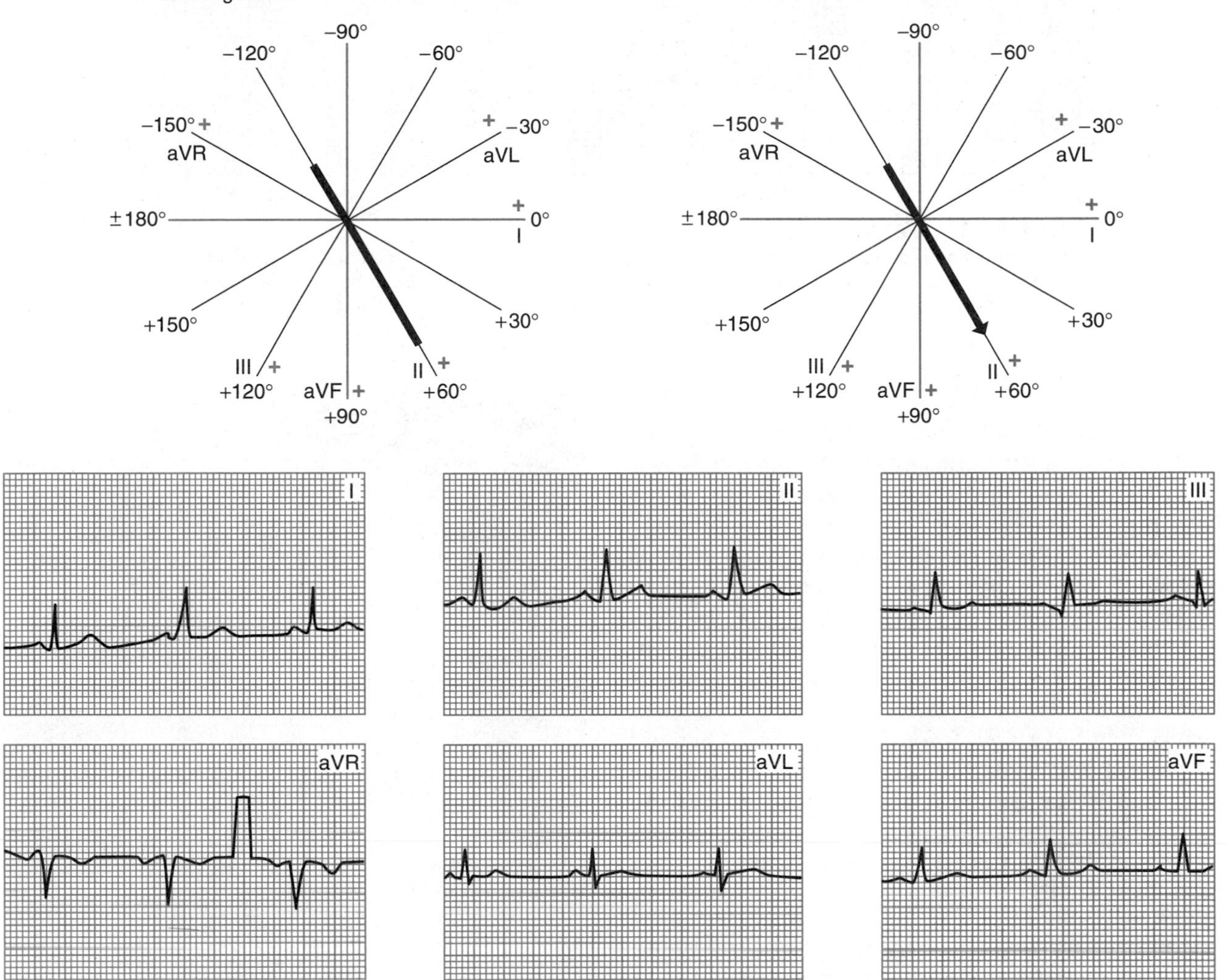

FIGURE 17–11

Determination of the cardiac axis. The six limb leads are examined. The lead with the most equiphasic QRS is noted. Current flow is perpendicular to the axis of this lead. Examination of the QRS in the perpendicular lead reveals the direction of flow. If the QRS is positive, current flow is toward the positive electrode; if the QRS is negative, current flow is away from the positive electrode.

Ischemic changes in the ST segment and T waves are seen at first. A further explanation of the ST changes of myocardial infarction may be found in the *current of injury* hypothesis, which holds that a gradient develops as injured cells leak negative ions. The exterior of these cells becomes more negative than that of adjacent normal cells, and current flows between the injured and normal areas. This results in depression of the ECG baseline in leads facing the injured area of myocardium; the ST segment then appears to be elevated.[7]

During the first 3 days after the acute episode, abnormally prominent Q waves usually develop in leads overlying the infarcted area. These are believed to result from the absence of depolarizations from the necrotic area, although the precise mechanism is unknown. In many subendocardial infarctions, Q-wave changes are not seen. The typical ECG findings in these non–Q-wave myocardial infarctions include ST-segment depression in all leads except aVR.[2] As the patient recovers, the ST segment returns to normal within 6 weeks, and the T wave returns to normal within several months. The Q-wave changes are usually permanent and allow detection of past myocardial infarction on subsequent ECGs. Table 17–2 indicates the leads in which ischemic evidence of myocardial infarction would be found with differing sites of infarction.

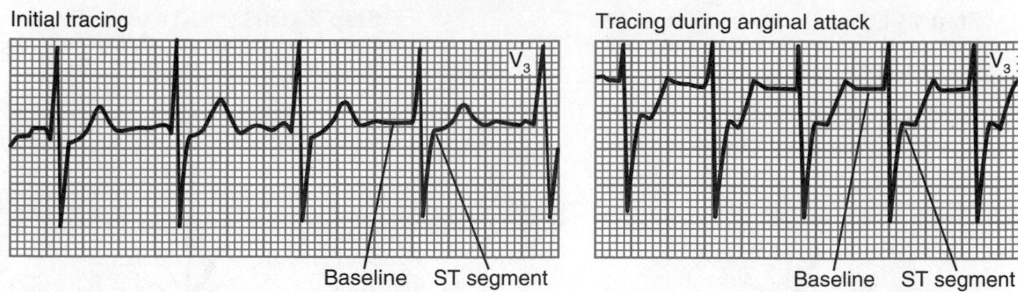

FIGURE 17–12

ECG signs of ischemia. During ischemic chest pain (angina), the ST segment may be elevated or depressed, and the T wave may be flattened or inverted owing to alterations in repolarization. In the example shown here, the ST segment is depressed, and the T wave is flattened.

Cardiomegaly. Atrial hypertrophy or dilation may cause an alteration in the shape of the P wave or the duration of the PRI. Ventricular enlargement is evidenced by changes in the shape and duration of the QRS complex.

Electrolyte Imbalance. Because action potentials are dependent on electrolyte gradients, imbalances may be detected by electrocardiography. Potassium and calcium imbalances are of particular clinical importance (Fig. 17–14). Hypokalemia causes prominent U waves, flat or inverted T waves, and peaked P waves. Hyperkalemia produces opposite changes: tall, peaked T waves and flat P waves. Hypocalcemia causes flattening of the T wave, similar to hypokalemia, whereas hypercalcemia causes a sagging depression of the ST segment, similar to that seen with digitalis therapy. Hypocalcemia lengthens, and hypercalcemia shortens, the QT interval. T-wave inversion may also occur with hypercalcemia. Magnesium imbalances do not result in clinically important ECG effects unless associated with Ca^{2+} or K^+ imbalances, which is the usual case. High Mg^{2+} correlates with low Ca^{2+} and high K^+; and low Mg^{2+} is seen with hypercalcemia and hypokalemia. As discussed later in this chapter, electrolyte imbalances may also trigger dysrhythmias in susceptible patients.

TABLE 17–2
ECG LOCATION OF MYOCARDIAL INFARCTION SITE

Infarction Site	Leads With Abnormal Q Waves
Inferior (right coronary artery occlusion)	II, III, aVF
Inferolateral (circumflex occlusion)	II, III, aVF, V_4–V_6
Anterior (left anterior descending artery occlusion)	I, aVL, V_1–V_6
Anterolateral (circumflex occlusion)	I, II, aVL, V_4–V_6
Anteroseptal (left anterior descending artery occlusion)	V_1–V_3
Posterolateral (right coronary artery occlusion)	V_1, V_4–V_6

Drug Effects. Drugs used in the treatment of cardiac and psychiatric disorders are most likely to affect the ECG by virtue of their effects on membrane permeability in excitable tissues (Table 17–3). Digi-

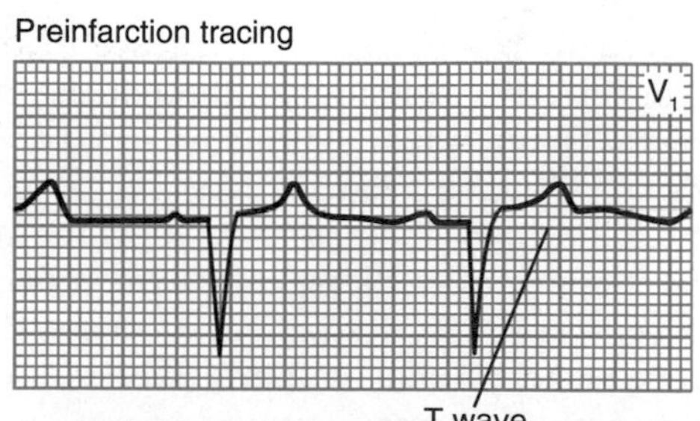

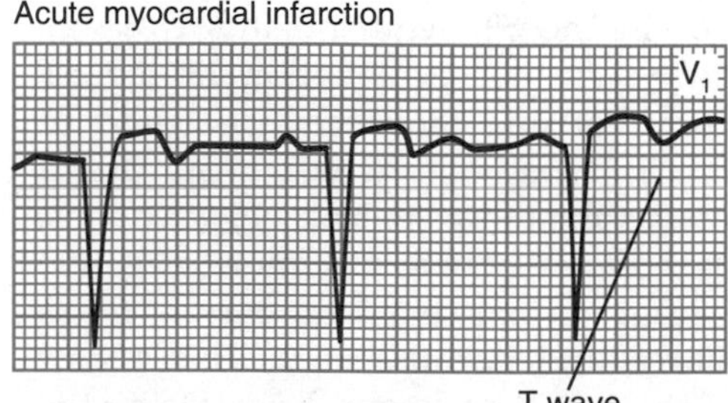

FIGURE 17–13

ECG evidence of myocardial infarction. In early myocardial infarction, a current of injury develops between injured myocardial cells (which leak negative ions) and more positive areas of the myocardium. This current depresses the ECG baseline in leads reflecting the injured areas, and the ST segment then appears to be elevated. Ischemic T-wave inversion is also seen here.

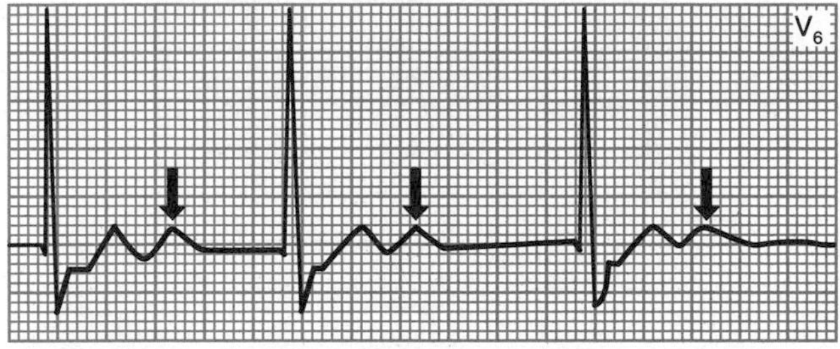

A

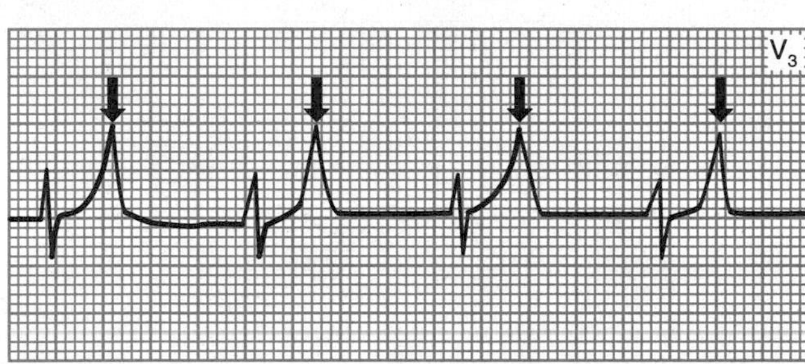

B

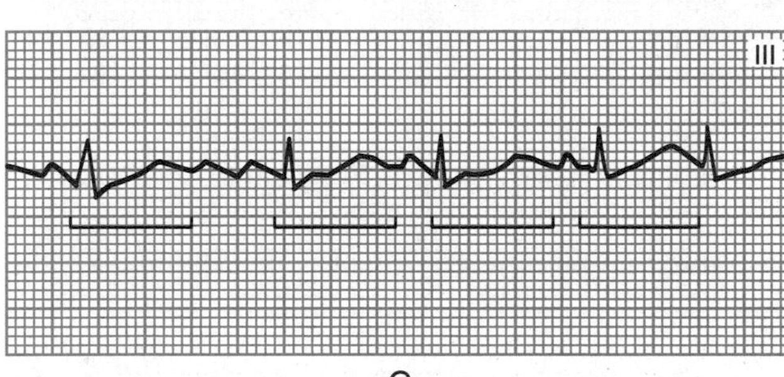

C

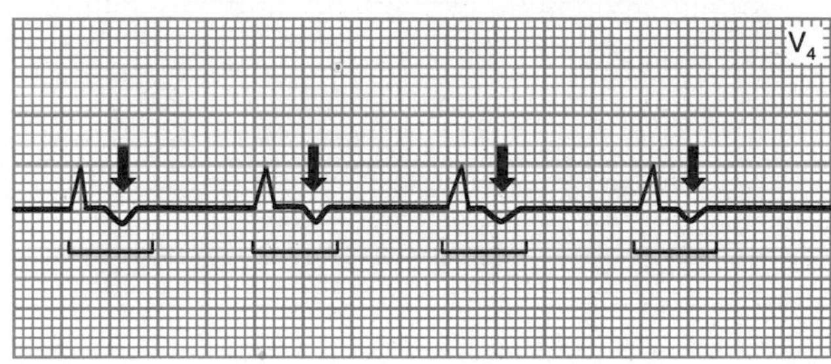

D

FIGURE 17–14

ECG evidence of electrolyte imbalance. *A*, Hypokalemia. Prominent U waves are indicated. *B*, Hyperkalemia. Flat P waves and tall, peaked T waves (indicated) are typical. *C*, Hypocalcemia. Flattening of the T wave and lengthening of the QT interval are seen. *D*, Hypercalcemia. T-wave inversion and shortening of the QT interval are apparent.

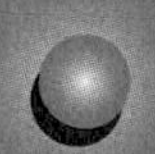

TABLE 17–3
DRUG EFFECTS ON THE ECG

DRUG	ECG EFFECTS
Cardiovascular Drugs	
Class Ia antiarrhythmics (quinidine, procainamide, disopyramide)	Widened QRS complex Increased PR interval Increased QT interval
Class Ib antiarrhythmics (phenytoin)	May increase PR interval May decrease QT interval
Class Ic antiarrhythmics (propafenone)	May increase PR interval Widened QRS complex
Class II antiarrhythmics (propranolol)	Decreased heart rate
Class III antiarrhythmics (amiodarone, sotalol, bretylium)	Increased PR interval May widen QRS complex May increase QT interval
Class IV antiarrhythmics (verapamil, nifedipine, diltiazem)	Increased PR interval May increase QT interval Decreased heart rate
Digitalis (positive inotropic agent)	Decreased heart rate Increased PR interval Increased QT interval ST depression Increased U-wave amplitude
Adenosine (antiarrhythmic)	Decreased heart rate AV block
Noncardiac Drugs	
Atropine (anticholinergic)	Increased heart rate Decreased PR interval
Antipsychotics (thorazine, chlorpromazine)	T-wave changes (widening, flattening, notching or inversion) Increased QT interval Increased U-wave amplitude
Tricyclic antidepressants (amitriptyline, desipramine, imipramine)	Increased heart rate Increased PR interval Increased QT interval Flattened T waves
Lithium (antimanic agent)	T-wave flattening or inversion
Cocaine (central nervous system stimulant)	Increased PR and QT intervals Widened QRS complex
Doxorubicin (antineoplastic)	Decreased QRS amplitude
Erythromycin (antibiotic)	Increased QT interval Increased U-wave amplitude
Pentamidine (antiprotozoal)	Increased QT interval T-wave inversion
Alcohol	Nonspecific ST segment and T-wave changes
Carbamazepine (antiepileptic)	SA block AV block
Probucol (antihyperlipidemic)	Increased QT interval
Epoprostenol (vasodilator)	Increased QT interval

talis, a cardiac glycoside long used in treatment of congestive heart failure, has characteristic effects on the ECG: shortened QT interval, sagging depression of the ST segment, and flattening of T waves. Ironically, many drugs used in the treatment of dysrhythmias may alter the ECG. Quinidine and procainamide (Pronestyl) cause prolongation of the PRI, widening of the QRS complex, and flattened or inverted T waves. *Proarrhythmia* refers to the initiation of a dysrhythmia, or the worsening of an existing one, by the administration of an antiarrhythmic drug, and is discussed further with specific dysrhythmias later in this chapter. Many psychotropic drugs, including phenothiazines, tricyclic antidepressants, and street drugs such as cocaine or methamphetamines, cause T-wave and U-wave changes and may alter the duration of the PRI, QT interval, or QRS complex to a lesser degree than the antiarrhythmic drugs.

Evaluation of the Cardiac Rhythm

The cardiac rhythm is best determined not from the 12-lead ECG but rather from a *rhythm strip*, a more prolonged recording of a single lead. Dysrhythmias are detected though examination of the heart rate, rhythm, P waves, PRI, and QRS complex.

Because the horizontal axis of the ECG graph represents time, heart rate can be determined from the recording. Several methods may be used, all of which essentially calculate the number of beats/minute from the number of seconds between beats (Fig. 17–15). A heart rate of less than 60 beats/minute indicates **bradycardia**, whereas a rate of more than 100 beats/minute signifies **tachycardia.**

Examination of the time intervals between beats reveals the rhythm. If the graphical distance (usually checked quickly with calipers) between beats is equal, or nearly so, the rhythm is regular. If the rhythm is irregular, the strip is inspected to see if the rhythm is totally (randomly) irregular, or if there is any pattern or predictability to the irregularity, such as coupled beats, cyclic acceleration, or slowing of the rhythm. The nature of any irregularity is an important cue in identifying many dysrhythmias.

P waves are examined for their presence, uniformity, and relationship to the QRS complex. The duration of the PRI is determined from the time graph and should not exceed 0.20 seconds. The QRS complex is examined for its duration and uniformity. Prolonged duration (widening) or distortion of the QRS complex signifies an abnormal or delayed current pathway through the ventricles.

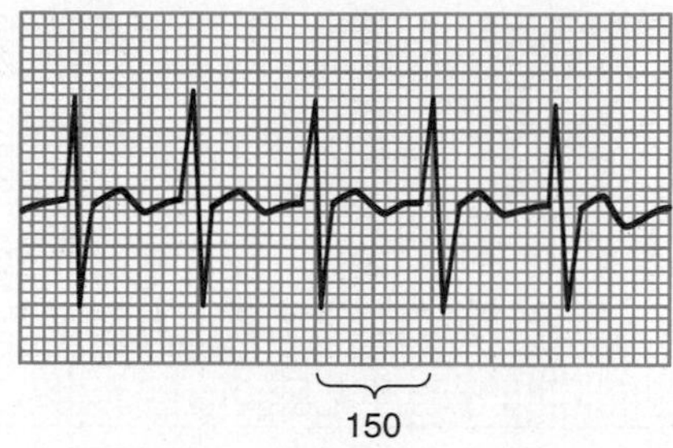

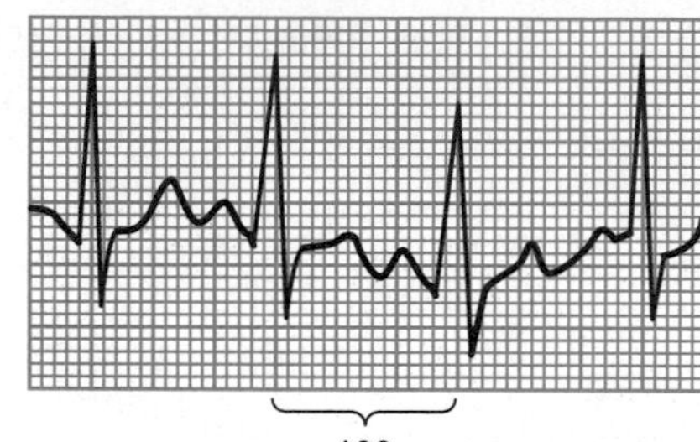

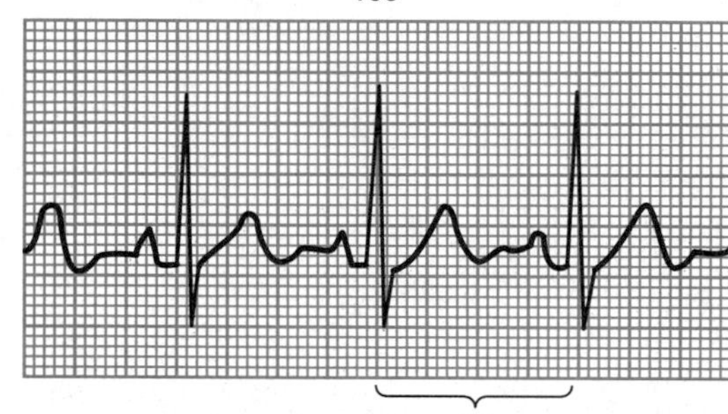

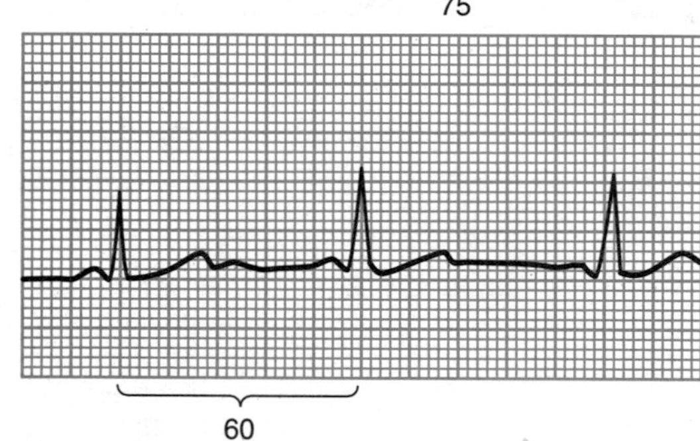

FIGURE 17–15

Determination of heart rate. Because each large square represents 0.20 seconds, the time interval between beats may be estimated in seconds. There are 60 seconds per minute, so the heart rate (beats/minute) may be calculated by dividing 60 by the time interval between beats. The heart rate is indicated below each example. (From Phillips, R.E., and Feeney, M.K. [1990]. *The Cardiac Rhythms: A Systematic Approach to Interpretation.* [3rd ed.]. Philadelphia: W.B. Saunders [p. 48].)

Figure 17–16 includes an example of **normal sinus rhythm (NSR)**, identified on the basis of a heart rate between 60 and 100 beats/minute, regular rhythm, consistent P waves preceding the QRS complex, PRI of less than 0.20 second, and normal configuration and narrow duration of the QRS complex. NSR denotes a normal origin of the cardiac rhythm and a normal conduction pathway through the heart. A variation of NSR often seen in young, well-conditioned adults is **sinus arrhythmia**. Evaluation of this rhythm reveals that all parameters are normal except the rhythm, which varies slightly in a cyclic increasing and decreasing (waxing and waning) pattern. The cyclic rhythm occurs in synchrony with the person's respirations and is due to autonomic reflex stimulation associated with intrathoracic pressure changes during ventilation. With the

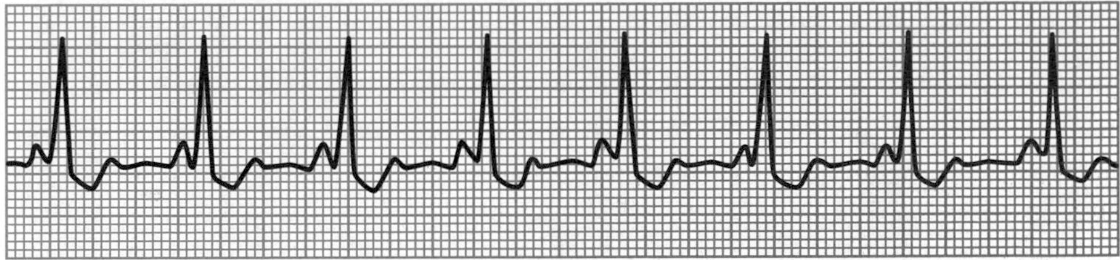

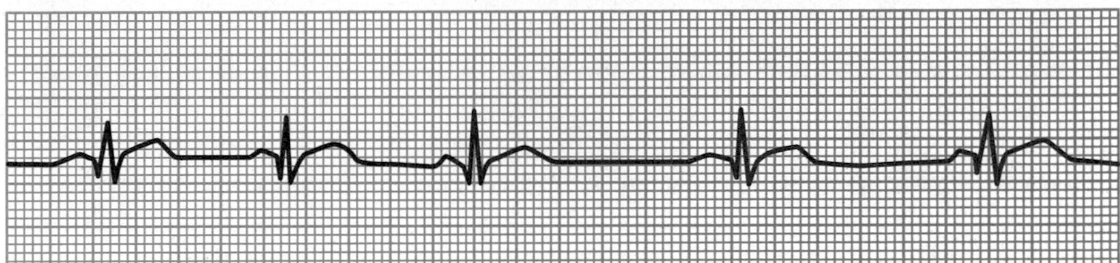

FIGURE 17–16
Normal rhythms. *A*, Normal sinus rhythm. *B*, Sinus arrhythmia. (Courtesy of M. Martha Vorvick, MS, RNC, Assistant Professor. Moorhead, MN: Tri-College University Nursing Program.)

exception of sinus arrhythmia, abnormality of any of the components of the rhythm strip indicates presence of a cardiac dysrhythmia.

CARDIAC DYSRHYTHMIAS

Cardiac dysrhythmias may be the result of: (1) altered automaticity, (2) **reentry**, or (3) **triggered activity**. These mechanisms are discussed below with the relevant dysrhythmias.

Tachycardias

Tachycardias are abnormally rapid rhythms. They are usually defined in reference to the normal sinus rate as exceeding 100 beats/minute, but the term is sometimes applied to rhythms paced by latent pacemakers with slower rates.

Sinus Tachycardia

Definition. Sinus tachycardia (Fig. 17–17) is a regular rhythm originating from the SA node with a usual rate between 100 and 150 beats/minute. The heart rate may approach 180 to 200 beats/minute with extreme stress or exertion, however.

Epidemiology. Sinus tachycardia is probably the most common of dysrhythmias because it is a normal manifestation of stress (see Chapter 1). Risk factors include emotional or physical stressors.

Etiology. The stress response, with its associated sympathetic stimulation and catecholamine release, is the most frequent etiologic mechanism. Activation of the baroreceptor reflex during low cardiac output states, such as cardiac failure or shock, also increases sympathetic stimulation of the SA node. Chemoreceptor mechanisms triggered by poor tissue perfusion (e.g., anemia) or hypermetabolic states (e.g., fever) also stimulate the vasomotor center, as do drugs that have a rate-accelerating (positive chronotropic) effect. These include sympathetic agonists such as epinephrine and ephedrine, anticholinergics such as atropine, social drugs such as caffeine, nicotine, and alcohol, and street drugs such as methamphetamines and cocaine.

Pathophysiology. Sinus tachycardia is usually an adaptive response to effect an increase in cardiac output. If exposure to the underlying stressor or condition is prolonged, however, persistent tachycar-

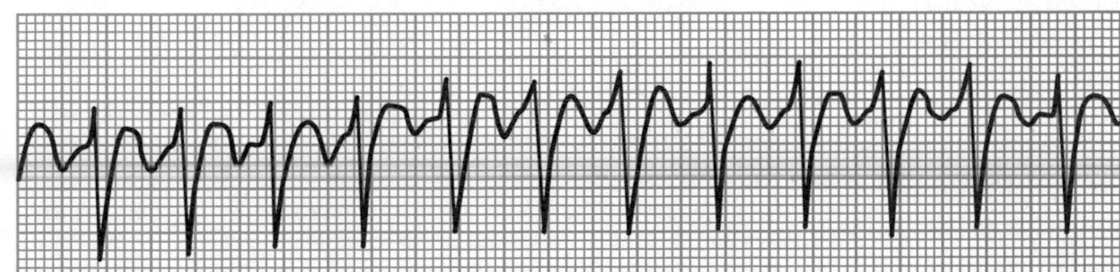

FIGURE 17–17
Sinus tachycardia. The heart rate is 150 beats/minute. (Courtesy of M. Martha Vorvick, MS, RNC, Assistant Professor. Moorhead, MN: Tri-College University Nursing Program.)

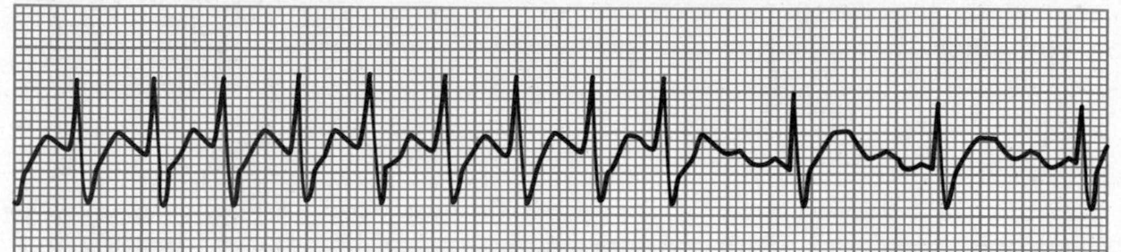

FIGURE 17–18
Paroxysmal supraventricular tachycardia (PSVT). Note the sudden cessation of the rapid rhythm. (Courtesy of M. Martha Vorvick, MS, RNC, Assistant Professor. Moorhead, MN: Tri-College University Nursing Program.)

dia may promote cardiac failure owing to depletion of sympathetic neurotransmitters or myocardial energy stores. At higher rates, stroke volume may be decreased owing to lack of diastolic filling time, and ischemia may result from decreased coronary perfusion.

Clinical Manifestations. The rapid heart rate may be perceived as palpitations or may be detectable only with monitoring of the pulse or ECG. Other manifestations of the stress response, such as diaphoresis, may be present. Manifestations of cardiac failure are uncommon except when the stressor or precipitating condition occurs in a person with limited cardiac reserve (see Chapter 16).

Prevention and Treatment. Stress management may be warranted. Underlying conditions, such as anemia or infection, should be treated. Drug therapy may be revised to exclude positive chronotropic agents. When sinus tachycardia occurs as a limited and appropriate response to stress, low-perfusion states, or hypermetabolism, no treatment is indicated.

Prognosis and Outcome. Sinus tachycardia is generally considered a benign dysrhythmia with a favorable outcome.

Supraventricular Tachycardia

Definition. Supraventricular tachycardia is a rapid rhythm (150 to 250 beats/minute) originating from one or more atrial locations or from within the AV junction.

Epidemiology. The most common form of supraventricular tachycardia occurs in sudden, brief episodes, or "runs," in young, healthy people (Fig. 17–18). Episodes of this **paroxysmal supraventricular tachycardia (PSVT)** are often triggered by excessive caffeine intake or tobacco use, especially in combination with stress and fatigue. Other supraventricular tachycardias may occur in patients with heart disease, when cell membranes within atrial and AV nodal conductive tissues are altered by ischemia, hypertrophy, or dilation.

Etiology. Supraventricular tachycardias may result from any of the three mechanisms of dysrhythmia, although 90% are believed to be due to reentry.[3]

Reentry. The reentry mechanism may originate in two ways. The most common form, *microreentry* (illustrated in Fig. 17–19), develops when ischemia or deformation creates an abnormal circuit within conductive fibers. Current flow is blocked in one direction within the circuit, but the descending impulse can travel in the other direction. By the time the impulse completes the circuit, the previously depolarized tissue within the circuit is no longer refractory to stimulation. That is, it has repolarized enough to respond to the stimulus with another depolarization.

In older people with heart disease, *AV nodal reentry* is the form of microreentry leading to PSVT. In this case, two separate conduction pathways develop within the AV junction: (1) a slow pathway with rapid repolarization (a short refractory period), through which current may pass in the anterograde direction from the atria to the ventricles; and (2) a fast pathway with a longer refractory period. Current passes in the normal (anterograde) direction through the slow pathway, and in the backward (retrograde) direction through the fast pathway, creating a reentry circuit (Fig. 17–20). PSVT by this mechanism begins with a **premature atrial contrac-**

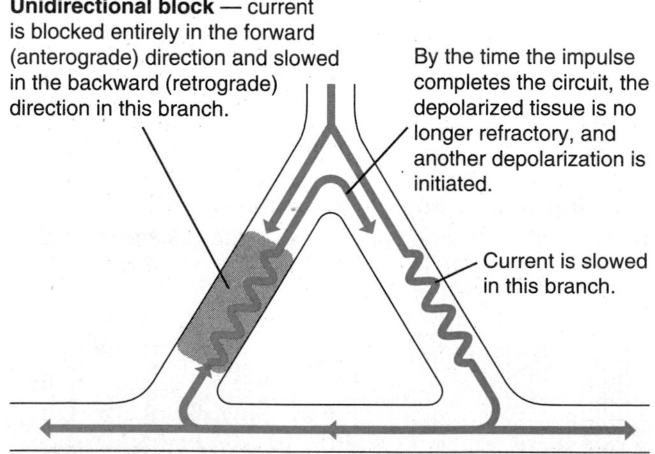
Unidirectional block — current is blocked entirely in the forward (anterograde) direction and slowed in the backward (retrograde) direction in this branch.
By the time the impulse completes the circuit, the depolarized tissue is no longer refractory, and another depolarization is initiated.
Current is slowed in this branch.

FIGURE 17–19
Microreentry. The most common mechanism of dysrhythmia originates when ischemia or deformation creates an abnormal short circuit within conductive fibers.

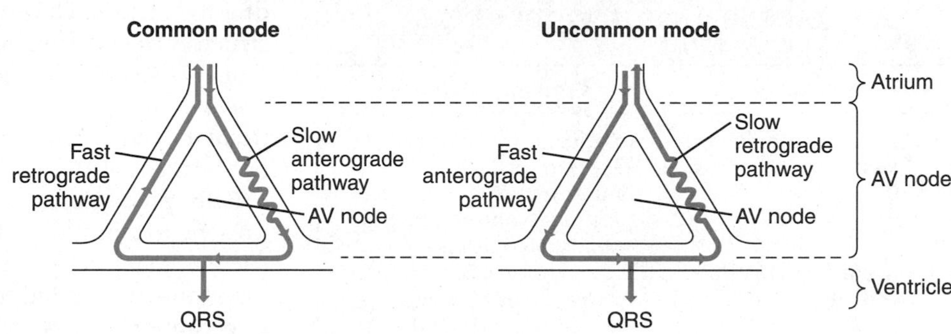

FIGURE 17–20
Atrioventricular (AV) nodal reentry. This mechanism of supraventricular tachycardia results from the development of separate pathways, one fast and one slow, *within* the AV node. In the most common form of this abnormality, current passes in the anterograde (forward) direction through the slow pathway, and in the retrograde (backward) direction through the fast pathway, creating a reentry circuit. Less commonly, the reentry circuit is reversed.

tion (PAC), which is blocked in the fast pathway because of its longer refractory period but is conducted slowly through the other pathway. By the time the impulse reaches the lower AV node, the fast pathway has recovered, and the impulse is conducted not only into the ventricles but also back to the atria, reentering the conductive circuit. In about 10% of cases of AV nodal reentry, the reentry circuit is reversed, with anterograde conduction through the fast pathway, and retrograde conduction through the slow pathway.

The second reentry mechanism, *macroreentry* (also known as *preexcitation*), depends on the presence of a congenital accessory pathway linking the atria and the ventricles outside the AV junction (Fig. 17–21). The most common of these conditions is **Wolff-Parkinson-White syndrome (WPW).** Others are summarized briefly in Table 17–4. In WPW, current usually descends from the atria to the ventricles through the accessory pathway because it offers less resistance than the AV junction. From high in the ventricles, current may ascend by retrograde conduction through the AV node, which slows the current enough to permit atrial repolarization. The ascending stimulus then re-excites the atria. The "short-circuit" of reentry allows rapid stimulation of atrial contraction. *Sinus node reentry* is an unusual mechanism of PSVT in which the reentry circuit includes the SA node. This differs from sinus tachycardia in that it begins and ends suddenly.

Enhanced Automaticity. Supraventricular tachycardias may also result from enhanced automaticity. Enhanced automaticity is the result of partial depolarization, which may increase the intrinsic rate of the SA node or of latent pacemakers, or may induce ectopic pacemakers to reach threshold and depolarize. Increased automaticity may occur with central nervous system stimulation or vasoconstriction, in electrolyte imbalance, or with use of positive chronotropic drugs. Myocardial ischemia often results in enhanced automaticity in patients with coronary artery disease, and myocardial dilation and hypertrophy may cause increased automaticity due to mechanical deformation of cell membranes.

Triggered Activity. Triggered activity refers to propagated impulses initiated by oscillations in membrane potential, or afterdepolarizations, which appear after the upstroke of the action potential. Early afterdepolarizations occur during plateau or early rapid repolarization, whereas delayed afterdepolarizations occur late in repolarization or immediately after repolarization. Early afterdepolarizations are more likely to occur when the heart rate is slow and may be induced by drugs that increase the duration of the action potential, presumably by slowing calcium flux. Delayed afterdepolarizations may be induced by rapid pacing, digitalis, or catecholamines, which increase intracellular calcium.

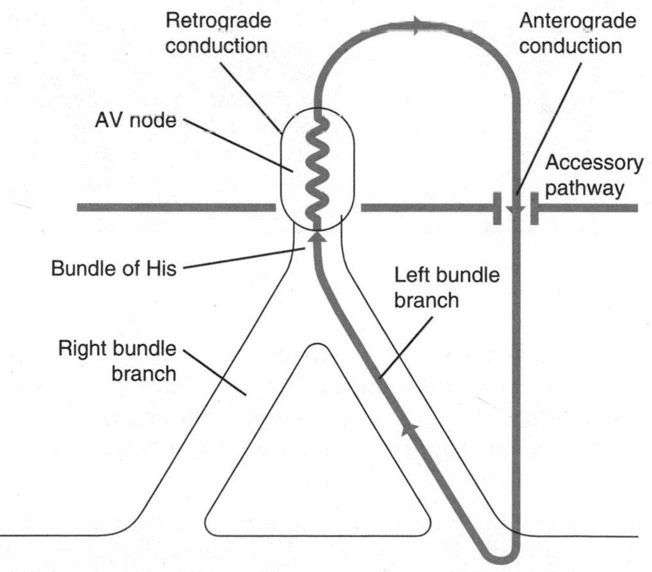

FIGURE 17–21
Macroreentry (pre-excitation). Supraventricular tachycardia in pre-excitation syndromes, such as Wolff-Parkinson-White syndrome, result from reentry due to the presence of an abnormal accessory pathway between the atria and ventricles, outside the atrioventricular (AV) node.

TABLE 17-4
CONGENITAL DISORDERS OF CARDIAC CONDUCTION

Disorder	Clinical Features
Congenital complete AV block	Absence of the lower atrial septum, or lack of continuity between a normal AV node and ventricular conductive tissues
Wolff-Parkinson-White syndrome	One or more accessory pathways (Kent bundles) between the atria and ventricles; the cardiac impulse may be conducted in the anterograde direction through the accessory pathway, then may reenter the atria by retrograde conduction through the AV node. Reentrant supraventricular tachycardia or atrial fibrillation results.
Mahaim's fibers	Presence of conductive fibers between the AV node and ventricular muscle, potentially causing reentrant supraventricular tachycardia.
Lown-Ganong-Levine syndrome	Presence of conductive fibers between the AV node and the bundle of His, potentially causing reentrant supraventricular tachycardia or atrial fibrillation.
False tendons	Presence of thin strands extending from the ventricular septum either to the left ventricular wall or to a papillary muscle; apparently triggering ventricular tachycardia with stretching of Purkinje fibers within them.

Atrial tachycardia, which arises from atrial myocardium, may be unifocal or multifocal. Unifocal atrial tachycardia usually results from enhanced automaticity or triggered activity originating from a single atrial site, although it may occasionally be due to reentry. These patients may or may not have structural heart disease. Multifocal atrial tachycardia (Fig. 17–22) results from the same mechanisms, involving multiple atrial sites. This type of supraventricular tachycardia occurs in acutely ill elderly patients, most of whom have pulmonary disease.[4]

Pathophysiology. Unless a degree of block is present to normalize the ventricular rate, supraventricular tachycardias result in decreased stroke volume due to limited diastolic filling. Because heart rate cannot be altered to compensate, some degree of cardiac failure is likely if the rhythm persists. Myocardial ischemia may result from decreased diastolic perfusion of the coronary arteries.

Clinical Manifestations. PSVT may manifest as palpitations, lightheadedness, and, less commonly, ischemic chest pain. Persistent supraventricular tachycardias may manifest as congestive heart failure. The rhythm strip reveals a rapid atrial (P wave) rate and a variable ventricular (QRS complex) rate, depending on the presence of **atrioventricular (AV) block**. P waves are abnormal in shape, except in SA nodal reentry, and vary from beat to beat if the rhythm is paced by multiple ectopic foci. WPW syndrome is also characterized by a slight alteration in the initial deflection of the QRS complex (known as a *delta wave*, see Fig. 17–23), caused by the abnormal route of entry of the current into the ventricles. In supraventricular tachycardia due to other causes, the QRS is usually normal, and these dysrhythmias may be referred to as *narrow complex tachycardias* to differentiate them from **ventricular tachycardia (VT)**. However, rate-dependent aberrant conduction of the impulse through the ventricles, with widening and distortion of the QRS, is occasionally seen. Aberrant conduction occurs when the atrial impulse reaches the bundle of His while it is still somewhat refractory, resulting in abnormal current flow within the ventricles.

Prevention and Treatment. PSVT may be prevented in some patients (e.g., those without structural heart disease) through stress management and reduction of caffeine intake and tobacco use. Acute episodes of PSVT may be interrupted in emergency settings with sedation and therapeutic vagal stimulation.

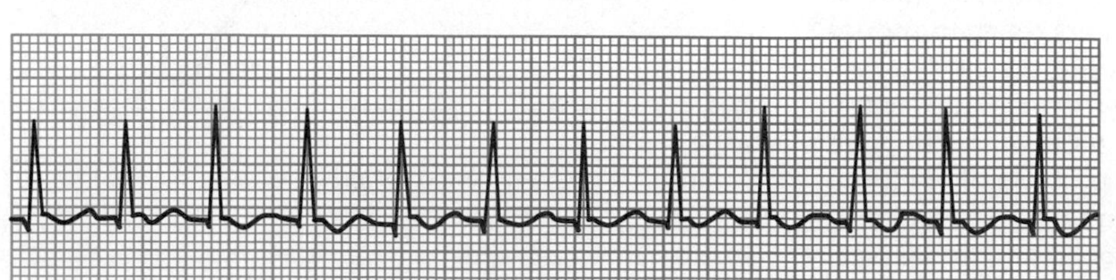

FIGURE 17–22
Atrial tachycardia. (Courtesy of M. Martha Vorvick, MS, RNC, Assistant Professor. Moorhead, MN: Tri-College University Nursing Program.)

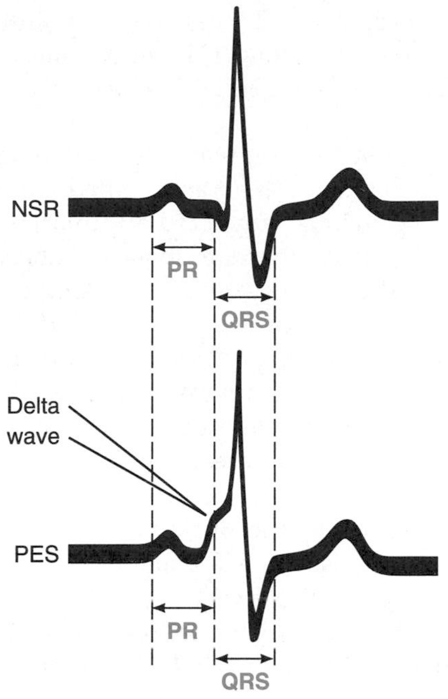

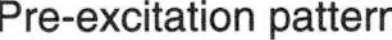

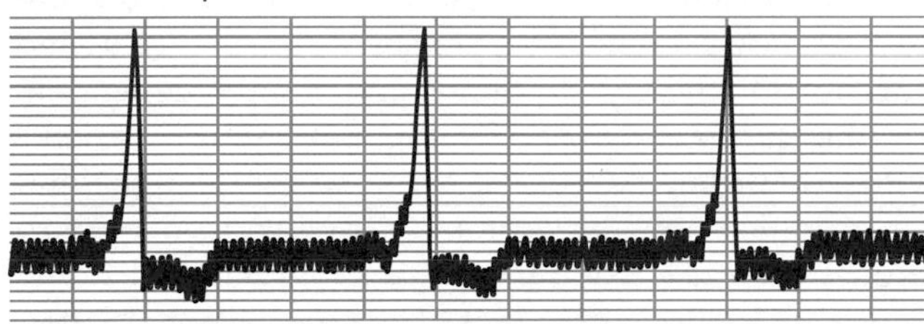

FIGURE 17–23

Wolff-Parkinson-White syndrome. This most common pre-excitation syndrome (PES) is characterized on the ECG by an alteration in the initial deflection of the QRS, known as the *delta wave*. The delta wave results from the abnormal route of current entry into the ventricles through the accessory pathway. NSR, normal sinus rhythm. The fine oscillation that widens the baseline in this tracing is due to external electrical interference. (From Phillips, R.E., and Feeney, M.K. [1973]. *The Cardiac Rhythms: A Systematic Approach to Interpretation*. Philadelphia: W.B. Saunders. [p. 141, 143].)

If vagal maneuvers, such as carotid sinus massage, do not terminate the tachycardia, antiarrhythmic drugs may be used (Table 17–5). According to the American Heart Association guidelines, adenosine (Adenocard), administered intravenously, is the drug of choice.[5] This agent binds to adenosine (A_1) receptors, opening potassium channels and hyperpolarizing AV nodal cells. This slows conduction through the AV node and interrupts the reentrant circuit.[6] Digitalis, verapamil, and quinidine may also be used to increase the degree of block at the AV node or to suppress myocardial irritability.

For persistent tachycardias with high ventricular rates, external electrical shock (synchronized cardioversion) may be used in an effort to depolarize all myocardial cells simultaneously, allowing the normal SA node pacemaker to resume its function (Fig. 17–24). WPW syndrome may be treated with surgical destruction or radiofrequency catheter ablation of the accessory pathway in some cases. Catheter ablation is done in the electrophysiology laboratory and involves the administration of a desiccating current by intracardiac catheters. This procedure is effective in destroying the accessory pathway in up to 90% of cases.[7] Treatment of any underlying cardiac disease is also warranted.

Prognosis and Outcome. Ninety-three per cent of supraventricular tachycardias may be successfully terminated with adenosine.[6] WPW syndrome demonstrates an annual rate of SCD of 0.1%.[4] Prognosis in supraventricular tachycardias associated with cardiac disease depends on the severity of the underlying condition. Most patients are at low risk of mortality due to the dysrhythmia but have significant morbidity and must be subjected to lifelong medical therapy.[8]

TABLE 17–5
ANTIARRHYTHMIC DRUGS (VAUGHAN WILLIAMS CLASSIFICATION)

Class	Examples of Drugs	Mechanism of Action
IA	Quinidine Procainamide Disopyramide Pirmenol	Potent blockade of inward sodium flux, increasing ventricular refractoriness
IB	Lidocaine Mexiletine Tocainide Aprindine	Moderate blockade of inward sodium flux; may shorten action potential duration and refractoriness in isolated tissues
IC	Flecainide Moricizine Propafenone Lorcainide	Most potent blockade of inward sodium flux, slowing conduction velocity with little effect on repolarization
II	Propranolol Timolol Metoprolol	β-Adrenergic antagonism
III	Amiodarone Bretylium *N*-acetyl-procainamide Sotalol	Prolongation of action potential duration and refractoriness
IV	Verapamil Diltiazem Nifedipine	Calcium-channel antagonism
V	Alinidine	Reduction of slope of depolarization of SA nodal cells, reducing heart rate

Data from Vaughan Williams, E.M. (1991). Significance of classifying antiarrhythmic actions since the Cardiac Arrhythmia Suppression Trial. *Journal of Clinical Pharmacology* 31, 123–135; and Vaughan Williams, E.M. (1992). Classifying antiarrhythmic actions: By facts or speculation. *Journal of Clinical Pharmacology* 32, 964–977.

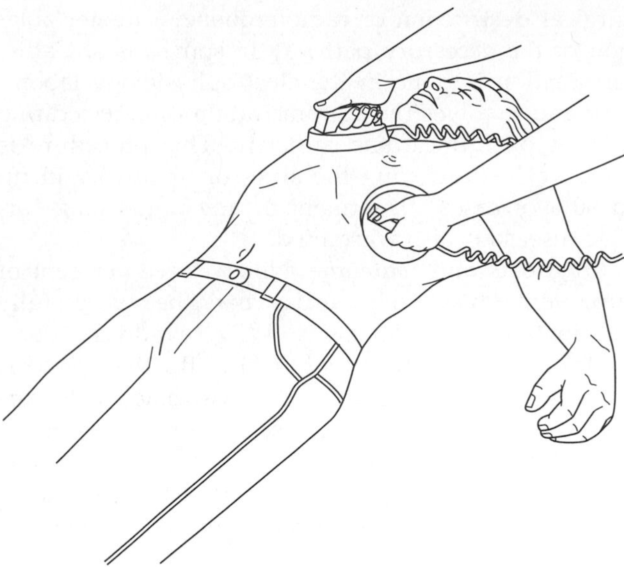

FIGURE 17–24

Placement of electrodes for cardioversion or defibrillation. An electrical shock is delivered across the heart to depolarize all cells simultaneously and facilitate the resumption of normal sinus rhythm. Synchronized cardioversion, used when the patient has an underlying rhythm such as atrial fibrillation, delivers the current at an optimal point within the cardiac cycle, preventing the initiation of ventricular fibrillation by a shock during the supernormal period (on or near the T wave). Defibrillation, used for ventricular fibrillation or ventricular tachycardia without effective perfusion, delivers the current immediately, regardless of the timing with respect to the cycle. (Redrawn from Black, J.M., and Matassarin-Jacobs, E. [1997]. *Medical-Surgical Nursing: Clinical Management for Continuity of Care.* [5th ed.] Philadelphia: W.B. Saunders. [p. 1312].)

Ventricular Tachycardia

Definition. Ventricular tachycardia is a rapid rhythm (100 to 200 beats/minute) originating from the ventricles. VT may be subclassified as *nonsustained,* in which there are between 3 and 30 consecutive beats of VT, or *sustained,* with more than 30 beats of VT.

Epidemiology. VT nearly always occurs in patients with heart disease, although a small number of otherwise healthy people have recurrent episodes of VT. Nonsustained VT is seen in up to 40% of patients during the first 48 hours after myocardial infarction, in 20% to 60% of those with idiopathic dilated cardiomyopathy, in 19% to 50% of those with hypertrophic cardiomyopathy, in 13% of those with mitral valve prolapse, and in up to 4% of those with no structural heart disease.[9]

Sustained VT is one mechanism of SCD, which occurs in 300,000 people per year in the United States.[10] Patients at highest risk for VT are those who have significant coronary artery disease and left ventricular damage due to previous myocardial infarction. A variant of VT, torsades de pointes, may occur in patients with long QT syndrome, a condition that may be congenital or associated with proarrhythmia.

Etiology. VT usually originates from damaged but viable myocardial cells that are embedded in scar tissue from previous myocardial infarction. At slower rates, VT may originate from enhanced automaticity and accelerated firing of a single ectopic focus, but most cases of VT are believed to result from formation of a reentry circuit within the ventricular myocardium, often surrounding a scar. Rare cases of VT in people without heart disease (idiopathic monomorphic VT) are believed to be caused by reentry circuits formed by congenital abnormalities in the structure of the Purkinje system or myocardial cells. The onset of VT is sudden; it probably begins with triggered activity in which a delayed afterdepolarization stimulates the cell during its supernormal period (see Chapter 4), facilitating the reentry circuit.

Pathophysiology. VT results in a degree of congestive heart failure proportional to the rate and duration of the dysrhythmia and highly dependent on the cardiac reserve of the patient. In patients with compromised hearts, acute cardiac failure and cardiogenic shock are common, owing to decreased stroke volume secondary to lack of diastolic filling time and loss of atrial kick. Impaired coronary perfusion during diastole may contribute to decreased contractility.

Clinical Manifestations. Slower rates of VT in otherwise healthy people may not be clinically detectable or may manifest as fatigue or dizziness. Patients with heart disease usually display manifestations of cardiogenic shock (see Chapter 15) and often lose consciousness rapidly owing to impaired cerebral perfusion.

The ECG reveals the rapid rate and is particularly identifiable because of the wide, bizarre QRS complex resulting from the ventricular origin and abnormal current pathway through the ventricles (Fig. 17–25). P waves are usually buried in the QRS complex, but if they can be seen, they bear no relationship to the QRS complex except for rare "capture" beats. VT may resemble atrial tachycardia with aberrant conduction when the latter occurs at rapid rates that obscure P waves. Examination of the cardiac axis often differentiates these dysrhythmias, however, because rhythms originating in the ventricles cause extreme right axis deviation owing to "backward" current vectors.

Death may occur within minutes if the dysrhythmia is not recognized and terminated. SCD occurs when VT degenerates into **ventricular fibrillation (VF)**, in which the myocardium is merely quivering,

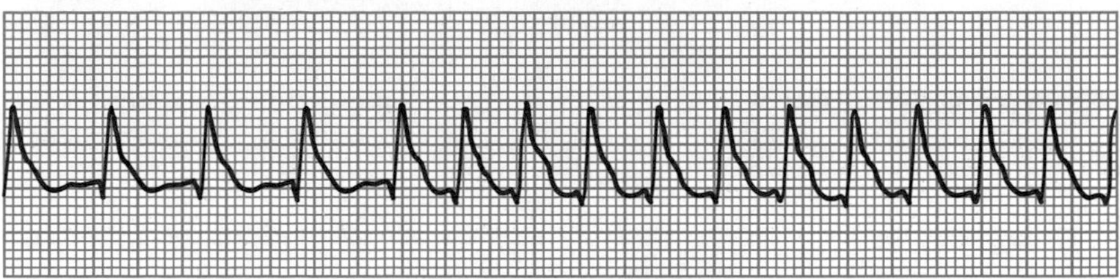

A Sustained ventricular tachycardia

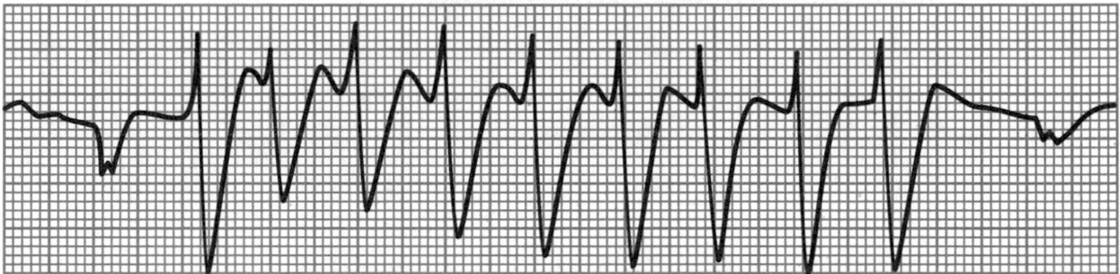

B Nonsustained ventricular tachycardia

FIGURE 17–25
Ventricular tachycardia. *A*, Sustained ventricular tachycardia (more than 30 consecutive beats). *B*, Nonsustained ventricular tachycardia (fewer than 30 beats). A nine-beat run is seen in this example. (Courtesy of M. Martha Vorvick, MS, RNC, Assistant Professor. Moorhead, MN: Tri-College University Nursing Program.)

resulting in no effective systemic perfusion. VF is discussed later in this chapter.

Prevention and Treatment. The risk associated with VT in patients with heart disease is variable, and the decision about whether and how to treat may be difficult given the proarrhythmic potential of antiarrhythmic drugs. Several large clinical trials are ongoing in an effort to determine optimal therapy of VT (see Focus of Current Research). There are no data to support preventive use of antiarrhythmic drugs or invasive measures in symptom-free patients with VT.[9] The risk of SCD due to sustained VT may be reduced with antiarrhythmic drug therapy (see Table 17–5). Amiodarone (Cordarone) has shown particularly promising results in early trials, but this drug has significant side effects and a significant rate of patient withdrawal.[9]

Acute, symptomatic episodes of VT may be treated electrically with cardioversion or defibrillation (see Fig. 17–24). These two procedures involve administration of an electrical shock between two paddle or adhesive pad electrodes placed on the chest, on either side of the heart. Cardioversion is performed on sedated conscious patients and is synchronized with the patient's underlying rhythm to deliver the impulse at a predetermined point within the PQRST cycle. Defibrillation delivers the shock immediately upon activation of the device by the operator, regardless of the status of the underlying cycle. Cardioversion cannot be set up as quickly as defibrillation but is preferred in nonemergent situations because there is no danger that the shock will be delivered during the supernormal period of the action potential (i.e., on or near the T wave). Defibrillation can be administered within seconds in an emergent situation. If the impulse is delivered during the supernormal period, VF can result; however, that rhythm usually can be converted with a second shock.

Ambulatory patients who suffer repeated episodes of symptomatic VT or VF may benefit from surgical or catheter ablation of the reentry circuit or from surgical implantation of an implantable cardioverter-defibrillator (ICD). An ICD consists of electrodes implanted on the myocardium and connected to a small impulse generator inserted into a pocket created beneath the skin of the chest or abdomen. This device senses and evaluates (by computer analysis of rate or waveform) the presence of VT or VF and automatically delivers a shock. Some ICDs also function as pacemakers, as discussed later.

Prognosis and Outcome. VT in the absence of heart disease is well tolerated. VT associated with significant heart disease is almost always responsive to preventive and emergency treatment in critical care units, although the significant coronary heart disease that often underlies VT carries a negative prognosis, as discussed in Chapter 16. Use of ICDs has decreased mortality in ambulatory patients. VT associated with VF and SCD has a high mortality rate, as discussed later in this chapter.

Flutter and Fibrillation

Flutter and fibrillation, the most rapid and disorganized of rhythms, may originate from either the atria or ventricles. Flutter is actually a subset of tachycardia, but because of its close association with fibrillation, it is considered separately here. Flutter often

Focus of Current Research

Study	Objective and Findings
Leor, et al. (1996) Sudden cardiac death triggered by an earthquake.	*Objective:* To examine the relation between emotional stress and sudden cardiac death *Findings:* On the day of the Northridge earthquake, there was a sharp increase in the number of sudden cardiac deaths related to coronary heart disease. Sixteen victims were affected during the first hour after the initial tremor.
Moss, et al. (1996) Improved survival with an implanted defibrillator in patients with coronary disease at high risk for ventricular arrhythmia.	*Objective:* To determine whether prophylactic therapy with an implanted cardioverter-defibrillator, as compared with conventional medical therapy, would improve survival *Findings:* Implanted defibrillator therapy leads to significantly improved survival in these high-risk patients.
Goyal, et al. (1996) Comparison of the ages of tachycardia onset in patients with atrioventricular nodal reentrant tachycardia and accessory pathway-mediated tachycardia.	*Objective:* To compare the ages at which tachycardia onset occurred in two types of supraventricular tachycardia *Findings:* A significantly greater proportion of patients (67%) with nodal reentrant tachycardia had the initial onset of symptoms after the age of 20 years, compared with 41% of those with accessory pathways.
Mathew, et al. (1996) Atrial fibrillation following coronary artery bypass graft surgery: Predictors, outcomes, and resource utilization.	*Objective:* To determine the incidence, predictors, and cost of atrial fibrillation and flutter after coronary artery bypass graft surgery *Findings:* Twenty-seven per cent of patients developed atrial fibrillation. Risk factors included male sex, history of congestive heart failure, preoperative heart rate > 100 beats/minute, postoperative pacing, and longer aortic cross-clamp time during surgery.
Tervahauta, et al. (1996) Resting electrocardiographic abnormalities as predictors of coronary events and total mortality among elderly men.	*Objective:* To examine the prognostic significance of ECG abnormalities among the elderly *Findings:* Higher risk was associated with Q waves, depressed ST interval, and atrial fibrillation.
Niebauer, et al. (1996) Atrioventricular node properties in patients with accessory pathways.	*Objective:* To compare AV nodal characteristics of patients with accessory pathways with those in controls *Findings:* AV nodal characteristics do not differ between the two groups.

Box continued on following page

Frishman, et al. (1996) Twenty-four-hour ambulatory electrocardiography in elderly subjects: Prevalence of various arrhythmias and prognostic implications (report from the Bronx Longitudinal Aging Study).	*Objective:* To identify risk factors and disease markers for cardiovascular, cerebrovascular, and dementia illness in old people *Findings:* Nonsustained ventricular tachycardia was an independent predictor of death and myocardial infarction. Transient AV block and sinus bradycardia were predictors of stroke.
Gallagher, et al. (1995) Effectiveness of bystander cardiopulmonary resuscitation and survival following out-of-hospital cardiac arrest.	*Objective:* To examine the relationship between effectiveness of bystander CPR and survival following cardiac arrest *Findings:* CPR was performed effectively in 32% of cases. Of those, 4.6% of patients survived, versus 1.4% of patients with ineffective CPR.

precedes fibrillation, and in the transitional state, the ECG may reveal aspects of both ("fib-flutter").

Atrial Flutter

Definition. Atrial flutter is a rapid rhythm of atrial origin in which the atrial rate is 250 to 350 beats/minute and the ventricular rate varies according to the degree of AV block. In most cases, the atrial rate is about 300 beats/minute, and the ventricular rate is 150 beats/minute (2:1 block).

Epidemiology. Atrial flutter is relatively uncommon but most often occurs in patients with coronary heart disease or congestive heart failure. Less commonly, atrial flutter occurs in the setting of rheumatic heart disease, thyroid crisis, or pneumonectomy.

Etiology. Atrial flutter is the result of a reentry circuit, confined to the atria, which develops as a result of ischemia or deformation of myocardial cells.

Pathophysiology. The atrial rate is so rapid that no effective atrial contraction occurs. Mural thrombi may form within the atria, and these may embolize, resulting in pulmonary emboli or stroke. Congestive heart failure nearly always occurs because the rapid ventricular rate diminishes ventricular filling, which is further compromised by loss of atrial kick.

Clinical Manifestations. Manifestations of congestive heart failure are present (see Chapter 16). Atrial flutter is distinguished on the ECG by the presence of rapidly firing peaked P waves, giving a saw-toothed appearance to the atrial activity (Fig. 17–26). QRS complexes follow some, but rarely all, P waves. The degree of AV block is usually regular at 2:1, 3:1, or 4:1, but may be variable in some cases. The QRS complex is normal unless aberrantly conducted.

Prevention and Treatment. Antiarrhythmic drugs and AV nodal depressant drugs (e.g., digitalis, quinidine, or procainamide) may be used to suppress automaticity in patients susceptible to this dysrhythmia. Therapy with oral antiarrhythmic drugs is rarely successful in terminating the dysrhythmia once it occurs, however. Use of adenosine (Adenocard), the treatment of choice in most supraventricular tachycardias, may induce life-threatening *increases* in heart rate in patients with atrial flutter due to reduction in the degree of AV block.[11] Cardioversion, overdrive pacing, and ablation of the reentrant circuit are the treatments of choice.[8] Implantable atrial defibrillators that also have antitachycardia pacing features are being evaluated in clinical trials.[12]

Prognosis and Outcome. Atrial flutter is often resistant to treatment. Prognosis depends on response to therapy and the degree of underlying heart disease.

Atrial Fibrillation

Definition. Atrial fibrillation is a totally irregular rhythm generated by disorganized atrial depolarization at a rate of 400 to 600 beats/minute, with random conduction of some impulses through the AV junction to the ventricles.

Epidemiology. Atrial fibrillation is the most common sustained dysrhythmia, occurring in 2% of the general population and in 5% of people older than 60 years.[13] Chronic congestive heart failure is most frequently associated with atrial fibrillation and may be due to coronary heart disease, hypertension, congenital heart disease, rheumatic heart disease, or pulmonary disease. The latter condition, known as

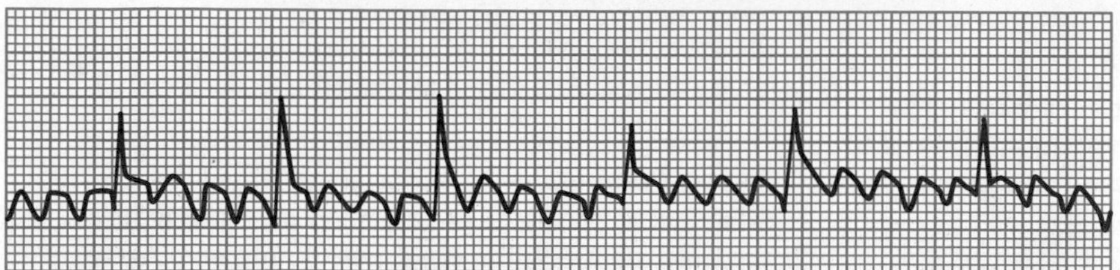

Atrial flutter with 3:1 block and 4:1 block

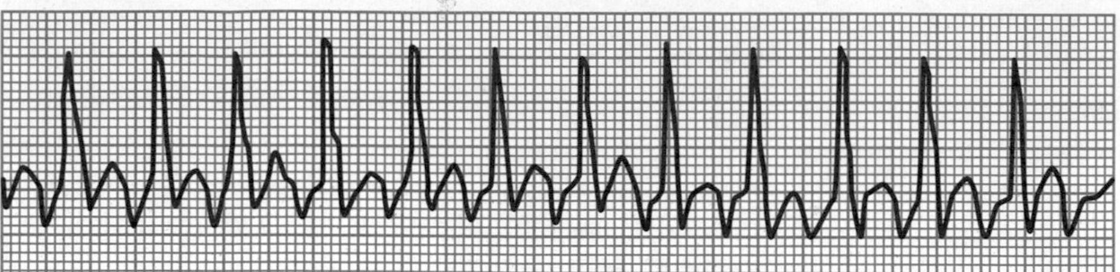

Atrial flutter with 2:1 block

FIGURE 17–26

Atrial flutter. Rapidly firing peaked P waves give a sawtooth appearance to the atrial activity. Atrioventricular (AV) block usually reduces the ventricular rate. (Courtesy of M. Martha Vorvick, MS, RNC, Assistant Professor. Moorhead, MN: Tri-College University Nursing Program.)

cor pulmonale, is discussed in Chapter 18. In the 10% of patients who have no known underlying condition, the dysrhythmia is referred to as *lone* atrial fibrillation.[13]

Etiology. Chaotic atrial depolarization probably results from the combination of enhanced automaticity and multiple reentry circuits created by atrial ischemia or deformation. The most prevalent hypothesis holds that multiple wandering "wavelets" of current are conducted through atrial tissue, extinguishing themselves, accelerating, or decelerating as they encounter cells in varying states of refractoriness. Because the degree of vagal stimulation of the heart influences refractoriness, changes in autonomic activity may precipitate the onset of atrial fibrillation. Resistance at the AV node blocks most atrial impulses, but the ventricular rate is still relatively rapid (usually 160 to 200 beats/minute).

Pathophysiology. As in atrial flutter, mural thrombosis may occur in atrial fibrillation, and congestive heart failure is probable due to loss of atrial kick. The more rapid the ventricular rate, the greater is the decrease in cardiac output, owing to diminished stroke volume and coronary perfusion.

Clinical Manifestations. Manifestations of congestive heart failure are usually present if the ventricular rate exceeds 100 beats/minute. The ECG demonstrates a totally irregular ventricular rhythm with no true P waves but rather with the characteristic wavy baseline (f waves) produced by the chaotic atrial activity (Fig. 17–27). The QRS complex is normal unless aberrantly conducted.

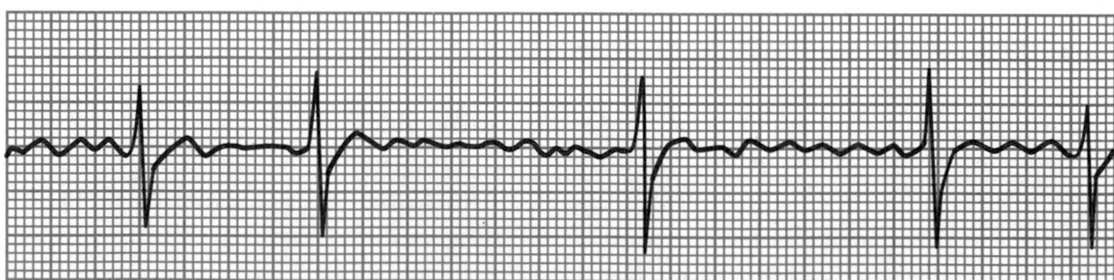

Atrial fibrillation with slow ventricular response

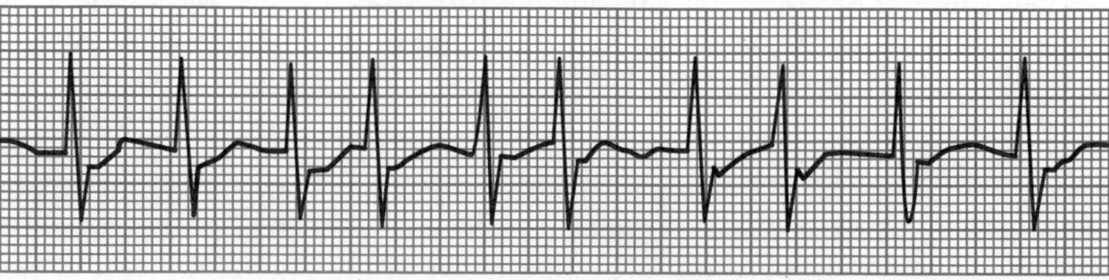

Atrial fibrillation with rapid ventricular response

FIGURE 17–27

Atrial fibrillation. Disorganized atrial depolarization results in an oscillating baseline without true P waves. Random conduction of current into the ventricles produces a totally irregular rhythm. (Courtesy of M. Martha Vorvick, MS, RNC, Assistant Professor. Moorhead, MN: Tri-College University Nursing Program.)

Prevention and Treatment. Prevention of atrial fibrillation involves appropriate management of the underlying cardiac disease. Treatment is primarily aimed at reducing atrial irritability and lowering the ventricular rate by increasing the degree of block at the AV junction. Digitalis, calcium-channel blockers, and β-blockers may be used either singularly or in combination to achieve these aims (see Table 17–5). If this "chemical cardioversion" is insufficient, direct current cardioversion may be used. Anticoagulants may be used in conjunction with these approaches to lower risks associated with mural thrombi. An imaging procedure, transesophageal echocardiography, has been used before electrical cardioversion to visualize any atrial thrombi, which could embolize with restoration of NSR.[14] If thrombi are apparent, the procedure is delayed until anticoagulation has been established. Radiofrequency ablation of the AV node may be employed in cases in which the ventricular rate cannot be controlled by pharmacologic therapy or cardioversion. This procedure involves induction of a permanent block at the AV node by means of radiofrequency energy delivered through a transvenous catheter. A ventricular pacemaker is then used to pace the cardiac rhythm.[13]

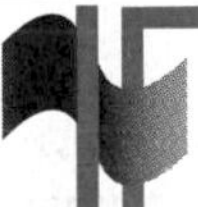

Clinical Scenario

F.F., a 60-year-old man with a history of myocardial infarction and congestive heart failure, is hospitalized for treatment of persistent atrial fibrillation. He has been treated with digoxin and diltiazem (Cardizem) during the past several weeks. On admission, F.F. complains of fatigue, loss of appetite, weight loss, and shortness of breath with exertion. His heart rate is rapid, ranging from 140 to 158 beats/minute. Echocardiography reveals an ejection fraction of 32%. Despite medical treatment of his congestive heart failure, F.F.'s clinical status worsens. Increasing pulmonary congestion and declining renal function are noted. Bedside monitoring demonstrates atrial fibrillation with a rapid ventricular response as well as intermittent periods of atrial flutter with 2 : 1 block.

1. Is F.F.'s dysrhythmia contributing to his worsening cardiac failure? Explain.
2. Could any of F.F.'s clinical manifestations be related to his therapy? Explain.

Prognosis and Outcome. Synchronized cardioversion is successful in restoring NSR in 70% to 85% of cases.[15] Continuous drug therapy is required to maintain this rhythm in three fourths of these patients. Prognosis depends primarily on the degree of underlying heart disease and on the incidence of embolic stroke associated with mural thrombi. Risk of stroke in patients with atrial fibrillation is sixfold, and these strokes are often severely debilitating.[16] Overall mortality in patients with atrial fibrillation is about twice that seen in healthy people.

Ventricular Flutter and Ventricular Fibrillation

Definitions. Ventricular flutter is a rapid rhythm (200 to 400 beats/minute) originating in the ventricles. Ventricular flutter often degenerates into VF, a totally chaotic rhythm of ventricular origin that results in ineffective quivering of the ventricles and SCD.

Epidemiology. The proportion of cardiac deaths that are sudden and unexpected has remained constant at 50% despite the overall decline in deaths due to cardiac disease. Overall incidence of SCD among the adult population of the United States is 0.1% to 0.2% per year.[17] Ventricular flutter and fibrillation are associated with myocardial ischemia due to the same causes as VT.

Patients at highest risk are those who have structural heart disease (e.g., myocardial infarction or cardiomyopathy) and who have evidence of: (1) history of a complicated clinical course in hospital, (2) ejection fraction less than 40%, (3) frequent **premature ventricular contractions (PVCs)** or episodes of nonsustained VT, (4) delayed afterdepolarizations, (5) reduced range of heart rate variability, and (6) depressed baroreceptor sensitivity.[18] Underlying risk associated with structural heart disease may be transiently increased by autonomic stimulation, reperfusion, or effects of proarrhythmic drugs.

Etiology. In ventricular flutter, a single reentry circuit, triggered by a PVC, results in cell-to-cell conduction within the ventricular myocardium. As the myocardium becomes even more ischemic, increased automaticity activates in additional reentry circuits and the multifocal, disorganized depolarizations of fibrillation.

Pathophysiology. Both dysrhythmias result in totally ineffective contraction, producing no cardiac output.

Clinical Manifestations. The clinical picture is of SCD. The patient is unconscious and pulseless, although a discernible rhythm is seen on the ECG. (The term **pulseless electrical activity** is used to denote a rhythm that does not result in perfusion.) In

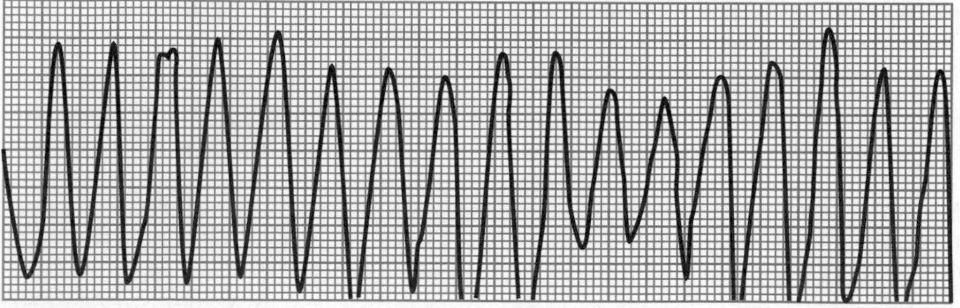

FIGURE 17–28
Ventricular flutter. The sine wave pattern is typical (Courtesy of M. Martha Vorvick, MS, RNC, Assistant Professor. Moorhead, MN: Tri-College University Nursing Program.)

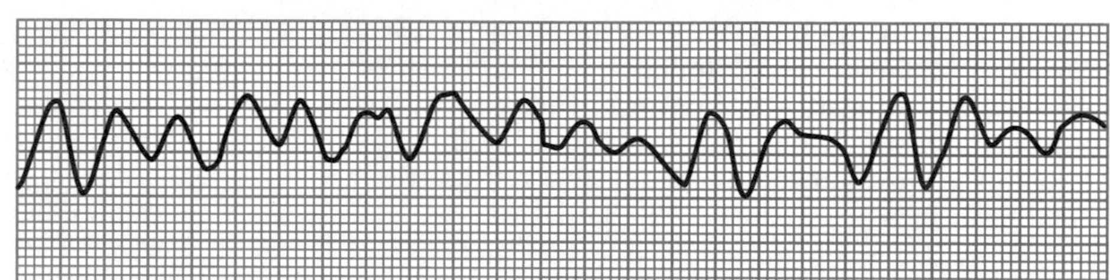

FIGURE 17–29
Ventricular fibrillation. Chaotic oscillation of the baseline is seen. A form of sudden cardiac death, this rhythm results in ineffective quivering of the ventricles and absence of cardiac output. (Courtesy of M. Martha Vorvick, MS, RNC, Assistant Professor. Moorhead, MN: Tri-College University Nursing Program.)

ventricular flutter, the ECG reveals a regular rapid rate and wide, bizarre ventricular complexes resembling a sine wave pattern (Fig. 17–28). VF (Fig. 17–29) is characterized by chaotic oscillation of the baseline, with no discernible PQRST complexes. As the heart becomes more ischemic, the frequency and amplitude of the oscillations decrease, and the ECG tracing reverts to a straight line **(asystole)**.

Prevention and Treatment. Prevention is similar to that in VT, with treatment of underlying cardiac disease, antiarrhythmic drug therapy (e.g., lidocaine, procainamide, β-blockers, amiodarone) to suppress ventricular irritability, possible surgical or catheter ablation of reentrant circuits, and possible use of an ICD. Defibrillation is essential to convert the dysrhythmia once it occurs, although **cardiopulmonary resuscitation (CPR)** should be initiated to provide some cardiac output until a defibrillator can be procured (Fig. 17–30). CPR consists of external cardiac compression to produce minimal perfusion and mouth-to-mouth, mouth-to-mask, or other means of artificial ventilation.

Prognosis and Outcome. Ventricular flutter and fibrillation result in death unless defibrillation is instituted. Defibrillation may be successful in terminating an acute episode, but the dysrhythmia usually signifies extensive myocardial damage with a grave prognosis. Survival rates average 25% to 30%.[18]

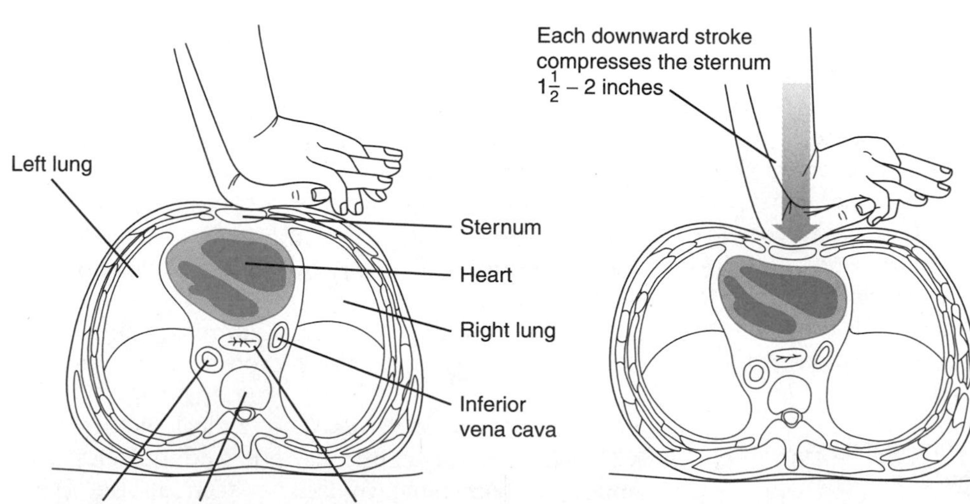

FIGURE 17–30
Cardiopulmonary resuscitation (CPR). CPR techniques include external cardiac compression, shown here, and artificial ventilation using mouth-to-mouth, mouth-to-mask, or a ventilatory assist device. (Redrawn from Black, J.M., and Matassarin-Jacobs, E. [1993]. *Luckmann and Sorensen's Medical-Surgical Nursing: A Psychophysiologic Approach.* [4th ed.]. Philadelphia: W.B. Saunders. [p. 1205].)

Bradycardias

A bradycardia is a rhythm with a ventricular rate of less than 60 beats/minute. Bradycardias result from slowing of the normal sinus node pacemaker (**sinus bradycardia**) or from pacing of the rhythm by latent pacemakers with slower intrinsic rates (**junctional rhythm** or **idioventricular rhythm**). AV blocks, discussed later in this chapter, may slow the ventricular rate owing to delay of the SA node impulse at the AV junction, or may be the cause of slow junctional or ventricular escape rhythms.

Sinus Bradycardia

Definition. Sinus bradycardia is a slow rhythm (less than 60 beats/minute) originating from the SA node.

Epidemiology. Sinus bradycardia is very common; it occurs normally during rest and sleep in many people. Aerobically conditioned athletes also have very slow resting heart rates. Any activity associated with vagal stimulation increases the risk of sinus bradycardia, and many drugs have a negative chronotropic effect (e.g., β-blockers, calcium-channel blockers, digitalis). Function of the SA node may be impaired in cardiac disease or in neurologic or systemic toxic conditions that affect autonomic nervous system function.

Etiology. Because sympathetic nervous system activity is minimized during rest and sleep, in people with normally low resting heart rates, sinus bradycardia may result. As discussed in Chapter 35, aerobically conditioned athletes have low resting heart rates owing to the efficiency of their cardiac muscle contraction in generating stroke volume as well as to the efficiency of their skeletal muscle energy metabolism. Increased parasympathetic activity induced by inappropriate or therapeutic vagal stimulation or by negative chronotropic agents slows the intrinsic SA node rate as well as the rate of conduction through the AV node. Ischemia or toxicity of the atrial myocardium or its autonomic innervation may impair SA node function by altering membrane transport in the pacemaker cells.

Pathophysiology. If adequate cardiac reserve is present, cardiac contractility increases to offset effects of the slowed heart rate. Because metabolic demands are decreased during rest and sleep, decreased cardiac output does not usually result in a perfusion deficit in these cases. With vagal stimulation, cardiac disease, or systemic toxicity, the SA node rate may decrease to the point at which cardiac output is insufficient, resulting in cardiac failure. The SA rate usually remains high enough to overdrive latent pacemakers.

Clinical Manifestations. Most cases of sinus bradycardia are asymptomatic. When the rate is very low, however, signs and symptoms of low cardiac output may be present, including confusion and hypotension. The ECG usually shows a rhythm that is normal in every aspect except for the slow rate (Fig. 17–31). In some very slow rhythms, escape beats originating from the AV junction or ventricles may be seen.

Prevention and Treatment. Inappropriate vagal stimulation should be prevented. Asymptomatic sinus bradycardia does not require treatment. Negative chronotropic drugs should be discontinued if the patient develops symptoms, and underlying cardiac, neurologic, or systemic disease should be managed. If signs of cardiac failure are present, the dysrhythmia is treated with an anticholinergic drug, such as atropine. In rare cases, pacing or positive inotropic agents may be required to maintain adequate cardiac output.

Prognosis and Outcome. Sinus bradycardia is usually a normal variant or a benign dysrhythmia that responds to treatment.

Junctional Rhythm

Definition. Junctional rhythm is a slow rhythm (40 to 60 beats/minute) originating in the AV junction.

Epidemiology. Junctional rhythm is relatively uncommon but may occur as an escape mechanism in conditions in which the SA node rate is decreased below the latent junctional rate by disease or drug

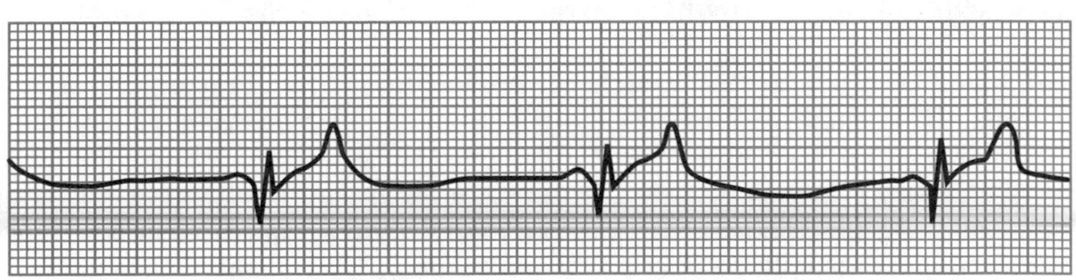

FIGURE 17–31
Sinus bradycardia. The heart rate is 38 beats/minute. Peaked T waves are also seen in this strip but are not relevant to identification of the rhythm. (Courtesy of M. Martha Vorvick, MS, RNC, Assistant Professor. Moorhead, MN: Tri-College University Nursing Program.)

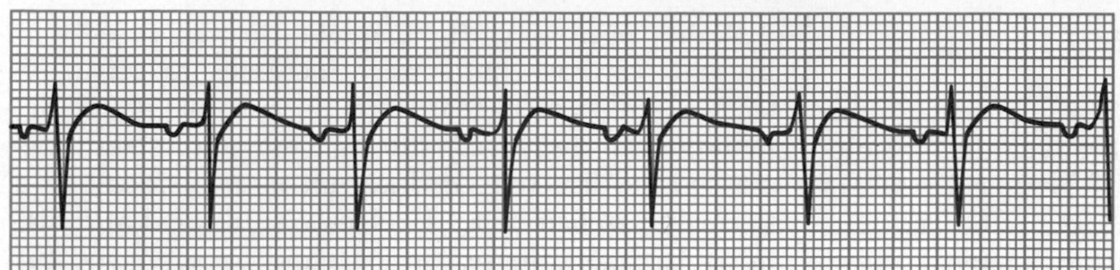

FIGURE 17–32
Junctional rhythm. Inverted P waves are typical. An accelerated junctional rhythm is seen here (heart rate, 86 beats/minute). (Courtesy of M. Martha Vorvick, MS, RNC, Assistant Professor. Moorhead, MN: Tri-College University Nursing Program.)

therapy. Alternatively, a lower junctional focus may pace the heart in cases of high AV block.

Etiology. The possible causes of slowed SA rate were discussed previously with sinus bradycardia. AV block is discussed later in this chapter.

Pathophysiology. Presence of junctional rhythm indicates loss of overdrive suppression by the SA node, or failure of the SA node impulse to reach the ventricles. If AV block is complete in the latter case, cardiac arrest occurs unless a junctional or ventricular escape rhythm ensues. Cardiac output depends primarily on the ventricular rate, with cardiac failure possible at very low or very high rates.

Clinical Manifestations. Junctional rhythm at relatively normal rates is asymptomatic. Manifestations of cardiac failure are present at very slow or very fast rates. The junctional rhythm usually displays the intrinsic rate of 40 to 60 beats/min, but neural stimulation or toxic alteration of the membranes of junctional cells may result in a more rapid rate (junctional tachycardia or accelerated junctional rhythm, Fig. 17–32). Because the rhythm originates in the junction, conduction through the atria is retrograde, resulting in abnormal P waves and PRI. A high junctional focus results in inverted P waves that precede the QRS complex, with a very short PRI. A mid-junctional focus may bury P waves in the QRS complex because atrial and ventricular conduction are occurring simultaneously. A low junctional focus may result in an inverted P wave that follows the QRS complex because the ventricles fire earlier than the atria. The impulse is conducted normally through the ventricles, resulting in a normal QRS complex.

Prevention and Treatment. Prevention is based on management of underlying cardiac or systemic disease predisposing to SA node dysfunction or AV block. Because drug toxicity (e.g., digitalis) is associated with junctional rhythm, therapy should be closely monitored. Symptomatic junctional rhythms are treated as bradycardias or tachycardias, with appropriate drug therapy (see Table 17–5).

Prognosis and Outcome. Junctional rhythms do not significantly impair function in most cases and are often adaptive. Those that negatively affect cardiac output are usually responsive to treatment.

Idioventricular Rhythm

Definition. Idioventricular rhythm is a slow rhythm paced by an ectopic focus in the ventricular myocardium. In most cases, the presence of ischemia induces the focus to fire at a rate higher than the intrinsic ventricular rate, at 50 to 100 beats/minute (accelerated idioventricular rhythm). A very slow idioventricular rhythm may precede asystole; this is often referred to as *agonal rhythm* or "dying heart."

Epidemiology. Idioventricular rhythm occurs only in the setting of significant myocardial disease, as a consequence of ischemia or reperfusion after interventions such as thrombolytic therapy (see Chapter 16). Inferior myocardial infarction imposes particularly high risk because of impaired perfusion of the conduction system secondary to right coronary artery occlusion.

Etiology. Ischemic or reperfusion injury may promote idioventricular rhythm by slowing the SA node rate, blocking impulses at the AV node, or increasing the automaticity of latent ventricular pacemakers.

Pathophysiology. Idioventricular rhythm may be well tolerated if the rate is near normal and may be an adaptive escape rhythm in SA node disease or AV block. Loss of atrial kick and low rates may result in heart failure, especially in patients with little or no reserve.

Clinical Manifestations. Idioventricular rhythm at normal rates may be asymptomatic. Accelerated idioventricular rhythm is usually seen transiently as a reperfusion dysrhythmia. Manifestations of congestive heart failure are present at very slow rates, and the rhythm may be a terminal event in a severely diseased heart that is unresponsive to treatment. The ECG reveals a slow rate and regular rhythm. P waves, if present, bear no relationship to the QRS complex, which is wide and distorted (Fig. 17–33).

Prevention and Treatment. Prevention involves management of underlying cardiac disease. Idioventricular rhythm at a normal rate may not require treatment if it is adaptive. In some cases, the rhythm is transient and unexplained, converting on its own. If the dysrhythmia precipitates cardiac failure, treat-

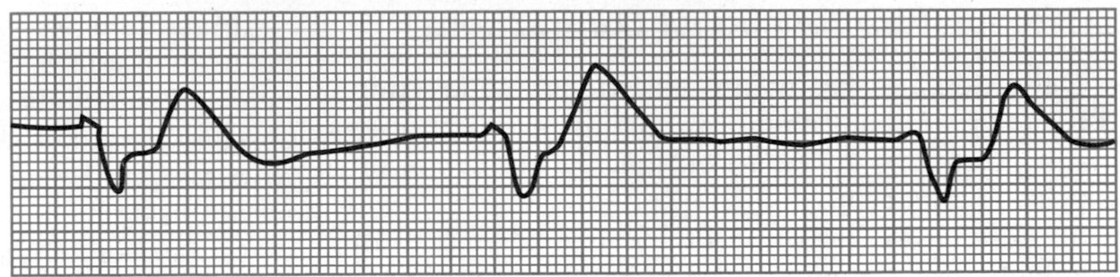

FIGURE 17–33
Idioventricular rhythm. An ectopic focus in the ventricles is pacing the heart at a slow rate. This example is of an agonal rhythm ("dying heart"). (Courtesy of M. Martha Vorvick, MS, RNC, Assistant Professor. Moorhead, MN: Tri-College University Nursing Program.)

ment is aimed at suppressing the irritable ventricular focus with drug therapy, and primary therapy of cardiac failure is instituted (see Chapter 16).

Prognosis and Outcome. Prognosis depends on the degree of myocardial disease. Idioventricular rhythm often signifies extensive myocardial damage associated with a poor prognosis.

Premature Contractions

Premature contractions, also known as *ectopic beats* or *extrasystoles,* are single or multiple beats paced by ectopic foci in the atria, AV junction, or ventricles. Premature beats do not, in themselves, define the cardiac rhythm; rather, they are superimposed on an underlying rhythm.

Premature Atrial Contractions

Definition. A PAC is a beat originating from an ectopic atrial focus that fires before an expected normal beat.

Epidemiology. PACs are common. They occur occasionally in normal hearts, particularly with excessive use of caffeine, alcohol, or tobacco. Fatigue, stress, and drugs containing theophylline may also increase risk.[19] PACs are most often associated with atrial dilation, as in congestive heart failure and cor pulmonale, or with myocardial ischemia, as in coronary artery disease or hypermetabolic states.

Etiology. One or more of the previously listed factors results in increased automaticity of one or more foci in the atrial myocardium, resulting in spontaneous depolarization before stimulation by the SA node impulse.

Pathophysiology. If it is conducted to the ventricles, the premature beat results in a weak contraction with decreased stroke volume due to decreased diastolic filling. PACs that occur very early, before the ventricles have repolarized, are nonconducted. In either case, the ectopic impulse depolarizes the SA node prematurely, and the SA node rhythm resets the pace after the PAC.

Clinical Manifestations. PACs are rarely frequent enough to compromise cardiac function significantly. They may be detectable to the patient as a "skipped" beat because the beat after the PAC is often slightly more forceful than normal. The PAC is usually audible with a stethoscope but may not result in a palpable pulsation. If conducted to the ventricles, the PAC is visible on the ECG as a beat occurring before the normal R-R interval, with a P wave that differs from normal (Fig. 17–34). The QRS complex of the premature beat is normal unless aberrantly conducted. The interval between the PAC and the following sinus beat is almost equal to the normal R-R interval, owing to resetting of the sinus rate. Nonconducted PACs are represented by a premature, abnormal P wave with no following QRS complex.

Prevention and Treatment. Reduction of risk factors, such as caffeine, alcohol, and tobacco use, is indicated. Treatment with antiarrhythmic drugs is not usually necessary, although drug therapy for congestive heart failure should be optimized. Because PACs can precede the onset of atrial fibrillation or flutter, they warrant careful monitoring, especially if they are frequent.

Prognosis and Outcome. PACs are benign and self-limited in most cases.

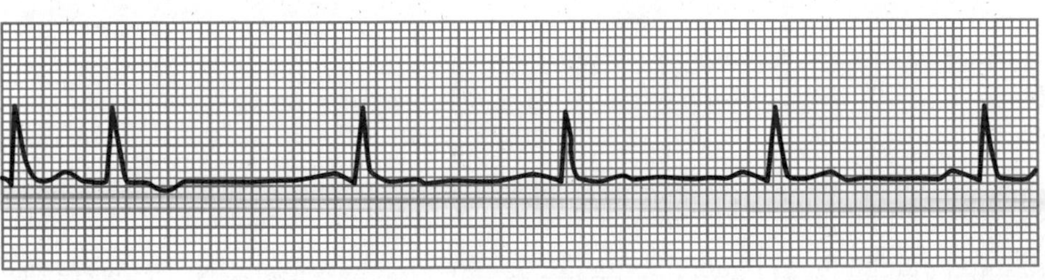

FIGURE 17–34
Premature atrial contraction (PAC). The second beat is a PAC. The underlying rhythm is normal sinus rhythm. (Courtesy of M. Martha Vorvick, MS, RNC, Assistant Professor. Moorhead, MN: Tri-College University Nursing Program.)

Premature Junctional Contractions

Definition. A **premature junctional contraction (PJC)**, or premature nodal contraction, is a beat originating from the AV junction that occurs before an expected sinus beat.

Epidemiology. Ischemia of the AV node is most frequently associated with PJCs. Drug toxicity (especially with digitalis) may also manifest as PJCs. PJCs may occur in normal hearts secondary to excessive use of caffeine or tobacco, or as a manifestation of emotional stress.

Etiology. Automaticity of an AV junctional focus is enhanced by any of the previously listed factors. Ischemia and digitalis toxicity may alter membrane transport characteristics. Nicotine may exacerbate ischemia due to vasoconstriction, and sympathetic activity is increased during stress or with caffeine use.

Pathophysiology. The irritable focus reaches threshold and depolarizes before its excitation by the SA node impulse. As with junctional rhythm, there is retrograde current flow through the atria, whereas excitation of the ventricles is usually normal. The premature beat produces a weak contraction, owing to lack of time for complete ventricular filling and loss of atrial kick.

Clinical Manifestations. As with PACs, the patient usually does not have symptoms, except for possible subjective awareness of skipped beats. As illustrated in Figure 17–35, the PJC has a normal QRS complex and P-wave characteristics that vary depending on whether a high, middle, or low junctional focus paces the beat (see previous discussion of junctional rhythm).

Prevention and Treatment. Risk reduction may be warranted if the rhythm is distressing to the patient. Treatment is unnecessary because cardiac function is not significantly compromised.

Prognosis and Outcome. PJCs are generally benign dysrhythmias.

Premature Ventricular Contractions

Definition. PVCs are premature beats that originate from one or more irritable foci in the ventricles.

Epidemiology. PVCs are the most common form of dysrhythmia.[20] They occur occasionally in normal hearts, particularly during exercise or stress. In the absence of cardiac disease, PVCs are most often due to potassium imbalance or acidosis. PVCs are commonly associated with ischemia and acute myocardial infarction. Digitalis toxicity is a common cause of PVCs in patients with chronic congestive heart failure.

Etiology. Myocardial cell membranes become unstable, owing to one or more of the previously listed factors, leading to enhanced automaticity. In rare cases, the ectopic focus is isolated from other electrical stimuli by entry and exit block, and fires at a regular ventricular rate that is independent of the underlying rhythm (parasystole). With digitalis toxicity, PVCs are often seen in a predictable pattern, owing to afterdepolarizations. *Bigeminy*, in which every other beat is a PVC, and *trigeminy*, in which every third beat is a PVC, are examples of such patterns. Bigeminy and trigeminy may also result from reentry circuits due to myocardial ischemia.

Pathophysiology. As with premature beats of atrial or junctional origin, stroke volume is decreased because of lack of filling time. Current flow originates abnormally in a ventricular focus and is conducted from cell to cell within the ventricles. Ventricular contraction resulting from this stimulation is usually ineffective; although in some cases, the beats produce enough stroke volume to generate a peripheral pulse. Some PVCs may be conducted through the AV node in a retrograde manner, resetting the SA node rate; but in most cases, the sinus rate is unaltered. A PVC may trigger a reentry circuit, producing VT or VF. PVCs that occur early in repolarization have been implicated most often in this case; however, late PVCs may also induce triggered activity.

Clinical Manifestations. Most PVCs are perceived by the patient as skipped beats, with an irregular pulse resulting from nonperfused PVCs. PVCs, in themselves, do not usually cause other clinical signs or symptoms. When PVCs occur in the setting of myocardial ischemia, they indicate significant membrane instability and may forewarn of SCD under any of the following circumstances: (1) more than

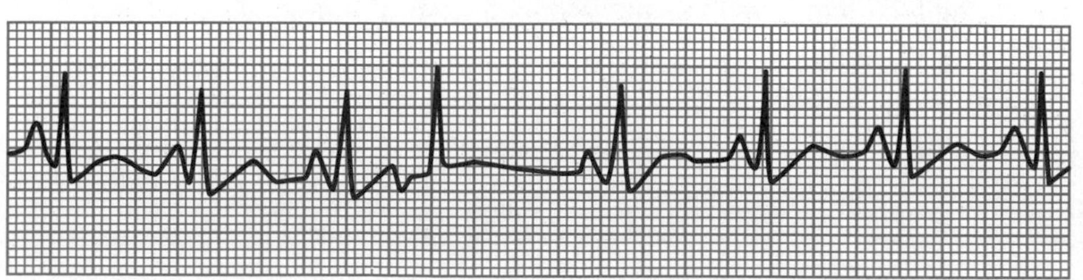

FIGURE 17–35
Premature junctional contraction (PJC). The fourth beat is a PJC. The underlying rhythm is normal sinus rhythm. (Courtesy of M. Martha Vorvick, MS, RNC, Assistant Professor. Moorhead, MN: Tri-College University Nursing Program.)

six PVCs per minute, (2) multifocal origin (more than one irritable focus), (3) couplets or triplets of PVCs, or (4) PVCs falling on or near the T wave of the preceding beat.

PVCs are readily identified on the ECG by their wide, bizarre QRS complexes (Fig. 17–36). If there is retrograde atrial conduction, an inverted P wave may follow the QRS complex. In most cases, however, the QRS complex of the premature beat is not associated with a visible P wave. The PVC is usually followed by a longer-than-normal R-R interval (compensatory pause), which results in the sinus rate resuming its previous cadence; that is, the R-R distance covered by three normal sinus beats is the same as that of two sinus beats with the PVC between them. Detection of the compensatory pause often permits differentiation of PVCs from PACs or PJCs with aberrant ventricular conduction. In the case of parasystole, however, the PVCs bear no consistent relationship to the preceding and following normal beats. Instead, a consistent interval between ectopic beats is seen.

Prevention and Treatment. In the absence of structural heart disease, treatment of PVCs is not warranted. Prevention of SCD is the impetus for detection and treatment of PVCs in patients at risk. Ventricular irritability is suppressed with antiarrhythmic drug therapy (e.g., lidocaine, procainamide, or quinidine). In the setting of acute myocardial infarction, intravenous lidocaine is usually the drug of choice for suppression of PVCs. Prophylactic therapy with lidocaine has not been shown to affect outcomes significantly, however.[21] If PVCs result from drug toxicity, electrolyte imbalance, or acidosis, these conditions are corrected.

Prognosis and Outcome. PVCs occurring in the absence of structural heart disease are generally benign. Prognosis in cardiac disease depends on the extent of myocardial damage.

Conduction Disturbances

Conduction disturbances are dysrhythmias that result from absence of normal impulse generation, excessive slowing of the impulse, or blockage of conduction of some or all impulses within the cardiac conduction system. Conduction disturbances may occur within the SA node, the AV junction, or the branches or fascicles of the bundle of His.

Sinus Arrest and Sinus Exit Block

Definitions. Sinus arrest is failure of the SA node to generate the cardiac impulse. (Failure of impulse generation of just one isolated beat is referred to as a **sinus pause.**) **Sinus exit block** is present when the SA node impulse is generated normally but is blocked (occasionally or consistently) from leaving the SA node to excite atrial tissues. The term **sick sinus syndrome** encompasses all of these findings.

Epidemiology. Abnormal SA node function is associated with ischemia of the node, excessive vagal stimulation, or toxicity due to therapy with negative chronotropic drugs (e.g., digitalis, β-blockers, or calcium-channel blockers).

Etiology. Normal automaticity is suppressed by any of the above factors, owing to either impaired membrane transport or abnormal autonomic stimulation of the SA node.

Pathophysiology. Each of these dysrhythmias results in absence of a P wave for one or more beats. There is no conduction of the sinus impulse and no atrial contraction. Unless a latent junctional or ventricular pacemaker fires, asystole occurs. Occasional asystoles (skipped beats) may not significantly impair cardiac function. Total asystole (cardiac standstill) is an uncommon mechanism of SCD.

Clinical Manifestations. The patient may be aware of the skipped beats, and the pulse is audibly and palpably irregular. Frequent asystoles or escape rhythms may result in symptoms of congestive heart failure due to slow rate and loss of atrial kick. SCD occurs rarely from this mechanism, but frequent asystoles may forewarn of its occurrence. The ECG reveals absence of P waves for one or more beats. With sinus pauses (Fig. 17–37), the sinus rate is reset when the rhythm resumes. As a result, the interval containing the skipped beat is different from the interval containing three normal beats. With sinus exit block, the SA node continues to fire regularly even though the impulse is occasionally

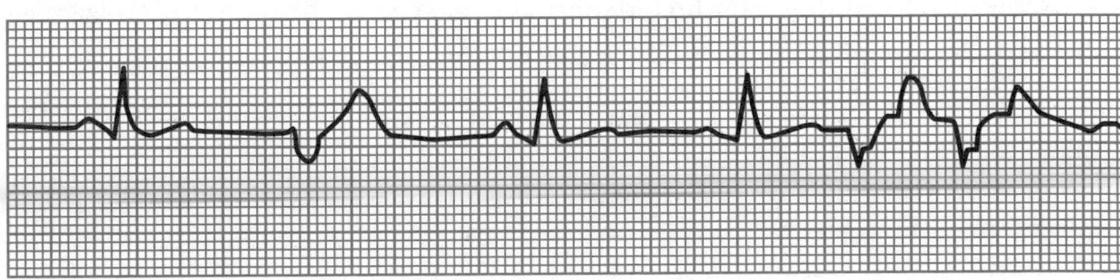

FIGURE 17–36
Premature ventricular contractions (PVCs). The second, fifth, and sixth beats are PVCs. (Courtesy of M. Martha Vorvick, MS, RNC, Assistant Professor. Moorhead, MN: Tri-College University Nursing Program.)

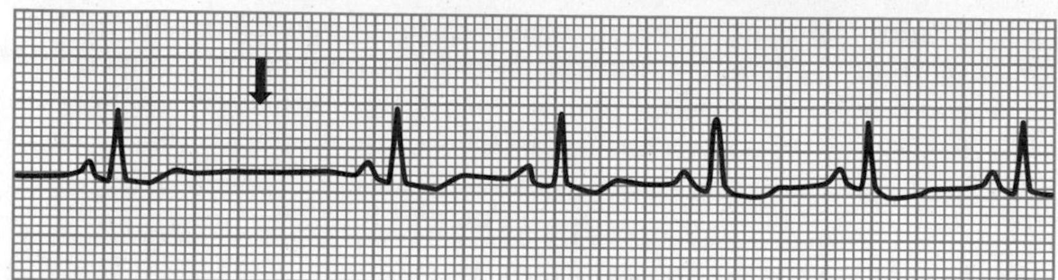

FIGURE 17–37
Sinus pause. After the first beat, the sinoatrial node fails to generate an impulse for one beat (indicated). The sinus rate is reset when the rhythm resumes. (Courtesy of M. Martha Vorvick, MS, RNC, Assistant Professor. Moorhead, MN: Tri-College University Nursing Program.)

blocked, and intervals containing skipped beats are exact multiples of the normal R-R interval.

Prevention and Treatment. Prevention of inappropriate vagal stimulation is important, as discussed with sinus bradycardia. Drug therapy should be altered to minimize negative chronotropic effects. Atropine may be administered to increase the rate of AV conduction in junctional escape. Artificial pacing may be instituted, either temporarily or permanently, if asystoles are frequent and escape rhythms do not produce an adequate cardiac output (Table 17–6; Fig. 17–38). CPR is initiated for cardiac arrest.

Prognosis and Outcome. Prognosis varies depending on the frequency of asystole, adequacy of escape rhythms, and degree of myocardial damage.

Wandering Atrial Pacemaker

Definition. Wandering atrial pacemaker is a conduction disturbance caused by competition among one or more ectopic atrial or junctional pacemakers and the SA node, with all pacemakers having nearly the same intrinsic rate.

Epidemiology. Wandering pacemaker is occasionally seen transiently in normal hearts and may be induced by vagal stimulation. Wandering pacemaker is most often seen with atrial ischemia, hypertrophy, or dilation, such as in chronic congestive heart failure.

Etiology. Because of slowing of the sinus rate by vagal stimulation or acceleration of latent pacemakers by ischemia or deformation, multiple pacemakers are active. Different pacemakers may pace different beats, or they may fire at the same time (atrial fusion). In any case, the resultant atrial depolarization has a slightly different sequence from beat to beat.

Pathophysiology. Because each impulse results in atrial contraction and is conducted normally in the ventricles, cardiac function is not significantly impaired unless the rate is very slow.

Clinical Manifestations. Manifestations of heart failure are rare. The ECG demonstrates differently shaped P waves among beats, with normal QRS configuration (Fig. 17–39).

Prevention and Treatment. Treatment is not usually necessary. Atropine may be used in treatment of symptomatic bradycardia.

Prognosis and Outcome. Wandering atrial pacemaker is considered a benign dysrhythmia.

TABLE 17–6
INDICATIONS FOR IMPLANTATION OF A PERMANENT CARDIAC PACEMAKER*

Indication Class	Description	Examples of Disorders
I	Conditions for which a permanent pacemaker should be implanted	Sick sinus syndrome with symptomatic bradycardia Symptomatic complete or second-degree AV block Fascicular block with intermittent symptomatic complete heart block Type II second-degree AV block
II	Conditions for which permanent pacemakers are frequently used but there is disagreement about need for use	Sick sinus syndrome with heart rate <40 beats/minute Asymptomatic second-degree AV block or complete heart block with heart rate >40 beats/minute Severely symptomatic patients with hypertrophic cardiomyopathy unresponsive to drug therapy
III	Conditions for which there is general agreement that a permanent pacemaker is not required	All other dysrhythmias

*Classes established by the Joint American College of Cardiology—American Heart Association Task Force.
Data from Kusumoto, F.M. (1996). Cardiac pacing. *New England Journal of Medicine* 334(2), 89–98.

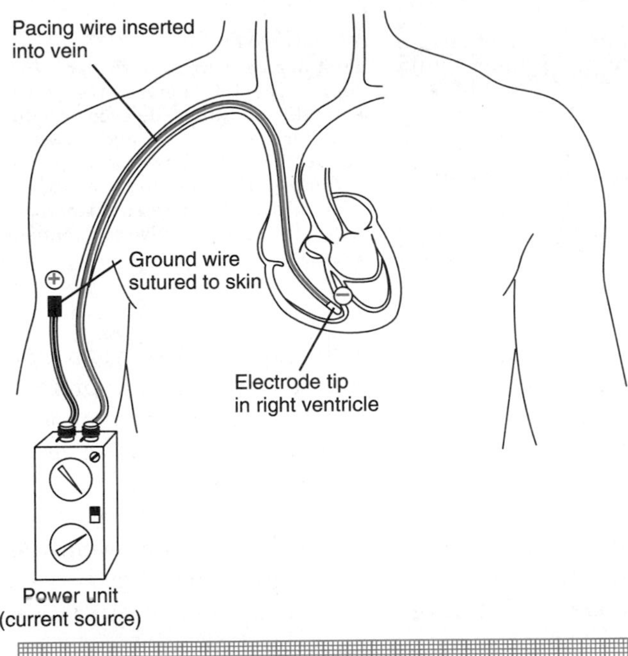

FIGURE 17–38

Transvenous pacemaker. In this form of temporary pacemaker, a wire tipped with a pacing electrode is advanced into the heart through a catheter inserted into a central vein. Electrical current is delivered to the myocardium at a rate and voltage regulated by an external power source. On the rhythm strip, the vertical deflection preceding each QRS complex represents the pacemaker current, or spike. Presence of the spike immediately before the QRS complex indicates that the electrode is in the ventricle and that the pacemaker is capturing the rhythm. (ECG tracing courtesy of M. Martha Vorvick, MS, RNC, Assistant Professor. Moorhead, MN: Tri-College University Nursing Program.)

Atrioventricular Blocks

Definition. AV block is present when the atrial impulse is slowed or prevented from being transmitted through the AV node to the ventricles. AV block may be physiologic if it is present during rapid atrial dysrhythmias (see discussion of atrial flutter and fibrillation). As discussed here, AV block indicates pathology of the AV node.

First-degree AV block is present when the atrial impulse is slowed but eventually conducted through the node to the ventricles. **Second-degree AV block** is present when some atrial impulses are blocked from transmission to the ventricles. **Third-degree AV block** (also known as *complete AV block*) results in blockage of all atrial impulses.

Epidemiology. About 1 million people in the United States have permanent pacemakers, and AV block is the usual indication for this intervention.[22] AV block is associated with drugs such as β-blockers and digitalis, which suppress conduction through the AV node. Blocks may also be associated with congenital heart defects affecting the conduction system (see Developmental Perspective). Most commonly, however, AV block occurs in the setting of anterior or inferior wall myocardial infarction due to ischemic damage of the node.

Etiology. Excitability of nodal tissue is suppressed, owing to lack of sympathetic stimulation or to membrane instability secondary to ischemia or drug effect.

Pathophysiology. Delayed AV conduction in first-degree block produces a regular rhythm of normal, or slightly slow, rate. Cardiac output is usually normal, although some patients may develop symptoms because of loss of optimal timing of the atrial and ventricular responses.

The three types of second-degree block are as follows: type I (**Wenckebach phenomenon**) is a progressively greater delay of the impulse with each beat, until one impulse is totally blocked. This cycle then repeats. Type II, a much less common type, produces intermittent dropped beats without any warning delays in conduction of previous beats. The block in type II is located low in the AV junction, indicating extensive damage to the ventricular muscle. Type II second-degree block may produce a rate low enough to precipitate congestive heart failure because cardiac reserve is likely to be severely limited by the degree of ventricular damage. It is also dangerous in that it often progresses to complete heart block. The third type, advanced second-degree AV block, is defined by the blocking of two or more consecutive P waves.[22]

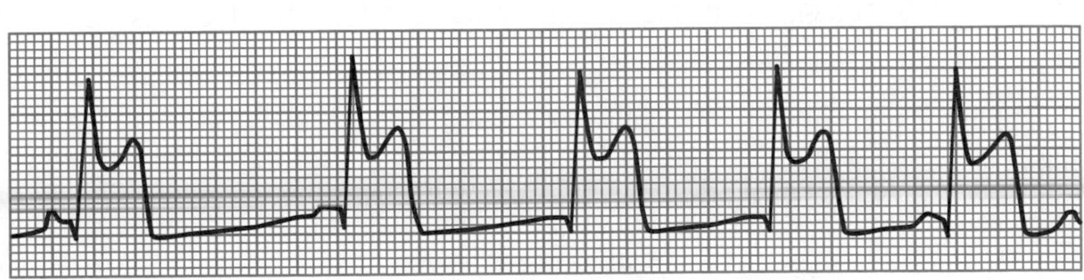

FIGURE 17–39

Wandering atrial pacemaker. This dysrhythmia is defined by the varying configuration of the P waves. The marked ST-segment elevation indicates ischemia but is not relevant to identification of the rhythm. (Courtesy of M. Martha Vorvick, MS, RNC, Assistant Professor. Moorhead, MN: Tri-College University Nursing Program.)

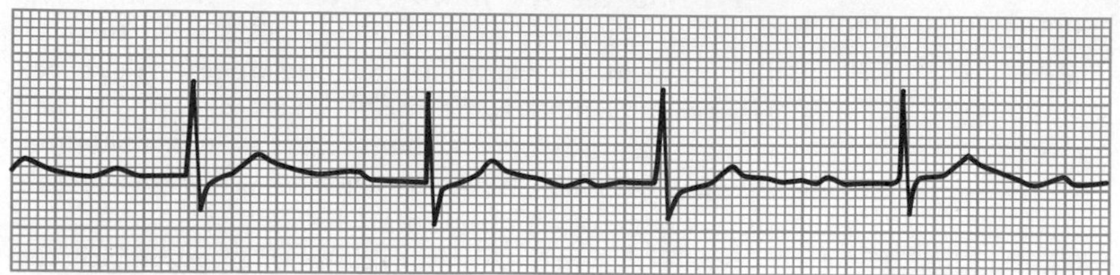

FIGURE 17–40

First-degree atrioventricular (AV) block. The PR interval exceeds 0.20 second, indicating delayed conduction through the AV node. Delayed conduction also slows the heart rate. (Courtesy of M. Martha Vorvick, MS, RNC, Assistant Professor. Moorhead, MN: Tri-College University Nursing Program.)

In third-degree block, all atrial impulses are prevented from entering the ventricles. If third-degree block occurs suddenly, as with acute myocardial infarction, SCD occurs unless a latent junctional or ventricular pacemaker paces an effective rhythm. Complete block often develops gradually, however, with a latent pacemaker producing at least a minimally effective rhythm and cardiac reserve mechanisms operating to increase contractility and stroke volume.

Clinical Manifestations. First-degree block is usually asymptomatic, with a normal ECG except for a PRI exceeding 0.2 second (Fig. 17–40). Clinical manifestations of second-degree block depend on the ventricular rate. Symptoms of congestive heart failure may develop at slow rates, especially if ischemic damage to the myocardium has produced the block. Type I is usually well tolerated. The ECG shows Wenckebach phenomenon: progressive lengthening of the PRI with successive beats, leading to a nonconducted P wave or dropped beat (Fig. 17–41). Type II and advanced second-degree blocks reveal dropped beats without progressive lengthening of the PRI and may be associated with abnormal configuration of the QRS complex due to **bundle branch block**, discussed later.

Third-degree block with junctional or ventricular escape is demonstrated on the ECG by the presence of AV dissociation (Fig. 17–42). Regular atrial activity is present, as manifested by regular P waves. A regular ventricular rhythm is present as well but bears no relationship to the P waves. An occasional fusion beat may be seen if the atria and ventricles fire simultaneously. Third-degree block may be well-tolerated if it develops gradually, but in most cases, it is symptomatic, owing to the slow ventricular rate superimposed on ventricular muscle damage. Sudden onset of complete block may produce transient unconsciousness (Stokes-Adams attacks) if there is a brief delay before a latent pacemaker takes over. Absence of a latent pacemaker response produces total asystole and SCD.

Prevention and Treatment. First-degree block and type I second-degree block usually require no treatment if they are asymptomatic. The patient is closely observed for progression of the block, particularly if there is other evidence of increasing ischemic damage, such as angina or heart failure. Type II second-degree block and complete block may be treated initially with atropine in an effort to increase AV node conduction. In most cases, however, temporary or permanent artificial pacing is indicated (see Table

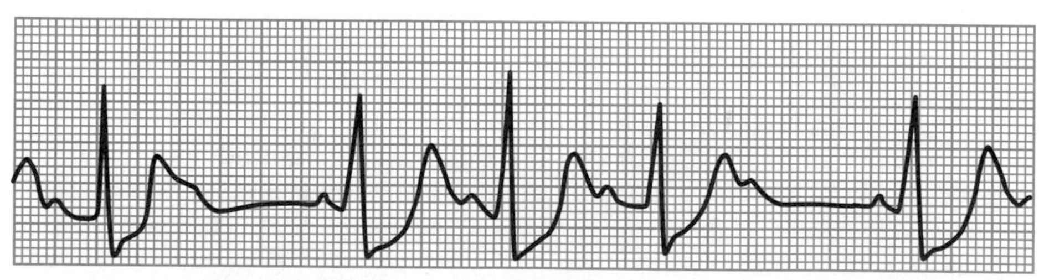

A Mobitz type I (Wenckebach's phenomenon)

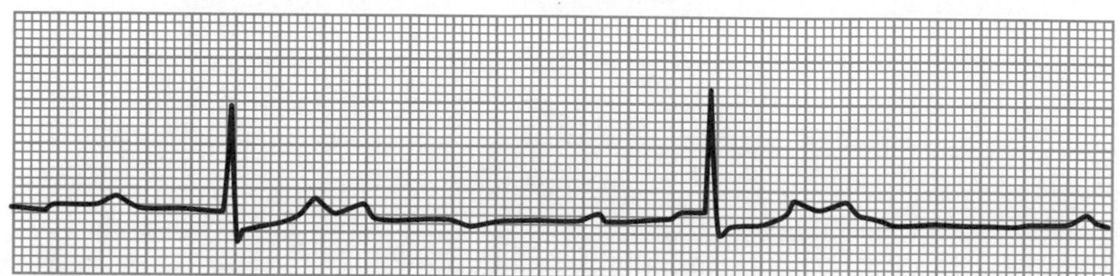

B Mobitz type II

FIGURE 17–41

Second-degree atrioventricular (AV) block. *A*, Mobitz type I. This type of second-degree block, known as the *Wenckebach phenomenon*, is most common. The atrial impulse is delayed longer with each successive beat, leading to total block of one beat. The cycle then repeats. *B*, Mobitz type II. Intermittent dropped beats are seen. The PR interval is uniformly increased, rather than progressively increased, as in the Wenckebach phenomenon. (Courtesy of M. Martha Vorvick, MS, RNC, Assistant Professor. Moorhead, MN: Tri-College University Nursing Program.)

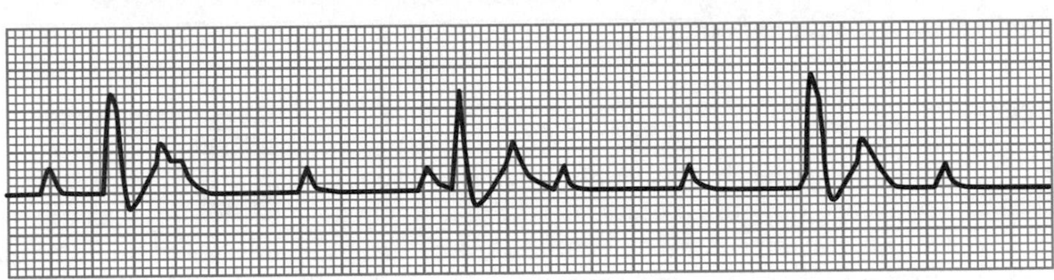

FIGURE 17–42
Third-degree atrioventricular (AV) block. There is complete blockade of atrial impulses at the AV node. Although P waves are occurring regularly owing to sinoatrial node firing, they bear no relationship to the ventricular escape rhythm, which is of junctional origin in this example. (Courtesy of M. Martha Vorvick, MS, RNC, Assistant Professor. Moorhead, MN: Tri-College University Nursing Program.)

17–6). In SCD, CPR is initiated until artificial pacing is available.

Prognosis and Outcome. Heart blocks can usually be effectively treated with artificial pacemakers, and permanent implantable pacemakers are in common use among patients with cardiac disease. The prognosis depends on the degree of myocardial damage.

Bundle Branch Block

Definition. Bundle branch block is delayed or blocked conduction through the right bundle branch, or through either or both fascicles of the left bundle branch.

Epidemiology. Bundle branch block is associated with ventricular ischemia or infarction.

Etiology. Cell membranes of bundle branch fibers in ischemic or infarcted myocardium are damaged, resulting in suppression of excitability and delayed or blocked conduction.

Pathophysiology. The area of myocardium served by the affected bundle branch or fascicle depolarizes later than the unaffected area, resulting in weak or uncoordinated contraction.

Clinical Manifestations. The patient usually manifests some degree of cardiac failure. The ECG shows a widened, distorted QRS complex. The cardiac axis and the configuration of the QRS complex reveal whether the block is in the right bundle, the left bundle, or one fascicle of the left bundle (called *fascicular block* or *hemiblock*). The differences in configuration are most evident in lead V_1 (Fig. 17–43). Normally, the QRS complex in this lead is negative and narrow, and the deflection represents activation of the right ventricle buried in the left ventricular depolarization. In right bundle branch block, depolarization of the right ventricle is delayed and becomes prominent on the ECG, resulting in a widened, M-shaped (rSR′) configuration. In left bundle branch block, the sequence of activation is appropriate, but left ventricular depolarization is delayed. A widened, negative complex results.

If myocardial ischemia is progressive, bundle branch block may also progress. If conduction through the right bundle branch and both fascicles of the left bundle slows, a prolonged PRI is also seen. If conduction is totally blocked, syncope (with transient block) or cardiac arrest occurs.

Prevention and Treatment. Treatment is aimed at management of congestive heart failure and other manifestations of myocardial ischemia or infarction.

Prognosis and Outcome. The prognosis depends on the degree of coronary heart disease and the extent of myocardial damage.

CLINICAL SIGNIFICANCE OF CARDIAC DYSRHYTHMIAS

Cardiac dysrhythmias usually occur in the setting of myocardial ischemia or infarction. Because their presence may signify the extent and location of myocardial damage, clinical monitoring of the cardiac rhythm provides valuable information on pathology

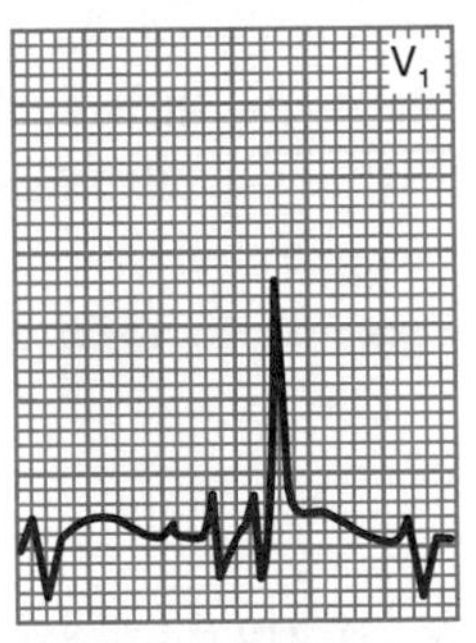

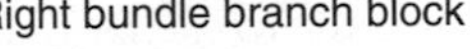

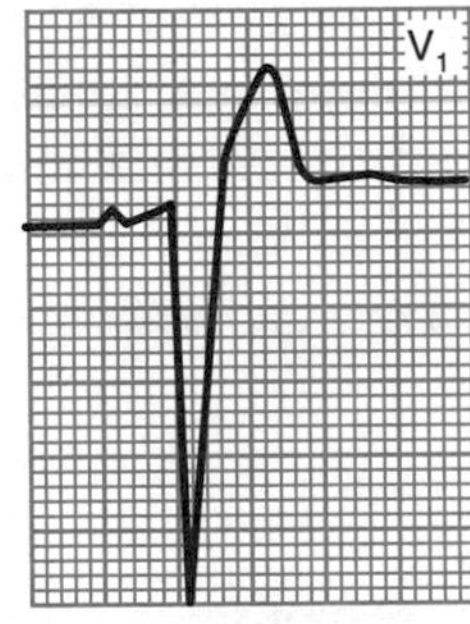

FIGURE 17–43
Bundle branch block. Delay of current flow through the ventricles is evidenced by widening and distortion of the QRS complex. In right bundle branch block, depolarization of the right ventricle is delayed. Right ventricular activation, which is normally buried in the left ventricular depolarization, is instead prominent, resulting in the M-shaped rSR′ configuration. In left bundle branch block, the activation sequence is normal, burying the right ventricular depolarization and permitting the normal negative deflection in lead V_1. Left ventricular depolarization is prolonged, however, widening the QRS complex. (Modified from Phillips, R.E., and Feeney, M.K. [1990]. *The Cardiac Rhythms*. [3rd ed.]. Philadelphia: W.B. Saunders. [pp. 329, 333].)

Developmental Perspective

Embryonic and Fetal Periods

The embryonic heart begins to beat on about the 22nd day of gestation. Intrinsic rate is set by the genetic direction of synthesis and insertion of protein channels and pumps into cardiac cells. The configuration of the action potential also changes developmentally because of the resulting changes in ion transport. Presence of conduction disturbances in several members of a family indicates a genetic basis for the abnormality. Congenital heart block and tachycardia due to macroreentry may manifest any time from the intrauterine period to adulthood. In mothers with systemic lupus erythematosus, antibodies may cross the placenta and damage the cardiac conduction system, producing fetal heart block.

Infancy and Childhood

In newborns, QRS duration is half that of adults. Dysrhythmias are uncommon during infancy and childhood. Isolated congenital heart block may have an autosomal dominant mode of inheritance and often manifests as sinus bradycardia progressing to advanced AV block. Another form, familial heart block, is often seen in association with conspicuous freckling. Familial tachycardias, atrial fibrillation, and nodal rhythm are also seen, either alone or in conjunction with structural heart defects, and are usually well-tolerated. Congenital long QT syndrome may manifest in childhood and may be associated with congenital deafness and increased risk of SCD.

Adolescence and Young Adulthood

Preexcitation syndromes such as WPW syndrome usually become apparent during adolescence. Familial SCD has been noted in teenage siblings after minimal psychological or physiologic stress and may be preceded by a tendency to faint with such stimuli. Pre-existing congenital valve disease and cardiomegaly related to athletic training may be associated with dysrhythmias that manifest during this period and that are usually benign.

Middle and Older Adulthood

In the absence of cardiac disease, cardiac rate and rhythm at rest remain unchanged with aging. The response of the heart to sympathetic stimulation by β-adrenergic receptors decreases with age, however, limiting this aspect of cardiac reserve. Loss of pacemaker and conducting cells is also seen, leading to a tendency to develop sick sinus syndrome, AV block, and bundle branch block. The incidence of supraventricular and ventricular dysrhythmias is also increased, even in the absence of structural heart disease. Because cardiac disease is most prevalent in this age group, the risk of dysrhythmia is doubly enhanced. In the setting of decreased renal or hepatic function, the use of antiarrhythmic drugs in treatment of dysrhythmia is associated with an increased risk of proarrhythmia in older people.

---

and response to therapy. Many dysrhythmias are relatively benign, but some can lead to SCD if not immediately interrupted.

Because dysrhythmias have their greatest impact on patients with heart disease, they are most prevalent among the middle-aged and elderly. Congenital heart defects or conditions producing electrolyte imbalance or systemic toxicity, however, may result in dysrhythmias in people of all ages (see Developmental Perspective).

The development of invasive electrophysiology studies has provided new insights into the cellular mechanisms of many dysrhythmias. Precise mechanisms of many dysrhythmias still remain uncertain, however, and the mechanisms of action of some antiarrhythmic drugs are still unknown. The degree to which antiarrhythmic therapy affects mortality from myocardial disease is also uncertain, and controversy surrounds the use of several of these agents. Clinical trials have resulted in discontinuation of use of some antiarrhythmic drugs. The effectiveness of surgical and catheter ablative treatments of dysrhythmias also remains to be established (see Focus of Current Research).

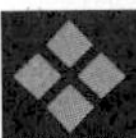

Summary of Key Points

- The electrical impulse that is essential to cardiac contraction originates and is conducted within the cardiac conduction system, a specialized network of noncontractile cells. The impulse normally originates within the SA node in the right atrium and is conducted quickly by internodal pathways and more slowly across the atrial myocardium to the AV node. Current flow is slowed at the AV junction until atrial contraction is complete, then is conducted to the ventricular myocardium through the bundle of His, bundle branches, and the Purkinje system.

- Cardiac cells that have membranes with sufficient leak channels are endowed with increased automaticity, the ability to self-generate action potentials and thus serve as pacemakers. Because the SA node has the highest rate of intrinsic automaticity, it normally paces the cardiac rhythm. Latent or ectopic pacemakers may pace one or more beats if their intrinsic rate exceeds that of the SA node. Autonomic nervous system reflexes influence automaticity through catecholamine effects on membrane ion channels. Sympathetic stimulation increases heart rate and AV nodal conductance, whereas parasympathetic stimulation decreases these. Cardiac axis, the mean vector of current flow through the heart, is influenced by individual current vectors and by the position of the heart in the chest.

- A positive deflection of the ECG waveform in a given lead results from current flowing toward the positive electrode of the lead, whereas a negative deflection results from current flow away from the positive electrode. The small positive deflection of the P wave represents atrial depolarization, followed by an isoelectric interval in which current flow is insufficient to be detected (AV node depolarization). The larger deflection of the QRS complex represents ventricular depolarization; the ST segment and T wave result from current flow during ventricular repolarization. The effects of cardiac disease, drug therapy, electrolyte imbalance, or other factors on ion flux across the myocardial membrane may be detected as alterations in heart rate, rhythm, or configuration of the PQRST complex.

- Cardiac axis may be determined by examination of the QRS configuration in the limb leads. Current flow is perpendicular to the axis of the lead in which the most equiphasic QRS complex is seen. Direction of flow along this axis is toward the positive end of the lead, which is perpendicular to the first lead identified, if the QRS configuration is upright; it is toward the negative end of this lead if the QRS configuration is downward. P waves should be present and uniform within a lead and should precede each QRS complex. The PRI should be no longer than 0.2 second. The QRS complexes should be narrow (no longer than 0.12 second), and the ST segment should be isoelectric. T waves should not be inverted, flattened, or peaked, and U waves, if seen, should not be prominent. The cardiac rhythm should be regular, and the rate should be between 60 and 100 beats/minute.

- Tachycardias are abnormally rapid rhythms and bradycardias are abnormally slow rhythms of SA nodal, atrial, junctional, or ventricular origin. Flutter results from extremely rapid impulse conduction from atrial or ventricular ectopic foci. In atrial flutter, conduction of the impulse to the ventricles is usually blocked by the AV node at regular intervals. Ventricular flutter usually precedes VF, a form of SCD. Atrial fibrillation results from multiple reentry circuits that generate competing wavefronts of current within the atria and random conduction into the ventricles. Premature contractions result from the firing of ectopic pacemakers in the atria, AV junction, or ventricles. Conduction disturbances are abnormalities of impulse generation at the SA node or conduction of the impulse through the AV junction. Because heart rate is a determinant of cardiac output, all dysrhythmias potentially induce heart failure.

REFERENCES

1. Creel, C.A. (1994). Silent myocardial ischemia and nursing implications. *Heart & Lung* 23(3), 218–227.
2. Castellanos, A., and Myerburg, R.J. (1990). The resting electrocardiogram. In: Hurst, J.W. (Ed.). *The Heart, Arteries, and Veins.* New York: McGraw-Hill Information Services (pp. 265–298).
3. Pieper, S.J., and Stanton, M.S. (1995). Narrow QRS complex tachycardias. *Mayo Clinic Proceedings* 70(4), 371–375.

4. Ganz, L.I., and Friedman, P.L. (1995). Supraventricular tachycardia. *New England Journal of Medicine* 332(3), 162–173.
5. Robinson, A.W. (1996). Common varieties of supraventricular tachycardia: Differentiation and dangers. *Heart & Lung* 25(5), 373–381.
6. Rankin, A.C., Brooks, R., Ruskin, J.N., *et al.* (1992). Adenosine and the treatment of supraventricular tachycardia. *American Journal of Medicine* 92(6), 655–664.
7. Berry, V.A. (1993). Wolff-Parkinson-White syndrome and the use of radiofrequency catheter ablation. *Heart & Lung* 22(1), 15–25.
8. Chun, H.M., and Sung, R.J. (1995). Supraventricular tachyarrhythmias: Pharmacologic versus nonpharmacologic approaches. *Medical Clinics of North America* 79(5), 1121–1134.
9. Hamdan, M., and Scheinman, M. (1995). Current approaches in patients with ventricular tachyarrhythmias. *Medical Clinics of North America* 79(5), 1097–1120.
10. Pires, L.A., and Huang, S.K.S. (1993). Nonsustained ventricular tachycardia: Identification and management of high-risk patients. *American Heart Journal* 126(1), 189–200.
11. Brodsky, M.A., Hwang, C., Hunter, D., *et al.* (1995). Life-threatening alterations in heart rate after the use of adenosine in atrial flutter. *American Heart Journal* 130(3 Pt. 1), 564–571.
12. Barold, S.S., and Falkoff, M.D. (1995). Treatment of atrial flutter by antitachycardia pacemaker: A 13-year follow-up. *American Heart Journal* 130(1), 187–191.
13. Baer, M., and Goldschlager, N. (1995). Atrial fibrillation: An update on new management strategies. *Geriatrics* 50(4), 22–29.
14. Prystowky, E.N. (1997). Management of atrial fibrillation: Simplicity surrounded by controversy. *Annals of Internal Medicine* (Editorial.) 126(3), 244–246.
15. Geraets, D.R., and Kienzle, M.G. (1993). Atrial fibrillation and atrial flutter. *Clinical Pharmacy* 12(10), 721–735.
16. Nelson, K.M., and Talbert, R.L. (1994). Preventing stroke in patients with nonrheumatic atrial fibrillation. *American Journal of Hospital Pharmacy* 51(9), 1175–1183.
17. Myerburg, R.J., Kessler, K.M., and Castellanos, A. (1993). Sudden cardiac death: Epidemiology, transient risk, and intervention assessment. *Annals of Internal Medicine* 119(2), 1187–1197.
18. Kolettis, T.M., and Saksena, S. (1994). Prophylactic implantable cardioverter defibrillator therapy in high-risk patients with coronary artery disease. *American Heart Journal* 127(4 Pt. 2), 1164–1170.
19. Snowberger, P. (1991). Premature atrial contractions. *RN* 54(6), 38–40.
20. Marriott, H.J.L., and Myerburg, R.J. (1990). Recognition of cardiac arrhythmias and conduction disturbances. In: Hurst, J.W. (Ed.). *The Heart, Arteries, and Veins.* New York: McGraw-Hill Information Services. (pp. 489–534).
21. Myerburg, R.J., and Kessler, K.M. (1990). Clinical assessment and management of arrhythmias and conduction disturbances. In: Hurst, J.W. (Ed.). *The Heart, Arteries, and Veins.* New York: McGraw-Hill Information Services. (pp. 535–560).
22. Kusumoto, F.M., and Goldschlager, N. (1996). Cardiac pacing. *New England Journal of Medicine* 334(2), 89–98.

SELECTED BIBLIOGRAPHY

Benditt, D.G., Mianulli, M., Lurie, K., *et al.* (1994). Multiple-sensor systems for physiologic cardiac pacing. *Annals of Internal Medicine* 121(12), 960–968.

Berntsen, R.F., Gunnes, P., and Rasmussen, K. (1995). Pattern of coronary artery disease in patients with ventricular tachycardia and fibrillation exposed by exercise-induced ischemia. *American Heart Journal* 129(4), 733–738.

Bhadha, K., Marchlinski, F.E., and Iskandrian, A.S. (1993). Ventricular tachycardia in patients without structural heart disease. *American Heart Journal* 126(5), 1194–1198.

Blanchard, S.M., and Ideker, R.E. (1994). Mechanisms of electrical defibrillation: Impact of new experimental defibrillator waveforms. *American Heart Journal* 127(4 Pt. 2), 970–977.

Blanck, Z., Dhala, A., Deshpande, S., *et al.* (1994). Catheter ablation of ventricular tachycardia. *American Heart Journal* 127(4 Pt. 2), 1126–1133.

Boisvert, J.T., Reidy, S.J., and Lulu, J. (1995). Overview of pediatric arrhythmias. *Nursing Clinics of North America* 30(2), 365–379.

Caruso, A.C. (1991). Supraventricular tachycardia: Changes in management. *Postgraduate Medicine* 90(2), 73–82.

Cohen, T.J., Goldner, B.G., Maccaro, P.C., *et al.* (1993). A comparison of active compression-decompression cardiopulmonary resuscitation with standard cardiopulmonary resuscitation for cardiac arrests occurring in the hospital. *New England Journal of Medicine* 329(26), 1918–1921.

Conover, M.B. (1988). *Understanding Electrocardiography: Arrhythmias and the 12-Lead EKG.* (5th ed.). St. Louis: C.V. Mosby.

Conti, J.B., and Curtis, A.B. (1993). Antiarrhythmic therapy in patients with congestive heart failure. *Postgraduate Medicine* 94(5), 121–137.

Coward, J.C., Coulshed, D.S., and Zaman, A.G. (1991). Antiarrhythmic therapy and survival following myocardial infarction. *Journal of Cardiovascular Pharmacology* 18(suppl. 2), S92–S98.

Davis, A.M., Gow, R.M., McCrindle, B.W., *et al.* (1996). Clinical spectrum, therapeutic management, and follow-up of ventricular tachycardia in infants and young children. *American Heart Journal* 131(1), 186–191.

Fowles, R.E. (1995). Myocardial infarction in the 1990s: Complications, prognosis, and changing patterns of management. *Postgraduate Medicine* 97(6), 155–168.

Frishman, W.H., Heiman, M., Karpenos, A., *et al.* (1996). Twenty-four-hour ambulatory electrocardiography in elderly subjects: Prevalence of various arrhythmias and prognostic implications (report from the Bronx Longitudinal Aging Study). *American Heart Journal* 132 (2 Pt. 1), 297–302.

Gallagher, E.J., Lombardi, G., and Gennis, P. (1995). Effectiveness of bystander cardiopulmonary resuscitation and survival following out-of-hospital cardiac arrest. *Journal of the American Medical Association* 274(24), 1922–1925.

Ganz, L.I., Andrews, T.C., Barry, J., *et al.* (1994). Silent ischemia preceding sudden cardiac death in a patient after vascular surgery. *American Heart Journal* 127(6), 1652–1654.

Glikson, M., Espinosa, R.E., and Hayes, D.L. (1995). Expanding indications for permanent pacemakers. *Annals of Internal Medicine* 123(6), 443–451.

Goyal, R., Zivin, A., Souza, J., *et al.* (1996). Comparison of the ages of tachycardia onset in patients with atrioventricular nodal reentrant tachycardia and accessory pathway-mediated tachycardia. *American Heart Journal* 132(4), 765–767.

Hohnloser, S.H., and Woosley, R.L. (1994). Sotalol. *New England Journal of Medicine* 331(1), 31–38.

Hurst, J.W. (Ed.). (1990). *The Heart, Arteries, and Veins.* (7th ed.). New York: McGraw-Hill Information Services.

Janeira, L.F. (1996). Wide-complex tachycardias: The importance of identifying the mechanism. *Postgraduate Medicine* 100(3), 259–278.

Kay, G.N., and Plumb, V.J. (1996). The present role of radiofrequency catheter ablation in the management of cardiac arrhythmias. *American Journal of Medicine* 100, 344–356.

Keller, C., and Williams, A. (1993). Cardiac dysrhythmias associated with central nervous system dysfunction. *Journal of Neuroscience Nursing* 25(6), 349–355.

Kendall, M.J., Lynch, K.P., Hjalmarson, A., *et al.* (1995). β-blockers and sudden cardiac death. *Annals of Internal Medicine* 123(5), 358–367.

Kerin, N.Z., and Somberg, J. (1994). Proarrhythmia: Definition, risk factors, causes, treatment, and controversies. *American Heart Journal* 128(3), 575–585.

Kinlay, S., Leitch, J.W., Neil, A., *et al.* (1996). Cardiac event recorders yield more diagnoses and are more cost-effective than

48-hour Holter monitoring in patients with palpitations: A controlled clinical trial. *Annals of Internal Medicine* 124(1 Pt. 1), 16–20.

Leor, J., Poole, W.K., and Kloner, R.A. (1996). Sudden cardiac death triggered by an earthquake. *New England Journal of Medicine* 334(7), 413–419.

Lessmeier, T.J., Lehmann, M.H., Steinman, R.T., *et al.* (1994). Implantable cardioverter-defibrillator therapy in 300 patients with coronary artery disease presenting exclusively with ventricular fibrillation. *American Heart Journal* 128(2), 211–218.

Levy, M., and Wiseman, M.N. (1991). Electrophysiologic mechanisms for ventricular arrhythmias in left ventricular dysfunction: Electrolytes, catecholamines, and drugs. *Journal of Clinical Pharmacology* 31(11), 1053–1060.

Levy, S. (1991). Diagnostic approach to cardiac arrhythmias. *Journal of Cardiovascular Pharmacology* 17(suppl. 6), S24–S31.

Liberthson, R.R. (1996). Sudden death from cardiac causes in children and young adults. *New England Journal of Medicine* 334(16), 1039–1044.

Lipka, L.J., Dizon, J.M., and Reiffel, J.A. (1995). Desired mechanisms of drugs for ventricular arrhythmia: Class III antiarrhythmic agents. *American Heart Journal* 130(3 Pt. 1), 632–640.

Lurie, K.G., Shultz, J.J., Callahan, M.L., *et al.* (1994). Evaluation of active compression-decompression CPR in victims of out-of-hospital cardiac arrest. *Journal of the American Medical Association* 271(18), 1405–1411.

Magdic, K.S., and Saul, L.M. (1997). ECG interpretation of chamber enlargement. *Critical Care Nurse* 17(1), 13–25.

Mathew, J.P., Parks, R., Savino, J.S., *et al.* (1996). Atrial fibrillation following coronary artery bypass graft surgery: Predictors, outcomes, and resource utilization. *Journal of the American Medical Association* 276(4), 300–306.

McCollam, P.L., and Parker, R.B. (1991). Evaluation and treatment of ventricular arrhythmias: An update. *Clinical Pharmacy* 10(3), 195–205.

Mont, L., Seixas, T., Brugada, P., *et al.* (1992). The electrocardiographic, clinical, and electrophysiologic spectrum of idiopathic monomorphic ventricular tachycardia. *American Heart Journal* 124(3), 746–753.

Moss, A.J., Hall, W.J., Cannom, D.S., *et al.* (1996). Improved survival with an implanted defibrillator in patients with coronary disease at high risk for ventricular arrhythmia. *New England Journal of Medicine* 335(26), 1933–1940.

Myerburg, R.J., Kessler, K.M., Chakko, S., *et al.* (1994). Future evaluation of antiarrhythmic therapy. *American Heart Journal* 127(4 Pt. 2), 1111–1118.

Myers, M.G. (1991). Caffeine and cardiac arrhythmias. *Annals of Internal Medicine* 114(2), 147–150.

Nattel, S. (1995). Newer developments in the management of atrial fibrillation. *American Heart Journal* 130(5), 1094–1106.

Niebauer, M.J., Daoud, E., Goyal, R., *et al.* (1996). Atrioventricular node properties in patients with accessory pathways. *American Heart Journal* 131(4), 716–719.

Patton, S.B., and Pacetti, P.E. (1995). Sudden cardiac death. *Critical Care Nursing Clinics of North America*. 7(3), 413–426.

Pires, L.A., Wagshal, A.B., Lancey, R., *et al.* (1995). Arrhythmias and conduction disturbances after coronary artery bypass graft surgery: Epidemiology, management, and prognosis. *American Heart Journal* 129(4), 799–808.

Pollak, A., and Falk, R.H. (1993). Pacemaker therapy in patients with atrial fibrillation. *American Heart Journal* 125(3), 824–830.

Rechavia, E., Strasberg, B., Mager, A., *et al.* (1992). The incidence of atrial arrhythmias during inferior wall myocardial infarction with and without right ventricular involvement. *American Heart Journal* 124(2), 387–391.

Reiffel, J.A., and Correia, J. (1994). "In the absence of structural heart disease. . . ." What is it, and why does it matter in antiarrhythmic drug therapy? *American Heart Journal* 128(3), 626–629.

Reimold, S.C., Lamas, G.A., Cantillon, C.O., *et al.* (1995). Risk factors for the development of recurrent atrial fibrillation: Role of pacing and clinical variables. *American Heart Journal* 129(6), 1127–1132.

Rich, B.S.E. (1994). Sudden death screening. *Medical Clinics of North America* 78(2), 267–288.

Roden, D.M. (1994). Risks and benefits of antiarrhythmic therapy. *New England Journal of Medicine* 331(12), 785–791.

Saver, C.L. (1994). Decoding the ACLS algorithms. *American Journal of Nursing* 94(1), 27–36.

Symanski, J.D., and Gettes, L.S. (1993). Drug effects on the electrocardiogram: A review of their clinical importance. *Drugs* 46(2), 219–248.

Tervahauta, M., Pekkanen, J., Punsar, S., *et al.* (1996). Resting electrocardiographic abnormalities as predictors of coronary events and total mortality among elderly men. *American Journal of Medicine* 100, 641–645.

Ukani, Z.A., and Ezekowitz, M.D. (1995). Contemporary management of atrial fibrillation. *Medical Clinics of North America* 79(5), 1135–1152.

Vaughan Williams, E.M. (1992). Classifying antiarrhythmic actions: By facts or speculation. *Journal of Clinical Pharmacology* 32(11), 964–977.

Vaughan Williams, E.M. (1991). Significance of classifying antiarrhythmic actions since the Cardiac Arrhythmia Suppression Trial. *Journal of Clinical Pharmacology* 31(2), 123–135.

Weindling, S.N., Saul, J.P., and Walsh, E.P. (1996). Efficacy and risks of medical therapy for supraventricular tachycardia in neonates and infants. *American Heart Journal* 131(1), 66–72.

Weitz, H.H., and Weinstock, P.J. (1995). Approach to the patient with palpitations. *Medical Clinics of North America* 79(2), 449–456.

Yabek, S.M. (1991). Ventricular arrhythmias in children with an apparently normal heart. *Journal of Pediatrics* 119(1 Pt. 1), 1–11.

Zuppiroli, A., Mori, F., Favilli, S., *et al.* (1994). Arrhythmias in mitral valve prolapse: Relation to anterior mitral leaflet thickening, clinical variables, and color Doppler echocardiographic parameters. *American Heart Journal* 128(5), 919–927.

Unit VI

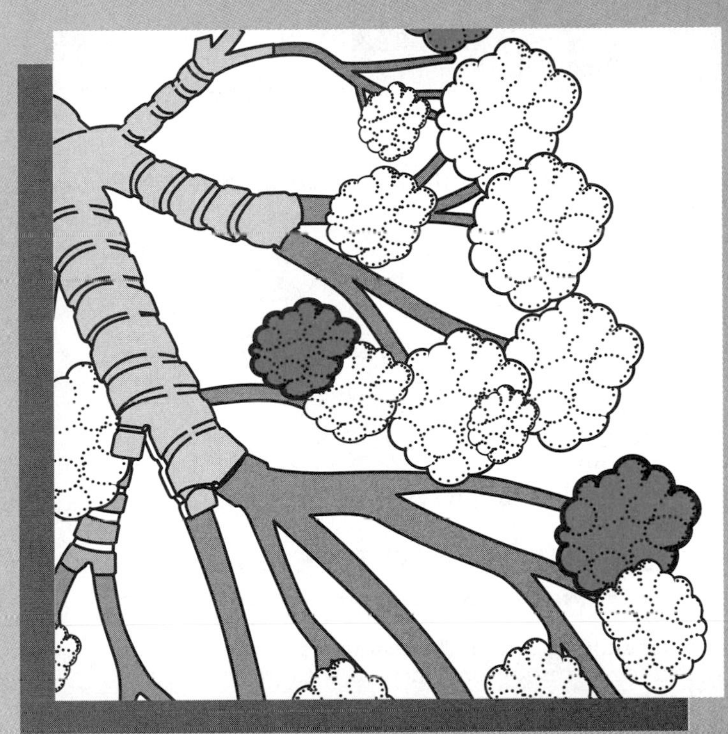

Chapter 18
Disorders of Pulmonary Ventilation

Chapter 19
Disorders of Gas Transport and Exchange

RESPIRATORY SYSTEM

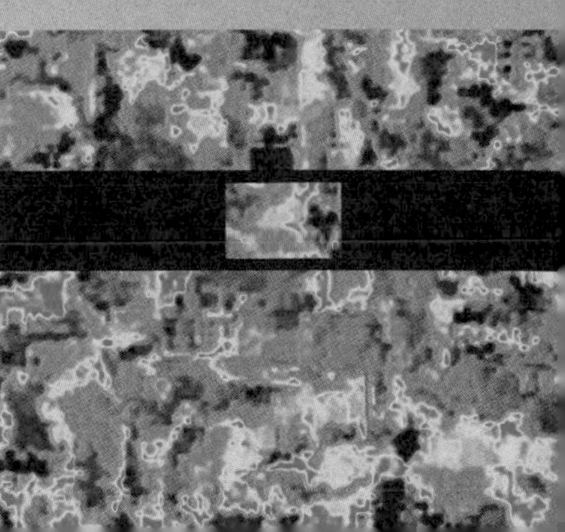

18 CHAPTER

Disorders of Pulmonary Ventilation

LEARNING OBJECTIVES

1. Relate the structural characteristics of the upper and lower respiratory tracts to their principal functions.
2. Describe the muscular effort and pressure gradients that result in inspiration and expiration.
3. Differentiate among the anatomic and physiologic factors that influence the work of breathing.
4. Summarize key aspects of the neural control of ventilation.
5. Rationalize the various modes of treatment of respiratory failure on the basis of the underlying etiology and pathophysiology.
6. Discuss clinical features of the more common upper respiratory infections.
7. Compare and contrast clinical features of the most prevalent forms of chronic obstructive pulmonary disease (chronic air flow limitation).
8. Discuss prevention and intervention related to laryngeal and lung cancers.
9. Relate the clinical manifestations of chest trauma to the underlying structural abnormalities.

key terms

acute bronchitis
alveolar hypoventilation
aspiration
asthma
atelectasis
bronchiectasis
cellular respiration
chest trauma
chronic bronchitis
chronic obstructive pulmonary disease (COPD)
common cold
croup (laryngotracheobronchitis)
cystic fibrosis
dead space
dyspnea
emphysema
epiglottitis
flail chest
hypercapnia
hyperventilation
hypoxemia
infant respiratory distress syndrome (IRDS)

laryngeal cancer
laryngitis
lung cancer (bronchogenic carcinoma)
obstructive sleep apnea
peak expiratory flow rate
pharyngitis
pneumothorax
reactive airways dysfunction syndrome (RADS)
respiration
respiratory center
respiratory failure
sinusitis
status asthmaticus
surfactant
tachypnea
tension pneumothorax
tidal volume (TV or V_T)
tonsillitis
ventilation
ventilation–perfusion ($\dot{V}/\dot{Q}$) abnormality
work of breathing

Ventilation is commonly understood to mean movement of air. In human physiology, its meaning is the same. Ventilation is accomplished by the pulmonary system, consisting of the airways and lungs, the blood vessels perfusing them, the muscles of the thorax and abdomen, and the innervation of these structures. Pulmonary ventilation, the movement of atmospheric air into and out of the lungs, depends on open airways and contraction of muscles to create pressure gradients for air flow. Ventilation is the critical first step in the complex process of **respiration,** the exchange of oxygen and carbon dioxide (CO_2) between the environment and the human system.

Ventilation, its regulation, and related disorders are detailed in this chapter. The multiple processes associated with pulmonary perfusion, transport of gases within the blood, and exchange of gases between the blood and body cells are discussed in Chapter 19, along with disorders primarily affecting pulmonary hemodynamics. It must be emphasized, however, that pulmonary ventilation and perfusion are interdependent processes, and the distinction between disorders of ventilation and perfusion is made for academic purposes. The pathophysiology and clinical manifestations of pulmonary disorders reflect abnormality of both processes. **Cellular respiration** refers to the use of oxygen and the production of CO_2 during cellular energy metabolism, which was discussed in detail in Chapter 3.

Even though cardiovascular disease accounts for the highest mortality in the United States, respiratory disease produces the most morbidity as defined by days lost from work or school (Fig. 18–1). Cardiovascular and respiratory functions are highly correlated in health and disease. Left ventricular failure, for example, results in increased pressure and volume in pulmonary capillaries, which impairs diffusion of oxygen from the airways to the blood. Conversely, mediators released during chronic inflammatory conditions of the lungs may impair perfusion, creating high resistance to blood flow and precipitating right ventricular failure (cor pulmonale).

The terms *pulmonary system* and *respiratory system* are generally used synonymously in clinical settings, although the former refers to anatomy and the latter to function. Respiration is the primary function of the pulmonary system, but this system is also essential to acid-base balance and fluid balance. Pulmonary regulation of CO_2 levels in the blood determines the amount of carbonic acid formed (see Chapter 10). Pulmonary disorders may cause either acidosis or alkalosis, and respiratory compensation is seen in acid-base disorders resulting from disease of other systems. As discussed in Chapter 8, pulmonary tissue is the principal source of angiotensin-converting enzyme, a critical component of the renin–angiotensin–aldosterone system. The empha-

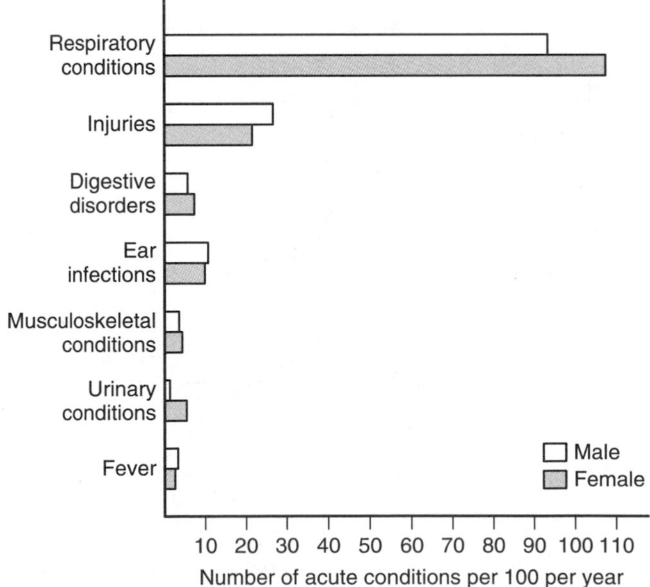

FIGURE 18–1
Morbidity due to respiratory disease. Acute respiratory disorders are significantly more prevalent than acute injuries or disorders of other systems. (Data from the National Health Survey, 1991. DHHS Publication No. (PHS) 93-1512.)

sis in this chapter is on the ventilatory function of the pulmonary system.

FUNCTIONAL ANATOMY OF THE PULMONARY SYSTEM

Gross anatomy of the pulmonary system is illustrated in Figure 18–2. The airways and lungs are divided into the *upper respiratory tract,* consisting of the nasopharynx, oropharynx, and larynx, and the *lower respiratory tract,* consisting of larger conducting airways and smaller exchange airways.

Upper Respiratory Tract

The upper respiratory tract structures serve as *conduits* for the intake, output, and conduction of air, and also as *conditioners* of that air (Fig. 18–3). The surfaces of these structures are highly vascular, ideally suited for warming and humidifying environmental air. Humans are obligate nose breathers, with most air intake alternating between nostril openings (nares) in 2- to 4-hour cycles. Each nostril contains three tissue protrusions *(turbinates),* which produce turbulent flow of air within the nasopharynx. This turbulent flow contributes to the quality of the voice and to the efficiency of humidification, warming, and filtration of the air. The nasopharynx is lined with hair and cilia to assist in filtering particles from inspired air, and its walls also contain olfactory receptors that mediate the sense of smell (see Chapter 23).

The frontal, maxillary, and ethmoid *sinuses* are air-filled spaces that are continuous with the nasopharynx and that normally provide resonance to the voice (Fig. 18–4). The *eustachian tubes* are passages between the middle ears and the posterior nasopharynx and are closed 99% of the time. When opened, typically during swallowing, they permit equilibration of atmospheric and middle ear pressures (see Chapter 23).

The larynx (Fig. 18–5) contains the vocal cords, thus serving the function of *phonation* (speech). Muscles of *deglutition* (swallowing) are also located in the larynx. These close the *epiglottis,* a flap of tissue that guards the entrance into the largest airway, the *trachea,* thus preventing the inappropriate **aspiration** of swallowed materials into the lungs. The upper respiratory tract contains *irritant receptors,* which initiate cough and sneeze reflexes, as discussed later.

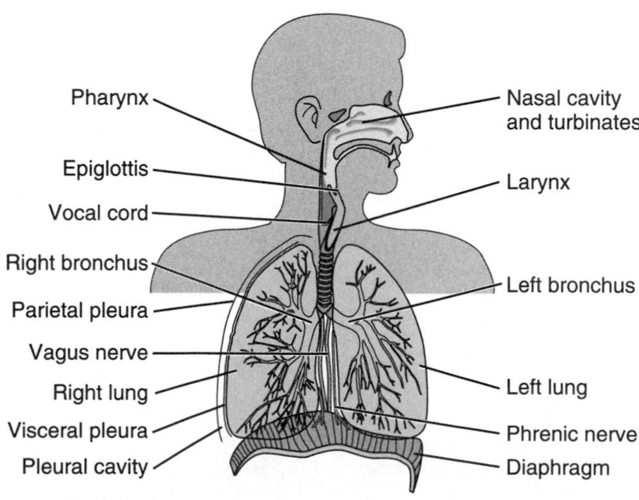

FIGURE 18–2
Anatomy of the pulmonary system. The larynx is the lowermost component of the upper respiratory tract. The lower respiratory tract consists of the larger conducting airways (trachea and bronchi) and the smaller exchange of airways of the lungs. Each lung is contained within a pleural cavity. The pleura is a two-layered membrane: the visceral pleura overlies the surface of the lungs, and the parietal pleura lines the pleural cavity. The principal muscle of inspiration, the diaphragm, is innervated by the phrenic nerve, whereas the airway smooth muscle is innervated by sympathetic and parasympathetic (vagal) nerve branches.

Lower Respiratory Tract

The lower respiratory tract is divided anatomically and functionally into the conducting airways, consisting of the trachea, the main-stem *bronchi,* and 16 successive generations (branchings) of these airways into smaller bronchi and *bronchioles;* and the exchange airways, collectively known as the *acinus* or respiratory unit (Fig. 18–6). The conducting airways move air in and out, with virtually no gas exchange occurring across airway walls. Larger airways are kept open by rigid cartilage in their walls, whereas connective tissue tethers provide external support for smaller ones (Fig. 18–7).

Conducting airways also contain smooth muscle, which responds to both autonomic and local stimuli, resulting in changes in airway diameter (bronchoconstriction or bronchodilation). Walls of the conducting airways contain irritant receptors, which initiate the cough reflex, and goblet cells, which secrete protective mucus. The epithelial cells lining these airways have cilia, which beat rhythmically upward to conduct mucus from the lower to the upper respiratory tract for expulsion. This *mucociliary escalator* constitutes one of several pulmonary defense mechanisms for removal of potentially harmful agents and maintenance of airway patency (Table 18–1).

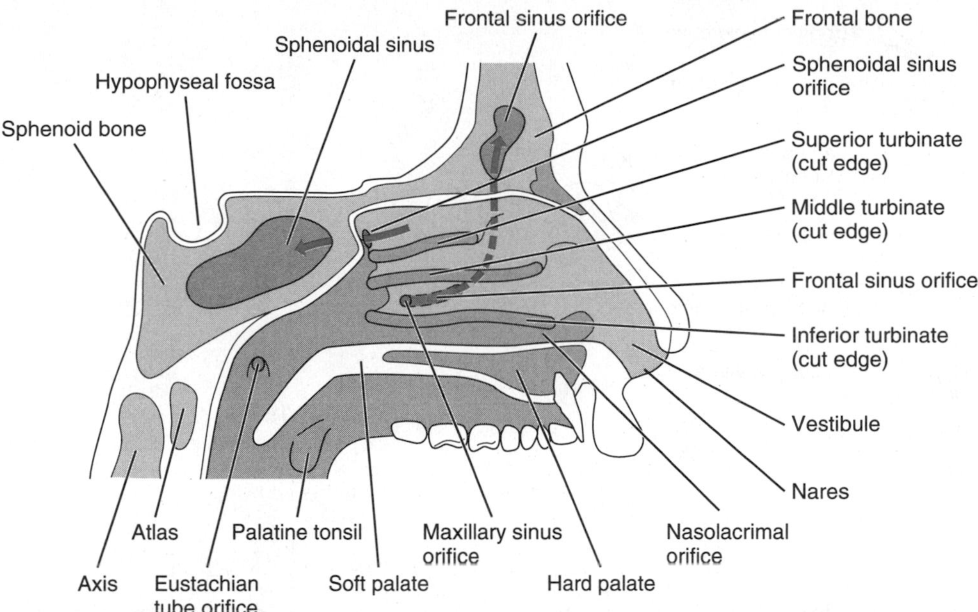

FIGURE 18–3

Structure of the nasopharynx. Air enters through the nares and is warmed, humidified, and filtered within the nasopharynx. The nasopharynx is lined with a highly vascular mucous membrane containing hair and cilia and is thus well suited to these functions. Olfactory receptors in the mucosa mediate the sense of smell. Tissue protrusions (turbinates) create turbulent air flow, contributing to the efficiency of humidification and warming and enhancing the resonance of the voice. Air-filled sinuses also contribute to voice quality. The eustachian tube, which connects the middle ear to the nasopharynx, permits equilibration of middle ear and atmospheric pressures.

The respiratory units, consisting of the *respiratory bronchioles, alveolar ducts,* and *alveoli,* are the terminal airway structures. Because of their thin walls and rich blood supply, they are ideally suited for their principal function of gas exchange between the air and the blood. The alveoli also contain fixed macrophages (designated type I alveolar cells) for defense against organisms invading through the respiratory route (see Chapter 13).

Lungs and Pleurae

The lower conducting airways and respiratory units are surrounded by the pulmonary vascular system and connective tissue, giving a sponge-like appearance to normal lung tissue. As shown in Figure 18–8, the right lung has three sections, or lobes, and the left lung has two. Each lung is covered by a membrane known as the *visceral pleura* and is contained within a space known as the *pleural space.* Each pleural space is lined with another layer of pleura, the *parietal pleura.* The *intrapleural space,* which lies between the two pleural layers, normally contains a small amount of fluid for lubrication. With cardiac or pulmonary disease, however, the intrapleural space may be a site of significant third spacing of fluid, which could impinge on ventilation (see *pleural effusion,* Chapter 19). Furthermore, the fluid pressure in the intrapleural space is slightly negative, possibly owing to lymphatic drainage or to offsetting elastic recoil forces between the lungs (which tend to collapse) and the chest wall (which tends to expand). This negative pressure, which helps to keep the lungs expanded, may be lost with **chest trauma,** leading to **pneumothorax,** or collapse

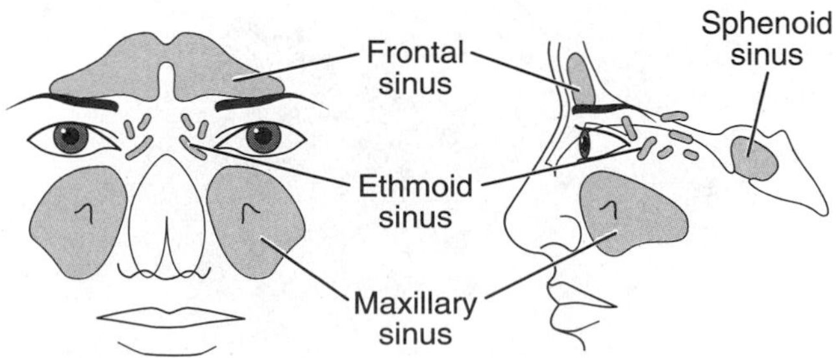

FIGURE 18–4

Sinus cavities. The frontal and maxillary sinuses lie immediately beneath facial structures and are readily accessible for clinical assessment. The smaller ethmoid and sphenoid sinuses lie posterior to the nasopharynx.

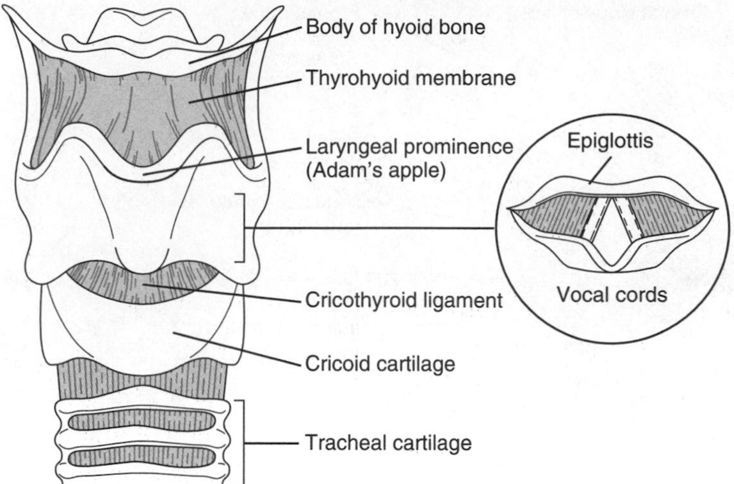

FIGURE 18–5
Laryngeal structures. The larynx contains the vocal cords and the epiglottis, a flap of tissue that closes the trachea during swallowing.

of the lung. These conditions are discussed subsequently.

PULMONARY VENTILATION

Pulmonary Volumes and Capacities

The parameters that define ventilatory function are four volumes, three of which may be directly measured in clinical settings, and four capacities, which are calculated from summed volumes (Fig. 18–9). **Tidal volume** (TV or V_T), the parameter most often referenced in clinical practice, is the volume of gas inspired and expired during a normal, relaxed breath (about 500 mL in a 70-kg adult). *Inspiratory reserve volume (IRV)* is the amount of gas that can be inhaled over and above the normal tidal volume (about 3000 mL). *Expiratory reserve volume (ERV)* is

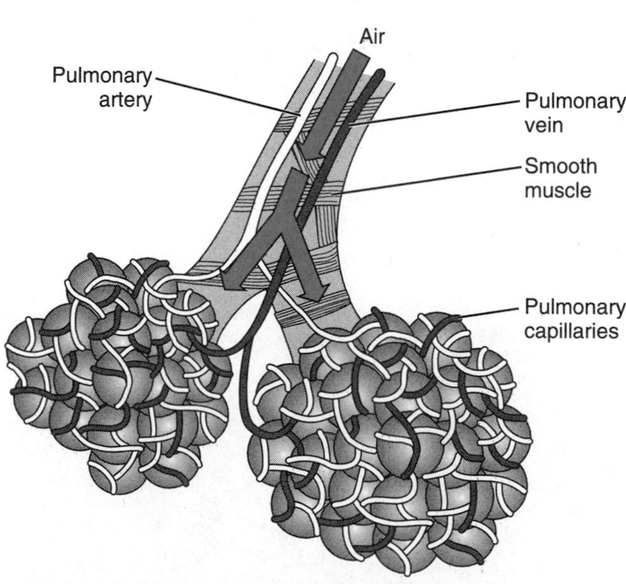

FIGURE 18–6
Respiratory unit (acinus). The respiratory unit consists of the respiratory bronchioles, alveolar ducts, and alveoli. These terminal air-filled structures are the site of pulmonary gas exchange, facilitated by the dense capillary network that surrounds them.

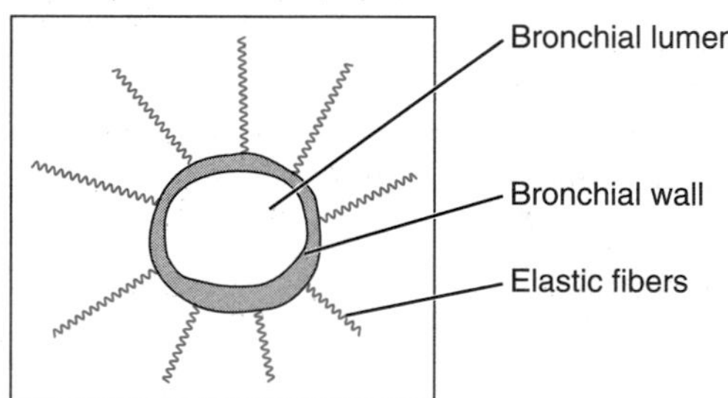

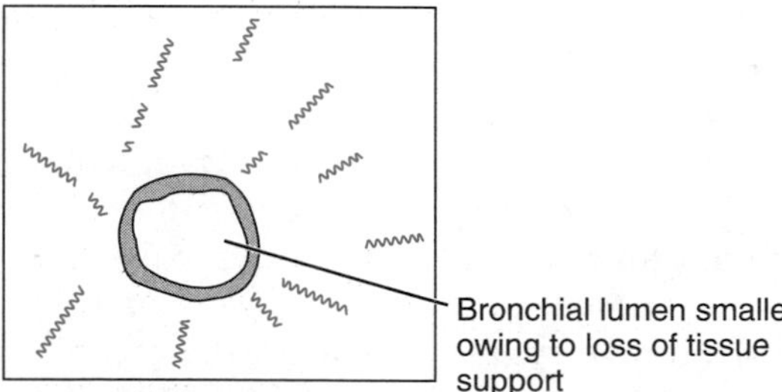

FIGURE 18–7
Connective tissue support of small airways. Smaller airways lack rigid cartilage in their walls and are kept open by the tethering forces that pull them open. These circumferential pulling forces are provided by elastic connective tissue.

TABLE 18–1
PULMONARY DEFENSE MECHANISMS

MECHANISM	DESCRIPTION
Secretory immunity (immunoglobulin A)	Antibody in respiratory mucosal secretions mounts a humoral immune response against antigens contacting the mucous barrier.
Particulate matter filtration	Hair and ciliated epithelium lining upper respiratory structures filter inhaled particles, trapping them in mucus.
Irritant reflex	Stimulation of irritant receptors by inhaled particles, cold air, or toxins initiates reflex bronchospasm to limit exposure and coughing or sneezing to expel the irritant.
Mucociliary escalator	Cilia of the respiratory epithelium beat rhythmically to conduct the mucus layer upward for swallowing or expulsion from the mouth or nose.
Alveolar macrophages	Type I alveolar cells (tissue macrophages) phagocytize organisms, toxins, and particles within the alveoli.
Glottic protective reflex	The epiglottis closes reflexively during swallowing to prevent aspiration of material into the trachea.

the amount of gas that can be forcibly exhaled beyond relaxed exhalation (about 1000 mL). The fourth volume, *residual volume (RV),* is the amount of gas remaining in the lungs after a maximal exhalation (about 1000 mL).

Total lung capacity (TLC) is the volume of air in the lungs after a maximal inspiration and is equal to the sum of all four volumes. *Vital capacity (VC)* is the maximal amount of gas expired after a maximal inhalation (IRV + TV + ERV). *Functional residual capacity (FRC)* is the amount of gas left in the lungs at the end of a normal, passive exhalation (ERV + RV). *Inspiratory capacity (IC)* is the amount of gas moved on maximal inspiration, beginning at FRC (TV + IRV).

Measurement or calculation of these volumes and capacities, as well as of air flow rates, is the basis of pulmonary function testing in clinical settings. TV, IRV, and ERV may be directly measured and are often decreased with pulmonary pathology. Flow–volume diagrams may also be generated from pulmonary function tests, indicating whether decreased pulmonary function is primarily due to airway obstruction *(obstructive pulmonary disease)* or lack of compliance of the airways or chest wall *(restrictive pulmonary disease)* (Fig. 18–10). Many ventilatory disorders have aspects of both obstruction and restriction.

Mechanics of Ventilation

Muscle Contraction

As illustrated in Figure 18–11, the major muscles of inspiration (air inflow) are the *diaphragm,* a dome-shaped muscle separating the thoracic and abdominal cavities, and the *external intercostal muscles* between the ribs. These muscles contract rhythmically in response to reflex stimuli from the brain stem. Contraction of the diaphragm moves it downward, and contraction of the external intercostals moves the anterior ribs upward and outward, increasing the volume of the thoracic cavity. During labored breathing, the sternocleidomastoid and scalenus muscles of the neck, and possibly muscles of the

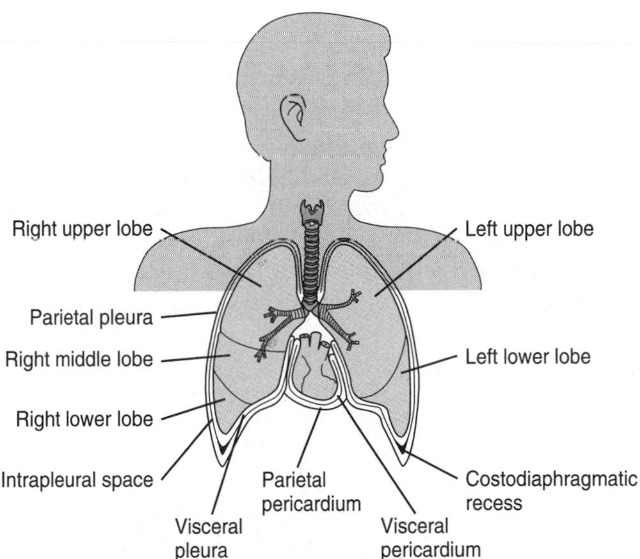

FIGURE 18–8
Structure of the lungs and pleurae. The right lung is divided into three segments, or lobes, whereas the left lung has two, yielding some thoracic space to the heart. Each lung is contained within a pleural space, separated by the mediastinal space containing the heart, trachea, esophagus, and great vessels. The intrapleural space, between the visceral pleura overlying the lung surface and the parietal pleura lining the cavity, contains a small amount of lubricating fluid, which facilitates smooth expansion of the lungs. The negative pressure of the intrapleural fluid contributes to maintenance of this expansion.

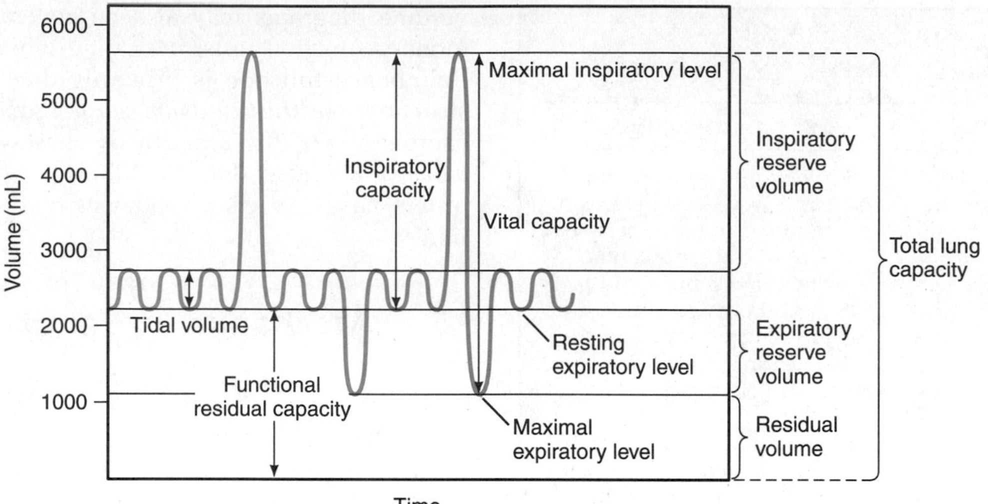

FIGURE 18–9

Pulmonary volumes and capacities. Ventilatory function may be quantified on the basis of four volumes (three of which are measurable) and four capacities calculated from summed volumes. *Tidal volume* (TV) is the volume of gas inspired and expired during a normal relaxed breath. *Inspiratory reserve volume* (IRV) is the volume of gas that can be inspired above the normal tidal volume, and *expiratory reserve volume* (ERV) is the volume that can be exhaled forcibly, beyond relaxed exhalation. The *residual volume* (RV) is the volume remaining at the end of a maximal exhalation; this volume cannot be measured directly with spirometry. The pulmonary capacities are calculated as follows: inspiratory capacity = TV + IRV; functional residual capacity = ERV + RV; vital capacity = IRV + TV + ERV; and total lung capacity = VC + IRV + TV + ERV.

face, may serve as accessory muscles of inspiration. Women normally rely more on external intercostal contraction, whereas men and children exhibit more diaphragmatic contraction. Because accessory muscles of ventilation are incompletely developed in infants and young children, head bobbing may be seen with labored breathing.

There are no major muscles of expiration (air outflow) because exhalation is normally a passive act. The diaphragm and external intercostals relax when the inspiratory signal ends, decreasing the size of the thoracic cavity. Accessory muscles do contract during labored breathing or in conditions in which outflow of air is obstructed. For example, the rectus abdominis assists in pushing up the diaphragm, and the internal intercostal muscles help to pull down the ribs.

Pressure Gradients for Air Flow

Air flow dynamics during ventilation are governed by gas laws derived from the study of physics. Figure 18–12 illustrates pressure changes during the inspiratory–expiratory cycle. In the resting state

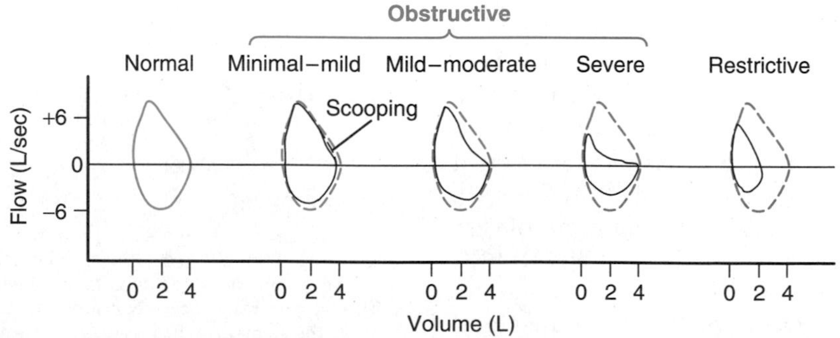

FIGURE 18–10

Obstructive and restrictive flow–volume curves. The normal curve is characterized by a rounded inspiratory curve and a straight expiratory curve after peak flow. In obstructive lung disease, lung volumes are lower, and scooping of the expiratory curve is caused by airway collapse during forced exhalation. Restrictive lung disease is demonstrated by normal inspiratory and expiratory curves but markedly reduced peak flow and lung volumes.

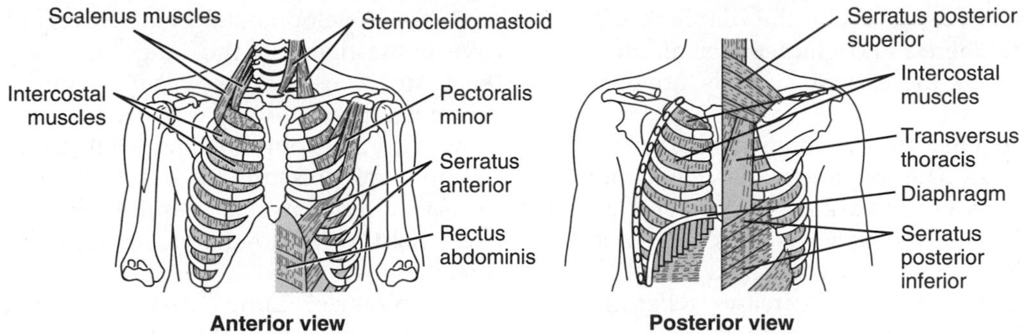

FIGURE 18–11

Muscles of ventilation. The major muscles of inspiration are the diaphragm and the external intercostal muscles. During labored inspiration, the sternocleidomastoid and scalenus muscles of the neck may serve as accessory muscles. There are no major muscles of expiration, which is normally a passive act. Accessory muscles that may assist forced exhalation include the rectus abdominis and external intercostal muscles.

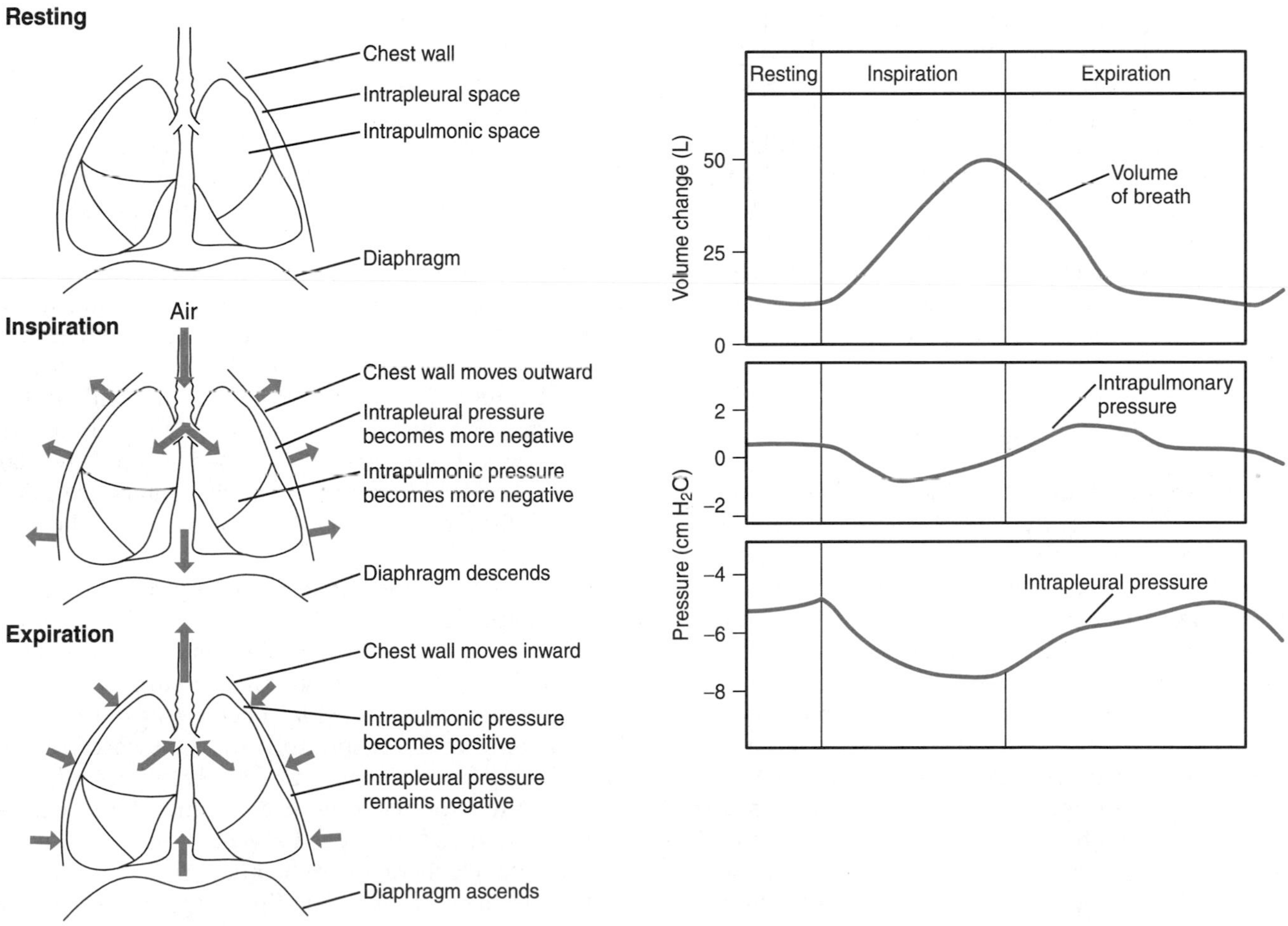

FIGURE 18–12

Pressure changes during the respiratory cycle. In the resting state, pressure in the airways is equal to atmospheric pressure, and no air flow occurs. During inspiration, the thoracic cavity is enlarged by muscle work, causing intrapleural and intrapulmonic pressures to decrease. Air flows inward along the resulting pressure gradient. During expiration, thoracic volume decreases because of relaxation of inspiratory muscles. Intrapleural and intrapulmonic pressures increase, and air flows outward. Intrapleural pressure remains negative throughout the cycle.

between breaths (i.e., at FRC), the diaphragm is relaxed upward. There is no gradient for air flow because pressure in the airways equals atmospheric pressure.

Inspiration begins with a neural signal to the inspiratory muscles. The diaphragm descends, and the chest wall moves out, enlarging the thoracic cavity. The pressure within the cavity is thus decreased because, according to the universal gas law (Boyle's law), the pressure of a gas decreases when a constant number of molecules of gas is contained within a larger space. Because intrathoracic pressure is less than atmospheric, a pressure gradient is created. The epiglottis opens, and atmospheric air flows into the lungs until the gradient is exhausted and the pressure in the airways is equal to atmospheric pressure.

When the inspiratory signal is removed, the diaphragm and intercostals relax, decreasing intrathoracic volume and creating higher airway pressure in accordance with Boyle's law. Air flows out of the lungs along this gradient until airway pressure equals atmospheric pressure. Effective development of intrathoracic pressure gradients depends on the relative rigidity of the thorax. Because the sternums and rib cages of infants are much more cartilaginous and pliable than those of adults, generation of negative pressure during inspiration may result in a slight degree of retraction of the sternum or intercostal tissues during inspiration. More marked retractions with inspiration, or intercostal bulging with forced expiration, indicate respiratory distress in children.

Work of Breathing

Work of breathing is defined as the amount of muscular effort required for inspiration and expiration. Work of breathing determines the oxygen consumption of the pulmonary system, which is normally low (about 5% of total oxygen consumption). If pulmonary disease increases significantly the work of breathing, metabolic demands increase concurrently, and positive feedback loops may result in **respiratory failure.** Respiratory failure, a common clinical syndrome associated with pulmonary, cardiovascular, and metabolic disorders, is discussed later in this chapter. Work of breathing may be increased as a consequence of several factors, including alteration of elastic recoil, compliance, alveolar surface tension, airway resistance, and **dead space.**

Elastic Recoil. Loss of elastic recoil of lung tissue may occur in **emphysema** and other conditions in which the lungs are chronically overinflated. Connective tissue changes associated with the normal aging process also contribute to reduced elastic recoil (see Developmental Perspective). Elastic connective tissue fibers in the lungs have a natural tendency to constrict or recoil. This elastic recoil promotes passive lung constriction and outward air flow during expiration and contributes to negative intrapleural pressure, as has been mentioned. Loss of elastic recoil usually requires that accessory muscles assist with exhalation, increasing the work of breathing.

Compliance. Lung tissue compliance is the amount of increase in lung volume per unit increase in airway pressure. Decreased lung tissue compliance (stiffening of the lungs) may occur with aging, with deposition of fibrin in inflammatory lung disorders, with accumulation of fluid in the interstitium (see *pulmonary edema,* Chapter 19), or with increased surface tension within the alveoli (discussed subsequently). Lungs with decreased compliance are difficult to inflate, resulting in increased work of breathing. In neonates, and particularly in premature infants, lung tissue is less compliant because it still conforms somewhat to its collapsed intrauterine state (see Chapter 33).

Decreased compliance of the chest wall also increases work of breathing because the thorax resists expansion. Abnormalities of the thoracic spine, such as scoliosis (see Chapter 34), or congenital deformities of the sternum may interfere with normal ventilation.

Alveolar Surface Tension. Increased alveolar surface tension is the most important mechanism of respiratory failure in premature infants with **infant respiratory distress syndrome (IRDS)** (see *prematurity,* Chapter 33). Surface tension is defined as the tendency for molecules on the surface of a liquid to adhere to each other when exposed to air. Alveolar sacs are lined with fluid, and their centers are filled with air. Surface tension thus promotes alveolar collapse.

Laplace's law holds that the pressure required to inflate a sphere is equal to twice the surface tension divided by the radius of the sphere; therefore, the smaller the sphere, the more air pressure is required to overcome surface tension. Because of the branching anatomy of the respiratory units, surface tension would tend to collapse smaller alveoli into larger alveoli if not for the presence of **surfactant,** a lipoprotein produced by type II alveolar cells. Surfactant molecules, which repel each other, separate the liquid molecules of alveolar fluid, opposing surface tension. The effect of surfactant is greatest in the smaller alveoli, where surfactant molecules are closer together. Premature infants suffer from a lack of surfactant, which is not produced until relatively late in gestation. Surfactant deficiency is also seen in adults due to destruction of alveoli, as in emphy-

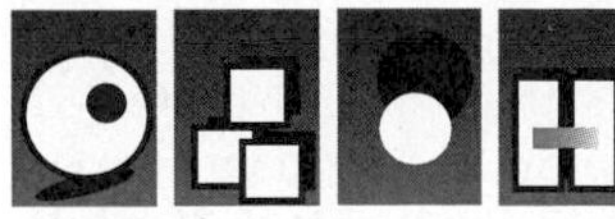

Developmental Perspective

Embryonic and Fetal Periods

Lung growth and development begins during the third week of gestation and continues until about 8 years of age. Differentiation of the conducting airways is complete by the end of the 16th week, but respiratory units continue to be added thereafter. Surfactant production begins at about 28 weeks' gestation. Prematurity is therefore characterized by abnormality of respiratory unit function. Congenital defects in pulmonary development include bronchogenic and pulmonary cysts, ectopic sequestrations of nonfunctional pulmonary tissue, bronchial obstruction, and various degrees of underdevelopment of the lung (pulmonary agenesis, aplasia, or hypoplasia). Cystic fibrosis, which primarily affects pulmonary ventilation, arises from a genetic defect in chloride transport.

Infancy and Childhood

The risk of airway obstruction is greater during this period because the airways are smaller and more flexible. The thorax is incompletely calcified, giving rise to more evident retraction with labored breathing. Asthma is prevalent in childhood, especially among boys, and is more often extrinsic in nature. URI is more frequent during childhood because of increased frequency of exposure and lack of acquired immunity to the common pathogens. Respiratory syncytial virus is the most significant pathogen in young children.

Adolescence and Young Adulthood

Cigarette smoking usually begins during this period, and occupational exposure to pulmonary irritants and carcinogens may predispose to COPD or cancer. Childhood asthma may be outgrown, although exercise-induced asthma is still prevalent. The risk of chest trauma is highest among this group.

Middle and Older Adulthood

The cumulative effects of long-term cigarette smoking frequently manifest as COPD or lung cancer. Most older adults demonstrate an age-related decline in pulmonary function, although this is widely variable, depending on lifestyle, exposure, and intercurrent illness. This senile emphysema is due to loss of elastic recoil and overstretching of airway structures rather than to destruction of alveolar walls. Some air trapping occurs, leading to increased residual volume and rounding of the thorax. A significant number of middle-aged adults, particularly obese men, suffer from obstructive sleep apnea, which is associated with increased risk of hypertension, dysrhythmia, congestive heart failure, myocardial infarction, and stroke.

sema. The tendency of alveoli to collapse from surface tension contributes to decreased compliance and thus increases the work of breathing.

Airway Resistance. Increased airway resistance is the most common cause of increased work of breathing. The smaller the lumen of the airway, the more resistance it offers to the flow of air within it. Airway resistance is higher in children than in adults, with the greatest resistance being provided by the upper airways. Airway resistance varies normally with residual volume and with autonomic input. Higher volumes within airways generate increased transmural pressure (internal pressure against airway walls). Sympathetic stimulation causes an increase in airway diameter (bronchodilation), whereas parasympathetic stimulation causes a decrease (bronchoconstriction). Autonomic nervous system function is detailed in Chapter 22.

Pulmonary disorders commonly result in increased airway resistance. Edema and inflammatory exudate may narrow airways in inflammatory conditions such as **chronic bronchitis** (discussed later in this chapter, and in lower respiratory tract infections such as pneumonia or bronchiolitis) (see Chapter 19). Congenital impairment of membrane transport obstructs airways with thick mucus in **cystic fibrosis,** as detailed subsequently.

Airway collapse during expiration greatly increases airway resistance in pulmonary diseases of children, who have less cartilage in their airways, and in adults with emphysema, owing to breakdown of connective tissue tethers holding small airways open (see Fig. 18–7). These patients must use accessory muscles to force air out during exhalation, and as air flows out and airway pressure falls, the pressure exerted by muscle contraction on the outside of the airway eventually exceeds the pressure within the airway. The airway then collapses, preventing any further increase in expiratory flow rate regardless of increased muscle work.

Dead-Space Ventilation. The final mechanism that can cause increased work of breathing is increased dead space. Dead space is the volume of air in the lungs that does not participate in gas exchange. Dead-space ventilation is thus "wasted" ventilation, which increases the work of breathing. There are two types of physiologic dead space: *anatomic dead space,* the volume of the conducting airways (normally about 150 mL in adults and proportionately greater in children), and *alveolar dead space,* the volume of any alveoli that are nonperfused or poorly perfused. Dead space may also vary iatrogenically with mechanical ventilation, in which case the volume of tubing connecting the patient to the ventilator must be added to the dead-space volume. An increase in physiologic dead space is often involved in respiratory failure, as discussed later, and may be associated with pulmonary emboli and other disorders of pulmonary perfusion (see Chapter 19).

Positional Variation in Ventilation

When lung volumes are normal, the dependent (lowermost) areas of the lung are better ventilated. When lung volumes are decreased, however, the opposite is true. The precise reasons for this positional variation are unknown. The healthy, ambulatory person normally changes positions frequently (even during sleep), facilitating normal ventilation and circulation. In hospitalized patients or in others with limited mobility, position changes initiated by health care personnel may be an important component of care.

Regulation of Ventilation

Regulation of pulmonary ventilation is complex, involving both neural and local mechanisms that affect the contraction of inspiratory and expiratory muscles as well as airway smooth muscle.

Regulation of the Central Respiratory Drive

The "central drive," or rhythmic neural signal that paces ventilation, resides primarily in the brain stem.

Reflex Versus Voluntary Control. The rate and duration of inspiration are primarily under automatic (reflex) regulation by respiratory control centers in the medulla oblongata, with potential modification of the basic ventilatory rhythm by inputs from higher centers, such as the cerebral cortex, or from multiple visceral receptors. Obviously, a person can voluntarily over-ride reflex control of ventilation *up to a point.* Voluntary holding of the breath soon results in acidosis due to CO_2 retention, and the person eventually loses consciousness due to central nervous system (CNS) depression. Reflex control would then prevail, with CO_2 levels driving increased ventilation to normalize blood gases.

Hyperventilation (increased rate or depth of ventilation) commonly occurs with extreme anxiety due to signals from the cerebral cortex or limbic system that modify reflex control. This response is also limited, however, because excess CO_2 would soon be exhaled. The resultant alkalosis would eventually impair neurotransmission within the CNS, leading to unconsciousness and restoration of normal reflex control.

Respiratory Control Centers. Figure 18–13 illustrates the multiple factors influencing ventilatory rate and rhythm. The neural stimulus for inspiration normally fires at a basal rate from pacemaker cells in the reticular formation of the medulla, in the lower brain stem. Pacemaker cells in this area are believed to function similarly to cardiac pacemakers, although this is still uncertain. This area, providing the central drive for ventilation, is known as the **respiratory center.** The respiratory center has two distinct clusters of neurons: the inspiratory area (dorsal respiratory group) and the expiratory area (ventral respiratory group). Only the inspiratory area fires during normal ventilation.

Neural impulses (action potentials) are conducted to the diaphragm and external intercostal muscles along the phrenic and intercostal nerves, initiating inspiration and sustaining it as long as the stimulus continues. The longer the inspiration, the greater the depth of ventilation. The expiratory area is probably important only during forceful exhalation, when it paces the contraction of accessory muscles such as the abdominals and internal intercostals. The rate and rhythm of normal ventilation *(eupnea)* and examples of altered ventilation are illustrated in Figure 18–14.

The intrinsic rate and duration of the inspiratory stimulus are subject to modification by descending signals from the limbic system and cerebral cortex, as has been mentioned, as well as from two areas located just above the respiratory center in the brain stem: the *apneustic center* in the lower pons, and the *pneumotaxic center* in the upper pons. The apneustic center probably plays no role in normal respiration, but it appears to drive a gasping type of ventilation when higher centers are depressed or damaged, as in head injury. The pneumotaxic center appears to

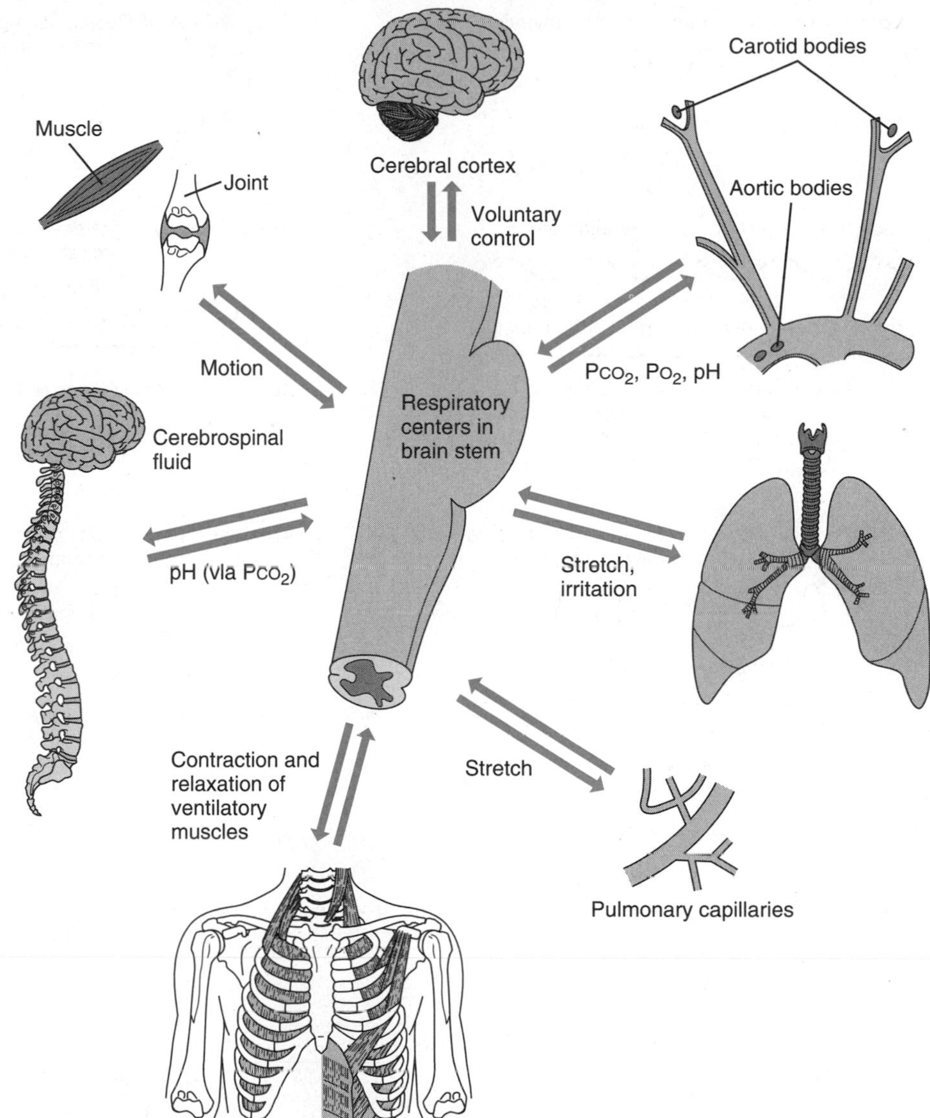

FIGURE 18–13
Regulation of ventilation. The respiratory centers in the medulla oblongata of the brain stem integrate sensory inputs from multiple central and peripheral receptors in pacing the rate and depth of ventilation. Regulation of ventilation is primarily reflex, although a limited degree of voluntary over-ride is possible.

influence the rate and depth of normal breathing by switching off the inspiratory signal when it reaches its peak. Normal ventilation can occur even in the absence of signals from the pneumotaxic center, however, so its precise role is uncertain.

Factors Influencing Ventilatory Rate and Depth. The medullary respiratory center receives and integrates inputs from chemoreceptors in the brain stem and in the carotid and aortic bodies, from stretch and irritant receptors in the airway walls, and from motion receptors in joints and muscles. These inputs comprise the afferent (ascending) signals of the visceral reflex arcs influencing ventilation.

Central Chemoreceptors. The central chemoreceptors are located in the medulla, near the subarachnoid space containing cerebrospinal fluid (CSF). They are activated by changes in the pH of CSF. An increase in acidity (i.e., a decrease in pH) of the CSF signals the respiratory center to increase rate and depth of ventilation. Because hydrogen ions do not readily diffuse into the CSF from the blood, the source of acidity in the CSF is CO_2, which easily crosses the blood–CSF barrier (see Chapter 21). CO_2 then enters the hydrolysis reaction (see Chapter 10), producing hydrogen ions and increasing acidity of the CSF.

In clinical settings, the serum Pa_{CO_2} is most closely monitored as the central stimulus for ventilation. CO_2 levels vary with the rate of metabolic production by cellular energy metabolism and with the rate of exhalation during ventilation. The proportionately greater heat loss and higher metabolic rates of children result in more rapid respiratory rates (up to 70 breaths/minute in active infants), whereas adults at rest normally breathe about 12 times per minute.

Peripheral Chemoreceptors. The peripheral chemoreceptors are located in the carotid and aortic bod-

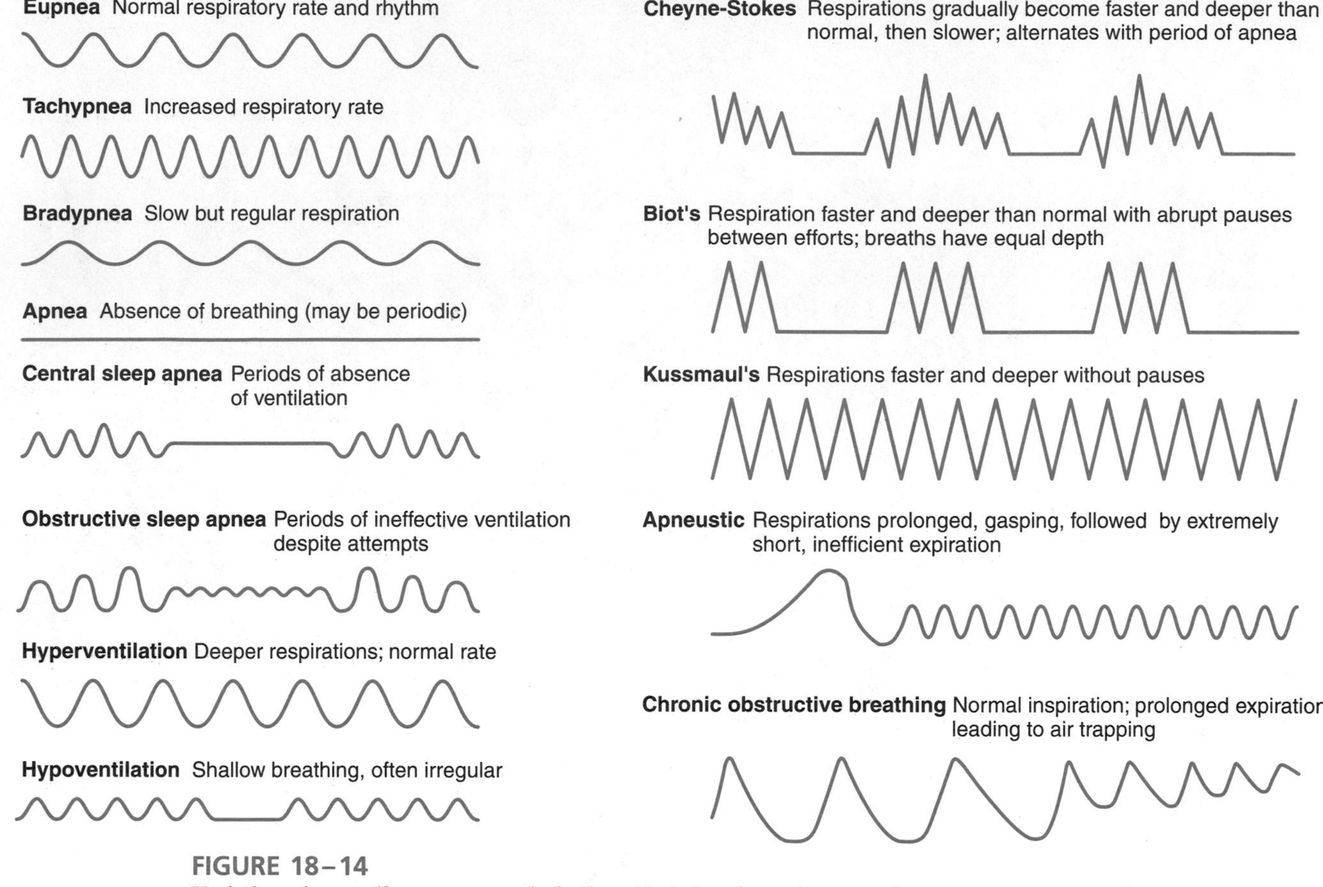
Eupnea Normal respiratory rate and rhythm
Tachypnea Increased respiratory rate
Bradypnea Slow but regular respiration
Apnea Absence of breathing (may be periodic)
Central sleep apnea Periods of absence of ventilation
Obstructive sleep apnea Periods of ineffective ventilation despite attempts
Hyperventilation Deeper respirations; normal rate
Hypoventilation Shallow breathing, often irregular
Cheyne-Stokes Respirations gradually become faster and deeper than normal, then slower; alternates with period of apnea
Biot's Respiration faster and deeper than normal with abrupt pauses between efforts; breaths have equal depth
Kussmaul's Respirations faster and deeper without pauses
Apneustic Respirations prolonged, gasping, followed by extremely short, inefficient expiration
Chronic obstructive breathing Normal inspiration; prolonged expiration leading to air trapping

FIGURE 18–14
Variations in ventilatory rate and rhythm. Variation from the normal eupneic pattern may be adaptive or may result from pathophysiologic processes affecting pulmonary structures or regulation of ventilation.

ies, near the baroreceptors within these large arteries. They respond to decreased PaO_2, increased $PaCO_2$, or decreased pH in arterial blood by signaling the respiratory center to increase the rate and depth of ventilation. Afferent signals travel to the respiratory center by the vagus and glossopharyngeal nerves. As discussed in Chapter 10, chemoreceptor-triggered reflex arcs initiate negative feedback loops, which are critical to regulation of levels of volatile acid in body fluids. Chemoreceptors also initiate reflex sighing and yawning, which intermittently ventilate all or most alveoli in the lungs.

Mechanoreceptors. Receptors sensing stretch or deformation play a minor role in the regulation of ventilation. Pulmonary stretch receptors located in the smooth muscle of airways mediate the *Hering-Breuer reflex,* which protects airways from excessive stretch during exercise. These receptors result in inhibition of further inspiration beyond a set point by the same pathways as chemoreceptor reflexes. Juxtacapillary receptors, located in alveolar walls near pulmonary capillaries, sense increased fluid pressure within the capillaries or interstitial space (as seen in pulmonary edema or inflammatory conditions). Stimulation of these receptors apparently drives a rapid, shallow ventilatory pattern. The irritant receptors that mediate cough and bronchoconstriction may also be stimulated by an increase in airway pressure, triggering rapid, shallow breathing. The mechanisms underlying the adaptive increase in ventilation that occurs during exercise are uncertain, as discussed in Chapter 35.

Regulation of Airway Diameter

Although airway diameter depends partly on the volume of gas contained within it (and therefore depends on central drive controlling depth of ventilation), many other factors may alter the size of the conducting airways. Irritant receptors in the pharynx and conducting airways respond to cold air or to irritants in inhaled dust or smoke by triggering a parasympathetic reflex. The resulting effect is bronchoconstriction (to limit further exposure to the irritant) and spasm of ventilatory muscles to expel the irritant with coughing or sneezing. During the stress response, sympathetic stimulation results in bronchodilation to maximize oxygen supply for the fight-

TABLE 18–2
CHEMICAL MEDIATORS OF AIRWAY DIAMETER

Mediator	Airway Effect	
	Bronchodilation	Bronchoconstriction
Neurotransmitters and Neuropeptides		
Acetylcholine		√
Epinephrine and norepinephrine	√	
Tachykinins (substance P, neurokinin A, neurokinin B)		√
Local Cellular Products		
Histamine		√
Prostaglandin E_2	√	
Prostaglandin $F_{2\alpha}$		√
Prostaglandin D_2		√
Thromboxane A_2		√
Leukotrienes C_4, D_4, and E_4		√
Platelet-activating factor		√
Drugs		
Methacholine		√
β-agonists (albuterol)	√	
Methylxanthines (theophylline)	√	
Anticholinergics (ipratropium)	√	
Mast cell stabilizers (cromolyn)	√	

or-flight response (see Chapter 1). Airway smooth muscle also responds to local mediators, such as histamine, prostaglandins, and leukotrienes; and a number of drugs affect airway diameter (Table 18–2).

VENTILATORY DISORDERS

The clinical syndrome of respiratory failure is discussed in this section, as are several disorders of ventilation that may manifest as respiratory failure.

Respiratory Failure

Definition. Respiratory failure is the inability of the pulmonary system to maintain adequate oxygenation of the blood, manifested clinically as **hypoxemia,** a PaO_2 of 50 mm Hg or less. In most cases, decreased ventilation is a component of respiratory failure, as manifested by **hypercapnia,** a $PaCO_2$ of 50 mm Hg or greater.

Epidemiology. Because respiratory failure is associated with numerous disorders of pulmonary, cardiovascular, and neuromuscular function, it is commonly encountered in clinical practice. Risk factors relate to the underlying conditions, discussed below and summarized in Table 18–3.

Etiology. Respiratory failure may develop as a result of (1) **alveolar hypoventilation,** (2) **ventilation–perfusion ($\dot{V}/\dot{Q}$) abnormality,** (3) decreased FIO_2 (fraction of inspired oxygen) in inspired air, or (4) impairment of diffusion of gases between the alveoli and the blood.

Alveolar Hypoventilation. Alveolar hypoventilation, a decrease in the rate of delivery of fresh atmospheric air to the alveoli for exchange, may result from a decrease in the rate or duration of the inspiratory signal from the respiratory center, as seen with CNS disease or trauma or with CNS depressant drugs such as anesthetics, sedatives, and hypnotics. Neuromuscular diseases, such as poliomyelitis or amyotrophic lateral sclerosis, may result in alveolar hypoventilation if they prevent normal contraction of respiratory muscles (see Chapter 22). The most common cause of alveolar hypoventilation is airway obstruction, seen in **chronic obstructive pulmonary disease** (COPD), also known as *chronic air flow limitation.* COPD includes chronic bronchitis, emphysema, and other disorders discussed later in this chapter.

Ventilation–Perfusion Abnormality. Ventilation–perfusion abnormality ($\dot{V}/\dot{Q}$ mismatch) occurs when, at the level of the alveoli, either ventilation ($\dot{V}$) or perfusion ($\dot{Q}$) is less than optimal (Fig. 18–15). Diffusion of oxygen and CO_2 between the alveolar air and the surrounding alveolar capillary blood is maximized when flow of air and blood is ideally matched. In adults, alveolar ventilation is about 4 L/minute, whereas perfusion is about 5 L/minute, yielding a $\dot{V}/\dot{Q}$ of 0.8.[1]

Low $\dot{V}/\dot{Q}$ states are common in pulmonary disease, resulting from intrapulmonary shunting or decreased ventilation secondary to airway obstruction when perfusion is normal. If the number of respiratory units with low $\dot{V}/\dot{Q}$ ratios is sufficient, oxygenation of the hemoglobin in the blood is impaired, resulting in hypoxemia. In health, as well as in pulmonary disease, not all respiratory units have the same $\dot{V}/\dot{Q}$, as discussed further in Chapter 19. Units with normal $\dot{V}/\dot{Q}$ ratios compensate for low $\dot{V}/\dot{Q}$ units to some extent by increasing their ventilation, but they cannot saturate hemoglobin beyond 100% of its oxygen-carrying capacity. The combination of the saturation of hemoglobin in low $\dot{V}/\dot{Q}$ units at, for example, 30%, and the saturation in normal units of 100% results in a net oxygenation of the blood that is still deficient.

TABLE 18–3
CONDITIONS PREDISPOSING TO RESPIRATORY FAILURE

Etiologic Mechanism	Examples
Alveolar hypoventilation	Central nervous system disease or trauma
	Stroke
	Brain tumor
	Head injury
	Spinal cord injury
	Central nervous system depressant drugs
	General anesthetics
	Sedative-hypnotics
	Neuromuscular disease
	Poliomyelitis
	Amyotrophic lateral sclerosis
	Guillain-Barré syndrome
	Muscular dystrophy
	Myasthenia gravis
	Airway obstruction
	Chronic obstructive pulmonary disease
	Pneumonia
	Laryngotracheobronchitis
	Lung cancer
	Acute epiglottitis
	Restrictive pulmonary disease
	Pulmonary fibrosis
	Pneumothorax
	Voluntary hypoventilation (as with pain of rib fractures)
	CO_2 narcosis
Ventilation–perfusion abnormality	Reduced ventilation (low $\dot{V}/\dot{Q}$)
	All conditions associated with hypoventilation (see above)
	Reduced perfusion (high $\dot{V}/\dot{Q}$)
	Pulmonary embolism
Decreased fraction of inspired oxygen	Consumption of ambient O_2 by fire or explosion
	Anesthesia error
	Mechanical ventilation error
Impaired diffusion	Adult respiratory distress syndrome
	Acute pulmonary edema

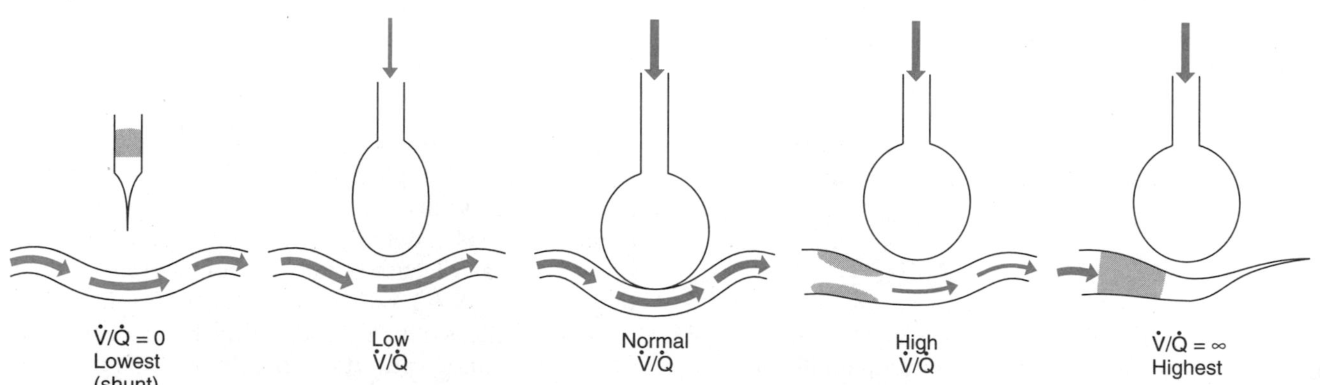

FIGURE 18–15
Ventilation–perfusion ($\dot{V}/\dot{Q}$) relationships. A normal $\dot{V}/\dot{Q}$ ratio results from optimal ventilation and perfusion of an alveolus. Abnormality of either ventilation (e.g., with airway obstruction) or perfusion (e.g., with pulmonary embolism) may result in suboptimal $\dot{V}/\dot{Q}$ ratios, which approach zero (low $\dot{V}/\dot{Q}$) or infinity (high $\dot{V}/\dot{Q}$). Gas exchange is impaired in either case.

TABLE 18–4
GAS COMPOSITION OF ATMOSPHERIC AIR*

GAS	PARTIAL PRESSURE (MM HG)	PERCENTAGE
Nitrogen	597.0	78.62%
Oxygen	159.0	20.84%
Carbon dioxide	0.3	0.04%
Water vapor	3.7	0.50%
TOTAL	760	100%

* Assuming moderate conditions of ambient temperature and humidity, at sea level.
Data from Guyton, A.C., and Hall, J.E. (1996). *Textbook of Medical Physiology*. (9th ed.). Philadelphia: W.B. Saunders.

High $\dot{V}/\dot{Q}$ states are much less common, resulting in most cases from decreased perfusion secondary to pulmonary emboli (see Chapter 19). High $\dot{V}/\dot{Q}$ is less likely to lead to hypoxemia because both affected and unaffected units can increase their ventilation to maximize the saturation percentage of the available hemoglobin.

Decreased Fraction of Inspired Oxygen. Decreased FIO_2, an uncommon cause of respiratory failure, results in hypoxemia when the inspired air does not contain sufficient oxygen to establish an adequate gradient for diffusion into the blood. As illustrated in Table 18–4, "room" air at sea level contains about 21% oxygen, with a partial pressure of about 159 mm Hg. This pressure decreases with increasing altitude, and such exposure may precipitate respiratory failure in unacclimated people or in those with compromised pulmonary systems. Decreased FIO_2 also occurs with consumption of ambient oxygen in enclosed spaces, more quickly in the presence of fire or explosion. In clinical settings, decreased FIO_2 may occur iatrogenically as a consequence of error in administration of anesthesia or mechanical ventilation.

Impaired Diffusion. Impaired diffusion refers to alteration of the tissues separating the alveolar air and the blood to the extent that diffusion of O_2 and CO_2 is slowed or prevented. These tissues, discussed further in Chapter 19 and known collectively as the *alveolar–capillary membrane,* must be severely damaged to impair diffusion because gases cross biologic membranes easily and because there is normally ample diffusion time available. At a normal heart rate of 60 beats/minute, for example, each pulsation of blood would dwell in the pulmonary capillaries for 1 second. Because of the high diffusibility of the blood gases, exchange is normally completed within 0.25 second. Even if thickening of the membrane slows diffusion, the extra time allows for complete exhaustion of the gradients in most cases. In some critical illnesses, such as adult respiratory distress syndrome or acute pulmonary edema, the membrane may be sufficiently impaired to cause respiratory failure (see Chapter 19).

Pathophysiology. Respiratory failure usually results in a combined metabolic and respiratory acidosis, affecting the function of all body systems (see Chapter 10). Tissue hypoxia is present due to hypoxemia, resulting in an increase in anaerobic metabolism and lactic acidosis. Respiratory acidosis may be present due to hypercapnia. The metabolic workload of the respiratory and cardiovascular systems is greatly increased in an effort to supply oxygen to tissues.

Clinical Manifestations. Arterial blood gases reveal the characteristic hypoxemia as well as possible hypercapnia and acidosis. Decreased saturation of hemoglobin with oxygen is probable, as demonstrated by blood testing or pulse oximetry. Increased work of breathing is often evidenced by **dyspnea,** the subjective sensation of difficult breathing, and by use of accessory muscles of ventilation. Depending on the mechanism of respiratory failure, ventilatory rate and depth are altered.

The heart rate and stroke volume are increased, evidenced by tachycardia and possible palpitations, and the metabolic demands imposed by hypoxic tissues and increased pulmonary workload may precipitate congestive heart failure, especially in those with limited cardiac reserve. Cyanosis of the skin, nailbeds, and mucous membranes may be seen owing to increased concentrations of unoxygenated hemoglobin. Clubbing of the fingers and toes occurs with chronic hypoxia of these tissues (Fig. 18–16).

Hypoxia of the kidneys causes release of the hormone erythropoietin from renal cells. Erythropoietin

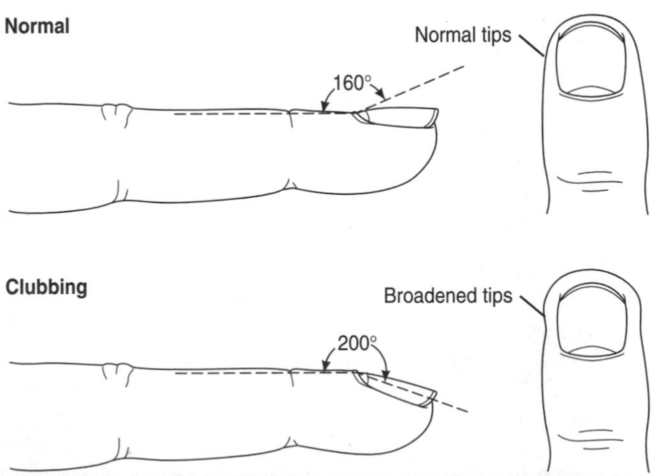

FIGURE 18–16
Clubbing. Chronic hypoxia disrupts tissue metabolism of the distal extremities, manifested by broadening of the tips of the fingers and toes. The nail angle exceeds the normal 160 degrees.

stimulates the bone marrow to increase its production of red blood cells in an adaptive effort to increase the oxygen-carrying capacity of the blood (see Chapter 12). The increase in circulating erythrocytes induced by this mechanism is known as *secondary polycythemia*.

Prevention and Treatment. Prevention depends on modification of factors such as exposure to inhaled toxins. Cigarette smoking is strongly associated with COPD and lung cancer, discussed later in this chapter. Treatment is aimed at removal of the specific cause, if possible, and at support of respiratory function with drug therapy, chest physiotherapy, oxygen therapy, or mechanical ventilation. Table 18–5 summarizes drugs commonly used in the treatment of respiratory failure. Bronchodilator drugs are commonly used, but their efficacy is unproved except in the treatment of **asthma.** Mucolytics and expectorants may be administered to decrease the viscosity of mucus, making it easier to expel. Cough suppressants may be used if persistent coughing is exhausting the patient or if the cough is ineffective in expelling mucus. As a general rule, however, a productive cough is considered to be adaptive and is not suppressed. Steroids may be employed to decrease airway edema but have potentially harmful side effects (see Chapter 29).

Chest physiotherapy includes a number of techniques designed to open airways obstructed with mucus. Postural drainage is done by sequentially

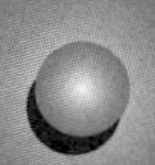

TABLE 18–5
DRUG THERAPY IN RESPIRATORY FAILURE

Drug Category and Examples	Effects
Anti-inflammatory Agents	
Glucocorticoids Beclomethasone (Vanceril) Betamethasone (Valisone) Triamcinolone acetonide (Azmacort)	Decrease the formation of inflammatory mediators from arachidonic acid, reducing airway edema and secretion
Mast cell stabilizers Cromolyn sodium (Intal)	Reduce mass cell permeability to calcium ions, inhibiting degranulation with release of inflammatory mediators
Antitussives	
Narcotic antitussives Codeine Methadone (Dolophine)	Increase the stimulation threshold of the neurons of the cough reflex, either centrally or locally
Nonnarcotic antitussives Dextromethorphan Diphenhydramine HCl (Benalyn)	Same as for narcotic antitussives
Bronchodilators	
β-agonists Terbutaline (Brethine) Metaproterenol (Alupent) Albuterol (Proventil, Ventolin)	Stimulate β_2-adrenergic receptors in bronchial smooth muscle, resulting in formation of cAMP, which relaxes the muscle
Theophylline derivatives Theophylline ethylenediamine (Aminophylline) Theophylline anhydrous (Theo-Dur)	Increase cAMP formation indirectly, probably through effects on intracellular calcium or adenosine
Anticholinergics Ipratropium bromide (Atrovent)	Decrease formation of cGMP, which opposes cAMP action
Respiratory Stimulants	
Analeptics Caffeine Doxapram (Dopram)	Stimulate the central nervous system, including the brain-stem respiratory centers
Carbon dioxide	Stimulates central and peripheral chemoreceptors
Mucolytics	
Acetylcysteine (Mucomyst)	Decreases viscosity of mucus by breaking bonds between mucoprotein molecules
Expectorants	
Guaifenesin Terpin hydrate Iodide preparations	Stimulates mucous glands to produce increased quantities of less viscous mucus

cAMP, cyclic adenosine monophosphate; cGMP, cyclic guanosine monophosphate.
Data from Kuhn, M.M. (1991). *Pharmacotherapeutics: A Nursing Process Approach* (2nd ed.). Philadelphia: F.A. Davis.

positioning the patient to facilitate gravitational drainage of the airways in various lung lobes. Manual or mechanical percussion (clapping over the thorax with cupped hands) or vibration may be used to loosen airway mucus to facilitate its expulsion by postural drainage or coughing.

Administration of oxygen may alleviate hypoxemia by increasing the diffusion gradient for oxygen. Several methods exist for the clinical administration of oxygen, which may be prescribed at a specific flow rate (1 to 15 L/minute) or FIO_2 (up to 100%). Oxygen therapy is associated with significant risks, however (Table 18–6).

Mechanical ventilation (artificial respiration) may provide assistance or totally over-ride the patient's own ventilatory function. The earliest ventilators were tanks ("iron lungs") that totally enclosed the patient's thorax and pulled air into the lungs by generating negative pressure outside the chest wall. The negative pressure principle has been adapted in the form of external shells or wraps, mainly for home use by patients requiring ventilatory assistance because of neuromuscular disorders. Most ventilators found in clinical settings are positive-pressure ventilators, which push air into the airways. This is an effective but nonphysiologic means of ventilation that may adversely affect cardiac function by altering intrathoracic pressures. Because these ventilators require a closed system, gas must be delivered through a cuffed endotracheal tube (Fig. 18–17) or, in short-term situations, a tight-fitting mask covering the mouth and nose. Several different modes of mechanical ventilation are available to provide varying degrees of control of respiratory rate, tidal volume, FIO_2, and airway pressure (Table 18–7).

Risks associated with mechanical ventilation include possible hypoxemia due to obstruction of the artificial airway (endotracheal tube) or machine gas source failure, infection due to instrumentation and bypass of upper airway defenses, failure to "wean" from the machine due to deconditioning of the diaphragm or psychological dependence, trauma of the airways due to high airway pressures (barotrauma) or volumes (volutrauma), and decreased venous return and diastolic filling of the heart due to high intrathoracic pressures. Patients may be psychologically distressed by their dependence on mechanical assistance for the essential function of respiration. Patients are unable to speak while intubated with a cuffed tube because the cuff surrounding the tube seals off the trachea below the vocal cords, preventing their vibration by upward currents of air.

Prognosis and Outcome. Despite advances in pulmonary medicine, treatment of acute hypoxemic respiratory failure is often unsuccessful. Mortality rates still range between 50% and 75%.[2]

Upper Respiratory Infection

Definition. Upper respiratory infections (URIs) include a number of inflammatory conditions of the upper airway, such as the **common cold, pharyngi-**

TABLE 18–6
RISKS ASSOCIATED WITH OXYGEN THERAPY

Detrimental Effect	Clinical Relevance
Combustibility	Oxygen is extremely flammable, thus care must be taken to eliminate sources of combustion (such as cigarette smoking and electrical shocks) while oxygen is in use.
CO_2 narcosis	In patients with chronic hypercapnia, it has been hypothesized that central chemoreceptors become desensitized to CO_2 as the primary stimulus for ventilation. Hypoxia then becomes the most important stimulus, and its removal by oxygen therapy may result in decreased ventilation and a rise in $PaCO_2$. Signs of CO_2 narcosis (lethargy progressing to coma) result from the central nervous system effects of acidosis and vasodilation.
Nitrogen washout	The greatest percentage of gas in the atmosphere and lungs is nitrogen. Because nitrogen is much less soluble than oxygen, its exchange between the alveoli and the blood is limited. Essentially, it moves in and out of the lungs and occupies space in the alveoli, helping to keep airways open. If 100% oxygen is administered, for example, the nitrogen in the airways is soon displaced by oxygen. Oxygen is absorbed readily, and airways collapse. Many low $\dot{V}/\dot{Q}$ areas are created, and hypoxemia may worsen.
Oxygen toxicity	In high doses, oxygen is toxic to body tissues because it promotes formation of reactive oxygen species, which may damage the DNA of cells. In *bronchopulmonary dysplasia*, oxygen damages alveoli, causing fluid exudation, airway scarring, and decreased surfactant production. *Retinopathy of prematurity* results from exposure of retinal tissues of premature infants to high oxygen concentrations. Overgrowth and tangling of retinal vessels occurs, with potential retinal detachment and blindness.

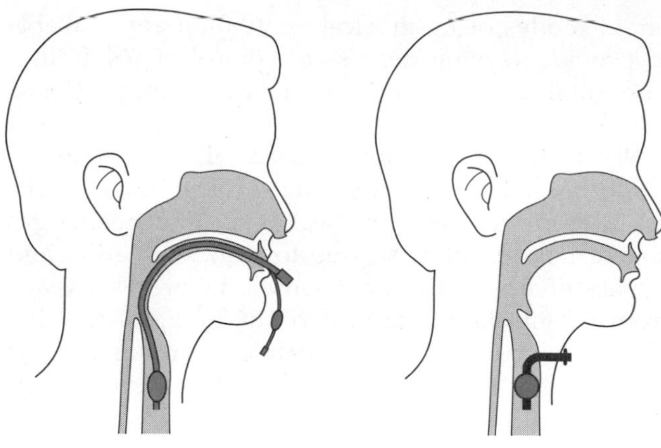

FIGURE 18–17
Endotracheal intubation. Mechanical ventilation requires a closed delivery system, which is usually established by means of a cuffed tube inserted into the trachea either orally, nasally, or transtracheally.

tis, laryngitis, croup (laryngotracheobronchitis), epiglottitis, tonsillitis, sinusitis, and **acute bronchitis.** Inflammation of these upper respiratory structures may also be entirely due to, or at least associated with, noninfectious causes (Table 18–8).

Epidemiology. URI is the most common of all diseases, afflicting adults 2 to 4 times per year and children 6 to 10 times per year in the United States.[3] Increased incidence of URI in children may be attributed to more frequent exposure to microorganisms causing URI and lack of acquired immunity to these agents. Children in day care centers experience more URIs than do those in the home, and children and spouses of those who smoke cigarettes, as well as smokers themselves, have a greater incidence.[4] A deficiency in secretory antibody (immunoglobulin A), whether hereditary or induced by cigarette smoking, may predispose to URI[5] (see Chapter 13). The risk of sinusitis is increased in people with chronic mucosal edema within the sinuses (e.g., due to allergy) or mechanical obstruction of sinus drainage (e.g., nasal polyps or deviated nasal septum).[6]

Etiology. Most URIs are due to viral infection, transmitted between people through direct contact with respiratory secretions containing the virus. Hundreds of causative agents have been identified to date (Table 18–9). Viruses may cause primary infection of either the upper or lower respiratory tracts. Bacterial infection may be the primary cause of URI but more often occurs secondarily to immunosuppression induced by the initial viral infection. Inflammation of the upper respiratory tract struc-

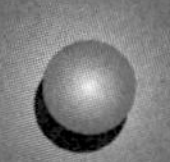

TABLE 18–7
MODES OF MECHANICAL VENTILATION

Mode	Description
Traditional Modes	
Volume-control	Ventilator settings determine rate and tidal volume; patient does not initiate ventilation.
Assist-control	Ventilator delivers a volume-controlled breath either when triggered by patient's inspiratory effort or when a preset interval passes without patient effort.
Synchronized intermittent mandatory ventilation (SIMV)	Ventilator delivers periodic breaths at a preset rate and volume; spontaneous breathing is also permitted.
Pressure-control	Ventilator delivers preset pressure to the airway for a preset time and at a guaranteed minimum rate; patient may breathe in excess of this rate.
Pressure-support	Each spontaneous breath is augmented by ventilator-delivered positive pressure up to a preset limit.
Positive end-expiratory pressure (PEEP)	Ventilator maintains some degree of positive airway pressure at the end of expiration in an effort to recruit collapsed alveoli and to prevent airway collapse due to dynamic airway compression.
Newer Alternative Modes	
Inverse ratio	Ventilator holds inspiratory positive pressure for a longer period during inspiration, achieving an inspiratory-to-expiratory time ratio of 1:1, 2:1, or 3:1. (The ratio for normal spontaneous breathing is about 1:2 or 1:3.)
High-frequency jet	Ventilator delivers breaths at low pressure but rapid rate in an effort to reduce barotrauma.
Liquid ventilation	Insufflation of the lungs with an oxygenated perfluorochemical liquid to support gas exchange, followed by active removal of the liquid.
Extracorporeal support	External membranes (e.g., cardiopulmonary bypass) are used to oxygenate the blood and to remove CO_2.

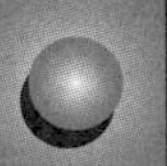

TABLE 18-8
NONINFECTIOUS SYNDROMES OF UPPER AIRWAY OBSTRUCTION

Syndrome	Clinical Features
Allergic rhinitis	Common familial condition that may be either seasonal (hay fever) or perennial (year-round). Usual allergens are pollens (tree and grass pollens in spring and summer; ragweed pollen in fall), dusts, molds, and animal danders. Inflammation results from immunoglobulin E–mediated mast cell degranulation
Nonallergic rhinitis with eosinophilia syndrome (NARES)	Resembles allergic rhinitis except that allergy tests are negative
Hormonally induced nasal congestion	About half of women have nasal congestion throughout most of pregnancy due to the vascular effects of estrogen and progesterone. Many patients with hypothyroidism have chronic nasal congestion, which subsides with thyroid replacement
Rhinitis medicamentosa	Nasal congestion due to rebound vasodilation occurring with overuse of nasal decongestant sprays
Vasomotor rhinitis	Nasal congestion due to excess parasympathetic tone causing local venous dilation and mucus secretion
Allergic sinusitis	Immunoglobulin E–mediated inflammation of the lining of the paranasal sinuses with clinical features similar to allergic rhinitis; may be seasonal or perennial
Mechanical laryngitis	Laryngeal inflammation secondary to trauma of overuse of the voice
Septal deviation	Abnormal position of the intranasal septum, which may be congenital or acquired (traumatic), obstructs nasal air flow
Nasal polyps	Obstructive protrusions of the nasal mucosa, associated with perennial rhinitis
Foreign bodies, tumors	May mechanically obstruct nasal passage or sinus outflow tracts (ostia)
Obstructive sleep apnea	Recurrent episodes of upper airway obstruction during sleep, usually occurring in obese, middle-aged men who are heavy snorers. The soft palate lengthens, owing to a chronic inflammatory response to vibratory trauma. Associated with increased risk of hypertension, dysrhythmias, congestive heart failure, myocardial infarction, and stroke

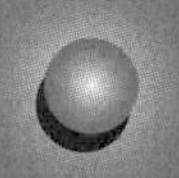

TABLE 18-9
CAUSATIVE AGENTS IN UPPER RESPIRATORY INFECTION

Viruses
Rhinovirus (more than 100 varieties)
Parainfluenza
Respiratory syncytial virus (RSV)
Coronavirus
Adenovirus
Enterovirus
Influenza A, B, or C
Reovirus
Varicella
Rubeola
Epstein-Barr virus (EBV)
Herpes simplex
Bacteria
Mycoplasma pneumoniae
Coccidioides immitis
Histoplasma capsulatum
Bordetella pertussis
Chlamydia psittaci
Streptococcus pneumoniae
Haemophilus influenzae
Moraxella (Branhamella) catarrhalis

tures may occur occasionally in the absence of infection, owing to irritation by inhaled toxins or, in the case of laryngitis, from mechanical irritation due to overuse of the voice.

Pathophysiology. The typical viral infection is mild and of limited duration. The inflammatory response to cell damage by viruses results in hyperemia and fluid exudation (see Chapter 13), and irritant receptors are triggered. Kinins and other inflammatory mediators may induce spasm of upper airway smooth muscle. Developmental differences in upper airway structures of young children may result in severe narrowing of the upper airways with inflammation, to the degree that respiratory failure may result from hypoventilation (see Developmental Perspective).

Clinical Manifestations. In the common cold, inflammation results in the cardinal symptoms of pain, redness, and swelling. Fluid exudation obstructs upper airways to some degree with mucus, resulting in drainage from the nares *(rhinorrhea)* and into the posterior pharynx (postnasal drainage). When purulent exudate persists for longer than 7 days, bacterial infection is likely.[7] Neonates breathe exclusively through the nose except when crying and so may be particularly distressed by any degree of nasal obstruction. In others, dyspnea is generally mild. The patient may run a low-grade fever, although children and the elderly may actually have a subnormal body temperature due to altered thermoregulation associated with immaturity or degenerative processes.

The tonsils or adenoids (pharyngeal tonsils), lymphatic tissues of the pharynx, may become painfully inflamed, producing profuse exudate and enlarging to the degree that they may obstruct the airway. Acute pharyngitis is manifested by scratchy pain of the throat, difficulty swallowing *(dysphagia)*, redness and swelling, and possible exudate formation. Inflammation involving the larynx may impair phonation.

Inflammation of the larynx, trachea, and upper bronchi in croup may result in significant airway obstruction, with labored breathing and *stridor*, a characteristic "crowing" sound produced on inspiration. Head bobbing may be seen in younger children, owing to use of immature accessory muscles of the neck during inspiration. The upper airway structures of infants and young children may become compressed during airway pressure changes with labored breathing. Stridor is produced by turbulent air flow past these compressed structures. Stridor may also signify epiglottitis, which is potentially the most dangerous manifestation of URI in children. The epiglottis is larger and shaped differently in young children, and further enlargement by inflammation may totally close the airway within 6 to 12 hours.

URIs are self-limited in most cases but may extend to the lower airways, causing acute bronchitis or pneumonia (discussed in Chapter 19). Many children are prone to otitis media (middle ear infection) as a complication of URI, due to ascending infection in the eustachian tube. Otitis media is discussed in Chapter 23. Infection may extend to the eyes, manifesting as conjunctivitis, and to the sinuses, causing acute sinusitis. URI rarely results in respiratory failure but may do so in children with epiglottitis. URI may precipitate respiratory failure if superimposed on chronically narrowed airways, such as those found in patients with emphysema or cystic fibrosis.

Prevention and Treatment. Childhood immunizations are critical in prevention of serious inflammatory disorders due to pathogenic bacteria and viruses (see Chapter 13). Prevention of exposure is warranted in vulnerable people with chronic cardiac or respiratory conditions or with immunodeficiency. Adherence to principles of hygiene, including frequent handwashing, decreases the risk of transmission. Because most URIs are self-limited, treatment is symptomatic and supportive of the inflammatory response. The time-honored regimen of fluids and rest is most effective. Anti-inflammatory drugs, such as aspirin or acetaminophen, may relieve fever and discomfort. Aspirin should not be administered to young children, however, because its use has been associated with risk of Reye's syndrome, a serious condition manifested by cerebral edema and liver failure (see Chapter 26). Over-the-counter decongestants may be used judiciously to manage symptoms, and cough suppressants may relieve a nonproductive cough and promote rest and sleep. Antihistamines may be useful in treatment of sinusitis or rhinitis that has an allergic cause (Table 18–10). There is no rationale for the use of antihistamines or

TABLE 18–10
CLINICAL USE OF ANTIHISTAMINES (H_1 ANTAGONISTS)

Category and Examples	Clinical Use	Side Effects
Classic (First-Generation) Brompheniramine (Dimetane) Chlorpheniramine (Chlor-Trimeton) Clemastine (Tavist) Dimenhydrinate (Dramamine) Diphenhydramine (Benadryl) Doxylamine (Unisom) Cyproheptadine (Periactin) Hydroxyzine HCl (Atarax) Meclizine (Antivert)	Allergic rhinitis; allergic conjunctivitis; urticarial reactions (hives); sleep induction; appetite stimulation; cough suppression; motion sickness; Meniere's disease; Parkinson's disease;	Dry mouth; urinary retention; weight gain; sedation; dizziness; tinnitus
Nonsedating (Second-Generation) Astemizole (Hismanal) Loratadine (Claritin) Terfenadine (Seldane)	Appetite stimulation; allergic rhinitis; asthma	Weight gain Cardiac dysrhythmia

Data from Peggs, J.F., Shimp, L.A., and Opdycke, R.A.C. (1995). Antihistamines: The old and the new. *American Family Physician* 52(2), 593–600.

expectorants in treatment of the common cold.[8] A number of studies have demonstrated that the administration of zinc (usually in lozenge form) reduces the time to resolution of cold symptoms, but side effects, such as nausea, were frequent[9] (see Focus of Current Research).

Inhalation of cool mist is commonly used in treatment of URI in infants and young children, but its benefit remains unproved.[10] Older children and adults may obtain substantial relief of throat edema and pain with salt-water gargles.

Treatment of recurrent tonsillitis is a matter of some controversy. Surgical removal (tonsillectomy and adenoidectomy) was common 25 years ago, but in recent decades, this procedure has been done far less frequently. Because the tonsils and adenoids normally begin to shrink on their own after the age of 10 years, exposure of a young child to the trauma of surgery may be unnecessary. Some children and young adults suffer repeated infections, however, and excessive morbidity, development of abscesses, or chronic association of tonsillitis with otitis media may justify surgery in these cases.

Development of acute upper airway obstruction in severe laryngotracheobronchitis or epiglottitis requires immediate recognition and intervention. If complete obstruction is imminent, an artificial airway is inserted and maintained until edema and spasm subside. If possible, an endotracheal tube is inserted through the nose or mouth, but if these tissues do not permit passage of the airway, a surgical opening into the trachea *(tracheostomy)* is done. If respiratory failure develops, it is managed with oxygen, bronchodilators, steroids, and possibly mechanical ventilation.

Antibiotics should be administered only in the presence of bacterial infection, as determined ideally by appropriate culture of inflamed surfaces or exudate. As discussed in Chapter 13, antibiotics are not helpful in treatment of viral infection, and their use may permit development of drug-resistant bacterial strains.

Prognosis and Outcome. Most manifestations of URI subside within 10 days to 2 weeks, with or without treatment. URI may pose significant risk to those with compromised cardiac, respiratory, or immune systems, however, and URIs in infants and young children pose greater risk, owing to smaller airways and limited immunity. Severe laryngotracheobronchitis and epiglottitis may be life-threatening, but recovery is usual with immediate diagnosis and appropriate airway management. Fortunately, routine pediatric immunizations have greatly reduced the incidence of these medical emergencies.[11] Pharyngitis due to group A β-hemolytic streptococcus (strep throat) may be followed by autoimmune disorders, such as glomerulonephritis and rheumatic fever, in susceptible patients (see Chapter 13).

Chronic Bronchitis

Definition. Chronic bronchitis is inflammation of bronchi with increased mucus production and chronic productive cough. It is differentiated from acute bronchitis by its persistence for at least 3 months of the year for 2 successive years, provided that other causes of chronic production of pulmonary secretions *(sputum)*, such as tuberculosis and bronchiectasis, are excluded.[12]

Epidemiology. Chronic bronchitis is the most common form of COPD, affecting up to 25% of adults in the United States.[13] Exposure to the numerous inhaled irritants present in cigarette smoke and air pollution substantially increases the risk of chronic bronchitis. Ninety per cent of patients with chronic bronchitis are current or former smokers. Clinically significant disease develops in only 15% of smokers, however, suggesting that other factors also contribute to risk.[14] COPD is more prevalent in urban versus rural environments and is clearly related to occupational factors (e.g., mineral and organic dusts) as well.[15]

Etiology. Repeated exposure of airways to irritants triggers an inflammatory response and chronically stimulates irritant receptors in airway walls, provoking sputum production and cough. Cigarette smoking is associated with impaired pulmonary defenses, with notable reduction in ciliary function, phagocytosis, and immunoglobulin A secretion. Bacterial colonization and susceptibility to infection are therefore increased.

Pathophysiology. Chronic inflammation results in mucous gland hyperplasia in the upper- and mid-level bronchi, manifesting as airway edema and increased mucus production. Irritant receptors trigger airway hyper-reactivity, with bronchoconstriction and chronic cough. Airway resistance is increased during both inspiration and expiration. Hypoxemia and hypercapnia occur secondary to hypoventilation because, for unknown reasons, the patient usually is unable to increase work of breathing enough to overcome the obstruction. The diameter of pulmonary blood vessels, quantified as pulmonary vascular resistance (PVR), is increased, owing to the presence of inflammation and to a compensatory vasoconstriction that occurs in areas of hypoventilation. This response, known as *hypoxic pulmonary vasoconstriction,* is designed to optimize $\dot{V}/\dot{Q}$ relationships and is discussed further in Chapter 19. Increased PVR constitutes increased afterload of the right ventricle (see Chapter 16). With repeated epi-

Focus of Current Research

Study	Objective and Findings
Adkinson, et al. (1997) A controlled trial of immunotherapy for asthma in allergic children.	*Objective:* to examine the effectiveness of immunotherapy in treatment of children with asthma *Findings:* Immunotherapy with injections for more than 2 years was of no apparent benefit in children who were receiving appropriate medical treatment.
Kudukis, et al. (1997) Inhaled helium-oxygen revisited: Effect of inhaled helium-oxygen during the treatment of status asthmaticus in children.	*Objective:* To assess the effects of breathing a low-density gas mixture on dyspnea and pulsus paradoxus in children with status asthmaticus *Findings:* The helium and oxygen mixture reduces the work of breathing and may forestall respiratory failure, preventing the need for mechanical ventilation.
Scherer & Schmieder (1997) The effect of a pulmonary rehabilitation program on self-efficacy, perception of dyspnea, and physical endurance.	*Objective:* To determine the effect of an outpatient pulmonary rehabilitation program in patients with chronic obstructive pulmonary disease *Findings:* The program improved self-efficacy and confidence, decreased perception of dyspnea, and increased exercise endurance.
Clemens, et al. (1997) Is an antihistamine-decongestant combination effective in temporarily relieving symptoms of the common cold in preschool children?	*Objective:* To determine whether an antihistamine and decongestant combination is superior to placebo in symptom relief for upper respiratory infection in preschool-aged children *Findings:* The medication regimen was equivalent to placebo and had significantly greater sedative side effects.
Mossad, et al. (1996) Zinc gluconate lozenges for treating the common cold.	*Objective:* To test the efficacy of zinc in reducing the duration of common cold symptoms *Findings:* The time to complete resolution of symptoms was significantly shorter in the zinc group (median 4.4 days versus 7.6 days). More patients in the zinc group had nausea and altered taste sensation.
Sciurba, et al. (1996) Improvement in pulmonary function and elastic recoil after lung reduction surgery for diffuse emphysema.	*Objective:* To assess the clinical benefit of lung reduction surgery in patients with severe emphysema *Findings:* Surgery increased the elastic recoil of the lungs in these patients, leading to short-term improvement in dyspnea and exercise tolerance.

Drazen, et al. (1996) Comparison of regularly scheduled with as-needed use of albuterol in mild asthma.	*Objective:* To compare the effects of regularly scheduled with as-needed use of albuterol in patients with mild, chronic, stable asthma *Findings:* Neither deleterious nor beneficial effects were derived from regularly scheduled use. Inhaled albuterol should be prescribed for patients with mild asthma on an as-needed basis.
Gold, et al. (1996) Effects of cigarette smoking on lung function in adolescent boys and girls.	*Objective:* To study the effects of smoking on the level and rate of growth of pulmonary function in boys and girls 10 to 18 years of age *Findings:* Cigarette smoking is associated with mild airway obstruction and slowed growth of lung function. Girls may be more vulnerable than boys to the effects of smoking.

sodes of inflammation, airway scarring and the permanent structural changes of emphysema develop. Respiratory infections may precipitate acute exacerbations, leading to respiratory failure. The pathogens most frequently implicated are *Haemophilus influenzae, Streptococcus pneumoniae, Moraxella (Branhamella) catarrhalis,* and *Chlamydia pneumoniae.*[12]

Clinical Manifestations. Pulmonary function testing reveals decreased air flow rates, most commonly evidenced as a decrease in FEV_1 (volume exhaled in one second of forced exhalation). Blood gas analysis shows respiratory acidosis with decreased PaO_2 and increased $PaCO_2$, possibly at levels consistent with respiratory failure (see Chapter 10). The patient may be dyspneic but usually does not appear to be working hard to breathe. Gurgling sounds *(rhonchi)* may be heard with a stethoscope over the larger airways, owing to the movement of exudate. Clinical signs of chronic hypoxemia are present, including cyanosis, clubbing, and secondary polycythemia. Right-sided heart failure, known as *cor pulmonale* when due to pulmonary disease, may result from high PVR, leading to increased venous congestion with associated jugular venous distention, hepatomegaly, and dependent edema (see Chapter 16).

Prevention and Treatment. Chronic bronchitis is largely preventable through individual abstention from tobacco abuse and community and legislative efforts to ensure clean environmental air. Immunization against influenza viruses and *Streptococcus pneumoniae* may reduce the risk of respiratory infections, preventing acute exacerbations. Bacterial infections are appropriately treated with antibiotics. Bronchodilators are usually administered by inhalation, which allows maximal bronchodilation while minimizing systemic effects. Ipratropium bromide (Atrovent), an anticholinergic agent, is the first-line agent most often used, although β-agonists such as albuterol (Proventil or Ventolin) are still frequently prescribed. The β-agonists have more significant side effects, however. Theophylline (aminophylline), once first-line therapy in COPD, has fallen from favor due to its narrow therapeutic index and significant cardiac side effects, which include cardiac dysrhythmias and seizures.[16] The use of steroid therapy is controversial, given the apparently small improvement when compared with placebo and the associated untoward effects.[17] Mucolytic agents, such as iodinated glycerol (Organidin), are beneficial to some in reducing the viscosity of sputum, easing its clearance with coughing or chest physiotherapy.[18] Cardiac failure is treated medically (see Chapter 16). Pulmonary rehabilitation programs incorporating supervised exercise training as well as education and psychosocial support have shown modest benefits with respect to exercise capacity and significant benefits with respect to perceived self-efficacy.[19] Respiratory failure may require treatment with oxygen or mechanical ventilation.

Prognosis and Outcome. The combination of chronic bronchitis and emphysema is the most common form of COPD, and outcome statistics usually reflect both disorders. COPD is the fifth leading cause of death in the United States, with 50% of patients surviving 5 years and 25% surviving 10 years after diagnosis.[18] The typical course is that of recurrent pneumonia and respiratory failure, with eventual inability to wean from mechanical ventilation.

Emphysema

Definition. Emphysema is defined anatomically as abnormal, permanent enlargement of alveoli and alveolar ducts, with destruction of alveolar walls and breakdown of connective tissue support of lower airways.

Epidemiology. Because emphysema most frequently occurs as a late manifestation of the repeated inflammatory episodes of chronic bronchitis, its epidemiology is similar. Up to 2.5 million Americans suffer from emphysema.[20] Cigarette smoking and air pollution are major risk factors for emphysema. In addition, an inherited (autosomal recessive) deficiency of the enzyme *α_1-antitrypsin (AAT)* may predispose some patients to earlier onset and more severe emphysema. An estimated 2% of cases of emphysema are caused by this disorder.[17] Aging constitutes an independent risk factor for emphysema, but this *senile emphysema* resulting from degenerative changes (stretching without destruction) in airway smooth muscle and connective tissue is not usually sufficient to impair pulmonary function to a significant degree.

Etiology. Most cases of emphysema are caused by the downward progression of inflammatory damage with repeated episodes of chronic bronchitis. In elderly people, the degenerative changes of senile emphysema may be superimposed on the inflammatory damage. In patients with AAT deficiency, destruction of airway tissue occurs due to unopposed activity of proteolytic enzymes such as trypsin. These enzymes are normally active in continuous tissue remodeling during growth and repair processes but are kept in check by the presence of antitrypsin. AAT deficiency allows trypsin and other proteolytic enzymes to destroy functional lung tissue.

Pathophysiology. Inflammation or proteolytic enzymes destroy lung tissue in one of two patterns (Fig. 18–18). *Centrilobular emphysema* mainly affects the respiratory bronchioles and is the type seen in association with chronic bronchitis. *Panlobular emphysema* affects the entire respiratory unit and is more closely associated with AAT deficiency and senile changes.

Destruction of alveolar walls results in loss of surface area for gas exchange and a decrease in surfactant production. Decreased surfactant produces areas of **atelectasis,** or alveolar collapse, further reducing the exchange area and decreasing lung tissue compliance. Loss of connective tissue tethering results in early airway collapse during forced exhalation. Air is trapped in the alveoli, leading to increased functional residual capacity. Under these conditions, length–tension relationships within respiratory muscles are less than optimal, promoting respiratory muscle inefficiency and fatigue.

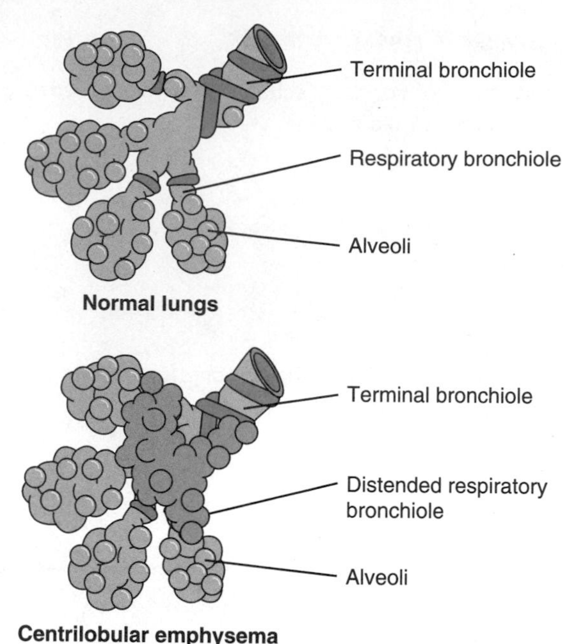

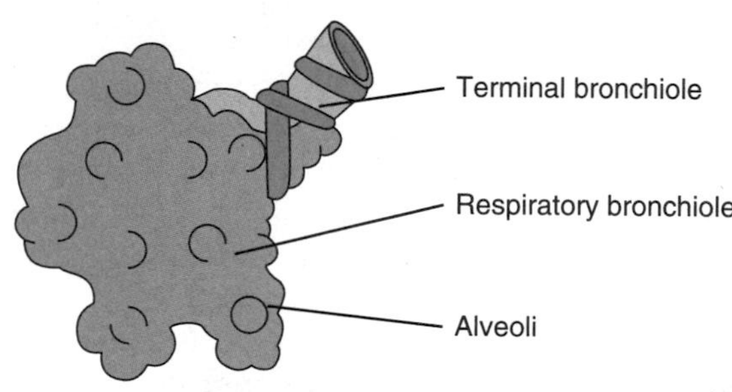

FIGURE 18–18

Patterns of emphysema. Centrilobular emphysema, which usually follows chronic bronchitis, is characterized by primary involvement of the respiratory bronchioles, sparing the alveoli. Panlobular emphysema, which is associated with α_1-antitrypsin deficiency and senile emphysema, affects the entire respiratory unit.

Proteolytic destruction of alveolar walls results in formation of large air spaces known as *bullae,* also referred to as *blebs* if they form on the outer surface of the lungs. Blebs are likely to rupture if air pressure inside them is increased (e.g., with mechanical ventilation), leading to loss of negativity in the intrapleural space and possible pneumothorax.

Clinical Manifestations. Like chronic bronchitis, emphysema results in decreased FEV_1. Altered flow rates in emphysema occur *only* during exhalation, however. Chronic air trapping results in rounding of the thorax (barrel chest) and increased functional residual capacity. Unlike in patients with chronic bronchitis, air flow on inspiration is not significantly impaired, and the patient usually works hard to ventilate. Dyspnea and use of accessory muscles are apparent, especially on expiration as the patient tries to overcome airway collapse. The patient often sits up to breathe *(orthopnea)*, so that diaphragmatic movement is unimpaired by the upward pressure of the abdominal viscera. Exhalation through pursed lips is a compensatory mechanism that may be instinctive or learned. Pursed-lip exhalation sustains transmural pressure during exhalation, postponing airway collapse. Nevertheless, exhalation is impaired, resulting in some degree of hypercapnia and respiratory acidosis. Hypoxemia occurs late in emphysema, after the patient becomes exhausted from increased work of breathing.

Prevention and Treatment. Emphysema is rare in those who abstain from cigarette smoking. AAT deficiency may now be treated with enzyme replacement, and those with known family history should be appropriately screened. Advanced emphysema is treated symptomatically and supportively, with oxygen therapy if hypoxemia is present. Pulmonary rehabilitation, based on exercise programs, may be of some benefit in increasing activity tolerance and self-esteem. Acute respiratory failure may occur with respiratory infections and is treated with drugs, chest physiotherapy, and oxygen therapy, as previously discussed. Mechanical ventilation is employed reluctantly in patients with advanced emphysema because of the risk of pneumothorax and diaphragmatic deconditioning.

The most recent advances in the treatment of emphysema are surgical. *Lung volume reduction*, which involves surgical resection of the most bullous lung segments, has been shown to restore some of the tethering forces on distal airways, thus decreasing air trapping and improving expiratory air flow.[21] In some cases, compression of pulmonary vessels is also lessened by this procedure, reducing PVR and right ventricular afterload.[22] Single and bilateral lung transplantations have been performed in selected cases of AAT deficiency and emphysema, resulting in improved quality of life and medium-term survival.[23]

Prognosis and Outcome. Tissue damage in emphysema is irreversible. It progresses most rapidly in patients who continue to smoke cigarettes. Supplemental oxygen therapy has been shown to improve quality of life and survival, especially when administered continuously[17] (see Table 18–6). Most patients with COPD have at least one acute exacerbation a year.[14] Mortality due to COPD is high, as discussed previously with chronic bronchitis. Patients admitted to intensive care units for acute exacerbations have a 24% hospital mortality rate.[24]

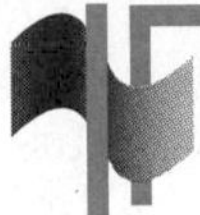

Clinical Scenario

J.B., a 61-year-old female, is admitted to the general medical unit after being brought to the emergency department by her daughter. J.B. has a history of emphysema and multiple sclerosis and now presents with cough, chills, weakness, and shortness of breath. She is a cigarette smoker, having smoked 1 to 2 packs per day for 40 years, and demonstrates a thin physique with a barrel chest. On examination, J.B.'s breath sounds are barely audible with a stethoscope. Prolonged expiration through pursed lips is noted. As measured while receiving oxygen at 2 L/minute by nasal cannula, her arterial blood gases are as follows: Pa_{O_2}, 60 mm Hg; Pa_{CO_2}, 56 mm Hg; and pH, 7.46.

1. What are the immediate priorities for intervention in J.B.'s case?
2. What probably caused this acute exacerbation of her condition?
3. What is the objective evidence of respiratory failure in this case?

Asthma

Definition. Asthma is an inflammatory airway disease characterized by increased airway responsiveness to a variety of stimuli, resulting in airway obstruction that is at least partially reversible.[25]

Epidemiology. Asthma affects an estimated 10 million people in the United States.[26] Childhood asthma occurs twice as often in males as females and is more often associated with an allergic response to extrinsic stimuli such as pollens from weeds or trees, dust, molds, food additives, animal dander, or drugs. Adult-onset asthma is equally prevalent in both sexes and is more often nonallergic, associated with intrinsic stimuli such as the cellular mediators released during stress, exercise, exposure to cold air, URI, and chronic bronchitis. A significant number of adults apparently acquire an allergic form of asthma, or exacerbate their existing asthma, from exposure to agents in the workplace. Allergens or irritants in flour, acid anhydrides, toluene di-isocyanates, and screwflies or river flies are among the agents associated with occupational asthma.[27]

Etiology. There are probably multiple mechanisms that induce airway spasm and increased mucus production in asthma. Many patients display a mixed etiology, responding to both intrinsic and extrinsic agents. The best-understood mechanism is immediate hypersensitivity, or true allergy, which occurs with inhaled extrinsic agents (see Chapter 13). Immunoglobulin E–mediated release of histamine and other local mediators from mast cells results in bronchospasm and inflammation. Other agents may induce mast cell degranulation by a nonimmunologic mechanism. Exercise-induced asthma is believed to be triggered by temperature changes in the airways during rapid breathing, although the cellular mechanism linking temperature and airway size is unknown.[28]

People with asthma have denser capillary beds and increased permeability of capillaries surrounding airways, but the significance of this is unknown. A genetic susceptibility to bronchial hyper-responsiveness may be coinherited, along with elevated levels of serum immunoglobulin E.[29] In many patients with asthma, neither the trigger nor the mechanism precipitating acute attacks is known.

Pathophysiology. Until recently, it was believed that airway hyper-responsiveness leading to bronchospasm was the underlying mechanism of asthma. It is now known, however, that airway inflammation with the release of cellular mediators precedes, and probably causes, the airway hyper-responsiveness. Mast cell mediators are dominant in allergic asthma. In nonallergic asthma, proteins, such as major basic protein, released from eosinophil granules may disrupt the integrity of airway epithelium. Inflammatory mediators released by lymphocytes, macrophages, and epithelial cells are also postulated to contribute to airway edema and spasm; these include adhesion molecules, interleukin-4, interleukin-5, granulocyte-macrophage colony-stimulating factor, leukotrienes, and platelet-activating factor.[17] These mediators induce the early, acute phase of an asthma attack, which peaks within 15 to 30 minutes and is primarily bronchospastic in nature, followed by a late phase peaking within 2 to 6 hours, which is primarily due to airway edema and increased mucus production.[30]

The role of neural stimuli in triggering asthmatic episodes is still uncertain. Abnormalities in autonomic reflex control of airway diameter remain unproved. A role for locally released neuromodulators, referred to as *tachykinins,* in the production of bronchospasm and increased mucus secretion is being investigated.[17]

Unlike other forms of COPD, asthma is characterized by intermittent, usually reversible, attacks during which airway resistance is markedly increased, increasing the work of breathing. Obstruction to air flow is usually greater during expiration, resulting in air trapping and alveolar hyperinflation. Worsening of symptoms at night is common and has been attributed to circadian variation in serum levels of cortisol and epinephrine and to nocturnal increases in cholinergic tone, vagal tone, histamine levels, and airway inflammation.[31]

Clinical Manifestations. The clinical picture depends on the degree of airway obstruction. Typically, the patient demonstrates anxiety, **tachypnea** (rapid breathing), wheezing, and cough that is productive of thick, ropy mucus containing casts of small bronchi. Wheezing subsides as the condition worsens, when edema and mucus severely diminish air movement. Pulmonary function testing reveals a decreased **peak expiratory flow rate** and FEV_1 (demonstrating reduced air flow rate). Blood gases show a decreased $Pa{CO_2}$ and respiratory alkalosis early, owing to hyperventilation, but hypercapnia and hypoxemia develop eventually due to exhaustion. **Status asthmaticus** refers to a severe, sustained asthmatic attack that is not responsive to first-line treatment. If not terminated, this medical emergency results in respiratory failure and possibly cardiac failure, owing to the extreme hypermetabolic state.

Prevention and Treatment. Prevention of exposure to known triggers is warranted. Hyposensitization may be beneficial if the asthma has an allergic mechanism (see Chapter 13). Drug therapy depends on the frequency and severity of attacks. For infrequent, mild, or predictable attacks, inhaled bronchodilator therapy, usually with a β-agonist, such as albuterol, may be sufficient to ward off or terminate bronchospasm. In patients with more severe disease, a maintenance regimen with an inhaled glucocorticoid, such as beclomethasone (Vanceril), is the treatment of choice for reduction of airway inflammation and hyper-responsiveness. Patients with a significant allergic component may benefit from a mast cell stabilizing agent, such as cromolyn sodium (Opticrom) or nedocromil sodium (Tilade). Systemic glucocorticoids are often prescribed for severe acute attacks.[32] Respiratory failure in status asthmaticus may necessitate endotracheal intubation and mechanical ventilation if blood gases continue to deteriorate despite drug therapy and if decreasing level of consciousness and impending respiratory arrest are apparent.

Prognosis and Outcome. The prognosis in most cases of asthma is positive, with survival rates not significantly different from rates for those without the disease.[33] Many children outgrow the condition, although in those with more severe disease, asthma may persist into adulthood. Since 1978, however, the mortality rate from asthma has increased significantly in the United States, particularly among residents of large cities, blacks, Hispanics, and those living under disadvantaged socioeconomic conditions.[34] In 1987, there were 4360 deaths due to asthma, up 31% from the death rate in 1980.[14] The increasing morbidity and mortality due to asthma during a time when air-quality standards have improved is of concern. Although the reasons for this trend are uncertain, the possibility of adverse effects of treatment with β-agonists has been raised and is under investigation.[35]

Reactive Airways Dysfunction Syndrome

Definition. Reactive airways dysfunction syndrome (RADS) is the development of asthma-like symptoms and airway hyper-responsiveness in a person with no previous history of respiratory problems after a single exposure to an inhaled toxin.[36]

Epidemiology. It has been estimated that about 60,000 cases of inhalation of irritant chemicals occur each year in the United States.[36] Risk factors include occupational and other environmental exposure to these chemicals.

Etiology. RADS is caused by acute exposure to a high concentration of an irritant gas, smoke, fume, or vapor. These agents include ammonia, chlorine, acetic acid, isocyanates, and other toxins. In contrast to asthma, immune mechanisms apparently do not play a role in RADS.

Pathophysiology. An inflammatory response results in airway injury proportionate to the degree of exposure. Injury ranges from mild irritation to extensive lesions. Some degree of airway remodeling is present, with sloughing and metaplasia of respiratory squamous epithelium typically seen. Moderate to severe fibrosis of the bronchial walls may be present. Release of inflammatory mediators induces airway edema and spasm. In the most severe cases, injury of the alveolar–capillary membrane leads to adult respiratory distress syndrome (see Chapter 19).

Clinical Manifestations. Within 24 hours of the exposure, symptoms of dyspnea, cough, and wheezing are present. The clinical picture is similar to that of chronic bronchitis with superimposed asthma. Acute exacerbations (e.g., status asthmaticus) do not occur.

Prevention and Treatment. Acute exposures occur as occupational accidents or, less commonly, as a consequence of the use of toxic gases in wartime. Occupational safety standards and wartime conventions may reduce these risks. Oxygen therapy and steroids have been used in treatment of RADS, but their efficacy is unproved.[36]

Prognosis and Outcome. Although resolution of inflammation and regeneration of epithelial cells may occur within a few months, in many cases, airway obstruction and hyper-responsiveness persist for years.

Obstructive Sleep Apnea

Definition. Obstructive sleep apnea, also known as upper airway resistance syndrome, is a syndrome of repeated episodes of obstructive cessation or reduction of ventilation during sleep.[37]

Epidemiology. Obstructive sleep apnea affects an estimated 5% of adults.[38] Most patients are middle-aged men, although the disorder also affects women and may be seen in adults of any age. Risk factors include craniofacial anatomic features that may be familial, habitual snoring, obesity (especially visceral obesity), hypertension, large neck circumference, cigarette smoking, and alcohol use.

Etiology. The precise cause is unknown, but anatomic and neuromuscular factors related to airway size are believed to interact with sleep stage to cause episodes of absent or decreased ventilation. In obese people, the airway may be narrowed by adipose tissue. Tonsillar hypertrophy or skeletal abnormalities may predispose to airway narrowing in people of normal body weight. The recurrent vibration of snoring, along with the more negative inspiratory pressures required to bypass airway obstruction, may cause edematous lengthening and thickening of the soft palate, thus worsening the degree of obstruction in a positive feedback loop. Upper airway muscles are most relaxed during the rapid eye movement stage of sleep (see Chapter 21).

Pathophysiology. Repetitive episodes of upper airway closure cause hypoxia and hypercapnia, which apparently influence autonomic nervous system regulation of ventilation and cardiovascular function. Sympathetic nervous system tone is increased, and sleep is fragmented and insufficient.

Clinical Manifestations. The patient's spouse may describe the patient's habitual snoring as well as apneic episodes followed by choking or snorting. Many patients exhibit signs of sleep deprivation, such as daytime sleepiness, morning headache, confusion, or depression. Hypertension is present in more than half of patients with sleep apnea syndrome and may be related to increased sympathetic tone.[39] Dysrhythmias are also more frequent in these people.

Prevention and Treatment. Factors that increase the severity of upper airway obstruction should be avoided. These include sleep deprivation; use of alcohol, sedatives, or hypnotic agents; and increased weight.[37] Significant sleep apnea is usually treated with application of continuous positive airway pressure, applied during sleep through nasal prongs, a nasal mask, or a mask covering the mouth and nose. Dental appliances are also available to help maintain patency of the airway. In some cases, surgical modification of the upper airway structures may be beneficial.

Prognosis and Outcome. Treatment with continuous positive airway pressure has been shown to decrease blood pressure in hypertensive patients, to reduce the incidence of dysrhythmias, to improve the arterial blood gas profile, and to improve cognitive function.[38]

Cystic Fibrosis

Definition. Cystic fibrosis is an inherited abnormality of exocrine gland function that affects the secretory surfaces of the respiratory, gastrointestinal, and genitourinary systems as well as the sweat glands. Respiratory function is most severely impaired by the presence of thick, obstructive mucus in airways.

Epidemiology. About 1000 new cases of cystic fibrosis are diagnosed in the United States each year, and about 30,000 Americans currently have the disease. About 5% of white Americans are symptom-free carriers of the genetic mutation that underlies the disorder.[40] Cystic fibrosis is usually inherited as an autosomal recessive defect but also occurs de novo in a significant number of cases (see Chapter 7). People of European descent are at highest risk.

Etiology. Cystic fibrosis results from a genetic abnormality on an autosome, chromosome 7. In 70% of patients, the defect is a deletion of a three-base-pair sequence that normally codes for the amino acid phenylalanine, but more than 300 different mutations have been identified.[41] All defects result in faulty synthesis or function of a membrane protein, cystic fibrosis transmembrane regulator (CFTR), which serves as a chloride channel.

Pathophysiology. Decreased chloride secretion results in mild secondary increases in sodium and water reabsorption, increasing the viscosity of exocrine secretions. In the airways, this leads to decreased mucociliary clearance and increased bacterial infection, most often with *H. influenzae, Staphylococcus aureus*, or *Pseudomonas* sp. Inflammatory damage to the airway epithelium further impairs pulmonary defenses in a positive feedback loop. Release of pancreatic enzymes into the small intestine is impaired by obstruction of pancreatic ducts with thick ductal secretions, leading to impaired absorption of nutrients. Blockage of secretion from the pancreas, gallbladder, and liver may lead to inflammation of these organs. About 10% of infants with cystic fibrosis have *meconium ileus* at birth. This is a congenital bowel obstruction due to the glue-like consistency of the stool formed in utero. Genitourinary manifestations include sterility in males due to blockage of the vas deferens, and decreased fertility in females due to abnormally thick cervical mucus. Abnormal reabsorption of chloride from sweat ducts leads to increased concentrations of chloride, sodium, and potassium in sweat.

Clinical Manifestations. Meconium ileus may be the initial sign of cystic fibrosis in some newborns. In others, the disorder may be detected by a parent who notes the salty taste of the infant's skin. In most cases, however, the disease is suspected later in childhood, owing to frequent respiratory infections, gastrointestinal problems, and general failure to thrive.

Airway obstruction with thick mucus leads to air trapping distal to the mucus plugs, with atelectasis occurring as trapped gases are absorbed into the blood. Increased work of breathing may be evidenced by head bobbing, retractions, and audible grunting on expiration. Grunting is an adaptive response (similar to pursed-lip breathing in adults) that prolongs airway resistance and delays airway collapse due to external compression. Airway obstruction and atelectasis lead to hypoxemia and hypercapnia. Hypoxemia may lead to secondary polycythemia, cyanosis, and clubbing of the fingers and toes. PVR is elevated to compensate for underventilation, and signs of cor pulmonale may be present. Overdistention of bronchioles may lead to a syndrome of emphysematous-type tissue damage referred to as **bronchiectasis**, manifested by barrel chest and increased functional residual capacity. (Bronchiectasis is discussed further in the next section.) Respiratory infections are common, and debris from the inflammatory process exacerbates the airway obstruction.

Meconium ileus leads to abdominal distention and absence of stools in the neonatal period. Later gastrointestinal manifestations include poor weight gain and copious, foul-smelling stools. The child's sweat may be collected for analysis, and increased electrolyte concentrations are diagnostic for cystic fibrosis.

Prevention and Treatment. Genetic screening tests are available that are highly reliable in detection of carrier status. Couples heterozygous for the CFTR mutation have a one in four risk of having an affected child with each pregnancy.[42] Prenatal diagnosis is also possible with genetic analysis.

Cystic fibrosis is treated symptomatically and supportively, with chest physiotherapy, appropriate fluid and electrolyte intake, and inhalation of mucolytic agents. Drugs used in treatment of respiratory manifestations of cystic fibrosis include amiloride (Midamor), a sodium-channel blocker that may decrease the reabsorption of sodium from secretions, thus improving viscosity. Uridine triphosphate, which stimulates chloride secretion by a non-CFTR channel, is also being studied.[42] Recombinant human DNase (Pulmozyme) is a DNA-splitting enzyme that assists in liquefying dense pulmonary mucus by breaking up the DNA strands that are a major component of inflammatory debris. Recombinant AAT has been administered to counteract the excessive proteolytic activity induced by neutrophil products during airway inflammation. None of these therapies is curative, but it is hoped that the clinical trials now in progress will demonstrate their benefit in managing the disease.

Nutritional manifestations are reduced with the replacement of vitamins and pancreatic enzymes. Management of cardiac or respiratory failure may be indicated during acute exacerbations. Gene therapy, involving the induced expression of normal CFTR into affected epithelial cells, is also under investigation.[43] Limited numbers of patients with severe respiratory failure have undergone organ transplantation, with heart and lung transplantation or, more recently, bilateral single lung transplantation.[42]

Prognosis and Outcome. Survival has increased from about 3 years in the early 1960s to nearly 30 years currently.[44] The usual cause of death is respiratory failure associated with recurrent infections and extensive bronchiectasis.

Bronchiectasis

Definition. Bronchiectasis is permanent dilation and distortion of the bronchi and bronchioles due to breakdown of airway smooth muscle and connective tissue support.

Epidemiology. The precise incidence of bronchiectasis is unknown, although it is believed to be declining, owing to earlier and more effective treatment of chronic bronchitis, asthma, and cystic fibrosis, the primary disorders that most often lead to bronchiectasis, and to immunization for childhood infections. Rarely, bronchiectasis follows an acute infection of the lower respiratory tract, such as pneumonia or bronchiolitis (see Chapter 19). Rare congenital disorders that may manifest as bronchiectasis include primary ciliary dyskinesia, Young's syndrome, and Kartagener's syndrome.[45]

Etiology. The structural damage results from chronic inflammation or pressure damage (barotrauma) secondary to overdistention of airways distal to persistent obstruction. Bronchiectasis may be confined to a small area of lung tissue if obstruction is localized, as could occur with aspiration of a foreign body or with presence of an obstructive tumor.

Pathophysiology. If obstruction is the initial stimulus, infection soon follows because of impaired pulmonary defenses. If infection is the stimulus, obstruction follows due to airway edema, spasm, and mucus plugging. Chronic inflammation and air trapping lead to scarring and weakening of airway walls, which become dilated to four times their normal diameters and collapse more readily on expiration. Damage may extend to the respiratory units, resulting in concurrent emphysema.

Clinical Manifestations. The clinical picture is similar to that of combined chronic bronchitis and emphysema, with chronic productive cough and increased work of breathing evidenced by tachypnea and use of accessory muscles. Hemoptysis is often seen, and retraction and grunting are common in children. Hypoxemia and hypercapnia are present, and signs of chronic hypoxia (clubbing and secondary polycythemia) are common. URIs may precipitate respiratory failure in these patients. Rare complications include formation of infectious abscesses, which may metastasize to distal locations such as the brain.

Prevention and Treatment. Bronchiectasis may be prevented by risk reduction measures for chronic bronchitis and asthma and by appropriate immunization, as previously discussed. Aggressive chest physiotherapy may reduce the risk of chronic airway obstruction and infection in cystic fibrosis, and appropriate therapy is warranted for infections of the lower respiratory tract (see Chapter 19). Localized bronchiectasis may be treated surgically, with segmental or lobar resection. Aspirated foreign bodies may be removed with *bronchoscopy,* which involves insertion of a tube into airways for removal of obstructions as well as sampling of tissue or secretions for diagnostic purposes. Once permanent airway damage has occurred, treatment is symptomatic and supportive, as in emphysema.

Prognosis and Outcome. Prognosis depends on the degree of airway damage and the severity of any underlying chronic lung disease.

Laryngeal Cancer

Definition. Laryngeal cancer is defined as the presence of a malignant neoplasm on, immediately above, or immediately below the vocal cords.

Epidemiology. In 1990, 12,300 new cases of laryngeal cancer were diagnosed, most often in men between 50 and 70 years of age.[46] Known risk factors for laryngeal cancer are cigarette smoking, alcohol abuse, vocal straining (chronic laryngitis), and occupational exposure to irritants. Laryngeal cancer also demonstrates a familial predisposition.

Etiology. Most laryngeal cancers arise from squamous epithelium. The precise etiology of laryngeal cancer is unknown. As is true of most cancers, multiple factors are probably involved (see Chapter 7).

Pathophysiology. Tumors of the glottis, involving the true vocal cords, are most common, followed by tumors in locations above the glottis (supraglottic tumors). Subglottic tumors are rare. An enlarging mass in the larynx obstructs swallowing and breathing to some degree. Decreased mobility of the vocal cords occurs if they are involved by the tumor. Laryngeal cancer may metastasize by the lymphatic route.

Clinical Manifestations. A palpable mass is present. Persistent hoarseness is the cardinal symptom of laryngeal cancer involving the vocal cords. Respiratory manifestations include dyspnea and possible stridor. Dysphagia is often present, accompanied by pain in the throat that may be referred to the ear. Coughing and hemoptysis may be seen, and the hyoid, thyroid, and cricoid cartilages may become fixed. Systemic manifestations, such as anorexia or weight loss, indicate advanced disease. Fifteen per cent of patients develop a second tumor within the respiratory or digestive tracts simultaneously with the laryngeal tumor or within the next 5 years.[46]

Prevention and Treatment. Modifiable risk factors should be removed or minimized. Early detection may allow treatment with radiation alone, which preserves the voice. More advanced laryngeal cancers must be treated surgically. If the tumor is limited to the vocal cords, partial laryngectomy may be done. In this case, a portion of the vocal cords may be retained, leaving the patient with a hoarse voice. Total laryngectomy, which involves removal of the larynx, vocal cords, and epiglottis, is indicated for tumors that extend above or below the vocal cords. Extensive dissection of the neck may be required for removal of adjacent lymph nodes, and a permanent tracheostomy is done to re-establish the airway and possibly to facilitate tracheoesophageal speech (Fig. 18–19).

Traditionally, laryngectomy patients have attempted to learn esophageal speech, in which the upper esophageal walls are vibrated by swallowing and eructation (belching) of boluses of air. Many fail at this because of the limited quantities of air that can be generated from the esophagus. With tracheoesophageal speech, a surgical shunt is created between the trachea and the esophagus to increase the flow of air. The voice may also be restored through use of an electronic larynx, a battery-powered vibratory source that may be placed in the mouth or against the neck. Chemotherapy protocols for adjunctive or palliative treatment of laryngeal cancer are under investigation.

Prognosis and Outcome. In most cases, laryngeal cancer involving the vocal cords is detected early enough to be surgically cured. Surgical disfigurement and loss of the natural voice may adversely impact quality of life. Subglottic tumors are usually clinically silent until advanced and are associated with an unfavorable prognosis. Five-year survival rate among those with early vocal cord lesions is 90%. With more advanced (stage III or IV) lesions, the 2-year survival rate ranges from 40% to 80%.[46]

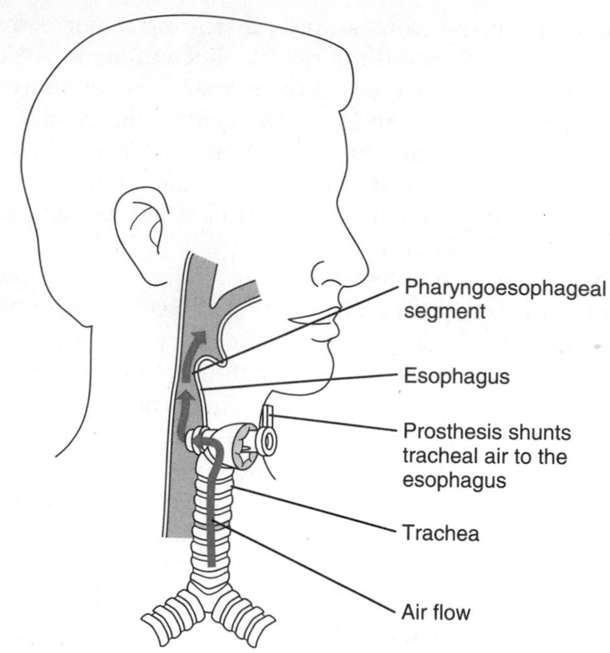

FIGURE 18–19
Tracheostomy with shunt for tracheoesophageal speech. After laryngectomy, a permanent tracheostomy establishes the airway. A prosthetic shunt device may permit vibration of esophageal walls, facilitating speech. (Redrawn from McKenna, J.P., Fornataro-Clerici, L.M., McManamin, P.C., *et al.* [1991]. Laryngeal cancer: Diagnosis, treatment, and speech rehabilitation. *American Family Physician* 44[1], 127. Published by the American Academy of Family Physicians.)

Lung Cancer (Bronchogenic Carcinoma)

Definition. Lung cancer is most precisely defined as a malignant neoplasm arising in lung tissue. The lung, however, is a frequent site of metastasis of tumors arising elsewhere in the body, with breast cancer being particularly prone to lung metastasis.

Epidemiology. Lung cancer is now the leading cause of cancer death in both men and women, with 160,000 new cases diagnosed each year.[47] Cigarette smoking accounts for 80% to 90% of lung cancers.[48] Passive exposure to environmental tobacco smoke, which includes the sidestream smoke emitted from burning tobacco products as well as exhaled tobacco smoke, also conveys increased risk and has been estimated to cause between 500 and 5000 cancer deaths per year. Occupational or residential exposure to inhaled carcinogens in asbestos, radon, radioactive dusts, arsenic, and plastics also increases the risk of lung cancer. Presence of chronic lung diseases, such as COPD, increases risk, probably owing to impaired mucociliary clearance of carcinogens and chronic inflammation. Aging also increases risk, and a familial predisposition is evident.

Etiology. As with most cancers, the precise etiology of lung cancer is unknown (see Chapter 7). The major carcinogen in cigarette smoke is benzopyrene. The incidence of lung cancer is directly correlated with the amount and duration of smoking in a dose–response relationship.

Pathophysiology. Ninety-five per cent of cases of lung cancer are bronchogenic carcinoma, arising from the bronchial epithelium, with a mixture of other types (e.g., adenoma, sarcoma, and melanoma) constituting the remaining 5%.[49] Classification of tumors is usually based on response to available treatments. *Non-small cell carcinoma* includes the epidermoid (squamous cell), large cell, and adenocarcinoma types, and *small cell carcinoma* includes oat cell and intermediate cell types. Squamous cell carcinoma usually manifests as a large, central mass, often involving local lymph nodes and the thoracic duct (Fig. 18–20). Cancer cells gradually invade the epithelium, connective tissue, pleurae, and chest wall. Significant tumor growth and lymphatic spread have usually occurred before the disease is diagnosed, with frequent involvement of the heart and other mediastinal structures. Hyperparathyroidism occurring as a paraneoplastic syndrome may induce hypercalcemia. Adenocarcinoma usually arises as a solitary peripheral lesion. Small cell carcinoma is considered a systemic disease at the time of clinical presentation, with early metastasis and significant paraneoplastic phenomena.[50]

Local tumor growth of central tumors may be invasive, eroding blood vessels and compressing adjacent structures, such as the heart, major vessels, esophagus, and trachea. Neurologic involvement may induce paralysis or pain. Peripheral tumors may involve the pleurae or chest wall. Metastasis may occur by the lymphatics or the bloodstream to the CNS, bone, bone marrow, liver, or adrenal glands.

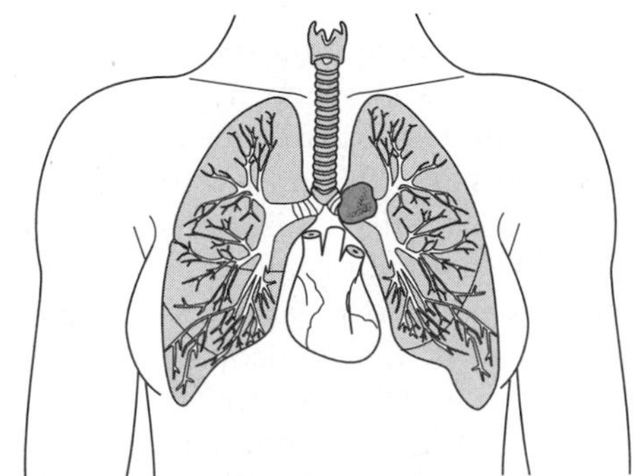

FIGURE 18–20
Bronchogenic carcinoma. Squamous cell cancer of the lung often involves central structures within the mediastinum, making surgical resection of the tumor difficult or impossible.

Clinical Manifestations. Cough is present early, owing to stimulation of irritant receptors, but it does not differ significantly from the "cigarette cough" that is persistently present in chronic smokers. Wheezing occurs later as airway obstruction increases. URIs are common because of impaired airway defenses, and blood-tinged sputum may be produced. Venous return to the right side of the heart may be impaired *(superior vena cava syndrome)*, resulting in headache, flushing, or upper extremity edema. Pleural involvement may result in third spacing (pleural effusion), which restricts ventilation. Shoulder and scapular pain may be due to Pancoast's syndrome, in which the brachial nerve plexus is compressed. This syndrome may also manifest as ulnar nerve tract pain or, with cervical nerve involvement, Horner's syndrome (eyelid droop, pupil constriction, and absence of sweating on one side of the face).[50] Pain also occurs with advanced lung cancer as the disease metastasizes to bone. Respiratory failure is usually a terminal event.

Prevention and Treatment. Cigarette smoking and occupational exposure to carcinogens are removable risk factors. Studies of the efficacy of dietary supplementation of antioxidant vitamins such as α-tocopherol and β-carotene in risk reduction have produced conflicting results (see Focus of Current Research). In a major Finnish study, β-carotene supplementation markedly *increased* the incidence of lung cancer among heavy smokers.[51]

In non-small cell cancer, the best chance for a cure is surgical treatment with removal of a lung (pneumonectomy) or lobe (lobectomy).[52] Lymph nodes may also be resected at the time of surgery. In some cases, bronchial structures may be salvaged with a more conservative approach, such as resection of the affected bronchial segment with reanastomosis of the airway ends (sleeve resection). Presence of distant metastasis at the time of cancer staging rules out surgical treatment. Patients with local lymph node involvement may be treated with a combination of surgical resection, chemotherapy, and radiation.

Surgical treatment is not an option in small cell lung cancer, which is treated with palliative chemotherapy and possibly radiation to reduce tumor mass and relieve airway obstruction. Newer therapies under investigation include immunotherapy,[53] photodynamic therapy and laser therapy through a bronchoscope for superficial squamous lesions, and endobronchial stents to maintain airway patency.[54]

Prognosis and Outcome. Unresectable lung cancer has a poor prognosis (5-year survival of less than 10%). In 20% to 25% of cases, lung cancer is unresectable at the time of diagnosis. Resection of stage I (localized) cancer with no nodal involvement yields a 5-year survival rate of 64% to 69%.[54] Small cell cancer of limited extent has a 50% initial remission rate, but few patients with advanced disease survive 5 years.[47]

Chest Trauma

Definition. Chest trauma is physical injury of the thorax by either a blunt or sharp force.

Epidemiology. Chest trauma is commonly associated with external forces, such as occur with motor vehicle accidents, sports injuries, gunshot wounds, or stab wounds, but it can also be caused by high airway pressures induced by violent coughing or mechanical ventilation. Weakening of the bony thorax by osteoporosis or metastatic cancer also increases the risk of chest trauma.

Etiology. Traumatic forces may result in loss of rigidity of the thorax or loss of negativity within the intrapleural space. Direct trauma to the mediastinal structures may also occur, with possible bruising or rupture of the heart, great vessels, esophagus, and large airways. Most cases of chest trauma impair only ventilation, however, as a result of rib fractures or pneumothorax.

Pathophysiology. Rib fractures usually affect the 4th through 12th ribs, resulting in hypoventilation due to severe pain. The first three ribs are protected by the clavicles and may be fractured only by significant force, placing the patient at risk for injuries to the trachea, main-stem bronchi, esophagus, aorta, and heart as well. In some cases, a section of ribs may be entirely detached from the sternum and thoracic spine, creating a free-floating segment and **flail chest** (Fig. 18–21). A displaced rib fragment or a penetrating object may puncture the chest wall, providing access of atmospheric air to the pleural space *(open pneumothorax)* and causing lung collapse due to unopposed elastic recoil forces. In the presence or absence of chest wall trauma, air may access the pleural space from *within* the airways *(closed pneumothorax).* This may occur with rib injuries or with rupture of alveoli on the lung surface due to high pressure generated when the person holds his or her breath in anticipation of impact. Blebs, enlarged alveoli on the lung surface, are most often associated with emphysema, as discussed previously. Spontaneous pneumothorax may occur due to rupture of a superficial bleb near the lung apex, usually in tall, slender young men. In this case, the blebs are believed to result from increased gravitational stress.[55] Closed pneumothorax may also occur in neonates who have experienced aspiration during delivery, creating a ball–valve effect on expiration, which traps air and increases airway pressure, rupturing alveoli.[56]

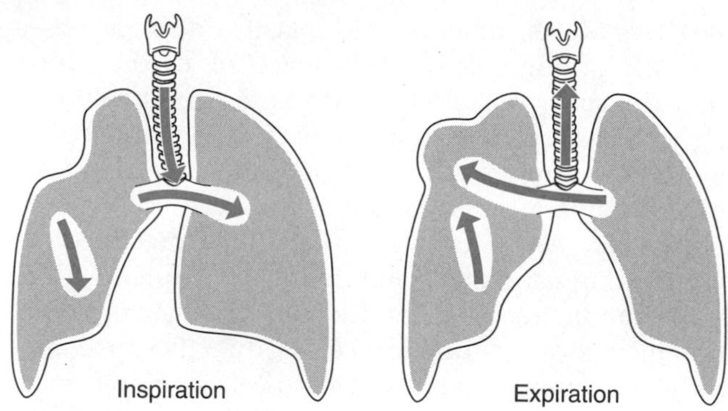

FIGURE 18–21

Flail chest. In some cases of chest trauma, rib fractures may result in a free-floating (flail) segment of the chest wall. Changes in intrathoracic pressure result in retraction of the flail segment with inspiration and bulging of the segment with expiration. This paradoxical ventilation is inefficient and results in increased work of breathing.

With chest trauma, blood vessels may be severed by rib fragments or pulled away from their points of attachment by great force, leading to hemorrhage within the airways, mediastinal space, pericardial space, or pleural space. *Pulmonary contusions,* bruises of lung tissue, often underlie rib fractures and may occur in children in the absence of fractures, owing to the flexibility of their ribcages. The inflammatory response to severe contusions resembles the pathologic response in adult respiratory distress syndrome, with critical impairment of blood gas diffusion (see Chapter 19).

Clinical Manifestations. Rib fractures are extremely painful with movement, resulting in the patient's voluntary hypoventilation to minimize pain. Hypoventilation may lead to hypoxemia and hypercapnia. Flail chest results in significant dyspnea and increased work of breathing because the isolated section of ribs moves *in* when negative intrathoracic pressure is generated during inspiration, and *out* with positive pressure during expiration. In the absence of thoracic rigidity, this *paradoxical ventilation* quickly leads to ventilatory failure.

An open chest wound creates a sucking sound as air is pulled in from the environment with inspiratory efforts. Lung collapse due to air (pneumothorax) or blood and air (hemopneumothorax) in the pleural space results in asymmetric ventilation and a shift in the position of the trachea, esophagus, and heart *(mediastinal shift).* **Tension pneumothorax** may develop if the chest wound has created a one-way

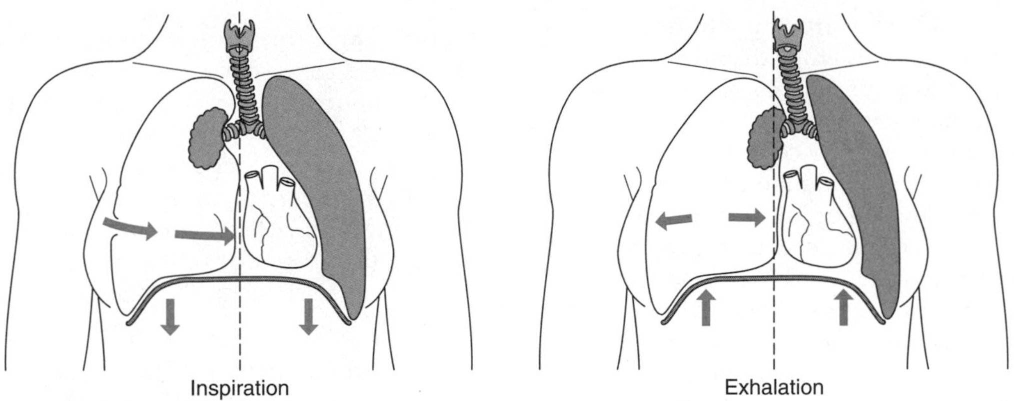

FIGURE 18–22
Tension pneumothorax. A one-way valve created by chest trauma may permit air to enter the pleural space during inspiration but prevent its exit during expiration. Pleural pressure rises with each ventilation, collapsing the lung on the affected side and imposing pressure on mediastinal structures.

valve effect (Fig. 18–22), allowing atmospheric air to enter the pleural space during inspiration, but preventing its escape during expiration. Pleural pressure thus rises with each respiratory effort, not only collapsing the lung on the affected side but also decreasing venous return to the heart. Open pneumothorax may result in rhythmic shifting of mediastinal structures from side to side as air moves in and out *(mediastinal flutter)*, potentially inducing cardiogenic shock and cardiac arrest.

Prevention and Treatment. Appropriate use of protective gear during contact sports has been shown to reduce the incidence of chest injuries. Seat belt use prevents chest injury due to impact with the steering wheel, although the shoulder strap may contribute to blunt cardiac trauma. A seat belt worn high on the abdomen may produce diaphragmatic rupture.[57]

Tears of great vessels or diaphragmatic ruptures are surgically repaired on an emergent basis. The primary goal in treatment of nondisplaced rib fractures is to manage pain, allowing the patient to ventilate normally. Analgesic drugs, such as meperidine (Demerol), that do not cause hypoventilation may be used, and in some cases nerve blocks (local injection of pain-transmitting nerves with anesthetic) may be employed. Flail chest is treated with positive-pressure mechanical ventilation if respiratory failure is present, and the flail segment may be surgically wired in place to restore thoracic rigidity.

A collapsed lung may be re-expanded with insertion of a noncollapsable chest tube into the pleural space. The tube is connected to an underwater seal or other one-way valve apparatus. The patient's inspiratory efforts gradually re-expand the lung and push pleural air into the tube. The one-way valve prevents atmospheric air from reentering during inspiration. The chest tube also allows drainage of any blood or inflammatory exudate from the pleural space. In patients with recurrent spontaneous pneumothorax or pleural effusion, a sclerosing agent may be administered into the chest tube, creating adhesions between the parietal and visceral pleurae. This *chest tube pleurodesis* seals the pleura, preventing the accumulation of excess fluid between the pleural layers.[58]

Prognosis and Outcome. Aortic rupture has an 80% to 90% mortality rate before the victim reaches the hospital.[57] In the absence of complicating injuries to the heart or great vessels, most chest trauma is effectively managed in clinical settings, resulting in no permanent impairment of ventilation.

CLINICAL SIGNIFICANCE OF VENTILATORY DISORDERS

Disorders of ventilation range in severity from the relatively benign but common URI to the most deadly form of neoplasia, lung cancer. Respiratory diseases significantly affect people of all ages (see Developmental Perspective), with the small, flexible airways of infants and young children being particularly vulnerable to obstruction with inflammatory conditions. The life-threatening ventilatory disorders affecting middle-aged and older adults are, to a great degree, *preventable*. Health care professionals have a primary responsibility for provision of public education and promotion of legislation aimed at cessation of cigarette smoking and maintenance of air-quality standards. Ventilatory function is potentially impaired in disorders of many systems, especially cardiac diseases, fluid imbalances, and acid-base abnormalities. Patients who are immobilized for any reason are at risk for ventilatory disorders.

Research efforts are ongoing to clarify the neural and cellular mechanisms involved in normal function of respiratory pacemaker cells as well as altered function in COPD. The epidemiologic link between cigarette smoking and lung disease is well established, but research continues with regard to identification of cocarcinogens and possible protective agents. Consistently effective methods for assisting nicotine-dependent people to quit smoking have not yet been found. Much research continues to focus on both behavioral and physiologic methods (e.g., nicotine patches and gums).

Identification and mapping of the cystic fibrosis gene has led to research aimed at development of gene replacement therapy that could eventually offer a cure for the disease. AAT, produced by recombinant DNA technology, is available for use in deficient patients who are at higher risk for emphysema, and the effectiveness of AAT screening and replacement therapy is under study. Drug therapy is minimally effective in treatment of chronic lung diseases and lung cancer, and clinical trials of new agents are in progress in an effort to develop curative and better palliative therapies. Bioengineering studies are aimed at developing methods of providing oxygenation and ventilatory support, with less risk of toxicity and adverse cardiopulmonary effects.

Clinical interventions successful in optimizing ventilation provide the "air side" diffusion gradients for gas exchange, a critical component of respiration. To ensure adequate oxygenation of cells and removal of CO_2, the "blood side" gradients must also be maintained within normal limits. Mechanisms for regulation of perfusion and disorders of gas transport and exchange are detailed in Chapter 19.

Summary of Key Points

- The upper respiratory tract, with its highly vascular surface, is ideally suited for warming and humidifying inspired air. The nasopharynx is lined with hair and cilia, which filter particulate matter from inspired air, and its walls contain irritant receptors, which initiate cough and sneeze reflexes to expel particles. Olfactory receptors in the mucosa mediate the sense of smell. Airway patency is ensured by the rigidity of cartilage in the walls in the largest airways and by connective tissue tethers in the smaller airways. The smooth muscle of the lower airways responds to a variety of stimuli to mediate changes in airway diameter, with bronchodilation permitting increased conduction of air on demand and bronchoconstriction restricting entry of air containing irritants or toxins. Goblet cells produce a protective layer of mucus, which is swept upward by beating cilia, clearing the airways of irritants and debris. Type I alveolar cells (macrophages) phagocytize foreign material that reaches the alveoli.
- Contraction of the major muscles of inspiration, the diaphragm and the internal intercostal muscles, enlarges the thoracic space, resulting in a reduction of intrathoracic pressure below atmospheric. This gradient mediates inflow of atmospheric air. With removal of the inspiratory signal, passive relaxation of these muscles decreases thoracic capacity, increasing intrathoracic pressure and reversing the gradient for air flow. Expiration then occurs.
- Work of breathing, the consumption of oxygen by the respiratory system during ventilation, is increased by conditions in which there is (1) loss of elastic recoil of lung tissue, (2) decreased lung tissue compliance, (3) decreased chest wall compliance, (4) increased alveolar surface tension, (5) increased airway resistance, or (6) increased dead space.
- Ventilation is normally under brain-stem reflex control, although limited over-ride by higher cortical centers is possible. The respiratory center in the medulla consists of two groups of neurons: the inspiratory area and the expiratory area. Normal ventilation is mediated by the inspiratory area in response to afferent signals from (1) central and peripheral chemoreceptors, (2) airway stretch and irritant receptors, and (3) motion receptors in joints and muscles. Efferent signals travel along the phrenic nerve to the diaphragm and the intercostal nerve to the intercostal muscles, resulting in inspiration. Expiration is a passive phenomenon under normal circumstances, but the expiratory center may drive forced exhalation during labored breathing.
- Treatment of respiratory failure is aimed at support of the processes of ventilation and gas exchange. Ventilation may be augmented with drug therapy (e.g., bronchodilators, anti-inflammatory agents, mucolytics, expectorants), chest physiotherapy (mechanical clearance of secretions), or mechanical ventilation. Gas exchange is supported indirectly

by measures that improve ventilation as well as directly by administration of supplemental oxygen to increase the gradient for diffusion.

- URIs are usually viral in origin. Bacterial infection, if present, may be primary but is more often secondary to immunosuppression induced by the initial viral agent. Inflammation is typically mild and self-limited, although acute upper airway obstruction and extension of the infection to lower airways may occasionally occur, particularly in children and the elderly. Usual manifestations are of rhinorrhea, postnasal drainage, nasal obstruction, and throat pain. Tonsils and adenoids, lymphatic tissues of the upper respiratory tract, may be enlarged and painful. Treatment of viral infections is symptomatic and supportive, whereas bacterial infections are also treated with appropriate antibiotics.

- COPD is a disease category inclusive of disorders characterized primarily by recurrent or persistent airway obstruction. Chronic bronchitis is airway inflammation associated with cigarette smoking and is defined by the presence of increased sputum and chronic productive cough for at least 3 months of the year for 2 successive years. Emphysema, usually secondary to chronic bronchitis but also associated with AAT deficiency, is present when alveolar walls are destroyed, along with the connective tissues supporting lower airways. Airways collapse on expiration, trapping air and further damaging alveolar walls, which in turn reduces surface area for gas exchange. Asthma is an inflammatory airway disease in which inflammatory mediators induce reversible airway obstruction due to increased mucus and bronchospasm.

- Cigarette smoking is the most important preventable risk factor for laryngeal and lung cancers. Treatment of laryngeal cancer is primarily surgical, with prognosis depending on the location of the lesion and stage at time of diagnosis. Most lung cancer is advanced when diagnosed. Surgical treatment is often not possible because of the proximity of tumors to vital mediastinal structures. Radiation and chemotherapy are palliative measures, but unresectable lung cancer demonstrates a 5-year survival of less than 10%.

- Chest trauma may manifest as rib fractures, flail chest, pneumothorax, and pulmonary contusions. The heart and great vessels may also be injured, leading to possible dysrhythmias, hemorrhage, or cardiac failure. Rib fractures are acutely painful, leading to voluntary hypoventilation. A free-floating segment of ribs results in ineffective paradoxical ventilation in flail chest because the flail segment moves in with inspiration and out with expiration. Pneumothorax may be open, collapsing the lung on the affected side because of loss of negativity in the pleural space. Tension pneumothorax results from a chest wound that creates a one-way tissue valve, permitting entry of atmospheric air during inspiratory effort, but preventing its expulsion with expiratory effort. A closed pneumothorax may lead to lung collapse in the absence of a chest wound, when atmospheric air enters the pleural space through a ruptured bleb or fracture-induced injury on the lung surface, resulting in loss of negativity of intrapleural pressure. Elastic recoil of lung tissue is then unopposed.

REFERENCES

1. Misasi, R.S., and Keyes, J.L. (1996). Matching and mismatching ventilation and perfusion in the lung. *Critical Care Nurse* 16(3), 23–38.
2. Abman, S.H., Griebel, J.L., Parker, D.K., *et al.* (1994). Acute effects of inhaled nitric oxide in children with severe hypoxemic respiratory failure. *Journal of Pediatrics* 124(6), 881–888.
3. Spector, S.L. (1995). The common cold: Current therapy and natural history. *Journal of Allergy and Clinical Immunology* 95(5 Pt. 2), 1133–1138.
4. Macknin, M.L. (1992). Respiratory infections in children: What helps and what doesn't? *Postgraduate Medicine* 92(2), 235–250.
5. Brandtzaeg, P. (1992). Humoral response patterns of human mucosae: Induction and relation to bacterial respiratory tract infections. *Journal of Infectious Diseases* 165(suppl. 1), S167–S176.
6. Williams, J.W., and Simel, D.L. (1993). Does this patient have sinusitis? Diagnosing acute sinusitis by history and physical examination. *Journal of the American Medical Association* 270(10), 1242–1246.
7. Ferguson, B.J. (1995). Acute and chronic sinusitis. *Postgraduate Medicine* 97(5), 45–57.
8. Hendeles, L. (1993). Efficacy and safety of antihistamines and expectorants in nonprescription cough and cold preparations. *Pharmacotherapy* 13(2), 154–158.
9. Mossad, S.B., Macknin, M.L., Medendorp, S.V., *et al.* (1996). Zinc gluconate lozenges for treating the common cold: A randomized, double-blind, placebo-controlled study. *Annals of Internal Medicine* 125(2), 81–88.
10. Quan, L. (1992). Diagnosis and treatment of croup. *American Family Physician* 46(3), 747–755.
11. Pryor, M.P. (1997). Noisy breathing in children. *Postgraduate Medicine* 101(2), 103–112.
12. Kronenberg, R.S., and Griffith, D.E. (1993). Chronic bronchitis: Key points in evaluation. *Postgraduate Medicine* 94(8), 84–90.
13. Verghese, A., and Ismail, H.M. (1994). Acute exacerbations of chronic bronchitis: Preventing treatment failures and early reinfection. *Postgraduate Medicine* 94(8), 75–89.
14. Subramanian, D., and Guntupalli, K.K. (1994). Diagnosing obstructive lung disease. *Postgraduate Medicine* 95(8), 69–85.

15. Garshick, E., Schenker, M.B., and Dosman, J.A. (1996). Occupationally induced airways obstruction. *Medical Clinics of North America* 80(4), 851–878.
16. Griffith, D.E., and Kronenberg, R.S. (1993). Chronic bronchitis: Choosing the optimal treatment. *Postgraduate Medicine* 94(8), 93–100.
17. Weinberger, S.E. (1993). Recent advances in pulmonary medicine (First of two parts). *New England Journal of Medicine* 328(19), 1389–1397.
18. Johannsen, J.M. (1994). Chronic obstructive pulmonary disease: Current comprehensive care for emphysema and bronchitis. *Nurse Practitioner* 19(1), 59–67.
19. Ries, A.L., Kaplan, R.M., Limberg, T.M., *et al.* (1995). Effects of pulmonary rehabilitation on physiologic and psychosocial outcomes in patients with chronic obstructive pulmonary disease. *Annals of Internal Medicine* 122(11), 823–832.
20. Wulfsberg, E.A., Hoffmann, D.E., and Cohen, M.M. (1994). α-1 Antitrypsin deficiency: Impact of a genetic discovery on medicine and society. *Journal of the American Medical Association*, 271(3), 217–222.
21. McGraw, L.R. (1997). Lung volume reduction surgery: An overview. *Heart & Lung* 26(2), 131–137.
22. Rogers, R.M., Sciurba, F.C., and Keenan, R.J. (1996). Lung reduction surgery in chronic obstructive lung disease. *Medical Clinics of North America* 80(3), 623–644.
23. Lynch, J.P., and Trulock, E.P. (1996). Lung transplantation in chronic airflow limitation. *Medical Clinics of North America* 80(3), 657–670.
24. Seneff, M.G., Wagner, D.P., Wagner, R.P., *et al.* (1995). Hospital and 1-year survival of patients admitted to intensive care units with acute exacerbation of chronic obstructive pulmonary disease. *Journal of the American Medical Association* 274(23), 1852–1857.
25. National Asthma Education Program. Expert Panel Report. (1991). Guidelines for the diagnosis and management of asthma. Bethesda: Department of Health and Human Services. DHHS Publication No. 19-3042.
26. Fromm, R.E., and Varon, J. (1994). Acute exacerbations of obstructive lung disease. *Postgraduate Medicine* 95(8), 101–106.
27. Alberts, W.M., and Brooks, S.M. (1995). Occupational asthma: Serious consequences for workers and employers. *Postgraduate Medicine* 97(6), 93–104.
28. McFadden, E.R., and Gilbert, I.A. (1994). Exercise-induced asthma. *New England Journal of Medicine* 330(19), 1362–1367.
29. Postma, D.S., Bleecker, E.R., Amelung, P.J., *et al.* (1995). Genetic susceptibility to asthma: Bronchial hyperresponsiveness coinherited with a major gene for atopy. *New England Journal of Medicine* 333(14), 894–900.
30. Levin, R.H. (1991). Advances in pediatric drug therapy of asthma. *Nursing Clinics of North America* 26(2), 263–272.
31. Wright, L. A., and Martin, R.J. (1995). Nocturnal asthma and exercise-induced bronchospasm: Why they occur and how they can be managed. *Postgraduate Medicine* 97(6), 83–90.
32. Jacobs, M. (1994). Maintenance therapy for obstructive lung disease. *Postgraduate Medicine* 95(8), 87–99.
33. Silverstein, M.D., Reed, C.E., O'Connell, E.J., *et al.* (1994). Long-term survival of a cohort of community residents with asthma. *New England Journal of Medicine* 331(23), 1537–1541.
34. Lang, D.M., and Polansky, M. (1994). Patterns of asthma mortality in Philadelphia from 1969–1991. *New England Journal of Medicine* 331(23), 1542–1546.
35. Taylor, D.R., Sears, M.R., and Cockcroft, D.W. (1996). The beta-agonist controversy. *Medical Clinics of North America* 80(4), 719–748.
36. Lemiere, C., Malo, J-L., and Gautrin, D. (1996). Nonsensitizing causes of occupational asthma. *Medical Clinics of North America* 80(4), 749–774.
37. Strollo, P.J., and Rogers, R.M. (1996). Obstructive sleep apnea. *New England Journal of Medicine* 334(2), 99–104.
38. Man, G.C.W. (1996). Obstructive sleep apnea: Diagnosis and treatment. *Medical Clinics of North America* 80(4), 803–820.
39. Fletcher, E.C. (1995). The relationship between systemic hypertension and obstructive sleep apnea: Facts and theory. *American Journal of Medicine* 98(2), 118–128.
40. Welsh, M.J., and Smith, A.E. (1995). Cystic fibrosis. *Scientific American* 273(6), 52–59.
41. Tizzano, E.F., and Buchwald, M. (1993). Recent advances in cystic fibrosis research. *Journal of Pediatrics* 122(6), 985–988.
42. Wilmott, R.W., and Fiedler, M.A. (1994). Recent advances in the treatment of cystic fibrosis. *Pediatric Clinics of North America* 41(3), 431–451.
43. Wagner, J.A., Chao, A.C., and Gardner, P. (1995). Molecular strategies for therapy of cystic fibrosis. *Annual Review of Pharmacology and Toxicology* 35, 257–276.
44. Wallace, C.S., Hall, M., and Kuhn, R.J. (1993). Pharmacologic management of cystic fibrosis. *Clinical Pharmacy* 12(9), 657–701.
45. Marwah, O.S., and Sharma, O.P. (1995). Bronchiectasis: How to identify, treat, and prevent. *Postgraduate Medicine* 97(2), 149–159.
46. McKenna, J.P., Fornataro-Clerici, L.M., McManamin, P.G., *et al.* (1991). Laryngeal cancer: Diagnosis, treatment and speech rehabilitation. *American Family Physician* 44(1), 123–129.
47. Jett, J.R. (1993). Current treatment of unresectable lung cancer. *Mayo Clinic Proceedings* 68(6), 603–611.
48. Davila, D.G., and Williams, D.E. (1993). The etiology of lung cancer. *Mayo Clinic Proceedings* 68(2), 170–182.
49. Cotran, R.S., Kumar, V., and Robbins, S.L. (1994). *Robbins Pathologic Basis of Disease.* (5th ed.). Philadelphia: W.B. Saunders. (pp. 720–725).
50. Patel, A.M., and Peters, S.G. (1993). Clinical manifestations of lung cancer. *Mayo Clinic Proceedings* 68(3), 273–277.
51. The Alpha-Tocopherol, Beta Carotene Cancer Prevention Study Group. (1994). The effect of vitamin E and beta carotene on the incidence of lung cancer and other cancers in male smokers. *New England Journal of Medicine* 330(15), 1029–1035.
52. Johnston, M.R. (1997). Curable lung cancer: How to find it and treat it. *Postgraduate Medicine* 101(3), 155–165.
53. Pisani, R.J. (1993). Bronchogenic carcinoma: Immunologic aspects. *Mayo Clinic Proceedings* 68(4), 386–392.
54. Edell, E.S., Cortese, D.A., and McDougall, J.C. (1993). Ancillary therapies in the management of lung cancer: Photodynamic therapy, laser therapy, and endobronchial prosthetic devices. *Mayo Clinic Proceedings* 68(7), 685–690.
55. Spillane, R.M., Shepard, J.O., and Deluca, S.A. (1995). Radiographic aspects of pneumothorax. *American Family Physician* 51(2), 459–464.
56. Wyatt, T.H. (1995). Pneumothorax in the neonate. *Journal of Obstetric, Gynecologic, and Neonatal Nursing* 24(3), 211–216.
57. Laskowski-Jones, L. (1995). Meeting the challenge of chest trauma. *American Journal of Nursing* 95(9), 23–30.
58. Samuel, J.R. (1997). Management of recurrent spontaneous pneumothorax and recurrent symptomatic pleural effusion with chest tube pleurodesis. *Critical Care Nurse* 17(1), 28–32.

SELECTED BIBLIOGRAPHY

Abou-Shala, N., and MacIntyre, N. (1996). Emergent management of acute asthma. *Medical Clinics of North America* 80(4), 677–699.

Adkinson, N.F., Jr., Eggleston, P.A., Eney, D., *et al.* (1997). A controlled trial of immunotherapy for asthma in allergic children. *New England Journal of Medicine* 336(5), 324–331.

Anderson, J.M. (1996). Management of four arterial blood gas problems in adult mechanical ventilation: Decision-making algorithms and rationale for their use. *Critical Care Nurse* 16(3), 62–73.

Anthonisen, N.R., Connett, J.E., Kiley, J.P., *et al.* (1994). Effects of smoking intervention and the use of an inhaled anticholinergic bronchodilator on the rate of decline of FEV_1: The Lung Health Study. *Journal of the American Medical Association* 272(19), 1497–1505.

Austan, F. (1996). Heliox inhalation in status asthmaticus and respiratory acidemia: A brief report. *Heart & Lung* 25(2), 155–157.

Barnes, P.J. (1995). Inhaled glucocorticoids for asthma. *New England Journal of Medicine* 332(13), 868–875.
Bartecchi, C.E., MacKenzie, T.D., and Schrier, R.W. (1994). The human costs of tobacco use (First of two parts). *New England Journal of Medicine* 330(13), 907–912.
Bechler-Karsch, A. (1994). Assessment and management of status asthmaticus. *Pediatric Nursing* 20(3), 217–223.
Bernstein, J.A. (1993). Allergic rhinitis: Helping patients lead an unrestricted life. *Postgraduate Medicine* 93(6), 124–132.
Bidani, A., Tzouanakis, A.E., Cardenas, V.J., *et al.* (1994). Permissive hypercapnia in acute respiratory failure. *Journal of the American Medical Association* 272(12), 957–962.
Breslin, E.H. (1996). Respiratory muscle function in patients with chronic obstructive pulmonary disease. *Heart & Lung* 25(4), 271–285.

Casey, K.R., and Winterbauer, R.H. (1995). Acute severe asthma: How to recognize and respond to a life-threatening attack. *Postgraduate Medicine* 97(6), 71–78.
Celli, B.R. (1996). Current thoughts regarding treatment of chronic obstructive pulmonary disease. *Medical Clinics of North America* 80(3), 589–609.
Chan-Yeung, M., and Malo, J-L. (1995). Occupational asthma. *New England Journal of Medicine* 333(2), 107–112.
Chapman, K.R. (1996a). An international perspective on anticholinergic therapy. *American Journal of Medicine* 100(suppl. 1A), 2S–4S.
Chapman, K.R. (1996b). Therapeutic approaches to chronic obstructive pulmonary disease: An emerging consensus. *American Journal of Medicine* 100(suppl. 1A), 5S–10S.
Clemens, C.J., Taylor, J.A., Almquist, J.R., *et al.* (1997). Is an antihistamine-decongestant combination effective in temporarily relieving symptoms of the common cold in preschool children? *Journal of Pediatrics* 130(3), 463–466.
Cockcroft, D.W., and Kalra, S. (1996). Outpatient asthma management. *Medical Clinics of North America* 80(4), 701–718.
Connors, C.A., and Rosenthal-Dichter, C. (1997). Components of breathing: Pediatric ventilatory challenges. *Critical Care Nurse* 17(1), 60–70.
Cressman, W.R., and Myer, C.M. (1994). Diagnosis and management of croup and epiglottitis. *Pediatric Clinics of North America* 41(2), 265–276.
Creticos, P.S., Reed, C.R., Norman, P.S., *et al.* (1996). Ragweed immunotherapy in adult asthma. *New England Journal of Medicine* 334(8), 501–506.

Dere, W.H. (1992). Acute bronchitis: Results of U.S. and European trials of antibiotic therapy. *American Journal of Medicine* 92(suppl. 6A), 53S–57S.
Dockery, D.W., Pope, C.A., Xu, X., *et al.* (1993). An association between air pollution and mortality in six U.S. cities. *New England Journal of Medicine* 329(24), 1753–1759.
Drazen, J.M., Israel, E., Boushey, H.A., *et al.* (1996). Comparison of regularly scheduled with as-needed use of albuterol in mild asthma. *New England Journal of Medicine* 335(12), 841–847.

Eanes, R. (1995). On the horizon: Liquid ventilation. *Journal of Obstetric, Gynecologic, and Neonatal Nursing* 24(2), 119–124.
Eigen, H., Rosenstein, B.J., FitzSimmons, S., *et al.* (1995). A multicenter study of alternate-day prednisone therapy in patients with cystic fibrosis. *Journal of Pediatrics* 126(4), 515–523.

Fireman, P. (1993). Pathophysiology and pharmacotherapy of common upper respiratory diseases. *Pharmacotherapy* 13(6 Pt. 2), 101S–109S.
Folland, D.S. (1997). Treatment of croup: Sending home an improved child and relieved parents. *Postgraduate Medicine* 101(3), 271–278.
Fontham, E.T.H., Correa, P., Reynolds, P., *et al.* (1994). Environmental tobacco smoke and lung cancer in nonsmoking women. *Journal of the American Medical Association* 271(22), 1752–1759.
Frantz, T.D., Rasgon, B.M., and Quesenberry, C.P. (1994). Acute epiglottitis in adults: Analysis of 129 cases. *Journal of the American Medical Association* 272(17), 1358–1360.

Gammon, R.B., Strickland, J.H., Kennedy, J.I., *et al.* (1995). Mechanical ventilation: A review for the internist. *American Journal of Medicine* 99(5), 553–562.
Gold, D.R., Wang, X., Wypij, D., *et al.* (1996). Effects of cigarette smoking on lung function in adolescent boys and girls. *New England Journal of Medicine* 335(13), 931–937.
Graft, D.F. (1996). Allergic and nonallergic rhinitis: Directing medical therapy at specific symptoms. *Postgraduate Medicine* 100(2), 64–74.
Grossbach, I. (1994). The COPD patient in acute respiratory failure. *Critical Care Nurse* 14(6), 32–38.
Guyton, A.C., and Hall, J.E. (1996). *Textbook of Medical Physiology.* (9th ed.). Philadelphia: W.B. Saunders.

Hayden, F.G., Diamond, L., Wood, P.B., *et al.* (1996). Effectiveness and safety of intranasal ipratropium bromide in common colds: A randomized, double-blind, placebo-controlled trial. *Annals of Internal Medicine* 125(2), 89–97.
Heath, J.M. (1993). Outpatient management of chronic bronchitis in the elderly. *American Family Physician* 48(5), 841–848.
Henderson, R.C., and Specter, B.B. (1994). Kyphosis and fractures in children and young adults with cystic fibrosis. *Journal of Pediatrics* 125(2), 208–212.
Henningfield, J.E. (1995). Nicotine medications for smoking cessation. *New England Journal of Medicine* 333(18), 1196–1203.

Jokic, R., and Fitzpatrick, M.F. (1996). Obstructive lung disease and sleep. *Medical Clinics of North America* 80(4), 821–850.

Kanner, R.E. (1996). Early intervention in chronic obstructive pulmonary disease: A review of the Lung Health Study Results. *Medical Clinics of North America* 80(3), 523–544.
Karsell, P.R., and McDougall, J.C. (1993). Diagnostic tests for lung cancer. *Mayo Clinic Proceedings* 68(3), 288–296.
Knight, A. (1995). The differential diagnosis of rhinorrhea. *Journal of Allergy and Clinical Immunology* 95(5 Pt. 2), 1081–1083.
Kravitz, R.M. (1994). Congenital malformations of the lung. *Pediatric Clinics of North America* 41(3), 453–472.
Kudikis, T.M., Manthous, C.A., Schmidt, G.A., *et al.* (1997). Inhaled helium-oxygen revisited: Effect of inhaled helium-oxygen during the treatment of status asthmaticus in children. *Journal of Pediatrics* 130(2), 217–224.
Kuhn, M.M. (1991). *Pharmacotherapeutics: A Nursing Process Approach.* Philadelphia: F.A. Davis.

Lauria, M.R., Gonik, B., and Romero, R. (1995). Pulmonary hypoplasia: Pathogenesis, diagnosis, and antenatal prediction. *Obstetrics & Gynecology* 86(3), 466–475.
Leiner, S. (1997). Acute bronchitis in adults: Commonly diagnosed but poorly defined. *Nurse Practitioner* 22(1), 104–117.
Lordi, G.M., and Reichman, L.B. (1993). Pulmonary complications of asbestos exposure. *American Family Physician* 48(8), 1471–1477.

Manning, H.L., and Schwartzstein, R.M. (1995). Pathophysiology of dyspnea. *New England Journal of Medicine* 333(23), 1547–1553.
Manthous, C.A. (1995). Management of severe exacerbations of asthma. *American Journal of Medicine* 99, 298–308.
Martinez, F.D., Wright, A.L., Taussig, L.M., *et al.* (1995). Asthma and wheezing in the first six years of life. *New England Journal of Medicine* 332(3), 133–138.
Maynard, L.C. (1994). Pediatric heart-lung transplantation for cystic fibrosis. *Heart & Lung* 23(4), 279–284.
McCaffrey, T.V. (1993). Functional endoscopic sinus surgery: An overview. *Mayo Clinic Proceedings* 68(6), 571–577.
McGinnis, J.M., and Foege, W.H. (1993). Actual causes of death in the United States. *Journal of the American Medical Association* 270(18), 2207–2212.
Meyer, T.J. (1994). Noninvasive positive pressure ventilation to treat respiratory failure. *Annals of Internal Medicine* 120(9), 760–770.
Midthun, D.E. (1997). Endobronchial techniques in lung cancer. *Postgraduate Medicine* 101(3), 169–178.

Midthun, D.E., McDougall, J.C., Peters, S.G., *et al.* (1997). Medical management and complications in the lung transplant recipient. *Mayo Clinic Proceedings* 72, 175–184.

Morris, R.J. (1996). Asthma: Specific preventive strategies. *Postgraduate Medicine* 100(2), 105–120.

Murphy, C.M., Coonce, S.L., and Simon, P.A. (1991). Treatment of asthma in children. *Clinical Pharmacology* 10(9), 685–703.

Newman, L.J., Platts-Millos, T.A., Phillips, C.D., *et al.* (1994). Chronic sinusitis: Relationship of computed tomographic findings to allergy, asthma, and eosinophilia. *Journal of the American Medical Association* 271(5), 363–367.

O'Donnell, D.E., Webb, K.A., and McGuire, M.A. (1993). Older patients with COPD: Benefits of exercise training. *Geriatrics* 48(1), 59–66.

O'Donohue, W.J., Jr. (1996). Home oxygen therapy. *Medical Clinics of North America* 80(4), 611–622.

Patel, A.M., Davila, D.G., and Peters, S.G. (1993). Paraneoplastic syndromes associated with lung cancer. *Mayo Clinic Proceedings* 68(3), 278–287.

Patel, A.M., Dunn, W.F., and Traster, V.F. (1993). Staging systems of lung cancer. *Mayo Clinic Proceedings* 68(5), 475–482.

Patrick, H., and Patrick, F. (1995). Chronic cough. *Medical Clinics of North America* 79(2), 361–372.

Peggs, J.F., Shimp, L.A., and Opdycke, R.A.C. (1995). Antihistamines: The old and the new. *American Family Physician* 52(2), 593–600.

Petty, T.L. (1996). Lung cancer and chronic obstructive pulmonary disease. *Medical Clinics of North America* 80(3), 645–655.

Pilmer, S.L. (1994). Prolonged mechanical ventilation in children. *Pediatric Clinics of North America* 41(3), 473–512.

Ramsey, B.W. (1996). Management of pulmonary disease in patients with cystic fibrosis. *New England Journal of Medicine* 335(3), 179–188.

Ruoff, G.E. (1996). Recurrent streptococcal pharyngitis: Using practical treatment options to interrupt the cycle. *Postgraduate Medicine* 99(2), 211–222.

Scherer, Y.K., and Schmieder, L.E. (1997). The effect of a pulmonary rehabilitation program on self-efficacy, perception of dyspnea, and physical endurance. *Heart & Lung* 26(1), 15–22.

Sciurba, F.C., Rogers, R.M., Keenan, R.J., *et al.* (1996). Improvement in pulmonary function and elastic recoil after lung reduction surgery for diffuse emphysema. *New England Journal of Medicine* 334(17), 1095–1099.

Shaw, E.G., Bonner, J.A., Foote, R.L., *et al.* (1993). Role of radiation therapy in the management of lung cancer. *Mayo Clinic Proceedings* 68(6), 593–602.

Shelhamer, J.H., Levine, S.J., Wu, T., *et al.* (1995). Airway inflammation. *Annals of Internal Medicine* 123(4), 288–304.

Sheth, R.D., Pryse-Phillips, W.E.M., Riggs, J.E., *et al.* (1995). Critical illness neuromuscular disease in children manifested as ventilatory dependence. *Journal of Pediatrics* 126(2), 259–261.

Siefkin, A.D. (1996). Optimal pharmacologic treatment of the critically ill patient with obstructive airways disease. *American Journal of Medicine* 100(suppl. 1A), 54S–61S.

Silverman, E.K., and Speizer, F.E. (1996). Risk factors for the development of chronic obstructive pulmonary disease. *Medical Clinics of North America* 80(3), 501–522.

Smith, M.B.H., and Feldman, W. (1993). Over-the-counter cold medications: A critical review of clinical trials between 1950 and 1991. *Journal of the American Medical Association* 269(17), 2258–2263.

Smoking Cessation Clinical Practice Guideline Panel and Staff. (1996). The Agency for Health Care Policy and Research Smoking Cessation Clinical Practice Guideline. *Journal of the American Medical Association* 275(16), 1270–1280.

Strollo, P.J., and Rogers, R.M. (1996). Obstructive sleep apnea. *New England Journal of Medicine* 334(2), 99–104.

Tobin, M.J. (1994). Mechanical ventilation. *New England Journal of Medicine* 330(15), 1056–1061.

van Schayck, C.P., van den Broek, P.J.J.A., den Otter, J.J., *et al.* (1995). Periodic treatment regimens with inhaled steroids in asthma or chronic obstructive pulmonary disease: Is it possible? *Journal of the American Medical Association* 274(2), 161–164.

Wald, E.R. (1995). Chronic sinusitis in children. *Journal of Pediatrics* 127(3), 339–347.

Weiss, S.M., and Petty, T.L. (1995). Physiologic evaluation of bronchial asthma: Why objective testing is essential. *Postgraduate Medicine* 97(6), 56–67.

Whitesell, P.L., and Drage, C.W. (1993). Occupational lung cancer. *Mayo Clinic Proceedings* 68(2), 183–188.

Disorders of Gas Transport and Exchange

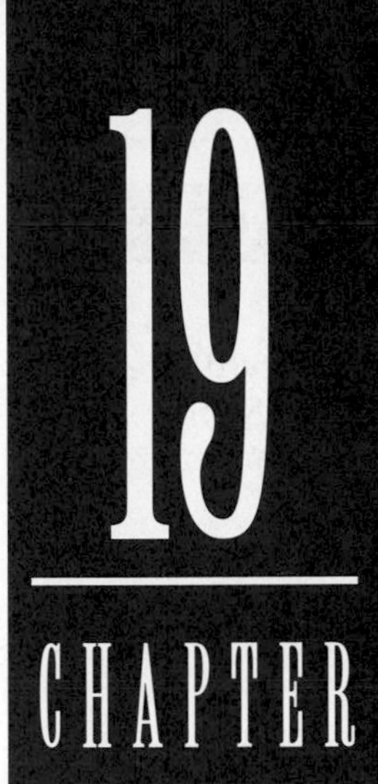

LEARNING OBJECTIVES

1. Explain the physiologic bases for the differences in pressure between the pulmonary and systemic vascular systems, including conditions that may alter this pressure gradient.
2. Discuss the cellular mechanism, adaptive purpose, and potential pathophysiologic consequences of hypoxic pulmonary vasoconstriction.
3. Identify the principal forms in which oxygen and carbon dioxide are transported in the blood.
4. Explain the physiologic basis of the shape of the oxyhemoglobin dissociation curve, including factors that may shift the curve to the right or left.
5. Discuss the relative importance of each of the following in determining the rate of gas diffusion across the alveolar–capillary membrane: membrane thickness, membrane surface area, diffusion coefficients of the gases, and pressure gradients.
6. Explain the pathophysiologic mechanisms that predict clinical manifestations and rationalize clinical intervention in selected disorders of blood gas transport and exchange.

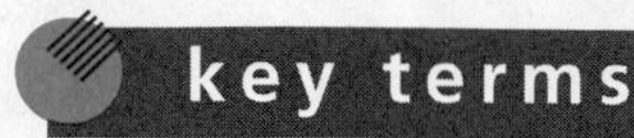

key terms

abscess
adult respiratory distress syndrome (ARDS)
alveolar–capillary membrane
anemia
aspiration pneumonia
atypical pneumonia
Bohr effect
bronchiolitis
bronchopneumonia
carbon monoxide intoxication
cor pulmonale
crackles
decompression disorder
diving reflex
empyema
environmental–occupational lung disease
Haldane effect
hemoptysis
hypercapnia
hypoxemia
hypoxic pulmonary vasoconstriction
idiopathic pulmonary fibrosis
lobar pneumonia
near-drowning
oxyhemoglobin dissociation curve
pleural effusion
pleurisy
pneumonia
primary pulmonary hypertension
pulmonary edema
pulmonary embolism
pulmonary fibrosis
pulmonary infarction
pulmonary vascular resistance (PVR)
respiratory syncytial virus (RSV)
rhonchi
sarcoidosis
sudden infant death syndrome (SIDS)
transudate
tuberculosis (TB)

Respiration, the exchange of oxygen and carbon dioxide between the human system and the environment, is the principal function of the pulmonary system. Normal respiration occurs as a result of exchange of these gases between the air and the blood in the respiratory units (i.e., alveoli, alveolar ducts, and respiratory bronchioles) of the lungs, a complex process that can be subdivided into three interdependent components: ventilation, blood gas transport, and diffusion. The physiologic processes related to ventilation were discussed in Chapter 18, along with disorders in which the initial or primary impact was due to alterations in ventilation. In this chapter, pulmonary perfusion is detailed, including pulmonary vascular anatomy, regulation of pulmonary perfusion, and disorders of pulmonary blood flow. Mechanisms of gas transport within the blood are reviewed, with emphasis on the role of hemoglobin. Factors affecting the simple diffusion of gases between alveolar air and pulmonary capillary blood are discussed. Clinical disorders that initially affect nonairway pulmonary tissues and manifest primarily as altered gas exchange are detailed. It must be understood, however, that these disorders ultimately affect *all* components of respiration.

Disorders of pulmonary transport or exchange may affect ventilation directly, as in the case of airway edema or fluid deposition, or indirectly, due to altered feedback to the respiratory control centers initiated by changes in the partial pressure of oxygen or carbon dioxide in the blood (see Chapter 18). Alterations in ventilation, pulmonary perfusion, gas transport, or exchange lead to variation in the amount of oxygen delivered to cells for use in oxidative energy metabolism, also known as *cellular respiration* (see Chapter 3). Alteration in the quantity and function of erythrocytes or hemoglobin has a significant impact on respiratory processes because, as discussed in this chapter, nearly all oxygen is transported in combination with hemoglobin. Erythrocyte disorders were detailed in Chapter 12. Separation of the respiratory processes is designed to facilitate more in-depth understanding of each, but their interdependence often is evident in the discussions of illustrative disorders.

Respiratory disorders account for the highest morbidity rates among all system disorders. The diseases discussed in this chapter contribute significantly to this morbidity. People of all ages are affected (see Developmental Perspective). **Pneumonia** is highly prevalent among the elderly, for example, whereas **bronchiolitis** affects a significant number of infants and children. **Pulmonary edema, pulmonary embolism,** and **adult respiratory distress syndrome** (ARDS) contribute to high mortality in critical illness originating from any body system. **Tuberculosis** (TB), once believed to be "under control" in the United States, is again increasing in incidence, and **environmental–occupational lung diseases** are contributing to increasing morbidity in the workplace. These and other, less common disorders of gas transport and exchange are examined in this chapter, following an overview of the pulmonary circulation and the processes mediating gas exchange between alveolar air and pulmonary capillary blood.

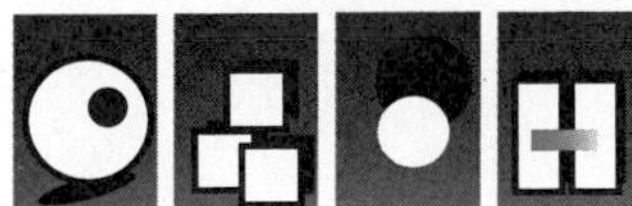

Developmental Perspective

Embryonic and Fetal Periods

By 22 weeks' gestation, respiration is possible because some primitive alveoli (terminal sacs), which are well vascularized, have formed. A small number of infants born at this time survive, but respiratory function is markedly impaired. The fetal lungs are collapsed in utero, with maternal–fetal gas exchange occurring across the placental villi. Fetal uptake of oxygen is favored by the 50% greater hemoglobin concentration in fetal than in maternal blood and by the higher affinity of Hb F, which shifts the oxyhemoglobin dissociation curve to the left. At term, the alveolar–capillary membrane has become thin to facilitate gas exchange after birth. Persistence of the ductus arteriosus and foramen ovale, fetal circulatory structures that bypass the lungs, may give rise to congenital heart defects. Fetal oxygenation may be compromised by maternal respiratory, circulatory, or hematopoietic disorders or by placental insufficiency.

Infancy and Childhood

The newborn infant has about 20 million alveoli, which are smaller than adult alveoli. Terminal bronchioles have not completed their branching. The number of alveoli increases until about 8 years of age, when the adult number of 300 to 600 million is attained. Collateral ventilation between alveoli and between terminal bronchioles develops throughout childhood and enhances ventilatory and exchange capacity. Structural changes in pulmonary perfusion are initiated with the first breath and continue during childhood with growth in diameter and reduction of muscularity of vessel walls. Infant respiratory distress syndrome occurs in many preterm and some full-term infants due to deficiency of surfactant production. Widespread atelectasis reduces the available surface area for gas exchange, and deposition of fibrin into the alveolar–capillary membrane impairs diffusion.

Adolescence and Young Adulthood

Working adults are at greater risk of occupational and other environmental exposures that may lead to pulmonary fibrosis and impaired diffusion. The risk of major trauma with subsequent hypovolemic shock and ARDS is also high in this group.

Middle and Older Adulthood

Most deaths due to complications of influenza occur in the elderly and may be attributed to exacerbation of underlying cardiac or pulmonary disease or to development of a secondary bacterial pneumonia. Pneumonia is the fourth leading cause of death in people older than 65 years, possibly owing to altered immunity, impaired swallowing leading to aspiration risk, underlying chronic disease, and increased colonization with upper respiratory pathogens.

ANATOMY OF THE PULMONARY CIRCULATION

Figure 19–1 illustrates the *pulmonary artery* and its branches as well as the *pulmonary veins.* As discussed in Chapter 16, the pulmonary artery receives blood from the venous system via the right ventricle. Although often referred to as *unoxygenated,* this venous blood actually contains some oxygen (its Po_2 is about 40 mm Hg), and lung tissue is able to extract a portion of this oxygen for its own metabolic use. The walls of conducting airways are also perfused by smaller *bronchial arteries,* which branch off the thoracic aorta. The bronchial circulation is of minor importance in pulmonary function, however, because its flow is normally 1/100 of that of the pulmonary arterial circulation. The bronchial circulation represents a physiologic left-to-right shunt of about 2% to 5% of cardiac output and may serve as an essential source of perfusion in the case of congenital abnormality of the pulmonary artery (see discussion of truncus arteriosus, Chapter 16) or obstruction due to pulmonary embolism, discussed later in this chapter.

The pulmonary capillary beds surrounding the alveoli and other respiratory unit structures are extremely dense, appearing under microscopy as a

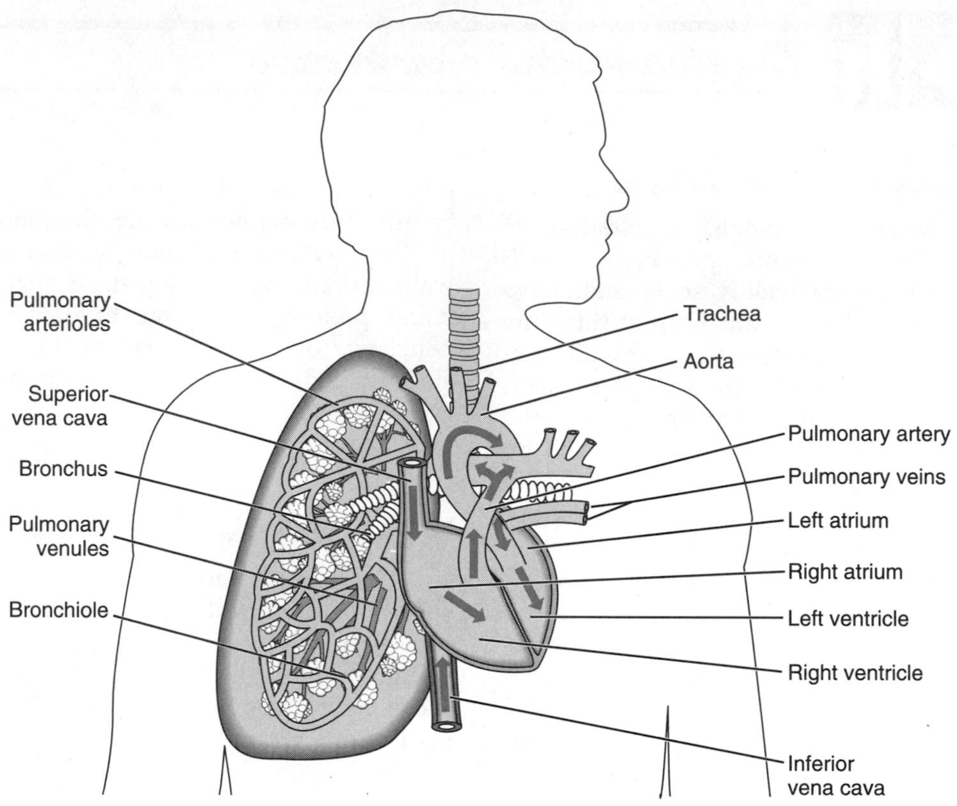

FIGURE 19–1
Pulmonary circulation. The pulmonary artery receives venous blood from the right ventricle. This blood is oxygenated within the pulmonary capillary beds, then returns to the left side of the heart through the pulmonary veins. Lung tissue extracts a small amount of oxygen from pulmonary arterial blood for its own metabolism.

nearly continuous sheet of blood. This rich perfusion, along with the normally thin, highly permeable structure of the **alveolar–capillary membrane**, creates an optimal anatomic configuration for gas exchange. As shown in Figure 19–2, the alveolar–capillary membrane actually consists of several layers. The alveolar and capillary walls are thin, however, and the interstitial space between them is normally small, containing little interstitial fluid or protein. Given the high lipid solubilities of oxygen and carbon dioxide, the membrane offers little resistance to diffusion unless it is thickened by abnormal fluid exudation or fibrin deposition.

REGULATION OF PULMONARY PERFUSION

Pulmonary blood flow is determined by the general resistance equation for circulation, as discussed in Chapter 15. The hemodynamic driving force is provided by right ventricular contraction, which depends on venous return and myocardial contractility. **Pulmonary vascular resistance** (PVR) is normally much less than resistance to flow in the systemic circulation because the pulmonary system is shorter, and its vessels are more compliant than the muscular arteries of the systemic circulation. As discussed later, conditions in which PVR is chronically increased result in increased resistance to outflow from the right ventricle (i.e., increased right ventricular afterload). Congestive heart failure resulting from this mechanism is known as **cor pulmonale**.

Hypoxic Pulmonary Vasoconstriction

PVR is regulated secondarily to ventilation by a local reflex mechanism known as **hypoxic pulmonary vasoconstriction**. Smooth muscle cells in the walls of pulmonary vessels respond to changes in the pressure of oxygen of the blood perfusing these vessels. **Hypoxemia** inhibits an outward potassium current from these cells, causing membrane depolarization and calcium entry through voltage-gated calcium channels.[1] Calcium entry mediates muscle cell contraction, resulting in vessel constriction, and PVR

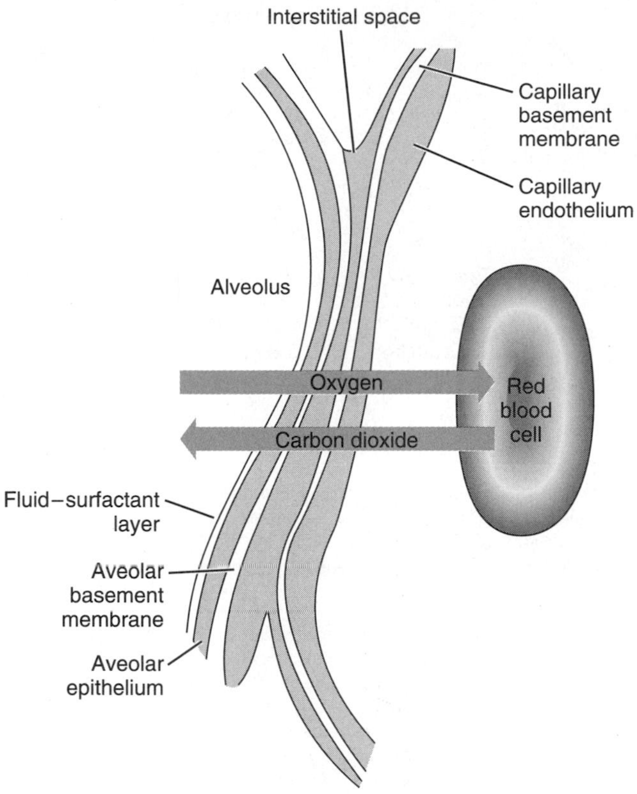

FIGURE 19–2

Alveolar–capillary membrane. The barrier through which the blood gases diffuse is thin and highly permeable despite its multilayered composition. Oxygen diffuses from alveolar air through (1) a fluid–surfactant layer, (2) the alveolar epithelium, (3) the alveolar basement membrane, (4) the interstitial space, (5) the capillary basement membrane, and (6) the capillary endothelium. Carbon dioxide diffuses from the pulmonary capillary blood to the alveolar air in reverse sequence through these structures. (Redrawn from Guyton, A.C., and Hall, J.E. [1996]. *Textbook of Medical Physiology*. [9th ed.]. Philadelphia: W.B. Saunders. [p. 508].)

increases. This is the same mechanism by which fetal lung vessels remain constricted in utero (see Chapter 33). With respect to pulmonary function after birth, the hypoxic pulmonary vasoconstriction response is adaptive in that it tends to optimize ventilation–perfusion ($\dot{V}/\dot{Q}$) relationships, redirecting blood flow to better-ventilated alveoli. As detailed in Chapter 18, $\dot{V}/\dot{Q}$ ratios reflect the relative flow rates of alveolar air and pulmonary capillary blood within the respiratory units of the lungs. The ideal $\dot{V}/\dot{Q}$ ratio ($\dot{V}/\dot{Q} = 0.8$) permits optimal gas exchange, whereas low or high $\dot{V}/\dot{Q}$ ratios reduce the efficiency of this exchange.

Autonomic Nervous System Effects

At the baseline state, sympathetic stimulation of the pulmonary circulation predominates over parasympathetic, maintaining basal vascular tone.[2] Sympathetic nerves originating from the thoracic region of the spinal cord secrete the neurotransmitter norepinephrine, which binds to β_2- and α_2-adrenergic receptors in vascular walls and induces vasodilation. In an opposing effect, binding of NE to α_1-adrenergic receptors results in vasoconstriction. The density and differential distribution of these various receptors determines the net effect. Increased parasympathetic stimulation, with release of acetylcholine, induces the pulmonary vascular endothelium to release the vasodilator nitric oxide (see Chapter 15).

Hormonal Regulation

Many circulating hormones affect PVR. Angiotensin II, for example, is a pulmonary vasoconstrictor, whereas arginine vasopressin (also known as antidiuretic hormone) and atrial natriuretic peptide dilate pulmonary vessels. The effects of numerous other mediators, including histamine, bradykinin, endothelin, serotonin, adenosine, prostaglandins, and thromboxanes depend on the initial level of pulmonary vascular tone. These usually exert a modulating effect, causing constriction when vascular tone is low and dilation when vascular tone is high.[2]

Physical and Mechanical Effects

As a result of hydrostatic pressure, pulmonary perfusion displays regional variation in the lungs, being greatest in the most dependent areas. In the upright lung, ventilation ($\dot{V}$) and perfusion ($\dot{Q}$) both increase from top to bottom, but they do not increase proportionately. As illustrated in Figure 19–3, $\dot{V}$ and $\dot{Q}$ are only well matched ($\dot{V}/\dot{Q} = 0.8$) in the middle regions (zone 2) of the lungs. In this area, blood flow is pulsatile. During systole, blood flows because arterial pressure is greater than alveolar pressure. During diastole, however, blood pressure cannot overcome the vessel compression resulting from alveolar air pressure. At the apices (zone 1) of the lungs, ventilation exceeds perfusion (high $\dot{V}/\dot{Q}$), and vessels are compressed by high alveolar air pressure. In the bases (zone 3), blood flow is continuous because perfusion pressure always exceeds alveolar pressure (low $\dot{V}/\dot{Q}$). The net $\dot{V}/\dot{Q}$ when all portions of the lung are considered still approaches the optimal ratio, however.

Ambulatory people normally change positions frequently, which assists in $\dot{V}/\dot{Q}$ matching. As discussed in Chapter 18, immobility, disease, and some forms of therapy may adversely affect $\dot{V}/\dot{Q}$ relationships by altering ventilation. Alteration of perfusion as a result of pulmonary embolism, right-sided heart

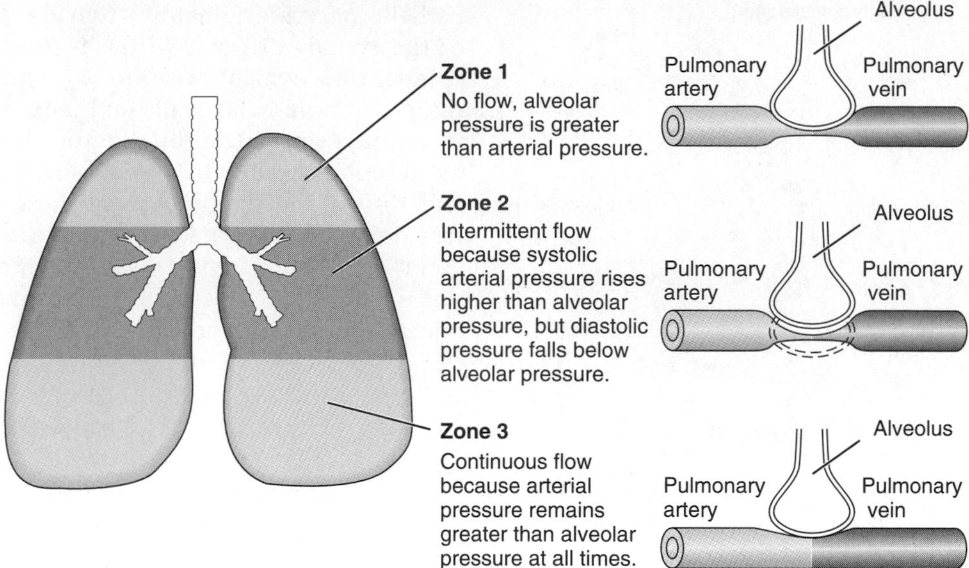

FIGURE 19–3

Regional variation in $\dot{V}/\dot{Q}$ relationships. Hydrostatic pressure due to gravitational forces is one of many factors contributing to variation in $\dot{V}/\dot{Q}$ ratios. Pulmonary capillary perfusion is greatest in the most dependent areas of the lung. In the lower areas (zone 3) of the upright lung, capillary hydrostatic pressure exceeds alveolar distending pressure throughout the cardiac cycle, and blood flow is continuous. Perfusion is increased relative to ventilation, and the $\dot{V}/\dot{Q}$ ratio is low. In the upper areas (zone 1), the opposite relationship exists, and the $\dot{V}/\dot{Q}$ ratio is high. The optimal $\dot{V}/\dot{Q}$ ratio is demonstrated in the middle regions (zone 2). The "net" $\dot{V}/\dot{Q}$ ratio, when all portions of the lung are considered, approaches the optimal ratio.

failure, or shock may also result in $\dot{V}/\dot{Q}$ mismatch and lead to respiratory failure. Mechanical ventilation at high airway pressures may totally compress pulmonary capillaries in some areas, preventing gas exchange and worsening respiratory failure.

BLOOD GAS TRANSPORT

Transport in Dissolved Form

The behavior of gases in solution is governed by Henry's law, which states that the concentration of a gas dissolved in a liquid depends on the partial pressure of the gas, its solubility, and the temperature of the liquid. In human physiology, body temperature does not vary enough to impact gas transport significantly. Solubility is constant for a given gas; carbon dioxide is about 20 times as soluble as oxygen, and both are much more soluble than nitrogen. The proportion of gas dissolved in blood is limited by relatively poor solubility in water. The amount of oxygen transported in this form is normally small (1% to 5%) but may be significantly increased with oxygen therapy in clinical settings. Normally, only about 10% of carbon dioxide is transported in dissolved form.

Transport in Combination With Hemoglobin

Binding of Oxygen to Hemoglobin

About 99% of oxygen and 20% of carbon dioxide are transported in combination with hemoglobin in red blood cells, as oxyhemoglobin and carbamino compounds, respectively. Hemoglobin is a protein composed of four polypeptide subunits (two α chains and two β chains folded in a globular, or *globin*, shape), each of which has an attached *heme* (iron-containing group) (see Chapter 12). Each heme contains a binding site for a molecule of oxygen, totaling four per hemoglobin molecule. The polypeptide chains contain separate binding sites for carbon dioxide, hydrogen ions, and a metabolite produced during glycolysis, 2,3-diphosphoglycerate (2,3-DPG).

The amount of oxygen that can be transported to cells thus depends not only on the partial pressure of oxygen (PaO_2) provided by ventilation but also on the quantity of hemoglobin and its affinity for oxygen, referred to as the *oxygen-carrying capacity* of the blood. Hemoglobin concentration, commonly measured in clinical settings, varies normally with age and sex and may also be altered by blood loss and disease, as discussed in Chapter 12.

Factors Affecting Affinity of Hemoglobin for Oxygen

Oxyhemoglobin Dissociation Curve. The affinity of a given oxygen-binding site decreases sequentially with binding of oxygen to the other three heme groups because this binding induces refolding of the polypeptide chains, decreasing accessibility of the site.[3] As a result, the relationship between PaO_2 and binding or saturation of hemoglobin with oxygen is nonlinear. Figure 19–4 illustrates the sigmoid (S-shaped) **oxyhemoglobin dissociation curve,** which characterizes this relationship. Of particular importance in clinical situations is the fact that, when PaO_2 drops below 50 mm Hg, oxygen saturation drops sharply, accounting for the potentially rapid onset of manifestations of respiratory failure.

Factors Altering the Shape of the Curve

Shift to the Right. The slope of the oxyhemoglobin dissociation curve may be altered (shifted to the left or right) adaptively or pathologically. A rightward shift of the curve signifies that, at a given PaO_2, hemoglobin has *less* affinity for oxygen, and a smaller percentage of total binding sites are occupied. This means that hemoglobin more readily releases its oxygen to tissues.

Increases in $PaCO_2$, hydrogen ions (H^+), 2,3-DPG, or temperature all induce refolding of globin proteins, shifting the curve to the right. Formation of carbamino compounds with carbon dioxide binding reduces the affinity of hemoglobin for oxygen. Binding of H^+ ions has a similar effect, and as discussed in Chapter 10, hemoglobin serves as an important intracellular buffer of H^+. These two factors are interrelated because increasing amounts of carbon dioxide in the blood lead to increased amounts of H^+ (acidosis) by the hydrolysis reaction. The rightward shift in the dissociation curve in acidosis, known as the **Bohr effect**, normally results in unloading of oxygen to tissues such as actively contracting muscle. The effects of temperature and 2,3-DPG are consistent with this adaptive purpose. Exercising muscle would also be generating more heat, and as discussed in Chapter 3, red blood cells would produce more 2,3-DPG during anaerobic metabolism.

Pathologic conditions that may result in rightward shift of the curve include hyperthyroidism, **anemia**, chronic hypoxia, and certain abnormalities of hemoglobin synthesis (see discussion of hemoglobinopathies, Chapter 12). Although the rightward shift enhances oxygen delivery to tissues, supplemental oxygen may be necessary in such cases to prevent tissue hypoxia due to the low PaO_2.

Although a decrease in affinity under these conditions is designed to be an adaptive response to increased metabolic demands of tissues, these same factors would theoretically result in decreased oxygen uptake at the alveolar capillary membrane, offsetting the beneficial tissue effects. This does not occur because the local diffusion of oxygen and carbon dioxide in the lungs normally prevents carbon dioxide accumulation and acidosis and limits anaerobic glycolysis. Also, pulmonary tissues have a lower metabolic rate than peripheral tissues; thus, the local temperature is lower. Because of these differences in local conditions, oxygen uptake is favored in the lungs, whereas oxygen release is favored in peripheral tissues.

Shift to the Left. A shift to the left of the dissociation curve indicates that hemoglobin has higher affinity for oxygen. Uptake of oxygen in the lungs is further enhanced, and release to tissues is inhibited. This configuration of the curve is appropriately induced by low metabolic rates in tissues, producing parameters opposite those discussed previously. Neonates normally have a leftward shift because their blood contains a significant amount of fetal hemoglobin (Hb F). The slightly altered shape of the globin subunits of Hb F confer a higher affinity than

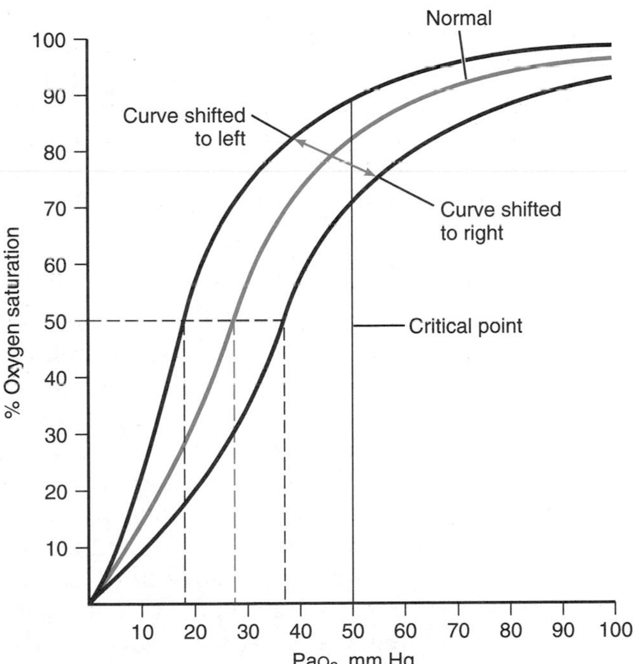

FIGURE 19–4

Oxyhemoglobin dissociation curve. The relationship between the partial pressure of oxygen in arterial blood (PaO_2) and the percentage of hemoglobin-binding sites occupied by oxygen is illustrated. The sigmoid shape of the curve results from variability in the affinity of remaining binding sites when one or more of the four sites on each hemoglobin molecule is occupied. The slope of the curve may be altered by numerous physiologic and pathologic factors. A shift to the left indicates higher affinity and, therefore, decreased oxygen release to tissues, whereas a shift to the right demonstrates the opposite condition. In clinical situations in which PaO_2 falls below 50 mm Hg, oxygen binding to hemoglobin drops sharply, and respiratory failure is imminent.

that of adult hemoglobin (Hb A). As discussed in Chapter 32, this arrangement favors oxygen transport from mother to fetus during pregnancy. Hb F is replaced by Hb A during the first few months of life.

A pathologic condition that may shift the curve to the left is **carbon monoxide intoxication**, detailed later in this chapter. Colorless, odorless carbon monoxide gas has a higher affinity for the heme site than does oxygen. With carbon monoxide poisoning, hemoglobin is well saturated, but tissues become hypoxic because the oxygen contained in carbon monoxide gas is not released from binding sites. At the same time, occupation of these sites prevents binding of oxygen. Massive transfusion of banked blood may also cause a leftward shift because 2,3-DPG leaves red blood cells during storage. Some hemoglobinopathies may also result in a shift to the left. **Methemoglobinemia**, in which heme iron is oxidized from the ferrous (Fe^{2+}) to the ferric (Fe^{3+}) state, is an uncommon disorder in which the affinity of any normal (Fe^{2+}) hemoglobin is increased. Methemoglobinemia is discussed later in this chapter.

Adaptive Alteration in Erythropoiesis

A rightward shift of the oxyhemoglobin dissociation curve in tissue hypoxia represents a short-term autoregulatory response to varying tissue needs for oxygen. A longer-term mechanism is activated with persistent tissue hypoxia, such as that seen with chronic lung disease or cyanotic heart defects. The hormone erythropoietin, released from hypoxic renal cells, stimulates the bone marrow to increase the rate of maturation and release of red blood cells. The erythropoietin response results in a detectable increase in oxygen-carrying capacity within 5 days. As discussed in Chapter 20, decreased erythropoietin production may result in anemia in patients with renal failure. Chronic activation of the erythropoietin mechanism may result in clinical manifestations of secondary polycythemia, in which red blood cell excess may compromise circulation because of increased blood viscosity (see Chapter 12).

Binding of Carbon Dioxide to Hemoglobin

As stated earlier, about 20% of carbon dioxide is normally transported in combination with hemoglobin. Carbon dioxide binds with high affinity in a linear relationship to the partial pressure of carbon dioxide in the blood ($PaCO_2$). Affinity for carbon dioxide is highest when hemoglobin is deoxygenated. This effect, known as the **Haldane effect**, favors loading of hemoglobin with carbon dioxide at the tissue level and unloading of carbon dioxide in the lungs, for excretion by ventilation.

Carbon Dioxide Transport Within the Bicarbonate Buffer System

As discussed in Chapter 10, most carbon dioxide travels in the blood in some stage of the carbonic acid–sodium bicarbonate buffer system. About 70% of carbon dioxide is transported as bicarbonate anion (HCO_3^-), which is reconstituted to carbon dioxide gas by reversal of the hydrolysis reaction (dehydration) in the pulmonary capillaries.

DIFFUSION OF GASES ACROSS THE ALVEOLAR–CAPILLARY MEMBRANE

Oxygen and carbon dioxide diffuse passively through the lipid portion of most biologic membranes, driven by pressure gradients (see Chapter 2). Simple diffusion predominates, although some oxygen transport may also be mediated by carrier proteins (facilitated diffusion). Pulmonary gas diffusion varies as a function of four factors: (1) membrane thickness, (2) membrane surface area, (3) diffusion coefficients of the gases, and (4) pressure gradients.

Membrane Thickness

As stated earlier, the alveolar–capillary membrane consists of several layers, all of which are highly permeable to the gases. Despite its multiple layers, the membrane is normally thin, such that the diffusion distance is about 0.6 μm. Accumulation of fluid in the interstitial spaces between alveoli and capillaries may occur in inflammatory conditions of the lung (e.g., pneumonia) or in congestive heart failure. Third-spacing of fluid into alveoli may occur with severe pulmonary edema, discussed later in this chapter. Severe or chronic inflammatory conditions may lead to fibrin deposition and scarring of membrane tissues.

Thickening of the alveolar capillary membrane is an uncommon cause of respiratory failure because the diffusion time available exceeds the usual equilibration time for the gases, as discussed in Chapter 18. This reserve diffusion time is lost at rapid heart rates, however, and if sufficiently thickened by fluid or fibrin, the membrane itself may impede diffusion. In such cases, oxygen diffusion is affected earlier and more severely because oxygen is less soluble in biologic membranes than is carbon dioxide.

Membrane Surface Area

The normal surface area available for gas exchange ranges from 50 to 100 m^2 in adults, up to 75% more than is needed for minimal function. Because of this pulmonary reserve, most people can tolerate loss of one entire lung. As discussed in Chapter 18, extensive loss of surface area may occur in advanced emphysema, resulting in decreased gas exchange owing to this mechanism.

Diffusion Coefficients

The diffusion coefficient of a gas is determined on the basis of its molecular weight and its solubility in water. Carbon dioxide is 20 times as soluble as oxygen, and oxygen is about twice as soluble as nitrogen (N_2). Oxygen and carbon dioxide are small enough and soluble enough to be readily transported by simple diffusion in healthy lungs. Nitrogen does not diffuse from the air to the blood in appreciable amounts except under nonphysiologic pressure conditions such as might be encountered by deep-sea divers or aviators. **Decompression disorders** are discussed later in this chapter.

Pressure Gradients

Under normal conditions, exchange of oxygen and carbon dioxide is driven by differences in partial pressures of the gases on either side of the alveolar–capillary membrane. These pressure gradients vary at different points within the airways and the circulation, as shown in Figure 19–5.

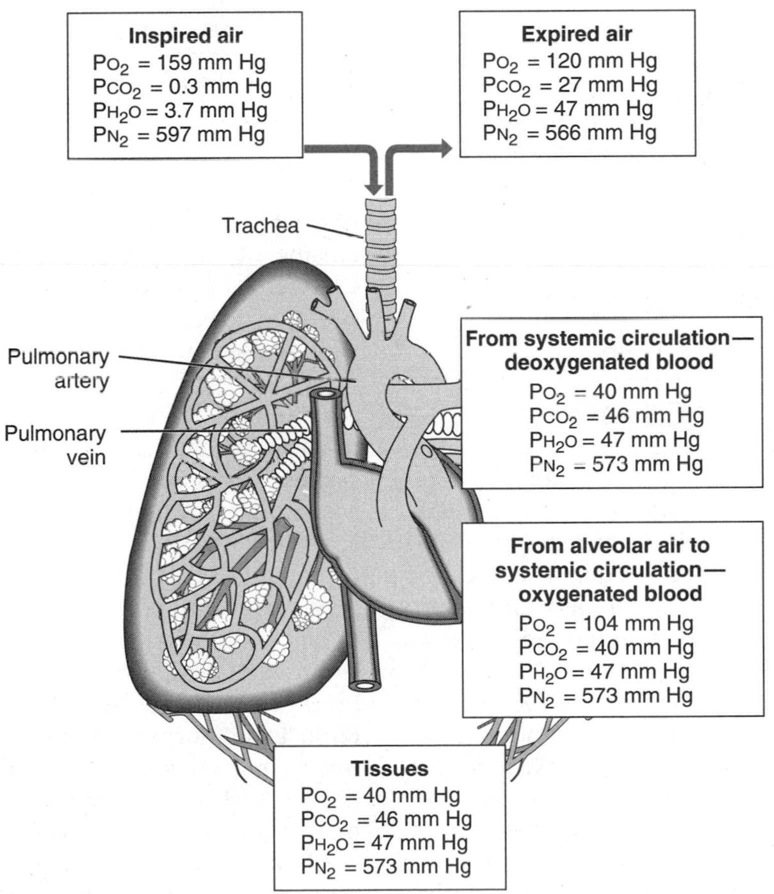

FIGURE 19–5

Pressure gradients for gas diffusion. Exchange of oxygen and carbon dioxide between the air and the blood is driven by pressure gradients, which vary at different levels of the pulmonary system. At the alveolar level, a gradient of about 104:40 promotes oxygen transport from alveolar air to pulmonary blood. A smaller gradient of about 46:40 drives carbon dioxide diffusion from pulmonary capillary blood to alveolar air. The smaller gradient for carbon dioxide transport is sufficient, given its higher diffusion coefficient. (Adapted from Thompson, J.M., McFarland, G.K., Hirsch, J.E., *et al.* [1993]. *Mosby's Clinical Nursing.* [3rd ed.]. St. Louis: Mosby–Year Book.)

Alveolar air has a PO_2 of about 104 mm Hg. This is less than the PO_2 of inspired air (as measured at the mouth) because inspired air is mixed with less-oxygenated dead-space air and residual air in the lungs, and because some inspired oxygen is constantly diffusing across the walls of respiratory units into the blood. The PCO_2 of 40 mm Hg in alveolar air originates almost entirely from diffusion of carbon dioxide from the blood because the amount of carbon dioxide in inspired air is negligible. Alveolar air has a water vapor pressure (PH_2O) of about 47 mm Hg, greater than that of the inspired air, owing to absorption of water from the walls of the upper humidifying airways. The nitrogen pressure (PN_2) is similar to that of inspired air and, because of its low solubility, remains relatively stable throughout respiration to assist in keeping airways open.

Pulmonary capillary blood ("venous" or "deoxygenated" blood) has a PO_2 of 40 mm Hg and a PCO_2 of 46 mm Hg. Comparison with values for alveolar air reveals gradients of 104:40 driving oxygen from alveoli into blood and 46:40 driving carbon dioxide from blood into alveolar air. The small gradient for carbon dioxide transport is more than adequate because of its higher solubility. Arterial blood gas values are achieved when gradients are exhausted, normally resulting in a $PaCO_2$ of 35 to 45 mm Hg and a PaO_2 of 80 to 100 mm Hg (see Chapter 10).

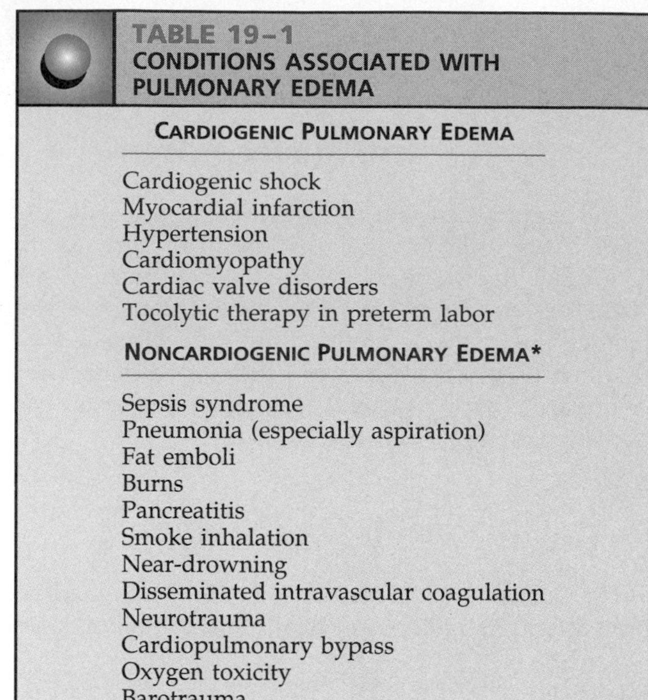

TABLE 19–1
CONDITIONS ASSOCIATED WITH PULMONARY EDEMA

Cardiogenic Pulmonary Edema
Cardiogenic shock
Myocardial infarction
Hypertension
Cardiomyopathy
Cardiac valve disorders
Tocolytic therapy in preterm labor
Noncardiogenic Pulmonary Edema*
Sepsis syndrome
Pneumonia (especially aspiration)
Fat emboli
Burns
Pancreatitis
Smoke inhalation
Near-drowning
Disseminated intravascular coagulation
Neurotrauma
Cardiopulmonary bypass
Oxygen toxicity
Barotrauma
Hantavirus pulmonary syndrome

*Noncardiogenic pulmonary edema is a component of adult respiratory distress syndrome, which may also result from many of these conditions (see Table 19–2).

DISORDERS OF GAS TRANSPORT AND EXCHANGE

Pulmonary Edema

Definition. Pulmonary edema is the abnormal accumulation of fluid in the interstitial spaces surrounding alveoli, with possible fluid exudation into alveolar air spaces. Pulmonary edema associated with cardiac failure is classified as *cardiogenic*, whereas that due to other causes is termed *noncardiogenic*.

Epidemiology. Cardiogenic pulmonary edema is a manifestation of left ventricular failure and is commonly encountered in clinical settings. Risk factors for cardiac failure are discussed in Chapter 16. Noncardiogenic pulmonary edema is associated with a variety of causes. Risk factors for the underlying conditions are relevant to the development of this form. Table 19–1 lists disorders associated with pulmonary edema.

Etiology. Pulmonary edema results from two mechanisms: (1) increased pulmonary capillary hydrostatic pressure (CHP), which favors net filtration of fluid from capillaries to the interstitium, and (2) abnormally increased capillary permeability. (Mechanisms of capillary fluid exchange are detailed in Chapter 8.) Cardiogenic pulmonary edema, the most common form, is the result of increased pulmonary CHP caused by the congestive effects of left ventricular failure (Fig. 19–6). Pulmonary lymphatic obstruction, which also increases CHP, may cause pulmonary edema in primary or metastatic lung cancers involving lymphatic vessels. The fluid that accumulates in the pulmonary interstitium as a consequence of increased CHP is a clear **transudate**, containing little protein.

Increased pulmonary capillary permeability occurs as an endothelial response to locally released and circulating mediators. Severe sepsis is characterized by the presence of such mediators (see Chapter 13). Fluid exudation in inflammation of the lower respiratory tract may produce pulmonary edema in conditions such as pneumonia or **pleurisy**. Both abnormal permeability of pulmonary capillaries and reactive systemic hypertension may occur with brain tumors or serious head injuries, causing *neurogenic pulmonary edema*. The causative mechanism of pulmonary edema in such cases is unknown.

Pathophysiology. Hypoxemia occurs if the alveolar–capillary membrane is thickened by fluid to the extent that gas diffusion is impaired. If fluid is third spaced into alveoli or into the intrapleural space,

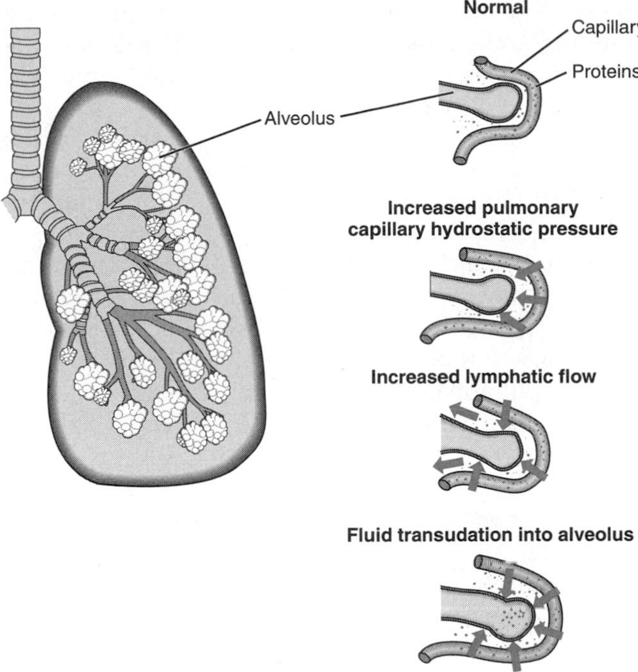

FIGURE 19–6

Progression of pulmonary edema. Pulmonary edema occurs when capillary hydrostatic pressure is increased, promoting transudation of fluid into the interstitial space of the alveolar–capillary membrane. Initially, increased lymphatic flow removes the excess interstitial fluid, but continued transudation eventually overwhelms this mechanism, and gas exchange is impaired by increased thickness of the membrane. Increasing interstitial fluid pressure ultimately results in the entry of fluid into alveolar air spaces, impeding ventilation and contributing to further impairment of gas exchange.

further detriment to gas exchange results from impaired ventilation. With respect to cardiac function, increased pulmonary artery pressure represents high right ventricular afterload, potentiating right ventricular failure (see Chapter 16). Because right ventricular failure may lead to left ventricular failure, the potential for development of a positive feedback loop exists. All organ systems potentially suffer hypoxemic effects associated with lack of both oxygenation and perfusion.

Clinical Manifestations. The respiratory system manifests effects of increased work of breathing, including dyspnea, use of accessory muscles, and potential respiratory failure. Pressure in the pulmonary microvasculature is measurable with use of a Swan-Ganz pulmonary artery catheter (see Chapter 16). Pulmonary artery wedge pressure is elevated when increased CHP is the causative mechanism but remains normal if increased permeability is the cause. Fluid transudation or exudation into the alveolar air spaces in severe pulmonary edema is evident as "whiteout" areas on the chest radiograph (Fig. 19–7) and results in frequent cough with production of thin, frothy sputum. Fluid in the airways is audible with a stethoscope, manifesting as **crackles** or **rhonchi**. If the CHP is very high, red blood cells may exude into the sputum, giving it a pink color. Right ventricular failure may manifest as jugular venous distention, hepatomegaly and splenomegaly, and dependent edema, as discussed in Chapter 16.

Prevention and Treatment. Prevention of pulmonary edema requires optimal management of the underlying causes. In many instances, this involves medical management of congestive heart failure. Maintenance of oxygen diffusion in severe pulmonary edema often requires oxygen therapy at high FIO_2 and mechanical ventilation using high driving pressures and positive end-expiratory pressure (PEEP). These measures impose a risk of iatrogenic complications, such as oxygen toxicity and barotrauma, as discussed in Chapter 18.

Prognosis and Outcome. Mild pulmonary edema is common with chronic congestive heart failure and usually responds to adjustment of diuretic or other drug therapy. Severe pulmonary edema culminating in respiratory failure carries a grave prognosis, owing to the usual severity of the underlying condition and the risks inherent in the therapy.

Adult Respiratory Distress Syndrome

Definition. ARDS, formerly known as *shock lung*, is a condition in which there is severe, diffuse injury of the alveolar–capillary membrane, resulting in in-

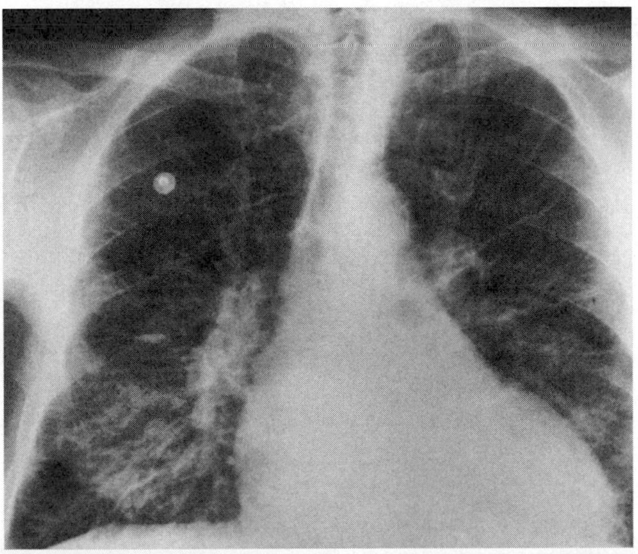

FIGURE 19–7

Pulmonary edema. (From Fraser, R.G., Paré, P., Paré, P.D., *et al.* [1988]. *Diagnosis of Diseases of the Chest.* [3rd ed.]. Philadelphia: W.B. Saunders. [p. 547].)

creased stiffness of the lungs and noncardiogenic pulmonary edema.

Epidemiology. An estimated 150,000 cases of ARDS occur annually in the United States.[4] ARDS is a complication of critical illness, most often trauma and sepsis. Because the disorder occurs in critically ill children as well as in adults, use of the more inclusive name, *acute respiratory distress syndrome*, has been suggested.[5] Conditions associated with ARDS are listed in Table 19–2 and discussed subsequently.

Etiology. The alveolar–capillary membrane injury that initiates ARDS may result from ischemia in shock, from oxygen toxicity (associated with bronchopulmonary dysplasia), from inhalation of toxic smoke, from aspiration of toxic substances (e.g., gastrointestinal contents containing enzymes or acids), or from inflammatory injury secondary to pneumonia or sepsis.

Pathophysiology. Mediators of the inflammatory response are produced in excess, leading to diffuse lung injury and greatly increased pulmonary capillary permeability. Four phases of the disorder have been characterized.[6] A *phase 1 injury* consists of damage to the pulmonary capillary endothelium mediated by increased adhesion of neutrophils, generation of reactive oxygen species, and induction of protease enzymes. With *phase 2 injury*, the damage extends to the basement membrane, interstitial space, and alveolar epithelium. Fluid, protein, blood cells, and fibrin exude into interstitial spaces around alveoli, increasing diffusion distance and lung stiffness. Impaired alveolar ventilation and increased work of breathing result from this intrapulmonary shunting and decreased compliance. *Phase 3 injury* is seen when the source of the sepsis persists and further mediator release occurs. The injured lung becomes a significant source of these mediators. *Phase 4 injury* is characterized by increasing pulmonary sepsis and irreversible deposition of fibrin, further reducing compliance.

Throughout this process, increasing damage to type II alveolar cells results in surfactant deficiency and alveolar collapse (atelectasis), which decreases pulmonary compliance. Reduced ventilation triggers hypoxic pulmonary vasoconstriction, increasing PVR and cardiac workload. Hemodynamic instability usually manifests as septic shock initially, with cardiogenic shock ultimately resulting from cardiac failure associated with hypoxemia and increased right ventricular afterload (see Chapter 15). Oxygen toxicity and barotrauma resulting from treatment of the disorder may contribute to further damage in a positive feedback loop.

Clinical Manifestations. The European-American Consensus Conference established objective criteria that define the diagnosis of ARDS: (1) impaired oxygenation, resulting in a PaO_2/FIO_2 ratio of 300 or less; (2) fluid exudation, evident as bilateral pulmonary infiltrates on chest radiographs; and (3) a noncardiogenic mechanism of pulmonary edema, demonstrated by a pulmonary artery wedge pressure of 18 mm Hg or less.[7]

Gas exchange is impaired as a consequence of the thickened membrane and impaired ventilation, resulting in severe hypoxemia early and **hypercapnia** later. Respiratory failure resulting from impaired diffusion and greatly decreased pulmonary compliance manifests as tachypnea and dyspnea. Crackles and rhonchi are audible secondary to pulmonary edema. Increased PVR leads to right-sided heart failure, manifested as jugular venous distention, hepatomegaly, and peripheral edema. Stress ulceration of the gastric mucosa occurs in most patients, leading to hemorrhage, which worsens the shock state (see Chapter 24). Multiple-system organ failure results from irreversible hypoxic injury in phase 4.

Prevention and Treatment. There are no specific preventive measures for ARDS, other than optimal treatment of conditions that may precede its development. The shock state, if present, is treated with cautious fluid replacement. Septicemia is treated with appropriate antibiotic therapy. Prophylactic use of antacids may reduce the risk of stress ulceration.

Treatment of the respiratory manifestations of ARDS is symptomatic and supportive. Steroid therapy was once considered detrimental but has been shown to be of benefit in halting the progression of late-phase fibrin deposition, thereby improving com-

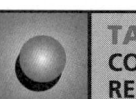

TABLE 19–2
CONDITIONS ASSOCIATED WITH ADULT RESPIRATORY DISTRESS SYNDROME

CONDITIONS CAUSING DIRECT INJURY TO ALVEOLAR–CAPILLARY MEMBRANE
Aspiration of gastric contents
Near-drowning
Smoke inhalation
Pneumonia
Barotrauma (mechanical ventilation)
Pulmonary embolism
SYSTEMIC DISORDERS CAUSING INDIRECT LUNG INJURY
Oxygen toxicity
Sepsis syndrome (especially gram-negative)
Shock
Pancreatitis
Disseminated intravascular coagulation
Cardiopulmonary bypass
Burns
Multiple trauma
Massive blood transfusion
Uremia

pliance.[6] Oxygen therapy and mechanical ventilation are mainstays of therapy. The goal is to use the lowest FIO_2 and the lowest tidal volumes and airway pressures possible while still achieving a reasonable PaO_2. The use of the PEEP mode of mechanical ventilation maintains some degree of positive pressure within the airways during expiration. PEEP results in the ventilation of additional alveoli, improving $\dot{V}/\dot{Q}$ relationships, but imposes the risk of volutrauma due to overdistention of previously ventilated alveoli. Several new modes of ventilatory support are in clinical trials, including inverse-ratio ventilation, high-frequency ventilation, and extracorporeal membrane oxygenation (see Chapter 18). Thus far, no one mode has been shown to be superior in the treatment of ARDS.[6] Administration of nitric oxide by inhalation is also under investigation for relief of hypoxemia.[8] This agent selectively dilates the pulmonary vasculature, improving $\dot{V}/\dot{Q}$ relationships.

Prognosis and Outcome. The mortality rate in ARDS is about 60%.[4] Patients who survive may have permanent lung dysfunction due to treatment-induced bronchopulmonary dysplasia (see Chapter 18).

Pulmonary Embolism

Definition. Pulmonary embolism is the occlusion of one or more pulmonary arterial vessels by a bolus of material (usually a blood clot) arising from a source outside the lung.

Epidemiology. The precise incidence of pulmonary emboli is unknown, but the condition is believed to be common. Pulmonary emboli are found at 64% of autopsies, regardless of the cause of death.[9] About 600,000 cases of major pulmonary embolism occur each year, and half of these individuals die within 2 hours. Risk factors for inappropriate thrombosis were detailed in Chapter 14. Predominant among these in adults is immobility, which promotes slow blood flow and venous clotting due to loss of the skeletal muscle pump. Atrial fibrillation is often associated with formation of mural thrombi due to ineffective atrial contraction (see Chapter 17). The incidence of pulmonary emboli in the pediatric population has been estimated at 3.7%.[10] In children, the presence of a central venous catheter imposes the greatest risk, followed by immobility and heart disease.

Etiology. Because small pulmonary emboli are common, it has been proposed that filtering such clots before their entry into the arterial circulation (where they could cause significant infarction) is a physiologic function of the lungs.[11] Although deep vein thrombosis most frequently affects the venous system of the calves, most emboli originate from venous clots in the pelvis. Untreated clots in the calves may propagate upward, increasing the likelihood of embolization. In a significant number of patients who have undergone general surgery or who have suffered skeletal trauma, clots originate in more proximal vessels.

Factors that promote mobilization of these clots are uncertain. As the clot retracts during normal hemostasis, the resulting increase in blood flow may cause the "tail" of the clot to break free into the bloodstream (see Chapter 14). Muscle contraction or manipulation of the tissues surrounding the clot may also promote embolization. Valsalva maneuver has also been associated with embolization, owing to increased thoracic pumping force and vagally induced vasodilation (see Chapter 15).

Mural thrombi in the atria may break free due to the hemodynamic effects of correction of an underlying atrial dysrhythmia. Clots in the right atrium would embolize to the lung. Less common causes of pulmonary emboli include clumps of bacterial "vegetations" formed on cardiac valves as a consequence of infective endocarditis (see Chapter 16), fat emboli originating from yellow bone marrow entering the bloodstream as a consequence of long bone fractures (see Chapter 34), and amniotic fluid emboli occurring as a complication of labor and delivery (see Chapter 32).

Pathophysiology. In most cases, large clots are broken up as they pass through the heart, resulting in the distribution of multiple small clots in the pulmonary vascular system. This creates several high $\dot{V}/\dot{Q}$ areas and potentially impairs gas exchange, with the extent of respiratory distress depending on the number of clots. If one or more large clots are passed into the pulmonary arterial system, an abrupt increase in PVR occurs, owing to occlusion of a major vessel. The abrupt increase in right ventricular afterload causes right ventricular pressure to rise suddenly, shifting the interventricular septum toward the left ventricle and impeding its filling.[12] Decreased coronary perfusion, myocardial ischemia, and cardiogenic shock may result. **Pulmonary infarction** occurs in about 10% of patients with massive embolism, when the bronchial circulation cannot compensate sufficiently for loss of pulmonary arterial perfusion.

Clinical Manifestations. It is believed that many pulmonary emboli result in no symptoms or very mild symptoms that may go unnoticed by the patient. Respiratory distress due to pulmonary emboli may range from mild dyspnea to overt respiratory failure, depending on the degree of occlusion and the state of the patient's pulmonary reserve. An imaging procedure, the ventilation–perfusion lung scan ($\dot{V}/\dot{Q}$ scan), may demonstrate lack of perfusion in normally ventilated areas, indicating that hypoxic pulmonary vasoconstriction is not the mechanism of vascular obstruction. With massive emboli, severe chest pain is present from ischemia associated with profound heart failure and possible pulmonary infarction. Electrocardiographic changes may reveal the increased strain on the right ventricle (see Chapter 17). Venous congestion behind the failing right ventricle is apparent as jugular venous distention. Sudden cardiac death is common with massive emboli. Patients who survive the acute episode may suffer from manifestations of multiple organ failure due to tissue hypoxia.

Prevention and Treatment. Prevention of inappropriate thrombosis involves risk reduction, as discussed in Chapter 14, with particular emphasis on optimal ambulation. In the presence of a high-risk state for thrombosis, anticoagulant therapy or use of an inferior vena cava filter may be indicated. The risk of inadvertent vagal stimulation may be reduced with antiemetic drug therapy to prevent nausea and vomiting and with stool softeners to prevent straining with defecation. Bedridden patients should be cautioned against straining with position changes or during use of an overhead trapeze and should be taught to breathe through all activities. If the patient has access to medical care soon after embolization has occurred, thrombolytic therapy (e.g., tissue plasminogen activator, streptokinase, urokinase) may be used to dissolve blood clots. Surgical embolectomy may be an option for some patients. Medical support of cardiac function and mechanical support of pulmonary function may also be required.

Prognosis and Outcome. Ten per cent of people with acute pulmonary embolism die within 1 hour of the event.[10] If diagnosis and treatment are delayed, symptomatic pulmonary embolism has a 35% mortality rate. With early recognition and appropriate therapy, mortality may be reduced to 8%.

Primary Pulmonary Hypertension

Definition. Primary pulmonary hypertension refers to sustained elevation of pulmonary artery pressure in the absence of a specific cause, such as congestive heart failure, congenital heart disease, or chronic respiratory disease.[13] In neonates, the disorder is known as persistent pulmonary hypertension of the newborn (PPHN).[14]

Epidemiology. The incidence of primary pulmonary hypertension within the general population has been estimated at 1 to 2 per million.[13] Among certain at-risk subgroups, however, the incidence is much higher. Patients with acquired immunodeficiency syndrome (AIDS) and adults with portal hypertension due to cirrhosis are at higher risk. Cocaine abuse, recent pregnancy, and use of oral contraceptives may also confer increased risk. Treatment of obesity with appetite suppressants such as fenfluramine and dexfenfluramine is also associated with increased risk[15] (see Focus of Current Research). A genetic predisposition is apparent in some cases, and a rare familial form demonstrates autosomal dominant inheritence.[13] Among neonates, the syndrome is often associated with lung hypoplasia, meconium aspiration, bacterial pneumonia, congenital diaphragmatic hernia, and surfactant deficiency.[14]

Etiology. In adults, increased PVR is the result of vasoconstriction, remodeling of the pulmonary vascular wall, and thrombosis, occurring in sequence.[13] Abnormal endothelial regulation of pulmonary vascular tone is believed to underlie the initial vasoconstriction, although the specific mediators are unknown. Proliferation of smooth muscle cells in the vessel wall follows, and thrombosis may then be triggered by endothelial injury or abnormality of coagulation or fibrinolytic processes.

In infants, the high PVR, which is the normal intrauterine state, persists abnormally. As discussed in Chapter 33, several factors inherent in the transition to extrauterine life normally result in greatly reduced PVR during the first few days of life. Increased pulmonary volumes with initial ventilatory efforts combine with changes in endogenous mediators of endothelial regulation to cause vasodilation. These mechanisms are impaired in PPHN. Vasoconstriction predominates, and ventilation is compromised.

Pathophysiology. Increased PVR results in right-sided heart failure (cor pulmonale) with compensatory dilation and hypertrophy of the right ventricle. Pressure of the enlarged right ventricle may eventually compress the left ventricle, limiting its filling and further reducing cardiac output. Ventilation–perfusion impairment is usually mild and patchy but results in some degree of hypoxemia. In neonates, increased PVR leads to right-to-left shunting through a patent ductus arteriosus and foramen ovale (see Chapter 16).

Clinical Manifestations. In adults, the onset of symptoms is gradual, with increasing dyspnea, fatigue, chest pain, edema, and possible syncope. Symptoms are consistent with class III or IV severity of heart failure according to the New York Heart Association classification (see Chapter 16). About 10% of patients report symptoms of digital vaso-

Focus of Current Research

Study	Objective and Findings
Markowitz, et al. (1997) Incidence of tuberculosis in the United States among HIV-infected persons.	*Objective:* To determine the incidence and predictors of tuberculosis in people infected with human immunodeficiency virus *Findings:* Incidence of tuberculosis was higher in the eastern United States in patients with CD4+ T-lymphocyte counts of less than 200 cells/mm^3 and in PPD-positive patients. Nonreactivity to mumps antigen indicated increased risk.
Anzueto, et al. (1996) Aerosolized surfactant in adults with sepsis-induced acute respiratory distress syndrome.	*Objective:* To evaluate the efficacy of surfactant replacement on mortality in adults with acute respiratory distress syndrome *Findings:* Continuous administration of aerosolized surfactant had no significant effect on survival, duration of mechanical ventilation, length of stay in intensive care, or physiologic function.
Hirsch, et al. (1996) Pulmonary embolism and deep venous thrombosis during pregnancy or oral contraceptive use: Prevalence of factor V Leiden.	*Objective:* To assess the frequency of a specific mutation in the gene coding for clotting factor V in women with venous thromboembolism during and after pregnancy or during use of oral contraceptives *Findings:* 10% of the women were heterozygous for the mutation, and 60% of this subgroup developed pulmonary embolism or deep venous thrombosis, as compared with 8% of women without the mutation.
Pouchot, et al. (1996) Reliability of tuberculin skin test measurement.	*Objective:* To ascertain the reliability of tuberculin skin test measurement *Findings:* Reading of skin tests may frequently result in misclassifications when measurements are close to the cutoff point that separates negative from positive results.
Robertson, et al. (1996) Delayed tuberculin reactivity in persons of Indochinese origin: Implications for preventive therapy.	*Objective:* To study a variant delayed reaction to tuberculin testing and to correlate the delayed reaction with lymphocyte blastogenesis *Findings:* Variant reactivity, an induration of less than 10 mm at 72 hours that increased in size after 6 days, was a predictor of positivity. An intermediate lymphocyte blastogenesis response also correlated with this finding.

Box continued on following page

continued from previous page

Study	Objective / Findings
Abenheim, et al. (1996) Appetite-suppressant drugs and the risk of primary pulmonary hypertension.	*Objective:* To investigate the potential role of anorexic agents in primary pulmonary hypertension *Findings:* The risk of pulmonary hypertension was more than six-fold in individuals who had used anorexic drugs such as fenfluramine, dexfenfluramine, and amphetamines.
Barnes, et al. (1996) Transmission of tuberculosis among the urban homeless.	*Objective:* To determine the percentages of primary versus reactivation tuberculosis in the urban homeless *Findings:* The percentage of cases due to primary tuberculosis was estimated to be 53%, as compared with a 10% estimate in the general population.
Kenyon, et al. (1996) Transmission of multidrug-resistant *Mycobacterium tuberculosis* during a long airplane flight.	*Objective:* To determine whether an infected passenger infected any of her contacts during an extensive trip *Findings:* On follow-up testing, 15 people were found to have positive skin tests and no other risk factors for tuberculosis. Six of these had sat in the same section of the plane as the infected patient.
Klonoff-Cohen and Edelstein (1995) A case-control study of routine and death scene sleep position and sudden infant death syndrome in Southern California.	*Objective:* To investigate whether infants who died of sudden infant death syndrome were routinely placed in different sleep positions than healthy infants *Findings:* Routine prone sleep position was not associated with an increased risk of sudden infant death syndrome in the study population.
Moser, et al. (1994) Frequent asymptomatic pulmonary embolism in patients with deep venous thrombosis.	*Objective:* To determine the frequency of pulmonary embolism in patients admitted for treatment of deep venous thrombosis *Findings:* Nearly 40% of patients who did not have symptoms had evidence of pulmonary embolism on chest radiograph and ventilation–perfusion scans.

spasm similar to Raynaud's phenomenon (see Chapter 15). Pulmonary artery pressure, measured with a Swan-Ganz catheter, may rise to more than three times normal.

Prevention and Treatment. Preventive measures are appropriately directly to associated disorders, when known. Reduction of the risks of AIDS, cirrhosis, and preterm delivery are discussed in Chapters 13, 26, and 32, respectively. In adults, primary pulmonary hypertension is treated supportively with vasodilators, including nitric oxide, prostacyclin, or adenosine. Calcium-channel blockers may also be used but may have detrimental effects on cardiac failure because of their negative inotropic effect. Vasodilator therapy also imposes a risk of worsening $\dot{V}/\dot{Q}$ relationships. Anticoagulant therapy is usually warranted to reduce pulmonary thrombosis. Creation of a channel (right-to-left shunt) between the atrial septa with a catheter-directed blade has been reported to reduce right ventricular dilation and improve cardiac output. Primary pulmonary hypertension is one of the more frequent disorders for which lung transplantation or combined heart and lung transplantation are indicated. Infants with PPHN may be treated with vasodilators, mechanical ventilation, and aerosolized surfactant therapy within the context of neonatal intensive care. Extracorporeal membrane oxygenation, a heart and lung bypass intervention, has been used in cases that were unresponsive to these measures (see Chapter 18).[16]

Prognosis and Outcome. In adults, the median survival after diagnosis is 2.5 years.[13] Most patients die of progressive right-sided cardiac failure, although some suffer sudden cardiac death due to dysrhythmia. Neonates with PPHN have less than a 20% chance of survival.

Pneumonia

Definition. Pneumonia is inflammation of the respiratory unit tissues (alveoli, alveolar ducts, and respiratory bronchioles). Two subclassifications are recognized: *community-acquired pneumonia* and *nosocomial pneumonia* (that acquired in a hospital or nursing home).

Epidemiology. About 4 million cases of pneumonia are diagnosed each year, and it is still the sixth leading cause of death in the United States and the leading cause of death due to infection.[17] Risk factors for development of pneumonia include immunosuppression (see Chapter 13), decreased level of consciousness, impaired pulmonary defenses (e.g., due to cigarette smoking), instrumentation of the pulmonary system (e.g., intubation, suctioning, or mechanical ventilation), immobility, aging, malnutrition, alcohol abuse, and presence of underlying chronic cardiac or pulmonary disease. Institutional care in a hospital or nursing home is an independent risk factor for pneumonia.

Etiology. Pneumonia is usually caused by a microorganism (Table 19–3), which may be inhaled, transmitted by the bloodstream in septicemia, or introduced iatrogenically by instrumentation. Virulent organisms may cause pneumonia in otherwise healthy people, but most cases occur in compromised people such as the elderly or others with chronic illness. In the absence of infection, inflammation may be triggered by smoke inhalation, inhalation of environmental or occupational toxins, or aspiration of toxic materials, such as foreign bodies or gastrointestinal contents. **Aspiration pneumonia** is common in people who have impaired swallowing or cough reflexes, including unconscious people and stroke patients. Presence of a nasogastric tube, often placed to decompress the stomach and reduce the risk of aspiration, may paradoxically contribute to aspiration by rendering the lower esophageal sphincter incompetent and allowing retrograde flow of gastric contents.[18] Thick respiratory secretions due to dehydration and ciliary damage due to cigarette smoking may impede the mucociliary escalator and provide an ideal medium for proliferation of microorganisms.

Pathophysiology. Inflammation involves the alveoli, alveolar ducts, and interstitial spaces surrounding alveolar walls. Fluid exudate and products of the breakdown of microorganisms and phagocytic cells form a gel-like substance that consolidates within lower airways and respiratory units. Inflammation spreads in one of three patterns (Fig. 19–8). In **lobar pneumonia**, typical of aspiration (of anaerobic organisms) or infection with a virulent organism such as pneumococcus, the process starts in one area and may extend to fill an entire lobe. In **bronchopneumonia**, the most common pattern, inflammation starts simultaneously in several areas, producing patchy, diffuse consolidations. Bronchopneumonia is usually seen with infection by less virulent organisms in debilitated patients. The third pattern, **atypical pneumonia**, is one of patchy, diffuse involvement that spares the alveoli. Only the alveolar ducts and interstitial spaces are inflamed. Atypical pneumonia is frequently caused by viruses such as type A or B influenza, or by *Mycoplasma* sp. or *Legionella* sp. bacteria. Gas exchange is impaired by low $\dot{V}/\dot{Q}$ areas, and diffusion impairment may be caused by consolidation and fluid exudation, resulting in hypoxemia and possible respiratory failure.

Abscesses (pus-filled or necrotic areas) may form if the organism is walled off but not destroyed. **Pleural effusion** may occur if fluid exudes into the intrapleural space. Third spacing of purulent fluid results in **empyema**. Significant effusion may impair ventilation. Failure to contain the infection within lung tissue may result in pleurisy, pericarditis or septicemia. (In critically ill patients with both pneumonia and septicemia, it is often impossible to determine which is cause and which is effect.) In bacterial infections, signs of metastatic infection may be apparent, including infective endocarditis, septic arthritis, or osteomyelitis.[19] Severe or recurrent pneumonia may result in permanent dilation of affected areas (see discussion of bronchiectasis, Chapter 18).

Clinical Manifestations. Systemic signs of infection are usually present and include fever and leukocytosis. Work of breathing is increased, as evidenced by dyspnea and tachypnea. Sputum production is increased, and sputum may be blood-tinged or colored and foul-smelling, depending on the causative organism. Movement of fluid in the airways is audible with a stethoscope. In larger airways, coarse rattling sounds (rhonchi) may be heard, whereas finer crackles may be heard over alveoli as they pop open with inspiration. Breath sounds may be inaudible over consolidated areas, and the area is dull to percussion.

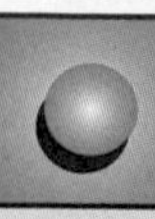

TABLE 19-3
CAUSATIVE ORGANISMS AND DRUG THERAPY OF PNEUMONIA*

Causative Organism	Drug Therapy
Bacteria (Typical Community-Acquired Pneumonia) *Streptococcus pneumoniae* Group A streptococci *Haemophilus influenzae* *Moraxella (Branhamella) catarrhalis* *Klebsiella* species *Staphylococcus aureus* *Pneumocystis carinii*	For outpatients without coexisting illness, age less than 60 years:* Erythromycin Azithromycin (Zithromax) Clarithromycin (Biaxin) Tetracycline For outpatients with coexisting illness, age 60 years or older:* Cefaclor (Ceclor) Cefpodoxime proxetil (Vantin) Cefuroxime (Ceftin, Kefurox) Loracarbef (Lorabid) Ceftriaxone (Rocephin) Trimethoprim, sulfamethoxazole (Bactrim, Septra) Amoxicillin, clavulanic acid (Augmentin)
Bacteria (Atypical Pneumonia) *Legionella* species *Mycoplasma pneumoniae* *Chlamydia pneumoniae*	Erythromycin Rifampin Doxycycline
Anaerobic Bacteria (Aspiration Pneumonia) Anaerobic cocci *Bacteroides fragilis* *Fusobacterium* species	Clindamycin Penicillin Metronidazole (Flagyl) Amoxicillin Cefoxitin (Mefoxin)
Bacteria (Nosocomial Pneumonia) *Pseudomonas aeruginosa* *Klebsiella pneumoniae* *Serratia marcescens*	Antipseudomonal penicillin Tobramycin Gentamycin Aztreonam Ceftazidime
Viruses Influenza Hantavirus	Amantadine Rimantadine Ribavirin (experimental)

* American Thoracic Society guidelines.

The chest radiograph reveals atelectasis, presence of consolidations, and the pattern of the pneumonia. Sputum culture may demonstrate presence of a causative organism. The cough reflex is stimulated by the presence of fluid in airways and by triggering of irritant receptors by the inflammatory process. Inflammation and muscle soreness due to frequent coughing result in dull chest pain.

Blood gases indicate hypoxemia and possibly respiratory failure (see Chapter 10). $PaCO_2$ is often low at first because the individual hyperventilates to compensate for low PaO_2. Hypercapnia occurs later in pneumonia, if at all, when the patient becomes too exhausted to ventilate adequately. Systemic signs of tissue hypoxia and acidosis depend on the degree and duration of impairment of gas exchange.

Prevention and Treatment. High-risk patients should be immunized against pneumococcus and influenza, and appropriate measures should be taken to limit their exposure to microorganisms. Hospital personnel must adhere to careful handwashing and other aseptic practices to reduce the risk of transmitting organisms among patients. Interventions such as turning, deep-breathing exercises, incentive spirometry, and early ambulation may be employed in the care of postoperative patients and others at risk for atelectasis and pneumonia (see Table 19–4).

Bacterial and fungal pneumonias are appropriately treated with antibiotic therapy (see Table 19–3). Supportive measures such as hydration and rest are important in facilitating an adaptive inflammatory response. Respiratory failure is treated with

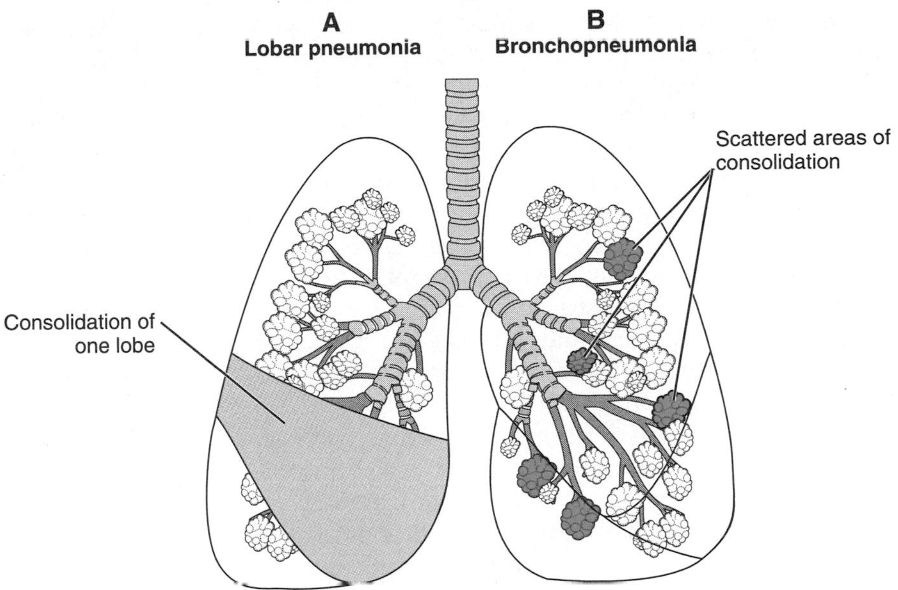

FIGURE 19–8

Patterns of pneumonia. The pattern of inflammatory consolidation in pneumonia may suggest the cause. In *lobar pneumonia,* inflammation begins in one area and may extend to fill an entire lobe. The lobar pattern is usually seen with aspiration or with infection by anaerobic or very virulent organisms. The most common pattern, *bronchopneumonia,* is characterized by the simultaneous development of inflammation in several areas, producing patchy, diffuse exudates. The involvement of alveoli often indicates infection with a less virulent organism in a debilitated patient (e.g., nosocomial pneumonia). Pneumonia producing scattered lesions similar to bronchopneumonia but sparing the alveoli is termed *atypical pneumonia* and is usually due to influenza viruses or to *Mycoplasma* or *Legionella* species of bacteria.

drug therapy, oxygen, and possibly mechanical ventilation, as discussed in Chapter 18.

Prognosis and Outcome. Uncomplicated, community-acquired pneumonias usually resolve completely within 6 weeks. Pneumonia occurring in debilitated people carries a poor prognosis. The mortality rate in hospitalized patients is 10% to 25%.[17] Pneumonia is often the terminal event in people with chronic cardiovascular or lung diseases.

Bronchiolitis

Definition. Bronchiolitis is inflammation of the bronchioles, typically occurring in infants under 2 years of age.

Epidemiology. The incidence in the first year of life is 11.4%, with peak incidence at 6 months of age.[20] Male infants, those of lower socioeconomic status, children in day care centers, children exposed

TABLE 19–4
PREVENTIVE MEASURES FOR ATELECTASIS AND PNEUMONIA

Intervention	Comments
Patient education	Methods by which risk factors, such as obesity and cigarette smoking, may be reduced should be stressed. Education may also promote patient compliance with therapy of underlying chronic respiratory disease.
Frequent change of position	Frequent turning and repositioning (every 2 hours) is effective in optimizing ventilation–perfusion relationships. Early and progressive ambulation stimulates ventilation and perfusion and promotes clearance of airway secretions. The risk of deep vein thrombosis and potential pulmonary embolism is reduced with activation of the skeletal muscle pump. Diaphragmatic deconditioning is minimized.
Pain management	Optimal management of postoperative or other pain enhances the effectiveness of position changes.
Deep-breathing exercises	Increased negativity of intrapleural pressure on inspiration enhances alveolar distention, reducing atelectasis. Deep-breathing exercises may be enhanced with use of an incentive spirometer, which provides feedback to the patient regarding the efficacy of inspiration. Deep-breathing exercises mimic the physiologic yawn and sigh reflexes.
Chest physiotherapy	Postural drainage, percussion, and vibration, done manually or mechanically, may enhance drainage of secretions.
Directed coughing	Spontaneous coughing is sufficient in many patients, but directed coughing (induced with deep breathing or "tracheal tickling") may be beneficial in those in whom the natural cough is inadequate. Incisions should be manually splinted to enhance patient comfort and security.

Data from Brooks-Brunn, J.A. (1995). Postoperative atelectasis and pneumonia. *Heart & Lung* 24(2), 94–115.

to environmental tobacco smoke, and those who were not breastfed (or breastfed for less than 1 month) are at higher risk. Bronchiolitis may also occur in children with congenital heart disease and in adults with chronic lung disease.

Etiology. Inflammation is usually triggered by a virus. **Respiratory syncytial virus** (RSV) is the major cause of lower respiratory tract infections in infants and children under the age of 3 years.[21] (RSV is much more likely to cause *upper* respiratory infections in older children and adults.) Outbreaks of RSV usually occur between November and April in the United States. Other microorganisms, including influenza viruses, mycoplasma, and other bacteria, may also cause bronchiolitis. Inhaled toxins in polluted air are less common causes of bronchiolitis.

Pathophysiology. In children with RSV infection, viral replication first occurs within the epithelium of the upper respiratory tract. Spread to the lower respiratory tract occurs in 40% to 50% of cases, causing either bronchiolitis or pneumonia.[22] Inflammation triggers necrosis of the respiratory epithelium and proliferation of goblet cells, increasing mucus production. Epithelium regenerates with nonciliated cells, impairing mucus clearance. Lymphocytic proliferation into the submucosa induces edema, which contributes to further obstruction of bronchioles. Air is trapped distal to the obstruction, and atelectasis occurs as this air is absorbed into pulmonary capillary blood. Low $\dot{V}/\dot{Q}$ units result and lead to impaired gas exchange.

Clinical Manifestations. Signs of both upper and lower respiratory infection may be apparent, and systemic signs of inflammation (fatigue, malaise, low-grade fever) are usually present to some degree. In infants, an acute phase may develop in which the child manifests significant respiratory distress, with tachypnea, retractions, crackles, wheezing, and cyanosis. Feeding is impaired by excessive mucus and malaise. The chest radiograph manifests areas of hyperinflation and atelectasis as well as diffuse interstitial fluid infiltration. Symptoms are not usually severe enough to require hospitalization, but overt respiratory failure may develop in some children. As is the case with pneumonia and upper respiratory infections, bronchiolitis in adults with chronic lung disease may trigger acute respiratory failure.

Prevention and Treatment. Because RSV is communicable by airborne droplets and may remain viable on the hands for 30 minutes or more, appropriate measures should be taken to prevent transmission. With community outbreaks of RSV, exposure should be prevented insofar as possible. Clinical testing of RSV vaccines is in progress, and passive immunization with RSV immune globulin (Respigam) has been shown to prevent lower respiratory tract infections in high-risk children.[23] Treatment of severe viral bronchiolitis with antiviral agents such as ribavirin may be indicated in some cases, but the high cost of these drugs prohibits their widespread use. Antibiotics are beneficial only if the primary infection is bacterial, which is uncommon in bronchiolitis, or if a secondary infection is present. The inflammatory response is supported with hydration. Cool-mist humidification may be used to offset fluid loss with tachypnea in children. Respiratory failure may require oxygen administration, bronchodilator drug therapy and ventilatory support, as discussed in Chapter 18.

Prognosis and Outcome. Bronchiolitis is usually self-limited, resolving completely within 5 to 7 days in most patients.[23] In severe cases, wheezing and cough may persist for several months. A significant number of patients have recurrent episodes and later develop asthma. The overall mortality rate is 1%, although in children with congenital heart disease, it approaches 37%.[22]

Tuberculosis

Definition. TB is a communicable infection of lung tissue *(pulmonary TB)* and potentially other tissues *(extrapulmonary* or *miliary TB)* caused by the bacillus *Mycobacterium tuberculosis.*

Epidemiology. TB is the most prevalent infectious disease in the world.[24] After the discovery of antituberculin drugs in the 1950s, the incidence of TB in the United States declined until 1979, when it began to increase again. Since 1985, the incidence of TB has increased 20%. In 1993, however, a 5.1% *decrease* in reported cases was noted in the United States, leading to speculation that the upward trend had ended. Still, one third of the world population has been infected with *M. tuberculosis,* and in the United States, an estimated 10 million people have been infected with the bacillus.[25]

Two significant risk factors account for the recent resurgence of TB: immigration and infection with human immunodeficiency virus. According to the Centers for Disease Control and Prevention, almost 30% of TB patients in the United States are foreign born.[26] Close, frequent, and prolonged contact between people and host debilitation due to malnutrition enhance the risk of transmission. These conditions often exist among refugees and others living in poverty. TB is often seen as an opportunistic infection in people whose immune systems are devastated by AIDS (see Chapter 13). Other risk factors for TB include alcoholism, age older than 50 years, diabetes, and environmental lung diseases.

Primary TB refers to overt disease occurring

within 2 years after infection, whereas disease that occurs later is known as *reactivation TB*. Research has revealed that, of cases accounting for the increased prevalence since the 1980s, about one third are due to primary disease, and two thirds represent reactivation.[27]

Etiology. Droplets of sputum containing the organism become airborne as a result of the coughing of an actively infected person (Fig. 19–9). If the pulmonary defenses of the host are not adequate in clearing the bacillus, the organism is inhaled and begins slowly multiplying at the site of deposition, usually the middle to lower lung zones because these areas receive most of the tidal volume.[24]

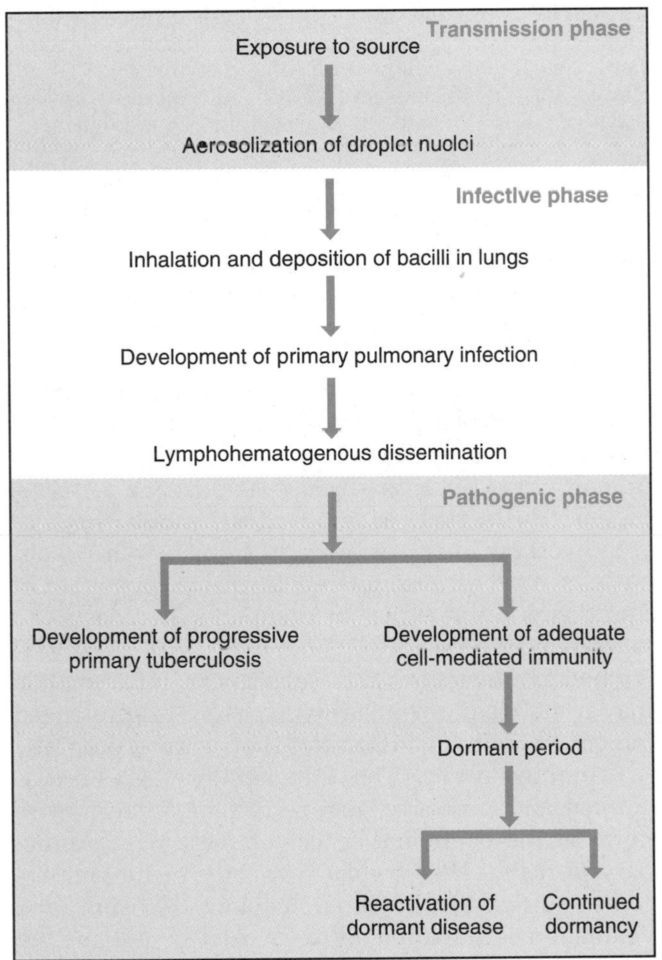

FIGURE 19–9

Phases of tuberculosis development. During the initial *transmission phase,* the patient is colonized with the tubercle bacillus through inhalation of the organism. During the *infective phase,* the organism multiplies within the lungs, triggering inflammatory and immune responses that may cause a mild pneumonia. These responses usually succeed in walling off the organism (granuloma formation), but viable bacilli persist within the granulomas. The nature of the *pathogenic phase* depends on the outcome of the inflammatory and immune responses. In most cases, a dormant period of several years follows. Less commonly, active tuberculosis develops from the initial exposure. If the patient's immune system later becomes compromised, dormant disease may be reactivated. (Redrawn from Colice, G.L. [1995]. Pulmonary tuberculosis: Is resurgence due to reactivation or new infection? *Postgraduate Medicine* 97[4], 37.)

Pathophysiology. The multiplying organism triggers a limited inflammatory response at the deposition site. A cell-mediated immune response develops and is usually successful in containing the infection within 4 to 6 weeks. The T-cell response results in the formation of granulomas around the bacilli, converting them to a dormant state. Although this response does not kill the initial infecting bacilli, it does confer immunity to a subsequent infection. Bacilli within granulomas may remain viable for many years and result in a positive purified protein derivative (PPD) or other skin test for TB (Table 19–5).

Active disease develops in 5% to 15% of those infected. The highest risk of active TB is present during the first 2 years after infection, but activation may occur anytime during the person's lifetime, particularly with debilitation and immunosuppression. In active TB, one or more of the granulomas breaks down, releasing bacilli, which multiply and trigger severe, destructive inflammation. Granulomas become necrotic and cheese-like in appearance, giving rise to the term *caseation* for this destructive process. Calcium may be deposited in necrotic areas. The apices of the lungs are most frequently damaged by necrosis.

Within pulmonary tissues, the bacillus initially spreads by the lymphatics, causing lymph node enlargements known as *Ghon complexes*. Eventually, the organism enters the bloodstream, which transmits it to other areas of the lung. Extrapulmonary tissues, such as the liver, spleen, kidneys, and adrenals, may be infected as well. Patients with AIDS may have an atypical pattern, demonstrating extrapulmonary TB without evident pulmonary involvement, and are also more likely to demonstrate progressive primary disease or the widely disseminated (miliary) form of TB.

Clinical Manifestations. During the initial infection and granuloma formation, the patient may be symptom free or may demonstrate mild bronchopneumonia. Skin tests convert to positive, and sputum culture confirms the presence of the organism. Granulomas may be visible on chest radiograph. Active TB is evidenced by the gradual onset of signs of chronic inflammation, including anorexia, weight loss, fatigue, low-grade fever, and night sweats. With advanced necrosis of pulmonary tissue, chest pain, cough, and **hemoptysis** are present. Necrotic areas and pleural effusions may be apparent on chest radiograph.

Prevention and Treatment. Prevention of TB involves education and screening to reduce the risk of infection and transmission. Tuberculin skin testing is routine in health assessment settings. People having

TABLE 19–5
TUBERCULIN SKIN TESTS

Test	Procedure	Results and Implications
PPD (Mantoux)	Single-needle intradermal injection of 0.1 mL (5 tuberculin units) of purified protein derivative (tuberculin antigen), forming a wheal. Area is evaluated after 48–72 hours for evidence of delayed hypersensitivity response.	Less than 5 mm induration—negative. 5 mm or more induration in an individual with close contact with infected person, positive chest radiograph, or human immunodeficiency virus–positive status—positive. 10 mm or more induration in a member of a high-risk group—positive. 15 mm or more induration in anyone—positive.
Multipuncture tests (Tine, Mono-Vacc, Aplitest)	Intradermal injection using a device that has tines impregnated with PPD or OT (old tuberculin antigen). Area is evaluated after 48–96 hours for evidence of delayed hypersensitivity.	Tine and Aplitest: vesicle formation at any puncture site—positive screen; follow with PPD to confirm. Mono-Vacc: any induration—positive screen; follow with PPD to confirm.

close or frequent contact with infected patients may undergo prophylactic therapy with antituberculin drugs. The infected person is taught to minimize the risk of airborne transmission by covering the mouth and nose when coughing.

TB is treated with appropriate antibiotics. Two first-line drugs, isoniazid (INH) and rifampin, have been most effective when used in combination for 1 to 3 years. Use of other antibiotics has become common in recent years, owing to the development of resistant strains of the bacillus. Because TB constitutes a risk to the public, antituberculin drugs are provided by the U.S. Public Health Service at no cost to the patient. Frequent follow-up of patients and their contacts is essential.

Prognosis and Outcome. With appropriate treatment and removal of risk factors, TB now has a favorable prognosis in the United States. The risk factor of AIDS is not yet removable, thus TB in these patients may trigger a terminal pneumonia. In developing countries, TB still kills 2.5 million people each year,[28] and concern is growing regarding the proliferation of resistant strains of the bacillus.[29]

Environmental–Occupational Lung Diseases

Definition. These lung diseases include a variety of inflammatory conditions of the lower respiratory tract that are triggered by inhaled toxins associated with a particular environment or occupation (Table 19–6). Environmental and occupational exposures are associated with 2% to 5% of all cases of asthma,[30] and because many of these inhaled irritants are carcinogenic, some cases of lung cancer may be classified as environmental lung diseases (see Chapter 18).

Epidemiology. The annual incidence of environmental lung diseases has been estimated at 400,000 in the United States, with 100,000 deaths annually.[31] Risk originates from environmental exposure to inorganic dusts such as silica, coal dust, or asbestos; organic dusts such as grain dust, moldy hay, or woodworking dust; or irritant gases or chemicals, such as may be encountered in plastic manufacturing, chemical industries, or occupational exposure to herbicides or pesticides.[32]

Etiology. Irritation and subsequent inflammation may result from low-intensity exposure for prolonged periods or from high-intensity, short-term exposure.

Pathophysiology. The inflammatory response is chronic and excessive and results in deposition of fibrin in the interstitial spaces of the lungs (**pulmonary fibrosis**). The alveolar–capillary membrane becomes sufficiently impaired to slow diffusion, and ventilation is impaired by decreased compliance of lung tissue.

Clinical Manifestations. The patient has no symptoms at first, although scattered inflammatory lesions may be seen on chest radiograph. Dyspnea with exertion is an early sign, followed by frequent cough productive of thick mucus. Hypoxemia and hypercapnia are evidenced by arterial blood gases, and respiratory failure eventually develops.

Prevention and Treatment. Exposure to pulmonary irritants must be prevented through appropriate industrial policies and practices. Treatment of lung damage and respiratory failure is symptomatic and supportive.

TABLE 19–6
ENVIRONMENTAL–OCCUPATIONAL LUNG DISEASES

Agent	Disease	Exposure
Mineral Dusts		
Coal dust	Anthracosis Macules Progressive massive fibrosis Caplan's syndrome	Coal mining (particularly hard coal)
Silica	Silicosis Caplan's syndrome	Foundry work, sandblasting, hard-rock mining, stone cutting, others
Asbestos	Asbestosis Pleural plaques Caplan's syndrome Mesothelioma Carcinoma of the lung, larynx, stomach, colon	Mining, milling, and fabrication, installation and removal of insulation
Beryllium	Acute berylliosis Beryllium granulomatosis ?Bronchogenic carcinoma	Mining, fabrication
Iron oxide	Siderosis	Welding
Barium sulfate	Baritosis	Mining
Tin oxide	Stannosis	Mining
Organic Dusts That Induce Hypersensitivity Pneumonitis		
Moldy hay	Farmer's lung	Farming
Bagasse	Bagassosis	Manufacturing wallboard, paper
Bird droppings	Bird-breeder's lung	Bird handling
Organic Dusts That Induce Asthma		
Cotton, flax, hemp	Byssinosis	Textile manufacturing
Red cedar dust	Asthma	Lumbering, carpentry
Chemical Fumes and Vapors		
Nitrous oxide, sulfur dioxide ammonia, benzene, certain insecticides (e.g., cyanate gases)	Bronchitis Asthma Pulmonary edema Respiratory distress syndrome Injury to exposed mucosa Fulminant poisoning	Occupational and accidental exposure

From Cotran, R.S., Kumar, V., and Robbins, S.L. (1994). *Robbins Pathological Basis of Disease.* (5th ed.). Philadelphia: W.B. Saunders. (p. 706).

Prognosis and Outcome. Environmental lung diseases are often detected at an advanced state, from which they progress to terminal respiratory failure.

Idiopathic Pulmonary Fibrosis

Definition. Idiopathic pulmonary fibrosis is a disorder characterized by inflammation and fibrosis of the pulmonary interstitium and respiratory units, for which a cause is unknown.

Epidemiology. The incidence of this disorder has been estimated at 5 per 100,000.[33] Specific risk factors are unknown.

Etiology. In response to an unknown triggering agent, local immunologic mechanisms are activated.

Pathophysiology. Within the respiratory units of the lungs, immunologic mechanisms result in an inflammatory response that has both cell-mediated and humoral components (see Chapter 13). Immune-mediated lung injury occurs, and proliferation of connective tissue matrix cells and protein deposition results in increased diffusion impairment and reduced lung compliance.[33] Elevated PVR develops as a consequence of hypoxic pulmonary vasoconstriction and may precipitate right-sided heart failure (cor pulmonale).

Clinical Manifestations. Typical clinical features include progressive dyspnea on exertion, digital clubbing, a restrictive ventilatory impairment, widespread shadowing on chest radiograph, and hypoxemia. Jugular venous distention, hepatomegaly, and edema may be seen, owing to cor pulmonale. Lung biopsy may demonstrate the fibrotic process, permitting definitive diagnosis and staging of the disease.

Prevention and Treatment. Specific preventive

measures are unknown. Standard treatment usually consists of corticosteroid and immunosuppressive drug therapy to suppress the immune and inflammatory responses. Cardiac failure and respiratory failure are treated supportively. Lung or heart and lung transplantation may be indicated in selected cases.

Prognosis and Outcome. Progression of the disease varies widely among patients, ranging from a chronic form persisting for many years to an acute form that progresses to respiratory failure within weeks. In most patients, death occurs within 2 years.[32]

Sarcoidosis

Definition. Sarcoidosis is a systemic disorder of unknown cause, characterized by noncaseating granulomatous lesions of multiple tissues, particularly the lungs and thoracic lymph nodes.[34]

Epidemiology. Sarcoidosis affects people of all races and ages, and is equally prevalent in males and females.[34] It is especially prevalent in blacks, in people of Irish and Scandinavian descent, and in adults younger than 40 years. The annual rate of incidence in the United States is 35.5 per 100,000 for blacks and 10.9 per 100,000 for whites. The disease is apparently transmitted by person-to-person contact or shared exposure to an environmental agent.

Etiology. The specific cause of sarcoidosis is unknown. Organic (e.g., microorganisms) or inorganic (e.g., dusts or toxins) agents may serve as specific antigens in triggering the immune response in sarcoidosis. A genetic predisposition may also be involved.

Pathophysiology. An excessive inflammatory response is initiated in the alveoli, bronchioles, and blood vessels of the lungs in nearly all patients. Other tissues that may be involved include thoracic lymph nodes (90%), heart (70%), liver (40% to 70%), skin (25%), eyes (25%), and nervous system (5%).[34] Monocyte-macrophages accumulate in the target tissue, where they differentiate into epithelioid and multinucleated giant cells and induce the inflammatory process (see Chapter 13). CD4+ T lymphocytes are also abundant, and sensitized immune cells form a ring around the inflamed area. Granuloma formation is complete when a dense band of fibroblasts, mast cells, collagen fibers, and proteoglycans encases the cluster of inflammatory and immune cells.

Clinical Manifestations. Pulmonary fibrosis results in increased thickness of the alveolar–capillary membrane, decreased compliance, and restrictive ventilatory impairment. Wheezing and stridor are common, and hypoxemia and hypercapnia are present to varying degrees. Lymph node enlargement is disfiguring, but nodes are not tender. Lymph node enlargement may obstruct blood vessels or encroach on other organs, inducing perfusion deficits or manifestations of organ dysfunction. Systemic effects depend on the extent of involvement of other organs. Cardiac failure is often present, and a wide variety of skin rashes may be seen. Lesions of the eyes may cause excess lacrimation, conjunctival nodules, and visual deficits ranging from blurred vision and photophobia to blindness. Significant hepatic dysfunction is uncommon, although the risk of cholestasis is increased (see Chapter 26). Hypercalciuria with increased risk of nephrolithiasis is also seen, owing to increased hepatic and renal activation of vitamin D (see Chapter 20).

Prevention and Treatment. Specific preventive measures are unknown. Because of the potential for spontaneous remission, those with mild disease are usually observed without therapy. Oral corticosteroids are indicated for treatment of significant organ dysfunction, to suppress the inflammatory and immune responses. Methotrexate, a cytotoxic agent, has been used to reduce the proliferation of immune cells in cases that do not respond to steroid therapy. Lung transplantation has been used, but the rate of rejection has been high, and the disease may recur in the grafted lung.[34] Treatment of other manifestations is specific to the involved system.

Prognosis and Outcome. For unknown reasons, some patients recover spontaneously, whereas others have a progressively worsening or relapsing course. For most, the prognosis is positive, although about half of patients have at least a mild degree of permanent organ dysfunction.[34]

Near-Drowning

Definition. Near-drowning is an acute episode in which respiration is prevented by submersion in water for a sufficient length of time to lead to significant morbidity and possibly to eventual mortality.

Epidemiology. Almost 9000 deaths due to drowning occur each year in the United States, and near-drowning occurs three to five times as frequently as drowning.[35] Two peaks of incidence are seen: young children, 1 to 2 years of age; and adolescents, 10 to 19 years of age. Among adolescents, 85% of deaths are in boys and are related to use of alcohol, "daredevil" behavior, water sports, and boating. Among young children, lack of adequate barriers around home pools is often implicated.

Etiology. Except in rare cases of homicide or suicide, drowning is accidental, associated with the identified risk factors.

Pathophysiology. In people older than 5 years, an initial period of voluntary apnea occurs immediately on submersion. The victim holds his or her breath, causing $PaCO_2$ levels to rise and PaO_2 levels to fall. A "break point" occurs when $PaCO_2$ rises to about 51 mm Hg and PaO_2 falls to about 73 mm Hg, and the person takes an involuntary breath.[35] In some people, hypoxemia causes loss of consciousness before the break point occurs. In young children, the **diving reflex** may be triggered. This primitive reflex is related to the startle response and is initiated by contact of the victim's face with cold water. Impulses carried by the trigeminal nerve stimulate brain-stem centers to slow the heart rate and to initiate selective vasoconstriction, which shunts blood from vessels of the skin and abdominal organs to the brain and heart.

The submerged breaths may result in either laryngospasm, which closes the airways, or aspiration of water (usually containing foreign matter) into the lungs. If sea water is aspirated, the hypertonic fluid in the airways pulls water from the pulmonary capillaries into the interstitium and alveoli, resulting in pulmonary edema. Aspirated fresh water is hypotonic to plasma and is thus absorbed into the circulation. In either case, surfactant is altered, leading to atelectasis and intrapulmonary shunting. Hypoxic pulmonary vasoconstriction follows, which increases pulmonary CHP and promotes pulmonary edema. The larger airways may become obstructed by laryngospasm, bronchoconstriction, foreign matter, foam, mucus, or aspirated gastric contents.

Hypoxemia and metabolic acidosis develop rapidly, leading to central nervous system depression and cerebral edema. Aspiration pneumonia occurs in those who aspirate significant amounts of foreign matter. Myocardial depression ensues, contributing to shock and organ failure. Brain death may result from cerebral hypoxia, carbon dioxide narcosis, laryngospasm, or vagally mediated cardiac arrest.

Clinical Manifestations. The near-drowning victim is usually unconscious due to cerebral edema and hypoxia, and the pupils may be fixed and dilated. The patient may be apneic or in severe respiratory distress due to laryngospasm or pulmonary edema. Cardiovascular manifestations range from full arrest (asystole or ventricular fibrillation) to bradycardia and other nonlethal dysrhythmias. Blood volume is usually normal. Renal ischemia may manifest as albuminuria, hemoglobinuria, or oliguria (see Chapter 20).

Prevention and Treatment. Prevention requires reduction of the associated risk factors, with measures such as pool safety covers, self latching gates, and public education and safety regulations regarding operation of water craft. Resuscitation of the near-drowning victim may require cardiopulmonary resuscitation, defibrillation, and mechanical ventilation. Oxygen therapy is instituted, and gastric contents are removed. Drug therapy may include antibiotics for aspiration pneumonia as well as positive inotropic agents and vasoactive agents, consistent with a cardiogenic shock state (see Chapters 15 and 16). Function of other organs is supported as indicated by laboratory values. Treatment of increased intracranial pressure is detailed in Chapter 21.

Prognosis and Outcome. Outcome is directly related to the length of the period of submersion and the resulting coma. Younger patient age and colder water temperatures promote more favorable outcomes. Those who are not comatose after the incident usually recover fully. Prolonged coma reduces the chance for recovery to about 10%, and residual effects such as blindness, decreased cognitive function, and seizure disorder are frequent.[35]

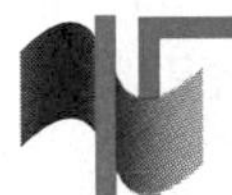

Clinical Scenario

W.J., a 5-year-old boy, is brought by ambulance to the emergency department following a near-drowning episode. After being submerged an estimated 3 minutes in a local lake, he was rescued by witnesses who initiated cardiopulmonary resuscitation. When paramedics arrived on the scene, they continued resuscitation, noted a pulse, and unsuccessfully attempted intubation. Spontaneous respirations returned, along with a productive cough. On arrival in the emergency department, W.J. is in severe respiratory distress. His eyes open occasionally, and he moves randomly but does not follow commands. Auscultation of the lungs reveals coarse crackles and wheezes. He is sedated and intubated, and mechanical ventilation is initiated. The chest radiograph demonstrates consolidated fluid infiltrations bilaterally.

1. W.J. demonstrates signs of fluid in his airways. What pathophysiologic processes may have contributed to this manifestation? Explain.
2. What factors in this situation suggest a positive prognosis?

Sudden Infant Death Syndrome

Definition. Sudden infant death syndrome (SIDS) is the sudden death of an infant who is younger than 1 year of age, which is unexplained after a thorough case investigation, including performance of a complete autopsy, examination of the death scene, and review of the clinical history.[36]

Epidemiology. In developed countries, SIDS is the most common cause of infant death between 1 month and 1 year of age. The incidence rate in the United States is less than 1.4 per 1000 live births.[37] Risk is highest among blacks and Native American infants and lowest among Asian infants. Maternal smoking during pregnancy, postnatal exposure of the infant to secondhand smoke, young maternal age, maternal drug addiction, low birth weight, routine abdominal sleep position, and lack of prenatal care are among the risk factors associated with SIDS (Table 19–7). Breastfeeding apparently conveys some degree of protection against SIDS. About two thirds of SIDS infants are boys.

Etiology. The etiology of SIDS is unknown. Several theories have been advanced, but none explains all cases. It is probable that more than one mechanism is operative. The *sleep apnea hypothesis* suggests that babies who die of SIDS have a chronic, subtle abnormality that predisposes them to transient episodes of airway obstruction and bradycardia, especially during sleep or nutritive sucking.[38] Such episodes, called *apparent life-threatening events*, may be observed by caregivers, who report them and seek intervention.

The role of prone position during sleep has received much scientific scrutiny. Carbon dioxide rebreathing and the limited ability of the infant to move while in the prone position have been implicated as possible causes of respiratory arrest leading to SIDS. Gastroesophageal reflux, which may or may not be associated with apnea, has also been proposed as a cause of SIDS. Refluxed acid may induce cessation of nasal airflow, laryngospasm, bronchoconstriction, and increased airway resistance as well as apnea and bradycardia. SIDS has also been attributed to a defect in β-oxidation of lipids in up to 3% of cases.[39]

Pathophysiology. Death almost always occurs during sleep, giving rise to the lay term *crib death* for SIDS. On autopsy, the infant typically appears to be normally hydrated and nourished. The airways, mouths, and noses of most infants are filled with blood-tinged fluid, indicating pulmonary edema. Thoracic organs are usually covered with petechiae, capillary hemorrhages indicating negative intrathoracic pressure before death. Inflammatory exudate is commonly found in the tissues of the upper airways.

Clinical Manifestations. Unexpected death of the infant is the only manifestation.

Prevention and Treatment. There is no certain prevention for SIDS. Reduction of modifiable risk factors is warranted. Maternal smoking during pregnancy or lactation should be curtailed, and infants should not be exposed to passive smoking after birth. The American Academy of Pediatrics recommends that healthy infants be positioned for sleep on their sides or backs.[38] Because the link between prone position and increased incidence of SIDS has not been consistently shown, and because there are known risks to the supine position (e.g., aspiration), this stance is controversial. Home apnea monitoring of high-risk infants may permit intervention in apparent life-threatening events. Autopsy serves to rule out other causes of death and may possibly lessen the guilt that parents may feel about "missing something" and failing to prevent the baby's death. Clinical intervention focuses on support of the grieving family.

Prognosis and Outcome. The parents and siblings of the SIDS infant require long-term support from health professionals, with continued reassurance that they did nothing to cause the infant's death. Mutual support groups composed of families of SIDS infants may be especially helpful.

TABLE 19–7
RISK FACTORS FOR SUDDEN INFANT DEATH SYNDROME

Risk Factors
Environmental
Cold weather season
Lower socioeconomic status of family
Prone sleeping position
Night or morning hours
Bundling or dressing too warmly
Secondhand tobacco smoke
Ethnic or Cultural
African American race
Native American race
Maternal
Lower age of mother
Prenatal and postnatal cigarette smoking by mother
Lack of prenatal care
Maternal drug use
Shorter interpregnancy interval
Infant
Age younger than 6 months
Prematurity
Twin or triplet birth
Low birth weight
Previous apparent life-threatening event
Male gender
Other
Sibling who suffered sudden infant death syndrome

From O'Donnell, J.K., and Gaedeke, M.K. (1995). Sudden infant death syndrome. *Critical Care Nursing Clinics of North America* 7(3), 474.

Methemoglobinemia

Definition. Methemoglobinemia is a disorder in which more than 2% of the iron in hemoglobin is oxidized from the normal ferrous (Fe^{2+}) state to the ferric (Fe^{3+}) state, in which it is incapable of binding oxygen.

Epidemiology. Methemoglobinemia is a rare disorder, which may be genetic or acquired. The genetic form is more common among people of Navajo, Athabascan, Cuban, Puerto Rican, or Japanese heritage.[40] Contact with exogenous agents that may induce the acquired disorder also constitutes a risk factor (see later).

Etiology. Congenital disorders that may result in methemoglobinemia include deficiency of glucose-6-phosphate dehydrogenase enzyme, deficiency of methemoglobin reductase enzymes, or abnormal hemoglobin structure (Hb M).[41] The more common, acquired form may be induced by exposure to exogenous oxidizing agents, including local anesthetics (benzocaine, lidocaine), nitrates and nitrites (nitroglycerin, nitroprusside, amyl nitrite, bismuth subnitrate, nitrate preservatives), other drugs (phenazopyridine, dapsone, antimalarials), or aniline dyes (ink, shoe polish).

Pathophysiology. Hereditary abnormality of one of the methemoglobin reduction pathways or overpowering of these pathways by exogenous oxidizing agents results in a rate of hemoglobin oxidation (electron removal or proton addition) that exceeds the rate of reduction (electron addition or proton removal). Large quantities of methemoglobin, containing Fe^{3+}, are produced. Inability of methemoglobin to bind oxygen increases the affinity of the remaining normal hemoglobin for oxygen, shifting the oxyhemoglobin dissociation curve to the left and depriving tissues of oxygen.

Clinical Manifestations. Cyanosis of the extremities despite a normal PaO_2 and a chocolate-brown appearance of both venous and arterial blood are the hallmarks of methemoglobinemia. The percentage of hemoglobin saturated with oxygen is low, and signs of tissue ischemia are apparent, including tachycardia, confusion, dyspnea with minimal exertion, fatigue, and nausea. Methemoglobin levels in patients with symptoms may range from 20% to 70%.[41]

Prevention and Treatment. Health care professionals should be aware of the risk of methemoglobinemia with use of the associated drugs and local anesthetics, and the patient should be closely monitored for development of the disorder. Methemoglobinemia is treated with administration of methylene blue, which acts as an electron donor in the reduction of methemoglobin to the ferrous form. Oxygen therapy is also required.

Prognosis and Outcome. With prompt recognition and treatment, methemoglobinemia may be resolved without complication.

Carbon Monoxide Intoxication

Definition. Carbon monoxide intoxication is the syndrome resulting from the inhalation of carbon monoxide gas in amounts sufficient to induce cerebral hypoxia.

Epidemiology. About 10,000 people are treated for carbon monoxide poisoning each year.[42] As many as one third of all cases are probably undiagnosed. Risk factors are inherent in situations in which carbon monoxide gas is present, particularly if ventilation is poor (see later).

Etiology. Carbon monoxide is a product of incomplete combustion of organic substances. A small amount is produced during normal metabolism, and about 0.5% of hemoglobin-binding sites are normally occupied by carbon monoxide. (The percentage is higher among cigarette smokers and those who live in urban areas.) Significant exogenous sources of carbon monoxide include motor vehicle exhaust, faulty heating systems, smoke inhalation (by fire victims or firefighters), and abuse or accidental inhalation of methylene chloride (paint stripper).[43] Inhalation is usually accidental but may be intentional in attempted suicide.

Pathophysiology. Carbon monoxide binds with high affinity to oxygen-binding sites on hemoglobin, forming carboxyhemoglobin. The resulting decrease in both oxygen-carrying capacity and oxygen release to tissues leads to tissue hypoxia. Binding of carbon monoxide to intracellular proteins, such as myoglobin and cytochrome oxidase, may contribute to toxicity. Compensatory increases in cardiac and respiratory workloads result in initial manifestations. Eventually, respiratory depression occurs, and death may occur from cerebral hypoxia or cardiac dysrhythmia.

Clinical Manifestations. Clinical features depend on the degree of carboxyhemoglobin formation and tissue hypoxia. They may include headache, dizziness, confusion, visual disturbance, weakness, fatigue, nausea, diarrhea, abdominal pain, and chest pain. Seizures and coma are seen in severe carbon monoxide poisoning. Cherry-red skin may be evident (due to the color of carboxyhemoglobin), but this sign, although highly specific, is not commonly seen.[42] Shock, cardiac dysrhythmia, and respiratory failure are usually associated with carboxyhemoglobin levels of greater than 50%.[43]

Prevention and Treatment. Prevention of carbon monoxide poisoning requires awareness of high-risk situations and appropriate behavioral intervention. Treatment begins with removal of the patient from the source of the gas. One hundred per cent oxygen is administered in an effort to displace carbon monoxide from hemoglobin-binding sites and to increase the fraction of dissolved oxygen gas, thus improving oxygenation. Hyperbaric oxygen therapy, available at specialized centers, reduces the elimination half-life of carboxyhemoglobin to less than 30 minutes.[43]

Prognosis and Outcome. Outcome depends on the degree of exposure. About 5600 deaths result from carbon monoxide poisoning each year, and these are usually associated with cardiac dysrhythmias.[42] Some who survive have permanent disorders due to cerebral injury, including dementia, psychosis, gait disorders, tremors, blindness, seizures, and peripheral neuropathy. A high rate of fetal death is evident among pregnant women who are exposed to carbon monoxide.

Decompression Disorder

Definition. Decompression disorder refers to any of a group of related disorders resulting from the entry of bubbles of nitrogen into body tissues as a result of exposure to an abnormal gas pressure environment.[44] The most important of these are *decompression sickness* ("the bends") and *arterial gas embolism.*

Epidemiology. Those at risk include divers, workers in caissons, pilots who experience low pressures at high altitudes, and astronauts wearing low-pressure space suits. Among recreational divers, 1 incident occurs per 5000 to 10,000 dives, whereas the risk among commercial divers is about 1 in 500 to 1000 dives.[44]

Etiology. Decompression sickness occurs in divers when an inert gas (nitrogen or helium) enters the body via the lungs during a dive and, at the elevated pressure of ocean depths, dissolves in the blood. Circulation carries the gas to the tissue capillaries, where it diffuses into tissues. Diffusion is quickest into the brain and spinal cord because of rich perfusion, variable in skeletal muscle depending on metabolism, and slowest in joints. During ascent and decompression, gas diffusion is in the opposite direction (from tissues back to blood and then to the alveoli for exhalation) at the same relative rates. Supersaturation of tissues with gas results in bubble formation. Arterial gas embolism occurs when an obstructed airway prevents gas that is expanding within the lungs during ascent from escaping. This usually results from a novice or panicky diver holding his or her breath during a rapid ascent. Airway rupture permits entry of the gas into the arterial blood.

Pathophysiology. In decompression sickness, nitrogen bubbles in tissues may expand under conditions of decreased pressure, rupturing capillaries and seeding bubbles in circulating blood. Direct tissue injury also results, and the hemostatic system may be activated, obstructing blood flow. Venous bubbles are normally filtered by the pulmonary capillary network and exhaled, but if present in excess, they may enter the arterial system. Alternatively, a congenital heart defect that permits a right-to-left shunt may permit entry into the arterial circulation, placing these people at higher risk. Arterial gas emboli reaching the brain result in stroke.

Clinical Manifestations. Signs of decompression sickness include headache, dizziness, nausea, visual disturbances, limb pain, numbness, paralysis, and cough. Signs of arterial gas embolism include loss of consciousness, seizures, hemiplegia, and possible sudden death.

Prevention and Treatment. Slower or interrupted ascent and breathing higher concentrations of oxygen may reduce the risk of decompression sickness in divers. Careful training in diving procedures and education to recognize the signs of the disorder are of obvious benefit. Treatment consists of administration of 100% oxygen under hyperbaric pressure, followed by slow decompression.

Prognosis and Outcome. In most cases, treatment of decompression disorder is effective. Arterial gas embolization to the brain results in stroke, manifested by sudden loss of consciousness, seizures, hemiplegia, and possibly death.

CLINICAL SIGNIFICANCE OF DISORDERS OF GAS TRANSPORT AND EXCHANGE

The importance of diseases that impair gas transport and exchange lies in the vital nature of these processes. Humans cannot survive without a continuous supply of oxygen. In a recent study, hypoxemia was shown to be inversely related to prognosis and survival, regardless of the mechanism and underlying disease.[45] Many of the disorders discussed in this chapter are both preventable and curable yet cause significant morbidity and mortality. Research is ongoing in an effort to improve clinical intervention in disorders of gas exchange because mechanical ventilation and oxygen therapy impose significant iatrogenic risk.

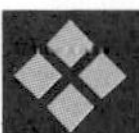

Summary of Key Points

- As a consequence of its shorter length and compliant vessels, the pulmonary circulation is a lower-pressure system than the systemic circulation. PVR is normally about one fifth of systemic vascular resistance; thus, the afterload of the right ventricle is normally much lower than that of the left. Conditions in which PVR is increased may precipitate right heart failure (cor pulmonale).

- Hypoxic pulmonary vasoconstriction is a local reflex mechanism that operates to maximize ventilation–perfusion matching. Smooth muscle cells in the walls of pulmonary vessels sense changes in the Po_2 of the blood perfusing them. Hypoxia inhibits an outward K^+ current from these cells, depolarizing them and opening Ca^{2+} channels. Ca^{2+} influx mediates smooth muscle contraction and vasoconstriction. Although beneficial in improving $\dot{V}/\dot{Q}$ relationships, hypoxic pulmonary vasoconstriction increases PVR, which may be detrimental in some cases.

- Although a small amount of oxygen is transported in dissolved form, nearly 99% is transported in reversible combination with hemoglobin. The affinity of oxygen for hemoglobin is widely variable under physiologic and pathologic conditions, represented by the oxyhemoglobin dissociation curve, and numerous factors influence the quantity of hemoglobin available. About 20% of carbon dioxide is transported in combination with hemoglobin at binding sites separate from those for oxygen. Most carbon dioxide is transported in some stage of the carbonic acid–bicarbonate buffer system.

- The oxyhemoglobin dissociation curve is sigmoid because the affinity of each of the four oxygen-binding sites on hemoglobin varies, owing to allosteric effects that depend on occupation of the other sites. The curve may shift to the right, indicating a lesser affinity at a given Pao_2, under physiologic conditions in which the peripheral tissues have a greater need for oxygen. Conversely, a leftward shift indicates a lesser tissue need for oxygen. A number of congenital and acquired disorders may shift the curve maladaptively.

- Pulmonary gas diffusion varies as a function of four factors: thickness of the alveolar–capillary membrane, membrane surface area, diffusion coefficients of the gases, and pressure gradients. Because of the solubility of oxygen and carbon dioxide in lipid and because equilibration time is ample at normal heart rates, membrane thickness must be greatly increased before any limitation in diffusion is clinically detectable. Similarly, adults possess up to 75% more exchange surface area than is required for normal function, constituting a large pulmonary reserve in this respect. The diffusion coefficient for a gas is a constant, determined by its solubility in water and its molecular weight. Because the exchangeable gases are very diffusible, with carbon dioxide being 20 times more soluble than oxygen, this is not a limiting factor. Deficient oxygen diffusion due to other factors, however, becomes apparent earlier than deficient carbon dioxide diffusion. Normal variation in gas diffusion results from alteration of the pressure gradients between the inspired air and the blood.

- Pulmonary disorders affecting gas exchange include those disorders in which ventilation is impaired because pressure gradients are altered. Pulmonary embolism abruptly reduces the gradients from the perfusion side. Pulmonary edema and ARDS result in impaired gas exchange, primarily owing to increased membrane thickness. Pneumonia and bronchiolitis affect both ventilation and diffusion.

REFERENCES

1. Weir, K.K., and Archer, S.L. (1995). The mechanism of acute hypoxic pulmonary vasoconstriction: The tale of two channels. *FASEB Journal* 9(2), 183–189.
2. Barnes, P.J., and Liu, S.F. (1995). Regulation of pulmonary vascular tone. *Pharmacological Reviews* 47(1), 87–131.
3. Dickson, S.L. (1995). Understanding the oxyhemoglobin dissociation curve. *Critical Care Nurse* 15(5), 54–58.
4. Hamner, J. (1995). Challenging diagnosis: Adult respiratory distress syndrome. *Critical Care Nurse* 15(5), 46–51.
5. Paulson, T.E., Spear, R.M., and Peterson, B.M. (1995). New concepts in the treatment of children with acute respiratory distress syndrome. *Journal of Pediatrics* 127(2), 163–175.
6. Brandstetter, R.D., Sharma, K.C., DellaBadia, M., *et al.* (1997). Adult respiratory distress syndrome: A disorder in need of improved outcome. *Heart & Lung* 26(1), 3–14.
7. Dirkes, S. (1996). Liquid ventilation: New frontiers in the treatment of ARDS. *Critical Care Nurse* 16(3), 53–58.
8. Lunn, R.J. (1995). Inhaled nitric oxide therapy. *Mayo Clinic Proceedings* 70(3), 247–255.
9. Weinmann, E.E., and Salzman, E.W. (1994). Deep-vein thrombosis. *New England Journal of Medicine* 331(24), 1630–1641.
10. Evans, D.A., and Wilmott, R.W. (1994). Pulmonary embolism in children. *Pediatric Clinics of North America* 41(3), 569–584.
11. Handler, J.A., and Feied, C.F. (1995). Acute pulmonary embo-

lism: Aggressive therapy with anticoagulants and thrombolytics. *Postgraduate Medicine* 97(1), 61–72.
12. Lualdi, J.C., and Goldhaber, S.Z. (1995). Right ventricular dysfunction after acute pulmonary embolism: Pathophysiologic factors, detection, and therapeutic implications. *American Heart Journal* 130(6), 1276–1282.
13. Rubin, L.J. (1997). Primary pulmonary hypertension. *New England Journal of Medicine* 336(2), 111–117.
14. Kinsella, J.P., and Abman, S.H. (1995). Recent developments in the pathophysiology and treatment of persistent pulmonary hypertension of the newborn. *Journal of Pediatrics* 126(6), 853–864.
15. Abenheim, L., Moride, Y., Brenot, F., *et al.* (1996). Appetite-suppressant drugs and the risk of primary pulmonary hypertension. *New England Journal of Medicine* 335(9), 609–616.
16. Roberts, J.D., and Shaul, P.W. (1993). Advances in the treatment of persistent pulmonary hypertension of the newborn. *Pediatric Clinics of North America* 40(5), 983–1004.
17. Bartlett, J.G., and Mundy, L.M. (1995). Community-acquired pneumonia. *New England Journal of Medicine* 333(24), 1618–1624.
18. Crowe, H.M. (1996). Nosocomial pneumonia: Problems and progress. *Heart & Lung* 25(5), 418–421.
19. Brown, R.B. (1993). Community-acquired pneumonia: Diagnosis and therapy of older adults. *Geriatrics* 48(2), 43–50.
20. Horst, P.S. (1994). Bronchiolitis. *American Family Physician* 49(6), 1449–1453.
21. Wright, S.A., and Bieluch, V.M. (1993). Selected nosocomial viral infections. *Heart & Lung* 22(2), 183–187.
22. Lugo, R.A., and Nahata, M.C. (1993). Pathogenesis and treatment of bronchiolitis. *Clinical Pharmacy* 12(2), 95–116.
23. Jeng, M-J., and Lemen, R.J. (1997). Respiratory syncytial virus bronchiolitis. *American Family Physician* 55(4), 1139–1146.
24. Colice, G.L. (1995). Pulmonary tuberculosis: Is resurgence due to reactivation or new infection? *Postgraduate Medicine* 97(4), 35–48.
25. Haas, D.W., and Des Prez, R.M. (1994). Tuberculosis and acquired immunodeficiency syndrome: A historical perspective on recent developments. *American Journal of Medicine* 96(5), 439–450.
26. Centers for Disease Control and Prevention. (1994). Expanded tuberculosis surveillance and tuberculosis morbidity: United States, 1993. *Journal of the American Medical Association* 272(4), 265–266.
27. Barnes, P.F., El-Hajj, H., Preston-Martin, S., *et al.* (1996). Transmission of tuberculosis among the urban homeless. *Journal of the American Medical Association* 275(4), 305–307.
28. Raviglione, M.C., Snider, D.E., and Kochi, A. (1995). Global epidemiology of tuberculosis: Morbidity and mortality of a worldwide epidemic. *Journal of the American Medical Association* 273(3), 220–226.
29. Moulding, T., Dutt, A.K., and Reichman, L.B. (1995). Fixed-dose combinations of antituberculous medications to prevent drug resistance. *Annals of Internal Medicine* 122(12), 951–954.
30. Smith, W. (1987). Chronic lung disease. In: *A Profile of Health and Disease in America: Respiratory and Infectious Diseases*. New York: Facts on File Publications. (pp. 88–98).
31. Alberts, W.M., and Brooks, S.M. (1995). Occupational asthma: Serious consequences for workers and employers. *Postgraduate Medicine* 97(6), 93–104.
32. Cotran, R.S., Kumar, V., and Robbins, S.L. (1994). *Robbins Pathologic Basis of Disease*. (5th ed.). Philadelphia: W.B. Saunders. (pp. 706–715).
33. duBois, R.M. (1993). Idiopathic pulmonary fibrosis. *Annual Review of Medicine* 44, 441–450.
34. Newman, L.S., Rose, C.S., and Maier, L.A. (1997). Sarcoidosis. *New England Journal of Medicine* 336(17), 1224–1234.
35. Levin, D.L., Morriss, F.C., Toro, L.O., *et al.* (1993). Drowning and near-drowning. *Pediatric Clinics of North America* 40(2), 321–336.
36. Willinger, M., James, L.S., and Catz, C. (1991). Defining the sudden infant death syndrome (SIDS): Deliberations of an expert panel convened by the National Institute of Child Health and Development. *Pediatric Pathology* 11, 677–684.
37. Klonoff-Cohen, H.S., and Edelstein, S.L. (1995). A case-control study of routine and death scene sleep position and sudden infant death syndrome in Southern California. *Journal of the American Medical Association* 273(10), 790–794.
38. Freed, G.E., Steinschneider, A., Glassman, M., *et al.* (1994). Sudden infant death syndrome prevention and an understanding of selected clinical issues. *Pediatric Clinics of North America* (41(5), 967–989.
39. Vockley, J. (1994). The changing face of disorders of fatty acid oxidation. *Mayo Clinic Proceedings* 69(3), 249–257.
40. Lukens, J. (1993). Methemoglobinemia and sulfhemoglobinemia. In: Williams, W., Buetler, E., Erslev, A., *et al.* (Eds.). *Wintrobe's Clinical Hematology*. (9th Ed.). Philadelphia: Lea & Febiger. (p. 1265).
41. deSolis, M.G-A., and Hendrix, L.Y. (1995). Acute methemoglobinemia: A nursing perspective. *Critical Care Nurse* 15(3), 33–38.
42. Hardy, K.R., and Thom, S.R. (1994). Pathophysiology and treatment of carbon monoxide poisoning. *Clinical Toxicology* 32(6), 613–629.
43. Kales, S.N. (1993). Carbon monoxide intoxication. *American Family Physician* 48(6), 1100–1104.
44. Moon, R.E., Vann, R.D., and Bennett, P.B. (1995). The physiology of decompression illness. *Scientific American* 273(2), 70–77.
45. Bowton, D.L., Suceri, P.E., and Haponik, E.F. (1994). The incidence and effect on outcome of hypoxemia in hospitalized medical patients. *American Journal of Medicine* 97(7), 38–46.

SELECTED BIBLIOGRAPHY

Anderson, J.M. (1996). Management of four arterial blood gas problems in adult mechanical ventilation: Decision-making algorithms and rationale for their use. *Critical Care Nurse* 16(3), 62–73.

Anzueto, A., Baughman, R.P., Guntupalli, K.K., *et al.* (1996). Aerosolized surfactant in adults with sepsis-induced acute respiratory distress syndrome. *New England Journal of Medicine* 334(22), 1417–1421.

Bradley, S.F. (1996). Influenza in the elderly: Prevention is the best strategy in high-risk populations. *Postgraduate Medicine* 99(2), 138–149.

Brooks-Brunn, J.A. (1995). Postoperative atelectasis and pneumonia. *Heart & Lung* 24(2), 94–115.

Cantwell, M.F., Snider, D.E., Cauthen, G.M., *et al.* (1994). Epidemiology of tuberculosis in the United States, 1985 through 1992. *Journal of the American Medical Association* 272(7), 535–539.

Carpenter, K.D. (1991). Oxygen transport in the blood. *Critical Care Nurse* 11(9), 20–33.

Centers for Disease Control. (1993). Update: Hantavirus pulmonary syndrome: United States, 1993. *Journal of the American Medical Association* 270(19), 2287–2288.

Chan-Yeung, M., and Malo, J-L. (1995). Occupational asthma. *New England Journal of Medicine* 333(2), 107–112.

Cohn, D.L. (1994). Treatment and prevention of tuberculosis in HIV-infected persons. *Infectious Disease Clinics of North America* 8(2), 399–412.

Colice, G.L. (1993). Detecting the presence and cause of pulmonary edema. *Postgraduate Medicine* 93(6), 161–170.

Craig, W.J. (1994). Iron status of vegetarians. *American Journal of Clinical Nutrition* 59(suppl.), 1233S–1237S.

Cunha, B.A. (1995). The antibiotic treatment of community-acquired, atypical, and nosocomial pneumonias. *Medical Clinics of North America* 79(3), 581–597.

Cunha, B.A., and Ortega, A.M. (1996). Atypical pneumonia: Extrapulmonary clues guide the way to diagnosis. *Postgraduate Medicine* 99(1), 123–132.

Dabbs, A.D., Kraemer, K.L., and Hoops, S. (1996). Pulmonary edema associated with the treatment of preterm labor: What critical care nurses need to know. *Critical Care Nurse* 16(3), 44–51.

Feied, C.F., Miller, G.H., Stephen, J.M., *et al.* (1995). Chronic pulmonary embolism: Often misdiagnosed, difficult to treat. *Postgraduate Medicine* 97(1), 75–84.

Fine, M.J., Smith, M.A., Carson, C.A., *et al.* (1995). Prognosis and outcomes of patients with community-acquired pneumonia: A meta-analysis. *Journal of the American Medical Association* 275(2), 134–141.

Gattinoni, L., Bombino, M., Pelosi, P., *et al.* (1994). Lung structure and function in different stages of severe adult respiratory distress syndrome. *Journal of the American Medical Association* 271(22), 1772–1779.

Gross, P.A., Hermogenes, A.W., Sacks, H.S., *et al.* (1995). The efficacy of influenza vaccine in elderly persons: A meta-analysis and review of the literature. *Annals of Internal Medicine* 123(7), 518–527.

Guyton, A.C., and Hall, J.E. (1996). *Textbook of Medical Physiology.* (9th ed.). Philadelphia: W.B. Saunders.

Hirsch, D.R., Middola, K.M., Marks, P.W., *et al.* (1996). Pulmonary embolism and deep venous thrombosis during pregnancy or oral contraceptive use: Prevalence of factor V Leiden. *American Heart Journal* 131, 1145–1148.

Kenyon, T.A., Valway, S.E., Ihle, W.W., *et al.* (1996) Transmission of multidrug-resistant *Mycobacterium tuberculosis* during a long airplane flight. *New England Journal of Medicine* 334(15), 933–938.

Kuhn, M.A. (1994). Multiple trauma with respiratory distress. *Critical Care Nurse* 14(2), 68–80.

Levy, D.L. (1995). Hantavirus pulmonary syndrome: Outbreak of a new disease caused by a new virus. *Postgraduate Medicine* 97(3), 127–139.

Lordi, G.M., and Reichman, L.B. (1993). Pulmonary complications of asbestos exposure. *American Family Physician* 48(8), 1471–1477.

Markowitz, N., Hansen, N.I., Hopewell, P.C., *et al.* (1997). Incidence of tuberculosis in the United States among HIV-infected persons. *Annals of Internal Medicine* 126(2), 123–132.

Menzies, D., Fanning, A., Yuan, L., *et al.* (1995). Tuberculosis among health care workers. *New England Journal of Medicine* 332(2), 92–98.

Misasi, R.S., and Keyes, J.L. (1996). Matching and mismatching ventilation and perfusion in the lung. *Critical Care Nurse* 16(3), 23–38.

Misasi, R.S., and Keyes, J.L. (1994). The pathophysiology of hypoxia. *Critical Care Nurse* 14(4), 55–63.

Moffitt, M.P., and Wisinger, D.B. (1996). Tuberculosis: Recommendations for screening, prevention, and treatment. *Postgraduate Medicine* 100(4), 201–220.

Moser, K.M., Fedullo, P.F., LitteJohn, J.K., *et al.* (1994). Frequent asymptomatic pulmonary embolism in patients with deep venous thrombosis. *Journal of the American Medical Association* 271(3), 223–225.

Odom, J.L. (1993). Airway emergencies in the post anesthesia care unit. *Nursing Clinics of North America* 28(3), 483–491.

O'Donnell, J.K., and Gaedeke, M.K. (1995). Sudden infant death syndrome. *Critical Care Nursing Clinics of North America* 7(3), 473–481.

Ortiz, C.R., and La Force, F.M. (1994). Prevention of community-acquired pneumonia. *Medical Clinics of North America* 78(5), 1173–1183.

Pickwell, S.M. (1995). Positive PPD and chemoprophylaxis for tuberculosis infection. *American Family Physician* 51(6), 1929–1934.

Pouchot, J., Grasland, A., Collet, C., *et al.* (1997). Reliability of tuberculin skin test measurement. *Annals of Internal Medicine* 126(3), 210–214.

Robertson, J.M., Burtt, D.S., Edmonds, K.L., *et al.* (1996). Delayed tuberculin reactivity in persons of Indochinese origin: Implications for preventive therapy. *Annals of Internal Medicine* 124(9), 779–784.

Rosen, M.J. (1994). Pneumonia in patients with HIV infection. *Medical Clinics of North America* 78(5), 1067–1079.

Rosenow, E.C. (1995). Venous and pulmonary thromboembolism: An algorithmic approach to diagnosis and management. *Mayo Clinic Proceedings* 70(1), 45–49.

Ruddy, R.M. (1994). Smoke inhalation injury. *Pediatric Clinics of North America* 41(2), 317–336.

Small, P.M., Hopewell, P.C., Singh, S.P., *et al.* (1994). The epidemiology of tuberculosis in San Francisco: A population-based study using conventional and molecular methods. *New England Journal of Medicine* 330(24), 1703–1709.

Smith, M.A., and Brennessel, D.J. (1994). Cytomegalovirus. *Infectious Disease Clinics of North America* 8(2), 427–438.

Snider, G.L. (1997). Tuberculosis then and now: A personal perspective on the last 50 years. *Annals of Internal Medicine* 126(3), 237–243.

Stead, W.W. (1995). Management of health care workers after inadvertent exposure to tuberculosis: A guide for the use of preventive therapy. *Annals of Internal Medicine* 122(12), 906–912.

Surratt, N., and Troino, N.H. (1993). Adult respiratory distress in pregnancy: Critical care issues. *Journal of Obstetrical, Gynecological, and Neonatal Nursing* 23(9), 773–780.

U.S. Public Health Service. (1994). Tuberculosis in adults. *American Family Physician* 50(4), 811–815.

Vincent, M.T., and Goldman, B.S. (1994). Anaerobic lung infections. *American Family Physician* 49(8), 1815–1820.

Vogel, F. (1995). A guide to the treatment of lower respiratory tract infections. *Drugs* 50(1), 62–72.

Vollman, K.M. (1994). Adult respiratory distress syndrome: Mediators on the run. *Critical Care Nursing Clinics of North America* 6(2), 341–358.

Weinberger, S.E. (1993). Recent advances in pulmonary medicine (Second of two parts). *New England Journal of Medicine* 328(20), 1462–1470.

Whitesell, P.L., and Drage, C.W. (1993). Occupational lung cancer. *Mayo Clinic Proceedings* 68, 183–188.

Whitson, B., and Campbell, G.D. (1994). Community-acquired pneumonia: New outpatient guidelines based on age, severity of illness. *Geriatrics* 49(3), 24–36.

Unit VII

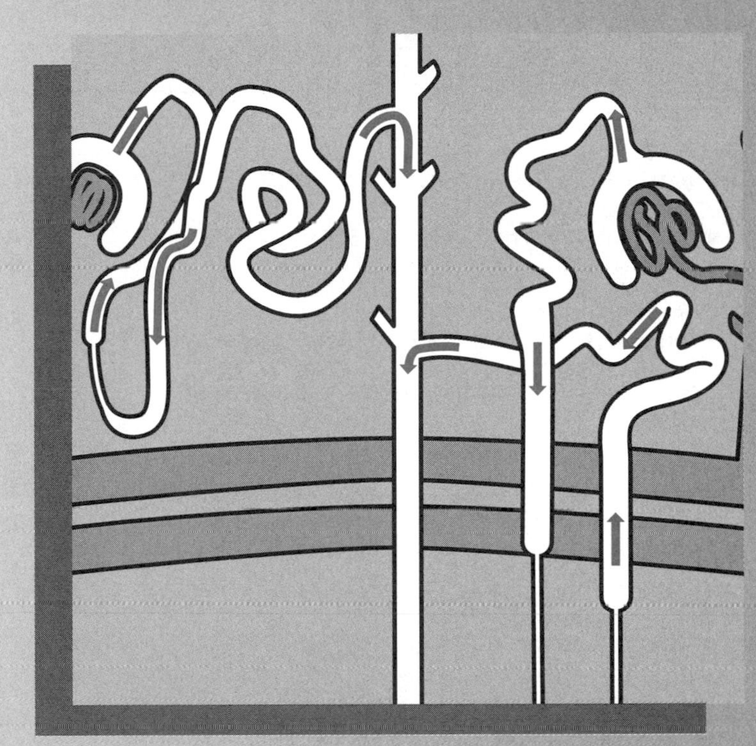

Chapter 20
Disorders of Renal and Urinary Function

RENAL-URINARY SYSTEM

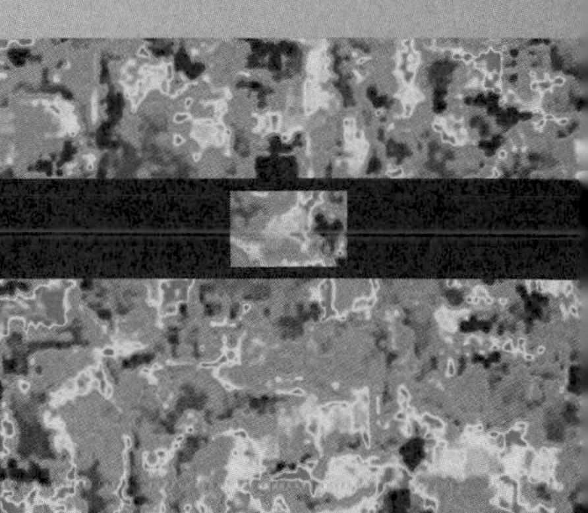

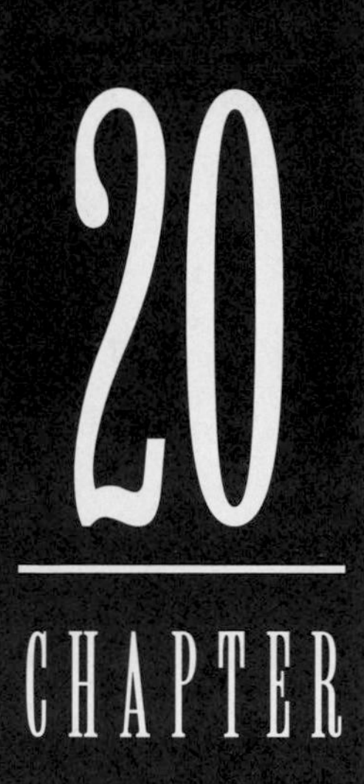

Disorders of Renal and Urinary Function

LEARNING OBJECTIVES

1. Identify the independent and interdependent functions of the renal-urinary system that may be compromised in renal-urinary disorders.
2. Relate the anatomy of the kidneys and lower urinary tract to their functions.
3. Discuss the principal modes of regulation of renal blood flow and glomerular filtration in the context of pathophysiologic processes that may disrupt this regulation.
4. Differentiate among the general transport processes in each segment of the renal tubule, along with clinical consequences of alteration of tubular transport.
5. Discuss the mechanisms by which the kidney may excrete a concentrated or a dilute urine, along with their potential alteration in acute and chronic renal failure.
6. Describe the normal micturition reflex and its possible alteration by developmental factors, neurologic factors, or disorders of the lower urinary tract.
7. Comprehend the pathophysiologic processes that underlie clinical manifestations and rationalize therapy in selected renal-urinary disorders.

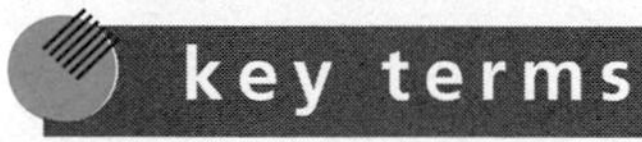

key terms

acute interstitial nephritis
acute renal failure (ARF)
acute tubular necrosis (ATN)
azotemia
chronic renal failure (CRF)
cystitis
dialysis
diuretic
end-stage renal disease (ESRD)
enuresis
functional incontinence
glomerular filtration rate (GFR)

glomerulonephritis
hematuria
hemolytic-uremic syndrome (HUS)
hepatorenal syndrome
interstitial cystitis
micturition
minimal lesion nephrotic syndrome (MLNS)
nephritic syndrome
nephrotic syndrome
overflow incontinence
polycystic kidney disease
proteinuria
pyelonephritis
reflex incontinence
renal adenocarcinoma
renal insufficiency
rhabdomyolysis
stress incontinence
uremia
ureteritis
urethritis
urge incontinence
urinary incontinence
urinary tract infection (UTI)
urolithiasis
von Hippel-Lindau disease
Wilms' tumor

The primary functions of the renal-urinary system are the regulation of the volume and composition of body fluids and the excretion of metabolic wastes. Formation of urine by the kidneys constitutes the first phase in accomplishing these functions. The second phase is completed when the postrenal components of the system appropriately store, transport, and excrete urine. These components are the organs of the lower urinary tract, namely the ureters, bladder, and urethra, along with the neurologic pathways regulating **micturition**, the reflex excretion of urine.

The kidney is also an endocrine organ, involved in the synthesis, release, or activation of the hormones erythropoietin, renin, and vitamin D. As discussed in Chapter 12, erythropoietin regulates the rate of red blood cell synthesis and maturation in response to tissue hypoxia. Renin is released by the juxtaglomerular cells of the kidney in response to a number of factors, setting off the regulatory cascade known as the renin–angiotensin–aldosterone system (RAAS). This system is integral to fluid volume homeostasis and to blood pressure regulation, and was discussed in detail in Chapter 8. The RAAS is revisited in this chapter, in the context of renal regulation. An essential step in the activation of the steroid hormone vitamin D (cholecalciferol) occurs in the kidney and is critical to calcium balance, as discussed in Chapter 9. The kidney also serves as a lesser site of gluconeogenesis, although most glucose formation from noncarbohydrate fuels occurs in the liver (see Chapter 29).

In volume regulation, the kidneys and the cardiovascular system work in concert, responding to a number of regulatory signals. The renal and respiratory systems function together with buffer systems in the regulation of the pH of body fluids (see Chapter 10).

Postrenal function is closely associated with reproductive function because of the anatomic proximity of the two systems. In males, the urethra transports both urine and semen. **Urinary tract infections (UTIs)** may ascend this duct and infect reproductive organs, and sexually transmitted diseases may manifest as difficulty in urination. The prostate gland, a reproductive organ, encircles the urethra in males, and prostate enlargement results in impairment of urination. Disorders of the male reproductive system are detailed in Chapter 30. In females, the orifices of the urethra and vagina are in close proximity. Sexual activity may be associated with ascending UTIs, a risk that is exacerbated by the short urethra in females. Gynecologic disorders such as pelvic inflammatory disease and trauma of childbearing may result in altered muscle tone, scarring, and adhesions affecting the bladder and urethra. Gynecologic disorders are discussed in Chapter 31.

In this chapter, the processes by which the kidneys regulate fluid volume and composition and the regulatory and transport processes resulting in urine formation and excretion are examined. **Acute renal failure (ARF)** occurs in an estimated 5% of all hospitalized patients and is associated with high mortality.[1] **Chronic renal failure (CRF)** has resulted in more than 172,000 people requiring **dialysis** treatment each year.[2] The costs associated with these conditions in terms of both human life and health care resources are considerable. These syndromes and the most prevalent renal disorders associated with renal failure are examined in this chapter. **Urinary incontinence**, which is believed to affect as many as 10 million people in the United States, is discussed, along with the specific urinary disorders of **urolithiasis,** UTI, **interstitial cystitis**, and bladder cancer. Congenital disorders of the urinary tract are briefly described.

RENAL-URINARY ANATOMY

The renal-urinary system is conventionally divided into the upper urinary tract, consisting of the kidneys, and the lower urinary tract, consisting of the ureters, bladder, and urethra. The structure of the nephron, the functional unit of the kidney, is integral to the regulatory and excretory functions of the system (Fig. 20–1).

Gross Anatomy

Kidneys

The kidneys are small, bean-shaped organs located bilaterally in the flank or lumbar areas. They are contained within the small retroperitoneal space, behind the abdominal cavity, and are perfused by branches of the two renal arteries that originate from the abdominal aorta. Each adult kidney is about 11 × 6 cm in size and is composed of an outer fibrous capsule, a cortex about 1-cm thick, an outer medulla, and an inner medulla. The location of nephron structures with respect to the cortical and medullary layers is a significant factor in renal function, as discussed later. The renal capsule restricts distention of the kidney by fluid, potentially contributing to high intrarenal pressures in disorders of obstructed urine outflow.

Lower Urinary Tract

Ureters. The ureters receive urine from the collecting ducts in the renal pelvis and transport it to the bladder. In adults, each ureter is about 30-cm long, with walls composed of smooth muscle. Urine is propelled by hydrostatic (gravitational) flow and by rhythmic contractions (peristalsis), which are self-paced but potentially influenced by neural or hormonal signals. Because ureter walls have a rich blood supply, irritation or obstruction frequently results in the microscopic or gross appearance of blood in the urine (**hematuria**). Receptors for pain are also present in ureter walls, and their stimulation by inflammation or obstruction may trigger neural reflexes, resulting in hyperperistalsis with crampy pain (*ureteral colic*) or decreased glomerular filtration and urine formation (*ureterorenal reflex*). The lower ends of the ureters are embedded within the bladder wall and are compressed when the blad-

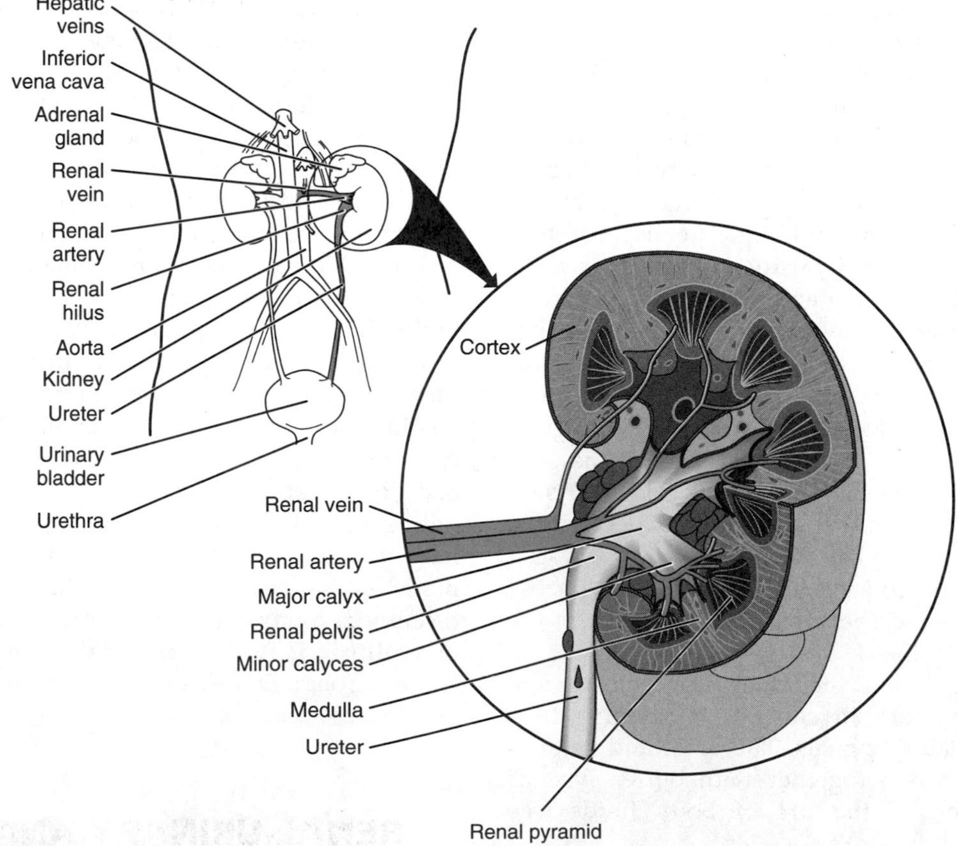

FIGURE 20–1
Renal and urinary anatomy. The kidneys are located bilaterally in the flank regions, within the retroperitoneal space. Each is composed of an outer capsule, a cortex, an outer medulla, and an inner medulla. The pelvis of each kidney leads to the lower urinary tract, consisting of the ureters, bladder, and urethra.

der contracts during micturition, normally preventing retrograde flow of urine.

Bladder. The bladder is a bag composed of smooth *detrusor* muscle, located above the prostate in males (Fig. 20–2) and in front of the uterus in females (Fig. 20–3). Bladder walls have a rich blood supply and may be the source of hematuria. The bladder is innervated by a parasympathetic reflex arc and contracts in response to stretch and other factors. This *micturition reflex* is detailed subsequently.

Urethra. The urethra, or outlet from the bladder, is about 3- to 4-cm long in females and 18- to 20-cm long in males. It has two sphincter muscles that control outflow of urine. The internal smooth muscle sphincter is under reflex control and opens automatically in response to stretch of bladder walls. The external skeletal muscle sphincter is innervated by a motor nerve (the pudendal nerve) and is under voluntary control. The capacity of the urethral sphincter to maintain a watertight seal during bladder filling depends not only on its muscle elements but also on its mucosal lining and underlying vascular cushion. The latter two elements are influenced by estrogen in premenopausal women (see Developmental Perspective). Furthermore, appropriate support of the bladder neck and urethra by pelvic floor muscles is necessary for maintenance of optimal sphincter muscle length and distribution of filling pressures.

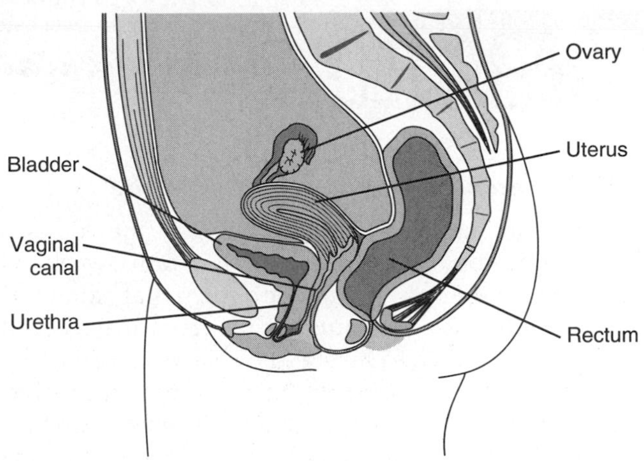

FIGURE 20–3
Female urinary tract. In females, the urinary bladder is located anterior to the uterus, and the urethra is located anterior to the vagina.

Microanatomy: The Nephron

Each kidney contains about 1 million nephrons, or functional units, of two types. As shown in Figure 20–4, the *cortical nephrons* lie more superficially and have more limited blood supplies. Because their loops of Henle are short, these nephrons do not play a major role in the concentration of urine, but they do function in glomerular filtration and in tubular transport, as detailed later. The long-looped *juxtamedullary nephrons* extend deep into the inner medulla and are surrounded by a capillary loop, the vasa recta. The juxtamedullary nephrons function in the concentration of urine and in fine regulation of serum volume and solute concentration.

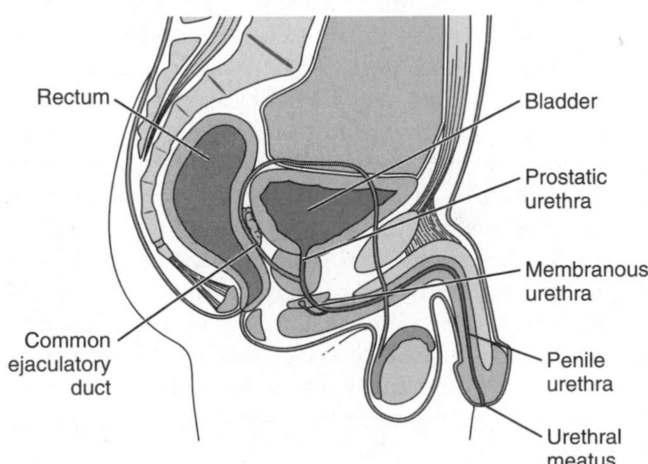

FIGURE 20–2
Male urinary tract. In males, the urinary bladder is located above the prostate gland, which encircles the proximal urethra. The urethra in males is about 18 to 20 cm in length and carries semen as well as urine.

Each nephron may be viewed as a vascular filter situated above a funnel-tipped tube. The filter is a capillary tuft, or glomerulus, which is unique in its permeability characteristics and in its placement between two arterioles. An *afferent arteriole* leads into the glomerulus, and an *efferent arteriole* leads out to a capillary network surrounding the tubular portion of the nephron. This network culminates in a typical venule.

As shown in Figure 20–5, glomerular capillary walls are three layers thick yet are more permeable than most capillaries because their endothelial cell walls contain holes (fenestra) and their epithelial cell layer has filtration slits, both covered by thin membranes. These slits are spaces between the epithelial cell extensions (foot processes), which make up the outer capillary wall. Negative surface charges on the protein coating of these foot processes interact with charged particles in the plasma, influencing their filtration and contributing to selective permeability. The glomerulus is permeable to virtually all components of plasma except for larger proteins, whose negative charges are repelled by the protein coat of the foot processes. In disorders such as glomerulonephritis and diabetic nephropathy, the foot processes may be blunted and the function of the pro-

Developmental Perspective

Embryonic and Fetal Periods

The metanephroi, from which the kidneys develop, arise during the fifth week of gestation. Nephron formation begins at about 8 weeks, with the adult number of nephrons reached at 35 to 36 weeks. During their development, the kidneys rotate and migrate upward from the pelvic area to the lumbar (flank) areas. The lower urinary tract structures begin to develop after division of the cloaca at about 5 weeks. The ability of the fetal kidneys to concentrate urine is about 20% to 30% of that of adult kidneys; however, fetal urine production forms the major portion of the amniotic fluid. During the first 5 months of gestation, renal growth occurs primarily in the inner medulla, whereas growth during the last 4 months is mainly in the outer medulla and cortex. Teratogenic insults during the first 5 weeks of gestation typically result in failure of renal development (renal agenesis or hypoplasia), whereas later insults produce horseshoe kidney, ectopic placement of the kidney, or cystic disease. Structural abnormalities of the lower urinary tract often result from insults during the second or third months of gestation.

Infancy and Childhood

At birth, 20% of nephrons have loops of Henle that are too short to reach the inner medulla, limiting renal concentrating ability. Tubular growth occurs rapidly after birth. Renal vascular resistance is high in newborns, limiting renal blood flow and GFR. Tubular thresholds for reabsorption of many solutes are reduced, leading to loss of these in the urine. Renal functional development is generally complete by the age of 3 months. The newborn's bladder is cigar-shaped and located in the abdominal cavity. During early childhood, the bladder sinks into the pelvis and assumes a pyramidal shape. The urethra in children is proportionately shorter, increasing the anatomic risk of UTI. Functional control of micturition is usually achieved by the age of 3 years, although enuresis is common. ARF in childhood is uncommon but may occur as a result of infectious or toxic disorders, such as acute postinfectious glomerulonephritis and hemolytic-uremic syndrome (HUS). Nephrotic syndrome in children is usually the result of MLNS (minimal change disease or lipoid nephrosis). Polycystic kidney disease and Wilms' tumor often become manifest during childhood.

Adolescence and Young Adulthood

UTI in this group may be associated with sexual activity or sexually transmitted disease. Young women are particularly prone to UTI. Abuse of drugs or exposure to nephrotoxins may predispose to renal failure. UTI during pregnancy imposes increased risk.

Middle and Older Adulthood

Anatomic changes in the aging kidney include loss of nephrons, loss of cortical mass, increased interstitial tissue, glomerular degeneration, thickening of glomerular and tubular basement membranes, and decrease in length and volume of the proximal and distal tubules. Cardiac output is typically decreased, and renal artery atherosclerosis is more prevalent with aging, leading to reduced renal blood flow. GFR is reduced to 60% to 70% of the normal adult value in most elderly people. Serum creatinine may rise in response to these changes. Because muscle tissue is the source of creatinine, however, the rate of rise is often limited by concurrent loss of muscle mass with aging. All of the events that may precipitate ARF and CRF (e.g., congestive heart failure, hypertension, diabetes mellitus) are more prevalent in the elderly. Compromise of lower urinary function is also more common. In men, prostatic enlargement may obstruct the bladder outlet. Lack of estrogen in postmenopausal women leads to a decline in bladder outlet and urethral resistance. These changes, along with weakening of pelvic support structures, predispose to urinary incontinence. Cognitive disorders or impaired mobility may preclude voluntary control of micturition. UTI is common in the elderly and is more likely to manifest atypically and to induce sepsis in older people than in younger people.

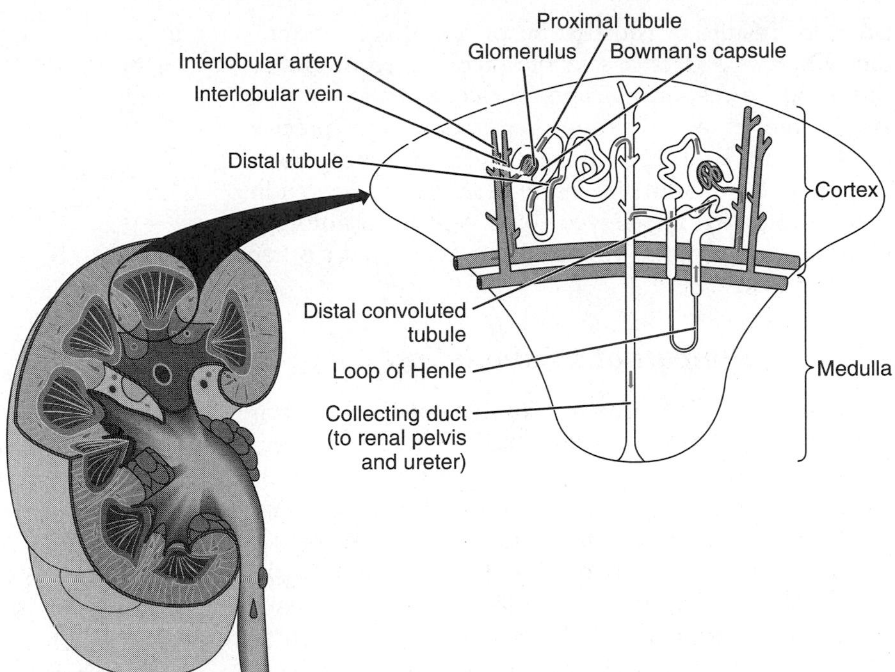

FIGURE 20–4
Anatomy of the nephron. Each nephron consists of a glomerular capillary tuft, which filters plasma constituents into a segmented tubule. From the glomerulus, the tubular structures are the Bowman's capsule, proximal convoluted tubule, loop of Henle, and distal convoluted tubule. The distal tubules of a number of nephrons enter each collecting duct. The two types of nephrons are differentiated on the basis of the length of the loop of Henle. The cortical nephrons have short loops contained within the cortex, whereas the juxtamedullary nephrons have long loops that extend into the medulla.

tein coat impaired, resulting in loss of selective permeability.

The receptacle portion of the nephron begins with Bowman's capsule, which receives the filtrate. Bowman's capsule leads into the convoluted tubule, which is divided functionally into the proximal convoluted tubule (PCT), the loop of Henle, and the distal convoluted tubule (DCT). As the filtrate flows through the tubule, it is altered by a variety of tightly regulated transport processes. The distal tubules of several nephrons lead into a smaller number of collecting ducts, in which further transformation of the filtrate occurs, and the final urine is directed from the collecting ducts into the ureters in the region of the renal pelvis.

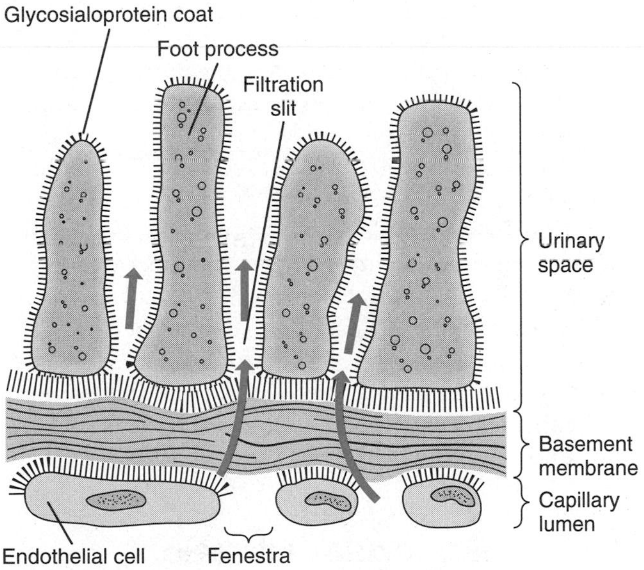

FIGURE 20–5
Structure of the glomerular capillary wall. Selective permeability of the glomerular capillaries is derived from their unique structure. Spaces (fenestra) between endothelial cells are covered by thin membranes. The capillary basement membrane constitutes the middle layer, and extensions (foot processes) of the epithelial layer create filtration slits. The foot processes are covered by a glycosialoprotein coat. The negative charges of this protein coat interact with charged particles, influencing their filtration. (From Cotran, R.S., Kumar, V., and Robbins, S.L. [1994]. *Robbins Pathologic Basis of Disease.* [5th ed.]. Philadelphia: W.B. Saunders. [p. 929].)

RENAL FUNCTION

Renal Perfusion

The glomeruli normally receive about 20% of the cardiac output, although the flow rate, quantified as the renal blood flow or renal plasma flow, varies in response to local, neural, and hormonal regulatory stimuli.

Local Autoregulation

Renal blood flow is autoregulated to a constant rate when the mean arterial pressure is within the range of 80 to 170 mm Hg.[3] As governed by the general resistance equation (see Chapter 15), maintenance of constant flow requires that changes in the pressure gradient be accompanied by proportional changes in resistance. In the kidney, a rise in blood pressure results in constriction of the afferent arteriole, whereas a decrease in blood pressure produces the opposite response, *within the autoregulatory range.* As is the case in all autoregulation, the precise mechanisms and regulatory factors are unknown. The role of endothelial regulation by nitric oxide and endothelins is believed to be central to autoregulation in the renal glomeruli as well as in other capillary beds.

Sympathetic Stimulation

The afferent and efferent arterioles of the nephron are innervated by the sympathetic nervous system (SNS). The nature of the renal response to SNS stimulation depends on the intensity of stimulation (Fig. 20–6). If SNS stimulation is moderate, as in the selective vasoconstriction of the stress state or early shock, both the afferent and efferent arterioles constrict. Renal plasma flow decreases, but glomerular filtration pressure is higher as a result of the efferent constriction. The *filtration fraction,* or percentage of renal blood flow that is filtered, increases. (The filtration fraction is normally about 20% of the volume flowing through the glomerulus.) This response is designed to maintain glomerular filtration as long as possible under conditions of decreased renal perfusion.

With stronger SNS stimulation, constriction of the afferent arteriole is greater than that of the efferent, and both renal plasma flow and **glomerular filtration rate (GFR)** decrease. SNS stimulation is also a secondary trigger of the RAAS, as discussed next.

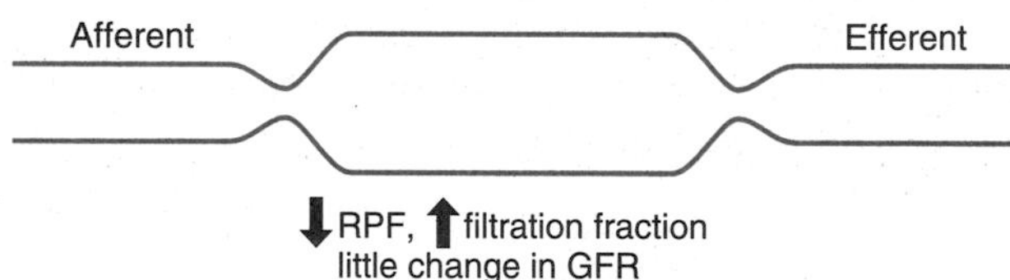

A Moderate SNS stimulation constricts both afferent and efferent arterioles; decreased renal plasma flow, increased filtration fraction, and little change in glomerular filtration rate.

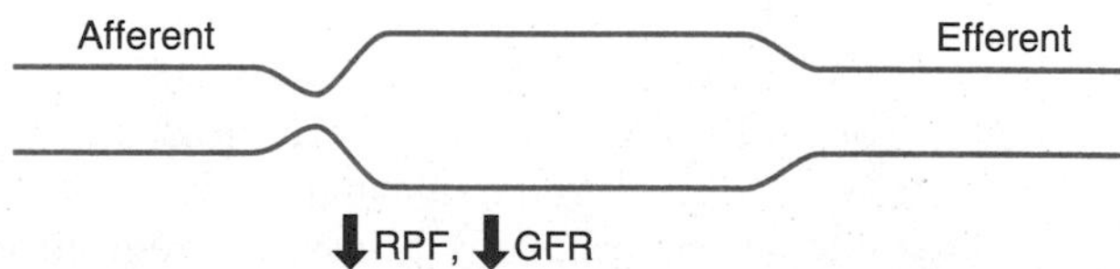

B Strong SNS stimulation constricts afferent more than efferent; decreased renal plasma flow and decreased glomerular filtration rate.

FIGURE 20–6

Effect of sympathetic stimulation on glomerular filtration. With moderate sympathetic nervous system (SNS) stimulation, as occurs in exercise, stress, or early shock, the glomerular filtration rate (GFR) is preserved. With strong sympathetic stimulation, as in progressive shock, the glomerular filtration rate decreases. RPF, renal plasma flow. (Adapted from Rose, B.D. [1994]. *Clinical Physiology of Acid-Base and Electrolyte Disorders* [4th ed.]. New York: McGraw-Hill. [p. 17]. Copyright 1994. Reproduced with permission of The McGraw-Hill Companies.)

Renin–Angiotensin–Aldosterone System

The RAAS, which affects both the pressure gradient and resistance components of renal perfusion, was illustrated in Chapter 8. The hormone renin is released from juxtaglomerular cells of the nephron in response to (1) decreased stretch of the afferent arteriole, reflecting decreased blood volume or pressure, (2) increased binding of SNS-mediated catecholamines to β-adrenergic receptors on juxtaglomerular cells, and (3) decreased serum sodium (Na^+), which is sensed by the macula densa as decreased Na^+ in the distal tubular fluid. Figure 20–7 illustrates the *juxtaglomerular apparatus* of the nephron, which encompasses the juxtaglomerular cells of the afferent arteriole, the macula densa cells of the distal tubule, and the mesangial cells, which are multifunctional cells that act as macrophages and also contract in response to varied stimuli to alter the glomerular surface area.

In the bloodstream, renin activates a circulating protein, angiotensinogen, to form angiotensin I (AGT I). As it circulates through the pulmonary system and other tissues, AGT I is converted to AGT II by angiotensin-converting enzyme (ACE). AGT II, a potent vasoconstrictor, increases mean arterial pressure, thereby decreasing SNS stimulation and inhibiting further renin release. AGT II constricts the efferent arteriole to a greater degree than the afferent, thus helping to maintain GFR. In the case of RAAS activation by a macula densa signal, dilation of the afferent arteriole occurs. Within the cascade of the RAAS, AGT II stimulates the adrenal cortex to release the hormone aldosterone, which increases the active reabsorption of sodium from the DCT. Water is reabsorbed passively along the resulting osmotic gradient, increasing blood volume and renal plasma flow, and completing the negative feedback loop.

Glomerular Filtration

The GFR is the volume filtered per unit time. The normal GFR in adults is 180 L/day or 125 mL/min, of which about 99% is normally returned to the blood by tubular transport processes.

Glomerular Capillary Dynamics

Glomerular filtration conforms to Starling's law of the capillary (see Chapter 8). As illustrated in Figure

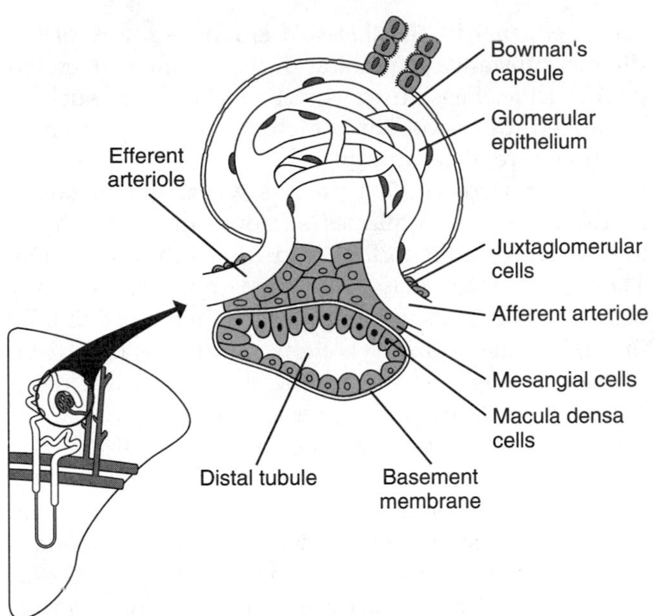

FIGURE 20–7
Juxtaglomerular apparatus. The juxtaglomerular apparatus includes the juxtaglomerular cells of the afferent arteriole, the macula densa cells of the distal tubule (which loops back in proximity to the glomerulus), and the mesangial cells.

20–8, the force favoring filtration, or outward movement of fluid from the capillary, is glomerular capillary hydrostatic pressure (GCHP), normally about 45 mm Hg. GCHP is derived from mean arterial pressure, renal plasma flow, and the resistance provided by the afferent and efferent arterioles. Conditions that alter blood volume, blood pressure, or SNS activity (e.g., shock or dehydration) may affect GCHP.

Forces opposing glomerular filtration are glomerular colloid osmotic pressure (GCOP) and Bowman's capsule hydrostatic pressure (BCHP). Colloid osmotic pressure in the glomerulus, as in all capillaries, is the osmotic pull of serum proteins such as albumin, which tends to keep fluid in the vascular compartment. GCOP may be decreased in protein malnutrition, liver disease, or glomerular loss of protein (**proteinuria**). BCHP, the fluid pressure in Bowman's capsule, is the glomerular equivalent of tissue interstitial fluid pressure in other capillaries. BCHP normally remains low because filtered fluid is immediately transported down the tubule. In cases of tubular obstruction by renal tubular disease or lower urinary tract obstruction (e.g., a stone or stricture), however, pressure may rise in Bowman's capsule, opposing further filtration.

Under normal circumstances, the GCHP of 45 mm Hg easily offsets the opposing forces, typically 25 mm Hg GCOP and 10 mm Hg BCHP, resulting in net forces favoring filtration. Excessive filtration may occur in glomerular diseases in which protein is filtered from the serum into Bowman's capsule. In the **nephrotic syndrome**, for example, proteinuria results in decreased plasma colloid osmotic pressure and increased Bowman's capsule colloid osmostic pressure. Filtered protein then creates an osmotic gradient that holds water in the tubules, resulting in dehydration, and lack of serum protein allows fluid to accumulate in the tissue interstitial spaces, resulting in edema.

Regulation of Glomerular Filtration Rate

Because glomerular filtration depends on renal plasma flow, GFR is regulated secondarily to the autoregulatory, neural, and hormonal stimuli governing renal perfusion. Perfusion is a critical determinant of glomerular filtration, which, in turn, influences tubular transport processes. The maintenance of a constant tubular flow rate is essential for optimal function of tubular transport processes, discussed next.

Tubular Transport

Epithelial Transport

Transport of water and solutes between the nephron tubules and the peritubular capillaries surrounding them is an example of epithelial transport. As discussed in Chapter 2, epithelial transport involves multiple channels and transport proteins as well as transport across more than one biologic membrane. The cells of the renal tubular walls form

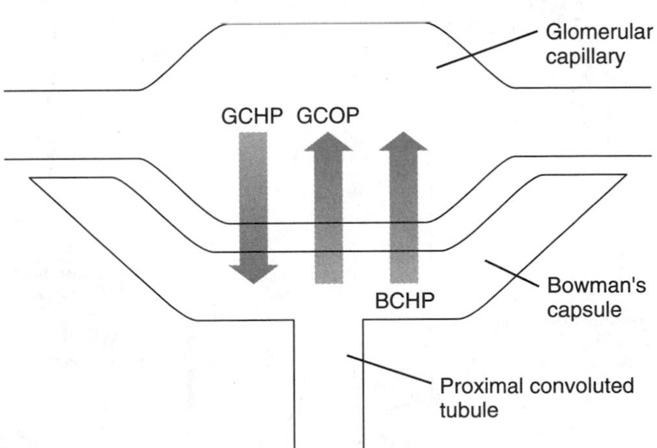

FIGURE 20–8
Glomerular capillary dynamics. Consistent with Starling's law of the capillary, the force favoring filtration from the glomerulus is glomerular capillary hydrostatic pressure (GCHP). Filtration is opposed by the colloid osmotic pressure within glomerular capillary blood (GCOP) and the hydrostatic pressure within Bowman's capsule (BCHP).

the barrier between the blood and the tubular filtrate, or potential urine. As shown in Figure 20–9, which depicts transport within the PCT, substances may be transported through the tubular cell membrane on both the tubular lumen (brush border or apical) side and the interstitial space (basolateral membrane) side. Because membrane lipids, protein channels, pumps, and carriers differ between the two sides, the epithelial cells are said to be *polarized.* Loss of this polarity may occur if renal tubular cells are damaged, resulting in impairment of transport functions. Substances may also be transported between tubular cells, with the permeability of these intercellular channels varying along the course of the tubule.

Transport Processes

Reabsorption and secretion are the two basic processes by which tubular cells modify the filtrate, so that the final urine is appropriate in its volume and constituency. Reabsorption, the recovery of filtered water and solutes from the tubular lumen for return to the plasma, may occur by both active and passive transport processes. Recall that active transport mechanisms require energy and also employ membrane protein pumps that are saturable; that is, they have a maximum rate of activity. This *tubular maximum,* or T_m, potentially limits the amount of a filtered substance that can be reabsorbed. If tubular flow rates are normal and the amount of a filtered substance does not exceed the T_m for that substance, then all of it will be reabsorbed. Once the system is saturated, that is, the *threshold* is reached, any of the filtered substance remaining in the tubule is excreted in the urine. Passive transport mechanisms, such as facilitated diffusion, in which a carrier protein is required, are also saturable.

Tubular secretion is a process whereby substances in the blood of capillaries surrounding the tubules are actively transported into the tubular lumen. These substances may have been unfiltered or may have been filtered and reabsorbed more proximally in the tubule. Most secretion occurs in the distal tubule, serving as a fine-tuning mechanism for regulation of potassium and other solutes.

Clinical evaluation of the efficiency of tubular transport is frequently based on the concept of *clearance.* Clearance is the ability of the kidneys to remove a specified substance from the blood within a given period of time. By comparing serum and urine levels of a substance (often creatinine, a product of protein metabolism), the status of renal function can be determined. Clearance of specific drugs is also of clinical importance, and dosages and administration intervals must often be adjusted in patients with renal disorders.

Transport in Specific Tubular Segments

Anatomic features, transport processes, and osmolarity of the filtrate in each segment of the tubule are summarized in Table 20–1.

Proximal Tubular Transport. The PCT is often called the "workhorse" of the nephron because

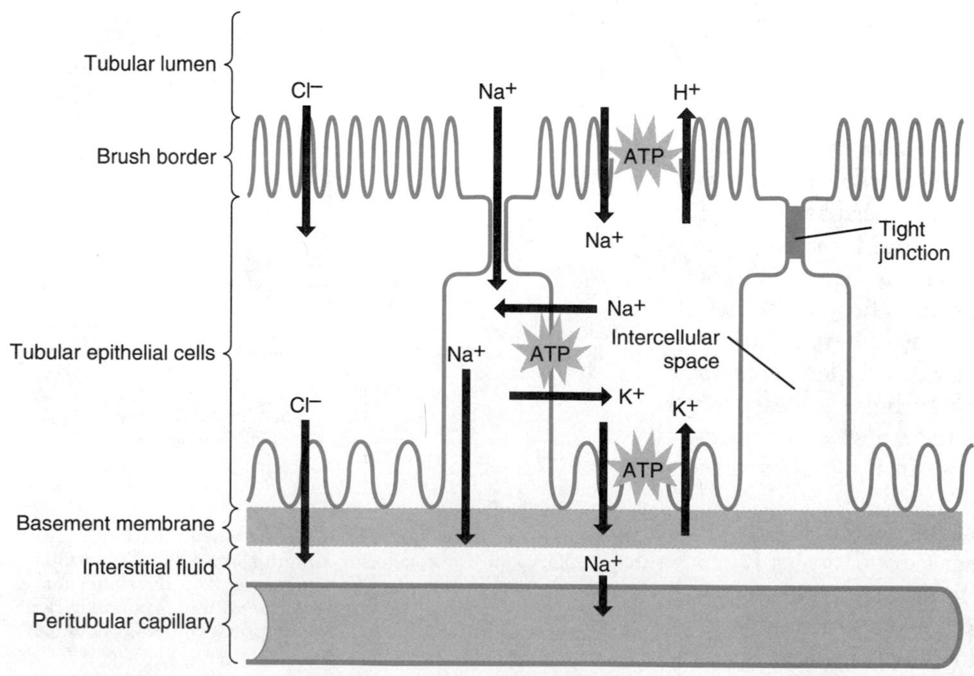

FIGURE 20–9
Transport across tubular cells. Tubular transport is an example of epithelial transport, involving multiple, polarized transport mechanisms and more than one biologic membrane. Principal methods of transport across the proximal convoluted tubule, between the tubular lumen and the capillary blood, are depicted. (Adapted from Guyton, A.C., and Hall, J.E. [1996]. *Textbook of Medical Physiology.* [9th ed.]. Philadelphia: W.B. Saunders. [p. 332].)

TABLE 20–1
SEGMENTAL VARIATION IN TUBULAR PERMEABILITY AND TRANSPORT

Tubular Segment	Structural Features	Transport Mechanisms
Proximal convoluted tubule	"Leaky" tight junctions between cells; many mitochondria to support active transport; extensive surface area on both brush border and basolateral membranes; water channels present. Proportional water and solute reabsorption; filtrate is isotonic.	Basolateral membrane: Na^+-K^+-ATPase (reabsorbs Na^+ in exchange for K^+) Passive reabsorption of Na^+ with HCO_3^- produced by hydrolysis Passive reabsorption of K^+ by K^+ channels Brush border: Na^+-solute cotransport for reabsorption Na^+-H^+ antiport (reabsorbs Na^+ and secretes H^+) Anion exchanger (reabsorbs Cl^- in exchange for formate) Water reabsorption by osmosis H^+-organic cation exchanger (secretes cations in exchange for H^+) Urate anion exchangers (urate reabsorption early, secretion late)
Descending loop of Henle	Highly permeable to water; moderately permeable to most solutes; few mitochondria (little or no active transport). More water leaves the tubule than solute; filtrate is hypertonic.	Passive reabsorption (minimal) Reabsorption of 20% of filtered water by osmosis
Ascending loop of Henle	Impermeable to water; passive diffusion of solutes in thin ascending segment; mitochondria to support active transport in thick ascending segment. Solute leaves tubule as filtrate ascends; filtrate becomes hypotonic.	Basolateral membrane: Na^+-K^+-ATPase Passive reabsorption of Cl^- by Cl^- channels Passive reabsorption of K^+ by K^+ channels Brush border: Na^+-K^+-$2Cl^-$ cotransporter (reabsorption) K^+ channels (secretion)
Early distal convoluted tubule (diluting segment)	Impermeable to water and urea; mitochondria to support active transport; macula densa cells for feedback control of renin secretion. Solute leaves tubule; filtrate is hypotonic.	Same as thick ascending loop of Henle
Late distal convoluted tubule and collecting duct	Two cell types: principal cells and intercalated cells. Permeability to water and urea variable with antidiuretic hormone (ADH) concentration. In the absence of ADH, NaCl reabsorption leaves filtrate increasingly hypotonic. If ADH is present, water is reabsorbed along the medullary gradient, and filtrate becomes increasingly hypertonic.	Basolateral membrane: Na^+-K^+-ATPase (in principal cells) H^+-ATPase (in intercalated cells; secretes H^+) K^+ channels (reabsorption) Cl^- channels (reabsorption)

nearly all of the filtrate is reabsorbed in this initial segment. The PCT is anatomically suited to reabsorption because it is highly permeable to water and most solutes. Much of the reabsorption is associated with gradients created by the active reabsorption of sodium. Most of the filtered sodium is reabsorbed here, by at least three mechanisms (see Fig. 20–9).

On the basolateral side of the tubular cell, an Na^+-K^+-ATPase pumps sodium out of the tubular cell, creating a concentration gradient for sodium to move from the tubular lumen brush border into the tubular cell, then into the blood, carrying with it other solutes, such as glucose, phosphate, or amino acids. The second mechanism begins with an antiport on the brush border side, which actively secretes hydrogen into the lumen in exchange for sodium, which is taken into the cell. A symport on the basolateral side then transports sodium into the blood, along with bicarbonate. The third mechanism involves the passive reabsorption of chloride, which occurs late in the PCT and creates an electrical gradient for additional sodium reabsorption.

Potassium and calcium are also actively reabsorbed in cotransport with Na^+, although the precise mechanisms are uncertain. About 40% of filtered urea, a waste product of protein metabolism, is first reabsorbed in the PCT, then secreted more distally as a component of the urine concentration mechanism, described later.

Secretion into the PCT does occur, although it is much more limited than reabsorption. Organic acids, such as bile acids, uric acid, and acidic drugs, are not filtered, but instead are secreted into the urine in the PCT. Organic bases are similarly secreted and include acetylcholine, creatinine, epinephrine, norepinephrine, dopamine, and basic drugs. The secretion of H^+ by the Na^+-H^+ antiport was discussed earlier with sodium transport. If serum pH is normal, about 95% of H^+ is secreted by this mechanism. In the lumen, this H^+ combines with filtered HCO_3^-, forming CO_2 and H_2O by reversal of the hydrolysis reaction (see Chapter 10). Because H^+ is not free in the lumen, proximal tubular pH is the same as that of the blood. PCT filtrate is also isotonic with the serum because water and solute are proportionately reabsorbed.

Loop of Henle Transport. Transport within the loop of Henle differs in each of its three sections, and these differences are critical to establishment of the hypertonic interstitial fluid gradient, a key component of the *countercurrent mechanism* for concentration of urine, detailed later in this section. As illustrated in Figure 20–10, the thin descending loop is permeable to water but impermeable to solutes. In this section, water is reabsorbed by osmosis along the hypertonic interstitial fluid gradient. The thin ascending loop, found only in juxtamedullary nephrons, is permeable to NaCl and urea, but not to water. Concentration gradients permit passive diffusion of NaCl from the tubule into the interstitium, and of urea from the interstitium to the tubule. There is a net *loss* of solute from this segment of the tubule, which is important to the countercurrent mechanism. The thick ascending loop is permeable *only* to Na^+, K^+, and Cl^-, which are actively reabsorbed by a symport as the initial step in the countercurrent mechanism. The thick ascending loop also secretes a mucoprotein (*Tamm-Horsfall protein*), which may serve an immune function within renal tissues.

Distal Tubular and Collecting Duct Transport. The proximal ("early") portion of the DCT, known

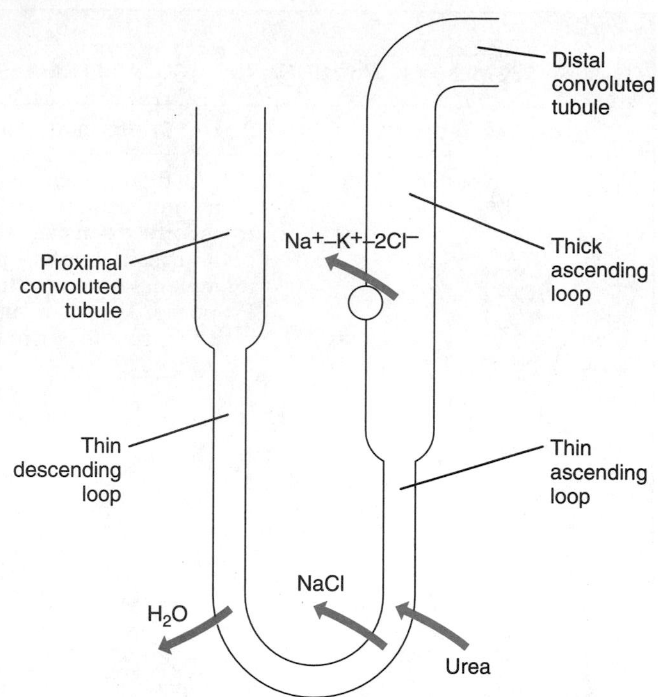

FIGURE 20–10
Transport in the loop of Henle. Water is reabsorbed from the thin descending loop, which is impermeable to solutes. The thin ascending loop, found only in juxtamedullary nephrons, is impermeable to water but permits diffusion of solutes such as NaCl and urea. The thick ascending loop is permeable only to Na^+, K^+, and Cl^-, which are actively reabsorbed.

as the diluting segment, is impermeable to both water and urea but is permeable to Na^+ and Cl^-, which are actively reabsorbed by a symport (Fig. 20–11). The "late" DCT and collecting duct are anatomically similar; they are relatively impermeable to Cl^- but permeable to Na^+, K^+, and H^+. As regulated by aldosterone, an Na^+-K^+-ATPase pump on the basolateral side pumps Na^+ from the tubular cell into the blood, creating a concentration gradient for Na^+ reabsorption from the tubular lumen. Cl^- remains in the lumen, and its negative charge tends to oppose Na^+ reabsorption.

The Na^+-K^+-ATPase antiport simultaneously secretes K^+ from the blood into the tubular cell, where its concentration rises, causing it to diffuse passively into the tubular lumen. Active transport of K^+ from the tubular cell into the lumen has also been postulated. High serum K^+ directly stimulates the adrenal cortex to secrete aldosterone, inducing the activity of the basolateral Na^+-K^+-ATPase. If serum K^+ is low, K^+ may back-leak by passive diffusion along its concentration gradient from the tubular cell into the blood. At high tubular flow rates, this back-leak does not occur, however, and K^+ may be lost in the urine even if serum levels are low.

On the brush border side, an antiport secretes H^+ into the tubule in exchange for K^+. If serum pH is

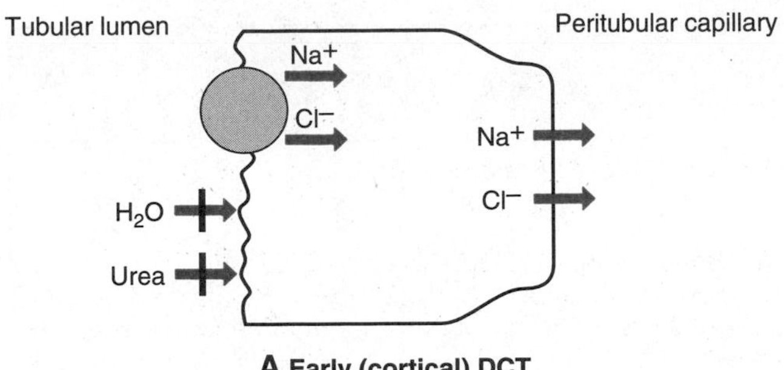

A Early (cortical) DCT

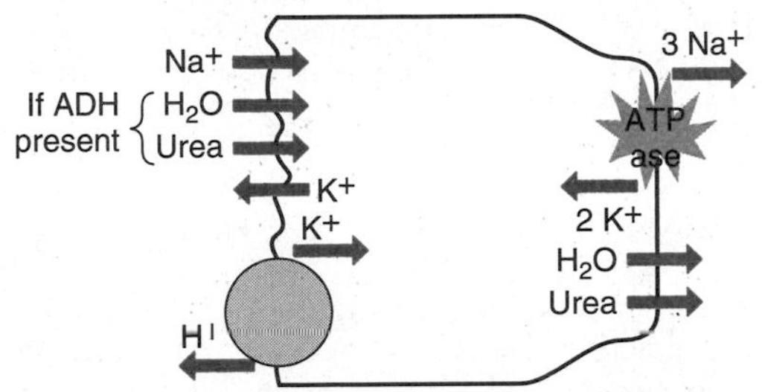

B Late (medullary) DCT and collecting duct

FIGURE 20–11

Transport in the distal tubule and collecting duct. The proximal portion of the distal convoluted tubule (DCT) is impermeable to water and urea but permits active reabsorption of Na^+ and Cl^-. The late distal tubule and cortical portion of the collecting duct have similar transport characteristics, and are permeable to Na^+, K^+, and H^+. Permeability to water and urea in this segment depends on the presence of antidiuretic hormone (ADH).

normal, only about 5% of H^+ is secreted in the DCT; however, much greater H^+ secretion can occur in cases of acidosis. As discussed in Chapter 10, urinary excretion of H^+ is limited by the capacity of urinary buffer systems. If both H^+ and K^+ are elevated, the kidney preferentially secretes H^+, promoting hyperkalemia. In alkalosis, bicarbonate filtration exceeds reabsorption in the PCT, and there is no DCT secretion of H^+.

Permeability of the late DCT and collecting duct to H_2O depends on the availability of antidiuretic hormone (ADH), synthesized by the hypothalamus and secreted by the posterior pituitary gland. As discussed in Chapter 8, the late DCT and collecting duct are impermeable to water in the absence of ADH, resulting in excretion of excess water in the urine. In the presence of ADH, water may be reabsorbed along the osmotic gradient created by Na^+ reabsorption by the Na^+-K^+-ATPase pump, under the influence of aldosterone. In addition, both water and urea may be passively reabsorbed from the DCT along the hypertonic interstitial fluid gradient, as part of the countercurrent mechanism.

Table 20–2 describes renal transport of specific constituents of tubular filtrate. Regulation of serum electrolyte concentrations is highly dependent on tubular transport processes. Excretion of metabolic wastes, including urea, a protein metabolite, creatinine, a muscle metabolite, and uric acid, a purine metabolite, is also dependent on tubular function. Accumulation of these wastes contributes to the development of **uremia**, a syndrome associated with renal failure.

Mechanisms for Concentration and Dilution of Urine

To fulfill its function of metabolic waste excretion, the kidney is obligated to excrete a minimal quantity of solute each day (about 900 mOsm in adults). If this solute were excreted in an isotonic solution, urinary fluid losses would approach 3 L/day. In fluid volume deficit or hyperosmolar imbalance, the kidney's mechanisms for concentration of urine permit excretion of hypertonic urine, conserving fluid when necessary while still excreting adequate amounts of urea, creatinine, and other solutes. Conversely, in fluid volume excess or hypo-osmolar imbalance, the kidney is able to excrete a dilute urine that is hypotonic to the serum.

Countercurrent Mechanisms for the Concentration of Urine

Concentration of urine requires the establishment and maintenance of a vertically graduated concentration gradient in the medullary interstitial fluid. As shown in Figure 20–12, the osmolarity of the interstitial fluid in the cortex, surrounding the PCT, is isotonic with the serum (approximately 300 mOsm/L). Within the medulla, however, interstitial fluid becomes increasingly hypertonic, to a maximum of about 1200 mOsm/L at the lower tip of the loop of Henle. Two mechanisms, the *countercurrent multiplier* in the loop of Henle and the *countercurrent exchanger* in the vasa recta, operate to create and maintain this gradient. Countercurrent mechanisms depend on an anatomic configuration that results in parallel flow in opposite directions.

Countercurrent Multiplier. In the loop of Henle, countercurrent flow occurs in the descending and ascending loops. Recall that the descending loop is permeable only to water, whereas the ascending loop is permeable only to solute. The countercurrent multiplier is a complex process that may be arbitrarily subdivided into three steps (Fig. 20–13). First, there is active transport of solute *out* of the ascending loop, creating a horizontal gradient between the tubular fluid in the descending limb and the interstitium. Second, because the descending loop is permeable only to H_2O, it moves out of the lumen along this gradient until tubular fluid and interstitial fluid

TABLE 20–2
TUBULAR TRANSPORT OF SELECTED SUBSTANCES

SUBSTANCE	TRANSPORT MECHANISMS AND SITES
Sodium	Freely filtered at glomerulus Reabsorbed in proximal convoluted tubule (PCT) by Na^+-K^+-ATPase in basolateral membrane; facilitated transport by symports (with glucose, PO_4^{3-}, and amino acids) in brush border and with HCO_3^- in basolateral membrane; antiport (with H^+ secretion) in brush border Reabsorbed passively with Cl^- and H_2O (via "leaky" tight junctions) Reabsorbed in thick ascending loop by active transport (Na^+-K^+-$2Cl^-$ symport) Reabsorbed in late distal convoluted tubule (DCT) and collecting duct by Na^+-K^+-ATPase (increased in response to aldosterone; decreased in response to atrial natriuretic peptide) Minimal active reabsorption by Na^+-Cl^- symport
Potassium	Freely filtered at glomerulus Reabsorbed passively in PCT (along gradients created by Na^+ and H_2O reabsorption) Reabsorbed actively in thick ascending loop (by Na^+-K^+-$2Cl^-$ symport) Reabsorbed or secreted in DCT and collecting by H^+-K^+-ATPase (secreted in exchange for H^+ if H^+ is low or K^+ is high; reabsorbed if K^+ is low or H^+ is high)
Chloride	Freely filtered at glomerulus Reabsorbed passively late in the PCT along concentration gradient created by earlier preferential reabsorption of HCO_3^- Active reabsorption in PCT by anion exchanger (antiport with formate) Active reabsorption in ascending loop of Henle by Na^+-K^+-$2Cl^-$ symport Active reabsorption in DCT by Na^+-Cl^- symport and Cl^--HCO_3^- antiport Passive reabsorption in DCT (along electrical gradient created by Na^+ reabsorption) through tight junctions
Hydrogen	Freely filtered at glomerulus Secreted into PCT by Na^+-H^+ antiport Reabsorbed from PCT by H^+ cation exchangers (e.g., creatinine, certain drugs) Secreted by H^+-K^+ antiport in DCT and collecting duct (when H^+ is high or K^+ is low)
Bicarbonate	Freely filtered at glomerulus Passive reabsorption in PCT and DCT (coupled with H^+ secretion)
Glucose	Freely filtered at glomerulus Entirely reabsorbed by Na^+-glucose symport (unless tubular maximum is exceeded)
Urea	Freely filtered at glomerulus

are in equilibrium at that level (hypertonic to the serum). Third, the addition of isotonic fluid from the PCT to the descending loop pushes the hypertonic tubular fluid downward around the hairpin turn. Continuous repetition of this sequence multiplies the single effect of the initial horizontal gradient and results in creation of the graduated vertical gradient. In this way, the gradient is established much more efficiently than would be possible with the operation of multiple active transport pumps along the loop. The countercurrent multiplier has its greatest effect in the long loops of Henle found in juxtamedullary nephrons, although a lesser gradient is established by this mechanism in cortical nephrons.

Countercurrent Exchanger. Countercurrent flow occurs simultaneously in the vasa recta of juxtamedullary nephrons (Fig. 20–14). In this capillary loop, which surrounds the loop of Henle, both ascending and descending limbs are freely permeable to both water and solute. Blood flow is normally slow, especially around the hairpin turn. The countercurrent exchange mechanism depends on this sluggish flow and on ease of exchange of substances between the two limbs. Because all transport between the medullary interstitium and the blood is passive, it would be expected that any movement of solute and water occurring in the descending limb would be offset by movement in the opposite direction in the ascending limb. Because of the flow dynamics, however, this is not the case. Solute uptake exceeds water efflux in the descending limb, and water uptake exceeds solute efflux in the ascending limb.

TABLE 20–2
TUBULAR TRANSPORT OF SELECTED SUBSTANCES *Continued*

SUBSTANCE	TRANSPORT MECHANISMS AND SITES
	Reabsorbed passively along its concentration gradient in PCT, late DCT, and collecting duct (baseline moderate permeability to urea is increased in the late tubule in the presence of antidiuretic hormone) May reenter descending and thin ascending loops of Henle from interstitium if concentration gradient is present
Calcium	60% (unbound fraction) is filtered at glomerulus Reabsorbed passively in PCT and thin loop of Henle (following NaCl and H_2O gradients) Reabsorbed actively in ascending thick loop of Henle and early DCT by hormone-sensitive carriers (increased by parathyroid hormone and vitamin D_3)
Phosphate	Freely filtered at glomerulus Reabsorbed in PCT by Na^+-PO_4^{3-} symport (decreased when PO_4^{3-} load is high, in response to parathyroid hormone, or when high H^+ secretion requires tubular buffering)
Magnesium	Unbound fraction (70%–80%) is filtered at glomerulus Most is reabsorbed in the thick ascending loop of Henle by both active and passive mechanisms (poorly understood)
Uric acid	Freely filtered at the glomerulus (mostly as urate anion) Reabsorbed early in PCT by urate-hydroxide anion exchanger driven by pH gradient created by Na^+-H^+ antiport Secreted by organic acid pump in mid-PCT (about 50% of filtered load) Reabsorption of secreted urate in late PCT possibly in an anion exchanger (typical net reabsorption of 90% of amount filtered; reabsorption is variable with Na^+ reabsorption)
Protein	Filtration depends on size and charge (high molecular weight and negative charge limit filtration of most serum proteins) Amino acids actively reabsorbed in PCT by symport with Na^+ across brush border, then by facilitated diffusion across basolateral membrane (by specific carriers) Small peptides hydrolyzed by brush border enzymes before reabsorption by amino acid carriers Larger peptides reabsorbed by receptor-mediated endocytosis into cell for entry into lysozomes, where they are metabolized into amino acids
Organic cations (creatinine, certain drugs)	Selectively filtered at glomerulus Secreted by H^+-organic cation antiport in PCT
Organic anions (urate, hippurate, ketoacid anions, certain drugs)	Secreted by multiple poorly understood mechanisms, including anion exchanger in PCT

The water reabsorbed from the collecting ducts in the presence of ADH is taken up by the ascending limb, which allows the medullary gradient to be maintained. If not for this mechanism, the water reabsorbed from the tubular filtrate in the DCT and collecting duct would soon dilute the hypertonic interstitial fluid and dissipate the gradient. Similarly, it is important that the accumulation of solute in the interstitium, resulting from the countercurrent multiplier in the loop of Henle, not be "washed out" by excessive uptake of solute by the vasa recta. This normally does not occur because the slow blood flow allows sufficient time for re-equilibration of solute loads between the ascending limb and the interstitium. At normal blood flow rates, there is a slight net uptake of solute from the vasa recta, but this is easily replenished by the active transport of solute from the ascending loop of Henle and by reabsorption of urea from the collecting duct, as discussed later. At increased blood flow rates, however, equilibration is incomplete, and solute is washed out of the interstitium.

Addition of Urea to the Medullary Interstitium

Maintenance of the medullary gradient depends not only on reabsorption of interstitial fluid and the addition and maintenance of NaCl in the interstitium but also on addition of another solute, urea, to the interstitium (Fig. 20–15). This occurs as a result of concentration of urea in the late DCT and collect-

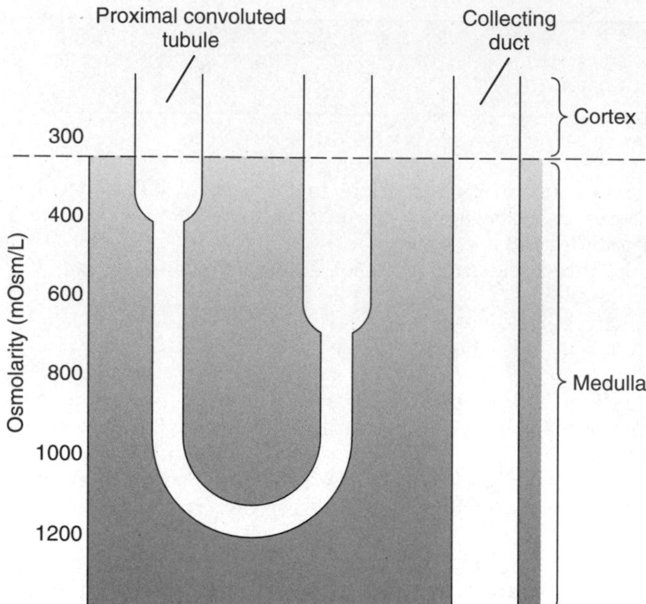

FIGURE 20–12

Medullary interstitial gradient. The interstitial fluid within the kidney becomes progressively more concentrated from the cortex to the inner medulla. Establishment and maintenance of this gradient is essential to mechanisms for concentration of urine.

ing duct, owing to reabsorption of Na^+ and H_2O by the Na^+-K^+-ATPase. A concentration gradient then exists for urea to diffuse from the collecting duct to the interstitium, a process that is facilitated by the presence of ADH.

Regulation by Antidiuretic Hormone

As detailed in Chapter 8, ADH is an important hormone in the regulation of fluid volume and osmolarity. When this peptide hormone binds to its receptors on the brush border side of tubular cells of the DCT and collecting duct, it activates cellular enzyme systems that insert (by exocytosis) protein water channels into the cell membranes, increasing their permeability. When the ADH is removed, channels are removed by endocytosis, packaged into vesicles, and internalized into the tubular cell.[4]

Although the primary stimulus for ADH release is increased serum osmolarity as sensed by osmoreceptors, decreased fluid volume (sensed by baroreceptors) also triggers ADH release. The response to ADH is concentration dependent. Assuming a normal medullary gradient, the amount of ADH present determines the degree of urine concentration (Fig. 20–16). The tubular fluid in the early DCT

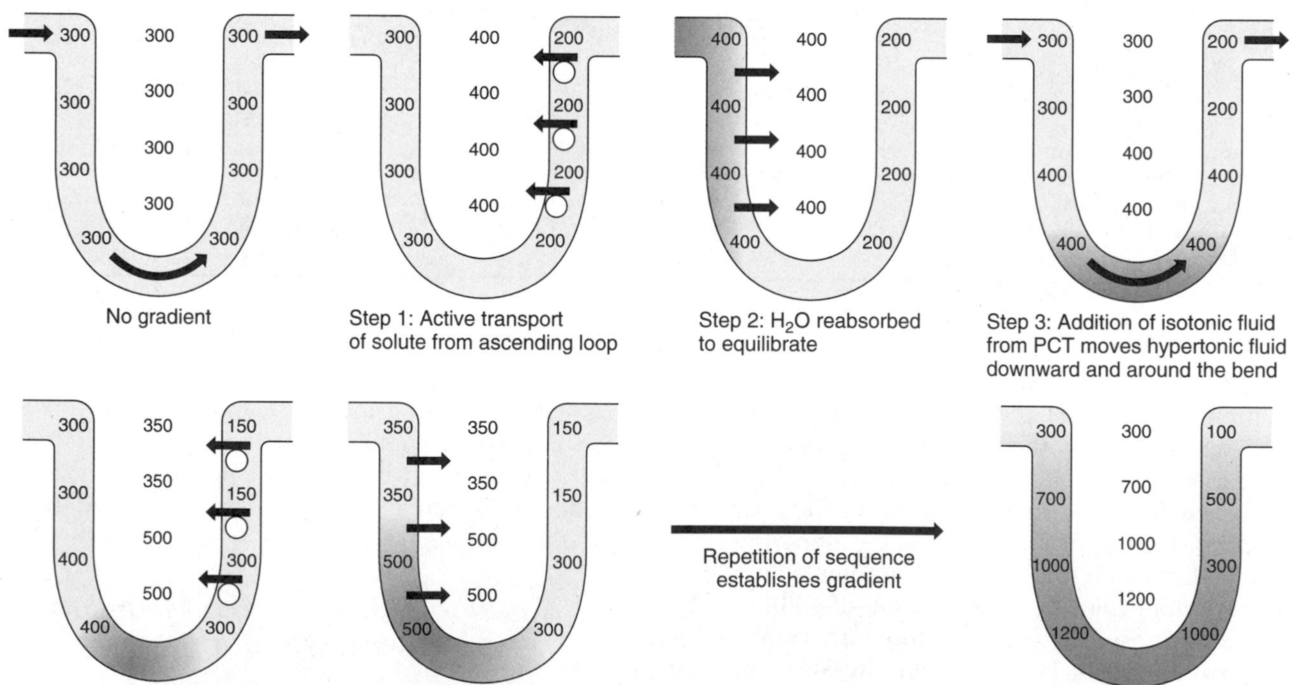

FIGURE 20–13

Countercurrent multiplier. The countercurrent multiplier mechanism, which establishes the vertical medullary interstitial gradient, operates most effectively in the long loops of Henle of juxtamedullary nephrons. The parallel alignment of the descending and ascending limbs, and the hairpin turn, contribute to the efficiency of this mechanism in amplifying the effects of active transport of solute from the thick ascending limb. PCT, proximal convoluted tubule. (Adapted from Guyton, A.C., and Hall, J.E. [1996]. *Textbook of Medical Physiology.* [9th ed.]. Philadelphia: W.B. Saunders. [p. 353].)

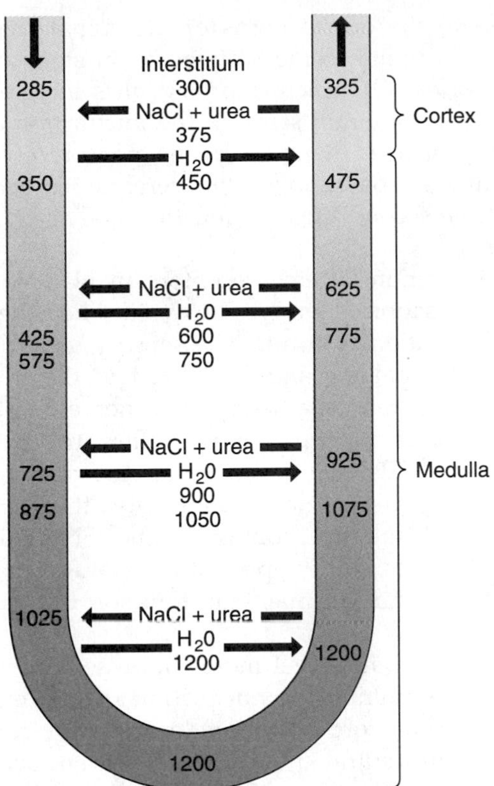

FIGURE 20–14

Countercurrent exchanger. Slow, countercurrent flow in the vasa recta permits reabsorption of water from the medullary interstitium into the capillary blood, preventing dilution of the medullary gradient. Slow flow also prevents washout of interstitial solutes.

(diluting segment) is hypotonic, owing to the active reabsorption of solute (without concurrent H_2O reabsorption) from the ascending loop of Henle. Without ADH, the late DCT and collecting duct are impermeable to water, and the hypotonic fluid is excreted as dilute urine. In the presence of ADH, water is reabsorbed from the tubular filtrate along the medullary gradient, and urine becomes hypertonic.

Effect of Diuretics on Renal Function

Diuretics are drugs that result in increased urine output. There are several diuretics in common use (Table 20–3), and they act by multiple mechanisms. *Osmotic diuretics,* such as mannitol (Osmitrol), are large molecules that are filtered but not reabsorbed. Within the tubular lumen, they exert osmotic pressure, which keeps water from being reabsorbed, and increased urine output occurs. *Loop diuretics,* such as furosemide (Lasix), inhibit the solute pump in the ascending loop of Henle. In the absence of initiation of the countercurrent multiplier mechanism, the hypertonic medullary gradient cannot be established, and water cannot be reabsorbed even if the tubule is permeable to it. Again, increased amounts of dilute urine are excreted. *Potassium-sparing diuretics,* such as spironolactone (Aldactone), are so named because they inhibit the Na^+-K^+-ATPase pump in the DCT, which prevents Na^+ and water reabsorption in that segment while simultaneously decreasing secretion

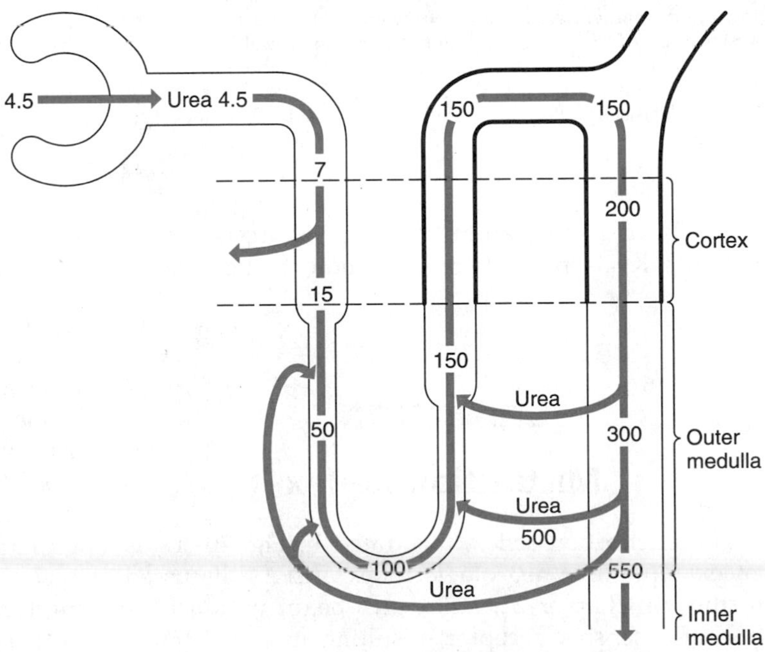

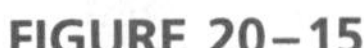

FIGURE 20–15

Addition of urea to the medullary interstitium. Urea, which is reabsorbed from the collecting duct in the presence of antidiuretic hormone, contributes to the osmolarity of the interstitital fluid. Urea is then reabsorbed into the thin loop of Henle. Although some urea is reabsorbed into the blood, most is "recycled" from the collecting duct back into the interstitium. (Adapted from Guyton, A.C., and Hall, J.E. [1996]. *Textbook of Medical Physiology.* [9th ed.]. Philadelphia: W.B. Saunders. [p. 355].)

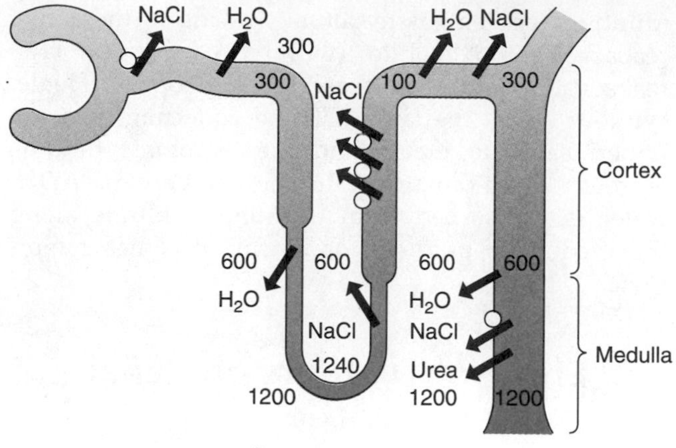

A ADH present

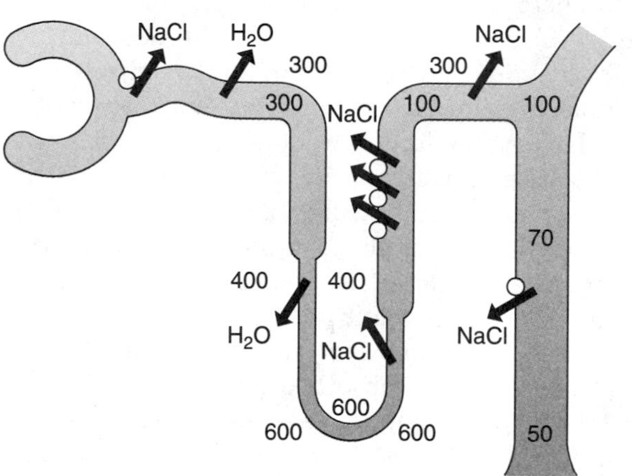

B ADH absent

FIGURE 20–16
Regulation of urine osmolarity by antidiuretic hormone. If the medullary interstitial gradient is normal, concentration of the urine is regulated by antidiuretic hormone (ADH) in a dose-dependent relationship. *A*, In the presence of ADH, the distal nephron is permeable to water, and its reabsorption along the medullary gradient results in concentration of the urine. *B*, In the absence of ADH, the distal nephron is impermeable to water. Water remains in the tubule, and a dilute urine is excreted. (Adapted from Guyton, A.C., and Hall, J.E. [1996]. *Textbook of Medical Physiology*. [9th ed.]. Philadelphia: W.B. Saunders. [pp. 351, 354].)

of K^+ by the same antiport pump. Diuresis occurs, but less K^+ is present in the tubule to be washed out.

URINATION

Micturition Reflex

The micturition reflex, illustrated in Fig. 20–17, is an example of a neurologic reflex arc. As discussed further in Chapter 22, reflex arcs begin with activation of a sensory receptor, resulting in signal transmission to the dorsal horns of the spinal cord and upward to higher centers of the brain stem and cerebral cortex. The micturition signal is integrated at the level of the brain stem, in the micturition center. These specialized neurons in the pons receive sensory inputs from above (the cerebral cortex) and below (the second through fourth sacral segments of the cord).

In micturition, stretch receptors in bladder walls initiate sensation of the need to void when the bladder fills to about 150 mL. The sensory signal enters the sacral segments and is relayed to the detrusor muscle by parasympathetic pelvic nerves, initiating contractions and completing the reflex arc. The more the bladder fills, the stronger are the contractions. Sympathetic nerves also innervate the detrusor muscle and internal sphincter, and SNS stimulation serves to block premature parasympathetic stimulation and to maintain tone of the internal sphincter.

Typically, higher-level motor impulses originating in the cortex inhibit the micturition reflex. Impulses from the sacral cord by the pudendal nerve constrict the external urethral sphincter and prevent urination except in socially acceptable situations. If the external sphincter is not released, the micturition reflex fatigues or dies out temporarily (from a few minutes to an hour), but signals begin again later as neurotransmitter stores and local factors governing smooth muscle contraction are replenished. Eventually, the bladder may fill to the point where reflex contraction is strong enough to overcome voluntary control, and incontinence of urine then occurs.

Neurologic inputs from higher centers of the brain may also be facilitative at times. That is, micturition may be initiated voluntarily, even in the absence of bladder wall stretch. As often experienced by patients asked to provide a urine specimen for laboratory analysis, the lower the bladder volume, the more difficult is this voluntary urination.

Factors That Can Impede Micturition

Reflex emptying of the bladder may be prevented pathologically by urinary tract obstruction (as in prostate enlargement or urolithiasis) or in neurogenic bladder syndromes, in which anesthesia or neurologic injuries impair neural control of micturition[5] (Table 20–4). Injury to the sacral levels of the cord interrupts the reflex arc and results in *detrusor areflexia*, or absence of bladder contraction. In such cases, the bladder will *not* fill indefinitely, until it ruptures, because rising fluid pressure in the lower urinary tract triggers the ureterorenal reflex, con-

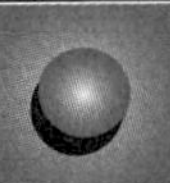

TABLE 20–3
MECHANISMS OF ACTION OF DIURETIC DRUGS

DIURETIC CLASS/EXAMPLES	MECHANISM OF ACTION
Osmotic Diuretics Mannitol (Osmitrol)	Filterable but nonabsorbable polysaccharide inhibits Na^+ and water reabsorption from the proximal convoluted tubule and loop of Henle
Loop Diuretics Furosemide (Lasix) Bumentanide (Bumex) Ethacrynic acid (Edecrin)	Compete for the Cl^- site on the Na^+-K^+-$2Cl^-$ pump in the thick ascending loop of Henle, inhibiting Na^+ reabsorption and establishment of the medullary gradient
Thiazide-Type Diuretics Chlorothiazide (Diuril) Hydrochlorothiazide (Esidrix) Bendroflumethiazide (Naturetin)	Compete for the Cl^- site on the Na^+-Cl^- symport in the distal convoluted tubule and early collecting duct, inhibiting Na^+ reabsorption and subsequent water reabsorption by osmosis
Potassium-Sparing Diuretics Spironolactone (Aldactone) Amiloride (Midamor) Tiamterene (Dyrenium)	Inhibit aldosterone-sensitive Na^+-K^+ antiport in the late distal convoluted tubule and early collecting duct, reducing Na^+ reabsorption (and osmotic water reabsorption provided antidiuretic hormone is present) as well as reducing secretion of K^+
Carbonic Anhydrase Inhibitors Acetazolamide (Diamox) Methazolamide (Neptazane) Dichlorphenamide (Daranide)	Inhibit carbonic anhydrase enzyme activity in proximal convoluted tubule cells, thereby reducing HCO_3^-, Na^+, and Cl^- reabsorption. NaCl and $NaHCO_3$ are lost in the urine, with water following by osmosis

Data from Rose, B.D. (1994). *Clinical Physiology of Acid-Base and Electrolyte Disorders.* (4th ed.). New York: McGraw-Hill, Inc.; and Kuhn, M.M. (1991). *Pharmacotherapeutics: A Nursing Process Approach.* (2nd ed.). Philadelphia: F. A. Davis.

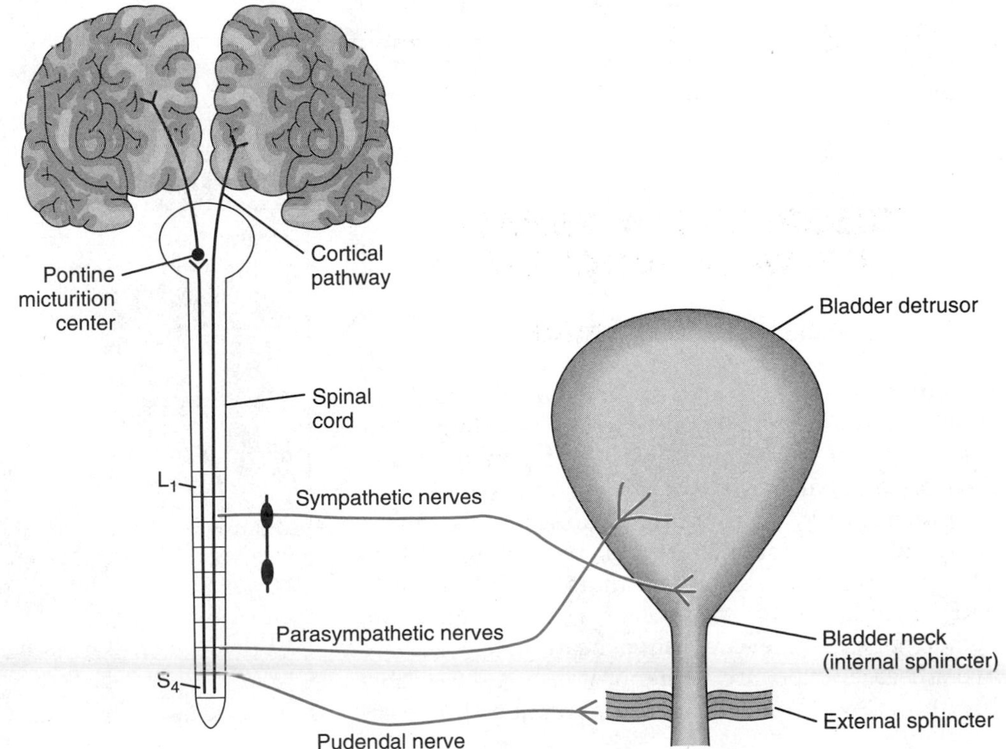

FIGURE 20–17
Micturition reflex. The signal to urinate begins with stimulation of stretch receptors in the bladder walls with filling. Neural impulses are generated, which ascend by sacral segments of the cord to the micturition center in the pons. Descending impulses from this center initiate contraction of the detrusor muscle and opening of the internal sphincter. Urination occurs with voluntary relaxation of the external urethral sphincter. Signals to the micturition center from the cerebral cortex may inhibit or facilitate the micturition reflex.

TABLE 20–4
NEUROGENIC BLADDER SYNDROMES

Syndrome	Etiology	Clinical Manifestations
Detrusor hyperreflexia	Incomplete or delayed maturation of inhibitory centers in brain, or cerebral cortical lesion	Urgency, urge incontinence
	Spinal cord lesion (above sacral level)	Detrusor–external sphincter dyssynergia (DESD)
Detrusor areflexia	Sacral reflex arc lesion	Overflow incontinence, poor voiding requiring increased abdominal pressure

Adapted from Amis, E.S., and Blaivas, J.G. (1991). Neurogenic bladder simplified. *Radiologic Clinics of North America* 29(3), 575.

stricting afferent arterioles of the nephron and decreasing GFR. Retention of urine, however, increases the risk of incontinence, UTI, and calculus (stone) formation, as discussed later in this chapter.

In the case of cerebral cortex injury, or in infants and young children who have not yet developmentally achieved controlled toileting, lack of the usual inhibition results in reflex urination each time the bladder fills sufficiently (*detrusor hyperreflexia*). Because the micturition center is intact, bladder contraction and external sphincter opening are coordinated. With spinal cord injuries above the sacral levels but below the pontine micturition center, a condition known as *detrusor–external sphincter dyssynergia* occurs, in which there is loss of coordination between bladder contraction and external sphincter opening. If the bladder contracts strongly against a closed sphincter, reflux of urine from the bladder into the ureters may occur, potentially damaging the kidneys. Spinal cord injuries and other disorders of motor function are detailed in Chapter 22.

DISORDERS OF RENAL-URINARY FUNCTION

Acute Renal Failure

Definition. ARF is the sudden (within hours to days) deterioration of renal function, resulting in accumulation of nitrogenous wastes and in fluid and electrolyte imbalance.

Epidemiology. ARF occurs in an estimated 5% of all hospitalized patients[1] and is present in 10% to 20% of those in intensive care units.[6] Risk factors for ARF include major trauma or surgery, infection, hemorrhage, severe congestive heart failure, severe liver disease, exposure to nephrotoxic agents (Table 20–5), or lower urinary tract obstruction. Pre-existing renal disease and extremes of age (i.e., neonates or elders) magnify the risk.

Etiology. ARF may be initiated by *prerenal, intrarenal (intrinsic),* or *postrenal* causes (Table 20–6). These categories are not mutually exclusive, however, because intrarenal failure results from prerenal or postrenal disorders if they are severe or prolonged.

Prerenal causes include vascular disorders upstream to the kidneys, which result in severe reduction of renal blood flow. Decreased renal perfusion may occur with shock, severe congestive heart failure, renal artery stenosis, or renal artery embolism, resulting in decreased GFR and tubular flow rates that alter tubular transport. In hepatic failure, altered renal blood flow may occur, leading to **hepatorenal syndrome** (see Chapter 26).

Intrinsic etiologies usually have an ischemic or

TABLE 20–5
NEPHROTOXIC AGENTS

Agent	Potential Renal Effects
Drugs	
Antibiotics (especially aminoglycosides)	Allergic acute interstitial nephritis Hypersensitivity vasculitis Acute renal failure Distal renal tubular acidosis (rare) Acute tubular necrosis
Nonsteroidal anti-inflammatory drugs	Acute interstitial nephritis
Loop and thiazide-type diuretics	Acute interstitial nephritis
Chemotherapy agents	Acute tubular necrosis
Heroin abuse	Acute tubular necrosis
Other Agents	
Radiographic contrast media	Acute tubular necrosis
Heavy metals, solvents	Acute tubular necrosis

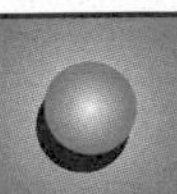

TABLE 20–6
ETIOLOGIC MECHANISMS IN ACUTE RENAL FAILURE

PRERENAL FAILURE
Mechanism: Reduced renal blood flow
Severe dehydration
Shock (all forms)
Cardiac failure
Renal artery stenosis
Renal artery embolism or thrombosis
Sickle cell crisis
INTRARENAL FAILURE
Mechanism: Renal parenchymal disease
Ischemic necrosis
Nephrotoxicity
Autoimmune or isoimmune disorders
Hypertensive nephropathy
Diabetic nephropathy
Renal trauma
Acute glomerulonephritis
Vasculitis
Acute interstitial nephritis
Rhabdomyolysis
POSTRENAL FAILURE
Mechanism: Prevention of Filtration Due to High Tubular Pressure (Obstructed Outflow)
Urolithiasis
Renal-urinary neoplasms
Congenital obstructive uropathies
Detrusor areflexia
Surgical trauma to ureters
Obstructive lymphadenopathy

toxic mechanism. Prolonged decreases in renal perfusion result in ischemic damage to tubular cells (**acute tubular necrosis [ATN]**). Nephrotoxic drugs and chemicals produce similar tubular damage. In such cases, tubules may become clogged with inflammatory and cellular debris, and further ischemia may result from increasing pressure due to this obstruction. **Acute interstitial nephritis,** detailed later, may result in ARF secondary to infection or, ironically, to the antibiotics used in treatment of the infection. In major trauma or systemic infections, muscle breakdown (**rhabdomyolysis**) may release myoglobin, which if filtered into the tubules, can cause obstruction (see Chapter 35). Massive hemolysis may release large quantities of hemoglobin into the blood, with similar effect. **Hemolytic-uremic syndrome (HUS),** the most common cause of ARF in childhood, is described later in this chapter.

Postrenal causes of ARF are the least common and include renal or ureteral stones (calculi), tumors, or strictures that obstruct the lower urinary tract. Lower urinary tract obstruction decreases GFR because of a rise in Bowman's capsule hydrostatic pressure and also by the ureterorenal reflex mechanism, which reduces glomerular capillary hydrostatic pressure. The rise in tubular pressure may result in ATN in rare cases. Lower urinary tract obstruction is detailed later in this chapter.

Pathophysiology. ARF typically displays three phases. The *oliguric phase,* which may last only a few days or several weeks, is characterized by oliguria (urine output of less than 30 mL/h or 400 mL/day), fluid volume excess, **azotemia** (elevated serum levels of urea, creatinine, and uric acid), and electrolyte imbalance. Ischemic or toxic injury causes the release of local mediators, which trigger intrarenal vasoconstriction.[7] Medullary hypoxia results in swelling of tubular and endothelial cells, in adherence of neutrophils to capillaries and venules, and in inappropriate platelet activation. These effects lead to further reduction in perfusion, amplifying the ischemic effects of vasoconstriction. Injury and death of tubular cells occurs by both necrosis and apoptosis. Injured cells lose their polarity, and disruption of tight junctions between cells may permit back-leak of filtrate. Ischemia impairs the function of energy-dependent membrane pumps, and calcium accumulates in cells, contributing to further vasoconstriction and to activation of proteases and other enzymes. With reperfusion, reactive oxygen species are formed, leading to further cell injury.

Because renal endothelial and tubular cells have the capacity to regenerate, the potential for recovery of renal function exists if the underlying cause is corrected. Those who recover renal function progress to the *diuretic (nonoliguric) phase,* characterized by a gradual increase in urine output. GFR is normal or increased, but tubular transport mechanisms are still abnormal. Urine is dilute, and high urine volumes may lead to dehydration and further electrolyte imbalance. The diuretic phase also lasts days to weeks. The *recovery phase* encompasses a gradual return to normal or near-normal renal function over a period of 3 to 12 months or longer.

Clinical Manifestations. Retention of nitrogenous wastes is apparent on laboratory testing of blood and urine (Table 20–7). Electrolyte imbalance is also evident, with hyperkalemia imposing significant risk of cardiac dysrhythmias. Metabolic acidosis occurs as a result of decreased excretion of H^+. Anemia may result from lack of erythropoietin release, glomerular filtration of erythrocytes, or bleeding associated with platelet dysfunction. Sepsis is common, owing to a decrease in cell-mediated immunity, although the precise mechanism accounting for this effect is unknown. The toxic syndrome resulting

TABLE 20–7
SELECTED DIAGNOSTIC TESTS OF RENAL-URINARY FUNCTION

Test	Purpose	Clinical Implications
Urinalysis	Screening of urine for evidence of renal-urinary disease or systemic disorders	Macroscopic examination detects changes in color, odor, appearance, specific gravity, and pH. Presence of significant glucose, protein, ketones, bilirubin, hemoglobin, blood cells, casts, or bacteria on microscopic examination suggests pathology.
Reagent strips (dipsticks)	Screening of urine for protein, ketones, glucose	Dipstick tests provide qualitative screening for proteinuria (indicating increased glomerular permeability), increased urinary glucose (indicating hyperglycemia), and increased urinary ketones (indicating ketosis). Increased alkalinity or use of certain drugs can alter the results.
Urine culture	Diagnosis of urinary tract infection	Urine should be obtained by catheterization or clean catch method to avoid contamination. Growth of a single microbe species in counts of >100,000/mL indicates infection.
Blood urea nitrogen (BUN)	Evaluation of renal function	BUN reflects the renal excretion of urea, an end product of protein metabolism. BUN begins to rise as the glomerular filtration rate (GFR) falls below 40%–60%, but factors such as volume status, protein intake or catabolism, gastrointestinal bleeding, exercise, and steroid therapy may affect results.
Serum creatinine	Evaluation of renal function	Creatinine, a product of muscle metabolism, is excreted through the kidneys. It is not affected by diet, fluid status, or normal activity. A rising serum creatinine indicates loss of functional nephrons.
BUN-to-creatinine ratio	Differentiation of etiology in renal failure	A ratio higher than 10:1 suggests a prerenal cause.
Creatinine clearance	Evaluation of renal function (especially GFR)	Urinary and blood values of creatinine are evaluated at prescribed intervals. Because creatinine is filtered but not secreted in significant amounts, creatinine clearance approximates GFR.
Fractional excretion of sodium (FENa)	Differentiation of etiology of renal failure	Urinary and blood values of sodium are evaluated in the context of GFR (estimated from creatinine clearance). FENa <1% indicates that the patient is reabsorbing sodium and suggests a prerenal cause. FENa >2% suggests that reabsorption of sodium is impaired by acute tubular necrosis.

from these combined renal effects is known as uremia.

Because of fluid overload and anemia, cardiac workload is increased during ARF, often precipitating cardiac failure in patients with limited reserve. Pericarditis may result from toxicity due to accumulated wastes. Anemia contributes to tissue hypoxia, which stimulates increased ventilation and work of breathing. Respiratory compensation for metabolic acidosis has a similar effect. A high percentage of patients with ARF develop gastrointestinal bleeding. In the uremic environment, abnormalities in quantity or function of anticoagulant proteins, coagulation factors, platelets, or endothelial mediators may lead to either a hypocoagulable or a hypercoagulable state. The uremic syndrome may also manifest as altered mental status and peripheral sensation, owing to effects on the highly sensitive cells of the nervous system secondary to retained toxins, hypoxia, electrolyte imbalance, and acidosis. The hypermetabolic state induced by this critical illness may promote tissue catabolism.

Prevention and Treatment. Careful monitoring of urinary output and laboratory values in patients at risk is essential to the earliest detection of impending renal failure. Maintenance of adequate intravascular volume and avoidance of nephrotoxic agents are important preventive measures. The priorities of treatment are to reverse the underlying cause, if possible, and to correct fluid and electrolyte imbalances. If ATN is suspected, loop diuretics may be used to increase tubular flow rates and wash out debris. Hyperkalemia is of immediate concern, owing to potential dysrhythmias, and may be corrected with exchange resins, glucose-insulin solution to promote cellular uptake of K^+, treatment of acidosis to promote K^+ excretion, or dialysis.

In many cases of ARF, continuous dialysis or other renal replacement therapies are employed to prevent fluid overload, accumulation of toxins, and critical electrolyte imbalances.[8] *Hemodialysis,* a process in which water and solute molecules are equilibrated across an artificial membrane, is illustrated in Fig. 20–18. Hemodialysis requires access to the patient's arterial blood, which is pumped through channels in the semipermeable dialyzing membrane, in countercurrent flow with a dialysate solution. The dialysate is formulated with specific osmolarity and concentrations of electrolytes and glucose to establish favorable gradients for transport of excess fluid, electrolytes, and wastes from the blood to the dialysate (Table 20–8). Countercurrent flow prevents the gradients from being quickly dissipated because the transported substances are immediately carried away in the dialysate. Negative hydrostatic pressure may be applied to the dialysate to pull excess water from the blood in patients who are hypervolemic. After exchange, the patient's blood is returned by venous access.

Continuous renal replacement therapies constitute a group of newer techniques that use the natural pressure gradient between the arterial and venous systems to facilitate filtration of solutes and water (Table 20–9). Usually employed on a short-term basis in critically ill patients, these procedures require vascular catheters (arterial and venous, or two venous), with a highly porous filter in line between them. Countercurrent flow of dialysate adjacent to the filter is a component of some systems. As blood flows through the filter, water and solutes are removed proportionately by the pressure gradient. Fluid and electrolytes are then selectively replaced until desired serum levels are achieved.

Dietary restriction of protein may be indicated to decrease urea production in patients with ARF, but this intervention must be balanced against increased

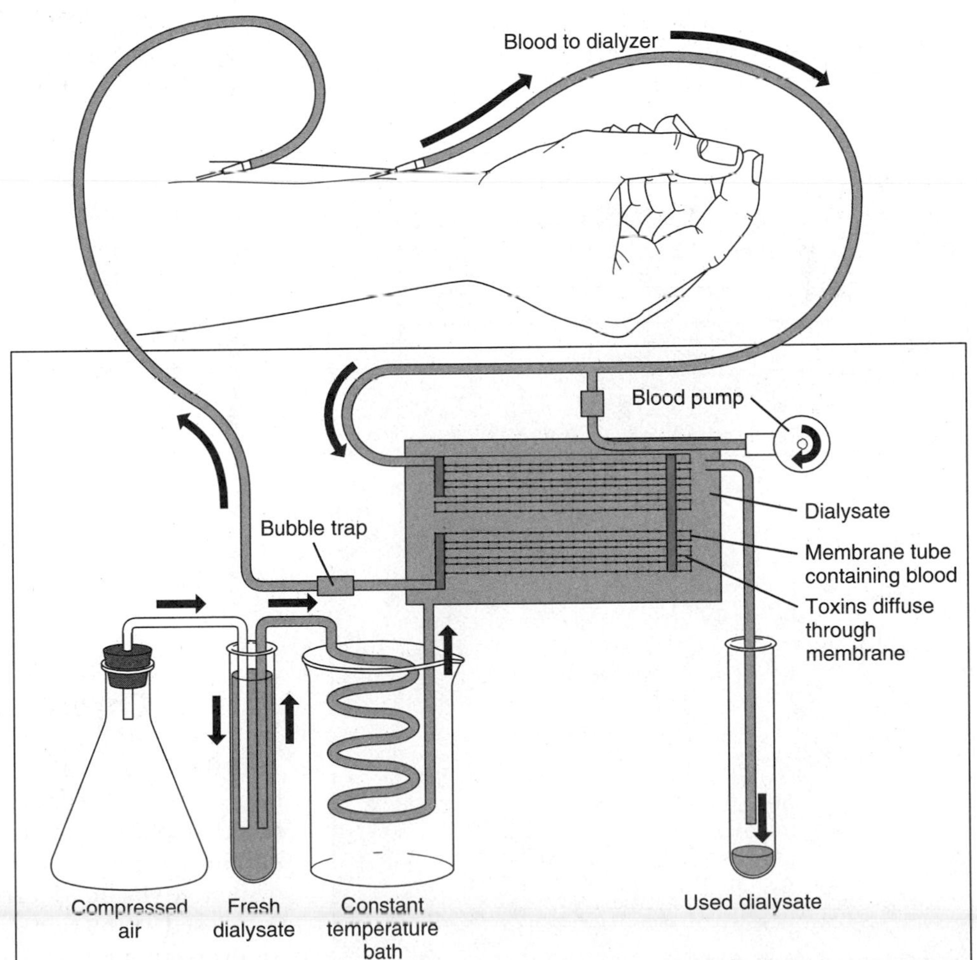

FIGURE 20–18

Principles of hemodialysis. The components of the artificial kidney (dialyzer) are illustrated schematically. The patient's arterial blood is pumped through channels in a semipermeable membrane, in countercurrent flow with a dialysate solution. Exchange between the blood and the dialysate results from gradients established by the composition of the dialysate and negative hydrostatic pressure applied to the solution. Countercurrent flow maintains the diffusion gradients because transported substances are immediately removed. When sufficient nitrogenous wastes have been removed and normal electrolyte composition is established, the patient's blood is returned by venous access. (Adapted from Rhoades, R., and Pflanzer, R. [1989]. *Human Physiology.* Philadelphia: Saunders College Publishing. [p. 776].)

TABLE 20-8
COMPARISON OF SERUM AND DIALYSATE CONSTITUENTS

Constituent	Dialysate Value	Diffusion Direction	Serum Value (Normal)
Glucose*	200 mg/dL or more	⟶	70–100 mg/dL
Sodium	132–141 mEq/L	⟷	135–145 mEq/L
Potassium	3 mEq/L	⟵	3.5–5 mEq/L
Calcium	3.5 mEq/L	⟷	4.5–5.5 mEq/L
Magnesium	0.5–1.5 mEq/L	⟷	1.5–2.5 mEq/L
Chloride	96–101 mEq/L	⟷	100–108 mEq/L
Bicarbonate	30 mEq/L	⟶	22–26 mEq/L

*Glucose is used primarily in peritoneal dialysis to provide osmotic pressure.

nutritional needs to offset catabolism. Infection, anemia, and hemorrhage are treated if present. The dosages of any drugs requiring renal metabolism or excretion must be adjusted to accommodate decreased renal function, dialysis, or continuous renal replacement therapy. A number of clinical trials are testing agents designed to mitigate the cellular mechanisms of ARF.[9]

Prognosis and Outcome. The mortality rate is greater than 50% during the oliguric phase, owing to sepsis, hyperkalemia, or hemorrhage. For patients requiring dialysis, mortality rates range from 60% to 90%.[6] For those in whom renal function does not improve after dialysis for more than 3 months, the condition is considered to be CRF.

TABLE 20-9
CONTINUOUS RENAL REPLACEMENT THERAPIES

Method	Description
Slow continuous ultrafiltration (SCUF)	Use of filter between arterial and venous lines, slowly removes excess fluid
Continuous arteriovenous hemofiltration (CAVH)	Use of filter between arterial and venous lines, removes fluid and uremic toxins; used with fluid and electrolyte replacement
Continuous arteriovenous hemodialysis (CAVHD)	Use of dialyzer membrane between arterial and venous access lines; dialysate solution runs countercurrent to blood; results in moderate fluid removal and increased removal of uremic toxins
Continuous venovenous hemofiltration (CVVH)	Similar to CAVH except that flow of venous blood is assisted by a pump
Continuous venovenous hemodialysis (CVVHD)	Similar to CAVHD except that flow of venous blood is assisted by a pump

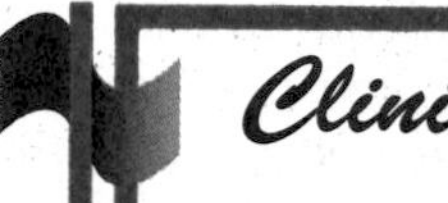

Clinical Scenario

K.B., a 37-year-old woman, is transferred from a small-town hospital for further evaluation of lower abdominal pain, nausea and vomiting, and progressive reduction in urine output, which began after a "drinking binge" 2 days ago. She reports a history of alcohol abuse as well as heavy use of nonsteroidal anti-inflammatory drugs for arthritis. She also has a history of hypertension and was diagnosed with insulin-dependent diabetes mellitus 2 years ago. During the past 2 days, her serum creatinine has risen to 9.6 mg/dL (normal is 0.4 to 1.2 mg/dL), and her blood urea nitrogen is 121 mg/dL (normal is 10 to 20 mg/dL). She is initially treated with diuretic therapy, but does not respond. Hemodialysis is instituted.

1. What risk factors for renal failure are apparent in this case?
2. What are the immediate priorities of treatment for K.B.?

Chronic Renal Failure

Definition. CRF is the progressive, irreversible loss of renal function due to replacement of functional nephrons with fibrous scar tissue. CRF first becomes clinically apparent as **renal insufficiency**, evidenced by mild azotemia and possibly polyuria (increased urination) and nocturia (urination at night) resulting from impaired tubular transport and concentration of urine. As the condition worsens, **end-stage renal disease (ESRD)** is manifested by a GFR consistently less than 10 mL/min,[6] a level that is not adequate for the homeostatic functions of the kidney to be served.

Epidemiology. According to 1990 statistics from the U.S. Renal Data System, more than 195,000 people had ESRD.[10] Fifty-five per cent of patients are male. Blacks and Native Americans are affected at higher rates than whites, owing to the higher rates of hypertension and diabetes in these groups.

Etiology. Renal insufficiency occurs when renal functional reserve is exhausted and GFR is reduced by 75%. ESRD is caused by loss of more than 90% of functional nephrons. Nephrons may be destroyed by toxic, inflammatory, ischemic, or degenerative processes. Diabetic nephropathy is the most prevalent cause of CRF in the United States, causing 36% of cases, whereas 30% of cases are due to hypertension.[11] Both type 1 and type 2 diabetes may be associated with nephropathy, owing to glycosylation of glomerular proteins and other factors (see Chapter 29). Hypertension may contribute to direct nephron injury (hypertensive nephropathy) or may result from renovascular disease, which also impairs renal perfusion (see Chapter 15). Diabetes and hypertension are particularly significant causes of CRF in that they are increasing in incidence, whereas primary renal causes have been relatively stable.

Primary disorders of the kidney that commonly lead to CRF include **glomerulonephritis** and **polycystic kidney disease.**[10] A variety of systemic disorders, including vasculitis, sickle cell disease, lupus erythematosus, and acquired immunodeficiency syndrome, may also manifest as nephropathy and renal failure. ARF leads to CRF in a minority of cases, and some cases are idiopathic.

Pathophysiology. In most patients, CRF develops gradually over a period of many years. Nephron damage (nephropathy) may take the form of glomerulosclerosis, tubulointerstitial injury, or vascular injury (Table 20–10). In glomerulosclerosis, filtration slits become distorted, and glomerular epithelial cells become eroded, leading to increased fluid transport across the glomerular wall. Large proteins may traverse the slits but often become trapped in the glomerular basement membrane, eventually obstructing the glomerular capillaries. Tubulointerstitial injury includes toxic or ischemic tubular damage such as occurs in ATN, with possible tubular obstruction with debris and deposition of calcium. The inflammatory response leads to fibrin deposition in tubules and surrounding interstitium. Microaneurysms may form as a result of vascular wall damage and increased pressure secondary to obstruction or hypertension. Loss of some nephrons leads to compensatory hyperfunction of others, increasing their vulnerability to damage in a positive feedback loop.

TABLE 20–10
MECHANISMS OF NEPHROPATHY IN CHRONIC RENAL FAILURE

Mechanism	Description
Glomerulosclerosis	Progressive, destructive hardening of glomerular capillaries initiated by adaptive changes in the nephrons, which are initially unaffected by a primary disease process. Epithelial and endothelial injury results in proteinuria. Hardening is due to mesangial cell proliferation, increased production of extracellular matrix, and intraglomerular coagulation.
Tubulointerstitial injury	Defects in tubular transport function associated with interstitial edema, leukocyte infiltration, and focal tubular necrosis
Vascular injury	Diffuse or focal ischemia of the renal parenchyma associated with thickening, fibrosis, or focal lesions of renal blood vessels. Reduced blood flow may result in tubular atrophy and interstitial fibrosis as well as functional disruption (e.g., reduced glomerular filtration rate, proteinuria, alteration of the medullary gradient with loss of concentrating ability).

Clinical Manifestations. Although their onset is gradual, manifestations of CRF are similar to those of ARF and include azotemia, fluid and electrolyte imbalance, metabolic acidosis, anemia, and bleeding or clotting disorders. In addition, effects resulting from long-term uremia are seen. Demineralization of bone (renal osteodystrophy) is due to three factors: decreased renal activation of vitamin D, which decreases absorption of dietary calcium; retention of phosphate, which leads to increased urinary loss of calcium; and increased circulating parathyroid hormone (due to decreased urinary excretion of this hormone), which promotes demineralization of the bones and teeth. Bone pain and pathogenic fractures are common because of this process.

Malnutrition occurs in patients with ESRD secondary to anorexia, malaise, and dietary restriction of protein. This leads to capillary fragility, decreased immune function, and poor wound healing. Patients with CRF have a characteristic grayish-yellow cast to the skin, secondary to retention of urinary pigments (urochromes). Pruritus is common, probably due to inflammatory mediators released by retained toxins in the skin, and a powdery white coating of the skin (uremic frost) may occur as a result of crystallization of uric acid and other substances in the sweat.

Peripheral neuropathy may result from toxic effects on sensitive nervous system cells (see Chapter 23). *Restless legs syndrome*, characterized by altered sensation and increased spontaneous movement of the feet and lower legs, is commonly seen, along with weakness and decreased deep tendon reflexes. Reproductive function is adversely affected in both males and females, owing to alteration of hormone levels by impaired excretion or activation. Females may not ovulate, menstruate, or be able to carry a pregnancy to term. Males have decreased sperm counts and are prone to impotence. The presence and severity of these manifestations depend on the duration of renal failure and the response to treatment.

Prevention and Treatment. Prevention of ESRD involves reduction of risk for ARF and optimal management of diabetes, hypertension, chronic renal diseases, and other systemic diseases associated with CRF. Three levels of treatment are available: conservative treatment, dialysis, and renal transplantation (Table 20–11). The choice depends on the degree of disease progression and the patient's underlying physical condition, lifestyle, and personal preferences.

Conservative treatment focuses on dietary restriction of fluid and protein, and of sodium if the patient is hypertensive. Potassium levels are appropriately monitored and treated (see Chapter 9). Treatment with ACE inhibitors has been shown to slow the progression of diabetic nephropathy in patients with proteinuria (see Chapter 29). The risk of renal osteodystrophy is reduced with the use of drugs such as calcium carbonate or calcium acetate, which bind phosphate and supplement calcium, and with replacement of vitamin D. Anemia, if present, may be treated with blood transfusion or, more commonly, by administration of synthetic erythropoietin (see Chapter 12).

If conservative therapy is not sufficient, as evidenced by worsening clinical manifestations, and a suitable donor kidney is not available for transplantation, dialysis is used to maintain body fluid homeostasis. For ESRD patients, hemodialysis is usually done about three times per week, with each "run" lasting about 4 hours. Hemodialysis was discussed earlier with ARF. *Peritoneal dialysis* is used in about 15% of patients with CRF. The peritoneum serves as

TABLE 20–11
LEVELS OF TREATMENT IN CHRONIC RENAL FAILURE

TREATMENT MODE	DESCRIPTION
Conservative Treatment	
Protein restriction	Protein intake restricted to 0.6–0.8 g/day
Tight glycemic control (in diabetics)	Frequent glucose testing with appropriate divided-dose insulin, oral hypoglycemic therapy, or dietary measures
Angiotensin-converting enzyme inhibitors (e.g., captopril)	Drug therapy to interrupt the renin–angiotensin–aldosterone system, improving renal blood flow and protecting against hypertensive nephropathy
Diuretics	Drug therapy to augment sodium and water excretion
Erythropoietin	Use of recombinant erythropoietin to treat anemia due to defective production of this hormone in renal disease
Low phosphate diet, calcium supplementation, vitamin D	Prevention and treatment of renal osteodystrophy
Renal Replacement Therapy	
Hemodialysis	Use of an extracorporeal circuit to create a blood flow rate of 200–400 mL/min through an artificial kidney (dialyzer). Patient's blood flows countercurrent to dialysate fluid, with exchange of water and solutes to effect normal fluid and electrolyte balance and removal of wastes.
Peritoneal dialysis	Use of the peritoneal membrane for exchange of water and solute between patient's blood (in abdominal wall and visceral capillaries) and dialysate instilled into peritoneal cavity
Renal Transplantation	Placement of a kidney from a living or cadaveric donor in the right or left iliac fossa, with anastomosis of the renal artery of the donor kidney to the hypogastric or common iliac artery of the recipient. The renal vein of the donor kidney is anastomosed to the iliac vein or inferior vena cava of the recipient.

the dialyzing membrane in this procedure, with equilibration occurring between the capillary blood and dialysate, which is periodically instilled into the peritoneal cavity. Access is provided by a catheter inserted through the abdominal wall and sutured in place. One to two liters of solution is instilled and allowed to dwell in the cavity until equilibration is complete. After equilibration, the dialysate is drained by gravity.

The frequency of peritoneal dialysis treatments and the dwell time are widely variable, depending on the individual patient's needs. Because the procedure can be done while the patient is ambulatory, peritoneal dialysis may allow a less-restricted lifestyle than hemodialysis. Catheter-induced peritonitis is a risk, however. In addition, because glucose must be used as a source of osmotic pressure in the dialysate, the absorption of glucose may contribute to hyperglycemia and hyperlipidemia. Finally, because the peritoneal membrane is somewhat permeable to protein, some degree of protein loss in the dialysate is common.

If a suitable donor kidney is available, the treatment of choice for CRF is renal transplantation. From 1988 to 1991, about 6500 transplantations using kidneys from living volunteer donors were done in the United States, and 33,000 cadaver kidneys were transplanted.[12] Tissue matching and other aspects of organ transplantation are discussed in Chapter 13.

Prognosis and Outcome. For the entire population of patients with ESRD, the 1-year survival rate is less than 80%. Five-year survival rates vary from 18% to 41%, depending on age, race, and specific etiology.[10] In patients undergoing renal transplantation, the 1-year graft survival rate for initial transplants is 80% to 95%. The original disease reoccurs in the graft in 10% to 20% of cases.[12]

Hemolytic-Uremic Syndrome

Definition. HUS is a systemic inflammatory disorder due to infectious and noninfectious processes in young children. HUS is characterized by endothelial damage and coagulopathy primarily affecting the kidneys, gastrointestinal system, and central nervous system.

Epidemiology. HUS is the most common cause of ARF in children younger than 5 years, affecting an estimated 5.8 per 100,000 each year in the United States.[13] Both epidemic and nonepidemic forms are seen, with the epidemic form transmitted through food and by person-to-person contact.

Etiology. Epidemic HUS has an infectious cause, with most cases occurring as a result of a verocytotoxin-producing *Escherichia coli*, transmitted by contaminated ground beef or unpasteurized milk or cheese. Other bacteria that can cause HUS include *Shigella dysenteriae, Salmonella typhimurium,* and *Campylobacter* and *Yersinia* spp. Nonepidemic HUS may be inherited or associated with nephrotoxic drugs, viral infections, Kawasaki disease, pregnancy, or rhabdomyolysis. The etiologic mechanism in such cases is often unclear.

Pathophysiology. The verocytotoxin (also known as Shiga-like toxin, or SLT) binds to receptors on the surfaces of sensitive cells in the kidney, gastrointestinal epithelium, and and central nervous system. The toxin is taken into the cell, where it inhibits protein synthesis, leading to cell damage and death. Pathogenic *E. coli* also release lipopolysaccharide, which is absorbed by lesions produced by the verocytotoxin. Lipopolysaccharide may initiate a cascade of responses that culminate in further endothelial cell damage, production of reactive oxygen species, and activation of the coagulation system. Platelets are consumed, and fibrin is deposited in renal vessels. Red blood cells are damaged as they pass through, inducing hemolysis.

Clinical Manifestations. Diarrhea (possibly bloody) is usually the initial manifestation, lasting 3 to 4 days. Pallor develops as a result of hemolytic anemia. Signs of renal failure become apparent as diarrhea subsides, and oliguria and fluid overload are typical. Seizures may occur with involvement of the central nervous system.

Prevention and Treatment. Poorly cooked beef and unpasteurized dairy products should be avoided, as should contact with people known to be infected. Treatment consists of fluid and electrolyte replacement, transfusion of packed red blood cells if anemia is severe, and support of other system functions as indicated. Dialysis is required in up to half of patients. Use of antibiotics for *E. coli* infection is controversial because bacterial cell death may cause increased release of toxins.

Prognosis and Outcome. ARF typically subsides within 2 weeks. Rarely, the disorder is complicated by thrombotic or hemorrhagic stroke, which may be fatal. Permanent, subtle cognitive deficits are believed to occur in a significant percentage of survivors of HUS. ESRD occurs in 10%.[13]

Glomerulonephritis

Definition. Glomerulonephritis is a general category that includes a number of primary and secondary disorders characterized by inflammation of the glomerular capillaries. In primary glomerulonephri-

TABLE 20–12
CLASSIFICATION OF GLOMERULONEPHRITIS

Classification	Etiology	Description
Acute, self-limited glomerulonephritis	Postinfectious (group A β-hemolytic streptococcus)	Immune complexes deposited in glomeruli
Subacute, rapidly progressive glomerulonephritis	Postinfectious Systemic diseases Systemic lupus erythematosus Goodpasture's syndrome Vasculitis Idiopathic	Immune-mediated glomerular injury characterized by accumulation of crescent-shaped accumulations of cells in Bowman's capsule, eventually obliterating the glomerular tuft
Chronic glomerulonephritis		
Membranous glomerulonephritis	Idiopathic (85%) Secondary (15%)	Deposition of immune complexes along the glomerular basement membrane
Membranoproliferative glomerulonephritis	Idiopathic	Alteration of glomerular basement membrane and proliferation of mesangial cells
Immunoglobulin A nephropathy (Berger's disease)	Genetic predisposition	Deposition of immunoglobulin A in mesangium
Focal sclerosis	Idiopathic or secondary	Destructive hardening of some glomeruli, involving only a portion of the capillary tuft

Data from Cotran, R.S., Kumar, V., and Robbins, S.L. (1994). *Robbins Pathologic Basis of Disease.* (5th ed.). Philadelphia: W.B. Saunders.

tis, the glomerulus is the initial site of the inflammatory process; in secondary glomerulonephritis, the kidney is one of several organs affected by systemic pathology.

Epidemiology. The incidence of acute glomerulonephritis is decreasing in the United States but the disorder is still common worldwide. More males than females are affected, for unknown reasons. Chronic glomerulonephritis is known to be a significant cause of CRF. Children between the ages of 6 and 10 years are at higher risk for development of acute postinfectious glomerulonephritis, although the condition may also affect adults of any age.[14] Streptococcal infection constitutes a risk factor for the postinfectious type of glomerulonephritis, whereas systemic lupus erythematosus, acquired immunodeficiency syndrome, and other systemic disorders increase the risk of secondary glomerular inflammation.

Etiology. Glomerulonephritis is descriptively classified as *acute but self-limited, subacute but rapidly progressive*, or *chronic*. As summarized in Table 20–12, the etiologies are usually different in each category. It is uncommon for acute forms to progress to subacute or chronic, or for subacute forms to progress to chronic, although this does occur. The postinfectious type of acute glomerulonephritis, which is by far the most common type, represents a maladaptive immune response, sometimes to a virus but usually to group A β-hemolytic streptococcal infection (e.g., "strep throat" or streptococcal skin infection). Subacute, rapidly progressive forms of glomerulonephritis are uncommon and usually accompany systemic autoimmune disorders or have an idiopathic etiology. This form often culminates in fatality due to ARF. Chronic glomerulonephritis rarely follows the acute or rapidly progressive forms, but instead represents an end-stage disorder associated with other, idiopathic glomerular disorders. The most common of these are membranous glomerulonephritis, membranoproliferative glomerulonephritis, immunoglobulin A (IgA) nephropathy, and focal sclerosis.

Pathophysiology. In acute postinfectious glomerulonephritis, viral or bacterial antigens stimulate increased IgG antibody production for 2 to 3 weeks after the initial infection. As discussed in Chapter 13, antigen–antibody complexes form in the blood and are deposited in the glomerular capillary wall (Fig. 20–19). Complement activation and an inflammatory response follow, and glomerular capillaries are damaged by edema, proliferation of endothelial and mesangial cells, and infiltration by leukocytes.

In the rapidly progressive form, autoantibodies resulting from pre-existing systemic disorders or developing idiopathically trigger glomerular inflammation. These disorders are particularly characterized by the extension of the inflammatory process into Bowman's capsule, resulting in crescent-shaped accumulations of fibrin, endothelial and mesangial cells, and phagocytic cells. The capsule space is obliterated, and glomerular capillaries are externally compressed.

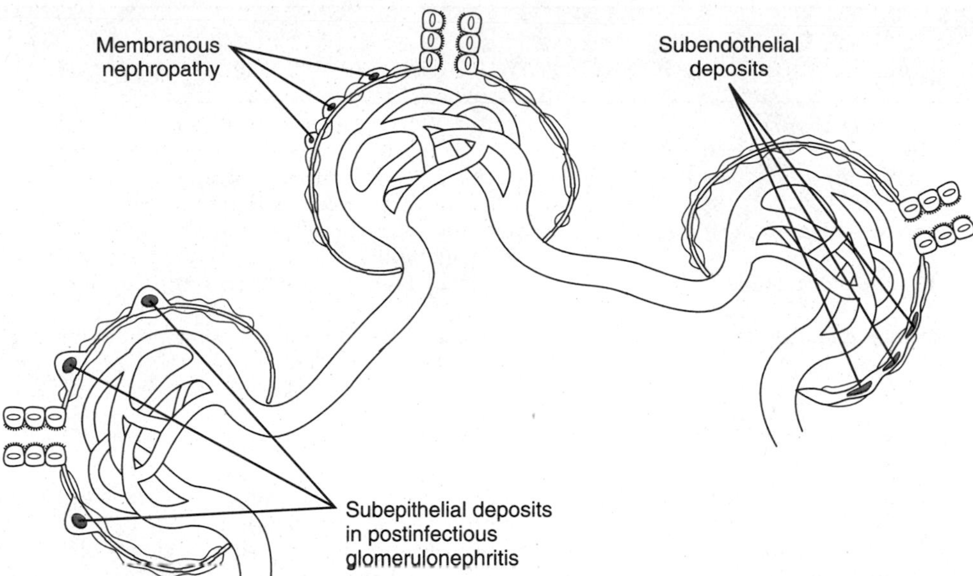

FIGURE 20–19
Immune complex deposition in glomerulonephritis. Subepithelial deposits are seen after postinfectious glomerulonephritis and membranous nephropathy. Subendothelial deposits are associated with postinfectious glomerulonephritis, immunoglobulin A nephropathy, or lupus glomerulonephritis. (Adapted from Rose, B.D., and Rennke, H.G. [1994]. *Renal Pathophysiology: The Essentials*. Baltimore: Williams & Wilkins. [p. 226].)

The "membranes" that characterize membranous glomerulonephritis develop gradually, owing to local antigen–antibody complex formation and deposition along the glomerular basement membrane. Capillary walls are thickened by cellular proliferation yet are more permeable than normal, probably owing to cell membrane damage by the membrane attack complex of complement. Membranoproliferative glomerulonephritis is similar in its pathophysiology, except that most proliferation occurs in the mesangial cells. In IgA nephropathy, abnormally increased serum levels of a form of IgA lead to IgA immune complex formation and deposition of these complexes in the mesangial cells. Inflammation and activation of the alternative complement pathway result in glomerular damage. Focal sclerosis is characterized by scattered areas of epithelial cell and basement membrane scarring, with deposition of IgM and the complement protein C_3. Tubular atrophy eventually occurs, and fibrin is deposited in the interstitium. In many cases, the course of these chronic disorders is so slow and insidious that the condition is not evident until the patient presents with CRF.

Secondary glomerular damage may result from a number of systemic disorders, most notably systemic lupus erythematosus, Henoch-Schönlein purpura, infective endocarditis, diabetes mellitus, amyloidosis, Goodpasture's syndrome, polyarteritis nodosa, and Wegener's granulomatosis. The glomerular lesions and mechanisms of their formation in these conditions are summarized in Table 20–13.

Clinical Manifestations. Acute and subacute glomerulonephritis typically manifest in some degree of the **nephritic syndrome**, in which urine contains red blood cells (which may be visible as hematuria), leukocytes, and casts. This urinary sediment is representative of the inflammatory process within the glomerulus and contains Tamm-Horsfall protein. Increased glomerular capillary permeability permits cellular loss in the urine. Proteinuria may also be present, and nonspecific signs of inflammation, including fever, headache, malaise, weakness, and anorexia, are common. Flank pain may result from increased pressure within the renal capsule due to edema, and vision may be disturbed by retinal edema. Oliguria may occur in more severe cases.

Conditions associated with chronic glomerulonephritis are more likely to manifest as the nephrotic syndrome, which is defined by more extensive proteinuria (greater than 3.5 g/day), low serum albumin secondary to renal loss, and edema (due to low serum colloid osmotic pressure). Low serum albumin leads to hypovolemia, with chronic stimulation of the RAAS, resulting in sodium and water retention. This, in turn, leads to some degree of hypertension and may precipitate congestive heart failure in compromised patients. Proteins lost in the urine include not only albumin but also immunoglobulins and hormones. Protein loss leads to increased synthesis of all classes of proteins by the liver, including lipoproteins and clotting factors. Clinical manifestations of renal failure become evident when renal function declines to 25%. Clinical features of the nephritic and nephrotic syndromes are contrasted in Table 20–14.

Prevention and Treatment. Streptococcal infections are appropriately treated with antibiotics. Diuretics and antihypertensive drugs may be employed, and corticosteroids may be used for their anti-in-

TABLE 20–13
CONDITIONS ASSOCIATED WITH SECONDARY GLOMERULAR DAMAGE

Disorder	Mechanism of Glomerular Injury
Systemic lupus erythematosus (SLE)	Autoimmune disorder in which immune complexes deposit in the glomeruli, mesangium, or tubular cells in either a focal or diffuse pattern
Henoch-Schönlein purpura	Immune-mediated vasculitis manifesting in the kidneys as deposits of complexes of immunoglobulins A and G and complement in the glomeruli
Infective endocarditis	Deposition of immune complexes initiated by antibody response to bacterial antigen
Diabetes mellitus	Thickening of the glomerular basement membrane, diffuse glomerulosclerosis, and nodular glomerulosclerosis, possibly due to metabolic end products resulting from hyperglycemia or insulin deficiency and to hypoxia secondary to microangiopathy
Amyloidosis	Deposition of amyloid (abnormal protein) in glomeruli, mesangium, and interstitium
Goodpasture's syndrome	Deposition of anti–basement membrane antibodies and complement along the glomerular basement membrane
Polyarteritis nodosa	Deposition of immune complexes in glomeruli
Wegener's granulomatosis	Acute focal proliferation and necrosis in glomeruli, with thrombosis of isolated glomerular capillaries, followed later by diffuse necrosis, proliferation, and crescent formation

Data from Cotran, R.S., Kumar, V., and Robbins, S.L. (1994). *Robbins Pathologic Basis of Disease.* (5th ed.). Philadelphia: W.B. Saunders.

flammatory effect in severe cases. Immunosuppressive agents and plasmapheresis (removal of immune complexes from the blood) have been used experimentally in the treatment of immune-mediated, rapidly progressive, and chronic forms of glomerulonephritis. Renal failure, if present, is treated as discussed earlier.

Prognosis and Outcome. Acute glomerulonephritis is self-limited in 95% of cases, with diuresis and relief of signs and symptoms occurring within 3 weeks.[14] Some degree of hematuria and proteinuria may persist for several months, however. Rapidly progressive glomerulonephritis often results in death due to ARF within 2 years. Chronic glomerulonephritis leads to CRF, usually over a period of several years.

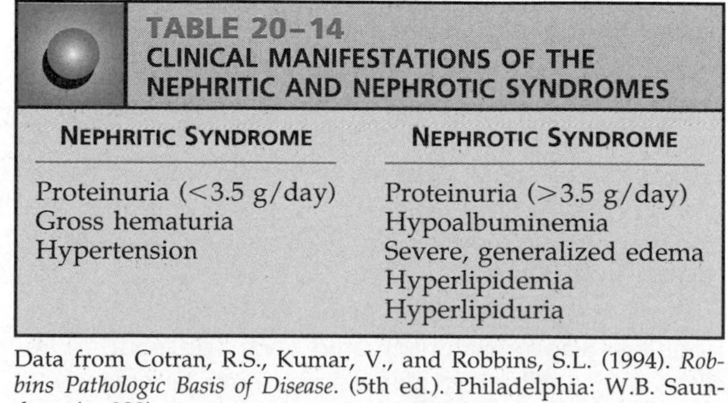

TABLE 20–14
CLINICAL MANIFESTATIONS OF THE NEPHRITIC AND NEPHROTIC SYNDROMES

Nephritic Syndrome	Nephrotic Syndrome
Proteinuria (<3.5 g/day)	Proteinuria (>3.5 g/day)
Gross hematuria	Hypoalbuminemia
Hypertension	Severe, generalized edema
	Hyperlipidemia
	Hyperlipiduria

Data from Cotran, R.S., Kumar, V., and Robbins, S.L. (1994). *Robbins Pathologic Basis of Disease.* (5th ed.). Philadelphia: W.B. Saunders. (p. 932).

Acute Interstitial Nephritis

Definition. Acute interstitial nephritis is a syndrome of abrupt onset of renal tubular and interstitial inflammation, potentially resulting in ARF.

Epidemiology. Acute interstitial nephritis accounts for 3% to 16% of all cases of ARF.[15] Risk factors are associated with exposure to certain drugs or infectious diseases.

Etiology. Although acute interstitial nephritis may be caused by bacterial or viral infection, it is more often induced by an allergic (hypersensitivity) reaction to a drug. Nonsteroidal anti-inflammatory drugs (NSAIDs) and antibiotics are the most common causes. NSAIDs implicated in causing acute interstitial nephritis include ibuprofen (Advil), fenuprofen (Nalfon), indomethacin (Indocin), naproxen (Anaprox), and others. Most categories of antibiotics may also cause the disorder, including penicillins, cephalosporins, vancomycin, tetracyclines, ciprofloxacin, sulfonamides, antiviral agents, and antituberculin drugs.[16]

Pathophysiology. An inflammatory reaction results from hypersensitivity or infection and involves the renal interstitium and tubules. These structures become infiltrated with mononuclear cells and eosinophils. Interstitial edema and altered tubular function result in ARF.

Clinical Manifestations. Clinical manifestations are usually nonspecific. Rash, painful joints, and fever may be present. Nephritic syndrome may be evident. Oliguria and azotemia manifest as renal function declines. Serum IgE levels may be elevated in the allergic type. Demonstration of tissue changes with renal biopsy may be required to confirm the diagnosis.

Prevention and Treatment. Nephrotoxic agents and infectious exposures should be avoided insofar as possible. Maintenance of optimal hydration may be protective. Infectious causes are treated with specific antibiotic therapy. Discontinuation of the use of offending drugs usually results in complete resolution of allergic interstitial nephritis. Short-term use of dialysis or other renal replacement therapy may be warranted in ARF.

Prognosis and Outcome. Complete resolution of the disorder is usual if it is promptly diagnosed and treated. Interstitial fibrosis and ESRD may result if the condition is untreated.

Minimal Lesion Nephrotic Syndrome

Definition. Minimal lesion nephrotic syndrome (MLNS), also known as lipoid nephrosis, is a relatively benign idiopathic disorder characterized by proteinuria due to reversible loss of foot processes of otherwise normal glomerular epithelial cells.

Epidemiology. MLNS is the most common cause of nephrotic syndrome in children, with a peak incidence between the ages of 2 and 6 years, although the disorder is seen in adults as well. Nephrotic syndrome in children demonstrates an annual incidence of about 2 cases per 100,000.[17] Respiratory infections and routine immunizations may be considered risk factors for MLNS because the disorder sometimes follows these. Associations with allergic disorders, such as eczema and hay fever, and with Hodgkin's disease have also been noted.

Etiology. The precise etiology is unknown. Although immune complexes do *not* form, an immunologic mechanism is suspected because of the associated conditions.

Pathophysiology. Damage to epithelial cells results in detachment of the glomerular basement membrane, leading to increased permeability and protein loss. It has also been postulated that loss of anionic membrane proteins contributes to increased permeability because these are no longer available to repel the transit of negatively charged serum proteins. Serum lipoproteins are increased and may accumulate in the walls of the proximal tubules.

Clinical Manifestations. The nephrotic syndrome is present to some degree, as described earlier with glomerulonephritis. Hypertension and hematuria are uncommon, however, and renal failure is rare.

Prevention and Treatment. Because the disorder is idiopathic, there are no known preventive measures. A high index of suspicion should be maintained in patients at risk, however, so that the disorder is detected and treated as early as possible. MLNS is effectively treated with corticosteroids in most cases. Long-term therapy is often necessary, which imposes risk of iatrogenic Cushing's syndrome (see Chapter 29).

Prognosis and Outcome. The long-term prognosis is excellent. In children, the condition is usually completely resolved by puberty. Adult forms also resolve over a period of several years of treatment.

Polycystic Kidney Disease

Definition. Polycystic kidney disease is an inherited disorder characterized by the development of multiple, bilateral, fluid-filled cysts throughout the kidneys as well as extrarenal manifestations. Cysts may occur in other ductal organs, including the liver and reproductive organs, and abnormalities of the cardiovascular, gastrointestinal, and musculoskeletal systems may be associated with the disorder.

Epidemiology. Polycystic kidney disease usually becomes apparent in adults older than 40 years, with an estimated prevalence of 1 in 400 to 1000 in whites.[18] An estimated 500,000 people in the United States have the disease. Polycystic kidney disease is less common in American blacks and is rare in Africa. A rare childhood form has also been reported. Although about 60% of patients are aware of a family history of the disorder, renal imaging techniques done on parents and other family members often reveal subclinical abnormalities.

Etiology. The adult form is inherited as an autosomal dominant trait, with nearly 100% penetrance (see Chapter 7). The genetic defect is located on either chromosome 16 or chromosome 4. The childhood form is autosomal recessive. De novo mutations account for about 10% of cases.[18]

Pathophysiology. Grape-like cysts develop over many years under defective regulation of cellular growth and differentiation. Normal nephrons interspersed between cysts are eventually obliterated by cystic development, and blood vessels may rupture. Renal tumors (adenomas) form in 21% of patients. The kidneys become greatly enlarged, often exceeding 40 cm in length and 8 kg in weight.[18] Defects in renal function include impairment of urine concentration and increased secretion of both renin and erythropoietin.

Clinical Manifestations. Manifestations are classified as cystic or noncystic, renal or extrarenal. Renal cysts display variable rates of progression and may manifest as hypertension, acute or chronic flank pain, hematuria, urolithiasis, and renal insufficiency progressing to ESRD. Extrarenal manifestations include liver cysts, ovarian cysts, pancreatic cysts, intracranial aneurysms, cardiac valve disease, diverticulosis of the colon, and inguinal hernia.

Prevention and Treatment. Prevention is limited to genetic counseling, although gene therapy may potentially prevent development of the disease. Cysts causing severe pain may be decompressed by percutaneous puncture or by surgical techniques. Cysts drained by puncture must be sclerosed with alcohol so that they do not refill. CRF is treated with conservative measures, dialysis, or transplantation.

Prognosis and Outcome. The rate of progression to renal failure is variable, with a small number of affected patients manifesting renal insufficiency in childhood. Up to half of cases do not manifest significant dysfunction and are diagnosed only at autopsy. Presence of hypertension is associated with a more aggressive course. Overall, 45% of patients have ESRD by the age of 60 years.[18]

Renal Cancers

Definition. Renal cancers are malignant tumors of the kidney. In adults, the most common type is **renal adenocarcinoma**, which accounts for 75% of cases. The most common childhood form is **Wilms' tumor** (nephroblastoma), which is also seen infrequently in adults.

Epidemiology. Renal cancers account for 2% of all malignancies in adults and for 20% of childhood cancers.[19] Adult tumors are slightly more common in men, with incidence increasing between the ages of 40 and 90 years. Wilms' tumor is most often seen in children between the ages of 2 and 5 years and affects 1 in 10,000 children worldwide.[20] Postulated risk factors for the development of adult renal cancers include cigarette smoking and excessive exposure to petrochemical products. A genetic predisposition is evident in people with **von Hippel-Lindau disease**, an autosomal dominant disorder characterized by multiple cancers. In children, Wilms' tumor often develops in association with congenital anomalies, including aniridia (absence of the iris of the eye), genitourinary malformations (e.g., hypospadias, cryptorchidism), and mental retardation. A familial predisposition is evident in some cases.

Etiology. The etiology of renal cancers is uncertain and is probably multifactorial, as discussed in Chapter 7. Specific genetic defects in Wilms' tumor have been identified at two loci and are known to give rise to three congenital syndromes (Table 20–15). In addition, the kidneys of nearly all children with Wilms' tumor contain *nephrogenic rests*, which are foci of primitive cells indicating a defect in embryonic development. These rests do not progress to tumor in all cases, however.

Pathophysiology. Painless renal enlargement occurs first as the cancer cells proliferate. Local extension may invade blood vessels, peripheral nerves, and lymphatics and may obstruct tubules. Excessive secretion of renin and erythropoietin are common. Metastasis to the lung, by the lymphatics, and direct invasion of bone may occur. Rupture of the tumor capsule may seed cancer cells within the peritoneal cavity.

Clinical Manifestations. Adult renal cancers usually present with pain and hematuria. In men, sudden development of varicocele (varicosity of scrotal veins) may occur as a result of venous obstruction. Evidence of paraneoplastic syndromes may be present, including hypertension due to renin excess or polycythemia due to erythropoietin excess.

In Wilms' tumor, an abdominal mass is often the first manifestation, discovered on routine physical examination or noted in children by parents. The nephritic syndrome may also be present to some degree. Later, manifestations of neoplasia are appar-

TABLE 20–15
SYNDROMES ASSOCIATED WITH WILMS' TUMOR

SYNDROME	DESCRIPTION
WAGR syndrome	Caused by allele deletion on the short arm of chromosome 11; clinical features of *W*ilms' tumor, *a*niridia, *g*enitourinary manifestations, and *r*etardation
Denys-Drash syndrome	Caused by point mutation of Wilms' tumor suppressor gene on chromosome 11; clinical features of Wilms' tumor, ambiguous genitalia, and nephropathy
Beckwith-Wiedemann syndrome	Caused by duplication of paternal allele on chromosome 11; clinical features of organomegaly, enlarged tongue, hemihypertrophy, neonatal hypoglycemia, and Wilms' tumor or other embryonal tumor

Adapted from Coppes, M.J., Haber, D.A., and Grundy, P.E. (1994). Genetic events in the development of Wilms' tumor. *New England Journal of Medicine* 331(9), 586–590.

ent, including fatigue, weight loss, and abdominal pain. Abnormal renin and erythropoietin levels may result in hypertension and polycythemia, although anemia is seen in some patients. Hypercalcemia may result from bone metastasis. Renal venous obstruction may lead to pulmonary embolism, and tubular obstruction may lead to hydronephrosis. The tumor is usually discovered and treated before development of renal failure.

Prevention and Treatment. Reduction of cancer risk is discussed in Chapter 7. Children who have aniridia should undergo frequent renal ultrasound examination for detection of Wilms' tumor. The treatment of choice in renal cancers is surgical resection of the involved kidney (nephrectomy), and resection of adjacent lymph nodes may be warranted. Radiation therapy is also used in treatment of unresectable tumors and advanced metastasis, or to reduce the risk of recurrence due to undetected seed sites. Hormonal therapy and conventional chemotherapy are not effective in treatment of renal cancers. Biologic response modifiers, such as α-interferon and interleukin-2, have been effective in debulking tumors in some unresectable cases and have occasionally induced extended remission.[21] Usually, the patient retains enough functional nephrons for normal renal function, although in some cases of unilateral tumor and in most cases of bilateral tumors, dialysis or transplantation is necessary.

Prognosis and Outcome. When the tumor is confined to the kidney (stage I disease), the 5-year survival rate after nephrectomy is about 65% in adults. In stage II disease, which extends beyond the kidney but is still resectable, the survival rate is 40%. More advanced disease is rapidly fatal. The outlook is more favorable in children with Wilms' tumor, with a more than 80% cure rate after appropriate multimodal treatment.[20]

Urinary Incontinence

Definition. Urinary incontinence is involuntary urination. Five types of urinary incontinence have been identified (Fig. 20–20). **Stress incontinence** is urination induced by increased bladder pressure due to an external force. **Urge incontinence** is associated with an unusually strong sensation of the need to urinate. **Reflex incontinence** is due to lack of normal inhibition of the micturition reflex. **Overflow incontinence** is associated with urinary retention and bladder distention. **Functional incontinence** is associated with lack of voluntary control of micturition due to developmental or environmental factors.

Epidemiology. An estimated 8 to 12 million people in the United States suffer from incontinence.[22] Risk factors have been identified for each type, as discussed next.

Etiology. Stress incontinence is associated with weakness of the external sphincter or pelvic floor muscles, which usually occurs in women, owing to the combined effects of aging and childbearing. Older men may have impaired sphincter control after prostate surgery or instrumentation of the urethra. Urge incontinence usually results from the irritation of UTI but may also occur with abnormal impulse conduction to the bladder in neurologic disorders, such as stroke, Parkinson's disease, or multiple sclerosis.

Reflex incontinence is associated with some neurogenic bladder syndromes, as previously discussed. Overflow incontinence is most commonly seen in older men with prostate enlargement, although detrusor areflexia, obstructive stones, or strictures could also cause this type. Functional incontinence is seen in infants and young children who have not yet achieved bladder control and in older people who have cognitive impairments that interfere with voluntary control of micturition. Functional incontinence may be secondary to impaired communication or mobility in older or disabled people, or may have an environmental cause (e.g., inattentive care or absence of toilets). **Enuresis**, which refers to urinary incontinence in a child older than 3 years, may have functional or physiologic causes. Enuresis may occur in the daytime but most often manifests as bedwetting during the night.

Pathophysiology. Stress incontinence is triggered by a sudden increase in intra-abdominal pressure, such as occurs with sneezing, coughing, laughing, walking, running, or jumping. In the presence of a weak external sphincter, pressure on the bladder results in loss of small amounts of urine. Urge incontinence results from strong, repetitive triggering of the micturition reflex, which eventually overcomes voluntary control of the external sphincter. Larger urine volumes are usually excreted with this type of incontinence. Reflex incontinence occurs due to lack of inhibition of the micturition reflex, producing a neurogenic bladder that frequently empties small amounts of urine. In overflow incontinence, the bladder becomes overdistended due to outlet obstruction or lack of detrusor muscle contraction, creating fluid pressure that results in continuous dribbling of urine. Mechanisms of functional incontinence are often multiple and complex. Most enuresis occurs in the absence of obvious precipitating factors, although emotional instability and family history may contribute in some cases.[23]

Clinical Manifestations. Urinary incontinence is associated with hygiene deficits that may contribute to increased incidence of genitourinary infections.

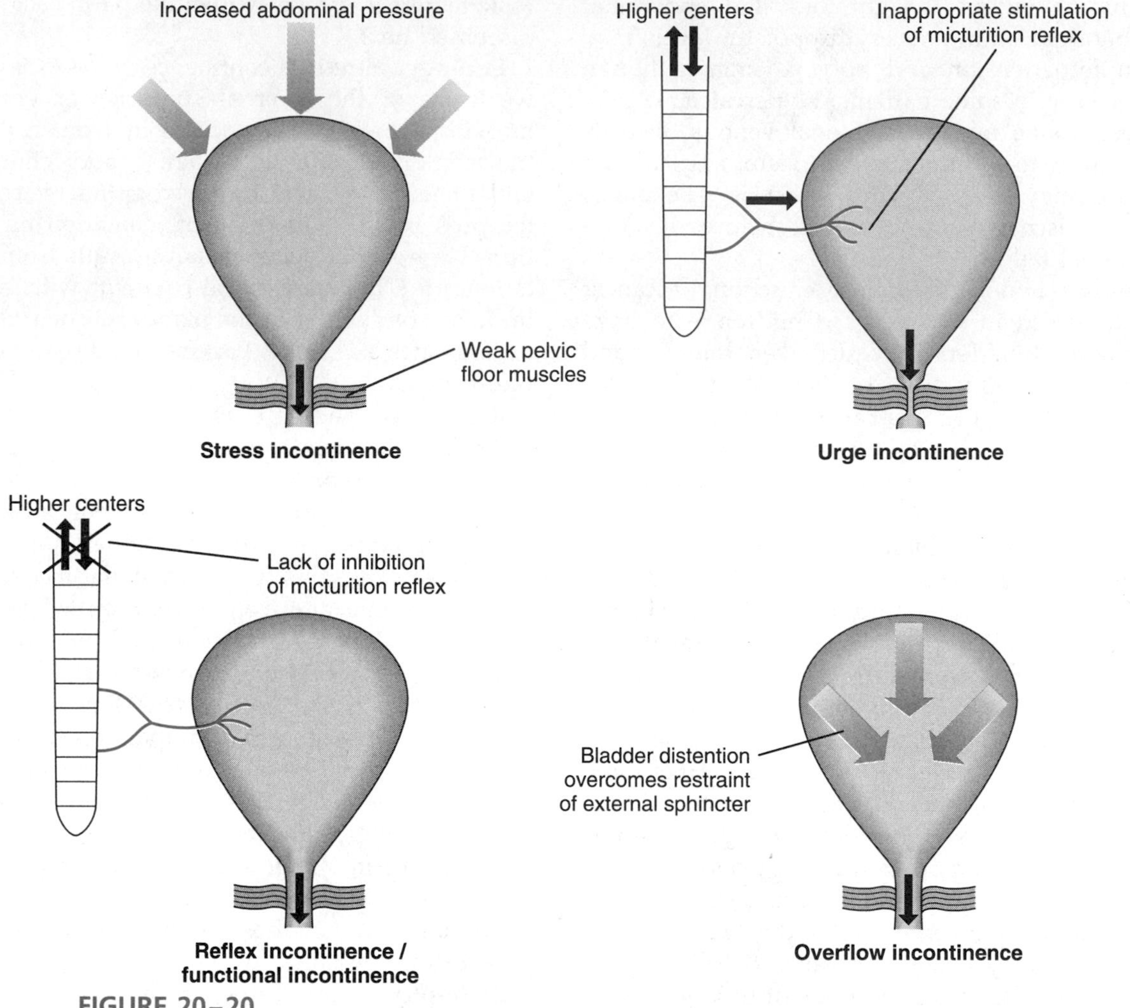

FIGURE 20–20

Types of urinary incontinence. *Stress incontinence* is induced by external pressure on the bladder, which overcomes a weak sphincter. *Urge incontinence* is associated with unusually strong neural stimulation of bladder contraction. *Reflex incontinence,* which includes functional incontinence, is due to lack of normal inhibition of the micturition reflex by higher centers. *Overflow incontinence* is due to increased internal pressure induced by a distended bladder.

Bladder and bowel incontinence may be associated with excoriation and ulceration of the skin of the perineal area. The emotional and social effects of the condition are often highly distressing to the affected person.

Prevention and Treatment. Medical, surgical, and behavioral interventions have been employed in the prevention and treatment of incontinence. Underlying conditions, such as UTI or neurologic disorders, should be addressed. Urinary collection devices, such as absorbent pads or undergarments and external or indwelling catheters, are effective in reducing distress due to odor and wetting of clothing. Indwelling catheters are associated with increased risk of UTI, however, and may damage urethral sphincters. Drug therapy of incontinence, summarized in Table 20–16, may enhance or inhibit detrusor muscle contraction or may increase the tone of the urethral sphincter. Surgical intervention may involve repair of pelvic floor musculature (see Chapter 31), removal of the prostate (see Chapter 30), or implantation of an artificial sphincter. Kegel exercises may help to strengthen the pelvic floor muscles and are often taught to women who have just given birth. Behavioral therapies for prevention and treatment of incontinence include bladder training (Table 20–17), biofeedback, and behavior modification. Factors associated with the physical or interpersonal environment that contribute to incontinence are altered if possible.

Prognosis and Outcome. Of children whose enuresis is purely functional, an estimated 15% stop wetting each year.[24] Interventions are often successful in treatment of incontinence, but in many cases

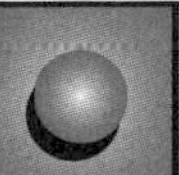

TABLE 20–16
DRUG THERAPY OF INCONTINENCE

DRUGS USED TO FACILITATE STORAGE OF URINE IN BLADDER
Drugs That Decrease Bladder Contractility
Oxybutynin chloride (Ditropan)
Flavoxate HCl (Urispas)
Propantheline bromide (Pro-Banthine)
Imipramine HCl (Tofranil)
Dicyclomine HCl (Bentyl)
Terodiline HCl (Micturin)
Hyoscyamine (Cystospaz)
Drugs That Increase Outflow Resistance
Ephedrine
Phenylephrine HCl
Phenylpropanolamine HCl (Propagest)
Estrogens
DRUGS USED TO FACILITATE BLADDER EMPTYING
Drugs That Increase Bladder Pressure
Bethanechol Cl (Duvoid, Urecholine)
Metoclopramide (Maxolon, Reglan), must be used with bethanechol
Drugs That Decrease Bladder Outlet Resistance
Phenoxybenzamine HCl (Dibenzyline)
Prazosin (Minipress)
Diazepam (Valium)
Dantrolene sodium (Dantrium)
Baclofen (Lioresal)

Adapted from Rosenthal, A.J., and McMurtry, C.T. (1995). Urinary incontinence in the elderly. *Postgraduate Medicine* 97(5), 109–121.

the disorder is neither diagnosed nor treated. About half of incontinent people do not seek treatment, believing that the condition is an inevitable consequence of aging.[25]

Urolithiasis

Definition. Urolithiasis is the formation of an obstructive solid mass (stone or calculus) within the urinary tract. Possible sites of stone formation are the renal pelvis, the ureters, and the bladder (Fig. 20–21).

Epidemiology. Calculi within the urinary system are believed to be common. The lifetime chance of a person having a stone is about 10% to 15%.[26] Any factor that promotes precipitation of solute out of the urine increases the risk of calculi. The major risk factors are concentration of urine, alkalinity of urine, UTI, and elevation of serum calcium or uric acid. Most people who seek treatment of urolithiasis are men, and the condition appears to have a familial predisposition. Examples of conditions associated with increased risk are listed in Table 20–18.

Etiology. The precise etiology of urolithiasis is unknown. Although many stone-forming patients have low urinary volumes, elevated urine solute, or both, many others do not form stones under these conditions. Still others have multiple stones despite no apparent risk factors, giving rise to the hypothesis that these people lack natural substances that inhibit crystallization. These inhibitors include citrate, magnesium, pyrophosphate, and proteins secreted by renal tubular cells (nephrocalcin, uropontin, and Tamm-Horsfall protein).[27]

Pathophysiology. The stone forms as a result of precipitation of solute around a nucleus (nidus) of sodium hydrogen urate, uric acid, or hydroxyapatite crystals. Calcium and oxalate ions then adhere to this nidus. Most stones (75%) are calcium based, 10% are uric acid based, 1% are cystine based, and the remainder are formed of magnesium ammonium phosphate (struvite), produced during UTI by urea-splitting bacteria.[27]

As the stone enlarges, it may obstruct urine flow. Ureteral or renal pelvic obstruction results in increased BCHP, which decreases GFR. Ureteral obstruction triggers the ureterorenal reflex, which also decreases GFR. Obstruction may result in engorgement of the proximal ureter and kidney with fluid (hydroureter or hydronephrosis) and may damage ureter walls and initiate an inflammatory response.

TABLE 20–17
BLADDER TRAINING PROGRAMS

PROGRAM	DESCRIPTION
Kegel exercises	Deliberate use of pelvic muscles to start and stop the urinary stream; regular repetitive exercises in which these muscles are contracted tightly for 3 seconds or more
Timed voiding regimen	Adherence to a voiding schedule based on frequency of urine leakage
Habit training	Use of a schedule of regular toileting, usually every 2 to 4 hours, with a gradual increase in the voiding interval
Prompted voiding	Patient is reminded every 2 hours to attempt voiding
Continence management	Consistent rewards or punishments are used to amend incontinence
Biofeedback	Training of bladder and pelvic floor muscle contraction using an electronic feedback signal

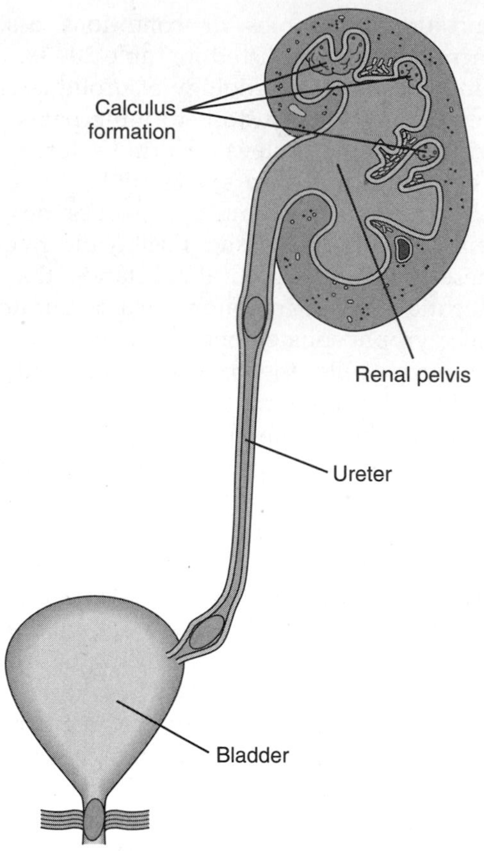

FIGURE 20–21
Sites of urolithiasis. Urinary tract stones may form at any level but are commonly found in the renal pelvis, ureters, and bladder. Urethral stones are less common.

In an effort to clear the obstruction or "pass" the stone, ureteral peristalsis increases to the point at which pain receptors are stimulated.

Clinical Manifestations. Urine output is decreased, and hematuria is common. The most distressing manifestation is renal colic, a severe, crampy pain in the flank area. Sediment or stones may be evident in the urine.

Prevention and Treatment. Known risk factors should be eliminated insofar as possible, through dietary adjustment or treatment of underlying conditions. Stones smaller than 5 mm usually pass spontaneously. Stones between 5 and 10 mm have a 50% chance of passing.[27] Analgesics, including narcotics, may be necessary for relief of severe pain. Fluid intake is increased in an effort to "flush out" stones and inhibit further precipitation.

Larger stones require intervention, usually performed on an outpatient basis but occasionally requiring hospitalization. In some cases, the stone may be accessed with a small ureteral catheter and either dislodged or crushed. Extracorporeal shock wave lithotripsy, a noninvasive therapy in which high-intensity shock waves are directed at the stone in an

TABLE 20–18
CONDITIONS ASSOCIATED WITH UROLITHIASIS

Risk Factors for Specific Stone Types	
Calcium oxalate	Hypercalcemia and hypercalciuria Hyperparathyroidism Diffuse bone disease Sarcoidosis Hypercalciuria without hypercalcemia Absorptive hypercalciuria Renal hypercalciuria Increased uric acid secretion Hyperoxaluria Hereditary hyperoxaluria Enteric disease Vegetarian diet Idiopathic
Struvite (Mg^{2+}, NH_4^+, PO_4^{3-})	Infection by urea-splitting organism, producing alkaline urine Some staphylococci *Proteus* sp.
Uric acid	Hyperuricemia and hyperuricosuria Gout High purine diet Rapid cell turnover (e.g., leukemia) Idiopathic (associated with increased acidity of urine)
Cystine	Genetic abnormality of renal transport of cystine and other amino acids
General Risk Factors	
Stagnation of urine	Detrusor areflexia Urinary tract obstruction
Urinary tract infection	Urinary tract instrumentation or catheterization Sexually transmitted disease Inadequate hygiene
Alteration of urine pH	Dietary factors Urinary tract infection Drug effects Acidosis or alkalosis
Deficiency of crystal inhibitory factors	Hereditary or acquired deficiency Diphosphonate Glycosaminoglycans Nephrocalcin Citrate Pyrophosphate
Supersaturation of urine	Excessive excretion of solute Dietary factors Renal disease Low urine volume Dehydration Oliguria Syndrome of inappropriate antidiuretic hormone (SIADH)

*Data from Cotran, R.S., Kumar, V., and Robbins, S.L. (1994). *Robbins Pathologic Basis of Disease.* (5th ed.). Philadelphia: W.B. Saunders.

TABLE 20–19
CLASSIFICATION AND TREATMENT OF URINARY TRACT INFECTIONS

CLASSIFICATION	DEFINING FEATURES	TREATMENT
Asymptomatic bacteriuria	Presence of at least 10^5 colony-forming units/mL on two successive cultures	No treatment except in pregnant women and before urologic surgery
Acute uncomplicated infection	Occurs in women 18–65 years old who have symptoms of frequency, dysuria, and urgency, with fever less than 101°F and no complicating factors	Empiric treatment with brief course of antibiotic, usually co-trimoxazole (Bactrim or Septra)
Complicated infection	Occurs in patients with functional, metabolic, or anatomic abnormalities of the urinary tract, e.g., symptoms or history of pyelonephritis or urinary obstruction; age under 18 or over 65 years; male sex, pregnancy; underlying systemic disease; immunosuppression; hospitalization; recent antibiotic use; recurrent urinary tract infection; persistent urinary tract infection symptoms; urinary tract instrumentation or catheterization	Specific oral or parenteral antibiotic therapy based on urine culture and antibiotic sensitivity testing; treatment for 7–14 days or longer; usual oral agents are co-trimoxazole, norfloxacin, ciprofloxacin, amoxicillin; usual parenteral agents are co-trimoxazole, ciprofloxacin, gentamicin, ceftriaxone, ampicillin, imipenem, ticarcillin, aztreonam

effort to pulverize it, has been beneficial to many. Surgical removal of calculi (lithotomy) may be used as a last resort.

Prognosis and Outcome. Patients who suffer two episodes of urolithiasis have a high rate of continued recurrence of the condition. Urolithiasis rarely progresses to renal failure because colic causes the patient to seek intervention before extensive nephron damage occurs.

Urinary Tract Infections

Definition. UTIs are inflammatory conditions of the urethra (**urethritis**), bladder (**cystitis**), or less commonly, ureter (**ureteritis**) or kidney (**pyelonephritis**).

Epidemiology. UTIs are extremely common, with an estimated 7 million people seeking treatment each year and countless others suffering untreated or self-treating the condition.[28] About 20% of women, 3% of girls, and 1% of boys are susceptible to recurrent infections. UTI is uncommon in adult males unless associated with sexually transmitted disease, structural deformity of the tract, or obstruction due to prostate enlargement. Hospitalization is an independent risk factor for UTI, with an estimated half-million patients each year acquiring the infection due to nosocomial transmission or presence of an indwelling catheter. Other risk factors include stasis of urine and alkalinity of urine, both of which are favorable to the growth of microorganisms, as well as urinary tract instrumentation and frequent or traumatic sexual intercourse, both of which may introduce organisms. The presence of genetically controlled blood group antigens on epithelial cells of the urinary tract has been associated with increased frequency of UTI, and the theory is that these antigens serve as receptors that bind bacteria to tract walls (see Focus of Current Research).[29]

Etiology. The causative organism is usually a gram-negative bacterium such as *E. coli*, *Pseudomonas* sp, or *Proteus* sp.

Pathophysiology. The organism triggers an inflammatory response within the lining of the urinary tract. This irritation inappropriately triggers the micturition reflex.

Clinical Manifestations. Clinical manifestations and host factors determine whether the UTI is complicated or uncomplicated, which in turn determines therapy (Table 20–19). Urine culture is not indicated in uncomplicated cystitis. The classic manifestations of UTI are frequency (frequent urination), urgency (strong sensation of need to urinate), and dysuria (burning pain with urination). Hematuria may be present but is usually microscopic. Pyuria (pus in the urine) may occur with severe infections. Because of decreased pain sensation and possible limitation of immune or inflammatory responses, the elderly often have no symptoms or exhibit increased confusion, which is not immediately apparent as associated with UTI. Urine may be foul smelling or foamy, owing to the presence of bacteria and inflammatory constituents, and urine culture reveals presence of the organism.

Focus of Current Research

Study	Objective and Findings
Klag, et al. (1997) End-stage renal disease in African-American and white men.	*Objective:* To determine reasons for the four-fold higher incidence of treated end-stage renal disease in African-American men compared with white men *Findings:* Both higher blood pressure and lower income are associated with a higher incidence of end-stage renal disease in both white and African-American men.
Curhan, et al. (1997) Comparison of dietary calcium with supplemental calcium and other nutrients as factors affecting the risk for kidney stones in women.	*Objective:* To examine the association between intake of dietary and supplemental calcium and the risk for kidney stones in women *Findings:* High intake of dietary calcium appears to decrease risk for symptomatic kidney stones, whereas intake of supplemental calcium may increase risk.
Chertow, et al. (1996) Is the administration of dopamine associated with adverse or favorable outcomes in acute renal failure?	*Objective:* To explore the relationship between the administration of low-dose dopamine and outcomes in renal failure *Findings:* There is insufficient evidence that the administration of low-dose dopamine increases survival or obviates the need for dialysis in patients with acute renal failure.
Levy, et al. (1996) The effect of acute renal failure on mortality: A cohort analysis.	*Objective:* To determine if the high mortality in acute renal failure is explained by underlying illnesses *Findings:* The mortality rate in subjects without renal failure was 7%, compared with 34% in the corresponding subjects with renal failure. Subjects who died after developing renal failure had complications such as sepsis, bleeding, delirium, and respiratory failure. The complications developed after the onset of renal failure.
Hooton, et al. (1996) A prospective study of risk factors for symptomatic urinary tract infection in young women.	*Objective:* To define prospectively risk factors for urinary tract infection in young women *Findings:* The strongest risk factors were recent use of a diaphragm with spermicide, recent sexual intercourse, and history of recurrent infection.
Terasaki, et al. (1995) High survival rates of kidney transplants from spousal and living unrelated donors.	*Objective:* To examine the factors influencing the high survival rates of spousal donor kidneys *Findings:* The high rate of survival, despite poor HLA matching, was due to the fact that the kidneys were uniformly healthy.

continued

Jantausch, et al. (1994) Association of Lewis blood group phenotypes with urinary tract infection in children.	*Objective:* To determine the relation between erythrocyte antigens and phenotypes and urinary tract infection in children *Findings:* The relative risk of urinary tract infection in children with specific Lewis antigens was more than three-fold.
Avorn, et al. (1994) Reduction of bacteriuria and pyuria after ingestion of cranberry juice.	*Objective:* To determine the effect of regular intake of cranberry juice on bacteriuria and pyuria in elderly women *Findings:* Use of cranberry juice reduced the frequency of bacteriuria with pyuria in this population by nearly half.

Prevention and Treatment. Prevention involves reduction of risk factors. Optimal hydration and hygiene are encouraged. Antibiotic treatment of asymptomatic bacteriuria is not warranted except in high-risk hosts. Cranberry juice has long been used as a home remedy for UTI because of its acidifying effect on the urine. There is some controversy about the extent of its effectiveness, however, and more recent evidence indicates that its apparent benefit results from inhibition of adhesion of bacteria to the bladder mucosa.[30] Surgical intervention may be indicated in cases of structural defects predisposing to infection. Definitive antibiotic therapy is detailed in Table 20–19.

Prognosis and Outcome. Uncomplicated UTIs usually respond quickly to a short-term course of antibiotics. In those with complicating factors, a 6- to 8-week course of therapy may be necessary. UTI of the lower tract uncommonly progresses to pyelonephritis and rarely progresses to renal failure.

Interstitial Cystitis

Definition. Interstitial cystitis is an idiopathic disorder characterized by chronic, unexplained irritative voiding symptoms, sterile urine, and specific changes within the bladder mucosa.[31]

Epidemiology. Ninety per cent of patients are women, with peak incidence between 30 and 59 years of age. Prevalence has been estimated at between 20,000 and 90,000 people in the United States.[32] Risk factors include a history of UTI and childhood bladder problems, hysterectomy, medication allergies, irritable bowel syndrome, paresthesias, abdominal complaints, sinusitis, frequent upper respiratory infections, and arthritis.[33]

Etiology. The etiology of interstitial cystitis is unknown. Hypothetical causes include subclinical infection, lymphovascular obstruction, inadequate secretion of the surface mucous coat of the bladder mucosa, *reflex sympathetic dystrophy* (a syndrome of excessive SNS activity), dietary toxins, and autoimmune phenomena.

Pathophysiology. Biopsy of the bladder reveals mild edema and hyperemia of the mucosa and elevation in the number of mast cells, consistent with inflammation. Increased permeability of the surface mucous coat lining the bladder has been demonstrated in patients with interstitial cystitis.[31] About 10% of patients have Hunner's ulcers, reddened mucosal patches with central ridges that may ooze blood when the bladder is distended. Ninety per cent have pinpoint hemorrhagic areas, known as glomerulations, which are believed to result from defects in cohesion of bladder epithelial cells.[32]

Clinical Manifestations. Patients with interstitial cystitis have signs and symptoms similar to UTI, including frequency, urgency, dysuria, and pain. Microscopic examination of the urine may reveal hematuria or pyuria, but urine cultures are usually sterile. Cystoscopy (endoscopic examination) of the bladder may reveal ulcers or pinpoint hemorrhages, but in most cases, the diagnosis of interstitial cystitis is made after exclusion of other causes of the manifestations. Depression is common among patients with interstitial cystitis, presumably owing to the chronicity of the disorder and the impact on quality of life.

Prevention and Treatment. Because the cause is unknown, there is no definitive prevention or treatment. The aim of empirical treatment is to relieve symptoms as much as possible, and includes oral medications such as anticholinergics, bladder analgesics, calcium-channel blockers, antidepressants, and antihistamines. Use of the fibrinolytic agent pentosan polysulfate (Elmiron) has been particularly effective. Rarely, surgical techniques, such as partial cystectomy or denervation of the bladder, are employed.

Prognosis and Outcome. Long-term remission of symptoms is accomplished in many, although this result cannot be attributed to any particular therapy.[33]

Bladder Cancer

Definition. Bladder cancer is a malignant neoplasm of the bladder epithelium.

Epidemiology. Carcinoma of the bladder accounts for 2% of all cancers, with 52,000 new cases diagnosed each year in the United States.[34] Incidence is highest among white men older than 50 years. Environmental risk factors include occupational chemical exposure (e.g., dry cleaners, beauticians, and painters), cigarette smoking, or previous exposure to chemotherapy or pelvic radiation.[35] Chronic UTI enhances risk of squamous cell carcinoma of the bladder, and a parasitic infection (schistosomiasis) is strongly associated with bladder cancer in Africa and Egypt. A relationship between bladder cancer and use of the artificial sweeteners saccharin and cyclamate in humans remains unproved.[34]

Etiology. The precise etiology of bladder cancer is unknown.

Pathophysiology. Two forms of bladder cancer are seen: a low-grade superficial type, which tends to be recurrent but not aggressively invasive; and high-grade invasive cancer. High-grade bladder cancer may be locally invasive to muscle or may metastasize to distant sites.

Clinical Manifestations. Painless hematuria is the presenting sign in 85% of cases.[35] Other signs are similar to those of UTI, including frequency, urgency, and dysuria. Flank pain may be present if the tumor is obstructive. Urine testing for nuclear matrix protein may reveal elevation of this tumor marker.[36] Cystoscopy may reveal tumors. Imaging studies in which dye is injected into the urinary tract may detect filling defects, which are indicative of malignancy. Metastasis may be apparent on systemic imaging studies.

Prevention and Treatment. Examination of the urine for nuclear matrix protein or suspicious cells is an effective screening tool for bladder cancer. Reduction of risk related to tobacco use or chemical exposure is warranted. Treatment of bladder cancer depends on the degree of invasiveness. Superficial tumors confined to the bladder mucosa may be removed by transurethral cystoscopy. Because the risk of recurrence is high, intravesical immunotherapy or chemotherapy (injection of drug into the bladder) is done in conjunction with therapeutic cystoscopy. Bacillus Calmette-Guérin is the most effective biologic

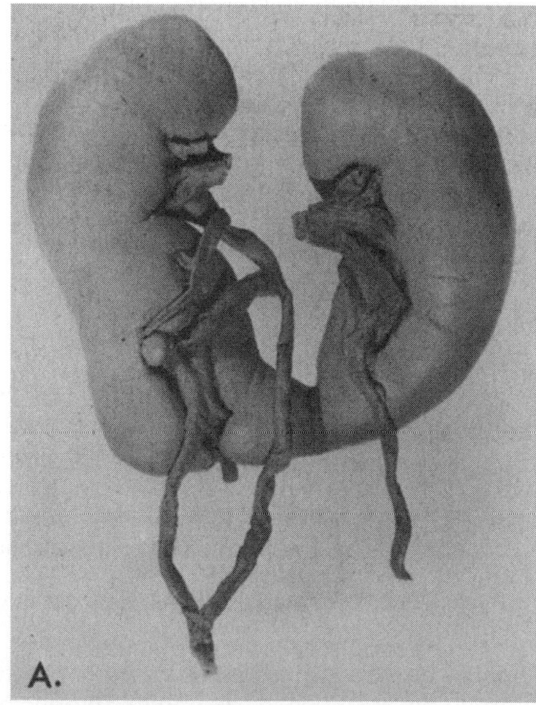

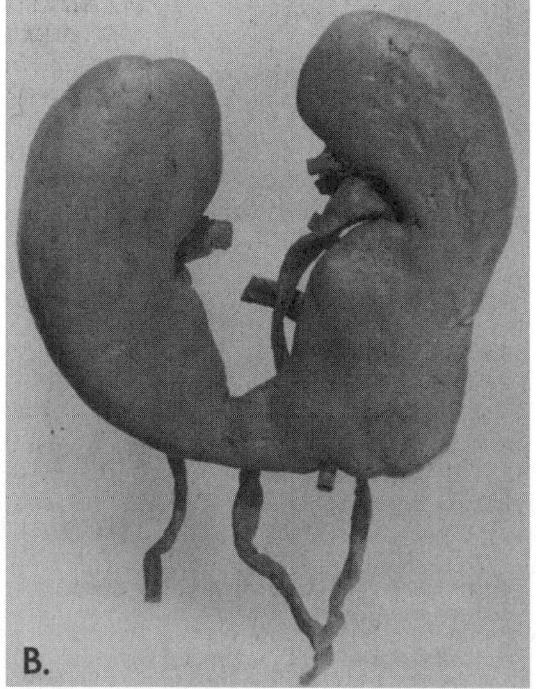

FIGURE 20–22

Horseshoe kidney. *A*, Anterior view. *B*, Posterior view. (From Moore, K.L., and Persaud, T.V.N. [1993]. *The Developing Human: Clinically Oriented Embryology.* (5th ed.). Philadelphia: W.B. Saunders. [p. 274].)

TABLE 20-20
CONGENITAL NEPHROPATHIES AND UROPATHIES

Disorder	Clinical Features
CONGENITAL NEPHROPATHIES	
Renal hypoplasia	The kidney is small, owing to reduction in the number of normally developed nephrons. The condition may be unilateral or bilateral; renal function is proportional to the degree of hypoplasia.
Renal dysplasia	The kidney is morphologically abnormal, owing to developmental arrest during metanephric stage; involved areas are nonfunctional. The most common congenital renal anomaly is *multicystic dysplastic kidney (MCDK)*, diagnosed in 1 in 4300 live births. MCDK is usually benign if unilateral.
Cystic diseases	Polycystic kidney disease, renal medullary cystic disease, and glomerular cystic disease may occur as hereditary or de novo defects.
Unilateral renal agenesis	One kidney fails to develop. One fourth of cases are associated with abnormalities of other systems. The condition is often familial and is asymptomatic.
Renal malrotation	The kidney is abnormally positioned. The condition is usually asymptomatic but may cause vague abdominal discomfort.
Ectopic kidney	The kidney is located in the pelvic or thoracic cavity, and abnormal placement usually causes reflux of urine from the bladder into the ureters.
Horseshoe kidney	The lower poles of the kidneys are fused by an isthmus of renal and fibrous tissue (see Fig. 20–22).
CONGENITAL UROPATHIES	
Disorder	**Clinical Features**
Obstructive uropathy	Forms of anatomic obstruction include ureteropelvic junction obstruction, megaureter, posterior urethral valves, and ureterovesical junction obstruction. Obstruction is due to abnormal vasculature, adhesions, kinks, or masses. Obstruction is usually left-sided and is more common in males. The clinical presentation is of hydronephrosis.
Prune belly syndrome	This syndrome is characterized by deficient abdominal musculature, bilateral cryptorchidism in males, and a dilated, nonobstructed urinary tract. The kidneys are dysplastic and cystic. Incidence is 1 in 29,000–40,000, and the syndrome is much more frequent in males.
Duplication of ureter or renal pelvis	These are the most common malformations of the urinary tract and are associated with increased risk of urinary tract infection, obstruction, or incontinence.
Ureterocele	A cystic dilation of the intravesicular ureter is often associated with duplication of the ureter. The condition may present as urinary tract infection or obstruction.
Vesicoureteral reflux	Retrograde flow of urine from the bladder into the ureter and possibly into the renal pelvis is usually associated with obstructive uropathy but may occur as an isolated functional defect.
Exstrophy of the bladder	The bladder appears in the suprapubic region as a protruding red mass that constantly seeps urine. The symphysis pubis is widely separated, and the hip sockets are rotated backward. Other genitourinary anomalies are usually associated. Exstrophy occurs in 1 in 30,000 live births and is three times more common in males.

Data from Becker, N., and Avner, E.D. (1995). Congenital nephropathies and uropathies. *Pediatric Clinics of North America* 42(6), 1319–1341; and Foster, R.L.R., Hunsberger, M.M., and Anderson, J.J.T. (1989). *Family-Centered Nursing Care of Children.* Philadelphia: W.B. Saunders.

response modifier for this purpose, although the chemotherapeutic agents mitomycin (Mutamycin), doxorubicin (Adriamycin), and thiotepa (Thioplex) have also been used.[36]

More extensive disease may require partial or complete removal of the bladder (cystectomy) and surrounding tissues. Complete (radical) cystectomy requires diversion of urinary flow to the abdominal surface or to a segment of ileum or colon. Patients who are not candidates for surgery are treated with immunotherapy, chemotherapy, radiation therapy, or a combination.

Prognosis and Outcome. The 5-year survival rate for bladder cancer ranges from 87% for patients with localized disease to 9% for those with distant metastasis.[37]

Congenital Defects of the Urinary Tract

Congenital defects of the urinary tract occur in 3% to 4% of newborns[38] and account for one third of cases of pediatric ESRD.[39] Table 20–20 lists clinical characteristics of the more common congenital nephropathies and uropathies. A rare disorder, horseshoe kidney, is illustrated (Fig. 20–22).

CLINICAL SIGNIFICANCE OF RENAL-URINARY DISORDERS

Renal failure is common and costly, and its impact on quality of life is inestimable. From the examples discussed in this chapter, it is evident that renal disorders affect people of all ages. The kidney may be adversely affected not only by primary renal disease but also by disorders of other systems, including hypertension and other circulatory disorders, diabetes mellitus, and connective tissue disorders such as systemic lupus erythematosus. Endocrine disorders affecting ADH and aldosterone also have a significant impact on renal function. Research is ongoing in an effort to identify etiologic mechanisms in the idiopathic disorders, to reduce nephrotoxicity of therapeutic agents, to determine the locations and mechanisms of genetic defects, and to develop modes of therapy that are more convenient and cost-effective.

Disorders of micturition also affect people of all ages but probably have their greatest impact on the elderly. Incontinence and its associated manifestations may severely impair self-esteem, social interaction, and self-care capacity. UTIs in the elderly impose high risk of sepsis, resulting in serious illness, hospitalization, and possible fatality. Disorders of the lower urinary tract may result in ascending infection or, in the case of obstruction, engorgement of the kidneys with fluid. Although renal failure is not commonly the result of lower tract disorders, it does occur. Current research related to these conditions is aimed at identification and reduction of risk factors for the common conditions of incontinence and UTI and at development of effective clinical interventions.

Summary of Key Points

- The primary functions of the renal-urinary system are the regulation of the volume and composition of body fluids and the excretion of metabolic wastes. Because renal perfusion is critical to these functions, the cardiovascular system functions in concert with the kidneys in this regard. Interdependence of renal and respiratory function is evident in regulation of acid-base balance. The kidney is also an endocrine organ, important in regulation of hematopoiesis (secretion of erythropoietin), blood pressure and electrolyte balance (secretion of renin), and calcium-phosphate homeostasis (activation of vitamin D_3).

- The dual-arteriolar perfusion of the glomerulus and the long loops of Henle of juxtamedullary nephrons are critical to the regulation of body fluids, as are the different permeabilities and transport mechanisms of renal tubular cells in various nephron segments. The smooth muscle of the bladder and ureters facilitates distention for storage and rhythmic contraction for propulsion and expulsion of urine, whereas the skeletal muscle of the external urinary sphincter permits voluntary control of micturition.

- Renal blood flow is subject to regulation by local, neural, and hormonal mechanisms. Because glomerular filtration is dependent on renal blood flow, the same factors apply. The precise mediators responsible for local autoregulation are uncertain but are believed to include endothelial vasoactive substances, such as endothelins and nitric oxide. Differential innervation of the afferent and efferent arterioles by the SNS permits fine regulation of glomerular capillary hydrostatic pressure and GFR. The RAAS impacts both blood volume and blood pressure, with secondary effects on renal blood flow and tubular transport of fluid and solutes.

- The PCT is permeable to water and most solutes. The bulk of the glomerular filtrate is reabsorbed in the PCT in association with gradients created by the active reabsorption of sodium. Secretion into the PCT is more limited but includes a number of organic acids and bases. The thin descending loop of Henle is permeable to water but impermeable to solutes. Its function is the reabsorption of water by osmosis, as governed by the hypertonic medullary interstitial gradient. The thin ascending loop (in juxtamedullary nephrons) is impermeable to water but permits the efflux of sodium and chloride from the tubule and the influx of urea from the interstitium. The thick ascending loop is permeable only to sodium, potassium, and chloride, and the active reabsorption of these ions is critical to the establishment of the medullary gradient. The DCT and collecting duct are permeable to sodium, potassium, hydrogen, and chloride (by active and passive transport mechanisms). Permeability to water depends on the concentration of antidiuretic hormone.

- The ability of the kidney to vary the concentration of urine initially depends on differential tubular transport and countercurrent mechanisms to establish and maintain a vertically graduated interstitial gradient in the inner medulla. The presence of antidiuretic hormone, which increases permeability of the DCT and collecting duct to water and urea, then governs the osmolarity of the urine by regulating water reabsorption in a dose-dependent manner.
- Micturition, the reflex act of urination, occurs when mechanoreceptors in the bladder wall sense stretch due to filling and initiate an afferent signal to the sacral segments of the spinal cord. Impulses are then conveyed back to the bladder along somatic and autonomic motor fibers, resulting in detrusor muscle contraction and expulsion of urine *if* the external urethral sphincter is relaxed. Descending impulses from higher centers in the pons and cerebral cortex further regulate the act of micturition, coordinating bladder contraction and sphincter relaxation and permitting urination at socially appropriate times.
- ARF may result from prerenal, intrarenal (renal parenchymal), or postrenal etiologies. CRF results from progressive, irreversible loss of functional nephrons due to primary renal disease or renal manifestations of systemic disorders, such as hypertension and diabetes mellitus. Lower urinary tract disorders may result from degenerative, infectious, or obstructive process within the tract, from congenital defects, or from impaired innervation of the micturition reflex. Intervention in these disorders involves resolution of the underlying etiology, if possible, as well as renal replacement therapies and occasionally surgical diversion or reconstruction of urinary tract structures.

REFERENCES

1. Rabkin, R. (1995). Insulin-like growth factor-1 treatment of acute renal failure. *Journal of Laboratory and Clinical Medicine* 125, 684–685.
2. Loghman-Adham, M. (1993). Role of phosphate retention in the progression of renal failure. *Journal of Laboratory and Clinical Medicine* 122, 15–25.
3. Guyton, A.C., and Hall, J.E. (1996). *Textbook of Medical Physiology*. (9th ed.). Philadelphia: W.B. Saunders. (p. 325).
4. Ausiello, D.A. (1993). Renal tubular transport mechanisms. *Seminars in Nephrology* 13(5), 472–478.
5. Amis, E.S., and Blaivas, J.G. (1991). Neurogenic bladder simplified. *Radiologic Clinics of North America* 29(3), 571–580.
6. Price, C.A. (1994). Acute renal failure: A sequelae of sepsis. *Critical Care Nursing Clinics of North America* 6(2), 359–372.
7. Thadhani, R., Pascual, M., and Bonventre, J.V. (1996). Acute renal failure. *New England Journal of Medicine* 334(22), 1448–1460.
8. Forni, L.G., and Hilton, P.J. (1997). Continuous hemofiltration in the treatment of acute renal failure. *New England Journal of Medicine* 336(18), 1303–1309.
9. Humes, H.D. (1997). Acute renal failure: The promise of new therapies. *New England Journal of Medicine* 336(12), 870–871.
10. Lafayette, R.A. (1995). Preventing disease progression in chronic renal failure. *American Family Physician* 52(6), 1783–1791.
11. Hood, V.L., and Gennari, F.J. (1996). End-stage renal disease: Measures to prevent it or slow its progression. *Postgraduate Medicine* 100(5), 163–176.
12. Suthanthiran, M., and Strom, T.B. (1994). Renal transplantation. *New England Journal of Medicine* 331(6), 365–376.
13. Grimm, P.C., and Ogborn, M.R. (1994). Hemolytic uremic syndrome: The most common cause of acute renal failure in childhood. *Pediatric Annals* 23(9), 505–511.
14. Cotran, R.S., Kumar, V., and Robbins, S.L. (1994). *Robbins Pathologic Basis of Disease*. (5th ed.). Philadelphia: W.B. Saunders. (pp. 945–959).
15. Kasama, R., and Sorbello, A. (1996). Renal and electrolyte complications associated with antibiotic therapy. *American Family Physician* 53(1), 227–232.
16. Fried, T. (1993). Acute interstitial nephritis: Why do the kidneys suddenly fail? *Postgraduate Medicine* 93(5), 105–120.
17. Warshaw, B.L. (1994). Nephrotic syndrome in children. *Pediatric Annals* 23(9), 495–504.
18. Gabow, P.A. (1993). Autosomal dominant polycystic kidney disease. *New England Journal of Medicine* 329(5), 332–342.
19. Davis, M. (1993). Renal cell carcinoma. *Seminars in Oncology Nursing* 9(4), 267–271.
20. Coppes, M.J., Haber, D.A., and Grundy, P.E. (1994). Genetic events in the development of Wilms' tumor. *New England Journal of Medicine* 331(9), 586–590.
21. Motzer, R.J., Bander, N.H., and Nanus, D.M. (1996). Renal-cell carcinoma. *New England Journal of Medicine* 335(12), 865–875.
22. Peggs, J.F. (1992). Urinary incontinence in the elderly: Pharmacologic therapies. *American Family Physician* 46(6), 1763–1769.
23. Rushton, H.G. (1995). Wetting and functional voiding disorders. *Urologic Clinics of North America* 22(1), 75–93.
24. Rosenfeld, J., and Jerkins, G.R. (1991). The bed-wetting child: Current managment of a frustrating problem. *Postgraduate Medicine* 89(2), 63–70.
25. Weiss, B.D. (1991). Nonpharmacologic treatment of urinary incontinence. *American Family Physician* 44(2), 579–586.
26. Resnick, M.I., and Persky, L. (1995). Summary of the National Institutes of Arthritis, Diabetes, Digestive and Kidney Diseases Conference of Urolithiasis: State of the art and future research needs. *Journal of Urology* 153(1), 4–9.
27. Trivedi, B.K. (1996). Nephrolithiasis: How it happens and what to do about it. *Postgraduate Medicine* 100(6), 63–78.
28. Hooton, T.M. (1995). A simplified approach to urinary tract infection. *Hospital Practice* 30(2), 23–30.
29. Jantausch, B.A., Criss, V.R., O'Donnell, R., *et al.* (1994). Association of Lewis blood group phenotypes with urinary tract infection in children. *Journal of Pediatrics* 124(6), 863–868.
30. Avorn, J., Monane, M., Gurwitz, J.H., *et al.* (1994). Reduction of bacteriuria and pyuria after ingestion of cranberry juice. *Journal of the American Medical Association* 271(10), 751–754.
31. Ratliff, T.L., Klutke, C.G., and McDougall, E.M. (1994). The etiology of interstitial cystitis. *Urologic Clinics of North America* 21(1), 21–30.
32. Warren, J.W. (1994). Interstitial cystitis as an infectious disease. *Urologic Clinics of North America* 21(1), 31–39.
33. Mobley, D.F., and Baum, N. (1996). Interstitial cystitis: When urgency and frequency mean more than routine inflammation. *Postgraduate Medicine* 99(5), 201–214.
34. Hossan, E., and Streigel, A. (1993). Carcinoma of the bladder. *Seminars in Oncology Nursing* 9(4), 252–266.

35. Moore, S., Newton, M., Grant, E.G., *et al.* (1993). Treating bladder cancer: New methods, new management. *American Journal of Nursing* 93(5), 32–39.
36. Badalament, R.A., and Schervish, E.W. (1996). Bladder cancer: Current diagnostic methods and treatment options. *Postgraduate Medicine* 100(2), 217–230.
37. Pack, R. (1993). Descriptive epidemiology of genitourinary cancers. *Seminars in Oncology Nursing* 9(4), 218–223.
38. Moore, K.L., and Persaud, T.V.N. (1993). *The Developing Human: Clinically Oriented Embryology*. (5th ed.). Philadelphia: W.B. Saunders. (p. 271).
39. Becker, N., and Avner, E.D. (1995). Congenital nephropathies and uropathies. *Pediatric Clinics of North America* 42(6), 1319–1341.

SELECTED BIBLIOGRAPHY

Abuelo, J.G. (1995). Diagnosing vascular causes of renal failure. *Annals of Internal Medicine* 123(8), 601–614.

Adler, S., Nast, C., and Artishevsky, A. (1993). Diabetic nephropathy: Pathogenesis and treatment. *Annual Review of Medicine* 44, 303–315.

Alaniz, C., Brosius, F.C., and Palmieri, J. (1993). Pharmacologic management of adult idiopathic nephrotic syndrome. *Clinical Pharmacy* 12(6), 429–439.

Allison, M.E.M., and Shilliday, I. (1993). Loop diuretic therapy in acute and chronic renal failure. *Journal of Cardiovascular Pharmacology* 22(suppl. 3), S59–S70.

Bailie, G.R., and Eisele, G. (1992). Continuous ambulatory peritoneal dialysis: A review of its mechanics, advantages, complications, and areas of controversy. *Annals of Pharmacotherapy* 26(11), 1409–1420.

Bakris, G.L. (1993). Diabetic nephropathy: What you need to know to preserve kidney function. *Postgraduate Medicine* 93(5), 89–100.

Bergeron, M.G. (1995). Treatment of pyelonephritis in adults. *Medical Clinics of North America* 79(3), 619–649.

Blantz, R.C., Gabbai, F.B., Tucker, B.J., *et al.* (1993). Role of mesangial cell in glomerular response to volume and angiotensin II. *American Journal of Physiology* 264(1 Pt. 2), F158–F165.

Boam, W.D., and Miser, W.F. (1995). Acute focal bacterial pyelonephritis. *American Family Physician* 52(3), 919–924.

Brezis, M., and Epstein, F.H. (1993). Cellular mechanisms of acute ischemic injury in the kidney. *Annual Review of Medicine* 44, 27–37.

Brezis, M., and Rosen, S. (1995). Hypoxia of the renal medulla: Its implications for disease. *New England Journal of Medicine* 332(10), 647–655.

Brown, W.W., and Wolfson, M. (1993). Diet as culprit or therapy: Stone disease, chronic renal failure, and nephrotic syndrome. *Medical Clinics of North America* 77(4), 783–794.

Burnett, A.L. (1995). Nitric oxide control of lower genitourinary tract functions: A review. *Urology* 45(6), 1071–1083.

Caty, M.G., and Shamberger, R.C. (1993). Abdominal tumors in infancy and childhood. *Pediatric Clinics of North America* 40(6), 1253–1271.

Chertow, G.M., Sayegh, M.H., Allgren, R.L., *et al.* (1996). Is the administration of dopamine associated with adverse or favorable outcomes in acute renal failure? *American Journal of Medicine* 101, 49–53.

Cleary, G.M., Higgins, S.T., Merton, D.A., *et al.* (1996). Developmental changes in renal artery blood flow velocity during the first three weeks of life in preterm neonates. *Journal of Pediatrics* 129(2), 251–257.

Cotran, R.S., Kumar, V., and Robbins, S.L. (1994). *Robbins Pathologic Basis of Disease*. (5th ed.). Philadelphia: W.B. Saunders.

Curhan, G.C., Willett, W.C., Speizer, F.E., *et al.* (1997). Comparison of dietary calcium with supplemental calcium and other nutrients as factors affecting the risk for kidney stones in women. *Annals of Internal Medicine* 126(7), 497–504.

Davda, R.K., and Guzman, N.J. (1994). Acute renal failure: Prompt diagnosis is key to effective management. *Postgraduate Medicine* 96(5), 89–101.

Dayer-Berenson, L. (1994). Rhabdomyolysis: A comprehensive guide. *American Nephrology Nurses Association Journal* 21(1), 15–18.

Eberst, M.E., and Berkowitz, L.R. (1994). Hemostasis in renal disease: Pathophysiology and management. *American Journal of Medicine* 96(2), 168–179.

Fernandes, E.T., Reinberg, Y., Vernier, R., *et al.* (1994). Neurogenic bladder dysfunction in children: Review of pathophysiology and current management. *Journal of Pediatrics* 124(1), 1–7.

Fick, G.M., and Gabow, P.A. (1994). Natural history of autosomal dominant polycystic kidney disease. *Annual Review of Medicine* 45, 23–29.

Forland, M. (1993). Urinary tract infection: How has its management changed? *Postgraduate Medicine* 93(5), 71–86.

Foster, R.L.R., Hunsberger, M.M., and Anderson, J.J.T. (1989). *Family-Centered Nursing Care of Children*. Philadelphia: W.B. Saunders.

Goligorsky, M.S., Lieberthal, W., Racusen, L., *et al.* (1993). Integrin receptors in renal tubular epithelium: New insights into pathophysiology of acute renal failure. *American Journal of Physiology* 264(1 Pt. 2), F1–F8.

Gray, M., Rayome, R., and Moore, K. (1995). The urethral sphincter: An update. *Urologic Nursing* 15(2), 40–53.

Guyton, A.C., and Hall, J.E. (1996). *Textbook of Medical Physiology*. (9th ed.). Philadelphia: W.B. Saunders.

Hassan, A. (1996). Renal disease in the elderly. *Postgraduate Medicine* 100(6), 44–57.

Hassan, A. (1997). Proteinuria: How much evaluation is appropriate? *Postgraduate Medicine* 101(4), 173–180.

Hooton, T.M., Scholes, D., Hughes, J.P., *et al.* (1996). A prospective study of risk factors for symptomatic urinary tract infection in young women. *New England Journal of Medicine* 335(7), 468–474.

Houshiar, A.M., and Ercole, C.J. (1996). Urinary calculi during pregnancy: When are they cause for concern? *Postgraduate Medicine* 100(4), 131–138.

Hruska, K., and Teitelbaum, S.L. (1995). Renal osteodystrophy. *New England Journal of Medicine* 333(3), 166–174.

Johnson, D.W., and Fleming, S.J. (1992). The use of vaccines in renal failure. *Clinical Pharmacokinetics* 22(6), 434–446.

Kaysen, G.A. (1994). Nonrenal complications of the nephrotic syndrome. *Annual Review of Medicine* 45, 201–210.

Kim, R., Rotnitzky, A., Sparrow, D., *et al.* (1996). A longitudinal study of low-level lead exposure and impairment of renal function: The Normative Aging Study. *Journal of the American Medical Association* 275(15), 1177–1181.

Kiningham, R.B. (1993). Asymptomatic bacteriuria in pregnancy. *American Family Physician* 47(5), 1232–1238.

Klag, M.J., Whelton, P.K., Randall, B.L., *et al.* (1996). Blood pressure and end-stage renal disease in men. *New England Journal of Medicine* 334(1), 13–18.

Klag, M.J., Whelton, P.K., Randall, B.L., *et al.* (1997). End-stage renal disease in African-American and white men. *Journal of the American Medical Association* 277(16), 1293–1298.

Klutke, J.J., and Bergman, A. (1995). Hormonal influence on the urinary tract. *Urologic Clinics of North America* 22(3), 629–639.

Kuhn, M.M. (1991). *Pharmacotherapeutics: A Nursing Process Approach*. (2nd ed.). Philadelphia: F.A. Davis.

Laffel, L.M.B., Gill, J.B., and Gans, D.J. (1995). The beneficial effect of antiotensin-converting enzyme inhibition with captopril on diabetic nephropathy in normotensive IDDM patients with microalbuminuria. *American Journal of Medicine* 99(11), 497–504.

Larsen, P.D., and Martin, J.H. (1994). Renal system changes in the elderly. *AORN Journal* 60(2), 298–301.

Lerner, G.R. (1994). Urinary tract infections in children. *Pediatric Annals* 23(9), 463–473.

Levy, E.M., Viscoli, C.M., and Horwitz, R.I. (1996). The effect of acute renal failure on mortality: A cohort analysis. *Journal of the American Medical Association* 275(19), 1489–1494.

Livornese, L.L., Benz, R.L., Ingerman, M.J., *et al.* (1995). Antibacterial agents in renal failure. *Infectious Disease Clinics of North America* 9(3), 591–614.

Mattana, J., Gibbons, N., and Singhal, P.C. (1994). Cocaine interacts with macrophages to modulate mesangial cell proliferation. *Journal of Pharmacology and Experimental Therapeutics* 271(1), 311–318.

McCarthy, J.J. (1997). Outpatient evaluation of hematuria: Locating the source of bleeding. *Postgraduate Medicine* 101(2), 125–180.

Moffatt, M.E.K., Harlos, S., Kirshen, A.J., *et al.* (1993). Desmopressin acetate and nocturnal enuresis: How much do we know? *Pediatrics* 92(3), 420–425.

Mojcik, C.F., and Klippel, J.H. (1996). End-stage renal disease and systemic lupus erythematosus. *American Journal of Medicine* 101, 100–107.

Moore, K.L., and Persaud, T.V.N. (1993). *The Developing Human: Clinically Oriented Embryology.* (5th ed.). Philadelphia: W.B. Saunders.

Nemes, J., and Donahue, M.C. (1994). Solid tumors in children. *Nursing Clinics of North America* 29(4), 585–598.

Nygaard, I.E., and Johnson, M. (1996). Urinary tract infections in elderly women. *American Family Physician* 53(1), 175–182.

Ouslander, J.G., and Schnelle, J.F. (1995). Incontinence in the nursing home. *Annals of Internal Medicine* 122(6), 438–449.

Ouslander, J.G., Schapira, M., Schnelle, J.F., *et al.* (1995). Does eradicating bacteriuria affect the severity of chronic urinary incontinence in nursing home residents? *Annals of Internal Medicine* 122(10), 749–754.

Patterson, J.E., and Andriole, V.T. (1995). Bacterial urinary tract infections in diabetes. *Infectious Disease Clinics of North America* 9(1), 25–51.

Pedrini, M.T., Levey, A.S., Lau, J., *et al.* (1996). The effect of dietary protein restriction on the progression of diabetic and nondiabetic renal diseases: A meta-analysis. *Annals of Internal Medicine* 124(7), 627–632.

Perdue, B.E., and Plaisance, K.I. (1995). Treatment of community-acquired urinary tract infections. *American Pharmacy* NS35(12), 37–45.

Peterson, J.C., Adler, S., Burkart, J.M., *et al.* (1995). Blood pressure control, proteinuria, and the progression of renal disease: The Modification of Diet in Renal Disease Study. *Annals of Internal Medicine* 123(10), 754–762.

Ritz, E. (1993). Hypertension in diabetic nephropathy: Prevention and treatment. *American Heart Journal* 125(5 Pt. 2), 1514–1519.

Ronald, A.R., and Pattullo, A.L.S. (1991). The natural history of urinary infection in adults. *Medical Clinics of North America* 75(2), 299–312.

Rose, B.D. (1994). *Clinical Physiology of Acid-Base and Electrolyte Disorders.* (4th ed.). New York: McGraw-Hill.

Rose, B.D., and Rennke, H.G. (1994). *Renal Pathophysiology: The Essentials.* Baltimore: Williams & Wilkins.

Rosenthal, A.J., and McMurtry, C.T. (1995). Urinary incontinence in the elderly: Often simple to treat when properly evaluated. *Postgraduate Medicine* 97(5), 109–121.

Rousseau, P., and Fuentevilla-Clifton, A. (1992). Urinary incontinence in the aged. Part 2: Management strategies. *Geriatrics* 47(6), 37–48.

Rush, C., and Entman, S.S. (1995). Pelvic organ prolapse and stress urinary incontinence. *Medical Clinics of North America* 79(6), 1473–1479.

Sakarcan, A., Timmons, C., and Seikaly, M.G. (1994). Reversible idiopathic acute renal failure in children with primary nephrotic syndrome. *Journal of Pediatrics* 125(5 Pt. 1), 723–727.

Samm, B.J., and Dmochowski, R.R. (1996). Urologic emergencies: Conditions affecting the kidney, ureter, bladder, prostate, and urethra. *Postgraduate Medicine* 100(4), 177–184.

Schmeider, R.E. (1994). Nephroprotection by antihypertensive agents. *Journal of Cardiovascular Pharmacology* 24(Suppl. 2), S55–S64.

Simonson, M.S., and Dunn, M.J. (1993). Endothelin peptides and the kidney. *Annual Review of Physiology* 55, 249–265.

Stamm, W.E., and Hooton, T.M. (1993). Management of urinary tract infections in adults. *New England Journal of Medicine* 329(18), 1328–1334.

Terasaki, P.I., Cecka, J.M., Gjertson, D.W., *et al.* (1995). High survival rates of kidney transplants from spousal and living unrelated donors. *New England Journal of Medicine* 333(6), 333–336.

Teschan, P.E. (1994). Uremia: An overview. *Seminars in Nephrology* 14(3), 199–204.

Thatte, L., and Vaamonde, C.A. (1996). Drug-induced nephrotoxicity: The crucial role of risk factors. *Postgraduate Medicine* 100(6), 83–100.

Tinetti, M.E., Inouye, S.K., Gill, T.M., *et al.* (1995). Shared risk factors for falls, incontinence, and functional dependence: Unifying the approach to geriatric syndromes. *Journal of the American Medical Association* 273(17), 1348–1353.

Trevisan, R., and Viberti, G. (1995). Genetic factors in the development of diabetic nephropathy. *Journal of Laboratory and Clinical Medicine* 126(4), 342–349.

Watson, A. (1993). Iron management during treatment with recombinant human erythropoietin in chronic renal failure. *Journal of Clinical Pharmacology* 33, 1134–1138.

Whelton, A. (1995). Renal effects of over-the-counter analgesics. *Journal of Clinical Pharmacology* 35, 454–463.

Williams, D.N. (1996). Urinary tract infection: Emerging insights into appropriate management. *Postgraduate Medicine* 99(4), 189–204.

Wisinger, D.B. (1996). Urinary tract infection: Current management strategies. *Postgraduate Medicine* 100(5), 229–239.

Woo, D. (1995). Apoptosis and loss of renal tissue in polycystic kidney diseases. *New England Journal of Medicine* 333(1), 18–25.

Wozniak-Petrofsky, J. (1997). Urodynamic tests: Client preparation, assessment, and follow-up. *Nurse Practitioner* 22(3), 70–89.

Yim, P.S., and Peterson, A.S. (1996). Urinary incontinence: Basic types and their management in older patients. *Postgraduate Medicine* 99(5), 137–150.

Unit VIII

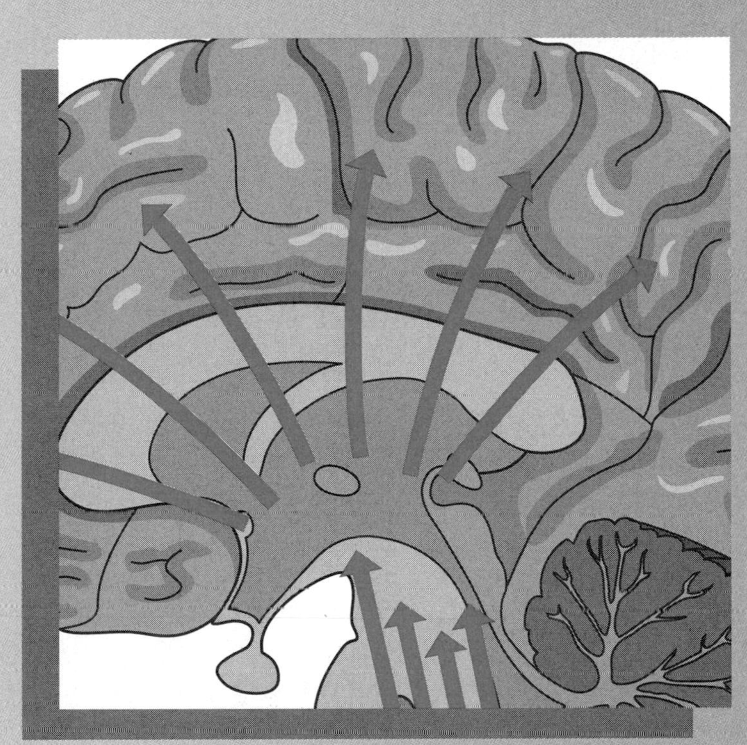

NEUROLOGIC SYSTEM

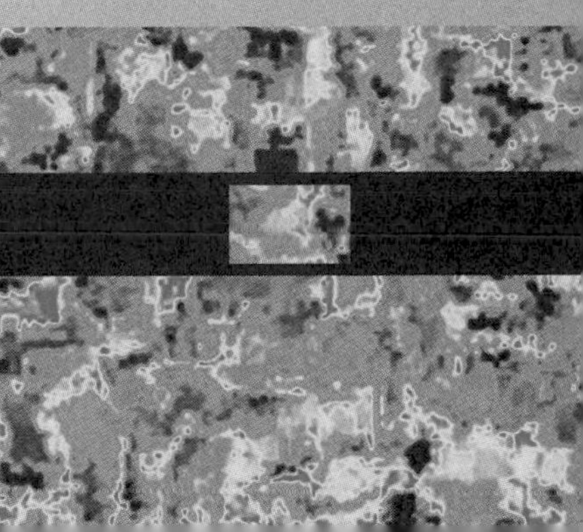

CHAPTER 21

Disorders of Cortical Function

LEARNING OBJECTIVES

1. Compare and contrast the components and principal functions of the central nervous system, peripheral nervous system, and autonomic nervous system.
2. Describe the cellular and molecular processes mediating neurotransmission.
3. Explain the role of the reticular activating system in regulation of consciousness and sleep.
4. Identify the components and functions of the limbic system.
5. Identify the cortical structures and processes that underlie the higher functions of cognition, memory, and language.
6. Comprehend the pathophysiologic mechanisms that underlie the clinical manifestations of clinically important cortical disorders and rationalize therapy for these disorders.

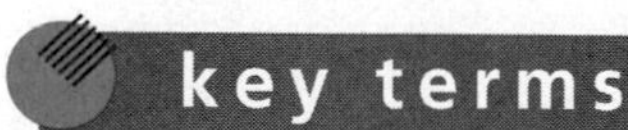

Alzheimer's disease
amnesia
anencephaly
aphasia
arteriovenous malformation (AVM)
brain death
coma
concussion
dementia
depression
dyslexia
dysphoria
encephalitis
encephalocele
encephalopathy
epidural hematoma
epilepsy
glioblastoma multiforme
hematoma
homonymous hemianopsia
hydrocephalus
hypersomnia
increased intracranial pressure (IICP)
insomnia
intracerebral hemorrhage

meningitis
meningocele
Monro-Kellie doctrine
myelomeningocele
neural tube defect (NTD)
normal-pressure hydrocephalus (NPH)
papilledema
parasomnia
psychosis
schizophrenia
seizure
spina bifida cystica
spina bifida occulta
status epilepticus
stroke
subarachnoid hemorrhage
subdural hematoma
traumatic brain injury
transient ischemic attack (TIA)
vegetative state

Among the hierarchy of subsystems in the human body, the nervous system ranks highest in regulation of system processes. Nearly all adaptive processes are either dependent on or potentially modified by neural inputs. The nervous system, consisting of the brain, spinal cord, and peripheral networks of nerves, directs or modulates the function of the other subsystems through the generation and transmission of action potentials and current flow (see Chapter 4). End-organ responses to neurologic stimuli are immediate but brief. Sustained responses require either repeated stimuli or neurologic activation of the other major regulatory system, the endocrine system. As discussed in Chapters 27 through 29, the effects of circulating hormones are of slower onset but are more prolonged. In addition, the critical importance of regulation at the local level (by cytokines and other mediators) is becoming increasingly apparent. Although these autoregulatory mechanisms do not *require* neurologic input, they do respond to it.

Because all organ subsystems depend on nervous system function, neurologic disorders may result in extensive functional impairment. Neurologic manifestations, such as headache, peripheral pain, confusion, anxiety, and depression, are among the most widely reported in clinical practice. Major neurologic disorders are not as common as cardiovascular and respiratory conditions, but their impact on quality of life and health care costs is arguably greater.

In this chapter, the general anatomy and function of the nervous system are reviewed, with a more detailed examination of the *cerebral cortex* and the structures that protect and perfuse the cortex. The highest level of hierarchic control within the nervous system resides in the *association areas* of the cerebral cortex, which receive modulatory inputs from the *limbic system* and the *reticular activating system* (RAS). These structures integrate signals from within the body and from the external environment and initiate descending neural transmissions that govern all human behavior.

Knowledge of the precise mechanisms of higher cortical function is limited, although research at the cellular and molecular levels has produced insights into the signal-transmission mechanisms that underlie higher cortical function. In most cases, the discrete functions of each cortical area are uncertain, and it is not known whether a specific anatomic area is the *only* area governing those functions. Classic studies of cortical function involved ablation experiments: studying the nature of function after the area under study had been destroyed. Unfortunately, loss of system integrity with this approach does not permit evaluation of the holistic processes critical to integrative function.

The higher cortical functions mediating intelligence, learning, memory, and language are explored in this chapter. The motivation and emotion that influence behavior are discussed, along with the mechanisms of brain activation associated with consciousness and sleep. The common disorders of higher cortical function detailed in this chapter include **schizophrenia, depression, Alzheimer's disease, epilepsy,** and brain tumors.

Disorders resulting from disruption of protective structures or neurocirculation also are discussed, including the general syndrome of **increased intracranial pressure (IICP)** and the specific disorders of **hydrocephalus, neural tube defects (NTDs), meningitis,** traumatic brain injury, and **stroke.** Disorders of motor, sensory, and autonomic function are detailed in Chapters 22 and 23.

OVERVIEW OF THE NERVOUS SYSTEM

Major Divisions

Traditionally, the nervous system is characterized as having three divisions: the *central nervous system* (CNS), the *peripheral nervous system,* and the *autonomic nervous system.* The CNS, consisting of the brain and spinal cord, has as its major function the *processing* of information. Ascending or sensory signals are received and integrated, and appropriate descending or motor signals are generated. The peripheral nervous system includes the paired cranial and spinal nerves, which function in the *transmission* of impulses between the CNS and peripheral organs. The autonomic nervous system is sometimes classified as part of the peripheral nervous system because it, too, performs a transmission function. This system is specialized, however, in that it transmits signals only to internal organs and generally operates automatically (by subconscious reflexes) for *maintenance of homeostasis.*

Anatomic Organization

Brain

The brain consists of the cerebrum, brain stem, and cerebellum.

Cerebrum. The cerebrum, illustrated in Figure 21–1, includes the cerebral cortex (outer gray matter), which is subdivided into bilateral lobes: the

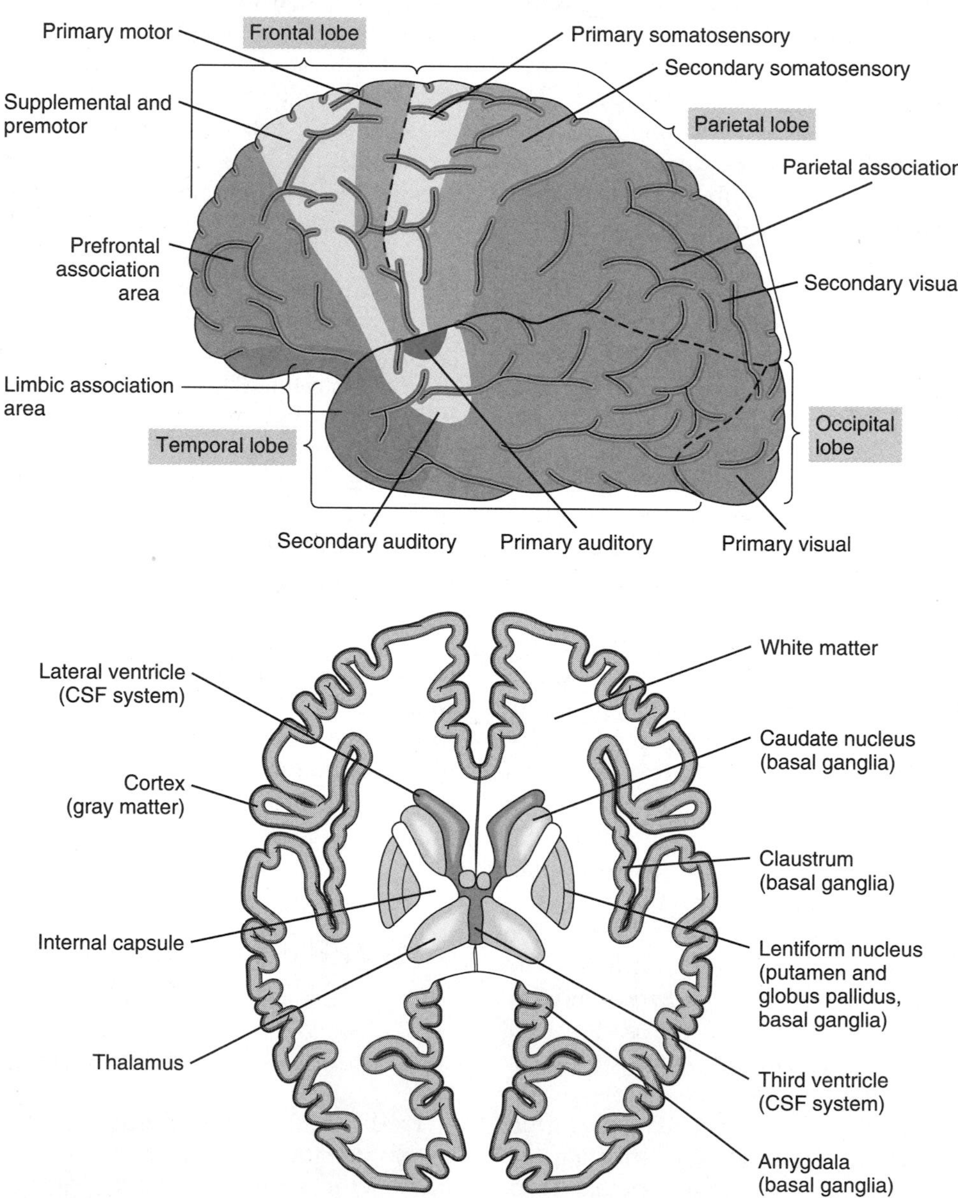

FIGURE 21–1

Lateral and horizontal views of the cerebrum. The outer gray matter (cerebral cortex) is subdivided into two hemispheres, each having four lobes: the *frontal, parietal, temporal,* and *occipital* lobes. Areas of gray matter deep within the cerebrum include the *basal ganglia, thalamus,* and *hypothalamus.* Because ascending and descending nerve fibers pass through the *internal capsule,* any injury to this area affects multiple functions. CSF, cerebrospinal fluid.

frontal, parietal, temporal, and *occipital* lobes. (Gray matter within the neurologic system consists of cell bodies of neurons, whereas white matter is made up primarily of nerve fibers extending from these cells, i.e., axons and dendrites.) Specialized areas within each cerebral lobe, along with their functions, are listed in Table 21–1. Areas of gray matter deep within the cerebrum include the *basal ganglia,* which function in fine motor control (see Chapter 22), the *thalamus,* an important relay station for sensory transmission (see Chapter 23), and the *hypothalamus,* which has both neurologic and endocrine functions (see Chapter 27). These deep areas of the cerebrum, sometimes known collectively as the *fifth lobe* or *limbic system* (Fig. 21–2), play a critical role in emotions as well as in higher functions, such as cognition and memory. An additional area of clinical importance within the cerebrum is the *internal capsule,* where many nerve fibers are tightly bundled. Even a small lesion (e.g., a tumor or stroke) affecting this region is likely to have a significant functional impact because of the multiple neural networks routed through this area.

Brain Stem. The brain stem, shown in Figure 21–3, consists of three regions: the *midbrain, pons,* and *medulla oblongata.* Many cranial nerves of the peripheral nervous system originate within the brain stem, and most sensory and motor nerve fibers decussate, or cross, at some level. The brain stem contains the neurons of the RAS, consisting of pacemaker cells that govern the level of consciousness and alertness of the cortex. Critical centers for homeostatic control of respiration, heart rate and contractile force, and blood vessel caliber are located in the brain stem.

Cerebellum. The cerebellum lies just below the cerebrum, under an inward fold of the brain covering (dura mater) known as the *tentorium* (see Fig. 21–3). The cerebellum has many neural interconnections with the cerebral cortex and brain stem and functions, along with the basal ganglia, in modification of movement, posture, and position sense (see Chapters 22 and 23).

TABLE 21–1
FUNCTIONS OF THE CEREBRAL LOBES

LOBE AND SPECIALIZED REGION	FUNCTIONS
Frontal Lobe	
Prefrontal association area	Cognition Implicit memory Language (Broca's area)
Limbic association area	Emotions, behavior, motivation
Supplemental and premotor areas	Planning of motor activity
Primary motor area (precentral gyrus)	Execution of motor activity
Parietal Lobe	
Primary somatosensory area (postcentral gyrus)	Reception of somatic sensory stimuli Localization of sensory information on body surface
Secondary somatosensory area	Interpretation of sensory inputs to primary area
Parietal association cortex	Recognition of objects by touch Understanding of the significance of sensory inputs
Occipital Lobe	
Primary visual cortex	Reception of visual stimuli
Secondary visual cortex (visual association area)	Interpretation of visual stimuli
Temporal Lobe	
Primary auditory cortex	Reception and processing of auditory stimuli
Secondary auditory cortex (auditory association area)	Interpretation of language (Wernicke's area)
Limbic association area	Emotions, behavior, motivation
Hippocampus	Emotions, libido, memory

Spinal Cord

The spinal cord, which extends downward through the bony *vertebral column* to the level of the first lumbar vertebra, consists of an inner core of gray matter surrounded by white matter. As shown in Figure 21–4, the gray matter is H-shaped or butterfly-shaped. The anterior or ventral extensions (horns) contain cells of the motor system, whereas the posterior or dorsal horns contain sensory neurons. At higher levels of the cord, intermediolateral horns are present, and these represent cells of the sympathetic division of the autonomic nervous system.

Peripheral Nerves

The peripheral nerves, consisting of bundled axons and dendrites of sensory neurons, motor neurons, autonomic neurons, or a combination of these, include the 12 pairs of *cranial nerves* and the 31 pairs of *spinal nerves.* The cranial nerves originate from either the cerebrum or the brain stem, as shown in

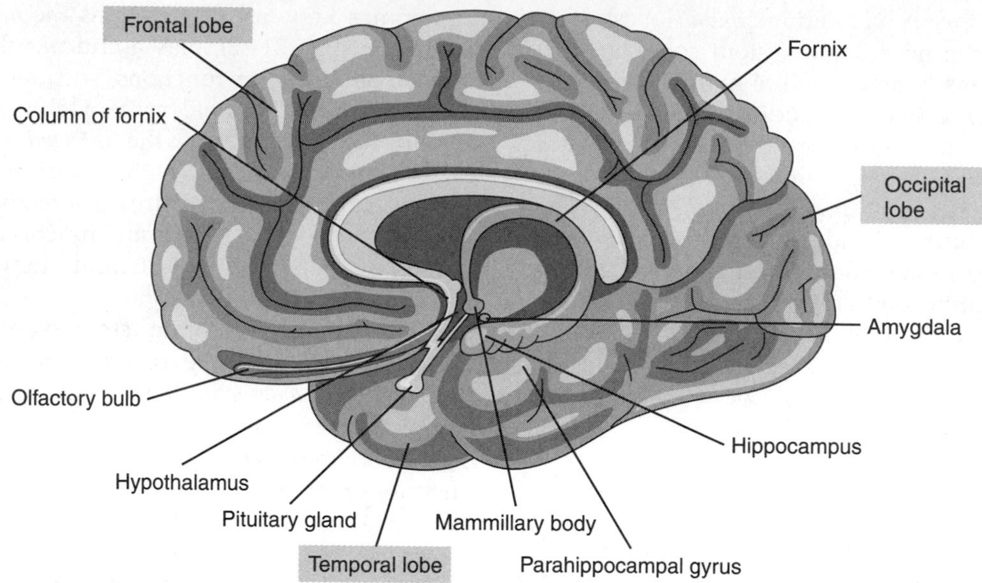

FIGURE 21–2
Limbic system. The limbic system is a functional system of gray matter located inferior to the cerebral lobes. Important structures within this system include the central *hypothalamus;* two nuclei, the *hippocampus* and *amygdala;* and portions of the *thalamus* and *basal ganglia.*

Figure 21–5. Designated by both Roman numerals and names, these nerves transmit impulses that mediate visceral reflexes and regulate sensation and movement of muscles of the face and neck (Table 21–2). The spinal nerves are classified according to the level of the cord from which they originate and include the eight pairs of cervical, 12 pairs of thoracic, five pairs of lumbar, five pairs of sacral, and one pair of coccygeal nerves. As shown in Figure 21–6, the spinal nerves extend below the level of the cord, forming a "horse's tail," or *cauda equina,* and interlace outside the cord to form networks, or

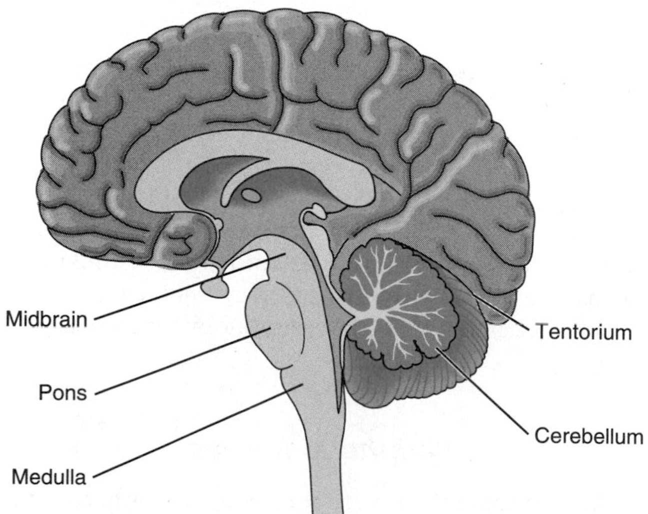

FIGURE 21–3
Relationships among the cerebrum, brain stem, and cerebellum. The brain stem is composed of three regions: the *midbrain, pons,* and *medulla oblongata.* The cerebellum lies posterior to the brain stem. An infolding of the dura, the tentorium, separates the cerebellum from the cerebrum above it.

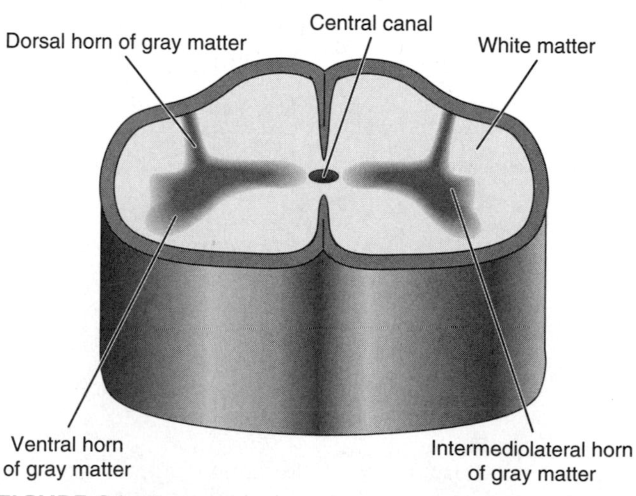

FIGURE 21–4
Spinal cord in cross-section. The spinal cord consists of an H-shaped core of gray matter surrounded by white matter. The ventral (anterior) horns contain neurons of the motor system, whereas the dorsal (posterior) horns contain sensory neurons. In the thoracic and lumbar regions, the cord gray matter also demonstrates the intermediolateral horns of the sympathetic division of the autonomic nervous system.

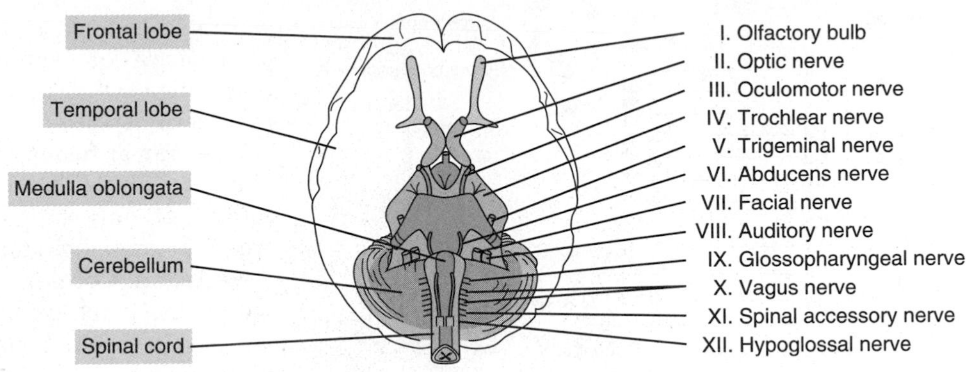

FIGURE 21–5
Cranial nerves. The 12 pairs of cranial nerves, which originate from the cerebrum and brain stem, mediate visceral reflexes and regulate sensation and movement of muscles of the face and neck. The Roman numeral designations of these nerves indicate their relative positions of origin, with the first cranial nerve (I) arising from the uppermost intracranial site and with cranial nerve XII originating from the lowest brain-stem site.

plexuses. Peripheral nerves terminate in end organs, such as muscle, skin, or viscera, and are critical to the function of sensory and motor reflex arcs.

The autonomic nerves are unique in that they transmit only motor (descending) impulses. They consist of two-neuron chains, with the sympathetic division *(sympathetic nervous system)* originating from the intermediolateral horns of the thoracic and lumbar segments of the cord and the parasympathetic division *(parasympathetic nervous system)* originating from the brain stem and sacral levels of the cord (see Chapter 22).

Protective and Supportive Structures

The protective and supportive structures of the nervous system include the cranium, vertebral column, and meninges.

Cranium. The cranium, illustrated in Figure 21–7, is composed of eight cranial bones, whose names

TABLE 21–2
CRANIAL NERVE FUNCTIONS

Cranial Nerve	Classification	Functions
I (olfactory)	Sensory	Smell
II (optic)	Sensory	Vision
III (oculomotor)	Motor	Movement of extraocular muscles
	Parasympathetic	Pupil constriction
IV (trochlear)	Motor	Movement of extraocular muscles
V (trigeminal)	Mixed	Facial sensation
		Jaw movement
VI (abducens)	Motor	Movement of extraocular muscles
VII (facial)	Mixed	Movement of facial muscles
	Parasympathetic	Taste (anterior two thirds of tongue)
		Secretion of saliva and tears
VIII (acoustic, auditory, or vestibulocochlear)	Sensory	Hearing
		Proprioception
IX (glossopharyngeal)	Mixed	Taste (posterior two thirds of tongue)
	Parasympathetic	Throat sensation (gag reflex)
		Voluntary swallowing and phonation
		Salivary secretion
		Carotid reflex for slowing of heart rate
X (vagus)	Mixed	Outer ear sensation
	Parasympathetic	Voluntary swallowing and phonation
		Reflex activity of cardiac muscle and visceral smooth muscle
XI (spinal accessory)	Motor	Shoulder elevation
		Head turning
		Swallowing
		Phonation
XII (hypoglossal)	Motor	Tongue movement

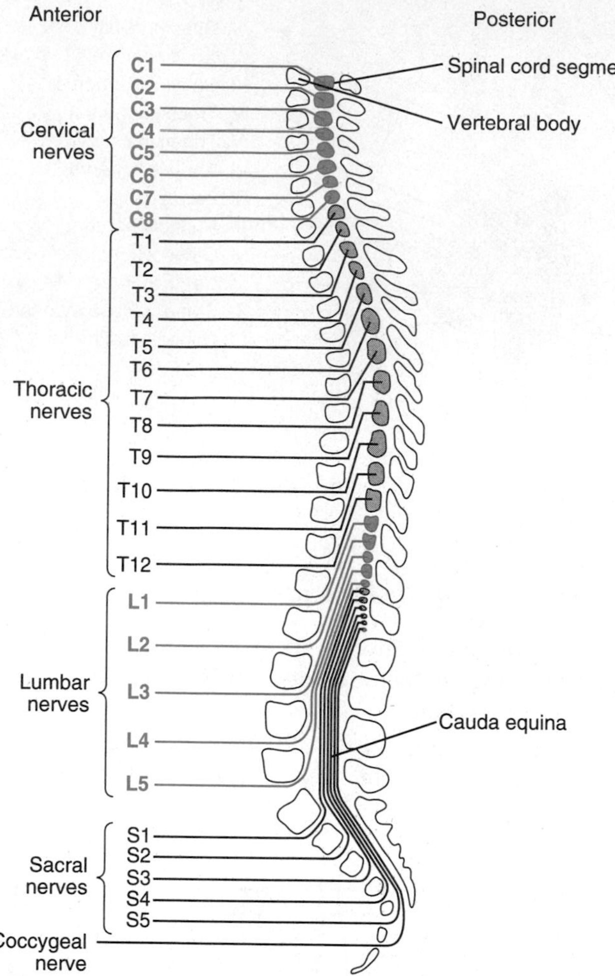

FIGURE 21–6

Spinal nerves. The 31 pairs of spinal nerves are classified according to the level of the spinal cord from which they originate. The spinal nerves extend below the level of the cord itself, forming a *cauda equina*, or "horse's tail." The spinal nerves mediate sensory and motor reflexes.

correspond to the lobes they cover, and the *sinuses* (air-filled spaces) that they enclose. Cranial bones extend downward and inward to form a base or floor under the cerebrum. The cranium has openings at the *orbits*, through which the optic nerve branches pass, and at the *foramen magnum*, through which the brain stem passes. In conditions manifested by IICP, brain tissue may herniate (bulge) through these openings. The interior surface of the cranium conforms to the many grooves on the surface of the cerebrum and is therefore rough. Traumatic injury to the head may cause brain tissue to be abraded against this rough surface, as discussed later in this chapter.

The joints at which cranial bones meet, known as *sutures*, fuse by about 18 months of age. In infancy, however, these joints are mobile, and the bones are separated to form membrane-covered spaces known as *fontanels*, or "soft spots" (Fig. 21–8). Fontanels may bulge when the infant is agitated or crying or may become sunken when the infant is dehydrated. Before cranial fusion, conditions such as hydrocephalus, in which intracranial pressure is increased, cause not only bulging fontanels but also an increase in cranial circumference.

Vertebral Column. The spinal cord is enclosed within the bony spine or vertebral column, consisting of 33 stacked bones: seven cervical, 12 thoracic, five lumbar, five sacral, and four coccygeal (Fig. 21–9). The sacral and coccygeal vertebrae are fused,

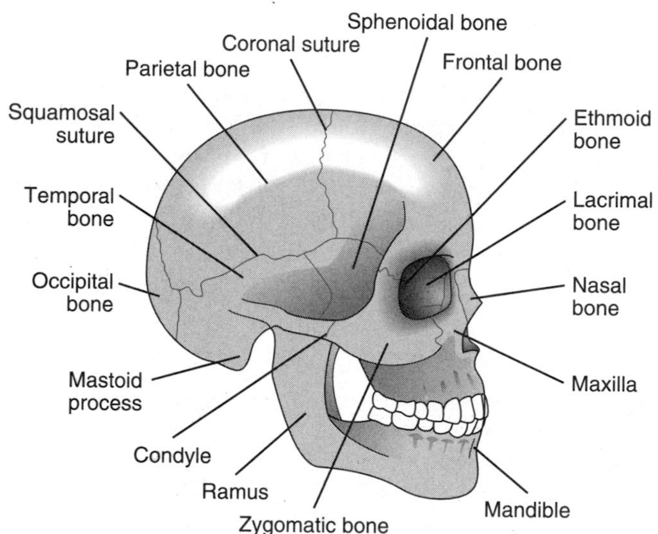

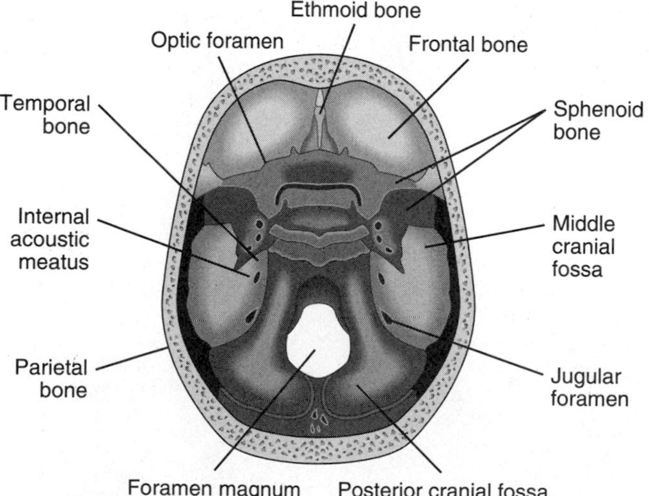

FIGURE 21–7

Cranium. The cranium (skull) is primarily composed of eight bones overlying the cerebral lobes for which they are named. Additional bones of the face and cranial floor are named for the sinuses they enclose. The mandible (jaw bone) articulates with the cranium. The rough interior of the cranium may abrade brain tissue in the case of head injury.

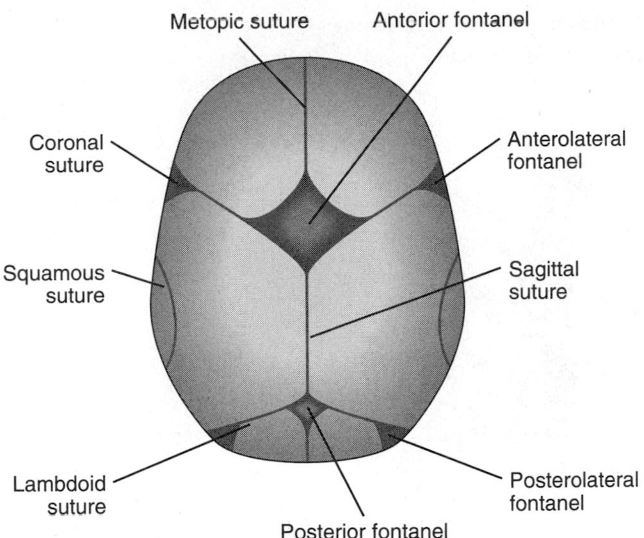

FIGURE 21–8
Fontanels. In infancy, the joints (sutures) between cranial bones are not fused, but rather are separated in places to form fontanels (soft spots). Fontanels may bulge with increased intracranial pressure or may be sunken with dehydration.

but the others are moved by intervertebral joints. Each vertebra has several openings, or *foramina,* through which the spinal cord, nerves, and blood vessels pass. Bony projections, or *spinous processes,* allow vertebral bones to articulate for stability and also form the points of attachment for longitudinal ligaments.

Cartilaginous *intervertebral disks* form joints between vertebrae and also serve as shock absorbers during movement. Acute trauma or chronic injury to the spine may cause disks to rupture or herniate out of position, putting pressure on nerves and causing a characteristic syndrome of shooting pain and numbness known as *radiculopathy* (see Chapter 23).

Meninges. The meninges are the fibrous coverings that surround the brain and spinal cord (Fig. 21–10). The tough outer layer, the *dura mater,* is characterized by many inward folds, including the tentorium between the cerebrum and cerebellum. The dura mater is composed of two fused layers that are separated in places to form dural sinuses. The *epidural space* between the dura mater and the interior of the cranium is not an actual space but rather is a potential space into which bleeding can occur with trauma, as discussed later in this chapter. The *subdural space,* between the dura mater and the middle meningeal layer, the *arachnoid,* is an actual space that can also be the site of bleeding. The arachnoid layer is named for its thin, delicate appearance, resembling a spider web. The *subarachnoid space,* between the arachnoid and the inner meningeal membrane, the *pia mater,* is an actual space through which cerebrospinal fluid (CSF) circulates. The pia mater, which directly overlies the brain and spinal cord, provides support for the blood vessels that penetrate the CNS. The pia mater and arachnoid membranes are the sites of inflammation in meningitis, as detailed later in this chapter.

Neurocirculatory Systems

The nervous system is perfused by two interconnected circulatory systems: the cerebrovascular system and the CSF circulation.

Cerebrovascular System. The cerebrovascular circulation differs from circulation to other organs in that both arteries and veins in the cerebrovascular circulation are thin walled and their distribution is unrelated. As illustrated in Figure 21–11, the principal arteries perfusing the brain are the *vertebral arteries,* which join to form the *basilar artery,* serving the posterior and lower parts of the brain; and the *carotid arteries,* which serve anterior and medial parts of the brain. Stroke patients typically manifest specific functional deficits that provide cues to the site of vascular occlusion or rupture. A clinically important structure within the cerebral arterial circulation is the *circle of Willis,* which interconnects the vertebral and carotid circulations and thus provides a collateral route for perfusion in the case of blockage in one system. Venous drainage from the brain is through the dural sinuses into the *jugular veins.* The *spinal arteries,* which branch off the vertebral artery, perfuse the cord (Fig. 21–12). *Spinal veins* drain into the vena cava. There are no true lymphatics in the CNS, but *perivascular spaces* between the pia mater and penetrating blood vessels remove excess fluid through the CSF circulation (Fig. 21–13).

Capillaries in most areas of the CNS are much less permeable than other capillaries because of their tight endothelial junctions and surrounding "foot" processes of astrocytes (Fig. 21–14). This *blood–brain barrier* protects the CNS from toxins carried in the bloodstream. Additional functions of astrocytes and other *glial cells* of the CNS are detailed later in this chapter.

Cerebrospinal Fluid Circulation. *Cerebrospinal fluid* is formed from blood primarily by *choroid plexuses* in the fluid-filled *ventricles* of the brain, but CSF is also formed by ependymal cells in ventricles and meningeal vessels and by endothelial cells of cerebral vessels. The choroid plexuses have specialized active transport systems that selectively remove certain substances from the CSF while pumping others from the blood into the CSF. This specialized trans-

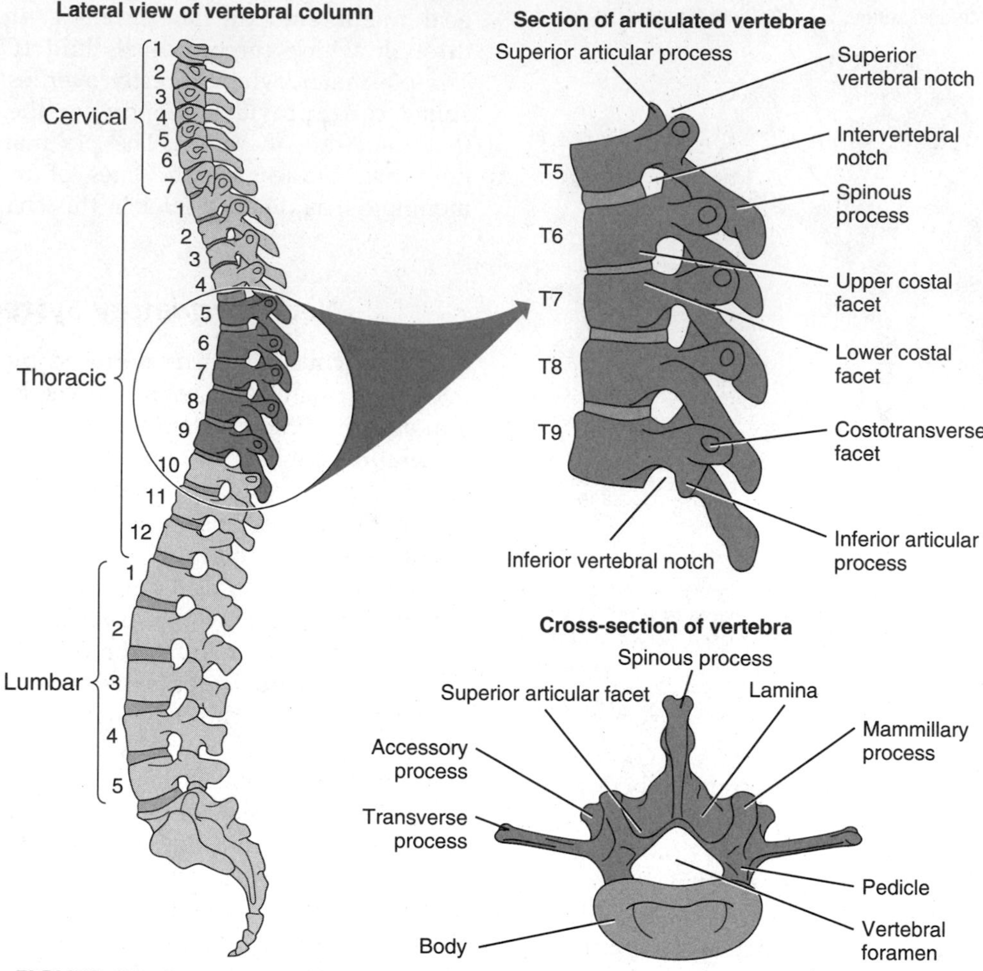

FIGURE 21–9
Vertebral column. The spinal cord is protected by its enclosure within the bony spine or vertebral column, which consists of 33 articulated bones (vertebrae). The spinal cord, nerves, and blood vessels pass through openings (foramina) in vertebrae. Spinal mobility and stability are mediated by intervertebral joints and by ligaments attached to vertebral processes.

port forms a functional barrier known as the *blood–CSF barrier.*

As shown in Figure 21–15, CSF flows between the ventricles, down the central canal of the cord (which may be normally absent), and through the subarachnoid space surrounding the brain and cord. CSF is reabsorbed by the *arachnoid villi,* extensions of the arachnoid that project into the dural sinuses, filtering the fluid before its entry into jugular veins.

CSF is normally clear, with constituents similar to plasma and a fluid pressure of 70 to 180 mm Hg (Table 21–3). With neurotrauma or stroke, CSF may be bloody. With neurologic infections such as meningitis, CSF may contain microorganisms or products of the inflammatory response. Leukocyte levels are elevated with inflammation, and protein content is increased because of increased capillary permeability, resulting in a cloudy appearance of the CSF. Glucose levels are typically low because of increased metabolism, impaired transport, or consumption by microorganisms. Obstruction of CSF circulation may result in increased CSF pressure and IICP, as discussed later.

CELLULAR STRUCTURE AND FUNCTION

Classification of Nervous System Cells

Specialized cells of the neurologic system include the information-processing and transmitting cells (neurons) and the supporting glial cells.

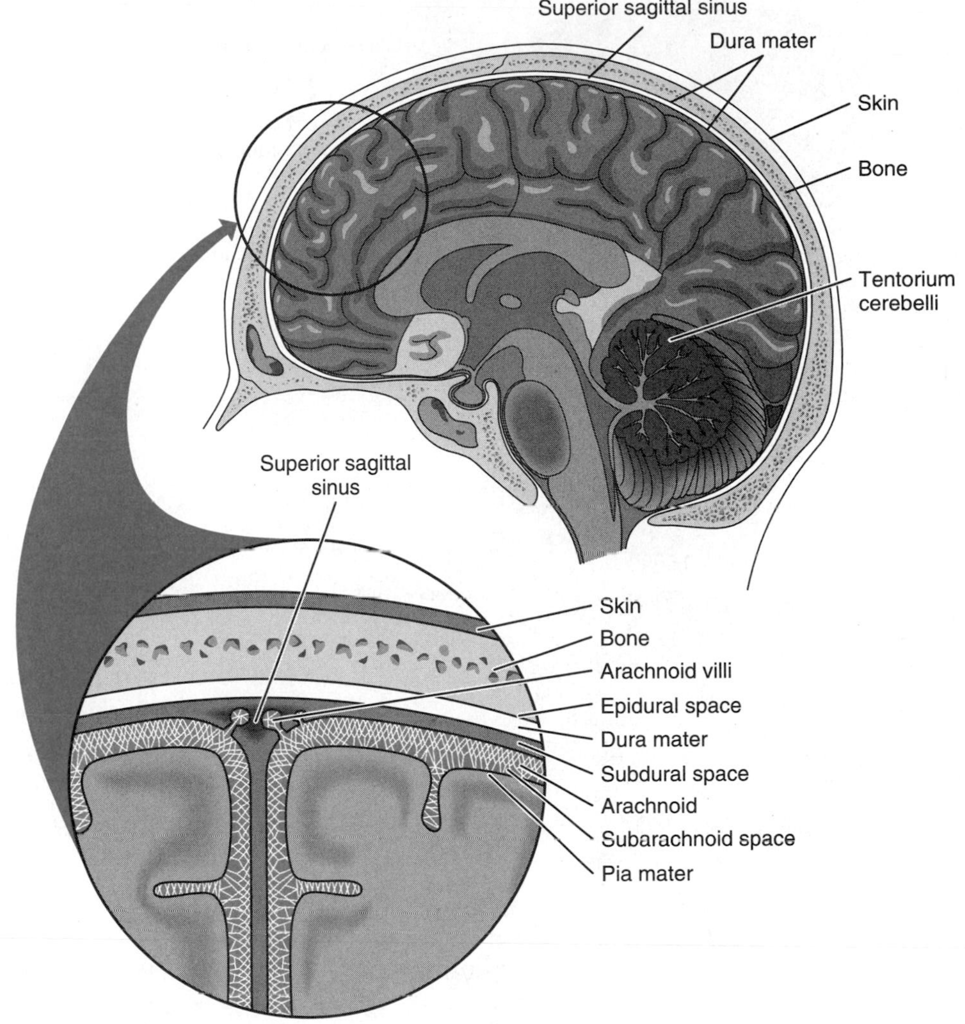

FIGURE 21–10
Meninges. The meninges are three fibrous membranes that cover the brain and spinal cord: the outer *dura mater,* middle *arachnoid,* and inner *pia mater*. Cerebrospinal fluid circulates beneath the arachnoid layer. Actual spaces between membranes (the *subdural* and *subarachnoid spaces*) and the potential space between the dura and the cranium *(epidural space)* may be sites of bleeding associated with head injury or cerebrovascular disease.

Neurons

There is much structural variability among neurons, but each type contains a cell body (soma), multiple afferent fibers (dendrites), and a single efferent fiber (axon). Figure 21–16 illustrates these structures on a typical motor neuron. Neurons are among the body cells that normally do not divide after reaching maturity, although severed axons may regenerate under ideal conditions.

Glial Cells

Glial cells (from Greek, meaning "glue") are supporting cells of connective tissue origin (Fig. 21–17). They include *oligodendrocytes,* which produce the lipid-based myelin sheath that surrounds many larger axonal fibers of the CNS; *Schwann cells,* which produce myelin for peripheral nerves; *astrocytes,* which protect and nourish adjacent neurons, contribute to the blood–brain barrier by their foot processes, and probably remove excess neurotransmitters and potassium from the surrounding extracellular fluid; *ependyma,* which participate in production and filtration of CSF; and *microglia,* which are phagocytic, antigen-presenting cells. Glial cells proliferate throughout life and, along with cells of cerebral blood vessels and connective tissue, are the usual source of neoplasia within the neurologic system.

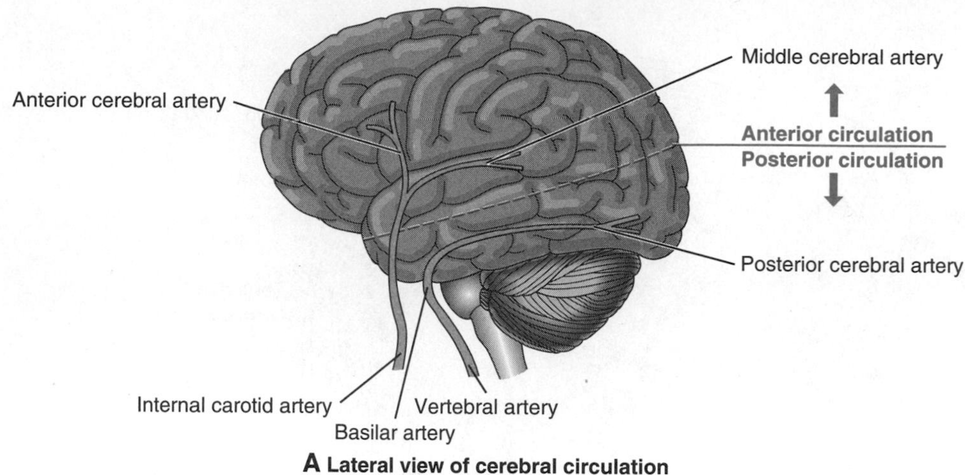

A Lateral view of cerebral circulation

Anterior communicating artery
Middle cerebral artery
Paramedian arteries
Basilar artery
Anterior inferior cerebellar artery
Posterior inferior cerebellar artery
Anterior spinal artery
Circle of Willis
Internal carotid artery
Posterior communicating artery
Posterior cerebral artery
Vertebral artery

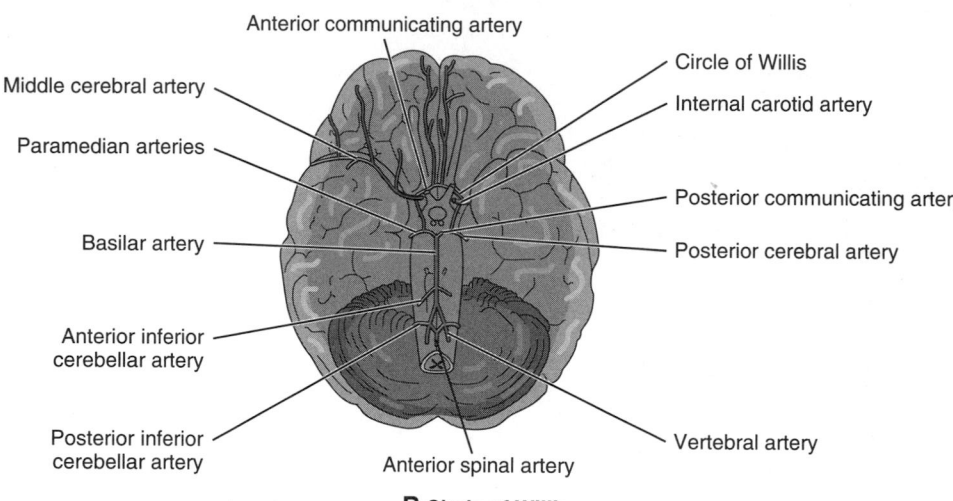

B Circle of Willis

FIGURE 21–11
Cerebrovascular circulation. The principal arteries of the central nervous system are the *vertebral arteries,* which join to form the *basilar artery,* serving the posterior and lower parts of the brain, and the *carotid arteries,* which perfuse the anterior and medial parts of the brain. The vertebral and carotid circulations are connected by communicating arteries to form the *circle of Willis,* providing potential collateral circulation in the event of blockage of one arterial system.

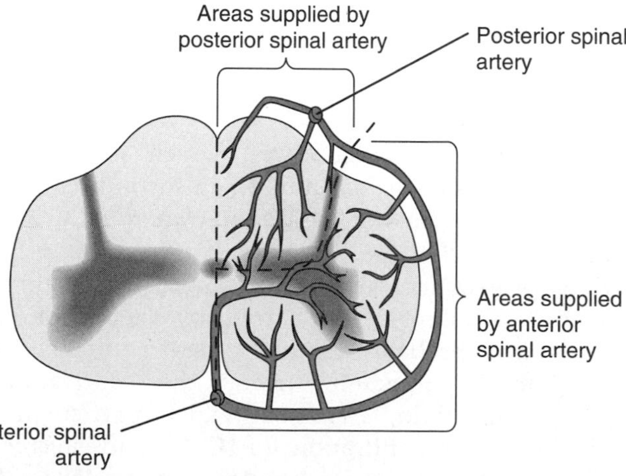

FIGURE 21–12
Arterial circulation of the spinal cord. The spinal cord (seen here in cross-section) is perfused by spinal arteries, which branch off the vertebral arteries.

Neurotransmission

As discussed in detail in Chapter 4, neurons, along with muscle cells, constitute the excitable tissues of the body. Neurons are capable of generating and conducting electrical current by means of both action potentials and electrotonic flow. This impulse conduction, along with specialized synaptic transmission between adjacent neurons and between neurons and end organs, is the basis of neural regulation of function.

Action Potential Generation in Neurons

Any stimulus that increases the permeability of the neuron plasma membrane to sodium results in a

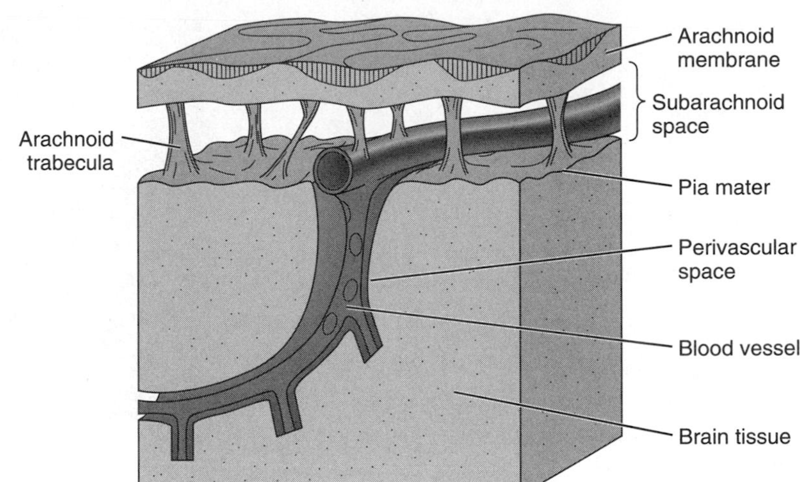

FIGURE 21–13
Perivascular spaces. Spaces created when penetrating blood vessels carry the pia mater inward serve a lymphatic-type function within the central nervous system. Excess fluid accumulating in perivascular spaces enters the cerebrospinal fluid within the subarachnoid space, which ultimately joins the venous system at the dural sinuses. (Redrawn from Guyton, A.C., and Hall, J.E. [1996]. *Textbook of Medical Physiology.* [9th ed]. Philadelphia: W.B. Saunders. [p. 787].)

rise in membrane potential that, if threshold is reached, gives rise to a full action potential. This stimulus may be an action potential from an adjacent neuron, an alteration in extracellular ion concentration, a mechanical disruption, or a receptor-mediated change in permeability. The nervous system, like the heart, contains some pacemaker cells, which have increased numbers of sodium "leak" channels and are thus capable of self-generation of action potentials (see later discussion of the RAS).

Because neuron cell bodies and dendrites have relatively few voltage-gated ion channels, most stimuli to these areas result in subthreshold membrane potentials and in electrotonic current flow through the cytoplasm. Because of increased numbers of voltage-gated channels in the area of the *axon hillock* (the point at which the axon is joined to the cell body), a full action potential is normally generated only in this area. The action potential is then conducted directionally down the length of the axonal fiber.

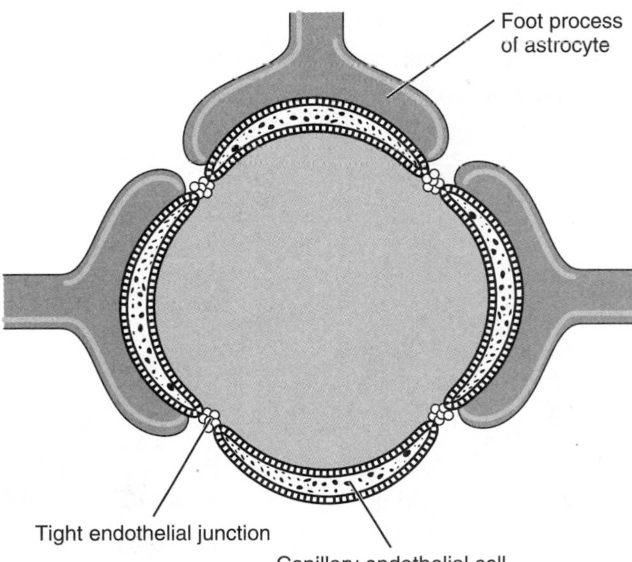

FIGURE 21–14
Anatomic basis of the blood–brain barrier. Capillaries in most areas of the brain are much less permeable than other capillaries because of their tight junctions between endothelial cells and surrounding foot processes of astrocytes. (Redrawn from Adams, R.D., and Victor, M. [1993]. *Principles of Neurology.* [5th ed]. New York: McGraw-Hill. [p. 558].)

Factors Influencing the Velocity of Impulse Conduction

Impulse conduction varies normally depending on the diameter of nerve fibers and whether they are myelinated. Axons that are insulated by myelin conduct the impulse faster because action potentials must be regenerated only at small unmyelinated areas (nodes of Ranvier) between myelin segments, whereas current flows electrotonically between (see Fig. 4–10). This saltatory ("dancing") conduction is present in most larger peripheral nerves and is about 50 times faster than conduction in unmyelinated nerves.

Transmission along unmyelinated fibers requires propagation of action potentials along the entire membrane, and the refractory periods during each repolarization require additional time. The larger the nerve diameter, the faster the conduction because less resistance is offered to electrotonic current flow in the cytoplasm. Table 21–4 compares conduction velocities of various classes of nerve fibers.

Conduction velocity also varies in response to extracellular conditions. Acidosis, for example, depresses nerve conduction, whereas alkalosis accelerates conduction (see Chapter 10). The mechanisms of

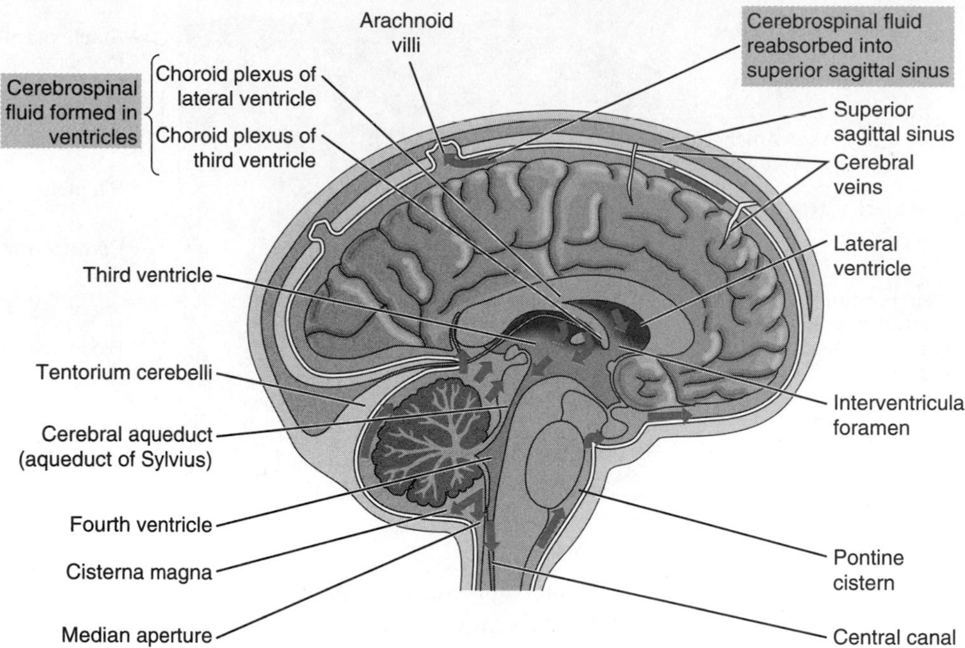

FIGURE 21–15

Cerebrospinal fluid (CSF) circulation. The CSF circulation is a one-way circulation originating at sites of CSF formation in the ventricles of the brain and ending with CSF absorption into the venous circulation at the arachnoid villi within the dural sinuses. CSF flows between the lateral, third, and fourth ventricles through various openings (foramina and apertures) and narrow channels (aqueducts) into the fluid-filled cisterns surrounding the cerebellum and brain stem. From the cisterns, CSF flows up and over the brain surface through the subarachnoid space. CSF flow down and around the cord through the central canal and subarachnoid space is facilitated by movement of the vertebral column.

this effect are uncertain but may involve adaptive changes in cation levels resulting from hydrogen ion imbalance, or pH-dependent effects on membrane permeability, active transport, or enzymatic activity. Hypoxia ultimately depresses the CNS, as it does other excitable cells, because of lack of adenosine triphosphate for active transport during repolarization. Sodium accumulates intracellularly, inhibiting

TABLE 21–3
COMPOSITION OF CEREBROSPINAL FLUID

COMPONENT	NORMAL VALUES
Color	Clear
Pressure	75–180 mm H_2O
Osmolarity	296 mOsm/L
pH	7.33
Red blood cells	None (unless traumatic lumbar puncture)
Leukocytes	0–5/μL (lymphocytes or monocytes; no granulocytes)
Glucose	50–75 mm/dL
Protein	15–45 mg/dL
Sodium	138 mEq/L
Potassium	2.8 mEq/L
Calcium	2.1 mEq/L
Magnesium	2.3 mEq/L
Chloride	119 mEq/L

Data from Kandel, E.R., and Schwartz, J.H. (1985). *Principles of Neural Science.* (2nd ed.). New York: Elsevier Science Publishing; Barker, E. (1994). *Neuroscience Nursing.* St. Louis: Mosby–Year Book; and Simon, R.P., Aminoff, M.J., and Greenberg, D.A. (1989). *Clinical Neurology.* Norwalk, CT: Appleton & Lange.

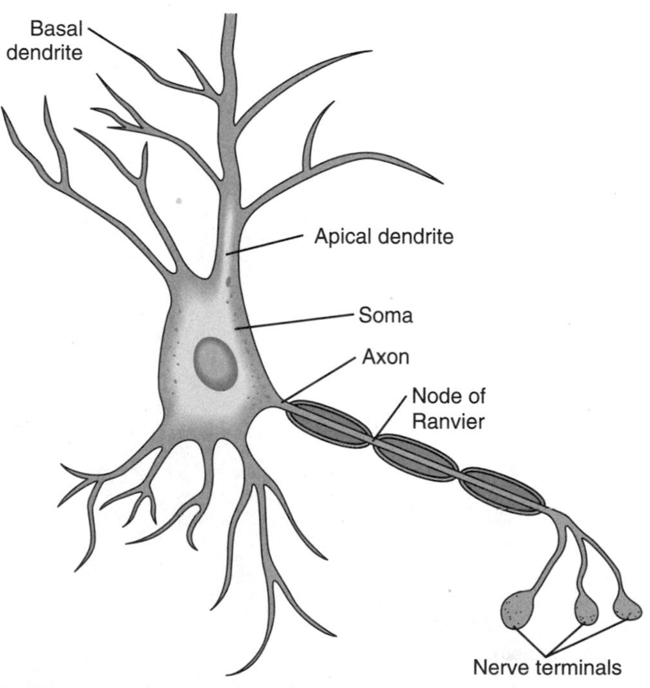

FIGURE 21–16

Typical motor neuron. The typical information-processing cell (neuron) consists of a *soma,* or cell body; multiple afferent (information-receiving) fibers, or *dendrites;* and a single efferent (transmitting) fiber, or *axon.* (With respect to the dimensions of the soma, the axon is proportionately much longer than it appears in this illustration.) Axons within larger nerves are myelinated, permitting rapid impulse transmission. Axon terminals establish contacts (synapses) with other neurons or with end organs.

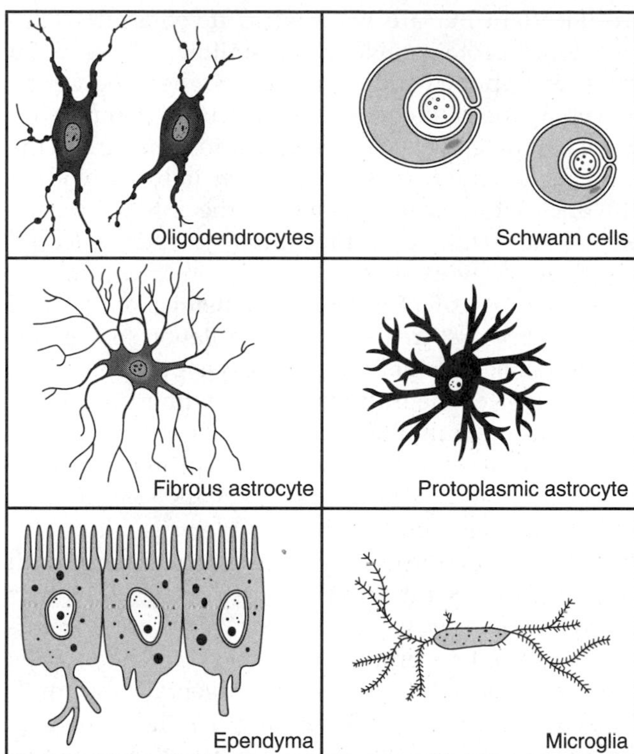

FIGURE 21–17

Glial cells. The glial cells serve a protective and supportive role within the nervous system. They include myelin-producing oligodendrocytes and Schwann cells, nutritive astrocytes, cerebrospinal fluid–producing ependyma, and phagocytic microglia.

repolarization and inducing osmolar gradients that result in cerebral edema. Local anesthetic drugs, such as procaine, prevent impulse conduction by dissolving in membrane lipids and impairing the operation of ion channels.

Synaptic Transmission

Impulse transmission within the nervous system requires conduction of impulses from the end of one axon, across a space (*synapse*), to some part of another neuron. Synaptic transmission permits the networking of multiple individual neurons into specialized functional pathways.

Synaptic Components. A typical synapse, illustrated in Figure 21–18 consists of a *presynaptic membrane,* which is actually the terminal end (*bouton,* or "knob") of an axon branch; a *postsynaptic membrane,* which is a part of the membrane of an adjacent neuron; and the space between these membranes, the *synaptic cleft.* The postsynaptic membrane on a neuron may be a dendrite *(axodendritic synapse),* a cell body *(axosomatic synapse),* or another axon *(axo-axonic* or *serial synapse).* Nearly all synapses within the nervous system are classified as chemical synapses because conduction of the electrical signal across the cleft requires the mediation of a chemical, or *neurotransmitter.* (Gap junctions, prevalent in cardiac and smooth muscle and discussed in Chapter 2, may permit direct transmission between adjacent cells and are sometimes referred to as *electrical synapses.* There are few of these in nervous tissue.)

Sequence of Events. Chemical synaptic transmission begins when depolarization of the presynaptic membrane initiates secretion of the neurotransmitter into the synaptic cleft. The neurotransmitter diffuses across the cleft and binds to an appropriate receptor on the postsynaptic membrane, opening ligand-gated channels and initiating ion flux. Depending on the nature of the receptor, the postsynaptic mem-

TABLE 21–4
CONDUCTION VELOCITIES OF VARIOUS NERVE FIBERS

CLASS	VELOCITY (M/SEC)	DIAMETER (μM)	MYELINATION	EXAMPLES
I/Aα	80–120	13–20	Yes	Sensory nerves from muscle spindles and Golgi tendon organs α-Motoneurons
II/Aβ	35–75	6–12	Yes	Sensory nerves from muscle spindles Sensory nerves for hearing and vestibular function Sensory nerves for fine touch
III/Aδ or Aγ	5–30	1–5	Yes	Sensory nerves for temperature, crude touch, sharp pain Motor nerves to muscle spindles
IV/C	0.5–2	0.2–1.5	No	Sympathetic nerves Sensory nerves for crude touch, pressure, tickle, itch, aching pain, temperature

Data from Guyton, A.C., and Hall, J.E. (1996). *Textbook of Medical Physiology.* (9th ed.). Philadelphia: W.B. Saunders; and Kandel, E.R., and Schwartz, J.H. (1985). *Principles of Neural Science.* (2nd ed.). New York: Elsevier Science Publishing.

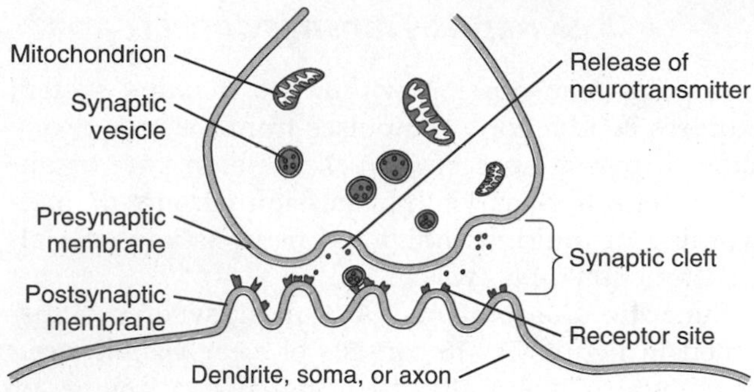

FIGURE 21–18

Typical synapse. The synapse consists of a *presynaptic membrane* (axon terminal), a *postsynaptic membrane* (area on the membrane of an adjacent neuron or end organ), and a *synaptic cleft* (actual space between the membranes). Synaptic transmission is mediated by release of a chemical neurotransmitter from the presynaptic membrane, diffusion of this chemical across the cleft, and binding to specific receptors on the postsynaptic membrane. Receptor binding initiates further transmission or end-organ activity.

brane may generate membrane potentials or action potentials or may be inhibited from doing so.

Neurotransmitters. Table 21–5 lists and classifies the major neurotransmitters of the CNS. The major neurotransmitters are small molecules, most of which contain nitrogen. The most prevalent of these are acetylcholine (ACh), norepinephrine (NE), epinephrine (EPI), dopamine, γ-aminobutyric acid (GABA), and glutamate. These chemicals are *essential* to neurotransmission from neurons that secrete them. The second class of neurotransmitters, the *neuromodulators,* includes a variety of substances widely distributed in body tissues. Although not essential to synaptic transmission, neuromodulators have an important signal-modifying effect. The neuromodulators located in the CNS are usually composed of peptides and are thus commonly known as *neuropeptides.*

The major neurotransmitters mediate rapid-onset effects, whereas neuropeptides influence slower-onset, longer-acting effects. A single neuron can synthesize and release just one major neurotransmitter but may also synthesize a number of neuropeptides. Each neuron, however, may have membrane receptors for a number of different neurotransmitters and neuropeptides. Synapses are classified on the basis of the neurotransmitter secreted by the presynaptic membrane and by the corresponding postsynaptic receptor for the chemical. *Cholinergic* synapses, for example, require ACh; *adrenergic* synapses may bind NE or EPI; *dopaminergic* synapses use dopamine; and *GABA-ergic* synapses use GABA.

Neurotransmitters are synthesized in the neuron soma, packaged into vesicles, and transported by the directional flow of cytoplasm toward the axon bouton. The mechanisms regulating this *axoplasmic flow* are uncertain but are believed to involve intracellular motor proteins. Neurotransmitter release from the presynaptic membrane occurs when the action potential opens voltage-gated calcium channels on the membrane. This allows calcium influx from the extracellular fluid, and the calcium induces binding of vesicles to release points on the interior of the membrane. The neurotransmitter is then released into the cleft by exocytosis.

Regulation of Synaptic Transmission. Three mechanisms are involved in regulation of neurotransmission: summation of postsynaptic potentials, inactivation of neurotransmitters within the cleft, and presynaptic inhibition.

Summation of Postsynaptic Potentials. A single neuron may have thousands of synapses at its dendrites and cell body and a few on its axon. Although each of these may deliver electrical stimuli to the neuron and produce membrane potentials (known as *postsynaptic potentials* [PSPs]) none is sufficient in itself to produce an action potential. PSPs must be *summated,* or added algebraically, until threshold is reached. Depending on the nature of the receptor at the synapse, a PSP is either *excitatory* or *inhibitory*. Excitatory PSPs open sodium channels and move the membrane potential closer to threshold, whereas inhibitory PSPs open potassium channels and lower the potential, hyperpolarizing the membrane (see Chapter 4). PSPs are summated both spatially and temporally. *Spatial summation* results from PSPs occurring at the same time over a speci-

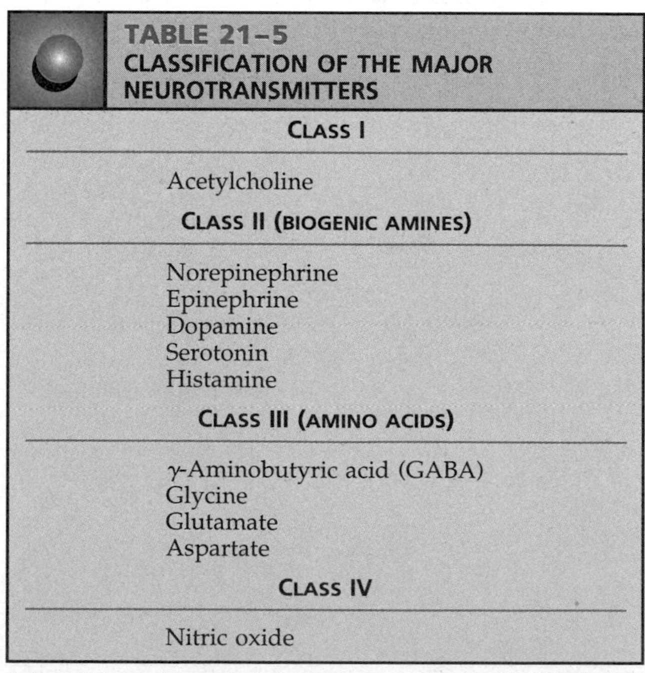

TABLE 21–5
CLASSIFICATION OF THE MAJOR NEUROTRANSMITTERS

CLASS I
Acetylcholine
CLASS II (BIOGENIC AMINES)
Norepinephrine Epinephrine Dopamine Serotonin Histamine
CLASS III (AMINO ACIDS)
γ-Aminobutyric acid (GABA) Glycine Glutamate Aspartate
CLASS IV
Nitric oxide

Adapted from Guyton, A.C., and Hall, J.E. (1996). *Textbook of Medical Physiology.* (9th ed.). Philadelphia: W.B. Saunders. (p. 572).

fied area of membrane, whereas *temporal summation* results from PSPs occurring close together in time.

Neurotransmitter Inactivation. Once secreted into the synaptic cleft, neurotransmitters may be inactivated by one or more of three mechanisms. *Reuptake* is a receptor-mediated mechanism by which the neurotransmitter is actively transported back into the presynaptic terminal. Catecholamine neurotransmitters (i.e., NE, EPI) are inactivated in this way. *Enzymatic degradation* inactivates some neurotransmitters (e.g., ACh) through chemical conversion to forms that cannot bind postsynaptic receptors. *Outward diffusion* from the synaptic cleft into the bloodstream reduces the activity of most neurotransmitters and accounts for the concurrent hormonal activity of many of these chemicals. Once in the blood, most neurotransmitters are metabolized by hepatic enzymes and excreted in the urine.

Presynaptic Inhibition. Synaptic transmission is also regulated by presynaptic inhibition, a negative feedback system that is incompletely understood. As the neurotransmitter accumulates in the synaptic cleft, the binding of some of the molecules to presynaptic receptors results in a reduction in neurotransmitter release. This mechanism is believed to involve specific subtypes of calcium channels in the presynaptic membrane.[1]

Neurochemical Pathways

The structures that mediate cortical function may be organized into pathways on the basis of the major neurotransmitter synthesized and released by neurons along the pathway.

The monoamine neurotransmitters are excitatory at most synapses. Dopaminergic pathways function in thermoregulation (see Chapter 11) and, along with norepinephrine, in motivational systems. The noradrenergic (NE) pathways are believed to be important in regulation of mood, learning, memory, motivational reinforcement, anxiety, hunger and satiety, and sleep. The role of adrenergic (EPI) pathways in cortical function is still uncertain. Serotonergic (5-hydroxytryptamine) pathways mediate many important cortical functions, including biorhythms, pain perception, sleep, and mood. Serotonin also participates in regulation of feeding, motor activity, and body temperature and modifies the effects of a number of classic hormones. Cholinergic (ACh) pathways regulate arousal, rapid eye movement (REM) sleep, pain perception, learning, memory, and thirst. Histaminergic (histamine) pathways are involved in sleep, feeding, and cardiovascular regulation.

Glutamate is the principal excitatory neurotransmitter in the brain, and glutamatergic pathways are known to be involved in cognition, memory, movement, and sensation. In addition, excessive activation of glutamate receptors may mediate neuronal injury in ischemic stroke and in neurodegenerative disorders.[1] The major inhibitory neurotransmitter is GABA, present at 60% of synapses within the CNS. GABA apparently influences eating behavior, anxiety, and intensity of emotion. The foundation of physiologic intervention in most disorders of higher cortical function is drug therapy; many drugs influence behavior by modifying specific neurochemical pathways.

The association between the major neurotransmitter synthesized by a neuron and the neuropeptides secreted is of apparent importance, and consistent patterns are seen. The clinical significance of this cotransmission is unknown. No clinical disorder has been specifically linked to deficiency of a neuropeptide. Neuropeptides have local synaptic effects similar to the major transmitters but may also enter the blood and diffuse to distant sites, where they exert neurohormonal effects. Neuropeptides, adrenal medullary function within the sympathetic nervous system (see Chapter 22), and the hypothalamic–pituitary axis (see Chapter 27) are examples of the many interactions between the nervous and endocrine systems in regulation of human function.

CORTICAL FUNCTION

Activation of the Brain

Reticular Activating System

The capacity of the cortical centers to respond to stimuli is governed by the RAS, which mediates *consciousness,* or the ability to experience the environment. The brain-stem nuclei that constitute the RAS are illustrated in Figure 21–19. This system of neurons is named for its net-like (reticular) histologic appearance and for its general function of pacing the rate of impulse transmission through the brain stem. The RAS has both ascending and descending projections from four areas: the *gigantocellular nucleus,* the *substantia nigra* (also associated with the basal ganglia), the *locus ceruleus,* and the *raphe nuclei.*

The ascending RAS extends from these brain-stem nuclei to the thalamus, basal ganglia, and cerebral cortex. The uppermost nuclei are apparently excitatory to these higher centers, resulting in increased level of cortical activity. The lower nuclei (below the middle pons) are inhibitory and function in sleep and decreased perception of pain (see Chapter 23). The anatomy of the descending RAS has not been

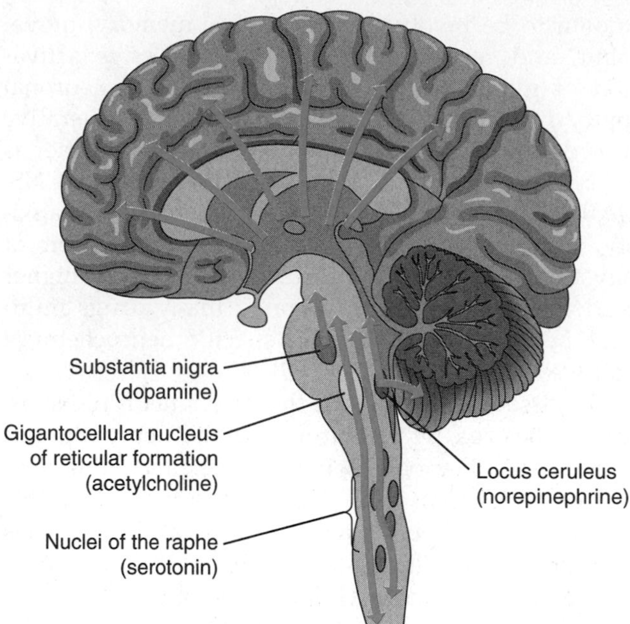

FIGURE 21–19
Reticular activating system (RAS). The brain-stem nuclei of the RAS serve a pacemaker function in governing the rate of impulse transmission to and from the brain. The RAS has both ascending and descending projections from four areas: the *gigantocellular nucleus, substantia nigra, locus ceruleus,* and *raphe nuclei.* Each of these pathways employs a different neurotransmitter.

precisely delineated, but RAS outputs are known to influence motor activity, vestibular and oculomotor function (for vision and position sense), respiration, and cardiovascular reflexes.

Clinical Parameters of Consciousness

Consciousness may be quantified in clinical settings through assessment of the level of stimulus to which the patient will respond. The Rancho Los Amigos Scale (Table 21–6), in common clinical use, details eight levels of consciousness (LOC), ranging from no response to any stimuli to purposeful and appropriate responses. Many descriptive terms are also used to describe states of reduced consciousness (Table 21–7).

Consciousness has two components: wakefulness and awareness. These states both require arousal, or increased activation of the cortex, governed by ascending impulses from the RAS. The patient who is in a **coma** is neither awake nor aware. The patient who is in a **vegetative state** has sleep–wake cycles but lacks awareness.

Sleep

Sleep may be thought of as arousable unconsciousness. There are two basic types of sleep, which normally occur in alternating cycles in a predictable pattern (Fig. 21–20). About 75% of the sleep period is spent in *slow-wave (non-REM)* sleep, a deep, restful sleep in which the person dreams but does not consolidate those dreams into memory. This type of sleep is regulated by the raphe nuclei along serotonergic pathways. At about 90-minute intervals, slow-wave sleep is interrupted by *REM sleep,* during which the person appears restless and agitated but is difficult to arouse. The eyes demonstrate rapid, fine movement, and dreams during this period are remembered on awakening. REM sleep is mediated by the locus ceruleus along noradrenergic pathways.

Electroencephalographic recording of brain electrical activity demonstrates predictable patterns during each sleep stage (see later). The precise mechanisms governing the rhythmic sleep–wake cycle are unknown. The physiologic purpose of sleep is also uncertain, but the prevalent hypothesis is that sleep is necessary for recalibration of homeostatic mechanisms. Sleep–wake cycles change over the lifetime of a person as the CNS matures during infancy

TABLE 21–6
LEVELS OF CONSCIOUSNESS (RANCHO LOS AMIGOS SCALE)

LEVEL	DESCRIPTION
I	No response: appears in deep sleep
II	Generalized response: displays reflex responses to deep pain
III	Localized response: has inconsistent responses, but reacts in a more specific manner to stimulus; might follow simple commands; responds purposefully to discomfort; visually tracks objects
IV	Confused, agitated: reacts to own inner confusion, fear, disorientation; excitable behavior may be aggressive or bizarre
V	Confused, inappropriate, nonagitated: displays gross attention to environment; is highly distractable; has difficulty learning new tasks; may engage in social conversation but with inappropriate verbalizations
VI	Confused, appropriate: is inconsistently oriented to time and place; has impaired recent memory; can consistently follow simple directions; goal-directed behavior with assistance
VII	Automatic, appropriate: performs daily routine without confusion, but in a robot-like manner; lacks realistic goals for the future
VIII	Purposeful, appropriate: is alert, oriented, able to form realistic goals for the future; is able to apply adequate judgment for daily living; may have decreased abilities relative to premorbid state.

Adapted from Rancho Los Amigos Medical Center, Downey, CA, Adult Brain Injury Service.

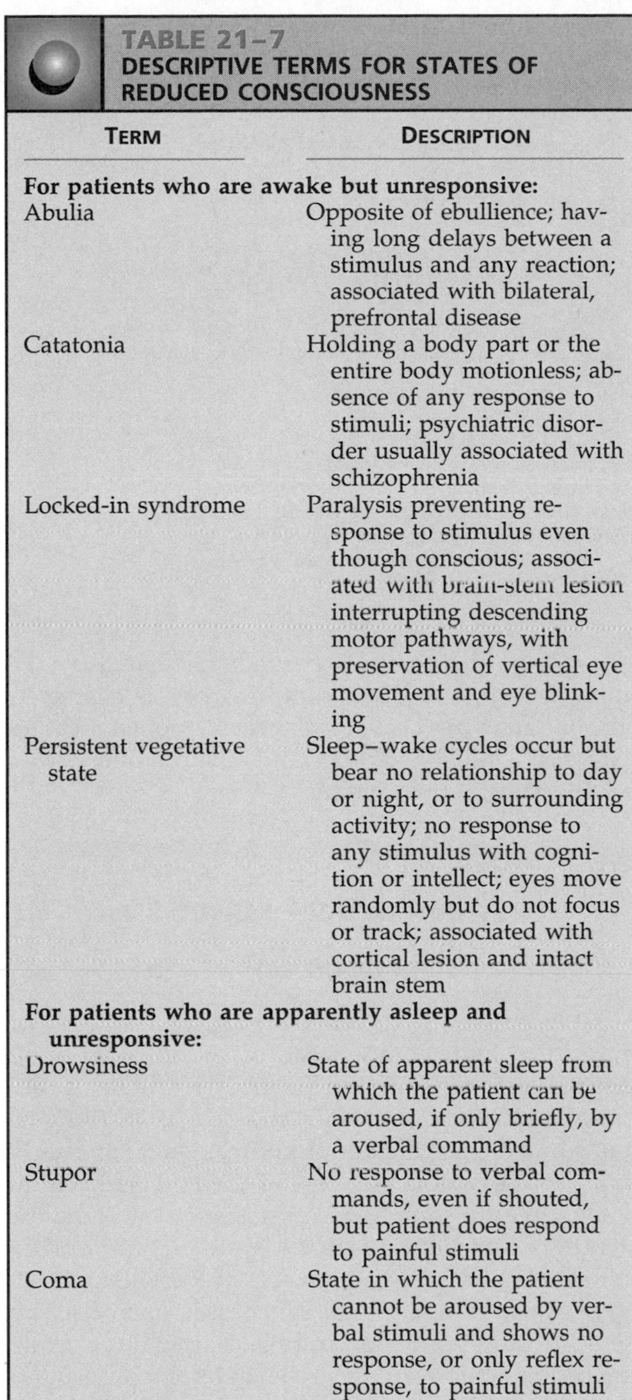

TABLE 21–7
DESCRIPTIVE TERMS FOR STATES OF REDUCED CONSCIOUSNESS

Term	Description
For patients who are awake but unresponsive:	
Abulia	Opposite of ebullience; having long delays between a stimulus and any reaction; associated with bilateral, prefrontal disease
Catatonia	Holding a body part or the entire body motionless; absence of any response to stimuli; psychiatric disorder usually associated with schizophrenia
Locked-in syndrome	Paralysis preventing response to stimulus even though conscious; associated with brain-stem lesion interrupting descending motor pathways, with preservation of vertical eye movement and eye blinking
Persistent vegetative state	Sleep–wake cycles occur but bear no relationship to day or night, or to surrounding activity; no response to any stimulus with cognition or intellect; eyes move randomly but do not focus or track; associated with cortical lesion and intact brain stem
For patients who are apparently asleep and unresponsive:	
Drowsiness	State of apparent sleep from which the patient can be aroused, if only briefly, by a verbal command
Stupor	No response to verbal commands, even if shouted, but patient does respond to painful stimuli
Coma	State in which the patient cannot be aroused by verbal stimuli and shows no response, or only reflex response, to painful stimuli

Data from Samuels, M.A. (1993). The evaluation of comatose patients. *Hospital Practice* 28(3), 165–182.

and childhood and degenerates with aging (Fig. 21–21 and see Developmental Perspective). Transient environmental influences, such as rotating work schedules and travel into different time zones, may also affect sleep. Sleep disorders include syndromes of insufficient sleep **(insomnias)** and excessive sleep **(hypersomnias)** and dysfunctional behaviors associated with sleep **(parasomnias)**. Clinical features of common sleep disorders are summarized in Table 21–8.

Electrophysiology

Electrodes may be placed over the surface of the brain to record summed membrane potentials generated during neurotransmission. The electroencephalogram (EEG) primarily detects inhibitory and excitatory postsynaptic potentials rather than action potentials because most of the latter are transmitted in a vertical direction, *perpendicular* to the scalp electrodes. As discussed in Chapter 17, waveforms of greatest amplitude are generated when current flow is *parallel* to the lead axis formed by two electrodes.

Figure 21–22 illustrates the four characteristic brain wave patterns: (1) alpha, associated with an awake but quiet brain; (2) beta, seen over areas of intense activity or REM sleep; (3) theta, associated with stress, frustration, and some sleep states; and (4) delta, seen during deep sleep. Dominant waveforms vary over different areas of the brain and during different stages of human development. In most cases, the significance of this variation is unknown. EEG waveforms may be used as a biofeedback signal in relaxation training for stress management. The EEG may also demonstrate pathology, with characteristic alterations in epilepsy, coma, and cortical or reticular lesions, such as tumors, infarcts, or hematomas. Absence of electrical activity (i.e., a "flat" EEG) has been used as a criterion for **brain death,** although absence of cerebral blood flow is considered to be a more reliable sign (Table 21–9). Any drug that affects neurotransmission also alters the EEG.

Limbic System Functions

The limbic system (see Fig. 21–2) is a functional system consisting of several nuclei located deep in the temporal lobes. These nuclei, which are also part of other anatomic and functional systems, include the hypothalamus, part of the thalamus, part of the basal ganglia, the hippocampus, the amygdala, and other nuclei. From the perspective of evolutionary development, the limbic system is considered to be the oldest part of the brain, concerned with basic and primitive motivations or drives.

The hypothalamus, which is central to the limbic system, is a critical organ that integrates neurologic and endocrine function. It is discussed in detail in Chapter 27. The nuclei of the limbic system are highly interconnected with other cortical and brain-

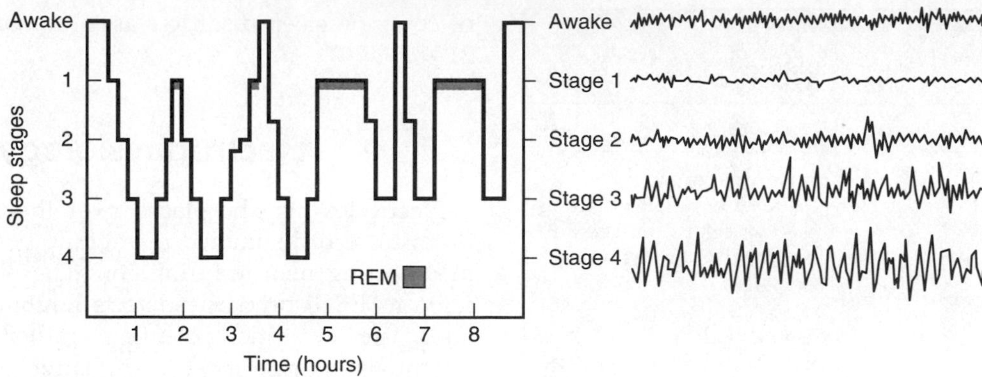

FIGURE 21–20
Brain activity during sleep. Normal sleep occurs in a typical pattern in which the person cycles between wakefulness, rapid eye movement (REM) sleep, and slow-wave (non-REM) sleep. Slow-wave sleep may be subdivided into four stages of increasing depth based on electroencephalographic recording of brain activity: stage 1 (alpha waves interspersed with theta waves), stage 2 (theta waves interspersed with sleep spindles), stage 3 (delta waves interspersed with sleep spindles), and stage 4 (delta waves). REM sleep resembles quiet wakefulness (alpha and beta waves).

stem areas, and most of these pathways are cholinergic. The limbic system is believed to link cortical perception of sensory inputs from the environment with stimuli originating from innate emotions and drives. Although the precise mechanisms and circuits are unknown in many cases, specific areas of the limbic system have been identified for the regulation of motivation (reward and punishment centers), emotion (rage and passivity centers), libido or sex drive, hunger and satiety, habituation and addiction, and consolidation of memory. The stress response (see Chapter 1) is partially mediated by the limbic system, and disruption of drives is characteristic of many psychiatric disorders, notably eating disorders (see Chapter 25) and clinical depression, detailed later in this chapter.

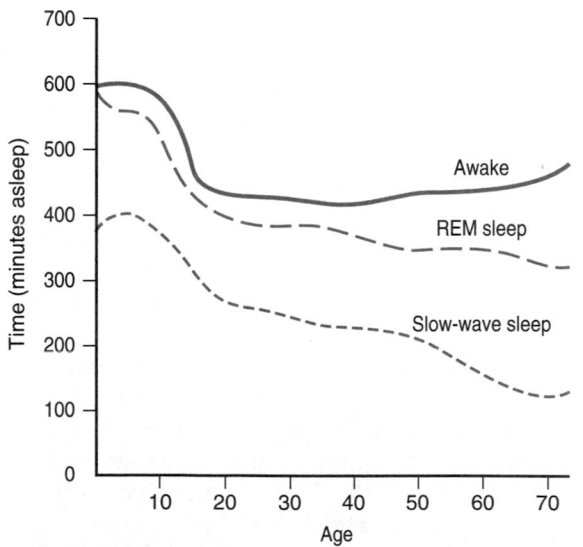

FIGURE 21–21
Changes in sleep patterns across the life span. During infancy and young childhood, rapid eye movement (REM) sleep predominates, but REM sleep declines and stabilizes at about 1 year of age. Awake time begins to increase during young adulthood. The elderly have longer sleep latency (awake time while trying to get to sleep) and more frequent, brief arousals.

Higher Cortical Functions

Cognition

The processes that convey the highest level of function to humans are those of cognitive or intellectual functioning. If intelligence is arbitrarily defined as the capacity to learn, and if learning is defined as the acquisition of knowledge, then clearly such processes as language and memory are central to cognitive function. One must also assume the existence of functional sensory systems, appropriate motivation, and access to sources of knowledge.

The study of intellectual function is hampered by the difficulty of demonstrating learning. Learning can be demonstrated by a behavioral change, but learning can also occur without observable change. The precise neural mechanisms of cognition are unknown, but these processes are believed to reside primarily in the *prefrontal association areas,* with multiple inputs from other cortical and subcortical regions. The evidence of this localization is derived from the increased prefrontal volume in humans as compared with lower animals, as well as from the observed behavior of humans who have undergone *frontal lobotomy.* Lobotomy, surgical interruption of frontal pathways, was once commonly used to control the behavior of people with schizophrenia and other psychiatric disorders. Destruction of these ar-

Developmental Perspective

Embryonic and Fetal Periods

The embryonic neural tube from which the nervous system develops is formed between days 21 and 26 of gestation. The first neurons appear as the tube closes, and by the second trimester, the glial cells are increasing in number. Electrical activity associated with sleep begins as early as the seventh day of life. Because the blood–brain barrier is not fully developed, the nervous system is vulnerable to teratogenic insults. Many agents are toxic to the developing CNS, and cortical dysfunction of varying degrees, from severe retardation to mild learning disabilities, is believed to be present in 10% to 20% of births. Teratogenic agents include rubella virus, lead and other metals, alcohol, pesticides, retinoids, and thalidomide. These may interfere with any of a number of developmental processes, including cellular proliferation, differentiation, migration, synapse formation, synthesis of neurotransmitters and receptors, myelination, and apoptosis. Failure of the neural tube to close occurs in about 1 in 1000 births in the United States. Many childhood brain tumors are of embryonic origin.

Infancy and Childhood

Ten per cent of young children manifest developmental delay, or failure to reach developmental milestones at the expected age. Such delay may have physiologic origins (e.g., prenatal or perinatal insult), environmental origins (e.g., poor caretaking environment), or both and may manifest as delays in motor, language, cognitive, or psychosocial development. In premature infants, the risk of intraventricular hemorrhage is increased as a result of the presence of an embryonic vascular structure, the subependymal germinal matrix. This thin-walled structure may rupture with increased blood pressure due to intrapartal or postnatal stress. Infants and young children are particularly vulnerable to meningitis because of incomplete development of the blood–brain barrier as well as more frequent exposure to pathogens. Children are also at risk for neurotrauma related to an unsafe or abusive environment. Infants and young children are at risk of Reye's syndrome, manifesting as hepatic failure and cerebral edema, after infection. The risk is believed to be exacerbated with administration of aspirin for treatment of a preceding fever. Term neonates and infants display two sleep stages: active sleep (REM sleep) and quiet sleep. Active sleep declines from 55% to 80% in neonates to 30% by the end of the first year, when it stabilizes. Girls demonstrate more sleep efficiency (time asleep divided by time in bed) than do boys. Childhood manifestations of altered cortical function include learning disorders, such as dyslexia; behavioral disorders, such as attention deficit disorder; sleep disorders; and epilepsy.

Adolescence and Young Adulthood

Growth of the brain continues until about 12 to 15 years of age. Adolescents have more homogeneous sleep patterns than people of any other stage. By early adulthood, there is a decrease in time in bed, percentage of sleep time, and total sleep time. Awake time rapidly increases after 29 years of age and is greater for men than for women. Most psychiatric disorders originate during the adolescent and young adult years. Eating disorders afflict significant numbers of adolescent girls, and childbearing women are prone to postpartum depression. Addiction to mood- and behavior-altering drugs usually begins in this stage, and the risk of traumatic brain injury associated with motor vehicle use and contact sports is highest in this group.

Middle and Older Adulthood

Cognitive functions, such as ability to memorize, to acquire and retain new information, and to recall names and dates, decline in most people after 70 years of age, although some retain exceptional cognitive function until much later in life. Personality changes are typical but not universal with aging; many older people manifest traits that are described as exaggerations of lifelong personality traits. The weight of the brain declines from the 3rd decade to the 10th, presumably because of neuronal atrophy and replacement with glial tissue. An increase in awake time is seen, and a trend toward more disturbed sleep is common, especially in men. Longer sleep latency (time to get to sleep) and decreased sleep efficiency are seen. Multiple short arousals occur during the night. Sleep cycles are distributed over the 24-hour period, with increased daytime napping. About to 25% to 40% of elderly people are diagnosed with sleep disorders. Agitated depression is the most frequent psychiatric illness during this period. Aging is the most significant risk factor for stroke and for Alzheimer's disease. The elderly are also at increased risk for traumatic brain injury due to falls.

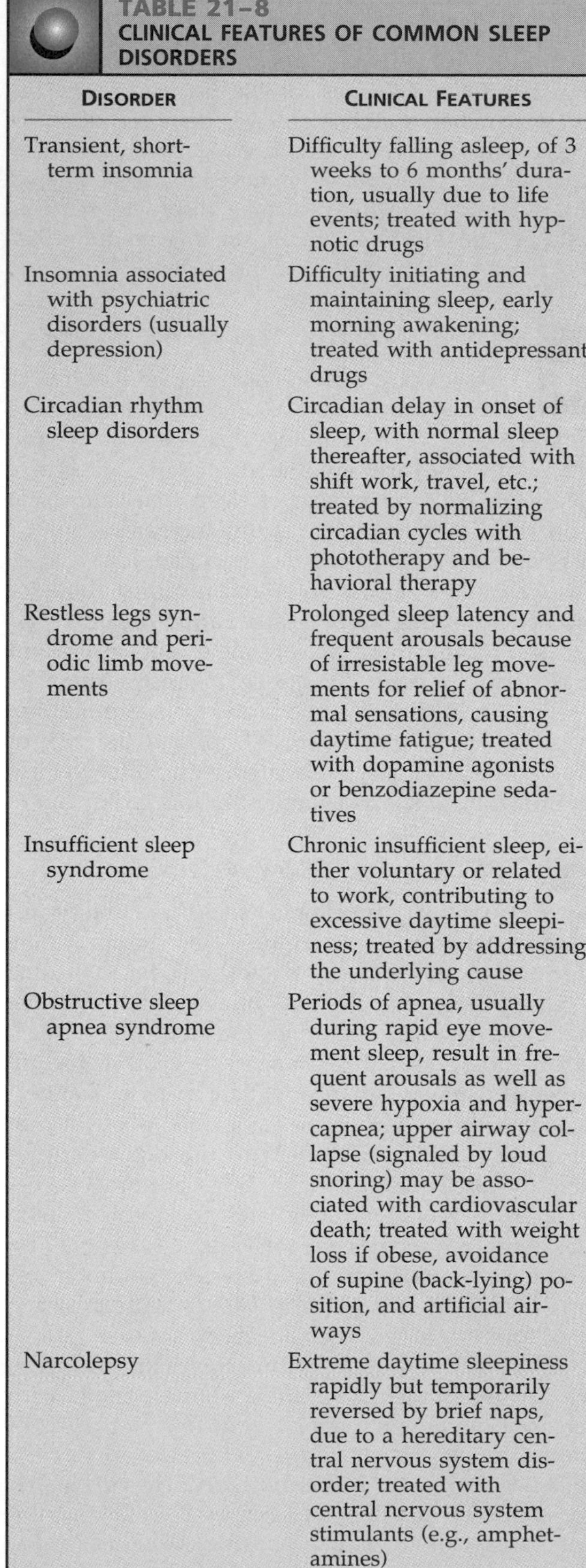

TABLE 21–8
CLINICAL FEATURES OF COMMON SLEEP DISORDERS

Disorder	Clinical Features
Transient, short-term insomnia	Difficulty falling asleep, of 3 weeks to 6 months' duration, usually due to life events; treated with hypnotic drugs
Insomnia associated with psychiatric disorders (usually depression)	Difficulty initiating and maintaining sleep, early morning awakening; treated with antidepressant drugs
Circadian rhythm sleep disorders	Circadian delay in onset of sleep, with normal sleep thereafter, associated with shift work, travel, etc.; treated by normalizing circadian cycles with phototherapy and behavioral therapy
Restless legs syndrome and periodic limb movements	Prolonged sleep latency and frequent arousals because of irresistable leg movements for relief of abnormal sensations, causing daytime fatigue; treated with dopamine agonists or benzodiazepine sedatives
Insufficient sleep syndrome	Chronic insufficient sleep, either voluntary or related to work, contributing to excessive daytime sleepiness; treated by addressing the underlying cause
Obstructive sleep apnea syndrome	Periods of apnea, usually during rapid eye movement sleep, result in frequent arousals as well as severe hypoxia and hypercapnea; upper airway collapse (signaled by loud snoring) may be associated with cardiovascular death; treated with weight loss if obese, avoidance of supine (back-lying) position, and artificial airways
Narcolepsy	Extreme daytime sleepiness rapidly but temporarily reversed by brief naps, due to a hereditary central nervous system disorder; treated with central nervous system stimulants (e.g., amphetamines)

Data from Farney, R.J., and Walker, J.M. (1995). Office management of common sleep-wake disorders. *Medical Clinics of North America* 79(2), 391–414.

eas leaves the patient quiet and docile, demonstrating neither spontaneity nor creativity.

Memory

The mechanisms of memory, the retention of learned knowledge, are also incompletely understood. At the cellular level, memory may involve a process known as *synaptic plasticity,* in which long-lasting modifications in synaptic strength occur.[2] The two components of synaptic plasticity are *long-term potentiation,* in which certain synapses are strengthened to provide functional links between neurons, and *long-term depression,* in which synaptic strength is decreased.[3] In theory, potentiated synapses facilitate more rapid retrieval of stored information, whereas depressed synapses suppress such retrieval. Induction of both long-term potentiation and depression is believed to result from activation of a subclass of glutamate receptors, the postsynaptic *N*-methyl-D-aspartic acid receptor, which then causes a rise in intracellular Ca^{2+}. Local mediators, including nitric oxide, may be important signaling molecules in this process. Facilitated memory circuits may be damaged with pathology or lost with age-related degeneration, resulting in memory loss (**amnesia**).

Explicit memory, also known as declarative memory, depends on an intact limbic system, particularly the hippocampus and its projections to the thalamus and medial cortical regions. This form of memory permits conscious recollection of facts and events. Three types of explicit memory are recognized: (1) *immediate memory,* lasting minutes; (2) *short-term* or *recent memory,* lasting hours to days; and (3) *long-term* or *remote memory,* lasting years. Memories are apparently encoded in some way by the hippocampus and adjacent cerebral cortices and stored with similar memories. Injury to hippocampal structures results in severe *anterograde amnesia* (difficulty in en-

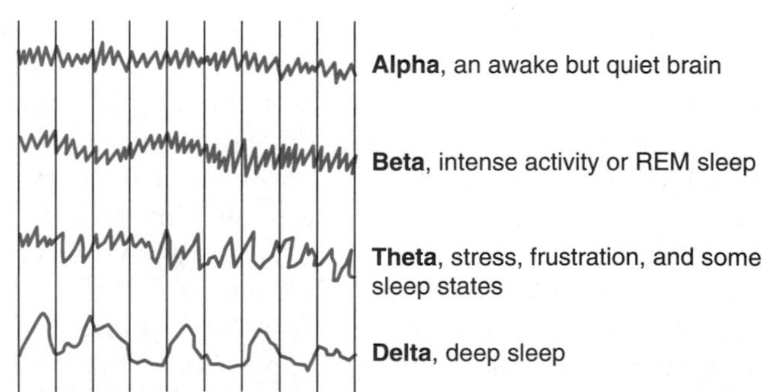

FIGURE 21–22
Normal brain wave patterns. The electroencephalogram uses scalp electrodes to record summed electrical activity generated by neurotransmission. Four characteristic patterns are discernible, each associated with different levels and types of activity of the underlying brain.

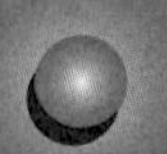

TABLE 21–9
CRITERIA FOR DETERMINATION OF BRAIN DEATH

UNIFORM DETERMINATION OF DEATH ACT CRITERIA*

An individual who has sustained either
(1) irreversible cessation of circulatory and respiratory functions, or
(2) irreversible cessation of all functions of the entire brain, including the brain stem,
is dead. A determination of death must be made in accordance with medical standards.

*Excludes children younger than 5 years.

HARVARD CRITERIA

Prerequisite: absence of hypothermia and drug intoxication
Criteria: unresponsive coma; apnea; absent reflexes
Confirmation: isoelectric electroencephalogram
Duration: 24 h

MINNESOTA CRITERIA

Prerequisite: irreparable intracranial lesion
Criteria: no spontaneous movement; apnea when off respirator for 4 min; absent brain-stem reflexes; including dilated and fixed pupils; absent corneal, ciliospinal, doll's head phenomenon, gag, vestibular, and tonic neck reflexes
Duration: 12 h

GUIDELINES FOR THE DETERMINATION OF BRAIN DEATH IN CHILDREN

Historical criteria
- Determination of the proximate cause of coma (absence of remediable or reversible conditions)

Physical examination criteria:
- Coexisting coma and apnea
- Absence of brain-stem function
- Absence of hypothermia or hypotension
- Flaccid tone or absence of spontaneous or induced movements (except spinal cord events)
- Consistent examination findings throughout observation and testing periods

Observation periods and laboratory testing
- Age 7 d–2 mo: two clinical examinations and apnea tests and two electroencephalograms 48 h apart
- Age 2–12 mo: two clinical examinations and apnea tests and two electroencephalograms at least 24 h apart
- Age >12 mo: two clinical examinations and apnea tests 12 h apart

Data from Walker, A.E. (1985). *Cerebral Death.* (3rd ed.). Baltimore: Urban & Schwarzenberg. (pp. 168–169); and Mejia, R.E., and Pollack, M.M. (1995). Variability in brain death determination practices in children. *Journal of the American Medical Association* 274(7), 550–553.

coding new memories) and lesser degrees of *retrograde amnesia* (difficulty in retrieving older memories).

Implicit memory (nondeclarative memory) refers to a nonconscious process that supports skill and habit learning, conditioned responses, and classification of experiences. Implicit memory apparently involves the prefrontal cortex and inferior temporal regions. The study of implicit memory is in its infancy, and the extent to which implicit memory depends on explicit memory is uncertain. Unlike explicit memory, implicit memory does not usually decline with aging.[4]

Language

Language is a complex process that resides in several areas of the cortex (Fig. 21–23). Although the language centers on both sides of the brain participate in speech, the left hemisphere is dominant in virtually all right-handed people and in 85% of left-handed people. The most important area for the interpretation of auditory and written language is *Wernicke's area* in the upper temporal lobe. This area is adjacent to, and receives inputs from, parietal *sensory association areas. Wernicke's aphasia* (receptive aphasia) is the inability to communicate coherently because of dominant-side damage to this area (e.g., by trauma, tumor, or stroke). The patient may be able to speak or write, but the message is garbled because of impaired language interpretation. *Broca's*

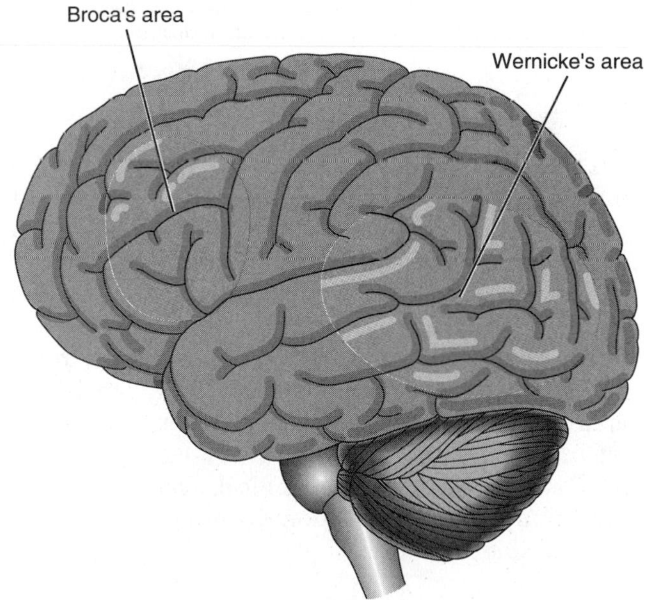

FIGURE 21–23
Cortical language areas. *Broca's area* in the frontal lobe is the motor area for speech. Injury to this area impairs speech but leaves language interpretation intact. *Wernicke's area* in the upper temporal lobe governs interpretation of spoken and written language. Injury to this area results in a garbled message, owing to faulty cognition, although individual words and phrases may be coherent. Nearly all right-handed people and 85% of left-handed people have their dominant speech centers in the left hemisphere. Bilateral activation of language areas is more pronounced in females than in males.

TABLE 21–10
COMMUNICATION DISORDERS

Classification	Clinical Features
Nonfluent cortical aphasia (e.g., Broca's aphasia)	Due to left anterior frontal lobe lesion; patient speaks slowly and effortfully, using key words only, or uses stereotyped verbal responses to everything; auditory comprehension of spoken language is intact
Nonfluent subcortical aphasia	Due to left thalamic or basal ganglia lesion; manifestations as with nonfluent cortical aphasia plus moderate to severe reading and written language impairments
Fluent cortical aphasia (e.g., Wernicke's aphasia)	Due to left posterior temporal or parietal lobe lesion; patient speaks effortlessly, but language is devoid of meaning
Fluent subcortical aphasia (e.g., anomic aphasia)	Comprehension may or may not be intact, depending on the location of the lesion; language characteristics similar to those of fluent cortical aphasia
Cognitive and communicative impairment	Due to focal damage to the nondominant (typically right) hemisphere, or to sudden or slow progressive widespread bilateral damage to both cerebral hemispheres; language skills appear to be intact, but pragmatic or social uses of language are impaired, e.g., disorganized conversation, focus on irrelevant details, confabulation, tangentiality, difficulty comprehending abstract or complex communication, failure to interpret nonverbal cues, speaking in a monotone
Dysarthria	Neurogenic voice and speech impairment due to damage to central and peripheral motor pathways for speech; patient exhibits weakness, slowness, lack of coordination, or altered tone of speech and voice muscles
Apraxia of speech	Inability to preplan, initiate, and accurately sequence speech movements, due to damage to Broca's area and the surrounding left frontal cortex
Conversion voice impairment	Psychogenic disorder; no underlying lesion

Data from Clark, L.W. (1994). Communication disorders: What to look for, and when to refer. *Geriatrics* 49(6), 51–55.

aphasia (motor or expressive aphasia) results from dominant-side damage to *Broca's area,* the motor area for speech in the frontal lobe. With this type of aphasia, the patient may interpret language correctly but is unable to speak. The angular gyrus, located near Wernicke's area, is believed to be involved in interpretation of visual language. **Dyslexia,** a reading disorder, has been associated with damage to this area; however, cortical lesions are often not demonstrable in patients with reading disabilities or other learning disorders.[5] Clinical features of the more common communication disorders are summarized in Table 21–10.

CORTICAL DISORDERS

The disorders discussed in the following sections include examples of mental illness (psychiatric disorders) as well as physiologic disorders (neurologic disorders). Because the distinction between these categories is often unclear, the term *neuropsychiatric disorder* is also in common use. **Encephalopathy** is a general term for degenerative disease of the brain, usually associated with disease of another system (e.g., acquired immunodeficiency syndrome encephalopathy). These syndromes are discussed in relevant systems chapters.

Psychiatric disorders are generally understood to involve cognitive or behavioral abnormalities that may or may not originate from pathophysiologic alterations; that is, they may include an aspect of disordered function that is derived solely from reactions to previous or present life experiences.[6] Common psychiatric disorders discussed in the following sections include schizophrenia, depression, and Alzheimer's disease. Other psychiatric disorders are described briefly in Table 21–11.

Neural tube defects, the most common congenital defects of the CNS, are discussed in detail, whereas less common congenital disorders are briefly summarized in Table 21–12. Meningitis is detailed as an example of inflammatory disease of the CNS, and epilepsy is discussed to illustrate altered CNS electrophysiology. IICP is described as a general syn-

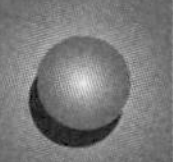

TABLE 21–11
OVERVIEW OF PSYCHIATRIC DISORDERS

Disorder	Clinical Characteristics
Psychoses	
Schizophrenia	Severe disorder characterized by dissociation of thought, emotion, and behavior, possibly due to dopamine imbalance; clinical signs include hallucination and delusions, cognitive impairment, and negative signs such as social withdrawal
Delusional (paranoid) disorder	Similar to schizophrenia except that delusions have a basis in reality, hallucinations are not dominant, and behavior unrelated to delusions is relatively normal
Brief reactive psychosis	Psychotic symptoms occurring in response to life events; symptoms last no longer than 1 mo
Schizophreniform disorder	Similar to brief reactive psychosis except there is no apparent precipitating event, and symptoms do not last longer than 6 mo
Induced psychotic disorder	Psychotic state related to association with another psychotic person and evidenced by a marked delusional system
Atypical psychosis	Psychotic symptoms other than the above
Mood Disorders	
Depression	Presence of depressed mood or loss of pleasure, accompanied by a change in appetite, weight, or sleep pattern; feelings of worthlessness or guilt; and possible suicidal ideation
Bipolar disorder (manic-depressive)	Mood swings encompassing both depressive and euphoric-hyperactive symptoms; manic symptoms include flight of ideas, insomnia, grandiosity, irritability, denial of illness, manipulativeness, and assaultive behavior
Anxiety Disorders	
Generalized anxiety disorder	Excessive worry about concrete issues that are not reality-based; symptoms of motor tension, autonomic hyperactivity, vigilance, and scanning of the environment
Panic disorder	Attacks of intense fear or discomfort lasting minutes to hours and occurring without apparent cause
Obsessive-compulsive disorder	Recurrent and persistent thoughts, ideas, impulses, or images that are experienced as intrusive and senseless (obsessions); repetitive behaviors (compulsions) performed in response to prevent or neutralize anxiety
Phobic disorder	Intense, irrational fear responses to an external object, activity, or situation
Post-traumatic stress disorder	Develops 1 mo or more after a life-threatening or traumatic event; major symptoms are numbing of responsiveness or reduced involvement with the external world; person also re-experiences the traumatic event as flashbacks, nightmares, or intrusive memories
Somatoform disorder	Patient has physical symptoms for which there is no known organic cause or physiologic mechanism
Dissociative disorder	Unconscious "splitting off" or removal from awareness of some information, feeling, or mental function; a mechanism for protection against repressed conflicts or experiences
Organic Mental Syndromes	
Delirium	Sudden onset of reduced awareness and attentiveness to the environment, disorganized thinking, and incoherent speech; due to cerebral dysfunction secondary to acute or chronic illness or to chemical agents
Dementia	Altered mental state due to cerebral disease; usually irreversible manifestations of intellectual decline, personality change, impaired judgment, and affective change
Personality Disorders	Personality traits are inflexible and maladaptive and cause either significant functional impairment or subjective distress
Sexual Disorders	
Paraphilia	Intense sexual urges focused on nonhuman objects, suffering or humiliation of self or partner, or of children or other nonconsenting people
Sexual dysfunction	Inhibition of sexual appetite or psychophysiologic changes that compromise sexual response
Eating Disorders	
Anorexia nervosa	Self-starvation due to fear of fatness and distorted body image; body weight is at least 15% below normal
Bulimia nervosa	Binge and purge syndrome in which periods of excessive food consumption are alternated with self-induced vomiting or abuse of laxatives and diuretics

Data from Keltner, N.L., Schwecke, L.H., and Bostrom, C.E. (1991). *Psychiatric Nursing: A Psychotherapeutic Management Approach.* St. Louis: Mosby–Year Book.

TABLE 21–12
CONGENITAL DISORDERS OF THE CENTRAL NERVOUS SYSTEM

Disorder	Clinical Features
Neural tube defects	Anomalies arising from failure of closure of the embryonic neural tube; may manifest as absence of brain tissue (anencephaly) or defects in closure of the vertebral column with protrusion of meninges, nerves, or cord
Cerebral palsy	Group of motor deficits of cerebral origin, usually due to damage at time of birth
Microcephaly	Small size of the brain and overlying cranium, associated with severe mental retardation
Agenesis of the corpus callosum	Complete or partial absence of the corpus callosum; may be asymptomatic or associated with seizures or mental retardation
Hydrocephalus	Congenital forms are more common than acquired; excessive volume or pressure of cerebrospinal fluid due to narrowing of cerebral aqueducts or obstruction of arachnoid villi
Arnold-Chiari malformation	Elongation of the medulla and herniation of the vermis cerebellum through the foramen magnum; often associated with spina bifida; results in communicating hydrocephalus
Mental retardation	Impairment of intelligence; may be due to genetic or chromosomal abnormality (e.g., Down syndrome), teratogenic insult (e.g., fetal alcohol syndrome), inborn errors of metabolism, or birth injury

Data from Moore, K.L., and Persaud, T.V.N. (1993). *The Developing Human: Clinically Oriented Embryology*. (5th ed.). Philadelphia: W.B. Saunders.

drome, along with the disorders that most frequently result in IICP, namely hydrocephalus, traumatic brain injury, stroke, and brain tumors.

Schizophrenia

Definition. Schizophrenia is a **psychosis** characterized by dissociation or disruption of thought processes and a split among thought, emotion, and behavior.[7] It is the most severe of mental illnesses.

Epidemiology. The prevalence of schizophrenia worldwide has been estimated at 0.85%.[7] Although the disorder is widely distributed in diverse populations, three risk factors have emerged from epidemiologic research: genetic characteristics, gestational and birth complications, and winter birth. It is clear that relatives of patients with schizophrenia are at increased risk for the disorder; however, neither the defective gene or genes nor the specific mode of inheritance is known. Schizophrenia is more prevalent among people who suffered gestational complications such as maternal infection or malnutrition. The observation that an excess of schizophrenic patients were born during winter months has not been explained.

Etiology. The precise cause of schizophrenia is unknown. Hypothetical mechanisms include inherited genetic defects and prenatal injury to the brain, consistent with the risk factors discussed previously. Postnatal injury to the developing brain by a viral or autoimmune mechanism has also been postulated, but no research evidence has definitely supported this etiology.[8] Psychosocial factors may play a causative role, but their impact is believed to be in modifying the course of the disease rather than in initiating the disorder.

Pathophysiology. The mechanisms that link cortical injury or abnormality to the disturbed behavior and thought that characterize schizophrenia are not known. The best-known hypothesis, the *dopamine hypothesis,* is based on the observed effects of administration of drugs that either block or stimulate dopaminergic pathways.[9] In many schizophrenic patients, blockade of one class of dopamine receptors (D_2) reduces symptoms, whereas dopamine agonists increase psychotic symptoms. Consistent structural abnormalities are seen at autopsy and with high-resolution imaging techniques in patients with schizophrenia, and these have led to the *neuroanatomic hypothesis* of schizophrenia.[7] Abnormalities of the ventricular system, temporal lobe abnormalities, decreased volume of the amygdala and hippocampus of the limbic system, structural changes in prefrontal white matter, and increased volume of the basal ganglia have been found. Cortical blood flow to prefrontal areas is typically decreased. It is unknown, however, whether these changes are due to primary pathology or are a response to drug treatment.

Clinical Manifestations. As is true for most psychiatric disorders, the diagnosis of schizophrenia is established on the basis of the behavioral manifestations and course of the disorder rather than on the presence of a characteristic anatomic lesion. Table 21–13 lists the accepted diagnostic criteria. Onset of the disorder may occur any time between the late

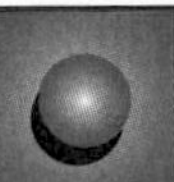

TABLE 21–13
CRITERIA FOR DIAGNOSING SCHIZOPHRENIA

CHARACTERISTIC SYMPTOMS

Two (or more) of the following, each present for a significant portion of time during a 1-mo period (or less if successfully treated):
(1) Delusions
(2) Hallucinations
(3) Disorganized speech
(4) Grossly disorganized or catatonic behavior
(5) Negative symptoms, i.e., affective flattening, alogia, or avolition

SOCIAL AND OCCUPATIONAL DYSFUNCTION

For a significant portion of the time, one or more major areas of functioning, such as work, interpersonal relations, or self-care, are markedly below the level achieved before onset.

DURATION

Continuous signs of disturbance persist for at least 6 mo.

Adapted and reprinted with permission from *Diagnostic and Statistical Manual of Mental Disorders.* (4th Ed.). Copyright 1994 American Psychiatric Association. Washington, DC: American Psychiatric Association.

teenage years and the early 40s and may be acute or gradual.

According to the *three compartment model,* symptoms of schizophrenia cluster into three domains: (1) positive symptoms (reflecting an excess or distortion of normal functions), such as hallucinations (false sensations) and delusions (false beliefs); (2) cognitive impairment, demonstrated by tangentiality (inability to stay "on message" with speech), loss of goals, incoherence, looseness of association, and neologisms (coining of new words); and (3) negative symptoms, reflecting a decline or loss of normal functions, such as flat affect (mask-like facial expression), diminished emotional range, poverty (slowness or hesitance) of speech, curbing of interests, diminished sense of purpose, and diminished social drive.[7] This model has been proposed to replace older descriptive classifications of schizophrenia (e.g., paranoid, hebephrenic, or simple schizophrenia). The three symptom clusters manifest in variable patterns among patients with all forms of schizophrenia.

Prevention and Treatment. There are no known measures for the prevention of schizophrenia. Treatment approaches aim to minimize symptoms and include drug therapy and psychosocial therapies. Antipsychotic (neuroleptic) drugs are the principal form of treatment for schizophrenia. These agents act by blocking dopamine receptors as well as cholinergic and adrenergic receptors to varying degrees (Table 21–14). Consequently, these drugs have significant side effects in most patients. Clozapine, an atypical antipsychotic drug, does not cause the *extrapyramidal symptoms* that occur with other agents (see Chapter 22) but does impose other risks, including a decrease in leukocytes *(agranulocytosis),* which predisposes the patient to infection. The most recently approved neuroleptic drug is risperidone (Risperdal), which is similar in action to clozapine but has not caused agranulocytosis is early studies.[10]

Psychosocial interventions in schizophrenia focus on practical behavioral approaches aimed at improving the patient's social and self-care skills, rather than the intensive psychotherapy that has been largely ineffective in the past. In recent years, care of patients with schizophrenia has shifted from custodial to community care, but in many cases, communities have been unprepared to provide adequate support. It has been estimated that one third to one half of homeless people in the United States have schizophrenia.[7]

Prognosis and Outcome. Functional impairment is lifelong and severe in most cases of schizophrenia. Deterioration is usually most severe during the first 5 years, after which the condition remains relatively stable. Nearly 25% of patients do not respond sufficiently to neuroleptic drugs and require custodial care.[10]

Depression

Definition. According to the accepted diagnostic criteria, *major depression* is defined as the presence of either depressed mood or loss of pleasure for at least 2 consecutive weeks, along with three of the following symptoms: change in appetite or weight, change in sleep pattern, psychomotor agitation or retardation, fatigue, feelings of worthlessness or excessive guilt, difficulty concentrating, or suicidal ideation.[11] *Chronic minor depression (dysthymia)* is defined as depressed mood for most of the day, more days than not, for at least 2 years, with presence while depressed of at least two of the following: appetite disturbance, sleep disturbance, fatigue, low self-esteem, poor concentration and difficulty making decisions, and feelings of hopelessness.[12]

Epidemiology. Major depression and dysthymia occur in about 6% of the adult population of the United States during any given 6-month period.[12] Major depression accounts for more days lost from work than does any chronic physiologic disorder.

TABLE 21–14
ANTIPSYCHOTIC (NEUROLEPTIC) DRUGS

Category and Examples	Potency	Mechanisms of Action
Phenothiazines		Dopamine receptor antagonism (therapeutic and side effects); low-potency agents also block α_1-adrenergic and cholinergic receptors (side effects)
Chlorpromazine (Thorazine)	Low	
Triflupromazine (Vesprin)	Low	
Thioridazine (Mellaril)	Low	
Mesoridazine (Serentil)	Low	
Perphenazine (Trilafon)	High	
Trifluoperazine (Stelazine)	High	
Fluphenazine (Permitil, Prolixin)	High	
Thioxanthenes		Same as phenothiazines
Chlorprothixene (Taractan)	Low	
Thiothixene (Navane)	High	
Butyrophenones		Same as phenothiazines
Haloperidol (Haldol)	High	
Droperidol (Inapsine)	High	
Dibenzodiazepine		Atypical agent; blocks dopamine receptors in selected areas, while increasing dopamine release in others; also blocks serotonin receptors
Clozapine (Clozaril)	Low	
Dibenzoxazepine		Same as phenothiazines
Loxapine (Loxitane)	Low	
Dihydroindolone		Same as phenothiazines
Molindone (Moban)	High	
Diphenylbutylpiperidine		Same as phenothiazines
Pimozide (Orap)	High	
Benzisoxazole		Same as clozapine
Risperidone (Risperdal)	Low	

Note: Low-potency drugs are administered in high daily doses and tend to have stronger sedative and hypotensive effects but fewer extrapyramidal (motor and autonomic) effects. High-potency drugs are given in low daily doses and cause less sedation and hypotension but tend to result in more extrapyramidal effects.

Furthermore, chronic medical disease and its treatment predispose to depression, and presence of depression is associated with more disability in those with medical disease.[13] According to the Agency for Health Care Policy and Research Clinical Practice Guideline, risk factors for depression are prior episodes of depression, prior suicide attempts, age less than 40 years, medical comorbidity, stressful life events, family history of depression, female sex, recent childbirth, lack of social support, and current substance abuse.[14]

Etiology and Pathophysiology. The precise etiology of depression and other mood disorders is unknown. The most widely accepted hypothesis is that of monoamine deficiency (e.g., norepinephrine and serotonin), but this may represent a final common pathway triggered by initial disorders involving other neurotransmitters or their receptors.[15] Autopsy examination of neural tissue of depressed people has shown significantly lower concentrations of serotonin metabolites, and other studies have shown reduced serotonin uptake by platelets in depressed people. Dietary restriction of L-tryptophan (an amino acid that is a serotonin precursor) also worsens depression in those with mood disorders. Psychosocial stress may play a role in depression by triggering major episodes or by determining the particular signs and symptoms that emerge, but environmental factors have not been shown to be independent causes of major depression.

Clinical Manifestations. The onset of depression is usually gradual, occurring over several days or weeks. Depression may or may not follow a stressful event or loss. Clinical features, discussed earlier related to definition, tend to cluster in four categories: (1) **dysphoria,** manifested as crying, pessimism, suicidal or homicidal tendency, or feelings of hopelessness, helplessness, worthlessness, self-reproach, or guilt; (2) activity impairment, manifested as loss of interest, lack of energy, decreased libido, increased fatigue, or social withdrawal; (3) vegetative symptoms, manifested as sleep disorder, appetite disorder, cyclic mood variations, agitation, or decreased cognitive ability; and (4) other psychiatric disturbances, such as anxiety, obsession, psychosis, hypochondria, or hysteria.[16]

Prevention and Treatment. Reduction in modifiable risk factors (e.g., lack of social support, substance abuse, stressful lifestyle) may reduce the frequency and severity of depressive episodes, but drug therapy and psychotherapy are required for treatment of most cases of depression. Five major classes of antidepressant drugs are in use. Examples of these agents and their mechanisms of action are listed in Table 21–15. Selective serotonin reuptake inhibitors (e.g., fluoxetine [Prozac]) are considered first-line treatment of depression.[17] Their mechanism is consistent with a serotonin deficiency etiology in that they increase the concentration of serotonin at the synapse.

Psychotherapy of depression emphasizes cognitive and behavioral techniques that are short-term, structured, and pragmatic. Regular exercise is strongly encouraged and has been shown to increase norepinephrine turnover, stabilize circadian rhythms, and increase output of mood-elevating endorphins and enkephalins (see Chapter 23).

Prognosis and Outcome. The likelihood of recovery from depression is inversely related to the duration and severity of the illness. An estimated 20% to 30% of patients do not respond to antidepressant drug therapy, and about one in four who do respond relapse within 2 months of discontinuance of therapy. About 60% of suicides are attributable to depression (about 18,000 people annually in the United States).[17]

Alzheimer's Disease

Definition. Alzheimer's disease is descriptively defined as primary degenerative **dementia,** one of a group of syndromes characterized by progressive decline in memory, judgment, intellectual function, and adaptive ability. The diagnosis of Alzheimer's disease is made after other, possibly reversible, causes of dementia have been ruled out and can often be confirmed only at autopsy. Table 21–16 lists potentially reversible forms of dementia.

Epidemiology. Alzheimer's disease is the most common cause of dementia, afflicting an estimated 4 million people in the United States.[18] Because the precise etiology is unknown, risk factors other than aging are uncertain. In a minority of cases, Alzheimer's disease is due to defects on chromosomes 14 and 21.[19] Patients with Down syndrome (trisomy 21) often develop manifestations of Alzheimer's disease if they survive to middle age (see Chapter 33). Women who give birth to infants with Down syndrome are five times more likely to develop Alzhei-

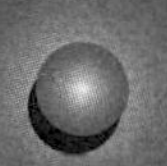

TABLE 21–15
ANTIDEPRESSANT DRUGS

Category and Examples	Mechanisms of Action
Selective serotonin reuptake inhibitors (SSRIs) Fluoxetine (Prozac) Paroxetine (Paxil) Sertraline (Zoloft)	Increase serotonin concentration at the synapse by blocking reuptake into the presynaptic terminal; little affinity for other receptors, thus few side effects
Heterocyclic antidepressants Amoxapine (Asendin) Maprotiline (Ludiomil) Nefazodone (Serdone) Trazodone (Desyrel) Venlafaxine (Effexor)	Inhibit serotonin reuptake and also block serotonin (5-hydroxytryptamine$_2$) receptors; active metabolites have serotonin agonist activity; venlafaxine also selectively inhibits norepinephrine reuptake.
Aminoketone antidepressants Bupropion (Wellbutrin)	Mechanism uncertain; exerts weak effects on norepinephrine, dopamine, and serotonin systems
Tricyclic antidepressants (TCAs) Amitriptyline (Elavil) Desipramine (Norpramin) Doxepin (Sinequan) Imipramine (Tofranil) Nortriptyline (Aventyl) Protriptyline (Vivactyl) Trimipramine maleate (Surmontil)	Inhibit norepinephrine and serotonin reuptake; may also influence release of corticotropin-releasing hormone (CRH)
Monamine oxidase inhibitors (MAOIs) Phenelzine (Nardil) Tranylcypromine (Parnate)	Inhibit monamine oxidase, a mitochondrial enzyme that catalyzes the deamination (and deactivation) of catecholamines and serotonin; the enzyme also metabolizes tyramine, a compound present in some cheeses and other foods, which must be avoided by patients taking MAOIs

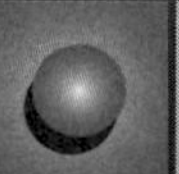

TABLE 21–16
POTENTIALLY REVERSIBLE CAUSES OF DEMENTIA

D — drugs
E — emotional illness (including depression)
M — metabolic and endocrine disorders
E — eye and ear problems
N — nutritional (e.g., anemia) or neurologic derangement
T — tumor or trauma (especially subdural hematoma)
I — infection
A — alcoholism

From Paist, S.S., III, and Martin, J.R. (1996). Brain failure in older patients. *Postgraduate Medicine* 99(5), 125–136.

mer's disease than other mothers. This early-onset form of dementia is known as *familial Alzheimer's disease.*

The more common forms of the disease, *late-onset familial* and *sporadic Alzheimer's disease,* have been linked to a specific gene encoding the synthesis of apolipoprotein E, located on chromosome 19. Those with the E4 allele of this gene are at higher risk for earlier onset of Alzheimer's disease, whereas those with the E2 allele are at lower risk. The E4 genotype confers increased risk of deposition of β-amyloid protein in the cerebral cortex.[20]

Environmental factors, such as repeated head trauma or exposure to such elements as aluminum, silicon, and iron, have been postulated as risk factors, although no direct causative link has been established. Occupational exposure to electromagnetic fields has also been proposed as a risk factor because electrical power line and cable workers, as well as dressmakers, tailors, and others who regularly use sewing machines, demonstrate an increased risk of developing Alzheimer's disease.[18]

Low attained education has also been associated with increased risk of Alzheimer's disease. It is uncertain whether this association is secondary to related environmental exposures or whether the lower neurocognitive reserve of these people increases the likelihood of their manifesting the cognitive symptoms of dementia. In a study of nuns, low linguistic ability in early life was a strong predictor of poor cognitive function and Alzheimer's disease in late life[21] (see Focus of Current Research).

Etiology. The causative mechanism of Alzheimer's disease is unknown.

Pathophysiology. Behavioral manifestations of progressive dementia are accompanied by characteristic structural changes, including cortical atrophy, ventricular dilation, formation of plaques composed of degenerating axons and dendrites, fibrous proteins (neurofibrillatory tangles) within the cytoplasm of neurons, and deposition of amyloid (glycoprotein) around cortical blood vessels. Brain volume is reduced, and the severity of dementia correlates with the degree of loss of cortical cells and synapses. There is selective loss of cholinergic neurons in pathways that project to the frontal lobes and hippocampus, areas critical to memory and cognitive functions.[22]

Clinical Manifestations. Alzheimer's disease usually progresses through three stages. The onset is gradual, with symptoms of random memory loss (both recent and remote), loss of the sense of smell, and flattening of the affect and personality gradually worsening over a 2- to 4-year period. A confusional state lasting several years follows and is typically characterized by lack of insight, decreased language ability, depression, wandering, and inability to manage activities of daily living. Some patients manifest hostile and abusive behavior during this stage. During the terminal stage, lasting 1 to 10 years, the patient is apathetic and unable to recognize family and friends. Motor deficits, such as weakness, rigidity, and spasticity, are seen. The patient becomes totally dependent and incontinent and may have seizure activity.

Prevention and Treatment. There is no known prevention for Alzheimer's disease. Tacrine hydrochloride (Cognex), which inhibits the breakdown of ACh at the synapse, was the first drug approved for the treatment of Alzheimer's disease. Early studies have shown some improvement in mental function with enhancement of cholinergic function by this drug, but its significant gastrointestinal side effects have limited its tolerance by many. Essentially, treatment of Alzheimer's disease is supportive and symptomatic, with emphasis on provision of a safe environment.

Prognosis and Outcome. Alzheimer's disease is fatal, usually within 6 to 15 years of diagnosis.[23]

Neural Tube Defects

Definition. Neural tube defects are congenital anomalies of the CNS arising from failure of dorsal induction of closure of the neural tube. The neural tube is an early embryonic structure that forms from folding of the ectodermal neural plate (see Chapter 6). The most common NTDs are **anencephaly, encephalocele, spina bifida cystica,** and **spina bifida occulta,** defined as follows:

Anencephaly: absence of brain tissue above a rudimentary brain stem and basal ganglia

Encephalocele: external sac or mass that may occur at any point over the vertex or base of the skull and that may be covered with either scalp or a transparent membrane

Focus of Current Research

Study	Objective and Findings
Marion, et al. (1997) Treatment of traumatic brain injury with moderate hypothermia.	*Objective:* To compare the effects of moderate hypothermia and normothermia in patients with severe closed head injuries *Findings:* Treatment with moderate hypothermia for 24 hours hastened neurologic recovery and may have improved the outcome.
King, et al. (1997) Moderate-intensity exercise and self-rated quality of sleep in older adults: A randomized controlled trial.	*Objective:* To determine the effects of moderate-intensity exercise training on subjective sleep quality among healthy, sedentary older adults reporting moderate sleep complaints *Findings:* Older adults with moderate sleep complaints can improve self-rated sleep quality by initiating a regular, moderate-intensity exercise program.
Snowdon, et al. (1997) Brain infarction and the clinical expression of Alzheimer disease: The Nun Study.	*Objective:* To determine the relationship of brain infarction to the clinical expression of Alzheimer's disease *Findings:* Cerebrovascular disease may play an important role in determining the presence and severity of the clinical symptoms of Alzheimer's disease.
Snowdon, et al. (1996) Linguistic ability in early life and cognitive function and Alzheimer's disease in late life: Findings from the Nun Study.	*Objective:* To determine if linguistic ability in early life is associated with cognitive function and Alzheimer's disease in late life *Findings:* Low linguistic ability in early life was a strong predictor of poor cognitive function and Alzheimer's disease in late life.
Kittner, et al. (1996) Pregnancy and the risk of stroke.	*Objective:* To quantify the risk of stroke associated with pregnancy *Findings:* The risks of both cerebral infarction and intracerebral hemorrhage are increased in the 6 weeks after delivery but not during pregnancy.
Thompson, et al. (1996) Effectiveness of bicycle safety helmets in preventing head injuries: A case-control study.	*Objective:* To examine the protective effectiveness of bicycle helmets in four different age groups of bicyclists, in crashes involving motor vehicles, and by helmet type and certification standards *Findings:* Bicycle helmets, regardless of type, provide substantial protection against head injuries for cyclists of all ages involved in crashes, including crashes involving motor vehicles.

Box continued on following page

Mejia & Pollack (1995) Variability in brain death determination practices in children.	*Objective:* To investigate variability in practices for determining brain death and organ procurement results in pediatric intensive care units *Findings:* Substantial variability exists in the criteria used by clinicians for the diagnosis of brain death. Some practices are contrary to the Guidelines for the Determination of Brain Death in Children and to recommendations for apnea testing.
Sosin, et al. (1995) Trends in death associated with traumatic brain injury, 1979–1992: Success and failure.	*Objective:* To report updates in national trends in traumatic brain injury deaths *Findings:* An average of 52,000 U.S. residents die each year with traumatic brain injury. The death rate declined 22% during the study period. Firearm-related deaths increased, whereas motor vehicle–related deaths decreased.
Andreasen, et al. (1994) Regional brain abnormalities in schizophrenia measured with magnetic resonance imaging.	*Objective:* To determine general and regional indices of structural brain abnormality in schizophrenia *Findings:* Compared with controls, the patients with schizophrenia had smaller average volume of frontal brain tissue and greater average volume of cerebrospinal fluid.
Amarenco, et al. (1994) Atherosclerotic disease of the aortic arch and the risk of ischemic stroke.	*Objective:* To quantify the risk of ischemic stroke associated with atherosclerotic disease of the aortic arch *Findings:* Patients with aortic arch plaques had a ninefold increased risk of ischemic stroke.
Rowe & Rowe (1994) Synthetic food coloring and behavior: A dose response effect in a double-blind, placebo-controlled, repeated-measures study.	*Objective:* To establish whether there is an association between the ingestion of synthetic food colorings and behavioral change in children referred for assessment of "hyperactivity" *Findings:* Behavioral changes in irritability, restlessness, and sleep disturbance are associated with the ingestion of tartrazine in some children.

Spina bifida cystica: incomplete fusion of one or more of the vertebrae, resulting in an external protrusion of the spinal tissue

Spina bifida occulta: incomplete fusion of one or more of the vertebrae, signaled only by an overlying dimple or tuft of hair[24]

Epidemiology. Anencephaly is the most frequently seen serious malformation, occurring in 0.1 to 0.7 cases per 1000 births. Females are affected three times more often than males, and the incidence is higher in certain geographic regions, including Ireland and England.[6] Encephalocele is the least common of the major NTDs, occurring one fifth as frequently as spina bifida cystica, which has an estimated incidence of 1 per 1000 births in the United States. Spina bifida occulta is believed to be common, occurring in as many as 25% of live births.

Family history, increased maternal age, poor prenatal care, and known exposure to teratogens increase the risk of birth defects in general. Studies have revealed an increased risk of NTDs in infants of women who are deficient in folic acid during early pregnancy[25] as well as in those of women who are obese.[26]

Etiology. The precise etiology of NTDs is unknown. Neural tube closure normally occurs first in the cranial region (at about 24 days' gestation), then more distally, closing finally in the lumbar region at about 26 days' gestation. Teratogenic insults occurring before 24 days could result in anencephaly or encephalocele, whereas those occurring before 26 days could also result in spina bifida.

Pathophysiology. Anencephalic infants lack any functional brain tissue, and scalp and cranial bones are absent. Although the brain stem, cerebellum, and spinal cord are present, they are abnormal. Low-level reflex function may be present but is insufficient to sustain life.

The degree of abnormality in patients with other NTDs varies widely. Encephalocele may present only as a small polyp, or it may be hidden in a nasal cavity, causing no dysfunction if the sac remains intact. Larger occipital encephaloceles may significantly disrupt CNS function, similarly to spina bifida cystica. In spina bifida occulta, the bony defect rarely affects the structure or function of the cord and peripheral nerve roots in the open segment (Fig. 21–24). Spina bifida cystica may manifest in two different forms: **meningocele,** in which only the meninges protrude in a CSF-filled sac; or **myelomeningocele,** in which peripheral nerves, their root segments, or the cord itself also protrudes. The abnormal configuration of the cord in myelomeningocele may result in varying degrees of sensory and motor dysfunction below the level of the lesion. The fluid-filled sac may rupture or leak, creating a route for the entry of microorganisms into the CSF.

Clinical Manifestations. Serum and amniotic fluid levels of α-fetoprotein and acetylcholinesterase are elevated in neural tube defects, serving as prenatal markers of the abnormal development (see Chapter 33). The anencephalic infant has a severe cranial abnormality that is immediately apparent at birth, and other organ development is also abnormal. Primitive reflexes may be present initially, but function deteriorates rapidly.

Clinical manifestations of encephalocele and spina bifida depend on the degree of disruption of neural tissue by the structural defect or associated infection. With larger encephaloceles, mental retardation, blindness, and motor disorders are usually seen. In spina bifida cystica, paralysis and loss of sensation below the level of the defect are common, as are associated bladder and bowel dysfunction. Skeletal abnormalities, such as developmental hip dysplasia, are frequently seen as a result of abnormal muscle stress on bones and joints. Spina bifida occulta may be detectable only on radiograph or may be noted as a dimple, small subcutaneous cyst, birthmark, or increased growth of hair in the lumbosacral region. Rarely, sensory or motor deficits, such as numbness, weakness, or gait disorders, may be present. Growth spurts may exacerbate symptoms during childhood.

Prevention and Treatment. Prevention of congenital disorders involves minimization of teratogenic exposure and optimal prenatal care. Dietary supplementation of folate is indicated, as is achievement of ideal body weight before pregnancy. Genetic testing is available for those with a family history of NTDs. Prenatal testing may confirm the presence of NTDs, leading to the possible option of termination of the pregnancy.

Treatment of anencephalic infants is supportive. Spina bifida occulta usually requires no intervention.

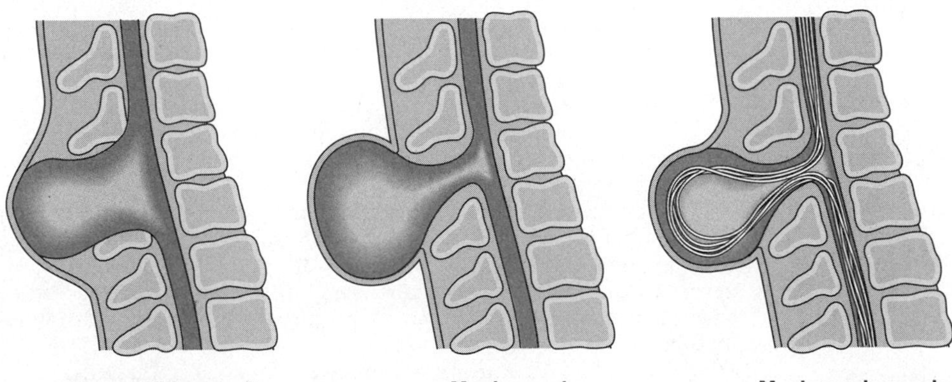

FIGURE 21–24

Forms of spina bifida. In *spina bifida occulta* (*A*), the vertebrae are incompletely fused, but no external sac is apparent, and functional deficits usually do not occur. The two forms of *spina bifida cystica* are meningocele (*B*) and myelomeningocele (*C*). In meningocele, an external sac is present, containing meninges and cerebrospinal fluid. In myelomeningocele, the protruding sac contains meninges, cerebrospinal fluid, peripheral nerves, and spinal cord tissue. Deficits in motor and sensory function below the level of the lesion are present to varying degrees in spina bifida cystica.

Encephalocele and spina bifida cystica are treated with surgical closure of the spine to reduce the risk of infection (e.g., **encephalitis** or meningitis) and with supportive and rehabilitative care related to motor and sensory deficits (see Chapter 22).

Prognosis and Outcome. Most anencephalic infants (65%) die in utero; those born alive die within a few days.[6] In patients with other types of NTD, outcome is variable depending on the extent of the functional deficits and the effectiveness of measures for prevention of associated risks.

Meningitis

Definition. Meningitis is acute or chronic inflammation of the pia mater and arachnoid membranes. Two principal forms are seen: *bacterial meningitis,* in which causative bacteria may be cultured from the CSF, and *aseptic meningitis,* in which the CSF culture is negative. Other, less common infectious disorders of the nervous system are briefly reviewed in Table 21–17.

Epidemiology. The incidence of bacterial meningitis is highest in children younger than 5 years and has been estimated to occur in 26 to 40 per 100,000 children per year in the United States.[27] Those at particular risk are infants with NTDs immunusuppressed patients, and those with neurotrauma. Healthy infants, children, adolescents, and young adults are most susceptible to *epidemic meningitis,* in which causative organisms are spread through contact with oral or respiratory secretions within day care centers, schools, and social settings. Chronic

TABLE 21–17
INFECTIOUS DISORDERS OF THE NERVOUS SYSTEM

Disorder	Clinical Features
Bacterial Infections	
Bacterial meningitis	Inflammation of pia mater and arachnoid membranes due to bacterial infection; highest incidence in children younger than 5 years; manifests as nuchal rigidity (stiff neck) and increased intracranial pressure
Tuberculous meningitis	May follow invasion of respiratory system by tubercle bacillus, especially in immunosuppressed patients (e.g., patients with acquired immunodeficiency syndrome)
Lyme disease	Infection of both peripheral and central nervous system by tick-borne bacterial spirochete *Borrelia burgdorferi;* endemic in Midwest, western wooded and coastal areas, and northeastern coast of United States; immune complex deposition in tissues and joints, causing inflammation; neural manifestations of meningitis, encephalitis, peripheral neuropathy, and radiculopathy
Brain abscess	Area of encapsulated or free pus in the brain parenchyma, between the bone and the dura mater, or in the subdural space; caused by infection entering through the blood, the sinuses, or a penetrating head wound
Viral Infections	
Aseptic meningitis	Inflammation of pia mater and arachnoid in which cerebrospinal fluid culture is negative; viral cause is usual, e.g., cytomegalovirus, enterovirus
Acute encephalitis	Acute viral infection of the brain parenchyma and meninges; usually caused by arthropod-borne arboviruses (e.g., St. Louis encephalitis, Eastern equine encephalitis) in epidemics; mild to severe inflammation without pus formation but causing edema, vascular lesions, myelin destruction, nerve cell degeneration or necrosis, and possibly hemorrhage
Herpes simplex encephalitis	Severe herpes simplex virus infection of the brain, usually transmitted intrapartally from mother to infant or occurring as an isolated infection
Creutzfeldt-Jakob disease	Rare disease caused by a "slow virus" or prion; rapidly fatal, causing progressive dementia and total incapacitation within weeks to months; cerebral cortex and basal ganglia are most affected, with atrophy occurring in the absence of inflammation
Rabies	Caused by highly neurotropic viruses, usually of the Rhabdovirus family, transmitted by the bites of infected animals; the virus enters the central nervous system unmyelinated nerve terminals and is sequestered from the immune system; encephalitis and peripheral neuropathy develop rapidly; peripheral nerves to salivary glands are also affected, and the virus is shed in the saliva; usual outcome without treatment is death within 2 weeks; vaccination of domestic animals has reduced incidence of rabies to almost negligible levels in the United States.

Data from Metcalf, J. (1994). Neurologic infections. In: Barker, E. *Neuroscience Nursing*. St. Louis: Mosby–Year Book; and Fishbein, D.B., and Robinson, L.E. (1993). Rabies. *New England Journal of Medicine* 329(22), 1632–1638.

middle ear, mastoid, and sinus infections predispose to meningitis because organisms may penetrate the bony barrier between these structures and the CNS. Encephalitis, inflammation of the brain tissue, may easily result in inflammation of adjacent meninges by direct extension.

Aseptic meningitis has an annual incidence of 11 to 27 cases per 100,000.[28] This syndrome is usually viral, most often transmitted by the fecal–oral route. Unusual bacteria may also cause aseptic meningitis, and the syndrome may be a component of rabies and Lyme disease, infections borne by animal vectors (Table 21–18). Risk factors for aseptic meningitis include young age, exposure to vectors (such as mosquitoes and ticks), immunosuppression, and prior history of meningitis.[29]

Etiology. Table 21–18 lists organisms most frequently implicated in causing bacterial and aseptic meningitis. In most cases, microorganisms enter the CNS through the blood. Less commonly, organisms gain entry by ascending infection of peripheral nerves or through erosion of bone. Penetrating trauma, such as skull fractures or cranial surgery, may allow direct access of microorganisms to the meninges. In some cases, meningitis may have a chemical rather than an infectious cause. Toxins, such as intrathecal drugs (which are injected into the CSF) or tumor cytokines, may directly trigger meningeal inflammation.

Pathophysiology. The route of entry of bloodborne organisms into the intact CNS is uncertain. Some studies indicate that invasion may occur through the choroid plexus (across the blood–CSF barrier) or within monocytes as a component of normal cellular movement.[30] Penetrating trauma facilitates direct entry of organisms. An inflammatory response occurs within the enclosed cranial vault. Usually, inflammation is much greater with bacterial infections than with viral infections. In accordance with the **Monro-Kellie doctrine** (discussed subsequently), intracranial pressure may ultimately rise. Pain receptors in the meninges are stimulated.

Clinical Manifestations. The classic manifestations of meningitis are nuchal rigidity (stiff neck), severe headache, and other manifestations of IICP. Visual deficits and seizures may be present as a consequence of inflammatory mediators, vascular deficiency, or direct pressure on cerebral structures. Examination of CSF reveals the presence of inflammation: increased leukocyte count, increased protein content, normal or decreased glucose content, increased CSF pressure, and in bacterial meningitis, increased lactate and presence of the causative organism. Some organisms, notably meningococcus and echovirus, are associated with characteristic skin rashes (meningitis streaks) because of involvement

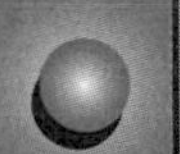

TABLE 21–18
USUAL CAUSES OF MENINGITIS

BACTERIAL MENINGITIS

In neonates: *Escherichia coli;* group B streptococci
In adolescents and young adults: *Neisseria meningitidis*
In the elderly: *Streptococcus pneumoniae; Listeria monocytogenes*

ASEPTIC MENINGITIS

Infectious Etiologies
Bacterial: *Mycobacterium tuberculosis,* brain abscess, bacterial endocarditis, *Brucella* and *Listeria* sp.
Fungal: *Candida albicans, Coccidioides immitis, Cryptococcus neoformans, Histoplasma capsulatum*
Mycoplasmal: *Mycoplasma pneumoniae, Mycoplasma hominis* (in neonates)
Nematodal: Eosinophilic meningitis due to rat worm larvae
Protozoal: *Toxoplasma gondii, Plasmodium* sp., amebae, visceral larva migrans
Rickettsial: Rocky Mountain spotted fever, Q fever, typhus
Spirochetal: Syphilis, leptospirosis, Lyme disease
Viral: Enteroviruses, mumps virus, lymphocytic choriomeningitis agent, Epstein-Barr virus, arboviruses, cytomegalovirus, varicella zoster virus, herpes simplex virus, human immunodeficiency virus

Malignant Etiologies
Primary medulloblastoma, metastatic leukemia, lymphoma, Hodgkin's disease, metastatic carcinomatosis, craniopharyngioma

Noninfectious Diseases Associated With Meningitis
Autoimmune disease: Guillain-Barré syndrome
Collagen-vascular disease: systemic lupus erythematosus, Sjögren's syndrome
Direct toxin exposure: intrathecal injections of contrast media, spinal anesthesia
Granulomatous disease: sarcoidosis
Poisoning: lead, mercury
Trauma: subarachnoid hemorrhage, traumatic lumbar puncture, neurosurgery

Medications
Sulfamethoxazole, trimethoprim, nonsteroidal anti-inflammatory agents, carbamazepine, isoniazid, penicillin

Vaccinations
Mumps, measles

Miscellaneous
Behçet's syndrome, Kawasaki disease, Mollaret's meningitis, multiple sclerosis, diseases of unknown etiology

Data on bacterial meningitis from Cotran, R.S., Kumar, V., and Robbins S.L. (Eds.). (1994). *Robbins Pathologic Basis of Disease.* (5th ed.). Philadelphia: W.B. Saunders.

Data on aseptic meningitis from Nelson, S., Sealy, D.P., and Schneider, E.F. (1993). The aseptic meningitis syndrome. *American Family Physician* 48(5), 809–815. Abstracted from Table 1, p. 812.

of peripheral blood vessels. Hydrocephalus may occur as a result of obstruction of CSF circulation or reabsorption, as discussed later.

Prevention and Treatment. Reduction of risk for meningitis involves limiting exposure to pathogens and providing optimal treatment of underlying conditions, such as chronic sinus infections, otitis media, and mastoiditis. Bacterial meningitis is treated with specific antibiotics. These drugs usually can penetrate the blood–brain barrier in the inflamed area because of the increased permeability induced by inflammation (see Chapter 13). Antibiotics are not effective in the treatment of viral meningitis; but in most cases, this disorder is less severe than the bacterial form and requires only supportive care until it runs its self-limited course. Intracranial pressure is usually not elevated to a degree requiring aggressive intervention. Persistent hydrocephalus is treated with shunting, as discussed later.

Prognosis and Outcome. If untreated, bacterial meningitis is usually fatal. Since the advent of antibiotic therapy, however, bacterial meningitis is not the deadly disease it once was. Although some patients have residual functional deficits or hydrocephalus, most recover fully. The mortality rate in patients who are optimally treated has been estimated at 5% to 15% for those infected with *Haemophilus influenzae* or meningococcus. Pneumococcal meningitis has a higher mortality rate of 15% to 30%. Mortality is highest among neonates and the elderly.[6]

Aseptic meningitis usually has a benign course, with full recovery. About 1% of cases are complicated by encephalitis, which may leave the patient with chronic fatigue syndrome, ataxia, muscle weakness, or language deficits.[29]

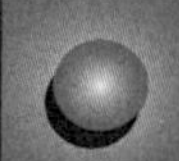

TABLE 21–19
REVERSIBLE CAUSES OF SEIZURES

Cerebral hypoperfusion or hypoxia
Cardiac arrest, cardiac dysrhythmia, severe hypotension
Meningitis or encephalitis
Bacterial or aseptic
Hyponatremia
Serum Na below 104–118 mEq/L, especially if rapid fall
Hypoglycemia
20–30 mg/dL
Hypernatremia, hyperosmolar nonketotic state
Serum osmolarity greater than 330 mOsm/L
Hypocalcemia
4.3–9.2 mg/dL
Encephalopathy
Associated with malignant hypertension, uremia, hepatic failure
Eclampsia
High-risk pregnancy; associated with hypertension and toxicity
Drug overdose
Tricyclic antidepressants, theophylline, aminophylline, phencyclidine, lidocaine, phenothiazines, isoniazid
Drug withdrawal
Antiepileptics, ethanol, sedative-hypnotics
Hyperthermia
Benign febrile seizures of childhood, temperature >107°F in adults

Data from Simon, R.P., Aminoff, M.J., and Greenberg, D.A. (1989). *Clinical Neurology*. Norwalk, CT: Appleton & Lange. Adapted from Table 9-1, p. 204.

Epilepsy

Definition. Epilepsy is a disorder characterized by recurrent **seizure** activity without reversible cause. Seizures (also referred to as *convulsions*) are paroxysmal episodes of spontaneous, uncontrolled neurotransmission evidenced on the EEG as well as by changes in motor, sensory, or behavioral activity. Seizures resulting from reversible causes are associated with a number of conditions (Table 21–19) and do not constitute epilepsy.

Epidemiology. An estimated 2 million people in the United States have been diagnosed with epilepsy.[31] The incidence is highest in childhood and old age. Risk factors for epilepsy include intracranial lesions or toxic conditions affecting cortical neurotransmission, such as birth trauma, head injury, brain tumor, stroke, and encephalitis. In many cases, however, there are no apparent risk factors.

Etiology. *Primary epilepsy,* in which there is no structural abnormality of the brain, is idiopathic. *Secondary epilepsy* is caused by structural or metabolic disruption of neuronal membranes, resulting in increased automaticity.

Pathophysiology. Individual neurons in the affected areas generate massive, excitatory depolarizations that are believed to result from failure of normal inhibitory mechanisms (decreased GABA activity) or local electrolyte shifts.

Clinical Manifestations. Epilepsies are classified based on the nature and patterns of abnormal activity that result from the abnormal neurotransmission (Table 21–20). *Generalized epilepsies* are characterized by widespread involvement of the brain, bilateral motor manifestations, and impaired consciousness during the seizure episode. *Partial epilepsies* demonstrate abnormal discharge limited to one hemisphere or to a focal area of the brain. With *simple partial* seizures, there is no impairment of consciousness; with *complex partial* seizures, consciousness is impaired to some degree. Figure 21–25 illustrates typi-

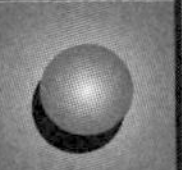

TABLE 21–20
INTERNATIONAL CLASSIFICATION OF EPILEPTIC SEIZURES

I. **Partial seizures (beginning locally):**
   A. Simple partial seizures: without impaired consciousness
      1. With motor symptoms: twitching of an arm or leg (formerly *jacksonian seizure*), speech arrest, vocalizations
      2. With somatosensory or special sensory symptoms: visual or auditory hallucinations, flashing lights
      3. With autonomic symptoms: pallor, sweating, flushing, piloerection
      4. With psychological symptoms: fear, sense of impending doom
   B. Complex partial seizures (with impaired consciousness; formerly *psychomotor* or *temporal lobe seizures*)
      1. Simple partial onset followed by impaired consciousness: automatisms (lip smacking, chewing, picking at clothes) possible; confusion after seizure (postictal confusion)
      2. Impaired consciousness at onset: automatisms possible; postictal confusion
   C. Partial seizures evolving into secondary generalized (tonic-clonic) seizures (see below)

II. **Generalized seizures (convulsive or nonconvulsive):** involve both hemispheres at outset; consciousness immediately impaired in most types
   A. Absence seizures (formerly *petit mal* seizures): brief loss of consciousness (10–15 s): possible automatisms or atony (loss of muscle tone)
   B. Myoclonic seizures: jerking of single or multiple muscle groups; consciousness usually preserved; occur early in the morning
   C. Atonic seizures (drop attacks): loss of muscle tone; brief impairment of consciousness
   D. Tonic-clonic seizures (formerly *grand mal* seizures): begin bilaterally; *tonic phase:* muscles become rigid, rigidity of respiratory muscles may cause a cry or moan, patient may stop breathing briefly and become cyanotic; *clonic phase:* rhythmic jerking of muscles, patient remains cyanotic but breathes deeply at end of seizure; tongue biting and incontinence may occur; confusion, headache, and sleep may follow seizure; tonic only, clonic only, and tonic-clonic-tonic patterns may also occur

III. **Unclassified seizures:** atypical nature; includes some neonatal seizures

Categories from the Commission on Classification and Terminology of the International League Against Epilepsy.

cal brain wave patterns seen with different forms of seizures.

Prevention and Treatment. Optimal management of the underlying causes of secondary epilepsies may reduce the frequency of seizures. The mainstay of therapy in all epilepsies is antiepileptic drug therapy (Table 21–21). Surgical treatment is limited to rare cases in which epilepsy is unresponsive to drug therapy and is severely disabling to function.[31] These operations include resection of the cortical region in which seizure activity originates, creation of an ablative lesion in the region of origin, and sectioning of the *corpus callosum* between the hemispheres to limit the spread of abnormal neurotransmission to one hemisphere. Intervention during seizures, particularly the generalized grand mal type, is aimed at protecting the patient from injury by turning the patient to the side so that oral secretions can drain and by gently restricting arm and leg movement to prevent injury during muscle contraction.

Prognosis and Outcome. Epilepsy is highly responsive to drug treatment in 80% of cases.[31] Surgery is curative in many other cases. **Status epilepticus,** a medical emergency in which seizure activity is continuous for a prolonged period, may prove fatal because of cardiac failure or stroke induced by the hypermetabolic state. This condition nearly always results from improper compliance with prescribed drug therapy.

Increased Intracranial Pressure

Definition. IICP (intracranial hypertension) is defined as the clinical syndrome resulting from interstitial and intraventricular fluid pressure in excess of 15 mm Hg within the cranial vault.

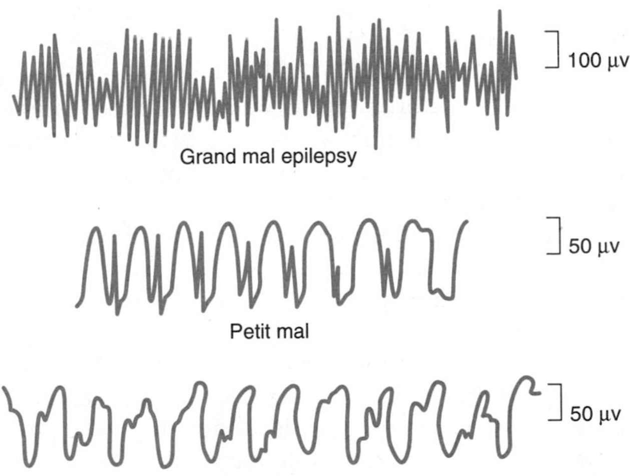

FIGURE 21–25
Brain wave patterns during seizures. During generalized tonic-clonic (grand mal) seizures, high-voltage, high-frequency activity is generated over the entire cortex. During generalized absence (petit mal) seizures, a spike-and-dome pattern is recorded over most or all of the cortex. Complex partial (psychomotor) seizures manifest as abnormal patterns originating from a localized region of the cortex. (From Guyton, A.C., and Hall, J.E. [1996]. *Textbook of Medical Physiology*. [9th ed.]. Philadelphia: W.B. Saunders. [p. 766].)

TABLE 21–21
ANTIEPILEPTIC DRUGS

Drug	Mechanism of Action	Clinical Use
Carbamazapine (Tegretol)	Prevents repetitive firing of action potentials in depolarized neurons through blockade of sodium channels	Partial and generalized tonic-clonic seizures
Phenytoin (Dilantin)	Induces blockade of sodium channels	Partial and generalized tonic-clonic seizures
Valproic acid (Depakene) Divalproex (Depakote)	Induces blockade of sodium channels; has other effects that are not well understood	All seizure types
Phenobarbital Primidone (Mysoline)	Prolongs inhibitory postsynaptic potentials by prolonging chloride channel opening, thus inducing GABA-ergic activity	Partial and generalized tonic-clonic seizures
Ethosuximide (Zarontin)	Reduces calcium conductance in thalamic neurons	Absence seizures
Clonazepam (Clonopin)	Enhances inhibitory effects at GABA-ergic synapses	Myoclonic seizures that do not respond to other agents
Gabapentin (Neurontin)	Uncertain; inhibits voltage-sodium currents and may enhance GABA actions	Partial seizures alone or with secondary generalized seizures; used as an add-on drug
Lamotrigine (Lamictal)	Inhibits sodium currents	Partial seizures alone or with secondary generalized seizures
Felbamate (Felbatol)	Incompletely understood; reduces sodium currents, enhances GABA actions, and blocks excitatory NMDA (glutamate) receptors.	Partial seizures alone or with secondary generalized seizures

GABA, γ-aminobutyric acid; NMDA, *N*-methyl-D-aspartate.
Data from Brodie, M.J., and Dichter, M.A. (1996). Antiepileptic drugs. *New England Journal of Medicine* 334(3), 168–175; and Dichter, M.A., and Brodie, M.J. (1996). New antiepileptic drugs. *New England Journal of Medicine* 334(24), 1583–1590.

Epidemiology. IICP is associated with a number of clinical conditions in which the intracranial volume of blood, CSF, or brain tissue is increased. Incidence and risk factors for IICP are those underlying the associated disorders (see later). The most important conditions potentially resulting in IICP are traumatic brain injury, brain tumors, and stroke, discussed later in this chapter.

Etiology. According to the Monro-Kellie doctrine, the volumes of blood, CSF, and brain tissue are at equilibrium within the closed cranial vault (Fig. 21–26). If any one of these components increases in volume, a rise in intracranial pressure occurs, unless another component is able to decrease its occupied space. Initially, as volume is added to the cranial vault, CSF moves from intracranial compartments into the subarachnoid space surrounding the spinal cord. Venous blood also shunts from the cerebral circulation to the systemic circulation. Once these compensatory mechanisms are exhausted, however, intracranial pressure begins to increase (Fig. 21–27). Although the precise mechanisms are incompletely understood, compensation for IICP is much more effective if the rise in intracranial volume occurs slowly rather than rapidly.[32]

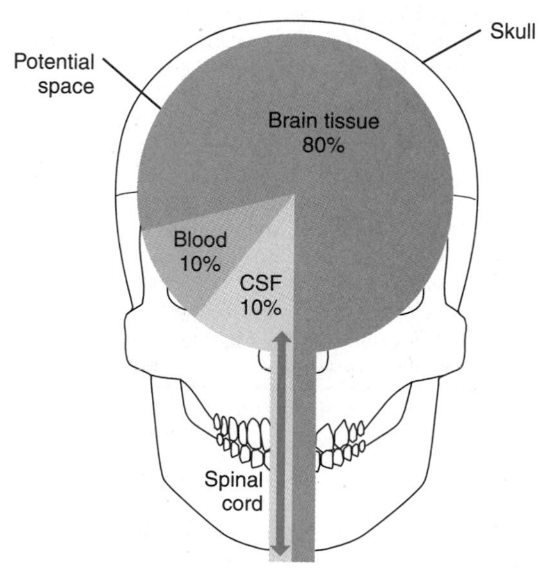

FIGURE 21–26
Monro-Kellie doctrine. Because the volumes of blood, cerebrospinal fluid, and brain tissue are at equilibrium within the closed cranial vault, an increase in any one of these compartments causes a rise in intracranial pressure unless the space occupied by another compartment decreases. CSF, cerebrospinal fluid. (Redrawn from Barker, E. [1994]. *Neuroscience Nursing*. St Louis: Mosby–Year Book. [p. 297].)

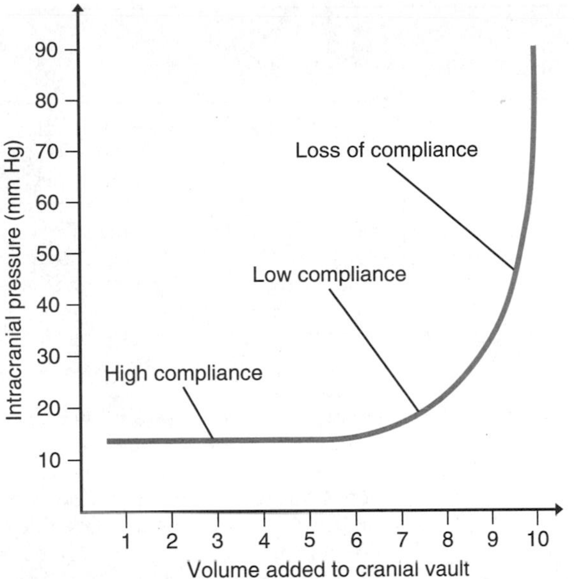

FIGURE 21–27

Cerebral compliance curve. When volume is added to the cranial vault, there is initially no change in intracranial pressure because of compensatory changes. As compensatory mechanisms are overcome (i.e., compliance is lost), intracranial pressure rises.

An increase in CSF volume usually results from abnormality of CSF circulation, as discussed further in the section on hydrocephalus. Blood volume may rise in conditions that impede venous outflow, in fluid overload states, with vascular lesions such as aneurysms or **arteriovenous malformations (AVMs),** or with intracranial hemorrhage and hematoma formation. Local autoregulatory factors resulting in vasodilation also increase cerebral blood volume. These include increased P_{CO_2}, decreased P_{O_2}, decreased pH, and endothelial regulators, such as nitric oxide (see Chapter 15). Brain tissue volume increases with inflammatory edema (see Chapter 13) or with space-occupying neoplasms.

Pathophysiology. Consistent with Starling's law of the capillary, intracranial pressure (positive tissue hydrostatic pressure) represents a force opposing capillary filtration, thus a rising intracranial pressure impedes *cerebral perfusion pressure* (CPP), which drives diffusion of nutrients and oxygen between the cerebral capillary blood and brain cells. Because the brain is incapable of storing large quantities of glycogen, it requires a continuous supply of oxygen and glucose through the bloodstream. Cerebral blood flow is therefore tightly autoregulated (see Chapter 15).

CPP may be calculated from mean arterial pressure (MAP) and intracranial pressure (ICP), as follows:

$$CPP = MAP - ICP$$

CPP is normally autoregulated by local mediators, remaining constant across an MAP range of 50 to 160 mm Hg. With CNS infection, neoplasia, or trauma, however, this local regulation is disrupted, and CPP fluctuates acutely with changes in MAP and ICP.[33] MAP may fall or ICP may rise to the point at which cerebral vessels are compressed and tissues are not adequately perfused with blood, resulting in ischemia.

With the exception of the fontanels in infants, the cranial vault is open only at the optic foramina and the foramen magnum. Brain tissue may be forced outward through these openings with IICP, resulting in damage to herniated brain tissue and pressure on adjacent structures. Figure 21–28 illustrates possible

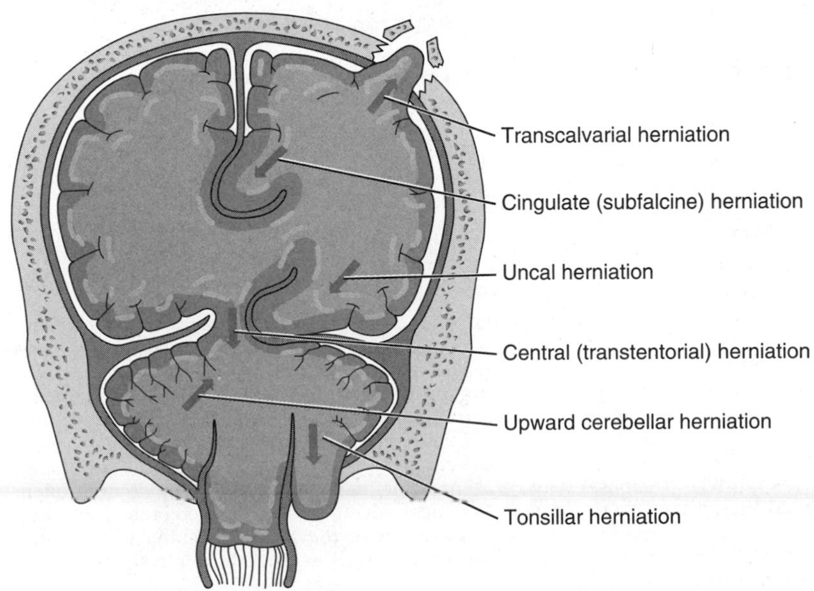

FIGURE 21–28

Cerebral herniation syndromes. Increasing intracranial pressure may induce shifting of brain tissue within the cranial vault, downward protrusion through the foramen magnum, or outward protrusion through defects in the cranium. *Transcalvarial herniation* occurs when severe intracranial pressure forces tissue through a skull fracture, craniotomy site, or fontanel. *Cingulate herniation* occurs when an expanding lesion of one hemisphere causes lateral shifting of the cingulate gyrus under the falx cerebri. *Uncal herniation* results from an expanding temporal lobe lesion, which causes the tip (uncus) of the lobe to be displaced laterally. In *central herniation,* an expanding midline mass causes downward displacement of cortical tissue, the basal ganglia, the hypothalamus, and the thalamus. In *upward cerebellar herniation,* a cerebellar mass causes upward protrusion of the central cerebellum and midbrain through the tentorial notch. *Downward (tonsillar) herniation* occurs when a cerebellar mass forces cerebellar tissue downward through the foramen magnum.

TABLE 21-22
ABNORMAL CRANIAL NERVE (CN) REFLEXES WITH INTRACRANIAL PATHOLOGY

REFLEX	NORMAL	ABNORMAL/SIGNIFICANCE
Pupillary (CN III)	Direct: Pupil constricts briskly in response to light. Consensual: opposite pupil also constricts.	Dilated, nonreactive pupil indicates CN III compression; pinpoint, nonreactive pupils indicate interruption of sympathetic pathways. (*Note:* Many drugs as well as direct eye trauma may also cause abnormal pupils.)
Corneal (CNs V and VII)	Corneal contact with wisp of cotton causes blink in both eyes.	Loss of the reflex indicates a lesion of the affected nerves or their central connections in the pons.
Oculocephalic ("doll's eyes"; CNs III, IV, VI, and medial longitudinal fasciculus of brain stem)	Both eyes deviate to the opposite direction when head is turned.	Eye roving or disconjugate movement of the eyes indicates some degree of brain-stem injury; absent reflex, in which eyes remain midline and move with the head, indicates significant brain-stem injury.
Oculovestibular (cold caloric; same structures as doll's eyes)	Rapid jerky eye movements (nystagmus) are in direction of ear irrigated with ice water.	Disconjugate eye movement indicates a brain-stem lesion; no response indicates little or no brain-stem function.

patterns of herniation. Of greatest concern are the herniation syndromes that affect the critical control centers in the medulla of the brain stem. These syndromes may culminate in respiratory arrest, cardiac arrest, or vascular collapse.

Clinical Manifestations. Neurologic effects of IICP include headache due to stimulation of pain receptors in cerebral vessels and meninges. Brain tissue does not contain pain receptors. Absent or abnormal reflexes may manifest as abnormal sensation or motor activity, owing to pressure on sensory or motor integrative areas. Because most pathways cross, manifestations such as weakness or paralysis frequently affect the side of the body opposite the cranial lesion. Primitive motor reflexes, which normally would be inhibited by higher-level function, may reemerge (see Chapter 22). Visual changes, such as *diplopia* (double vision), loss of visual activity, and pupil dilation, may result from pressure on cranial nerves II, III, IV, and VI, which regulate vision. Other cranial nerve reflexes, including the corneal, oculocephalic, and oculovestibular reflexes, may eventually be lost (see Fig. 23-17). Table 21-22 summarizes the effects of IICP on cranial nerve reflexes.

Impaired spinal reflexes may manifest as abnormal postural responses (Fig. 21-29). Abnormal body temperature (usually hyperthermia) is common because of disruption of hypothalamic thermoregulation (see Chapter 11). Level of consciousness and orientation may be decreased if pressure affects integrative areas of the cerebrum or the RAS of the brain stem. Pressure behind the optic foramina may

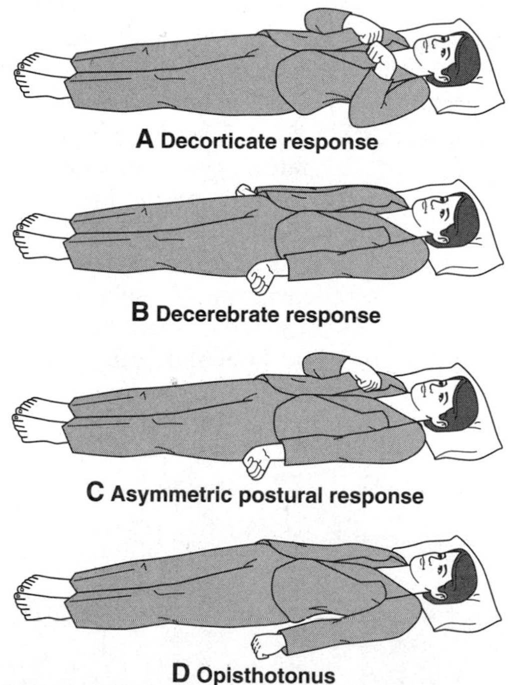

FIGURE 21-29
Abnormal postural responses. Increased intracranial pressure and other brain injury may manifest as abnormal postural responses due to loss of higher level regulation of motor activity. *A, Decorticate (flexor) posturing* results from injury or metabolic abnormality affecting the cerebral hemispheres, basal ganglia, hypothalamus, and thalamus. *B, Decerebrate (extensor) posturing* indicates more extensive injury affecting the midbrain and pons. *C,* Postural responses may be asymmetric, depending on the underlying lesion. *D, Opisthotonos,* the most severe form of decerebrate posturing, manifests as rigid extension of the head, clenching of the teeth, and arching of the back as well as an extensor response of the extremities.

cause orbital edema (swelling around the eyes) and **papilledema** (edema of the optic disc of the retina). If cranial bones are not fused, fontanels bulge.

The cardiovascular and respiratory systems are potentially affected by pressure on medullary control centers and by autoregulatory mechanisms. Bradycardia, widened pulse pressure, and slow, deep respirations are typical signs of IICP and are collectively termed *Cushing's triad.* Bradycardia and altered respiratory patterns are believed to result from pressure on the cardioregulatory center and respiratory centers in the medulla and pons (Fig. 21–30). Widened pulse pressure is the result of a rise in systolic blood pressure due to the CNS ischemic response (see Chapter 15). Neurogenic pulmonary edema may contribute to respiratory failure (see Chapter 19).

Although vomiting often occurs as a gastrointestinal manifestation of IICP, it is atypical in that it is not preceded by nausea. Rather, it is believed to result from disruption of the vomiting reflex, which involves chemoreceptor trigger zones (receptor areas for drugs and toxins) and the brain-stem neurons that constitute the vomiting center (see Chapter 24). Stress ulceration with gastrointestinal bleeding frequently accompanies IICP.

Prevention and Treatment. Prevention depends on risk reduction for contributing conditions and, in clinical settings, careful monitoring of patients who may develop IICP. Such monitoring includes physical assessment to detect any of the manifestations described previously. Interstitial fluid pressure in the brain may be monitored invasively using mechanical sensors placed on the dural surface or catheters placed beneath the dura. CSF pressure may be measured by a catheter placed in a ventricle. Some monitoring systems allow manual or automatic drainage of CSF if pressure rises above a certain threshold point. Lumbar puncture ("spinal tap"), in which a needle is inserted into the subarachnoid space of the cord, allows direct measurement of CSF pressure. This procedure must be done with extreme caution when IICP is suspected, however, because sudden drainage of CSF may potentiate tonsillar herniation and even hemorrhage (if brain tissue pulls away from the dura mater as pressure suddenly drops).

Patients with significant IICP are usually mechanically ventilated to maintain tight control of PO_2 and PCO_2. Oxygenation is maximized, and the patient is usually hyperventilated to produce a low PCO_2, theoretically preventing cerebral vasodilation by autoregulatory mechanisms. Because the ability of the cerebrovascular system to respond to CO_2 is reduced in cerebral injury, however, the efficacy of this intervention has been questioned.[34] Furthermore, when hyperventilation does result in reduced cerebral blood flow, it is uncertain whether this decreased flow worsens cerebral hypoxia or is protective against the ischemic pressure effects.

Care is taken to prevent sudden increases in blood pressure, such as might occur with Valsalva maneuver (see Chapter 15) or with pain and stress. If necessary, the patient is sedated or given neuromuscular blocking drugs to induce paralysis. In patients in whom intracranial pressure rises rapidly,

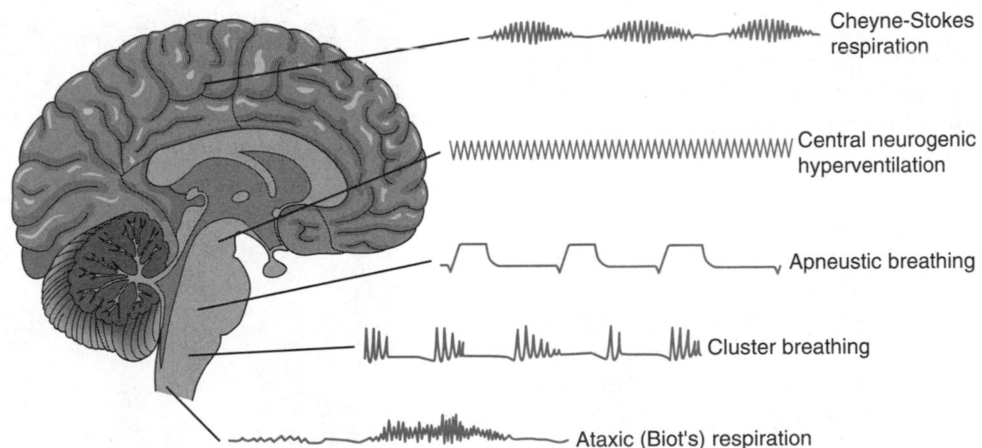

FIGURE 21–30
Altered ventilation in central nervous system dysfunction. *Cheyne-Stokes ventilation,* a waxing and waning pattern with brief apneic periods, is typical with bilateral deep cerebral lesions or cerebellar lesions. *Central neurogenic hyperventilation,* manifested by rapid, deep breathing, is usually seen with lesions of the midbrain and pons. *Apneustic breathing,* with prolonged inspiratory and expiratory pauses, is typical of pontine lesions. *Cluster breathing,* with alternating periods of apnea and gasping respirations, is typical of lesions of the lower pons and upper medulla. *Ataxic (Biot's) respirations* are totally irregular and result from medullary lesions. (Redrawn from Barker, E. [1994]. *Neuroscience Nursing.* St. Louis: Mosby–Year Book. [p. 305].)

coma may be therapeutically induced with barbiturate drugs to minimize the cerebral metabolic demands. Osmotic diuretics are used to increase serum osmolarity, inducing an interstitial-to-plasma fluid shift and dehydrating the brain. Loop diuretics decrease fluid volume and also have a direct effect on the choroid plexus to decrease CSF production. Replacement of fluid losses with isotonic or hypertonic saline maintains the osmolar effect.

Burr holes may be drilled in the patient's skull, or a flap of cranial bone may be removed to create space for the edematous brain to expand. *Craniotomy* (surgical incision of the cranial vault) may be done to remove a space-occupying lesion such as a tumor, aneurysm, or **hematoma.** Therapy appropriate to the patient's underlying condition is instituted, and the patient is supported until IICP subsides.

Prognosis and Outcome. Outcome is determined by the severity of the underlying disorder and the efficacy of treatment in restoring and maintaining cerebral perfusion. Without intervention, a sustained IICP above 20 mm Hg triggers a positive feedback loop that culminates in death due to herniation.[33]

Hydrocephalus

Definition. Hydrocephalus is an excessive volume of CSF, resulting in increased intracranial volume or pressure. Hydrocephalus is classified as *noncommunicating (obstructive)* if CSF circulation is blocked or as *communicating (nonobstructive)* if CSF is overproduced or if CSF outflow is deficient.

Epidemiology. Congenital hydrocephalus occurs in 0.5% to 1.8% of live births.[35] The precise incidence of acquired hydrocephalus is uncertain. Risk factors in infants include intrauterine infection and intracranial hemorrhage associated with birth trauma or prematurity. Meningitis, mastoiditis, and chronic otitis media are risk factors in older children and adults. Aging is associated with an increased incidence of an idiopathic type of hydrocephalus known as **normal-pressure hydrocephalus (NPH).** NPH may also follow subarachoid hemorrhage, meningitis, head trauma, Paget's disease of the skull, and mucopolysaccharidosis of the meninges.[36] Patients of any age with brain tumors or intracranial hemorrhage are at risk for hydrocephalus due to obstruction.

Etiology. Hydrocephalus may result from either genetic or acquired mechanisms. Congenital narrowing of a circulatory channel (aqueductal stenosis) may be due to X-linked recessive inheritance, and failure of development (agenesis) of the arachnoid villi has also been linked to a genetic defect. Nongenetic causes include obstruction of CSF flow between the ventricles and the subarachnoid space and plugging of arachnoid villi by blood clots, fibrin, or tumor cells (as in CNS hemorrhage, infection, or neoplasia). Venous insufficiency associated with otitis media or mastoiditis may result in venous clots obstructing the dural sinuses. Oversecretion of CSF is an uncommon cause of hydrocephalus but may occur with tumors affecting the choroid plexus.

Pathophysiology. In most cases of hydrocephalus, both CSF volume and pressure are increased. Consistent with the Monro-Kellie doctrine, brain tissue and cerebral blood vessels are compressed. In NPH, CSF volume is increased, but CSF pressure is, at least intermittently, normal. In some cases, the normal pressure may be attributed to a concurrent decrease in brain volume (i.e., neuronal atrophy).

Clinical Manifestations. Except in NPH, clinical manifestations are those of IICP. In infants, the cranial circumference is enlarged, the eyes are turned downward ("sunset" sign), the scalp is thin with prominent veins, and the sutures are separated (Fig. 21–31). A "cracked pot" sound (Macewen's sign) is elicited with percussion of the head. NPH usually is accompanied by dementia, gait disorder (ataxia), and urinary incontinence. Although overt signs of IICP are absent in NPH, papilledema may be present.

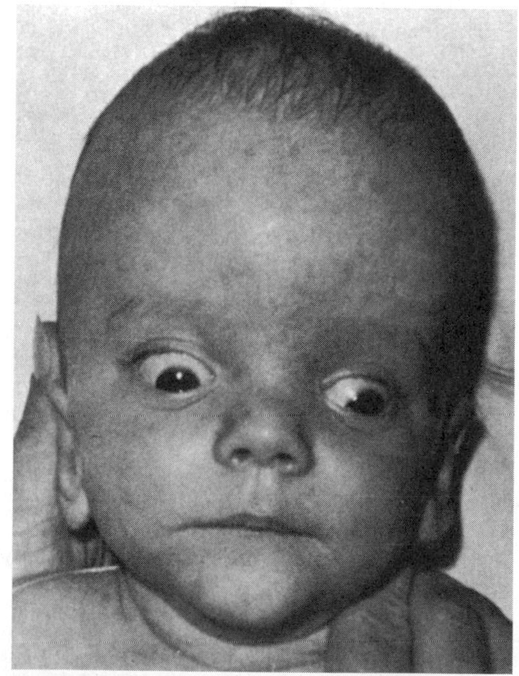

FIGURE 21–31
Infant with hydrocephalus. Increased head circumference and "sunset" eyes are apparent. (From Youmans, J.R. [1982]. *Neurological Surgery.* [2nd ed.]. Volume 3. Philadelphia: W.B. Saunders. [p. 1384].)

Prevention and Treatment. Patients with underlying conditions associated with hydrocephalus should be treated appropriately and must be monitored closely to detect IICP at an early stage, before the development of pressure trauma or ischemia affecting brain structures. The treatment of choice for hydrocephalus is surgical shunting of CSF from the ventricles of the brain to a reservoir implanted beneath the scalp. This reservoir then may empty in response to CSF pressure or manual pumping into the heart, jugular vein, or peritoneal cavity (Fig. 21–32).

Prognosis and Outcome. In untreated infants, hydrocephalus is associated with a 50% mortality rate by 1 year of age and a 75% mortality rate by 10 years of age. In cases in which hydrocephalus is optimally treated with shunting, mortality varies depending on the underlying condition and on the development of shunt-related complications, such as intracranial hemorrhage or infection. About 15% of children suffer associated developmental disabilities. Sixty percent of patients with NPH improve with treatment.[35]

Traumatic Brain Injury

Definition. Traumatic brain injury is physical damage to, or functional impairment of, the cranial contents from acute mechanical energy exchange.[37]

Epidemiology. Head injury is the third leading cause of death and the most common cause of brain damage in people younger than 40 years in the United States.[38] Two million Americans suffer head injuries each year, leading to 100,000 deaths, 750,000 hospitalizations, and 50,000 chronic disabilities. Risk factors are derived from participation in activities such as contact sports or use of motor vehicles, particularly if adequate safety measures (e.g., helmets and other protective equipment, seat belts, child restraint devices, and air bags) are not employed. Aging increases the risk of head injury due to falls. Use of alcohol or other mind-altering drugs amplifies the risk of injury in each case. Other high-risk environments are those in which assault or physical abuse are likely.

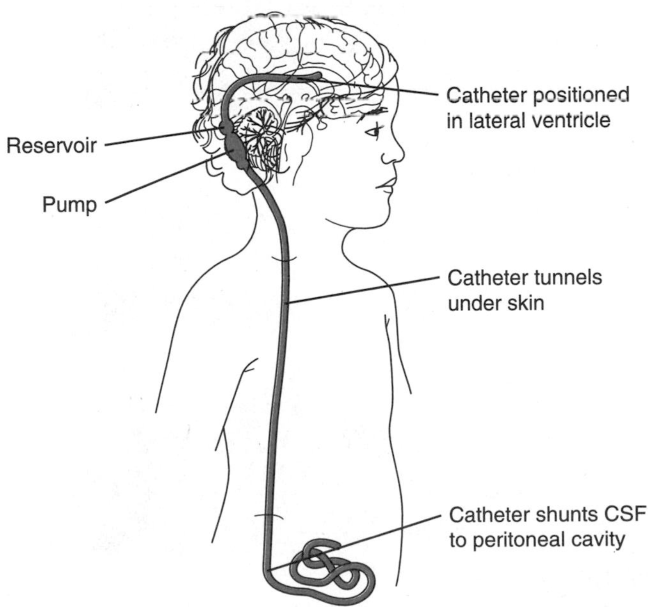

FIGURE 21–32
Ventriculoperitoneal shunt. Treatment of hydrocephalus usually entails surgical implantation of a shunt to divert excess cerebrospinal fluid from the ventricles to the peritoneal cavity, from which it is reabsorbed into the venous system.

Etiology. Two types of force may result in head injury: impact force and inertial force.[37] Impact force occurs when the head strikes a surface, resulting in focal injuries, such as scalp vessel bleeding, skull fracture, **epidural hematoma,** and contusions (bruising) or lacerations (cutting) of brain tissue. Inertial forces are derived from violent motion of the brain inside the skull, resulting in **concussion, subdural hematoma,** and diffuse injury.

Head injuries may also be classified according to the traumatic mechanism, which allows prediction of the nature and site of injury (Fig. 21–33). In most cases, both impact and inertial forces are involved. *Acceleration (coup) injury* occurs when the stationary head is struck by a moving object, resulting in impact injury to the area of the brain underlying the contact site. *Deceleration (contrecoup) injury* occurs when the moving head strikes a stationary object and frequently results not only in injury at the site of impact but also in inertial injury to the opposite side of the brain as it rebounds against the cranial vault. Penetrating trauma, such as that due to gunshot wounds or skull fragments, may directly damage cerebral structures. (Craniotomy may also be classified as a form of penetrating craniocerebral trauma.) Finally, shearing or tearing of cerebral tissues (diffuse brain injury) may result from acceleration or deceleration trauma due to the movement of brain tissue against the rough inner cranial surface and rigid cartilagenous support structures within the cerebrum.

Pathophysiology. Damage to cerebral and cranial structures includes that due to the blow itself (primary injury) and secondary injury due to inflammation or hemorrhage. Types of soft tissue damage due to impact include concussion; diffuse brain injury in which structural damage is usually minimal and functional disruption (e.g., seizures, confusion, or loss of consciousness) is transient; contusion, in which visible bruising of the brain is evident and functional disruption is more extensive and pro-

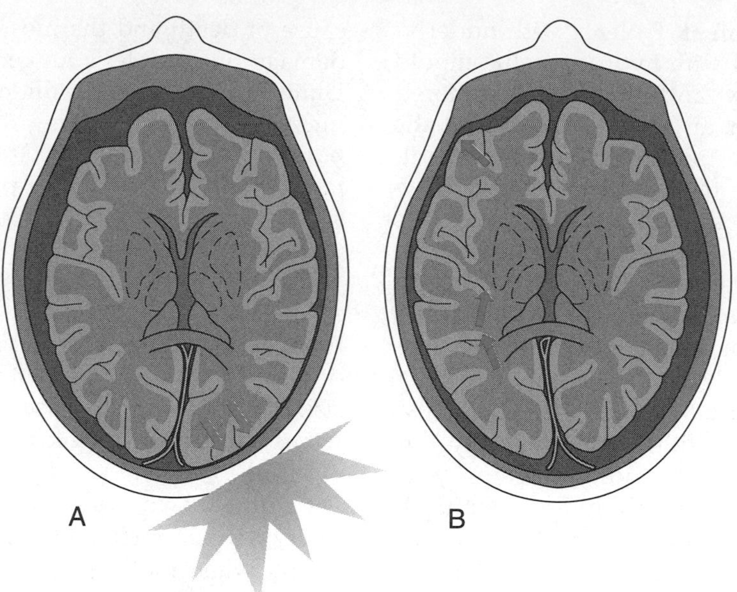

FIGURE 21–33
Mechanisms of brain injury. *A, Acceleration (coup) injury* results when the stationary head is struck by a moving object, producing impact injury at the point of contact. *B, Deceleration (contrecoup) injury* occurs when the moving head strikes a stationary object and results not only in impact injury but also in injury due to rebound of brain tissue against the opposite side of the cranium. *Diffuse brain injury* may also occur with acceleration and deceleration injuries as a result of movement of brain tissue against rough intracranial structures. (From Foster, R.L.R., Hunsberger, M.M., and Anderson, J.J.T. [1989]. *Family-Centered Nursing Care of Children.* Philadelphia: W.B. Saunders. [p. 1769].)

longed; and laceration, in which brain structures are cut or torn and in which immediate neurologic deficits may result from interruption of neural pathways.

Skull fracture may occur with head injury and, like other bone fractures, may be closed (nondisplaced) or open (depressed). Bone fragments may lacerate the dura mater, leading to hemorrhage and possible entry of microorganisms. Fracture of the bones of the floor of the cranium are especially common with blows to the nose or face and may allow communication between the pharynx or sinuses and the brain.

Secondary injury frequently results in more severe manifestations than those due to the impact itself. The inflammatory response to the injury is often maladaptive because it occurs within an enclosed space, leading to cerebral edema and IICP. Cerebral tissue may become hypoxic if cerebral vessels are compressed. Presence of a skull fracture may attenuate these effects because edema may be displaced outward rather than downward onto critical control centers in the medulla. Hemorrhage secondary to head injury may be diffuse, especially if it involves tearing of multiple small vessels as a result of movement of the brain within the cranium. More often, however, bleeding is limited to a discrete area and results in a growing clot or hematoma (Fig. 21–34).

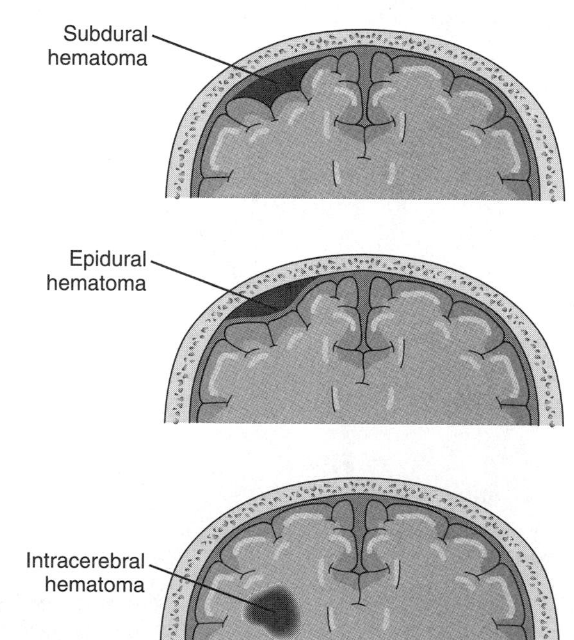

FIGURE 21–34
Intracranial hematomas. A *subdural hematoma* results from venous bleeding and thus grows slowly, whereas an *epidural hematoma* is of arterial origin and grows quickly. Diffuse brain injury or stroke may cause accumulation of blood within brain tissue (*intracerebral hematoma*). (From Barker, E. [1994]. *Neuroscience Nursing.* St. Louis: Mosby–Year Book. [p. 332].)

Subdural hematomas usually are due to a venous source of bleeding and grow slowly, whereas epidural hematomas are usually of arterial origin and may grow quickly. Hematomas constitute space-occupying masses within the cranium and may cause rapid increases in intracranial pressure as well as focal deficits (specific abnormalities that depend on the location of the clot). Bleeding into the subarachnoid space may also occur with head injury but is much more common with ruptured cerebral aneurysms (see later discussion of stroke).

Clinical Manifestations. Signs and symptoms of head injury are those of IICP. Seizures may result from alteration of membrane transport in the area of injury. Ecchymosis around the eyes ("raccoon eyes") and leakage of blood or CSF from the nose or ears are signs of possible cranial floor fracture. Focal deficits involving motor and sensory areas of the brain may produce alterations in speech, movement, or sensation, whereas frontal or limbic lesions may produce alterations in cognition, memory, or consciousness. Vision or other special senses may be impaired by lesions affecting these regulatory pathways (see Chapter 23).

Prevention and Treatment. Prevention of head injury depends on public education and legislation to enforce safety standards in operation of motor vehicles and participation in contact sports. Such measures include mandated standards for equipment and behavior as well as environmental design to maximize safety in the home and workplace. Treatment of head injuries may include craniotomy to ligate any bleeding vessels or to evacuate hematomas or penetrating objects. Prevention of acutely increased intracranial pressure is a high priority. Research indicates that maintenance of a moderate degree of hypothermia (32° to 33°C) may hasten recovery and improve outcomes in selected patients[39] (see Focus of Current Research). This intervention appears to suppress the inflammatory response and reduce CSF concentrations of excitatory neurotransmitters.

Once intracranial pressure has returned to normal and cerebral perfusion has maximized, displaced skull fractures are surgically reduced (restored to normal bone configuration) with procedures that may involve use of wires, plates, or screws. Rehabilitative measures, such as physical, speech, or vocational therapies, are often required during long-term recovery from more severe injuries.

Prognosis and Outcome. Outcome of head injury is widely variable in both duration of recovery and functional results, depending on the location and severity of the impact injury and the nature of any secondary injury. The most widely used index of severity of traumatic brain injury, the Glasgow Coma Scale (Table 21–23), quantifies coma depth and also correlates with prognosis. The longer the duration of coma, the less favorable the outcome. In moderate to severe brain injuries, more than 90% of survivors are left with significant disability.[37]

TABLE 21–23
GLASGOW COMA SCALE

Response*	Coma Scale Score
Best Motor Response	
Obeys (normal spontaneous movements)	6
Localizes (withdraws to touch)	5
Withdraws (withdraws to pain)	4
Abnormal flexion	3
Extensor response	2
Nil	1
Verbal Response	
Oriented (coos, babbles)	5
Confused conversation (irritable, cries spontaneously)	4
Inappropriate words (cries to pain)	3
Incomprehensible sounds (moans to pain)	2
Nil	1
Eye Opening	
Spontaneous	4
To speech	3
To pain	2
Nil	1
Total score: Sum of best eye opening, verbal, and motor response scores	
Maximum score: 15	
Minimum score: 3	

*Modifications for infants given in parentheses.

Reprinted with permission from Teasdale, G., and Jennett, B. (1974). Assessment of coma and impaired consciousness: A practical scale. *Lancet* 2, 81; and James, H.E. (1993). Emergency management of acute coma in children. *American Family Physician* 48(3), 473–478. Published by the American Academy of Family Physicians.

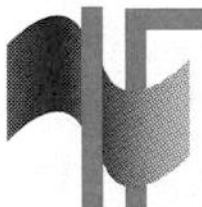

Clinical Scenario

J.T., a 23-year-old woman, is taken to the emergency department by ambulance after a motor vehicle accident. She was the unrestrained driver of a small car that was hit on the passenger side by a pickup truck after sliding through a stop sign. On admission, J.T. has labored respirations and is unconscious, responding only to painful stimuli. Her blood pressure is 158/88 mm Hg; her temperature is 96.8°F, pulse is 115 beats/min, and respirations are 28 breaths/min. She has multiple facial abrasions, contusions, and lacerations to the right forehead area and a laceration under her right eye. Her pupils are unreactive. Clinical assessment reveals a Glasgow Coma Scale score of 3.

1. What is the pathophysiologic basis of J.T.'s altered vital signs?
2. What degree of severity is indicated by the Glasgow Coma Scale score?

Stroke

Definition. Stroke, also known as *cerebrovascular accident,* is descriptively defined as a persistent focal neurologic deficit of acute onset that is not associated with head trauma. Strokes are classified on the basis of their etiology as *hemorrhagic* (due to bleeding) or *ischemic* (due to occlusion of arterial circulation to the brain).

Epidemiology. Stroke is the third leading cause of death in the United States, occurring in an estimated 500,000 people each year.[40] It is the most common serious neurologic disorder seen in hospitalized patients. Risk factors include hypertension (a factor in 70% of strokes), cigarette smoking, diabetes mellitus, obesity, sedentary lifestyle, increased serum cholesterol (in ischemic stroke), alcohol abuse, and use of high-dose oral contraceptives.[41] About 70% of stroke patients are older than 65 years, and 60% are men. Blacks in the United States have a mortality rate due to stroke that is twice that of whites. Risk factors are discussed further with etiology.

Etiology. Hemorrhagic strokes may result from bleeding into the interstitium of the brain **(intracerebral hemorrhage)** or bleeding into the subarachnoid space **(subarachnoid hemorrhage)**. Ischemic strokes are most often the result of atherosclerotic occlusion of neck or cerebral vessels, which triggers local thrombosis, but they may also be caused by blood clots originating from the left side of the heart and embolizing to these vessels. Risk factors and mechanisms of atherosclerosis and of inappropriate clotting and embolization are discussed in Chapters 14 and 15. Atrial fibrillation is strongly associated with the development of atrial clots and thus constitutes a risk factor for ischemic stroke (see Chapter 17).

Hemorrhagic strokes are associated with hypertension (see Chapter 15), bleeding disorders (see Chapter 14), and vessel defects such as AVMs and aneurysms (see Chapter 15). Cerebrovascular defects are usually congenital, but their growth and potential rupture may be related to underlying hypertension or bleeding disorders. Common types and locations of lesions associated with stroke are illustrated in Figure 21–35.

Pathophysiology. The region of the brain served by the occluded or ruptured vessel is deprived of its normal perfusion. This perfusion deficit may develop immediately (e.g., in the case of emboli or hemorrhage) or over a few days (e.g., in the case of thrombotic strokes). Thrombotic strokes, the most common type, are often preceded by focal neurologic deficits that simulate the manifestations of stroke but that last less than 24 hours. These **transient ischemic attacks (TIAs)** may result from spasm at sites of plaque or from miniemboli composed of plaque fragments or blood clots. TIAs signal impending stroke by atherosclerotic and thrombotic occlusion.

In ischemic strokes, some of the neurons normally served by occluded vessels die from lack of oxygen and nutrients, resulting in cerebral infarction. The inflammatory response is triggered by the cellular injury and may result in IICP. In cells sustaining nonlethal ischemic injury, oxidative metabolism is

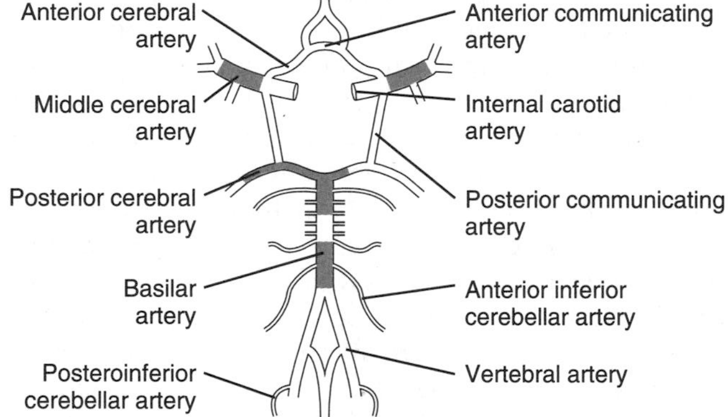

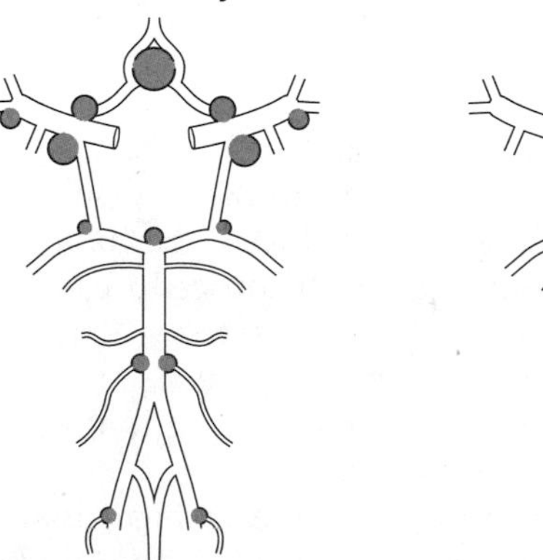

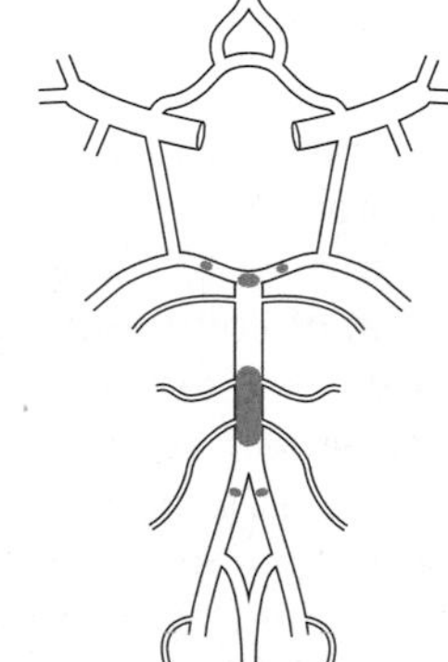

FIGURE 21–35
Lesions associated with stroke. Branch points of the major arteries are the usual sites of atherosclerotic occlusions, thromboemboli, or aneurysms resulting in stroke. Most lesions are in the anterior circulation.

disrupted, leading to altered ion transport, localized acidosis, and formation of reactive oxygen species. Injured cells accumulate calcium, sodium, and water, and the release of excitatory neurotransmitters (e.g., glutamate and aspartate) promotes further cellular injury in a positive feedback loop.

In hemorrhagic strokes, cells are also hypoxic because of lack of perfusion. In addition, a growing intracerebral hematoma may constitute a space-occupying lesion and result in pressure trauma or herniation. Subarachnoid hemorrhage irritates the meninges, and products of blood breakdown may occlude the arachnoid villi, promoting hydrocephalus. As discussed in Chapter 14, ruptured blood vessels tend to constrict initially to limit blood loss. When this vasospasm occurs within cerebral vessels, it may further exacerbate ischemia and neurologic damage. Formation of a clot within a bleeding vessel may stop the bleeding for a time but also decreases normal perfusion and may worsen ischemia. Rebleeding may occur when the fibrinolytic system breaks down the clot to restore perfusion, and this secondary hemorrhage is a frequent complication of subarachnoid hemorrhage.

Clinical Manifestations. The specific manifestations of stroke depend on the mechanism (ischemic or hemorrhagic) and the area and extent of the brain affected. Hemorrhagic strokes typically result in the most extensive functional deficits. About half of cases involve bleeding into the internal capsule area, resulting in severe motor and sensory deficits and potential cardiac or respiratory arrest due to brainstem failure. Signs of meningeal irritation, including severe headache and nuchal rigidity, are common with subarachnoid hemorrhage, and hydrocephalus may develop as a result of occlusion of arachnoid villi.

In ischemic strokes, preliminary TIAs are common, and each episode is more severe and prolonged than the previous. If clinical manifestations do not subside after 24 hours, a stroke is said to have occurred. Typical manifestations of an ischemic stroke involving sensory and motor areas of one hemisphere include flaccid paralysis (hemiplegia) of the side of the body opposite the lesion, disruption of language ability **(aphasia),** loss of part of the visual field **(homonymous hemianopsia),** and loss of sensation on the paralyzed side, resulting in a syndrome of unilateral neglect (lack of awareness or acknowledgment of the affected side). Cognitive ability, memory, and personality may be affected in the case of frontal or limbic lesions. Signs of IICP, including decreased level of consciousness, are present to varying degrees. Seizures may originate from marginal areas surrounding infarcts.

Prevention and Treatment. Prevention of stroke depends on optimal treatment of underlying conditions, such as hypertension and atrial fibrillation, as well as on reduction of modifiable risk factors for atherosclerosis. Patients demonstrating TIAs may be candidates for carotid endarterectomy, the surgical removal of atherosclerotic plaque from carotid arteries, or extracranial–intracranial bypass, in which a scalp artery is anastomosed to a cerebral artery, creating collateral circulation around an obstructed area. Antiplatelet agents, such as low-dose aspirin, may be prescribed to prevent thrombosis in areas of plaque deposition. If the presence of cerebral aneurysm or AVM results in warning manifestations of IICP or subarachnoid hemorrhage, surgical intervention may prevent later bleeding from these defects.

Treatment of stroke depends on the classification and underlying pathophysiology. Thrombotic and embolic strokes may resolve without extensive deficits if thrombolytic agents such as tissue plasminogen activator or streptokinase are administered soon after the onset of stroke (see Chapter 14). Anticoagulants, such as warfarin sodium, may prevent further clotting, and surgical endarterectomy or vascular bypass procedures may also be of benefit in restoring perfusion. In hemorrhagic strokes, craniotomy is warranted as soon as the patient is stable enough to undergo surgery. Bleeding aneurysms are clipped, AVMs are excised or sclerosed, and hematomas are evacuated. A newer endovascular technique for treatment of intracranial aneurysms involves insertion of soft metallic coils within the lumen of the aneurysm, followed by electrical induction of thrombosis around the coils, obliterating the aneurysmal sac.[42] Hydrocephalus is treated with shunting, if necessary.

IICP is carefully monitored and treated appropriately to optimize cerebral perfusion. Clinical trials of a number of cytoprotective interventions designed to interrupt the ischemic cellular responses are ongoing. These include the use of calcium-channel blockers, glutamate receptor blockers, oxygen free radical scavengers, and adhesion molecule inhibitors.[43] Rehabilitative measures are instituted as soon as the patient is stabilized and intracranial pressure is normal (i.e., the stroke is completed).

Prognosis and Outcome. Nearly one third of stroke victims die during the first 3 weeks after the event.[40] Those who are initially comatose are at highest risk of early mortality. Hemorrhagic strokes are associated with higher mortality and worse functional outcomes than ischemic strokes. Most recovery of functional ability occurs during the first 30 to 60 days, with limited improvement thereafter. Long-term survivors of stroke often suffer decreased quality of life; 15% require institutional care, 30% require assistance in their activities of daily living, and 60% are essentially home-bound.

Brain Tumors

Definition. Brain tumors are benign and malignant intracranial neoplasms that may arise as either primary tumors (from cells of the brain or its coverings) or metastatic lesions (originating from primary lesions outside the cranial vault). Table 21–24 lists the most clinically important primary brain tumors along with their tissues of origin.

Epidemiology. Brain tumors are diagnosed in about 35,000 adults[44] and 1500 to 2000 children[45] each year in the United States. The number of metastatic tumors is roughly equal to the primary incidence, with most of the metastatic tumors arising from cancers of the breast or lung. Incidence of primary tumors is equal in both sexes. Risk factors for brain tumors are obscure. Cigarette smoking, dietary factors, alcohol abuse, and history of head injury do *not* correlate with incidence of brain tumors.[46] Cranial irradiation and family history of cancer *do* correlate with CNS neoplasia, and certain rare, genetically transmitted diseases are also associated with increased risk. These include neurofibromatosis, tuberous sclerosis, Turcot's syndrome, Li-Fraumeni cancer syndrome, and von Hippel-Lindau disease.

TABLE 21–24
TYPES AND ORIGINS OF BRAIN TUMORS

TUMOR	TISSUE OF ORIGIN
Benign Tumors	
Meningioma	Arachnoid
Pituitary adenoma	Secretory or nonsecretory cells of the anterior pituitary gland
Acoustic neuroma	Sheath of the vestibular nerve
Craniopharyngioma	Pharyngeal epithelium
Epidermoid tumor	Squamous epithelium
Hemangioblastoma	Blood vessels, usually of cerebellum
Malignant Tumors	
Astroglial neoplasms	Astrocytes
Astrocytoma (low-grade)	
Anaplastic astrocytoma (moderate-grade)	
Glioblastoma multiforme (high-grade)	
Oligodendroglioma	Oligodendrocytes
Ganglioglioma	Astrocytes and neurons of the temporal or frontal lobe
Ependymoma	Ependymal cells
Medulloblastoma	Primitive undifferentiated neuroectodermal cell, arising in the cerebellum
Primitive neuroectodermal tumor	Primitive undifferentiated neuroectodermal cell, arising in the cerebral hemispheres
Pineal region tumor	Usually germ cells
Primary cerebral lymphoma	Lymphocytes

Data from Black, P.M. (1991). Brain tumors. Part 2. *New England Journal of Medicine* 324(22), 1555–1564.

Etiology. The precise etiology of primary intracranial tumors is unknown. Molecular alterations in tumor suppressor genes, proto-oncogenes, or both are believed to underlie neoplastic transformation. CNS tumors usually arise from glial cells but may also originate from neurons, embryonic neuroectoderm, and meningeal or lymphatic tissues.

Pathophysiology. As with other neoplasms, tumor cell division and growth may invade and compress surrounding tissues. Within the limited space of the cranial vault, growth of the space-occupying lesion (whether benign or malignant) results in IICP. Blood vessels and nerve sheaths may be invaded. Focal deficits specific to the site of the tumor are also seen. Tumors arising within the cranial vault rarely metastasize to other parts of the body.

Clinical Manifestations. Manifestations of IICP may include headache, dizziness or vertigo, nausea and vomiting, and papilledema. Herniation syndromes may result in dysfunction of cranial nerve reflexes and brain-stem control centers for cardiovascular and respiratory function. Focal deficits may include motor deficits, such as weakness, paralysis, or gait disorders; sensory disturbances, such as anesthesia, paresthesia, or deficits in vision or hearing; and disturbances of higher functions, such as cognition, memory, or language. Table 21–25 lists manifestations typical of tumors in specific cranial locations.

Prevention and Treatment. Specific preventive measures have not been identified. Intracranial tumors are treated with surgery, radiation therapy, and chemotherapy, with the specific mode or combination of modes depending on tumor size, tumor site, and tissue of origin. Surgical excision is often difficult or impossible because of the proximity of the tumor to vital tissues. Presence of the blood–brain barrier may limit access of drugs to tumor cells. Hyperthermia has been employed as adjuvant therapy in treatment of malignant brain tumors.[47] Heat is a sensitizing agent that may render neoplastic cells more vulnerable to the effects of radiation or chemotherapy by inhibiting DNA repair mechanisms.

TABLE 21-25
FOCAL MANIFESTATIONS OF PRIMARY BRAIN TUMORS

Tumor Location	Neurologic Signs
Frontal lobe	Dementia, personality changes, gait disturbances, generalized or focal seizures, expressive aphasia
Parietal lobe	Receptive aphasia, sensory loss, hemianopia, spatial disorientation
Temporal lobe	Complex partial or generalized seizures, quadrantanopia, behavioral alterations
Occipital lobe	Contralateral hemianopia
Thalamus	Contralateral sensory loss, behavioral changes, language disorder
Cerebellum	Ataxia, dysmetria, nystagmus
Brain stem	Cranial nerve dysfunction, ataxia, pupillary abnormalities, nystagmus, hemiparesis, autonomic dysfunction

Reprinted with permission from Newton, H.B. (1994). Primary brain tumors: Review of etiology, diagnosis, and treatment. *American Family Physician* 49(4), 787–797. Published by the American Academy of Family Physicians.

Prognosis and Outcome. Prognosis depends on tumor location, tumor grade, and cell of origin. Malignant tumors arising in astrocytes are associated with the poorest prognosis; the 2-year survival rate for the high-grade **glioblastoma multiforme** is only 5%.[48] Prognosis in other tumors may be much more favorable, and total surgical cure is possible. Craniotomy for the purpose of tumor removal or reduction of tumor mass may be thought of as an intentional head injury and as such is associated with potentially significant complications.

CLINICAL SIGNIFICANCE OF CORTICAL DISORDERS

The individuality or personhood of human beings resides in higher cortical function. Any disruption of that function by trauma or disease therefore has the potential to significantly impair function and may threaten the life of the patient. The diseases discussed in this chapter illustrate the commonality of such disorders among people of all ages. Prevention and treatment of cortical disorders is limited by both anatomic considerations and lack of basic knowledge regarding etiologic and pathophysiologic mechanisms.

Intracranial lesions affecting higher cortical functions may disrupt motor, autonomic, and sensory function as well. Because motor function (muscle contraction and glandular secretion) is under hierarchic neural regulation, disorders such as stroke, brain tumor, or traumatic brain injury, affecting the motor cortex, premotor, and association areas of the brain, may have devastating effects on these processes. In Chapter 22, normal motor and autonomic function are examined, with emphasis on the neuromuscular junction, motor reflexes, motor pathways, and higher-level integrative centers. Common disorders affecting these systems are discussed in detail.

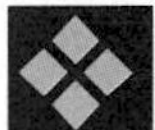

Summary of Key Points

- The nervous system is traditionally characterized as having three divisions. The CNS, consisting of the brain and spinal cord, has as its major function the processing of information. The peripheral nervous system, consisting of the paired cranial and spinal nerves, functions in the transmission of impulses between the CNS and peripheral organs. The autonomic nervous system, consisting of the sympathetic and parasympathetic motor nerve networks, functions in the reflex regulation of homeostasis.
- Neurotransmission is mediated by action potential formation and conduction along nerve fibers. Transmission along myelinated nerves is faster because full action potentials are generated only at nodes of Ranvier, between myelin segments, with electrotonic flow between. Transmission along unmyelinated fibers is slower because action potentials must be propagated along the entire membrane surface. Transmission between neurons or between a neuron and an end organ requires the synthesis and release of a chemical signaling molecule (neurotransmitter), which diffuses across an actual space (synaptic cleft), then binds to a postsynaptic receptor. The resulting action depends on the receptor type.
- The capacity of the cerebral cortex to respond to stimuli is governed by the RAS, which mediates consciousness and sleep (arousable unconsciousness). This system resides in four areas of the brain stem that have pacemaker function and both ascending and descending projections.
- The limbic system is a functional system con-

Summary continued on next page

sisting of several nuclei located deep in the temporal lobes. Components include the hypothalamus, part of the thalamus, the hippocampus, and other nuclei. The limbic system is involved in autonomic regulation, cognitive function and memory, and linkage of cortical perception of environmental inputs with stimuli originating from emotions and drives.

- The neural mechanisms of cognition are believed to reside primarily in the prefrontal association areas, with multiple inputs from other cortical and subcortical regions. Memory involves the hippocampus, thalamus, medial cortex, prefrontal cortex, and inferior temporal regions and is mediated at the molecular level by synaptic plasticity. Language resides in several cortical areas, most notably Broca's area in the frontal lobe, mediating motor function, and Wernicke's area in the temporal lobe, the receptive area for language.
- Cortical disorders include disorders of thought and behavior (psychiatric illnesses), physiologic disorders (neurologic disorders), and neuropsychiatric disorders, which have aspects of the first two types. Pathophysiologic mechanisms affecting cortical function include disordered environmental stimuli (e.g., pathologic relationships or stressful events), neurotrauma, infection, neoplasia, congenital abnormalities, and degeneration. A significant number of neurologic disorders are idiopathic. Therapy of cortical disorders aims to remove the underlying causes, to minimize behavioral or somatic clinical manifestations, and to optimize the patient's functional status.

REFERENCES

1. Lipton, S.A., and Rosenberg, P.A. (1994). Excitatory amino acids as a final common pathway for neurologic disorders. *New England Journal of Medicine* 330(9), 613–622.
2. Malenka, R.C. (1994). Synaptic plasticity in the hippocampus: LTP and LTD. *Cell* 78, 535–538.
3. Schacter, D.L. (1992). Understanding implicit memory: A cognitive neuroscience approach. *American Psychologist* 47(4), 559–569.
4. Grady, C.L., McIntosh, A.R., Horwitz, B., *et al.* (1995). Age-related reductions in human recognition memory due to impaired encoding. *Science* 269, 218–221.
5. Galaburda, A.M. (1993). Neuroanatomic basis of developmental dyslexia. *Neurologic Clinics* 11(1), 161–171.
6. Adams, R.D., and Victor, M. (1993). *Principles of Neurology.* (5th ed.). New York: McGraw-Hill. (pp. 607, 1014, 1287).
7. Carpenter, W.T., and Buchanan, R.W. (1994). Schizophrenia. *New England Journal of Medicine* 220(10), 681–690.
8. Kirch, D.G. (1993). Infection and autoimmunity as etiologic factors in schizophrenia: A review and reappraisal. *Schizophrenia Bulletin* 19(2), 355–370.
9. Kane, J.M. (1996). Schizophrenia. *New England Journal of Medicine* 334(1), 34–41.
10. Pary, R., Tobias, C.R., and Lippmann, S. (1995). Chronic schizophrenia: Options for pharmacologic management. *Postgraduate Medicine* 98(5), 163–173.
11. Goldberg, R.J. (1995). Diagnostic dilemmas presented by patients with anxiety and depression. *American Journal of Medicine* 98(3), 278–284.
12. Goodwin, F. (1996). A 47-year-old man with chronic depression. *Journal of the American Medical Association* 275(6), 479–485.
13. Ormel, J., VonKorff, M., Uston, B., *et al.* (1994). Common mental disorders and disability across cultures: Results from the WHO Collaborative Study on Psychological Problems in General Health Care. *Journal of the American Medical Association* 272(22), 1741–1748.
14. Depression Guideline Panel. (1993). *Depression in Primary Care. Volume 1: Detection and Diagnosis.* Rockville, MD: Department of Health and Human Services. AHCPR Publication No. 93-0550.
15. Finley, P.R. (1994). Selective serotonin reuptake inhibitors: Pharmacologic profiles and potential therapeutic distinctions. *Annals of Pharmacotherapy* 28(12), 1359–1369.
16. Brodaty, H. (1993). Think of depression: Atypical presentations in the elderly. *Australian Family Physician* 22(7), 1195–1203.
17. Kuzel, R. (1996). Management of depression: Current trends in primary care. *Postgraduate Medicine* 99(5), 179–195.
18. Golden, R. (1995). Dementia and Alzheimer's disease: Indications, diagnosis, and treatment. *Minnesota Medicine* 78(1), 25–29.
19. Sandson, T.A., Sperling, R.A., and Price, B.H. (1995). Alzheimer's disease: An update. *Comprehensive Therapy* 21(9), 480–485.
20. Polvikoski, T., Sulkava, R., Haltia, M., *et al.* (1995). Apolipoprotein E, dementia, and cortical deposition of β-amyloid protein. *New England Journal of Medicine* 333(19), 1242–1247.
21. Snowdon, D.A., Kemper, S.J., Mortimer, J.A., *et al.* (1996). Linguistic ability in early life and cognitive function and Alzheimer's disease in late life: Findings from the Nun Study. *Journal of the American Medical Association* 275(7), 528–532.
22. Filley, C.M. (1995). Alzheimer's disease: It's irreversible but not untreatable. *Geriatrics* 50(7), 18–23.
23. O'Brien, M.E. (1994). The dementia syndromes: Distinguishing their clinical differences. *Postgraduate Medicine* 95(5), 91–101.
24. Disabato, J., and Wulf, J. (1989). Nursing strategies: Altered neurologic function. In: Foster, R.L.R., Hunsberger, M.M., and Anderson, J.J.T. (Eds.). *Family-Centered Nursing Care of Children.* Philadelphia: W.B. Saunders. (p. 1734).
25. Daly, L.E., Kirke, P.N., Molloy, A., *et al.* (1995). Folate levels and neural tube defects. *Journal of the American Medical Association* 274 (21), 1698–1702.
26. Shaw, G.M., Velie, E.M., and Schaffer, D. (1996). Risk of neural tube defect-affected pregnancies among obese women. *Journal of the American Medical Association* 275(14), 1093–1096.
27. Swaiman, K., and Wright, F. (1982). *The Practice of Pediatric Neurology.* (2nd ed.). St. Louis: C.V. Mosby.
28. Beghi, E., Nicolosi, A., Kurland, L.T., *et al.* (1984). Encephalitis and aseptic meningitis, Olmstead County, Minnesota, 1950–1981: Epidemiology. *Annals of Neurology* 16, 283.
29. Nelson, S., Sealy, D.P., and Schneider, E.F. (1993). The aseptic meningitis syndrome. *American Family Physician* 48(5), 809–815.
30. Tunkel, A.R., and Scheld, W.M. (1993). Pathogenesis and pathophysiology of bacterial meningitis. *Annual Review of Medicine* 44, 103–120.
31. Engel, J. (1996). Surgery for seizures. *New England Journal of Medicine* 334(10), 647–652.
32. Diringer, M.N. (1993). Intracerebral hemorrhage: Pathophysiology and management. *Critical Care Medicine* 21(10), 1591–1603.

33. Vos, H.R. (1993). Making headway with intracranial hypertension. *American Journal of Nursing* 93(2), 28–35.
34. Kerr, M.E., and Brucia, J. (1993). Hyperventilation in the head-injured patient: An effective treatment modality? *Heart & Lung* 22(6), 516–522.
35. Prockop, L.D., and Shah, C.P. (1989). Hydrocephalus. In: Rowland, L.P. (Ed.). *Merritt's Textbook of Neurology.* (8th ed.). Philadelphia: Lea & Febiger. (p. 253).
36. Evidente, V.H., and Gwinn, K.A. (1997). 73-year-old man with gait disturbance and imbalance. *Mayo Clinic Proceedings* 72, 165–168.
37. Michaud, L.J., Duhaime, A-C., and Batshaw, M.L. (1993). Traumatic brain injury in children. *Pediatric Clinics of North America* 40(3), 553–565.
38. Sullivan, T.E., Schefft, B.K., Warm, J.S., *et al.* (1994). Closed head injury assessment and research methodology. *Journal of Neuroscience Nursing* 26(1), 24–29.
39. Marion, D.W., Penrod, L.E., Kelsey, S.F., *et al.* (1997). Treatment of traumatic brain injury with moderate hypothermia. *New England Journal of Medicine* 336(8), 540–546.
40. Goldstein, L.B., and Matcher, D.B. (1994). Clinical assessment of stroke. *Journal of the American Medical Association* 271(14), 1114–1120.
41. Bronner, L.L., Kanter, D.S., and Manson, J.E. (1995). Primary prevention of stroke. *New England Journal of Medicine* 333(21), 1392–1400.
42. Schievink, W.I. (1997). Intracranial aneurysms. *New England Journal of Medicine* 336(1), 28–40.
43. Fisher, M., and Bobousslavsky, J. (1993). Evolving toward effective therapy for acute ischemic stroke. *Journal of the American Medical Association* 270(3), 360–364.
44. Black, P.M. (1991). Brain tumors. Part 1. *New England Journal of Medicine* 324(21), 1471–1476.
45. Pollack, I.F. (1994). Brain tumors in children. *New England Journal of Medicine* 331(22), 1500–1507.
46. Newton, H.B. (1994). Primary brain tumors: Review of etiology, diagnosis, and treatment. *American Family Physician* 49(4), 787–797.
47. Welsh, D.M. (1995). Hyperthermia treatment of malignant brain tumors. *Critical Care Nursing Clinics of North America* 7(1), 115–124.
48. Black, P.M. (1991). Brain tumors. Part 2. *New England Journal of Medicine* 324(22), 1555–1564.

SELECTED BIBLIOGRAPHY

Amarenco, P., Cohen, A., Tzourie, C., *et al.* (1994). Atherosclerotic disease of the aortic arch and the risk of ischemic stroke. *New England Journal of Medicine* 331(22), 1474–1479.

Andreasen, N.C., Flashman, L., Flaum, M., *et al.* (1994). Regional brain abnormalities in schizophrenia measured with magnetic resonance imaging. *Journal of the American Medical Association* 272(22), 1763–1769.

Andrews, J.M., and Nemeroff, C.B. (1994). Contemporary management of depression. *American Journal of Medicine* 97(suppl. 6A), 24S–32S.

Barker, E. (1994). *Neuroscience Nursing.* St. Louis: Mosby–Year Book.

Barker, F.G., and Israel, M.A. (1995). The molecular biology of brain tumors. *Neurologic Clinics* 13(4), 701–715.

Barnett, H.J.M., Eliasziw, M., and Meldrum, H.E. (1995). Drugs and surgery in the prevention of ischemic stroke. *New England Journal of Medicine* 332(4), 238–248.

Bootzin, R.R., Quan, S.F., Bamford, C.R., *et al.* (1995). Sleep disorders. *Comprehensive Therapy* 21(8), 401–406.

Boswell, E.B., and Stoudemire, A. (1966). Major depression in the primary care setting. *American Journal of Medicine* 101(suppl. 6A), 3S–9S.

Bright, D.A. (1994). Postpartum mental disorders. *American Family Physician* 50(3), 595–598.

Broderson, J.M. (1995). Surgical options for brain tumor treatment. *Critical Care Clinics of North America* 7(1), 91–102.

Brodie, M.J., and Dichter, M.A. (1996). Antiepileptic drugs. *New England Journal of Medicine* 334(3), 168–175.

Casey, D.A., DeFazio, J.V., Jr., Vansickle, K., *et al.* (1996). Delirium: Quick recognition, careful evaluation, and appropriate treatment. *Postgraduate Medicine* 100(1), 121–134.

Chalmers, D.J. (1995). The puzzle of conscious experience. *Scientific American* 236(6), 80–86.

Chua, W., and Chediak, A.D. (1994). Obstructive sleep apnea: Treatment improves quality of life—and may prevent death. *Postgraduate Medicine* 95(2), 123–138.

Clark, L.W. (1994). Communication disorders: What to look for, and when to refer. *Geriatrics* 49(6), 51–55.

Cole, S., and Raju, M. (1996). Making the diagnosis of depression in the primary care setting. *American Journal of Medicine* 101 (suppl. 6A), 10S–17S.

Cotran, R.S., Kumar, V., and Robbins, S.L. (Eds.). (1994). *Robbins Pathologic Basis of Disease.* (5th ed.). Philadelphia: W.B. Saunders.

Coull, B.M., and Clark, W.M. (1993). Abnormalities of hemostasis in ischemic stroke. *Medical Clinics of North America* 77(1), 77–94.

Cravatt, B.F., Prospero-Garcia, O., Siuzdak, G., *et al.* (1995). Chemical characterization of a family of brain lipids that induce sleep. *Science* 268, 1506–1509.

Daffner, K.R., Schomer, D.L., Cosgrove, R., *et al.* (1991). Broca's aphasia following damage to Wernicke's area: For or against traditional aphasiology. *Archives of Neurology* 48, 766–768.

Diagnostic and Statistical Manual of Mental Disorders. (4th ed.) (DSM-IV). (1994). Washington, DC: American Psychiatric Association.

Dichter, M.A., and Brodie, M.J. (1996). New antiepileptic drugs. *New England Journal of Medicine* 334(24), 1583–1590.

Dilsaver, S.C. (1993). Antipsychotic agents: A review. *American Family Physician* 47(1), 199–204.

Early Identification of Alzheimer's Disease and Related Dementias Panel. (1997). Early identification of Alzheimer's disease and related dementias. *American Family Physician* 55(4), 1303–1314.

El-Mallakh, R.S., Wright, J.C., Breen, K.J., *et al.* (1996). Clues to depression in primary care practice. *Postgraduate Medicine* 100(1), 85–96.

Engstrom, F., and Hong, K.L. (1997). Psychotropic drugs: Modern medicine's alternatives to purgatives, straitjackets, and asylums. *Postgraduate Medicine* 101(3), 198–211.

Executive Committee for the Asymptomatic Carotid Atherosclerosis Study. (1995). Endarterectomy for asymptomatic carotid artery stenosis. *Journal of the American Medical Association* 273(18), 1421–1428.

Fallon, B.A., and Nields, J.A. (1994). Lyme disease: A neuropsychiatric illness. *American Journal of Psychiatry* 151(11), 1571–1582.

Farney, R.J., and Walker, J.M. (1995). Office management of common sleep-wake disorders. *Medical Clinics of North America* 79(2), 391–414.

Ferster, D., and Spruston, N. (1995). Cracking the neuronal code. *Science* 270, 756–757.

Fine, H.A., and Mayer, R.J. (1993). Primary central nervous system lymphoma. *Annals of Internal Medicine* 119(11), 1093–1104.

First, L.R., and Palfrey, J.S. (1994). The infant or young child with developmental delay. *New England Journal of Medicine* 330(7), 478–483.

Fishbein, D.B., and Robinson, L.E. (1993). Rabies. *New England Journal of Medicine* 329(22), 1632–1638.

Fowler, S.B., Hertzog, J., and Wagner, B.K.J. (1995). Pharmacological interventions for agitation in head-injured patients in the acute care setting. *Journal of Neuroscience Nursing* 27(2), 119–123.

Geldmacher, D.S., and Whitehouse, P.J. (1996). Evaluation of dementia. *New England Journal of Medicine* 335(5), 330–336.

Gilman, J.T., and Tuchman, R.F. (1995). Autism and associated behavioral disorders: Pharmacotherapeutic intervention. *Annals of Pharmacotherapy* 29, 47–56.

Golding, D.W. (1994). A pattern confirmed and refined: Synaptic, nonsynaptic and parasynaptic exocytosis. *Bioessays* 16(7), 503–508.

Goldman, H.H. (1992). *Review of General Psychiatry.* (3rd ed.). Norwalk, CT: Appleton & Lange.

Graves, V.B., and Duff, T.A. (1990). Intracranial arteriovenous malformations: Current imaging and treatment. *Investigative Radiology* 25(8), 952–960.

Greenamyre, J.T., and Porter, R.H.P. (1994). Anatomy and physiology of glutamate in the CNS. *Neurology* 44(suppl. 8), S7–S13.

Guyton, A.C., and Hall, J.E. (1996). *Textbook of Medical Physiology.* (9th ed.). Philadelphia: W.B. Saunders.

Hebert, L.E., Scherr, P.A., Beckett, L.A., *et al.* (1995). Age-specific incidence of Alzheimer's disease in a community population. *Journal of the American Medical Association* 273(17), 1354–1359.

Hilton, G. (1994). Secondary brain injury and the role of neuroprotective agents. *Journal of Neuroscience Nursing* 26(4), 251–255.

Hirschfeld, R.M.A., Keller, M.B., Panico, S., *et al.* (1997). The national depressive and manic-depressive association consensus statement on the undertreatment of depression. *Journal of the American Medical Association* 277(4), 333–340.

Hoffman, R.S., and Goldfrank, L.R. (1995). The poisoned patient with altered consciousness: Controversies in the use of a "coma cocktail." *Journal of the American Medical Association* 274(7), 562–569.

James, H.E. (1993). Emergency management of acute coma in children. *American Family Physician* 48(3), 473–478.

Jamison, K.R. (1995). Manic-depressive illness and creativity. *Scientific American* 272(2), 62–67.

Jensen, D.P., and Herr, K.A. (1993). Sleeplessness. *Nursing Clinics of North America* 28(2), 385–405.

Jermain, D.M. (1995). Treatment of postpartum depression. *American Pharmacy* NS35(1), 33–38.

Jokic, R., and Fitzpatrick, M.F. (1996). Obstructive lung disease and sleep. *Medical Clinics of North America* 80(4), 821–850.

Kandel, E.R., and Schwartz, J.H. (1985). *Principles of Neural Science.* (2nd ed.). New York: Elsevier Science Publishing.

Kaufman, H.H., Timberlake, G., Voelker, J., *et al.* (1993). Medical complications of head injury. *Medical Clinics of North America* 77(1), 43–60.

Keltner, N.L., Schwecke, L.H., and Bostrom, C.E. (1991). *Psychiatric Nursing: A Psychotherapeutic Management Approach.* St. Louis: Mosby–Year Book.

Kennedy, M.B. (1994). The biochemistry of synaptic regulation in the central nervous system. *Annual Review of Biochemistry* 63, 571–600.

Keys, M.P. (1993). The pediatrician's role in reading disorders. *Pediatric Clinics of North America* 40(4), 869–879.

King, A.C., Oman, R.F., Brassington, G.S., *et al.* (1997). Moderate-intensity exercise and self-rated quality of sleep in older adults: A randomized controlled trial. *Journal of the American Medical Association* 277(1), 32–37.

Kinney, H.C., Korein, J., Panigrahy, A., *et al.* (1994). Neuropathological findings in the brain of Karen Ann Quinlan: The role of the thalamus in the persistent vegetative state. *New England Journal of Medicine* 330(21), 1469–1475.

Kittner, S.J., Stern, B.J., Feeser, B.R., *et al.* (1996). Pregnancy and the risk of stroke. *New England Journal of Medicine* 335(11), 768–774.

Knapp, M.J., Knopman, D.S., Solomon, P.R., *et al.* (1994). A 30-week randomized controlled trial of high-dose Tacrine in patients with Alzheimer's disease. *Journal of the American Medical Association* 271(13), 985–991.

Knowlton, B.J., and Squire, L.R. (1993). The learning of categories: Parallel brain systems for item memory and category knowledge. *Science* 262, 1747–1749.

Koenig, H.L., Schumacher, M., Ferzaz, *et al.* (1995). Progesterone synthesis and myelin formation by Schwann cells. *Science* 268, 1500–1503.

Kraus, J.F., Peek, C., McArthur, D.L., *et al.* (1994). The effect of the 1992 California motorcycle helmet use law on motorcycle crash fatalities and injuries. *Journal of the American Medical Association* 272(19), 1506–1511.

Kupfer, D.J., and Reynolds, C.F., III. (1997). Management of insomnia. *New England Journal of Medicine* 336(5), 341–346.

Lamb, S.A. (1995). Radiation therapy options for management of the brain tumor patient. *Critical Care Nursing Clinics of North America* 7(1), 103–114.

LeBlanc, K.E. (1994). Concussion in sports: Guidelines for return to competition. *American Family Physician* 50(4), 801–806.

Lendon, C.L., Ashall, F., and Goate, A.M. (1997). Exploring the etiology of Alzheimer disease using molecular genetics. *Journal of the American Medical Association* 277(10), 825–831.

Marchello, V., Boczki, F., and Shelkey, M. (1995). Progressive dementia: Strategies to manage new problem behaviors. *Geriatrics* 50(3), 40–43.

Masand, P. (1995). Sleepwalking. *American Family Physician* 51(3), 649–653.

Mejia, R.E., and Pollack, M.M. (1995). Variability in brain death determination practices in children. *Journal of the American Medical Association* 274(7), 550–553.

Moore, K.L., and Persaud, T.V.N. (1993). *The Developing Human: Clinically Oriented Embryology.* (5th Ed.). Philadelphia: W.B. Saunders.

Moore, P.S., and Broome, C.V. (1994). Cerebrospinal meningitis epidemics. *Scientific American* 271(5), 38–45.

Meyer, F.B., Morita, A., Puumala, M.R., *et al.* (1995). Medical and surgical management of intracranial aneurysms. *Mayo Clinic Proceedings* 70(2), 153–172.

Multi-Society Task Force on PVS. (1994). Medical aspects of the persistent vegetative state. *New England Journal of Medicine* 330(21), 1499–1508.

Multi-Society Task Force on PVS. (1994). Medical aspects of the persistent vegetative state. *New England Journal of Medicine* 330(22), 1572–1579.

National Institute of Neurological Disorders and Stroke rt-PA Stroke Study Group. (1995). Tissue plasminogen activator for acute ischemic stroke. *New England Journal of Medicine* 333(24), 1581–1587.

Nichols, D.A., Meyer, F.B., Piepgras, D.G., *et al.* (1994). Endovascular treatment of intracranial aneurysms. *Mayo Clinic Proceedings* 69(3), 272–285.

Oldham, J.M. (1994). Personality disorders: Current perspectives. 272(22), 1770–1776.

Pachner, A.R. (1995). Early disseminated Lyme disease: Lyme meningitis. *American Journal of Medicine* 98 (suppl. 4A), 30S–43S.

Pagel, J.F. (1994). Treatment of insomnia. *American Family Physician* 49(6), 1417–1421.

Paist, S.S., III, and Martin, J.R. (1996). Brain failure in older patients. *Postgraduate Medicine* 99(5), 125–136.

Pary, R., Lippmann, S., and Tobias, C.R. (1994). Obsessive-compulsive disorder: How to free patients from intrusive thoughts and rituals. *Postgraduate Medicine* 96(8), 119–125.

Peden, J.G., Jr., and Lichstein, P.R. (1996). Management strategies for depression in primary care. *American Journal of Medicine* 101(suppl. 6A), 18S–25S.

Petronis, A., and Kennedy, J.L. (1995). Unstable genes: Unstable mind? *American Journal of Psychiatry* 152(2), 164–172.

Pickar, D., and Hsaio, J.K. (1995). Clozapine treatment of schizophrenia. *Journal of the American Medical Association* 274(12), 981–983.

Post, S.G., Whitehouse, P.J., Binstock, R.H., *et al.* (1997). The clinical introduction of genetic testing for Alzheimer disease: An ethical perspective. *Journal of the American Medical Association* 277(10), 832–836.

Price, L.H., and Heninger, G.R. (1994). Lithium in the treatment of mood disorders. *New England Journal of Medicine* 331(9), 591–598.

Prociuk, J.L. (1995). Management of cerebral oxygen supply–demand balance in blunt head injury. *Critical Care Nurse* 15(4), 38–45.

Prusiner, S.B. (1995). The prion diseases. *Scientific American* 272(1), 48–57.

Regestein, Q.R., and Monk, T.H. (1995). Delayed sleep phase syndrome: A review of its clinical aspects. *American Journal of Psychiatry* 152(4), 602–608.

Robinson, C.R. (1993). Impaired sleep. In: Carrieri-Kohlman, V., Lindsey, A.M., and West, C.M. (Eds.). *Pathophysiological Phenomena in Nursing: Human Responses to Illnesses.* Philadelphia: W.B. Saunders.

Rodier, P.M. (1995). Developing brain as a target of toxicity. *Environmental Health Perspectives* 103(suppl. 6), 73–76.

Rodier, P.M. (1994). Vulnerable periods and processes during central nervous system development. *Environmental Health Perspectives* 102(suppl. 2), 121–124.

Rogers, S.J., and Sherman, D.G. (1993). Pathophysiology and treatment of acute ischemic stroke. *Clinical Pharmacology* 12(5), 359–376.

Rowe, K.S., and Rowe, K.J. (1994). Synthetic food coloring and behavior: A dose response effect in a double-blind, placebo-controlled, repeated-measures study. *Journal of Pediatrics* 125(5 Pt. 1), 691–698.

Rusy, K.L. (1996). Rebleeding and vasospasm after subarachnoid hemorrhage: A critical care challenge. *Critical Care Nurse* 16(1), 41–48.

Samuels, M.A. (1993). The evaluation of comatose patients. *Hospital Practice* 28(3), 165–182.

Sansone, R.A., and Sansone, L.A. (1995). Borderline personality disorder: Interpersonal and behavioral problems that sabotage treatment success. *Postgraduate Medicine* 97(6), 169–179.

Schachter, S. (1994). Neuroendocrine aspects of epilepsy. *Neurologic Clinics* 12(1), 31–37.

Schachter, S.C., and Yerby, M.S. (1997). Management of epilepsy: Pharmacologic therapy and quality-of-life issues. *Postgraduate Medicine* 101(2), 133–153.

Shaywitz, S.E. (1996). Dyslexia. *Scientific American* 275(5), 98–104.

Simon, R.P., Aminoff, M.J., and Greenberg, D.A. (1989). *Clinical Neurology*. Norwalk, CT: Appleton & Lange.

Snowdon, D.A., Greiner, L.H., Mortimer, J.A., *et al.* (1997). Brain infarction and the clinical expression of Alzheimer disease: The Nun Study. *Journal of the American Medical Association* 277(10), 813–817.

Sosin, D.M., Sniezek, J.E., and Waxweiler, R.J. (1995). Trends in death associated with traumatic brain injury, 1979–1992: Success and failure. *Journal of the American Medical Association* 273(22), 1778–1780.

Sosnowski, C., and Ustik, M. (1994). Early intervention: Coma stimulation in the intensive care unit. *Journal of Neuroscience Nursing* 26(6), 336–341.

Steriade, M. (1996). Arousal: Revisiting the reticular activating system. *Science* 272, 225–226.

Stern, Y., Tang, M-X., Albert, M.S., *et al.* (1997). Predicting time to nursing home care and death in individuals with Alzheimer disease. *Journal of the American Medical Association* 277(10), 806–812.

Streit, W.J., and Kincaid-Colton, C.A. (1995). The brain's immune system. *Scientific American* 273(5), 54–61.

Strollo, P.J., and Rogers, R.M. (1996). Obstructive sleep apnea. *New England Journal of Medicine* 334(2), 99–104.

Thelan, L.A., Davie, J.K., and Urden, L.D. (1994). *Textbook of Critical Care Nursing: Diagnosis and Management.* (2nd ed.). St. Louis: Mosby–Year Book.

Thompson, D.C., Rivara, F.P., and Thompson, R.S. (1996). Effectiveness of bicycle safety helmets in preventing head injuries: A case-control study. *Journal of the American Medical Association* 276(24), 1968–1973.

Tinkle, M. (1997). Folic acid and food fortification: Implications for the primary care practitioner. *Nurse Practitioner* 22(3), 105–114.

Tuomanen, E. (1993). Breaching the blood-brain barrier. *Scientific American* 268(2), 80–84.

Welty, T.E., and Horner, T.G. (1990). Pathophysiology and treatment of subarachnoid hemorrhage. *Clinical Pharmacy* 9(1), 35–39.

Werler, M.M., Louik, C., Shapiro, S., *et al.* (1996). Prepregnant weight in relation to risk of neural tube defects. *Journal of the American Medical Association* 275(14), 1089–1092.

Whiting, A.S., and Johnson, L.N. (1992). Papilledema: Clinical cues and differential diagnosis. *American Family Physician* 45(3), 1125–1134.

Young, B., Runge, J.W., Waxman, K.S., *et al.* (1996). Effects of pegorgotein on neurologic outcome of patients with severe head injury: A multicenter, randomized controlled trial. *Journal of the American Medical Association* 276(7), 538–543.

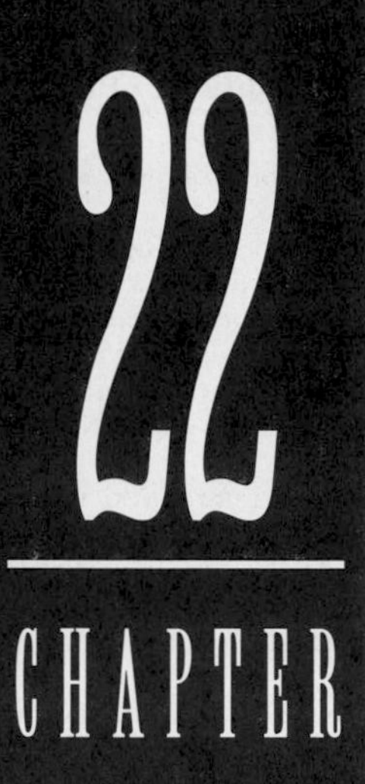

Disorders of Somatic Motor and Autonomic Function

LEARNING OBJECTIVES

1. Differentiate between the anatomic characteristics and general motor functions of the somatic motor system and the autonomic nervous system.
2. Discuss the basis and importance of hierarchic control of motor function.
3. Describe the processes involved in neurotransmission at the neuromuscular junction.
4. Identify the essential components of the motor reflex arc.
5. Differentiate between the pyramidal and extrapyramidal motor pathways.
6. Discuss the roles of the cerebellum and basal ganglia in modulation of motor function.
7. Differentiate between the distributions, neurotransmitters, receptors, and functions of the sympathetic and parasympathetic divisions of the autonomic nervous system.
8. Discuss the influences of cortical and brainstem inputs and endocrine factors in the integration of autonomic activity.
9. Identify the opposing effects of sympathetic and parasympathetic innervation on specific end organs.
10. Comprehend the pathophysiologic bases of the clinical manifestations and treatment of the more prevalent disorders of somatic motor and autonomic function.

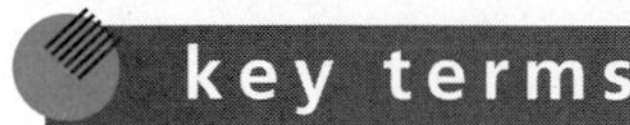

akinesia
amyotrophic lateral sclerosis (ALS)
anhidrosis
atonia
autonomic hyper-reflexia
autonomic neuropathy
Bell's palsy
bradykinesia
cerebral palsy
cutaneous reflex
deep tendon reflex
dyskinesia
dystonia
extrapyramidal symptoms
Guillain-Barré syndrome
hemiplegia
hemiparesis

Huntington's disease
hyperhidrosis
hyperkinesia
hypertonia
hypokinesia
hypotonia
lower motor neuron disease
multiple sclerosis (MS)
myasthenia gravis (MG)
myasthenic crisis
neuroblastoma
optic neuritis
paralysis
paraplegia
paresis
parkinsonism
Parkinson's disease
pathologic reflex
pheochromocytoma
physiologic reflex
poliomyelitis
polyneuropathy
primitive reflex
quadriplegia
spinal cord injury
spinal shock
syringomyelia
upper motor neuron disease

The *motor system* includes the components of the nervous system that initiate or modify all expressed behavior. Behavior results from the activity of skeletal, smooth, and cardiac muscle as well as secretory glands. The most obvious motor activity is the skeletal muscle contraction essential to functions such as movement, posture, respiration, affect (facial expression), speech, and manipulative skills. Skeletal muscle contraction is dependent on innervation by the *somatic motor system*. Motor activity also includes *visceral behavior:* (1) the cardiac contraction essential to circulation; (2) the smooth muscle contraction that is the basis of numerous functions, including motility of the gastrointestinal and urinary tracts, vasomotion, and alterations in airway diameter; and (3) regulated secretion by glands. These actions are largely under regulation by the *autonomic nervous system (ANS)*.

Motor activity of all kinds and at all levels requires not only intact motor systems but also appropriate sensory input. Sensory receptors in muscles and joints inform cortical sensory areas about the contractile state and position of skeletal muscle groups before, during, and after contraction. The special senses of vision and hearing provide input from the external environment, and sensory receptors in internal organs provide feedback on the state of visceral function. Sensory function is detailed in Chapter 23.

In this chapter, the anatomy and functions of the somatic motor and autonomic nervous systems are discussed, along with the most prevalent disorders of these systems.

SOMATIC MOTOR SYSTEM

Components of the System

The somatic motor system may be subdivided into (1) the *primary* motor system, whose neuron cell bodies are found in the spinal cord, brain stem, *primary motor cortex,* and *premotor* or *supplemental areas,* and (2) the accessory motor systems, consisting of neurons in the *cerebellum* and *basal ganglia.* Primary motor system components are involved in selecting and initiating motor activity, whereas accessory systems evaluate and modify the activity. The accessory systems are not essential to motor activity, but without their inputs, such activity would be crude, inaccurate, and graceless.

Hierarchic Motor Control

The primary motor system exhibits hierarchic control, as illustrated in Figure 22–1. The lowest level of regulation is demonstrated by the automatic activity (motor reflexes) mediated by spinal cord neurons and peripheral nerves. These stereotyped muscle contractions occur in response to stimulation of sensors in muscles, and although they do not *require* higher-level input, they are potentially (and usually) modified by such input. The next level of motor

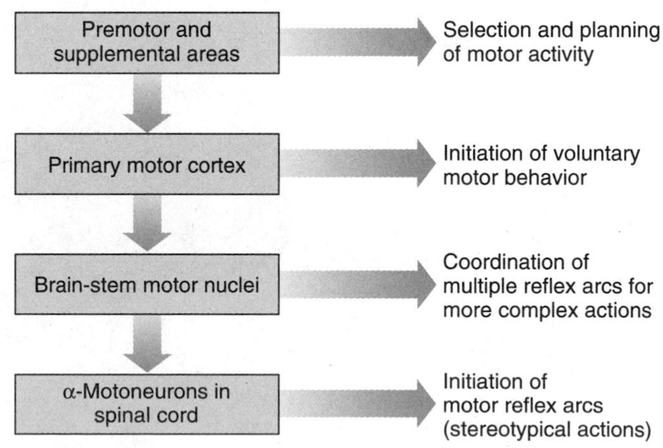

FIGURE 22–1
Hierarchic control of motor function. The premotor and supplemental areas exert the highest level of motor control. The lowest level is the spinal cord α-motoneuron, which mediates the motor reflexes that are the building blocks of more complex motor activity.

regulation occurs within specific brain-stem *nuclei* (neuron cell bodies), which subconsciously integrate multiple spinal cord reflexes, resulting in more complex behaviors. The neurons of the primary motor cortex ("motor strip") in the cerebral cortex initiate voluntary behavior by signaling the brain-stem motor nuclei and the motor neurons in the cord. The highest level of motor regulation occurs in the premotor and supplemental areas of the cortex (Fig. 22–2), which select a course of action based on multiple sensory inputs. These neurons then program and initiate this action through signals to the primary motor cortex and lower motor areas.

The accessory motor systems, although not a part of the chain of command, are essential to the quality of the resulting behavior. The person throwing a ball, for example, could propel the ball through space without the input of the accessory systems. The throw would be inaccurate in direction and distance, however, and the throwing movement would be uncoordinated, lacking a smooth follow-through. Cerebellar neurons receive continuous sensory inputs from muscles and joints, which allow them to compare intended actions with actual motor activity and to make adjustments in descending signals when necessary. The basal ganglia refine cortical motor outputs before their descent to the cord, so that activities are smooth, coordinated, and graceful.

Neurotransmission at the Neuromuscular Junction

As discussed in Chapter 21, impulse transmission within the nervous system requires conduction of impulses from the end of one axon, across a space (synapse), to some part of another neuron. Synaptic transmission permits the networking of multiple individual neurons into specialized functional pathways. Within the somatic motor system, the axons involved are those of motor neurons, and the final motor neuron in a pathway culminates in a specialized synapse *(neuromuscular junction)* between an axon branch and a discrete area of a skeletal muscle fiber known as the *motor end plate.*

The neurotransmitter at the neuromuscular junction is acetylcholine (ACh), and the ACh receptors of the motor end plate are ligand-gated sodium channels that induce action potentials and subsequent contraction of the muscle fiber (see Chapters 4 and 5). ACh is inactivated within the synaptic cleft by the activity of the enzyme acetylcholinesterase, which is synthesized by the muscle cell and released

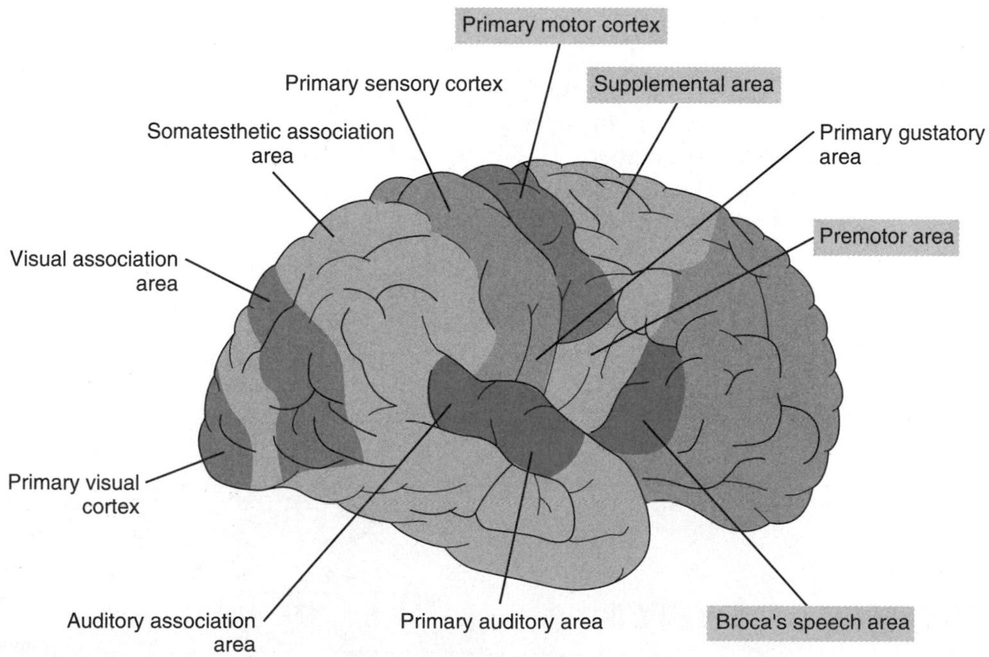

FIGURE 22–2
Cortical motor areas. The premotor and supplemental areas interact with the primary motor cortex in planning and directing motor activity. Broca's area, the motor area for speech, is also shown. The position of the cortical motor areas relative to several sensory areas is illustrated. All motor activity depends on sensory input.

from grooves in the motor end plate. **Myasthenia gravis (MG),** the prototype disorder of neuromuscular junction transmission, is detailed later in this chapter. Patients with MG demonstrate muscle weakness due to lack of ACh effect at the neuromuscular junction.

Lower Motor Neuron Function

Classification

The neurons from which the motor cranial nerves originate and those found in anterior horns of the spinal cord are known as *lower motor neurons (LMNs),* in contrast to the *upper motor neurons (UMNs)* found in the cortical motor regions and the brain stem. LMNs include *α-motoneurons, γ-motoneurons,* and *interneurons.*

α-Motoneurons represent the final neuron in each motor pathway, the lowest level of hierarchic motor control. The axons of these neurons directly innervate skeletal muscles at neuromuscular junctions. Axons of α-motoneurons are branched, allowing a single neuron to innervate 10 to 2000 muscle fibers. Muscle groups involved in precise, or fine, motor activities (such as manipulative skills of the hands) receive innervation from a greater number of α-motoneurons, whereas muscles involved in less precise activity (such as the antigravity muscles of the lower extremities and trunk) are innervated by fewer α-motoneurons.

γ-Motoneurons are smaller than α-motoneurons and are fewer in number. These neurons innervate the *muscle spindles,* sensory receptors arranged parallel to muscle fibers (Fig. 22–3). γ-Motoneurons regulate the sensitivity of the muscle to stretch, that is, the ease of muscle response during the stretch reflex (discussed in the next section).

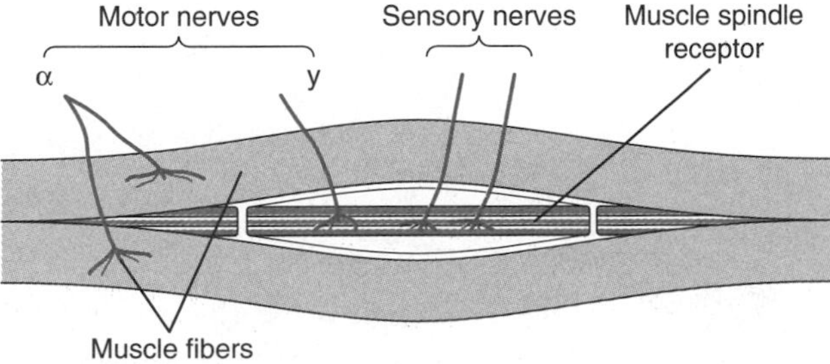

FIGURE 22–3
Muscle spindle receptors. Muscle spindles are sensory receptors that lie parallel to muscle fibers. Muscle spindles are innervated by γ-motoneurons, which regulate the sensitivity of the muscle to stretch. (Redrawn from Guyton, A.C., and Hall, J.E. [1996]. *Textbook of Medical Physiology.* [9th ed.]. Philadelphia: W.B. Saunders. [p. 686].)

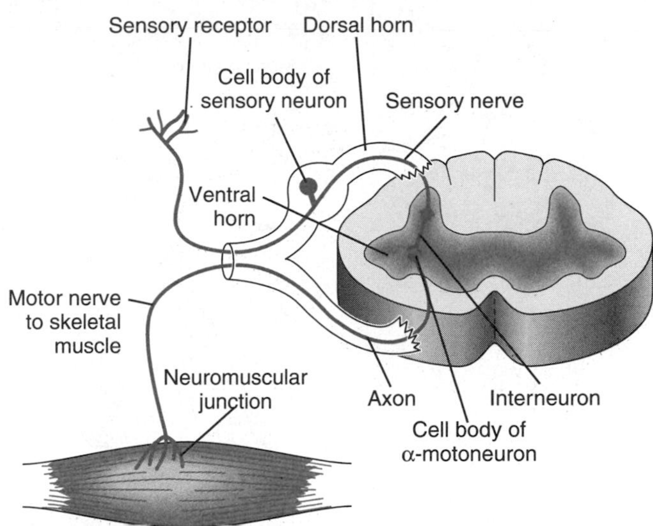

FIGURE 22–4
Essential components of a reflex arc. The reflex arc consists of a sensory receptor, its sensory nerve, a synapse between the sensory nerve and an α-motoneuron, a motor nerve, and the neuromuscular junction between this nerve and a muscle fiber.

Interneurons, also known as *internuncial* or *central neurons,* are small neurons with short axons. Interneurons may serve as interconnections between sequential motor neurons and between motor and sensory neurons. Most descending motor signals are transmitted by a number of interneurons before reaching α-motoneurons.

Reflex Arcs

The simplest neural pathways resulting in motor activity are known as *reflex arcs.* As illustrated in Figure 22–4, the neural pathway consists of (1) a sensory receptor (a specialized dendritic terminal), (2) a sensory nerve (the dendritic fiber leading from the receptor to the cell body of the sensory neuron, in the dorsal horn of the cord), (3) a synapse between the sensory nerve axon and an α-motoneuron, (4) a motor nerve (axon of the α-motoneuron), and (5) the neuromuscular junction between motor nerve and muscle fiber. The classic knee-jerk response (patellar reflex) is an example of a motor reflex (Fig. 22–5). Striking of the patellar tendon below the kneecap stretches the quadriceps muscle. This stretch is sensed by muscle spindles, which initiate automatic contraction of the quadriceps, and the lower leg moves outward.

Descending motor pathways (from UMNs) ultimately synapse on α-motoneurons and influence reflex activity. Because these synapses may result in either excitatory or inhibitory postsynaptic potentials (see Chapter 21), higher-level input may be either

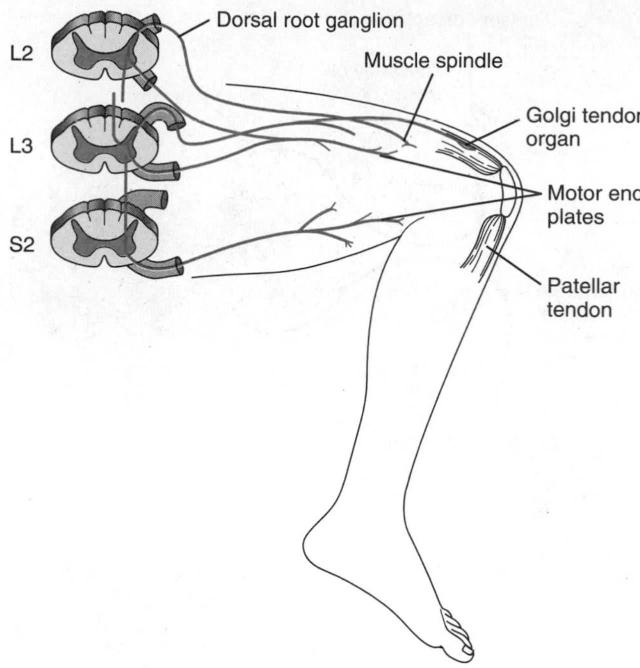

FIGURE 22–5

Patellar reflex. The patellar (knee-jerk) reflex is an example of a deep tendon reflex. Striking the patellar tendon stretches the quadriceps muscle. This stretch is sensed by muscle spindles, which initiate quadriceps contraction. The patellar reflex restores the original length of the quadriceps and causes the lower leg to move outward. A normal patellar reflex demonstrates intact reflex arc components in the lumbar and sacral segments of the cord as well as appropriate descending signals. (Redrawn from Carpenter, M.B., and Sutin, J. [1983]. *Human Neuroanatomy.* [8th ed.]. Baltimore: Williams & Wilkins.)

facilitative or inhibitory. Most reflexes can be voluntarily suppressed or induced to some extent, allowing conscious control of somatic motor activity. An example of subconscious regulation is the inhibition of contraction of one set of muscles (e.g., extensors such as the triceps) when an opposing muscle group (e.g., flexors such as the biceps) is contracting. This coordination of motor activity is possible because of interneuronal connections between the motor pathways leading to these muscle groups. This *reciprocal inhibition* may be clinically useful in relieving muscle cramps through voluntary contraction of opposing muscle groups. A calf muscle cramp (charley horse) may often be relieved by pulling the toes toward the nose, thus contracting opposing muscles.

Physiologic Reflexes

The reflexes that form the basis of normal activity are categorized as **physiologic reflexes** and include the muscle stretch (myotatic) reflex, the inverse myotatic reflex, the withdrawal (flexor) reflex, and the superficial **cutaneous reflexes.** In clinical settings, the integrity of reflex arcs is assessed by testing **deep tendon reflexes** (such as the patellar reflex) and cutaneous reflexes (superficial muscle contraction in response to stroking of the skin of the umbilical or anogenital areas).

The stretch (myotatic) reflex, initiated by muscle spindles, has been discussed. The inverse myotatic reflex begins with stimulation of a second type of muscle receptor, the *Golgi tendon organ.* Illustrated in Figure 22–6, this receptor is situated in series between muscle fibers and the tendon that attaches the muscle to bone. Whereas the muscle spindle responds to *stretch,* the Golgi tendon organ responds to an increase in muscle *tension,* initiating a reflex arc that inhibits excessive muscle contraction. Because this reflex is in opposition to the myotatic reflex, it protects muscle fibers from damage due to excessive tension.

The withdrawal (flexor) reflex also serves a protective function. This reflex arc is initiated with the stimulation of pain receptors in the skin or other tissues. Touching the finger to a candle flame, for example, results in a reflex motor response that withdraws the finger from the source of pain. The withdrawal reflex requires an interneuronal connection between sensory and motor neurons in the cord. Postural reflexes include those mediating the activities of running, walking, and standing. These involve several interneuronal connections along the length of the cord and are elicited by various stimuli, such as presssure on the foot, contraction of specific muscle groups, and relaxation of others.

Primitive and Pathologic Reflexes

Reflexes that are normally present during infancy but that are suppressed later in life are known as **primitive reflexes,** and those that appear only with neurologic disease or trauma are known as **pathologic reflexes.** Infants normally display reflexes

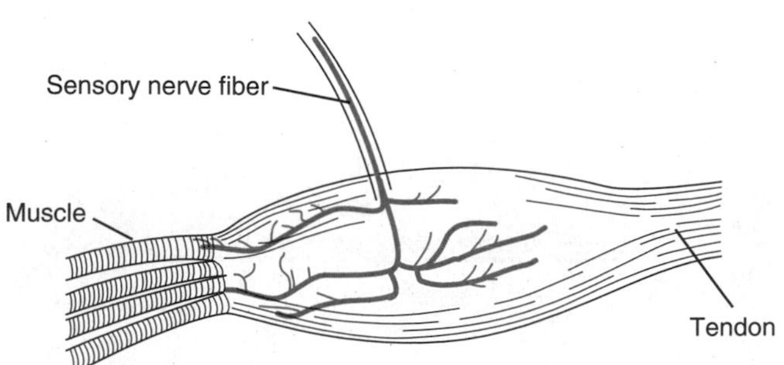

FIGURE 22–6

Golgi tendon organ. The Golgi tendon organ receptor is situated in series between muscle fibers and the tendon that connects the muscle to bone. This sensory receptor detects increases in muscle tension, initiating reflex inhibition of excessive muscle contraction. (Redrawn from Guyton, A.C., and Hall, J.E. [1996]. *Textbook of Medical Physiology.* [9th ed.]. Philadelphia: W.B. Saunders. [p. 691].)

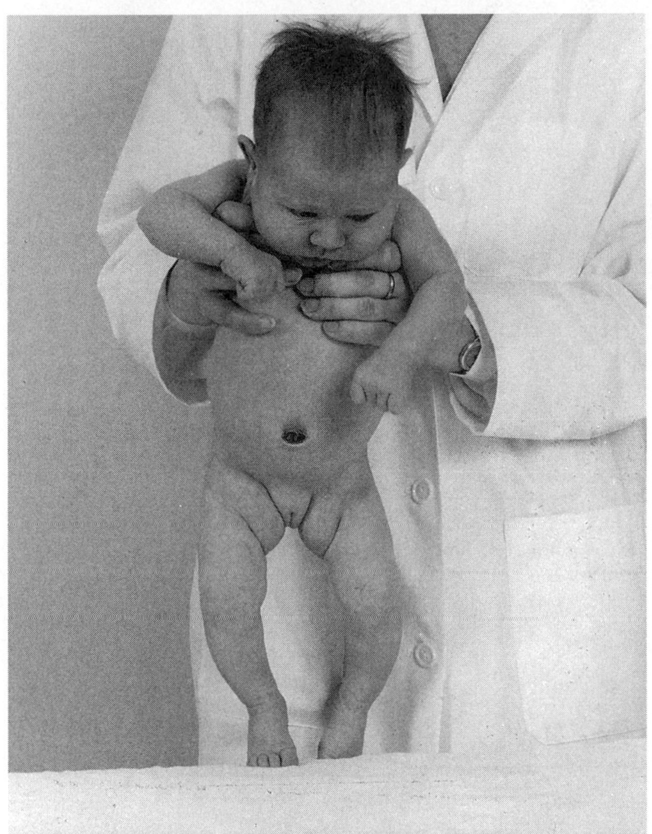

FIGURE 22–7
Primitive stepping reflex. Infants display motor reflexes such as stepping motions with pressure of the feet on a surface. These reflexes are normally inhibited as the central nervous system matures but may reemerge later in life with central nervous system pathology. (From Jarvis, C. [1996]. *Physical Examination and Health Assessment.* [2nd ed.]. Philadelphia: W.B. Saunders. [p. 747].)

which are inhibited with later maturation of motor pathways. Clinical assessment of these reflexes, such as sucking, grasping, startle, and stepping (Fig. 22–7), is a component of evaluation of developmental status of infants (see Chapter 33). In older children or adults with damage to higher motor centers, these primitive reflexes may be disinhibited. The patient may reflexively suck on a suction catheter or mouth swab, for example, or may grasp an object reflexively but be unable to release it on command. When primitive reflexes re-emerge in such cases, they are considered pathologic.

Other pathologic reflexes are those seen only with neuropathology, providing clinical evidence of the degree of damage. *Decorticate* and *decerebrate posturing* may be seen in patients with head injury, for example, when damage to cortical motor areas permits inappropriate postural reflexes (see Fig. 21–29 in Chapter 21). *Babinski's sign* (plantar reflex), a pathologic extension of the toes when the sole of the foot is stroked, usually indicates **upper motor neuron disease,** although it may be normally present in infants and young children. *Ankle clonus,* a sustained, rhythmic sequence of flexion and extension at the ankle, may be elicited with forceful dorsiflexion of the foot in patients with motor system disorders.

Upper Motor Neuron Function

Upper motor neurons are those of the primary motor cortex, premotor and supplemental areas, and brain stem.

Cortical Motor Areas

The primary motor cortex lies in the most posterior aspect of the frontal lobe (see Fig. 22–2). Its cells are arranged in vertical columns, and it is widely, although not universally, believed that each column regulates a single function. Fine motor activity (such as precise hand skills) requires more cortical input than does gross movement (such as standing upright or walking). Areas of the cortex that regulate specific activities have been accurately mapped and are illustrated in the *motor homunculus* (Fig. 22–8), a classic figure in which body parts

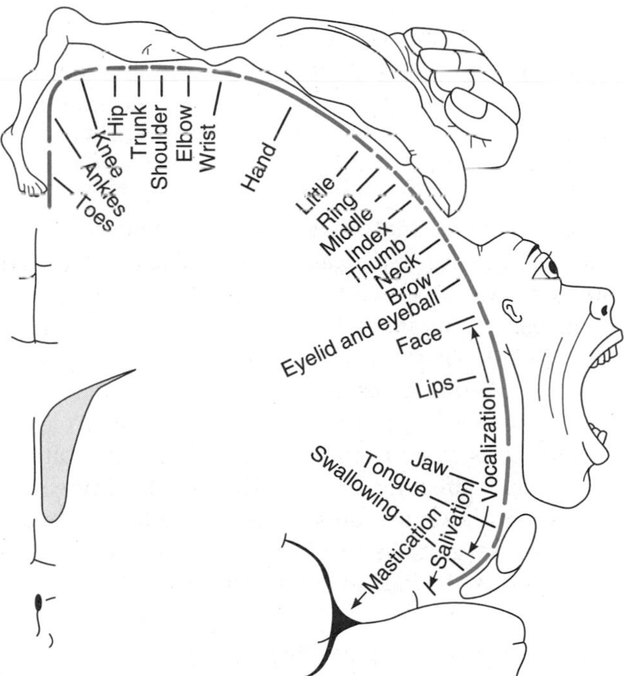

FIGURE 22–8
Motor homunculus. In this classic figure, the size of the body part is proportionate to the density of innervation required for its activity. The motor strip (right hemisphere) location of neurons governing these activities is also represented. (Redrawn from Penfield, W., and Rasmussen, T. [1950]. *The Cerebral Cortex of Man.* Indianapolis: Macmillan Publishing. Reprinted with the permission of Simon & Schuster. Copyright 1950 Macmillan Publishing Company; copyright renewed © 1978 Theodore Rasmussen.)

demanding more motor input are displayed proportionately larger. The fine movement of the hands, thumbs, and muscles of speech, for example, is prominently represented.

The premotor area lies anterior to the primary motor cortex and sends signals to it by direct axonal connections or by synapses with basal ganglia or thalamic nuclei. The premotor cortex contains specialized functional areas such as Broca's area, the motor area for speech (see Chapter 21), and a hand skills area that is essential to the planning and execution of manipulative activities. The supplemental area is located anterior to the premotor area and is believed to function similarly, although its function is not as well understood.

Major Motor Pathways

The major motor pathways descending from the cortical motor areas are the bilateral *corticospinal (pyramidal) tracts,* which originate in the primary motor cortex and pass through the internal capsule (Fig. 22–9). Some axons (corticobulbar fibers) then synapse on motor nuclei in the brain stem, but most (corticospinal fibers) continue downward. Most corticospinal fibers decussate (cross) in an area of the medulla oblongata known as the *pyramids,* then travel downward in lateral regions of the anterior horns (the lateral corticospinal tracts), eventually synapsing on LMNs. A few corticospinal fibers do not cross in the pyramids, but instead continue downward more medially (the ventral corticospinal tracts), not crossing until just before they synapse on LMNs.

The remaining motor pathways are known collectively as the *extrapyramidal tracts.* These pathways also originate in the motor cortex, but they project to the basal ganglia and cerebellum before descent (Fig. 22–10). They are involved in the "fine-tuning" activities of the accessory motor systems, as discussed later in this section. The effects of neuroleptic drugs on this system and the clinical manifestations of disorders affecting these pathways are known as **extrapyramidal symptoms.** These include such manifestations as gait disturbances and tremors, as discussed later with **Parkinson's disease.**

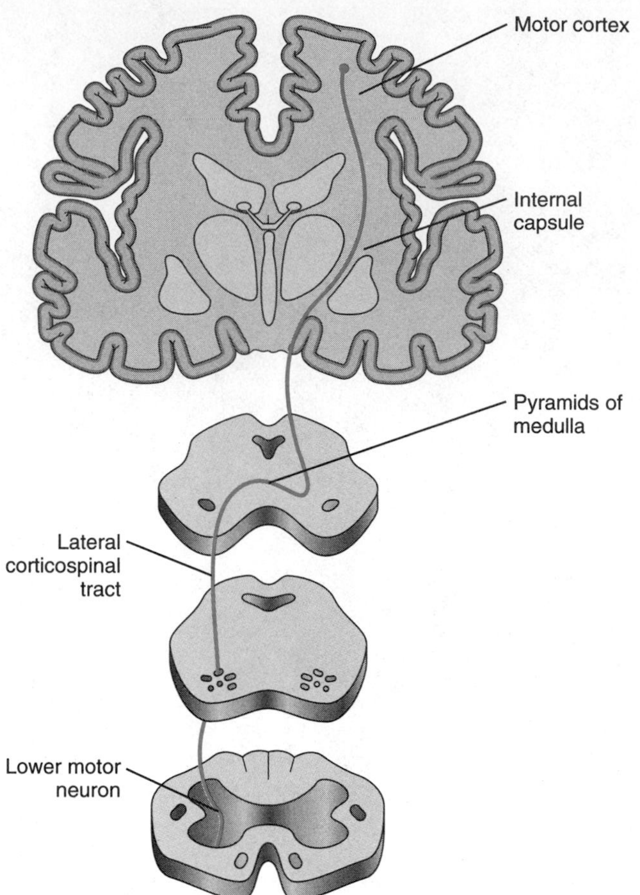

FIGURE 22–9

Corticospinal (pyramidal) tract. The bilateral corticospinal tracts originate in the primary motor cortex (one tract is shown here). Fibers from the primary motor cortex descend through the internal capsule and cross at the pyramids of the medulla oblongata. Most corticospinal fibers continue downward in the lateral regions of the anterior horns, eventually synapsing on lower motor neurons.

Brain-Stem Motor Nuclei and Pathways

The motor areas of the brain stem are illustrated in Figure 22–11. Fibers from the primary motor cortex and the cerebellum synapse on the *red nucleus,* located in the midbrain, which gives rise to the descending fibers of the *rubrospinal tract.* This tract lies slightly anterior to the corticospinal tract fibers in the cord, and it may serve as a backup motor pathway in the event of damage to the corticospinal tract. Movements executed by this tract are not as well coordinated, however.

The reticular nuclei of the cord constitute the motor portion of the reticular activating system, pacemaker neurons of the central nervous system (CNS) that can spontaneously generate impulses (see Chapter 21). These neurons include the *pontine reticular nuclei,* located in the pons, and the *medullary reticular nuclei,* located in the medulla. The pontine nuclei transmit *excitatory* impulses through the *pontine reticulospinal tract* to the LMNs of antigravity muscles. The medullary nuclei transmit *inhibitory* impulses to antigravity muscles through the *medullary reticulospinal tract.* The *vestibular nuclei,* located in the medulla and pons, constitute the motor portion of the proprioceptive (position sense) system (see Chapter 23). When cortical motor areas are damaged (e.g., by

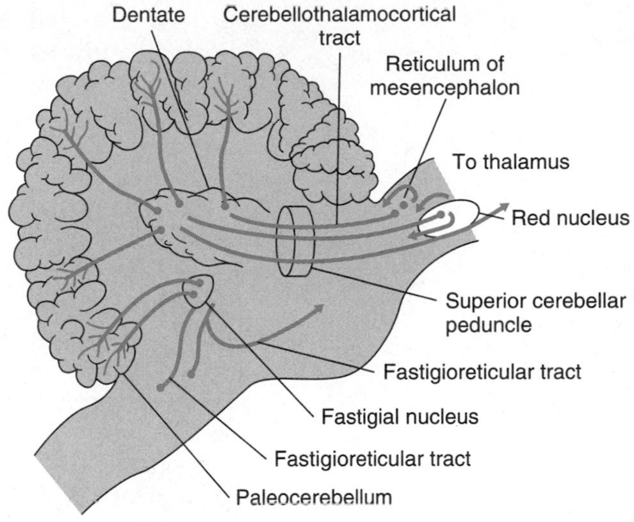

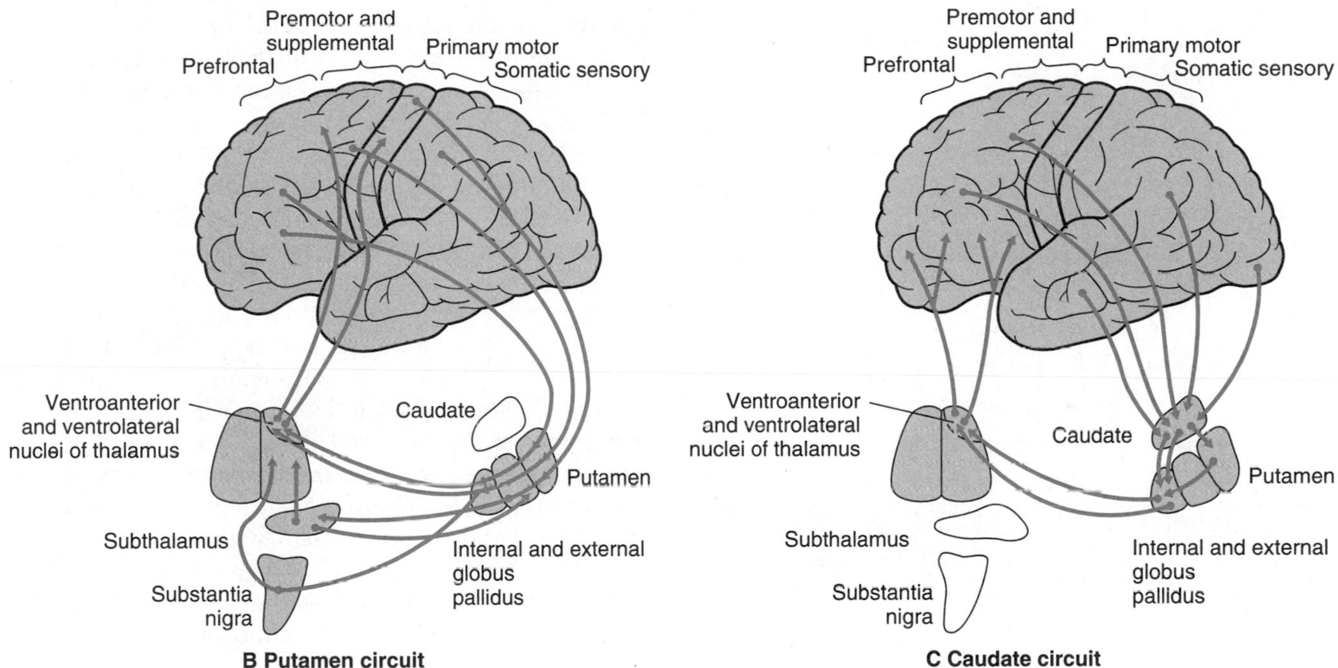

FIGURE 22–10

Extrapyramidal tracts. The principal motor pathways outside the corticospinal (pyramidal) tracts are the *cerebellar circuit* and the two primary circuits of the basal ganglia (the *putamen* and *caudate circuits*). These pathways are involved in fine control of motor activity. (Redrawn from Guyton, A.C., and Hall, J.E. [1996]. *Textbook of Medical Physiology.* [9th ed.]. Philadelphia: W.B. Saunders. [pp. 718, 726–727].)

stroke or head injury), brain-stem motor nuclei independently initiate abnormal motor reflexes, such as decerebrate and decorticate posturing.

Fibers from cranial nerves III, IV, and IX emerge from the midbrain; V, VI, VII exit the pons; and X, XI, and XII arise from the medulla. All of these cranial nerves have motor functions, detailed in Chapter 21. **Bell's palsy,** a common disorder in which facial paralysis results from cranial nerve VII dysfunction, is discussed later in this chapter. Motor disorders associated with cranial nerve dysfunction also include impairment of phonation (voice) and deglutition (swallowing), discussed in Chapters 18 and 24.

Role of the Cerebellum and Basal Ganglia

The cerebellum ("little brain") is anatomically similar to the cerebrum in that it has an outer cortex of

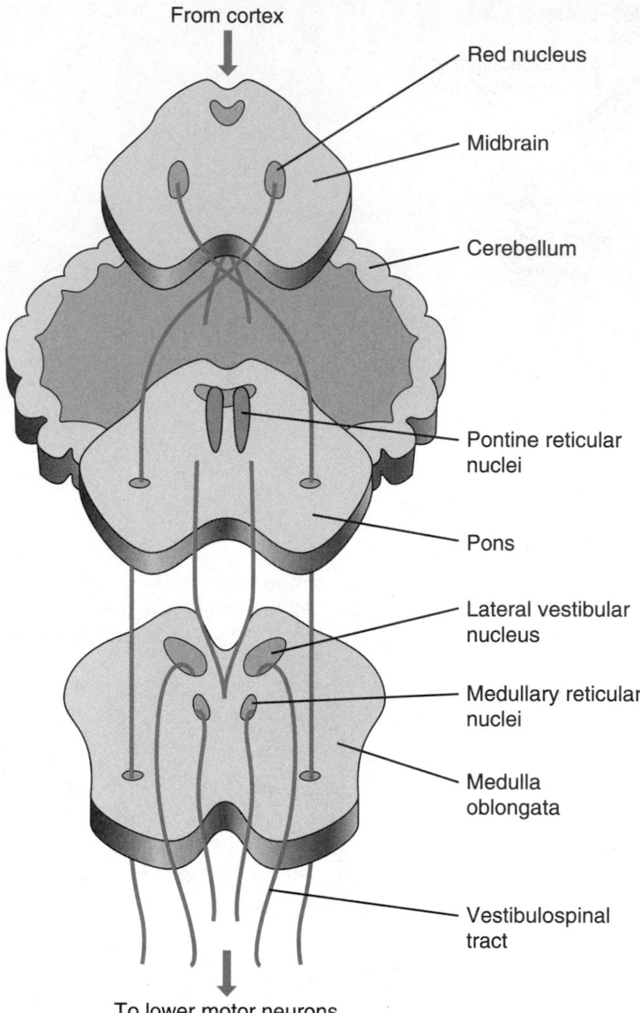

FIGURE 22–11

Motor areas of the brain stem. Descending nerve fibers from the *red nucleus* of the midbrain form the *rubrospinal tract,* which may mediate crude movement. The *reticular nuclei* signal the lower motor neurons serving the antigravity muscles. The *vestibular nuclei* mediate motor responses to proprioceptive (position sense) signals.

gray matter and also contains deep nuclei, the most important of which are the *dentate* and *fastigial* nuclei (see Fig. 22–10*A*). Each nucleus is part of a different motor pathway that projects upward to the cortical motor areas. Motor neurons in the cerebellum receive input from sensors of the proprioceptive system. Descending fibers from the motor cortex also synapse on cerebellar neurons, and the signal is modified based on proprioceptive input. In addition to its proprioceptive function, the cerebellum is important in coordination and appropriate sequencing of skilled motor acts ("cerebellar learning") and in damping of muscle movements to prevent inaccuracies, such as over-reaching a target due to momentum. An example of cerebellar learning is the coordinated handwork and footwork involved in driving a car with a standard transmission. Initially, one must think through and voluntarily initiate every movement, but with experience, these actions become automatic.

The basal ganglia consist of pairs of deep cerebral nuclei, located just above the brain stem (see Fig. 21–1). These include the *corpus striatum,* with its two component nuclei, the *lentiform* and *caudate* nuclei, and the *claustrum.* The *amygdala* is often considered to be a part of the basal ganglia, but its functions are more consistent with those of the limbic system (see Chapter 21). The lentiform nucleus has two components, the *globus pallidus* and the *putamen.* The function of the claustrum is uncertain. The internal capsule lies between the two nuclei most important in motor function, the caudate and the putamen. Neurons of the *subthalamus* and the *substantia nigra,* located in the upper midbrain, are considered to be a functional component of the basal ganglia because their axonal fibers project to these nuclei.

The basal ganglia receive inputs from the premotor and supplemental areas as well as from the primary sensory and sensorimotor association areas in the cortex. Output signals are relayed to the primary motor cortex by the thalamus. The neural interconnections are complex, and their function is not well understood. γ-Aminobutyric acid (GABA) and dopamine are the primary neurotransmitters at inhibitory synapses, whereas ACh is employed at excitatory synapses within the basal ganglia. The caudate circuit is believed to mediate fine regulation of the timing and scale of movement, whereas the putamen circuit endows movement with smoothness and grace (see Fig. 22–10*B*, *C*). Degeneration of dopaminergic neurons of the basal ganglia results in the tremor and gait disorder of Parkinson's disease.

AUTONOMIC NERVOUS SYSTEM

The ANS is so named because it regulates visceral functions that were long believed to be automatic. Although autonomic activity is principally reflex in nature, classification of ANS-mediated activity as involuntary is not strictly accurate. Higher-level inputs may facilitate or inhibit the activity of this visceral motor system similarly to the hierarchic control of the somatic motor system, although to a more limited degree.

Disorders originating from primary autonomic pathology are not common. Although three conditions are discussed later in this chapter to illustrate consequences of inappropriate autonomic stimulation, the greater clinical significance of the ANS is derived from its mediation of *adaptive responses* in disorders resulting from other pathologic mechanisms. The clinical manifestations of virtually any disorder include those indicating adaptive responses as well as those attributable to the specific pathology.

Anatomy and General Functions

The ANS is a motor system in that the axons of its neurons carry descending impulses to effector organs. Like the somatic motor system, the basic mechanism of regulation is the reflex arc, and the sensory or afferent arm of ANS reflexes consists of somatic sensory pathways. The ANS differs from the somatic motor system in that its effector organs are cardiac and smooth muscle rather than skeletal muscle. Secretory glands, such as the sweat glands and the adrenal medulla, are also ANS effectors.

Although some ANS reflexes are mediated within the spinal cord, similarly to the somatic motor system, most are integrated within specialized nuclei in the brain stem. Autonomic function also overlaps endocrine function in that (1) autonomic neurotransmitters function as hormones when they enter the bloodstream; (2) the hypothalamus, a neuroendocrine organ, is the central integrative organ of the ANS; and (3) the adrenal medulla, an endocrine organ, functions as a "giant sympathetic ganglion" in autonomic function.

Autonomic Nervous System Divisions and Their Distribution

The ANS has two principal subdivisions: the *sympathetic nervous system* (SNS) and the *parasympathetic nervous system* (PNS), which are anatomically and functionally distinct. Generally, their effects are in opposition, with the homeostatic balance between SNS and PNS stimulation determining the state of visceral function.

As shown in Figure 22–12, the ANS motor pathways are (with one exception) two-neuron relays. Axons of the primary neurons (first ones in each pathway) of the SNS exit the spinal cord between the first thoracic and second lumbar vertebrae. Axons from primary PNS neurons exit the brain stem with specific cranial nerves and also emerge from sacral segments of the cord. The two subdivisions thus differ in distribution: the SNS is *thoracolumbar*, whereas the PNS is *craniosacral*.

The SNS and PNS also differ in the configuration of their pathways. With one exception, the primary neurons of the SNS have short axons (preganglionic fibers) that synapse just outside the cord with secondary neurons, forming the "sympathetic chain." (Note that the term *ganglion* generally refers to any neuron cell body located outside the CNS.) The single exception occurs in the SNS innervation of the adrenal medulla. In this case, long preganglionic fibers do not synapse until they reach the adrenal medulla, and this organ functions as the secondary "neuron" in the pathway. The secondary neurons of the sympathetic chain send long axons (postganglionic fibers) to target organs. A few of these fibers reenter the cord and exit on the opposite side before traveling to target organs.

Most primary neurons of the PNS send long axonal (preganglionic) fibers to the walls of their target organs, where they synapse with secondary neurons. These in turn send short postganglionic fibers into the organ walls. A few primary neurons synapse with ganglia near the cord. Because 75% of all PNS impulses travel along the vagus nerve (cranial nerve X), the term *vagal stimulation* is often used clinically in reference to parasympathetic stimulation.

End-Organ Synapses

In smooth muscle and cardiac muscle, neuromuscular junctions are more diffusely distributed than in skeletal muscle. The autonomic motor nerves end in branches embedded within muscle or gland. Axonal branches have swellings, known as *varicosities*, that contain neurotransmitters within vesicles. The neurotransmitter released from a single presynaptic membrane may bind receptors on several target organ cells. The postsynaptic effect may be either excitatory or inhibitory, depending on the nature of the receptor, as discussed next.

Autonomic Receptors

The receptors within autonomic motor pathways are of two types: *adrenergic* and *cholinergic*, with each of these having subclasses. Adrenergic receptors bind the catecholamines norepinephrine (NE) and epinephrine (EPI). Cholinergic receptors bind ACh. Within the SNS, all primary (preganglionic) synapses are cholinergic, whereas most postganglionic synapses are adrenergic. The few SNS fibers that reenter the cord and exit again with motor nerves culminate in cholinergic synapses, affecting sweat glands, piloerector muscles, and some blood vessels. Within the PNS, all synapses are cholinergic.

Table 22–1 illustrates characteristics of receptor

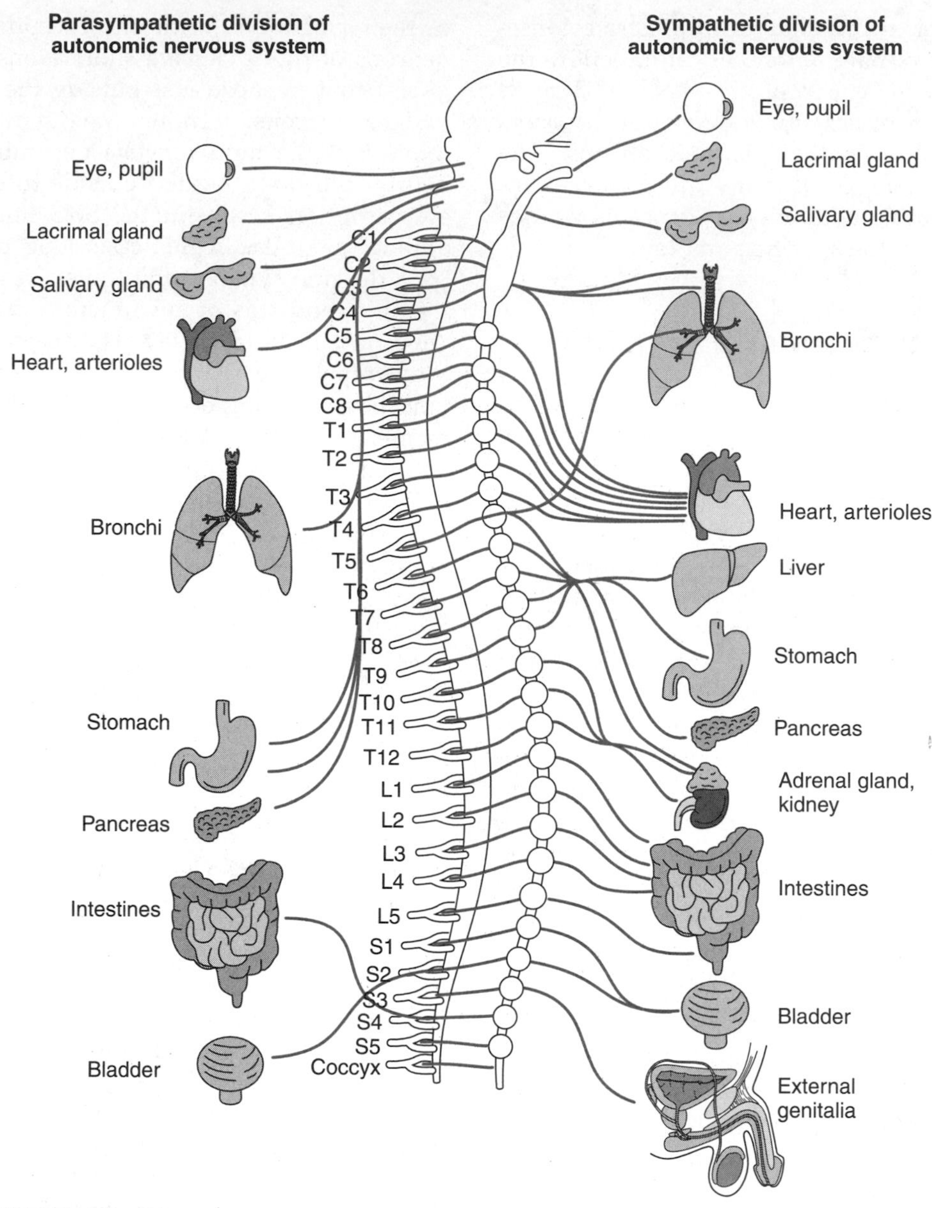

FIGURE 22–12

Autonomic nervous system. The *sympathetic division* has a thoracolumbar distribution, whereas the *parasympathetic division* has a craniosacral distribution. With few exceptions, these divisions innervate the same end organs, mediating opposing effects.

subtypes. Adrenergic receptors include two major classes, α and β, with each of these also having subdivisions based on their microanatomy, their effects on specific tissues, and their preference for NE or EPI. Cholinergic receptor subtypes are classified as muscarinic or nicotinic, based on the ligands (muscarine or nicotine) used to differentiate their functions in laboratory testing.

Role of the Adrenal Medulla

The adrenal medulla constitutes the inner portion of the adrenal gland. The anatomy and physiology of this endocrine organ are further detailed in Chapter 29, along with the function of the hormones of its outer zone, the adrenal cortex. The adrenal medulla arises from the same embryonic tissue as the ANS and is functionally integrated with the SNS. SNS stimulation of the adrenal medulla results in the secretion of the catecholamines EPI (80%) and NE (20%) into the bloodstream, where they circulate until binding to adrenergic receptors on target organs. Because sympathetic neurons also secrete norepinephrine, these regulatory chemicals act as both neurotransmitters and hormones in SNS function. The hormonal effects are more widespread and of longer duration, however, amplifying the neurotransmitter effects.

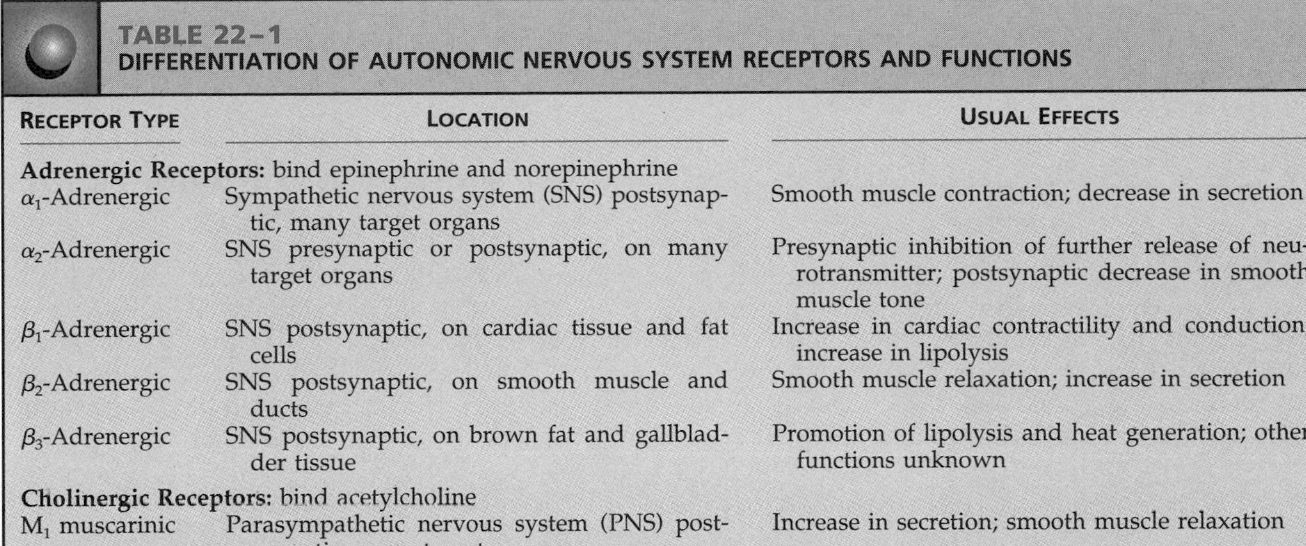

TABLE 22–1
DIFFERENTIATION OF AUTONOMIC NERVOUS SYSTEM RECEPTORS AND FUNCTIONS

Receptor Type	Location	Usual Effects
Adrenergic Receptors: bind epinephrine and norepinephrine		
α_1-Adrenergic	Sympathetic nervous system (SNS) postsynaptic, many target organs	Smooth muscle contraction; decrease in secretion
α_2-Adrenergic	SNS presynaptic or postsynaptic, on many target organs	Presynaptic inhibition of further release of neurotransmitter; postsynaptic decrease in smooth muscle tone
β_1-Adrenergic	SNS postsynaptic, on cardiac tissue and fat cells	Increase in cardiac contractility and conduction; increase in lipolysis
β_2-Adrenergic	SNS postsynaptic, on smooth muscle and ducts	Smooth muscle relaxation; increase in secretion
β_3-Adrenergic	SNS postsynaptic, on brown fat and gallbladder tissue	Promotion of lipolysis and heat generation; other functions unknown
Cholinergic Receptors: bind acetylcholine		
M_1 muscarinic	Parasympathetic nervous system (PNS) postsynaptic, many target organs	Increase in secretion; smooth muscle relaxation
M_2 muscarinic	PNS postsynaptic, in heart; smooth muscle	Decrease in heart rate; decrease in conduction; smooth muscle relaxation
M_4 muscarinic	PNS postsynaptic; in smooth muscle pancreatic acinar and islet cells	Increase in pancreatic secretion of insulin and enzymes
Nicotinic	Sympathetic ganglia	Indirect mediation of most SNS effects; direct mediation of sweating, piloerection

Data from Berne, R.M., and Levy, M.N. (1993). *Physiology*. (3rd ed.). St. Louis: Mosby–Year Book. (pp. 249–252); Ganong, W.F. (1995). *Review of Medical Physiology*. (17th ed.). Norwalk, CT: Appleton & Lange. (pp. 204–209); and Flier, J.S., and Underhill, L.H. (1996). Adrenergic receptors: Evolving concepts and clinical implications. *New England Journal of Medicine* 334(9), 580–585.

Regulation of Autonomic Function

Central Integration of Autonomic Nervous System Activity

Figure 22–13 illustrates a typical autonomic (visceral) reflex arc, which is triggered by stimulation of a visceral sensory receptor. The impulse travels along a somatic sensory (visceral afferent) fiber to a synapse with an autonomic neuron in the brain stem or cord. Autonomic efferent fibers then transmit the signal back to the organ that initiated the signal.

Consistent with the principle of hierarchic control that characterizes all neural regulation, the basic reflex arc may be facilitated or inhibited by higher-level input to the autonomic neurons in the brain stem or cord. Specialized brain-stem nuclei (visceral regulatory centers) constitute the next level of control, and these are influenced in turn by hypothalamic nuclei. The hypothalamus, in response to inputs from the cerebral cortex and limbic system, signals the brain stem or cord centers to facilitate or inhibit visceral reflexes, thus adjusting cardiovascular and respiratory function, bladder contraction, gastrointestinal motility and secretion, and many other homeostatic functions. Because of this hierarchic control, conscious thoughts and subconscious

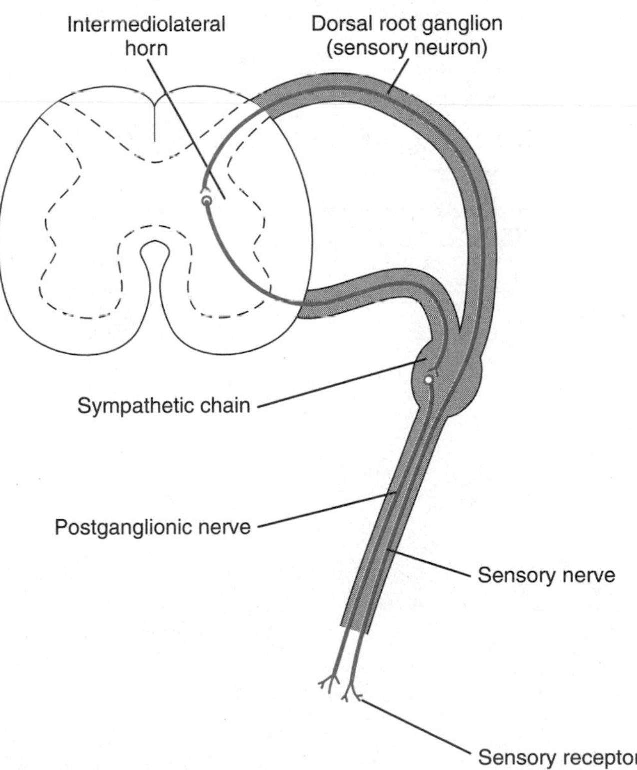

FIGURE 22–13
Autonomic reflex arc. Stimulation of a sensory receptor in an internal organ initiates impulse transmission along a somatic sensory nerve to a synapse with an autonomic neuron in the brain stem or spinal cord. Autonomic efferent fibers then transmit the signal back to the target organ.

emotions may regulate visceral activity to some degree; and the end point may or may not be beneficial, as discussed in reference to the stress response (see Chapter 1).

Influence of Drugs on Autonomic Function

Many drugs are chemically similar to catecholamines, acetylcholine, or their precursors. Binding of these ligands to autonomic receptors may either mimic the action of the natural neurotransmitter (i.e., act as agonists) or block the normal effect by preventing the natural ligand from binding (i.e., act as antagonists or blockers). Table 22–2 summarizes the actions of such agents in common clinical use.

Organ-Specific Autonomic Effects

Table 22–3 summarizes the effects of SNS and PNS stimulation on the various target organs. In many cases, the effect is predictable if SNS effects are considered to benefit the human during stress (see Chapter 1) and PNS effects to be beneficial during relaxation or restorative states.

TABLE 22–2
DRUGS INFLUENCING AUTONOMIC FUNCTION

Classification	Examples	Clinical Use
Cholinergic agonists (parasympathomimetics)	Carbachol (Isopto)	Treatment of glaucoma
	Bethanechol (Urecholine)	Treatment of urinary stasis or abdominal distention
	Pilocarpine	Treatment of glaucoma
Neuromuscular blocking agents	Succinylcholine (Anectine)	Muscle relaxation during surgery or mechanical ventilation
Acetylcholinesterase inhibitors (anticholinesterases)	Ambenonium (Mytelase)	Treatment of myasthenia gravis
	Pyridostigmine (Mestinon)	Treatment of myasthenia gravis
	Edrophonium (Tensilon)	Treatment of myasthenia gravis, paralytic ileus, dysrhythmias
Muscarinic antagonists (anticholinergics)	Atropine	Treatment of bradycardia
	Scopolamine	Treatment of motion sickness and enhancement of effectiveness of preoperative analgesics and sedatives in obstetrics
	Glycopyrrolate (Robinul)	To decrease secretions before anesthesia
Ganglionic agonists	Nicotine	To produce controlled hypotension during surgery; treatment of ulcerative colitis; treatment of tobacco withdrawal
Ganglionic blocking agents	Mecamylamine (Inversine)	Treatment of autonomic hyper-reflexia
Adrenergic agonists (sympathomimetics)	Epinephrine (Adrenalin)	Treatment of cardiac arrest, shock, bronchospasm (as in asthma or anaphylaxis)
	Dopamine (Intropin)	Treatment of shock and poor renal perfusion
	Norepinephrine (Levophed)	Treatment of hypotension
	Isoproterenol (Isuprel)	Treatment of cardiac conduction disturbances and blocks
	Ephedrine (Vatronol)	Treatment of nasal congestion
α-Adrenergic antagonists	Phenoxybenzamine (Dibenzyline)	Treatment of peripheral vascular spasm, e.g., Raynaud's disease
	Ergot alkaloids (Ergomar)	Treatment of confusion and vascular headaches
β-Adrenergic antagonists	Propranolol (Inderal)	Treatment of hypertension, dysrhythmias, migraine
	Metoprolol (Lopressor)	Treatment of hypertension
	Timolol (Timoptic)	Treatment of glaucoma

Data from Lehne, R.A. (1994). *Pharmacology for Nursing Care.* (2nd ed.). Philadelphia: W.B. Saunders. (pp. 109–204).

TABLE 22–3
AUTONOMIC EFFECTS ON SPECIFIC ORGAN SYSTEMS

Organ	Effect of Sympathetic Stimulation	Effect of Parasympathetic Stimulation
Eye		
Pupil	Dilated	Constricted
Ciliary muscle	Slight relaxation (far vision)	Constricted (near vision)
Glands Nasal Lacrimal Parotid Submandibular Gastric Pancreatic	Vasoconstriction and slight secretion	Stimulation of copious secretion (containing many enzymes for enzyme-secreting glands)
Sweat glands	Copious sweating (cholinergic)	Sweating on palms of hands
Apocrine glands	Thick, odoriferous secretion	None
Blood vessels	Most often constricted	Most often little or no effect
Heart		
Muscle	Increased rate Increased force of contraction	Slowed rate Decreased force of contraction (especially of atria)
Coronaries	Dilated (β_2); constricted (α)	Dilated
Lungs		
Bronchi	Dilated	Constricted
Blood vessels	Mildly constricted	? Dilated
Gut		
Lumen	Decreased peristalsis and tone	Increased peristalsis and tone
Sphincter	Increased tone (most times)	Relaxed (most times)
Liver	Glucose released	Slight glycogen synthesis
Gallbladder and bile ducts	Relaxed	Contracted
Kidney	Decreased output and renin secretion	None
Bladder		
Detrusor	Relaxed (slight)	Contracted
Trigone	Contracted	Relaxed
Penis	Ejaculation	Erection
Systemic arterioles		
Abdominal viscera	Constricted	None
Muscle	Constricted (adrenergic α) Dilated (adrenergic β_2) Dilated (cholinergic)	None
Skin	Constricted	None
Blood		
Coagulation	Increased	None
Glucose	Increased	None
Lipids	Increased	None
Basal metabolism	Increased up to 100%	None
Adrenal medullary secretion	Increased	None
Mental activity	Increased	None
Piloerector muscles	Contracted	None
Skeletal muscle	Increased glycogenolysis Increased strength	None
Fat cells	Lipolysis	None

From Guyton, A.C., and Hall, J.E. (1996). *Textbook of Medical Physiology*. (9th ed.). Philadelphia: W.B. Saunders. (p. 775).

DISORDERS OF MOTOR FUNCTION

Somatic motor system disorders may originate from abnormality of motor neurons, the neuromuscular junction, or the muscle. Primary muscle disorders are discussed in Chapter 35. Although "pure" autonomic disorders are rare, autonomic dysfunction may contribute to, or result from, disorders of virtually every system (Table 22–4). Frequently, disease or trauma affecting somatic motor function also affects autonomic function.

TABLE 22–4
CLINICAL DISORDERS OF THE AUTONOMIC NERVOUS SYSTEM

Disorder	Clinical Features
Complete autonomic paralysis (dysautonomic polyneuropathy)	Loss of autonomic regulation of sweating, blood pressure, pupillary reflexes, lacrimation, salivation, bowel and bladder function, and sexual function occurring gradually over a period of weeks; affects both adults and children; most recover completely; believed to be an autoimmune disorder similar to Guillain-Barré syndrome
Botulism	Clostridial toxin interferes with release of acetylcholine at the neuromuscular junction and at cholinergic synapses in the autonomic nervous system. Acute paralysis is the major effect; autonomic effects include dryness of eyes and mouth and paralytic ileus.
Orthostatic hypotension	Blunting of the baroreceptor response causes a postural drop in blood pressure with change from a lying position to a sitting or standing position; common with aging; may be associated with spinal cord injury and with other neuromuscular disorders (see Chapter 15)
Riley-Day syndrome	Autosomal recessive disorder in which there is a deficiency of autonomic neurons, resulting in blood pressure fluctuation, alteration in temperature regulation, hearing loss, hyperhidrosis, blotchiness of skin, emotional lability, insensitivity to pain, and vomiting
Horner's syndrome	Syndrome of pupil constriction, eyelid drooping, and absence of sweating on one side of the face, due to interruption of preganglionic fibers by tumors or trauma
Autonomic hyper-reflexia	Rise in blood pressure, bradycardia, sweating, and piloerection in regions below the level of spinal cord injury
Disorders of sweating	Hyperhidrosis (increased sweating) and anhidrosis (absence of sweating) may be associated with injury or degeneration of postganglionic sympathetic nervous system (SNS) fibers.
Raynaud's syndrome	Episodic spasm of arteries in fingers, resulting in blanching; triggered by local trauma or exposure to cold; most common in young women who have connective tissue disease; considered to be an idiopathic disorder. The role of the SNS, which innervates digital arteries, is uncertain (see Chapter 15).
Bladder incontinence	Interruption of parasympathetic nervous system (PNS) innervation of bladder smooth muscle or somatic motor fibers to skeletal muscle of sphincter results in loss of regulation of micturition (see Chapter 20).
Congenital megacolon (Hirschsprung's disease)	Congenital absence of PNS innervation of the rectosigmoid area of the colon and the internal anal sphincter; this segment is constricted, leading to retention of feces and massive distention of the colon above the affected segment (see Chapter 24).
Priapism	Sustained painful penile erection due to disinhibition of the PNS reflex, secondary to injury or disease of the spinal cord above the sacral levels (see Chapter 30)

Data from Adams, R.D., and Victor, M. (1993). *Principles of Neurology.* (5th ed.). New York: McGraw-Hill. (pp. 468–478).

Dystonia

Definition. Dystonia is a general term encompassing disorders of muscle tone, including **atonia** (absence of muscle tone), **hypotonia** (decreased tone), and **hypertonia** (excessively increased muscle tone).

Epidemiology. Because it is associated with many common disorders, dystonia is common. Risk factors are those related to the underlying disorders.

Etiology. Abnormalities of muscle tone may result from trauma to motor system components (including damage to the sensory arm of reflex arcs). High-risk behaviors include use (especially careless use) of motor vehicles and participation in contact sports. Disorders resulting in decreased perfusion of nerves also impair motor neurotransmission and include atherosclerosis, abnormal blood clotting, and hypoxic disorders. Metabolic disorders, such as diabetes mellitus, may result in damage to peripheral nerves, and renal disease or other disorders producing electrolyte imbalance may impair action potential formation and conduction (see Chapter 9). Drugs (especially antipsychotics and antiarrhythmics) and circulating toxins may have similar effects. Primary or metastatic tumors may directly damage nervous tissue or may interfere with its perfusion (see Chapter 21).

Pathophysiology. Muscle tone is detected as a slight resistance to passive movement or attempts to deform muscle. It normally results from baseline activity of the motor system, in which the myotatic and inverse myotatic reflexes are in equilibrium, as mediated by balanced excitatory and inhibitory inputs from higher centers. The elastic recoil of the muscle protein connectin (titin) also contributes to tone (see Chapter 5).

Atonia results from total absence of motor input to muscle, as in the case of severing or atrophy of a peripheral motor nerve. The muscle is totally limp and flaccid, offering no resistance. Hypotonia is manifested as little resistance and is seen in corticospinal tract or cerebellar motor pathway disorders. Hypertonia occurs when LMN reflex arcs are not appropriately inhibited by higher centers, resulting in rigidity or spasticity of muscles. Hypertonia is common in spinal cord disorders and lesions of the cortical and subcortical motor areas. Table 22–5 describes patterns of dystonia seen with common motor disorders.

Clinical Manifestations. The most striking manifestations of dystonia of skeletal muscle are muscle flaccidity and weakness, or spasticity (see Chapter 35). Abnormal tone of smooth muscle may manifest in the vascular system as vasospasm, vasodilation, or vasoconstriction (see Chapter 15); in the gastrointestinal system as increased motility (diarrhea and malabsorption) or lack of peristalsis (paralytic ileus), with resultant obstruction (see Chapter 24); and in the genitourinary system as ureteral colic, atonic bladder, or bladder spasms (see Chapter 20).

Prevention and Treatment. Reduction of risk factors for dystonia involves safety measures and optimal treatment of underlying disorders. Treatment may include compensating for decreased skeletal muscle tone with bracing or other adjunctive devices. Drug therapy, surgical ablation of nerve pathways, or avoidance of triggering stimuli also may be used in specific disorders.

Prognosis and Outcome. Outcome depends on the nature and severity of the underlying disorder.

TABLE 22–5
COMMON PATTERNS OF DYSTONIA AND ASSOCIATED CAUSES

Pattern	Description	Usual Causes
Atonia		
Flaccidity	Muscle is paralyzed and offers no resistance to stretch; muscle atrophy ensues; absence of all movement	Lower motor neuron disease, e.g., spinal cord injury, peripheral nerve injury, or peripheral neuropathy
Hypertonia		
Spasticity	Muscle exhibits lack of reflex control, with continuous or intermittent increase in tone, spasm, clonus, and hyperactive deep tendon reflexes	Upper motor neuron disease, e.g., stroke, brain tumor, cerebral palsy, traumatic brain injury
Rigidity	Muscles are continuously firm and tense, usually most pronounced in flexor muscles; no hyper-reflexia	Extrapyramidal disorders, e.g., Parkinson's disease

Data from Adams, R.D., and Victor, M. (1993). *Principles of Neurology.* (5th ed.). New York: McGraw-Hill. (pp. 41, 65–66).

Dyskinesia

Definition. Dyskinesia is abnormal muscle movement. Movement may be excessive and abnormal in character *(hyperkinetic)* or decreased *(hypokinetic)*. An absence of movement is described as an *akinetic* state.

Epidemiology. Dyskinesia is a common component of neuromuscular disorders, such as Parkinson's disease, **multiple sclerosis (MS), Huntington's disease,** and **cerebral palsy,** and may also result from systemic toxicity as in dystonia. Risk factors are the same as those for dystonia.

Etiology. Dyskinesias may originate from traumatic, hypoxic, degenerative, or metabolic damage to UMNs, from imbalance in the production or removal of excitatory versus inhibitory neurotransmitters, or from interruption of LMN reflex arcs.

Pathophysiology. Damage to UMNs removes the normal descending regulatory inputs to the motor reflex arc. The motor response is thus uncontrolled and inaccurate. Similarly, imbalance of excitatory and inhibitory neurotransmitters impairs fine-tuning of motor responses. Inhibition or interruption of LMN reflex arcs, or **lower motor neuron disease,** results in diminished or absent activity.

Clinical Manifestations. Table 22–6 describes the characteristics and causes of the more common types of dyskinesia. **Hyperkinesia** may manifest as tremors, tics, gait disturbances, and other involuntary movements. **Hypokinesia** may manifest as muscle weakness **(paresis)** or slowed movement **(bradykinesia)** and may result from either UMN or LMN dysfunction.

Akinesia (paralysis) may also result from either UMN or LMN dysfunction, with varying patterns of muscle group involvement, depending on the location of the lesion within the motor system. Characteristics of UMN and LMN disorders are contrasted in Table 22–7. In the case of a stroke involving the

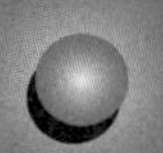

TABLE 22–6
COMMON PATTERNS OF DYSKINESIA AND ASSOCIATED CAUSES

Pattern	Description	Usual Causes
Hypokinesia		
Monoplegia or monoparesis	Paralysis or weakness of all muscles of one leg or arm	Lesion of the cerebral cortex (if muscular atrophy is absent) Disuse, partial spinal cord injury, peripheral nerve plexus injury (if muscular atrophy is apparent)
Hemiplegia or hemiparesis	Paralysis or weakness of the arm, leg, and sometimes the face on one side of the body	Lesion of the corticospinal pathway on one side, e.g., stroke, partial spinal cord injury, cortical or brain-stem injury
Paraplegia or paraparesis	Paralysis or weakness of both legs	Spinal cord injury at thoracic or lumbar levels, spina bifida, multiple sclerosis
Diplegia	Weakness predominantly in both legs but also affecting the arms to a minimal extent	Cerebral palsy
Quadriplegia or tetraplegia	Weakness or paralysis of all four extremities	Lesions of the spinal cord at the cervical level
Isolated paralysis	Weakness or paralysis of one or more isolated muscle groups	Peripheral nerve or nerve root injury; idiopathic, e.g., Bell's palsy of the facial nerve
Hysterical paralysis	Weakness in any pattern, with intact deep tendon reflexes and absence of atrophy	Psychiatric disorder
Bradykinesia	Slowness of movement	Extrapyramidal disorder, e.g., Parkinson's disease
Akinesia or hypokinesia	Disinclination to use an affected part ("poverty of movement")	Extrapyramidal disorder
Hyperkinesia		
Tremor	Rhythmic movements due to alternating contraction of antagonist muscles; may occur when muscle is at rest, or with activity (intention)	Parkinson's disease (rest tremor); cerebellar disorder (intention tremor); intense activity, fright, metabolic disturbance, e.g., alcohol withdrawal; familial inheritance (essential tremor)
Asterixis	Irregular interruptions in sustained muscle contraction	Encephalopathy due to liver or kidney disease; drug effect
Clonus	Series of brief muscle contractions of a single muscle group	Central nervous system (CNS) disease, e.g., head injury, seizure disorder; drug effect
Tics	Irresistable, stereotyped movements, actions, or spasms	Habit; neuropsychiatric disorder, e.g., Tourette's syndrome
Limited dystonias	Involuntary spasms of specific muscle groups	Often idiopathic, e.g., torticollis (neck muscle spasm); blepharospasm (eyelid spasm)
Chorea	Involuntary jerky movements, e.g., grimacing; forcible limb movements	Varied CNS lesions, e.g., Huntington's chorea, Sydenham's chorea
Ballismus	Flinging movements due to involuntary contraction of proximal limb muscles	Subthalamic lesion
Athetosis	Inability to sustain body parts in one position; interruption of posture with slow, sinuous movements (often combined with chorea as choreoathetosis)	Huntington's disease, familial encephalopathies, drug effect
Tardive dyskinesias	Patterned, repetitive movements	Iatrogenic disorder due to use of dopamine receptor–blocking agents, e.g., phenothiazines for psychosis

Data from Adams, R.D., and Victor, M. (1993). *Principles of Neurology.* (5th ed.). New York: McGraw-Hill. (pp. 51–54, 64–73, 934–935).

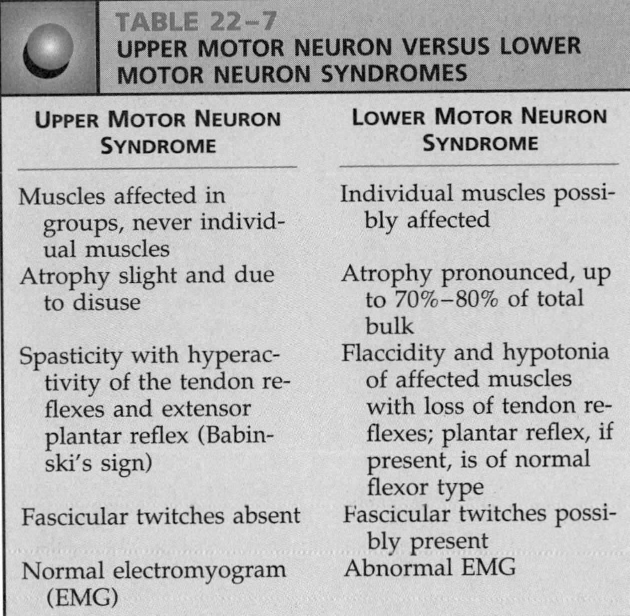

TABLE 22–7
UPPER MOTOR NEURON VERSUS LOWER MOTOR NEURON SYNDROMES

Upper Motor Neuron Syndrome	Lower Motor Neuron Syndrome
Muscles affected in groups, never individual muscles	Individual muscles possibly affected
Atrophy slight and due to disuse	Atrophy pronounced, up to 70%–80% of total bulk
Spasticity with hyperactivity of the tendon reflexes and extensor plantar reflex (Babinski's sign)	Flaccidity and hypotonia of affected muscles with loss of tendon reflexes; plantar reflex, if present, is of normal flexor type
Fascicular twitches absent	Fascicular twitches possibly present
Normal electromyogram (EMG)	Abnormal EMG

Adapted from Adams, R.D., and Victor, M. (1993). *Principles of Neurology*. (5th ed.). New York: McGraw-Hill. (p. 49).

motor cortex of one hemisphere, the muscles of the opposite side of the body are typically weakened **(hemiparesis)** or paralyzed **(hemiplegia).** With **spinal cord injury,** the pattern of involvement depends on the level of the injury, as described next.

Prevention and Treatment. Intervention in dyskinesias involves compensation for abnormal motor function and specific treatment of the underlying disorder.

Prognosis and Outcome. Outcome is highly variable, depending on the specific disorder.

Spinal Cord Injury

Definition. Spinal cord injury is the traumatic complete or partial transection of the cord.

Epidemiology. The estimated annual incidence of spinal cord injury is 10,000 in the United States.[1] The risk is highest in young males aged 15 to 30, owing to their involvement in motor vehicle use, contact sports, and alcohol consumption. Diving accidents causing spinal cord injury are often associated with alcohol use, which impairs the person's judgment regarding water of unknown depth; alcohol is a frequent contributor to motor vehicle accidents as well.

Etiology. Spinal cord injury is caused by (1) primary (force-induced or mechanical) injury and (2) secondary injury induced by the primary insult. Four types of forces may injure the spinal cord: acceleration–deceleration, rotation with deformation, axial loading (compression), and penetration. Acceleration–deceleration injury occurs in motor vehicle collisions, when the sudden cessation of movement results in hyperflexion, then hyperextension, of the spine (Fig. 22–14). The degree of damage depends on the speed at which the collision occurred. Whiplash injuries are mildest and involve strain of muscles and ligaments of the spine with no direct damage to the cord. With more forceful collisions, vertebral fractures may occur, and the cord may be damaged by bone fragments or overstretching.

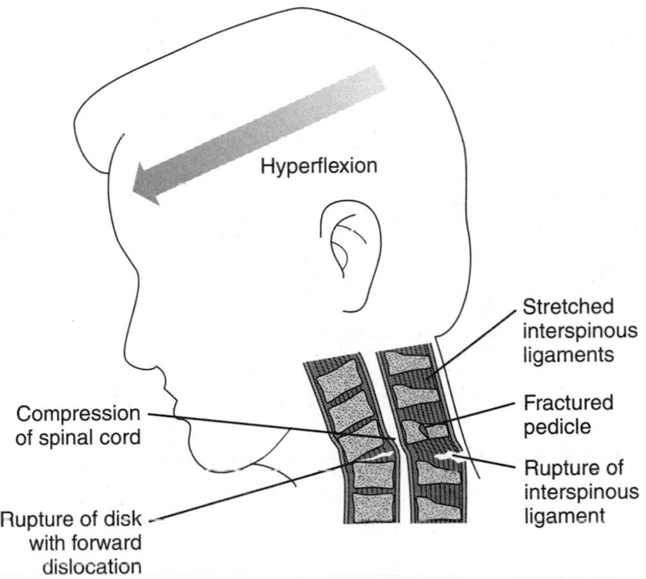

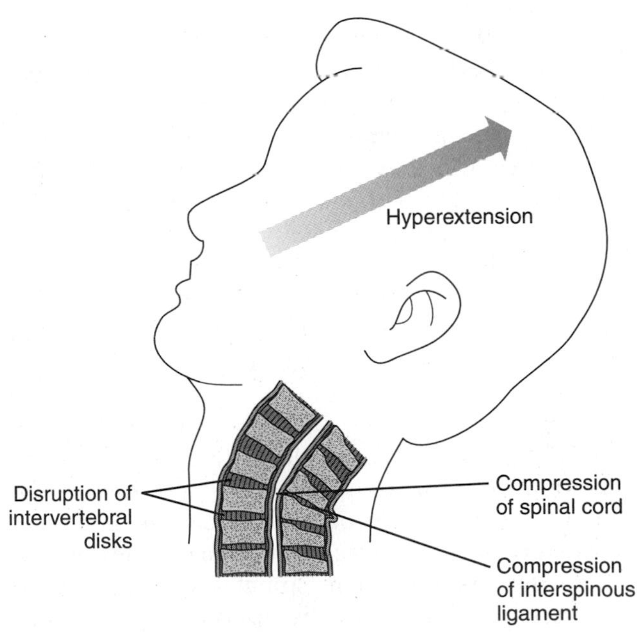

FIGURE 22–14

Acceleration–deceleration injury of the spinal cord. Sudden cessation of movement (as in a motor vehicle collision) causes hyperflexion, then hyperextension, of the spine. Potential injuries include strain or rupture of ligaments, fracture of vertebrae, and stretch or penetration of the spinal cord.

Excessive rotation of the head may also rupture ligaments, fracture vertebrae, or cause tension trauma to the cord. Axial loading is the usual mechanism of injury in diving accidents and sports injuries. A severe compressive force shatters vertebrae and damages the cord. Penetrating trauma (other than bone fragments) is an uncommon cause of spinal cord injury, but bullets, knives, and other penetrating objects may result in direct damage to the cord.

The etiology of secondary injury is uncertain but may include alterations in cellular and mitochondrial metabolism induced by the impact. Ischemia, release of excitatory amino acids (e.g., glutamate), formation of reactive oxygen species, peroxidation of cell membrane lipids, or a rise in intracellular calcium may underlie secondary cord damage after spinal cord injury.

Pathophysiology. The initial lesion of spinal cord injury may be a concussion, contusion, or laceration of the cord and may be complicated by fracture of the bones of the spine. Concussion of the cord results in temporary motor dysfunction and may be seen in cases of child abuse when the child has been violently shaken. Contusion or bruising of the cord results from blunt trauma or stretching, whereas laceration results from sharp trauma. Transection, or severing of the cord, is rarely complete as a result of direct damage to the cord.

In most cases, secondary injury extends the lesion. Edema occurring in the relatively enclosed space of the injury creates additional pressure that may impede blood flow and cause tissue hypoxia. The presence of hemorrhage may further exacerbate the necrotic process, resulting in extension of the lesion. Within the lesion, hemorrhagic necrosis usually destroys the central gray matter and most of the adjacent white matter within 24 hours.[2] A cord that is partially transected by the injuring force may thus be completely transected as a result of horizontal extension of the lesion by hemorrhage or inflammation. Furthermore, the spinal cord lesion may extend vertically, interrupting a larger number of LMN reflex arcs.

Complete transection blocks neurotransmission from UMNs to LMNs, resulting in lack of normal facilitation or inhibition of reflex arcs below the level of the injury. **Spinal shock** ensues and may persist for days to weeks. Although the precise mechanisms are unknown, spinal shock is believed to represent a functional disruption of neurotransmission in structurally intact reflex arcs below the level of the injury, related to the lack of descending inputs from higher centers.

As spinal shock subsides, intact reflexes return and may be hyper-reflexic because of absence of in-

TABLE 22–8
LEVEL-DEPENDENT FUNCTIONAL STATUS IN SPINAL CORD INJURY

Neurologic Level of Complete Injury (Vertebrae)	Functional Ability
C-1–C-2	Limited movement of head and neck Ventilator dependent Dependent in all ADLs Requires electric wheelchair with breath, head, or shoulder controls
C-3–C-4	Good head and neck control Some diaphragm control, may need ventilatory support Dependent in ADLs Requires electric wheelchair with breath, head, or shoulder controls
C5	Full head, neck, shoulder, and diaphragm control, with some elbow flexion Able to feed and groom self with adaptive devices Requires major assistance with ADLs Needs electric wheelchair with hand control or manual wheelchair with rim projections
C6	Strong elbow flexion with some wrist extension (tenodesis) Independent in eating, grooming, bathing, bowel and bladder care with adaptive devices Requires minor assistance with dressing and transfers Independent in manual wheelchair on level surface; able to drive with hand controls
C7	Full elbow flexion with elbow extension, wrist flexion, and some finger control Independent in ADLs with aids Manual wheelchair on most surfaces
C-8–T-1	Moderate to full arm, wrist, and finger control Independent in all ADLs; may need adaptive devices
T-2–L-2	Full use of arms Independent in ADLs May have limited ability to ambulate short distances with crutches and orthoses Needs wheelchair
L2 and below	Full use of arms Independent in ADLs Good candidate for ambulation with or without orthoses

ADLs, activities of daily living.
Modified from Wirtz, K.M., La Favor, K.M., and Ang, R. (1996). Managing chronic spinal cord injury: Issues in critical care. *Critical Care Nurse* 16(4), 25. Reprinted with permission of *Critical Care Nurse*.

hibitory inputs from higher centers. Muscle spasms and bladder spasms are common. A potentially fatal complication, **autonomic hyper-reflexia,** may also occur. Also known as autonomic dysreflexia, this syndrome results from an excessive and uncoordinated autonomic response resulting from injury to the spinal cord above the level of T-7. Highest risk is present just after spinal shock subsides (1 to 12 weeks after injury), and the risk may persist for up to 6 years.

Autonomic hyper-reflexia requires a triggering stimulus, intact autonomic reflex arcs, and impaired communication with higher integrative centers. Possible stimuli include bladder distention, fecal impaction (or its manual removal), muscle spasms, or pain. Because of impaired integration, the sympathetic response to the triggering stimulus is exaggerated, causing massive reflex vasoconstriction of vessels below the level of the injury, pupillary dilation, nausea, and sweating and piloerection above the level of the injury. Hypertension resulting from the vasoconstriction then triggers the PNS through activation of the baroreceptor reflex (see Chapter 15). The heart rate decreases in response to vagal impulses (which descend outside the cord), but blood vessels below the level of injury remain constricted because efferent impulses cannot descend through the injured cord.

Years after the initial injury, some patients may develop post-traumatic **syringomyelia,** in which a fluid-filled cavity forms and extends within the central part of the lesion.[3] This complication extends the spinal lesion and results in additional function deficits.

Clinical Manifestations. If cord transection interrupts motor pathways, paralysis occurs below the level of the injury. Complete transection above the third cervical vertebra is rapidly fatal because of paralysis of respiratory muscles. Transection at other cervical levels results in **quadriplegia** (paralysis of all extremities); whereas damage below this level produces **paraplegia** (paralysis of both legs). Table 22–8 describes specific motor manifestations of injuries at various levels of the cord. Complete transection of sensory pathways produces anesthesia (loss of sensation) below the level of the injury. Partial transection produces a wide variety of clinical manifestations ("cord syndromes"), depending on the specific pathways involved (Table 22–9).

During the period of spinal shock, all motor reflexes below the level of injury are absent, resulting in flaccid paralysis. Autonomic reflexes are also absent, resulting in vasodilation, orthostatic hypotension (see Chapter 15), and absence of bladder and bowel function.

Autonomic hyper-reflexia is characterized by sudden onset of hypertension (systolic blood pressure as high as 300 mm Hg), blurred vision, severe headache, nausea, nasal congestion, and flushing and piloerection above the level of injury due to SNS-mediated hyperactivity. Bradycardia (heart rate 30 to 40 beats/min) results from the parasympathetic

TABLE 22–9
SPINAL CORD SYNDROMES ASSOCIATED WITH INCOMPLETE TRANSECTION

SYNDROME	NATURE OF INJURY	CLINICAL FEATURES
Central cord syndrome Microscopic hemorrhage and edema in central gray matter of spinal cord	Microscopic damage to central gray matter, associated with hyperextension or stenosis of the spinal canal	Motor weakness of all extremities but greater in upper Variable bowel and bladder dysfunction
Anterior cord injury Compressed anterior portion of cord	Acute compression of anterior portion of cord, associated with flexion injury, spinal artery thrombosis, or herniated intervertebral disk	Immediate loss of motor function below level of injury Decreased or absent pain and temperature sensation below level of injury Intact proprioceptive, touch, and vibration sensation
Brown-Séquard syndrome Hemisection of cord	Transection of half of the cord, associated with penetrating injury	Loss of motor function on same side as lesion Loss of pain and temperature sensation on opposite side

Data from Barker, E. (1994). *Neuroscience Nursing*. St. Louis: Mosby–Year Book. (p. 356). Illustrations from same.

response that follows. Unless interrupted, autonomic hyper-reflexia may lead to cardiac failure (see Chapter 16) or stroke (see Chapter 21).

Chronic and "phantom" pain are common among spinal cord injury patients, usually developing months to years after the injury. Pain is experienced despite loss of the integrity of sensory pathways and may be due to realignment of structural and synaptic connections, release of excitatory or accessory pain pathways, or dendritic "sprouting" in the area of injury as tissues heal.[3] Pain mechanisms are detailed in Chapter 23.

Prevention and Treatment. Prevention of spinal cord injury involves the same measures as those employed in the prevention of head injury (see Chapter 21). Prevention of associated autonomic hyper-reflexia involves identification and removal of triggering stimuli. Preventive measures are also taken to reduce the risk of urinary tract infection (see Chapter 20).

Immediate treatment of SCI is aimed at preventing extension of the force-induced injury by stabilizing any fractures and minimizing hypoxic trauma secondary to inflammation or hemorrhage. The spine is initially immobilized with bracing, and traction may be applied using a halo apparatus (Fig. 22–15) or weights suspended from pins or tongs inserted into the skull. Surgical fusion may be performed to stabilize the spine when edema has subsided and bone fragments are in normal apposition. Hemorrhage and shock are treated with fluid resuscitation and other measures, as discussed in Chapter 15. Injuries to the cervical spine may result in the need for ventilatory assistance (see Chapter 18). Corticosteroids may be used to decrease inflammation.

For autonomic hyper-reflexia, the head of the bed is elevated, and vasodilating drugs that act peripherally, such as calcium-channel blockers or α-adrenergic antagonists, may be administered. Muscle spasticity is usually treated with baclofen (Lioresol), which potentiates the inhibitory neurotransmitter, GABA.

When the patient is stable, rehabilitation is initiated, including physical therapy, bladder and bowel retraining, use of adjunctive devices such as braces, crutches, and wheelchairs, and possibly psychological counseling or vocational rehabilitation.

Prognosis and Outcome. Patients with spinal cord injury usually regain some degree of function after spinal shock and edema subside but permanently lose those functions mediated by reflex arcs in the damaged segment of the cord. Reflexes below the level of injury are intact but cannot be voluntarily facilitated or inhibited. The outlook is most favorable for patients with paraplegia, with most recovering a high degree of independent function. Life expectancy is lower than that for the general population but is increasing.[4] More than 88% survive 12 years or more after injury. Because of their limited mobility, spinal cord injury patients are at higher risk for pneumonia, deep vein thrombosis, urinary tract disorders, and decubitus ulcers of the skin. Septicemia secondary to one or more of these disorders is the leading cause of death.

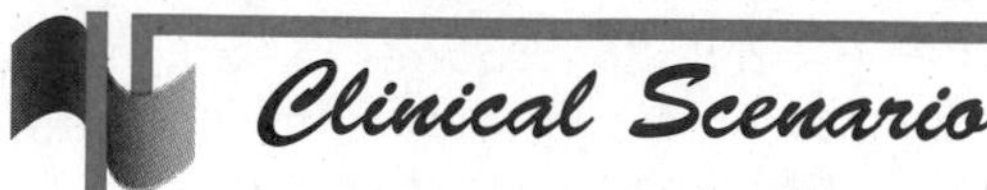

P.R., a 22-year-old male college student, was partying with some friends when he sustained a cervical fracture as a consequence of diving into the shallow end of a swimming pool. His spinal cord was completely transected at the C-6 level. He underwent surgery to fuse the cervical spine, and after his condition stabilized, entered a specialized rehabilitation program. About 4 weeks after his injury, P.R. developed severe spasticity, especially in his legs, which responded to treatment with baclofen. While in rehabilitation, P.R. developed a severe decubitus ulcer over his coccyx. He requires a permanent indwelling urinary catheter.

1. Given the level of his injury, what degree of motor function can P.R. expect to regain? What interventions may be employed to maximize his recovered function?
2. Explain the physiologic basis of spasticity in P.R.'s case. Why was it not apparent immediately after his injury?

Myasthenia Gravis

Definition. MG is an autoimmune disorder characterized by progressive muscular weakness and fatigue with repetitive activity.

Epidemiology. The prevalence of MG has been estimated at 50 to 125 cases per million people in the United States.[5] Two peaks in incidence are apparent: women in their teens and 20s, and men in their 70s and 80s.[6] Risk factors for development of the disorder include hyperactivity or persistent activity of the thymus gland (possibly due to a benign or malignant thymic tumor), patient or family history of autoimmune disorders, and demonstration of specific human leukocyte antigen genotypes (see Chapter 13).

Etiology. MG is caused by autoimmune attack against ACh receptors at the neuromuscular junc-

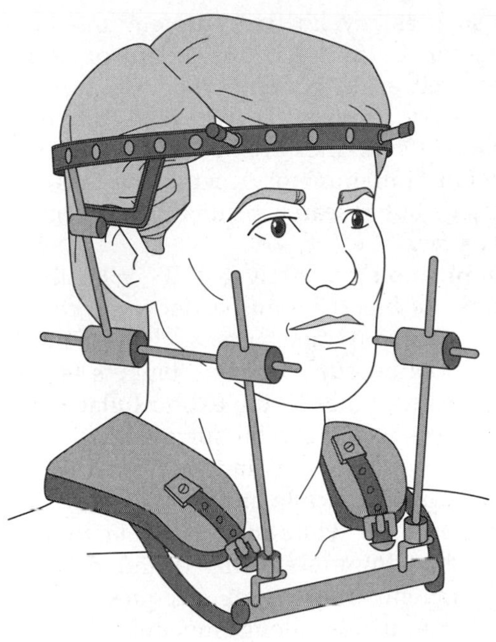

FIGURE 22–15
Halo apparatus for immobilization of cervical spine injury. The metal halo (ring) is fixed to the cranium with pins and connected to a rigid jacket or vest by adjustable rods.

tion. The precise trigger of autoantibody production is unknown, although infection with a microorganism similar in molecular structure to the acetylcholine receptor has been hypothesized. Autoantibodies may destroy ACh receptors or may compete with the natural ligand for receptor binding.

Pathophysiology. Autoimmune attack against ACh receptors results in (1) destruction of about one third of receptors at all neuromuscular junctions of skeletal muscles, (2) flattening of the postsynaptic folds, and (3) widening of the synaptic cleft (Fig. 22–16). The motor nerve terminal is normal, and there is no deficiency of acetylcholine secretion.[7] Failure of neurotransmission is progressively greater with repeated neural stimulation of the muscle because of the combined effects of reduced receptors and the normal decline ("rundown") of ACh release from motor nerve fibers with successive depolarizations.

Clinical Manifestations. Table 22–10 summarizes clinical stages of MG. The characteristic features of the disorder are muscle weakness and fatigability, which tend to become worse with repeated or sustained activity and to improve with rest. Muscle weakness is generalized in 85% of patients and limited to the extraocular (external eye) muscles in 15%.[6] Muscles of the face and eye are usually affected first, resulting in ptosis (eyelid droop) and diplopia (double vision). Patients may display a flat affect (bland facial expression), slurred speech, and difficulty swallowing (dysphagia). Weakness of respiratory muscles indicates **myasthenic crisis.**

Prevention and Treatment. There are no known preventive measures for MG. Four treatment modalities are in use: anticholinesterase drugs, surgical thymectomy (removal of the thymus gland), immunosuppression, and short-term immunotherapies. Anticholinesterase drugs, such as pyridostigmine (Mestinon), delay the enzymatic inactivation of ACh at the neuromuscular junction. Thymectomy is indicated in cases of known thymic neoplasia and has resulted in clinical improvement in younger MG patients with no evidence of thymic tumor or hyperplasia. The therapeutic mechanism in the latter case is unknown. Because of associated risks, immunosuppressive drugs, such as cyclosporine and corticosteroids, are used only if adequate control of weakness is not achieved with anticholinesterase drugs. In the case of myasthenic crisis, circulating antibodies may be removed with plasmapheresis to effect a short-term improvement (see Chapter 13). Intravenous administration of immunoglobulin has resulted in short-term benefits for some patients, although the mechanism is unknown.

Prognosis and Outcome. With optimal treatment,

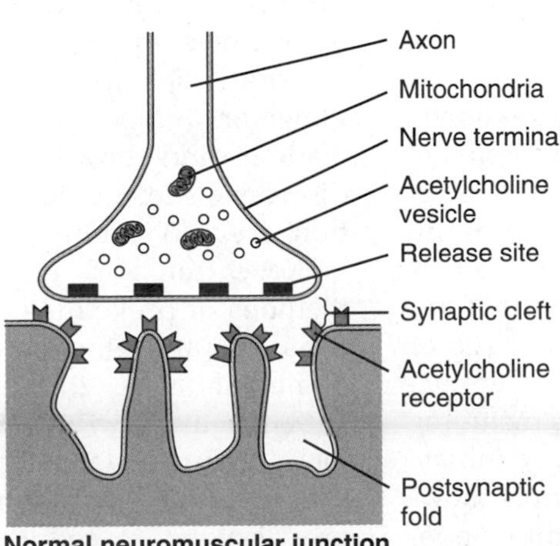

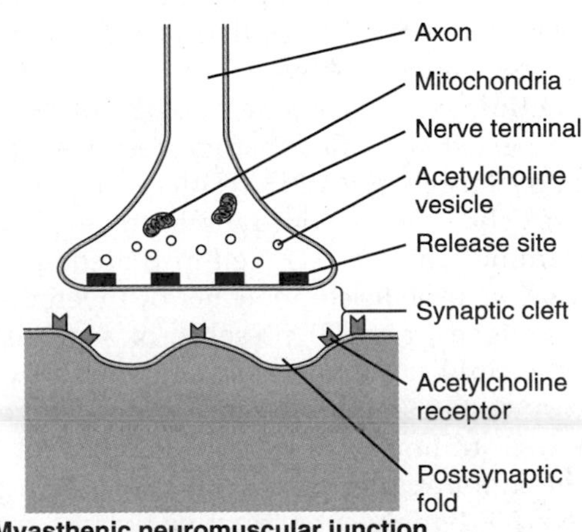

FIGURE 22–16
Normal and myasthenic neuromuscular junctions. In contrast to the normal structure, the myasthenic neuromuscular junction demonstrates flattened postsynaptic folds and widening of the synaptic cleft. About one third of all postsynaptic receptors are destroyed.

TABLE 22–10
CLINICAL STAGES OF MYASTHENIA GRAVIS

STAGE	DISTRIBUTION AND SEVERITY OF SYMPTOMS
I	Ocular myasthenia
IIA	Mild generalized myasthenia; drug response good
IIB	Moderate generalized myasthenia; drug response less than satisfactory
III	Acute fulminating myasthenia with respiratory crisis; poor drug response
IV	Late severe myasthenia; same as stage III, but takes 2 years to progress from stage I or stage II

Based on Osserman, K.E. (1958). *Myasthenia Gravis*. New York: Grune & Stratton. (pp. 78–80), as cited in Juhn, M.S. (1993). Myasthenia gravis: Diagnostic methods and control measures for a chronic disease. *Postgraduate Medicine* 94(5), 163.

the mortality rate due to the disease itself is essentially zero, and most patients may lead normal lives. Patients who must undergo immunosuppression are at increased risk of infection and neoplasia.

Multiple Sclerosis

Definition. MS is a disorder of neurotransmission resulting from demyelination and ultimate destruction of axons of motor, sensory, and autonomic nerves.

Epidemiology. About 250,000 people in the United States have been diagnosed with MS.[8] People between the ages of 20 and 40 years are at highest risk, as are those with a family history of the disorder and those living in temperate climates. Twice as many women are diagnosed with the disorder as men, but men tend to have more severe disease. A genetic susceptibility is apparent, demonstrated by a 10-fold higher incidence among identical twins than among nonidentical twins or other close relatives.[8] Whites of northern European descent demonstrate a risk that is four times that of the general population in the United States.

Etiology. The precise etiology of MS is unknown. A persistent inflammatory response that preferentially targets the CNS results in destruction of myelin. The two major hypotheses explaining this inflammation are (1) cell-mediated immune attack against protein components of myelin and other autoantigens, and (2) presence of a persistent virus or other infectious process against which the inflammatory response is directed. Various triggers, including stress, trauma, pregnancy, or infection, may initiate the autoimmune process in susceptible people; however, T lymphocytes reactive against myelin components, such as myelin basic protein and proteolipid protein, can be found in the serum of normal subjects as well as in patients with MS. An abnormal inflammatory response, in which destructive (proinflammatory) cytokines are secreted in excess of protective (anti-inflammatory) cytokines, has also been postulated, but research results have been inconclusive thus far.[9]

Pathophysiology. Activated T cells are able to penetrate the blood–brain barrier in a process mediated by adhesion molecules such as integrins and immunoglobulin superfamily members (see Chapter 2). Protease enzymes in the extracellular matrix then permit access to the myelin surrounding nerves. The inflammatory response is initiated, with activation of the complement cascade and phagocytosis of myelin segments in CNS white matter by macrophages (see Chapter 13). Immune-mediated inflammation produces demyelinating lesions (plaques) and disrupts impulse conduction along myelinated nerves. Lesions are separated by areas of normal myelin and may occur in any myelinated nervous tissue within the somatic motor, autonomic, and sensory systems. Lesions may also occur in gray matter and in tissues outside the CNS, notably the retinas. After each acute exacerbation, lesions heal and myelin regenerates, but not completely. Ultimately, myelin destruction is permanent, and axons then "drop out," or degenerate. The pattern and rate of progression of the disease to this end stage are highly variable among patients.[10]

Clinical Manifestations. The typical course of MS is of an initial episode that may last several years, followed by episodes of remission and relapse. Table 22–11 compares the various patterns of progression. Specific clinical manifestations are variable, depending on the location and extent of the lesions.

Many patients present with unilateral visual impairment due to involvement of the optic nerve **(optic neuritis).** Many of these patients do not develop any additional lesions, although some have motor problems, such as fatigue, paresis or paralysis, gait disturbance, spasticity, tremors, and slurred speech; sensory problems, such as pain, numbness, and tingling; or autonomic problems, such as neurogenic bladder and bowel dysfunction. Neurobehavioral disorders, such as depression and cognitive dysfunction, are also common.

Prevention and Treatment. There are no known methods of preventing MS. Therapy of MS has three aims: to prevent ongoing inflammatory destruction of neural tissue, to manage symptoms so that the patient may function at a higher level, and to promote repair of damaged myelin.[11] Acute attacks are usually treated with corticosteroids such as methylprednisolone, to reduce inflammation. Recombinant

TABLE 22–11
CLINICAL COURSE OF MULTIPLE SCLEROSIS

Type	Frequency (%)	Clinical Features
Relapsing and remitting	65	Exacerbations due to CNS lesions or plaques develop subacutely and resolve over weeks to months
Relapsing and progressive	15	Exacerbations similar to relapsing and remitting form except less complete recovery between flare-ups
Chronic progressive	20	Absence of remission; progressive spinal cord and cerebellar dysfunction; may be initial pattern or may develop out of relapsing and remitting form over time

Data from Mitchell, G. (1993). Update on multiple sclerosis therapy. *Medical Clinics of North America* 77(1), 231.

β-interferons (Betaseron and Avonex) were recently approved by the Food and Drug Administration for use in the treatment of the relapsing and remitting form of MS and have been effective in reducing the frequency of relapses and the accumulation of plaques.[11] β-Interferons have not been shown to affect clinical disability caused by the disease, however, and are of no benefit in patients with progressive MS. Glatiramer (Copaxone), a synthetic polypeptide, has also been approved and may provide modest benefits to those patients who do not respond to β-interferons. The mechanism of action of these drugs is unknown. Treatment with oral myelin, intended to hyposensitize the patient against autoimmune attack, is being investigated in clinical trials.[11]

Treatment of progressive MS emphasizes immunosuppressive measures, such as cytotoxic drugs (e.g., azathioprine, cyclophosphamide, cyclosporine, methotrexate, and cladribine), and total lymphoid irradiation. Experimental therapy includes lymphocytophoresis (removal of lymphocytes from the plasma) and monoclonal antibodies against T cells or their receptors.[12]

Symptomatic and supportive measures are also instituted. Fatigue may respond to periodic rest or to medications such as the anti–Parkinson's disease drug selegiline (Eldepryl) or the antidepressant fluoxetine (Prozac). Spasticity may be treated with baclofen or with physical therapy. Tremors may be lessened with the use of weighted bracelets or with drug therapy. A number of agents are used, including benzodiazepines (e.g., diazepam [Valium]) and tetrahydrocannabinol (in marijuana).[9] Intervention in bladder and bowel dysfunction is discussed in detail in Chapters 20 and 24. Management of chronic pain is discussed in Chapter 23.

Prognosis and Outcome. Most cases persist chronically for many years. The rapidly progressive form of MS leads to death within 1 to 2 years. Complications such as pneumonia and septicemia cause most deaths. The suicide rate for patients with MS is 7.5 times that for similar age groups among the general population.[13]

Guillain-Barré Syndrome

Definition. Guillain-Barré syndrome is the most common form of acute inflammatory demyelinating polyneuropathy (AIDP), a group of demyelinating disorders of peripheral nerves.

Epidemiology. The estimated annual incidence of Guillain-Barré syndrome is 1.5 to 2.0 per 100,000 U.S. population.[14] Incidence increases with advancing age. Guillain-Barré syndrome has replaced **poliomyelitis** as the most common cause of flaccid paralysis in otherwise-healthy adults. Most cases are preceded by an infection with a virus (e.g., Epstein-Barr virus, human immunodeficiency virus, or cytomegalovirus) or a bacterium (e.g., *Campylobacter jejuni*). Less common associated conditions include immunization, pregnancy, surgery, Hodgkin's disease, hepatitis B, and chlamydial infection.[15]

Etiology. Although the precise etiology is unknown, an autoimmune mechanism is the probable cause. A severe infection precedes development of manifestations of Guillain-Barré syndrome in about two thirds of cases.[15] *C. jejuni* infection is the most common illness preceding Guillain-Barré syndrome, especially in children.[16] This infectious trigger apparently initiates autoimmune attack against the myelin of cranial and spinal nerves, with motor nerve roots sustaining the greatest injury.

Pathophysiology. Autoantibody-initiated inflammation is apparent, with infiltration of monocyte-macrophages into nerve roots, ganglia, and distal nerves. Macrophages penetrate and strip myelin, phagocytizing the debris (Fig. 22–17). Complement activation occurs, contributing to inflammatory injury (see Chapter 13). In some cases, inflammatory injury detaches the axon from the cell body, resulting in permanent loss of conduction. *Nissl bodies*, granular components that are sites of protein synthesis and metabolism in neurons, may dissolve, in a process known as *chromatolysis*. Destruction of the basement membrane of myelin-producing Schwann cells may also occur, inhibiting myelin repair and healing of the lesions. Schwann cells are believed to

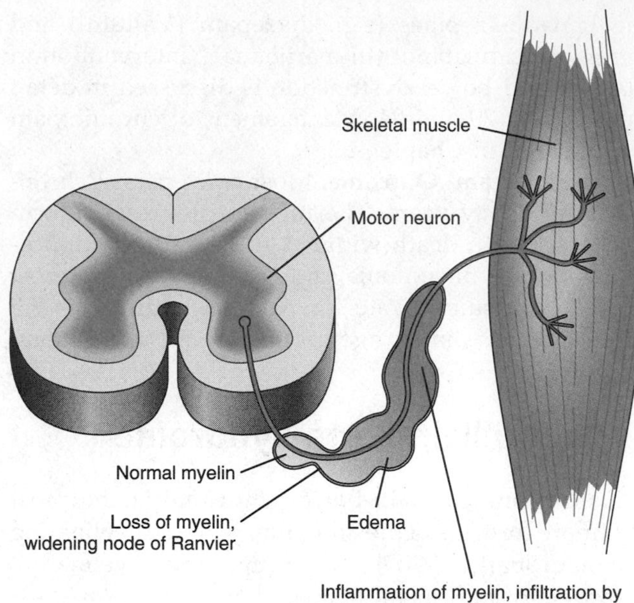

FIGURE 22–17
Neural lesions in Guillain-Barré syndrome. Degeneration of the myelin sheath is apparent, with local inflammation and edema. Loss of myelin impairs saltatory conduction of nerve impulses. Motor neurons are affected most commonly, but sensory and autonomic dysfunction may also occur. (From Murray, D.P. [1993]. Impaired mobility: Guillain-Barré syndrome. *Journal of Neuroscience Nursing* 25[2], 100.)

be the primary target of immune attack in Guillain-Barré syndrome.[14]

Both cranial and spinal nerves may be involved. Although somatic motor dysfunction usually predominates, sensory and autonomic dysfunction are often affected as well. Involvement of the CNS is rare. For unknown reasons, the disorder is usually self-limiting, with lesions subsiding in reverse order of their initiation.

Clinical Manifestations. Guillain-Barré syndrome typically begins with symmetric weakness of the lower extremities. Deep tendon reflexes are usually lost. Flaccid paralysis consistent with interruption of the reflex arc develops and ascends rapidly, possibly affecting autonomic function and muscles of respiration. Paraplegia and quadriplegia are common, and respiratory arrest is possible. Peripheral sensation may be intact or decreased. Autonomic dysfunction has replaced respiratory failure as the leading cause of death in patients with Guillain-Barré syndrome.[15] Clinical signs include cardiac dysrhythmias, extreme hypertension or circulatory collapse, hyperthermia or hypothermia, and impaired bowel and bladder function.

Laboratory findings include elevated serum levels of immunoglobulins. Cerebrospinal fluid demonstrates increased protein levels consistent with inflammation. Electromyography reveals abnormal generation and conduction of action potentials in skeletal muscles served by affected motor nerves. After 2 to 4 weeks, clinical manifestations usually begin to subside.

Prevention and Treatment. There are no known preventive measures. Early recognition and prompt treatment may prevent a more severe course. Treatment of Guillain-Barré syndrome is symptomatic and supportive. During the period of paralysis, the patient may require total care. Mechanical ventilation is required in 20% to 30% of cases.[15] The two principal modes of therapy are plasmapheresis to remove circulating antibodies and corticosteroid therapy to suppress the inflammatory and immune responses.

Prognosis and Treatment. Half of patients recover completely, and about 35% have permanent deficits in neurologic function. About 10% experience relapse after apparent recovery.[15]

Amyotrophic Lateral Sclerosis

Definition. Amyotrophic lateral sclerosis (ALS), also known as Lou Gehrig's disease, is a motor disorder resulting from progressive degeneration of the anterior horn cells and the corticospinal tracts.

Epidemiology. ALS demonstrates an annual incidence of 0.4 to 1.76 per 100,000 U.S. population.[17] Peak incidence is in the early 50s, and males are affected two to three times as often as females. Of all cases, 5% to 10% are familial, and the remainder are designated as sporadic ALS.[18]

Etiology. The etiology of ALS is unknown. Genetic, viral, metabolic, and autoimmune mechanisms have been hypothesized. Some familial cases have been linked to a defect in the gene encoding superoxide dismutase, an antioxidant enzyme. It is unknown why motor neurons should be selectively vulnerable to this defect, however.[18] Another theory holds that glutamate, the primary excitatory neurotransmitter in the CNS, accumulates to toxic concentrations at synapses.[19] Environmental toxins have been implicated in the unusually high incidence of ALS in Guam.[20] Immune complexes are elevated in the serum of patients with ALS, but their clinical significance is unknown.

Pathophysiology. A noninflammatory degenerative process leads to progressive destruction of both UMNs and LMNs. Cranial nerves III, IV, and VI, which innervate extraocular muscles, are spared. Neuronal tissue is replaced by nonfunctional scar tissue, leaving affected motor units without innervation. Sprouting of axons from adjacent motor nerves may maintain some degree of function for a time, but the precision of activity is impaired because of the decrease in number of motor units.

Clinical Manifestations. Manifestations of both UMN and LMN dysfunction are gradually, but asymmetrically, progressive. Paresis degenerates to paralysis, which is usually flaccid but occasionally spastic. Muscle atrophy is secondary to denervation. Dysphagia and dysarthria are particular problems. Bladder, bowel, and respiratory function are usually spared until late in the disease. Sensory function and intellectual function are not impaired.

Prevention and Treatment. There is no known prevention for ALS and no definitive treatment. In early 1996, the drug riluzole (Rilutek) was approved for use in patients with ALS.[19] Riluzole, which modulates the activity of glutamate, has been shown to slow the progression of ALS (see Focus of Current Research). Symptomatic and supportive care measures are instituted, including speech, respiratory and physical therapies.

Prognosis and Outcome. ALS is a fatal disease. The average life expectancy from the time of diagnosis is 2 to 5 years, although as many as 10% of patients survive longer than 10 years.[20]

Huntington's Disease

Definition. Huntington's disease, also known as Huntington's chorea, is an autosomal dominant disorder characterized by a delayed onset of progressive degeneration of neurons of the basal ganglia, cerebral cortex, and cerebellum.

Epidemiology. The prevalence of Huntington's disease in North America and Europe has been estimated at 7 to 10 per 100,000 population.[21] Risk is derived from autosomal dominant inheritance: 50% of the offspring of affected people manifest the disease in midlife. All races and both sexes are equally affected.

Etiology. Huntington's disease is an autosomal dominant genetic disorder displaying a high degree of penetrance (see Chapter 7). The abnormal gene is located on the short arm of chromosome 4.[22]

Pathophysiology. GABA-ergic neurons of the basal ganglia, frontal cortex, and cerebellum are preferentially destroyed, and glial cells proliferate. Deficiency of GABA, the primary inhibitory neurotransmitter within the CNS, creates a relative excess of dopamine, resulting in abnormal neurotransmission within the affected neural pathways.

Clinical Manifestations. Clinical manifestations are usually not apparent until the patient reaches 40 to 50 years of age. Progressive dementia and hyperkinesia (chorea) are then seen. Signs become relentlessly worse over a 15- to 20-year course.

Prevention and Treatment. The only available prevention is genetic testing of people from affected families who are contemplating childbearing. The ethical implications of such testing are considerable. There is no definitive treatment of the disorder. Neurotropic drugs, such as haloperidol (Haldol) and diazepam, may be used to modify abnormal movements and behavioral manifestations.[22]

Prognosis and Outcome. Huntington's disease is incurable. Death usually occurs after 15 to 20 years of symptoms, often due to respiratory failure secondary to aspiration. Gene therapy may offer some hope to patients in the future.

Parkinson's Disease

Definition. Parkinson's disease is a slowly progressive dyskinetic disorder caused by degeneration of dopaminergic neurons of the substantia nigra of the brain stem, which project to the basal ganglia. The term **parkinsonism** is frequently used to describe a syndrome of extrapyramidal motor system dysfunction characterized by muscle rigidity leading to flat affect and gait disturbance and by a characteristic "pill-rolling" tremor of the hands. Parkinsonism is a component of Parkinson's disease as well as other disorders of the basal ganglia, and a potentially reversible form may result from use of street drugs or antipsychotic drugs, such as phenothiazines.

Epidemiology. Parkinson's disease affects 1% of the population older than 60 years, with males and females equally affected.[23] In rare cases, Parkinson's disease is inherited as an autosomal dominant condition, but in most cases, there is no apparent familial pattern. Aging is considered to be a risk factor because the incidence increases proportionately to age after 40 years of age.

Etiology. The etiology of Parkinson's disease is unknown. Viral, toxic, metabolic, genetic, and vascular mechanisms have been hypothesized. The most widely accepted theory of pathogenesis is the *oxidative stress hypothesis,* which proposes that reactive oxygen species are produced in increased amounts in dopaminergic neurons of the substantia nigra and that these are ultimately toxic in susceptible patients (see Chapter 3). Unusually active microglia are seen in patients with Parkinson's disease, and these may stimulate oxidative damage.[24] Brain cells are less capable of repair of oxidative damage than are other tissues.

Pathophysiology. The degenerative process destroys dopaminergic neurons of the substantia nigra, the axons of which normally project to the corpus striatum. Aging enhances the degenerative process; about 4% of dopamine-producing neurons are normally lost during each decade of adulthood.[24] Defi-

Focus of Current Research

Study	Objective and Findings
Goldstein, et al. (1997) Sympathetic cardioneuropathy in dysautonomias.	*Objective:* To classify dysautonomias on the basis of positron emission tomography scanning and other assessments *Findings:* Mechanisms of dysautonomia include loss of myocardial sympathetic nerve terminals, intact nerve terminals but no neurotransmission, and dysautonomia with normal sympathetic stimulation of the myocardium.
Burke, et al. (1996) Gender differences in heart rate before and after autonomic blockade: Evidence against an intrinsic gender effect.	*Objectives:* To document gender differences in heart rate in healthy young men and women and to examine variables that may be associated with gender differences in heart rate *Findings:* Sinus cycle length is longer in men than in women, owing to a gender difference in exercise capacity rather than differences in autonomic stimulation.
Schendel, et al. (1996) Prenatal magnesium sulfate exposure and the risk for cerebral palsy or mental retardation among very-low-birth-weight children aged 3 to 5 years.	*Objective:* To examine the relationship between prenatal magnesium sulfate exposure and the risk of cerebral palsy or mental retardation in very-low-birth-weight children *Findings:* Prenatal magnesium sulfate exposure is associated with reduced risk of cerebral palsy and possibly with reduced risk of mental retardation.

Continued

ciency of dopamine, which is inhibitory at these synapses, permits excessive excitatory neurotransmission at cholinergic synapses and impairs normal modulation of motor function by the basal ganglia. In addition to substantia nigra neurons, other brainstem nuclei (e.g., the raphe nuclei and locus ceruleus) secreting different neurotransmitters are also lost. Loss of these nondopaminergic neurons may contribute to depression and other nonmotor manifestations of Parkinson's disease. As a component of the limbic system, the basal ganglia also interconnect with the hypothalamus. Abnormal neurotransmission thus potentially affects the autonomic and endocrine functions mediated by the hypothalamus as well.

Clinical Manifestations. Progressive stages of Parkinson's disease are described in Table 22–12. The first manifestations of the disorder, which occur

TABLE 22–12
HOEHN-YAHR CLASSIFICATION OF PARKINSON'S DISEASE

STAGE	DISTRIBUTION AND SEVERITY OF SYMPTOMS
I	Unilateral tremor, rigidity, akinesia, or postural abnormalities only
II	Bilateral tremor, rigidity, akinesia, or postural abnormalities
III	First signs of deteriorating balance, but still fully independent
IV	Requires help with some or all activities of daily living; unable to live alone without assistance
V	Confined to wheelchair or bed unless assisted

From Hoehn, M.M., and Yahr, M.D. (1967). Parkinsonism: Onset, progression, and mortality. *Neurology* 17, 427–442, as cited in Beizer, J.L. (1995). Treatment options in Parkinson's disease. *American Pharmacy* NS35(1), 22.

Jansen, et al. (1995) Central command neurons of the sympathetic nervous system: Basis of the fight-or-flight response.	*Objective:* To define the neurons and central nervous system circuits responsible for the fight-or-flight response in stress *Findings:* By using a new labeling technique, the existence of a set of central autonomic neurons in the brain stem and hypothalamus was demonstrated. These neurons innervate both the sympathetic chain and the adrenal medulla.
Kordower, et al. (1995) Neuropathological evidence of graft survival and striatal reinnervation after the transplantation of fetal mesencephalic tissue in a patient with Parkinson's disease.	*Objective:* To provide evidence that grafts of fetal tissue can survive and innervate the corpus striatum *Findings:* In a single patient, scanning of the brain demonstrated survival of two large grafts. Neural process had grown out of the grafts and reinnervated the striatum after 18 months.
Rees, et al. (1995) *Campylobacter jejuni* infection and Guillain-Barré syndrome.	*Objective:* To examine the association between *C. jejuni* infection and subsequent development of Guillain-Barré syndrome *Findings:* 26% of Guillain-Barré syndrome patients had evidence of preceding *C. jejuni* infection, as compared with 2% of household controls and 1% of age-matched hospital controls.
Bensimon, et al. (1994) A controlled trial of riluzole in amyotrophic lateral sclerosis.	*Objective:* To evaluate the efficacy and safety of the antiglutamate agent riluzole in treatment of amyotrophic lateral sclerosis *Findings:* Riluzole appears to slow the progression of the disease, and it may improve survival in some patients.

when dopamine is depleted by 80%, are of motor dysfunction, including the pill-rolling tremor at rest, muscle rigidity, and postural instability. Rigid muscles lead to a mask-like facial expression, absent or slowed movement (bradykinesia or "poverty" of movement), a bent-forward (simian) posture, and a gradually accelerating gait known as a *festination gait* (Fig. 22–18). Autonomic manifestations of Parkinson's disease include excessive sweating and decreased motility of the gastrointestinal and genitourinary smooth muscle, possibly leading to constipation and urinary retention. Orthostatic hypotension may result from impairment of the vascular smooth muscle response to baroreceptor signals. Oily skin is commonly present as a result of inappropriate androgen production mediated by the hypothalamic–pituitary axis (see Chapter 27). Most patients develop some degree of impairment of higher cognitive function later in the course of the disease. Some develop severe dementia, similar to that seen in patients with Alzheimer's disease (see Chapter 21).

Prevention and Treatment. Parkinson's disease has no known prevention or cure. When motor symptoms become severe, dopamine replacement therapy may be instituted. Because dopamine does not cross the blood–brain barrier, drug therapy includes dopamine precursors such as levodopa (Sinemet), dopamine agonists such as bromocriptine (Parlodel), and dopamine reuptake inhibitors such as amantadine (Symmetrel). The mainstay of therapy has been levodopa, but its effectiveness is dependent on the presence of *some* normal dopaminergic neurons in the basal ganglia that can convert the precursor to dopamine. Anticholinergics such as benztropine mesylate (Cogentin) are also employed in an

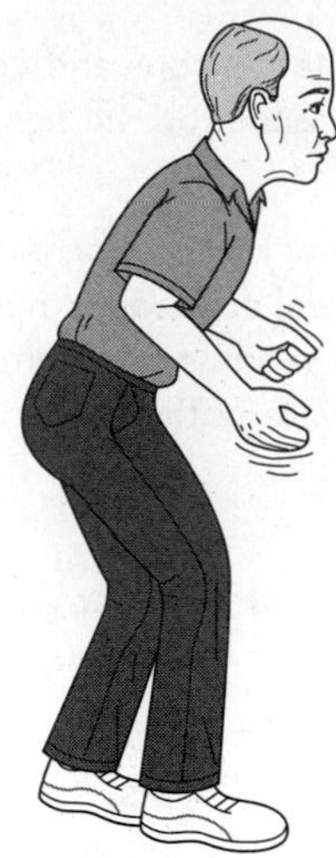

FIGURE 22–18
Manifestations of Parkinson's disease. The affected person demonstrates a mask-like facial expression, bent-forward (simian) posture, muscle rigidity, and a gradually accelerating gait known as a *festination gait.* A "pill-rolling" tremor of the hands is apparent at rest.

effort to restore the dopamine–ACh balance. A large clinical trial evaluating the effectiveness of neuroprotective drugs such as selegiline, which inhibits the formation of reactive oxygen species, suggested but did not prove that such agents may slow the progression of the disorder.[25] Experimental therapies include neural pacing, stereotactic destruction of excitatory pathways in the basal ganglia, use of gangliosides (glial-derived neurotrophic factors that promote sprouting of axons), and transplantation of fetal dopaminergic tissue (see Focus of Current Research).[26, 27]

Prognosis and Outcome. The rate of disease progression varies widely among patients. With optimal therapy, some patients continue working and leading relatively normal lives for 10 years or more after diagnosis.[28]

Bell's Palsy

Definition. Bell's palsy, or peripheral facial nerve paralysis, is an idiopathic disorder in which an inflammatory process leads to dysfunction of cranial nerve VII.

Epidemiology. Bell's palsy is the most common peripheral nerve paralysis. It affects males and females of all age groups, but usually occurs between the ages of 20 and 40 years.[22] Specific risk factors are unknown.

Etiology. The precise etiology of Bell's palsy is unknown. Infection, local ischemia, and emotional distress have been considered possible causes. Neural involvement is usually unilateral but may be bilateral in some cases.

Pathophysiology. Facial paralysis occurs as a result of lack of appropriate neural stimulation by motor fibers of the facial nerve. Paralysis is on the same side of the face as the affected nerve in cases of unilateral involvement.

Clinical Manifestations. The onset of manifestations is abrupt, with unilateral signs of facial paralysis, upward movement of the eyeball when the eye is closed *(Bell's phenomenon)*, drooping of the mouth, flattening of the nasolabial fold, widening of the palpebral fissure, and lid lag.[22] Loss of taste sensation and reduction of salivation may result in difficulty eating. The patient may also experience ear pain, tinnitus, or hearing loss on the affected side.

Prevention and Treatment. There is no known prevention nor definitive treatment of Bell's palsy. Treatment is symptomatic and supportive, including such measures as analgesics, application of warm, moist heat, massage of affected areas, and use of artificial tears and an eye patch. Corticosteroids may be beneficial in reducing inflammatory edema.

Prognosis and Outcome. Most patients recover spontaneously within a few weeks to a year. Rarely, the paralysis is permanent.

Cerebral Palsy

Definition. Cerebral palsy is a symptom complex, covering a group of nonprogressive motor impairment syndromes that may result from lesions or anomalies of the brain arising in the early stages of its development.[29]

Epidemiology. The prevalence of the disorder is 1.5 to 2.5 per 1000 live births.[29] In the United States, an estimated 100,000 people younger than 18 years have been diagnosed with cerebral palsy. Low birth weight, prematurity, twin gestations, nonvertex presentation, and presence of congenital defects are known risk factors for cerebral palsy. Maternal factors include history of long intervals between menses, hyperthyroidism, and estrogen therapy. Breathing impairment during delivery (birth asphyxia) is weakly associated with development of cerebral palsy, but it is not certain whether this represents a cause or a consequence of the disorder.[29]

Etiology. A strong association has been found between cerebral palsy and low birth weight and severe birth asphyxia.[30] It is a matter of controversy whether cerebral palsy develops as a consequence of difficulties in the birth process or whether difficult birth results from pre-existing abnormalities in the fetus. A minority of children with cerebral palsy develop the condition *after* birth as a result of meningitis, encephalitis, neurotrauma, or neurovascular occlusion. In most, however, the precise etiologic mechanism is unclear.

The primary lesion of cerebral palsy is *periventricular leukomalacia,* an abnormality of the white matter surrounding the ventricles of the brain, which is believed to be the result of a hypoxic or ischemic process. Other theories attribute this lesion to toxic cytokines associated with infection, oxidative damage, or an excess of excitatory neurotransmitters during the perinatal period. Presence of overt intracranial hemorrhage is less commonly associated with eventual development of cerebral palsy. Intraventricular hemorrhage is a relatively common complication of prematurity[29] (see Chapter 33). Very high levels of serum bilirubin, once seen with Rh incompatibility, may cause cerebral palsy as a consequence of bilirubin deposition in the basal ganglia. Because of Rh immunization and improved treatment of elevated serum bilirubin, this form of encephalopathy is now rare (see Chapters 13 and 26). Rarely, cerebral palsy is inherited as an autosomal recessive disorder.[30]

Pathophysiology. Abnormality of the structure and function of cerebral nerve tracts results in impairment of motor function and cognition. Manifestations of this impairment may not be apparent until months after birth, apparently because myelination of axons and maturation of basal ganglia neurons must first be completed. As CNS tissues continue to mature, manifestations may increase in severity, or they may decrease.

Clinical Manifestations. Soon after birth, cerebral palsy may manifest as excessive lethargy or irritability, high-pitched cry, poor head control, weak sucking, unusual posturing, or asymmetric movements. Later, it becomes apparent that gross and fine motor movement are impaired. One or more of the extremities exhibits paralysis, spasticity, extrapyramidal syndromes, or other dystonia or dyskinesia. Epilepsy, visual problems, mental retardation, and learning disorders are common. Because there is no specific diagnostic test for cerebral palsy, the diagnosis is established by excluding other causes.[30]

Prevention and Treatment. Reduction of perinatal risk involves optimal care during the prenatal and perinatal periods. Reduction of risk for congenital defects is discussed in Chapter 7. Reduction of risk of prematurity and low birth weight are discussed in Chapter 33. There is no definitive care for children with cerebral palsy. Supportive and rehabilitative measures are instituted. Medications may be used to intervene in seizures, spasticity, and gastrointestinal problems as necessary. Casting, bracing, or corrective surgery of the extremities may improve function in some cases. Occupational and physical therapy may also be indicated. Mobility devices, such as walkers, scooters, or wheelchairs, are frequently needed.

Prognosis and Outcome. A small number of mildly affected children outgrow the disorder, but most are permanently impaired. More than 90% live to adulthood, but their life expectancy is significantly less than that of the general population.[30]

Autonomic Neuropathy

Definition. Autonomic neuropathy, also known as *dysautonomia,* is the clinical syndrome resulting from hypofunction or hyperfunction of the ANS.

Epidemiology. Autonomic neuropathy is usually a component of **polyneuropathy,** that is, a disorder of more than one category of peripheral nerve. The leading cause of polyneuropathy is diabetic neuropathy, discussed in Chapter 29. Reliable estimates of incidence are not available.[31] Risk factors are those for diabetes and for other underlying disorders.

Etiology. Although some disorders affect motor, sensory, *and* autonomic nerves, the most common syndrome affects smaller nerve fibers, which are predominantly sensory and autonomic. These fibers may be damaged by many different inflammatory, metabolic, and toxic agents (Table 22–13), and a rare familial dysautonomia has been reported.[17] Autonomic neuropathy is most often associated with diabetes mellitus, Guillain-Barré syndrome, and chronic alcoholism.

Pathophysiology. The common denominator in all forms of neuropathy is hypoxic or toxic damage to the neuronal membrane, which impairs selective membrane transport and leads to altered ion flux and impulse conduction.

Clinical Manifestations. The effects of autonomic neuropathy are manifested in all organs served by the ANS. In most cases, clinical signs demonstrate hypofunction rather than hyperfunction. Neurologic manifestations include syncope (fainting) secondary to impairment of the baroreceptor reflex and hypothermia secondary to impaired thermoregulation. The cardiovascular system manifests the altered baroreceptor reflex as orthostatic hypotension, and either tachycardia or bradycardia may be seen. Gastrointestinal motility and secretion are usually decreased, leading to dry mouth, abdominal distention, and constipation, although diarrhea may occur in some patients. Effects on the urinary system include urinary retention or incontinence. Reproductive system effects include impotence in the male

TABLE 22–13
TOXIC NEUROPATHIES CAUSED BY ORGANIC COMPOUNDS

Toxic Agent	Source of Exposure	Molecular Basis	Clinical Findings	Pathologic Findings
Ethanol	Alcoholic beverages	Probable superimposed nutritional deficiencies	Slowly progressive distal sensorimotor neuropathy	Axonal degeneration (myelinated and unmyelinated fibers)
Acrylamide	Industry (polymerizing agent used as flocculant and for grouting)	Unknown	Numbness and sweating of hands and feet, progressing to distal sensorimotor neuropathy	Axonal degeneration, most pronounced in distal nerves (large-caliber fibers most affected)
Hexane	Industry (solvent) and inhalant abuse (glue sniffing)	Protein alkylation; impaired intermediate filament transport	Distal symmetric sensorimotor polyneuropathy	Enlarged axons filled with neurofilaments; axonal degeneration predominantly affecting large-caliber axons
Organophosphorus esters	Industry (pesticides, petroleum additives, plasticizers) and contaminated food products	Induction of esterase activity (neurotoxic esterase); altered protein phosphorylation	Rapidly progressive distal sensorimotor polyneuropathy after latent phase (7–21 days)	Axonal degeneration affecting long axons of the peripheral and central nervous systems
Vinca alkaloids	Medicine (vincristine used in cancer chemotherapy)	Impaired assembly of microtubules	Diminished ankle jerk earliest sign; subsequent progression to sensorimotor neuropathy	Axonal degeneration; large intravenous doses may cause accumulation of filaments in cell bodies

From Cotran, R.S., Kumar, V., and Robbins, S.L. (1994). *Robbins Pathologic Basis of Disease.* (5th ed.). Philadelphia: W.B. Saunders. (p. 1284).

and vaginal dryness in the female. Decreased sweating **(anhidrosis)** is usually seen, but increased sweating **(hyperhidrosis)** is also possible. The eyes may be dry because of decreased lacrimation, and vision may be blurred because of impairment of iridic and ciliary muscle contraction.

Prevention and Treatment. Prevention of neuropathy depends on prevention or optimal management of underlying conditions. In most cases, removal of the damaging stimulus allows the peripheral nerve fibers to regenerate, restoring impulse transmission and normal function. Treatment in these cases is essentially supportive. In cases of hyperfunction, clinical improvement may be obtained with selective use of autonomic drugs to block receptors mediating distressing symptoms.

Prognosis and Outcome. Outcome depends on the severity of the underlying disorder.

Pheochromocytoma

Definition. Pheochromocytoma is a catecholamine-secreting tumor originating in chromaffin cells. These cells are found primarily in tissues of embryonic neural crest origin, namely the SNS and adrenal medulla. More than 90% of pheochromocytomas are located in the adrenal medulla.[32] Pheochromocytomas outside the adrenal medulla are most likely to occur in sympathetic ganglia.

Epidemiology. Pheochromocytomas are rare but are clinically important in that they constitute a curable cause of hypertension. Fewer than 1 in 1000 cases of hypertension is due to pheochromocytoma, however.[33] About 5% of pheochromocytomas are inherited as an autosomal dominant trait, and half of these are bilateral.[32] Women are at slightly higher risk than men, and the tumor is most common in middle age.

Etiology. Except in the rare case of inheritance, the etiology of pheochromocytoma is unknown.

Pathophysiology. The tumor is usually fairly large and encapsulated. Ninety per cent are benign.[32] For those that do metastasize, the lymph nodes, skeleton, lung, liver, brain, and omentum have been reported as secondary sites. The neoplastic cells of the tumor synthesize and store catecholamines normally but release the hormones in increased amounts. Because adrenal pheochromocytomas are not innervated, catecholamine release is not triggered by SNS stimulation. The usual trigger of increased stimulation is displacement of abdominal contents, although many other triggers have been identified, including a number of drugs. In contrast to normal secretion by the adrenal medulla, the tumor usually secretes more norepinephrine than epinephrine.

Clinical Manifestations. Hypertension is the cardinal sign. Patients usually have sustained hypertension that does not respond to usual drug therapy. Patients may also have paroxysmal hypertensive attacks during which their blood pressures rise even higher. Hypertension manifests as a severe headache; other sympathetic manifestations include sweating, tachycardia, palpitations, and apprehension. Increased urinary excretion of catecholamines and catecholamine metabolites (metanephrines and vanillylmandelic acid) establishes the diagnosis. The tumor mass also is often evident on radiograph.

Prevention and Treatment. There is no known prevention for pheochromocytoma. Acute attacks of hypertension may be prevented by identifying and avoiding triggers. Drug therapy with α-adrenergic antagonists or nitroprusside may be used preoperatively to prevent severe hypertension. The definitive treatment of the tumor is surgical excision.

Prognosis and Outcome. Pheochromocytoma is associated with high mortality and morbidity if not recognized and treated. The surgical mortality rate is 2% to 4%.[32] No other forms of therapy are curative. Some degree of hypertension persists in about one fourth of patients, but this is usually well managed with standard antihypertensive therapy (see Chapter 15). Lifelong follow-up is necessary to detect recurrence of benign tumors or malignancy.

Neuroblastoma

Definition. Neuroblastoma is a malignant tumor of embryonic neural crest origin, most frequently located in the adrenal medulla, but also found anywhere along the sympathetic chain and within the cranial vault.

Epidemiology. Neuroblastoma demonstrates an annual incidence of 1 in 100,000 children under the age of 15 years.[34] Because the cell of origin is a primitive embryologic cell, the disease is most frequently diagnosed in children younger than 5 years. In a minority of cases, an autosomal dominant pattern of inheritance is evident, but in most cases, there is no clear familial predisposition.

Etiology. The precise etiology of neuroblastoma, except in known cases of inheritance, is unclear. The genetic defect manifested by tumor cells is usually a deletion on chromosome 1.

Pathophysiology. The growing tumor mass is obstructive, with precise manifestations depending on the locations of the primary and metastatic tumors. The metabolic demands of the tumor are high. Hypermetabolism is exacerbated in most patients by excessive catecholamines secreted by the tumor.

Clinical Manifestations. A growing mass may be evident and may compress the gastrointestinal or genitourinary tracts, causing obstruction, or the spinal cord, causing sensory loss or paralysis. Mediastinal tumors may obstruct bronchi, causing respiratory distress, or neck vessels, causing facial edema and other manifestations of superior vena cava syndrome (see Chapter 18). Intracranial tumors cause focal deficits and manifestations of increased intracranial pressure (see Chapter 21). Anemia is often present with or without bone marrow metastasis. Increased levels of catecholamines and their metabolites, as well as certain enzymes, are evident in serum and urine. Hypertension may or may not be present.

Prevention and Treatment. There is no known primary prevention for neuroblastoma. Treatment depends on the extent of the disease (Table 22–14). Surgical resection of the tumor is the treatment of choice for stages I and II disease. Radiation therapy may be used for treatment of any residual tumor in stage II and is the primary mode of therapy in more advanced stages. Several chemotherapy regimens have been employed in advanced disease.

Prognosis and Outcome. Young children with stage I disease have nearly a 100% survival rate. Stage II and III disease is associated with 50% to 80% survival rates, whereas only 10% of patients survive stage IV disease.[35]

TABLE 22–14
STAGES OF NEUROBLASTOMA

STAGE	DESCRIPTION
I	Tumor is confined to the organ of origin.
II	Tumor extends in continuity beyond organ of origin but does not cross the midline; lymph nodes on same side of the body may or may not be involved.
III	Tumor extends in continuity beyond the midline; lymph nodes on same side of the body may or may not be involved.
IV	Metastatic disease to the viscera, distal lymph nodes, soft tissue, and skeleton.
IV-S	(Special class.) Patients whose disease would be classified as stage I or II but who have distant disease of the liver, skin, or bone marrow.

Data from Cotran, R.S., Kumar, V., and Robbins, S.L. (1994). *Robbins Pathologic Basis of Disease.* (5th ed.). Philadelphia: W.B. Saunders. (p. 460).

Developmental Perspective

Embryonic and Fetal Periods

In response to stimuli (e.g., maternal movement), the embryo demonstrates slow, patterned movements of the head, trunk, and extremities as early as 5 weeks' postconception. As nerves continue to develop and become myelinated, these movements differentiate into discrete reflexes. Blinking, sucking, grasping, visceral reflexes, and deep tendon and plantar reflexes may be elicited by the 24th week. The nature of reflexes elicited in preterm infants may be used in determining gestational age. Prenatal insults may contribute to difficult birth and the development of cerebral palsy. The ANS begins to differentiate during the fifth week of gestation. Failure of migration of neural crest cells into the walls of the colon may result in dilation and hypertrophy (congenital megacolon, or Hirschsprung's disease) as a result of lack of parasympathetic innervation.

Infancy and Childhood

Autonomic regulation of homeostatic functions relative to respiration, circulation, temperature regulation, and feeding begins at birth. Movements of the neonate are often weak or erratic because the extremities are no longer buoyed by amniotic fluid. Cerebellar development continues during infancy, as does neuronal branching and development of synapses. The bulk of myelination is completed during infancy, but some continues into adulthood. Neonatal (primitive) reflexes, such as the Moro reflex, grasping, sucking, and rooting, are present at term but disappear gradually with continued development of voluntary motor control. Neural tube defects and other congenital anomalies, as well as birth trauma and perinatal hypoxia, may adversely affect motor function as well as cognitive development. The achievement of age-specific milestones in motor development may be delayed by illnesses such as congenital heart disease, cystic fibrosis, renal and hepatic diseases, severe infections, or major surgeries. Neuroblastoma usually manifests during childhood.

Adolescence and Young Adulthood

Adolescents and young adults are at highest risk for spinal cord injury, and the onset of autoimmune disorders such as MG and MS frequently occurs during this period. Motor agility begins to decline in early adulthood, owing to a gradual decrease in neuromuscular control as well as to changes in joints and muscles.

Middle and Older Adulthood

Motor signs of advancing age include reduced rate and amount of motor activity, slowed reaction time, decreased agility and fine motor coordination, and changes in posture and gait. Handwriting often deteriorates, and choking on food occurs more frequently. Stress incontinence is common as a result of a decrease in pelvic muscle strength and voluntary sphincter control. Loss of muscle mass may relate to decreased neural stimulation. Dystonias and dyskinesias are more frequent in the elderly because of neural deterioration. Autonomic failure in the elderly may manifest as orthostatic (postural) hypotension, impaired thermoregulation, decreased sweating of the lower body and increased sweating of the upper body, and impotence. Degenerative motor diseases, such as Parkinson's disease and ALS, are associated with advancing age.

CLINICAL SIGNIFICANCE OF SOMATIC MOTOR AND AUTONOMIC DISORDERS

The disorders described in this chapter evidence the impact of motor dysfunction on people of all ages (see Developmental Perspective). The impact on society is incalculable from the perspective of lost productivity, consumption of health care resources, and cost of supportive care. Evidence of ANS-mediated homeostatic activity is a component of the clinical picture in disorders of all systems. The most recognizable autonomic syndrome is the initial "fight-or-flight" stage of the stress response, discussed in Chapter 1. Disorders that originate in structural or functional pathology of the ANS or its "accessory" organ, the adrenal medulla, impair homeostatic function and may threaten the life of the patient.

Examples of research related to motor disorders are displayed in the Focus of Current Research. Spinal cord injury and Parkinson's disease are priority areas for research funding at this time, and it is hoped that intervention beyond supportive care can soon be offered to patients with degenerative motor disorders. Research is also ongoing in an effort to clarify mechanisms of autonomic regulation. Many drugs in clinical use act by blocking or facilitating autonomic function, and a critical goal of pharmacologic research is to increase the selectivity, safety, and efficacy of these agents.

As was stated early in this chapter, somatic motor function and autonomic function are dependent on appropriate afferent inputs from the somatic and special senses. Sensory function and related disorders are detailed in Chapter 23.

Summary of Key Points

- Both the somatic motor system and the ANS are involved in regulation of motor activity; that is, they modify all expressed behavior. The somatic motor system, which regulates skeletal muscle contraction, consists of motor neurons in the cortex and brain stem, with descending pathways traversing all levels of the spinal cord. The ANS, which regulates the contraction of smooth and cardiac muscle and the secretion of glands, consists of two divisions with opposing actions. Nuclei of the sympathetic division are located near the thoracic and lumbar regions of the cord, whereas those of the parasympathetic division are located in subcortical regions within the cranial vault and near the sacral levels of the cord.
- Hierarchic control of motor function permits the construction of complex activities from basic LMN reflex arcs. The primary motor cortex initiates somatic motor activity based on modulatory inputs from the premotor and supplemental areas as well as basal ganglia and cerebellar circuits. These higher-level signals are relayed to the brain-stem nuclei, where integration of reflex activity occurs.
- The neuromuscular junction is the specialized synapse between motor nerve and skeletal muscle. The neurotransmitter at the neuromuscular junction is ACh, and the ACh receptors at the motor end plate on the muscle fiber are ligand-gated sodium channels that induce action potentials and subsequent contraction. ACh is inactivated by the enzyme acetylcholinesterase, found in grooves in the motor end plate.
- The essential components of a motor reflex arc are (1) a sensory receptor, (2) a sensory nerve, (3) a synapse between a sensory nerve and an α-motoneuron, (4) a motor nerve, and (5) the neuromuscular junction.
- The corticospinal (pyramidal) motor pathway originates in the primary motor cortex and descends through the internal capsule to synapse on brain-stem nuclei or motor neurons in the anterior horns of the spinal cord. Disturbance of the pyramidal system may result in absence of movement (paralysis). This pathway is the major motor tract, directly influencing the initiation of somatic motor activity. Collectively, the other motor pathways are known as the extrapyramidal system, encompassing circuits through the cerebellum and basal ganglia before descent. These tracts are involved in modulation of motor activity to ensure that movement is accurate, efficient, smooth, and graceful.
- The cerebellum modifies the descending cortical motor signal based on inputs from peripheral proprioceptors, increasing the accuracy and optimizing the sequencing of activities. The basal ganglia receive multiple cortical inputs from the premotor and supplemental areas as well as from sensory areas of the cortex. Extrapyramidal lesions do not cause paralysis, but may cause weakness or lack of coordination of activity. Efferent signals are relayed by the thalamus to the primary motor cortex, modifying the descending signal to imbue activities with smoothness and grace.
- The SNS has a thoracolumbar distribution and, in most cases, short preganglionic fibers synapsing on nuclei located just outside the cord and long postganglionic fibers synapsing on target organs. Its neurotransmitters are ACh at preganglionic synapses and NE and EPI at postganglionic synapses. ACh binds to cholinergic receptors, whereas NE and EPI bind to adrenergic receptors. The PNS has a craniosacral distribution and, in most cases, long preganglionic fibers synapsing on nuclei in the walls of target organs. ACh is the neu-

Summary continued on following page

rotransmitter at all synapses. The sympathetic system mediates arousal (fight or flight), whereas the parasympathetic system mediates more restorative functions.

- Descending cortical and brain-stem tracts may influence the basic reflex arcs of the ANS, permitting conscious thoughts and subconscious emotions to influence visceral behavior to some degree. Brain-stem regulatory centers are interconnected anatomically and functionally with hypothalamic centers, facilitating neuroendocrine control of homeostatic functions.
- In general, the sympathetic and parasympathetic systems have opposing functions on target systems. In the cardiovascular system, for example, SNS stimulation causes increased heart rate and contractility as well as vasoconstriction. PNS stimulation results in decreased heart rate, decreased conduction, and dilation of some vessels. SNS stimulation results in bronchodilation, whereas the PNS mediates bronchoconstriction. SNS stimulation decreases gastrointestinal motility and constricts sphincters, whereas PNS stimulation increases motility and relaxes sphincters.
- Disorders of somatic motor function manifest as alterations in skeletal muscle contraction, such as weakness, paralysis, and other dystonias and dyskinesias. Disorders of autonomic function result in impaired homeostatic mechanisms and visceral dysfunction.

REFERENCES

1. Fehlings, M.G., and Louw, D. (1996). Initial stabilization and medical management of acute spinal cord injury. *American Family Physician* 54(1), 155–162.
2. Atkinson, P.P., and Atkinson, J.L.D. (1996). Spinal shock. *Mayo Clinic Proceedings* 71, 384–389.
3. Wirtz, K.M., La Favor, K.M., and Ang, R. (1996). Managing chronic spinal cord injury: Issues in critical care. *Critical Care Nurse* 16(4), 24–35.
4. Dittuno, J.F., and Formal, C.S. (1994). Chronic spinal cord injury. *New England Journal of Medicine* 330(8), 550–556.
5. Kernich, K.A., and Kaminski, H.J. 91995). Myasthenia gravis: Pathophysiology, diagnosis, and collaborative care. *Journal of Neuroscience Nursing* 27(4), 207–215.
6. Drachman, D.B. (1994). Myasthenia gravis. *New England Journal of Medicine* 330(25), 1797–1810.
7. Juhn, M.S. (1993). Myasthenia gravis: Diagnostic methods and control measures for a chronic disease. *Postgraduate Medicine* 94(5), 161–174.
8. Steinman, L. (1996). Multiple sclerosis: A coordinated immunological attack against myelin in the central nervous system. *Cell* 85, 299–302.
9. Arnason, B. (1995). The role of cytokines in multiple sclerosis. *Neurology* 45(suppl. 6), S54–S55.
10. Sobel, R.A. (1995). The pathology of multiple sclerosis. *Neurology Clinics* 13(1), 1–21.
11. Weiner, H.L., Hohol, M.J., Khoury, S.J., *et al.* (1995). Therapy for multiple sclerosis. *Neurologic Clinics* 13(1), 173–196.
12. Mitchell, G. (1993). Update on multiple sclerosis therapy. *Medical Clinics of North America* 77(1), 231–249.
13. Miller, C.M., and Hens, M. (1993). Multiple sclerosis: A literature review. *Journal of Neuroscience Nursing* 25(3), 174–179.
14. Murray, D.P. (1993). Impaired mobility: Guillain-Barré syndrome. *Journal of Neuroscience Nursing* 25(2), 100–104.
15. Dematteis, J.A. (1996). Guillain-Barré syndrome: A team approach to diagnosis and treatment. *American Family Physician* 54(1), 197–200.
16. Kankam, C.G., and Sallis, R. (1997). Guillain-Barré syndrome. *Postgraduate Medicine* 101(3), 279–290.
17. Adams, R.D., and Victor, M. (1993). *Principles of Neurology.* (5th ed.). New York: McGraw-Hill. (pp. 994, 1152).
18. Rowland, L.P. (1995). Amyotrophic lateral sclerosis: Human challenge for neuroscience. *Proceedings of the National Academy of Science, U.S.A.* 92, 1251–1253.
19. Bensimon, G., Lacomblez, L., Meininger, V., *et al.* (1994). A controlled trial of riluzole in amyotrophic lateral sclerosis. *New England Journal of Medicine* 330(9), 585–591.
20. Barker, E. (1994). *Neuroscience Nursing.* St. Louis: Mosby–Year Book. (p. 592).
21. Braunwald, E., Isselbacher, K.J., Petersdorf, R.G., *et al.* (1987). *Harrison's Principles of Internal Medicine.* (11th ed.). New York: McGraw-Hill. (p. 2015).
22. Black, J.M., and Matassarin-Jacobs, E. (1997). *Medical-Surgical Nursing: Clinical Management for Continuity of Care.* (5th ed.). Philadelphia: W.B. Saunders. (pp. 883, 930–931).
23. Ahlskog, J.E. (1994). Treatment of Parkinson's disease: From theory to practice. *Postgraduate Medicine* 95(5), 52–69.
24. Youdim, M.B.H., and Riederer, P. (1997). Understanding Parkinson's disease. *Scientific American* 276(1), 52–59.
25. Stacy, M., and Brownlee, H.J. (1996). Treatment options for early Parkinson's disease. *American Family Physician* 53(4), 1281–1287.
26. Kordower, J.H., Freeman, T.B., Snow, B.J., *et al.* (1995). Neuropathological evidence of graft survival and striatal reinnervation after the transplantation of fetal mesencephalic tissue in a patient with Parkinson's disease. *New England Journal of Medicine* 332(17), 1118–1124.
27. Calne, D.B. (1993). Treatment of Parkinson's disease. *New England Journal of Medicine* 329(14), 1021–1027.
28. Silverstein, P.M. (1996). Moderate Parkinson's disease. *Postgraduate Medicine* 99(1), 52–68, 204.
29. Kuban, K.C.K., and Leviton, A. (1994). Cerebral palsy. *New England Journal of Medicine* 330(3), 188–195.
30. Eicher, P.S., and Batshaw, M.L. (1993). Cerebral palsy. *Pediatric Clinics of North America* 40(3), 537–551.
31. Ross, M.A. (1993). Neuropathies associated with diabetes. *Medical Clinics of North America* 77(1), 111–124.
32. Werbel, S.S., and Ober, K.P. (1995). Pheochromocytoma: Update on diagnosis, localization, and management. *Medical Clinics of North America* 79(1), 131–153.
33. Cryer, P., Glazer, H., Clifford, D., *et al.* (Discussants). (1996). Hypertension and myocardial and cerebral infarctions. *American Journal of Medicine* 100, 357–364.
34. Behrman, R.E., Kliegman, R.M., Nelson, W.E., *et al.* (Eds.). (1992). *Nelson Textbook of Pediatrics.* (14th ed.). Philadelphia: W.B. Saunders. (p. 1304).
35. Cotran, R.S., Kumar, V., and Robbins, S.L. (1994). *Robbins Pathologic Basis of Disease.* (5th ed.). Philadelphia: W.B. Saunders. (p. 460).

SELECTED BIBLIOGRAPHY

Ahlskog, J.E. (1996). Treatment of early Parkinson's disease: Are complicated strategies justified? *Mayo Clinic Proceedings* 71, 659–670.

Beck, R.W., Cleary, P.A., Trobe, J.D., *et al.* (1993). The effect of corticosteroids for acute optic neuritis on the subsequent development of multiple sclerosis. *New England Journal of Medicine* 329(24), 1764–1769.

Beizer, J.L. (1995). Treatment options in Parkinson's disease. *American Pharmacy* NS35(1), 20–32.

Berne, R.M., and Levy, M.N. (1993). *Physiology*. (3rd ed.). St. Louis: Mosby–Year Book.

Bhushan, V., Paneth, N., and Kiely, J.L. (1993). Impact of improved survival of very low birth weight infants on recent secular trends in the prevalence of cerebral palsy. *Pediatrics* 91(6), 1094–1100.

Billiau, A. (1995). Interferons in multiple sclerosis: Warnings from experiences. *Neurology* 45(suppl. 6), S50–S53.

Brady, S.T. (1993). Motor neurons and neurofilaments in sickness and in health. *Cell* 73, 1–3.

Burke, J.H., Goldberger, J.J., Ehlert, F.A., *et al.* (1996). Gender differences in heart rate before and after autonomic blockade: Evidence against an intrinsic gender effect. *American Journal of Medicine* 100, 537–543.

Chiles, B.W., and Cooper, P.R. (1996). Acute spinal injury. *New England Journal of Medicine* 334(8), 514–520.

Coyle, P.K., Krupp, L.B., and Doscher, C. (1993). Significance of reactive Lyme serology in multiple sclerosis. *Annals of Neurology* 34(5), 745–747.

Eisen, A. (1995). Amyotrophic lateral sclerosis is a multifactorial disease. *Muscle & Nerve* 18, 741–752.

Ganong, W.F. (1995). *Review of Medical Physiology*. (17th ed.). Norwalk, CT: Appleton & Lange.

Georgopoulos, A.P. (1994). Behavioral neurophysiology of the motor cortex. *Journal of Laboratory and Clinical Medicine* 124(6), 766–774.

Goldstein, D.S., Holmes, C., Cannon, R.O., III, *et al.* (1997). Sympathetic cardioneuropathy in dysautonomias. *New England Journal of Medicine* 336(10), 696–702.

Graybiel, A.M., Aosaki, T., Flaherty, A.W., *et al.* (1994). The basal ganglia and adaptive motor control. *Science* 265, 1826–1831.

Guyton, A.C., and Hall, J.E. (1996). *Textbook of Medical Physiology*. (9th ed.). Philadelphia: W.B. Saunders.

Herbison, G.J., and Graziani, V. (1995). Neuromuscular disease: Rehabilitation and electrodiagnosis. 1. Anatomy and physiology of nerve and muscle. *Archives of Physical Medicine and Rehabilitation* 76, S3–S9.

Hohlfeld, R., Meinl, E., Weber, F., *et al.* (1995). The role of autoimmune T lymphocytes in the pathogenesis of multiple sclerosis. *Neurology* 45(suppl. 6), S33–S38.

Hugon, J. (1996). ALS therapy: Targets for the future. *Neurology* 47(suppl. 4), S251–S254.

Hyde, T.M., and Weinberger, D.R. (1995). Tourette's syndrome: A model neuropsychiatric disorder. *Journal of the American Medical Association* 273(6), 498–501.

Insel, P.A. (1996). Adrenergic receptors: Evolving concepts and clinical implications. *New England Journal of Medicine* 334(9), 580–585.

Jansen, A.S.P., Van Nguyen, X., Karpitskiy, V., *et al.* (1995). Central command neurons of the sympathetic nervous system: Basis of the fight-or-flight response. *Science* 270, 644–646.

Jerusalem, F., Pohl, C., Karitzky, J., *et al.* (1996). ALS. *Neurology* 47(suppl. 4), S218–S220.

Lehne, R.A. (1994). *Pharmacology for Nursing Care*. (2nd ed.). Philadelphia: W.B. Saunders.

Leigh, P.N., and Meldrum, B.S. (1996). Excitotoxicity in ALS. *Neurology* 47(suppl. 4), S221–S227.

Lucas, K., and Hohlfeld, R. (1995). Differential aspects of cytokines in the immunotherapy of multiple sclerosis. *Neurology* 45(suppl. 6), S4–S5.

Oksenberg, J.R., Begovich, A.B., Erlich, H.A., *et al.* (1993). Genetic factors in multiple sclerosis. *Journal of the American Medical Association* 270(19), 2362–2369.

Olanow, C.W. (Discussant). (1996). A 61-year-old man with Parkinson's disease. *Journal of the American Medical Association* 275(9), 716–722.

Raymond, J.L., Lisberger, S.G., and Mauk, M.D. (1996). The cerebellum: A neuronal learning machine? *Science* 272, 1126–1131.

Rees, J.H., Soudain, S.E., Gregson, N.A., *et al.* (1995). *Campylobacter jejuni* infection and Guillain-Barré syndrome. *New England Journal of Medicine* 333(21), 1374–1379.

Schendel, D.E., Berg, C.J., Yeargin-Allsopp, M., *et al.* (1996). Prenatal magnesium sulfate exposure and the risk for cerebral palsy or mental retardation among very-low-birth weight children aged 3 to 5 years. *Journal of the American Medical Association* 276(22), 1805–1810.

Scott, T.F. (1991). Diseases that mimic multiple sclerosis. *Postgraduate Medicine* 89(8), 187–191.

Stein, P.K., Bosner, M.S., and Kleiger, R.E. (1994). Heart rate variability: A measure of cardiac autonomic tone. *American Heart Journal* 127(5), 1376–1381.

St. George, C.L. (1993). Spasticity: Mechanisms and nursing care. *Nursing Clinics of North America* 28(4), 819–827.

Taylor, A.A. (1994). Autonomic control of cardiovascular function: Clinical evaluation in health and disease. *Journal of Clinical Pharmacology* 34, 363–374.

Tidwell, J. (1993). Pulmonary management of the ALS patient. *Journal of Neuroscience Nursing* 25(6), 337–342.

Weinshenker, B.G. (1995). The natural history of multiple sclerosis. *Neurologic Clinics* 119–146.

Young, W. (1996). Spinal cord regeneration. *Science* 273, 451.

Young, W.F. Jr., and Maddox, D.E. (1995). Spells: In search of a cause. *Mayo Clinic Proceedings* 70, 757–765.

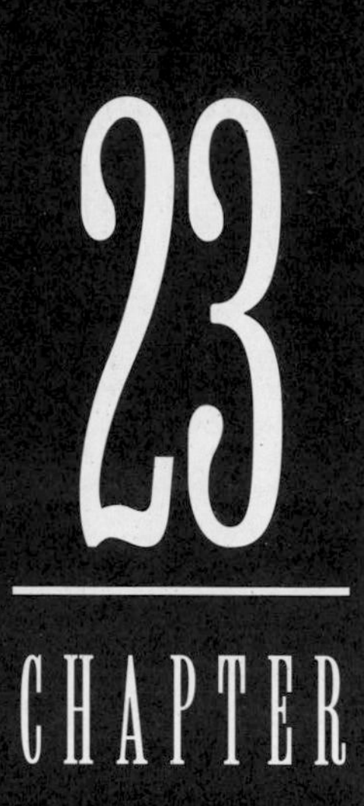

Disorders of Sensory Function

LEARNING OBJECTIVES

1. Discuss the importance of the somatic and special sensory systems in regulation of motor activity.
2. Identify the essential components of the sensory functional unit.
3. Differentiate between the the dorsal column–medial lemniscus and anterolateral pathways with respect to anatomy and function.
4. Identify the cortical areas involved in reception and perception of sensation.
5. Compare and contrast the four principal theories of pain sensation.
6. Discuss the contribution of each of the components of the proprioceptive system.
7. Describe the three physiologic processes essential to vision.
8. Describe the conductive and sensorineural processes essential to auditory function.
9. Discuss the physiology and clinical importance of the chemical senses of taste (gustation) and smell (olfaction).
10. Comprehend the pathophysiologic bases of the clinical manifestations and treatment of the more prevalent disorders of the somatic and special senses.

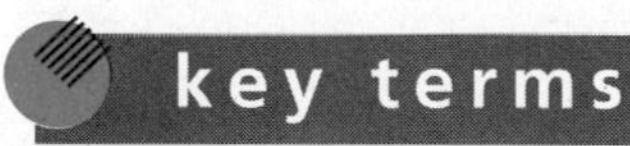

allodynia
analgesia
anesthesia
ankylosing spondylitis
aphakia
benign positional vertigo
carpal tunnel syndrome (CTS)
cataract
cauda equina syndrome

cervical radiculopathy
cholesteatoma
color blindness
conductive hearing loss
conjunctivitis
corneal opacity
corneal reflex
diplopia
fibromyalgia
glaucoma
hyperalgesia
hyperopia
intervertebral disk disease
macular degeneration
mastoiditis
Meniere's disease
myopia
nystagmus
otitis media
otosclerosis
peripheral neuropathy
phantom pain
presbycusis
presbyopia
radiculopathy
referred pain
retinal detachment
retinitis
retinopathy
sciatica
sensorineural hearing loss
spinal stenosis
tinnitus
trigeminal neuralgia
uveitis
vertigo

The critical nature of sensory input to motor function is established in Chapter 22. In this chapter, the sensory pathways and mechanisms that provide continuous information to the integrative areas of the central nervous system (CNS) are discussed in detail. The *somatic sensory system,* which provides information about the status of the body through the function of peripheral and visceral receptors for touch, pain, temperature, vibration, and proprioception, is discussed, and illustrative disorders are reviewed. The function of the *special sensory systems,* which collect environmental information, also is examined, along with disorders of vision, hearing, taste, and smell.

In the language of general systems theory (see Chapter 1), the sensory systems facilitate the inputs critical to human function. Disorders of sensory function are common manifestations of diseases of all body systems. Pain is particularly widespread, and there is growing evidence that it is inadequately treated in many patients.[1] Although the pathophysiology of pain is incompletely understood, the prevalent theories are discussed in this chapter. Transmission of pain and other sensory impulses occurs through action potential formation and conduction, discussed in Chapter 4, and through the mechanisms of neurotransmission, discussed in Chapter 21.

The special senses are so named because each subsystem is highly specialized in terms of its anatomy, receptor function, and signal processing. Disorders of the special senses, particularly vision and hearing, are common among people of all ages (see Developmental Perspective). Screening programs and treatment of these disorders are a major component of pediatric and gerontologic practices and a primary focus of school health and allied medical professions.

SOMATIC SENSATION

Sensory Functional Unit

Organization of the sensory functional unit is illustrated schematically in Figure 23–1. The following structures are essential to sensation: (1) a sensory receptor (specialized ending of a dendritic fiber) in skin, muscle, or viscera; (2) a sensory nerve (afferent or dendritic fiber); (3) a sensory neuron (cell body or dorsal root ganglion); (4) another sensory nerve (efferent fiber or axon); and (5) a synapse with another neuron, which may be either a motor or sensory neuron. Somatic sensory pathways consist of three types of neurons, classified as first, second, or third order. The neuron whose dendritic fiber contains the peripheral sensory receptor is designated as the first-order neuron. Its axonal fibers synapse on a second-order neuron (also known as an *association neuron*) located in the dorsal horn gray matter of the spinal cord or the medulla oblongata of the brain stem. Axonal fibers from second-order neurons synapse on a third-order neuron in the thalamus, which in turn signals the sensory areas of the cerebral cortex.

Sensory Receptors

Classification of Receptors

The five types of sensory receptors are *mechanoreceptors,* which detect physical deformation of their membranes; *thermoreceptors,* which detect alteration in the temperature of the surrounding extracellular fluid; *nociceptors* (pain receptors), which detect mechanical stimuli and cytokines associated with tissue trauma or toxicity; *chemoreceptors,* which detect

Developmental Perspective

Embryonic and Fetal Periods

The intrauterine environment is a source of varied, rhythmic sensory stimulation to the developing human. The somatic sensory and special sensory systems develop in the following order: touch, smell, vestibular function, taste, hearing, and vision. Peripheral sensory fibers myelinate after motor fibers, whereas central sensory fibers myelinate before motor fibers. Fetal responsivity to touch is present before 32 weeks' gestation, and maternal movement provides stimulation to the fetal vestibular system. The structures of the inner ear and cochlea mature at about 20 weeks' gestation, and the fetus is observed to respond to sounds in the external environment at 25 to 28 weeks' gestation. Development of the eye is apparent early in the embryonic period. By 22 weeks, the retinal layers have formed, and rods and cones develop soon after. Preterm infants display visual attentiveness at 30 to 32 weeks' gestation, but myelination of the optic nerve is incomplete at birth. Congenital inequality of pupil size (anisocoria) is common. Many other congenital defects of the sensory system are associated with genetic defects and teratogenesis. These conditions, which are rare, include glaucoma, cataracts, aniridia (absence of the iris), aphakia (absence of the lens), microphthalmos (small, undeveloped eyes), cholesteatoma, and deafness.

Infancy and Childhood

Sprouting and myelination of sensory nerves continue slowly throughout this period. Pain and touch sensations are highly developed in the newborn. Ophthalmia neonatorum, conjunctivitis occurring within the first 10 days of life, is a reportable communicable disease for which prophylactic antibiotic therapy is routine in newborn nurseries. By 3 months of age, the infant is able to fixate visually and follow an object, demonstrating macular development. After a few weeks of life, the infant normally startles in response to loud noises and responds with visual searching to other sounds. Auditory sensations are important in the development of language, beginning at 2 to 3 months of age, and delays in language development may be the initial signs of auditory disorder. Failure of the child to see and hear are more often due to cerebral defects than to problems with the sensory systems. Recurrent otitis media may impose risk of conductive hearing loss during this period.

Adolescence and Young Adulthood

Adolescents and young adults are at risk for a number of sensory disorders, including headaches, low back pain, carpal tunnel syndrome, Meniere's syndrome, and benign positional vertigo. Occupational or recreational exposure to loud noise may predispose to sensorineural hearing loss. AIDS-related retinopathy and traumatic retinal detachment are also more prevalent during this developmental stage. Pregnancy imposes increased risk of carpal tunnel syndrome due to increased fluid volume.

Middle and Older Adulthood

Neurologic signs indicative of subclinical peripheral neuropathy are often found in apparently healthy elderly people and may predispose these people to falls. Peripheral neuropathy secondary to diabetes, hypertension, or cardiovascular disease has its highest incidence in this age group. Sensory changes typical of aging include impairment of vibratory sense, especially in the feet and ankles, and a diminished sense of touch. Compression fractures related to osteoporosis may result in low back pain and headaches. Hormonal changes during menopause may trigger headaches. Proprioception is impaired little or not at all. Pupils are smaller and more sluggish in reflex responses to light and accommodation. Presbyopia of the lens also impairs accommodation, and vision may be further impaired by senile cataracts and age-related macular degeneration. Presbycusis manifests as progressive hearing loss, especially for high tones. The senses of smell and taste are diminished. Stroke is most prevalent in this age group and manifests as sensory disorder.

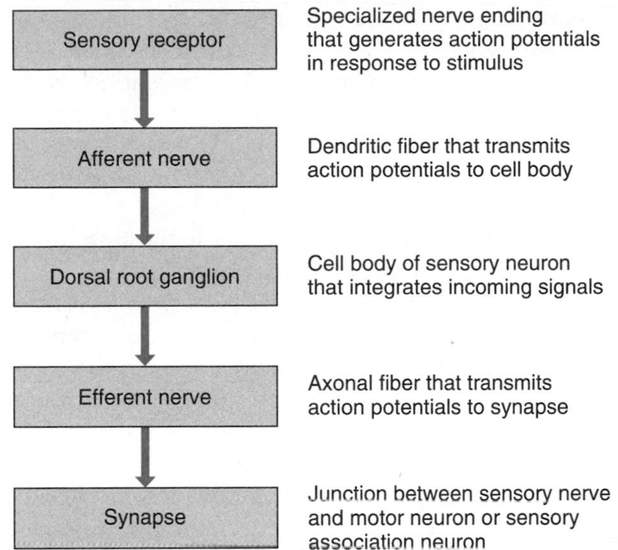
Sensory receptor
Specialized nerve ending that generates action potentials in response to stimulus
Afferent nerve
Dendritic fiber that transmits action potentials to cell body
Dorsal root ganglion
Cell body of sensory neuron that integrates incoming signals
Efferent nerve
Axonal fiber that transmits action potentials to synapse
Synapse
Junction between sensory nerve and motor neuron or sensory association neuron

FIGURE 23–1
Sensory functional unit. The structures essential to sensory transmission are illustrated. Sensation normally originates within a peripheral sensory receptor, initiating an impulse that is relayed to a motor neuron or to a higher-order sensory neuron.

changes in the extracellular concentration of ions or other molecules; and *electromagnetic receptors,* which detect light on the retina of the eye. Table 23–1 lists examples of each class of receptor, along with the specific functions of each. Peripheral receptors have different anatomic configurations, depending on their location and function. Figure 23–2 illustrates an example of each class of sensory receptor.

Mechanism of Receptor Activation

The common denominator in the function of all classes of sensory receptors is alteration of the receptor membrane by a physical, thermal, or chemical stimulus. Sodium influx follows, generating an action potential (receptor potential) if threshold is reached (see Chapter 4). This impulse is then conducted along the myelinated or unmyelinated fibers of the sensory pathway.

Factors Affecting Intensity of Sensation

Several factors can affect the intensity of sensation, including receptor density, threshold variation, stimulus intensity, and receptor adaptation. The greater the number of sensory receptors within a given area, the more intense the sensation. Tissues of the fingertips and lips, for example, have high receptor density. The membrane potential at which an action potential is generated by a sensory recep-

TABLE 23–1
CLASSIFICATION OF SENSORY RECEPTORS

Class	Functions	Examples
Mechanoreceptors	Tactile sensation of skin	Free nerve endings Merkel's disks Ruffini's endings Meissner's corpuscles Krause's corpuscles Hair end organs
	Deep tissue sensation	Free nerve endings Ruffini's endings Pacini's corpuscles Muscle spindles Golgi tendon organs
	Hearing	Cochlear sound receptors
	Proprioception	Vestibular receptors
	Arterial pressure regulation	Baroreceptors
Thermoreceptors	Temperature sensation	Cutaneous and visceral thermoreceptors
Nociceptors	Pain sensation	Free nerve endings
Electromagnetic receptors	Vision	Rods Cones
Chemoreceptors	Taste	Taste bud receptors
	Smell	Receptors of olfactory epithelium
	PaO_2 regulation	Aortic body and carotid body receptors
	Osmolarity regulation	Osmoreceptors of hypothalamus
	$PaCO_2$ regulation	Aortic body and carotid body receptors, receptors in respiratory center in medulla

Adapted from Guyton, A.C., and Hall, J.E. (1996). *Textbook of Medical Physiology.* (9th ed.). Philadelphia: W.B. Saunders. (p. 584).

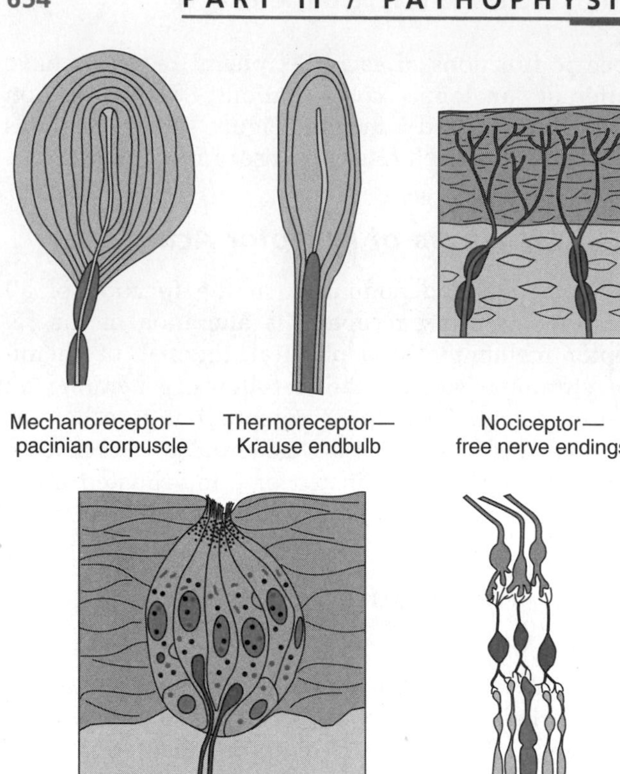

FIGURE 23–2
Sensory receptors. An example of each class of sensory receptor is illustrated.

tor is known as its *afferent threshold.* This threshold is fairly constant within receptor types and determines the amount of stimulation necessary to cause the receptor to "fire." Most sensation demonstrates a *subjective threshold* as well, which is the level of stimulation necessary for perception of sensation by the cerebral cortex. The subjective threshold normally is near the afferent threshold but may vary with cortical modulation based on level of consciousness, previous experience with the sensation, or the concurrent presence of other stimuli, such as attention distractors, fatigue, or strong emotion. This phenomenon is readily apparent in clinical practice; patients manifest widely variable responses to similar levels of painful stimuli.

Receptor Adaptation

As the intensity of the stimulus increases, the rate of action potential generation at first increases proportionately, then levels off at a maximal point. This pattern apparently allows receptors to be sensitive at low levels of stimulation yet protects them against extreme stimulus intensity. Receptor adaptation is evidenced by an eventual decline in action potential generation and finally by a total lack of receptor response when a continuous stimulus is applied. The precise mechanism of this adaptation is unknown but is believed to be a structural change in the receptor membrane related to continuous ion flux.

With respect to adaptation, receptors are of two types: (1) slowly adapting or nonadapting (tonic) receptors and (2) rapidly adapting (phasic) receptors. Tonic receptors keep firing persistently or indefinitely in response to continuous stimuli, whereas phasic receptors respond quickly and strongly, but briefly. Tonic receptors include the Golgi tendon organs and vestibular receptors for position sense, pain receptors, arterial baroreceptors, and some tactile receptors (e.g., Ruffini's endings and Merkel's disks). Pacini's corpuscles and motion receptors in joints and in the semicircular canals of the inner ear are examples of phasic receptors.[2]

Sensory Pathways

The two principal somatic sensory pathways are the *dorsal column–medial lemniscus pathway* (DCML), also known as the discriminative pathway, and the *anterolateral pathway.* As illustrated in Figure 23–3, the DCML is a three-neuron pathway whose fibers ascend within the dorsal horns of the cord, cross at the medulla, ascend to the thalamus by the medial lemniscus tract, and finally project through the internal capsule to the primary sensory cortex in the parietal lobe. Its nerves are large and myelinated; thus, transmission is rapid. The DCML mediates the delicate and discrete sensations of light touch, vibration, and proprioception.

The anterolateral pathway, illustrated in Figure 23–4, has two main divisions based on point of termination: the anterior *spinothalamic* (also known as neospinothalamic) and the lateral *spinoreticular* (also known as paleospinothalamic) divisions. From second-order neurons in the dorsal horns, the fibers of both divisions cross immediately before ascending. The thalamus is the termination point for the spinothalamic division, which mediates fast transmission of sharp pain sensation. Spinoreticular fibers ascend to the reticular activating system (RAS), limbic system, and pain reception areas, such as the periaquaductal gray region, as well as to the thalamus. The spinoreticular tract transmits impulses for sensation of dull or pressure-type pain, temperature, and crude or heavy touch. These tracts also mediate complex sensations, such as tickle, itch, and sexual sensation, and are believed to integrate the emotional content of sensation.

Because the DCML is a more discrete pathway

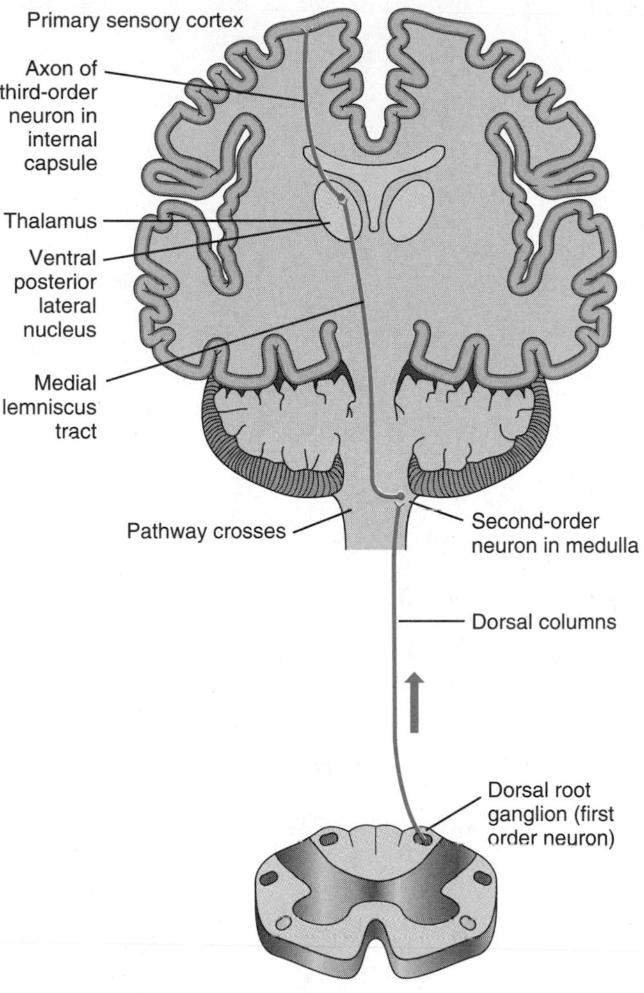

FIGURE 23–3
Dorsal column–medial lemniscus pathway. This pathway is also known as the *discriminative pathway* because it carries subtle sensations such as fine touch, vibration, and proprioception. Fibers ascend through the dorsal columns (posterior gray matter) of the spinal cord, cross at the medulla, and ascend to the thalamus through the medial lemniscus tract. (The pathway is present bilaterally. One tract is shown here.)

than the anterolateral system, it is more often damaged with neurotrauma such as spinal cord injury. The many branches and collateral pathways of the anterolateral system make it more resistant to destruction and may allow it to function as a limited backup system in the event of DCML dysfunction.

Peripheral Distribution of Sensory Nerves

Somatic sensory nerve fibers exit each level of the cord from the dorsal root ganglia, then interlace with motor, autonomic, and other sensory nerves outside the cord. This interlacing, or *plexus* formation, allows development of collateral sensory pathways in the event of peripheral nerve damage, provided that the sensory neuron cell bodies (dorsal root ganglia) remain intact. Such sensation would not be as accurate or discriminating, however. The region of the body served by a single pair of dorsal root ganglia is known as a *dermatome.* The dermatomes have been mapped accurately (Fig. 23–5), which allows localization of sensory deficits in clinical practice. Lack of sensation in certain skin areas provides evidence regarding the level of the lesion in spinal cord injury, for example (see Chapter 22). Herpes zoster virus (shingles) is a common dermato-

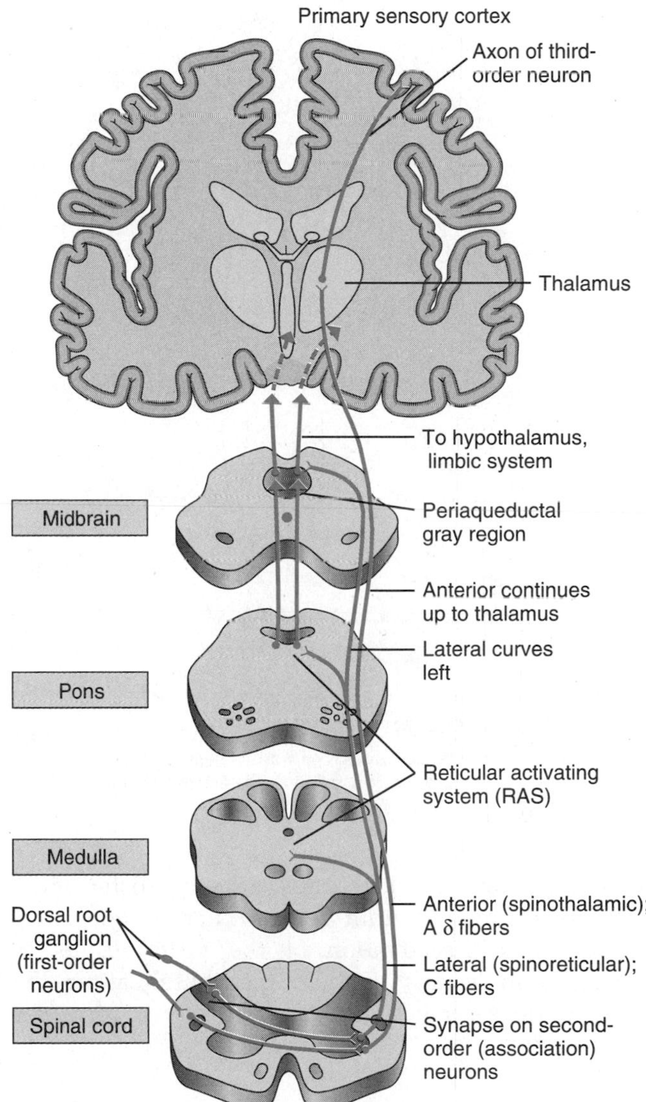

FIGURE 23–4
Anterolateral pathway. The anterolateral pathway has two divisions: the anterior *spinothalamic* and lateral *spinoreticular* tracts. Fibers of both tracts cross at entry into the cord. The spinothalamic fibers, which mediate acute pain sensation, ascend in the anterior gray matter, terminating in the thalamus. The spinoreticular fibers, which transmit dull pain, pressure, temperature, and crude touch, ascend in the lateral gray matter and project to brain stem and limbic nuclei as well as the thalamus.

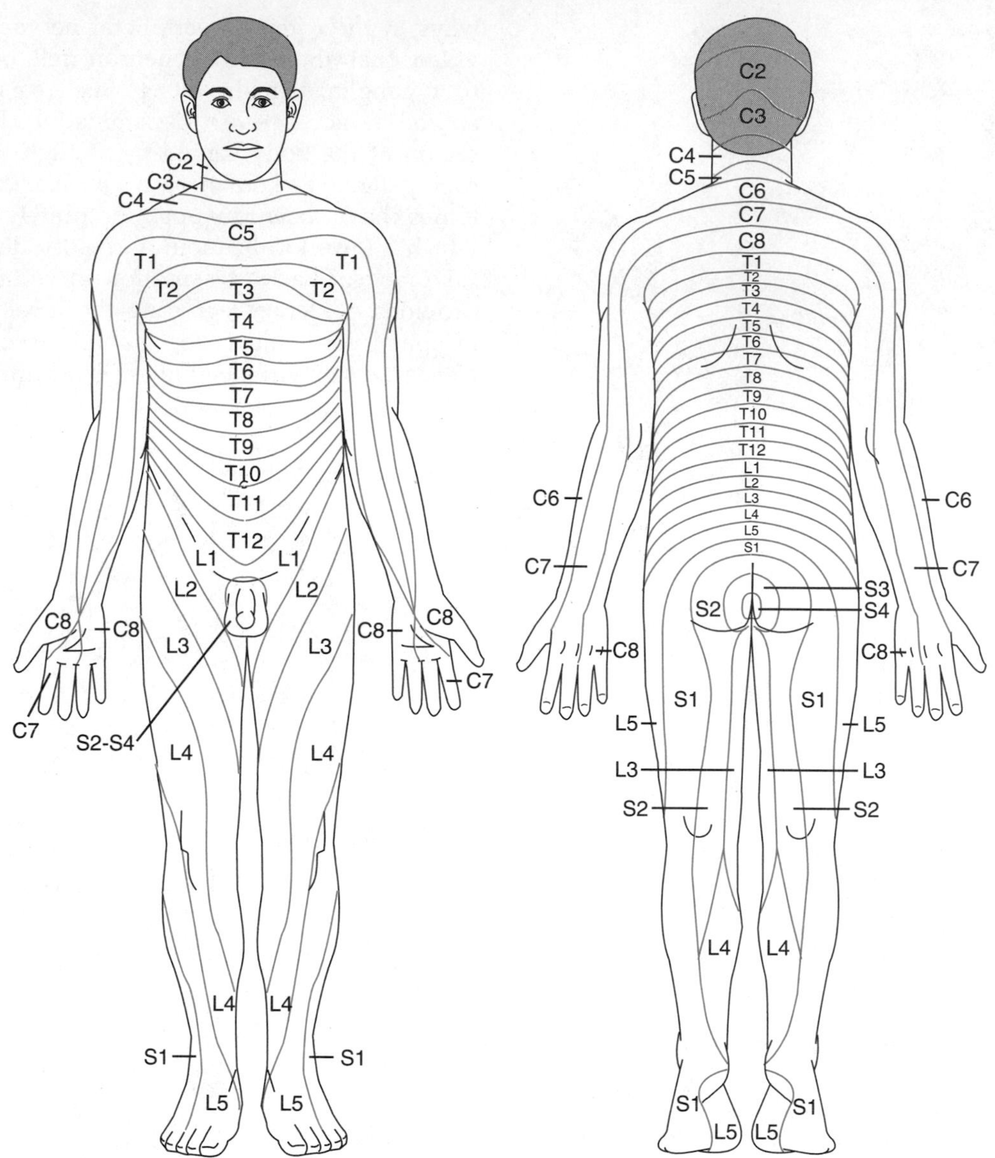

FIGURE 23–5
Dermatomes. Skin areas served by specific sensory nerves *(dorsal root ganglia)* have been accurately mapped, providing a basis for clinical localization of neural lesions.

logic disorder in which the varicella zoster virus remains dormant within sensory nerve roots after chicken pox. Reactivation of the virus results in painful skin lesions that are distributed along the dermatome served by the affected nerve root (see Chapter 36).

Cortical Sensory Areas

Ascending sensory impulses terminate in the *primary sensory cortex* in the parietal lobe (Fig. 23–6). This area, located just posterior to the motor cortex of the frontal lobe, functions in the *reception* of ascending sensory impulses. The number of cortical neurons involved depends on the density of receptors in the tissue from which the impulses originate. The *sensory homunculus* (Fig. 23–7) illustrates the proportionate distribution of neurons involved with reception of sensation from various tissues. Tissues demonstrating fine touch sensation have greater representation on the cortex. The primary sensory cortex is able to localize (determine the source of) incoming impulses and determine their intensity. The *meaning* of the sensory impulses is determined by an adjacent cortical area, the *sensory association area.* This area *perceives* sensation by integrating multiple inputs from the primary sensory cortex and other areas and by comparing incoming sensory input to "stored" sensations. Cortical areas involved in the

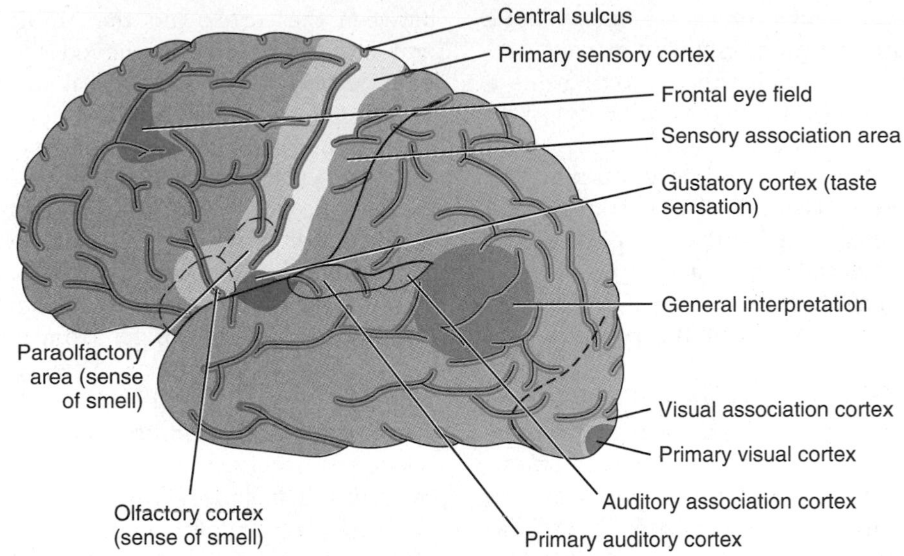

FIGURE 23–6
Cortical sensory areas. The highest level of sensory integration occurs in the *sensory association area,* which interprets the meaning of sensory stimuli from adjacent sensory areas. The *primary sensory cortex* of the parietal lobe receives somatic sensory inputs, whereas other cortical areas are dedicated to the special senses.

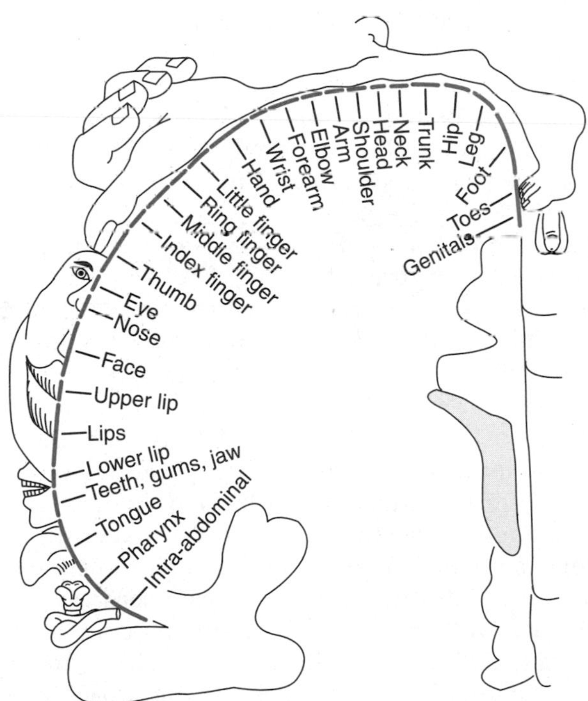

FIGURE 23–7
Sensory homunculus. This classic figure illustrates the proportionate distribution of neurons of the primary sensory cortex dedicated to reception of sensory input from specific body areas. Tissues that have a high density of sensory receptors have greater representation on the cortex. (Redrawn from Penfield, E., and Rasmussen, T. [1955]. *The Cerebral Cortex of Man.* New York: Macmillan Publishing. Reprinted with the permission of Simon & Schuster. Copyright 1950 Macmillan Publishing Company; renewed © 1978 Theodore Rasmussen.)

special senses of taste, smell, vision, and hearing are also shown. Their functions are detailed later in this chapter.

Specific Sensory Modalities

Touch (Tactile Sensation)

Tactile receptors are located in both superficial (skin) and deep (visceral) tissues. (Examples were detailed in Table 23–1 and illustrated in Fig. 23–2.) Transmission of tactile stimuli occurs along both somatic sensory pathways; fine touch is mediated quickly by the large fibers of the DCML system, and crude touch or pressure is conducted along the smaller fibers of the anterolateral pathway. Because of its collateral fibers projecting to the limbic system, the anterolateral pathway is important in the transmission of tactile sensations (e.g., sexual touch) associated with emotional content.

Pain (Nociception)

Theories of Pain. Pain is a complex, poorly understood sensory modality. Pain sensation clearly has psychological and sociocultural components as well as a physiologic basis, resulting in variation among people with respect to pain perception and behavioral response. The precise mechanisms involved in pain sensation have not yet been fully established. Four principal theories underlie clinical management of pain: the *specificity theory, pattern the-*

ory, gate control theory, and *neuromatrix theory.* None of these fully explains all manifestations of pain.

Specificity Theory. Specificity theory represents a rigid application of the *labeled line principle,* whereby any sensation requires a specific type of receptor (a nociceptor in the case of pain) and a neural pathway dedicated *only* to transmission of that particular sensation. According to specificity theory, pain occurs only when action potentials generated at nociceptors are transmitted along anterolateral system fibers to specialized pain receptor areas in the primary sensory cortex.

Pattern Theory. In contrast, pattern theory holds that pain may also occur as a result of high stimulus *intensity,* regardless of the type of receptor stimulated and the particular ascending pathway involved. High-intensity touch (deep pressure) could be perceived as pain, as could intense vibration, loud noise, or intense heat or cold, even if there were no actual tissue damage. Several different theories attempt to explain the anatomic and physiologic interactions among nervous system components that could result in the perception of pain by the pattern mechanism, including summation of incoming impulses by dorsal horn neurons, inhibition of small-fiber transmission by large-fiber transmission, and a particular role for the substantia gelatinosa of the dorsal horns in modulation of pain impulses at the level of the cord.[3]

Gate Control Theory. The gate control theory, put forth by Melzack and Wall in 1965, proposes that interneuronal connections are present between pain pathways and other sensory pathways.[3] Simultaneous firing of two pathways (e. g., touch and pain) "closes the gate" on pain transmission by both dorsal horn and cortical mechanisms, resulting in the perception of touch alone. This theory provides the rationale for such nontraditional pain interventions as transcutaneous electrical nerve stimulation and brushing or rubbing of tissues from which pain originates.

Neuromatrix Theory. Based on observations of **phantom pain** in patients with paraplegia or amputation, Melzack has proposed a more comprehensive theory of sensation in general, and of pain in particular, termed the neuromatrix theory.[3] This theory holds that all sensation is imprinted by processes in the brain. Although these processes are normally activated and modulated by inputs from the body, they can act in the absence of any such inputs. In other words, all sensory experience lies in neural networks (the neuromatrix) of the brain. Stimuli may trigger the patterns of sensation but do not produce them. Melzack proposed that the neuromatrix is a widespread network of neurons consisting of loops between the thalamus and cortex as well as between the cortex and the limbic system. The lateral hypothalamus is believed to be critical to the pain perception aspect of the neuromatrix.

These theories of pain are not necessarily mutually exclusive. Pain is no longer considered to be a unitary symptom but rather a sensory end point that can be generated by a number of different processes under different clinical conditions.

Physiologic Versus Clinical Pain. Physiologic (acute) pain is a protective mechanism, designed to warn of impending danger from injurious stimuli in the external environment. This type of pain is explained by the specificity theory. That is, it is sensed by nociceptors, transmitted by dedicated pain pathways, and received and interpreted by specific cortical areas. Transmission is rapid, and the excitatory neurotransmitter glutamate is predominant within synapses. Efferent outputs from these areas then trigger the withdrawal reflex[4] (see Chapter 22).

Clinical (chronic) pain, on the other hand, is characterized by the onset of dull, burning, or stabbing pain in response to normally nonpainful stimuli or to no apparent stimuli. Clinical pain is further defined by the presence of sensory hypersensitivity, consisting of **hyperalgesia,** an exaggerated or increased response to a noxious stimulus, and **allodynia,** the production of pain by low-intensity stimuli.[4] Sensory hypersensitivity may be induced by the presence of inflammatory mediators or by lesions of the neurons of the sensory pathways. Under these conditions, intense or repeated stimuli from tissue damage results in lowering of the threshold for activation of the nociceptors.[5]

Pain Reception and Transmission. Nociceptors, illustrated in Figure 23–2, are free nerve endings found in skin, viscera, blood vessels, muscle, fascia, and joint capsules. They are stimulated by noxious (unpleasant) stimuli, either by mechanical or chemical means. That is, the receptor membrane may depolarize in response to physical deformation or by receptor-mediated changes in permeability. The inflammatory mediators prostaglandin, bradykinin, and histamine are among the local cytokines known to mediate pain sensation. Both divisions of the anterolateral pathway can transmit pain sensation. The fast track, with its Aδ fibers, is the anterior (spinothalamic) division, mediating acute, sharp pain such as that induced by a pinprick or pinch. The lateral (spinoreticular) division is the slow track because of its unmyelinated C fibers and many side projections. It transmits impulses perceived as dull, achy, diffuse, or unpleasant pain. During pain transmission, the cell bodies of the dorsal root ganglia release a number of neuropeptides (notably substance P and calcitonin gene–related peptide) that amplify the intensity of the ascending transmission.

As with other sensations, pain is localized in the primary sensory cortex and perceived in the adjacent sensory association areas. In some cases of pain originating in deep organs, however, pain is inaccurately localized as originating from certain areas of the skin surface. Examples of this **referred pain** are described in Table 23–2. Referred pain is possible when primary sensory neurons from both the skin and the viscera synapse on the same second-order neurons in the cord. Phantom pain is perceived as originating from a limb that has been amputated or paralyzed. This sensation may occur even in people who were born with missing or paralyzed limbs, a phenomenon that is unexplained except by the neuromatrix theory, discussed earlier. Pain is perceived as *radiating* when it extends superficially along the skin surface in a dermatomal pattern. Thus, stimulation of a pain pathway at points proximal to the sensory receptor may result in the perception of pain as originating from peripheral nociceptors.

Endogenous Modulation of Pain

Hyperalgesia. Hyperalgesia, or increased sensitivity to pain, is characteristic of chronic pain, as discussed earlier, and is incompletely understood. This phenomenon may originate from the presence of inflammatory mediators that amplify the afferent signal, from lesions within the pain pathways (e.g., compression of nerves or nerve roots), or from lowering of nociceptor thresholds by repeated stimulation. Psychological factors, such as mood, personality, and attitude, as well as culture and social support, clearly influence the perception of chronic pain, possibly by influencing the balance of excitatory and inhibitory neurotransmitters.[5] Increased sympathetic nervous system activity *(reflex sympathetic dystrophy)* in response to the stressor of pain may contribute to hyperalgesia by inducing muscle spasm, peripheral vasoconstriction, and ischemia. Ischemia may result in the local release of mediators that amplify the pain signal (see Chapter 15).

Analgesia. The intensity of pain sensation may be reduced by the *endogenous analgesia system,* a specialized descending pathway originating in two areas of the brain stem, the periaqueductal gray area of the midbrain and the raphe nucleus of the descending reticuloendothelial system or RAS (see Chapter 21). These areas have a high density of receptors for endogenous opioids, neuropeptides of the endorphin, enkephalin, and dynorphin families that bind to the same opioid receptors as narcotic analgesics, such as heroin and morphine. Many types of cells produce these peptides, but serotonergic neurons are a particularly important source within the CNS. (The "runner's high," or exercise-induced euphoria, experienced by sustained aerobic exercise is mediated by release of these same neuromodulators.)

The periaqueductal gray and raphe areas of the brain stem receive inputs from many areas, including the cerebral cortex, hypothalamus, anterolateral tract, and limbic system. Motor axons descend from these areas to the dorsal horns, where they synapse on second-order neurons of the pain pathways. Binding of endogenous opiates to receptors in the analgesia system blocks some ascending pain transmission at these second-order sensory neurons. Table 23–3 summarizes common therapeutic modalities for the reduction of pain **(analgesia)** and reduction of all sensation **(anesthesia)**.

TABLE 23–2
CLINICAL EXAMPLES OF REFERRED PAIN

Source of Pain	Typical Region of Referral
Sinus	Teeth
Jaw	Ear, temple, teeth
Neck muscles	Head
Myocardium	Inner aspect of the left arm, jaw
Diaphragm	Tip of the shoulder
Gallbladder, liver	Tip of the right shoulder, lower point of the scapula
Pancreas	Lower back
Kidney	Costovertebral angle, flank, inguinal area, scrotum
Appendix	Umbilicus
Ureter	Back, flank, genitalia, anterior thigh
Bladder	Sacrum, genitalia, inner thighs
Rectum	Sacrum

Temperature (Thermosensation)

Temperature sensation is transmitted along the same pathway as "slow" pain (the lateral branch of the anterolateral pathway). Thermoreceptors resemble nociceptors in that they are free nerve endings, and there may be separate receptors for heat and cold stimuli.[2] Cold sensation is transmitted by $A\delta$ and C fibers, with the frequency of action potential transmission proportional to the rate and extent of temperature reduction. Some receptors are most sensitive to a cold stimulus, between 30° and 10°C; above this range, they also respond to a heat stimulus. Warmth is transmitted by C fibers, whereas intense heat is mediated by $A\delta$ pain fibers.[6]

Vibration

Vibration (tested clinically using a tuning fork on a bony prominence) is perceived by two types of receptors: Meissner's corpuscles for slow-frequency

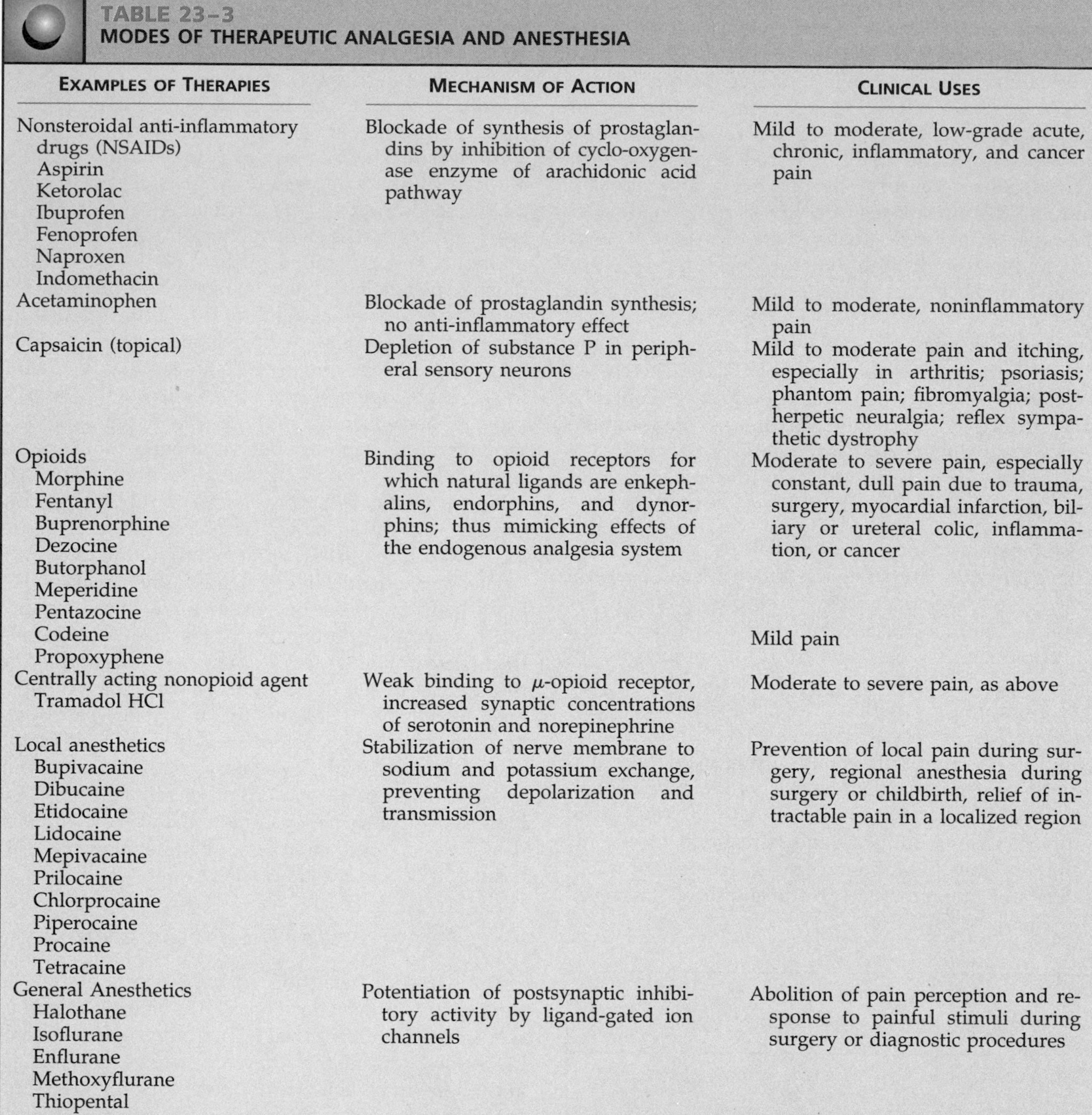

TABLE 23–3
MODES OF THERAPEUTIC ANALGESIA AND ANESTHESIA

Examples of Therapies	Mechanism of Action	Clinical Uses
Nonsteroidal anti-inflammatory drugs (NSAIDs)	Blockade of synthesis of prostaglandins by inhibition of cyclo-oxygenase enzyme of arachidonic acid pathway	Mild to moderate, low-grade acute, chronic, inflammatory, and cancer pain
Aspirin		
Ketorolac		
Ibuprofen		
Fenoprofen		
Naproxen		
Indomethacin		
Acetaminophen	Blockade of prostaglandin synthesis; no anti-inflammatory effect	Mild to moderate, noninflammatory pain
Capsaicin (topical)	Depletion of substance P in peripheral sensory neurons	Mild to moderate pain and itching, especially in arthritis; psoriasis; phantom pain; fibromyalgia; postherpetic neuralgia; reflex sympathetic dystrophy
Opioids	Binding to opioid receptors for which natural ligands are enkephalins, endorphins, and dynorphins; thus mimicking effects of the endogenous analgesia system	Moderate to severe pain, especially constant, dull pain due to trauma, surgery, myocardial infarction, biliary or ureteral colic, inflammation, or cancer
Morphine		
Fentanyl		
Buprenorphine		
Dezocine		
Butorphanol		
Meperidine		
Pentazocine		
Codeine		Mild pain
Propoxyphene		
Centrally acting nonopioid agent	Weak binding to μ-opioid receptor, increased synaptic concentrations of serotonin and norepinephrine	Moderate to severe pain, as above
Tramadol HCl		
Local anesthetics	Stabilization of nerve membrane to sodium and potassium exchange, preventing depolarization and transmission	Prevention of local pain during surgery, regional anesthesia during surgery or childbirth, relief of intractable pain in a localized region
Bupivacaine		
Dibucaine		
Etidocaine		
Lidocaine		
Mepivacaine		
Prilocaine		
Chlorprocaine		
Piperocaine		
Procaine		
Tetracaine		
General Anesthetics	Potentiation of postsynaptic inhibitory activity by ligand-gated ion channels	Abolition of pain perception and response to painful stimuli during surgery or diagnostic procedures
Halothane		
Isoflurane		
Enflurane		
Methoxyflurane		
Thiopental		
Pentobarbital		
Propofol		
Nitrous oxide		

vibration and Pacini's corpuscles for high-frequency vibration. Vibration is transmitted by the same pathway as fine touch (the DCML).[2]

Proprioception (Position Sense)

Proprioception is the sensory modality that informs the cerebral cortex of the position of the body at rest *(static position sense)* or in motion *(kinesthetic sensation)*. The proprioceptive system is complex and involves not only the DCML pathway of the somatic sensory system but also important side projections to the vestibular system of the inner ear and brain stem and to the cerebellum. The receptors of this system (proprioceptors) include the muscle spindle receptors and Golgi tendon organs of muscle, Ruf-

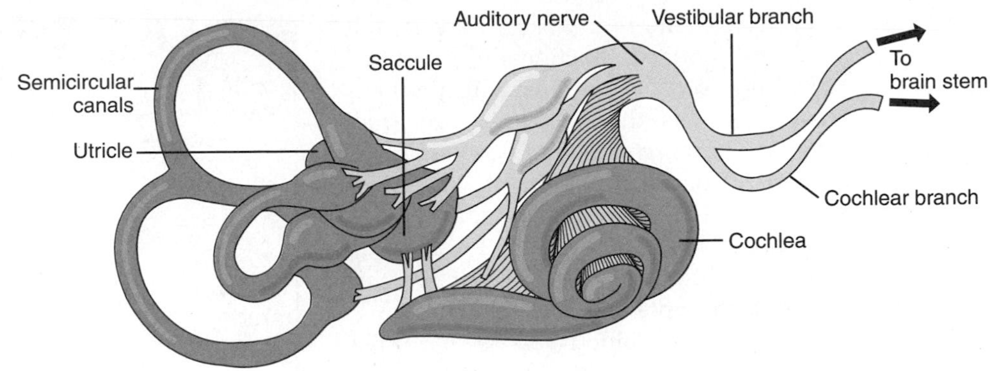

FIGURE 23–8
Vestibular system of the inner ear. Hair cell receptors in the fluid-filled semicircular canals, utricle, and saccule are deformed with movement of the head. Signals initiated by these mechanoreceptors are transmitted to the vestibular nuclei of the brain stem, then to the vestibular area of the primary sensory cortex by the auditory nerve (cranial nerve VIII). The auditory apparatus (cochlea) is also illustrated.

fini's receptors in deep tissues, and hair cells in the vestibular system (Fig. 23–8).

As discussed in Chapter 22, the muscle spindle receptors and Golgi tendon organs sense the state of muscle tone or contraction. The cerebellum receives this input by connections with the DCML and vestibular system, and its simultaneous motor system inputs allow comparison and correction of motor outputs so that actual position and motion are equal to intended position and motion. The vestibular apparatus of the inner ear, shown in Figure 23–8, consists of: (1) hair cell receptors located in the three semicircular canals, the utricle, and the saccule, and (2) the neural interconnections between these receptors and the vestibular nuclei of the brain-stem RAS, the cerebellum, the thalamus, and the vestibular area of the primary sensory cortex.

The hair cells are contained within enclosed cavities that are filled with fluid *(endolymph)*. Movement of this fluid with motion of the head deforms the receptors and initiates impulses to the vestibular nuclei, from which they are transmitted to other parts of the vestibular system. Most proprioception is subconscious, mediated by postural reflexes coordinated at the level of the hypothalamus. Disorders of proprioception often manifest as abnormal movement or gait (see Chapter 22) or as **vertigo** or **nystagmus,** discussed later in this chapter.

SPECIAL SENSES

The special senses of vision, hearing, taste, and smell operate in conjunction with the somatic senses in the detection and processing of stimuli from the internal and external environments.

Vision

The visual system consists of the eyeballs, protective orbital bones, lids and lashes, lacrimal apparatus, extraocular muscles, intraocular fluid system, and neural pathways that mediate vision.

Anatomy of the Visual System

Eyeball. The eyeball, illustrated in Figure 23–9, consists of three layers: the outer *sclera,* the middle *choroid,* and the inner *retina.* The sclera is normally white, except for a few tiny blood vessels and the transparent *cornea* that overlies the fluid-filled *anterior chamber.* The sclera is a tough, fibrous layer that functions in the protection of internal structures. The choroid contains the colored *iris* and the *lens* that refracts or bends the light rays entering through the aperture in the iris, the *pupil.* The choroid supports the numerous blood vessels that perfuse the eye, and contains single-unit smooth muscles (*circular* and *ciliary* muscles) that alter pupil size and lens

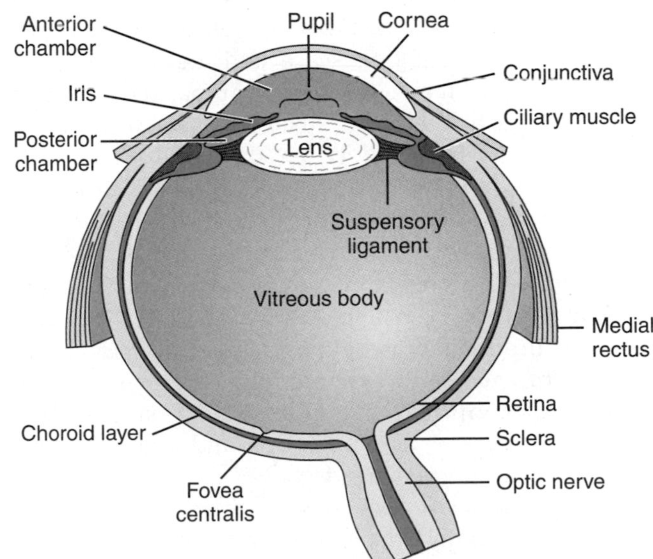

FIGURE 23–9
The eye. The principal structures of the eyeball are shown in cross-section, including the three layers, the *sclera, choroid,* and *retina.* The *optic nerve* (cranial nerve II) exits at the back of the eyeball.

curvature, respectively. The retina has 10 layers, but these are usually categorized functionally into just 2 layers: the *retinal pigmented epithelium*, which adjoins the choroid and contains the photoreceptors (*rods* and *cones*); and the *neural retina*, which contains converging nerve fibers for transmission of visual signals. Between these two layers is a potential space, the subretinal space, which is the point of separation in a pathologic condition discussed later in this chapter, **retinal detachment.**

The retina is perfused by blood vessels that originate from the *optic disk* (the point of exit of the optic nerve) and also by the *choriocapillaris*, specialized exchange vessels that originate from the choroid. Retinal vessels are readily visible with ophthalmoscopic (funduscopic) examination and reflect the status of the systemic vascular system. Color Figure 23–1 illustrates the normal retina as viewed through the ophthalmoscope. The optic disk may be swollen ("choked disk" or papilledema) in cases of increased intracranial pressure (Color Fig. 23–2). The disk may be sunken, or "cupped," in glaucoma, as discussed later in this chapter (Color Fig. 23–3). Evidence of vascular changes in the retina may be apparent (Color Figs. 23–4 through 23–6). The retina also contains glial cells, which sustain retinal metabolism. The central area of the retina is known as the *macula*, and the core of this area, the *fovea centralis*, is the area of highest visual acuity. **Macular degeneration,** a common age-related disorder that may lead to blindness, is discussed later in this chapter, along with other forms of **retinopathy** (Color Figs. 23–7 and 23–8).

Protective Structures. The eyeball is recessed within a cavity formed by the orbital bones (see Chapter 21). These bones are delicate and may be fractured with facial or head trauma. The eyelids and their particle-filtering lashes protect the eyeball from airborne irritants. When the cornea is stimulated by an irritant, the lids close as a result of the **corneal reflex,** mediated by cranial nerves V and VII. The vascular lining of the upper and lower lids is known as the *palpebral conjunctiva*, and the clear covering of the eyeball is known as the *bulbar conjunctiva*. Inflammation of these protective tissues as a result of chemical irritation, infection, or allergy is known as **conjunctivitis.** Table 23–4 summarizes clinical features of conjunctivitis and other inflammatory disorders of the external eye.

The *lacrimal apparatus* consists of the tear-forming lacrimal glands and their outflow structures, the lacrimal sac and nasolacrimal duct (Fig. 23–10). Tears flow through 12 ducts in the upper palpebral conjunctiva across the bulbar conjunctiva to lubricate the eye for lid movement and to wash out particulate matter. Tears contain an antibacterial lysozyme

TABLE 23–4
INFLAMMATORY DISORDERS OF THE EYE

Disorder	Description
Blepharitis	Chronic inflammation of the eyelid margins, usually beginning in childhood and continuing throughout life; usually caused by staphylococcal infection or seborrheic dermatitis
Hordeolum	Also known as stye, an acute inflammation of the follicle of an eyelash or its associated sebaceous or sweat gland
Chalazion	Chronic inflammatory lipogranuloma of a meibomian (sebaceous) gland of the eyelid margin
Conjunctivitis	Inflammation of the conjunctiva due to a microorganism (usually staphylococcus), foreign material (drugs, smoke, smog, chemical fumes, contact lenses), or allergy
Keratitis	Inflammation of the cornea due to microorganisms, tear deficiency, denervation, exposure, immune reactions, ischemia, or trauma; ulcerative keratitis may lead to corneal scarring or perforation
Dacryocystitis	Acute or chronic inflammation of the lacrimal sac due to obstruction of the lacrimal sac or nasolacrimal duct; normal drainage is impaired, leading to microbial infection
Episcleritis	Recurrent, noninfectious inflammation of the superficial layer of the sclera
Scleritis	Recurrent inflammation of the sclera often associated with systemic disorders such as systemic lupus erythematosus or rheumatoid arthritis
Uveitis	Inflammation of the middle coat of the eye, including the choroid, ciliary body, and iris
Retinal vasculitis	Inflammation of retinal veins, usually associated with systemic disease such as multiple sclerosis, tuberculosis, or sarcoidosis
Cytomegalovirus retinitis	Intraocular infection with cytomegalovirus, usually secondary to acquired immunodeficiency syndrome
Optic neuritis	Inflammation of the optic nerve, usually due to viral infection, demyelination (multiple sclerosis), or autoimmune disease

Data from Newell, F.W. (1992). *Ophthalmology: Principles and Concepts.* (7th ed.). St. Louis: Mosby–Year Book.

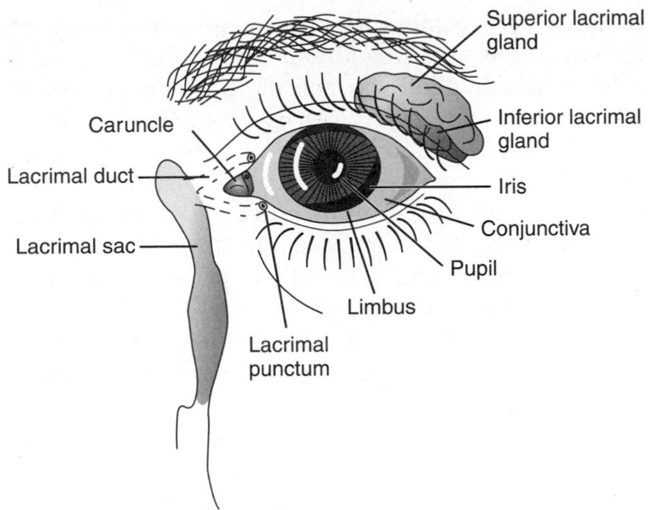

FIGURE 23–10

Lacrimal apparatus. Tears formed in the lacrimal glands flow through ducts in the upper palpebral conjunctiva over the scleral surface. Outflow is into the nasal cavity through the lacrimal ducts in the inner aspect of the eye.

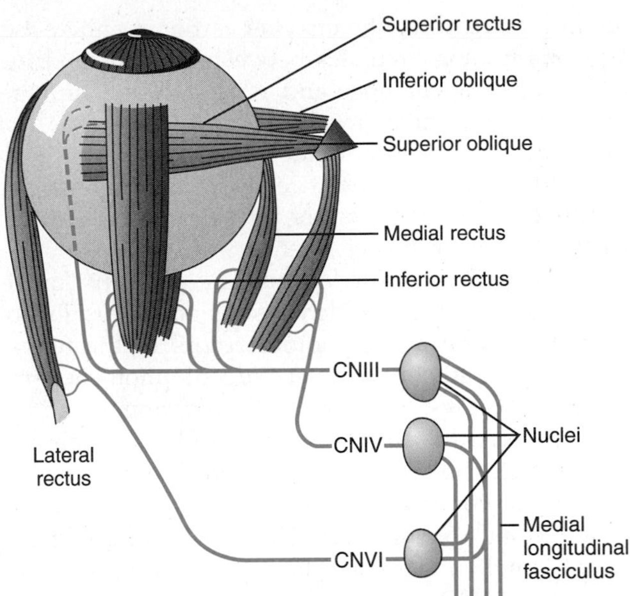

FIGURE 23–11

Extraocular muscles. Six pairs of muscles, innervated by cranial nerves III, IV, and VI, move both eyeballs in synchrony for binocular vision. (Redrawn from Guyton, A.C., and Hall, J.E. [1996]. *Textbook of Medical Physiology.* [9th ed.]. Philadelphia: W.B. Saunders. [p. 656].)

and thus also supply a protective bacteriostatic barrier. Lacrimation is regulated by the autonomic nervous system and may be increased in response to emotional stimuli as well as irritants. Decreased lacrimation is characteristic of Sjögren's syndrome, a connective tissue disorder that often accompanies rheumatoid arthritis (see Chapter 34). Decreased lacrimation is also typical of normal aging and occurs as a side effect of anticholinergic drug therapy (see Chapter 22).

Extraocular Muscles. As illustrated in Figure 23–11, six pairs of extraocular muscles move both eyeballs in synchrony for binocular vision. These muscles are innervated by cranial nerves III, IV, and VI. Loss of synchronous or conjugate eye movement may occur with unilateral weakness or impaired innervation of these muscles and may manifest as **diplopia** (double vision), *strabismus* (misaligned eye), or *amblyopia* ("lazy" eye). Nystagmus, a rhythmic contraction–relaxation sequence of these muscles that produces a visible jerking of the eye within the orbit, may be seen in association with proprioceptive disorders. Presence of a few beats of nystagmus in the horizontal plane with extreme lateral gaze is considered normal. Sustained nystagmus in vertical, horizontal, or rotary planes is abnormal and indicates some disruption of impulse conduction by cortical or vestibular system pathology. Nystagmus often accompanies the vertigo of **Meniere's disease,** discussed later in this chapter, or may signify a brain-stem or cerebellar lesion (see Chapter 21).

Intraocular Fluid System. The eye contains two types of fluid: *vitreous humor,* a gel-like fluid that provides shape to the posterior eyeball (posterior chamber) and serves as a nutritive and refractive medium; and *aqueous humor,* a clear fluid formed by active transport of selected components of plasma by the ciliary body (Fig. 23–12). Formation of aque-

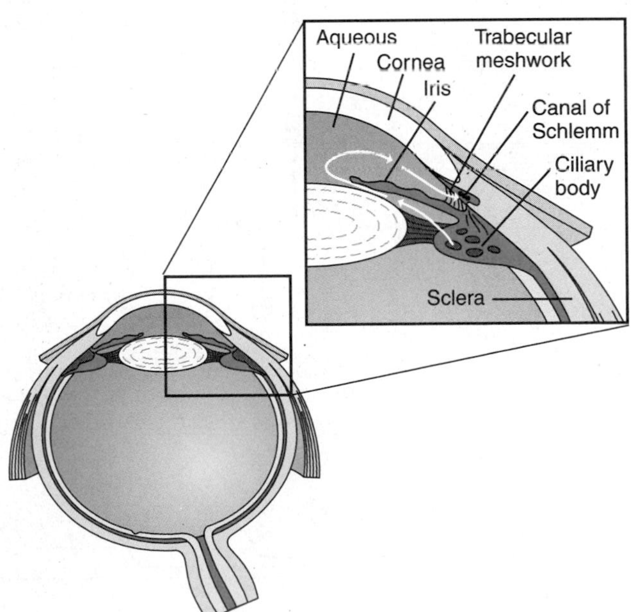

FIGURE 23–12

Intraocular fluid circulation. Clear aqueous humor, formed from plasma by the *ciliary body,* circulates between the lens and iris to the anterior chamber. This fluid is then filtered through the bony *trabecular meshwork* into the *canal of Schlemm,* from which it is reabsorbed into the venous circulation.

ous humor requires the enzyme carbonic anhydrase. Aqueous humor circulates between the lens and iris to the anterior chamber and is reabsorbed through the bony trabecular meshwork into the canal of Schlemm. Intraocular fluid pressure is routinely screened in clinical practice. An elevation above 20 mm Hg may indicate the presence of **glaucoma,** discussed later in this chapter.

Neural Pathways for Vision. The stimulus for vision is light energy, which results in disruption of the membranes of the photoreceptors in the retinal pigmented epithelium. A cascade of photochemical reactions follows, resulting in generation of action potentials conducted along axonal fibers of bipolar cells, which then synapse on a smaller number of retinal ganglion cells via converging synapses in the neural retina (Fig. 23–13). The axonal fibers of the retinal ganglion cells exit the eye as the optic nerve (cranial nerve II).

The intracranial visual pathways are illustrated in Figure 23–14. Axons from the nasal fields cross at the *optic chiasm,* then synapse with the *lateral geniculate nucleus* in the thalamus before terminating in the *visual cortex* of the opposite occipital lobe. Axons from the temporal fields do not cross but rather terminate in the occipital lobe on the same side. This complex arrangement results in a wide variety of patterns of visual loss (blind spots or visual field cuts), depending on the specific location of lesions within the pathway. As discussed in Chapter 21, a common clinical manifestation of stroke is homonymous hemianopsia, loss of half the visual field because of a unilateral lesion affecting a segment of the visual pathway. Figure 23–15 illustrates homonymous hemianopsia and other visual field cuts, along with the usual causes of each. The visual cortex receives and localizes the stimulus, then transmits it to the parietal association cortex for interpretation.

Physiology of Vision

Vision is mediated by three processes: refraction, the photochemical cascade, and visual reflexes.

Refraction. *Refraction* is the bending of light as it passes at an angle through eye structures of differing densities. The refractive surfaces of the eye are the cornea, the lens, and the vitreous and aqueous humors. Of these, the only one that varies normally is the lens. For near vision, the ciliary muscles contract to increase the curvature of the lens, making it more concave or rounded. For distance vision, the

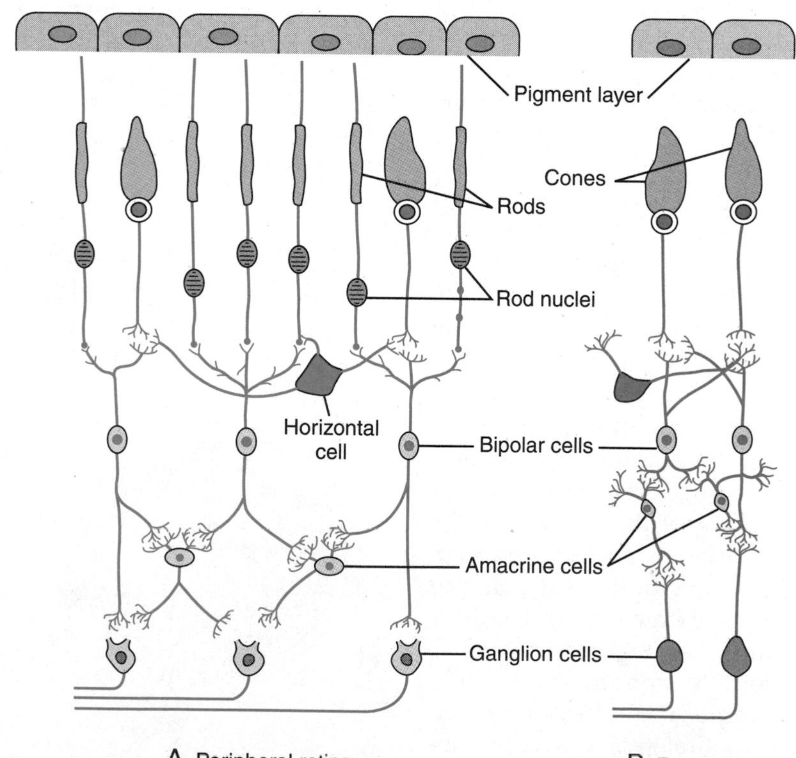

FIGURE 23–13
Neural organization of the retina. Action potentials generated by retinal photoreceptors (*rods* and *cones*) are transmitted by converging synapses, exiting the eye as the optic nerve (cranial nerve II). (Redrawn from Guyton, A.C., and Hall, J.E. [1996]. *Textbook of Medical Physiology.* [9th ed.]. Philadelphia: W.B. Saunders. [p. 646].)

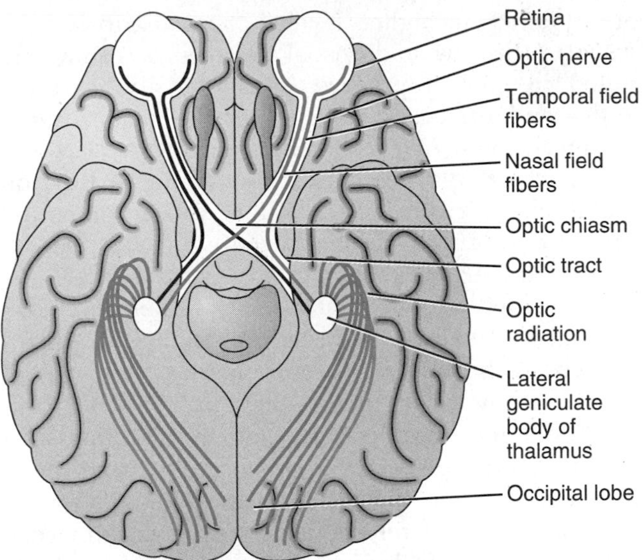

FIGURE 23–14
Intracranial visual pathways. Axonal fibers of the optic nerve separate into two tracts. Those of the *nasal fields* cross at the optic chiasm, synapse in the thalamus, then terminate in the visual cortex of the occipital lobe. Axons from the *temporal fields* do not cross.

ciliary muscles relax, flattening the lens. This process of *accommodation,* which keeps objects in sharp focus on the retina, also involves reflex constriction or dilation of the pupil by iris muscles and slight adjustments in eyeball position by the extraocular muscles. **Presbyopia,** thickening and loss of elasticity of the lens with age, results in impairment of accommodation in many elderly people.

Abnormal refraction (refractive errors) may decrease visual acuity as a consequence of opacity of the cornea or lens, altered shape of the eyeball or cornea, or abnormal density of the humors. Light waves are slowed or incorrectly refracted as they pass through the eyeball, and the resulting image is not sharply focused on the retina (Fig. 23–16). **Hyperopia** (farsightedness) results from an abnormally short eyeball or an abnormally flat lens, whereas **myopia** (nearsightedness) is caused by a long eyeball or an abnormally convex lens. *Astigmatism* is a nonuniform curvature of the cornea or lens. These are congenital conditions of unknown cause, which display a familial predisposition. They may be treated with corrective lenses or, in some cases, with corrective surgery.[7] **Corneal opacity** may occur as a result of traumatic abrasion or toxic injury of the cornea or may be the result of rare congenital disorders. Refraction is also impaired with opacity of the lens (**cataract;** Color Fig. 23–9), discussed later in this chapter.

Photochemical Cascade. The transduction of light energy into action potentials occurs in the retinal pigmented epithelium and is the function of two types of photoreceptors, the rods and cones (see Fig. 23–13). These primary sensory neurons contain the visual pigments packaged into disk-shaped, membrane-bound vesicles at the end of their dendritic fibers, which are embedded in the epithelium. At the other end of the receptor cell, axonal fibers project into the neural layer and synapse with bipolar cells. The rods are important to night vision and black and white vision. They are highly sensitive in detection of outlines and movement in low-light conditions but not in color vision or detail. Cones are more important in daylight or high-light conditions, for the detection of detail and color.

The visual pigments are formed from *retinal,* a light-absorbing molecule synthesized from vitamin A, in combination with proteins known as *opsins.* Black and white vision, night vision, and peripheral vision are transduced by a chemical cascade reaction in which light energy is absorbed by the pigment *rhodopsin* in rods. Rhodopsin undergoes a rapid series of chemical transformations that ultimately generate graded potentials. These subthreshold potentials converge on bipolar cells, where they are summated to generate action potentials for transmission of the visual impulse. The molecular mechanism of this signal transduction is still poorly understood but involves the operation of light-sensitive membrane channels, calcium flux, and a cyclic guanosine monophosphate second-messenger system.[8] In the absence of light, rhodopsin re-forms. Perception of the image depends on differential light activation of specific retinal areas.

The mechanism of central vision and color vision mediated by cones is similar, involving retinal and opsins. There are three different types of cones, each using different opsins, with electrical charges facili-

Etiology	Left	Right	Clinical manifestation
Complete lesion of right optic nerve			Total blindness in right eye
Pressure on chiasm (such as a pituitary tumor)			Visual loss in temporal half of each eye (bitemporal hemianopsia)
Complete lesion of right optic tract (such as in stroke)			Visual loss in the same half of each eye (left homonymous hemianopsia)
Partial lesion of right optic tract (such as parietal lesion)			Visual loss in lower left quadrant of each eye (homonymous left lower hemianopsia)

FIGURE 23–15
Visual field deficits. Loss of a portion of the field of vision occurs with lesions of the visual pathways. The pattern of visual field deficit indicates the location of the lesion.

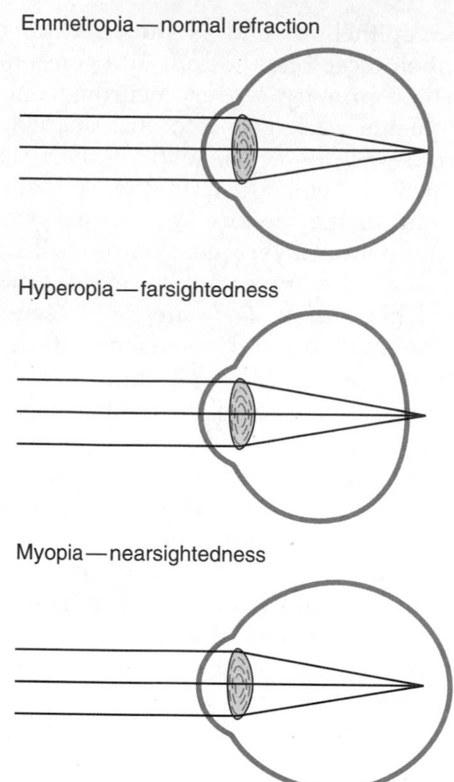

FIGURE 23–16
Errors of refraction. Abnormal shape of the eyeball or lens results in decreased visual acuity because the image is not sharply focused on the retina. *Hyperopia* results from a short eyeball or a flat lens, whereas *myopia* is caused by a long eyeball or an abnormally convex lens.

tating the absorption of specific wavelengths of light. Blue cones thus *maximally* absorb blue light (wavelength, 455 nm), green cones absorb green light (530 nm), and red cones absorb red light (625 nm). Other colors are perceived by the simultaneous stimulation of these three types, and those closest in wavelength are stimulated most strongly. Central vision is also mediated by cones, and the center of highest visual acuity, the fovea, contains only cones. The ratio of foveal cones to bipolar cells approaches 1:1, accounting for the increased acuity over rod-mediated vision, in which axons from many photoreceptors converge on a small number of bipolar cells. **Color blindness** is an inherited disorder in which the person lacks one or more of the cone types.[9] Most afflicted people are males who cannot distinguish red from green because of an X-linked recessive deficiency of either red or green cones. Lack of blue cones, an autosomal recessive trait, is rare.

Visual Reflexes. The dependence of vision on the visual pathways has been discussed. As is the case with other systems, vision is regulated by reflexes that are potentially integrated and either facilitated or inhibited at higher levels. The integrity of the visual pathways and visual reflexes is commonly tested in clinical practice. Visual acuity is tested with standardized charts, such as the Snellen chart, or simply with object identification or reading. *Pupillary reflexes* may be elicited by shining a light on the pupil. If cranial nerve III is intact, the pupil constricts in *direct response* to the light, and the opposite pupil also constricts in *consensual response.* Accommodation requires intact cranial nerves II, III, IV, and VI and may be tested by asking the person to focus with both eyes on an object as it is moved closer. As the object nears, the pupils should constrict and the eyes converge, or cross. Intracranial lesions, brain-stem lesions, or increased intracranial pressure affecting the visual pathways may impair the normal visual reflexes and may elicit abnormal visual reflexes, including the oculovestibular and oculocephalic reflexes (Fig. 23–17).

Visual signals from the retina are normally integrated at the level of the thalamus, by the lateral geniculate nucleus, before terminating in the visual cortex and association areas. Visual interpretation depends on inputs from the motor cortex for conscious focus on objects, the brain-stem RAS for visual attentiveness, and the limbic system for integration of the emotional content of vision. Common disorders of vision are discussed later in this chapter.

Hearing (Auditory Sensation)

Anatomy of the Auditory System

The auditory system consists of the external ear, the middle ear, and the auditory apparatus *(cochlea)* of the inner ear or *labyrinth* as well as the neural pathways and auditory areas of the cortex.

As illustrated in Figure 23–18, the external ear consists of the *auricle (pinna),* which funnels sound into the *auditory canal.* Sound is conducted inward through this canal, and protection of inner structures is facilitated by the fine hairs that line the canal and by the secretion of waxy *cerumen,* which traps particles and may serve an antibacterial function.

The middle ear begins at the *tympanic membrane* (eardrum), which vibrates in response to the sound waves reaching it through the canal. Three delicate bones or ossicles, the *malleus* (hammer), *incus* (anvil), and *stapes* (stirrup), connect the tympanic membrane to the *oval window* of the inner ear, transducing the vibration. The middle ear is connected to the oropharynx by the *eustachian tube,* which allows equalization of middle ear and atmospheric pressures as

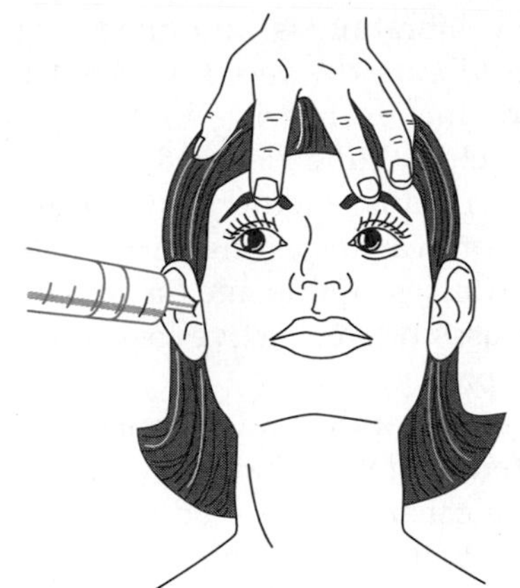

FIGURE 23–17
Visual reflexes. The *oculovestibular* and *oculocephalic* reflexes may be evaluated clinically and should be normal if the brain-stem centers that coordinate eye movement by cranial nerves III, IV, and VI are intact. The oculovestibular reflex is tested with injection of ice water into the external ear, which should elicit rapid nystagmus in the direction of the tested ear. The oculocephalic reflex is tested with brisk movement of the head while the eyes are held open. Head movement should cause the eyes to deviate together in the opposite direction. Absent or abnormal response to these maneuvers usually indicates impaired brain-stem function. (From Thelan, L.A., Davie, J.K., *et al.* [1994]. *Textbook of Critical Care Nursing.* [2nd ed.]. St. Louis: C.V. Mosby. [pp. 510–511].)

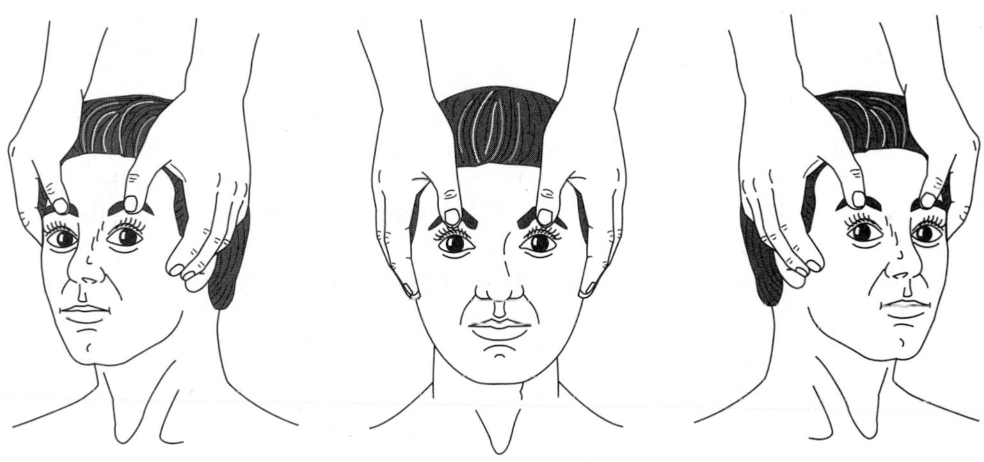

well as drainage of any middle ear fluid. Occlusion of this tube secondary to inflammation or collapse may lead to **otitis media,** discussed later in this chapter. Otoscopic examination permits visualization of the auditory canal and tympanic membrane. The normal membrane is translucent and pearly gray in color, with the underlying ossicles barely visible (Color Fig. 23–10). A wedge-shaped reflection of the otoscope light indicates normal contour of the tympanic membrane, and there should be no suggestion of fluid in the middle ear.

The fluid-filled inner ear, contained within a cavity in the temporal bone, consists of the vestibular apparatus for proprioception, discussed earlier, as well as the auditory apparatus or cochlea. The oval window and *round window* vibrate with opposing in-and-out motions, resulting in cyclic fluid movement detected by the cochlear *organ of Corti.* This organ contains the hair cell auditory receptors.

Impulses generated at the hair cells are conducted along the cochlear branch of cranial nerve VIII, the *auditory nerve* (also known as the *vestibulocochlear* or *acoustic nerve*) to the cochlear nucleus in the pons. The signal then ascends to the *primary auditory cortex* in the upper temporal lobe, and from there to the surrounding *auditory association areas.* As is the case with the visual pathways, some auditory fibers cross, whereas others do not, leading to variable effects of unilateral lesions.

Auditory Function

Conductive Versus Sensorineural Mechanisms. The conversion of sound energy to action potentials initially depends on conduction of sound waves through air to the tympanic membrane, with amplification of resulting tympanic membrane vibrations by the middle ear ossicles, which connect the membrane to the oval window. The processes that begin at the oval window and result in transduction of

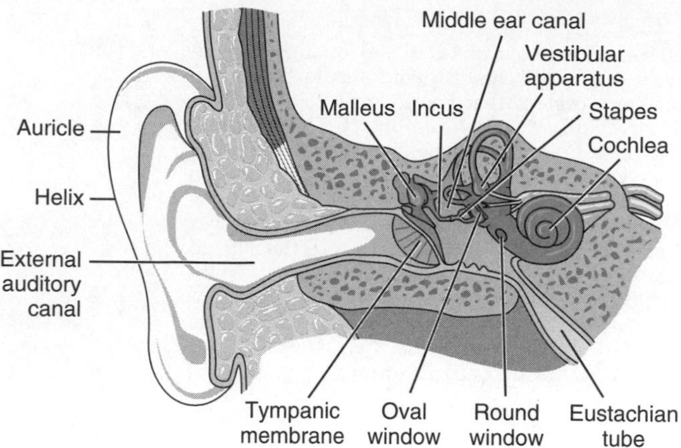

FIGURE 23–18

The external ear and auditory system. The external ear *(auricle)* conducts sound inward through the *auditory canal.* The *tympanic membrane* vibrates on stimulation by sound waves, and this vibration is transduced to the *oval window* of the inner ear by the middle ear bones *(ossicles).* The fluid-filled inner ear contains the vestibular system and the auditory apparatus, or *cochlea.*

fluid waves to action potentials by hair cells and the regulation of these processes by neural reflexes and higher cortical processes are known collectively as *sensorineural mechanisms* of hearing. Hearing loss resulting from defects in sound transmission through the auditory canal or middle ear is thus termed **conductive hearing loss,** whereas that due to inner ear or neural pathway disorders is termed **sensorineural hearing loss**. Conditions associated with both forms of hearing loss are listed in Table 23–5.

Conduction of Sound. Sound waves travel through air or other media by causing periodic increases and decreases in the density of the medium. These cyclic sound waves are characterized by *amplitude* (the magnitude of the change in density), perceived as intensity or loudness of sound; and *frequency* (the rate of density change), perceived as pitch. The greater the initial density of the medium, the greater the velocity of sound transmission through it. Although it is possible to bypass the auditory canal and cause oval window vibration by applying a sound source to bone (e.g., a tuning fork to the mastoid process behind the ear), most sound first reaches the auditory apparatus by being conducted through the air of the auditory canal. One mechanism of conductive hearing loss, then, is obstruction of the canal, as with a foreign body or impacted cerumen.

Tympanic membrane vibration in response to sound waves requires the potential for free movement of the membrane and middle ear ossicles. This in turn requires middle ear pressures equal to atmospheric and anatomic integrity of these structures. Because the tympanic membrane is much larger in area than the oval window, the intensity of oval window vibration is amplified to the extent necessary to vibrate the more resistant fluid of the inner ear. Conductive hearing loss may occur as a result of eustachian tube obstruction or structural defects of the tympanic membrane or ossicles from inflammation or scarring, congenital defects, or degenerative processes. Otitis media and **otosclerosis,** common causes of conductive loss, are discussed later in this chapter.

Sound Reception and Transmission. Vibration of fluid (endolymph and perilymph) in the cochlea causes mechanical disruption of the auditory receptors, the hair cells of the organ of Corti. Membrane disruption gives rise to action potentials, which are conducted along afferent fibers to the primary auditory cortex and association areas for reception and interpretation. Similarly to the strings of a piano, certain regions of the organ contain hair cells that are "tuned" to particular frequencies or pitches, based on their different anatomic and functional characteristics. Hair cells nearest the oval window respond preferentially to high-frequency sounds, and these are the first to be lost with traumatic exposure to excessive noise. Hair cells farthest away from the oval window respond to low-frequency sounds. Ascending auditory signals travel through brain-stem and thalamic relays to the auditory cortex in the temporal lobe.

Neural regulation of auditory sensation is limited and is protective in nature. Two tiny muscles under reflex neural control modify conduction to some extent. The *tensor tympani,* attached to the tympanic membrane, and the *stapedius,* attached to the stapes,

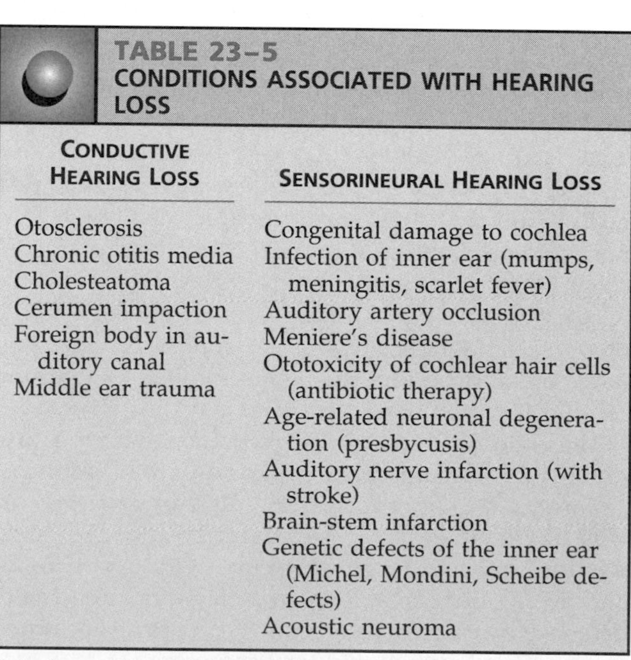

TABLE 23–5
CONDITIONS ASSOCIATED WITH HEARING LOSS

Conductive Hearing Loss	Sensorineural Hearing Loss
Otosclerosis	Congenital damage to cochlea
Chronic otitis media	Infection of inner ear (mumps, meningitis, scarlet fever)
Cholesteatoma	Auditory artery occlusion
Cerumen impaction	Meniere's disease
Foreign body in auditory canal	Ototoxicity of cochlear hair cells (antibiotic therapy)
Middle ear trauma	Age-related neuronal degeneration (presbycusis)
	Auditory nerve infarction (with stroke)
	Brain-stem infarction
	Genetic defects of the inner ear (Michel, Mondini, Scheibe defects)
	Acoustic neuroma

Data from Adams, R.D., and Victor, M. (1993). *Principles of Neurology.* (5th ed.). New York: McGraw-Hill.

constrict in a reflex response to loud sounds, limiting vibration and decreasing sound conduction. This reflex response is slow in onset, however, so cannot protect the auditory apparatus from sudden, loud sounds, and its limited scope cannot protect against prolonged exposure to loud sounds. Hair cell damage due to such traumatic sound is a common mechanism of sensorineural hearing loss in people exposed to noisy environments.

Nearly all elderly people experience some degree of sensorineural hearing loss due to degenerative changes in hair cells. This condition, known as **presbycusis,** may be related to reduced perfusion of the auditory apparatus and is often accompanied by **tinnitus,** described by patients as a "ringing," "buzzing," or "roaring" in the ears. There is no known prevention for presbycusis, and unfortunately, the manifestations of hearing loss in the elderly may extend to social withdrawal and personality changes. Some are helped marginally by hearing aids, which amplify conducted sound and reduce background noise, and a few may be candidates for surgical treatment with cochlear implants.[10]

The integrity of cranial nerve VIII and the auditory cortices may be congenitally abnormal or disrupted by intracranial trauma, infections, tumors, ischemia, or toxicity, resulting in sensorineural hearing loss. Several drugs are classified as ototoxic because of their untoward effects on auditory function (Table 23–6).

TABLE 23–6
OTOTOXIC DRUGS

Drug	Vestibular Effects	Auditory Effects
Aminoglycoside Antibiotics		
Amikacin	Uncommon	3% to 11% of patients
Gentamicin	2% of patients	Uncommon
Kanamycin	7% of patients	30% of patients
Neomycin	Uncommon	Common, irreversible, severe
Streptomycin	25% to 75% of patients	4% to 15% of patients
Tobramycin	1% to 11% of patients	1% to 11% of patients
Antineoplastic Agent		
Cisplatin	—	Progressive hearing loss, tinnitus
Diuretic		
Ethacrynic acid	—	Transient or permanent deafness

Adapted from Clark, J.B.F., Queener, S.F., and Karb, V.B. (1993). *Pharmacologic Basis of Nursing Practice.* (4th ed.)., St. Louis. Mosby–Year Book. (p. 485).

Taste (Gustation)

Taste is a complex sensation directly mediated by chemoreceptors in the *taste buds* of the oral cavity and indirectly influenced by other sensations, especially the other chemical sense, smell. Taste buds are globular structures consisting of three types of epithelial cells: supporting cells, taste cells, and basal cells (see Fig. 23–2). Supporting cells surround and nourish the taste cells, which are the sensory receptors. Basal cells are precursor cells to taste cells, which have a rapid cell cycle. Surface taste cells are sloughed every 7 to 10 days and are replaced by continuous division of basal cells. Most taste buds are found on the tongue, although a few are scattered elsewhere in the oral cavity.

Four basic tastes are sensed by taste buds: sweet, sour, salty, and bitter. Although taste buds can respond to stimuli representative of all four types, taste buds in certain regions of the tongue are most sensitive to one type. Sweet taste is best detected by the tip of the tongue, with salty, sour, and bitter tastes best perceived in sequentially more posterior regions of the tongue. Many substances elicit a taste that is a combination of types.

For a substance to trigger a gustatory response, it must first be dissolved in saliva so that it can penetrate the pore in the surface of the taste bud and bind to receptors on the *gustatory hairs* of the taste cells. This ligand binding alters the taste cell membrane and generates action potentials conducted along the associated dendritic fibers. The impulses are primarily transmitted along cranial nerves VII (facial nerve) and IX (glossopharyngeal nerve), although cranial nerve X (vagus nerve) carries some impulses originating from the epiglottis and pharynx. These nerves synapse in the medulla and the thalamus before ascending to the gustatory cortex in the parietal lobe. Interneuronal connections between taste pathways and other visceral reflexes result in simultaneous triggering of digestive reflexes and may initiate retching or vomiting with ingestion of noxious substances (see Chapter 24).

The sensation of taste would be limited if not for the facilitating influences of other senses. Food that looks good usually "tastes" better, and the appropriate stimulation of thermoreceptors by food temperature and even pain receptors by spicy foods add to the sensation of taste. Of greatest importance is the ability to smell the food. The subtlety of taste perception clearly depends on concurrent stimulation of olfactory receptors.[11] Furthermore, the concept of "acquired taste" applies. A person may learn to perceive as pleasant tasting substances that are bitter or sour.

Many clinical factors can influence the sense of taste. The four "pure" tastes may be triggered by a number of different molecules. Sweet taste is elicited by sugars, saccharin, and some amino acids. Sour taste is normally elicited by hydrogen ions in acids. Salty taste is triggered most strongly by sodium chloride but also by other inorganic salts. Bitter taste is stimulated by alkaloids (e.g., quinine, caffeine) and by some nonalkaloid substances, such as aspirin and other drugs. As is the case with other rapidly cycling cells, taste cells are potentially affected by therapies (such as cancer chemotherapy) that target such cells. Because taste receptors adapt rapidly, they may become insensitive with prolonged stimulation, as evidenced by the diminished taste sensation of long-time cigarette smokers. Table 23–7 summarizes clinical conditions and drug reactions that can manifest as altered sense of taste.

Smell (Olfaction)

The second chemical sense, olfaction, or smell, also detects molecules in solution. Millions of olfactory receptors (about 1000 different types), with their supporting cells, make up the olfactory epithelium in the roof of each nasal cavity[12] (Fig. 23–19). Olfactory receptor cells are actually bipolar neurons. At one end are the olfactory hairs, which protrude through the nasal epithelium. These hairs are covered by a protective coat of mucus, which also serves as a solvent for odor-producing molecules. At the other end of each olfactory cell is an unmyelinated axon. These axons converge to form the *olfactory nerve* (cranial nerve I), which synapses on a structure known as the *olfactory bulb.* Higher-level

TABLE 23–7
CONDITIONS ASSOCIATED WITH ALTERED TASTE SENSATION

Etiologic Category	Examples
Congenital or genetic	Familial dysautonomia Turner's syndrome
Endocrine or metabolic	Adrenal insufficiency Diabetes mellitus Hypothyroidism Hyperthyroidism Pregnancy Pseudohypoparathyroidism
Exposure	Lead Smokeless tobacco Cigarette smoke
Gastrointestinal or liver disease	Acute hepatitis Chronic liver disease Crohn's disease Cronkhite-Canada syndrome Obstructive jaundice
Cardiovascular disease	Hypertension
Drug therapy	Penicillin Metronidazole Sulfasalazine Tetracycline Amphotericin B Carbamazepine Aspirin Cholestyramine Methotrexate Cisplatin Lithium Allopurinol β-Blockers Angiotensin-converting enzyme inhibitors
	Calcium-channel blockers Nitroglycerine Spironolactone D-Amphetamine Baclofen
Iatrogenic disorders	Craniotomy Dialysis Laryngectomy Radiation therapy Tonsillectomy
Infection	Upper respiratory infection
Local effects	Hansen's disease Submandibular gland carcinoma Sjögren's syndrome Parotid infection or tumor Glossitis Oral mycosis
Miscellaneous disorders	Cancer Sarcoidosis
Neurologic disorders	Bell's palsy Brain tumor Guillain-Barré syndrome Head trauma High-altitude syndrome Migraine Multiple sclerosis Seizure disorder
Psychiatric disorder	Bulimia
Renal disorder	Uremia

Adapted from Mott, A.E., and Leopold, D.A. (1991). Disorders in taste and smell. *Medical Clinics of North America* 75(6), 1321–1353.

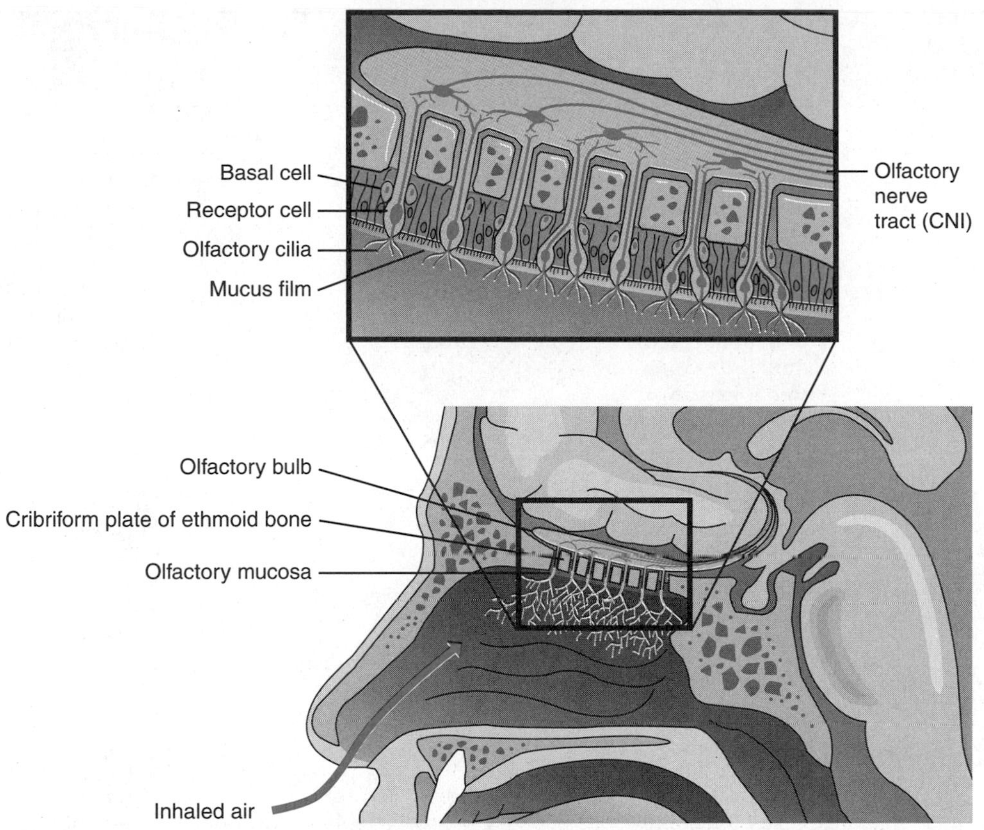

FIGURE 23–19

Olfactory system. Olfactory receptors in the roof of each nasal cavity are bipolar neurons, with hair cell receptors that detect odor molecules dissolved in mucus. Impulses are conducted along pathways with converging synapses, culminating in the *olfactory nerve* (cranial nerve I), which synapses on the *olfactory bulb.*

inputs to these synapses may inhibit or facilitate the sense of smell. From the olfactory bulbs, afferent fibers ascend to the *olfactory cortex,* which receives and interprets olfactory sensation. Interconnections with the limbic system contribute to the emotional response to certain smells. Disorders of olfactory sensation are common but usually of minor significance. Table 23–8 summarizes these conditions.

SENSORY DISORDERS

Peripheral Neuropathy

Definition. Peripheral neuropathy, also known as *diffuse peripheral polyneuropathy,* is a general term for dysfunction of the peripheral nervous system. Although the autonomic and motor systems may be affected (see Chapter 22), function of the somatosensory system is usually disturbed to the greatest extent.

Epidemiology. The overall prevalence of this disorder is not precisely known, but it has been estimated to affect as many as 20% of older adults.[13] The most significant risk factor is diabetes mellitus, although other systemic illnesses also increase the risk. These include chronic obstructive pulmonary disease, cancer, alcohol abuse, vitamin B_{12} deficiency, renal failure, and thyroid disease. Long-term use of certain drugs is also associated with peripheral neuropathy (Table 23–9). A decline in peripheral nerve function is also present in otherwise healthy elderly people.[13]

Etiology. Metabolic derangement results in a toxic insult to the cell bodies of peripheral nerves. The affected neurons then have difficulty supporting their extensions.

Pathophysiology. The longest fibers, typically those of the somatic sensory nerves with their long intraspinal fibers, lose function first. Because lower extremities are longer than upper extremities, distal sensory function in the feet and lower legs is most impaired. Impairment of other peripheral nerves follows, manifesting first as disorder of distal motor function, then upper extremity sensory function, and finally upper extremity motor function.

Clinical Manifestations. Loss of lower extremity

TABLE 23–8
OLFACTORY DISORDERS

Etiologic Category	Examples	Etiologic Category	Examples
Inflammation	Upper respiratory infection Allergic rhinitis Postviral anosmia		Multiple sclerosis Meningioma Migraine
Congenital	Congenital anosmia or dysosmia Cleft lip or palate Down syndrome Familial dysautonomia Hypogonadism Turner's syndrome		Parkinson's disease Seizure disorder Temporal lobe tumor
		Toxicity	Acrylate, methacrylate vapor Ammonia Benzine Cadmium dust Chalk dust Chestnut wood dust Cigarette smoke Formaldehyde Oil of peppermint Potash Solvents Sulfuric acid
Endocrine or metabolic	Adrenal insufficiency Diabetes mellitus Hypothyroidism Pseudohypoparathyroidism	Psychiatric disorders	Hypochondriasis Major depression Post-traumatic stress disorder Schizophrenia
Iatrogenic	Ethmoidectomy Frontal lobectomy Laryngectomy Rhinoplasty Submucous resection Temporal lobectomy Dialysis	Renal disorder	Uremia
Infection	Herpes simplex meningitis or encephalitis Human immunodeficiency virus infection	Miscellaneous disorders	Cystic fibrosis Giant cell arteritis Sarcoidosis
Liver disease	Acute viral hepatitis Cirrhosis	Drug therapy	Opioids Scopolamine β-Blockers Calcium-channel blockers D-Amphetamine Isotretinoin Cocaine Menthol Zinc sulfate
Local processes	Hansen's disease Adenoid hypertrophy Nasal polyps Sinusitis Sjögren's syndrome Olfactory tumor		
Neurologic disease	Alzheimer's disease Head trauma Huntington's disease Korsakoff's syndrome		

Adapted from Mott, A.E., and Leopold, D.A. (1991). Disorders in taste and smell. *Medical Clinics of North America* 75(6), 1321–1353.

TABLE 23–9
DRUGS ASSOCIATED WITH NEUROTOXICITY

- Ethanol abuse
- Nitrofurantoin (Macrodantin)
- Phenytoin (Dilantin)
- Lithium
- Gold compounds
- Vincristine (Oncovin)
- Isoniazid
- Ethambutol (Myambutol)
- Disulfiram (Antabuse)
- Amiodarone (Cordarone)

Adapted from Richardson, J.K., and Ashton-Miller, J.A. (1996). Peripheral neuropathy: An often-overlooked cause of falls in the elderly. *Postgraduate Medicine* 99(6), 162.

distal sensation is the hallmark of peripheral neuropathy. Loss of vibratory sensation is particularly apparent. Foot deformities and calluses (e.g., claw toes and depressed metatarsal heads) are commonly seen because lack of neural stimulation leads to muscle atrophy and skin changes. The Achilles tendon (heel-jerk) reflex is usually absent bilaterally. Proprioception is impaired, and the risk of falling is increased.

Prevention and Treatment. Optimal treatment of the underlying disorder is warranted. Prevention of falls and other injuries involves educating patients about the risks inherent in loss of sensation. Because vision is important in compensation for somatosensory loss, any prescriptions for eyewear should be current, and adequate lighting in the home should be ensured. Support during ambulation may take the form of a cane or a walker. The patient should wear well-fitting shoes to reduce the risk of callous formation and foot injury. Exercises that improve balance and extremity strength may also reduce the risk of injury.

Prognosis and Outcome. Outcome is associated with the severity of the underlying disorder and the adequacy of compensation.

Headache

Definition. *Headache* is acute or chronic pain occurring in various patterns over the face, scalp, or neck. Most cases of headache are benign, primary disorders, unrelated to a specific underlying cause. A small percentage are secondary manifestations of identifiable disorders, such as intracranial tumors, strokes, sinus infections, meningitis, or vasculitis. Although classification systems are somewhat arbitrary because of overlap between types, the International Headache Society classification recognizes the following types of primary headache: migraine, cluster, and tension-type.[14] Table 23–10 lists examples of primary and secondary headaches. Primary headaches are the focus of this discussion.

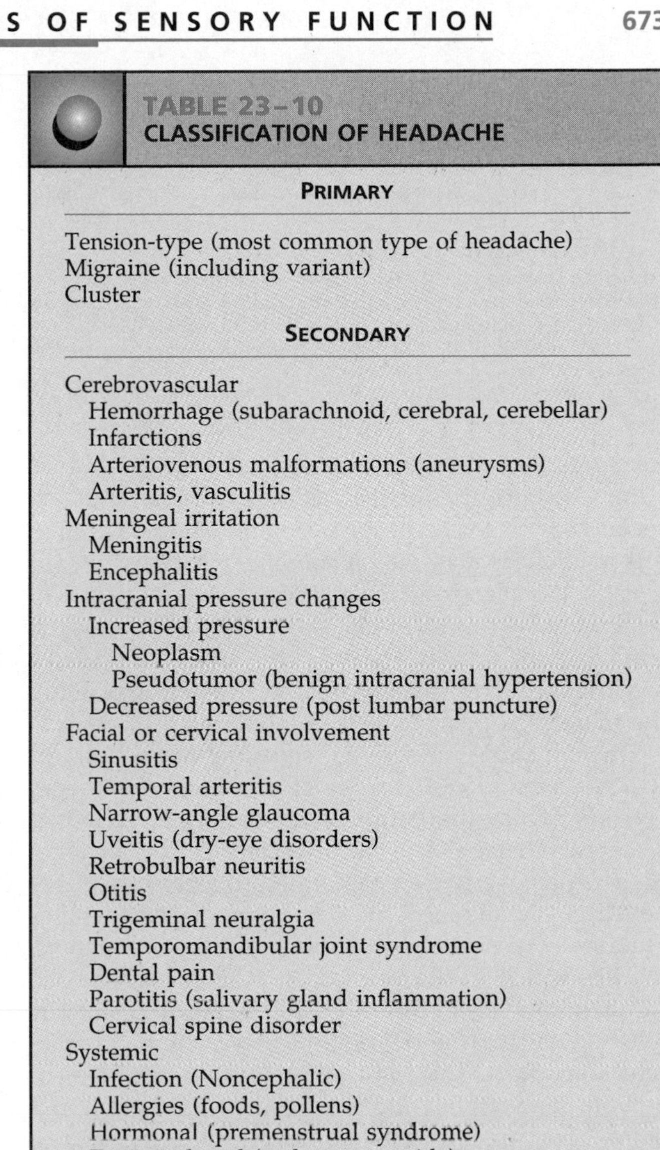

TABLE 23–10
CLASSIFICATION OF HEADACHE

PRIMARY

- Tension-type (most common type of headache)
- Migraine (including variant)
- Cluster

SECONDARY

- Cerebrovascular
  - Hemorrhage (subarachnoid, cerebral, cerebellar)
  - Infarctions
  - Arteriovenous malformations (aneurysms)
  - Arteritis, vasculitis
- Meningeal irritation
  - Meningitis
  - Encephalitis
- Intracranial pressure changes
  - Increased pressure
    - Neoplasm
    - Pseudotumor (benign intracranial hypertension)
  - Decreased pressure (post lumbar puncture)
- Facial or cervical involvement
  - Sinusitis
  - Temporal arteritis
  - Narrow-angle glaucoma
  - Uveitis (dry-eye disorders)
  - Retrobulbar neuritis
  - Otitis
  - Trigeminal neuralgia
  - Temporomandibular joint syndrome
  - Dental pain
  - Parotitis (salivary gland inflammation)
  - Cervical spine disorder
- Systemic
  - Infection (Noncephalic)
  - Allergies (foods, pollens)
  - Hormonal (premenstrual syndrome)
  - Toxin-induced (carbon monoxide)
  - Drug-induced (including cocaine, alcohol)
  - Caffeine withdrawal
  - Exertional (coital, cough)
- Traumatic
  - Concussion, postconcussion
  - Hematomas (subdural, epidural)

Used with permission from Weiss, J. (1993). Assessment and management of the client with headaches. *Nurse Practitioner* 18(4), 47. © 1993 Springhouse Corporation.

Epidemiology. Headache is the most common type of pain. About 73% of adults in the United States report experiencing headache in the past year.[14] Headache accounts for 18 million outpatient visits each year. Risk factors include stress, depression, sinus inflammation, fatigue, hypertension, constipation, caffeine intake, hormonal cycles or therapy, cigarette smoking, alcohol use, and in some people, foods such as cheese and chocolate or foods containing nitrates or monosodium glutamate.

Etiology. The etiology of primary headache is still uncertain. Headache pain has been thought to result from either sustained contraction of neck or scalp muscles (tension-type headaches) or from vasomotor changes (migraine or cluster headaches), or both. Electromyographic studies, however, do not consistently show findings of muscle contraction in patients with tension-type headaches.[15] In migraine, changes in cerebral blood flow are known to be modest and to follow a surface distribution rather than a vascular distribution.[16] Furthermore, the timing of vascular changes is not associated with the symptoms of migraine. Although migraine and tension-type headaches have been considered to be separate entities, mixed types are frequently seen, and both types occur with frequency in headache-prone patients.[14] Many researchers believe migraine and tension headaches represent a clinical continuum (Fig. 23–20).

Pathophysiology. Neural tissue does not contain pain receptors, but there are many receptors in the meninges, skull, and blood vessels and in the muscles of the face, scalp, and neck. In tension-type headaches, sustained muscle contraction, associated with stress or activities such as assembly line, sewing, or keyboard work, may directly deform pain receptors or may compress blood vessels, leading to

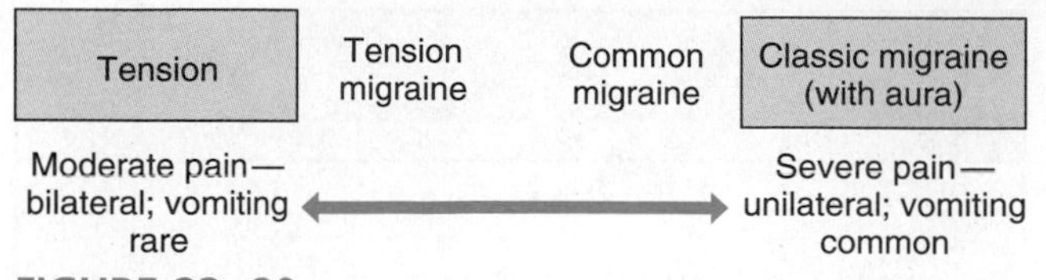

FIGURE 23–20

Headache continuum. Migraine and tension headaches may represent the extremes of a clinical continuum because many patients have mixed symptomatology. (From Weiss, J. [1993]. Assessment and management of the client with headaches. *Nurse Practitioner* 18[4], 47.)

ischemia. Either or both mechanisms may produce pain. Osteoarthritis of the cervical spine is often associated with this type of headache, and inflammatory mediators may play a role in such cases.

With vascular headaches, there is some degree of hyperemia within cerebral and scalp vessels, which may or may not be preceded by a period of vasoconstriction. The most prevalent theory explaining the manifestations of migraine holds that it is due to a phenomenon known as *spreading depression,* in which a wavefront of hyperactive neuron discharges spreads across the cortex, followed by a period of electrical silence that is followed in turn by recovery of neuronal activity.[16] Spreading depression is believed to be induced by activation of serotonin or glutamate receptors in people who have a genetic predisposition to the phenomenon. Pain may be the result of the *axon reflex,* in which neurotransmitters released during the depression wave stimulate adjacent somatic sensory and autonomic nerves that innervate intracranial vessels, causing vasomotion and pain. This process may continue until the neurotransmitters are depleted.

Clinical Manifestations. The pain of tension-type headaches is usually aching or tight in character and is felt in a hatband-like pattern around the head as well as down the back of the neck. Migraine is typically unilateral and throbbing and is accompanied by nausea and photophobia. Migraine may or may not be preceded by an *aura,* an episode of focal neurologic deficit that is usually visual. Cluster headaches are characterized by exacerbations in which headaches occur daily over periods of several weeks or months, followed by periods of remission for months or years. Pain is excruciating and unilateral over the eye or temporal area and is associated with other facial manifestations, such as ptosis or nasal congestion on the affected side.

Prevention and Treatment. Identification and avoidance of triggering agents is warranted in all primary types of headache. Tension-type headaches are usually responsive to simple analgesics, (e.g., acetaminophen), or nonsteroidal anti-inflammatory drugs (NSAIDs) (e.g., aspirin, ibuprofen, and naproxen sodium; see Chapter 13). Antidepressants, such as amitriptyline and doxepin, may be used preventively for those with chronic tension-type headaches, and antistress interventions, such as psychotherapy, relaxation therapy, and biofeedback, may be helpful.[14]

Symptomatic treatment of migraine headaches includes NSAIDs for milder forms. Ergotamine preparations have long been used for their vasoconstrictive effect, but these have toxic effects, including nausea and muscle cramping. Sumatriptan (Imitrex), a serotonin derivative, is used in the treatment of migraine and cluster headaches and has been shown

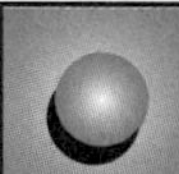

TABLE 23–11
CONDITIONS ASSOCIATED WITH LOW BACK PAIN

MECHANICAL OR ACTIVITY-RELATED CAUSES
Segmental and disk degeneration
Myofascial or soft tissue injury or disorder
Disk herniation with possible radiculopathy
Spinal instability with possible spondylolisthesis or fracture
Vertebral body fracture
Spinal canal or lateral recess stenosis
Arachnoiditis, including postoperative scarring
SYSTEMIC DISORDERS
Primary or metastatic neoplasm, including myeloma
Osseous, disk, or epidural infection
Inflammatory spondyloarthropathy
Metabolic bone disease, including osteoporosis
Vascular disorders such as atherosclerosis or vasculitis
NEUROLOGIC SYNDROMES
Myelopathy from intrinsic or extrinsic processes
Lumbosacral plexopathy, especially from diabetes
Neuropathy, including inflammatory demyelinating type (i.e., Guillain-Barré)
Mononeuropathy, including causalgia
Myopathy, including myositis and metabolic causes
REFERRED PAIN
Gastrointestinal disorders
Genitourinary disorders, including nephrolithiasis, prostatitis, and pyelonephritis
Gynecologic disorders, including ectopic pregnancy and pelvic inflammatory disease
Abdominal aortic aneurysm
Hip pathology
Psychosocial causes
Compensable injury
Somatoform pain disorder
Psychiatric syndromes, including delusional pain
Drug seeking
Abusive relationships
Seeking disability or out-of-work status

From Wheeler, A. (1995). Diagnosis and management of low back pain and sciatica. *American Family Physician* 52(5), 1334.

to be effective in 75% of patients.[17] Nasal instillation of the local anesthetic lidocaine has also been effective.[18] Some patients with chronic migraines may benefit from prophylactic therapy with β-blockers or calcium-channel blockers to reduce vasomotion or with selective serotonin reuptake inhibitors (e.g., fluoxetine [Prozac]).

Acute attacks of cluster headaches may be aborted with ergotamine preparations, inhalation of 100% oxygen, or nasal instillation of cocaine, lidocaine, or capsaicin (a substance P releaser).[14] Preventive therapy includes calcium-channel blockers, steroid therapy, lithium, or methysergide (Sansert), agents that influence vasomotion or neurotransmission. In cases that do not respond to medical therapy, anesthetic injection and surgical section of the trigeminal nerve have been used with some success.[14]

Prognosis and Outcome. Headaches are a major cause of morbidity in the United States but are not usually indicative of life-threatening disorders. Headache-prone people generally have recurrent episodes, but acute pain is preventable in many cases and nearly always amenable to treatment.

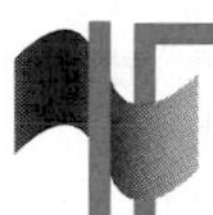

Clinical Scenario

F.V., a 29-year-old man, has recently been seen frequently in the walk-in clinic complaining of severe headache. Ten months ago, F.V. fell from a ladder while working at his construction job. He sustained a skull fracture and was hospitalized for 10 days without complication. Since that time, he has been unable to work and has become irritable and depressed. He says his headache is "constant," and describes it as left-sided and associated with nasal congestion, sensitivity to light, dizziness, and nausea and vomiting. A computed tomography scan was done, ruling out the presence of an intracranial hematoma. F.V.'s wife has taken a part-time job, leaving F.V. to care for the couple's two young children.

1. What factors in this situation may relate to F.V.'s headache?
2. What are the priorities for intervention in this case? Are any measures other than analgesia warranted?

Low Back Pain

Definition. *Low back pain* is a syndrome that includes aching discomfort in the lower back that may or may not be accompanied by signs of systemic disease, **sciatica** (radiating pain down the buttock and leg), or neurologic deficits. Low back pain may be classified as *simple,* if there are no risk factors or signs of underlying pathology, or *complex,* if underlying disorders are suspected.[19]

Epidemiology. At some time in their lives, 75% of adults have low back pain, although only 1.5% experience sciatica.[20] The overall annual prevalence in the United States is 15% to 20%. Ninety-eight per cent of cases are associated with mechanical conditions of the spine, such as **intervertebral disk disease, spinal stenosis,** ligament strains, or spinal fractures, whereas the remainder are due to systemic and vascular diseases (Table 23–11). Risk factors for lumbar disk disease include advanced age, vigorous exercise, sedentary work, history of back trauma, male sex, obesity, and cigarette smoking.[21] Spinal stenosis, in which the spinal canal is degeneratively or congenitally narrowed, may cause nerve entrapment, which contributes to pain. Spinal fractures may be associated with acute trauma (see Chapter 22) but are more often due to osteoporosis with advancing age (see Chapter 34). **Fibromyalgia** is a disorder of muscle in which deconditioning or repeated microtrauma causes pain triggered by mechanical stimulation of tender points (see Chapter 35). This syndrome may also affect the lower back. **Ankylosing spondylitis** is an inflammatory disease of unknown cause that commonly involves the spine and hip joints (see Chapter 34). Spinal cord tumors (primary or metastatic) may also cause low back pain. The following discussion focuses on lumbar disk disease and ligament strains, the most common structural abnormalities of the lower back.

Etiology. The risk of pain is highest with activities in which there is static loading of the spine (e.g., prolonged sitting or standing), long-levered activities (e.g., vacuuming), or levered postures (e.g., bending forward). The degree of anatomic abnormality does not correlate well with the degree of pain or disability. Many adults have some degree of disk abnormality evident on imaging studies, but most do not have symptoms.[22]

Pathophysiology. Disk herniation is the protrusion of the gelatinous material of the disk (nucleus pulposus) through the outer annulus fibrosis (Fig. 23–21). If the disk compresses a spinal nerve root, sciatic pain and paresthesia **(radiculopathy)** occur in the sensory distribution of the nerve. Chronic inflammation in low back disorders may also contribute to pain. As the nucleus pulposus becomes accessible to the vascular system, an autoimmune response may occur, triggering inflammation. Alternatively, release of local cytokines and lipid mediators may promote inflammation[21] (see Chapter 13).

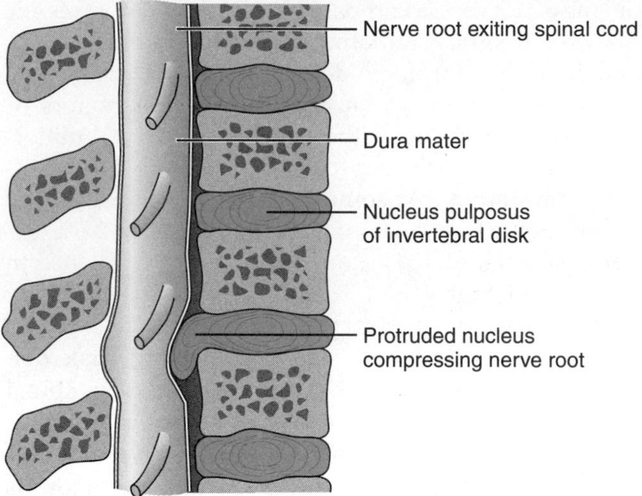

FIGURE 23–21
Herniated intervertebral disk. The *nucleus pulposus* (gelatinous material in the interior of the intervertebral disk) may protrude through the outer fibrous layer, compressing a dorsal nerve root. Pain and abnormal sensation occur in the dermatomal distribution of the sensory nerve.

Disk herniation associated with low back pain is most common between the L-3 and S-1 levels. (**Cervical radiculopathy,** which occurs with herniation of disks in the lower cervical region of the spine, manifests as neck pain and upper extremity paresthesias.) Protruding disk material may be reabsorbed over time. The posterior longitudinal ligament of the spine has nociceptors, which may give rise to pain with stretch injury.

Clinical Manifestations. Sciatica is present in cases of nerve root compression. Pain radiates down the leg below the knee, with numbness often extending to the lower leg and foot in a dermatomal distribution. Regional back pain, without sciatica, is confined to the area of inflammation and exacerbated by activity. Patients with disk herniation often have great difficulty sitting or bending, whereas those with ligament strain need to change position frequently to relieve the pain.[22] Continuous pain at rest is suggestive of a nonmechanical cause of back pain.

Prevention and Treatment. Prevention of mechanical back injury involves attention to the ergonomic aspects of activity (i.e., maintenance of appropriate body posture and mechanics) as well as achievement and maintenance of optimal fitness. As a result of a lack of controlled studies, the relative effectiveness of different treatments for low back pain are unknown. Bed rest in a supine position is known to decrease pressure within disks; however prolonged bed rest is not recommended because of the associated risk of deconditioning, deep vein thrombosis, and muscle atrophy. Medications for relief of pain include NSAIDs, muscle relaxants, antidepressants, and if necessary, short-term use of opioids. Physical therapy measures, such as ultrasound and deep heat, may provide symptomatic relief. Traction, back braces, and transcutaneous electrical nerve stimulation have not been shown to be of benefit.[20] Exercises that include both flexion and extension movements may reduce chronic pain and improve range of motion but are contraindicated during acute pain.

The benefits of osteopathic and chiropractic manipulation are unproved. Injection therapies include epidural analgesia and steroid therapy to relieve pain and inflammation, prolotherapy (injection of glycerin or phenol to promote fibrous tissue proliferation), and chemonucleolysis (injection of chymopapain enzyme to digest the disk). These treatments are of uncertain benefit and are not widely used. Surgical treatment of disk disease is controversial. Laminectomy (disk removal) and spinal fusion (bone grafts to stabilize the spine) are done with much greater frequency in the United States than in other developed countries, with the rates of surgery varying 15-fold in different areas of the United States. Surgery for back pain is considered to be elective, except in the unusual cases of unstable spinal fracture, or **cauda equina syndrome,** characterized by urinary retention, radiculopathy, and anesthesia of the *saddle region* (areas served by sacral nerves).

Prognosis and Outcome. Ninety per cent of cases of low back pain due to disk disease or other mechanical disorder resolve within 6 weeks, regardless of treatment, and another 5% resolve within 12 weeks.[22] In 5% of cases, back pain persists and becomes a chronic condition.

Carpal Tunnel Syndrome

Definition. Carpal tunnel syndrome (CTS) is a neuropathy syndrome resulting from entrapment of the median nerve within a narrowed carpal tunnel.

Epidemiology. CTS is the most common nerve entrapment syndrome, affecting nearly 1% of the general population of the United States.[23] Table 23–12 describes other nerve entrapment syndromes and disorders associated with repetitive motion injury. Risk factors for CTS include repetitive use of the wrists, female gender, use of oral contraceptives, pregnancy, prior surgical removal of the ovaries (oophorectomy), myxedema (hypothyroidism), diabetes mellitus, rheumatoid arthritis, prior wrist fracture (Colles' fracture) or other wrist trauma, and occupations characterized by repetitive motions of the wrist.[24]

Etiology. Many cases are idiopathic. Irritation of the medial nerve may result from acute trauma or

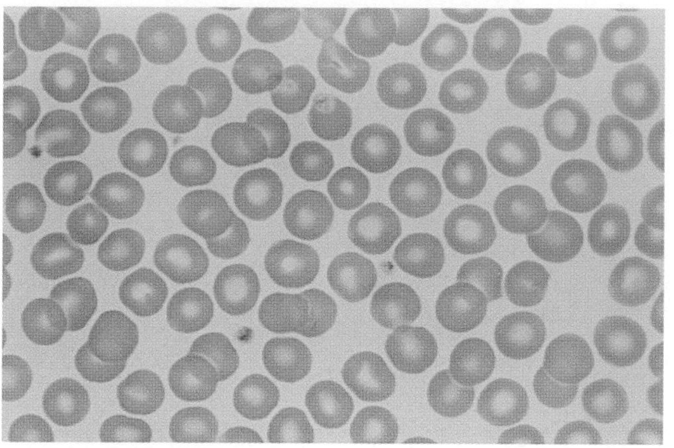

COLOR FIGURE 12–1
Normal peripheral blood smear. (From Rodak, B.F. [1995]. *Diagnostic Hematology.* Philadelphia: W.B. Saunders. [p. 154.].)

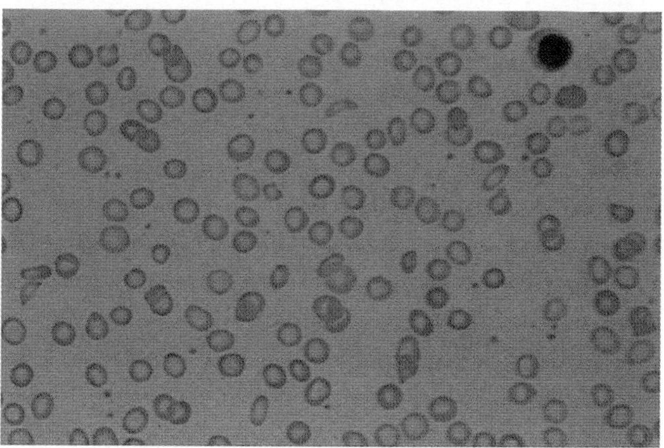

COLOR FIGURE 12–2
Iron deficiency anemia. (From Rodak, B.F. [1995]. *Diagnostic Hematology.* Philadelphia: W.B. Saunders. [p. 183.].)

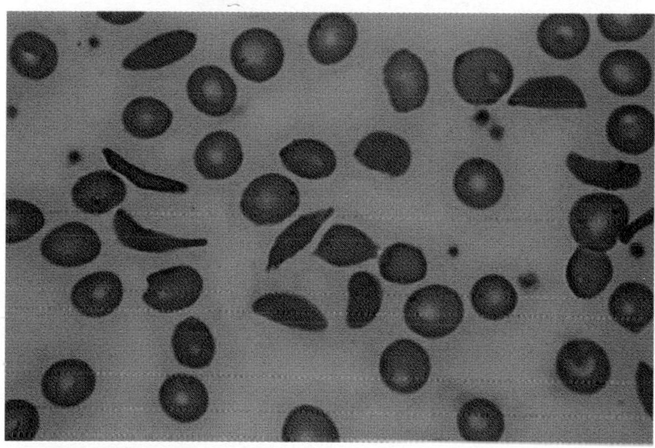

COLOR FIGURE 12–3
Sickle cell anemia. (From Rodak, B.F. [1995]. *Diagnostic Hematology.* Philadelphia: W.B. Saunders. [p. 257.].)

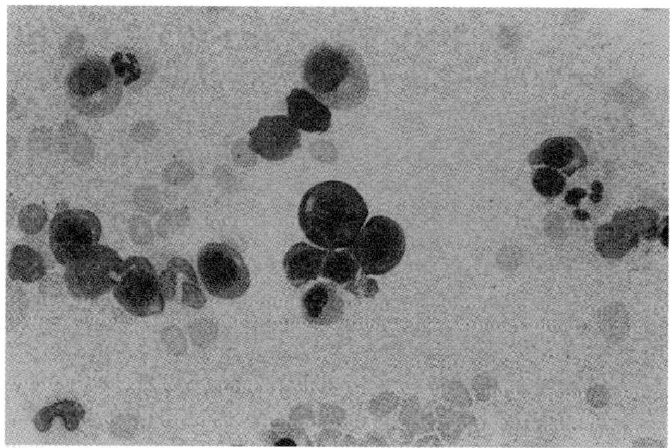

COLOR FIGURE 12–4
Pernicious anemia. (From Rodak, B.F. [1995]. *Diagnostic Hematology.* Philadelphia: W.B. Saunders. [p. 187.].)

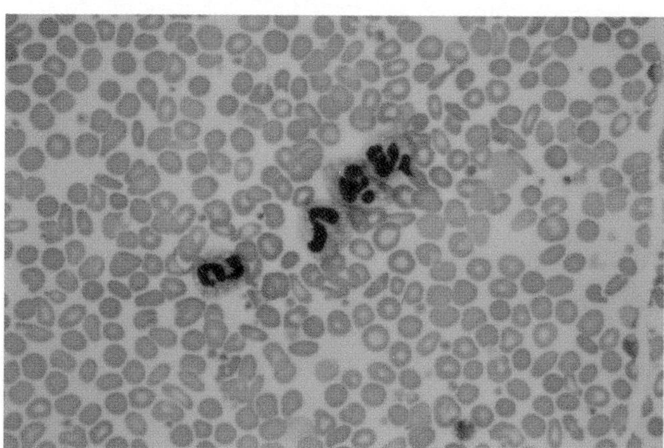

COLOR FIGURE 12–5
Polycythemia vera. (From Rodak, B.F. [1995]. *Diagnostic Hematology.* Philadelphia: W.B. Saunders. [p. 366.].)

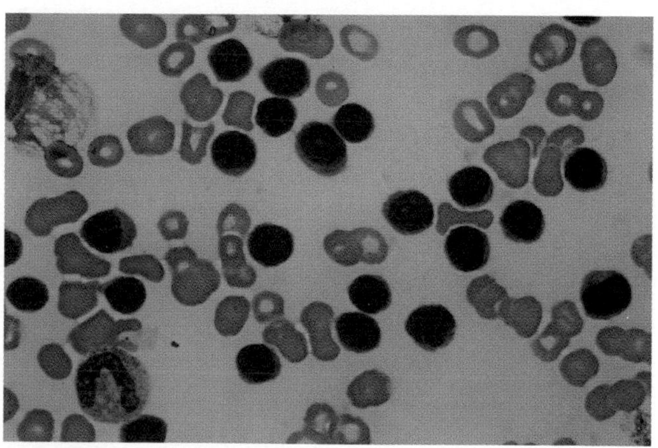

COLOR FIGURE 12–6
Chronic lymphocytic leukemia. (From Rodak, B.F. [1995]. *Diagnostic Hematology.* Philadelphia: W.B. Saunders. [p. 352.].)

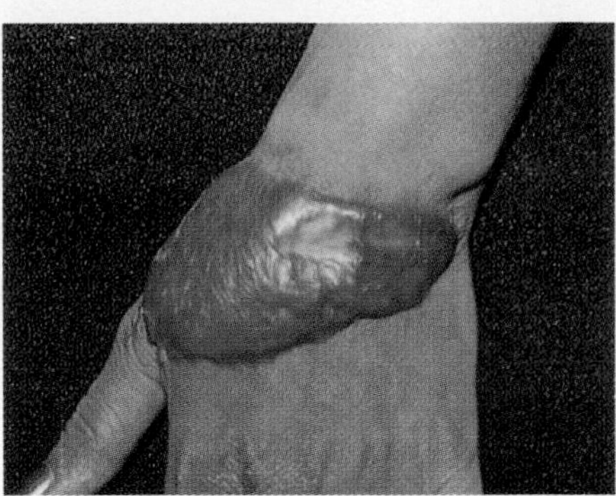

COLOR FIGURE 13–1
Keloid. (From Lookingbill, D.P., and Marks, J.G. [1993]. *Dermatology*. [2nd ed.]. Philadelphia: W.B. Saunders. [p. 106].)

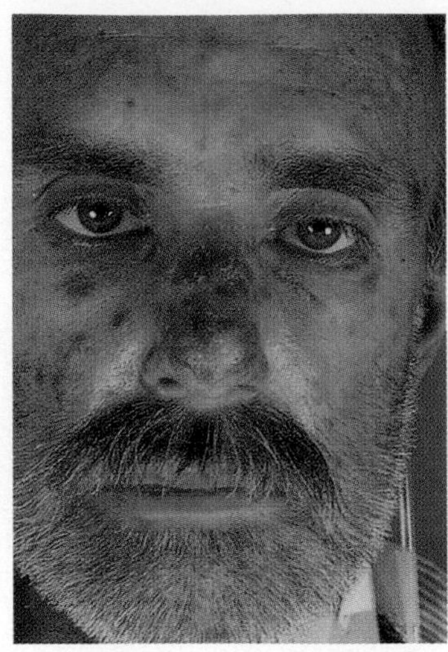

COLOR FIGURE 13–2
Kaposi's sarcoma. (From Friedman-Kien, A.E., and Cockerell, C.J. [1996]. *Color Atlas of AIDS*. [2nd ed.]. Philadelphia: W.B. Saunders. [p. 58.].)

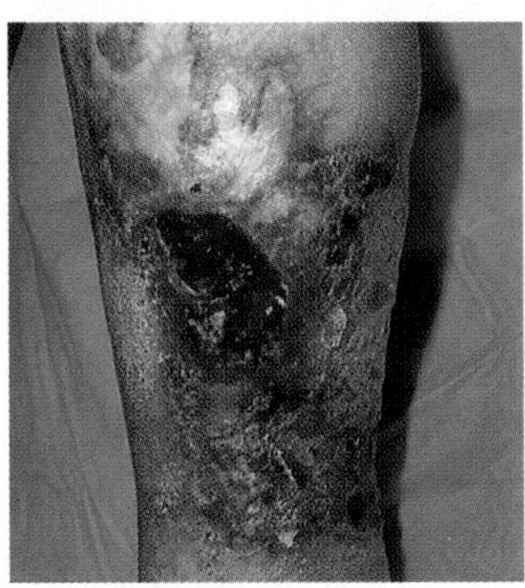

COLOR FIGURE 14–1
Venous stasis ulcer. (From Lookingbill, D.P., and Marks, J.G. [1993]. *Principles of Dermatology*. [2nd ed.]. Philadelphia: W.B. Saunders. [p. 267.].)

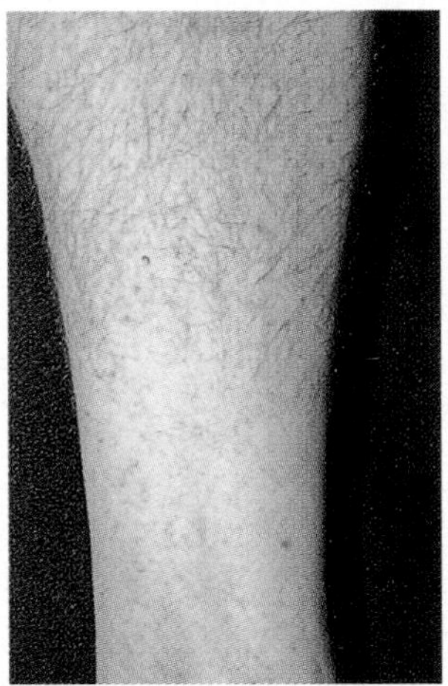

COLOR FIGURE 14–2
Petechiae. (From Lookingbill, D.P., and Marks, J.G. [1993]. *Principles of Dermatology*. [2nd ed.]. Philadelphia: W.B. Saunders. [p. 251.].)

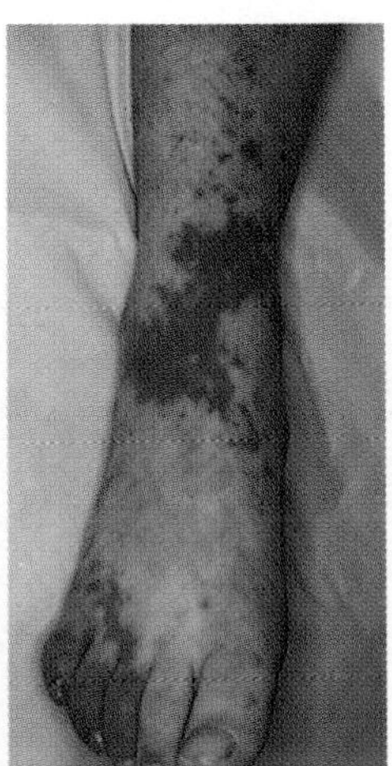

COLOR FIGURE 14–3
Purpura. (From Hurwitz, S. [1993]. *Clinical Pediatric Dermatology: A Textbook of Skin Disorders of Childhood and Adolescence*. [2nd ed.]. Philadelphia: W.B. Saunders. [p. 269.].)

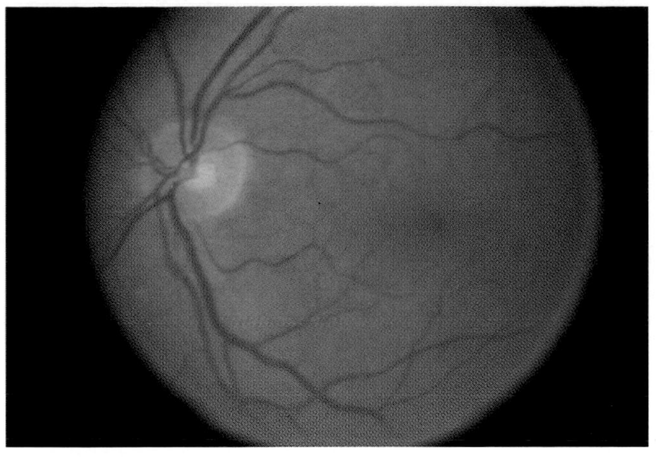

COLOR FIGURE 23–1
Normal retina. (From Swartz, M.H. [1998]. *Textbook of Physical Diagnosis.* [3rd ed.]. Philadelphia: W.B. Saunders. [Fig. 8-33*A*.].)

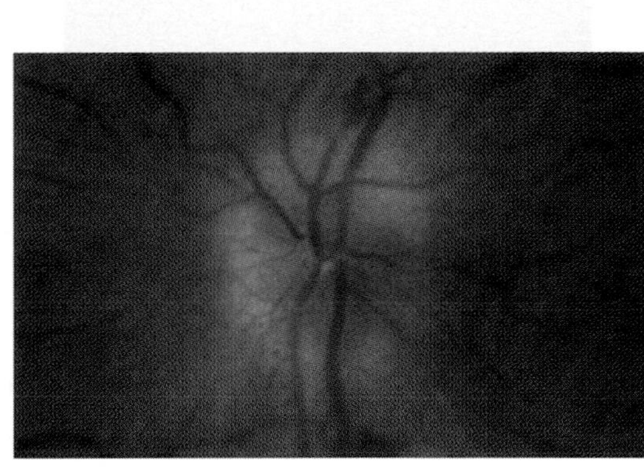

COLOR FIGURE 23–2
Papilledema (choked disc). (From Albert, D.M., and Jakobiec, F.A. [1995]. *Atlas of Clinical Ophthalmology.* Philadelphia: W.B. Saunders. [p. 452.].)

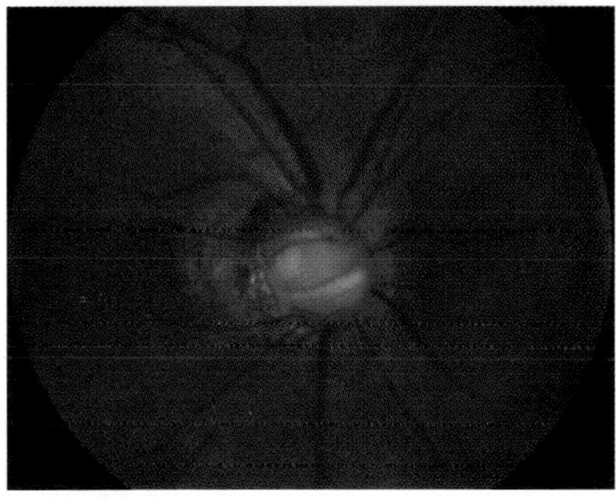

COLOR FIGURE 23–3
Glaucoma (cupped disc). (From Albert, D.M., and Jakobiec, F.A. [1995]. *Atlas of Clinical Ophthalmology.* Philadelphia: W.B. Saunders. [p. 279.].)

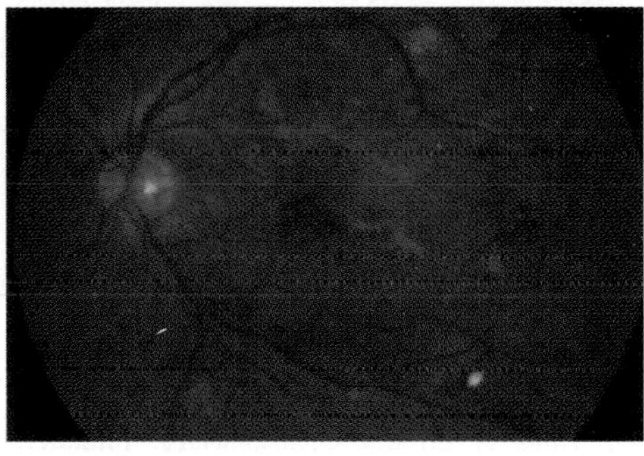

COLOR FIGURE 23–4
Diabetic retinopathy. (From Albert, D.M., and Jakobiec, F.A. [1995]. *Atlas of Clinical Ophthalmology.* Philadelphia: W.B. Saunders. [p. 179.].)

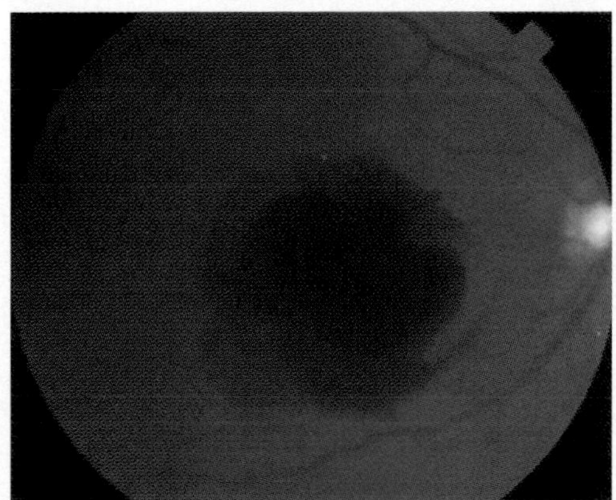

COLOR FIGURE 23–5
Hypertensive retinopathy. (From Albert, D.M., and Jakobiec, F.A. [1995]. *Atlas of Clinical Ophthalmology.* Philadelphia: W.B. Saunders. [p. 186.].)

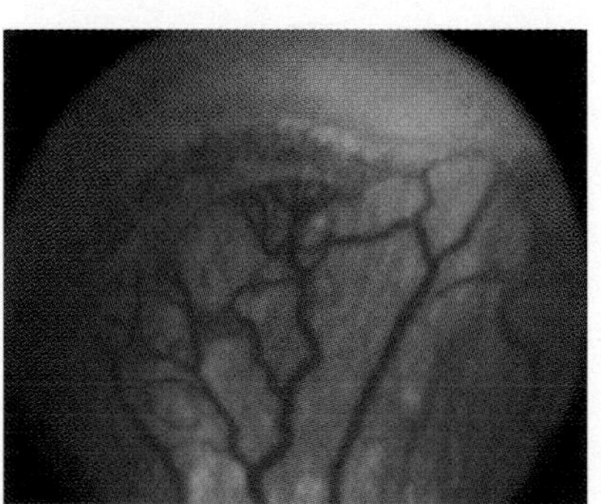

COLOR FIGURE 23–6
Retinopathy of prematurity. (From the Committee for Classification of Retinopathy of Prematurity. [1984]. An international classification of retinopathy of prematurity. *Arch Ophthalmol* 102, 1131. 1984. Copyright 1984, American Medical Association.)

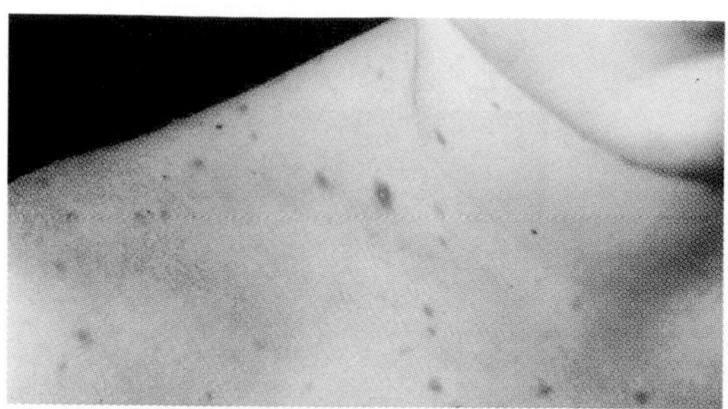

COLOR FIGURE 36–4
Varicella zoster virus (chickenpox). (From Lookingbill, D.P., and Marks, J.G. [1993]. *Principles of Dermatology.* [2nd ed.]. Philadelphia: W.B. Saunders. [p. 167.].)

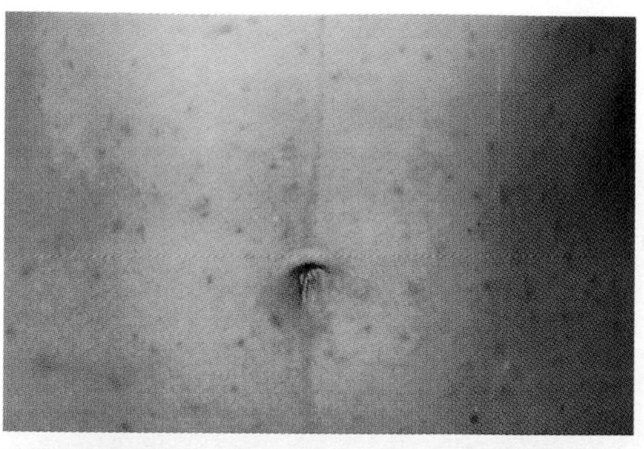

COLOR FIGURE 36–5
Scabies. (From Lookingbill, D.P., and Marks, J.G. [1993]. *Principles of Dermatology.* [2nd ed.]. Philadelphia: W.B. Saunders. [p. 180.].)

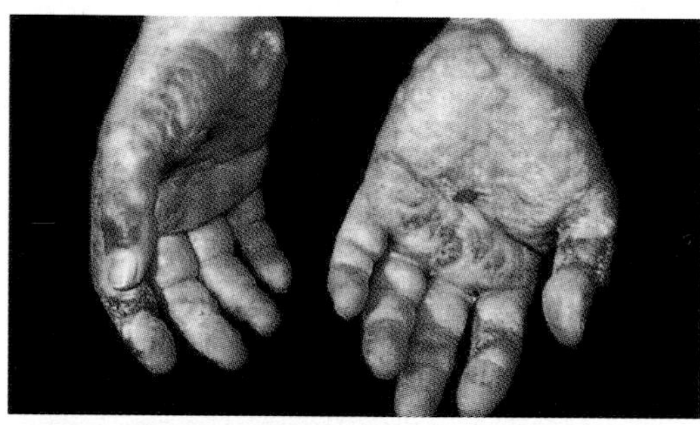

COLOR FIGURE 36–6
Atopic dermatitis (eczema). (From Lookingbill, D.P., and Marks, J.G. [1993]. *Principles of Dermatology.* [2nd ed.]. Philadelphia: W.B. Saunders. [p. 122.].)

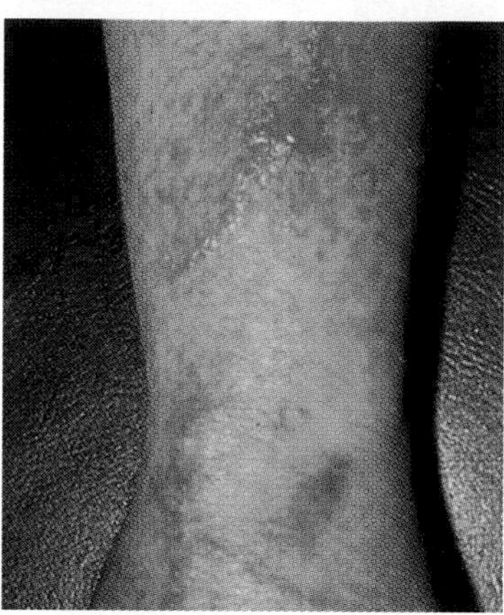

COLOR FIGURE 36–7
Contact dermatitis. (From Lookingbill, D.P., and Marks, J.G. [1993]. *Principles of Dermatology.* [2nd ed.]. Philadelphia: W.B. Saunders. [p. 124.].)

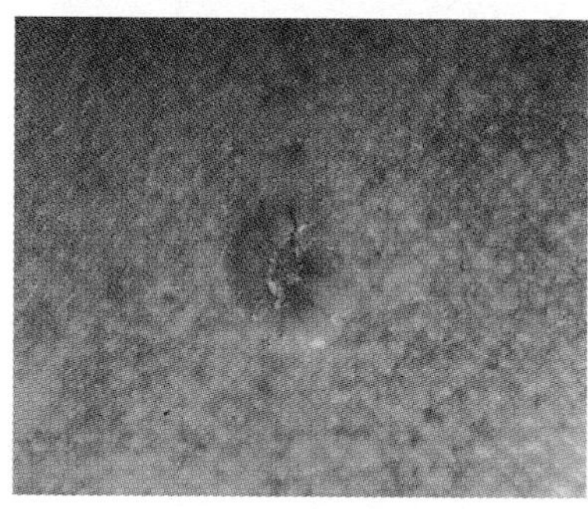

COLOR FIGURE 36–8
Basal cell carcinoma. (From Lookingbill, D.P., and Marks, J.G. [1993]. *Principles of Dermatology.* [2nd ed.]. Philadelphia: W.B. Saunders. [p. 81.].)

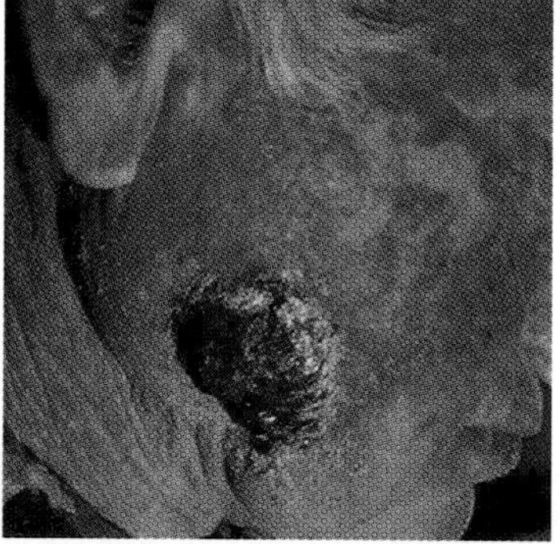

COLOR FIGURE 36–9
Squamous cell carcinoma. (From Lookingbill, D.P., and Marks, J.G. [1993]. *Principles of Dermatology.* [2nd ed.]. Philadelphia: W.B. Saunders. [p. 79.].)

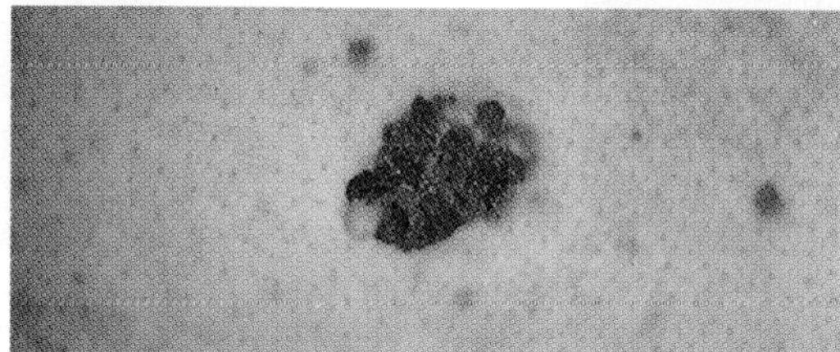

COLOR FIGURE 36–10
Malignant melanoma. (From Lookingbill, D.P., and Marks, J.G. [1993]. *Principles of Dermatology.* [2nd ed.]. Philadelphia: W.B. Saunders. [p. 94.].)

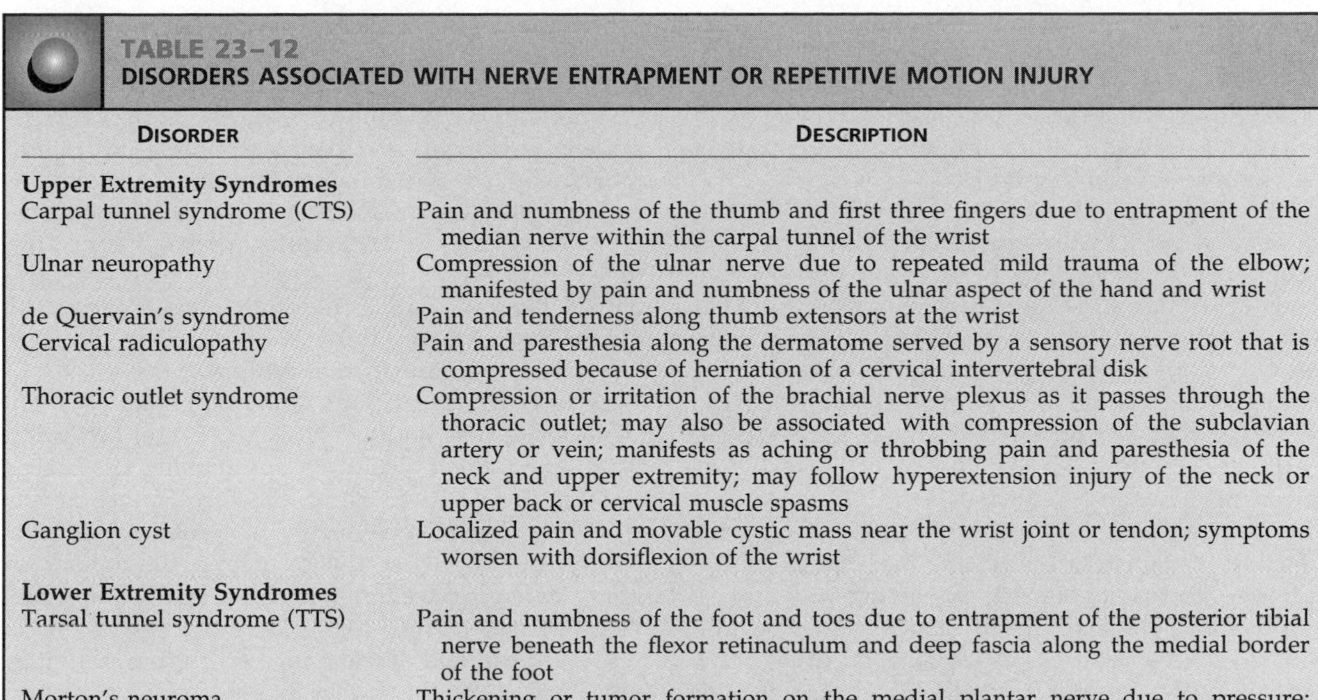

TABLE 23–12
DISORDERS ASSOCIATED WITH NERVE ENTRAPMENT OR REPETITIVE MOTION INJURY

Disorder	Description
Upper Extremity Syndromes	
Carpal tunnel syndrome (CTS)	Pain and numbness of the thumb and first three fingers due to entrapment of the median nerve within the carpal tunnel of the wrist
Ulnar neuropathy	Compression of the ulnar nerve due to repeated mild trauma of the elbow; manifested by pain and numbness of the ulnar aspect of the hand and wrist
de Quervain's syndrome	Pain and tenderness along thumb extensors at the wrist
Cervical radiculopathy	Pain and paresthesia along the dermatome served by a sensory nerve root that is compressed because of herniation of a cervical intervertebral disk
Thoracic outlet syndrome	Compression or irritation of the brachial nerve plexus as it passes through the thoracic outlet; may also be associated with compression of the subclavian artery or vein; manifests as aching or throbbing pain and paresthesia of the neck and upper extremity; may follow hyperextension injury of the neck or upper back or cervical muscle spasms
Ganglion cyst	Localized pain and movable cystic mass near the wrist joint or tendon; symptoms worsen with dorsiflexion of the wrist
Lower Extremity Syndromes	
Tarsal tunnel syndrome (TTS)	Pain and numbness of the foot and toes due to entrapment of the posterior tibial nerve beneath the flexor retinaculum and deep fascia along the medial border of the foot
Morton's neuroma	Thickening or tumor formation on the medial plantar nerve due to pressure; manifests as severe burning in web space between third and fourth toes

repetitive motion of the wrists. The carpal tunnel of the wrist is a narrow channel created by the stiff transverse carpal ligament on the palm side of the wrist and by the carpal bones on the dorsal side (Fig. 23–22). Nine tendons and the median nerve pass through the carpal tunnel. Any condition in which the tunnel is narrowed or fluid pressure within the tunnel is increased might compress the median nerve. Alterations of the endocrine or immune systems may increase the fluid pressure within the tunnel.

Pathophysiology. Compression of the median nerve initially impairs sensory transmission to the thumb, index finger, second finger, and inner aspect of the third finger (median nerve distribution). If the condition becomes chronic, motor function may also be impaired. In many cases, pain receptors are also stimulated.

Clinical Manifestations. Sensory loss is manifested as numbness and tingling, often occurring at night. Shaking the fingers and hand (like shaking down the mercury in a thermometer) often relieves the symptoms. Although numbness may present acutely with trauma, more often it is of gradual onset and intermittent. Motor deficits may take the form of clumsiness or weakness. Pain may be limited to the fingers and wrist, or may be referred to the elbow and shoulder. Atrophy of the thenar muscle at the base of the thumb may become evident in chronic cases. Several tests for CTS may be em-

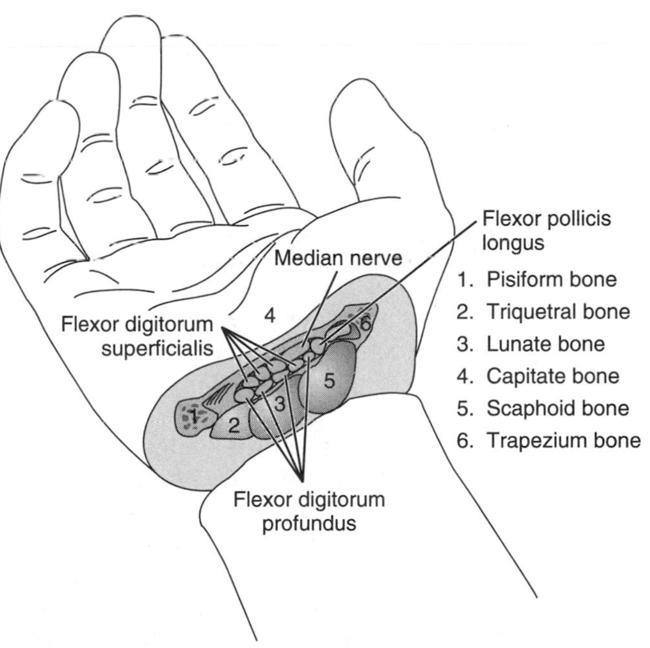

FIGURE 23–22

Carpal tunnel syndrome. The carpal tunnel is a narrow channel in the wrist, through which the median nerve and nine tendons pass. Structural changes or edema may compress the nerve, resulting in numbness, tingling, and often pain of the thumb and first three fingers. (With permission from Katz, R.T. [1994]. Carpal tunnel syndrome: A practical review. *American Family Physician* 49[6], 1372. Published by the American Academy of Family Physicians.)

ployed on diagnostic examination. Phalen's test suggests CTS if forceful flexion of the wrist for 20 to 30 seconds produces numbness and tingling. The newer carpal compression test is similar, except that pressure is applied with the examiner's thumbs over the median nerve in the tunnel.

Prevention and Treatment. Prevention involves avoidance of risk factors insofar as possible. A lightweight plastic splint may be worn to prevent constant wrist flexion. Ergonomic measures, such as repositioning of computer keyboards, may be indicated. Underlying disorders, such as diabetes or hypothyroidism, should be optimally managed. Fluid retention related to hormonal changes may respond to diuretic therapy. CTS in pregnancy usually resolves spontaneously after delivery. Oral corticosteroids may be used in the treatment of arthritis affecting the wrist, but cortisone injection is contraindicated because of the risk of scarring.[25]

Splinting alone may be sufficient to relieve symptoms in mild disease. NSAIDs may be used. Some patients report symptomatic relief with use of pyridoxine (vitamin B_6), but its therapeutic effect remains unproved.[25] If medical therapy is ineffective, surgical release (enlargement) of the carpal tunnel may be performed, using either an open incision or an endoscopic procedure.

Prognosis and Outcome. As many as 75% of patients obtain relief of pain and improvement in sensory and motor function with conservative measures.[25] The success rate for surgery is 80% to 95%. Success with either approach is enhanced if the patient is able to remove associated risk factors as well.

Trigeminal Neuralgia

Definition. Trigeminal neuralgia, also known as *tic douloureux,* is a syndrome of excruciating facial pain due to disease of the fifth cranial nerve.

Epidemiology. An estimated 15,000 cases are diagnosed each year in the United States.[7] Although most patients are between 50 and 70 years of age, the disorder may affect adults of any age. Females are affected slightly more often than males. Risk factors for the development of trigeminal neuralgia are unknown but may be derived from previous nerve injury or from a vascular or demyelinating disorder affecting cranial nerve V. A familial predisposition has been reported in some cases.[26]

Etiology. The precise etiology is unknown. Stimuli that may trigger acute attacks include certain foods, such as chocolate or vinegar, which initiate salivation. Touching the face, eating, brushing the teeth, or talking may induce an attack in some cases.

Pathophysiology. There is usually no identifiable nerve lesion, although in younger adults with multiple sclerosis, plaques may affect cranial nerve V (see Chapter 22). Hyperactivity of trigeminal nerve transmission is present, and the right side is most commonly affected. Some patients experience a preliminary syndrome consisting of episodes of toothache or sinus-type pain lasting for several hours at a time.[26] Pain occurs in the area of the face served by one of the three divisions of the facial nerve: the ophthalmic division (forehead), maxillary division (cheek), or mandibular division (jaw).

Clinical Manifestations. Intermittent attacks are characterized by sudden onset of severe, throbbing pain. The patient usually stops moving or talking and refrains from touching the face during an attack. The affected side of the face contorts. Attacks are infrequent at first, but over time, the periods of remission become shorter and the attacks more severe.

Prevention and Treatment. Triggering activities are avoided to the extent possible. Drug therapy with carbamazepine (Tegretol), an antiepileptic, is the treatment of choice. This drug may act by reducing impulse transmission along cranial nerve V. Initial response to carbamazapine confirms the diagnosis, but many patients eventually become unresponsive to the drug. The antiepileptic drug phenytoin (Dilantin) and the antispasmodic drug baclofen (Lioresal) may also be used in an effort to prevent attacks. When medications are no longer effective in controlling pain, or when drug therapy is intolerable because of adverse effects, neurosurgical procedures may be used. These techniques selectively destroy portions of cranial nerve V or decompress the surrounding lesions.

Prognosis and Outcome. Although this syndrome is well controlled in some patients by medication only, many patients find the adverse effects of the drugs debilitating. Surgery provides permanent relief of pain for many, although facial numbness results from most techniques. For others, surgery provides only temporary relief of pain.[7]

Meniere's Disease

Definition. Meniere's disease, also known as *Meniere's syndrome* or *endolymphatic hydrops,* is a chronic disorder of hearing and proprioception in which function of the auditory nerve (cranial nerve VIII) is impaired by excessive endolymphatic fluid pressure.

Epidemiology. An estimated 300,000 new cases are diagnosed each year in the United States.[27] Meniere's disease is most common among adults 40 to 60 years of age but is also seen in younger adults and in the elderly. Men are affected more often than women. Risk factors are unknown.

Etiology. The precise cause is unknown. The diagnosis of Meniere's disease is made after excluding other etiologies. Endolymph may accumulate as a result of either hypersecretion or hypoabsorption. Acute attacks are believed to be precipitated when the labyrinth ruptures, allowing potassium-containing endolymph to leak into surrounding structures and disrupt neurotransmission.[28]

Pathophysiology. The condition is unilateral in 70% of cases.[27] Excessive endolymph dilates the semicircular canals, utricle, and saccule and leads to degeneration of hair cell receptors and impaired proprioception. Excessive or abnormal stimulus transmission along the vestibular branch of cranial nerve VIII impairs postural reflexes and inappropriately stimulates the vomiting reflex (see Chapter 24). Sound perception is abnormal because of this stimulation, and auditory acuity may be permanently affected because of pressure trauma to sensory receptors for hearing.

Clinical Manifestations. Clinical manifestations are variable in severity but typically include vertigo (a sense that one's environment is spinning, usually accompanied by nausea and vomiting), nystagmus, tinnitus (usually described as roaring in the ear), a sense of fullness in the ear, and sensorineural hearing loss.[28] Vertigo is usually so severe that the patient cannot stand or walk. Nystagmus is seen on the affected side and is of the horizontal or rotary type. Cold caloric testing reveals abnormality of the oculovestibular reflex in that nystagmus is absent or diminished. Acute attacks of vertigo and tinnitus are episodic, followed by periods of remission that may last several months or only a few days. Some degree of hearing loss persists throughout remission.

Prevention and Treatment. There is no specific prevention for Meniere's disease, although restriction of caffeine, alcohol, and tobacco is often advised. Low-sodium diet, ammonium chloride, and diuretics have been used empirically in prevention of acute attacks, but there are no clinical trials establishing their effectiveness.[29] Treatment during acute attacks consists of CNS depressants such as diazepam (Valium) to decrease the excitability of vestibular nuclei, diuretics to decrease endolymph pressure, and bed rest to minimize head movement. Between attacks, an empiric medical regimen, including agents such as diuretics, CNS depressants, antivertigo antihistamines such as meclizine (Antivert) or dimenhydrinate (Dramamine), and vasolidators (e.g., calcium-channel blockers, β-blockers) may control the condition and preserve some auditory function. For severe attacks not responsive to medical therapy, surgical shunting of endolymph or ablation of sensory pathways may be warranted. Such surgery may result in deafness in the affected ear.

Prognosis and Outcome. Medical management is successful in reducing the severity of attacks and preserving some hearing in most patients. Except in cases of surgical ablation, the possibility of acute vertigo persists and may require the patient to curtail activities during which such attacks could threaten the safety of self or others (e.g., driving or operating machinery). Most middle-aged patients with Meniere's disease recover spontaneously within a few years.[29]

Benign Positional Vertigo

Definition. Benign positional vertigo is a peripheral vestibular disorder affecting the posterior semicircular canal and resulting in episodic vertigo with assumption of certain head positions.

Epidemiology. Benign positional vertigo and Meniere's disease are the most common causes of vertigo. (Other causes of dizziness and vertigo are summarized in Table 23–13.) In middle-aged people, benign positional vertigo is often idiopathic, with no apparent risk factors. In younger people,

TABLE 23–13
CONDITIONS ASSOCIATED WITH DIZZINESS AND VERTIGO

Etiologic Category	Examples
Nonvertiginous dizziness	Orthostatic hypotension
	Ataxia due to cerebellar, degenerative, neoplastic, vascular, or metabolic disorder
	Psychiatric disorder
Vertigo	
Central vertigo	Vertebrobasilar artery insufficiency
	Cerebellar tumor
	Vestibular tumor
	Migraine
	Multiple sclerosis
Peripheral vertigo	Benign positional vertigo
	Meniere's disease
	Recurrent vestibulopathy
	Vestibular neuronitis
	Labyrinthitis
	Cholesteatoma
	Perilymphatic fistula
	Inner ear trauma
	Ototoxicity
	Acoustic neuroma (vestibular schwannoma)

Data from Ruckenstein, M.J. (1995). A practical approach to dizziness: Questions to bring vertigo and other causes into focus. *Postgraduate Medicine* 97(3), 70–81.

the disorder may be associated with prior head injury. Basilar artery insufficiency and viral neuronitis may also contribute to the disorder.

Etiology. Symptoms of the disorder are believed to be caused by the development of basophilic deposits (otoliths), either freely floating within the endolymph or attached to the cupula of the posterior semicircular canal.[30]

Pathophysiology. As the patient moves, the basophilic deposits also move, resulting in abnormal deflection of the cupula and inappropriate stimulation of proprioceptors.

Clinical Manifestations. A few seconds after a certain movement of the head, the patient is afflicted with vertigo, dizziness, and nystagmus, which increase in intensity, then disappear after about 1 minute. Hearing is not affected. The diagnosis is confirmed with the Hallpike-Dix maneuver, in which the patient lies down with the head turned to the affected side and with the ear 30 to 45 degrees below the horizontal plane. This position triggers the typical clinical signs of the disorder.[30]

Prevention and Treatment. There is no specific prevention for benign positional vertigo. The condition may be treated conservatively with canalith repositioning procedures, in which the patient is positioned in such a way as to move the otolith out of the posterior semicircular canal. The application of vibration to the mastoid process on the affected side may facilitate breakup of debris. Habituation exercises, in which the patient deliberatively assumes the offending head position several times a day, have the same clinical objective. Surgical occlusion of the semicircular canal may also be performed.

Prognosis and Outcome. In most patients, the disorder is self-limited, with manifestations subsiding spontaneously after a few weeks or months.[30] Others have alternating periods of exacerbation and remission of the disorder. In patients who have manifestations persisting for more than 1 year, the disorder usually does not subside without surgery. Surgical occlusion of the semicircular canal is usually curative, and hearing is preserved.

Retinopathy

Definition. Retinopathy is a general term that is inclusive of visual deficits resulting from primary or secondary retinal disease. The most common forms of retinopathy are diabetic retinopathy, hypertensive retinopathy, retinopathy of prematurity (ROP), acquired immunodeficiency syndrome (AIDS)–related retinopathy, retinal detachment, and macular degeneration.

Epidemiology. Diabetic retinopathy is the leading cause of blindness in patients 25 to 74 years of age and is responsible for up to 24,000 new cases of blindness each year in the United States.[31] The overall prevalence of macular degeneration is 1.2% in patients 52 to 64 years old and 19.7% in those 75 to 85 years old. ROP occurs in an estimated 47% of infants weighing 1000 to 1250 g at birth, 78% of those weighing 750 to 999 g, and 90% of those weighing less than 750 g.

Aging and cigarette smoking are independent risk factors for macular degeneration, and prematurity is the definitive risk factor for ROP. Retinal detachment is more likely to occur in myopic people. Other risk factors are related to the underlying disorders.

Etiology. Retinal detachment may be caused by trauma to the eye (e.g., a blow to the head or intraocular surgery); but in many cases, this condition is idiopathic. Systemic disorders, such as atherosclerosis, hypertension, diabetes, and AIDS, commonly damage the retina as a result of ischemic, hypoxic, toxic, infectious, or vascular pressure trauma. Retinal damage may also result from the increased intraocular pressure of glaucoma, discussed later in this chapter. Less common disorders associated with retinopathy are described in Table 23–14.

Pathophysiology. Diabetic retinopathy, discussed further in Chapter 29, is subdivided into two forms. In the nonproliferative, or background, type, retinal vessels develop microaneurysms secondary to glycosylation of proteins of the vessel endothelium. These aneurysms may hemorrhage, leading to retinal nerve infarcts and exudates (see Color Fig. 23–4). In the proliferative type, a tangled overgrowth of new retinal vessels is believed to result from release of angiogenic factors from chronically hypoxic retinal cells. The vitreous humor apparently causes traction on these new vessels and, consequently, on the retina, potentially causing detachment or vitreous hemorrhage.

Atherosclerosis and hypertension damage retinal vessels similarly to the effects of these often-concurrent conditions on other arteries. Aneurysms and plaques may cause retinal hypoxia (see Color Fig. 23–5).

The pathophysiology of ROP is incompletely understood (see Chapter 33). Prolonged oxygen therapy, shock, sepsis, asphyxia, and other perinatal stressors may injure the developing retinal capillary bed in the premature infant. After a variable delay, the vessels begin to regrow, but growth is excessive in many cases, leading to hemorrhage, retinal scarring, or retinal detachment (see Color Fig. 23–6). Prolonged oxygen therapy has been associated with tissue injury from oxidative stress, but use of antioxidants has not been shown to be beneficial in prevention and treatment of ROP.[32]

TABLE 23-14
LESS COMMON DISORDERS ASSOCIATED WITH RETINOPATHY

DISORDER	DESCRIPTION
Melanosis of the retina	Nonfamilial, nonprogressive disorder characterized by small grayish-black spots (accumulations of retinal pigmented epithelial cells); minute visual field defects correspond to these areas
Retinal dysplasia	Congenital disorder (possibly hereditary) in which outer nuclear retinal cells are arranged in a radiating pattern around a central ocular space; retina is detached, and eye is microphthalmic with white lesion in pupil; patient is blind
Phakomatosis	Group of disorders in which there are congenital benign tumors of blood vessels or neural tissues of the retina; associated with a number of intracranial and ocular tumors and vascular disorders
Coats' disease	Chronic, progressive, vascular disorder in which retinal vessels leak fluid; results in an exudative retinal detachment that decreases central or peripheral vision
Retinal artery occlusion	Obstruction of a central or peripheral retinal artery by embolus or thrombosis, leading to sudden, painless loss of vision; usually associated with atherosclerosis, cardiac valve disease, or arteriosclerosis
Retinal vein occlusion	Obstruction of a central or peripheral retinal vein by external compression, venous stasis, or degeneration of the endothelium; associated with atherosclerosis or arteriosclerosis; leads to immediate vision loss of varying degree
Eales' disease	Phlebitis of retinal veins, leading to recurrent retinal hemorrhage and loss of vision; may be autoimmune in origin; usually affects men 15–30 years of age
Retinal edema	Increase of extracellular fluid within the sensory retina because of failure of the retinal pigmented epithelium to limit plasma flux; associated with diabetes, uveitis, cataract extraction, and retinitis pigmentosa
Macular edema	Increase in fluid leakage into the sensory retina because of abnormal permeability of capillary beds surrounding the fovea; reduces vision to 20/200; associated with many vascular, inflammatory, and degenerative conditions
Retinitis pigmentosa	Hereditary group of progressive disorders of rods and cones due to genetic defect; night blindness is apparent during adolescence, and visual loss is progressive until only a small, tubular visual field remains; this is also lost eventually
Leber's congenital amaurosis	Autosomal recessive disorder in which there is either no light perception or near blindness from birth; may be associated with mental retardation, epilepsy, congenital cataract or glaucoma, or albinism
Best's disease	Autosomal dominant disorder in which central retinal region is occupied by a bright orange deposit; vision is normal until later childhood or adolescence, when the deposited material scatters, leading to scarring and pigmentary changes and loss of central vision
Retinoschisis	Splitting of the sensory retina due to either a genetic defect or to a degenerative process; manifests as light flashes or floaters; vision gradually decreases in the genetic form to about 20/200 at puberty
Retinoblastoma	Neuroblastic neoplasm of the outer nuclear layer of the retina; genetically transmitted, similarly to Wilms' tumor and neuroblastoma

Data from Newell, F.W. (1992). *Ophthalmology: Principles and Concepts.* (7th ed.). St. Louis: Mosby–Year Book. (pp. 284–317).

The precise mechanism of age-related macular degeneration is unknown. Oxidative stress or reduced levels of antioxidant enzymes are possible factors, along with vascular insufficiency typical of aging[33] (see Focus of Current Research). Loss of vision is primarily due to proliferation of choroidal vessels into the retina, which may lead to retinal detachment, hemorrhage, and scarring in the area of the macula (see Fig. 23–7). Patients with this condition also accumulate deposits of a yellow material *(drusen)*, which is believed to consist of lipofuscin and other debris from degenerating retinal pigmented epithelial cells.

Retinal detachment occurs when the subretinal space, a potential fluid space between the pigmented and neural layers, fills with fluid or blood (see Color Fig. 23–8). Normally, this is prevented by the continuous reabsorption of fluid by the choroid. Detachment may occur as a consequence of a hole or break in the retina that allows vitreous fluid to enter the subretinal space. Traction on retinal vessels by the vitreous fluid or traction due to scarring of the retinal membrane may elevate the intact neural layer, enlarging the subretinal space and impairing fluid reabsorption.

Retinal inflammation in AIDS may be due to di-

Focus of Current Research

Study	Objective and Findings
Maizels, et al. (1996) Intranasal lidocaine for treatment of migraine.	*Objective:* to evaluate the effectiveness of intranasal lidocaine for treatment of acute migraine headache *Findings:* Intranasal lidocaine provides relief in about 55% of patients with migraine. Relapse is common and occurs early after treatment.
Seddon, et al. (1996) A prospective study of cigarette smoking and age-related macular degeneration in women.	*Objective:* To evaluate the relationship between smoking and incidence of age-related macular degeneration (AMD) among women *Findings:* Women who smoked 25 or more cigarettes per day had a relative risk of 2.4 when compared with nonsmokers. Past smokers had a two-fold risk of developing AMD.
Christen, et al. (1996) A prospective study of cigarette smoking and risk of age-related macular degeneration in men.	*Objective:* To examine the association between smoking and incidence of AMD in men *Findings:* Relative risk among those who smoked 20 or more cigarettes per day was 2.46. Past smokers had a relative risk of 1.30.
Brook, et al. (1996) Microbial dynamics of persistent purulent otitis media in children.	*Objective:* To investigate the flora of patients with acute otitis media and spontaneous perforation of the tympanic membrane who were unresponsive to initial antibiotic therapy *Findings:* Penicillin-resistant organisms were isolated in all seven cases.
Johnson, et al. (1995) Severe retinopathy of prematurity in infants with birth weights less than 1250 grams: Incidence and outcome of treatment with pharmacologic serum levels of vitamin E in addition to cryotherapy from 1985 to 1991.	*Objective:* To determine the effect of vitamin E prophylaxis and treatment on the sequelae of severe retinopathy of prematurity (ROP) in infants treated with cryotherapy *Findings:* Severe ROP developed in 22 of 450 infants who were alive at 3 months. The combination of vitamin E and cryotherapy appeared to decrease the severity of ROP.
Kleinman, et al. (1994) The medical appropriateness of tympanostomy tubes proposed for children younger than 16 years in the United States.	*Objective:* To describe clinical reasons that tympanostomy (or T) tubes are proposed for children and to assess their appropriateness *Findings:* About one fourth of T-tube insertions were proposed for inappropriate indications, and another one third for equivocal indications.

Continued

Study	*Objective and Findings*
Rosenfeld, et al. (1994) Clinical efficacy of antimicrobial drugs for acute otitis media: Meta-analysis of 5400 children from thirty-three randomized trials.	*Objective:* To reconcile conflicting reports about the comparative efficacy of antimicrobial drugs for acute otitis media (AOM) in children *Findings:* Drugs have a modest but significant impact on the primary control of AOM. The spontaneous rate of resolution of AOM, without antibiotics or tympanocentesis, was 81%.
Zadnik, et al. (1994) The effect of parental history of myopia on children's eye size.	*Objective:* To evaluate whether eye size and shape are different in children based on their parental history of myopia *Findings:* Even before the onset of juvenile myopia, children of myopic parents have longer eyes. Risk is greatest for those with two myopic parents.
Cleeland, et al. (1994) Pain and its treatment in outpatients with metastatic cancer.	*Objective:* To assess the adequacy of prescribed analgesic drugs using World Health Organization guidelines *Findings:* 42% of patients did not receive adequate analgesia.

rect invasion of human immunodeficiency virus or may be the result of opportunistic infection, often with cytomegalovirus. Infarcts of the neural layer are common with **retinitis** and may lead to retinal detachment.

Clinical Manifestations. The manifestations of retinopathy are limited to the eye and the visual sense and depend on the degree of retinal damage. Early signs are detected with funduscopic (ophthalmoscopic) examination, in which the retina is directly examined under magnification by a light shined through the dilated pupil. Hemorrhages, aneurysms, atherosclerosis, vascular overgrowth, infarcts, and exudates may be visible before any detectable loss of visual acuity is experienced. Visual acuity is referenced to a normal of 20/20, meaning that the patient sees at 20 feet what a "normal" person sees at 20 feet. *Legal blindness* is defined as 20/200. *Ambulatory blindness* (loss of visual acuity to the extent that vision can no longer guide ambulation) is defined as 20/800.[30] Loss of visual acuity may occur with lesions of the optic nerve, occipital cortex, or visual pathways as well as with retinopathy. In the case of retinal detachment due to formation of holes or tears, the patient may perceive flashing lights or "floaters"—bright spots in the field of vision, or a "curtain" going down over a portion of the visual field. Funduscopic examination reveals grayness or opacity of the detached region (see Color Fig. 23–8).

Prevention and Treatment. Secondary retinopathy may be prevented with risk reduction measures and optimal treatment of diabetes, prematurity, atherosclerosis, hypertension, and AIDS. Retinal hemorrhages and aneurysms may be repaired with laser photocoagulation or ablation of damaged or hypervascular areas of the retina. Retinal detachment is traditionally treated surgically with scleral buckling, in which the sclera and choroid are folded in under retinal holes and secured with silicone straps. More recently, retinal detachment has been treated with pneumatic retinopexy, involving injection of a gas bubble to tamponade retinal holes while subretinal fluid reabsorbs. Laser photocoagulation is used to close the defects.[31]

Prognosis and Outcome. Prognosis is variable depending on the cause and degree of retinopathy. Timely treatment may reduce the severity, but some loss in acuity nearly always occurs and is permanent.

Cataracts

Definition. A cataract is an opacity of the lens (see Color Fig. 23–9). Cataracts may be congenital or acquired.

Epidemiology. About 5 to 10 million people in the United States become visually disabled each year because of cataracts.[34] Most cataracts are associated with advancing age and are known as *senile cataracts*. Nearly all people older than 70 years have some degree of cataract formation.[35] *Congenital cataracts* may be hereditary or may result from prenatal toxicity. A number of genetic, traumatic, inflammatory, and metabolic disorders are also associated with cataract formation (Table 23–15).

Etiology. The precise etiologic mechanism leading to lens opacification is uncertain and may vary with different forms. The defect lies in abnormal biochemical reactions and transport within the lens. With aging, protein aggregation and oxidative injury are evident, along with increased pigmentation in the central region (nucleus) of the lens. With trauma, rupture of the lens capsule may lead to phagocytosis of lens material or to chronic inflammation. Foreign bodies within the lens may also lead to inflammation and opacity. Diabetic cataract is uncommon but may occur in patients with poorly controlled type 1 diabetes. In this type, the opacity is bilateral and of rapid onset. In these cases, excess glucose in the lens is reduced by the enzyme aldose reductase to its alcohol, sorbitol, which accumulates. Excess water is absorbed along the osmotic gradient created by sorbitol.[34]

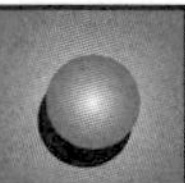

TABLE 23–15
CONDITIONS ASSOCIATED WITH CATARACT FORMATION

CATARACT WITH SYSTEMIC DISORDER
Generalized
Intrauterine infection (rubella, cytomegalovirus, toxoplasmosis)
Retinal pigmented epithelium degeneration
Systemic infection
Cutaneous
Atopic dermatitis
Ectodermal dysplasia
Metabolic
Diabetes mellitus
Galactosemia
Hypocalcemia
Fabry's disease
Glucose-6-phosphatase deficiency
Chromosomal Abnormality
Down syndrome
Marfan syndrome
CATARACT WITHOUT SYSTEMIC DISORDER
Otherwise Healthy Eye
Senile cataract
Many congenital cataracts
Combined With Other Ocular Disorders
Congenital defects (microphthalmia, coloboma, aniridia)
Glaucoma
Uveitis
Retinal detachment
Myopia
Ocular neoplasm
Retinopathy of prematurity
Ocular toxicity (corticosteroids, phenothiazines)
Ocular trauma

Adapted from Newell, F.W. (1996). *Ophthalmology: Principles and Concepts.* (8th ed.). St. Louis: Mosby–Year Book. (p. 370).

Pathophysiology. The lens typically becomes swollen at first, then dehydrated. Cataracts develop through four stages of decreasing opacity of the lens: (1) immature cataracts, which allow some vision because opacity is not complete; (2) mature or "ripe" cataracts, which are completely opaque and severely impair vision; (3) intumescent cataracts, in which the lens is swollen with water, often resulting in glaucoma because of obstructed outflow of intraocular fluid; and (4) hypermature cataracts, in which lens proteins break down, leaking peptides through the lens capsule.[34] These peptides undergo phagocytosis and may also contribute to intraocular fluid obstruction and glaucoma.

Clinical Manifestations. Visual acuity decreases gradually, although there is no pain or inflammation in the eye. Transient double vision (diplopia) in one eye may occur as a result of splitting of light by the lens opacity, and lights may appear to be surrounded by a colored halo. Vision is improved in dim lighting at first, as the pupil dilates. Fixed spots in the visual field and a temporary improvement in vision are also typical as the cataract develops.[34] Cataracts are apparent on funduscopic examination because of absence of the *red reflex,* a reflection of the vascular retinal grounds that causes the pupil to appear red (as often accidentally captured on flash photographs). Further inspection of the lens reveals the opacity (see Color Fig. 23–9).

Prevention and Treatment. Congenital and metabolic cataracts may be prevented with reduction of prenatal risk factors and optimal management of conditions such as diabetes mellitus. Removal of toxins may prevent or reverse cataract development in some cases. There is no known prevention of senile cataracts. Cataracts are usually treated surgically by removal of the entire lens and its capsule (intracapsular extraction) or by removal of the anterior lens capsule, nucleus, and cortex, with retention of the posterior capsule (extracapsular extraction). The latter method is generally preferred because it provides more support for an implanted lens. Removal of the lens results in markedly reduced refractive power **(aphakia)**, which may then be treated with eyeglasses, an implanted artificial lens, a contact lens, or corneal surgery.

Prognosis and Outcome. Surgical treatment is successful in most cases. Postoperative glaucoma is common for the first 24 to 72 hours, but this usually responds to medical management. Patients have an increased risk of retinal detachment for the first year after the procedure. About 35% of patients with congenital cataracts have an associated eye defect that impairs vision, even after successful surgery.[34]

Glaucoma

Definition. Glaucoma encompasses a group of disorders characterized by progressive damage to the optic nerve, with a characteristic loss of vision.[36] Types of glaucoma include open-angle (70% of cases), angle-closure, secondary, congenital, and childhood forms. The angle of reference is the *iridic angle,* the angle formed by the iris and lens at the corner of the anterior chamber (see Fig. 23–12).

Epidemiology. An estimated 2 million people in the United States have glaucoma; half of these cases are undiagnosed.[37] Risk factors for open-angle glaucoma include increased intraocular fluid pressure, aging, black race, severe myopia, and a family history. Concurrent illnesses, including cardiovascular disease, diabetes mellitus, migraine headaches, and vasospasm, are also associated with increased risk.[36, 37] Angle-closure glaucoma is more prevalent in people with narrow iridic angles (e.g., Asians, Eskimos, and hyperopic people), in the elderly, and in those with a familial predisposition.[36] Trauma or surgery of the eye, **uveitis,** diabetic retinopathy, venous occlusion, and long-term steroid use may predispose to edematous obstruction of intraocular fluid outflow, which may result in secondary glaucoma. In primary congenital glaucoma, an abnormality of the trabecular meshwork results in increased intraocular fluid pressure. About 10% of cases are inherited through an autosomal recessive pattern, but most congenital glaucomas demonstrate multifactorial inheritance.[34]

Etiology. Theoretically, glaucoma results from an imbalance between intraocular fluid production and outflow. Primary open-angle glaucoma occurs in the absence of a known cause of either increased production or obstructed outflow. There may be increased resistance to flow of aqueous humor through the trabecular meshwork, resulting in gradually increasing intraocular fluid pressure and damage to the optic nerve head. In cases in which the iridic angle is anatomically narrow, acute onset of glaucoma may occur if pupil dilation (due to contraction of iridic muscles) further narrows the angle, obstructing outflow of intraocular fluid. In some cases, glaucomatous damage occurs in people with normal angle *and* normal intraocular fluid pressure.

Pathophysiology. Two mechanisms have been proposed to account for optic nerve damage in glaucoma. The *vascular theory* holds that increased intraocular fluid pressure may inhibit perfusion of the optic nerve and retina, resulting in ischemic damage. The level of pressure resulting in optic nerve injury is known to vary among patients. The *mechanical theory* suggests that mechanical distortion and displacement of the lamina cribrosa, the sieve-like structure that bridges the posterior opening through which the optic nerve leaves the eye, causes damage to axons of the nerve.[37]

Clinical Manifestations. Elevation of intraocular fluid pressure is common but not essential to the diagnosis of glaucoma. More than half of patients have normal pressure readings (10 to 21 mm Hg).[34] Acute attacks of closed-angle glaucoma are painful, but the more common open-angle type is painless. Visual impairment may take various forms, including blurring and seeing halos around objects. The most typical pattern is loss of peripheral vision, occurring so gradually that it is not noticed until far advanced. Funduscopic examination reveals a cupped disk, thinning of the neuroretinal rim, occasional disk hemorrhages, and pallor of remaining neural tissue (see Color Fig. 23–3). Progressive optic nerve damage may lead to blindness if the condition is not treated.

Prevention and Treatment. Because the onset of glaucoma is insidious in most cases, routine funduscopic examination and screening of intraocular fluid pressure is warranted as a means of early detection. Medical treatment is aimed at lowering pressure and involves instillation of eye drops, including miotics (e.g., pilocarpine) to constrict the pupil and maintain the iridic angle, and β-blockers (e.g., timolol) or carbonic anhydrase inhibitors (e.g., acetazolamide) to reduce intraocular fluid production. Laser therapy applied to the trabecular meshwork increases aqueous outflow, although the precise mechanism is unknown. Surgical therapy (glaucoma filtration treatment) is based on the creation of additional outflow channels for intraocular fluid.

Prognosis and Outcome. If detected and treated early, optic nerve injury and vision loss may be minimized. An estimated one third of patients fail to comply with medical treatment, reducing its effectiveness. Laser and surgical treatment substantially reduce pressure in 75% of patients, but 50% of these have recurrence within 5 years.[37] Glaucomatous injury to the optic nerve is irreversible.

Otitis Media

Definition. Otitis media is inflammation of the middle ear. Two clinical forms are recognized: acute otitis media (AOM), and otitis media with effusion (OME).

Epidemiology. Otitis media is the most common diagnosis of childhood and the second most common diagnosis in medical practice.[38] Two thirds of children in the United States are affected before the age of 2 years. Risk declines significantly after the age of 5 years because of development of the immune system and normal changes in the angle, shape, and function of the eustachian tube. General risk factors for AOM are upper respiratory infection, which precedes most cases, and abnormal eustachian tube function, which contributes to recurrent forms. Other risk factors include male gender, history of otitis in siblings, bottle feeding, group day care, exposure to tobacco smoke, family history of allergy, and Native American or Eskimo race.[39] OME is also seen in adults, usually after pressure-induced trauma to the tympanic membrane.

Etiology. In AOM, an upper respiratory infection is the source of organisms that ascend the eustachian tube to the middle ear. This process is facilitated by a pressure gradient (middle ear pressure negative to pharyngeal) that develops with crying, nose-blowing, or swallowing when the nose is obstructed with secretions. The usual causative organisms are bacteria, with *Streptococcus pneumoniae, Haemophilus influenzae,* and *Moraxella catarrhalis* accounting for most cases.[40] In OME, the primary cause is chronic blockage of the eustachian tube. This blockage may be functional, due to immature cartilage development leading to ease of collapse of the tube, or mechanical, due to inflammation, obstructive adenoids, barotrauma, or tumor. Blockage of the tube impairs drainage from the middle ear and results in negative pressure development when trapped air is reabsorbed.

Pathophysiology. Middle ear fluid accumulation, or effusion, is present in both forms. In AOM, the effusion is composed of purulent inflammatory exudate (Color Fig. 23–11). In OME, the effusion is nonpurulent (Color Fig. 23–12). Middle ear pressure impedes vibration of the tympanic membrane and ossicles and may rupture the tympanic membrane. An inflammatory process is present in either case, and recurrent inflammation may lead to scarring and fixation of middle ear structures. Inflammation may extend to surrounding lymph nodes, bony structures (e.g., **mastoiditis**), or rarely, to the meninges or other intracranial structures.

Clinical Manifestations. Acute forms are accompanied by manifestations of upper respiratory infection (see Chapter 18). AOM is acutely painful because of stretching of the tympanic membrane, and young children often demonstrate their discomfort by pulling at the ear, irritability, and restlessness. Hearing loss may be evident. Chronic forms are usually not as painful because the membrane apparently becomes more distensible. Internal examination with an otoscope reveals variable signs of inflammation, including redness of the membrane, bulging due to middle ear fluid (with a possible fluid level visible behind the membrane), possible drainage of exudate through tympanic membrane perforations, or in recurrent cases, retraction of the membrane over the ossicles because of scarring. With chronic inflammation and perforation of the tympanic membrane, cystic lesions known as **cholesteatomas** may develop in rare cases as a result of ingrowth of epithelial cells into the middle ear. These lesions may enlarge to the point at which they erode the ossicles and inner ear structures.

Prevention and Treatment. Management of otitis media is a matter of some controversy. AOM is usually treated with appropriate antibiotic therapy, but there is a growing body of evidence that these drugs have only a modest effect on resolution in most cases[41] (see Focus of Current Research). In most uncomplicated cases, the inflammatory response is apparently sufficient, and nonessential use of such drugs may increase the development of resistant strains of microorganisms (see Chapter 13). Analgesics and antipyretics may be used to ease discomfort and limit fever. Tympanocentesis, the surgical incision of the tympanic membrane to facilitate drainage of the effusion, is also controversial. Simple incision (myringotomy) or insertion of indwelling drainage tubes (tympanoplasty, or T, tubes) is commonly done. In 1988, about 670,000 of these operations were done in the United States, although the effectiveness of the procedure in reducing the frequency of recurrent attacks and in minimizing hearing loss is questionable.[38] Surgical removal of the adenoids (adenoidectomy) nearly always results in clinical improvement when enlargement of these lymphatic tissues compresses the eustachian tube. Surgical removal of lymphatic tissues is controversial, however (see Chapter 18).

Prognosis and Outcome. Hearing loss associated with acute attacks of otitis media is usually temporary, with auditory acuity returning to normal after resolution of the episode. Recurrent otitis may result in some degree of permanent conductive loss, and this may impair cognitive and social development of children. Extension of middle ear infection to the mastoid or intracranial structures is uncommon.

Otosclerosis

Definition. Otosclerosis is a genetic disorder in which focal areas of the bony capsule of the inner ear remodel and harden.[42]

Epidemiology. Severe otosclerosis is uncommon, and the disorder is usually inherited as an autosomal dominant trait with variable penetrance. Mild otosclerosis has been common in young to middle-aged adults, although its incidence is declining.

Etiology. The specific mechanism producing bony overgrowth is unknown. Apparently, there is an imbalance between normal bone formation and bone resorption (see Chapter 34).

Pathophysiology. Abnormal bone may fuse the stapes to the oval window, limiting the mobility of these structures. The degree of immobilization determines the degree of conductive hearing loss. Usually, both ears are equally affected.

Clinical Manifestations. Otosclerosis causes slowly progressive hearing loss over several decades.

Prevention and Treatment. There is no known prevention for this condition. Surgical reconstruction or prosthetic replacement of the ossicles may restore mobility of the stapes and oval window to some extent.

Prognosis and Outcome. If untreated, severe otosclerosis leads to marked conductive hearing loss. The outcome of surgical reconstructive procedures is usually positive.

CLINICAL SIGNIFICANCE OF SENSORY DISORDERS

Sensory disturbance is a component of many traumatic and degenerative disorders of the nervous system, with head injury, spinal cord injury, and CNS tumors or cerebrovascular disorders often resulting in permanent abnormality or loss of all somatic sensation in a part of the body. The phenomenon of pain is associated with all mechanisms of cellular injury and with disorders of all body systems. Pain may be present even in the absence of demonstrable pathology. The impact of chronic pain syndromes on productivity and quality of life is inestimable, and management of acute pain is one of the foremost challenges of the health care professions. Research aimed at clarification of the mechanisms of pain and its modulation by physiologic, psychological, or pharmacologic means is ongoing.

Disorders of the special senses are, with few exceptions, not life-threatening. Loss of vision and hearing have a profound impact on quality of life, however. Research in this area is primarily focused on molecular mechanisms of sensation and evaluation of experimental forms of therapy.

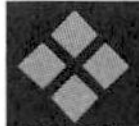

Summary of Key Points

- Accurate, appropriate motor activity is dependent on the integration of sensory information. The somatic sensory system provides information about the current status of the body through the senses of touch, pain, temperature, vibration, and proprioception. The special senses of vision, hearing, taste, and smell provide information about the status of the environment.
- The essential components of the sensory functional unit are the sensory receptor, afferent sensory nerve fiber, dorsal root ganglion, efferent sensory nerve fiber, and a synapse with another nerve or end organ.
- The DCML pathway ascends along the dorsal horns of the cord, crosses at the medulla, and ascends to the thalamus along the medial lemniscus tract to the primary sensory cortex. Its nerves are large and myelinated, permitting rapid transmission. The DCML mediates the delicate and discrete sensations of light touch, vibration, and proprioception. The anterolateral pathway has anterior (spinothalamic) and posterior (spinoreticular) divisions that cross at the dorsal horns and ascend to the thalamus and reticular formations, respectively. These tracts mediate pain, temperature, heavy touch, and complex sensations, such as tickle and itch and sexual sensation.
- Ascending somatic sensory impulses are received and localized in the primary sensory cortex in the parietal lobe. Perception of these impulses requires integration in adjacent sensory association areas. The special senses are mediated by the visual cortex in the occipital lobe, the auditory cortex in the temporal lobe and surrounding auditory association areas, the gustatory cortex, the olfactory bulb, and the olfactory cortex.
- Four principal theories of pain have been proposed. The specificity theory holds that pain sensation requires activation of specific pain receptors, ascending transmission along

Continued

dedicated pain pathways, and perception by specific cortical pain areas. The pattern theory proposes that pain may also occur as a result of high-intensity stimulation of any type of sensory receptor. The gate control theory proposes that simultaneous transmission along a pain pathway and another sensory pathway closes an interneuronal "gate" between them, resulting in perception of the nonpain stimulus only. The neuromatrix theory holds that all sensation, including pain, is imprinted by processes in the brain that can be triggered by sensory input but that are not dependent on such input.

- The proprioceptive system depends on somatic sensory input by the DCML to provide information about the position of the muscles and joints. The vestibular system of the inner ear and brain stem provides data about head position. The cerebellum receives inputs from both the DCML and vestibular system and functions in the continuous comparison of actual and intended motor outputs, fine-tuning the accuracy of motor activity related to position.

- Vision is mediated by three processes: refraction, the photochemical cascade, and visual reflexes. Refraction, the bending of light as it passes at an angle through eye structures of different densities, normally focuses the image sharply on the retina. Rod and cone receptors transduce the light signal to neural signals by the photochemical cascade, a series of chemical transformations of receptor visual pigments that open membrane channels in neurons. Visual reflexes are mediated by cranial nerves and, like motor reflexes, are potentially integrated at higher cortical levels. Visual interpretation depends on inputs from the motor cortex, RAS, and limbic system.

- The conversion of sound energy to action potentials first depends on conductive processes, which include conduction of sound waves through air to the tympanic membrane and amplification of membrane vibrations by the middle ear ossicles connected to the oval window. Oscillating movement of the oval and round windows results in cyclic fluid movement detected by hair cell receptors in the organ of Corti. The sensorineural mechanisms of hearing require that these mechanoreceptors transduce the movement to action potentials, which are conducted along the cochlear branch of cranial nerve VIII to the auditory areas of the cortex.

- Intact gustatory and olfactory sensations are necessary for protection and for complete appreciation of the range of environmental experience. Clinical disorders of chemosensation are believed to be common and may be associated with neurotrauma, neoplasia, drug effects, and genetic defects.

- Disorders of the senses manifest as increased, decreased, or abnormally triggered sensation as well as alteration of related motor activity. Sensory neuropathies and pain syndromes are common components of systemic disorders. Disorders of the special senses are also common and may significantly impact human function. Treatment modalities in sensory disorders are aimed at resolution of underlying systemic diseases, compensation for sensory losses, and minimization of distressing sensory abnormalities such as vertigo and pain.

REFERENCES

1. Jacox, A., Carr, D.B., and Payne, R. (1994). New clinical-practice guidelines for the management of pain in patients with cancer. *New England Journal of Medicine* 330(9), 651–655.
2. Guyton, A.C., and Hall, J.E. (1996). *Textbook of Medical Physiology*. (9th ed.). Philadelphia: W.B. Saunders. (pp. 583–584, 587, 603).
3. Melzack, R. (1993). Pain: Past, present, and future. *Canadian Journal of Experimental Psychology* 47(4), 615–629.
4. Woolf, C.J. (1994). A new strategy for the treatment of inflammatory pain. *Drugs* 47 (suppl. 5), 1–9.
5. Markenson, J.A. (1996). Mechanisms of chronic pain. *American Journal of Medicine* 101 (suppl. 1A), 6S–18S.
6. Kandel, E.R., and Schwartz, J.H. (1985). *Principles of Neural Science*. (2nd ed.). New York: Elsevier Science Publishing. (pp. 295–296).
7. Black, J.M., and Matassarin-Jacobs, E. (1997). *Textbook of Medical-Surgical Nursing: Clinical Management for Continuity of Care.* Philadelphia: W.B. Saunders. (pp. 929, 976).
8. Lagnado, L., and Baylor, D.A. (1994). Calcium controls light-triggered formation of catalytically active rhodopsin. *Nature* 367, 273–277.
9. Hunt, D.M., Dulai, K.S., Bowmaker, J.K., *et al.* (1995). The chemistry of John Dalton's color blindness. *Science* 267, 984–988.
10. NIH Consensus Development Panel on Cochlear Implants in Adults and Children. (1995). Cochlear implants in adults and children. *Journal of the American Medical Association.* 274(24), 1955–1961.
11. Davidson, T.M., Murphy, C., and Jalowayski, A.A. (1995). Smell impairment: Can it be reversed? *Postgraduate Medicine* 98(1), 107–118.
12. Axel, R. (1995). The molecular logic of smell. *Scientific American* October, 154–159.
13. Richardson, J.K., and Ashton-Miller, J.A. (1996). Peripheral neuropathy: An often-overlooked cause of falls in the elderly. *Postgraduate Medicine* 99(6), 161–172.

14. Kumar, K.L., and Cooney, T.G. (1995). Headaches. *Medical Clinics of North America* 79(2), 261–286.
15. Trachtenberg, D.E. (1994). Tension headaches: Relieving pain without creating dependence. *Postgraduate Medicine* 95(6), 44–56.
16. Hoffert, M.J. (1994). Treatment of migraine: A new era. *American Family Physician* 49(3), 633–638.
17. Plosker, G.L., and McTavish, D. (1994). Sumatriptan: A reappraisal of its pharmacology and therapeutic efficacy in the treatment of migraine and cluster headache. *Drugs* 47(4), 622–651.
18. Maizels, M., Scott, B., Cohen, W., *et al.* (1996). Intranasal lidocaine for treatment of migraine. *Journal of the American Medical Association* 276(4), 319–321.
19. Wipf, J.E., and Deyo, R.A. (1995). Low back pain. *Medical Clinics of North America* 79(2), 231–246.
20. Margo, K. (1994). Diagnosis, treatment and prognosis in patients with low back pain. *American Family Physician* 49(1), 171–179.
21. Gilmer, H.S., Papadopoulos, S.M., and Tuite, G.F. (1993). Lumbar disk disease: Pathophysiology, management and prevention. *American Family Physician* 47(5), 1141–1152.
22. Wheeler, A.H. (1995). Diagnosis and management of low back pain and sciatica. *American Family Physician* 52(5), 1333–1341.
23. Whitley, J.M., and McDonnell, D.E. (1995). Carpal tunnel syndrome: A guide to prompt intervention. *Postgraduate Medicine* 97(1), 89–96.
24. Stevens, J.C., Beard, C.M., O'Fallon, W.M., *et al.* (1992). Conditions associated with carpal tunnel syndrome. *Mayo Clinic Proceedings* 67, 541–548.
25. Miller, B.K. (1993). Carpal tunnel syndrome: A frequently misdiagnosed common hand problem. *Nurse Practitioner* 18(12), 52–56.
26. McConaghy, D.J. (1994). Trigeminal neuralgia: A personal review and nursing implications. *Journal of Neuroscience Nursing* 26(2), 85–90.
27. Knox, G.W., and McPherson, A. (1997). Meniere's disease: Differential diagnosis and treatment. *American Family Physician* 55(4), 1185–1190.
28. Barker, E. (1994). *Neuroscience Nursing.* St. Louis: Mosby–Year Book. (p. 460).
29. Adams, R.D., and Victor, M. (1993). *Principles of Neurology.* (5th ed.). New York: McGraw-Hill. (pp. 263–265).
30. Neatherlin, J.S., and Egan, J. (1994). Benign paroxysmal positional vertigo. *Journal of Neuroscience Nursing* 26(6), 330–335.
31. D'Amico, D.J. (1994). Diseases of the retina. *New England Journal of Medicine* 331(2), 95–106.
32. Phelps, D.L. (1993). Retinopathy of prematurity. *Pediatric Clinics of North America* 40(4), 705–714.
33. Seddon, J.M., Willett, W.C., Speizer, F.E., *et al.* (1996). A prospective study of cigarette smoking and age-related macular degeneration in women. *Journal of the American Medical Association* 276(14), 1141–1146.
34. Newell, F.W. (1992). *Ophthalmology: Principles and Concepts.* (7th ed.). St. Louis: Mosby–Year Book. (pp. 81, 358, 368–389).
35. Walter, J.B. (1992). *An Introduction to the Principles of Disease.* (3rd ed.). Philadelphia: W.B. Saunders. (p. 598).
36. Chaudhry, I., and Wong, S. (1996). Recognizing glaucoma: A guide for the primary care physician. *Postgraduate Medicine* 99(5), 247–264.
37. Liesegang, T.J. (1996). Glaucoma: Changing concepts and future directions. *Mayo Clinic Proceedings* 71, 689–694.
38. Kleinman, L.C., Kosecoff, J., Dubois, R.W., *et al.* (1994). The medical appropriateness of tympanostomy tubes proposed for children younger than 16 years in the United States. *Journal of the American Medical Association* 271(16), 1250–1255.
39. Swanson, J.A., and Hoeker, J.L. (1996). Otitis media in young children. *Mayo Clinic Proceedings* 71, 179–183.
40. Barnett, E.D., and Klein, J.O. (1995). The problem of resistant bacteria for the management of acute otitis media. *Pediatric Clinics of North America* 42(3), 509–517.
41. Rosenfeld, R.M., Vertrees, J.E., Carr, J., *et al.* (1994). Clinical efficacy of antimicrobial drugs for acute otitis media: Metaanalysis of 5400 children from thirty-three randomized trials. *Journal of Pediatrics* 124(3), 355–367.
42. Ruckenstein, M.J. (1995). Hearing loss: A plan for individualized management. *Postgraduate Medicine* 98(4), 197–214.

SELECTED BIBLIOGRAPHY

Allegrante, J.P. (1996). The role of adjunctive therapy in the management of chronic nonmalignant pain. *American Journal of Medicine* 101 (suppl. 1A), 33S–39S.

Aniansson, G., Alm, B., Andersson, B., *et al.* (1994). A prospective cohort study on breast-feeding and otitis media in Swedish infants. *Pediatric Infectious Disease Journal* 13(3), 183–188.

Bargmann, C.I. (1994). Molecular mechanisms of mechanosensation? *Cell* 78, 729–731.

Berman, S. (1995). Otitis media in children. *New England Journal of Medicine* 332(23), 1560–1565.

Blackburn, S.T., and Loper, D.L. (1992). *Maternal, Fetal, and Neonatal Physiology: A Clinical Perspective.* Philadelphia: W.B. Saunders.

Bracker, M.D., and Ralph, L.P. (1995). The numb arm and hand. *American Family Physician* 51(1), 103–116.

Brook, I., and Frazier, E.H. (1996). Microbial dynamics of persistent purulent otitis media in children. *Journal of Pediatrics* 128(2), 237–240.

Carter, T.L. (1994). Age-related vision changes: A primary care guide. *Geriatrics* 49(9), 37–47.

Casey, K.L. (1996). Match and mismatch: Identifying the neuronal determinants of pain. *Annals of Internal Medicine* 124(11), 995–998.

Christen, W.G., Glynn, R.J., Manson, J.E., *et al.* (1996). A prospective study of cigarette smoking and risk of age-related macular degeneration in men. *Journal of the American Medical Association* 276(14), 1147–1151.

Clark, J.B.F., Queener, S.F., and Karb, V.B. (1993). *Pharmacologic Basis of Nursing Practice.* (4th ed.). St. Louis: Mosby–Year Book.

Cleeland, C.S., Gonin, R., Hatfield, A.K., *et al.* (1994). Pain and its treatment in outpatients with metastatic cancer. *New England Journal of Medicine* 330(9), 592–596.

Daniels, J.M. (1997). Treatment of occupationally acquired low back pain. *American Family Physician* 55(2), 596–597.

Dawson, D.M. (1993). Entrapment neuropathies of the upper extremities. *New England Journal of Medicine* 329(27), 2013–2018.

The Diabetes Control and Complications Trial Research Group. (1995). The effect of intensive diabetes therapy on the development and progression of neuropathy. *Annals of Internal Medicine* 122(8), 561–568.

Downs, D.G. (1997). Nonspecific work-related upper extremity disorders. *American Family Physician* 55(4), 1296–1302.

Escalante, A. (1993). Ankylosing spondylitis: A common cause of low back pain. *Postgraduate Medicine* 94(1), 153–166.

Franks, N.P., and Lieb, W.R. (1994). Molecular and cellular mechanisms of general anesthesia. *Nature* 367, 607–614.

French, A.S. (1992). Mechanotransduction. *Annual Review of Physiology* 54, 135–152.

Friendly, D.S. (1993). Development of vision in infants and young children. *Pediatric Clinics of North America* 40(4), 693–703.

Froehling, D.A., Silverstein, M.D., Mohr, D.N., *et al.* (1994). Does this patient have a serious form of vertigo? *Journal of the American Medical Association* 271(5), 385–388.

Guyton, A.C., and Hall, J.E. (1996). *Textbook of Medical Physiology.* (9th ed.). Philadelphia: W.B. Saunders.

Johnson, L., Quinn, G.E., Abbasi, S., *et al.* (1995). Severe retinopathy of prematurity in infants with birth weights less than 1250 grams: Incidence and outcome of treatment with pharmacologic serum levels of vitamin E in addition to cryotherapy from 1985 to 1991. *Journal of Pediatrics* 127(4), 632–639.

Katz, R.T. (1994). Carpal tunnel syndrome: A practical review. *American Family Physician* 49(6), 1371–1379.

Katz, W.A. (1996). Approach to the management of nonmalignant pain. *American Journal of Medicine* 101 (suppl. 1A), 54S–63S.

Kennedy, D., and Barter, R. (1994). Outpatient care of the headache client: A challenging specialty. *Journal of Neuroscience Nursing* 26(2), 73–77.

King, R.A. (1993). Common ocular signs and symptoms in childhood. *Pediatric Clinics of North America* 40(4), 753–766.

Lazaro, L., and Quinet, R.J. (1994). Low back pain: How to make the diagnosis in the older patient. *Geriatrics* 49(9), 48–53.

Levy, M.H. (1996). Pharmacologic treatment of cancer pain. *New England Journal of Medicine* 335(15), 1124–1132.

Malmivaara, A., Hakkinen, U., Aro, T., *et al.* (1995). The treatment of acute low back pain: Bed rest, exercises, or ordinary activity? *New England Journal of Medicine* 332(6), 351–355.

McClaflin, R.R. (1994). Myofascial pain syndrome: Primary care strategies for early intervention. *Postgraduate Medicine* 96(2), 56–73.

Mirza, N. (1996). Otitis externa: Management in the primary care office. *Postgraduate Medicine* 99(5), 153–158.

Mogil, J.S., Sternberg, W.F., Marek, P., *et al.* (1996). The genetics of pain and pain inhibition. *Proceedings of the National Academy of Sciences, U.S.A.* 93, 3048–3055.

Montauk, S.L., and Martin, J. (1997). Treating chronic pain. *American Family Physician* 55(4), 1151–1160.

Moore, K.L., and Persaud, T.V.N. (1993). *The Developing Human: Clinically Oriented Embryology.* (5th ed.). Philadelphia: W.B. Saunders.

Mott, A.E., and Leopold, D.A. (1991). Disorders in taste and smell. *Medical Clinics of North America* 75(6), 1321–1353.

Ostrowski, V.B., and Wiet, R.J. (1996). Pathologic conditions of the external ear and auditory canal. *Postgraduate Medicine* 100(3), 223–237.

Page, J.M., Schneeweiss, S., Whyte, H.E.A., *et al.* Ocular sequelae in premature infants. *Pediatrics* 92(6), 787–790.

Perkins, A.T., and Ondo, W. (1995). When to worry about headache: Head pain as a clue to intracranial disease. *Postgraduate Medicine* 98(2), 197–208.

Potter, W.S. (1993). Pediatric cataracts. *Pediatric Clinics of North America* 40(4), 841–853.

Quigley, H.A. (1993). Open-angle glaucoma. *New England Journal of Medicine* 328(15), 1097–1106.

Radhakrishnan, K., Ahlskog, E., Garrity, J.A., *et al.* (1994). Idiopathic intracranial hypertension. *Mayo Clinic Proceedings* 69, 169–180.

Raffa, R.B. (1996). A novel approach to the pharmacology of analgesics. *American Journal of Medicine* 101(suppl. 1A), 40S–46S.

Reichel, E. (1995). Vitreoretinal emergencies. *American Family Physician* 52(5), 1415–1419.

Repka, M.X. (1993). Common pediatric neuro-ophthalmologic conditions. *Pediatric Clinics of North America* 40(4), 777–788.

Rook, J.L. (1997). Wound care pain management. *Nurse Practitioner* 22(3), 122–136.

Ruckenstein, M.J. (1995). A practical approach to dizziness: Questions to bring vertigo and other causes into focus. *Postgraduate Medicine* 97(3), 70–81.

Ruoff, G.E. (1993). Headache in elderly patients: How to recognize and manage benign types. *Postgraduate Medicine* 94(8), 109–121.

Schiffman, S. (1994). Changes in taste and smell: Drug interactions and food preferences. *Nutrition Reviews* 52(8), S11–S14.

Shapiro, A.M., and Bluestone, C.D. (1995). Otitis media reassessed: Up-to-date answers to some basic questions. *Postgraduate Medicine* 97(5), 73–82.

Silberstein, S.D. (1995). Migraine and women: The link between headache and hormones. *Postgraduate Medicine* 97(4), 147–153.

Spoelhof, G.D. (1995). When to suspect an acoustic neuroma. *American Family Physician* 52(6), 1768–1774.

Stein, C. (1995). The control of pain in peripheral tissue by opioids. *New England Journal of Medicine* 332(25), 1685–1690.

Stevens, J.C., and Cain, W.S. (1993). Changes in taste and flavor in aging. *Clinical Reviews in Food Science and Nutrition* 33(1), 27–37.

Wagner, R.S. (1993). Glaucoma in children. *Pediatric Clinics of North America* 40(4), 855–867.

Weinstock, F.J., and Weinstock, M.B. (1996). Common eye disorders: Six patients to treat, pitfalls to avoid. *Postgraduate Medicine* 99(4), 119–123.

Weinstock, F.J., and Weinstock, M.B. (1996). Common eye disorders: Six patients to refer. *Postgraduate Medicine* 99(4), 107–116.

Weiss, J. (1993). Assessment and management of the client with headaches. *Nurse Practitioner* 18(4), 46–57.

Weiss, J.C., Yates, G.R., and Quinn, L.D. (1996). Acute otitis media: Making an accurate diagnosis. *American Family Physician* 53(4), 1200–1206.

Wintermeyer, S.M., and Nahata, M.C. (1994). Chronic suppurative otitis media. *Annals of Pharmacotherapy* 28, 1089–1099.

Zadnik, K., Satariano, W.A., Mutti, D.O., *et al.* (1994). The effect of parental history of myopia on children's eye size. *Journal of the American Medical Association* 271(17), 1323–1327.

Unit IX

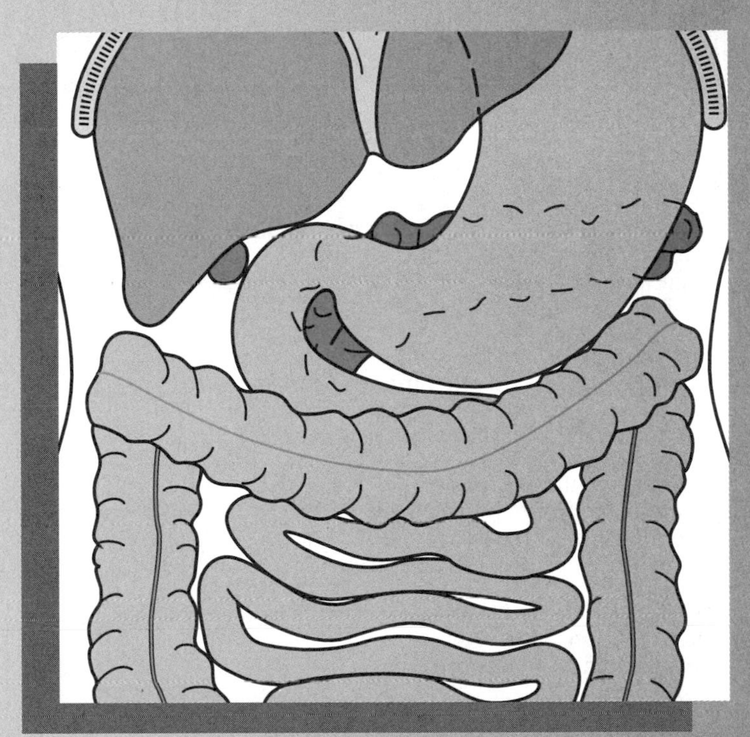

GASTRO-INTESTINAL SYSTEM

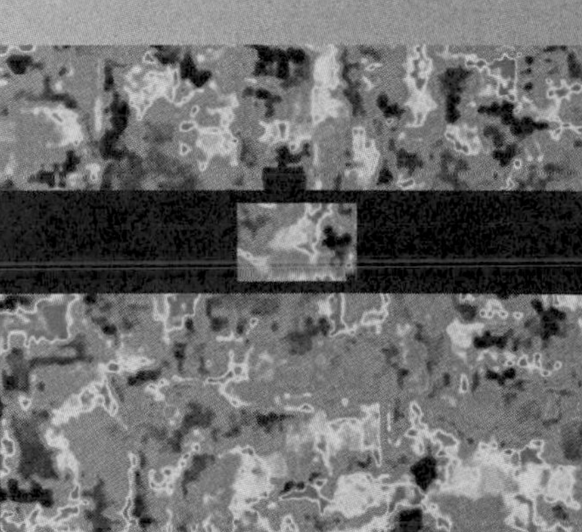

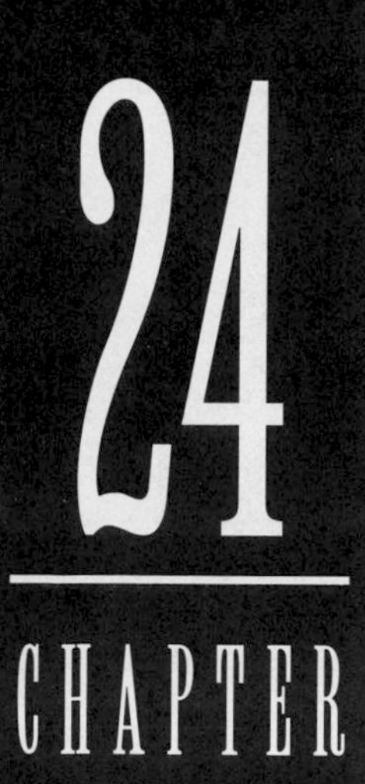

24 CHAPTER Disorders of Gastrointestinal Motility and Secretion

LEARNING OBJECTIVES

1. Identify the principal functions of each component of the gastrointestinal system.
2. Identify the regulatory factors that influence visceral smooth muscle contraction and gastrointestinal motility.
3. Discuss the importance of each type of gastrointestinal motility to gastrointestinal function.
4. Differentiate among the types of gastrointestinal secretion in terms of source and function.
5. Describe the mechanisms of the six most common manifestations of altered gastrointestinal motility and secretion.
6. Comprehend the physiologic basis of the clinical manifestations and treatment of representative disorders of each segment of the alimentary canal.
7. Appreciate the clinical significance of disorders of gastrointestinal motility and secretion.

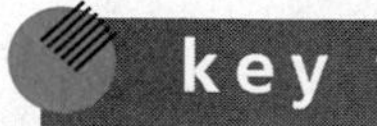

key terms

achalasia
achlorhydria
adhesions
appendicitis
Barrett's metaplasia
bowel obstruction
colorectal cancer
constipation
Crohn's disease (CD)
diarrhea
diverticulitis
diverticulosis

dumping syndrome
dysentery
dysphagia
emesis
eructation
esophageal atresia
esophageal cancer
esophageal varices
esophagitis
fecal incontinence
gastric cancer
gastritis
gastroenteritis
gastroesophageal reflux disease (GERD)
hematemesis
hematochezia
hemorrhoids
hiatal hernia
Hirschsprung's disease
hypertrophic pyloric stenosis (HPS)
inflammatory bowel disease (IBD)
irritable bowel syndrome (IBS)
lower gastrointestinal bleeding
melena
occult bleeding
paralytic ileus
peptic ulcer disease (PUD)
peritonitis
polyps
pseudomembranous colitis
stress ulceration
tracheoesophageal (TE) fistula
ulcerative colitis (UC)
upper gastrointestinal bleeding
Zollinger-Ellison syndrome (ZES)

The gastrointestinal (GI) system consists of the organs of the alimentary canal and the accessory organs that secrete substances into the canal. The canal, extending from the mouth to the anus, functions in the ingestion, digestion, and absorption of the nutrients that supply the energy fuel for all body systems and in the elimination of solid metabolic wastes. The exocrine pancreas, salivary glands, liver, and gallbladder secrete fluids containing enzymes and ions that are essential to the functions of the canal.

It has been said that "the gut is the mirror of the soul," and, indeed, alterations in GI function often reflect stress, anxiety, or depression. GI motility and secretion are dependent on innervation and perfusion as well as endocrine regulation, and numerous disorders of these and other systems may first be seen as alterations in GI function.

In Chapter 25, the mechanisms by which nutrients are ingested, mechanically and chemically degraded, and subsequently absorbed into the blood will be examined, and selected disorders affecting nutrient ingestion, digestion, and absorption will be discussed. Chapter 26 focuses on the structure, function, and common disorders of the liver and biliary systems.

In this chapter, the anatomy and general functions of the alimentary canal will be reviewed, with particular emphasis on mechanisms that govern GI motility and secretion in health and disease. Several clinical syndromes that illustrate abnormal motility and secretion will be examined, including nausea and vomiting, **diarrhea, constipation, fecal incontinence, bowel obstruction,** and gastrointestinal bleeding. Representative disorders of motility and secretion effecting each level of the alimentary canal will also be discussed.

FUNCTIONAL ANATOMY OF THE GASTROINTESTINAL SYSTEM

The GI system is illustrated in Figure 24–1. The alimentary canal begins at the mouth and ends at the anus. A general overview of GI anatomy and function is provided in this section; a more thorough exploration of specific processes may be found in subsequent sections.

Alimentary Canal

Mouth

Gastrointestinal functions of the mouth consist of ingestion (intake of food) and beginning digestion (breakdown of food). Although ingestion and digestion are detailed in other chapters in this unit, it should be noted that motility and secretion are integral to these processes. Contraction of the skeletal muscles of the mandible (jaw) and tongue contributes to the initial digestion of nutrients by mechanically breaking down nutrients and mixing them with saliva. Salivary glands, including the *parotid*, *submandibular*, and *sublingual* glands, secrete saliva into the mouth.

Esophagus

The esophagus functions in deglutition (swallowing) of food from the mouth and propulsion of this food to the stomach. The skeletal muscle of the *upper esophageal sphincter* (UES) first relaxes to permit entry of food, then contracts during deglutition to

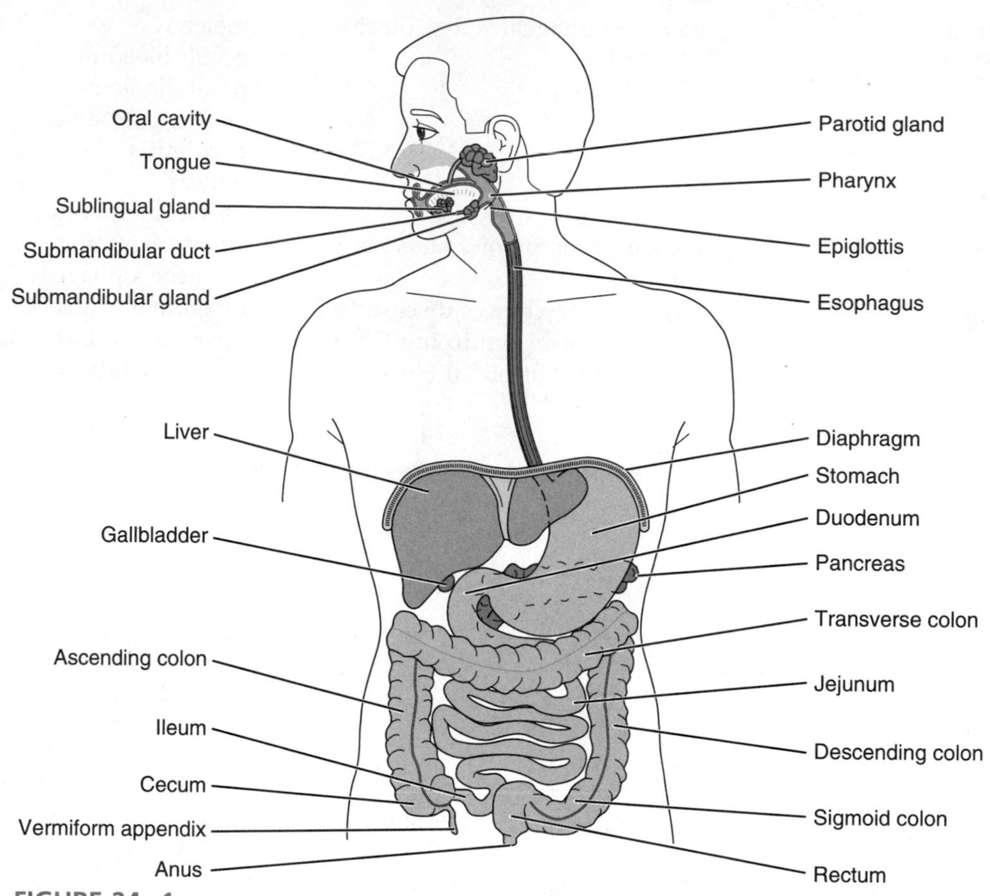

FIGURE 24–1

Gastrointestinal system. The gastrointestinal system includes the alimentary canal (mouth, esophagus, stomach, small intestine, and large intestine) and its associated secretory organs (liver, gallbladder, and pancreas).

propel food downward and prevent its regurgitation into the mouth. The *lower esophageal sphincter* (LES or cardiac sphincter), located at the junction of the esophagus and the upper portion (cardia) of the stomach, is composed of thick longitudinal smooth muscle. This sphincter passes through an opening in the diaphragm known as the *esophageal hiatus.* Relaxation of the LES permits food to pass into the stomach. The LES and the skeletal muscle of the diaphragm in the hiatal region then contract to prevent reflux of food and stomach acids into the lower esophagus.[1]

Stomach

The three anatomic regions of the stomach are the upper *fundus,* middle *body,* and lower *antrum.* The stomach functions primarily in the digestion of food, mechanically via muscle contraction and mixing and chemically via a number of gastric secretions. These secretions are of particular importance in the digestion of proteins, as discussed in Chapter 25. Food that has been mixed and acted on by gastric secretions is known as *chyme.* The stomach also has a limited absorptive function. Water and some dissolved substances may be absorbed from the stomach wall into the blood. The antrum ends in the *pyloric sphincter,* which leads into the small intestine and prevents reflux of intestinal contents into the stomach.

Small Intestine

The small intestine is about 5 m long and consists of the proximal *duodenum,* the middle *jejunum,* and the distal *ileum.* It is this portion of the canal in which digestion is completed and most absorption occurs. Secretions from the liver and pancreas into the duodenum and from intestinal wall cells into the lumen of the gut contain digestive enzymes for the complete breakdown of carbohydrates, proteins, and fats. As the chyme is propelled along the small intestine by smooth muscle contraction, the digested nutrients, along with water, electrolytes, vitamins,

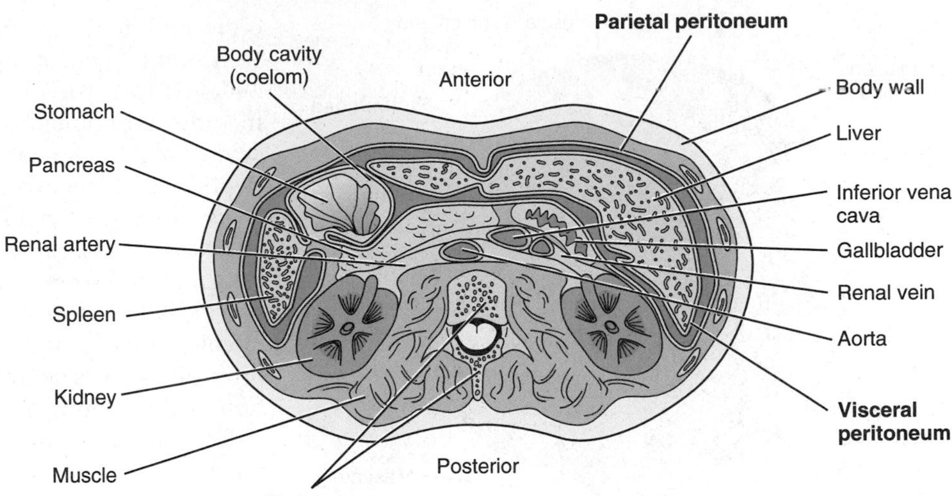

FIGURE 24–2
Peritoneal cavity. The stomach, intestines, and accessory organs of the GI system are contained within the peritoneal cavity. This cavity lies between two layers of membrane: the *parietal peritoneum,* which lines the anterior portion of the abdominal cavity, and the *visceral peritoneum,* which overlies the abdominal organs.

and minerals, are absorbed into the blood. The *ileocecal valve,* which leads from the terminal ileum into the large intestine, functions with other sphincters in promoting directional flow at an optimal rate for absorption of nutrients and water.

Large Intestine

The large intestine is about 1.5 m in length and consists of the proximal *cecum* with its attached *vermiform appendix;* the *colon,* with its ascending, transverse, descending, and sigmoid (S-shaped) segments; the *rectum;* and the *anus* with its internal smooth muscle sphincter and external skeletal muscle sphincter. The large intestine contains microorganisms (the intestinal flora), which have a minor role in completing the digestion of nutrients. The large intestine absorbs water from the chyme, along with some electrolytes. The unabsorbed portion of the chyme as well as electrolytes and other substances secreted into the lumen constitutes solid waste (feces or stool). The most important function of the large intestine is defecation, the expulsion of feces. Alimentary canal function is effectively modeled by general systems theory (see Chapter 1), in which environmental matter is taken into the system (input), processed and expelled from the system back into the environment (output).

Peritoneal Cavity

The organs of the alimentary canal and its accessory organs are contained within the peritoneal cavity. As illustrated in Figure 24–2, this cavity lies between two layers of membrane: the *visceral peritoneum,* which overlies the abdominal organs, and the *parietal peritoneum,* which lines the anterior portion of the abdominal cavity. Another membrane, the *mesentery,* supports the coiled lengths of the jejunum and ileum. The peritoneal cavity normally contains a small amount of lubricating fluid to facilitate mobility of organs. In inflammatory or obstructive conditions, however, significant amounts of fluid may be third spaced here, resulting in ascites (see Chapter 8). The smaller *retroperitoneal space,* which lies behind the peritoneal cavity, contains the lumbosacral spine, kidneys, and adrenals.

GASTROINTESTINAL MOTILITY

Contraction of Visceral Smooth Muscle

Structure of the Intestinal Wall

Figure 24–3 illustrates the cross-sectional structure of the intestinal wall as it exists between the lower two thirds of the esophagus and the anus. (The upper esophagus contains skeletal muscle.) The gut wall consists of five layers. The inner *mucosa* contains cells that produce mucus for lubrication of chyme and protection of the wall. Because mucosal cells have a short cell cycle, they are potentially affected by radiation therapy and cancer chemotherapy (see Chapter 7). The *submucosa* consists of connective tissue supporting blood vessels, nerves, and cells that secrete digestive enzymes. Two layers of smooth muscle adjoin the submucosa: one of circular muscle and one of longitudinal muscle. Contraction of these muscle layers underlies the mixing and propulsive moments of the gut. The outer *serosa* consists of the visceral peritoneum as it overlies the canal. Inflammatory processes that involve this layer

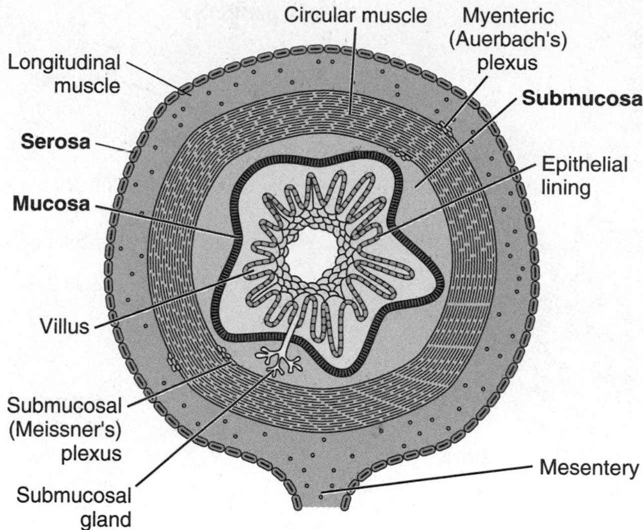

FIGURE 24–3

Structure of the intestinal wall. The intestinal wall consists of five layers: (1) the inner *mucosa,* which contains mucus-producing cells; (2) the *submucosa,* a connective tissue layer that supports blood vessels, nerves, and secretory cells; (3) a circular muscle layer; (4) a longitudinal muscle layer; and (5) the *serosa,* or visceral peritoneum.

may result in bands of scar tissue **(adhesions),** a common cause of **bowel obstruction.**

Regulation of Smooth Muscle Contraction

Enteric Nervous System. The cellular mechanism of smooth muscle contraction is the sliding filament mechanism, as discussed in Chapter 5. The smooth muscle cells of the gut are capable of pacing their own contractions via *interstitial cells of Cajal,* nonneural cells that are similar to cardiac pacemaker cells (see Chapter 17). Although contraction is not *dependent* on neural input, it is potentially affected by signals from the autonomic nervous system. These signals are relayed to the gut smooth muscle via a specialized *enteric nervous system,* consisting of two networks of neurons (Fig. 24–4). This system, the "brain of the gut,"[2] contains more than 100 million neurons that regulate motility, secretion, and perfusion of the alimentary canal and that are involved in modulation of immune and inflammatory responses.

Two main types of neurons make up the system: Type I neurons are motor neurons that may either excite or inhibit contraction of smooth muscle, and type II neurons are the sensory limbs of the reflexes that mediate GI motility and secretion. The principal neurotransmitters at type I excitatory synapses are acetylcholine and substance P, whereas vasoactive intestinal polypeptide and nitric oxide are found at inhibitory synapses. All sensory neurons are cholinergic and may or may not secrete substance P as well. Other neurotransmitters and neuromodulators believed to be involved in enteric neurotransmission include norepinephrine, serotonin, γ-aminobutyric acid (GABA), somatostatin, calcitonin gene-related peptide, endogenous opioids, and neuropeptide Y.[2]

As illustrated in Figure 24–4, the neurons of the *myenteric (Auerbach's) plexus* are located between the two muscle layers of the gut wall, and those of the *submucosal (Meissner's)* plexus are found between the circular muscle and submucosal layers. Stimulation of either plexus affects muscle contraction; stimulation of the submucosal plexus affects secretion also.

The parasympathetic nerves that synapse with the plexuses of the enteric nervous system include the vagus nerve (CN X), which innervates the stomach, small intestine, cecum, ascending colon, and transverse colon, and the pelvic nerve, which innervates the rest of the colon and the rectum. In some cases, PNS nerves synapse directly on smooth muscle cells. A number of autonomic reflex arcs affect GI function, and PNS inputs are excitatory in most cases. Triggered by mechanoreceptors or chemoreceptors in the gut wall, enteric reflexes comprise the basic level of neural regulation of GI function. These reflexes, summarized in Table 24–1, are discussed in greater detail in subsequent sections pertaining to specific types of GI movement and secretion. Sympathetic nervous system (SNS) stimulation of visceral smooth muscle is mainly inhibitory. Most SNS impulses are transmitted along the splanchnic nerves, which synapse on neurons of the enteric nervous system.

Hormonal Regulation. Endocrine regulation of gastrointestinal motility and secretion originates from the diffuse endocrine system rather than the classic endocrine system (see Chapter 27). The hormones of the diffuse system consist primarily of peptides secreted into the blood from a variety of tissues that are not anatomically classified as components of the endocrine system. Many of these peptides also serve as neuromodulators within the enteric nervous system.

Three hormones of particular importance in the regulation of GI motility are released from small intestine mucosal cells: *cholecystokinin (CCK), secretin,* and *gastric inhibitory peptide* (enterogastrone). Secretin and CCK are released in response to chyme in the duodenum. Secretin decreases the motility of the stomach and intestine, and CCK decreases gastric (stomach) motility. Gastric inhibitory peptide, which is released in response to fat in the duodenum, decreases gastric motility. Hormonal inhibition of motility under these circumstances has the effect of allowing sufficient time for digestive enzymes to work on chyme.

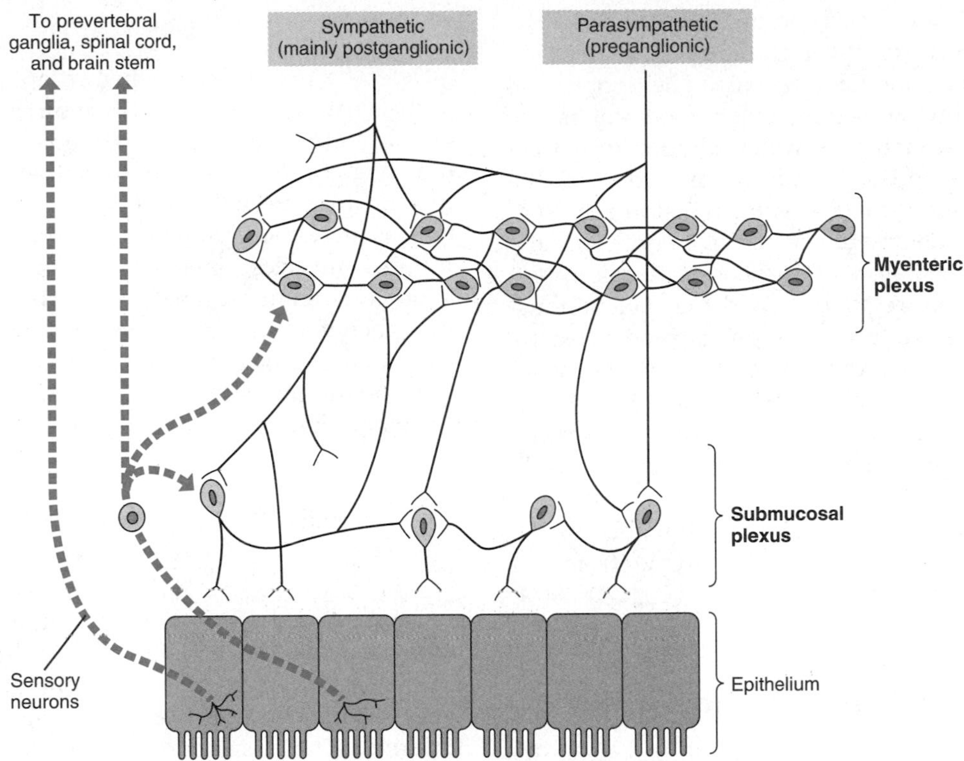

FIGURE 24–4

Enteric nervous system. Two networks of motor and sensory neurons regulate contraction and secretion by the intestinal wall. The *myenteric (Auerbach's) plexus* is located between the two muscle layers of the gut wall, and the *submucosal (Meissner's) plexus* is found between the circular muscle and submucosal layers. Neurons of the autonomic nervous system may synapse on neurons of these plexuses or directly on smooth muscle cells. (Redrawn from Guyton, A.C., and Hall, J.E. [1996]. *Textbook of Medical Physiology.* [9th Ed.]. Philadelphia: W.B. Saunders. [p. 796].)

TABLE 24–1
EXAMPLES OF ENTERIC REFLEXES

Reflex	Function
Receptive relaxation	Relaxation of the fundus of the stomach in response to swallowing of food
Enterogastric	Inhibition of gastric emptying in response to acid and protein in the duodenum
Gastrocolic	Increase in motility of the ileum, cecum, and colon in response to distention of the stomach and duodenum
Gastroileal	Opening of the ileocecal valve in response to gastric emptying
Intestinointestinal	Relaxation of intestinal smooth muscle in response to overdistention of one segment of the intestine
Ileogastric	Decrease in gastric motility in response to distention of the illeum

Specific Types of Gastrointestinal Motility

Deglutition

Swallowing typically occurs without conscious effort about 600 times during a 24-hour period.[3] Deglutition is accomplished through a four-phase series of events: oral preparation, oral phase, pharyngeal phase, and esophageal phase. Oral preparation is voluntary and reflex and consists of manipulation of masticated food and fluids in the mouth by the lips, cheeks, and tongue, mixing with saliva, and formation of a cohesive mass or bolus. The oral phase of swallowing moves the bolus of food to the back of the throat, stimulating stretch receptors. Afferent signals from these receptors ascend to the swallowing centers in the medulla and pons of the brain stem. Descending signals along the vagus nerve result in coordination of swallowing and breathing so that aspiration of food into the trachea is normally prevented.

The efferent vagal signal initiates the pharyngeal phase, in which constriction of the pharynx causes backward and downward propulsion of food. The epiglottis contracts to cover the trachea, inspiration is inhibited, and the UES relaxes. The esophageal phase of swallowing begins when food enters the esophagus and stretches its walls. Rhythmic contractions ensue that propel food downward, and the LES relaxes to allow food to enter the stomach. Regulation of LES tone is the result of neural stimulation and local mediators. The smooth muscle of the LES is under vagal regulation, and the skeletal muscle of the surrounding diaphragm is innervated by the phrenic nerve. Esophageal distention and swallowing initiate reflex relaxation of the LES smooth muscle and inhibit contraction of the diaphragm. *Gastrin,* a hormone secreted by the stomach wall, and high levels of parasympathetic stimulation inhibit the relaxation of the LES, presumably to decrease the risk of reflux of acid chyme from the stomach into the esophagus.

Mixing and Propulsive Movements

In the stomach, muscle contraction mechanically digests food, forming chyme. Contractions are paced from the middle (body) of the stomach, propelling food downward toward the antrum. If the pyloric sphincter is closed, contraction of the antrum pushes chyme back upward, "churning" it. Between contractions, the pyloric sphincter is open, and the more liquid chyme flows by gravity into the duodenum.

In the small intestine, locally paced *segmentation waves* (slow contractions of circular muscle) move chyme forward and backward. Such movement mixes the chyme with pancreatic juice and bile and ensures adequate exposure of chyme to the intestinal wall for absorption. As regulated by a PNS reflex (the *gastroenteric reflex*), segmentation waves increase after a meal. *Peristalsis,* the sequential contraction of circular and longitudinal muscles behind the bolus of chyme, propels the chyme along the canal. Collection of chyme in the terminal ileum creates a pressure gradient that opens the ileocecal valve, allowing entry of liquid chyme into the cecum. Opening of this valve is inhibited by a SNS reflex in cases of cecal distention or irritation, as in constipation or appendicitis.

In the large intestine, segmental contractions known as *haustral movements* churn the chyme to expose all surfaces to the wall for absorption of water. Propulsive *mass movements* occur when a large section of the colon contracts as a unit. These movements occur in series lasting 10 to 30 minutes, several times each day, and trigger the *defecation reflex.*

Defecation

Defecation is initiated when receptors in the rectal walls sense irritation or distention (Fig. 24–5). Sensory signals enter the sacral segments of the cord and synapse on PNS neurons that mediate relaxation of the internal sphincter. An interneuron synapse initiates simultaneous contraction of the abdominal muscles, increasing pressure outside the colon. Descending signals from the cerebral cortex may facilitate defecation by opening the external anal sphincter or may inhibit its relaxation until an appropriate time and place. Voluntary contraction of the abdominal muscles may also initiate the reflex.

Function of Valves and Sphincters

The rate and timing of ingestion, motility, and defecation are dependent on the function of the sphincters of the esophagus, stomach, and anus as well as the ileocecal valve leading into the large intestine. These structures also ensure directional flow, normally preventing reflux that could damage more proximal organs. As discussed in subsequent

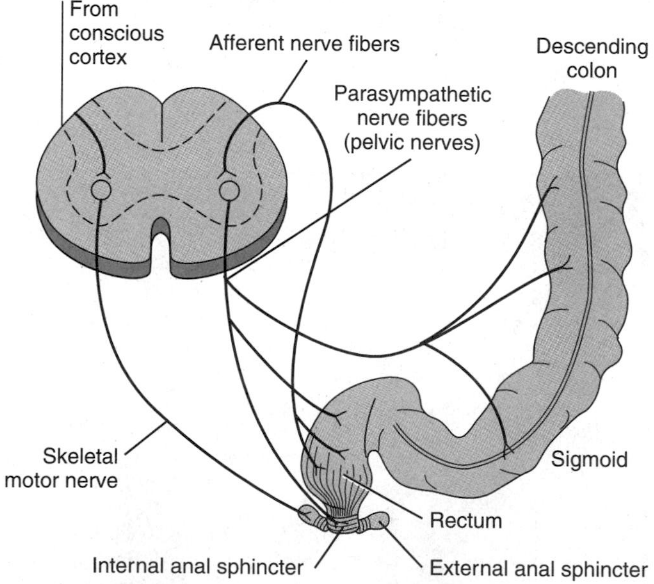

FIGURE 24–5

Defecation reflex. Elimination of feces is initiated when receptors in the rectal walls sense irritation or distention. Sensory impulses are transmitted to sacral levels of the cord, where the sensory neurons synapse on parasympathetic neurons that then induce relaxation of the internal (smooth muscle) anal sphincter. Contraction of the abdominal muscles is stimulated simultaneously via an interneuronal synapse, and defecation occurs if descending signals from higher centers relax the external (skeletal muscle) anal sphincter. (Redrawn from Guyton, A.C., and Hall, J.E. [1996]. *Textbook of Medical Physiology.* [9th Ed.]. Philadelphia: W.B. Saunders. [p. 812].)

sections, conditions that increase the rate of flow of chyme through the gut may result in inadequate absorption of nutrients and disrupt virtually all homeostatic mechanisms. Decreased or absent GI motility leads to distention of the bowel, retention of wastes, and possible obstruction or pressure-driven reflux.

GASTROINTESTINAL SECRETION

Gastrointestinal Fluid Balance

Approximately 7000 mL of fluid are secreted into the GI tract each day. Normally, all but 50 to 200 mL are reabsorbed. Gastrointestinal fluids are similar in composition to the plasma with regard to water and electrolytes, although the precise concentrations are flow rate–dependent.

Regulation of Secretion

The basic mechanism of secretion from cells of the GI tract is exocytosis, as discussed in Chapter 2. Local stimuli such as changes in lumen pH, stretch, or presence of toxins may trigger autonomic reflexes that alter the rate of secretion. Typically, parasympathetic stimulation increases secretion, and sympathetic stimulation decreases secretion.

Three hormones released from cells of the alimentary canal are most important in stimulation of secretion. Cholecystokinin and secretin, discussed in the section on regulation of motility, affect secretion as well. Amino acids in the duodenum result in the release of CCK into the blood, with the resulting effect of initiation of gallbladder contraction and pancreatic secretion. The enzymes contained in bile and pancreatic juice thus enter the duodenum, where they act to chemically digest the chyme. Secretin is released in response to an acid chyme ($pH < 3.0$) and causes increased bicarbonate secretion in pancreatic juice. Gastrin, released from the antrum of the stomach and from the duodenum in the presence of chyme, causes increased secretion of hydrochloric acid and an enzyme precursor, *pepsinogen,* from the stomach. Release of gastrin is facilitated by parasympathetic stimulation and by amino acids and calcium in the chyme. A number of other substances, including alcohol, caffeine, and histamine, may trigger gastrin secretion with potentially detrimental effects on the gastric and duodenal mucosa.

Specific Types of Gastrointestinal Secretion

Salivation

The salivary glands (Fig. 24–6) secrete approximately 1000 mL of saliva per day. Parasympathetic stimulation increases salivation, and sympathetic stimulation decreases it (as evidenced by the characteristic dry mouth during stress). Saliva is composed of water and electrolytes, mucous glycoprotein, antibacterial enzymes, and the enzyme salivary amylase (ptyalin) for initial carbohydrate digestion. The salivary glands may become obstructed with calculi or may become inflamed. Viral infection of the parotid glands (*parotitis* or "mumps") was common in the United States before the current immunization program was instituted. Clinical features of these and other disorders caused by alterations in salivation are summarized in Table 24–2.

Gastric Secretion

Figure 24–7 illustrates the locations of the five types of secretory cells within the gastric mucosa. Mucous cells throughout the stomach secrete mucus that forms a protective coating against hydrochloric acid (HCl) and proteolytic enzymes. This mucoid barrier may break down under ischemic or inflammatory conditions or with excessive ingestion of aspirin or alcohol.

The *oxyntic cells* (also known as parietal cells) secrete HCl and intrinsic factor. These cells have receptors for histamine, acetylcholine, and gastrin.[4]

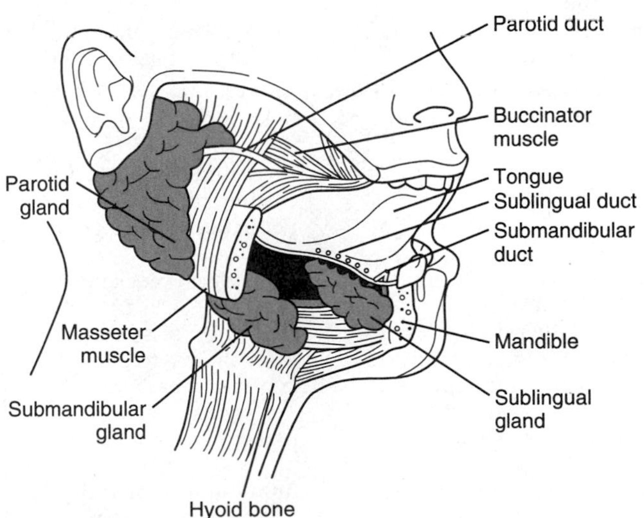

FIGURE 24–6
Salivary glands. The three pairs of salivary glands are the parotid, submandibular, and sublingual glands, which secrete about 1000 mL of saliva per day.

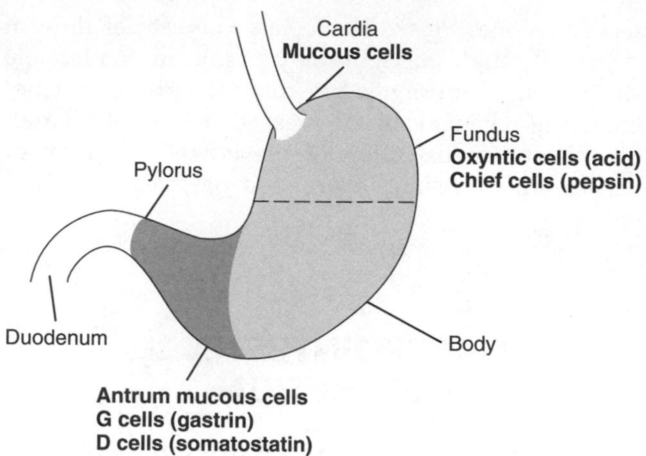

FIGURE 24–7

Gastric secretory cells. Gastric secretions originate from five cell types. *Mucous cells* located throughout the stomach secrete a mucus barrier that protects the mucosa against damage by acid and proteolytic enzymes. *Oxyntic (parietal) cells* secrete hydrochloric acid and intrinsic factor. *Chief (zymogen) cells* secrete pepsinogen, which is converted to the proteolytic enzyme pepsin when gastric pH is below 5.0. Oxyntic and chief cells are located in the fundus and body of the stomach. In the antrum, *G cells* secrete gastrin, mucus, and serotonin, and *D cells* secrete somatostatin. (Redrawn from Cotran, R.S., Kumar, V., and Robbins, S.L. [1994]. *Robbins Pathologic Basis of Disease.* [5th Ed.]. Philadelphia: W.B. Saunders. [p. 767].)

Binding of any of these ligands to their receptors initiates a series of intracellular reactions that culminate in the secretion of hydrogen ions against a huge concentration gradient to produce an acid gastric pH. The active transport mechanism that accomplishes this is an H^+-K^+-ATPase known as the *proton pump.* Secreted HCl dissolves fibrous proteins, acts as a bacteriocide against swallowed organisms, and converts the precursor pepsinogen to the proteolytic enzyme *pepsin.* Intrinsic factor is a glycoprotein carrier that facilitates the absorption of vitamin B_{12} from the ileum. This vitamin is necessary for erythrocyte synthesis. Lack of intrinsic factor usually occurs as a consequence of atrophy of gastric cells (as with chronic gastritis) and results in pernicious anemia (see Chapter 12).

Chief cells (also known as zymogen cells) secrete pepsinogen, which is converted to pepsin when the gastric pH is less than 5.0. Optimal gastric pH for pepsin activity is 2.0. The proteolytic activity of pepsin breaks down proteins into polypeptides (shorter chains of amino acids linked by peptide bonds). Pepsin within the gastric chyme is inactivated when the chyme enters the alkaline pH of the duodenum.

The *G cells* (also known as gastrin cells, argentaffin cells, or pyloric glands) secrete serotonin (5-hydroxytryptamine), mucus, and gastrin. As discussed earlier, gastrin stimulates the release of HCl and pepsinogen. The significance of serotonin, a chemical that serves as a major neurotransmitter within the central nervous system (CNS), is unknown with respect to GI function. Antral *D cells* secrete the hormone somatostatin, which opposes the production and secretion of gastrin.

Pancreatic Secretion

Although the pancreas is perhaps best appreciated for its endocrine role in the regulation of serum glucose, the exocrine cells of the pancreas comprise the bulk of this gland. The endocrine pancreas is detailed in Chapter 29. Figure 24–8 illustrates the anatomic relationship of the pancreas, liver, gallbladder, and biliary tract to the alimentary canal. Secretions from these accessory organs enter the duodenum.

The exocrine cells of the pancreas are the *acinar cells,* which synthesize and secrete digestive enzymes

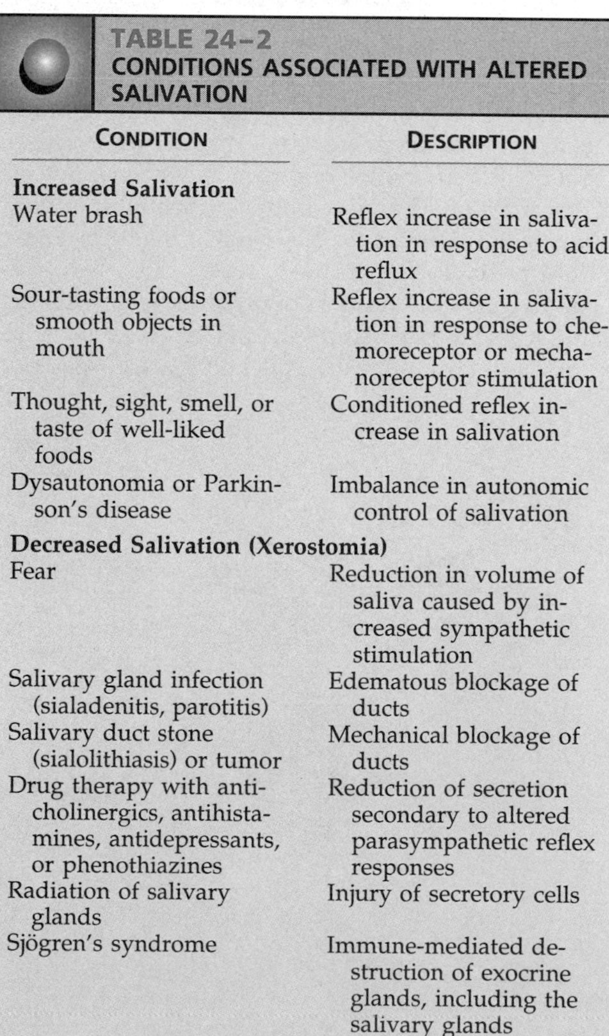

TABLE 24–2
CONDITIONS ASSOCIATED WITH ALTERED SALIVATION

Condition	Description
Increased Salivation	
Water brash	Reflex increase in salivation in response to acid reflux
Sour-tasting foods or smooth objects in mouth	Reflex increase in salivation in response to chemoreceptor or mechanoreceptor stimulation
Thought, sight, smell, or taste of well-liked foods	Conditioned reflex increase in salivation
Dysautonomia or Parkinson's disease	Imbalance in autonomic control of salivation
Decreased Salivation (Xerostomia)	
Fear	Reduction in volume of saliva caused by increased sympathetic stimulation
Salivary gland infection (sialadenitis, parotitis)	Edematous blockage of ducts
Salivary duct stone (sialolithiasis) or tumor	Mechanical blockage of ducts
Drug therapy with anticholinergics, antihistamines, antidepressants, or phenothiazines	Reduction of secretion secondary to altered parasympathetic reflex responses
Radiation of salivary glands	Injury of secretory cells
Sjögren's syndrome	Immune-mediated destruction of exocrine glands, including the salivary glands

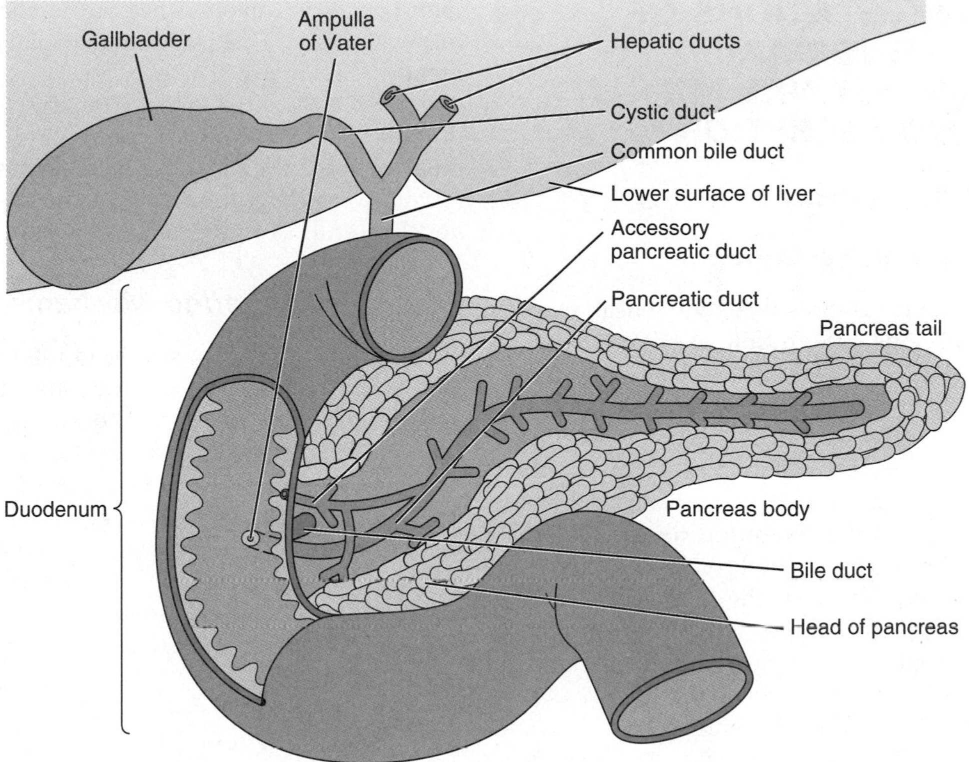

FIGURE 24–8

Gastrointestinal organs. The anatomic relationship of the pancreas, liver, gallbladder, and biliary tract to the duodenum is illustrated. Pancreatic juice, containing digestive enzymes and bicarbonate, and bile, containing bile acids for emulsification of dietary fats, are secreted into the duodenum in response to stimuli in chyme.

into ducts within the gland. The epithelial cells lining these ducts secrete bicarbonate and water into the ducts as well, resulting in an alkaline pH of the pancreatic juice. Bicarbonate is derived from a hydrolysis reaction within these cells (see Chapter 10).

Pancreatic enzymes include three proteolytic enzymes that are secreted as inactive proenzymes and activated by *enterokinase,* an enzyme released by cells of the duodenal mucosa. The proteolytic enzymes are *trypsin, chymotrypsin,* and *carboxypeptidase.* A trypsin inhibitor that prevents activation of the proenzymes while still in the pancreatic ducts is released simultaneously. The acinar cells also secrete *pancreatic amylase,* which cleaves bonds in carbohydrates, and *pancreatic lipase,* which breaks down lipids. Pancreatic secretion is stimulated by parasympathetic stimulation as well as by gastrin, CCK, and secretin.

Biliary Secretion

The liver secretes bile, a green-yellow fluid containing bile salts, cholesterol, bilirubin pigment, electrolytes, and water. Bile salts are necessary for the intestinal absorption of fats. Hepatic synthesis of bile, gallbladder storage, and biliary recycling mechanisms are detailed in Chapter 26. Action of bile salts on fats are discussed with lipid absorption in Chapter 25. Bile enters the duodenum in response to CCK and another duodenal hormone, *motilin,* which are released in response to the presence of fat in the duodenum.

Intestinal Secretion

Protective, lubricating mucus is secreted from cells of the small and large intestines. In addition, the small intestine surface cells secrete intestinal juices containing *peptidases* and *disaccharidases,* which complete the digestion of proteins and carbohydrates, respectively. As previously mentioned, the duodenum also secretes enterokinase, which activates pancreatic proenzymes. Cells located below the intestinal wall surface in the crypts of Lieberkühn secrete a serous fluid that acts as a diluent to facilitate absorption of nutrients (see Chapter 25). Intestinal secretion is largely under autonomic control, with PNS stimuli increasing secretion and SNS stimuli decreasing secretion.

MANIFESTATIONS OF ABNORMAL GASTROINTESTINAL MOTILITY AND SECRETION

Nausea and Vomiting

Vomiting Reflex

Nausea is an unpleasant subjective sensation resulting from conscious recognition of stimulation of the *vomiting centers* in the medulla. Vomiting, also known as **emesis,** is the sudden, forceful expulsion of the stomach contents (vomitus). Figure 24–9 illustrates the vomiting reflex. Sensory receptors in the duodenum are stimulated with distention or irritation. Afferent signals are transmitted to the bilateral vomiting centers in the medulla. From there, efferent signals are transmitted back to the alimentary canal, abdominal muscles, and diaphragm. The vomiting centers receive input from higher centers, including the cerebral cortex and the *chemoreceptor trigger zones* (CTZ) on the floor of the fourth ventricle.

Vomiting is usually, but not always, preceded by nausea. In response to the efferent signals, *antiperistalsis* (retrograde peristaltic contraction) pushes the contents of the stomach (and possibly the small intestine) up toward the fundus of the stomach. An increase in salivation is usually noted. Vomiting then occurs via events that are in the reverse order of swallowing. The individual usually takes a deep breath reflexively, the UES opens, and the glottis and posterior nares close. The diaphragm and abdominal muscles contract, producing *retching*. Relaxation of the LES allows the vomitus to be expelled. *Projectile vomiting* occurs when muscle contraction is very forceful, as in the case of intestinal obstruction.

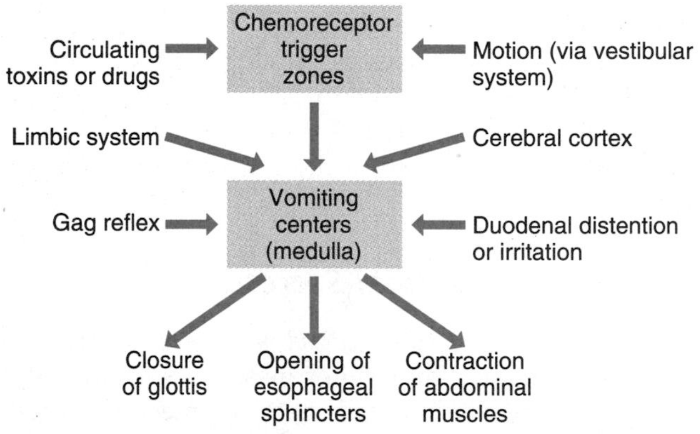

FIGURE 24–9
Vomiting reflex. Vomiting may be triggered by a number of different stimuli, all of which are integrated in the bilateral vomiting centers of the medulla. Initiation of the gag reflex or distention or irritation of the duodenum may signal the vomiting centers directly, resulting in reflex closure of the glottis (to prevent aspiration into the trachea), opening of the esophageal sphincters, and contraction of the abdominal muscles to expel gastric contents. Stimuli from higher centers may also trigger vomiting. The cerebral cortex and limbic system may initiate vomiting by an unknown mechanism, in response to noxious stimuli or extreme stress. Neurons of the chemoreceptor trigger zones of the fourth ventricle may be stimulated by endogenous toxins, drugs, or motion (via the vestibular system). The trigger zones then signal the vomiting centers, inducing vomiting.

Triggering Mechanisms

The vomiting reflex, which is intended to be protective in that it expels irritants, may be triggered by a variety of mechanisms. The strongest stimulation for vomiting, distention or irritation of the duodenum, is consistent with the adaptive purpose. Vomiting may be voluntarily triggered by initiation of the *gag reflex* with manual stimulation of the posterior wall of the pharynx. Neurons of the CTZ may be stimulated by endogenous toxins or by drugs such as morphine, digitalis, and several general anesthetics. The CTZ may also receive signals from the vestibular system, resulting in vomiting associated with motion sickness (see Chapter 23). Stimulation of the cerebral cortex by distressing sights or odors or by extreme stress may trigger vomiting by an unknown mechanism.

Clinical Effects and Management

The vagal vomiting reflex is followed by a rebound sympathetic nervous system response manifested by sweating and tachycardia. Loss of fluid and electrolytes may lead to dehydration, electrolyte imbalance, and acid-base imbalance (usually alkalosis caused by HCl loss). Gastrointestinal bleeding may result from **esophagitis** or ulceration as a result of reflux of acid and bile during frequent or prolonged vomiting. Removal of the irritant may prevent further vomiting in a negative feedback loop. If vomiting is maladaptive, antiemetic drugs such as ondansetron (Zofran) or prochlorperazine (Compazine) may be used to decrease the sensitivity of the CTZ neurons. Drugs such as dimenhydrinate (Dramamine), used in the treatment of motion sickness, decrease the sensitivity of the vestibular nuclei in the brain stem. Resolution of the underlying cause is the principal form of treatment of nausea and vomiting.

Diarrhea

Definition and Mechanisms

Diarrhea is increased frequency, fluidity, and volume of stools. Diarrheal diseases can be objectively defined by daily stool weights greater than 200 g.[5] Diarrhea may be acute or chronic, and it is associated with three causative mechanisms. In *osmotic diarrhea,* the osmotic pressure exerted by nonabsorbable substances in the gut or by increased numbers of osmotic particles in the gut draws water into the stool. *Secretory diarrhea* results from excessive secretion of water and electrolytes into the bowel. Increased secretion may be triggered by bacterial toxins, locally irritating substances (including some drugs) in chyme, or by tumors that produce peptides similar to CCK or secretin. In *motile diarrhea,* a reflex increase in motility is stimulated by inflammation, neuropathy, or obstruction. In the case of inflammation or obstruction, the increased motility represents an adaptive attempt to expel the irritant or clear the obstruction, whereas in neuropathy the stimulus is maladaptive. Table 24–3 lists examples of conditions associated with each of these mechanisms.

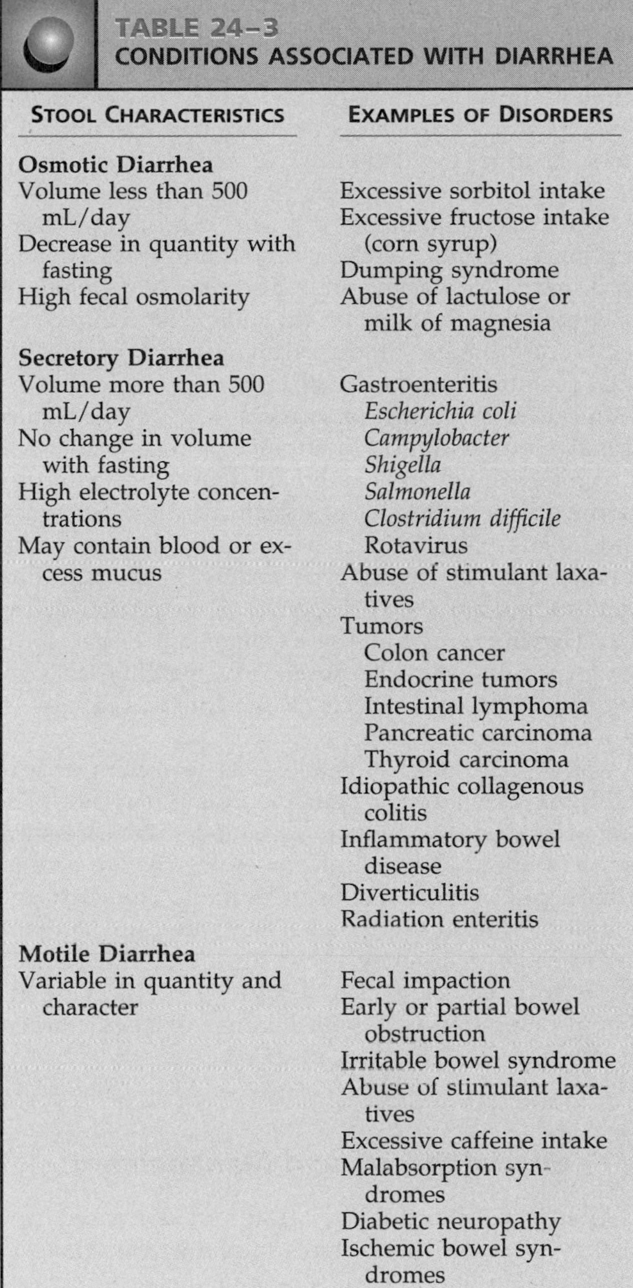

TABLE 24–3
CONDITIONS ASSOCIATED WITH DIARRHEA

STOOL CHARACTERISTICS	EXAMPLES OF DISORDERS
Osmotic Diarrhea	
Volume less than 500 mL/day	Excessive sorbitol intake
Decrease in quantity with fasting	Excessive fructose intake (corn syrup)
High fecal osmolarity	Dumping syndrome
	Abuse of lactulose or milk of magnesia
Secretory Diarrhea	
Volume more than 500 mL/day	Gastroenteritis *Escherichia coli* *Campylobacter* *Shigella* *Salmonella* *Clostridium difficile* Rotavirus
No change in volume with fasting	Abuse of stimulant laxatives
High electrolyte concentrations	Tumors Colon cancer Endocrine tumors Intestinal lymphoma Pancreatic carcinoma Thyroid carcinoma
May contain blood or excess mucus	Idiopathic collagenous colitis
	Inflammatory bowel disease
	Diverticulitis
	Radiation enteritis
Motile Diarrhea	
Variable in quantity and character	Fecal impaction
	Early or partial bowel obstruction
	Irritable bowel syndrome
	Abuse of stimulant laxatives
	Excessive caffeine intake
	Malabsorption syndromes
	Diabetic neuropathy
	Ischemic bowel syndromes

Clinical Effects and Management

Crampy abdominal pain (*colic*) may be evident as a result of increased peristalsis, and bowel sounds may be increased in frequency and amplitude. Very loud sounds, audible without a stethoscope, are known as *borborygmi.* Increased mucus may be evident in the stool, and stools may be bloody if an inflammatory process is asssociated with the underlying condition. Prolonged diarrhea leads to dehydration as well as electrolyte and acid-base imbalance.

Most cases of irritant-induced diarrhea are self-limiting, because increased stools clear the irritant. These cases are managed with replacement of water, electrolytes, and nutrients as necessary. Bulk-forming drugs such as psyllium (Metamucil) may be used to decrease the fluidity of the stool. Drugs such as loperamide (Imodium) and diphenoxylate HCl (Lomotil) are commonly used to decrease motility. Definitive therapy is directed at the underlying cause.

Constipation

Definition

Constipation, defined as infrequent or difficult defecation, is the most common digestive complaint in the United States, accounting for an estimated 2.5 million physician visits each year.[6] Incidence is particularly high among elderly persons. Although normal bowel frequency is highly variable among individuals, constipation has been defined by the International Workshop on Constipation as occurrence of two or more of the following for at least 12 months: (1) fewer than three bowel movements per week, (2) excessive straining with at least 25% of bowel movements, (3) a feeling of incomplete evacuation at least 25% of the time, and (4) passage of hard or pellet-like stools at least 25% of the time.[7]

Mechanisms

Constipation is usually considered to be a functional disorder of bowel motility, associated with slow transit of food residues through the colon, difficulty in expulsion of stool from the rectosigmoid region, or both. In addition to aging, factors such as anatomic lesions, metabolic disorders, diet, and drug therapy may contribute to constipation by one or more of four mechanisms.

Constipation may result from decreased neural stimulation of GI motility, abdominal muscle weakness, bowel obstruction, or voluntary retention of stool. Neural stimulation of GI smooth muscle may be decreased because of inactivity or immobility, lack of bulk to stimulate the defecation reflex, interruption of neural pathways by trauma (e.g., spinal cord injury), or degenerative disorders (e.g., multiple sclerosis). Interruption of the reflex arc caused by sacral cord injury produces an atonic bowel, with fecal retention and potential impaction. Loss of communication with higher centers (e.g., with higher spinal cord injury or brain injury) results in fecal incontinence, which is automatic emptying with triggering of the reflex. Drugs such as anticholinergics and opiates also impair neural stimulation of the canal. Abuse of irritant-type laxatives may also impair the normal reflex response. A congenital disorder, **Hirschsprung's disease** (congenital megacolon), which results from the absence of ganglion cells in the enteric nervous system of the colon, is discussed in a subsequent section.

Abdominal muscle weakness, as seen with deconditioning or neuromuscular disorders, may not permit generation of adequate intra-abdominal pressure for defecation. Mechanical bowel obstruction results from a physical barrier to defecation. Voluntary retention is due to higher level inhibition of the defecation reflex. This may occur in young children, in those with psychological disorders, or in those in whom defecation is painful because of **hemorrhoids** or anal lesions.

Clinical Effects and Management

Altered GI function can result in decreased frequency of stools, hard stools, painful defecation, or abdominal fullness. Headache and malaise may accompany chronic constipation. Vagal stimulation with straining at stool may result in reflex fluctuation in blood pressure and pulse (an initial decrease followed by a rebound increase), which could be detrimental to individuals with underlying cardiovascular disease.

Prevention of constipation involves removal of the underlying risk factors and causes, if possible. Bowel retraining, based on dietary management; regular timing of defecation; and manual stimulation of the defecation reflex may be possible in those with neurologic impairment. Tap water enemas, in which water is instilled into the rectum to stretch the walls and trigger the defecation reflex, impose some risk of fluid-electrolyte imbalance and are now used infrequently in clinical practice. Small-volume enemas containing bowel irritants such as phosphate to stimulate defecation are more often used. Laxative and cathartic drugs that promote normal defecation include bulk-formers, stool softeners, lubricants, prokinetic agents, and (as a last resort) irritants. Table 24–4 lists agents in common use. Digital disimpaction (manual removal of impacted stool) may be necessary in severe constipation. Treatment of secondary disorders contributing to constipation is also warranted.

Fecal Incontinence

Definition and Mechanisms

Fecal incontinence, or deficient control of defecation in a mature person, may vary in severity from

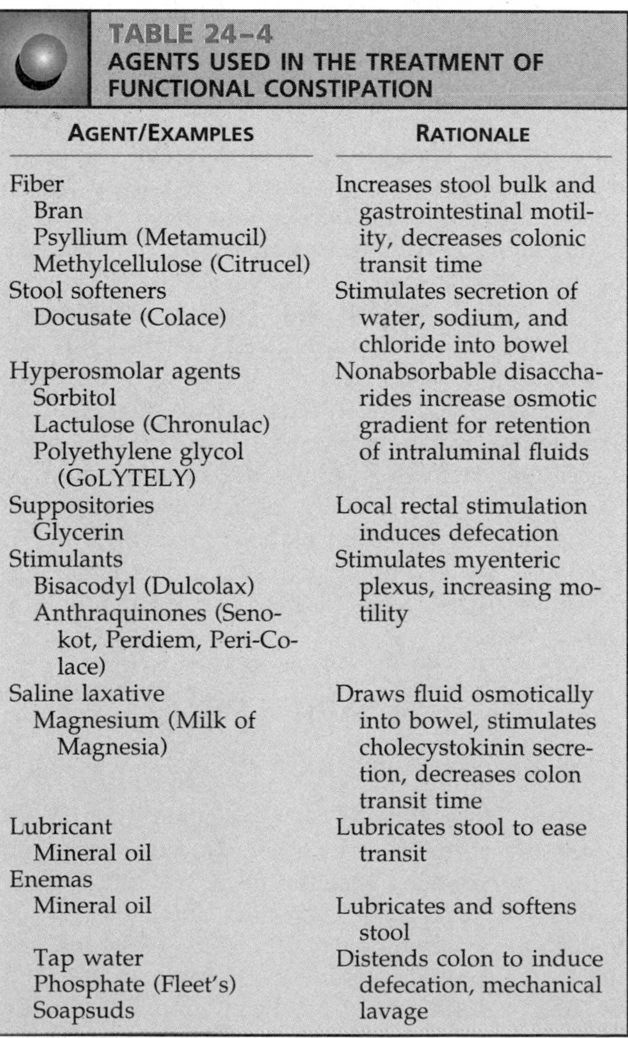

TABLE 24–4
AGENTS USED IN THE TREATMENT OF FUNCTIONAL CONSTIPATION

AGENT/EXAMPLES	RATIONALE
Fiber Bran Psyllium (Metamucil) Methylcellulose (Citrucel)	Increases stool bulk and gastrointestinal motility, decreases colonic transit time
Stool softeners Docusate (Colace)	Stimulates secretion of water, sodium, and chloride into bowel
Hyperosmolar agents Sorbitol Lactulose (Chronulac) Polyethylene glycol (GoLYTELY)	Nonabsorbable disaccharides increase osmotic gradient for retention of intraluminal fluids
Suppositories Glycerin	Local rectal stimulation induces defecation
Stimulants Bisacodyl (Dulcolax) Anthraquinones (Senokot, Perdiem, Peri-Colace)	Stimulates myenteric plexus, increasing motility
Saline laxative Magnesium (Milk of Magnesia)	Draws fluid osmotically into bowel, stimulates cholecystokinin secretion, decreases colon transit time
Lubricant Mineral oil	Lubricates stool to ease transit
Enemas Mineral oil	Lubricates and softens stool
Tap water Phosphate (Fleet's) Soapsuds	Distends colon to induce defecation, mechanical lavage

Adapted with permission from Romero, Y., Evans, J.M., Fleming, K.C., et al. (1996). Constipation and fecal incontinence in the elderly population. *Mayo Clinic Proceedings* 71, 81–92.

minor incontinence (partial soiling or incontinence of flatus or liquid stool) to major incontinence (involuntary defecation of stool of normal consistency).[8] The condition is particularly prevalent among elderly individuals, especially those in nursing homes. The most common causes are constipation (in which liquid stool leaks around an impaction), improper use of laxatives, hyperosmolar enteral feedings, neurologic disorders, colorectal disorders, and functional dependence that impairs toileting.[9]

Normal continence requires a balance between expelling and resisting forces for defecation. Weakness of the external anal sphincter (as with pudendal neuropathy) impairs voluntary resistance, as does a weak pelvic floor (often associated with obstetrical trauma). Rectal sensation may also be impaired with neuropathy, and the individual may thus not be "warned" of impending reflex defecation. Diarrheal disorders or a very large volume of stool may overwhelm continence mechanisms in some cases.

Clinical Management

Attention to diet and toileting needs, along with preventive measures for constipation or diarrhea, are beneficial to most individuals. Pelvic floor disorders may be amenable to surgical repair (see Chapter 31). Definitive treatment of any associated colorectal disorders may also be required.

Bowel Obstruction

Definition and Mechanisms

Bowel obstruction is blockade of chyme transport along the alimentary canal. Obstruction may be congenital or acquired, complete or partial, mechanical (caused by an obstructive mass, constriction, or lesion), or functional (caused by impaired neural stimulation of motility).

Figure 24–10 illustrates common forms of bowel obstruction. **Hypertrophic pyloric stenosis (HPS)** is particularly prevalent and is discussed in the section on GI disorders. Congenital obstruction of the esophagus may take the form of **esophageal atresia** (also discussed in the GI disorders section). Hernias, in which a loop of bowel may protrude through the muscle of the abdominal wall (e.g., the inguinal canal, the umbilicus, or an incisional scar), may be related to congenital or acquired wall weakness. Herniation is often induced by increased intra-abdominal pressure, as with lifting, straining, or violent coughing. Inguinal hernia, the most common form, primarily affects males and is discussed in Chapter 30. Other lesions that may mechanically obstruct the bowel are tumors, **polyps,** and scar tissue adhesions. **Colorectal cancer** and its associated risk factors are discussed in the section on GI disorders.

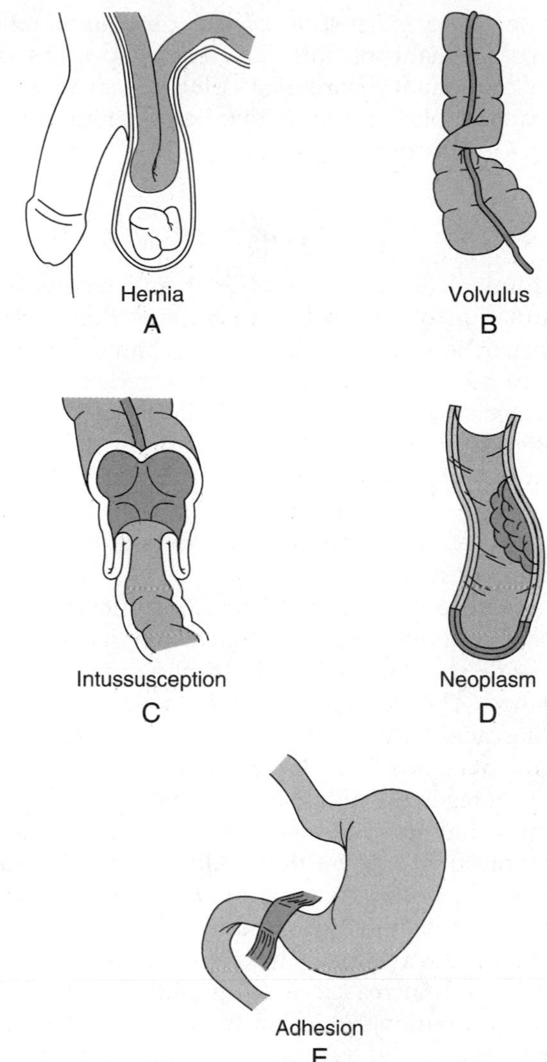

FIGURE 24–10

Forms of bowel obstruction. *A,* With hernia, a loop of bowel protrudes through a weakness in the abdominal wall and may become obstructed with incarceration or strangulation. *B,* Obstruction in volvulus is caused by twisting of the bowel, which may occur congenitally or around a lesion such as a tumor. *C,* Intussusception, or telescoping of the bowel into itself, may also be congenital or acquired as a result of an obstructive lesion. *D,* Benign or malignant neoplasms may obstruct the lumen of the bowel. *E,* Fibrous membranes within the peritoneal cavity may fuse together after inflammation, forming obstructive bands or adhesions.

Paralytic ileus is a transient form of functional bowel obstruction seen after general anesthesia, particularly with abdominal surgery in which the bowel is manipulated. For a period of several hours to days postoperatively, bowel motility may be absent because of a lack of neural stimuli. Because functional obstruction leads to mechanical obstruction as feces accumulate, and mechanical obstruction eventually leads to exhaustion of the defecation reflex, the two mechanisms intersect. Hirschsprung's disease, a congenital disorder of colon innervation that also leads to obstruction, is detailed later in the section on GI disorders.

Clinical Effects and Management

Abdominal distention is evident and results from accumulation of gas, solid waste, and fluid behind the obstruction. Motility behind mechanical obstructions may be increased at first in a reflex adaptive effort to clear the obstruction. This increased motility may be perceived as a crampy pain or colic. In mechanical obstruction, bowel sounds are increased at first, but are absent later when GI reflexes are exhausted. Bowel sounds are absent throughout functional obstruction.

As pressure behind the obstruction increases, distention of the intestine or stomach may induce vomiting, with resultant fluid, electrolyte, and acid-base imbalance. The pH of the vomitus determines the resulting acid-base abnormality. Loss of acidic gastric contents leads to metabolic alkalosis, and loss of alkaline intestinal fluids leads to metabolic acidosis. Vomiting may include bile or even fecal material in lower intestinal obstruction. Altered motility and impaction of bowel contents may lead to decreased absorption, inflammation, and possible ischemia at the site of obstruction. The combination of bowel ischemia and increased intraluminal pressure may lead to perforation, which in turn causes shock due to hemorrhage and sepsis. Ventilation may be impaired because of upward pressure on the diaphragm by abdominal distention.

Mechanical obstruction often requires surgical relief. Acquired functional obstruction is usually self-limited and requires only decompression of the bowel with nasogastric suction until neural reflexes resume. Fluid, electrolyte, and acid-base imbalances are treated with appropriate replacement or other therapy (see Chapters 8, 9, and 10).

Gastrointestinal Bleeding

Definition and Mechanisms

Gastrointestinal bleeding is hemorrhage into the alimentary canal. Bleeding from the esophagus, stomach, or duodenum is classified as **upper GI bleeding,** and bleeding from the jejunum, ileum, colon, or rectum is classified as **lower GI bleeding.** Figure 24–11 illustrates the more common sites of GI bleeding.

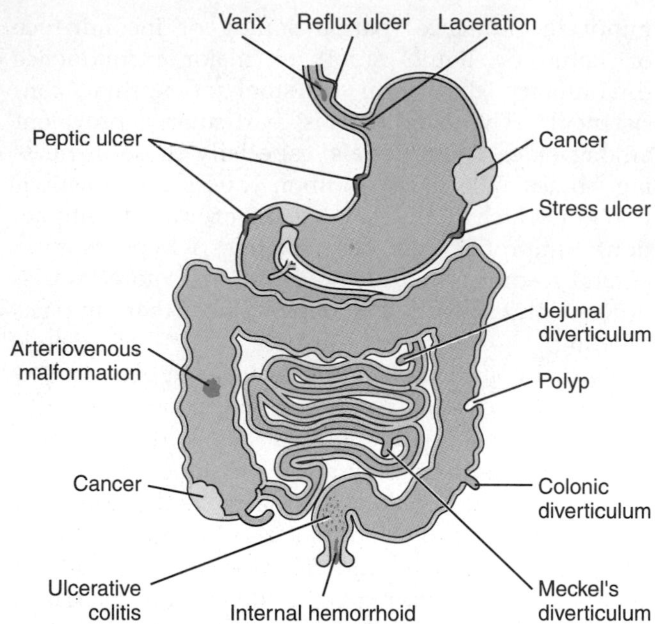

FIGURE 24–11

Bleeding lesions of the gastrointestinal tract. Bleeding from the esophagus, stomach, or duodenum is categorized as *upper GI bleeding*. Bleeding from below the duodenum is called *lower GI bleeding*. Bleeding lesions may be ulcers, lacerations, vascular defects, or bowel wall defects.

Table 24–5 describes common disorders associated with upper and lower GI bleeding. Selected disorders associated with bleeding are detailed in the next section. Upper GI bleeding may be caused by injury to the gut wall or excessive pressure within upper GI vessels. Mechanisms of wall injury and associated vessel erosion may be toxic, infectious, autoimmune, neoplastic, or ischemic. Injury to the gastric wall requires that the protective mucous barrier be breached. Gastrointestinal ischemia, as seen in selective SNS-mediated vasoconstriction with extreme stress (see Chapter 1), may reduce the mucous barrier and lead to bleeding from **stress ulceration.** Gastritis may lead to bleeding from superficial vessels. Bleeding in those with **peptic ulcer disease (PUD)** is often more severe because of the deeper erosion of tissues in this condition. Elevated pressure in the portal venous system engorges vessels of the esophagus and increases the risk of hemorrhage. This condition, **esophageal varices,** is associated with portal venous hypertension in hepatic cirrhosis (see Chapter 26).

Bleeding from the lower bowel is associated with inflammatory conditions such as **Crohn's disease, ulcerative colitis,** and **diverticulitis** and with ischemic and vascular disorders affecting the bowel. Hemorrhoids of the rectum are a potential source of bleeding from the rectum. Colorectal cancer results in bleeding when the neoplastic process invades

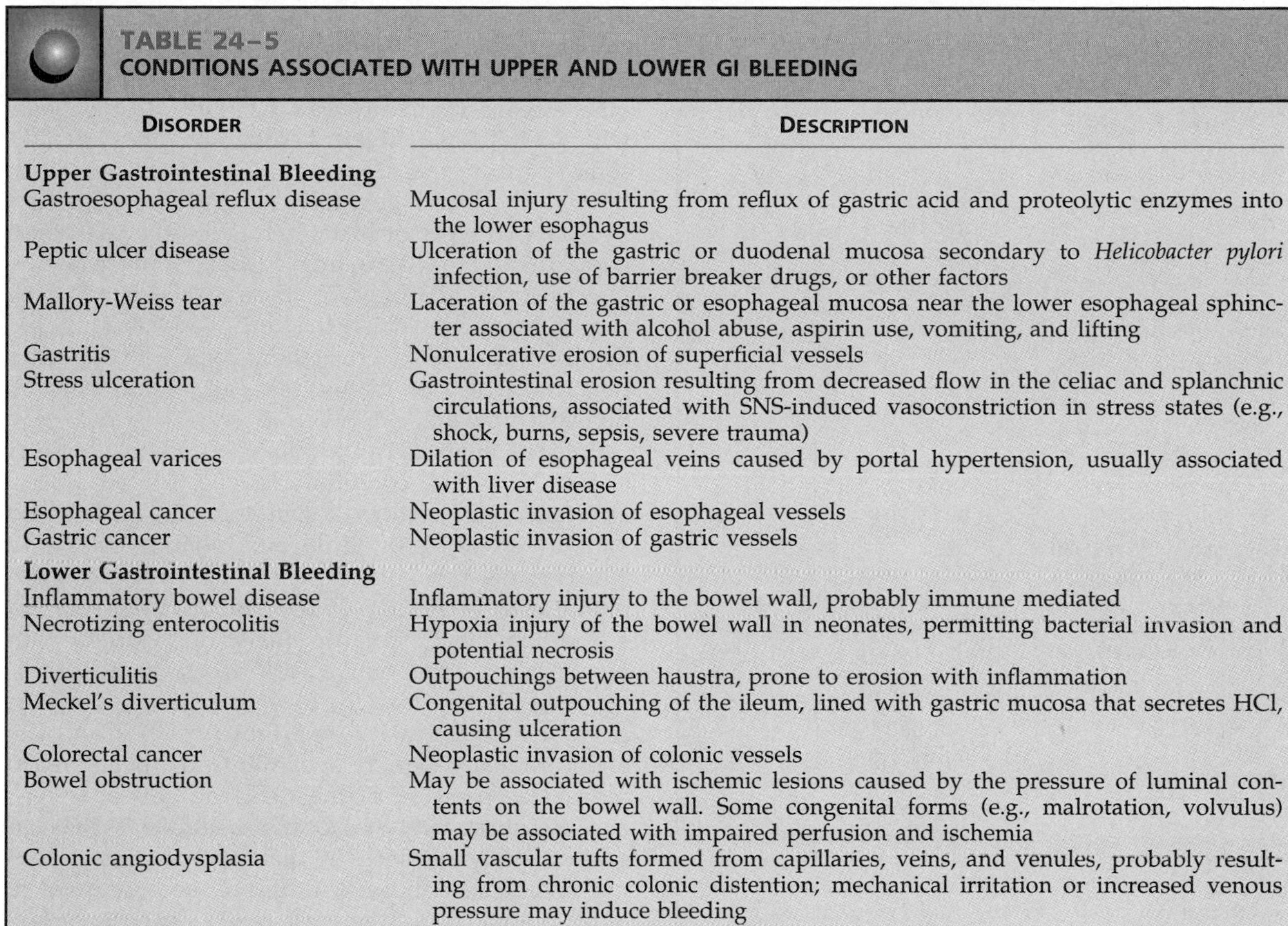
TABLE 24–5
CONDITIONS ASSOCIATED WITH UPPER AND LOWER GI BLEEDING

DISORDER	DESCRIPTION
Upper Gastrointestinal Bleeding	
Gastroesophageal reflux disease	Mucosal injury resulting from reflux of gastric acid and proteolytic enzymes into the lower esophagus
Peptic ulcer disease	Ulceration of the gastric or duodenal mucosa secondary to *Helicobacter pylori* infection, use of barrier breaker drugs, or other factors
Mallory-Weiss tear	Laceration of the gastric or esophageal mucosa near the lower esophageal sphincter associated with alcohol abuse, aspirin use, vomiting, and lifting
Gastritis	Nonulcerative erosion of superficial vessels
Stress ulceration	Gastrointestinal erosion resulting from decreased flow in the celiac and splanchnic circulations, associated with SNS-induced vasoconstriction in stress states (e.g., shock, burns, sepsis, severe trauma)
Esophageal varices	Dilation of esophageal veins caused by portal hypertension, usually associated with liver disease
Esophageal cancer	Neoplastic invasion of esophageal vessels
Gastric cancer	Neoplastic invasion of gastric vessels
Lower Gastrointestinal Bleeding	
Inflammatory bowel disease	Inflammatory injury to the bowel wall, probably immune mediated
Necrotizing enterocolitis	Hypoxia injury of the bowel wall in neonates, permitting bacterial invasion and potential necrosis
Diverticulitis	Outpouchings between haustra, prone to erosion with inflammation
Meckel's diverticulum	Congenital outpouching of the ileum, lined with gastric mucosa that secretes HCl, causing ulceration
Colorectal cancer	Neoplastic invasion of colonic vessels
Bowel obstruction	May be associated with ischemic lesions caused by the pressure of luminal contents on the bowel wall. Some congenital forms (e.g., malrotation, volvulus) may be associated with impaired perfusion and ischemia
Colonic angiodysplasia	Small vascular tufts formed from capillaries, veins, and venules, probably resulting from chronic colonic distention; mechanical irritation or increased venous pressure may induce bleeding
Hemorrhoids	Mechanical irritation or luminal pressure may induce rupture
Anal fissure	Linear ulceration, usually in the posterior midline, caused by trauma to the anal canal during defecation

blood vessels of the large intestine. These conditions are detailed in the next section.

Clinical Effects and Management

Gastrointestinal bleeding may manifest as **hematemesis** (vomiting of blood), **hematochezia** (bright red blood in the stool), **melena** (black, tarry stools), or **occult bleeding** (blood in stools not visible to the eye). The nature of the bleeding depends on the source and rate of bleeding. Hematemesis may be bright red if bleeding is recent or rapid, or it may have a "coffee grounds" appearance if blood remains in the stomach long enough for gastric juices to chemically act on it. Likewise, with rapid bleeding and rapid transit of blood through the bowel, blood in the stool is bright red. Black stools indicate that blood has been in the bowel for some time and that GI acid has altered it. Minimal bleeding results in occult blood, detectable only with chemical testing (e.g., Hemoccult or Hematest) for its presence. Epigastric pain and fullness result from local irritation and distention with blood, and vomiting may be triggered by these same factors. Chronic, slow blood loss leads to iron-deficiency anemia (see Chapter 12), and severe hemorrhage leads to hypovolemic shock (see Chapter 15).

Treatment of GI bleeding depends on the source and severity and may involve fluid resuscitation in cases of shock. The specific source of bleeding may be identified, and sometimes treated, with endoscopy. Endoscopic procedures are accomplished through the insertion of a tube into the GI tract, either orally or rectally (Table 24–6). The scope permits visualization and biopsy of the mucosa (Color Figs. 24–1 to 24–6), and a number of therapeutic interventions may be performed endoscopically. Specific medical and surgical interventions are described in the next section with the disorders for which they are implemented.

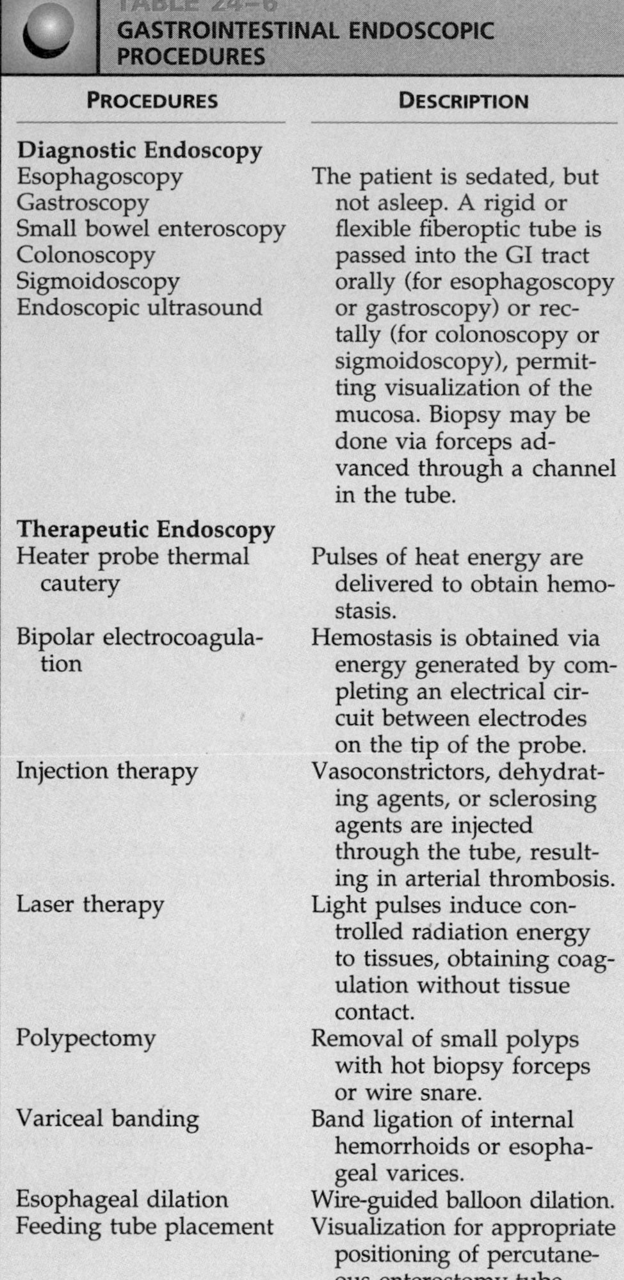

TABLE 24-6 GASTROINTESTINAL ENDOSCOPIC PROCEDURES

Procedures	Description
Diagnostic Endoscopy	
Esophagoscopy Gastroscopy Small bowel enteroscopy Colonoscopy Sigmoidoscopy Endoscopic ultrasound	The patient is sedated, but not asleep. A rigid or flexible fiberoptic tube is passed into the GI tract orally (for esophagoscopy or gastroscopy) or rectally (for colonoscopy or sigmoidoscopy), permitting visualization of the mucosa. Biopsy may be done via forceps advanced through a channel in the tube.
Therapeutic Endoscopy	
Heater probe thermal cautery	Pulses of heat energy are delivered to obtain hemostasis.
Bipolar electrocoagulation	Hemostasis is obtained via energy generated by completing an electrical circuit between electrodes on the tip of the probe.
Injection therapy	Vasoconstrictors, dehydrating agents, or sclerosing agents are injected through the tube, resulting in arterial thrombosis.
Laser therapy	Light pulses induce controlled radiation energy to tissues, obtaining coagulation without tissue contact.
Polypectomy	Removal of small polyps with hot biopsy forceps or wire snare.
Variceal banding	Band ligation of internal hemorrhoids or esophageal varices.
Esophageal dilation	Wire-guided balloon dilation.
Feeding tube placement	Visualization for appropriate positioning of percutaneous enterostomy tube.

Data from Gupta, P.K., and Fleischer, D.E. (1993). Nonvariceal upper gastrointestinal bleeding. *Medical Clinics of North America* 77(5), 973–992.

DISORDERS OF GASTROINTESTINAL MOTILITY AND SECRETION

Gastroesophageal Reflux Disease

Definition. Gastroesophageal reflux disease (GERD) includes a group of disorders in which reflux of gastric contents into the lower esophagus results in clinical symptoms or structural alterations in the tissue of the esophagus (*reflux esophagitis*) or other organs (*extraesophageal GERD*).[9] Most patients with GERD have **hiatal hernia,** the protrusion of some part of the upper portion of the stomach through the esophageal hiatus into the thoracic cavity. The two types of hiatal hernia are type I (sliding hernia) and type II (rolling or paraesophageal hernia) (Fig. 24–12). In 90% of cases, the hernia is a sliding hernia, in which the cardia and the LES are displaced upward. In the rolling type, the sphincter remains below the hiatus, but part of the stomach herniates upward.

Epidemiology. Gastroesophageal reflux disease is a very common condition in the United States. Heartburn, its principal symptom, is experienced daily by 4% to 7% of adults and monthly by 15% to 40%.[10] Hiatal hernia is present in up to 94% of these individuals. However, GERD and hiatal hernia are not synonymous, because many individuals with hernia are asymptomatic. Risk is also increased in cigarette smokers and in other conditions in which salivation is decreased (see Table 24–2). Chocolate and carminatives (e.g., spearmint and peppermint) reduce the pressure of the LES, and coffee, onions, and tomatoes may be locally irritating.[11] Delayed gastric emptying, seen in diabetes, cigarette smoking, and alcohol abuse; with use of medications such as theophylline and progesterone; and after ingestion of high-fat meals, may also predispose to reflux. Incidence of hiatal hernia increases with age, and women are more often affected than men. Risk fac-

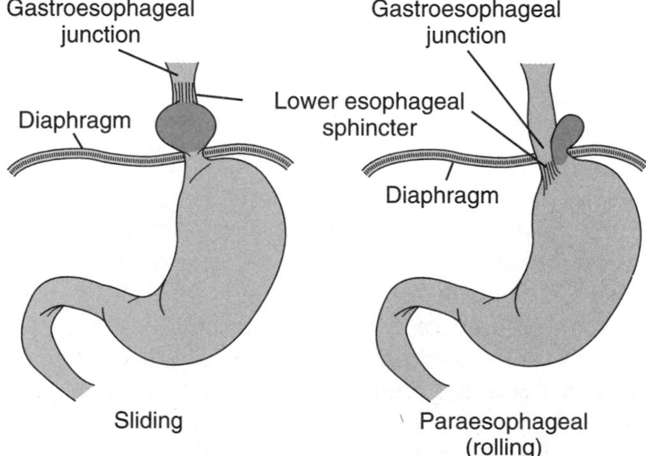

FIGURE 24–12
Hiatal hernia. Type I (sliding) hernia, in which the cardia and lower esophageal sphincter (LES) are displaced upward through the esophageal hiatus, is present in 90% of cases. In type II (rolling) hernia, the sphincter remains below the hiatus, but a portion of the cardia herniates upward.

tors for hiatal hernia are conditions that increase intra-abdominal pressure, including obesity, ascites, and pregnancy.

Etiology. Gastroesophageal reflux disease is caused by a combination of reflux-promoting factors that overcome the acid reflux barrier of the LES and surrounding diaphragmatic muscle. Abnormal function of the LES may play an important role. In most patients with GERD, frequent transient episodes of inappropriate relaxation of the LES (i.e., not triggered by swallowing) occur, either spontaneously or induced by diet, medications, smoking, or alcohol use. Concurrent presence of hiatal hernia impairs LES function and may serve as a local reservoir of gastric acid that may be pushed upward by recumbent position or increased intra-abdominal pressure. About 25% of patients with GERD have abnormal peristalsis within the esophagus, and many others have delayed gastric emptying, both of which promote acid reflux.

The factors that normally inhibit reflux include (1) high basal pressure of the LES, (2) the normal intra-abdominal location of the LES, (3) external pressure on the LES by diaphragmatic contraction during inspiration, and (4) the acute angle of entry of the esophagus into the stomach.[12] Mucus secreted by submucosal cells also provides a barrier against acid, and epithelial cell membranes and tight intercellular junctions provide further mechanical barriers. Despite the anatomic and functional barrier of the LES, some reflux occurs normally in all individuals. This acid is normally cleared efficiently by reflex swallowing and neutralized by bicarbonate-rich saliva. Conditions that impair these defenses also contribute to the development of GERD.

Pathophysiology. The degree of esophageal injury is variable, depending on the amount and concentration of refluxed gastric acid, proteolytic enzymes, and bile acids. In mild mucosal injury, the resulting inflammatory response may culminate in tissue healing (resolution). More severe or chronic injury may induce impaired swallowing (**dysphagia**) with possible aspiration, upper GI bleeding with possible ulceration and perforation, or scarring with possible obstructive stricture. The most severe consequence of GERD is **Barrett's metaplasia** (Barrett's esophagus), in which chronic epithelial injury induces metaplastic transformation of the native squamous epithelium into columnar epithelium. Barrett's metaplasia is considered to be a premalignant condition; the risk of development of adenocarcinoma of the esophagus in these individuals is much higher than that of the general population.[13]

Extraesophageal manifestations of GERD are summarized in Table 24–7. The association between acid reflux and asthma is particularly strong, with up to 89% of asthmatics also having GERD.[14] Whether direct or indirect irritation of the bronchial mucosa occurs because of reflux is unknown.

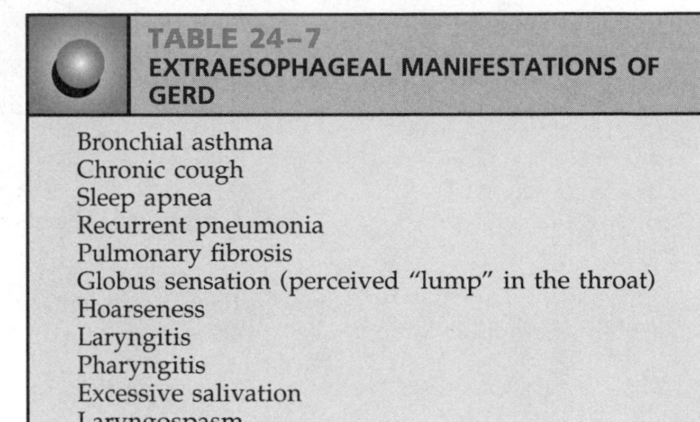
TABLE 24–7
EXTRAESOPHAGEAL MANIFESTATIONS OF GERD

Bronchial asthma
Chronic cough
Sleep apnea
Recurrent pneumonia
Pulmonary fibrosis
Globus sensation (perceived "lump" in the throat)
Hoarseness
Laryngitis
Pharyngitis
Excessive salivation
Laryngospasm
Chest pain
Dental erosion

Adapted with permission from Weinberg, D.S., and Kadish, S.L. (1996). The diagnosis and management of gastroesophageal reflux disease. *Medical Clinics of North America* 80(2), 412.

Clinical Manifestations. The patient may experience dysphagia, heartburn (a burning irritation in the epigastric area), hypersalivation, and **eructation** (belching) caused by acid reflux. Obstruction may result in a feeling of substernal fullness. In some cases, substernal pain is severe and may radiate to the back, neck, or jaw, simulating manifestations of angina pectoris. Discomfort is usually worse when the patient is lying down, because the upward pressure of the abdominal viscera is greater in this position. Some individuals have upper GI bleeding. Dyspnea may be noted because of ventilatory impairment.

Prevention and Treatment. Prevention may involve weight reduction, cessation of cigarette smoking, modification of alcohol use, avoidance of foods that increase acid secretion, or avoidance of activities that increase intra-abdominal pressure. Elevation of the upper body while sleeping may also be beneficial. Acid reflux may be treated medically with antacids to buffer HCl, histamine (H_2) blocking agents to decrease gastrin-mediated HCl release, prokinetic agents to enhance LES pressure and promote gastric emptying, or proton pump inhibitors to decrease gastric acid secretion. Acid-suppressive drug therapy is summarized in Table 24–8.

Antireflux surgery may be used in those who do not achieve satisfactory outcomes with the medical approach. *Nissen fundoplication, Hill posterior gastropexy,* and *Belsey Mark IV repair* are examples of procedures used to strengthen the anatomic barrier at the LES. Nissen fundoplication, in which the fundus of the stomach is wrapped around the distal esopha-

TABLE 24–8
ACID-SUPPRESSIVE DRUG THERAPY

Class	Drugs	Mechanism of Action
Antisecretory agents		
H_2-receptor antagonists	Cimetidine (Tagamet) Famotidine (Pepcid) Nizatidine (Axid) Ranitidine (Zantac)	Suppresses acid secretion by blocking H_2 receptors on parietal cells
Proton pump inhibitors	Omeprazole (Prilosec)	Suppresses acid secretion by inhibiting H^+-K^+-ATPase, the enzyme that makes gastric acid
Muscarinic antagonists	Pirenzepine (Gastrozepine)	Suppresses acid secretion by blocking muscarinic-cholinergic receptors (on parietal cells?)
Mucosal protectants	Sucralfate (Carafate)	Forms a barrier over the ulcer crater that protects against acid and pepsin
	Bismuth (Pepto-Bismol)	Forms a barrier over the ulcer crater that protects against acid and pepsin; reduces colonization with *Helicobacter pylori*
Antisecretory agents that enhance mucosal defenses	Misoprostol (Cytotec)	Protects against NSAID-induced ulcers by stimulating secretion of mucus and bicarbonate, maintaining submucosal blood flow, and suppressing secretion of gastric acid
Antacids	Aluminum hydroxide Magnesium hydroxide Calcium carbonate	Converts gastric acid to neutral salts
Antibiotics	Metronidazole (Flagyl) Tetracycline Amoxicillin	Eradicates *H. pylori* infection

H_2, type 2 histamine receptor; NSAID, nonsteroidal anti-inflammatory drug.
From Lehne, R.A. (1994). *Pharmacology for Nursing Care.* (2nd ed.). Philadelphia: W.B. Saunders. (p. 844).

gus and sutured to itself, is now done laparoscopically in many centers.[1]

Prognosis and Outcome. In mild GERD, 45% of patients experience spontaneous healing, and 50% have chronic symptoms but no progression of the disorder. Five percent progress to severe GERD, with complications of stricture, ulceration, or Barrett's metaplasia.[15] Long-term medical therapy is often effective in the management of GERD, but symptoms tend to recur within 6 months of discontinuation.[12] An estimated 70% to 90% of patients undergoing antireflux surgery maintain good results for 10 years; however, about one third of operations may fail to control the disorder after 20 years.[12]

Achalasia

Definition. Achalasia is a motor disorder of the esophagus characterized by absence of esophageal peristalsis and impaired relaxation of the LES during swallowing.

Epidemiology. The precise incidence of achalasia has not been reported. The disorder occurs most often in middle-aged adults and affects men and women equally.[1] A familial predisposition is apparent in some cases.[16]

Etiology. The etiology of achalasia is unknown. Two thirds of patients have autoantibodies against a dopamine-carrying protein on the surface of cells in the myenteric plexus, suggesting an autoimmune etiology in these cases.[1]

Pathophysiology. Impaired neural stimulation of the lower esophagus underlies the clinical manifestations of the disorder. Degeneration of the myenteric plexus is apparent, with nitric oxide–containing neurons preferentially lost.[1]

Clinical Manifestations. Patients have dysphagia, chest pain, and weight loss. Regurgitation of undigested food and mucus hours after eating is also common.[16]

Prevention and Treatment. There is no specific prevention for achalasia. The goal of treatment is to reduce the constriction at the LES. Nitroglycerin and calcium-channel blocking drugs may relax esophageal smooth muscle and relieve symptoms of dysphagia temporarily. Definitive treatment consists of balloon dilation of the LES or surgical esophagomyotomy, in which sphincter smooth muscle is incised down to the mucosal layer to enlarge the passage. These procedures impose risk of esophageal perforation and may predispose to acid reflux, however. Endoscopic injection of botulinum toxin into the LES has recently been shown to be effective in reducing sphincter pressure in achalasia.[1] Botulinum toxin blocks the release of acetylcholine from the myenteric plexus, impeding smooth muscle constriction.

Prognosis and Outcome. Achalasia is successfully managed with recurrent treatment in most patients. Botulinum treatment induces esophageal dilation lasting 6 months or more, with no apparent toxicity.[1] The outcome of balloon dilation is similar, with an estimated 5% risk of esophageal perforation. Esophagomyotomy may result in permanent relief of constriction, but restenosis is possible and acid reflux is common.

Esophageal Atresia

Definition. Esophageal atresia is a congenital abnormality of the esophagus usually associated with concurrent abnormality of the trachea. Figure 24–13 illustrates the three most common forms of the defect: type I (80% to 90%), in which the esophagus ends in a blind pouch and a distal **tracheoesophageal (TE) fistula** leads from the trachea to the stomach; type II (5% to 8%), in which the esophagus ends in a blind pouch but there is no TE fistula; and type III (2% to 5%), in which the esophagus is patent but a TE fistula is present.

Epidemiology. The overall prevalence is 1 in 3000 to 4000 live births.[17] The condition is associated with other congenital anomalies in nearly 50% of cases, and one third of affected infants are born prematurely. A prenatal history of polyhydramnios (excess amniotic fluid) is common, suggesting that swallowing of amniotic fluid is impaired in utero.

Etiology. The teratogenic factors specific to esophageal atresia are unknown. Factors associated with teratogenesis are discussed in Chapter 7.

Pathophysiology. Type I and type III atresia permit aspiration of oral secretions and feedings into the respiratory system, resulting in airway obstruction, ventilatory impairment, and possible pneumonia. Tracheal air is shunted into the stomach, leading to abdominal distention. Transport of ingested nutrients from the esophagus to the stomach is impaired in types I and III and prevented in type II, leading to malnutrition if alternative feeding methods are not instituted.

Clinical Manifestations. Except in type III, increased pharyngeal secretions are apparent. If feeding is attempted, the infant coughs and regurgitates and may become cyanotic. If a small fistula is present in type III, signs may be less obvious; however, recurrent pneumonia is likely during the first few months.

Prevention and Treatment. There is no known primary prevention for the anomaly. Early detection and intervention are essential to prevent aspiration pneumonia and malnutrition. Treatment consists of surgical anastomosis (connection) of the upper and lower portions of the esophagus in the case of atresia, with closure of the fistula, if present.

Prognosis and Outcome. Surgical repair is usually successful, although some individuals require periodic dilation of the esophagus at the point of anastomosis to prevent reflux. The overall survival rate is 85% to 90%.[17] Mortality is usually from associated cardiac defects.

Esophageal Cancer

Definition. Esophageal cancer includes two types of malignant tumors of the esophagus: squamous cell carcinoma and adenocarcinoma.

Epidemiology. Carcinomas of the esophagus are relatively uncommon, but are associated with high mortality. Squamous cell carcinoma of the esophagus represents 75% of cases. The estimated annual

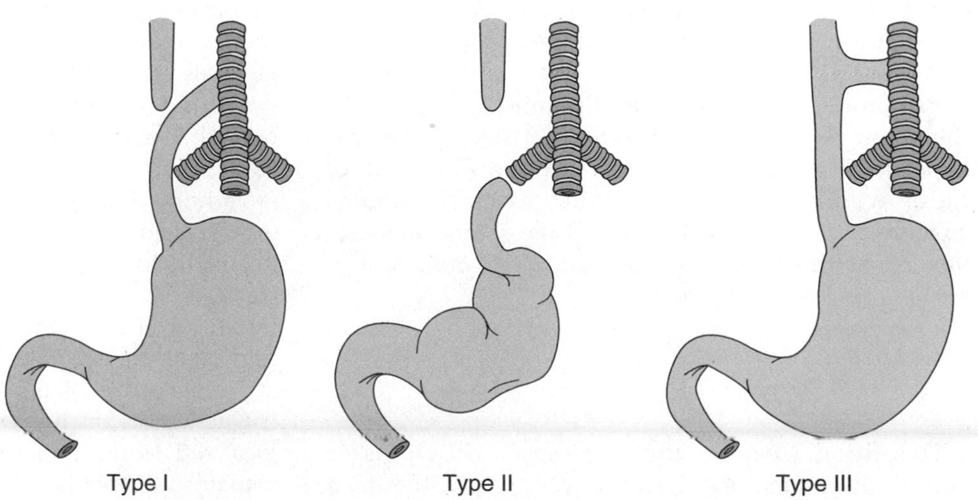

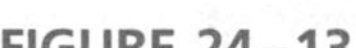
FIGURE 24–13

Forms of esophageal atresia. In type I, the esophagus ends in a blind pouch, and a distal tracheoesophageal (TE) fistula leads from the trachea to the stomach. In type II, the esophagus ends in a blind pouch, but there is no TE fistula. In type III, the esophagus is patent, but a TE fistula is present.

incidence is 4 per 100,000 males in the United States and less than half as many females.[18] Most affected individuals are older than age 50 years. Risk factors include alcohol and tobacco abuse, malnutrition, and chronic esophagitis. Adenocarcinoma comprises the remaining 25% of cases and is associated with neoplastic progression of Barrett's metaplasia of the esophagus, seen in chronic GERD. Adenocarcinoma is usually seen in those older than age 40 years, and it is more common in whites than blacks.[18]

Etiology. The precise etiology is unknown, but probably involves the combined effects of chronic tissue trauma, prolonged exposure to carcinogens, and environmental promoting agents (see Chapter 7).

Pathophysiology. Chronic esophagitis leads to progressive neoplastic transformation of epithelial and glandular tissue. Most squamous cell tumors are located in the upper or middle third of the esophagus. Growth of the tumor may become obstructive or may cause ulceration of the esophageal and tracheal walls, with bleeding and possible fistula formation. Lymphatic spread is common. Adenocarcinomas are usually found in the lower third of the esophagus and may extend locally into the gastric cardia.

Clinical Manifestations. Unfortunately, there are no early symptoms, and the tumor is usually well advanced when discovered. Signs of GERD may or may not be evident. Dysphagia is a late symptom, followed by weight loss associated with tumor growth and impaired nutrition. Ulceration may lead to hemorrhage or sepsis. Fistula formation is accompanied by aspiration.

Prevention and Treatment. Abuse of tobacco or alcohol should be curtailed, and nutritional status should be optimized. Gastroesophageal reflux disease should be managed, although there is no evidence that medical therapy decreases the risk of progression of Barrett's metaplasia to cancer.[18] Patients at risk should be screened endoscopically for the development of lesions. Surgical resection is the treatment of choice, but may not be curative in cases of advanced lesions.

Prognosis and Outcome. Prognosis varies with the stage of the disease. The 5-year survival rate for superficial squamous cell carcinoma is 75%; 25% of those with more advanced but resectable tumors survive 5 years. Because many tumors are very advanced at the time of diagnosis, the overall rate of survival is less than 15%.[18]

Peptic Ulcer Disease

Definition. Peptic ulcer disease (PUD) is a chronic inflammatory disorder resulting in the deep erosion of the mucosa of the stomach or duodenum by acid and pepsin (see Color Fig. 24–1).

Epidemiology. Approximately 10% of persons in the U.S. are affected by PUD at some time in their lives.[19] Bleeding peptic ulcers account for approximately 150,000 hospitalizations per year.[20] Risk factors include colonization of the upper GI tract with *Helicobacter pylori,* chronic use of nonsteroidal anti-inflammatory drugs (NSAIDs), and pathologically high secretion of gastric acid, as in **Zollinger-Ellison syndrome (ZES).**[21] This syndrome is caused by a gastrin-secreting tumor, usually located in the duodenum, which induces hypersecretion of gastric HCl.[22] As many as half the world's population may be infected with *H. pylori.* Crowded living conditions and poor sanitation exacerbate the risk of infection. An estimated 10% to 20% of infected individuals will develop a duodenal ulcer within 10 to 20 years of infection.[23] Risk of ulceration also increases with age, family history, and blood type O.

Etiology. The etiology of PUD is multifactoral, involving factors that promote inflammation and acid secretion as well as those that decrease the protective mucous barrier. Acid and pepsinogen secretion may be increased with the chronic vagal stimulation of a prolonged stress response. Some individuals may have congenitally increased numbers of gastric secretory cells, or these cells may be unusually sensitive to triggering stimuli. Increased acid and pepsinogen are not consistently seen in those with bleeding peptic ulcers, however. Damage to the protective mucosal barrier may occur with alcohol abuse, cigarette smoking, or chronic use of "barrier breaker" drugs, including aspirin and other NSAIDs. Infection with *H. pylori* may result in direct inflammatory injury to the mucosa or may alter the hormonal regulation of gastric acid production. Particular strains of the bacterium are associated with ulceration, whereas others produce nonulcerative gastritis.[20] Lewis antigens, expressed more frequently in those with type O blood, facilitate the attachment of *H. pylori* to the mucosa, and certain HLA subtypes apparently influence the immune response to infection (see Chapter 13).

Pathophysiology. Infection with *H. pylori* alters gastric acid secretion through a variety of mechanisms, including increased gastrin production by antral G cells and decreased somatostatin production by antral D cells. In gastric ulcer, diffuse inflammation leads to atrophic changes and decreased parietal cell mass, which reduces output of acid and intrinsic factor. In duodenal ulcer, the inflammation is localized to the antrum of the stomach, and loss of somatostatin leads to increased acid output. *Helico-*

Focus of Current Research

Study	Objective and Findings
Khuroo, et al. (1997) A comparison of omeprazole and placebo for bleeding peptic ulcer.	*Objective:* To compare the efficacy of omeprazole versus placebo in control of bleeding in peptic ulcer disease *Findings:* 10.9% of patients treated with omeprazole continued to bleed, compared with 36.4% of those treated with placebo.
Hansson, et al. (1996) The risk of stomach cancer in patients with gastric or duodenal ulcer disease.	*Objective:* To investigate the risk of gastric cancer during long-term follow-up of patients with gastric or duodenal ulcers *Findings:* Gastric ulcer patients are at increased risk of gastric cancer (relative risk, 1.8), whereas those with duodenal ulcer are at significantly *lower* risk than the general population.
Giovannucci, et al. (1995) Aspirin and the risk of colorectal cancer in women.	*Objective:* To investigate the relationship between regular use of aspirin and development of colorectal cancer among women participants in the Nurses' Health Study *Findings:* Regular use of two or more tablets of aspirin per week for at least a decade is associated with significantly decreased risk of colorectal cancer. After 20 years of use, risk was one-half that of the general population.
Macarthur, et al. (1995) *Helicobacter pylori,* gastroduodenal disease, and recurrent abdominal pain in children.	*Objective:* To assess the evidence for a causal relationship between *H. pylori* infection and antral gastritis, abdominal pain, and peptic ulcer disease in children *Findings: H. pylori* infection is strongly associated with antral gastritis and duodenal ulcer in children. The association with gastric ulcer and abdominal pain is weak.
Owens, et al. (1995) The irritable bowel syndrome: Long-term prognosis and the physician-patient interaction.	*Objective:* To evaluate the long-term course and prognosis associated with IBS and to determine the effect of an effective physician-patient relationship on health care use *Findings:* IBS is associated with a good prognosis, which is unlikely to change to that of an organic disorder. An effective relationship may decrease health care use.
Thomas, et al. (1995) Transdermal nicotine as maintenance therapy for ulcerative colitis.	*Objective:* To examine the value of transdermal nicotine for the maintenance of remission in UC *Findings:* Nicotine alone was no better than placebo in maintaining remission.

Box continued on following page

continued from previous page

Pullan, et al. (1994) Transdermal nicotine for active ulcerative colitis.	*Objective:* To examine the effect of nicotine as a supplemental treatment for ulcerative colitis *Findings:* The addition of transdermal nicotine to conventional therapy improves symptoms in UC.
Greenberg, et al. (1994) A clinical trial of antioxidant vitamins to prevent colorectal cancer.	*Objective:* To test the efficacy of β-carotene and vitamins C and E in preventing colorectal adenoma *Findings:* None of these treatments appeared to be effective in prevention.
Pahor, et al. (1994) Physical activity and risk of severe gastrointestinal hemorrhage in older persons.	*Objective:* To assess whether regular physical activity is associated with decreased risk of severe GI hemorrhage in older persons *Findings:* Activity is associated with reduced risk (relative risk, 0.6 to 0.7).

bacter pylori is not an invasive organism, but instead produces cellular injury through the release of mucolytic enzymes and toxins such as ammonia. The organism penetrates the mucus layer and adheres to glycolipids and phospholipids on the surface of epithelial cells, disrupting their membranes and permitting access of toxins to mucosal cells. The local immune response induces and sustains an inflammatory process that produces ulcerative lesions of the mucosa, possibly extending to the muscle layers. Blood vessels are eroded in about 15%, resulting in bleeding. Ulcers heal with scarring, which may lead to pyloric obstruction. Severe ulceration may perforate the bowel, leading to peritonitis.

Clinical Manifestations. Bleeding may be evident as hematemesis or melena, or it may be insidious (occult). Detection of occult blood in a stool sample requires that the patient be on a diet free of meats, certain vegetables, and medications such as iron preparations that could cause inaccurate results. If hemorrhage is severe, signs of shock are apparent (see Chapter 15). The inflammatory process results in crampy epigastric pain. Pain is often relieved with eating, which dilutes irritants; however, protein, calcium, or other components of the diet may stimulate further secretion, causing pain to recur soon thereafter. Pyloric obstruction leads to a feeling of fullness after meals, and in severe cases, may lead to projectile vomiting. Perforation is acutely painful, and peritonitis is evidenced as abdominal distention and septic shock. Over the long term, chronic PUD may lead to mucosal dysplasia, which predisposes to cancer. Those with significant atrophic changes may develop pernicious anemia as a result of lack of intrinsic factor (see Chapter 12).

Prevention and Treatment. Reduction of stress, abstinence from alcohol use, and discontinuation of use of barrier breaker drugs are indicated for the prevention of PUD in those at risk. Two noninvasive screening tests for *H. pylori* are now in use: the ^{13}C-urea breath test and measurement of serum immunoglobulin *H. pylori* antibody titers.[24] Conservative management of PUD consists of frequent small meals, which may reduce fullness; augmenting the acid barrier; and minimizing fluctuations in acid secretion. Milk-based ("sippy") diets are no longer advocated for ulcer prevention or treatment, because their high calcium content stimulates a rebound increase in gastrin release. Calcium-based antacids are also avoided for this reason.

Acid-suppressive drug therapy (see Table 24–8) is the mainstay of treatment in PUD. Magnesium and aluminum-based antacids are used to increase gastric pH and inactivate pepsin. H_2-receptor blockade with drugs such as cimetidine (Tagamet) and ranitidine (Zantac) decreases histamine-mediated gastrin release. Proton pump inhibitors such as omeprazole (Prilosec) may also be used to decrease acidity and have recently been shown to decrease the rate of active bleeding (see Focus of Current Research).[25] Coating agents such as sucralfate (Carafate) bind to ulcerated tissue in an acid pH, augmenting the bar-

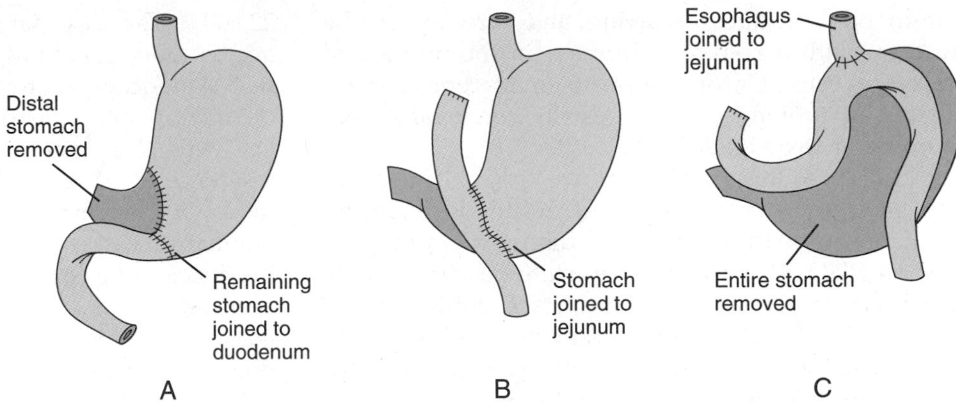

FIGURE 24–14
Surgical treatment of peptic ulcer disease. *A,* In the Billroth I procedure, the distal stomach is removed and the remaining portion is sutured to the duodenum. *B,* In the Billroth II procedure, the stomach remnant is sutured to the proximal jejunum. *C,* In total gastrectomy, the entire stomach is resected and the esophagus is sutured to the jejunum.

rier. Eradication of *H. pylori* infection with antibiotic therapy prevents the recurrence of peptic ulcer disease in up to 96% of patients,[26] and is the ultimate goal of treatment. The optimum combination of drugs is still uncertain. "Triple therapies" with antibiotics (e.g., metronidazole, tetracycline) and acid-suppressive drugs (H_2 blockers or proton pump inhibitors) have been most effective.

Significant bleeding may require nasogastric suction via a flexible tube inserted into the stomach or duodenum. Iced saline irrigation (*lavage*) and instillation of vasoconstrictor substances have been used to constrict surface vessels and lessen bleeding, but the efficacy of these measures is unproved.[20] Lavage may be used before endoscopy to cleanse the stomach and improve visualization of the mucosa. Endoscopic therapies such as laser therapy, thermal electrocoagulation, and sclerotherapy may be beneficial in those with substantial bleeding (see Table 24–6).

Surgery is usually performed only when endoscopic procedures are unsuccessful or unavailable, such as in cases of severe hemorrhage or perforation (Fig. 24–14). Surgical techniques include Billroth procedures, in which the lower portion of the stomach and part of the duodenum are removed; total or subtotal gastrectomy, to remove the affected gastric mucosa; and vagotomy, to eliminate the autonomic stimulus for secretion. A complication of such procedures is **dumping syndrome,** in which rapid emptying of gastric contents into the small intestine creates a high osmotic gradient in the lumen of the bowel, resulting in hypovolemia caused by fluid shifts from the surrounding vessels into the GI tract.

Prognosis and Outcome. If *H. pylori* infection can be eradicated, PUD is curable. Most patients with PUD respond well to risk reduction and medical therapy, but they do have recurrence of disease if therapy is stopped. Mortality is associated with bleeding and perforation.

Clinical Scenario

V.K., a 61-year-old male with a history of peptic ulcer disease, undergoes endoscopic evaluation for recurrent GI bleeding, evidenced by mahogany-colored stools. He has been taking H_2 antagonists for several years, which have been effective in reducing symptoms of epigastric pain and fullness. It is determined with endoscopy that he has a small, actively bleeding duodenal ulcer and several scarred areas near the pylorus. Biopsy and serum testing confirm the presence of *Helicobacter pylori.*

1. Is V.K.'s rectal bleeding typical of peptic ulcer disease? Explain.
2. Is V.K.'s condition curable? If so, how?

Gastritis

Definition. Gastritis is acute or chronic inflammation of the gastric mucosa (see Color Fig. 24–2).

Epidemiology. Acute gastritis is most common in individuals aged 40 to 50 years. Chronic gastritis is most common in those older than 60 years. Men are more prone to gastritis than women. Cigarette smoking, high caffeine intake, alcohol abuse, frequent intake of spicy foods, use of aspirin and other NSAIDs, and *H. pylori* infection increase the risk of gastritis. Gastritis may be associated with endogenous toxins in the case of shock, hepatic failure, or renal failure.

Etiology. In acute gastritis, increased acid and pepsinogen secretion and barrier breakdown promote inflammation. In chronic gastritis, barrier breakdown is the more prevalent factor. Chronic inflammation produces scarring and atrophy of the mucosa, with a resultant decrease in the number of secretory cells. Chronic gastritis may represent recurrent or prolonged acute gastritis, or it may have immune or toxic etiology.[18]

Pathophysiology. *Helicobacter pylori* infection, present in the majority of cases, results in impaired regulation of acid secretion, as discussed in the section on PUD. Inflammation in acute gastritis results in superficial erosion of the surface epithelium of the stomach, with healing occurring within a few days, usually by regeneration. In chronic gastritis, there is progressive, permanent thinning and degeneration of the gastric mucosa. Atrophy of chief cells and oxyntic cells causes impaired digestion of protein and lack of intrinsic factor impedes vitamin B_{12} absorption.

Clinical Manifestations. A significant number of patients are asymptomatic. In others, the clinical manifestations of acute gastritis are of epigastric pain and hematemesis, usually less severe than in the case of PUD. In chronic gastritis, **achlorhydria** (lack of HCl secretion) is usually present rather than hyperacidity, and pernicious anemia may be evident on hematology studies.

Prevention and Treatment. Prevention consists of removing the causative agents or risk factors, if possible. Acid-suppressive therapy may be instituted in those who have hypersecretion. For those with chronic gastritis, frequent, small meals are better tolerated, and replacement of vitamin B_{12} is indicated for pernicious anemia (see Chapter 12). If chronic gastritis results in severe erosion of the gastric mucosa, surgical resection (Billroth or gastrectomy) might be required.

Prognosis and Outcome. Acute gastritis is usually self-limited and subsides with removal of the offending agent. Chronic gastritis is usually well managed with medical therapy; however, affected individuals have a two-fold to three-fold risk of developing gastric cancer.[27]

Gastric Cancer

Definition. Gastric cancer is a primary malignant neoplasm of the stomach. Ninety percent are adenocarcinomas (see Color Fig. 24–3); the remainder are primarily non-Hodgkin's lymphomas or leiomyosarcomas.[27]

Epidemiology. Gastric cancer is still the eighth leading cause of cancer death in the United States, despite decreasing incidence during the past four decades.[28] The average age at diagnosis is 55 to 60 years. Annual incidence is currently estimated at 22,800.[27] The disorder is twice as common in men and is more common in blacks, Hispanics, and Native Americans than in whites. Associated factors include atrophic gastritis, colonization of the stomach with *H. pylori*, low socioeconomic status, urban residence, frequent eating of smoked or pickled foods, and exposure to radiation or trace metals. A familial predisposition is evident. The decline in the incidence of gastric cancer in recent decades has been attributed to a reduction in the distal (intestinal) type, which is most strongly associated with poor refrigeration and storage of foods.

Etiology. The precise etiology is unknown. As with most cancers, multiple factors are probably involved (see Chapter 7). Gastric disorders in which chronic inflammation induces metaplastic changes in mucosal cells are strongly associated, along with dietary, genetic, and environmental factors that promote the progression of such changes.

Pathophysiology. Most gastric cancers are adenocarcinomas, arising from the mucosal layer. The antral and pyloric areas are most often affected. The neoplasm spreads by direct extension (often to the pancreas), seeding to peritoneal surfaces, or by lymphatic or blood-borne infiltration of the liver, lungs, and bones.

Clinical Manifestations. Because early signs of gastric cancer are vague, the disease is often not diagnosed until the neoplasm has invaded the stomach wall and spread to other organs. The patient may report weight loss, indigestion, or a feeling of fullness. Mild discomfort may be present, which is either induced or relieved by eating. More obvious obstructive manifestations occur if the tumor impedes esophageal emptying in the area of the cardia or pyloric emptying into the duodenum. Chronic blood loss leads to anemia, but bleeding into the stool is usually occult. The tumor marker alpha-fetoprotein is elevated in the serum of 30% of patients with gastric cancer.[27]

Prevention and Treatment. Reduction of risk is warranted for prevention of gastric cancer. Those at risk should be carefully monitored for early signs, possibly with screening endoscopy. The treatment of choice for resectable cancer is surgery, either total or partial gastrectomy (see Fig. 24–14). Adjacent lymph nodes are usually resected as well. If the tumor is unresectable and metastasis has occurred, surgery may be done palliatively, and a combination of chemotherapy and radiation therapy may be used to slow the spread of the cancer.

Prognosis and Outcome. Five-year survival after resection of tumors is variable depending on the stage at diagnosis. The overall 5-year survival rate is approximately 15%.[28]

Hypertrophic Pyloric Stenosis

Definition. Hypertrophic pyloric stenosis (HPS) is a congenital obstructive disorder of the gastric outlet, resulting from hypertrophy of the circular musculature surrounding the pylorus.

Epidemiology. This disorder occurs in about 3 per 1000 infants, affecting four times as many males as females. A genetic predisposition is apparent.[29]

Etiology. The precise etiology of the congenital form of HPS is uncertain, but multifactorial inheritance is a contributing factor. (It may also be acquired later in life as a consequence of PUD or gastric cancers affecting the pylorus.)

Pathophysiology. Hypertrophy may develop as a consequence of faulty genetic control of development or lack of innervation. Local edema and inflammatory changes in the mucosa may aggravate the obstruction. Decreased levels of *nitric oxide synthase* enzyme have also been noted in HPS patients.[29] Lack of nitric oxide, which relaxes smooth muscle, may contribute to pyloric obstruction. Obstruction impedes gastric emptying and rising epigastric pressure induces vomiting.

Clinical Manifestations. The condition usually becomes evident within 3 to 10 weeks after birth.[29] Vomiting is usually projectile, but may occasionally be nonprojectile. Vomitus does not contain bile. Prolonged vomiting may result in dehydration and metabolic alkalosis (see Chapter 10). The pylorus can often be palpated as an olive-shaped mass in the right epigastrium. After ingestion of contrast media, the obstruction can be seen radiographically.

Prevention and Treatment. There is no known prevention for congenital HPS. Surgical correction with pyloromyotomy (Fredet-Ramstedt procedure) is the definitive treatment. This operation consists of a longitudinal incision down the mucosa, with splitting of the hypertrophied muscle to enlarge the outlet.[30]

Prognosis and Outcome. Prognosis is excellent with prompt recognition of the disorder, correction of fluid and acid-base disorders, and surgical intervention. Patients can usually begin unrestricted feeding within hours after surgery.

Gastroenteritis

Definition. **Gastroenteritis** is inflammation of the stomach, intestines, or both.

Epidemiology. Viral gastroenteritis is very common throughout the world, often occurring in epidemics and referred to as the "stomach flu." Inflammation caused by bacterial toxins or irritants in food ("food poisoning") is also believed to be common, with *Salmonella* and *Escherichia coli* often implicated. Bacterial gastroenteritis is more prevalent in those living in unsanitary conditions, in young children, and in homosexual males. Improper handling and cooking of food may increase risk. Infection of the colon with *Clostridium difficile* is common among hospitalized patients on prolonged therapy with multiple antibiotics.

Etiology. Inflammation in gastroenteritis is caused by viruses, toxins, or bacteria.

Pathophysiology. Organisms multiply rapidly within the bowel, producing manifestations of the disease within about 16 hours. Endotoxins cause local inflammation and stimulate GI smooth muscle and secretory cells. These may induce vomiting and may lead to diarrhea by motile and secretory mechanisms. Bacterial infection of the colon is often referred to as **dysentery.** *Clostridium difficile* colitis results from overgrowth of this organism when the normal flora of the colon is lost with antibiotic therapy. This superinfection produces characteristic patchy lesions of the lower bowel (**pseudomembranous colitis**).

Clinical Manifestations. Systemic signs of inflammation are present to varying degrees (see Chapter 13). Crampy pain results from increased motility. Vomiting and diarrhea may lead to dehydration, electrolyte imbalance, and acid-base imbalance. Some bleeding into the stool may be evident as a result of inflammatory erosion of superficial vessels in the GI wall. Pseudomembranous colitis is associated with significant rectal bleeding in some cases.

Prevention and Treatment. Prevention involves reduction of risk factors, proper sanitation measures, and limitation of exposure, especially for infants, elderly persons, and debilitated individuals. The need to prevent imprudent use of antibiotics is discussed in Chapter 13. Treatment consists of replacement of fluid and electrolytes and appropriate antibiotics for bacterial infection. Antidiarrheal agents, which decrease bowel motility, are usually contraindicated because they allow the causative agent to remain in the bowel for a longer period of time.

Prognosis and Outcome. If detected early and treated with appropriate fluid and electrolyte replacement, gastroenteritis is usually self-limited and resolves fully.

Irritable Bowel Syndrome

Definition. **Irritable bowel syndrome (IBS)** includes a number of chronic functional bowel disorders characterized by persistence or recurrence of the following symptoms for a period of at least 3 months[31]:

1. Abdominal pain or discomfort, relieved with defecation or associated with a change in frequency or consistency of stool
2. An irregular pattern of defecation at least 25% of the time, with two or more of the following:

   - Altered stool frequency
   - Hard, loose, or watery stool
   - Straining or sense of urgency, feeling of incomplete evacuation
   - Passage of mucus
   - Bloating or abdominal distention

Epidemiology. Symptoms typical of IBS are reported in 10% to 22% of adults, with slightly more women affected than men.[31] Symptoms usually begin in young adulthood, but persist throughout the life span. An etiologic link between stress and IBS has been postulated, but remains unproved. An increased incidence of psychological disorders, such as personality disorders, anxiety, and depression, is seen among those who seek medical attention for IBS.

Etiology. The precise etiology of IBS is unknown. Whether the defect lies in abnormal innervation of the gut or in the GI smooth muscle itself is unknown. Visceral sensation is also altered, suggesting a neural mechanism.

Pathophysiology. Most dysfunction is at the level of the colon, in which altered neural stimulation results in nonpropulsive segmentation waves, promoting constipation. In those with abdominal pain, paroxysmal contractions of the duodenum and jejunum are noted in the fasting state. Patients have demonstrated a lower pain threshold in response to distention of the bowel with gas while having a normal threshold to other forms of somatic pain. Patients with IBS often have concurrent noncardiac chest pain as well as dysfunction of esophageal, pulmonary, and urologic smooth muscle. This suggests that the syndrome is a systemic, rather than a single-organ, disorder.

Clinical Manifestations. The typical clinical manifestations are those that establish the diagnosis. It may manifest primarily as either diarrhea or constipation. In many cases, the diagnosis is one of exclusion of GI disorders in which a specific cause, defect, or lesion can be demonstrated.

Prevention and Treatment. The patient is usually advised to avoid dairy products and other gas-forming foods and to optimize dietary fiber. Although no single drug has proven effective in all cases, the usual approach is to treat the predominant symptom. Psychosocial factors that may be contributing to the condition may be addressed through psychotherapy or biofeedback.

Prognosis and Outcome. Most patients continue to have symptoms, regardless of treatment. Although quality of life is undoubtably compromised by IBS, life expectancy is normal and the condition does not result in significant GI dysfunction.

Inflammatory Bowel Disease

Definition. Inflammatory bowel disease (IBD) encompasses a number of chronic conditions of the intestine, of which the most common are Crohn's disease (CD) and ulcerative colitis (UC). Crohn's disease is granulomatous, transmural inflammation of discontinuous segments of bowel, usually confined to the terminal ileum and proximal colon but potentially affecting any portion of the GI tract. Ulcerative colitis is demonstrated by inflammation of the mucosa and submucosa, first involving the rectum and potentially ascending upward through the entire colon.[32]

Epidemiology. Both UC and CD display a familial incidence and an onset in young adulthood. Incidence is highest in whites and in Jewish persons. Although CD is equally distributed among males and females, UC is more prevalent in females. Ulcerative colitis is the most common cause of chronic colitis, with an incidence of 4 to 15 cases per 100,000. The incidence of CD varies geographically from 1 to 10 cases per 100,000.[32] Although cigarette smoking is a risk factor for CD, smoking is associated with *lower* risk of UC. Indeed, nicotine has been used in the treatment of UC (see Focus of Current Research).

Etiology. The precise etiology of these disorders is unknown, although genetic and autoimmune mechanisms have been proposed. In many but not all cases, the patient demonstrates other immune pathology such as systemic lupus erythematosus or rheumatoid arthritis (see Chapter 34). Emotional disturbances or stress may exacerbate symptoms, but they are not known to cause IBD.

Pathophysiology. The location and appearance of inflammatory lesions differs between the two forms. In CD, inflammatory lesions extend through the bowel wall and develop simultaneously in separate areas. Granuloma formation occurs first, followed by ulceration and abscess formation. Fistulas may form between the affected areas and the bladder, vagina, or rectum. With repeated episodes, the gut wall assumes a cobblestone appearance, with permanent scarring and constriction. The characteristic lesion of UC is the crypt abscess, a pus-filled, necrotic lesion that starts at the bases of the crypts of Lieberkühn.

These lesions ulcerate and bleed during flares, then heal with scarring and constriction. Perforation of the bowel and peritonitis are possible.

Clinical Manifestations. Both conditions are characterized by rectal bleeding, diarrhea, weight loss, and abdominal pain. Pain of CD is usually located in the right lower quadrant or periumbilical region of the abdomen, and UC is manifested by crampy pain of the left lower quadrant. Consistent with autoimmune etiology, extraintestinal manifestations of IBD may be seen. These include iritis, uveitis, conjunctivitis, erythema nodosum, migratory arthritis, ankylosing spondylitis, chronic hepatitis, and sclerosing cholangitis.[33]

Prevention and Treatment. There is no known primary prevention for IBD. Stress management and avoidance of factors that promote GI secretion may help minimize exacerbations. Drug therapy in mild IBD consists of sulfasalazine and other anti-inflammatory aminosalicylates. Steroids may be used in more severe disease. Immunosuppressive agents such as azathioprine, methotrexate, and cyclosporine may be used to suppress the immune response when anti-inflammatory therapy is insufficient, and antidiarrheals may be used to reduce diarrhea. Nicotine patches, nicotine gum, and cigarette smoking appear to have a beneficial effect on symptoms of UC, possibly because of induced changes in the colonic mucosa or suppression of inflammatory mediators.[34] Fluids and electrolytes are replaced as necessary, and total parenteral nutrition (see Chapter 25) may be used to rest the bowel. Small bowel resection with possible ileostomy may be needed to prevent or treat perforation.

Prognosis and Outcome. Although most patients with IBD can be managed with current therapy, it does not seem to alter the natural course of the disease.[35] Most patients demonstrate recurrent relapse. The risk of colorectal cancer is increased in patients with UC, and patients with CD involving the small intestine are at increased risk of developing adenocarcinoma of the small bowel.[36]

Appendicitis

Definition. Appendicitis is inflammation of the vermiform appendix.

Epidemiology. The estimated annual incidence of appendicitis in the United States is 11 cases per 10,000.[37] Appendicitis is most common among those aged 10 to 19 years, but it occasionally occurs in older adults. There are usually no apparent risk factors, although presence of chronic inflammation or intra-abdominal adhesions is associated with the disorder in older persons. Recently, the role of dietary, hereditary, and social influences on the disorder have been investigated. Western housing, rather than Western diet (e.g., low fiber, high fat), has been associated with increased risk, and a familial predisposition is apparent.[37]

Etiology. Appendicitis is caused by obstruction of the appendix by a *fecolith* (pellet of impacted stool) occluding the lumen, by torsion or kinking of the appendix, or by inflammatory or fibrotic conditions that obstuct the appendix internally or externally.

Pathophysiology. Once luminal obstruction has occurred, continued production of mucus increases pressure and distends the appendix. Pressure decreases perfusion and leads to ischemic injury, inflammation, and possible perforation. Visceral afferent nerves are stimulated, resulting in pain that is referred to the epigastric and umbilical areas at first. Perforation allows entry of bowel contents into the peritoneal cavity, precipitating peritonitis that is localized to the right lower quadrant of the abdomen and possible septic shock.

Clinical Manifestations. The classic abdominal pain of appendicitis begins with intermittent discomfort in the epigastric or periumbilical regions related to bowel obstruction and distention. As the inflammation spreads to involve the peritoneum, the pain becomes continuous and is perceived in the right lower quadrant. The patient may vomit, and typically draws the legs upward to guard the painful area and reduce abdominal tension. Palpation of the abdomen reveals muscle rigidity and rebound tenderness (acute pain with release of pressure) over the right lower quadrant. *Psoas sign* is present if passive extension or active flexion of the hip elicits pain, indicating irritation of the psoas muscle. If inflammation extends to the obturator internus muscle, the *obturator sign* may be positive. In this case, pain is elicited with passive internal rotation of the flexed thigh. Systemic signs of inflammation, including low-grade fever and mild leukocytosis, may be present.

Prevention and Treatment. There is no known prevention for appendicitis. Early detection is critical to prevention of perforation, peritonitis, and septic shock (see Chapter 15). Uncomplicated acute appendicitis is treated with surgical removal of the appendix and inversion of the stump (appendectomy). The patient is supported with fluid and electrolyte replacement and antibiotic therapy. In cases of perforation, the condition is usually treated nonoperatively at first, with parenteral fluids and antibiotic therapy. Presence of a palpable right lower quadrant mass after 2 to 5 days indicates an abscess that must be drained. Six weeks after resolution of symptoms, appendectomy is performed, possibly using a laparoscopic approach.

Prognosis and Outcome. Prognosis after early appendectomy is excellent. Mortality is associated with unrecognized perforation and peritonitis.

Peritonitis

Definition. Peritonitis is inflammation of the peritoneal membrane. It may be sterile, resulting from noninfectious irritants, or infectious.

Epidemiology. The precise incidence of peritonitis is unknown. Risk is derived from the presence of disorders in which bacteria or chemical irritants may access the peritoneum.

Etiology. Sterile peritonitis is usually caused by: (1) rupture of the biliary system, permitting the entry of bile into the peritoneal cavity; (2) acute hemorrhagic pancreatitis, in which pancreatic enzymes leak into the cavity; (3) endometriosis, in which blood enters the cavity during the menstrual cycle; or (4) surgical procedures, in which mechanical abrasion of surfaces may lead to inflammation. Infectious peritonitis is usually caused by: (1) extension of bacteria through the wall of a ruptured or compromised bowel, gallbladder, or fallopian tube, or (2) entry of bacteria from the environment via abdominal trauma or invasive procedures such as peritoneal dialysis.[18]

Pathophysiology. Inflammation results in loss of peritoneal integrity, with third spacing of exudate into the cavity. Involvement of the bowel with the inflammatory process results in increased secretion, increasing intraluminal pressure and resulting in a reflex decrease in motility (paralytic ileus). Abdominal distention may mechanically impair ventilation.

Clinical Manifestations. Signs of decreased circulatory volume are evident to some degree and may indicate the presence of septic shock (see Chapter 15). Bowel sounds are absent, and abdominal pain and rigidity are typical. Functional bowel obstruction may result in nausea and vomiting. Respirations are usually shallow because of abdominal pain and distention.

Prevention and Treatment. Patients at risk for peritonitis should be carefully monitored with frequent assessment of bowel sounds. Distention is treated with insertion of an intestinal tube for decompression and drainage of the bowel. Fluids are replaced intravenously. Infectious peritonitis is treated with appropriate antibiotic therapy. Surgical repair of underlying bowel disorders may be warranted when the patient's condition stabilizes.

Prognosis and Outcome. Prognosis is variable depending on the underlying disorder and the degree of circulatory failure. Mortality is high in septic shock associated with peritonitis.

Diverticulitis

Definition. Diverticulitis is inflammation of a diverticulum, a ballooned segment of the colon wall created by herniation of the mucosal layer outward through the muscular layers (Fig. 24–15). The term that applies to presence, but not inflammation, of diverticula is **diverticulosis.**

Epidemiology. Diverticula occur in one third of persons older than age 50 and two thirds of those older than age 80 in the United States and other developed countries.[38] Of these individuals, 10% to 20% will develop diverticulitis. Diverticulitis is rare in undeveloped countries, where the typical diet is much higher in fiber and where defecation is accomplished in a knee-chest position. Risk factors for the condition are those associated with chronic constipation, including lack of dietary fiber, lack of physical activity, and poor bowel habits. Use of Western

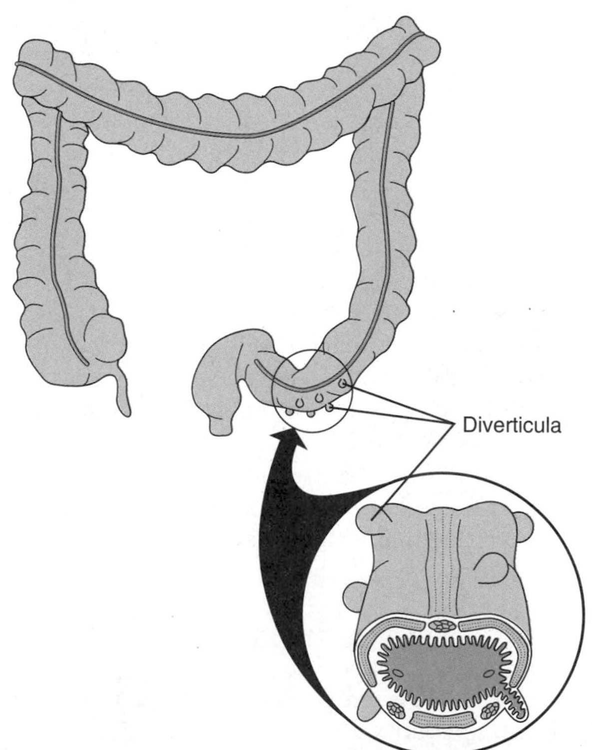

FIGURE 24–15

Diverticulosis. Diverticula are areas of the colon wall in which the mucosal layer herniates outward through the muscular layers, creating ballooned segments. Diverticula are prone to inflammation and bleeding caused by mechanical or chemical irritation. (From Ignatavicius, D.D., Workman, M.L., and Misher, M.A. [Eds.]. [1995]. Medical-Surgical Nursing: A Nursing Process Approach. [2nd Ed.]. Philadelphia: W.B. Saunders. [p. 1651].)

toilets is also believed to increase risk, because high intracolonic pressures are generated during defecation.[38] Genetic factors are also believed to be important in the location and timing of onset of diverticular disease.

Etiology. Although the precise etiology is unknown, the increased intraluminal pressure may predispose to formation of diverticula in areas where the colonic wall is weakest, that is, where nutrient arteries penetrate the muscle layers.

Pathophysiology. Diverticula usually occur in the sigmoid colon, where the longitudinal muscle is separated into segments (*haustra*). Herniation occurs between these haustra because of the increased intraluminal force generated in this area, which has a smaller diameter than other segments of the colon. These weakened areas are then prone to inflammation caused by mechanical or chemical irritation, with perforation and hemorrhage possible. Chronic diverticular disease may also be associated with the formation of fistulas between the colon and the vagina, occurring almost exclusively in women who have had hysterectomies.

Clinical Manifestations. Abrupt onset of abdominal pain and alteration in bowel pattern are common initial signs.[38] Pain is often localized to the left lower quadrant and is sometimes referred to as "left-sided appendicitis." Colovaginal fistulas manifest as vaginitis. Diverticular disease is a common cause of acute lower GI bleeding, but it is not seen in all patients. When bleeding does occur, it is usually from diverticula located in the *right* colon, for unknown reasons.[39] Bleeding is from an arterial source and tends to be massive.

Prevention and Treatment. Adoption of a healthy lifestyle with proper dietary and bowel habits as well as optimal exercise may prevent the condition. Most acute episodes require only bowel rest (clear liquid diet or nothing by mouth) until inflammation subsides. More severe or prolonged episodes are treated with antibiotics and steroids. Hemorrhage and perforation are indications for surgical resection of the diseased colon with possible diversion of the fecal stream through the abdominal wall via a colostomy (Fig. 24–16).

Prognosis and Outcome. Most cases of diverticulitis are mild and respond well to conservative measures. About 20% of patients eventually require surgery.[38]

Colorectal Cancer

Definition. Colorectal cancer is a primary malignant neoplasm of the colon or rectum.

Epidemiology. Colorectal cancer is the second most frequent cause of cancer death in the United States (approximately 57,000 deaths per year). An estimated 138,000 new cases are diagnosed each year.[40] Incidence increases sharply with age older than 50 years, and some forms are familial. Presence of adenomatous polyps or IBD is associated with increased risk. The United States is among several nations (e.g., New Zealand, Australia, and many European countries) with the highest death rates from colorectal cancer in the world. Japan and other Asian and South American countries have the lowest death rates, suggesting that a diet high in fat and low in fiber may convey significant risk. Although studies are still inconclusive, associations have been noted between colorectal cancer and ethanol intake, refined sugar consumption, calcium and folate deficiencies, cigarette smoking, sedentary lifestyle, and obesity.[41]

Etiology. The precise etiology of most cases of colorectal cancer is unknown. Hereditary nonpolyposis colon cancer (HNPCC) and hereditary GI polyposis syndrome, known to be caused by inherited genetic defects, account for about 6% and 1% of colorectal cancers, respectively.[41] Factors involved in the process of carcinogenesis are reviewed in Chapter 7.

Pathophysiology. Colorectal cancer usually begins with the development of polyps or luminal projections from the mucosa (see Color Fig. 24–4). Although most polyps remain benign and limited in

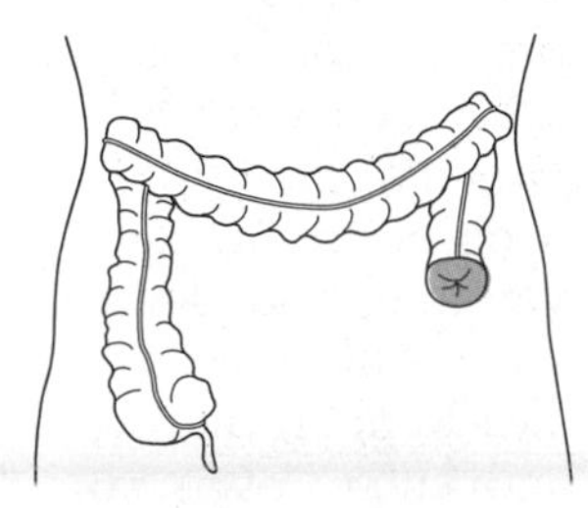

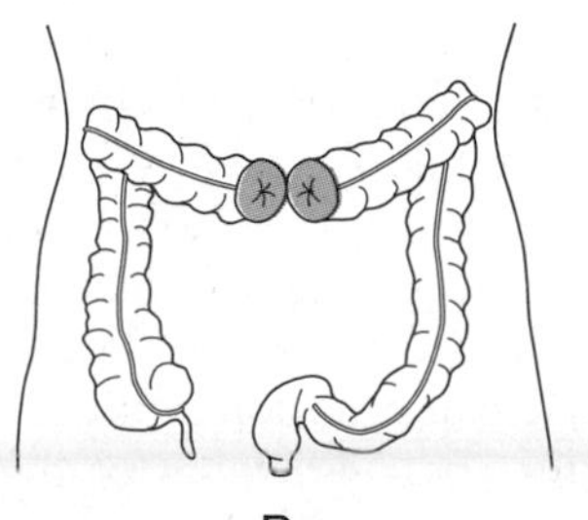

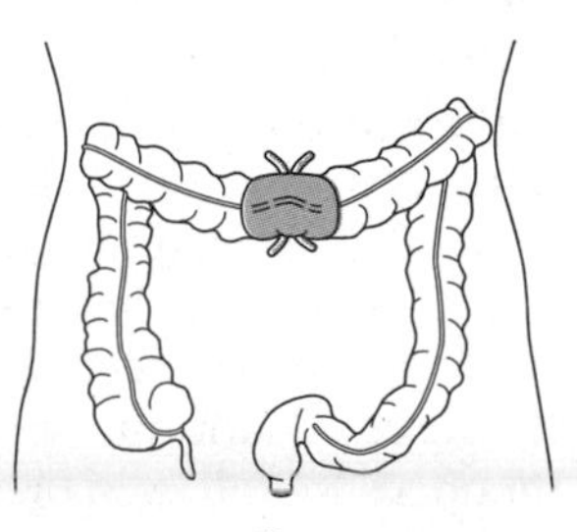

FIGURE 24–16
Types of colostomies. *A,* Single-barrel colostomy. *B,* Double-barreled colostomy. *C,* Loop colostomy.

extent, in some cases they continue to grow, invading the glands of the mucosa. Once the neoplasm enters the lymphatics, it metastasizes rapidly. Tumors of the ascending colon tend to manifest as polyps along one side of the wall, which tend to ulcerate and bleed rather than to become obstructive. Tumors of the descending colon tend to form button-like lesions that encircle the wall and become obstructive as well as ulcerative (see Color Fig. 24–5).

Colorectal tumor cells undergo a predictable genetic alteration that forms the basis of staging and prognosis. These genetic defects involve mutational activation of the *ras* oncogene on chromosome 12, plus inactivation or loss of tumor suppressor genes *mcc* on chromosome 5, *p53* on chromosome 17, and *dcc* on chromosome 18.[40] Tumors also express tumor antigens such as carcinoembryonic antigen (CEA), which may be detectable in the blood as tumor markers. Carcinoembryonic antigen is a glycoprotein normally produced during early fetal life but not after birth. Its reappearance in the blood may be related to heavy cigarette smoking or may signify the presence of colorectal or other cancers, hepatic cirrhosis, pancreatitis, or other disorders.[16] Because of this lack of specificity, CEA is not useful as a screening test for colorectal cancer, but it may be of benefit in preoperative staging of the disease or in monitoring for response to therapy or disease recurrence.

Clinical Manifestations. Most tumors are initially asymptomatic and are detected with routine endoscopic examination or fecal occult blood testing. Ulcerative lesions manifest as anemia and rectal bleeding. Right-sided (ascending and transverse colon) lesions tend to produce a dark red to mahogany-colored blood mixed with the stool, and left-sided (descending colon and rectum) lesions usually produce bright red blood coating the stool. Signs of bowel obstruction accompany left-sided lesions, including crampy abdominal pain, distention, vomiting, and constipation. An abdominal mass may be palpable. Metastasis results in signs specific to the location as well as systemic signs such as weight loss and anorexia. Direct visualization and biopsy of the lesion on colonoscopy or sigmoidoscopy confirms the diagnosis.

Prevention and Treatment. Reduction of dietary risk seems warranted, although additional research is needed to validate dietary prevention. Recent research suggests that regular use of aspirin may be associated with decreased risk (see Focus of Current Research).[42] Routine screening examination is recommended for all persons older than 40 years of age and may include testing for fecal occult blood, rectal examination, barium enema, or endoscopy, depending on individual risk. Colorectal cancer is treated with surgical resection to remove tumors or to relieve obstruction or hemorrhage. If the tumor is located in the rectum, a permanent colostomy is required.

Prognosis and Outcome. Outcome depends on the extent of cancer at the time of treatment. Bowel wall tumors that have not metastasized to lymph nodes or adjacent organs are curable with surgery. Overall 5-year survival is about 50%, reflecting the advanced stage of many cancers at the time of diagnosis.[41]

Hirschsprung's Disease

Definition. Hirschsprung's disease, also known as congenital megacolon, is an obstructive disorder of the colon resulting from absence of intramural ganglionic cells of the enteric nervous system.

Epidemiology. The disorder is present in 1 in 5000 to 8000 live births, with males affected three to four times as often as females.[43] Genetic transmission of the disease is variable. Aganglionosis (absence of neural innervation) affecting the entire bowel often displays an autosomal recessive pattern. When Hirschsprung's disease is associated with other anomalies, an autosomal dominant pattern is sometimes evident. Specific environmental teratogens associated with the disorder have not been identified.

Etiology. The precise etiology is unknown in most cases and is probably multifactorial. Genetic and environmental factors apparently interfere with the migration and development of neuroblasts from the neural crest to the distal colon during the seventh week of gestation.[43]

Pathophysiology. Absence of ganglion cells prevents the normal relaxation of peristalsis in the bowel wall and internal anal sphincter, creating a functional obstruction. The affected segment hypertrophies, and the proximal bowel becomes dilated and filled with feces and gas. This segment may dilate to 15 to 20 cm in diameter and may perforate if stretched very thinly. Mucosal ulceration may result from the pressure of impacted stool.[18]

Clinical Manifestations. Five different patterns of presentation are seen: (1) complete obstruction evident soon after birth, with vomiting and failure to pass *meconium* (the first stool); (2) repeated, spontaneously resolving episodes of obstruction, with vomiting and delay of meconium passage; (3) persistent mild constipation leading to complete obstruction; (4) diarrhea followed by obstruction, fever, and enterocolitis; and (5) persistent mild constipation that never results in complete obstruction.[43] The infant often fails to gain weight and may appear pale and listless. Perforation leads to manifestations of peritonitis and sepsis.

Prevention and Treatment. Prenatal testing and genetic counseling may be indicated in families at risk. Neonates are routinely screened for passage of meconium, which usually occurs within the first 24 hours after birth. The definitive treatment of Hirschsprung's disease is surgical, with resection or bypass of the aganglionic segment.

Prognosis and Outcome. With early recognition and treatment, the prognosis is favorable. Untreated, the disease is associated with 50% mortality by age 1 year.[43]

Hemorrhoids

Definition. Hemorrhoids are dilated vascular channels (arteriovenous complexes) located beneath the lining of the anal canal (see Color Fig. 24–6).[44] They may be internal (originating in the upper anal canal, above the pink dentate line and covered with mucosa) or external (originating in the lower canal, covered with skin).

Epidemiology. Hemorrhoids occur in more than 75% of individuals at some time during their life. In 50% of affected persons older than age 50 years, they are severe enough to require treatment.[45] Heredity and conditions in which pressure in rectal vessels is increased predispose to development of hemorrhoids. Such conditions include constipation, lifting and straining, pregnancy, portal hypertension with liver disease, and occupations that require prolonged sitting or standing.

Etiology. The precise etiology is unknown. The commonality of hemorrhoids among asymptomatic persons, including neonates, has led to the suggestion that they may be normal features of the anal canal.[45]

Pathophysiology. Bulging rectal vessels are irritated by mechanical and chemical stimuli, resulting in inflammation and possible perforation. Thrombosis occurs within hemorrhoids because of stasis of blood, but these clots do not embolize. In severe cases, hemorrhoids may prolapse through the anus and become strangulated with contraction of the anal sphincter. Lack of perfusion may lead to necrosis and gangrene in such cases.

Clinical Manifestations. Internal hemorrhoids are graded according to descent and ease of replacement (Table 24–9). Internal hemorrhoids are painless, because there are no pain fibers above the dentate line. The usual clinical signs are of rectal bleeding (hematochezia), usually after defecation, and a palpable mass. The patient may also report a feeling of fullness after defecation. Itching is an unusual manifestation. Thrombosed external hemorrhoids are acutely painful and may interfere with walking or sitting.

TABLE 24–9
GRADING OF INTERNAL HEMORRHOIDS

Grade	Description
Grade I	Hemorrhoids are present and identifiable. Although usually asymptomatic, they may bleed if irritated.
Grade II	Hemorrhoids prolapse from the sphincter with bowel movements, but return spontaneously.
Grade III	Hemorrhoids prolapse with bowel movements and require manual replacement.
Grade IV	Hemorrhoids prolapse with bowel movements and remain outside the anus despite efforts to replace them. In extreme cases, strangulation may occur.

Data from Pfenninger, J.L., and Surrell, J. (1995). Nonsurgical treatment options for internal hemorrhoids. *American Family Physician* 52(3), 821–834.

Prevention and Treatment. Reduction of risk factors is warranted. The diet should be high in fiber with adequate fluid intake. Stool softeners may facilitate defecation. Sitz baths and ointments containing anti-inflammatory agents and local analgesics may provide some symptomatic relief. Ligation of hemorrhoids with high-tension rubber bands is the most common form of treatment and may be done on an outpatient basis. This method is highly effective in inducing strangulation. The hemorrhoid sloughs off, leaving an ulcer that heals gradually. Newer endoscopic therapies include infrared coagulation, electrocoagulation, low-voltage direct current, sclerotherapy, cryotherapy, and laser therapy. Severe hemorrhoids (grades III or IV) may be surgically ligated and removed (hemorrhoidectomy).

Prognosis and Outcome. Hemorrhoids are a distressing but benign condition that usually responds to preventive measures and treatment. Recurrence rates vary from 10% to 50% over 5 years.[45]

CLINICAL SIGNIFICANCE OF DISORDERS OF GASTROINTESTINAL MOTILITY AND SECRETION

Gastrointestinal disorders are among the most commonly reported in clinical practice. Because many GI conditions are not immediately life-threat-

Developmental Perspective

Embryonic and Fetal Periods

The primitive alimentary canal forms during the fourth week of gestation. The esophagus, stomach, and duodenum originate from the same structures as the trachea, and anomalies may involve respiratory and digestive structures, for example, esophageal atresia with tracheoesophageal fistula. Development of the small intestine and the ascending and transverse segments of the colon involves herniation of these structures from the abdominal cavity to the extraembryonic coelom of the proximal umbilical cord at about the sixth week. The bowel elongates and rotates, then retracts into the abdominal cavity by the 10th week. Abnormalities of these processes may give rise to congenital herniation or bowel obstruction. During weeks 5 to 7, abnormal development of the urorectal septum, which forms the perineum, may result in imperforate anus or other anomalies of the lower GI system. Swallowing of amniotic fluid normally begins at 10 to 13 weeks. Its failure results in polyhydramnios and is associated with bowel obstruction. Meconium passage in utero indicates fetal distress and is thought to be caused by an excess of hormones such as motilin.

Infancy and Childhood

Gastrointestinal motility and secretion are immature at birth. The mucosal barrier is immature during the first 4 to 6 months of life, increasing the risk of infection. Initiation of feeding stimulates the development of neural and hormonal reflexes for regulation of motility and secretion. Passage of meconium, consisting of swallowed constituents of amniotic fluid as well as intestinal secretions, usually indicates bowel patency and motility. Esophageal motility is decreased in the newborn, and LES tone is reduced, predisposing to reflux and regurgitation of feedings. Gastric tone is also decreased, and gastric emptying is delayed. Intestinal motility is poorly coordinated in infancy. High levels of secretion of gastrin and HCl are seen during the first few days of life, and stress ulceration may develop. By 2 years of age, GI motility and secretion have matured to patterns similar to those in adults.

Adolescence and Young Adulthood

Inflammatory bowel disease has its onset during this age group, and appendicitis is common. Disturbances of GI motility are common during pregnancy, caused by mechanical and hormonal factors.

Middle and Older Adulthood

Age-related changes occur in epithelial cells lining the GI tract, in secretory cells, and in visceral smooth muscle. Salivation is decreased. Esophageal motility is slower and more disorganized, giving rise to dysphagia. The incidence of reflux increases, and hiatal hernia is much more common in older persons. Gastric volume is decreased and gastric emptying is delayed. Atrophy of antral cells is commonly seen, resulting in decreased secretion of HCl and intrinsic factor with the possibility of impaired protein digestion and vitamin B_{12} absorption. The risk of PUD, gastritis, diverticulitis, and GI cancers is increased with aging. Intestinal motility is slowed and secretion of intestinal juices is decreased. Constipation and fecal incontinence are especially common in the elderly, as a result of physiologic, dietary, and lifestyle factors.

---

ening and may have manifestations not deemed appropriate for discussion in social settings, they often do not receive the same media attention as that afforded disorders of other systems. The disorders discussed in this chapter illustrate the prevalence of GI disorders in individuals of all ages (see Developmental Perspective). The essential nature of the nutritive and eliminative functions of the GI system attests to its critical importance. Research is ongoing to examine the etiologic mechanisms of IBD, IBS, and cancers of the alimentary tract. In recent years, much has been learned about the etiology and pathophysiology of PUD, and treatment of this disorder has been radically altered. Disorders of GI motility and secretion inevitably alter digestion and absorption of nutrients, as discussed in Chapter 25.

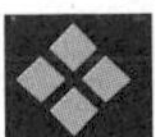

Summary of Key Points

- The GI system consists of the alimentary canal and its accessory organs, contained within the peritoneal cavity. Functions of the mouth include ingestion and digestion. The esophagus functions in deglutition. The stomach is of particular importance to digestion, although some substances are also absorbed from the gastric mucosa. Most absorption takes place in the small intestine. The large intestine also functions in absorption; however, its primary function is defecation.

- Smooth muscle contraction, the basis of GI motility, is regulated by neural and hormonal factors. The enteric nervous system innervates the alimentary canal. This system is not dependent on higher level neural input but is often modulated by such input. A number of hormones of the diffuse endocrine system also regulate GI motility, including CCK, secretin, and gastric inhibitory peptide.

- Deglutition is critical to the ingestion and initial propulsion of food. It also prevents aspiration into the tracheobronchial tree. Contraction of gastric smooth muscle serves to mechanically digest chyme and mix it with digestive enzymes and HCl. Peristaltic contractions in the small and large intestines serve to propel chyme down the canal and to expose nutrients to the intestinal wall for absorption. Defecation from the large bowel eliminates unabsorbed nutrients and wastes.

- Five types of secretion occur within the GI system. (1) Salivation, from the salivary glands that open into the mouth, dilutes and lubricates the food bolus and supplies an enzyme for initial digestion of carbohydrates. (2) Gastric secretions include (a) mucus (from mucous cells), which serves as a protective barrier to the mucosa; (b) HCl and intrinsic factor (from oxyntic cells), which serve in protein digestion and vitamin B_{12} absorption, respectively; (c) pepsinogen (from chief cells), which is activated to the proteolytic enzyme pepsin in the acid environment of the stomach; (d) gastrin (from G cells), which triggers the release of HCl and pepsinogen; and (e) somatostatin (from D cells), which opposes gastrin secretion. (3) Pancreatic secretions contain bicarbonate, to neutralize gastric acid in the small intestine, and enzymes for the digestion of all three nutrient types. (4) Bile, secreted by the liver and released from the gallbladder, contains acids that are necessary for the intestinal absorption of fats. (5) Intestinal cells secrete protective mucus and enzymes for the complete digestion of proteins and fats.

- A number of manifestations are common to many forms of GI disease. Vomiting is a protective reflex triggered by epigastric irritation or pressure as well as proprioceptive and toxic stimuli. Diarrhea is a protective response aimed to clear irritants from the bowel, and it may result from osmotic, secretory, or motile mechanisms. Constipation results from slowed motility or difficulty in expulsion of feces, or both. Fecal incontinence results from imbalance in the expelling and resisting forces for defecation. Bowel obstruction may result from mechanical or functional mechanisms. Gastrointestinal bleeding results from inflammatory, ischemic, or invasive disorders of the upper or lower alimentary canal.

- Most disorders of the alimentary canal impair motility and secretion. Esophageal disorders result in impaired swallowing and in bleeding, if invasive cancer or acid reflux are present. Gastric disorders are also associated with bleeding caused by disruption of the mucous barrier, invasion of the mucosa, or increased secretion or acid or proteolytic enzymes. Inflammatory disorders of the lower bowel may be infectious or autoimmune in nature, and they may result in increased motility and secretion as well as bleeding in cases where vessels are eroded. Obstruction may occur at any level of the canal, impeding absorption and secretion. Treatment is aimed at relief of the underlying cause as well as restoration of normal motility and secretory functions.

- Gastrointestinal disorders are among the most commonly reported in clinical practice. Disorders of other systems may be demonstrated as alterations of GI function. These disorders have a significant impact on quality of life of individuals of all ages, and they may be life threatening in some cases because of neoplastic invasion, hemorrhage, or sepsis. The integrity of GI motility and secretory processes has a direct impact on the ability of the individual to ingest and absorb the nutrients essential to energy metabolism.

REFERENCES

1. Mittal, R.K., and Balaban, D.H. (1997). The esophagogastric junction. *New England Journal of Medicine* 336(13), 924–932.
2. Goyal, R.K., and Hirano, I. (1996). The enteric nervous system. *New England Journal of Medicine* 334(17), 1106–1115.
3. Baker, D.M. (1993). Assessment and management of impairments in swallowing. *Nursing Clinics of North America* 28(4), 793–805.
4. Parent, K. (1994). Acid reduction in peptic ulcer disease. *Postgraduate Medicine* 95(6), 53–59.
5. Donowitz, M., Kokke, F.T., and Saidi, R. (1995). Evaluation of patients with chronic diarrhea. *New England Journal of Medicine* 332(11), 725–729.
6. Romero, Y., Evans, J.M., Fleming, K.C., and Phillips, S.F. (1996). Constipation and fecal incontinence in the elderly population. *Mayo Clinic Proceedings* 71, 81–92.
7. Rao, S.S.C. (1995). Functional colonic and anorectal disorders: Detecting and overcoming causes of constipation and fecal incontinence. *Postgraduate Medicine* 98(5), 115–126.
8. Ouslander, J.G., and Schnelle, J.F. (1995). Incontinence in the nursing home. *Annals of Internal Medicine* 122, 438–449.
9. Kahrilas, P.J. (1996). Gastroesophageal reflux disease. *Journal of the American Medical Association* 276(12), 983–988.
10. Weinberg, D.S., and Kadish, S.L. (1996). The diagnosis and management of gastroesophageal reflux disease. *Medical Clinics of North America* 80(2), 411–429.
11. Robinson, M. (1994). Gastroesophageal reflux disease: Selecting optimal therapy. *Postgraduate Medicine* 95(2), 88–102.
12. Marshall, J.B. (1995). Severe gastroesophageal reflux disease: Medical and surgical options for long-term care. *Postgraduate Medicine* 97(5), 98–106.
13. Bozymski, E.M. (1993). Pathophysiology and diagnosis of gastroesophageal reflux disease. *American Journal of Hospital Pharmacy* 50(1 suppl.), S4–S6.
14. Harding, S.M., Richter, J.E., Guzzo, M.R., *et al.* (1996). Asthma and gastroesophageal reflux: Acid suppressive therapy improves asthma outcome. *American Journal of Medicine* 100, 395–405.
15. DeVault, K.R., and Castell, D.O. (1994). Current diagnosis and treatment of gastroesophageal reflux disease. *Mayo Clinic Proceedings* 69, 867–876.
16. Black, J.M., and Matassarin-Jacobs, E. (1997). *Medical-Surgical Nursing: Clinical Management for Continuity of Care.* (5th ed.). Philadelphia: W.B. Saunders. (pp. 1710, 1733–1737).
17. Dillon, P.W., and Cilley, R.E. (1993). Newborn surgical emergencies: Gastrointestinal anomalies, abdominal wall defects. *Pediatric Clinics of North America* 40(6), 1289–1314.
18. Cotran, R.S., Kumar, V., and Robbins, S.L. (1994). *Robbins Pathologic Basis of Disease.* (5th ed.). Philadelphia: W.B. Saunders. pp. 746–766, 770–773, 786–787, 825–826.
19. The Consensus Development Panel on *Helicobacter pylori* in Peptic Ulcer Disease. (1994). *Helicobacter pylori* in peptic ulcer disease. *Journal of the American Medical Association* 272(1), 65–69.
20. Laine, L., and Peterson, W.L. (1994). Bleeding peptic ulcer. *New England Journal of Medicine* 331(11), 717–727.
21. Anderson, M.L. (1994). *Helicobacter pylori* infection: When and in whom is treatment important? *Postgraduate Medicine* 96(6), 40–50.
22. Meko, J.B., and Norton, J.A. (1995). Management of patients with Zollinger-Ellison syndrome. *Annual Review of Medicine* 46, 395–411.
23. Peura, D.A. (1996). *Helicobacter pylori* and ulcerogenesis. *American Journal of Medicine* 100 (5A suppl.), 5A-19S–5A-26S.
24. Cutler, A.F., Havstad, S., Ma C.K., *et al.* (1995). Accuracy of invasive and noninvasive tests to diagnose *Helicobacter pylori* infection. *Gastroenterology* 109, 136–141.
25. Khuroo, M.S., Yattoo, G.N., Javid, G., *et al.* (1997). A comparison of omeprazole and placebo for bleeding peptic ulcer. *New England Journal of Medicine* 336(15), 1054–1058.
26. Hunt, R.H. (1996). Eradication of *Helicobacter pylori* infection. *American Journal of Medicine* 100 (5A suppl.), 5A-42S–5A-51S.
27. Fuchs, C.S., and Mayer, R.J. (1995). Gastric carcinoma. *New England Journal of Medicine* 333(1), 32–41.
28. Onishi, K., and Miaskowski, C. (1996). Mechanisms and management of gastric cancer: A comparison between the Japanese and U.S. experiences. *Cancer Nursing* 19(3), 187–196.
29. Deluca, S.A. (1993). Hypertrophic pyloric stenosis. *American Family Physician* 47(9), 1771–1773.
30. Borkowski, S. (1994). Common pediatric surgical problems. *Nursing Clinics of North America* 29(4), 551–562.
31. Bonis, P.A.L., and Norton, R.A. (1996). The challenge of irritable bowel syndrome. *American Family Physician* 53(4), 1229–1236.
32. Tooson, J.D., and Varilek, G.W. (1995). Inflammatory diseases of the colon: Narrowing a wide field of symptoms and possible causes. *Postgraduate Medicine* 98(5), 46–78.
33. Doughty, D.B. (1994). What you need to know about inflammatory bowel disease. *American Journal of Nursing* July 1994, 24–31.
34. Pullan, R.D., Rhodes, J., Ganesh, S., *et al.* (1994). Transdermal nicotine for active ulcerative colitis. *New England Journal of Medicine* 330(12), 811–815.
35. Elson, C.O. (1996). The basis of current and future therapy for inflammatory bowel disease. *American Journal of Medicine* 100, 656–662.
36. Statter, M.B., Hirschl, R.B., and Coran, A.C. (1993). Inflammatory bowel disease. *Pediatric Clinics of North America* 40(6), 1213–1231.
37. Silen, M., and Tracy, T.F., Jr. (1993). The right lower quadrant "revisited". *Pediatric Clinics of North America* 40(6), 1201–1211.
38. Freeman, S.R., and McNally, P.R. (1993). Diverticulitis. *Medical Clinics of North America* 77(5), 1149–1167.
39. Manten, H.D., and Green, J.A. (1995). Acute lower gastrointestinal bleeding: A guide to initial management. *Postgraduate Medicine* 97(4), 154–157.
40. Truszkowski, J.A., and Summers, R.W. (1995). Colorectal neoplasms: Screening can save lives. *Postgraduate Medicine* 98(5), 97–112.
41. Marshall, J.B. (1996). Colorectal cancer screening: Present strategies and future prospects. *Postgraduate Medicine* 99(3), 253–264.
42. Giovannucci, E., Egan, K.M., Hunter, D.J., *et al.* (1995). Aspirin and the risk of colorectal cancer in women. *New England Journal of Medicine* 333(10), 609–614.
43. Worman, S., and Ganiats, T.G. (1995). Hirschsprung's disease: A cause of chronic constipation in children. *American Family Physician* 51(2), 487–494.
44. Metcalf, A. (1995). Anorectal disorders: Five common causes of pain, itching, and bleeding. *Postgraduate Medicine* 98(5), 81–94.
45. Pfenninger, J.L., and Surrell, J. (1995). Nonsurgical treatment options for internal hemorrhoids. *American Family Physician* 52(3), 821–834.

SELECTED BIBLIOGRAPHY

Abell, T.L., and Werkman, R.F. (1996). Gastrointestinal motility disorders. *American Family Physician* 53(3), 895–902.

Beluzzi, A., Brignola, C., Campieri, M., *et al.* (1996). Effect of an enteric-coated fish-oil preparation on relapses in Crohn's disease. *New England Journal of Medicine* 334(24), 1557–1560.

Bennett, W.G., and Cerda, J.J. (1996). Benefits of dietary fiber: Myth or medicine? *Postgraduate Medicine* 99(2), 153–175.

Boren, T., Falk, P., Roth, K.A., *et al.* (1993). Attachment of *Helicobacter pylori* to human gastric epithelium mediated by blood group antigens. *Science* 262, 1892–1895.

Brady, S.K., and McKee, D.D. (1993). Collagenous colitis: A cause of chronic diarrhea. *American Family Physician* 48(6), 1081–1084.

Butcher, J.D. (1993). Runner's diarrhea and other intestinal problems of athletes. *American Family Physician* 48(4), 623–627.

Cave, D.R. (1996). Transmission and epidemiology of *Helicobacter pylori*. *American Journal of Medicine* 100 (5A suppl.), 5A-12S–5A-18S.

Cheney, C.P., and Wong, R.K.H. (1993). Acute infectious diarrhea. *Medical Clinics of North America* 77(5), 1169–1196.

Cook, D.J., Fuller, H.D., Guyatt, G.H., *et al.* (1994). Risk factors for gastrointestinal bleeding in critically ill patients. *New England Journal of Medicine* 330(6), 377–381.

DeMarkles, M.P., and Murphy, J.R. (1993). Acute lower gastrointestinal bleeding. *Medical Clinics of North America* 77(5), 1085–1100.

Egan, L.J., and Sandborn, W.J. (1996). Methotrexate for inflammatory bowel disease: Pharmacology and preliminary results. *Mayo Clinic Proceedings* 71, 69–80.

Ferrante, J.M. (1996). Colorectal cancer screening. *Medical Clinics of North America* 80(1), 27–43.

Gormally, S.M., Prakash, N., Durnin, M.T., *et al.* (1995). Association of symptoms with *Helicobacter pylori* infection in children. *Journal of Pediatrics* 126(5 Pt. 1), 753–756.

Greenberg, E.R., Baron, J.A., Tosteson, T.D., *et al.* (1994). A clinical trial of antioxidant vitamins to prevent colorectal adenoma. *New England Journal of Medicine* 331(3), 141–147.

Hanauer, S.B. (1996). Inflammatory bowel disease. *New England Journal of Medicine* 334(13), 841–848.

Hansson, L-E., Nuren, O., Hsing, A.W., *et al.* (1996). The risk of stomach cancer in patients with gastric or duodenal ulcer disease. *New England Journal of Medicine* 335(4), 242–249.

Heigh, R.I. (1994). Use of NSAIDs: An assault on the upper gastrointestinal tract. *Postgraduate Medicine* 96(6), 63–68.

Hirschfeld, S., and Clearfield, H.R. (1995). Pharmacologic therapy for inflammatory bowel disease. *American Family Physician* 51(9), 1971–1975.

Howden, C.W. (1996). Clinical expressions of *Helicobacter pylori* infection. *American Journal of Medicine* 100 (5A suppl.), 5A-27S–5A-34S.

Jen, J., Kim, H., Piantadosi, S., *et al.* (1994). Allelic loss of chromosome 18q and prognosis in colorectal cancer. *New England Journal of Medicine* 331(4), 213–221.

Jensen, D.M., Cheng, S., Kovacs, T.O.G., *et al.* (1994). A controlled study of ranitidine for the prevention of recurrent hemorrhage from duodenal ulcer. *New England Journal of Medicine* 330(6), 382–386.

Juckett, G. (1995). Common intestinal helminths. *American Family Physician* 52(7), 2039–2048.

Kelly, C.P., Pothoulakis, C., and LaMont, J.T. (1994). *Clostridium difficile* colitis. *New England Journal of Medicine* 330(4), 257–262.

Kilgore, P.E., Holman, R.C., Clarke, M.J., *et al.* (1995). Trends in diarrheal disease-associated mortality in U.S. children, 1968 through 1991. *Journal of the American Medical Association* 274(14), 1143–1148.

Koch, W.M. (1993). Swallowing disorders. *Medical Clinics of North America* 77(3), 571–582.

Laine, L.A. (1996). *Helicobacter pylori* and complicated ulcer disease. *American Journal of Medicine* 100(5A suppl.), 5A-52S–5A-59S.

Lang, C.A., and Ransohoff, D.F. (1994). Fecal occult blood screening for colorectal cancer: Is mortality reduced by chance selection for screening colonoscopy? *Journal of the American Medical Association* 271(13), 1011–1013.

Lipsky, M.S., and Adelman, M. (1993). Chronic diarrhea: Evaluation and treatment. *American Family Physician* 48(8), 1461–1466.

Loening-Baucke, V. (1994). Management of chronic constipation in infants and toddlers. *American Family Physician* 49(2), 397–406.

Lynn, R.B., and Friedman, L.S. (1993). Irritable bowel syndrome. *New England Journal of Medicine* 329(26), 1940–1945.

Lynn, R.B., and Friedman, L.S. (1995). Irritable bowel syndrome: Managing the patient with abdominal pain and altered bowel habits. *Medical Clinics of North America* 79(2), 373–390.

Macarthur, C., Saunders, N., and Feldman, W. (1995). *Helicobacter pylori*, gastroduodenal disease, and recurrent abdominal pain in children. *Journal of the American Medical Association* 273(9), 729–734.

Mathias, J.R., and Clench, M.H. (1995). Neuromuscular diseases of the gastrointestinal tract: Specific disorders that often get a nonspecific diagnosis. *Postgraduate Medicine* 97(3), 95–108.

McKenna, C.J. (1994). Gastrointestinal bleeding in children. *Nursing Clinics of North America* 29(4), 599–613.

Oureshi, W.A., and Netchvolodoff, C.V. (1993). Acute bleeding from peptic ulcers. *Postgraduate Medicine* 93(4), 167–178.

Owens, D.M., Nelson, D.K., and Talley, N.J. (1995). The irritable bowel syndrome: Long-term prognosis and the physician-patient interaction. *Annals of Internal Medicine* 122, 107–112.

Pahor, M., Guralnik, J.M., Salive, M.E., *et al.* (1994). Physical activity and risk of severe gastrointestinal hemorrhage in older persons. *Journal of the American Medical Association* 272(8), 595–599.

Parsonnet, J., Hansen, S., Rodriguez, L., *et al.* (1994). *Helicobacter pylori* infection and gastric lymphoma. *New England Journal of Medicine* 330(18), 1267–1271.

Pope, C.E. II. (1994). Acid-reflux disorders. *New England Journal of Medicine* 331(10), 656–660.

Rae, S.S.C. (1997). Belching, bloating, and flatulence: How to help patients who have troublesome abdominal gas. *Postgraduate Medicine* 101(4), 263–278.

Sackier, J.M. (1996). New applications of laparoscopy in gastrointestinal surgery. *American Family Physician* 53(1), 237–242.

Slutsker, L., Ries, A.A., Greene, K.D., *et al.* (1997). *Escherichia coli* 0157:H7 diarrhea in the United States: Clinical and epidemiologic features. *Annals of Internal Medicine* 126(7), 505–513.

Soll, A.H. (1996). Medical treatment of peptic ulcer disease. *Journal of the American Medical Association* 275(8), 622–629.

Talley, N.J. (1993). Nonulcer dyspepsia: Current approaches to diagnosis and management. *American Family Physician* 47(6), 1407–1416.

Thomas, G.A.O., Rhodes, J., Mani, V., *et al.* (1995). Transdermal nicotine as maintenance therapy for ulcerative colitis. *New England Journal of Medicine* 332(15), 988–992.

Toribara, N.W., and Sleisenger, M.H. (1995). Screening for colorectal cancer. *New England Journal of Medicine* 332(13), 861–867.

Vigneri, S., Termini, R., Leandro, G., *et al.* (1995). A comparison of five maintenance therapies for reflux esophagitis. *New England Journal of Medicine* 333(17), 1106–1110.

Walsh, J.H., and Peterson, W.L. (1995). The treatment of *Helicobacter pylori* infection in the management of peptic ulcer disease. *New England Journal of Medicine* 333(15), 984–991.

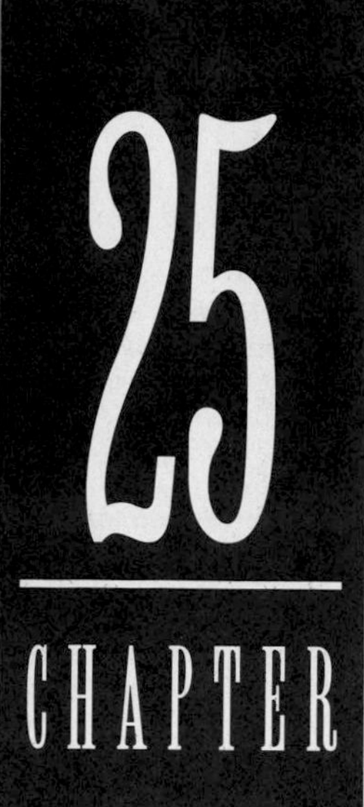

Disorders of Ingestion, Digestion, and Absorption

LEARNING OBJECTIVES

1. Discuss the anatomic structures and physiologic processes influencing the ingestion of nutrients.
2. Describe the biochemical processes by which carbohydrates, proteins, and fats are digested.
3. Discuss the characteristics of the intestinal microstructure that facilitate the absorption of nutrients.
4. Compare and contrast the transport processes that underlie the absorption of specific nutrients.
5. Identify the pathophysiologic mechanisms that may result in nutrient malabsorption.
6. Comprehend the pathophysiologic bases of the clinical manifestations and treatment of the more prevalent disorders of nutrient ingestion, digestion, and absorption.

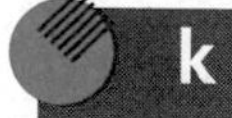

key terms

anorexia
anorexia nervosa
body mass index (BMI)
bulimia nervosa
cachexia
celiac disease
cleft lip and palate
dyslipidemia
dysphagia
eating disorder
erythroplasia
familial hypercholesterolemia
first-pass effect
flatulence
gingivitis
gluten-sensitive enteropathy
hypercarotenemia
hyperinsulinemia
hyperlipidemia
hyperlipoproteinemia
inborn error of metabolism
insulin resistance
jaundice
lactose intolerance
leukoplakia
obesity
oral cancer

pancreatic cancer
pancreatitis
periodontal disease
pickwickian syndrome
primary hyperalphalipoproteinemia
pseudocysts
steatorrhea
tropical sprue
Trousseau's syndrome
xanthomata

The most important function of the gastrointestinal (GI) system is the conversion of ingested nutrients to substrates for energy metabolism. This "food processor" function depends in part on GI motility and secretion, detailed in Chapter 24. The transformation of nutrients into energy substrates was introduced in Chapter 3, with emphasis on the cellular generation of adenosine triphosphate (ATP). In this chapter, the processes involved in the ingestion of food, the chemical digestion of nutrients, and the transport of these nutrients from the alimentary canal into the blood are detailed. The unique aspects of the GI circulation that facilitate absorption of nutrients are also described. Disorders addressed in this chapter illustrate alterations of these processes and include **oral cancer, cleft lip and palate, periodontal disease, eating disorders, obesity, gluten-sensitive enteropathy, lactose intolerance, hyperlipidemia, pancreatitis,** and **pancreatic cancer.**

NUTRIENT INGESTION

Patterns of Ingestion

Nutrient ingestion (food intake or feeding) may be conceptualized as a three-stage process: (1) recognition of hunger or appetite, acquisition of food, and bringing of food into the mouth; (2) preparation of ingested food for swallowing, and (3) swallowing, or passage of food from the mouth through the esophagus and into the stomach.[1] Human beings normally ingest three or four meals a day, separated by periods of 3 to 4 hours during which little or no food is taken in. This pattern corresponds with the time necessary for the GI tract to process nutrients for absorption.

Hunger and Satiety

Regulation of food intake is complex, involving psychosocial and cultural factors as well as physiologic mechanisms (see Chapter 3). Local, neural, and hormonal GI mechanisms apparently participate in triggering the initiation and termination of eating behaviors.[2] Definitions of satiety must account not only for gastric fullness but also for the pleasant feeling of satisfaction that usually accompanies eating. The size and frequency of meals is primarily regulated by nutrient receptors in the GI tract, and metabolic signals regulate overall energy demands.

Hunger is apparently triggered by receptors in the upper small intestine that signal the hypothalamus and other areas of the brain. Chemoreceptors of a different type in intestinal cells are believed to sense the presence of specific nutrients in the gut, activating the release of local chemicals that induce a feeling of satiety and a reduction in food intake. These chemicals may act as neurotransmitters, stimulating afferent nerves, or may circulate in the blood, acting as hormones. Reduction in stimulation of these receptors may disinhibit appetite centers, inducing hunger and food intake.

Fat intake is more effective than carbohydrate intake in inducing a feeling of satiety, and it has the additional effect of slowing the rate at which the food moves through the alimentary canal. Carbohydrate intake induces a more effective metabolic signal for satiety and reduction of energy intake than does dietary fat. The probable reason for this is that glycogen stores in the liver have a finite capacity, whereas adipose tissue storage of fat is virtually unlimited. Filling of glycogen stores may signal satiety centers in the brain via vagal impulses, and rising serum glucose may initiate an endocrine signal for appetite suppression.[2]

A number of GI hormones have been implicated in the regulation of hunger and satiety (see Chapter 3). Cholecystokinin (CCK), released primarily from the duodenal mucosa, may act as a hunger suppressant, but research findings have been inconsistent in this regard.[2] Gastric distention is also sensed with the intake of food, but this mechanical factor is believed to be less important than neural or hormonal mediators of appetite.

Adaptation to Altered Intake

Humans have demonstrated the capacity to adapt to changes in usual dietary intake over time. The individual who is dieting, for example, often feels very hungry for the first few days, but this sensation gradually subsides. After prolonged dieting, ingestion of larger meals and more calories may cause the dieter to feel uncomfortably full. On the other hand, prolonged ingestion of larger meals, higher in fat or calories, also induces adaptation. Over time, gastric emptying and small bowel transit time increase adaptively to process these nutrients, and the small intestine hypertrophies to provide more surface area for absorption. During illness, hunger is suppressed and aversion to food (**anorexia**) is common. Nutrient adaptation in these cases does not involve actual shrinkage or expansion of the stomach, but rather appears to be caused by hormonally mediated up- or down-regulation of nutrient receptors in response to prolonged alterations in customary intake.[2] Down-regulation of nutrient receptors in response to high food intake may play a role in obesity, as discussed later in this chapter.

Anatomic Factors Influencing Ingestion

The oropharynx, a component of the respiratory and GI systems, functions in the formation of ingested food into a bolus and in passage of this bolus into the esophagus while preventing aspiration into the trachea (see Chapter 18). The anatomy of the oropharynx favors nipple feeding and sucking in infants, but by the age of 2 years structures have developed to favor chewing and drinking from a cup (Fig. 25–1). To suck, the lips are closed around the nipple and the tongue seals against the posterior pharynx. Depression of the tongue and jaw creates negative pressure that moves liquid into the oral cavity. The infant with cleft lip or palate may not be able to produce an effective seal, as discussed later in this chapter. During the first year of development, tongue movement becomes more controlled and the oral cavity enlarges, permitting bolus formation and manipulation. The development of teeth allows biting and mastication (see Developmental Perspective).

In infants, the larynx is situated high in the neck, enabling the passage of liquids over the tongue, around the epiglottis, and into the esophagus, reducing the risk of aspiration. After 2 or 3 years of age, however, the larynx descends, and the anatomic risk of aspiration increases. Neural reflex coordination of the phases of swallowing is then essential to prevent aspiration of food into the airways.[1]

Regulation of Deglutition (Swallowing)

Swallowing occurs without conscious thought about 600 times during each 24-hour period.[3] The process of deglutition occurs in four phases:[3,4]

1. *Oral Preparation:* Solid food particles are broken down and mixed with saliva during mastication. Movements of the lips, cheeks, and tongue form food into a bolus within the anterior oral cavity. Cerebellar coordination of motor inputs from cranial nerves (CNs) V, VII, and XII is essential to regulation of this phase.

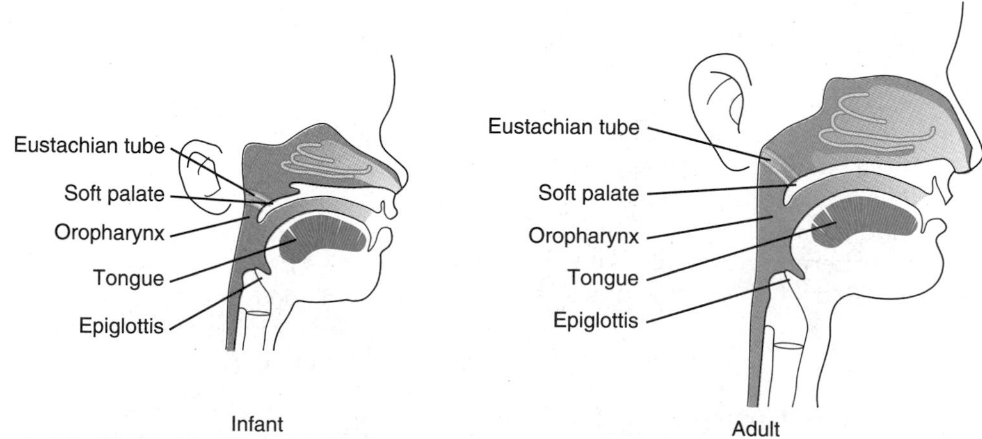

FIGURE 25–1
Structure of the oropharynx. In infants, the structure of the oropharynx favors nipple feeding and sucking. The larynx is situated high in the neck, enabling passage of liquids over the tongue and into the esophagus, reducing the risk of aspiration. The oral cavity is much smaller than in the adult, with virtually no space for manipulation of a solid food bolus. In adults, the lower position of the larynx provides for more space for manipulation of a food bolus, but increases the risk of aspiration of liquids.

Developmental Perspective

Embryonic and Fetal Periods

Because fetal nutritional needs are met by placental transfer, optimal maternal nutrition is critical to prenatal development. Glucose, amino acids, and free fatty acids readily cross the placenta. Development of digestive enzyme systems begins by 6 to 16 weeks, but lactase levels do not reach peak levels until 36 to 40 weeks. Appetite regulation and adipocyte numbers are believed to be established during the fetal period. Intestinal villi are well developed by 19 weeks of gestation. Swallowing begins at 10 to 14 weeks, and effective sucking develops over weeks 15 to 32. Intrauterine growth retardation or macrosomia may be associated with impaired fetal nutrition. Genetic defects or teratogenic insults may lead to congenital defects such as inborn errors of metabolism, pancreatic anomalies, cleft lip and palate, esophageal atresia, or cystic fibrosis. Maternal obesity is associated with an increased incidence of perinatal mortality.

Infancy and Childhood

The infant's intestinal mucosal barrier is immature for 4 to 6 months after birth, predisposing to the absorption of antigenic proteins and microorganisms. Immaturity of gastrointestinal function at birth increases the risk of malabsorption and malnutrition, especially in preterm infants. Decreased turnover of intestinal epithelial cells decreases absorptive surface area in infants. Exocrine pancreatic function is also immature, but enzymes in human milk and in oral and intestinal secretions normally compensate for this lack. Feeding induces maturation of digestive enzyme systems and intestinal villi during the first 6 months to 2 years of life. The oropharyngeal anatomy adapts to the transition from nipple feeding to chewing and drinking. Development of the teeth facilitates the ingestion of solid foods. Obesity in the first year of life is caused by an increase in size of adipose cells and does not correlate with later development of obesity in adulthood. Obesity developing between the ages of 4 and 11 is associated with an increase in number of adipocytes and is usually lifelong. Body mass index normally increases during the first year of life and then decreases until the age of about 5 years, when it again increases. Cholesterol levels are much higher in newborn infants than in older children. Adolescent levels are normally reached by 3 years of age. High cholesterol levels in children older than age 2 years tend to persist into adulthood.

Adolescence and Young Adulthood

Adolescence is a period of increased obesity risk, especially in females. Ironically, this period also represents the highest-risk period for the development of anorexia nervosa and bulimia nervosa. Periodontal disease and associated gingivitis often manifest during this stage. Gums may bleed easily and cause discomfort with chewing. During pregnancy, progesterone enhances the height of intestinal villi, increasing absorptive surface area, and also induces increased lactase and maltase activity. Excessive weight gain during pregnancy is common and may contribute to lifelong obesity. Familial hyperlipidemias usually manifest during young adulthood, as do acquired dyslipidemias caused by dietary factors or systemic diseases. Lipid disorders may be exacerbated by the use of steroids, such as corticosteroids, estrogen-containing oral contraceptives, or anabolic steroids.

Middle and Older Adulthood

Ingestion may be impaired as a consequence of dental problems, decline in the senses of taste and smell, decreased salivary secretion, or impaired swallowing because of stroke or other neuromuscular disorder. Nutrient absorption is often diminished as a consequence of decreased secretion of pancreatic and intestinal digestive enzymes, blunting of the intestinal villi, and decreased perfusion of the gastrointestinal tract. Conversely, an increasingly sedentary lifestyle may promote the development of obesity. Risks associated with insulin resistance and hyperlipidemia are highest during middle age, possibly contributing to systemic disorders such as atherosclerosis, hypertension, and type 2 diabetes mellitus.

2. *Oral Phase:* The tongue shapes the bolus and pushes it posteriorly into the oropharynx. When the bolus touches sensory receptors near the anterior tonsillar pillars, the involuntary swallowing reflex is triggered (afferent stimuli via CNs VII, IX, and X to the brain stem).
3. *Pharyngeal Phase:* The soft palate elevates, preventing reflux through the nasopharynx. The tongue provides a downward pumping force, and the larynx elevates and moves forward under the base of the tongue. The airway is protected by closure of the vocal cords and covering of the laryngeal vestibule by the epiglottis, and the upper esophageal sphincter relaxes to permit passage of the bolus (CNs V, VII, IX, X, and XII).
4. *Esophageal Phase:* During a period of 8 to 20 seconds, peristalsis carries the bolus through the esophagus and past the relaxed lower esophageal sphincter into the stomach.

Disorders of the mouth, oropharynx, and larynx are common in clinical settings, and are associated with impairment of ingestion as well as risk of aspiration into respiratory passages. Conditions associated with impaired swallowing (**dysphagia**) are summarized in Table 25–1. Disorders of esophageal motility are detailed in Chapter 24. Aspiration pneumonia is discussed in Chapter 19. Disorders of the oropharynx that may impair ingestion are discussed later in this chapter.

TABLE 25–1
CONDITIONS ASSOCIATED WITH IMPAIRED SWALLOWING

CATEGORY/MECHANISM	EXAMPLES
Neoplasia Pain Disruption of cranial nerve function Mechanical obstruction	Benign or malignant tumors in the lower cranial vault, pharynx, or mediastinum
Neuromuscular disease Disruption of cranial nerve function	Stroke Closed head injury Poliomyelitis Cerebral palsy Parkinson's disease Amyotrophic lateral sclerosis Multiple sclerosis Myasthenia gravis Huntington's disease
Metabolic disorders Peripheral neuropathy Electrolyte imbalance	Diabetes mellitus Hypercalcemia
Infectious disease Pain	*Candida* and other agents
Iatrogenic causes Disruption of cranial nerve function Decreased salivation Mucosal injury	Surgery of the thyroid, cranial vault, head, neck, or thorax Radiation therapy of oral cavity, neck, larynx, or pharynx
Anatomic abnormalities Disruption of laryngeal nerve function Extrinsic esophageal compression	Cervical bone spurs Mitral valve disease Thoracic aortic aneurysm Esophageal atresia Zenker's diverticulum Schatzki ring
Autoimmune disease Connective tissue disruption Decreased salivation	Scleroderma Dermatomyositis Sjögren's syndrome
Other Globus sensation ("lump" in throat) Mechanical obstruction	Stress and anxiety Foreign body ingestion

Data from Koch, W.M. (1993). Swallowing disorders: Diagnosis and therapy. *Medical Clinics of North America* 77(3), 574–575.

NUTRIENT DIGESTION

Digestion was defined in Chapter 24 as the breakdown of food into particles small enough to be absorbed. Digestive processes are mechanical (physical breakdown from motility and mastication) and biochemical (catabolic reactions). (NOTE: The molecular structure and dietary sources of the nutrients [carbohydrates, proteins, and fats] were introduced in Chapter 3 in the context of energy metabolism. Emphasis here is on the processing of these nutrients by the GI tract and the mechanisms of their absorption and transport in the blood.)

Biochemistry of Digestion

Nutrients are formed by condensation reactions in which H^+ and OH^- are successively removed from constituent molecules (e.g., monosaccharides, amino acids, or fatty acids) with linkages formed at removal sites. The chemical breakdown (catabolism) or digestion of these nutrients requires an opposite reaction: the *addition* of H^+ and OH^-, that is, the addition of water. These catabolic reactions are classified as hydrolysis reactions. Specific digestive enzymes act as catalysts for the reactions, with different enzymes involved in the chemical digestion of each class of nutrient. Numerous genetic disorders may result in deficiency or defective function of these enzymes, resulting in clinical syndromes known collectively as **inborn errors of metabolism.** Clinical features of the most common of these disorders are summarized in Table 25–2.

TABLE 25–2
INBORN ERRORS OF METABOLISM

Disorder	Clinical Features
Galactosemia	The absence of an enzyme that converts galactose 1-phosphate to glucose 1-phosphate results in accumulation of galactose. Manifestations are failure to thrive in infancy, mental retardation, cataract, and cirrhosis of the liver.
Glucose-6-phosphate dehydrogenase deficiency	This X-linked disorder is common in African and American blacks. Lack of this enzyme in red blood cells causes acute hemolytic anemia when certain drugs (e.g., primaquine or sulfonamides) are taken.
Phenylketonuria (PKU)	This autosomal recessive disorder is caused by lack of the enzyme that converts phenylalanine to tyrosine. Phenylalanine accumulates, causing mental retardation.
Alpha$_1$-antitrypsin deficiency	Lack of this protease inhibitor leads to panacinar emphysema.
Lysosomal storage disease	Absence of any of the lysosomal enzymes leads to accumulation of its natural substrate in cellular lysosomes. Examples include Tay-Sachs disease (see Table 2 2).
Glycogen storage disease	Defective activity of any of the enzymes involved in synthesis or degradation of glycogen leads to its accumulation in various tissues.
Ehlers-Danlos syndrome	Abnormal collagen synthesis is caused by any of several biochemical defects. Collagen is easily stretched, leading to joint hyperextension, hypermobility of skin, and fragility of blood vessels and intestinal tissues.

Data from Walter, J.B. (1992). *An Introduction to the Principles of Disease.* (3rd ed.). Philadelphia: W.B. Saunders. (pp. 270–272).

Digestion of Carbohydrates

The initial chemical digestion of carbohydrates, catalized by salivary amylase and pancreatic amylase, breaks down complex carbohydrates (polysaccharides) to double sugars (disaccharides). A number of small intestinal surface enzymes (disaccharidases) then split disaccharides into simple sugars (monosaccharides) for absorption into the venous blood. These enzymes include *lactase, sucrase, maltase,* and *α-dextrinase.* Table 25–3 summarizes enzymatic actions in the chemical digestion of carbohydrates. About 80% of carbohydrate is absorbed as glucose, 10% as fructose, and 10% as galactose. Some dietary carbohydrate is undigestable fiber that is not available for absorption. This carbohydrate is important in modifying the viscosity of the intestinal contents, which affects absorption of other nutrients, as detailed later. Some of this fiber is degraded by the bacterial flora in the large intestine, yielding gases that may be reabsorbed or passed as flatus. Undigestible carbohydrate also provides bulk to the feces, increasing their water-holding capacity and facilitating defecation.[5] Carbohydrate malabsorption is common in clinical practice, with lactose intolerance (discussed later in this chapter) being particularly prevalent.

Digestion of Proteins

Nearly all dietary protein is absorbed in the form of single amino acids, after digestive processes have

TABLE 25–3
DIGESTION OF CARBOHYDRATES

Enzyme	Action
Enzymes in Exocrine Secretions	
α-amylase (in saliva, pancreatic juice, and breast milk)	Splits starches into small glucose polymers (maltose, maltotriose, and α-branched dextrins)
Intestinal Mucosal Enzymes	
Lactase	Hydrolyzes lactose (milk sugar) to glucose and galactose
Sucrase-isomaltase	Hydrolyzes sucrose (table sugar), maltose, and isomaltose to glucose and fructose
Trehalase	Hydrolizes trehalose (in fungi) to glucose
Glucoamylase	Hydrolizes α-1,4 glycosidic bonds in maltotriose and other oligosaccharides originating from starch

Data from Ushijima, K., Riby, J.E., and Kretchmer, N. (1995). Carbohydrate malabsorption. *Pediatric Clinics of North America* 42(4), 899–915; and Branski, D., Lerner, A., and Lebenthal, E. (1996). Chronic diarrhea and malabsorption. *Pediatric Clinics of North America* 43(2), 317.

cleaved the peptide bonds between them. Although only 1% of protein is absorbed as peptides (linked chains of amino acids) or whole proteins, this form is of clinical importance because these proteins are antigenic, resulting in possible food allergies (see Chapter 13). The enzymes involved in protein digestion include the gastric enzyme *pepsin,* which initiates hydrolysis of peptide bonds; the pancreatic proteolytic enzymes *trypsin* and *chymotrypsin,* which split larger peptides into smaller ones, and *carboxypeptidase,* which cleaves single amino acids from one end of the peptide chain; and intestinal cell peptidases that complete peptide breakdown to single amino acids.

Digestion of Fats

Ninety-nine percent of dietary fat is absorbed in the form of triglyceride, a molecule consisting of three fatty acids bound to a carbohydrate (glycerol) backbone (see Chapter 3). The remaining absorbed lipid is in the form of phospholipid, cholesterol, or cholesteryl ester (a fatty acid connected to cholesterol with ester linkage). Nearly all lipid digestion occurs in the small intestine.

Lipid digestion begins with emulsification, the breakdown of fats into small particles. This process depends on the detergent action of bile, which facilitates fragmentation of larger fat particles. Emulsification increases the total surface area of fat particles that is accessible by digestive enzymes. Lipids then assemble in the form of *micelles,* small spheres in which the sterol (fat-soluble) portions are oriented inward and the polar (water-soluble) groups are oriented to the outside of the sphere. This form facilitates the stability of lipids in solution within the intestinal fluids.

Triglycerides are hydrolyzed by *pancreatic lipase,* which splits the molecules into free fatty acids (FFAs) and monoglycerides. These are then taken up by micelles and transported to the intestinal wall for absorption. Two other pancreatic enzymes, *cholesteryl ester hydrolase* and *phospholipase A_2,* hydrolize cholesteryl ester and phospholipid, respectively. The released fatty acids are also packaged into micelles.

NUTRIENT ABSORPTION

Absorption is the transport of water, ions, minerals, vitamins, and digested nutrients from the intestinal lumen into the blood, either directly or via the lymph. Active and passive transport mechanisms are involved, and the membrane to be traversed consists of polarized epithelial cells (see Chapter 2).

Anatomy of the Intestinal Epithelium

The luminal surface of the small intestine consists of epithelial cells (*enterocytes*) and has numerous finger-like projections known as *villi* (Fig. 25–2). This anatomic arrangement greatly increases the available surface area for absorption. Within each villus, an arteriole leads into a capillary bed surrounding a

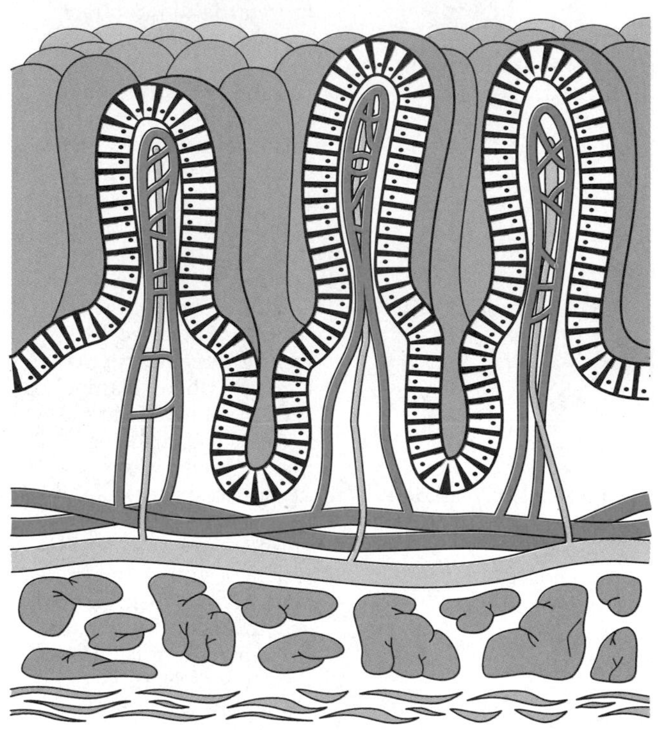

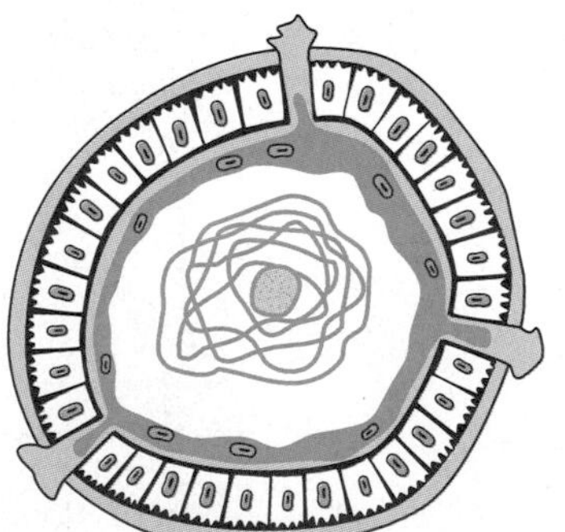
Cross-section of a villus, showing epithelial cells and basement membrane

FIGURE 25–2
Absorptive surface of the small intestine. The epithelial lining of the small intestine demonstrates numerous projections (*villi*). Within each villus an arteriole leads into a capillary bed surrounding a central *lacteal,* or lymphatic capillary. A venule leads out of the capillary bed into the portal venous circulation. The villous structure greatly increases the available surface area for absorption of nutrients, and the countercurrent blood flow within villi maintains gradients for absorption.

central *lacteal,* or lymphatic capillary. A venule leads out of the capillary bed into the portal venous circulation. Arterial and venous blood are in *countercurrent* flow within the villus, which facilitates maintenance of gradients for exchange (see Chapter 20). A potentially detrimental aspect of this arrangement, however, is that oxygen may diffuse from the arteriole to the venule at the base of the villus, depriving the tips of the villi and making these tissues highly vulnerable to ischemic damage under conditions of decreased perfusion or decreased oxygenation of the blood.

Perfusion of the Gastrointestinal Tract

Figure 25–3 illustrates the *splanchnic circulation,* including the major branches of the abdominal aorta that perfuse the alimentary canal and accessory organs. Nutrients are absorbed primarily from the small intestine into the *portal vein,* which then flows through the liver in a unique series configuration before entering the inferior vena cava. This circuit through the liver is essential to hepatic biotransformation of ingested nutrients before their entry into the general circulation, and it also allows the removal of ingested bacteria or their toxins by phagocytic cells of the liver (see Chapter 26). Drugs taken by the oral route must pass through the liver before being delivered to their target sites, and this **first-pass effect** may either inactivate much of the drug (the usual case) or activate the drug through hepatic metabolism.

Blood flow within the intestinal villi is autoregulated, with perfusion increasing in direct proportion to motility, secretion, and absorption. The precise mechanism of this autoregulation is unknown, but it is believed to involve local peptides such as CCK and kinins and may be based on the degree of oxy-

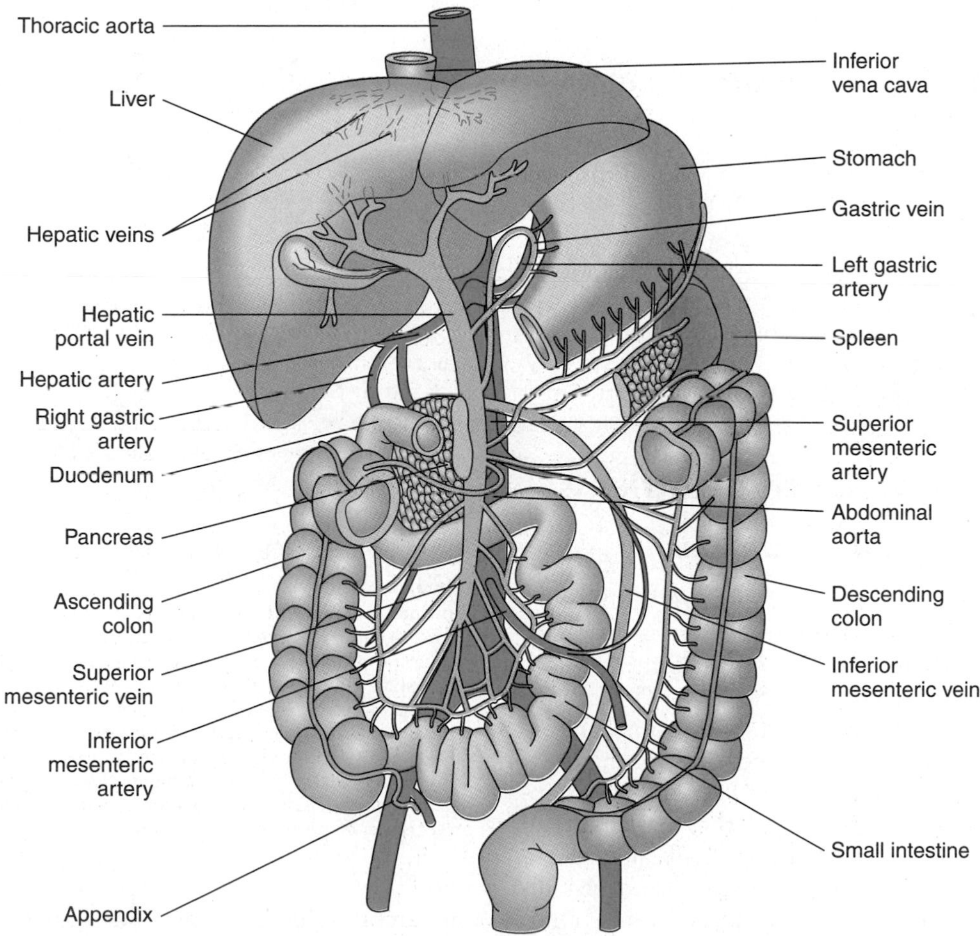

FIGURE 25–3

Splanchnic circulation. The alimentary canal and its accessory organs are perfused by arteries that branch off the thoracic aorta. Nutrients absorbed from the intestine enter the portal vein, which then flows through the liver before entering the vena cava. The connection of the intestine and liver in series is the basis of the *first-pass effect,* by which drugs taken orally are inactivated to a significant extent by the liver before circulating to their target sites.

genation or metabolic demand of GI cells (see Chapter 15). After a standard meal, blood flow to the gut increases 100% to 150%, and this effect persists for 3 to 6 hours. Because blood is temporarily diverted from other systems, ingestion of a large meal may precipitate an acute ischemic event such as angina pectoris, myocardial infarction, or stroke in those with limited cardiovascular reserve.

Gastrointestinal vessels are innervated by the sympathetic nervous system (SNS), with increased SNS stimulation constricting arterioles and venules. During stress states, arteriolar constriction is adaptive in that it shunts more blood to critical systems, that is, the brain, heart, respiratory system, and muscles (see Chapter 1). SNS-mediated constriction of the GI veins, an important blood reservoir, shunts an additional 200 to 300 mL of blood into the central circulation. The alimentary canal is prone to ischemic damage with prolonged sympathetic stimulation, however, and stress ulceration and bacterial translocation are common complications of prolonged stress or shock states (see Chapter 15).

Function of the Unstirred Layer

Adjacent to the luminal surface of the intestinal epithelium is an *unstirred layer* of fluid through which solutes must pass (Fig. 25–4). The viscosity of this fluid varies depending on the constituents of the diet. A diet rich in polysaccharides, for example, increases the viscosity of the unstirred layer and may slow the absorption of carbohydrate and lipid.[6] This effect may be beneficial in modulating fluctuations in blood glucose or lipids between meals.

Absorption of Specific Nutrients

Water and Electrolytes

The walls of the alimentary canal are highly permeable to water and electrolytes. Water is absorbed by osmosis as particles are absorbed from the stomach, small intestine, and large intestine. The cations sodium, potassium, calcium, and magnesium are actively absorbed from the gut lumen, by mechanisms which parallel reabsorption in the kidney (see Chapter 20). Sodium is pumped from the intestinal cell into the plasma, creating an intracellular concentration gradient for passive diffusion from the intestinal lumen into the cell. The sodium pump is stimulated by aldosterone via the renin-angiotensin-aldosterone system in volume-depleted states (see Chapter 8). The sodium gradient created by the initial active transport also drives most carbohydrate and protein absorption by cotransport, and

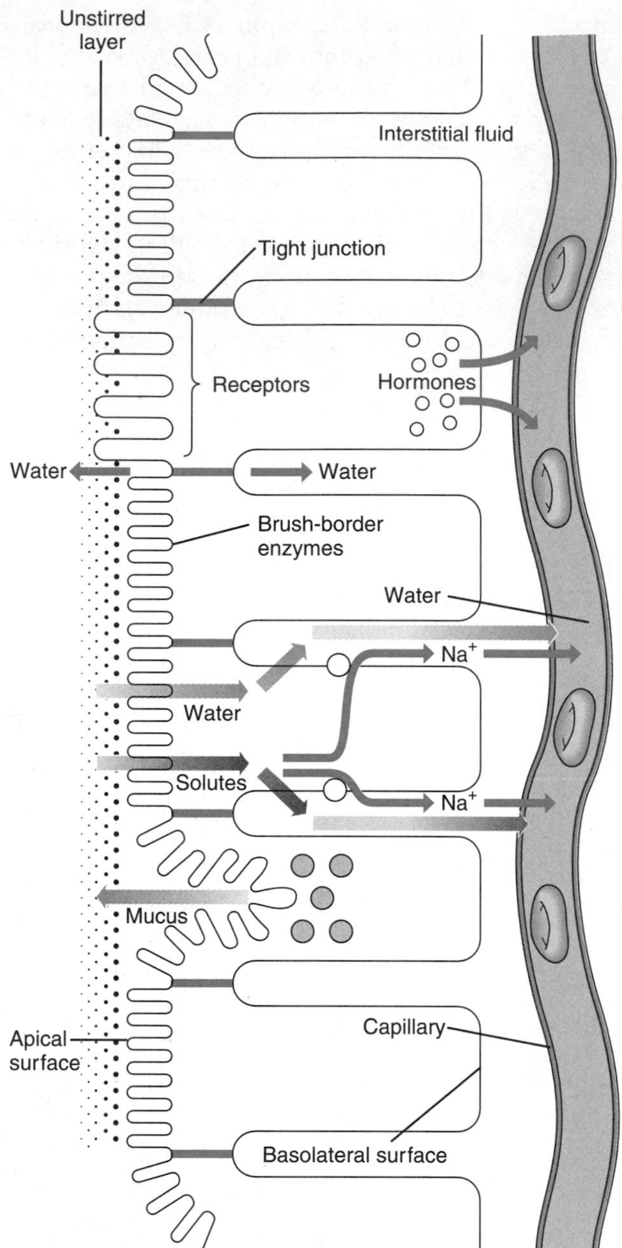

FIGURE 25–4

Luminal transport of nutrients. Nutrient molecules are absorbed by active and passive transport mechanisms from the intestinal lumen into the blood or lymph. Adjacent to the luminal surface is an unstirred layer of fluid through which solutes must pass before encountering the apical surface of intestinal epithelial cells. Absorption may be slowed if this layer is highly viscous because of a diet high in polysaccharides. Epithelial cells are polarized, with different transport mechanisms operating on each side of the cell. Some epithelial cells are specialized for function as receptors or secretion of hormones or mucus.

the anions chloride and bicarbonate are absorbed passively along the electrical gradient. Calcium and phosphate absorption are regulated by parathyroid hormone and vitamin D_3, as discussed in Chapter 9. Hydrogen ions are secreted into the gut lumen in countertransport with sodium. Fine regulation of electrolyte levels occurs in the large intestine, analogous to the function of the distal convoluted tubule of the kidney.

Carbohydrates and Proteins

Most carbohydrates and proteins are absorbed by active cotransport with sodium. Because these systems are saturable, the quantity of nutrient particles and the rate at which they are propelled along the alimentary canal are important determinents of absorption. Glucose and galactose are actively cotransported with sodium to the interior of the intestinal cell, from which they are absorbed into the blood by facilitated diffusion. In contrast, fructose absorption is entirely passive, mediated by facilitated diffusion. Amino acids and peptides are actively absorbed with sodium.

Lipids

Lipid levels in the blood originate from two intersecting metabolic pathways, the *exogenous pathway* and the *endogenous pathway,* illustrated in Figure 25–5. Lipids in the blood are transported in complex with protein. Figure 25–6 illustrates a typical *lipoprotein.* Lipoproteins are classified on the basis of their size, lipid composition, and specific membrane proteins that serve as markers or receptors (Table 25–4).

Exogenous Pathway. In the exogenous pathway, dietary lipids are transported to the intestinal wall in micelles and enter the epithelial cells of the small intestine by dissolving in membrane lipids. The epithelial cells then package the dietary lipids into *chylomicrons,* large lipoprotein particles containing 90% triglyceride and a small amount of cholesterol and protein. Chylomicrons first enter the lymphatics, which join the venous circulation at the thoracic duct (see Chapter 15). A very few short-chain triglycerides and FFAs may be absorbed directly into the blood. As they travel in the bloodstream, chylomicrons encounter the enzyme *lipoprotein lipase,* released by endothelial cells of peripheral capillaries. This enzyme cleaves FFA and glycerol from chylomicron triglycerides, and these substrates may then

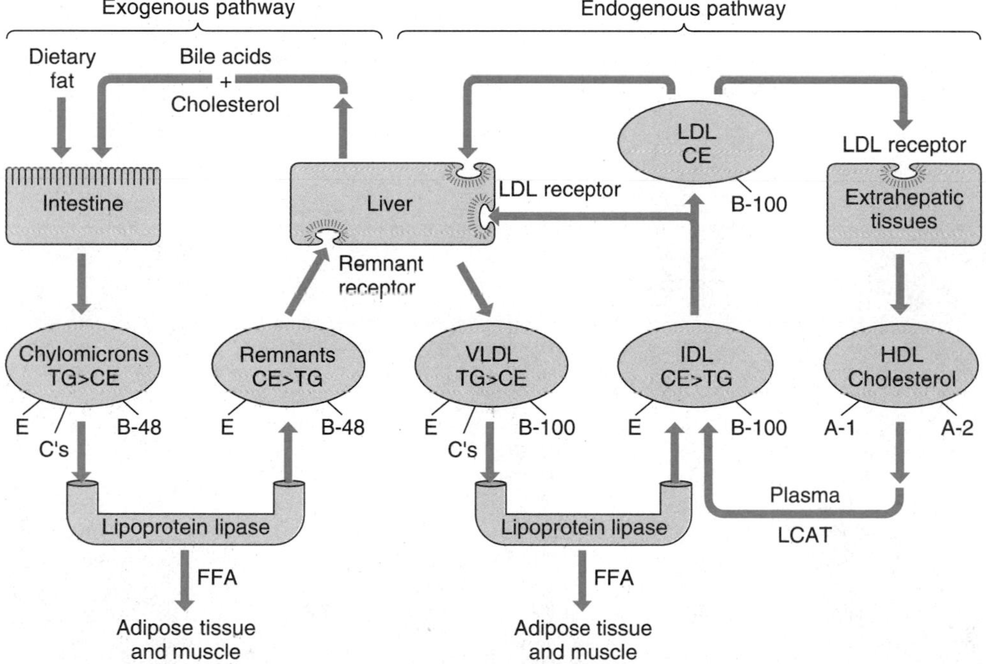

FIGURE 25–5

Lipid absorption and transport. The intersecting endogenous and exogenous pathways for lipid metabolism are shown. The exogenous pathway begins with the ingestion of dietary fats, which are absorbed into intestinal epithelial cells and complexed with protein to form *chylomicrons.* These large lipoproteins are then released into the blood. The endogenous pathway begins with synthesis of very-low-density lipoproteins (VLDLs) from dietary carbohydrates and cholesterol. Circulating VLDLs are metabolized to smaller, more atherogenic low-density lipoproteins (LDLs). *Reverse cholesterol transport* by high-density lipoprotein (HDL) is also illustrated. This transport removes LDL from the circulation. TG, triglyceride; CE, cholesteryl ester; E, apo E; C, apo C's; B-48, apo B-48; B-100; apo B-100; FFA, free fatty acids; LCAT, lecithin cholesterol acyltransferase; IDL, intermediate-density lipoprotein. (From Goldstein, J.L., Kita, T., and Brown, M.S. [1983]. Defective lipoprotein receptors and atherosclerosis. *New England Journal of Medicine* 309, 288.)

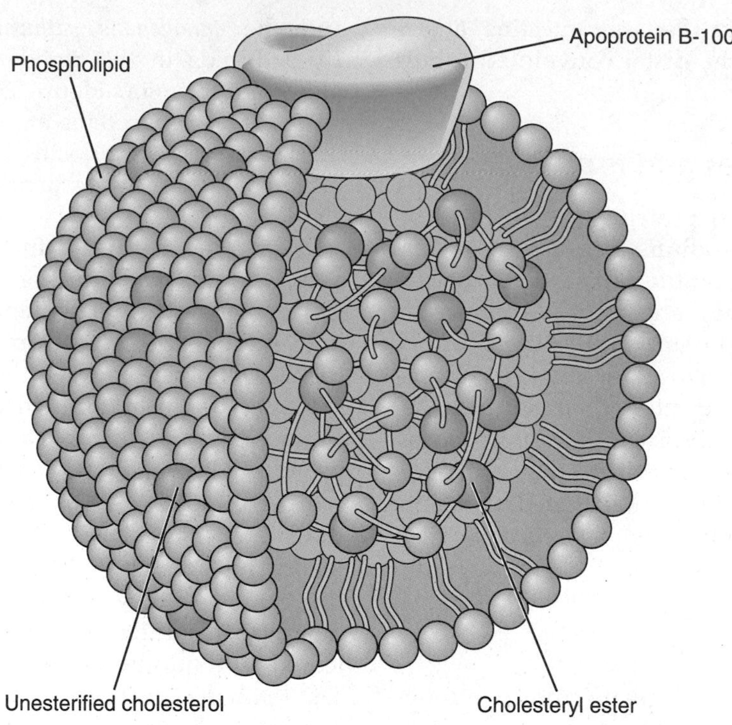

FIGURE 25–6

Structure of low-density lipoprotein. Low-density lipoproteins (LDLs) are spherical particles with an oily core of cholesteryl esters and an outer coat composed of phospholipids, cholesterol, and a protein (apoprotein B-100), which serves as a recognition site.

TABLE 25–4
CLASSIFICATION OF LIPOPROTEINS

LIPOPROTEIN	SIZE (NM)	COMPOSITION	APOPROTEINS	ATHEROGENICITY
Chylomicron	75–1000	85% TG 6% C 8% PL 2% Pro	Apo A=IV Apo B=48 Apo C=II Apo C=III	Nonatherogenic
Very-low-density lipoproteins (VLDL)	30–80	55% TG 20% C 17% PL 8% Pro	Apo B=100 Apo C=II Apo C=III Apo E	Nonatherogenic when newly synthesized; remnants are atherogenic
Intermediate-density lipoproteins (IDL, also known as VLDL remnants)	25–40	30% TG 30% C 22% PL 18% Pro	Apo B=100	Atherogenic
Low-density lipoproteins (LDL)	20	7% TG 53% C 20% PL 20% Pro	Apo B=100 Apo E	Atherogenic
High-density lipoproteins (HDL)	7.5–10	5% TG 20% C 25% PL 50% Pro	Apo A=I Apo A=II Apo A=IV Apo C=III Apo E	Antiatherogenic

TG, triglycerides; C, cholesterol; PL, phospholipid; Pro, protein; Apo, apoprotein.

diffuse into muscle cells for energy metabolism or into fat (adipose tissue) cells for storage. The *chylomicron remnant* that remains is composed primarily of cholesterol. This particle is transported to the liver, where it is taken up by endocytosis via a chylomicron remnant receptor. The liver may store this cholesterol or may use it in the synthesis of other lipoproteins or bile.

Endogenous Pathway. The endogenous pathway begins in the liver, with the synthesis of another lipoprotein, *very-low-density lipoprotein (VLDL),* from dietary carbohydrates and cholesterol. VLDLs, containing mostly triglyceride but some cholesterol, are released into the blood. In peripheral capillaries, lipoprotein lipase releases FFA and glycerol, leaving a VLDL remnant rich in cholesterol. These remnants, also known as *intermediate-density lipoproteins (IDLs),* may be removed from the blood by the liver or may remain in the blood. If they continue to circulate, lipoprotein lipase removes more and more triglyceride from them until a particle consisting of mostly cholesterol is formed. This particle, *low-density lipoprotein (LDL),* constitutes 75% of circulating cholesterol. Some LDL is removed from the blood via receptor-mediated endocytosis by the liver or by other cells that express the LDL receptor on their membranes. These are cells that need cholesterol for synthesis of plasma membranes, organelle membranes, or steroid hormones (see Chapter 29).

Regulation of Serum Lipid Levels. Low-density lipoprotein cholesterol is often referred to as "bad" cholesterol because elevated serum levels confer independent risk of atherosclerosis (see Chapter 15). Mechanisms by which serum LDL levels are lowered are of considerable clinical importance, and drug therapies have been designed to augment these mechanisms (see later discussion of hyperlipidemia). Cells that require cholesterol have intracellular enzyme systems for its synthesis, but these cells more readily take up LDL from the blood (Fig. 25–7). The more cholesterol they are able to take up and store, the fewer LDL receptors they express on their membranes. When serum LDL is elevated, it is also taken up by phagocytic cells of the monocyte-macrophage system via their "scavenger" receptors. This uptake contributes to the formation of cholesterol deposits in the skin and tendons (**xanthomata**), and it is an important component of the lipid infiltration hypothesis of atherosclerosis.

Another mechanism by which LDL levels may be lowered is by *reverse cholesterol transport,* mediated by the "good" cholesterol particle *high-density lipo-*

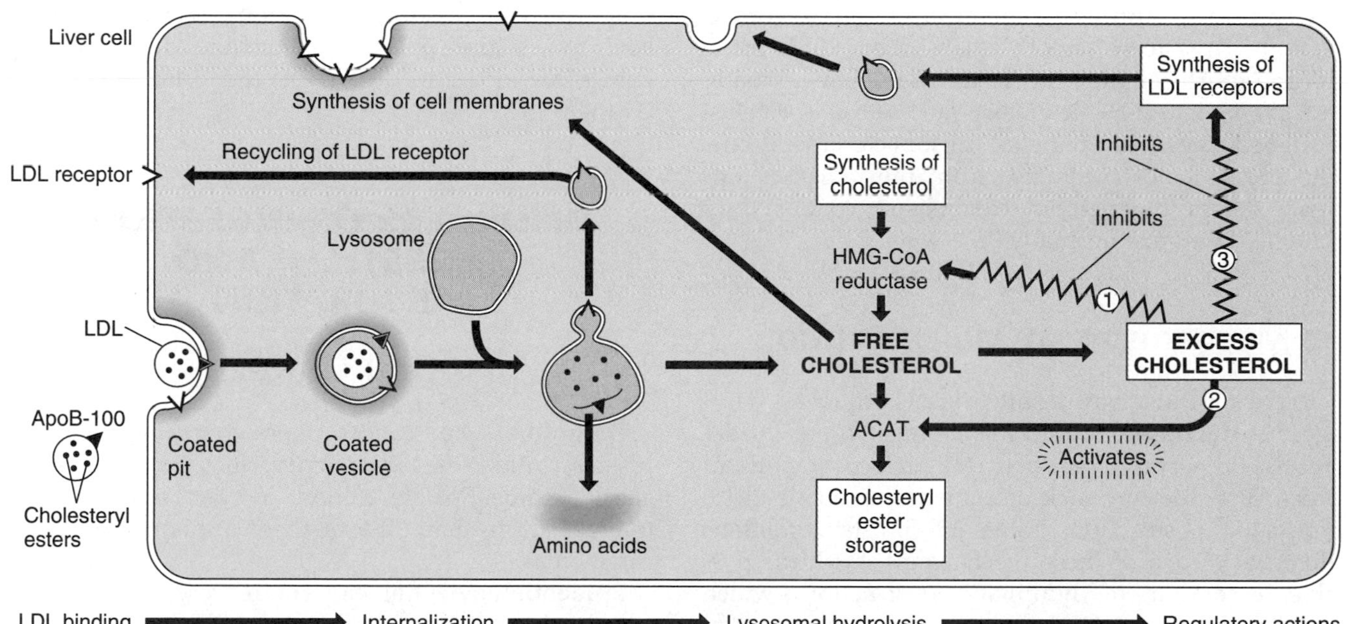

FIGURE 25–7

Cellular uptake and metabolism of low-density lipoprotein cholesterol. Cells that require cholesterol for the synthesis of membranes or hormones express low-density lipoprotein (LDL) receptors on their surfaces. These receptors recognize and bind apoprotein B-100 (apo B-100), and receptors and LDLs are taken in by receptor-mediated endocytosis. Lysosomal enzymes release the cholesterol and recycle the receptor to the membrane. Cholesterol uptake from the blood: (1) inhibits 3-hydroxy-3-methylglutaryl coenzyme A (HMG-CoA) reductase, a key enzyme in the pathway for intracellular synthesis of cholesterol; (2) activates ACAT enzyme, promoting storage of cholesteryl esters, and (3) down-regulates LDL receptor synthesis. Normal turnover of these cells may release free cholesterol into the blood. ACAT, acyl CoA:cholesterol acyltransferase.

protein (HDL). HDLs, which are synthesized by the liver and by intestinal epithelial cells, are flat, rigid disks composed of 50% protein and 50% lipids. Their role in lipid metabolism is to attract the free cholesterol in the blood that originates from normal cell membrane turnover. This cholesterol adsorbs to the surface of the HDLs, which then transfer it to IDLs or LDLs for transport to the liver, from which most of it is excreted in the bile. HDLs apparently inhibit subsequent reuptake of this cholesterol into the blood and into cells, and they also may remove cholesterol from atherosclerotic lesions. High HDL levels are an "antirisk" factor for atherosclerosis and are associated with regression or stabilization of existing plaque. Aerobic exercise, *moderate* alcohol intake, and estrogen have been shown to promote increased HDL levels, whereas cigarette smoking and elevated VLDLs decrease HDL levels.

The LDL and IDL cholesterol that is taken up by the liver may be used in the synthesis of bile, which enters the duodenum in response to fat in the chyme. Once in the gut, this cholesterol may be reabsorbed into the bloodstream or excreted in the feces (see Chapter 26).

TABLE 25–5
MALABSORPTIVE DISORDERS

Mechanism	Examples of Disorders
Damage to the intestinal mucosa	Gastroenteritis, inflammatory bowel disease, gluten-sensitive enteropathy, radiation enteritis, amyloidosis, protein-losing enteropathy
Decreased transit time	Inflammatory disorders (see above), endocrine diseases, hormone-secreting tumors
Decreased absorptive surface	Short bowel syndrome (surgical resection or bypass), gluten-sensitive enteropathy
Insufficient digestive enzymes or bile	Chronic pancreatitis, pancreatic cancer, biliary tract disease, inborn errors of metabolism, lactose intolerance, cystic fibrosis
Lymphatic obstruction	Small bowel lymphoma, Whipple's disease

Formation of the Feces

Unabsorbed nutrients remain in the bowel for excretion in the feces (stool). Unabsorbed solids make up one fourth of the bulk of the stool and normally include 10% to 20% of dietary fats, fibrous proteins, sloughed intestinal epithelial cells, bacteria, and bile. The brown color originates from the bilirubin pigments (from hemoglobin catabolism) contained in the bile. Feces are normally 75% water.

Mechanisms of Malabsorption

Malabsorption may result from: (1) mucosal damage, (2) decreased intraluminal transit time, (3) decreased absorptive surface, (4) defective nutrient processing due to a lack of enzymes or bile, and (5) lymphatic obstruction. Table 25–5 lists conditions illustrating each of these mechanisms. With the possible exception of lymphatic obstruction, which could result from neoplasia, inflammation is a common denominator in most forms of malabsorption. Diarrhea, which results in malabsorption as a consequence of altered motility, secretion, or intestinal osmotic gradients, is detailed in Chapter 24. Gluten-sensitive enteropathy and lactose intolerance, discussed later in this chapter, are other common disorders characterized by malabsorption. Cystic fibrosis, a genetic disorder in which exocrine glands become plugged with abnormally viscous secretions, may lead to malabsorption if pancreatic digestive enzymes are not able to access the duodenum (see Chapter 18).

DISORDERS OF INGESTION, DIGESTION, AND ABSORPTION

Oral Cancer

Definition. Oral cancer refers to malignant neoplasms within the oral cavity, including the lips, cheek, gums, palate, floor of the mouth, and tongue.[7] More than 90% of these are squamous cell carcinomas.

Epidemiology. Oral cancers represent 6% of all cancers diagnosed annually in the U.S.[7] The greatest risk factor for development of oral cancer is cigarette smoking, present in approximately 90% of cases. Use of smokeless tobacco (snuff) is also associated with the disorder and may account for the rising incidence of oral cancer in adolescent and young adult males. Use of alcohol increases the tobacco-associated risk, because alcohol facilitates absorption of tobacco by the oral mucosa. Other reported risk factors include oral viral infection (e.g., herpes simplex virus, human papilloma virus), sunlight exposure, poor dentition, and betel-nut chewing.[7]

Etiology. As is true of most cancers, the precise etiology is unknown (see Chapter 7). A multifactorial etiology is probable.

Pathophysiology. The condition usually begins with the appearance of a precancerous oral lesion, **leukoplakia** (Color Fig. 25–1). These white patches undergo malignant transformation in 4% to 18% of individuals.[7] The appearance of red mucosal plaques having no inflammatory cause (**erythroplasia**) is even more ominous, increasing the risk of malignant transformation sevenfold. Cancerous lesions are usually ulcerated, with a discolored base (Color Fig. 25–2). Lesions may penetrate to involve nerves, and oral cancer may metastasize to cervical lymph nodes.

Clinical Manifestations. Appearance of precancerous and malignant lesions signals the presence of neoplasia. Lesions may bleed easily. Mouth pain, sore throat, and poorly fitting dentures or loosening of teeth are commonly seen. Neck masses and weight loss are evidence of more advanced cancer.

Prevention and Treatment. Cessation of smoking and use of smokeless tobacco have been shown to reduce the incidence of oral cancer.[7] Alcohol use should also be limited. Treatment depends on the site and stage of the tumor. Small, localized lesions may be treated with surgical excision or, in some cases, with radiation alone. Dissection of neck lymph nodes may be warranted in more advanced tumors, and chemotherapy may be used adjunctively.

Prognosis and Outcome. Prognosis depends on the site of the tumor and its stage at time of diagnosis. The overall 5-year survival rate is 53%, suggesting that the disease is often advanced when diagnosed.[7] An estimated 8000 deaths result from oral cancer in the United States each year.

Cleft Lip and Palate

Definition. Cleft lip (harelip) is a congenital splitting or defect in the integrity of the lip. It may occur with or without concurrent splitting of the palate (cleft palate).

Epidemiology. The estimated incidence of cleft lip with or without cleft palate is 1 in 1000 births. Cleft palate alone occurs in an estimated 1 in 2500 births.[8] Risk is increased in those with a positive family history, but environmental factors are also believed to be involved. Isolated cleft palate is more common in females, probably because structures of the developing palate close about a week later in females. Individuals of Japanese ancestry are at highest risk, and whites are at greater risk than blacks. Specific environmental teratogens associated with cleft lip and palate are uncertain. Use of the antiepileptic drug phenytoin (Dilantin) has been implicated in some cases.[8]

Etiology. Cleft lip and palate demonstrate multifactorial inheritance, with genetic factors probably of greater importance in the development of cleft lip (with or without cleft palate) than that of cleft palate alone.[9] Some clefts occur as part of single-gene defect syndromes, whereas others are part of chromosomal defects, such as trisomy 13.

Pathophysiology. The disorder may take various forms. Cleft lip is disfiguring and may affect early parental bonding and later speech and social interaction. Ingestion may be impaired to varying degrees in cleft lip and palate if the infant is unable to seal the oropharynx. Aspiration risk may be increased. Cleft palate may also impair normal function of the eustachian tube, increasing the risk of otitis media (see Chapter 23).

Clinical Manifestations. Facial deformity is evident with cleft lip, which may be unilateral or bilateral (Fig. 25–8). Oral inspection reveals cleft palate. Radiographic examination may reveal associated bony deformities. Some infants may have difficulty feeding. If the defect is not repaired, development of the teeth may be affected, and speech may be abnormal or delayed.

Prevention and Treatment. Exposure to teratogenic agents should be limited insofar as possible during pregnancy. Use of large, soft nipples or prosthetic devices may aid feeding before repair. Surgical correction is the treatment of choice, and it is

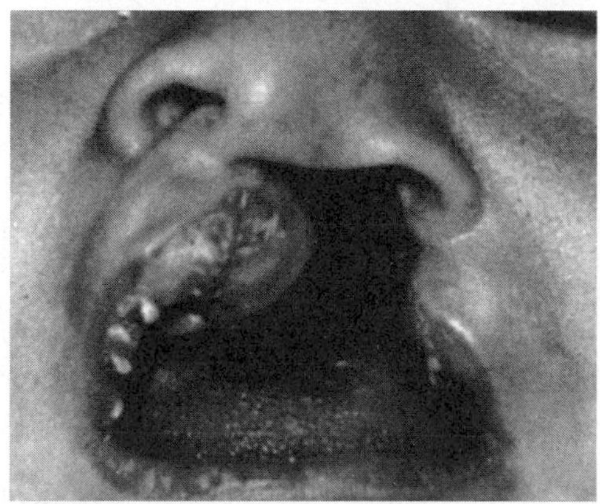

FIGURE 25–8
Cleft lip and palate. Complete unilateral cleft of the lip and palate is illustrated. (From Moore, K.L., and Persaud, T.V.N. [1993]. *The Developing Human: Clinically Oriented Embryology.* Philadelphia: W.B. Saunders. [p. 221].)

often done in stages over the first 4 or 5 years of life. Speech therapy and orthodontic care are often required as well.

Prognosis and Outcome. Appropriate and timely surgical treatment is associated with optimal cosmetic and functional outcomes. These children continue to be at increased risk of dental caries, sinus infections, and otitis media, however.[8]

Periodontal Disease

Definition. Periodontal disease includes a number of inflammatory disorders of the *gingiva* (gums) that may lead to tooth loss.

Epidemiology. Periodontal disease is common, affecting more than 90% of the population of the United States.[10] Risk factors include poor dental hygiene and a high dietary intake of sugar.

Etiology. Accumulation of plaque and colonization with bacteria lead to dental caries and inflammation of the gums.

Pathophysiology. Plaque formation is initiated by oral bacteria from substrates in dietary carbohydrates and saliva. Bacteria are enveloped within a sticky film that accumulates on the teeth, usually near the interface with the gums. Superficial inflammation (**gingivitis**) is evident at first. Dental caries may occur. As inflammation extends to deeper tissues, the gums separate from the teeth, and teeth loosen when supporting alveolar bone and ligaments degenerate (Fig. 25–9).

Clinical Manifestations. Inflammation of the gums is evidenced as redness, swelling, and possible ulceration. Teeth are loose and gums bleed easily with brushing or minor trauma. Plaque deposition is apparent, and caries (cavities) in the teeth are common. Impaired nutrition in the elderly is often associated with tooth loss or poorly fitted dentures.

Prevention and Treatment. Prevention involves plaque removal with brushing and flossing and regular dental cleaning and examination. Supplemental fluoride treatments may help to strengthen the tooth enamel, and sealing of molar surfaces may help prevent cavities during childhood. Reduction of dietary sugars, especially sticky foods that adhere to the teeth, may also be beneficial in reducing plaque formation and bacterial growth. Dental caries are filled as necessary, and tooth extraction may be required in some cases. Abscesses may require drainage and appropriate antibiotic therapy.

Prognosis and Outcome. Tooth loss is no longer considered to be a normal part of the aging process. With early and regular dental hygiene, most individuals should have healthy teeth and gums for a lifetime.

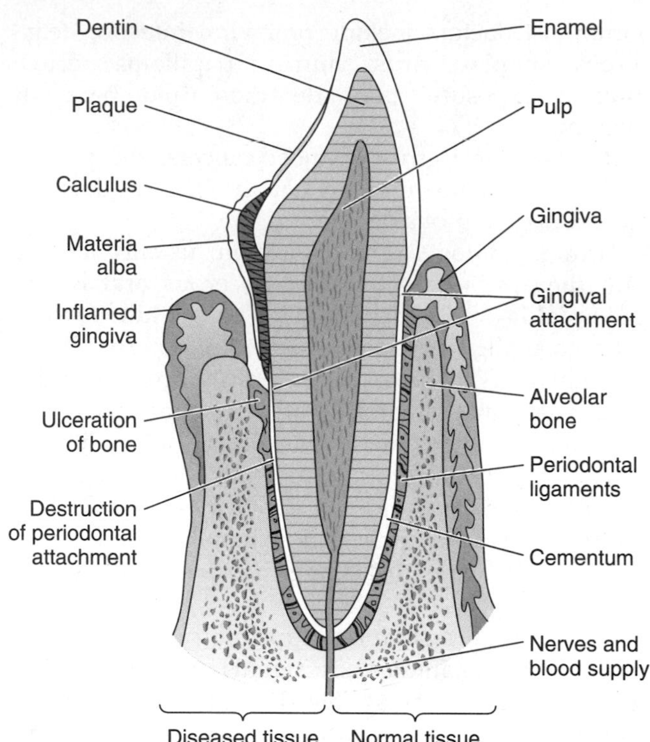

FIGURE 25–9

Periodontal disease. Accumulation of plaque leads to gingival inflammation and destruction of alveolar bone and periodontal fibers, leading to loosening of the tooth. (From Black, J.M., and Matassarin-Jacobs, E. [1997]. *Medical-Surgical Nursing: Clinical Management for Continuity of Care.* (5th Ed.). Philadelphia: W.B. Saunders. [p. 1721].)

Eating Disorders

Definition. Anorexia nervosa is a psychological and physiologic disorder of self-starvation defined by four criteria: failure to maintain a minimal weight for height and age, fear of fatness, distorted body image, and absence of menstruation in females. **Bulimia nervosa,** or binge-purge syndrome, is a disorder characterized by periods of excessive consumption of high-calorie foods followed by purging behaviors, including self-induced vomiting as well as abuse of diuretics and laxatives.[11]

Epidemiology. Anorexia and bulimia are the most prevalent psychiatric disorders in adolescents, particularly females. Together, these eating disorders afflict about 1.2 million young women in the U.S.[11] Bulimia is more prevalent than anorexia; however, the two conditions commonly coexist. Although females between the ages of 12 and 25 are at highest risk, increasing numbers of young children and older individuals are also developing these disorders. The current sociocultural emphasis on thinness and physical fitness as symbols of beauty and success is believed to underlie these trends. Young men are uncommonly afflicted, although athletes trying to "make weight" (e.g., wrestlers, gymnasts) may indulge in binge-purge behavior as an isolated, usually benign, instance.[12] Male homosexuals display an increased incidence, as do males with chemical dependency. Individuals who have a history of physical and sexual abuse are also at higher risk.[11] A genetic predisposition has been hypothesized but remains unproved.

Etiology. No single cause has been found for either of these disorders. Emotional, physical, sociologic, and family factors apparently contribute to the multifactorial etiology.

Pathophysiology. Patients with anorexia nervosa believe themselves to be obese, and they severely decrease caloric intake until their weight drops to at least 15% below ideal body weight. Body fat and protein stores are depleted and muscle wasting is seen. Young women become deficient in estrogen as a result of lack of lipid substrate for synthesis of the hormone as well as decreased levels of the gonadotropins luteinizing hormone and follicle-stimulating hormone (see Chapter 31). In males, testosterone levels fluctuate, but decreased erectile function and sperm production are seen. Thyroid function is reduced in about 10% of those with anorexia nervosa. Electrolyte imbalances occur in about 40% of anorexics because of volume depletion and inadequate intake. In the absence of carbohydrate intake, ketoacidosis results from increased use of fat as energy fuel (see Chapter 3). Rhabdomyolysis and renal failure are possible with severe protein catabolism (see Chapter 20). Red blood cell (RBC) function may be abnormal because of the lack of ATP and 2,3-diphosphoglycerate (see Chapter 12). Brain parenchymal tissue is reversibly lost, and dilation of the cerebral ventricles is seen.[13] Insulin-like growth factors (IGFs) are reduced, contributing to growth deficiency in children and adolescents.

In bulimia, repeated vomiting and abuse of laxatives may result in structural and functional disorders of the GI tract. Electrolyte imbalance and acid-base imbalance may also result from these purging behaviors, as well as from abuse of diuretics. Weight loss is not as great as that in anorexia nervosa, and tissue loss is not life-threatening. Chronic use of laxatives may impair bowel motility and lead to constipation. Frequent vomiting of acid-containing stomach contents may cause tooth decay and irritation of the esophagus. Gastric bleeding may result from traumatic tears at the junction of the stomach and esophagus.

Clinical Manifestations. In anorexics, **cachexia** is evident to others, but not to the patient (Fig. 25–10). "Paradoxic satiety" is commonly seen, in which the patient reports no hunger when fasting and feels bloated although she does not eat. When she does eat, she feels more hungry with each mouthful. Menstruation is absent, and secondary sex characteristics are suppressed. Hair loss, cold intolerance, frequent upper respiratory infections, and constipation are typical, and edema and **hypercarotenemia** may be seen. Laboratory findings include decreased serum albumin, globulin, calcium, potassium, and sodium as well as reduced RBC and WBC counts.[14]

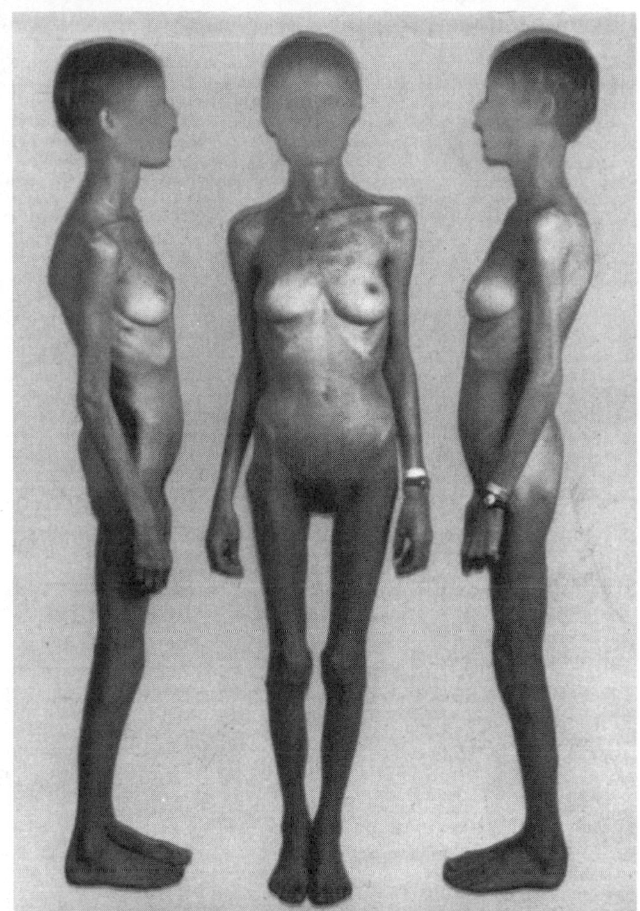

FIGURE 25–10

Cachexia in anorexia nervosa. Body weight in anorexia nervosa is less than 85% of normal for height and age and may be severely decreased, as illustrated here. (From Comerci, G.D. [1990]. Medical complications of anorexia nervosa and bulimia nervosa. *Medical Clinics of North America* 74(5), 1293–1310.)

Bulimics often have a "chipmunk-like" facial appearance because of swelling of the parotid glands that results from contact with acidic gastric contents. Etching and decay of the teeth are common for the same reason. Those who induce vomiting with a finger in the throat may display scarring on the dorsal surface of the hand. Weight fluctuations are common, but cachexia is not seen. Abdominal distention is a frequent finding, and abdominal striae ("stretch marks") may be seen because of weight fluctuation. Laboratory findings typical of bulimia include hypokalemia, metabolic alkalosis, and an elevated level of CCK.

Complications of eating disorders and their treatment affect nearly every body system. These are summarized in Table 25–6.

Prevention and Treatment. Intervention in eating disorders consists of psychological counseling and education and, if necessary, hospitalization with enforced refeeding. Patients with anorexia nervosa are often unwilling to voluntarily accept treatment, because they deny the extent of their illness. Hospitalization is necessary for those with medical complications (e.g., severe emaciation, hypokalemia, hyponatremia, cardiac dysrhythmia) or psychiatric complications (e.g., depression and suicide risk). Nutritional rehabilitation and weight restoration are priorities and may necessitate supervised intake, assistance with meal planning, or, in some cases, enforced enteral or parenteral nutrition. (A comparison of these methods of supplemental nutrition is shown in Table 25–7.) Use of antidepressant medication may be warranted.

Bulimic patients are usually more amenable to treatment because they have more insight into their disturbed behavior. Use of antidepressant medication is highly effective in most cases, probably because of its effects on multiple neurotransmitters, on receptors affecting appetite, and directly on the depression that frequently accompanies eating disorders.

Psychotherapy is an important mode of therapy in eating disorders and may take the form of short-term cognitive therapy; long-term, insight-oriented therapy; or family therapy.[14] Complications are treated appropriately, with particular attention given to life-threatening manifestations of cardiac dysrhythmia (see Chapter 17).

Prognosis and Outcome. With psychiatric intervention, as many as 75% of patients with eating disorders improve significantly over time.[11] Outcome is least favorable in those in whom the conditions become chronic. Overall mortality in anorexia nervosa is estimated to be 5% in the first 2 years after diagnosis and may approach 20% in those who are untreated.[14] Mortality in bulimia nervosa is rare and usually results from aspiration of vomitus.

TABLE 25–6
MEDICAL COMPLICATIONS OF ANOREXIA NERVOSA AND BULIMIA NERVOSA

Cardiovascular
- Arrhythmia
- Bradycardia
- Cardiomyopathy
- Congestive heart failure
- Edema
- Hypotension
- Peripheral cyanosis

Dermatologic
- Callus formation on hands
- Carotene pigmentation
- Dry skin and nails
- Irritation at corners of mouth
- Lanugo hair
- Thinning scalp hair

Endocrine
- Amenorrhea
- Decreased tri-iodothyronine and thyroxine levels
- Increased cortisol level
- Increased growth hormone level

Gastrointestinal
- Bloating and early satiety
- Constipation
- Dental caries
- Diarrhea
- Esophageal or gastric dilation or rupture
- Pancreatitis
- Parotitis and hyperamylasemia

Hematologic
- Low erythrocyte sedimentation rate
- Low white blood cell count
- Mild anemia

Metabolic
- Hypokalemia
- Hypomagnesemia
- Hyponatremia
- Increased blood urea nitrogen level

Musculoskeletal
- Delayed bone maturation
- Osteoporosis
- Reduced stature

Neurologic
- Seizures

From Zerbe, K.J. (1996). Anorexia nervosa and bulimia nervosa: When the pursuit of bodily 'perfection' becomes a killer. *Postgraduate Medicine* 99(1), 167. Used with permission.

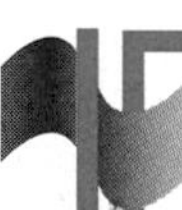

Clinical Scenario

T.J., a 19-year-old college student, is admitted to the Medical Unit after what was described as a possible seizure. She had been having breakfast at a restaurant with her parents, after which she went to the restroom and returned feeling "dizzy." Her parents reported that she looked "grayish," and that after sitting down "her arms and legs began jerking" and she "didn't respond when we talked to her." The incident lasted about 5 minutes. Physical examination on admission reveals a slightly low blood pressure (90/50) and a pulse of 120. T.J. is 5 feet, 6 inches tall and weighs 98 lb. Her skin is dry, and her hair appears very brittle. Neurologic testing is normal. T.J.'s serum electrolytes are abnormal, with sodium, potassium, calcium, and chloride levels all low.

1. What additional information should be sought in obtaining the medical history in T.J.'s case?
2. What is the pathophysiologic explanation for T.J.'s "episode"?

TABLE 25–7
COMPARISON OF ENTERAL AND PARENTERAL NUTRITION

Parameter	Total Enteral Nutrition (TEN)	Total Parenteral Nutrition (TPN)
Clinical indications for use	Inability to voluntarily ingest adequate diet to prevent catabolism for a period longer than 7 days; adequate digestive and absorptive function	Same as TEN, but GI tract function is not adequate because of malabsorptive disorder or extreme hypermetabolic state
Method of providing access	Feeding tube placed in the stomach, duodenum, or jejunum via nasogastric insertion, percutaneous puncture, or surgical incision	Large-bore catheter placed in a central vein
Form of nutrient administration	Liquid formulas ranging from blenderized foods to elemental diets consisting of dextrose, amino acids, and fatty acids	Intravenous fluids containing amino acids, dextrose, and emulsified fats with added electrolytes and trace elements
Advantages	Reduced risk of bacterial translocation across the gut wall, maintenance of GI-mediated immune and hormonal functions, maintenance of villus height, reduced risk of catheter-associated complications (sepsis, pneumothorax, hyperglycemia)	The enteral route is preferred when it is available—"If the gut works, use it"; TPN may represent the only route of nutrition in selected cases

GI, gastrointestinal.

Obesity

Definition. Obesity, the accumulation of an abnormally large quantity of adipose tissue, may be defined quantitatively with reference to ideal body weight (IBW), fraction of body fat, or **body mass index (BMI).** Ideal body weight has long been derived from standard height-weight formulas or tables such as the Metropolitan Life Insurance Company standards of desirable weights; however, these are believed to underestimate obesity-related mortality because they do not account for cigarette smokers, who tend to be thin but unhealthy.[15] On the basis of body fat percentage, obesity may be defined as a body fat percentage of greater than 25% in men and 30% in women.[16] Accurate measurement of body fat is cumbersome, however, and the percentage does not account for differences in risk associated with *distribution* of fat (see pathophysiology section). The BMI is now the preferred means of quantifying obesity-related risk in epidemiologic studies. BMI has been shown to correlate with body fat and is calculated from height and weight as follows:

$$BMI = w/h^2$$

where w = weight in kilograms (pounds divided by 2.2) and h = height in meters (inches divided by 39.4). According to the 1995 guidelines issued by the National Institutes of Health and the American Health Foundation, a BMI of less than 25 is desirable.[15] According to the World Health Organization, a BMI of 30 or higher places an individual at major health risk because of obesity.

Epidemiology. In the United States, 31% of men and 24% of women are overweight (BMI = 25–30), and 12% of men and women are at high risk because of obesity (BMI > 30).[17] Factors that may contribute to the development of obesity are hereditary and environmental. At least five genes have been shown to influence the development of obesity in laboratory animals, but no mutations of these genes have as yet been found in humans.[15] Research has also shown that the role of shared environmental effects in development of obesity is minimal. High-fat diets and low levels of physical activity, common in the Western world, clearly predispose many individuals to weight gain. In the United States, the prevalence of obesity increases with age until about 55 to 65 years, after which it levels off. Black women are at particularly high risk. Higher socioeconomic status correlates with obesity in men, whereas lower status correlates with obesity in women.[16] Childhood obesity demonstrates a low correlation with later obesity in adulthood.[18] Unusual factors that may contribute to obesity include hypothalamic lesions affecting appetite control centers (e.g., with head injury, stroke, or tumor) and endocrine disorders such as Cushing's syndrome or hypothyroidism. Smoking cessation is associated with a minor risk of weight gain (see Focus of Current Research).

Focus of Current Research

Study	*Objectives and Findings*
Heini and Weinsier (1997) Divergent trends in obesity and fat intake patterns: The American paradox.	*Objective:* To compare recent changes in diet and physical activity trends in body weight and obesity prevalence *Findings:* Reduced fat and calorie intake and frequent use of low-calorie food products have been associated with a paradoxical increase in the prevalence of obesity.
Ronnemaa, et al. (1997) Relation between plasma leptin levels and measures of body fat in identical twins discordant for obesity.	*Objective:* To determine whether genetic factors or body fat distribution affect the association between leptin levels and obesity *Findings:* Plasma levels of leptin, the normal product of the *ob* gene, are increased in obese persons, but are not caused by genetic factors. Visceral fat may be important in regulation of leptin levels in men.
Newman and Hulley (1996) Carcinogenicity of lipid-lowering drugs.	*Objective:* To review the findings of studies of rodent carcinogenicity of lipid-lowering drugs *Findings:* Lipid-lowering drug treatment, especially with fibrates and statins, should be avoided except in patients at high short-term risk of coronary heart disease.
Himeno, et al. (1996) Weight reduction regresses left ventricular mass regardless of blood pressure level in obese subjects.	*Objective:* To investigate the effects of weight reduction on left ventricular mass in obese normotensive and hypertensive subjects *Findings:* Weight reduction by mild exercise and caloric restriction can reduce left ventricular mass, whether or not subjects have high blood pressure.
Rensch, et al. (1996) Gluten-sensitive enteropathy in patients with insulin-dependent diabetes mellitus.	*Objective:* To determine the prevalence of celiac disease in a cohort of patients with insulin-dependent diabetes *Findings:* Prevalence of celiac disease in the study group was 6.4%, significantly greater than the prevalence in the general population (estimated at 0.02% to 0.1% in the United States).

continued

Study	*Objectives and Findings*
Flegal, et al. (1995) The influence of smoking cessation on the prevalence of overweight in the United States.	*Objective:* To estimate the influence of smoking cessation on the increase in the prevalence of overweight in the United States *Findings:* Smoking cessation is associated with a small increase in the prevalence of overweight (about one fourth of the increase in men and one sixth of the increase in women).
Young and Gelskey (1995) Is noncentral obesity metabolically benign?	*Objective:* To determine if individuals who are overall obese but have low waist-to-hip ratios have unfavorable lipid profiles *Findings:* Individuals with noncentral obesity have lipid profiles that are in between those of centrally obese and nonobese individuals.
Manson, et al. (1995) Body weight and mortality among women.	*Objective:* To examine the association between body mass index and mortality in a cohort of U.S. women enrolled in the Nurses' Health Study *Findings:* Body weight and mortality from all causes were directly related among these middle-aged women. Lowest mortality was observed in those who weighed at least 15% less than the U.S. average for women of this age group.
Writing Group for the DISC Collaborative Research Group (1995) Efficacy and safety of lowering dietary intake of fat and cholesterol in children with elevated low-density lipoprotein cholesterol.	*Objective:* To assess the effect of dietary intervention in children ages 8 to 10 years during 3 years of treatment *Findings:* Modest lowering of LDL cholesterol was achieved while maintaining adequate growth, iron stores, nutritional adequacy, and psychological well-being during adolescent growth.
Suarez, et al. (1995) A comparison of symptoms after the consumption of milk or lactose-hydrolyzed milk by people with self-reported severe lactose intolerance.	*Objective:* To evaluate gastrointestinal symptoms in a group of people claiming to be severely lactose intolerant after drinking 240 mL of milk daily for 1 week *Findings:* Gastrointestinal symptoms were minimal, and there were no significant differences in symptoms when patients consumed regular milk versus lactose-hydrolyzed milk.
Everhart and Wright (1995) Diabetes mellitus as a risk factor for pancreatic cancer.	*Objective:* To evaluate whether diabetes is a risk factor for pancreatic cancer or a consequence of pancreatic cancer *Findings:* Persons with long-standing diabetes have double the usual risk of pancreatic cancer.

Etiology. Obesity is a multifactorial disorder. Theoretically, three mechanisms could lead to obesity: (1) excess lipid deposition in fat cells (adipocytes), (2) reduction of mobilization of lipids from adipocytes, or (3) decreased utilization of lipids.[19] The second mechanism, reduced lipid mobilization, has not yet been shown to contribute to human obesity. The first and third mechanisms are implicated in most cases. Excess lipid deposition occurs when a state of positive energy balance exists, that is, calories are consumed in excess of utilization. An eating pattern of fewer, larger meals and a higher composition of fat in the diet further contributes to this deposition. Controversy exists as to whether genetic alterations in physiologic appetite-regulatory systems contribute to excess intake. Decreased lipid utilization may result from lack of physical activity or from hereditary differences in metabolic rates and thermogenesis.

Pathophysiology. Two patterns of obesity are observed: visceral (also known as abdominal, central, or android obesity—the "apple-shaped" pattern) and peripheral (also known as gluteofemoral or gynoid obesity—the "pear-shaped" pattern). Visceral obesity, associated with greater morbidity, is present when the individual's waist measurement divided by the hip measurement (waist:hip ratio) is greater than 1.0 in men or 0.8 in women.[16] The enzyme lipoprotein lipase, which regulates peripheral lipolysis and conversion of dietary lipids into triglycerides for adipose storage, is much more active in abdominal fat than in hip fat.

Obesity induces several endocrine abnormalities, including increased cortisol secretion, low secretion of sex steroid hormones and growth hormone, and cellular resistance to insulin.[20] These abnormalities are most severe in visceral obesity, but they also affect those with peripheral obesity to a greater degree than nonobese individuals. Sympathetic nervous system function is also impaired, indicating a general disturbance of the stress response system in obesity.

The phenomenon of **insulin resistance** is central to the major pathophysiologic effects of obesity. Obese persons often have normal or elevated blood sugar levels despite the presence of **hyperinsulinemia,** or excess insulin in the blood. Lipolysis in abdominal fat releases FFAs into the portal circulation. When these are deposited in the liver, they interfere with hepatic uptake of insulin. Normally, the liver removes up to 80% of the insulin secreted by the pancreas by the first-pass effect, but this is diminished in visceral obesity. As detailed in Chapter 29, insulin normally promotes the uptake of glucose from most tissues. This effect is blunted in obesity because enlarged adipocytes have decreased numbers of insulin receptors and a reduced response to insulin after receptor binding.[16]

Clinical Manifestations. Insulin resistance predisposes to the development of type 2 diabetes mellitus, which in turn promotes atherosclerosis (see Chapters 15 and 29). Hyperlipidemia in obese persons is associated with hyperinsulinemia, which promotes increased hepatic production of VLDLs. Furthermore, total body cholesterol is increased because of storage of cholesterol in adipose tissues. The LDL fraction is increased and HDL is decreased.[16] Hypertension is often, but not universally, present in obese individuals, and is associated with increased blood volume but normal peripheral vascular resistance (see Chapter 15). Hyperinsulinemia may contribute to hypertension by increasing sodium retention, stimulating the sympathetic nervous system, or stimulating the proliferation of vascular smooth muscle cells.[16]

Obesity is a risk factor for cardiac disease even if diabetes, hypertension, and hyperlipidemia are excluded. The workload of the left ventricle is increased, leading to left ventricular hypertrophy. In extremely obese individuals, respiratory failure may result from the increased ventilatory work imposed by thoracic body fat (see Chapter 18). This **pickwickian syndrome** may lead to secondary polycythemia and right-sided cardiac failure (cor pulmonale).

Hypersecretion of cholesterol in the bile may promote the formation of gallstones (see Chapter 26). Deregulation of the hypothalamic–pituitary axis manifests as altered cortisol, sex steroid, and growth hormone secretion, which may lead to erectile dysfunction in males and alterations in the menstrual cycle in females. The risk of estrogen-sensitive malignancies, including endometrial, breast, cervical, ovarian, gallbladder, colorectal, prostatic, pancreatic, and gastric cancers, is increased in obese individuals. Obesity is associated with increased complications of osteoarthritis because of stress on weight-bearing joints (see Chapter 34), increased obstetrical complications (see Chapter 32), and higher surgical risk.

Prevention and Treatment. Prevention of obesity involves measures to monitor and ensure energy balance. Periodic assessment of energy balance includes not only body weight but also body fat percentage and distribution. Maintenance of a dietary program consisting of low-fat, high-fiber foods and calorie-restricted but frequent meals is advisable for most individuals. Optimal physical activity should also be undertaken, because exercise prevents the adaptive decrease in resting metabolic rate that accompanies caloric restriction (see Chapter 3). Exercise also promotes the loss of fat rather than muscle in such cases and induces a more favorable serum lipid profile. Aerobic exercise is particularly beneficial (see Chapter 35). Behavioral modification, in which lifestyle habits promoting obesity are altered through education and reinforcement, is known to enhance the success of diet and exercise programs in the prevention and treatment of obesity.

Adjunctive treatments for high-risk obesity include anorectic (appetite-suppressant) drugs (Table 25–8) and surgery (Table 25–9). Short-term (less than 6 months) drug therapy has been shown to induce an additional weight loss of about 0.23 kg per week when combined with diet and exercise.[21] Weight tends to be regained when drug therapy is discontinued, however, and some agents have been associated with the development of significant toxic effects such as pulmonary hypertension (see Chapter 19). Long-term studies of pharmacologic agents in the treatment of obesity are ongoing. Surgical procedures ranging from jaw-wiring to intestinal bypass have resulted in weight loss; however, metabolic complications may be significant, and weight loss tends to plateau if diet, exercise, and behavioral interventions are not undertaken.[22]

Prognosis and Outcome. Excess weight brings excess morbidity and mortality. There is considerable evidence that maintenance of stable body weight at least 15% below the national average in the United States is associated with reduced mortality and increased longevity.[23,24] Permanent reversal of obesity with conventional treatment is achieved in fewer than 10% of patients after 10 years.[19] Weight loss has been shown to reduce blood pressure, cardiac risk, glucose control, and serum lipid profiles. The risk of cancer is also lowered.[16] The risk of death from all causes is 60% greater in those with a BMI of 27 to 29, 110% greater in those with a BMI of 29 to 32, and 120% greater in those with a BMI of 32 to 35, as compared with those having a BMI of less than 19.[15] There is no consistent evidence that weight cycling ("yo-yo dieting") increases risk.[25]

Gluten-Sensitive Enteropathy

Definition. Gluten-sensitive enteropathy is a disorder characterized by malabsorption, abnormal small bowel structure, and intolerance of *gluten* (α-gliadin and related proteins) found in wheat, barley, rye, malt, and possibly oats. The disorder under consideration here is also known as *nontropical sprue,* which is different from **tropical sprue,** a bacterial infection of the small bowel that affects persons living in or visiting certain tropical countries. Gluten-sensitive enteropathy in children is known as **celiac disease.**

Epidemiology. The prevalence of gluten-sensitive enteropathy has been estimated at 1 in 1000 in Europe, North Africa, and South America, but this is believed to be a conservative estimate because many others probably have minor disease or clinically si-

TABLE 25–8
PHARMACOLOGIC TREATMENT OF OBESITY

Drug	Mechanism of Action	Comments
Phenylpropanolamine HCl (Acutrim, Dexatrim)	Catecholamine-like; suppression of hypothalamic appetite centers	Nonprescription; low abuse potential; may increase heart rate and blood pressure
Diethylpropion HCl (Tepanil, Tenuate)	Catecholamine-like; mild CNS stimulant; suppression of hypothalamic appetite centers	Controlled substance; low abuse potential; mood-elevating; few adverse effects
Mazindol (Mazanor, Sanorex)	Catecholamine-like; CNS stimulant; suppression of hypothalamic appetite centers	Controlled substance; high abuse potential; mood-elevating; may increase heart rate
Phentermine (Adipex, Fastin, Ionamin, Zantryl)*	Catecholamine-like; CNS stimulant; suppression of hypothalamic appetite centers	Controlled substance; low abuse potential; increases heart rate and blood pressure; no effect on mood
Fenfluramine HCl (Pondimin)*	CNS depressant; stimulation of satiety centers	Controlled substance; may cause depression or sedation; may increase blood pressure; low abuse potential
Dexfenfluramine (Redux)	Increases serotonin release, stimulating satiety centers	Approved by the FDA in April 1996; may cause drowsiness, dry mouth, headache

CNS, central nervous system; FDA, Food and Drug Administration.

*Use of phentermine and fenfluramine in combination may impose high risk of pulmonary hypertension and cardiac valve disease. This "phen-fen" combination was not approved by the FDA; rather, the drugs were approved separately. Fenfluramine and dexfenfluramine were withdrawn from the market in September, 1997.

TABLE 25-9
PROCEDURAL AND SURGICAL TREATMENTS FOR OBESITY

Procedure	Description	Comments
Gastric bubble or balloon	Insertion and temporary inflation of a balloon in the stomach limits gastric capacity	Weight is regained after removal of the balloon
Waist cord or abdominal belt	Constrictive apparatus limits gastric capacity	Many patients do not tolerate the procedure, but it may be effective when combined with jaw wiring
Mandibular fixation (jaw wiring)	Jaw wiring limits ingestion of solids	Weight is often regained after wire removal
Intestinal bypass	Surgical bypass of a portion of the small intestine limits absorptive capacity	This procedure results in significant weight loss in morbidly obese individuals but is no longer recommended because of life-threatening metabolic complications
Gastroplasty	Vertical bands of staples limit gastric capacity	Weight loss tends to plateau at about 30% after 18 months; procedure is well tolerated

Data from Caterson, I.D. (1990). Management strategies for weight control: Eating, exercise and behavior. *Drugs* 39 (3 suppl.), 20–32.

lent disease that is undiagnosed. Curiously, the disorder is rarely diagnosed in the United States.[26] Gluten-sensitive enteropathy usually has its onset in childhood, but clinical manifestations may be so mild or vague that the diagnosis is not made until adulthood, or not made at all. Seventy percent of diagnosed patients are female, and a strong genetic influence is evident, involving both the HLA genes of the major histocompatibility complex (see Chapter 13) and non-HLA genes. Individuals with autoimmune disorders such as thyroid disease, Addison's disease, pernicious anemia, type 1 diabetes mellitus, and immunoglobulin A nephropathy are also at increased risk.

Etiology. The autoimmune etiology of the disorder is now well accepted. Immune attack against enterocytes of the small intestine occurs by humoral and cell-mediated mechanisms (see Chapter 13). Gluten serves as the antigenic protein in triggering this inappropriate and excessive response in genetically predisposed individuals.

Pathophysiology. The villi of the small intestine are damaged by this response, resulting in flattening of the mucosal surface and loss of surface area for absorption. Decreased secretion of CCK and secretin from these cells leads to a reduction in pancreatic secretion, which impairs chemical digestion and subsequent absorption of nutrients. Complications of this enteropathy include possible ulceration of the mucosa of the jejunum and ileum and neoplastic transformation of lymphatic cells. The relative risk of non-Hodgkin's lymphoma is greatly increased in patients with gluten-sensitive enteropathy (see Chapter 13).[26]

Clinical Manifestations. The patient has malnutrition and weight loss. Affected children typically have short stature, and adult patients are thin. Crampy abdominal pain, distention, diarrhea, and **steatorrhea** (fatty stools) are typical, with stools frequently having the consistency and color of oatmeal. In a variant form of celiac disease, patients may demonstrate a symmetric skin rash, *dermatitis herpetiformis,* as their major clinical manifestation, with relatively mild intestinal symptoms.[26]

Prevention and Treatment. In most patients, acute episodes may be prevented with strict, lifelong adherence to a gluten-free diet, which excludes wheat, rye, and barley products. Rice, soybean, and corn products are well tolerated as substitutes, and most patients may ingest moderate amounts of oats with no ill effects.[27] Corticosteroids may be used in the treatment of acute inflammatory episodes.

Prognosis and Outcome. Most patients respond to a gluten-free diet with greatly reduced frequency and severity of diarrhea episodes. In a recent study done in Scotland, overall mortality was reported to be 1.9 times that of the general population.[28] Mortality resulted from lymphoma of intestinal origin rather than from malabsorption.

Lactose Intolerance

Definition. Lactose intolerance is the impaired ability to absorb lactose, a carbohydrate found in dairy products, caused by lack of activity of the enzyme *lactase,* normally found in the brush border of the luminal surface of the small intestine. Many other carbohydrate intolerances are also encountered in clinical practice, resulting in similar clinical manifestations (Table 25–10).

Epidemiology. An estimated 25% of adults in the United States and 75% of the population worldwide have some degree of lactose intolerance.[29] Risk of the disorder is highest after childhood, among individuals of racial origins other than northern European, and in some African tribes.[30] Lactase activity reaches its maximum point during the perinatal period, then, in most races, it declines to about 10% of this level by age 5 to 7. Lactase activity persists into adulthood among races in which dairy products constitute a significant portion of the diet.

TABLE 25–10
DISORDERS LEADING TO CARBOHYDRATE MALABSORPTION

Mechanism	Examples of Disorders
Primary Carbohydrate Malabsorption Syndromes	
Genetic defect of the Na^+/glucose cotransporter in the brush border (SGLT1) on chromosome 22	Glucose-galactose malabsorption
Genetic defect of the carrier protein (GLUT5) for fructose absorption by facilitated diffusion	Fructose malabsorption (irritable colon of childhood or toddler's diarrhea)
Primary deficiency of a brush border disaccharidase enzyme, impairing digestion of monosaccharides	Lactose intolerance (lactase deficiency) Sucrose intolerance (sucrase-isomaltase deficiency) Trehalose intolerance (trehalase deficiency)
Primary deficiency of amylase enzyme in secretions	Intolerance of dietary starch
Primary deficiency of glucoamylase in the brush border	Intolerance of dietary starch
Secondary Carbohydrate Malabsorption Syndromes	
Lack of absorptive surface area	Gastrointestinal surgery Inflammatory bowel disease
Transient injury to intestinal epithelium	Infective gastroenteritis Necrotizing enterocolitis Acquired immunodeficiency syndrome Immune-mediated enteropathy (e.g., sensitivity to gluten, cow's milk protein, soy protein) Laxative abuse Cytotoxic drugs Radiation enteritis

Data from Ushijima, K., Riby, J.E., and Kretchmer, N. (1995). Carbohydrate malabsorption. *Pediatric Clinics of North America* 42(4), 899–915.

Etiology. The gene for lactase is on chromosome 2. Rarely, lactose intolerance is inherited as an autosomal recessive defect. With this *congenital lactase deficiency,* clinical manifestations are apparent immediately after birth. *Secondary lactose malabsorption* can occur at any age and is caused by an insult to the GI tract, such as GI surgery, inflammatory bowel disease, gastroenteritis, or necrotizing enterocolitis (see Chapter 24). Most lactose intolerance is associated with the natural absence or decline of lactase activity coupled with high dietary intake of dairy products.

Pathophysiology. The mechanism is similar in all forms of carbohydrate malabsorption. Malabsorption results in lack of the carbohydrate in the bloodstream as well as its accumulation in the lumen of the bowel. When unabsorbed carbohydrate reaches the large intestine, it exerts osmotic pressure, pulling water into the bowel. Bacteria act on the carbohydrate, producing acids as fermentation products. Hydrogen and methane gases are produced as byproducts.

Clinical Manifestations. The primary signs and symptoms are similar for all forms of carbohydrate malabsorption. Gas in the bowel contributes to bloating, hyperactive bowel sounds, **flatulence,** and crampy abdominal pain. Absorbed gases may be detected in the breath. Watery diarrhea results from osmotic factors as well as the irritation of acids. Secondary manifestations associated with diarrhea may include dehydration, electrolyte imbalance, metabolic acidosis, failure to thrive in infancy, anorexia, vomiting, edema, and irritability (see Chapter 24).[30]

Prevention and Treatment. Exclusion of dairy products from the diet prevents manifestations of lactose intolerance in most people. Recent research has shown that most individuals with lactose intolerance can ingest up to 8 ounces of milk per day with little or no distress.[29] Soy-based or casein-based formulas should be substituted for milk-based products in infants with congenital lactase deficiency. Many lactose-free dairy products are now available. Lactaid, a fungal lactase, may also be used to increase lactose absorption.

Prognosis and Outcome. The disorder is successfully managed in most cases, causing little inconvenience or distress and no long-term effects.

Hyperlipidemia

Definition. Hyperlipidemia is the elevation of serum lipids, specifically cholesterol and triglycerides. A related term is **hyperlipoproteinemia,** elevation of any class of lipoprotein, either singly, or more usu-

TABLE 25–11
CLASSIFICATION OF THE HYPERLIPIDEMIAS

DISORDER	PREVALENCE	LIPID PROFILE	COMMENTS
Familial hypercholesterolemia	1 in 500 are heterozygous 1 in 1 million are homozygous Polygenic in 1% of those with coronary artery disease	Increased LDL (type IIA pattern): >190 mg/dL in polygenic; >250 mg/dL in heterozygous; >600 mg/dL in homozygous	Defective LDL receptors result in decreased LDL clearance; xanthomata are seen, except in the polygenic form
Familial combined hyperlipidemia	14% of survivors of myocardial infarction	Increased LDL and VLDL (type IIB pattern); triglycerides 1 to 3 times higher than cholesterol	Diabetes is often present in this type; HDL may or may not be reduced
Dysbetalipoproteinemia	0.5% of patients with premature coronary heart disease	Increased chylomicron remnants and VLDL remnants (IDLs; type III pattern)	Lipoproteins are abnormally rich in cholesterol and thus are atherogenic
Familial hypertriglyceridemia	5% of survivors of myocardial infarction	Increased VLDLs (type IV pattern) or increased VLDLs and chylomicrons (type V pattern) or increased chylomicrons	Triglyceride levels higher than 1000 are associated with increased risk of pancreatitis, splenomegaly, and hepatomegaly; HDL is often reduced also; this type is common in obesity and in lipoprotein lipase deficiency
Familial hypoalphalipoproteinemia	4% of patients with premature coronary heart disease	Decreased HDL (<10 mg/dL)	Either synthesis or catabolism of HDL may be abnormal; genetic apo A-1 deficiency is rare
Familial Lp(a) excess	15% of patients with premature coronary heart disease	Increased Lp(a) (>40 mg/dL)	Lp(a) is LDL with one molecule of apo(a) attached; patients do not have xanthomata

LDL, low-density lipoprotein; IDL, intermediate-density lipoprotein; VLDL, very-low-density lipoprotein; HDL, high-density lipoprotein; apo, apolipoprotein; Lp(a), lipoprotein(a).

Data from Schaefer, E.J. (1994). Familial lipoprotein disorders and premature coronary artery disease. *Medical Clinics of North America* 78(1), 21–39; and Larsen, M.L., and Illingworth, D.R. (1994). Drug treatment of dyslipoproteinemia. *Medical Clinics of North America* 78(1), 225–245.

ally, in combination. Table 25–11 illustrates the classification of hyperlipoproteinemias based on the pattern of elevation of certain lipoprotein classes. The term **dyslipidemia** is the most inclusive in describing lipid abnormalities, because it also incorporates reduction of HDL.

Epidemiology. Prevalence of the more common hyperlipoproteinemias is included in Table 25–11. Studies of middle-aged men with premature coronary heart disease have demonstrated that an estimated 26% have LDL cholesterol levels greater than 160 mg/dL and 63% have HDL cholesterol below 35 mg/dL.[31] Some hyperlipidemias are known to be genetic disorders, with an autosomal dominant mode of inheritance. A familial predisposition is evident in all forms. Most hyperlipidemias are considered to be multifactorial, however, with risk also originating from (1) dietary intake of fat and cholesterol; (2) visceral obesity; (3) systemic diseases, including pancreatitis, type 2 diabetes mellitus, and chronic renal failure (Table 25–12) and use of certain drugs (Table 25–13). Familial and diet-induced hyperlipidemias are classified as *primary hyperlipidemias* and those caused by other systemic disease or to drugs are classified as *secondary hyperlipidemias.* Lifestyle factors other than diet are important risk factors as well, primarily because of their effects on HDL cholesterol. Tobacco abuse reduces HDL cholesterol, whereas exercise and moderate use of alcohol increase HDL cholesterol.

Etiology. Five mechanisms contribute to development of hyperlipidemia: (1) dietary intake of lipoprotein precursors; (2) genetic defects in LDL receptor structure or function; (3) defective hepatic

TABLE 25–12
SECONDARY CAUSES OF HYPERLIPIDEMIA

Condition	Predominant Lipid Abnormality	Change in High Density Lipoprotein
Acromegaly	Hypertriglyceridemia	
Acute intermittent porphyria	Hypercholesterolemia	Normal HDL
Alcohol excess	Hypertriglyceridemia	Elevated HDL
Amiodarone	Hypercholesterolemia	
Anabolic steroids	Hypercholesterolemia	Low HDL
Anorexia nervosa	Hypercholesterolemia	
Alpha blockers		Increased HDL
Antiepileptics		Increased HDL
Beta blockers	Hypertriglyceridemia	Low HDL
Burns	Hypertriglyceridemia	
Chlorinated hydrocarbon insecticides	Hypercholesterolemia	Increased HDL
Cholestasis (e.g., primary biliary cirrhosis)	Hypercholesterolemia (Lp-X)	
Chronic renal failure	Hypertriglyceridemia	Low HDL
Cyclosporine therapy	Hypercholesterolemia	
Diabetes	Hypertriglyceridemia	Low HDL in NIDDM
Estrogen therapy	Hypertriglyceridemia	Increased HDL
Glucocorticoids	Hypertriglyceridemia	Increased HDL
Glycogen storage diseases	Hypertriglyceridemia	
Growth hormone deficiency	Hypercholesterolemia	
Hyperandrogenism in women	Hypertriglyceridemia	Low HDL
Hypothyroidism	Hypercholesterolemia	
Isotretinoin	Hypertriglyceridemia	Low HDL
Lipodystrophy	Hypertriglyceridemia	
Myelomatosis (IgA, IgG)	Hypercholesterolemia	
Nephrotic syndrome	Hypercholesterolemia	Low HDL
Progestins	Hypercholesterolemia	Low HDL
Systemic lupus and polyclonal gammopathy	Hypertriglyceridemia	
Syndrome X	Hypertriglyceridemia	Low HDL
Thiazide diuretics	Hypercholesterolemia/hypertriglyceridemia	Low HDL
Weight gain	Hypertriglyceridemia	Low HDL

HDL, High-density lipoprotein; NIDDM, noninsulin-dependent diabetes mellitus; Lp-X, special lipoprotein seen in obstructive liver disease.

From Stone, N.J. (1994). Secondary causes of hyperlipidemia. *Medical Clinics of North America* 78(1), 119. Used with permission.

metabolism of lipids; (4) deficiency or defect of apoproteins; and (5) hormonal influences.

Individuals who ingest large quantities of saturated fats, *trans* polyunsaturated fats, and cholesterol tend to have elevated levels of LDL. Butter and other dairy fats high in the fatty acid myristic acid strongly increase LDL levels.[32] Beef fat (containing palmitic and stearic acids) increases LDL to a lesser degree, and cocoa butter (containing stearic acid) slightly increases LDL. Omega-3 polyunsaturated fatty acids, found primarily in fish oils, decrease triglyceride levels but increase LDL cholesterol. *Trans* polyunsaturated fats, formed by partial hydrogenation of liquid vegetable oils in shortening and margarine, increase LDL and *lipoprotein (a)* and reduce HDL. Lipoprotein (a) is a recently discovered, highly atherogenic particle similar in structure to LDL but also containing a unique glycoprotein, apo (a).[33] *Cis* polyunsaturated fats decrease serum cholesterol, and monounsaturated fats such as those in olive and canola oil do not influence serum cholesterol. Increased carbohydrate intake promotes increased VLDL synthesis by the liver.

In **familial hypercholesterolemia,** associated with the highest risk of atherosclerosis, an autosomal dominant, single-gene defect results in dysfunction of LDL receptors and decreased cellular uptake of LDL. **Primary hypoalphalipoproteinemia** is a genetic disorder manifested by a deficiency of apoprotein A-1, necessary for the synthesis of HDL. Other primary hyperlipidemias are multifactorial, having genetic and environmental components.

The link between secondary hyperlipidemias and atherosclerosis risk is less certain. Type 2 diabetes mellitus is usually associated with increased VLDLs; however, concurrent decreases in HDL and increases in LDL are also seen. These individuals are often obese as well, and glycosylation of apoproteins may be a factor in producing the lipid abnormalities. Elevation of LDL is common in individuals with end-

TABLE 25–13
DRUGS AFFECTING THE LIPID PROFILE

Drug	Effect on Serum Lipids	Comments
Corticosteroids Prednisone Cortisone	↑ VLDL, ↑ HDL	Effects result from increased insulin resistance; patients with diabetes or uremia are at highest risk because of impaired triglyceride uptake
Anabolic Steroids Stanozolol (Winstrol) Oxymetholone (Anadrol) Injectable testosterone	↓ HDL, ↑ VLDL ↑ LDL with stanozolol	Effects are seen within 1 to 2 weeks of drug use; HDL catabolism is increased
Female Hormones Oral contraceptives Hormone replacement therapy	Estrogens increase LDL, HDL, and triglycerides; Progesterone has opposing effects	Effects vary depending on the combination of hormones, whether they are natural or synthetic, and whether they are administered orally or transdermally
Diuretics Thiazides	↑ LDL, total cholesterol, and triglycerides	Thiazides blunt the efficacy of a low-fat diet
Alpha Blockers Prazosin (Minipress)	↑ HDL, no effect on LDL	These agents may decrease the clearance of HDL; hypertensives with visceral obesity may benefit from these agents
Beta Blockers Propranolol (Inderal) Atenolol (Tenormin) Timolol (Blocadren)	↑ triglycerides, ↓ HDL	Effects may be reduced with diet, exercise, and concurrent use of lipid-lowering drugs
Retinoids Isotretinoin (Accutane)	↑ triglycerides, ↑ VLDL, ↓ HDL	Lipid changes are reversed with cessation of this anti-acne agent
Cyclosporine	↑ LDL, Lp(a), and triglycerides	This immunosuppressive agent may cause myositis if used with HMG-CoA reductase inhibitors (lipid-lowering drugs)
H_2 Blockers Cimetidine (Tagamet) Ranitidine (Zantac)	↑ HDL in women	Cimetidine has greater effect than ranitidine
Antiepileptics Phenobarbital Phenytoin (Dilantin) Carbamazepine (Tegretol)	↑ HDL	Effects are greater in women
Tamoxifen (Tamofen)	↑ HDL, ↓ LDL	This agent, used in treatment of breast cancer, is not indicated for use as a lipid-lowering agent
Amiodarone (Cordarone)	↑ cholesterol	Effects of this antiarrhythmic are independent of its effect on thyroid hormone

VLDL, very-low-density lipoprotein; HDL, high-density lipoprotein; LDL, low-density lipoprotein; HMG-CoA, 3-hydroxy-3-methylglutaryl–coenzyme A.

Data from Stone, N.J. (1994). Secondary causes of hyperlipidemia. *Medical Clinics of North America* 78(1), 121–127.

stage renal disease, possibly because of alteration of apoprotein synthesis. Patients with hypothyroidism often have increased LDL levels, which may be caused by decreased cellular uptake of LDL or associated with the obesity that often accompanies this disorder (see Chapter 28).

Because the liver is the primary site of nutrient biotransformation, including the synthesis of lipoproteins, hepatic disease often manifests as dyslipidemia (see Chapter 26). Hormones, whether natural or synthetic, have been shown to influence serum lipid levels. Natural estrogens, which are synthesized from cholesterol, promote increased HDL levels in premenopausal women. Progesterone, in contrast, tends to increase LDL and decrease HDL. Synthetic estrogens found in some oral contraceptives tend to increase VLDL. The protective effect of hormone replacement therapy in postmenopausal women depends on the specific agents used and the length of therapy (see Chapter 31). Prolonged steroid therapy and abuse of anabolic steroids are associated with decreased HDL levels and increased risk of atherosclerosis (see Chapter 29).

Pathophysiology. Increased LDL levels and decreased HDL levels are associated with accelerated development of atherosclerosis, which manifests as coronary heart disease, cerebrovascular disease, peripheral vascular disease, and hypertension (see Chapters 15, 16, and 21). Individuals with elevated lipoprotein(a) levels and with LDL subsets in which LDL particles are smaller are at particular risk. Increased VLDL levels are associated with smaller LDL particle size and may contribute to atherosclerosis. Increased VLDL levels are also known to be associated with the development of pancreatitis (discussed in next section).

Clinical Manifestations. Xanthomata may be evident because of precipitation of cholesterol in the skin, tendons, or other tissues (Color Fig. 25–3). The serum lipid profile demonstrates the particular lipid disorder. Ideally, blood is drawn after a 12-hour period of fasting. Total cholesterol (TC), HDL, and triglycerides are measured directly. VLDL is estimated by dividing the triglyceride value by 5 (if triglycerides are less than 400 mg/dL). VLDL cannot be calculated from a nonfasting sample, because triglycerides are then carried by chylomicrons as well as VLDLs.[33] LDL is calculated by the formula:

$$LDL = TC - (HDL + VLDL)$$

The atherosclerotic risk associated with the lipid profile depends less on specific values of the components than on the *ratio* of total cholesterol to HDL cholesterol. For adults, the TC:HDL ratio should be less than 3.0, and for children this ratio should be less than 3.5.[34] Levels of specific apolipoproteins are not routinely screened, but they may be measured in individuals with early atherosclerotic disease in whom the lipid profile is normal. Lipoprotein(a) has recently been shown to be an independent risk factor for coronary heart disease when elevated.[35] Measurement of this particle may also be warranted in some cases.

Prevention and Treatment. Primary prevention of hyperlipidemias depends on minimizing nongenetic risk factors. This involves a diet limited in saturated fat and cholesterol (Table 25–14) and an active lifestyle that includes aerobic exercise. Consideration should be given to hormone replacement therapy for postmenopausal women, especially if they have other risk factors for atherosclerosis. Drug treatment of dyslipidemias depends on the particular class or classes of lipoproteins that are abnormal (Table 25–15). In rare instances of homozygous familial hyperlipoproteinemia, plasmapheresis at regular intervals may be used to directly remove lipid from the blood.

Prognosis and Outcome. Except in individuals over the age of 70, lowering of LDL cholesterol and raising of HDL cholesterol by dietary, pharmacologic, or other means has been shown to decrease the risk of adverse events caused by coronary heart disease.[36] Atherosclerotic plaque has been shown to regress with improvement in the lipid profile. In the Multiple Risk Factor Intervention Trial (MRFIT), mortality from all causes in men was lowest among those whose total cholesterol was 120 to 140 mg/dL.[37]

Pancreatitis

Definition. Pancreatitis is acute or chronic inflammation of the pancreas.

Epidemiology. The annual incidence of acute pancreatitis is about 100,000 in the United States, and the incidence has been steadily increasing during the past three decades. The prevalence of pancreatitis among patients with acquired immunodeficiency

TABLE 25–14
DIETARY TREATMENT OF HYPERLIPIDEMIA

NUTRIENT	AVERAGE AMERICAN DIET	STEP ONE	STEP TWO
Total fat	35% to 40%	<30%	<30%
Saturated fat	13% of calories	<10%	<7%
Cholesterol	380 mg/day	<300 mg	<200 mg

Adherence to a Step One diet reduces serum cholesterol by an average of 3% to 4% within 3 months. More significant reduction may occur with the Step Two diet. Because of their greater lipid requirements for growth, children should not be restricted beyond the Step One recommendations.

From the National Cholesterol Education Program, National Institutes of Health. Adapted with permission from Baker, A.L., Roberts, C., and Gothing, C. (1995). Dyslipidemias in childhood. *Nursing Clinics of North America* 30(2), 243–259.

TABLE 25–15
DRUG THERAPY OF HYPERLIPIDEMIA

Drug Category/Examples	Mechanism of Action	Indications
Bile acid sequestrants Cholestyramine (Questran) Colestipol (Colestid)	Bile acids are bound in the gut lumen, preventing their absorption; depletion of the bile acid pool stimulates hepatic uptake and use of LDL	LDL reduction
Nicotinic acid (niacin)	Reduced lipolysis in adipose tissue and inhibition of hepatic synthesis of apolipoprotein B and lipoprotein(a) are possible mechanisms	LDL reduction
HMG-CoA reductase inhibitors Lovastatin (Mevacor) Simvastatin (Zocor) Pravastatin (Pravachol)	Blockade of the enzyme HMG-CoA reductase interferes with hepatic cholesterol synthesis	Reduction in LDL and VLDL
Fibrates Clofibrate (Atromid-S) Gemfibrozil (Lopid)	Mechanisms may include activation of lipoprotein lipase, suppression of free fatty acid release from adipose tissue, inhibition of hepatic triglyceride synthesis, and increased secretion of cholesterol into the bile	LDL and VLDL reduction, and elevation of HDL
Probucol (Lorelco)	Increased nonreceptor-mediated catabolism of LDL may occur, and the drug may reduce the oxidation of LDL	LDL reduction (but lowers HDL also)

VLDL, very-low-density lipoprotein; HDL, high-density lipoprotein; LDL, low-density lipoprotein; HMG-CoA, 3-hydroxy-3-methylglutaryl–coenzyme A.

Data from Larsen, M.L., and Illingworth, D.R. (1994). Drug treatment of dyslipoproteinemia. *Medical Clinics of North America* 78(1), 225–245.

syndrome is 4 to 22 per 100.[38] Pancreatitis rarely occurs in children, but the most common cause in this group is pancreatic trauma associated with child abuse. Known risk factors for pancreatitis in adults include obesity, gallbladder disease, alcohol abuse, elevated levels of VLDL, exposure to toxins (including some drugs), and immunosuppression. A rare hereditary form of chronic pancreatitis is also seen.

Etiology. Four major etiologic theories have been proposed: (1) obstruction of pancreatic ducts; (2) reflux of bile into pancreatic ducts; (3) reflux of duodenal contents into pancreatic ducts; and (4) inappropriate activation of proteolytic enzymes within pancreatic acinar cells. None of these theories is fully supported by research data.[39]

In patients with gallstones, obstruction of the ampulla of Vater by a stone may prevent outflow of pancreatic juice from the gland or may permit reflux of bile into the pancreatic ducts (Figure 25–11). Ductal obstruction caused by pancreatic tumors or benign strictures is rarely found in pancreatitis. In less than 20% of the population, a common channel distal to the pancreatic and common bile ducts permits reflux of bile into the pancreatic ducts. Bile does not trigger activation of proteolytic enzymes, however. Duodenal obstruction could permit activated enzymes to reenter the pancreas, leading to proteolytic damage of glandular tissue. Activation of proteolytic enzymes within the pancreas is believed to be an etiologic mechanism in many cases; however, the mechanism by which this occurs is unknown. A significant number of cases of pancreatitis are classified as idiopathic. Table 25–16 lists specific conditions associated with the development of acute or chronic pancreatitis.

Pathophysiology. An autodigestive process leads to destruction of pancreatic exocrine and endocrine tissue to varying degrees. Pancreatic enzyme precursors become activated within the gland, leading to inflammation with possible necrosis and cyst formation. Small amounts of activated trypsin may be inactivated by trypsin inhibitor, but large amounts of activated enzyme apparently overwhelm this protective mechanism. Pancreatic enzymes may digest blood vessels within the gland, leading to hemorrhage. Release of trypsin activates the complement and kinin cascades, leading to possible disseminated intravascular coagulation and shock; and phospholipase A_2 activation is believed to degrade lung surfactant, leading to atelectasis and possible respiratory failure. Lipase release leads to fatty necrosis and predisposes to secondary infection of the pancreas by bacteria that may be translocated from the gut during shock. Superimposed viral, bacterial, or fungal infection may contribute to the pathogenesis of acute pancreatitis, especially in immunosuppressed persons.[38]

Hypersecretion of protein is a factor in the pathogenesis of chronic pancreatitis.[40] This protein precipitates in ducts, forming plugs that may promote re-

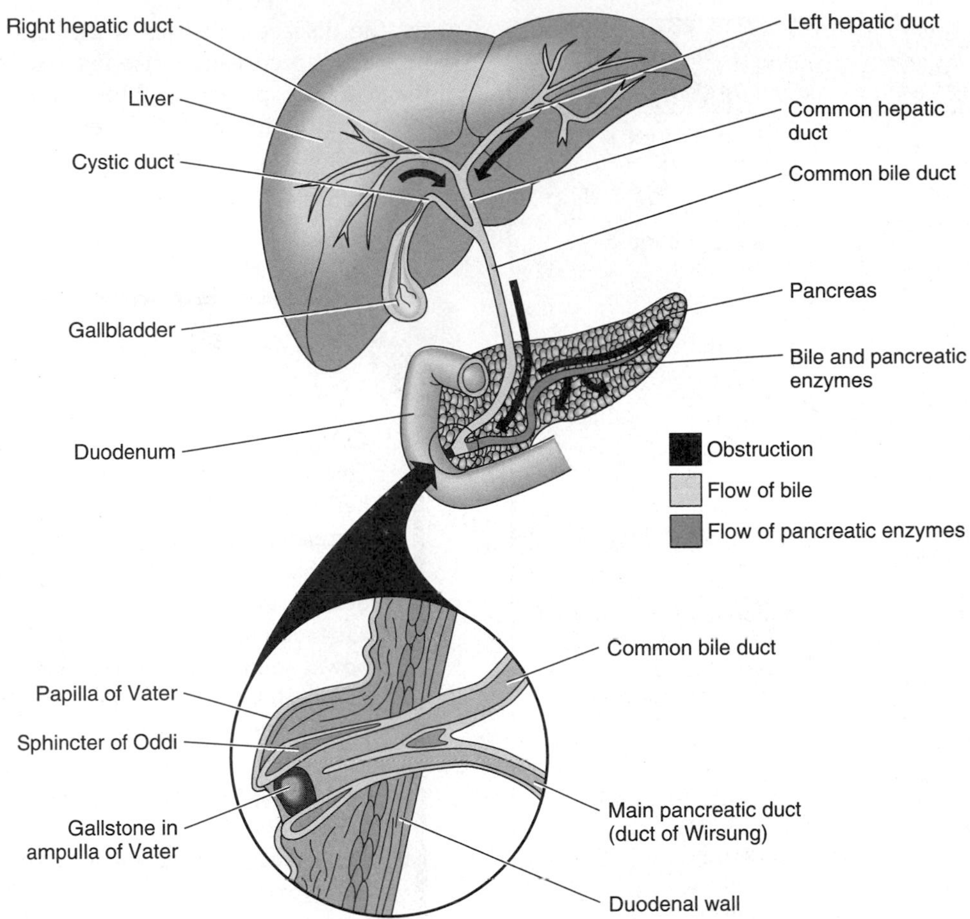

FIGURE 25–11
Pancreatic duct obstruction. Obstruction of the ampulla of Vater by a gallstone may obstruct outflow of pancreatic juices from the gland or may permit reflux of bile into the pancreatic ducts.

current episodes of acute inflammation. Fibrosis and destruction of pancreatic exocrine and endocrine tissue is progressive in such cases. Toxic effects of alcohol or other drugs may promote the formation of plugs, but because pancreatitis develops in only 5% of individuals who abuse alcohol, other factors must also be involved.[38] **Pseudocysts,** collections of pancreatic enzymes contained within fibrous walls of granulation tissue, develop in approximately 10% of patients with chronic pancreatitis.[40]

Clinical Manifestations. Although it is sometimes clinically silent, pancreatitis usually causes continuous epigastric pain that is described by many patients as excruciating. Pain is worse when the patient is in a supine position. Manifestations of shock, disseminated intravascular coagulation, peritonitis, and respiratory failure may be present. Serum levels of amylase and other enzymes are elevated. Ductal obstruction may be demonstrated with endosocopic retrograde cholangiopancreatography (ERCP). Hyperglycemia may be present if the endocrine portion of the pancreas is affected (see Chapter 29). Manifestations of malabsorption (e.g., diarrhea, steatorrhea) and weight loss are evident when less than 10% of exocrine function remains in those with chronic pancreatitis.

Prevention and Treatment. Prevention involves abstinence from alcohol and other toxic agents. Gallbladder disease is treated as discussed in Chapter 26. Treatment of acute episodes is primarily supportive, including elimination of oral intake, replacement of fluids and electrolytes, adequate analgesia for relief of pain, and nasogastric suction if distention is present. Removal of factors such as alcohol or drugs that might have precipitated the attack is also warranted. "Bowel rest" programs using drugs that inhibit pancreatic secretion or enzyme activation have not been proven beneficial in most cases.[40] Early treatment of alcohol-induced pancreatitis with antibiotic therapy (cefuroxime) has recently been shown to improve outcomes.[41] The cardiovascular, respiratory, and renal systems are supported as necessary. Surgical removal of necrotic tissue may be indicated in some cases.

Prognosis and Outcome. Approximately 25% of attacks of acute pancreatitis are severe, leading to

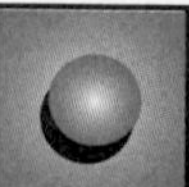

TABLE 25–16
CONDITIONS ASSOCIATED WITH THE DEVELOPMENT OF PANCREATITIS

In Adults	In Children
Acute Pancreatitis	
Obstruction	Obstruction
Gallstones	Congenital anomaly
Pancreatic cancer	Gallstones
Hypertensive sphincter of Oddi	Pseudocyst
Toxins and drugs	Toxins and drugs
Ethyl alcohol	Drug hypersensitivity
Drug hypersensitivity	Drug toxicity
Drug toxicity	
Trauma	Trauma
Blunt abdominal trauma	Abdominal trauma with abuse
Iatrogenic injury with ERCP or cardiopulmonary bypass	Iatrogenic injury
Metabolic abnormalities	Metabolic abnormalities
Hypertriglyceridemia	Hypertriglyceridemia
Hypercalcemia	Hypercalcemia
	Hemochromatosis
	Uremia
	Anorexia nervosa
Infections	Infections
Hepatitis	Childhood viral infections
Cytomegalovirus	Enterovirus
	Epstein-Barr virus
	Hepatitis
	Hereditary diseases
	Cystic fibrosis
	Familial pancreatitis
	$Alpha_1$-antitrypsin deficiency
	Systemic disorders
	Diabetes mellitus
	Henoch-Schönlein purpura
	Systemic lupus erythematosus
	Reye's syndrome
	Kawasaki disease
Chronic Pancreatitis	
Alcohol abuse	Cystic fibrosis
Obstruction	Hereditary pancreatitis
Idiopathic	

ERCP, endoscopic retrograde cholangiopancreatography.

Data from Steinberg, W., and Tenner, S. (1994). Acute pancreatitis. *New England Journal of Medicine* 330(17), 1198–1210; Steer, M.L., Waxman, I., and Freedman, S. (1995). Chronic pancreatitis. *New England Journal of Medicine* 332(22), 1482–1490; and Lerner, A.L., Branski, D., and Lebenthal, E. (1996). Pancreatic diseases in children. *Pediatric Clinics of North America* 43(1), 125–156.

complications. These episodes result in 9% mortality. The mortality rate in children is 20% to 25%.[38] In 85% to 90% of uncomplicated cases of acute pancreatitis, the disease subsides within a week. In chronic pancreatitis, recurrent episodes result in permanent damage to the pancreas. Most of these patients become diabetic and will also require lifelong replacement of pancreatic enzymes to prevent malabsorption.

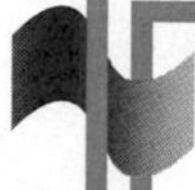

Clinical Scenario

O.N., a 71-year-old woman, is brought to the Emergency Department in the early morning by her worried husband, who says his wife has been "screaming in pain" for the past 2 hours. The pain had started before eating dinner the evening before and had progressively worsened. O.N. has abdominal distention on examination, but bowel sounds are audible. She indicates the right upper abdominal quadrant as the source of her pain, which is "like being stabbed." O.N.'s medical history includes type 2 diabetes, gastroesophageal reflux disease, peptic ulcer disease, gallbladder disease, hypothyroidism, and hypertension. She takes a diuretic (hydrochlorothiazide) for her hypertension. O.N. denies abusing alcohol or tobacco. She is 5 feet, 2 inches tall and weighs 145 lb. Computed tomography of the abdomen suggests the presence of pancreatitis, which is confirmed by a serum amylase level of 1182 U/L (normal range, 30 to 220).

1. What etiologic factors are apparent that may have contributed to the onset of O.N.'s disease?
2. How does the pain of pancreatitis differ from that which might result from other disorders in O.N.'s history?

Pancreatic Cancer

Definition. Nearly all pancreatic cancers are carcinomas arising in the ductal epithelial cells of the exocrine pancreas. Carcinomas of the acinar cells of the exocrine pancreas and of the islet cells of the endocrine pancreas are rare.[41] Islet cell tumors are discussed in Chapter 29 with disorders of the endocrine pancreas.

Epidemiology. Pancreatic cancer accounts for 5% of all cancer deaths in the United States, with 26,000 deaths each year. Each year, 28,000 new cases are diagnosed.[42] Most patients are older than age 50 years, and blacks are more often affected than whites. Individuals with diabetes mellitus and those with hereditary chronic pancreatitis are also at higher risk. Smokers and those whose diets are high in fats and meats are at higher risk, and those who undergo partial gastrectomy are at higher long-term risk.

Etiology. The precise etiology of pancreatic cancer is unknown. General mechanisms and theories of carcinogenesis are discussed in Chapter 7.

Pathophysiology. The course of the disease depends on the location of the tumor. The head of the pancreas is involved in 60% of cases, and such lesions often obstruct the ampulla of Vater, common bile duct, and duodenum. These tumors are often diagnosed earlier because manifestations of bowel obstruction and biliary tract obstruction are apparent. Tumors of the body or tail of the pancreas usually grow silently, and these cancers may not be diagnosed until the tumor has invaded adjacent structures and metastasized widely.

Clinical Manifestations. **Jaundice** is present in 90% of patients with carcinoma of the head of the pancreas and may be seen in other forms as well. About 10% of patients are prone to recurrent thrombophlebitis (**Trousseau's syndrome**) because of tumor cytokines that act as platelet-aggregating factors.[42] Duodenal obstruction may result in nausea and vomiting. Other manifestations are typical of many cancers and include weight loss, pain (abdominal or back pain), anorexia, and malaise. Once symptoms become apparent, they usually become rapidly worse.

Prevention and Treatment. Reduction of risk factors such as smoking is warranted. The treatment of choice is surgical resection, which may be curative in localized lesions. The Whipple procedure, in which the pancreas, duodenum, and antrum of the stomach are removed, is a common approach. In other cases, pancreatectomy may be done palliatively, and obstruction of the bowel or biliary tract may be surgically relieved. Radiation and chemotherapy are not curative, but they may be used in an effort to slow the progression of the disease. Other treatment is symptomatic and supportive, with control of pain being a major objective. Replacement of fluids, electrolytes, and pancreatic enzymes and hormones is required for treatment of the malabsorption that results from pancreatic dysfunction or removal.

Prognosis and Outcome. Fewer than 15% of pancreatic tumors are resectable when diagnosed. One-year survival is less than 20%, and 5-year survival is 3%.[42]

CLINICAL SIGNIFICANCE OF DISORDERS OF NUTRIENT ABSORPTION

The significance of the disorders discussed in this chapter is evident from their commonality among individuals of all ages. Nutrients and oxygen are the essential elements that fuel the human system. Although their lack is incompatible with life itself, excessive intake of nutrients may also contribute to significant disorders. Hyperlipidemias, discussed in this chapter, may contribute to development of atherosclerosis. Excess intake of carbohydrates, proteins, and fats promotes obesity and insulin resistance, which in turn are associated with life-threatening cardiovascular and endocrine disorders. Research is ongoing in an effort to clarify basic mechanisms by which nutrient absorption and transport occur, to identify risk factors contributing to nutritional disorders, and to develop rational strategies for prevention and treatment.

The roles of the liver and biliary system in GI function have been described superficially in Chapters 24 and 25. These functions are described in more detail in Chapter 26. The extensive metabolic processes through which hepatic function and dysfunction affect other systems will also be detailed.

Summary of Key Points

- Regulation of food intake is complex, involving psychosocial and cultural factors as well as physiologic mechanisms. Processes by which hunger and satiety are mediated are incompletely understood, but are known to involve hypothalamic and other brain centers and peripheral chemoreceptors that respond to a number of neurotransmitters and hormones. Receptors also sense gastric pressure and serum levels of absorbed nutrients. Structures of the oropharynx function in formation of ingested food into a bolus and in passage of this bolus into the esophagus while preventing aspiration into the trachea.
- Digestion includes mechanical and biochemical processes that break down ingested food into particles small enough to be absorbed. Catabolism of ingested nutrients occurs via hydrolysis reactions that split nutrients into their constituent molecules (usually monosaccharides, amino acids, and triglycerides).

Summary continued on next page

These reactions are catalyzed by intestinal surface enzymes (disaccharidases, proteolytic enzymes and peptidases, and pancreatic lipases).

- The luminal surface of the small intestine provides an ideal anatomic arrangement for absorption of nutrients. Numerous finger-like projections (villi) increase the available surface area, and each villus is perfused by vascular and lymphatic capillaries that receive absorbed nutrients. The countercurrent flow of arterial and venous blood within the villus maintains gradients for nutrient absorption. An unstirred layer of fluid lines the intestinal wall and functions in modulation of absorption rates.
- Water is absorbed from the entire intestinal surface, along the osmotic gradients created by particle absorption. Electrolytes are actively absorbed, in conjunction with sodium transport in most cases, and may also be actively secreted into the gut lumen. Most carbohydrates (except fructose) and proteins are absorbed by active cotransport with sodium. Fructose absorption occurs by facilitated diffusion. Lipid absorption and transport is complex, occurring along exogenous and endogenous pathways. In the exogenous pathway, dietary lipids (primarily triglycerides) are first packaged into micelles for transport to the gut wall, then enter intestinal epithelial cells by dissolving in membrane lipids. These lipids are then incorporated into chylomicrons, which enter the lymphatics. The endogenous pathway begins in the liver, which synthesizes VLDLs from dietary carbohydrate and cholesterol. VLDLs are released into the blood. In peripheral capillaries, the enzyme lipoprotein lipase releases FFAs and glycerol from the triglycerides in circulating lipoproteins, leaving progressively smaller, cholesterol-rich particles that may be atherogenic.
- Malabsorption may result from defective intraluminal processing of nutrients, impairment of transport across the intestinal surface, lymphatic obstruction, or decreased transit time within the lumen of the gut.
- Clinical disorders that impair ingestion, digestion, or absorption result in malnutrition with impairment of energy balance. Energy imbalance ultimately affects the function of all body systems. Alteration in the serum levels of particular nutrients or regulatory hormones may also increase the risk of developing cardiovascular and endocrine disorders such as coronary heart disease and type 2 diabetes mellitus. Although genetic factors play a role in etiology, many nutritional disorders may be prevented or reversed to a significant extent by lifestyle and dietary modifications.

REFERENCES

1. Rudolph, C.D. (1994). Feeding disorders in infants and children. *Journal of Pediatrics* 125(6 Pt. 2), S116–S124.
2. Read, N., French, S., and Cunningham, K. (1994). The role of the gut in regulating food intake in man. *Nutrition Reviews* 52(1), 1–10.
3. Baker, D.M. (1993). Assessment and management of impairments in swallowing. *Nursing Clinics of North America* 28(4), 793–805.
4. Koch, W.M. (1993). Swallowing disorders. *Medical Clinics of North America* 77(3), 571–582.
5. Cerda, J.J. (1993). Diet and gastrointestinal disease. *Medical Clinics of North America* 77(4), 881–886.
6. Schneeman, B.O. (1994). Carbohydrates: Significance for energy balance and gastrointestinal function. *Journal of Nutrition* 124, 1747S–1753S.
7. Alvi, A. (1996). Oral cancer: How to recognize the danger signs. *Postgraduate Medicine* 99(4), 149–156.
8. Hunsberger, M., and Issenman, R. (1989). Nursing strategies: Altered digestive function. In: Foster, R.L., Hunsberger, M., and Anderson, J. (Eds.). *Family-Centered Nursing Care of Children*. Philadelphia: W.B. Saunders. (pp. 1398–1405).
9. Moore, K.L., and Persaud, T.V.N. (1993). *The Developing Human: Clinically Oriented Embryology*. (5th ed.). Philadelphia: W.B. Saunders. (pp. 216–223).
10. Black, J.M., and Matassarin-Jacobs, E. (Eds.). (1993). *Luckmann and Sorensen's Medical-Surgical Nursing*. (4th ed.). Philadelphia: W.B. Saunders. (pp. 1573–1575).
11. Zerbe, K.J. (1996). Anorexia nervosa and bulimia nervosa: When the pursuit of bodily 'perfection' becomes a killer. *Postgraduate Medicine* 99(1), 161–169.
12. Commerci, G.D. (1990). Medical complications of anorexia nervosa and bulimia nervosa. *Medical Clinics of North America* 74(5), 1293–1310.
13. Golden, R. (1995). Dementia and Alzheimer's disease: Implications, diagnosis, and treatment. *Minnesota Medicine* 78(1), 25–29.
14. Giannini, A.J., Newman, M., and Gold, M. (1990). Anorexia and bulimia. *American Family Physician* 41(4), 1169–1176.
15. Gibbs, W.W. (1996). Gaining on fat. *Scientific American* August, 88–94.
16. Skelton, N.K., and Skelton III, W.P. (1992). Medical implications of obesity. *Postgraduate Medicine* 92(1), 151–162.
17. Brownell, K.D., and Rodin, J. (1994). The dieting maelstrom: Is it possible and advisable to lose weight? *American Psychologist* 49(9), 781–791.
18. Dietz, W.H. (1994). Critical periods in childhood for the development of obesity. *American Journal of Clinical Nutrition* 59, 955–959.
19. Wilber, J.F. (1991). Neuropeptides, appetite regulation, and human obesity. *Journal of the American Medical Association* 266(2), 257–259.
20. Bjorntorp, P. (1995). Neuroendocrine abnormalities in human obesity. *Metabolism* 44(2 suppl.), 38–41.
21. Goldstein, D.J., and Potvin, J.H. (1994). Long-term weight loss: The effect of pharmacologic agents. *American Journal of Clinical Nutrition* 60, 647–657.
22. Caterson, I.D. (1990). Management strategies for weight control: Eating, Exercise and Behavior. *Drugs* 39(3 suppl.), 20–32.

23. Manson, J.E., Willett, W.C., Stampfer, M.J., *et al.* (1995). Body weight and mortality among women. *New England Journal of Medicine* 333(11), 677–685.
24. Sohal, R.S., and Weindruch, R. (1996). Oxidative stress, caloric restriction, and aging. *Science* 273, 59–63.
25. National Task Force on the Prevention and Treatment of Obesity. (1994). Weight cycling. *Journal of the American Medical Association* 272(15), 1196–1202.
26. Troncone, R., Greco, L., and Auricchio, S. (1996). Gluten-sensitive enteropathy. *Pediatric Clinics of North America* 43(2), 355–373.
27. Janatuinen, E.K., Pikkarainen, P.H., Kemppainen, T.A., *et al.* (1995). A comparison of diets with and without oats in adults with celiac disease. *New England Journal of Medicine* 333(16), 1033–1037.
28. Logan, R.F.A., Rifkind, E.A., Turner, I.D., *et al.* (1989). Mortality in celiac disease. *Gastroenterology* 97, 265.
29. Suarez, F.L., Savaiano, D.A., and Levitt, M.D. (1995). A comparison of symptoms after the consumption of milk or lactose-hydrolyzed milk by people with self-reported severe lactose intolerance. *New England Journal of Medicine* 333(1), 1–4.
30. Ushijima, K., Riby, J.E., and Kretchmer, N. (1995). Carbohydrate malabsorption. *Pediatric Clinics of North America* 42(4), 899–915.
31. Schaefer, E.J. (1994). Familial lipoprotein disorders and premature coronary artery disease. *Medical Clinics of North America* 78(1), 21–39.
32. Willett, W.C. (1994). Diet and health: What should we eat? *Science* 264, 532–537.
33. Bostom, A.G., Cupples, L.A., Jenner, J.L., *et al.* (1996). Elevated plasma lipoprotein(a) and coronary heart disease in men aged 55 years and younger. *Journal of the American Medical Association* 276(7), 544–548.
34. Baker, A.L., Roberts, C., and Gothing, C. (1995). Dyslipidemias in childhood. *Nursing Clinics of North America* 30(2), 243–259.
35. Schaefer, E.J., Lamon-Fava, S., Jenner, J.L., *et al.* (1994). Lipoprotein (a) levels and risk of coronary heart disease in men. *Journal of the American Medical Association* 271(13), 999–1003.
36. Krumholz, H.M., Seeman, T.E., Merrill, S.S., *et al.* (1994). Lack of association between cholesterol and coronary heart disease mortality and morbidity and all-cause mortality in persons older than 70 years. *Journal of the American Medical Association* 272(17), 1335–1340.
37. Neaton, J.D., Blackburn, H., Jacobs, D., *et al.* (1992). Serum cholesterol level and mortality findings for men screened in the Multiple Risk Factor Intervention Trial. *Archives of Internal Medicine* 152, 1490–1500.
38. Steinberg, W., and Tenner, S. (1994). Acute pancreatitis. *New England Journal of Medicine* 330(17), 1198–1210.
39. Calleja, G.A., and Barkin, J.S. (1993). Acute pancreatitis. *Medical Clinics of North America* 77(5), 1037–1056.
40. Steer, M.L., Waxman, I., and Freedman, S. (1995). Chronic pancreatitis. *New England Journal of Medicine* 332(22), 1482–1490.
41. Sainio, V., Kemppainen, E., Puolakkainen, P., *et al.* (1995). Early antibiotic treatment in acute necrotizing pancreatitis. *Lancet* 346, 663–667.
42. Cotran, R.S., Kumar, V., and Robbins, S.L. (Eds.). (1994). *Robbins Pathologic Basis of Disease.* (5th ed.). Philadelphia: W.B. Saunders. (pp. 905–907).

SELECTED BIBLIOGRAPHY

Bakker-Arkema, R.G., Davidson, M.H., Goldstein, R.J., *et al.* (1996). Efficacy and safety of a new HMG-CoA reductase inhibitor, atorvastatin, in patients with hypertriglyceridemia. *Journal of the American Medical Association* 275(2), 128–133.

Benlian, P., De Gennes, J.L., Foubert, L., *et al.* (1996). Premature atherosclerosis in patients with familial chylomicronemia caused by mutations in the lipoprotein lipase gene. *New England Journal of Medicine* 335(12), 848–854.

Branski, D., Lerner, A., and Lebenthal, E. (1996). Chronic diarrhea and malabsorption. *Pediatric Clinics of North America* 43(2), 307–331.

Cappell, M.S., and Marks, M. (1995). Acute pancreatitis in HIV-seropositive patients: A case control study of 44 patients. *American Journal of Medicine* 98, 243–248.

Carek, P.J., Sherer, J.T., and Cardon, D.S. (1997). Management of obesity: Medical treatment options. *American Family Physician* 55(2), 551–558.

Denke, M.A. (1995). Effects of continuous combined hormone-replacement therapy on lipid levels in hypercholesterolemic postmenopausal women. *American Journal of Medicine* 99, 29–35.

Everhart, J., and Wright, D. (1995). Diabetes mellitus as a risk factor for pancreatic cancer. *Journal of the American Medical Association* 273(20), 1605–1609.

Flegal, K.M., Troiano, R.P., Pamuk, E.R., *et al.* (1995). The influence of smoking cessation on the prevalence of overweight in the United States. *New England Journal of Medicine* 333(18), 1165–1170.

Furberg, C. (1994). Lipid-lowering trials: Results and limitations. *American Heart Journal* 128(6 pt. 2), 1304–1308.

Ganz, P., Creager, M.A., Fang, J.C., *et al.* (1996). Pathogenetic mechanisms of atherosclerosis: Effect of lipid lowering on the biology of atherosclerosis. *American Journal of Medicine* 101 (4A suppl.), 10S–16S.

Garg, A. (1994). Efficacy of dietary fiber in lowering serum cholesterol. *American Journal of Medicine* 97, 501–503.

Gasiano, J.M., Buring, J.E., Breslow, J.L., *et al.* (1993). Moderate alcohol intake, increased levels of high-density lipoprotein and its subfractions, and decreased risk of myocardial infarction. *New England Journal of Medicine* 329(25), 1829–1834.

Gasiano, J.M., Hebert, P.R., and Hennekens, C.H. (1996). Cholesterol reduction: Weighing the benefits and risks. *Annals of Internal Medicine* 124(10), 914–918.

George, E.K., Mearin, M.L., Bouquet, J., *et al.* (1996). High frequency of celiac disease in Down syndrome. *Journal of Pediatrics* 128(4), 555–557.

Gotto, A.M. (1994). Heart disease in the assessment and treatment of hypercholesterolemia: Coronary artery disease and other atherosclerotic disease, family history, and left ventricular hypertrophy. *American Journal of Medicine* 96(6A suppl.), 6A-9S–6A-18S.

Hardy, S.C., and Kleinman, R.E. (1994). Fat and cholesterol in the diet of infants and young children: Implications for growth, development, and long-term health. *Journal of Pediatrics* 125 (5 Pt. 2), S69–S77.

Havel, R.J., and Rapaport, E. (1995). Management of primary hyperlipidemia. *New England Journal of Medicine* 332(22), 1491–1498.

Heini, A.F., and Weinsier, R.L. (1997). Divergent trends in obesity and fat intake patterns: The American paradox. *American Journal of Medicine* 102, 259–264.

Himeno, E., Nishino, K., Nakashima, Y., *et al.* (1996). Weight reduction regresses left ventricular mass regardless of blood pressure level in obese subjects. *American Heart Journal* 131(2), 313–319.

Hoeg, J.M. (1994). Familial hypercholesterolemia: What the zebra can teach us about the horse. *Journal of the American Medical Association* 271(7), 543–546.

Hunninghake, D.B., LaRosa, J.C., Kinosian, B., *et al.* (1994). Long-term treatment of hypercholesterolemia with dietary fiber. *American Journal of Medicine* 97, 504–508.

Johnson, K., and Kligman, E.W. (1992). Preventive nutrition: Disease-specific dietary interventions for older adults. *Geriatrics* 47(11), 39–49.

Katan, M.B., Zock, P.L., and Mensink, R.P. (1994). Effects of fats and fatty acids on blood lipids in humans: An overview. *American Journal of Clinical Nutrition* 60(suppl.), 1017S–1022S.

Kottke, B.A. (1994). Lipoproteins and apolipoproteins: Making use of their metabolic properties to individualize therapy. *Postgraduate Medicine* 95(2), 51–65.

Kuczmarski, R.J., Flegal, K.M., Campbell, S., *et al.* (1994). Increasing prevalence of overweight among U.S. adults. *Journal of the American Medical Association* 272(3), 205–211.

Larsen, M.L., and Illingworth, D.R. (1994). Drug treatment of dyslipoproteinemia. *Medical Clinics of North America* 78(1), 225–245.

Lehne, R.A. (1994). *Pharmacology for Nursing Care.* (2nd ed.). Philadelphia: W.B. Saunders.

Lentze, M.J. (1995). Molecular and cellular aspects of hydrolysis and absorption. *American Journal of Clinical Nutrition* 61(suppl.), 946S–951S.

Lerner, A., Branski, D., and Lebenthal, E. (1996). Pancreatic diseases in children. *Pediatric Clinics of North America* 43(1), 125–156.

Levine, G. N., Keaney, J.F., and Vita, J.A. (1995). Cholesterol reduction in cardiovascular disease. *New England Journal of Medicine* 332(8), 512–521.

Lindpaintner, K. (1995). Finding an obesity gene: A tale of mice and man. *New England Journal of Medicine* 332(10), 679–680.

McClain, C.J., Humphries, L.L., Hill, K.K., *et al.* (1993). Gastrointestinal and nutritional aspects of eating disorders. *Journal of the American College of Nutrition* 12(4), 466–474.

Moore, E.E., and Moore, F.A. (1991). Immediate enteral nutrition following multisystem trauma: A decade perspective. *Journal of the American College of Nutrition* 10(6), 633–648.

Newman, T.B., and Hulley, S.B. (1996). Carcinogenicity of lipid-lowering drugs. *New England Journal of Medicine* 275(1), 55–60.

Rader, D.J., Hoeg, J.M., and Brewer, H.B. (1994). Quantitation of plasma apolipoproteins in the primary and secondary prevention of coronary artery disease. *Annals of Internal Medicine* 120(12), 1012–1025.

Rao, S.S.C. (1997). Belching, bloating, and flatulence: How to help patients who have troublesome abdominal gas. *Postgraduate Medicine* 101(4), 263–278.

Rensch, M.J., Merenich, J.A., Lieberman, M., *et al.* (1996). Gluten-sensitive enteropathy in patients with insulin-dependent diabetes mellitus. *Annals of Internal Medicine* 124(6), 564–567.

Ribera, M., Pinto, X., Argimon, J.M., *et al.* (1995). Lipid metabolism and apolipoprotein E phenotypes in patients with xanthelasma. *American Journal of Medicine* 99, 485–490.

Ronnemaa, T., Karonen, S-L., Rissanen, A., *et al.* (1997). Relation between plasma leptin levels and measures of body fat in identical twins discordant for obesity. *Annals of Internal Medicine* 126(1), 26–31.

Sax, H.C., and Souba, W.W. (1993). Enteral and parenteral feedings. *Medical Clinics of North America* 77(4), 863–880.

Schaefer, E.J., Lichtenstein, A.H., Lamon-Fava, S., *et al.* (1995). Body weight and low-density lipoprotein cholesterol changes after consumption of a low-fat ad libitum diet. *Journal of the American Medical Association* 274(18), 1450–1455.

Seed, M. (1994). Postmenopausal hormone replacement therapy, coronary heart disease and plasma lipoproteins. *Drugs* 47(2 suppl.), 25–34.

Shepherd, J., Cobbe, S.M., Ford, I., *et al.* (1995). Prevention of coronary heart disease with prevastatin in men with hypercholesterolemia. *New England Journal of Medicine* 333(20), 1301–1307.

Slyper, A.H. (1994). Low-density lipoprotein density and atherosclerosis. *Journal of the American Medical Association* 272(4), 305–308.

Souba, W.W. (1997). Nutritional Support. *New England Journal of Medicine* 336(1), 41–48.

Stone, N.J. (1994). Secondary causes of hyperlipidemia. *Medical Clinics of North America* 78(1), 117–141.

Verschuren, W.M.M., Jacobs, D.R., Bloemberg, B.P.M., *et al.* (1995). Serum total cholesterol and long-term coronary heart disease mortality in different cultures. *Journal of the American Medical Association* 274(2), 131–136.

Walsh, J.M.E., and Grady, D. (1995). Treatment of hyperlipidemia in women. *Journal of the American Medical Association* 274(14), 1152–1158.

Walter, J.B. (1992). *An Introduction to the Principles of Disease.* (3rd ed.). Philadelphia: W.B. Saunders.

Walton, C., Lees, B., Crook, D., *et al.* (1995). Body fat distribution, rather than overall adiposity, influences serum lipids and lipoproteins in healthy men independently of age. *American Journal of Medicine* 99, 459–464.

Weinsier, R.L., Wilson, L.J., and Lee, J. (1995). Medically safe rate of weight loss for the treatment of obesity: A guideline based on risk of gallstone formation. *American Journal of Medicine* 98, 115–117.

Wise, G.R., and Schultz, T.T. (1996). Hyperlipidemia: When does treatment make a difference? *Postgraduate Medicine* 100(1), 138–149.

Writing Group for the DISC Collaborative Research Group. (1995). Efficacy and safety of lowering dietary intake of fat and cholesterol in children with elevated low-density lipoprotein cholesterol. *Journal of the American Medical Association* 273(18), 1429–1435.

Young, T.K., and Gelskey, D.E. (1995). Is noncentral obesity metabolically benign? *Journal of the American Medical Association* 274(24), 1939–1941.

Disorders of the Liver and Biliary System

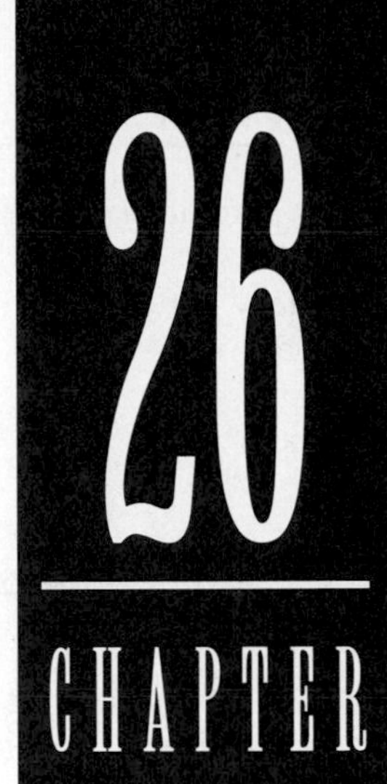

LEARNING OBJECTIVES

1. Relate the anatomy of the hepatic lobule to hepatobiliary function and manifestations of hepatic disorders.
2. Describe the hepatic processes of bilirubin metabolism and their potential disruption in hyperbilirubinemia.
3. Discuss the roles of the liver and gallbladder in bile synthesis, storage, and secretion.
4. Discuss the importance of the liver's function as a vascular reservoir.
5. Summarize the multiple metabolic functions of the liver.
6. Relate the storage functions of the liver to the potential for hepatotoxicity.
7. Discuss the possible consequences of impaired hepatic synthesis of serum proteins.
8. Discuss the possible consequences of impaired hepatic biotransformation of drugs and hormones.
9. Comprehend the pathophysiologic processes that predict clinical manifestations and rationalize intervention in selected hepatobiliary disorders.

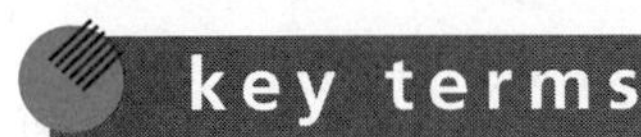

alcoholism
ascites
asterixis
biliary cirrhosis
cardiac cirrhosis
cholecystitis
cholelithiasis
cholestasis
cirrhosis
esophageal varices
extrahepatic biliary atresia
fetor hepaticus
fulminant hepatitis
fulminant liver failure
gallbladder cancer
hepatic coma
hepatic encephalopathy
hepatic failure
hepatic steatosis
hepatoblastoma
hepatocytes

hepatocellular carcinoma
hepatomegaly
hepatopulmonary syndrome
hepatorenal syndrome
hepatotoxicity
hyperbilirubinemia
jaundice
kernicterus
Laënnec's cirrhosis
nonalcoholic steatohepatitis
pathologic jaundice
physiologic jaundice
portal hypertension
postnecrotic cirrhosis
primary biliary cirrhosis
primary sclerosing cholangitis
splenomegaly
spontaneous bacterial peritonitis
steatorrhea
viral hepatitis

Because of its diversity of function, the liver defies classification with any one of the anatomic subsystems of the body. The nutritional functions of the liver were briefly discussed in Chapter 25. Along with the pancreas, the liver and gallbladder serve as accessory organs of digestion and absorption. The synthesis of bile by the liver, the storage of bile in the gallbladder, the mechanisms that regulate the release of bile, and the recycling of biliary constituents will be detailed in this chapter. The additional functions of the liver as a vascular reservoir and in the biochemical synthesis, storage, and biotransformation of endogenous and exogenous substances will also be discussed.

Disorders of the liver and biliary system are common, and they account for significant morbidity and mortality in the United States. Those disorders of greatest clinical importance are detailed in this chapter and include the syndromes of **hepatic failure, cirrhosis,** and **hyperbilirubinemia** as well as these specific disorders: **cholelithiasis, viral hepatitis, alcoholism, primary biliary cirrhosis, primary sclerosing cholangitis, extrahepatic biliary atresia, gallbladder cancer,** and **hepatocellular carcinoma.** Clinical features of other, less-common hepatobiliary disorders are briefly summarized.

FUNCTIONAL ANATOMY OF THE BILIARY SYSTEM

Gross Anatomy

The Liver

As shown in Figure 26–1, the liver lies primarily in the right upper quadrant of the abdominal cavity, extending no more than 5 to 6 cm across the midline. The largest glandular organ in the body, the liver is contained within the peritoneal space, with its upper edge pushing the diaphragm slightly upward on the right side. The lower edge of the liver is concave, creating a space for the gallbladder, and lies roughly parallel to the lower border of the rib cage (costal margin).

The Gallbladder

The gallbladder is a thin-walled sac, about 10 cm long, composed primarily of smooth muscle. Bile leaves the liver via the *hepatic duct* and enters the gallbladder via the *cystic duct.* The gallbladder normally stores about 30 to 60 mL of bile, which becomes concentrated as water is absorbed by gallbladder mucosal cells. Within about 30 minutes of ingestion of a meal (especially a fatty meal), gallbladder contraction is mediated by parasympathetic reflex stimulation as well as by the duodenal hormones cholecystokinin (CCK) and motilin (see Chapters 24 and 25). Opening of the cystic duct

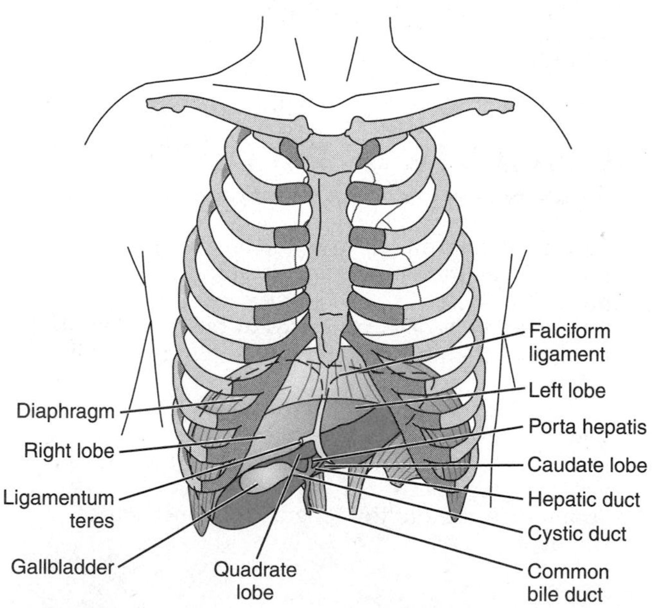

FIGURE 26–1
Location and structure of the liver and gallbladder. The liver occupies much of the right upper abdominal cavity. It is attached to the underside of the diaphragm and moves with respiration. The *falciform ligament* divides the liver into a large right lobe and smaller left lobe. The inferior surface of the right lobe is subdivided into the anterior quadrate lobe and the posterior caudate lobe. A depression between the quadrate and caudate lobes, the *porta hepatis* ("door to the liver"), is the site of entry of the hepatic artery and portal vein and the site of exit for the hepatic vein and *hepatic ducts.* The gallbladder is nestled into the underside of the liver in its own depression, or fossa. Its duct, the *cystic duct,* joins the hepatic ducts to form the *common bile duct.*

sphincter allows bile to enter the duodenum via the *common bile duct,* which also transports pancreatic juices.

Perfusion of the Biliary System

The liver has a dual blood supply (Fig. 26–2). The *hepatic artery,* which branches off the abdominal aorta, accounts for one fourth of the blood entering the liver and serves to supply the hepatic tissues with oxygen and nutrients. Three fourths of the volume of blood entering the liver is venous blood, from the *portal vein.* With respect to circulation, the liver is situated in series with the alimentary canal (see Chapter 15). Thus, all nutrients (and potentially drugs, toxins, or other absorbed substances) pass through the liver immediately after being absorbed from the intestinal lumen. Venous outflow from the liver is via *hepatic veins,* which enter the inferior vena cava.

Microanatomy

The functional unit of the liver is the *lobule,* illustrated in Figure 26–3. The hepatic lobules are composed of **hepatocytes** (functional liver cells) arranged in stacked double rows that radiate outward from a *central vein.* Hepatocytes are surrounded by porous exchange vessels known as *sinusoids.* These vessels, which receive hepatic arterial and portal ve-

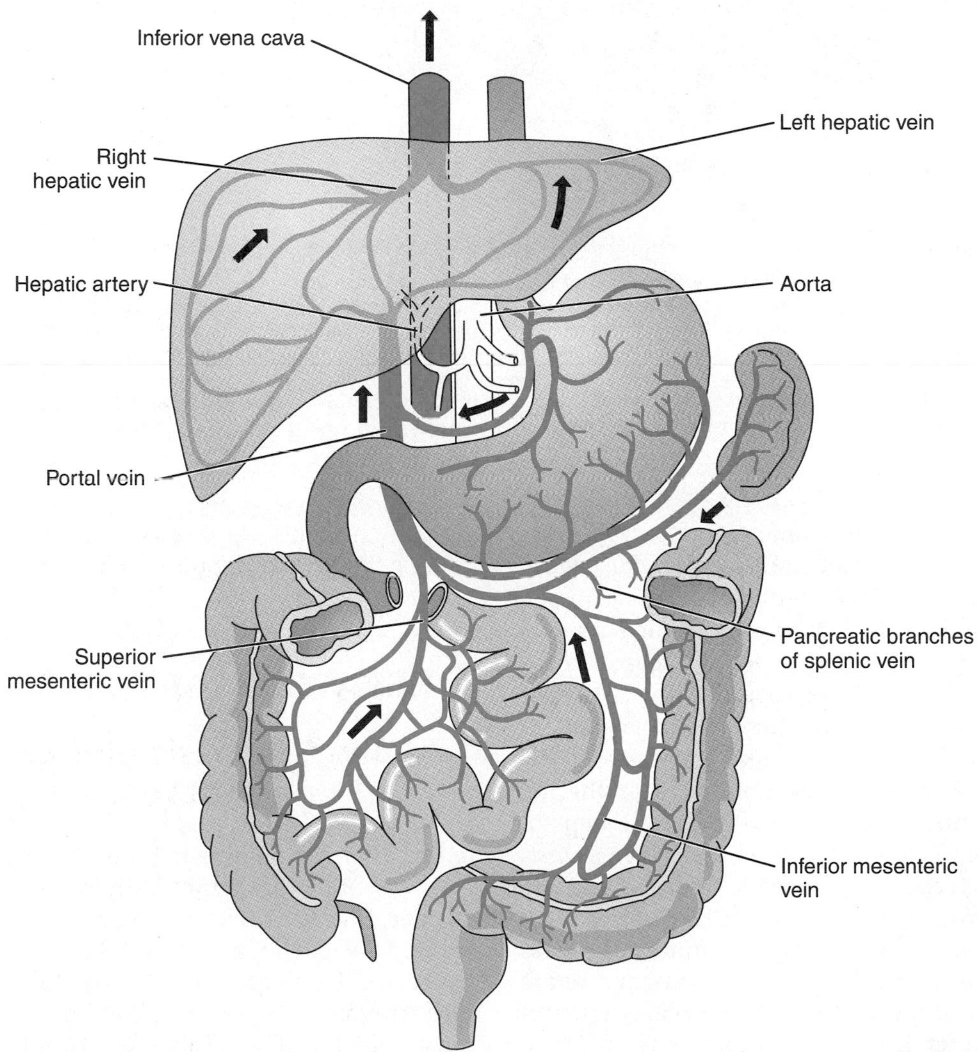

FIGURE 26–2
Perfusion of the liver. The liver has a dual blood supply, with the hepatic artery supplying one fourth and the portal vein supplying three fourths of hepatic perfusion. Portal venous blood is rich in nutrients absorbed from the intestinal lumen. Venous outflow is via the hepatic veins, which enter the inferior vena cava.

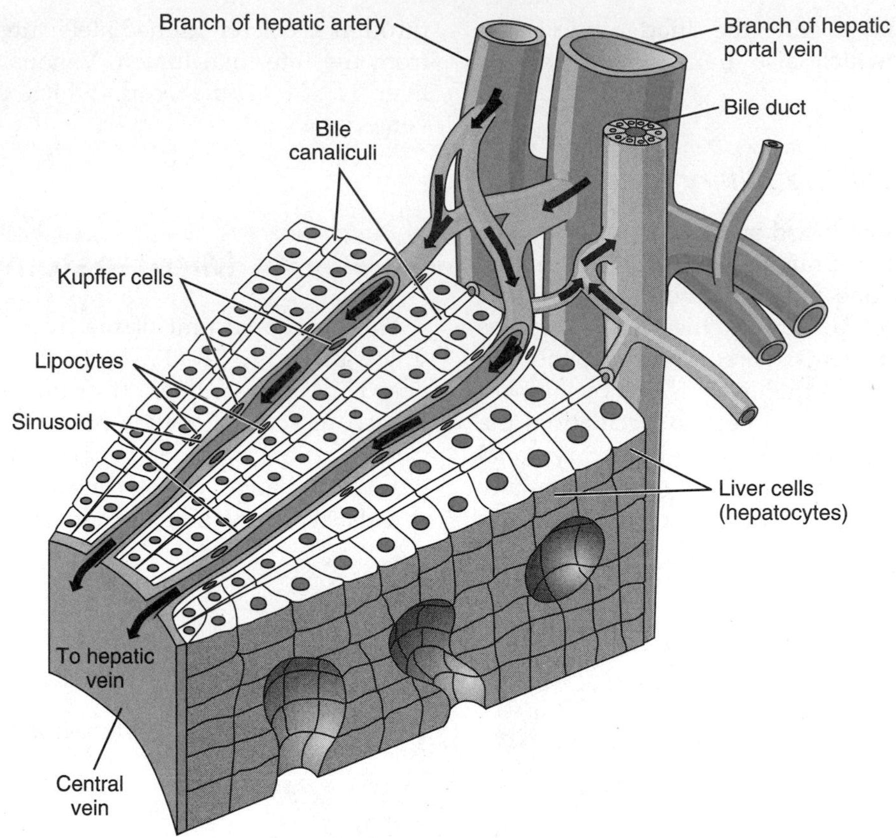

FIGURE 26–3

The hepatic lobule. The functional unit of the liver is the lobule, composed of *hepatocytes* arranged in stacked double rows that radiate outward from a *central vein.* Porous exchange vessels (*sinusoids*) surround the hepatocytes and receive hepartic arterial and portal venous blood. Sinusoids are lined with phagocytic *Kupffer cells.* Tiny channels (*bile canaliculi*) between the rows of hepatocytes receive newly synthesized bile and drain into the hepatic duct. The interstitial space between the hepatocytes and sinusoids (*space of Disse*) is drained by terminal lymphatic vessels. Fat-storing *lipocytes* are found around the circumference of this space.

nous blood, are functionally analogous to capillaries. Venous drainage from sinusoids is via the central vein. Sinusoids are lined with phagocytic tissue macrophages known as *Kupffer cells,* which remove 99% of the bacteria and other foreign particles ingested in the typical diet. Between the rows of hepatocytes are the *bile canaliculi,* tiny channels that receive the bile as it is synthesized and released by hepatocytes. The canaliculi eventually enter the hepatic duct. The interstitial space between the hepatocytes and the sinusoids, known as the *space of Disse,* is drained by terminal lymphatic vessels that remove excess fluid and protein from the lobules. Approximately half of all lymphatic fluid originates from within the liver lobules, and lymphatic tissue of the liver is an important site of lymphocyte maturation (see Chapter 13). *Lipocytes* (also known as Ito cells) are found around the circumference of the space of Disse. These cells normally serve an adipose storage function but may undergo transformation in chronic liver disease, contributing to disruption of the normal lobular architecture in cirrhosis.

HEPATOBILIARY PHYSIOLOGY

Bile Synthesis and Bilirubin Metabolism

Bile is a yellow-green fluid that contains the *bile salts* essential to chemical digestion and absorption of fats. Bile salts are bile acids (e.g., cholic acid or chenodeoxycholic acid) that have been chemically combined (conjugated) with glycine or taurine. Bile also contains water, electrolytes, proteins, cholesterol, and bilirubin (Table 26–1). An estimated 500 to 1000 mL of bile is produced each day.

Bilirubin, a pigment that imparts color to the bile, urine, and stool, is derived from the breakdown of

TABLE 26–1
COMPOSITION OF BILE

	Liver Bile	Gallbladder Bile
Water	97.5 g/dL	92 g/dL
Bile salts	1.1 g/dL	6 g/dL
Bilirubin	0.04 g/dL	0.3 g/dL
Cholesterol	0.1 g/dL	0.3 to 0.9 g/dL
Fatty acids	0.12 g/dL	0.3 to 1.2 g/dL
Lecithin	0.04 g/dL	0.3 g/dL
Na^+	145 mEq/L	130 mEq/L
K^+	5 mEq/L	12 mEq/L
Ca^+	5 mEq/L	23 mEq/L
Cl^-	100 mEq/L	25 mEq/L
HCO_3^-	28 mEq/L	10 mEq/L

From Guyton, A.C., and Hall, J.E. (1996). *Textbook of Medical Physiology.* (9th ed.) Philadelphia: W.B. Saunders. (p. 828). Used with permission.

heme proteins, 80% of which are found in the hemoglobin of red blood cells (RBCs). The remaining 20% of circulating heme originates from RBC precursors and nonhemoglobin heme proteins.[1] Normal RBC turnover or increased RBC breakdown (hemolysis) releases heme into the blood (see Chapter 12). The enzyme heme oxygenase then removes a carbon atom as well as the iron from the heme, forming biliverdin, which is then reduced to form bilirubin (Fig. 26–4).

In the plasma, free (unconjugated) bilirubin binds reversibly to albumin and is transported to the liver. There, it dissociates from albumin and is taken into hepatocytes by one of two carrier proteins, Y protein (ligandin) or Z protein. In the endoplasmic reticulum of hepatocytes, bilirubin is conjugated, or rendered more water-soluble by the addition of two molecules of glucuronic acid. The enzyme glucuronosyl transferase catalyzes this reaction.

Conjugated bilirubin then enters the bile canaliculus and is excreted into the small intestine for potential elimination in the feces. About half of the conjugated bilirubin is converted by bacterial action to *urobilinogen,* some of which is reabsorbed into the blood for recycling by the liver. About 5% of reabsorbed urobilinogen is excreted by the kidneys, imparting color to the urine. Exposure of urobilinogen in urine or feces to air results in its oxidation to *urobilin* or *stercobilin,* respectively.

Some of the conjugated bilirubin within the intestine may be hydrolyzed back to the unconjugated form by the enzyme β-glucuronidase, and in this form it may be reabsorbed into the portal venous circulation. Unconjugated bilirubin is lipid soluble and tends to accumulate in lipid tissues when serum

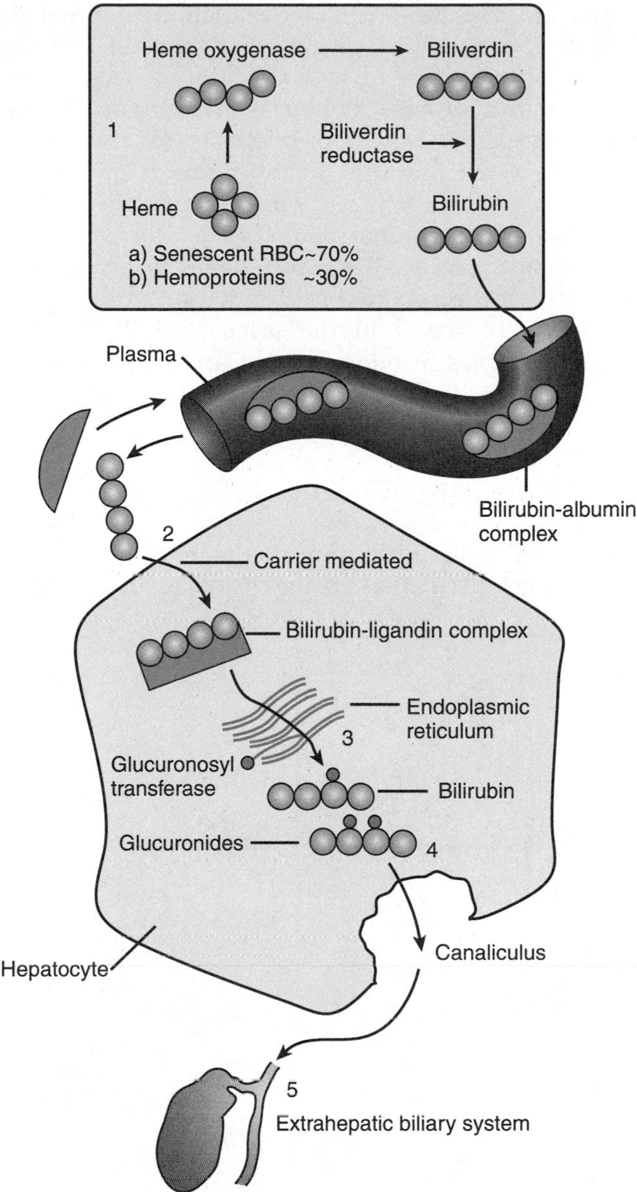

FIGURE 26–4

Bilirubin metabolism. Normal turnover of senescent red blood cells (RBCs) releases hemoglobin, and other heme-containing proteins are derived from enzymes such as cytochrome P-450. The enzyme *heme oxygenase,* contained within monocytes and macrophages, converts heme to *biliverdin,* which is then reduced to *bilirubin* by the enzyme *biliverdin reductase.* Bilirubin is transported to the liver bound to albumin, then dissociates from albumin and is taken into hepatocytes by carrier proteins (e.g., *ligandin*). In the endoplasmic reticulum of hepatocyes, bilirubin is conjugated with glucuronic acid to render it more water soluble. Conjugated bilirubin then enters the bile canaliculus and hepatic duct. Potential mechanisms leading to jaundice include (1) excessive release of heme (with hemolysis), (2) reduced hepatic uptake, (3) impaired conjugation, (4) impaired excretion by hepatocytes, or (5) obstruction of biliary canaliculi or ducts. (From Cotran, R.S., Kumar, V., and Robbins, S.L. [1994]. *Robbins Pathologic Basis of Disease.* [5th Ed.]. Philadelphia: W.B. Saunders. [p. 837].)

levels are elevated. This accumulation is noted as **jaundice,** a yellow appearance of the skin and the sclerae of the eyes.

Through a process known as *enterohepatic circulation,* approximately 95% of bile salts are reabsorbed from the small intestine. Reabsorption is by passive diffusion in the early portions and by active transport from the terminal ileum. From the portal venous blood, nearly all the bile salts are returned to the liver for reuse in bile synthesis, and a small amount is excreted in the urine (Fig. 26–5). The small quantities of bile salts that are not reabsorbed but lost in the feces are replenished by hepatocytes.

Vascular Reservoir Function

Because of the position of the liver with respect to the venous circulation, rising pressure in the vena cava opposes outflow from the hepatic veins and results in "storage" of 300 to 400 mL of blood in the liver. This causes some degree of enlargement (**hepatomegaly**) and is a typical clinical manifestation of congestive heart failure (see Chapter 16). The ability of the liver to serve as a vascular reservoir is adaptive in the case of hemorrhage, when contraction of the liver (along with the systemic veins and spleen) shunts more blood into the effective circulation in an effort to preserve perfusion to vital organs (see Chapter 15).

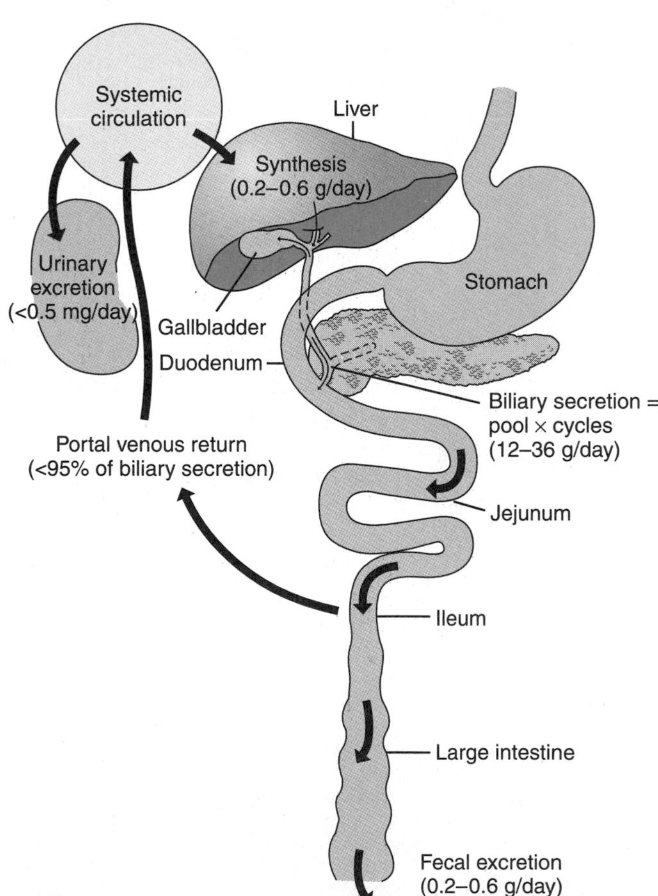

FIGURE 26–5
Enterohepatic circulation of bile salts. Nearly 95% of the bile salts entering the duodenum are reabsorbed by active and passive mechanisms. Portal venous blood carries the bile salts back to the liver for reuse in bile synthesis. A small fraction of bilirubin in the circulation is excreted in the urine, and a small amount is not reabsorbed but rather excreted in the feces. Fecal and urinary losses of bile salts are easily replenished by hepatocyte synthesis. The pool of bile salts is recycled several times per day.

Metabolism of Carbohydrates, Lipids, and Proteins

Carbohydrates

The liver serves as a "glucose buffer" in the maintenance of serum glucose levels. Under endocrine regulation, the liver removes glucose from the blood when serum levels are high, and stores it as glycogen (glycogenesis). When glucose levels are low, the liver produces glucose by two mechanisms: (1) glycogenolysis, the catabolism of stored glycogen to glucose and subsequent release of this glucose into the blood and (2) gluconeogenesis, the synthesis of glucose from amino acids. Glucose metabolism is discussed in detail in Chapter 29.

Lipids

As discussed in Chapter 25, the liver is central to the endogenous pathway of lipoprotein synthesis and transport. Hepatocytes also contain the enzymes for β-oxidation of fatty acids for energy metabolism (see Chapter 3). Faulty metabolism of fatty acids may lead to accumulation of fat in the liver (**hepatic steatosis**), which may precede the development of cirrhosis.

Proteins

In addition to its ability to convert amino acids into glucose, the liver also has enzymatic pathways for the synthesis of nonessential amino acids. Hepatocytes convert ammonia (a product of protein catabolism) into urea for excretion by the kidneys. Failure of this conversion in liver disease may result in the accumulation of ammonia in the blood.

The many metabolic functions of the liver potentially give rise to a large number of congenital and acquired metabolic liver diseases, resulting in abnormal hepatic function as well as impaired nutrition, energy metabolism, and cellular development. These include heavy-metal storage diseases (e.g., hemochromatosis, Wilson's disease), protoporphyria, tyrosinemia, α_1-antitrypsin deficiency, Reye's syndrome, and Niemann-Pick disease. Clinical features of these disorders are summarized in Table 26–2. Hemochromatosis and porphyrias were discussed in detail in Chapter 12. The altered metabolism of pregnancy may also be associated with liver dysfunction (see Chapter 32).

Vitamin and Mineral Metabolism

The liver normally stores several months' supply of vitamins B_{12} and D and several years' supply of vitamin A. Excessive intake of fat-soluble vitamins may be toxic to the liver. Along with the kidneys, the liver is important in the activation of vitamin D_3, a steroid hormone essential to calcium homeostasis and bone metabolism (see Chapter 9). As discussed in Chapter 12, much of the body's iron stores are in the form of ferratin in the liver. The "iron buffering" function of the liver permits storage and release of iron as needed for hematopoiesis.

Synthesis of Serum Proteins

Protein clotting factors are synthesized by the liver, and their lack in hepatic failure may contribute to bleeding (see Chapter 14). The liver synthesizes other plasma proteins also, notably albumin and transferrin. Transferrin binds iron for plasma transport. Albumin is important in serum binding and transport of electrolytes and drugs, and it is the particle that generates colloid osmotic pressure essential to capillary exchange and fluid compartment balance (see Chapter 8). Deficiency of albumin contributes to edema and may predispose some individuals to drug toxicity related to an increase in the unbound (active) fraction of drugs. Hepatic synthesis of the apoprotein portion of lipoproteins may be genetically impaired, contributing to dyslipidemia (see Chapter 25).

Biotransformation of Drugs and Hormones

As they pass through the liver, nearly all circulating drugs are inactivated by hepatic enzymes that

TABLE 26–2
METABOLIC LIVER DISEASES

DISORDER	CLINICAL FEATURES
Wilson's disease	Autosomal recessive disorder in which the liver is unable to transport and store normally absorbed dietary copper. Hepatocytes become overloaded with copper, and cirrhosis develops. Penicillamine, a copper chelating agent, is the treatment of choice.
Hemochromatosis	Autosomal recessive disorder seen earlier in males. Increased iron absorption leads to cirrhosis, diabetes, and a gray, metallic cast to the skin. Hepatocellular carcinoma often develops in untreated disease. Phlebotomy is the treatment of choice.
Protoporphyria	Inherited disorder that is usually autosomal dominant. An enzymatic defect in heme synthesis leads to photosensitivity of the skin and, in a small number of patients, fatal black liver disease. Gene therapy is experimental.
Tyrosinemia	Autosomal recessive disorder characterized by progressive liver failure and renal tubular dysfunction causing rickets. Deficiency of the enzyme fumarylacetoacetase (FAH) prevents metabolism of tyrosine, phenylalanine, and methionine, and their accumulation is toxic to hepatic and renal cells. Dietary restriction is used in treatment.
α_1-Antitrypsin deficiency	Deficiency of a protease inhibitor, presenting as liver disease in children or early emphysema in adults. An autosomal recessive pattern is seen, with homozygous individuals more often affected by liver disease. Only a small number develop cirrhosis, which is treated with liver transplantation.
Reye's syndrome	Acquired disorder of hepatic mitochondrial function usually associated with administration of aspirin to young children during a viral illness. Lipid deposition is seen in hepatocytes as well as in cells of the nervous system and other organs. Liver failure and cerebral edema are the most evident effects. Treatment is supportive.
Niemann-Pick disease type C	Autosomal recessive disorder in which intracellular cholesterol transport is impaired. Cells accumulate cholesterol in unesterified form within lysosomes of the liver, brain, bone marrow, spleen, eye, skin, and skeletal muscle. Clinical onset and severity are variable. No definitive treatment is available.

Data from Schwarzenberg, S.J., and Sharp, H.L. (1996). Update on metabolic liver disease. *Pediatric Clinics of North America* 43(1), 27–56; Quam, D.A. (1994). Recognizing a case of Reye's syndrome. *American Family Physician* 50(7), 1491–1496; and Schiffmann, R. (1996). Niemann-Pick disease type C. *Journal of the American Medical Association* 276(7), 561–564.

conjugate, oxidize, reduce, or hydrolyze them. (A few drugs are *activated* by hepatic enzymes.) Some circulating hormones, including antidiuretic hormone, aldosterone, and estrogen, are also inactivated in this way. "Overdose" or toxic effects of these agents may be seen as a consequence of hepatic failure or, in the case of neonates, hepatic immaturity (see Developmental Perspective).

DISORDERS OF HEPATIC AND BILIARY SYSTEM FUNCTION

Hepatic Failure

Definition. Hepatic failure is impairment of liver function to a degree resulting in a predictable syndrome of observable clinical effects. *Acute hepatic failure* becomes evident within 6 weeks to 6 months of onset of illness.[2] Hepatic failure may also occur as an end-stage syndrome in those with chronic, progressive liver diseases.

Epidemiology. An estimated 2000 cases of acute liver failure are diagnosed in the United States each year.[3] Risk factors are specific to each of the etiologic mechanisms discussed in the next section.

Etiology. Hepatic failure may result from traumatic, toxic, viral, or ischemic injury to liver lobules (Table 26–3). The liver is easily injured by physical trauma, with displaced rib fractures often causing hepatic perforation. Because the liver is a highly vascular organ, hepatic trauma may lead to significant intra-abdominal hemorrhage. Drug and alcohol-related toxicity and viral hepatitis are the most common causes of hepatic failure.[4] **Hepatotoxicity** may occur as a consequence of any drug or foreign substance that is metabolized by the liver (Table 26–4). A few hepatotoxins produce metabolic products that are uniformly toxic in a dose-dependent manner, but others are injurious only in rare persons who metabolize them abnormally because of genetic defects of hepatic enzymes. Acetaminophen (Tylenol) overdose is particularly toxic in persons who also abuse alcohol or are malnourished.[5] In such cases, acetaminophen metabolism produces reactive oxygen species, and alcohol abuse or malnutrition results in deficiency of glutathione, a peptide that normally binds and inactivates harmful oxygen radicals. Congenital and acquired defects that obstruct the outflow of bile are a rare cause of hepatotoxicity. Inflammation of hepatic tissue in biliary atresia and cholelithiasis may result from the toxic action of retained biliary constituents as well as from pressure-induced damage to hepatic tissue.

Viral hepatitis may cause rapidly progressive **fulminant liver failure** at the time of initial infection in a small number of cases. Hepatic failure is much more likely in cases of chronic hepatitis associated with hepatitis B or C, however.

Prolonged states of decreased perfusion may lead to ischemic liver failure ("shock liver") as a result of catecholamine-mediated selective vasoconstriction, which shunts circulation away from the abdominal organs and skin to perfuse the brain, heart, and lungs (see Chapter 15).

Pathophysiology. The liver has much functional reserve and can maintain basal function with as few as 10% intact lobules. Trauma may directly destroy hepatic lobules or may induce profound ischemia secondary to hemorrhage. Toxicity resulting from drugs, viruses, or other agents may lead to necrosis of hepatocytes as metabolites such as reactive oxygen species form covalent bonds with cellular proteins, lipids, or DNA (see Chapter 3). In addition, toxic agents may induce hepatic enzyme systems, altering the metabolism of other substances. Combination of drug metabolites with hepatocellular proteins may trigger a hypersensitivity reaction (see Chapter 13). Some agents may directly damage bile canaliculi, leading to intrahepatic obstruction of bile flow (**cholestasis**). Tissue changes may reflect inflammation (hepatitis), accumulation of fat within hepatocytes (hepatic steatosis), deposition of scar tissue (hepatic fibrosis), or abnormal collagen deposition and disruption of lobular structure (cirrhosis).

Clinical Manifestations. Nearly all body systems are affected by hepatic failure, as detailed in the following sections.

Biliary System. Within the liver, the inflammatory response leads to tenderness and enlargement (hepatomegaly) at first, possibly followed by atrophy when scar tissue begins to contract. Damage and death of hepatocytes results in spilling of hepatic enzymes into the blood, with alteration in serum levels of L-lactate dehydrogenase, aspartate transaminase, alanine aminotransferase, alkaline phosphatase, and gamma-glutamyl transpeptidase (Table 26–5). Loss of Kupffer cell function may lead to sepsis if ingested bacteria are not cleared. Loss of functional hepatocytes leads to impairment of all hepatic functions.

Protein synthesis, lipid metabolism, and glucose buffering functions may all be impaired, leading to malnutrition and fatigue as well as manifestations related to deficits of specific nutrients. Abnormal metabolism of an amino acid, methionine, may lead to **fetor hepaticus,** an acetone-like, "old wine" odor of the breath. Impaired absorption, storage, or activation of fat-soluble vitamins may lead to deficiency syndromes including night blindness (vitamin A), osteoporosis (vitamin D_3), coagulopathy (vitamin K),

Developmental Perspective

Embryonic and Fetal Periods

Development of the liver, gallbladder, and biliary ducts begins during the 4th week of gestation. The liver grows rapidly, filling much of the abdominal cavity by the end of the 10th week. Hematopoiesis begins during the 6th week, and bile formation begins during the 12th week. Bile enters the duodenum through patent ducts by the 13th week, giving color to the fetal stool (meconium). As a site of B lymphocyte maturation, the liver is important in the development of immune competence. Most metabolic functions are performed by the maternal liver, however, and the ductus venosus shunts most blood past the fetal liver during gestation. Although minor abnormalities in the structure of hepatic lobules and ducts are common, most are clinically insignificant. Extrahepatic biliary atresia, a notable exception, may arise when the ductal system fails to reopen after the normal period of obliteration by proliferating epithelial tissues.

Infancy and Childhood

With removal of the placenta at birth, blood flow through the ductus venosus ceases, and permanent closure of the ductus is evident after a few weeks. The newborn liver is proportionately large, accounting for about 5% of the infant's weight. Hematopoiesis continues for a few weeks, then ceases as metabolic functions gradually increase. Function of liver enzyme systems is immature in neonates, contributing to physiologic jaundice and diminished ability to metabolize some nutrients and to biotransform drugs. Normal growth and development may be retarded in children with chronic liver disease. Obstruction of biliary ducts may occur in children with cystic fibrosis. Hepatic tumors are rare during childhood. Cholelithiasis is uncommon in otherwise healthy children, but it may occur in those with risk factors.

Adolescence and Young Adulthood

Alcohol abuse often begins during adolescence. Consequences of alcohol abuse usually manifest during this period, not only as liver disease but also as increased risk of accidents, suicide, or homicide. Abuse of other hepatotoxins is also prevalent among this age group and may contribute to direct injury of the liver and to risk-taking behaviors that can result in viral hepatitis. Cholelithiasis and related disorders are common among younger adults. Young adults with inflammatory bowel disease are at increased risk of primary sclerosing cholangitis. A number of hepatobiliary disorders are unique to pregnancy, including cholestasis of pregnancy, HELLP (*h*emolysis, *e*levated *l*iver enzymes, *l*ow *p*latelet count) syndrome, and acute fatty liver of pregnancy. In addition, many hepatobiliary disorders are exacerbated by the altered metabolic demands of pregnancy.

Middle and Older Adulthood

Hepatic blood flow decreases with advancing age, and the liver decreases in size. Liver function tests usually remain within the normal range, but differences in drug metabolism may be apparent. Alcohol abuse is as prevalent among the elderly as in younger adults, contributing to hepatic cirrhosis and risk of injury. Elderly individuals attain higher blood alcohol concentrations per quantity ingested, probably because of their lower fluid volumes. Alcohol-drug interactions are more frequent in older individuals because of their greater use of prescription drugs. Gallbladder function does not decline with normal aging. Hepatocellular carcinoma may arise during this period as a consequence of previous cirrhosis.

---

and decreased RBC survival (vitamin E). B-vitamin deficiencies may be manifested as anemia, inflammation of the tongue (glossitis) and lips (cheilitis), and peripheral neuropathy.

Decreased conjugation of bilirubin and decreased biliary excretion may lead to deposition of bilirubin and other bile constituents in the skin, resulting in jaundice and pruritus (itching). Stools may be clay-colored because of the lack of bilirubin pigment, and **steatorrhea** (fatty stools) may result from impairment of fat absorption. Urine is typically dark in cases of biliary obstruction because of the increased

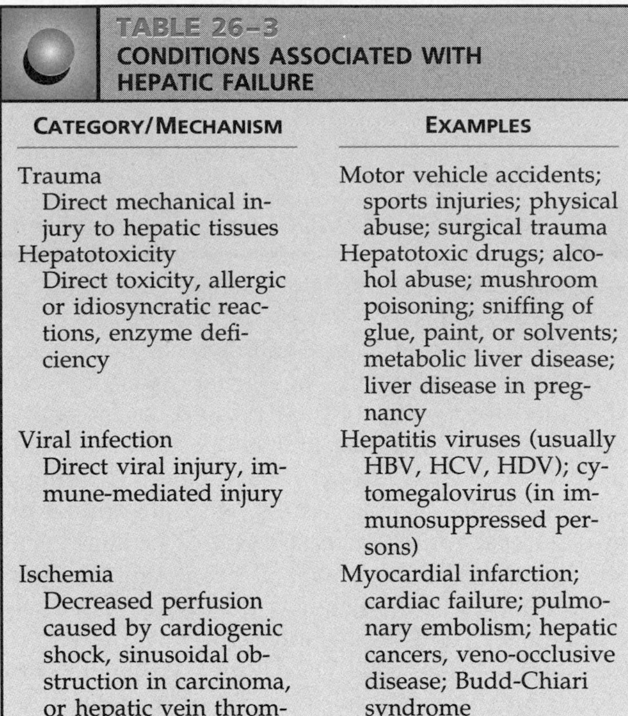

TABLE 26–3
CONDITIONS ASSOCIATED WITH HEPATIC FAILURE

CATEGORY/MECHANISM	EXAMPLES
Trauma Direct mechanical injury to hepatic tissues	Motor vehicle accidents; sports injuries; physical abuse; surgical trauma
Hepatotoxicity Direct toxicity, allergic or idiosyncratic reactions, enzyme deficiency	Hepatotoxic drugs; alcohol abuse; mushroom poisoning; sniffing of glue, paint, or solvents; metabolic liver disease; liver disease in pregnancy
Viral infection Direct viral injury, immune-mediated injury	Hepatitis viruses (usually HBV, HCV, HDV); cytomegalovirus (in immunosuppressed persons)
Ischemia Decreased perfusion caused by cardiogenic shock, sinusoidal obstruction in carcinoma, or hepatic vein thrombosis	Myocardial infarction; cardiac failure; pulmonary embolism; hepatic cancers, veno-occlusive disease; Budd-Chiari syndrome

Data from Lee, W.M. (1993). Acute liver failure. *New England Journal of Medicine* 329(25), 1862–1872.

TABLE 26–4
TOXIC REACTIONS OCCURRING IN THE LIVER

TYPE OF REACTION	EXAMPLES OF AGENTS
Direct reaction	Acetaminophen, carbon tetrachloride, mushrooms, phosphorus
Idiosyncratic reaction	Isoniazid, disulfiram, propylthiouracil*
Toxic–allergic reaction	Halothane, isoflurane, ticrynafen
Allergic hepatitis	Phenytoin, amoxicillin–clavulanic acid, sulfonamides
Cholestatic reaction	Chlorpromazine, erythromycin estolate, estradiol, captopril, sulfonamides
Granulomatous reaction	Diltiazem, quinidine, phenytoin, procainamide
Chronic hepatitis	Nitrofurantoin, methyldopa, isoniazid, trazodone
Alcoholic hepatitis–like reaction	Amiodarone, perhexiline maleate, valproic acid
Microvesicular steatosis	Tetracyclines, aspirin, zidovudine, didanosine, fialuridine
Fibrosis or cirrhosis alone	Methotrexate, vitamin A, methyldopa
Veno-occlusive disease	Cyclophosphamide, other chemotherapeutic agents, herbal teas
Ischemic damage	Cocaine, sustained-release nicotinic acid, methylenedioxyamphetamine

*There are hundreds of other agents that can cause idiosyncratic reactions.

From Lee, W.M. (1995). Drug-induced hepatotoxicity. *New England Journal of Medicine* 333(17), 1119.

fraction of bilirubin that must be excreted by this route. Hyperbilirubinemia, which may also result from nonhepatic causes, is detailed later in this chapter.

Drug toxicity is common as a result of impaired biotransformation. Elevated levels of hormones such as antidiuretic hormone and aldosterone may contribute to fluid overload and electrolyte imbalance. Serum levels of estrogens may be elevated, resulting in vascular changes (e.g., angiomata, redness of the nose, and palmar erythema, or redness of the hands) and feminization in males (e.g., gynecomastia, decreased pubic and axillary hair, testicular atrophy, and decreased libido).

Cardiovascular and Hematopoietic Systems. Cardiovascular effects may include edema and bleeding tendencies as a result of decreased synthesis of clotting factors and albumin. Anemia in hepatic failure is caused by decreased storage of vitamin B_{12} and iron and by increased removal of RBCs from the circulation by the engorged spleen (see Chapter 12). Splenomegaly may also result in leukopenia and thrombocytopenia.

If inflammation or scarring of the liver is obstructive to portal venous inflow, **portal hypertension** results, leading in turn to engorgement of the spleen and collateral veins, including those of the esophagus, gastric fundus, and rectum (Fig. 26–6). High venous pressure leads to twisting and bulging of these veins, producing **esophageal varices** or hemorrhoids. Increased esophageal venous pressure (above 12 mm Hg) may lead to significant gastrointestinal bleeding with rupture of varices.

Elevated portal venous pressure also leads to **ascites** (Fig. 26–7). Ascites is third spacing of vascular fluid into the peritoneal cavity that results from altered capillary dynamics (see Chapter 8). Increased capillary hydrostatic pressure in hepatic failure results from several factors, including high venous pressure and dilation of the splanchnic circulation in response to local mediators such as glucagon, prostaglandins, endotoxins, and nitric oxide.[6] Peripheral vasodilation also occurs, leading to decreased systemic vascular resistance and stimulation of the renin–angiotensin–aldosterone system (RAAS). RAAS activation results in renal retention of sodium

TABLE 26-5
LIVER FUNCTION TESTS

SERUM PARAMETER	NORMAL RANGE	SIGNIFICANCE OF ABNORMALITY
Bilirubin	Total: 0.5–1.2 mg/dL Unconjugated (indirect): <1.1 mg/dL Conjugated (direct): <0.5 mg/dL	Elevation may indicate: Physiologic jaundice (in newborns) Hemolysis Cholestasis Hepatocellular disease
Serum aminotransferase enzymes	Alanine aminotransferase (ALT): 0–50 U/L (formerly SGPT) Aspartate aminotransferase (AST): 0–50 U/L (formerly SGOT)	Elevated in hepatocellular disease and disease of other organs; ALT is more specific for liver and has a longer serum half-life; ALT:AST ratio >2 may indicate alcoholic hepatitis Depression in patients with end-stage renal disease caused by endogenous inhibitors or vitamin B_6 deficiency may mask presence of liver disease
L-Lactate dehydrogenase (LDH)	Total: 45–90 U/L LD1: 14%–26% LD2: 29%–39% LD3: 20%–26% LD4: 8%–16% LD5: 6%–16%	LD4 and LD5 are more specific for liver disease; elevation may also indicate hemolysis
Alkaline phosphatase (ALP)	0–250 U/L	Low normal (<100 U/L) in Wilson's disease; elevation in cholestatic liver disease, bone turnover, and pregnancy; enzyme source may be determined by heat fractionation
Gamma-glutamyl transpeptidase (GGT or GGTP)	0–250 U/L	Elevation indicates cholestatic liver disease or acute pancreatitis

Data from Neuschwander-Tetri, B.A. (1995). Common blood tests for liver disease: Which ones are most useful? *Postgraduate Medicine* 98(1), 49–63.

and water, which further increases capillary hydrostatic pressure in a positive feedback loop. Patients with ascites are prone to develop **spontaneous bacterial peritonitis,** in which there is no obvious intra-abdominal source of infection (see Chapter 24).[7] Bacteremia is believed to be the route of infection and may be associated with invasive procedures, leukopenia, complement deficiency, impaired monocyte-macrophage function, and impaired opsonization of bacteria caused by protein deficiency in ascitic fluid.[6]

Respiratory System. Respiratory function may be impaired in hepatic failure because of ascites, which impedes ventilation, or because of adult respiratory distress syndrome resulting from sepsis (see Chapter 19). **Hepatopulmonary syndrome,** manifested by pulmonary microvascular dilation and oxygen diffusion impairment, may lead to acute respiratory failure.[8] In this syndrome, hypoxemia occurs because oxygen cannot effectively diffuse across the increased distance to the center stream of dilated capillaries, where most RBCs normally flow.

Renal System. Renal failure may occur because of **hepatorenal syndrome,** in which renal perfusion is decreased as a result of vascular consequences of portal hypertension. Decreased renal perfusion and glomerular filtration lead to oliguria and azotemia (see Chapter 20). The failing kidneys are structurally intact during this syndrome, and renal failure subsides if hepatic function can be restored. Hepatorenal syndrome may be triggered by overaggressive diuretic therapy, GI bleeding, or use of aminoglycoside antibiotics (e.g., gentamicin or tobramycin) or nonsteroidal anti-inflammatory drugs (NSAIDs), which are hepatotoxic and nephrotoxic.[6]

Nervous System. Neurologic effects of hepatic failure include peripheral neuropathy caused by deficiency of vitamins B_6 and B_{12} (see Chapter 23) and **hepatic encephalopathy** (also known as portal systemic encephalopathy). Encephalopathy manifests early as degeneration of handwriting ability, **asterixis** (a characteristic tremor of the upper extremity often referred to as "liver flap"), increased disorientation, agitation, combativeness, and later as **hepatic coma.**

The precise etiologic mechanism of hepatic en-

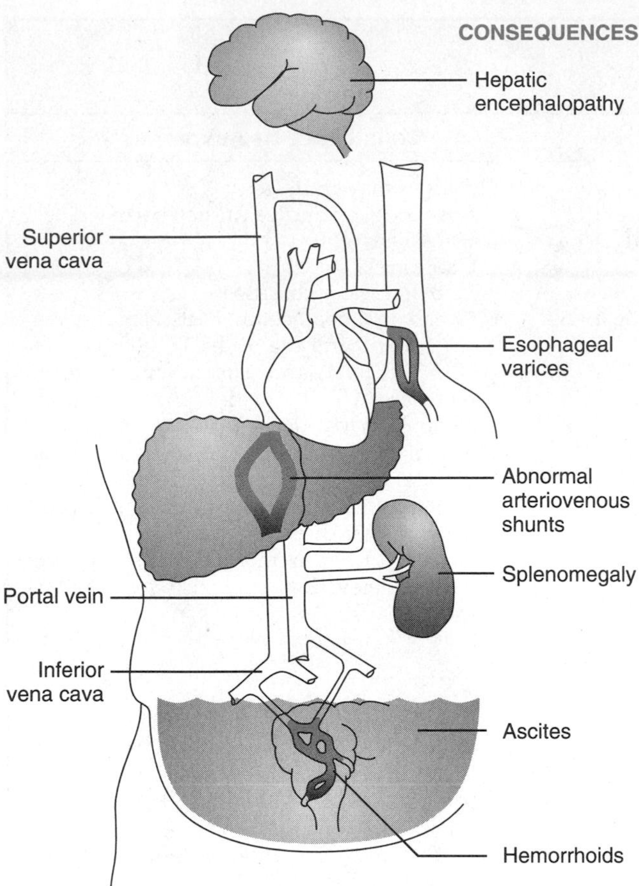

FIGURE 26–6

Consequences of portal hypertension. Elevation of portal venous pressure results from increased resistance to blood flow within the liver caused by fibrosis and cirrhotic disruption of lobular structure. Portal hypertension leads to pressure-induced varicosity of collateral veins in the alimentary canal (e.g., *esophageal varices* and *hemorrhoids*), third spacing of fluid into the peritoneal cavity (*ascites*), engorgement of the spleen (*splenomegaly*), and development of arterovenous connections within scar tissue (*portosystemic venous shunts*). *Hepatic encephalopathy* often accompanies portal hypertension, because of the toxic effects of altered metabolism as blood bypasses the liver. (From Cotran, R.S., Kumar, V., and Robbins, S.L. [1994]. *Robbins Pathologic Basis of Disease.* [5th Ed.]. Philadelphia: W.B. Saunders. [p. 836].)

cephalopathy is unknown, but the principal hypothesis, the *ammonia intoxication hypothesis,* holds that accumulation of ammonia (NH_3) results in toxicity to central nervous system cells. Elevation of serum ammonia levels may be caused by (1) failure of hepatocytes to convert ammonia to urea for renal excretion; (2) bypass of the scarred, obstructive liver by collateral veins in the gut, leaving more NH_3 in the general circulation; and (3) GI bleeding, in which blood proteins in the bowel are converted to NH_3 by intestinal bacteria. An acute episode of GI bleeding is often the precipitating event in hepatic encephalopathy. Because serum ammonia levels often do not correlate well with the degree of encephalopathy, the ammonia hypothesis has been increasingly questioned.[2]

A second hypothesis, the *false neurotransmitter hypothesis,* suggests that encephalopathy results from a reduction in the ratio of branched-chain amino acids (e.g., valine, leucine, and isoleucine) to aromatic amino acids (e.g., methionine, phenylalanine, and tyrosine) in the plasma. This abnormality may lead to the synthesis of nonfunctional or "false" neurotransmitters and depletion of true neurotransmitters such as dopamine and norepinephrine. This hypothesis also lacks research evidence of its validity.

Newer hypotheses include the *multifactorial hypothesis,* which proposes that circulating neurotoxins such as mercaptans, fatty acids, and ammonia act together to induce encephalopathy. The *γ-aminobutyric acid (GABA) hypothesis* suggests that increased activity of the inhibitory neurotransmitter GABA mediates encephalopathy. The newest proposal, the *benzodiazepine hypothesis,* holds that endogenous benzodiazepines (similar in structure to diazepam) are increased in encephalopathy.[6] In severe encephalopathy, cerebral edema may be present, causing increased intracranial pressure (see Chapter 21).

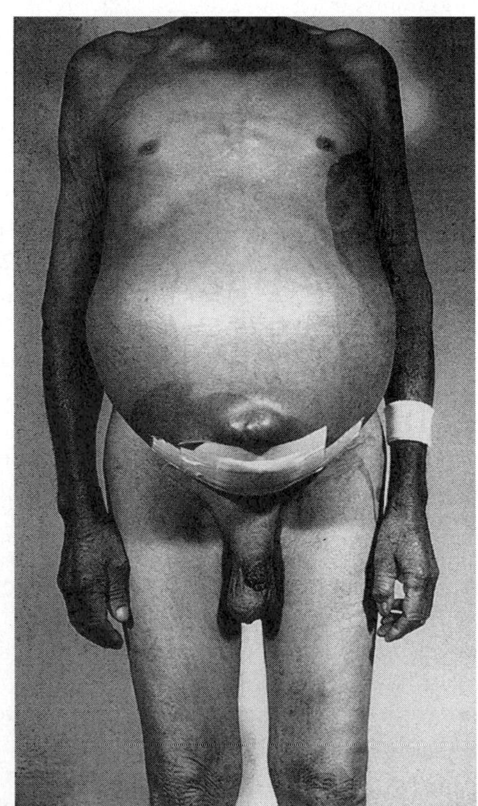

FIGURE 26–7

Ascites. Abdominal distention is caused by third spacing of fluid into the peritoneal cavity. (From Heuman, D.M., Scott Mills, A., and McGuire, H.H. [1997]. *Gastroenterology.* Philadelphia: W.B. Saunders. [p. 170].)

Prevention and Treatment. Prevention of hepatic failure depends on minimization of risk and optimal treatment of underlying conditions. Restriction of sodium and use of diuretics and β-blockers is standard therapy for minimizing portal hypertension. Elimination of precipitating factors for hepatic encephalopathy might involve prevention and treatment of GI bleeding, restriction of dietary protein, normalization of circulating blood volume and electrolyte status, discontinuation of hepatotoxic drugs or alcohol, or treatment of infection.

Treatment of hepatic failure is largely symptomatic and supportive and is focused on identification and management of the specific cause as well as general support of the patient, who may be critically ill. Nutritional supplementation and circulatory support are paramount. If serum ammonia levels are elevated, the antibiotic neomycin (Mycifradin) may be administered to decrease NH_3 production by intestinal bacteria. Lactulose (Cephulac, Chronulac), an osmotic agent that also lowers intestinal pH, may be administered orally or rectally to convert ammonia to ammonium (NH_4^+), which cannot be absorbed from the gut.

The treatment of choice for bleeding esophageal varices is now endoscopic rubber-band ligation, similar to the treatment of hemorrhoids (see Chapter 24).[9] Injection of sclerosing agents such as sodium tetradecyl sulfate has also been widely used. Other methods, including administration of vasoconstrictor agents (e.g., arginine vasopressin or octreotide, a somastatin analog) and balloon tamponade of bleeding vessels are now less frequently used.

Ascites may be treated with dietary sodium restriction, diuretic therapy, or therapeutic paracentesis (removal of ascitic fluid via a catheter inserted into the peritoneal cavity). Paracentesis may lead to protein depletion, however, and the resulting complement deficiency may predispose the patient to bacterial infection. Surgical shunting of ascitic fluid from the peritoneal cavity to the venous system (e.g., LeVeen or Denver shunts) are now less frequently used than they were in the 1980s, because of the frequency of shunt malfunctions and surgical complications.[10] Transjugular intrahepatic postosystemic shunt (TIPS) is a procedure in which a catheter is placed in the right hepatic vein via a jugular approach and advanced through the liver parenchyma to the main branch of the portal vein. A tubular stent is then deployed to maintain a tract between the two vessels.[11] TIPS may be used as a salvage procedure when other interventions for portal hypertension and bleeding varices fail or as a bridge to liver transplantation.

Liver transplantation offers the best survival rates in hepatic failure, but because of its significant risk, it is generally pursued only after all available therapies have been exhausted and spontaneous recovery of the patient is doubtful.[6] Indications for liver transplantation are listed in Table 26–6. Absolute contraindications to the procedure include malignancy or infection outside the biliary system, acquired immunodeficiency syndrome (AIDS), and severe cardiorespiratory compromise. Complications of organ transplantation are discussed in Chapter 13. Experimental therapies in which the failing liver is supported temporarily with artificial assist devices, porcine grafts, or partial grafts from living donors have shown some promise (See Focus of Current Research).

Prognosis and Outcome. Outcomes of treatment in hepatic failure have generally been very poor. The overall mortality rate in those with acute liver failure approaches 80%.[3] In those undergoing liver transplantation, 1-year survival now exceeds 75%.[10] Lifelong immunosuppression is required to prevent graft rejection.

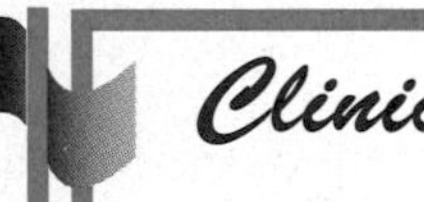

Clinical Scenario

J.S., a 22-year-old female, is admitted to the Emergency Department after the intentional ingestion of 60 acetominophen (Tylenol) tablets. On admission, she is responsive but seems very depressed. She admits having been despondent over a recent breakup with her boyfriend. J.S.'s vital signs were normal on admission. Blood was drawn for laboratory testing. J.S. is treated with administration of N-acetylcysteine (Mucomyst).

1. What additional information should be obtained through interviewing J.S. or family members or friends?
2. What are the physiologic consequences of acetaminophen toxicity?

Cirrhosis

Definition. Cirrhosis refers to a progressive tissue response to chronic (never acute) liver injury resulting in extensive hepatic fibrosis and regenerative nodules disrupting the parenchymal architecture of the entire liver.[11]

Epidemiology. Cirrhosis, which culminates in hepatic failure, is the ninth leading cause of death in the United States, with an age-adjusted death rate of 10.4 per 100,000.[12] Alcohol abuse is associated with 45% of deaths caused by cirrhosis. **Laënnec's cirrho-**

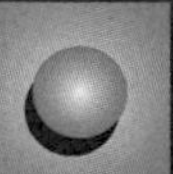

TABLE 26-6
INDICATIONS FOR LIVER TRANSPLANTATION

- Diseases associated with fulminant hepatic failure
  - Viral hepatitis, A, B, B+D; and unknown viruses
  - Drug or toxin-induced liver injury
  - Wilson's disease
  - Acute fatty liver of pregnancy
- End-stage liver disease
  - Hepatocellular disease
    - Autoimmune chronic hepatitis
    - Chronic viral hepatitis
    - Chronic drug-induced hepatitis
    - Alcoholic cirrhosis
    - α_1-antitrypsin deficiency
    - Wilson's disease
  - Cholestatic disorders
    - Primary biliary cirrhosis
    - Sclerosing cholangitis
    - Secondary biliary cirrhosis
    - Arteriohepatic dysplasia
    - Cystic fibrosis
  - Vascular disorders
    - Budd-Chiari syndrome
    - Veno-occlusive disease
  - Miscellaneous
    - Polycystic liver disease
    - Congenital hepatic fibrosis
  - Metabolic disorders
    - Hemochromatosis
    - Tyrosinemia
    - Glycogen storage disease
    - Familial hypercholesterolemia
- Malignancy
  - Primary hepatic malignancy
    - Some hepatocellular carcinomas
    - Fibrolamellar hepatocellular carcinomas
    - Some cholangiocarcinomas
    - Some hemangioendotheliomas
    - Some angiosarcomas
  - Selected metastatic disorders
    - Gastrinomas
    - Carcinoid tumors

Reprinted from Zetterman, R.K. (1994). Primary care management of the liver transplant patient. *American Journal of Medicine* 96(1A suppl.), 1A-11S. Copyright 1994, with permission from Excerpta Medica, Inc.

sis occurs in 25% of the more than 15 million persons in the United States who abuse alcohol. Cirrhosis and alcoholic liver disease are not synonymous, however. **Biliary cirrhosis** results from either prolonged obstruction of biliary ducts (caused by such disorders as congenital biliary atresia or common bile duct stones) or from ascending infection of gallbladder origin (**cholecystitis**). **Postnecrotic cirrhosis** is an increasingly common complication of hepatitis, most often chronic hepatitis B or C infection, but also seen occasionally with exposure to hepatotoxic drugs or chemicals. **Cardiac cirrhosis** is an uncommon complication of chronic hepatomegaly associated with cardiac failure (see Chapter 16).

Etiology. The precise mechanisms by which chronic hepatic injury progresses to cirrhosis are not well understood. The degree of hepatic tissue disruption does not correlate well with the magnitude of exposure to the toxic agent, and in some cases there is no known exposure to such an agent. The toxic effects of alcohol on the liver are the result of alteration of metabolic pathways, direct effects on cell and organelle membranes and on mitochondrial function, generation of reactive oxygen species, and induction of autoimmune attack on hepatic proteins (see later discussion of alcoholism). Concurrent presence of malnutrition, common in those who abuse alcohol, exacerbates the disease process. In cardiac cirrhosis, the mechanism of injury is pressure trauma caused by chronic engorgement of the liver with blood, a "backward" effect of right ventricular failure.

Pathophysiology. Hepatic fibrosis, or scarring, is the initial process in the development of cirrhosis. The scar is formed from an increase in extracellular matrix components consisting of fibril-forming collagens, proteoglycans, fibronectin, and hyaluronic acid (see Chapter 2).[13] The predominant site of collagen deposition within the liver varies depending on the etiologic agent. The amount of collagen in the cirrhotic liver may approach six times normal. In addition, the composition of the matrix within the space of Disse is altered, eventually impairing the function of hepatocytes because of altered membrane transport and tissue matrix signaling. The risk of neoplastic transformation of hepatocytes is increased under these conditions.

Fat-storing cells (lipocytes or Ito cells) found around the circumference of the space of Disse are believed to be the source of the altered matrix components (Fig. 26–8). When activated, these cells undergo transformation to smooth-muscle–like, protein-secreting cells. Contraction of these cells may also contribute to disruption of the lobular architecture and obstruction of the flow of blood or bile. Lipocyte activation is preceded by macrophage infiltration, and this response may be triggered by inflammation or cellular necrosis induced by oxidative injury. Activated lipocytes also express receptors for stimulatory cytokines, which promote fibrin formation and deposition. Vitamin A derivatives (retinoids) and tissue matrix proteins may also play a role in the regulation of the cascade of cellular events that results in cirrhosis.

Cellular changes in cirrhosis lead to bands of scar tissue that disrupt the lobular structure. Regenerative processes produce nodules of functional hepatocytes interspersed within scar tissue (Fig. 26–9). Bili-

Focus of Current Research

Study	Objective and Findings
Zein, et al. (1996) Hepatitis C virus genotypes in the United States: Epidemiology, pathogenicity, and response to interferon therapy.	*Objective:* To determine the geographic distribution and clinical significance of hepatitis C (HCV) genotypes in the United States and the influence of these on response to interferon therapy *Findings:* Genotypes 1a and 1b are most prevalent and are associated with more severe liver disease and lower rates of response to therapy.
Tanaka, et al. (1996) Effect of hepatitis G virus infection on chronic hepatitis C.	*Objective:* To clarify the effect of hepatitis G virus (HGV) infection on chronic HCV *Findings:* Patients who had only HCV infection did not differ from those with HCV and HGV coinfection. HGV, a newly cloned virus, closely resembles HCV.
Gane, et al. (1996) Long-term outcome of hepatitis C infection after liver transplantation.	*Objective:* To investigate the impact of persistent HCV infection after liver transplantation *Findings:* After 5 years, the rates of graft and overall survival are similar between patients with and those without HCV infection.
Besson, et al. (1995) Sclerotherapy with or without octreotide for acute variceal bleeding.	*Objective:* To compare sclerotherapy alone with sclerotherapy and octreotide, a splanchnic vasoconstrictor agent, in control of acute bleeding and prevention of early rebleeding in patients with cirrhosis and esophageal varices *Findings:* Combination treatment is more effective than sclerotherapy alone in controlling acute bleeding, but there is no difference in overall mortality with the two approaches to treatment.
Gejman, et al. (1994) No structural mutation in the dopamine D_2 receptor gene in alcoholism or schizophrenia.	*Objective:* To examine the dopamine D_2 receptor (*DRD2*) gene coding sequences for abnormalities associated with schizophrenia or alcoholism *Findings:* No coding abnormalities were found using denaturing gradient gel electrophoresis.
Miller (1994) Hemochromatosis, multiorgan hemosiderosis, and coronary artery disease.	*Objective:* To examine the prevalence of coronary artery disease in autopsies of patients with iron-overload syndromes *Findings:* Iron overload is not associated with an increased prevalence of coronary artery disease.

Box continued on following page

Study	*Objective and Findings*
Sempos, et al. (1994) Body iron stores and the risk of coronary heart disease.	*Objective:* To assess the association between higher body iron stores and the risk of coronary heart disease *Findings:* There may be an inverse association of iron stores with overall mortality and with mortality from cardiovascular causes.
Chari, et al. (1994) Brief report: Treatment of hepatic failure with ex vivo pig-liver perfusion followed by liver transplantation.	*Objective:* To describe the use of an artificial liver combining synthetic material and active pig hepatocytes *Findings:* In four critically ill patients, the artificial liver was used successfully as a bridge to transplantation in one patient. Three patients died.

ary outflow and portal venous inflow may be obstructed. Hepatic failure occurs with end-stage cirrhosis.

Clinical Manifestations. Manifestations are those of hepatic failure.

Prevention and Treatment. Abstinence from alcohol and attention to optimal nutrition constitute prevention of Laënnec's cirrhosis. Intervention in alcoholism is discussed subsequently. Similarly, in other forms of cirrhosis, reduction of risk factors and treatment of the underlying condition are warranted. Hepatic failure is treated as discussed in the preceding section.

Prognosis and Outcome. Outcome of cirrhosis depends on its severity and the responsiveness of the underlying condition to treatment. Fibrotic damage in cirrhosis is irreversible. Hepatic failure, with ascites, variceal bleeding, and hepatic encephalothy develops in a significant number of patients with cirrhosis. In a few cases, hepatocellular carcinoma is the cause of death.

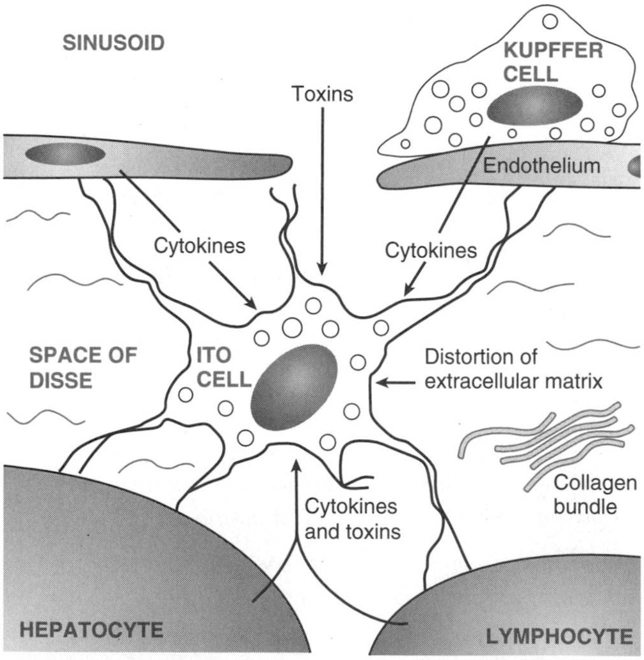

FIGURE 26–8
Increased collagen production in cirrhosis. Hepatic lipocytes (*Ito cells*), which normally store fats within the liver, become transformed to collagen-producing cells in cirrhosis. Possible mechanisms of this transformation include signals from disrupted extracellular matrix proteins, endothelial cytokines, Kupffer cells, hepatocytes, toxins, and inflammatory cells such as lymphocytes. (From Cotran, R.S., Kumar, V., and Robbins, S.L. [1994]. *Robbins Pathologic Basis of Disease.* [5th Ed.]. Philadelphia: W.B. Saunders, [p. 835].)

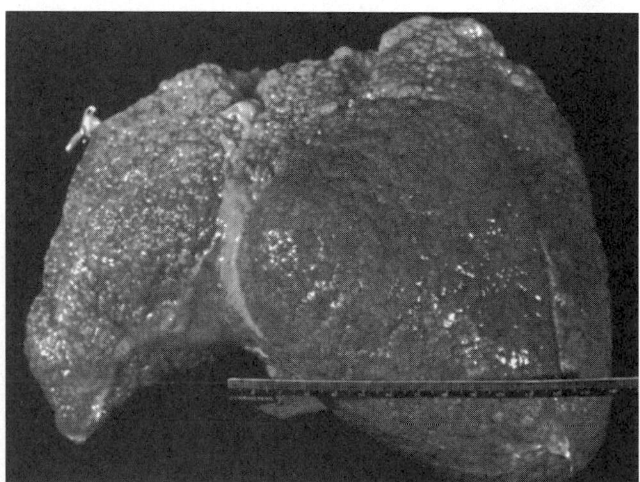

FIGURE 26–9
Alcoholic (Laënnec's) cirrhosis. Diffuse nodularity is evident, induced by underlying fibrous scarring. (From Cotran, R.S., Kumar, V., and Robbins, S.L. [1994]. *Robbins Pathologic Basis of Disease.* [5th Ed.]. Philadelphia: W.B. Saunders. [p. 859].)

Hyperbilirubinemia

Definition. Hyperbilirubinemia is elevation of total serum bilirubin above 1.2 mg/dL.[14] Jaundice is apparent when levels rise above 2.0 to 2.5 mg/dL, and hyperbilirubinemia is considered to be significant when serum bilirubin levels exceed 15 mg/dL.[1]

Epidemiology. Jaundice develops in more than 50% of newborns.[1] Many normal newborns develop **physiologic jaundice** as a consequence of developmental factors, and risk is even higher among premature infants. Breast feeding is also associated with higher bilirubin levels, as is Asian heritage. Other maternal and neonatal risk factors for significant jaundice are listed in Table 26–7. Risk factors for **pathologic jaundice,** which is hyperbilirubinemia persisting beyond the neonatal period or developing in older children or adults, are those related to the specific underlying conditions, are listed in Table 26–8.

Etiology. Hyperbilirubinemia results from increased bilirubin production, decreased bilirubin excretion, or a combination of these two mechanisms. Measurable bilirubin in the blood consists of unconjugated (termed *indirect* because of the assay method) and conjugated (*direct*) forms. Unconju-

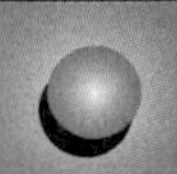

TABLE 26–7
RISK FACTORS FOR NEONATAL JAUNDICE

Infant History
Abdominal distention
Delayed passage of meconium
Lethargy
Light stools, dark urine
Low Apgar scores
Poor feeding, weight loss
Vomiting

Infant Physical Examination
Bruising
Cephalhematoma
Congenital anomalies
Hepatosplenomegaly
Pallor, petechiae
Small or large for gestational age

Maternal History
Chorioamnionitis
Delivery by forceps or vacuum extraction
Diabetes mellitus
Difficult delivery
Exposure to certain drugs during pregnancy
Failure to receive immune globulin in previous pregnancy or abortion that involved risk of isoimmunization
Family history of jaundice, anemia, liver disease, or splenectomy
Greek or Asian
Pre-eclampsia
Unexplained illness during pregnancy

From Lasker, M.R., and Holzman, I.R. (1996). Neonatal jaundice: When to treat, when to watch and wait. *Postgraduate Medicine* 99(3), 191. Used with permission.

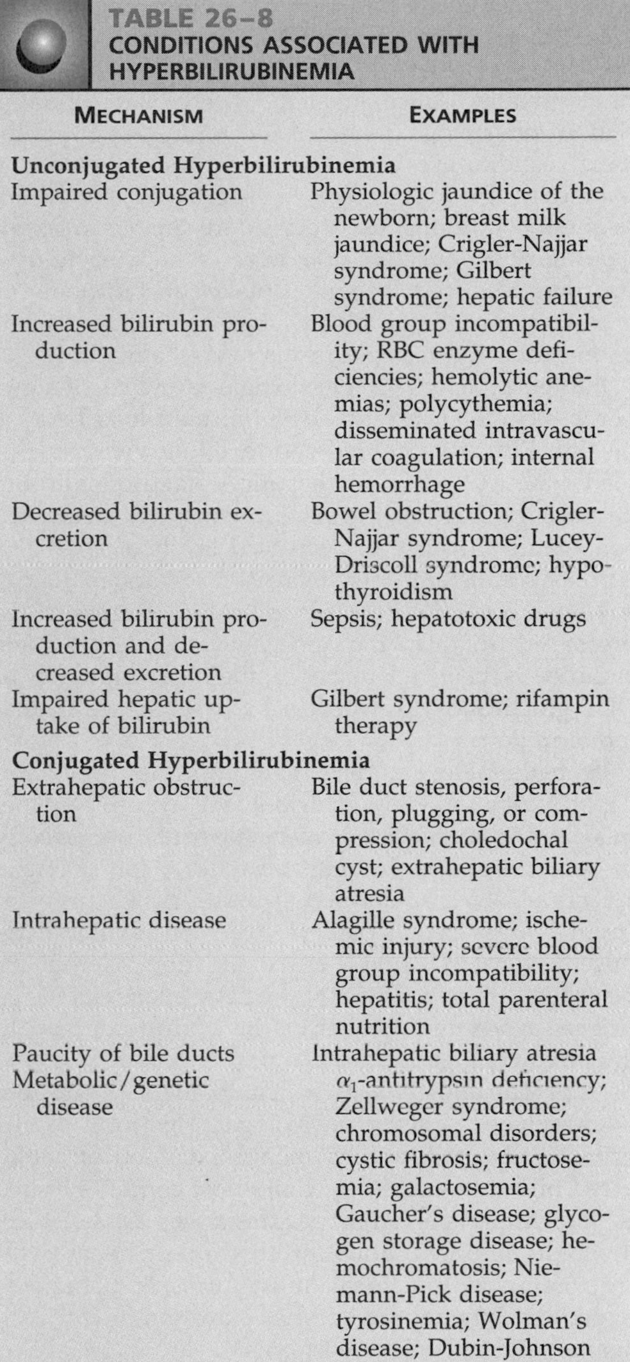

TABLE 26–8
CONDITIONS ASSOCIATED WITH HYPERBILIRUBINEMIA

MECHANISM	EXAMPLES
Unconjugated Hyperbilirubinemia	
Impaired conjugation	Physiologic jaundice of the newborn; breast milk jaundice; Crigler-Najjar syndrome; Gilbert syndrome; hepatic failure
Increased bilirubin production	Blood group incompatibility; RBC enzyme deficiencies; hemolytic anemias; polycythemia; disseminated intravascular coagulation; internal hemorrhage
Decreased bilirubin excretion	Bowel obstruction; Crigler-Najjar syndrome; Lucey-Driscoll syndrome; hypothyroidism
Increased bilirubin production and decreased excretion	Sepsis; hepatotoxic drugs
Impaired hepatic uptake of bilirubin	Gilbert syndrome; rifampin therapy
Conjugated Hyperbilirubinemia	
Extrahepatic obstruction	Bile duct stenosis, perforation, plugging, or compression; choledochal cyst; extrahepatic biliary atresia
Intrahepatic disease	Alagille syndrome; ischemic injury; severe blood group incompatibility; hepatitis; total parenteral nutrition
Paucity of bile ducts	Intrahepatic biliary atresia
Metabolic/genetic disease	α_1-antitrypsin deficiency; Zellweger syndrome; chromosomal disorders; cystic fibrosis; fructosemia; galactosemia; Gaucher's disease; glycogen storage disease; hemochromatosis; Niemann-Pick disease; tyrosinemia; Wolman's disease; Dubin-Johnson syndrome; Rotor's syndrome

Adapted with permission from Lasker, M.R., and Holzman, I.R. (1996). Neonatal jaundice: When to treat, when to watch and wait. *Postgraduate Medicine* 99(3), 189–190. Additional data from Cotran, R.S., Kumar, V., and Robbins, S.L. (1994). *Robbins Pathologic Basis of Disease.* (5th Ed.). Philadelphia: W.B. Saunders. (p. 840).

gated bilirubin not bound to albumin is not measurable, but represents a small fraction of serum bilirubin. In most cases of hyperbilirubinemia, one form predominates. Unconjugated hyperbilirubinemia is seen in physiologic jaundice and a number of pathologic conditions, including hemolysis, hereditary liver diseases, and hepatic failure (see Table 26–8). In these conditions, hepatocytes are unable to conjugate bilirubin effectively because of hepatocyte dysfunction, reduced hepatic uptake of bilirubin, or excessive production of bilirubin, so that the conjugation capacity of hepocytes is overwhelmed.

Etiologic factors in physiologic jaundice of newborns include (1) an increased bilirubin load because of high RBC volume and shortened survival time of fetal RBCs; (2) deficient hepatic uptake of bilirubin because of lack of carrier proteins; (3) decreased conjugation because of decreased levels of UDP-glucuronosyltransferase; (4) increased enterohepatic circulation; and (5) deficient bilirubin excretion.[1] In breast-fed infants, the mechanism of physiologic jaundice is believed to be competitive inhibition of UDP-glucuronosyltransferase by a substance in maternal milk.[15]

In pathologic jaundice, hemolysis and impaired hepatic function may contribute to hyperbilirubinemia, and both factors may be present concurrently in some etiologies. In hepatic failure, for example, splenomegaly may induce increased RBC turnover, whereas impaired hepatocyte function results in reduced bilirubin uptake or conjugation. Hereditary disorders of glucuronosyltransferase activity (e.g., Gilbert syndrome, Crigler-Najjar syndrome) lead to impaired conjugation.

Hyperbilirubinemia in which conjugated bilirubin predominates is never physiologic. This form results primarily from decreased biliary excretion of conjugated bilirubin caused by cholestatic conditions such as cholelithiasis and biliary atresia (see Table 26–8). It should be noted, however, that unless hepatocytes are totally nonfunctional, most forms of pathologic hyperbilirubinemia manifest as elevation of *both* conjugated and unconjugated forms.

Pathophysiology. Bilirubin accumulates in the blood because of increased production within the plasma or because impaired biliary secretion promotes hepatic excretion into the blood rather than into the bile. Unconjugated bilirubin is lipid soluble and primarily bound to albumin. In this form, it cannot be excreted in the urine. The small fraction of free bilirubin is able to cross the immature blood–brain barrier of neonates, potentially damaging brain tissue. The adult brain is normally protected from bilirubin toxicity. Deposition of unconjugated bilirubin in the lipid tissues of the skin and the sclerae of the eyes occurs, producing visible jaundice. Intestinal malabsorption of lipids and fat-soluble vitamins may be present in cases of impaired biliary excretion (see Chapter 25). Hemolytic conditions are accompanied by anemia and impaired tissue oxygenation (see Chapter 12).

Clinical Manifestations. With physiologic jaundice, serum bilirubin rarely exceeds 15 mg/dL before returning to normal levels within 7 to 10 days.[15] In breast-fed babies, some degree of jaundice persists as long as the baby is breast-fed. Jaundice of severe intensity or extending to the baby's feet warrants checking of the serum bilirubin level and possible exploration for pathologic factors.

In severe pathologic jaundice, bilirubin levels may rise as high as 30 to 40 mg/dL.[12] In unconjugated hyperbilirubinemia, the urine is pale, whereas in predominantly conjugated hyperbilirubinemia, it is dark (tea-colored). Stool is pale in hyperbilirubinemia because of impaired biliary excretion, and steatorrhea may be present as a result of fat malabsorption. Pruritus often accompanies jaundice, probably because of retained bile acids, and cholesterol deposits (xanthomata) may also form in the skin. Hepatic enzymes may be altered in a pattern characteristic of the underlying disorder (see Table 26–5). Bilirubin-induced brain injury (**kernicterus** or bilirubin encephalopathy) in newborns may manifest as seizures, spasticity or hypotonia, high-pitched cry, paresis of upward gaze, and hearing loss.

Prevention and Treatment. Prevention of hyperbilirubinemia requires reduction of risk factors for the underlying conditions. Physiologic jaundice in term newborns is not preventable, and discontinuation of breast feeding is usually not warranted.[1] Phenobarbital, which induces UDP-glucuronosyltransferase, may be used to decrease conjugated bilirubin concentrations. Periodic exposure of the infant to blue light (wavelength of 430 to 500 nm) reduces bilirubin levels by converting bilirubin to a more water-soluble structure, enhancing its excretion. Phototherapy may be done in the hospital nursery or at home. Emergent treatment of severe hyperbilirubinemia in infants requires exchange transfusion to remove bilirubin and its RBC sources (see Chapter 12). Pruritus is treated supportively (see Chapter 36), and, in pathologic jaundice, definitive treatment of the underlying disorder is of primary importance.

Prognosis and Outcome. Physiologic jaundice of the newborn is a benign condition. Bilirubin encephalopathy in otherwise healthy infants is not associated with long-term neurologic deficits. This condition in premature or otherwise at-risk infants may result in severe dysfunction or death.[1] Prognosis in pathologic jaundice depends on the nature and severity of the underlying disorder.

Cholelithiasis

Definition. Cholelithiasis is the disorder resulting from formation of obstructive stones (gallstones) within the gallbladder, cystic duct, or common bile duct.

Epidemiology. Cholelithiasis is very common, diagnosed in 10% to 20% of the U.S. population.[16] Many more individuals are believed to have asymptomatic stones. Gallstones are more common in women, and risk increases with age. Specific risk factors vary depending on the major constituent of the stones. For the more common cholesterol stones, individuals at highest risk are white, middle aged or older, viscerally obese, multiparous females. Persons of Native American and Mexican-American ancestry, those experiencing rapid weight loss or pregnancy, or those diagnosed with diabetes mellitus or Crohn's disease are also at higher risk. Iatrogenic factors increasing risk include major abdominal surgery, heart transplantation, and total parenteral nutrition.[17] Risk is also increased with increased triglyceride levels or decreased levels of high-density lipoprotein (HDL).[18] Pigmented stones are more common in individuals with cirrhosis of the liver, hemolytic disorders, and in those of Asian or African descent.

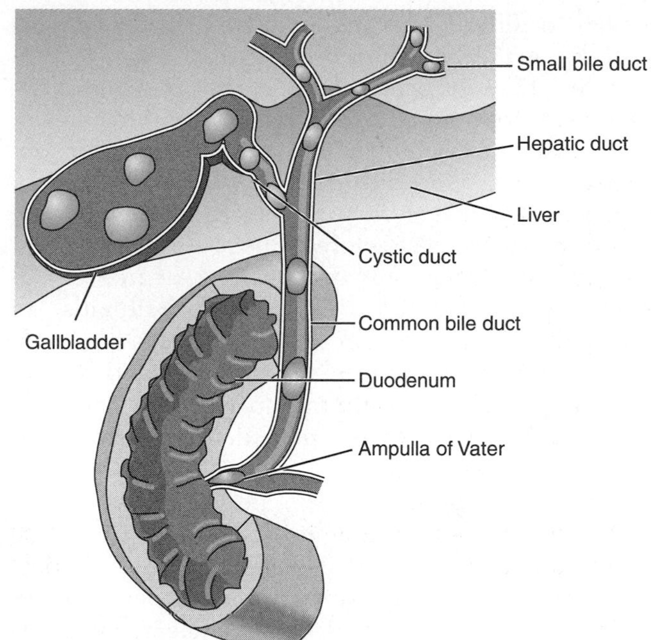

FIGURE 26–10

Common locations of gallstones. Gallstones are most commonly found within the gallbladder but pass into the common bile duct in 10% to 15% of cases. Stones obstructing the cystic, hepatic, or common bile ducts create obstruction to entry of bile into the duodenum, leading to cholestasis and malabsorption of lipids. A stone obstructing the ampulla of Vater may prevent passage of pancreatic enzymes into the duodenum, promoting malabsorption and increasing the risk of pancreatitis.

Etiology. In aqueous solutions such as bile, cholesterol will remain soluble as long as the concentration of bile salts and lecithin is adequate to sustain micelle formation.[19] Cholesterol stones form when bile becomes supersaturated with cholesterol. In the presence of a nucleating factor (probably gallbladder mucin or a lipoprotein) as well as a relative deficiency of antinucleating factors, insoluble crystals of cholesterol form and precipitate out of solution, forming "sludge." Stasis of bile then promotes growth of the crystals, forming cholesterol stones. The factors leading to supersaturation of bile with cholesterol are uncertain; however, increased biliary secretion is implicated in many associated conditions.

In pigmented stones, the unconjugated bilirubin content of the bile is increased as a result of impaired hepatic conjugation (as in cirrhosis), increased serum levels (as in hemolysis), or bacterial deconjugation (as in biliary tract infection). Because unconjugated bilirubin is less water soluble, it tends to precipitate out of solution in the bile, forming complexes with calcium (calcium bilirubinate).

Pathophysiology. Figure 26–10 illustrates usual locations of stones within the biliary system. Obstruction of the hepatic duct by stones leads to intrahepatic retention of bile and increased release of bilirubin into the bloodstream for eventual urinary excretion. Increased serum bilirubin levels lead to deposition of the pigment in lipid tissues. Cystic duct obstruction leads to inflammation of the gallbladder (cholecystitis) and a compensatory increase in gallbladder contraction and peristalsis within the duct. The inflamed, obstructed gallbladder may become greatly distended and ischemic, and it may perforate, leading to peritonitis. A gallstone obstructing the opening of the pancreatic duct into the common bile duct leads to retention of pancreatic enzymes within the gland, which may contribute to pancreatitis (see Chapter 25). Biliary obstruction prevents bile from entering the duodenum, resulting in impairment of the digestion and absorption of lipids.

Clinical Manifestations. Although many cases are asymptomatic, the most typical manifestation of cholelithiasis is steady pain in the right upper quadrant of the abdomen, particularly after ingestion of a high-fat meal. Pain will usually increase over 30 to 60 minutes, plateau over approximately 60 minutes, then gradually subside.[19] Careful assessment is essential to differentiate this pain from that of angina pectoris, hiatal hernia, and other conditions. Typical manifestations of acute cholecystitis are acute onset of severe abdominal pain, nausea, vomiting, fever, and leukocytosis. Jaundice is evident if stones obstruct the common bile duct (about 10% of cases). Other obstructive symptoms, such as elevation of serum bilirubin, clay-colored stools, steatorrhea, and dark urine, depend on the site and degree of obstruction and are not always seen. Peritonitis, an unusual complication of acute cholecystitis, may lead to septic shock (see Chapters 15 and 24). A minority of gallstones are radiopaque and visible on radiographs. Because of their density, most gallstones may be detected with ultrasonography, confirming the diagnosis.

Prevention and Treatment. Risk factors should be minimized as much possible. Maintenance of ideal body weight and adherence to a low-fat diet are known to reduce the incidence of cholelithiasis. Surgical and nonsurgical treatments may be used in the treatment of cholecystitis and symptomatic gallstones. Removal of the gallbladder (cholecystectomy) may be done with an open abdominal incision or through a laparoscope. Laparoscopic surgery is accomplished through very small incisions in the abdomen, through which specialized instruments are passed.[20] The abdominal cavity is inflated with carbon dioxide, allowing visualization of structures through the laparoscope, which is passed through another small incision. Such "Bandaid" surgery allows for shorter hospital stays and more rapid recovery; it may be done as an outpatient procedure in some cases. Obstructive stones in the ducts may be removed or crushed via laparoscopic procedures, dissolved with acidic drugs such as ursodeoxycholic acid (ursodiol), or mechanically fragmented with shock waves (extracorporeal shock wave lithotripsy).

Prognosis and Outcome. Surgical intervention in cholelithiasis is usually successful in reducing symptoms. Biliary function is usually normal, although some patients experience postcholecystectomy diarrhea or symptoms attributed to abnormal peristalsis within the biliary system (**biliary dyskinesia**).[21] When the gallbladder is removed, the liver contracts in response to hormonal and parasympathetic stimulation to release bile when fat is present in the duodenum. Pain similar to but usually much milder than that experienced in the preoperative state may persist. Signs such as belching, bloating, chronic pain, or intolerance of fatty foods are not attributable to removal of the gallbladder. The need for dietary modification may be lifelong. The rate of postoperative complications of laparoscopic surgery is approximately 0.5%,[20] and such complications include bile duct injury with possible obstruction or perforation. Oral dissolution therapy (e.g., ursodiol) has an 80% success rate with small (<5 mm in diameter) stones.[19]

Viral Hepatitis

Definition. Viral hepatitis is inflammation of the liver with necrosis of liver cells, caused by infection with one or more hepatoviruses, classified as hepatitis A, B, C, D, and E. Infection with hepatis G virus has recently been described; however, little is known as yet about this blood-borne virus.[22] Viral hepatitis is the most common form of hepatitis, although hepatitic inflammation may also result from other infectious agents, toxins, autoimmune phenomena, and metabolic defects. Less common forms of hepatitis are described in Table 26–9.

Epidemiology. Viral hepatitis is a reportable disease, with approximately 50,000 cases reported annually to the Centers for Disease Control and Prevention (see Chapter 1).[23] Because viral hepatitis is often asymptomatic, it is likely that many more cases are undiagnosed. Risk factors are specific to each class of virus (see next section).

Etiology. Hepatitis A (HAV), formerly known as infectious hepatitis, is found in contaminated food and water and is usually communicated via the enteric (fecal-oral) route. Poor handwashing technique or deficient food preparation or sanitation procedures increase the risk of transmission. Because the virus is in the serum briefly, it could also be transmitted through contact with the blood or other body fluids of an infected person, but this is believed to be unusual. Hepatitis B (HBV), formerly known as serum hepatitis, is transmitted via blood and body fluids, similarly to AIDS. Hepatitis C (HCV), "classic" hepatitis, is a blood-borne type of hepatitis formerly classified as non-A, non-B hepatitis. This form is common among treated hemophiliacs and individuals who abuse injectible drugs. Up to 40% of cases of HCV are idiopathic. Hepatitis D (HDV), delta hepatitis, is a blood-borne form that must coexist with HBV to exert its viral activity. This covirus worsens the course and outcome of illness with HBV. Hepatitis E (HEV), the enteric form of non-A, non-B hepatitis, is primarily seen in underdeveloped countries. Risk factors and modes of transmission of the hepatitis viruses are summarized in Table 26–10.

Pathophysiology. Hepatovirus infection results in one of five clinical syndromes: (1) carrier state; (2) asymptomatic infection; (3) acute hepatitis; (4) chronic hepatitis; or (5) fulminant hepatitis. Carriers harbor the virus and may transmit it, whether or not they are symptomatic. The carrier state is most

TABLE 26–9
LESS COMMON FORMS OF HEPATITIS

Disorder	Description
Alcoholic hepatitis	Usually induced acutely after a bout of heavy drinking in a patient who chronically abuses alcohol; often follows hepatic steatosis and precedes cirrhosis but may occur independently of either; cholestasis and jaundice are common; fibrosis is progressive with repeated attacks
Autoimmune hepatitis	Unresolving hepatocellular inflammation of unknown cause; associated with liver-associated autoantibodies in the serum and hypergammaglobulinemia
Toxic hepatitis	Results from exposure to a toxin or drug that causes direct injury or acts as a hapten and initiates immune-mediated injury
Nonalcoholic steatohepatitis	Histologic features similar to alcoholic hepatitis but no history of alcohol abuse; may be associated with toxicity from elevation of free fatty acids; most common in obese, middle-aged women
Neonatal hepatitis	General term for any disorder causing conjugated hyperbilirubinemia in neonates; idiopathic if toxic, metabolic, and infectious causes are ruled out
Liver abscesses	Manifestation of systemic parasitic infection; common in developing countries; highest risk in those who are immunosuppressed

often seen in children born of HBV-infected mothers and in HCV infection. Acute hepatitis may result from infection by any of the hepatoviruses. Virally induced inflammation leads to diffuse injury and necrosis of hepatocytes, hypertrophy and hyperplasia of Kuppfer cells and sinusoidal lining cells, and intrahepatic exudation of inflammatory fluid. In some patients, circulating immune complexes lead to systemic manifestations of inflammation. Hepatocytes usually retain the capacity to conjugate bilirubin, but its excretion in the bile may be obstructed.

Chronic hepatitis, defined by the continuous or recurrent evidence of hepatic inflammation for more than 6 months, is a common outcome of HBV and HCV infections. Chronic hepatitis imposes significant risk for later development of cirrhosis or hepatocellular carcinoma. Inflammation in chronic hepatitis is highly variable in severity. In some cases, the only evidence of inflammation is the spilling of hepatic enzymes into the blood, whereas in others the integrity of lobular structures is greatly disrupted. With extensive inflammation, fibrous scarring leads to cirrhosis. Fulminant hepatitis, which is rare, is defined by rapid progression from the onset of symptoms to overt liver failure within 2 to 3 weeks.

Clinical Manifestations. Except in HEV, viral hepatitis is evidenced by antigenic markers in the serum (Table 26–11). Detection of viral antigen or antibodies demonstrates exposure. However, because levels of these markers may be very low at times, failure to detect them does not necessarily rule out the disease. In most cases of hepatitis, clinical manifestations are mild. Fatigue, malaise, and anorexia are common systemic signs of hepatic inflammation. Jaundice may be present because of intrahepatic obstruction of bile caniliculi, and impaired hepatocyte function may lead to angiomata and palmar erythema. Signs of hepatic failure, including encephalopathy, are seen only with fulminant hepatitis.

Prevention and Treatment. Prevention of hepatitis is based on reduction of exposure risk with sanitation measures for enterically transmitted forms. Standard precautions are indicated to reduce risk of transmission of blood-borne forms (see Chapter 13). Intervention in high-risk behaviors is indicated. Active immunization against HAV has recently become available, and it is recommended for frequent international travelers, children in communities with high rates of HAV infection, male homosexuals with multiple partners, illicit drug users, patients with chronic liver disease, and those with clotting factor disorders.[24] Active immunization against HBV is advocated for those at risk of exposure to contaminated blood and body fluids. The Advisory Committee on Immunization Practices (ACIP) of the Centers for Disease Control and Prevention recommends the following: (1) routine vaccination of all infants; (2) screening for hepatitis B antigen (HBsAg) in pregnant women; and (3) vaccination of adolescents and adults at risk.[25] HAV immune globulin may be administered preventively to persons with known recent exposure or those traveling on short notice to areas where the virus is endemic. HBV immune globulin is used to convey some degree of passive immunity after known exposure to the virus.

Most cases of hepatitis are treated with rest and

TABLE 26-10
RISK FACTORS AND MODES OF TRANSMISSION IN VIRAL HEPATITIS

Virus	Risk Factors	Modes of Transmission
Hepatitis A (HAV)	Poor personal hygiene Poor sanitation Household contact Sexual contact Employment or attendance at a day care center International travel	Fecal-oral transmission via person-to-person contact Ingestion of contaminated food (e.g., raw shellfish or frozen foods) or water Parenteral transmission (rare)
Hepatitis B (HBV)	Homosexual contact Heterosexual contact Intravenous drug abuse Work in health care environment Transfusion of blood products Dialysis Tattooing or body piercing Forty per cent of those infected have no known risk factors	Exposure to infected blood or other body fluids Perinatal transmission (rare)
Hepatitis C (HCV)	Same as HBV	Exposure to infected blood or other body fluids Fecal-oral transmission (rare) Perinatal transmission (rare)
Hepatitis D (HDV)	Same as HBV HBV infection	Exposure to infected blood or other body fluids Perinatal transmission (rare)
Hepatitis E (HEV)	Same as HAV (in endemic regions)	Fecal-oral transmission Ingestion of contaminated drinking water

supportive care, because the illness is generally self-limited. α-Interferon may be used in the treatment of chronic HBV or HCV infections to stimulate the immune response and inhibit viral replication (see Chapter 13), and other antiviral agents are under development.[26] Liver transplantation may be beneficial in some cases of fulminant hepatitis with hepatic failure.

Prognosis and Outcome. Prognosis is favorable in most cases of hepatitis. HDV superinfection is associated with more severe HBV disease and higher mortality, as is the chronic hepatitis that may develop in a significant number of patients with HBV and HCV infections. Mortality in fulminant hepatitis is high because of complications of hepatic failure. Liver transplantation is frequently used in the treatment of chronic and fulminant hepatitis to reduce the risk of subsequent cirrhosis and hepatocellular carcinoma. Hepatitis may recur in the grafted liver, eventually resulting in rejection (see Chapter 13).

Alcoholism

Definition. Alcoholism is excessive or prolonged abuse of alcohol, resulting in dependence and impairment of biologic, interpersonal, or occupational function.[27]

Epidemiology. Alcohol (ethanol) is the drug most frequently abused throughout the world.[28] An estimated 15 to 20 million persons in the United States are alcoholics, and 20% to 40% of all individuals admitted to general hospitals have alcohol-related problems. Alcoholism affects adolescents to a significant degree, with an estimated 3 million abusers among this age group.[29] Prevalence among the elderly is similar to that of the general adult population, approximately 2% to 10%.[30]

Although women have traditionally consumed less alcohol than men, this gap is narrowing among younger drinkers. In women, smaller body size and a higher proportion of body fat promote higher blood alcohol levels than those in men who consume equal quantities. Younger women also have less activity of the enzyme alcohol dehydrogenase, and with less alcohol broken down in the stomach, more enters the bloodstream.[28] Heredity is a factor in the predisposition to alcoholism, accounting for individual differences in the rate of metabolism of alcohol as well as the severity of alcoholic liver disease. A consistent pattern of inheritance has not been observed, however. A genetic defect in the dopaminergic system has been hypothesized; however, recent research has failed to substantiate this (see Focus of Current Research).[31] In addition to family history, risk factors for the development of alcoholism include extreme poverty, family dysfunction, learning disability, and peer abuse of alcohol.[32]

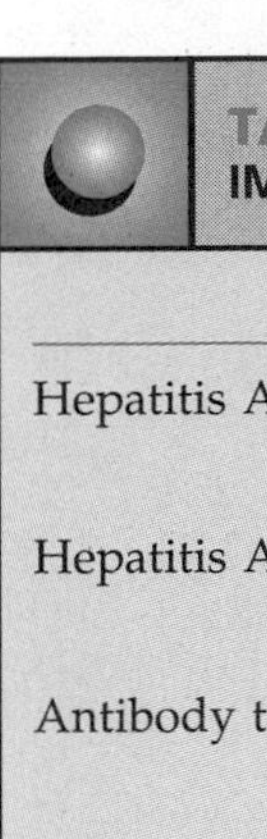

TABLE 26–11
IMMUNOLOGIC MARKERS OF HEPATITIS

Test	Interpretation of Positive Result
Hepatitis A IgM antibody (IgM anti-HAV)	Current or recent acute hepatitis A; detectable IgM typically persists for 4 to 6 months after infection but can persist for up to 12 months
Hepatitis A total antibody (total anti-HAV)	Current or previous HAV infection; test detects IgM and IgA early in course and predominantly IgG thereafter (little indication for use in individual patients)
Antibody to hepatitis B surface antigen (anti-HBs)	One of the following: • Previous exposure to hepatitis B and no active liver disease at present • Previous hepatitis B vaccination • Recent hepatitis B immune globulin prophylaxis • When present with HBsAg (unusual), indicates ineffective antibody and chronic hepatitis B
Hepatitis B surface antigen (HBsAg)	Acute or chronic hepatitis B; patient is infectious through sexual contact and blood exposure
Hepatitis B e antigen (HBeAg)	Acute or chronic hepatitis B with active viral replication
Antibody to hepatitis B e antigen (anti-HBe)	Suppression of hepatitis B viral replication
Hepatitis B core IgM antibody (IgM anti-HBc)	One of the following: • Current or recent hepatitis B (past 4 to 6 months) • Chronic hepatitis B with active viral replication (less common)
Hepatitis B core total antibody (total anti-HBc)	Previous hepatitis B; timing and chronicity unknown if both HBsAg and anti-HBs are not detected
Hepatitis B DNA (HBV DNA)	Acute or chronic hepatitis B
Hepatitis C antibody by enzyme immunoassay (anti-HCV by EIA)	Chronic hepatitis C (rarely detectable in acute hepatitis C)
Hepatitis C antibody by recombinant immunoblot assay (anti-HCV by RIBA)	Chronic hepatitis C (useful for evaluating suspected false-positive anti-HCV by EIA)
Hepatitis C RNA by polymerase chain reaction (HCV RNA by PCR)	Acute or chronic hepatitis C

Ig, immunoglobulin.
From Neuschwander-Tetri, B.A. (1995). Common blood tests for liver disease: Which ones are most useful? *Postgraduate Medicine* 98(1), 55. Used with permission.

Etiology. The precise etiology of alcoholism is unknown. It is likely that the disorder is multifactorial, with environmental and psychological factors superimposed on an inherited predisposition. Although individuals vary in their susceptibility to alcohol, most require an intake in excess of 80 g per day (i.e., eight 12-ounce beers, a liter of wine, or a half-pint of 80 proof whiskey).[33]

Pathophysiology. Alcoholism typically has a gradual onset and progresses for 10 to 20 years before severe manifestations are evident.[32] Because it is a small molecule that is soluble in water and lipids, alcohol permeates all body tissues.[28] Alcohol abuse contributes to diseases affecting all body systems (Table 26–12). The liver, which metabolizes 90% of the alcohol absorbed, is the organ most severely affected. Hepatic steatosis, followed by hepatic fibrosis, may be evident within days after heavy drinking.[28] Laënnec's cirrhosis may develop after an inflammatory response (*alcoholic hepatitis*) or in the absence of inflammation. In the latter case, cirrhosis apparently develops as a consequence of direct activation of lipocytes (Ito cells).

When present, ethanol becomes the primary metabolic fuel for the liver, completely suppressing the intermediary metabolism of other nutrients. Ethanol is metabolized by two pathways: (1) a primary pathway catalized by alcohol dehydrogenase, which produces acetaldehyde and reduces nicotinamide adenine dinucleotide (NAD) to $NADH_2$, and (2) a secondary pathway involving a system of ethanol-oxidizing enzymes and producing acetaldehyde and reactive oxygen species.[33] Excess $NADH_2$ promotes lactic acidosis and excess of uric acid and opposes gluconeogenesis, β-oxidation of fatty acids, and the Krebs cycle (see Chapter 3), thereby favoring the development of hypoglycemia and hyperlipidemia. Acetaldehyde is toxic to cells of the liver and other organs in a number of ways, including reduction of mitochondrial oxygen utilization, depletion of DNA

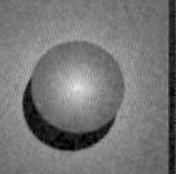

TABLE 26–12
SYSTEMIC EFFECTS OF ALCOHOLISM

Skin
Pellagra dermatitis
Signs of trauma
Infestation (lice)

Head
Fracture
Subdural hematoma
Other trauma

Mouth
Nutritional stomatitis
Cheilosis
Increased incidence of cancer

Eyes
"Tobacco-alcohol" amblyopia
Ophthalmoplegia

Genitourinary
Hypogonadism in men
Impotence
Infertility in women

Gastrointestinal
Esophagitis
Esophageal spasm
Mallory-Weiss tear
Esophageal rupture
Esophageal cancer
Erosive gastritis
Chronic hypertrophic gastritis
Peptic ulcer
Stomach cancer
Malabsorption
Alcoholic diarrhea
Hepatic steatosis
Alcoholic hepatitis
Cirrhosis
Acute pancreatitis

Cardiovascular
Cardiomyopathy
Beriberi (high-output cardiac failure)

Neurologic
Alcohol withdrawal syndrome
Amblyopia
Wernicke-Korsakoff syndrome
Cerebellar degeneration
Polyneuropathy
Central pontine myelinolysis
Cerebral atrophy
Dementia
Myopathy

Respiratory
Increased susceptibility to infection
Fractured ribs
Atelectasis
Pneumothorax
Respiratory depression
High prevalence of smoking

Endocrine and Metabolic
Decreased testosterone level
Hyperglycemia
Hypoglycemia
Hyperlacticemia
Hyperuricemia
Metabolic acidosis
Respiratory acidosis
Alcoholic ketoacidosis
Hypophosphatemia
Hypermetabolism
Hypokalemia
Hypomagnesemia
Hypercholesterolemia
Hypertriglyceridemia
Protein malabsorption
Hypotransferrinemia
Vitamin B deficiencies

From West, L.J., Maxwell, D.S., Noble, E.P., *et al.* (1984). Alcoholism. *Annals of Internal Medicine* 100, 405–416.

repair systems and glutathione (a free radical scavenger), inducing lipid peroxidation, and potentially damaging cellular DNA and proteins. Acetaldehyde is able to cross the placenta, and its toxic effects may contribute to fetal alcohol syndrome (see Chapter 33). Activation of ethanol-oxidizing enzymes contributes to alcohol tolerance and affects the metabolism of tobacco and other drugs, contributing to further toxicity. Reactive oxygen species are toxic and potentially carcinogenic, as discussed in Chapter 7.

Alcohol affects plasma membranes of cells within the central nervous system, depressing neurotransmission, although chronic alcohol abusers are able to compensate for this effect over time. Exciteability resurfaces when alcohol is withdrawn, producing the syndrome of withdrawal (Table 26–13).

Clinical Manifestations. Clinical findings are variable, depending on the severity of liver involvement and effects on other body systems. In milder forms, hepatomegaly and abnormality in serum levels of hepatic enzymes may be the only physiologic findings. Psychological and behavioral problems are frequently reported as well. Anorexia, weight loss, and fatigue are often seen as the disease progresses. If the individual is deprived of alcohol for a time, signs of autonomic hyperactivity caused by alcohol withdrawal may be apparent (see Table 26–13). Severe alcoholic liver disease manifests as hepatic failure, often complicated by jaundice, ascites, bleeding esophageal varices, and hepatic encephalopathy.

Prevention and Treatment. All individuals should be educated regarding the importance of moderation in alcohol consumption. Total abstinence should be recommended for those at high risk, including those with a positive family history of alcoholism, all adolescents, pregnant women or those trying to conceive, persons with chronic illnesses such as congestive heart failure or chronic hepatitis, or those taking drugs that might interact with alcohol.

For those with acute alcoholism, the detoxification process involves stopping the alcohol intake and supporting the patient through the withdrawal syndrome. Drug therapy with magnesium sulfate, clonidine (Catapres), benzodiazepines and other central nervous system depressants may modulate the neuromuscular exciteability associated with withdrawal. Nutritional status is monitored, and supplements of vitamins and minerals are used as necessary.

Once the individual is stable and abstinent, psychotherapy and support groups (e.g., Alcoholics Anonymous) may be of benefit. Drugs that induce an aversion to drinking have also been used. These include disulfiram (Antabuse), which causes unpleasant sensations when alcohol is ingested, and naltrexone HCl (ReVia), which reduces the craving for alcohol.[32]

Systemic disorders are treated supportively. Hepatic failure may necessitate liver transplantation. Most centers require a documented period of abstinence from alcohol before the individual may be a candidate for transplant.

Prognosis and Outcome. Relapsing is common in those who undergo detoxification. Cirrhosis develops in only 10% to 30% of heavy drinkers. These individuals are at high risk for hepatic failure and hepatocellular carcinoma. Alcoholism is frequently associated with morbidity and mortality from accidents, homicides, and suicides, and it is believed to claim an estimated 100,000 lives annually in the United States.[28]

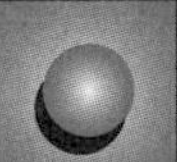

TABLE 26–13
CLINICAL MANIFESTATIONS OF ALCOHOL WITHDRAWAL

Early Signs (Seen 24–48 Hours After Termination of Consumption)
Low-grade fever
Insomnia
Restlessness
Agitation
Nausea and vomiting
Headache and muscle aches
Tremors
Systolic hypertension
Tachycardia
Possible grand mal seizures
Visual or auditory hallucinations but otherwise clear sensorium
Late Signs (More Than 48 Hours After Termination of Consumption)
Cognitive impairment (delirium)
Persistent tremor (tremens)
Decreasing restlessness and agitation
Decreasing hallucinations

Data from Lohr, R.H. (1995). Treatment of alcohol withdrawal in hospitalized patients. *Mayo Clinic Proceedings* 70, 777–782.

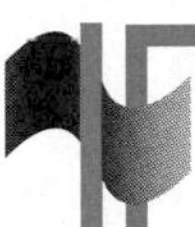

Clinical Scenario

R.G., a 58-year-old college administrator, underwent routine surgery for repair of an inguinal hernia. The morning after surgery, he is observed to be increasingly agitated, tossing and turning in his bed. He is responsive but irritable. He denies incisional pain, but insists on getting "something for his nerves." He has a noticeable tremor of his hands, which becomes worse when he tries to reach objects on the bedside table. His blood pressure and pulse are slightly elevated. His incision is dry and his abdomen is soft. R.G.'s chart indicates that he has a history of "social drinking."

1. What postoperative complications could account for R.G.'s behavior? What clinical findings support or refute these?
2. Could R.G. be experiencing alcohol withdrawal? What evidence suggests this?

Primary Biliary Cirrhosis

Definition. Primary biliary cirrhosis (PBC) is a disease characterized by the destruction of small intrahepatic bile ducts by an immune-mediated inflammatory reaction.

Epidemiology. The prevalence of PBC is uncertain, because there are believed to be many undiagnosed, asymptomatic cases. Prevalence is known to vary in different countries, but PBC has been reported from all parts of the world.[34] Ninety per cent of patients are females, and a familial predisposition has been noted. The usual age of onset of clinical manifestations is 40 to 60 years. Individuals often have other autoimmune disorders such as rheumatoid arthritis, scleroderma, Sjögren's syndrome, dermatomyositis, or systemic lupus erythematosus. Autoimmune thyroiditis and a syndrome resembling gluten-sensitive enteropathy are also frequently present. About a third of patients have gallstones.

Etiology. The precise etiology of primary biliary cirrhosis is unknown, but an autoimmune mechanism is suspected. More than 95% of patients have circulating antibodies to mitochondrial antigens, smooth muscle antigens, and nuclear antigens.[35]

Pathophysiology. Stasis of bile within the liver leads to hepatic injury with destruction and abnormal proliferation of bile ducts. Inflammation is associated with granuloma formation, fibrosis, and the lobular disruption characteristic of cirrhosis. Extrahepatic bile ducts are not involved.

Clinical Manifestations. Liver enzymes are elevated in the cholestatic pattern (see Table 26–5). The course of the disease is variable and unpredictable. Some patients remain asymptomatic, but most experience a gradual onset of pruritus, followed by jaundice within 2 to 3 years. Liver biopsy, in which a sample of liver tissue is obtained by fine-needle aspiration, establishes the diagnosis. Some patients experience a progressive downhill course to hepatic failure.

Prevention and Treatment. There is no known

prevention for PBC. Pruritus is treated with cholestyramine (Questran) or naloxone (Narcan). Supplementation of fat-soluble vitamins is often warranted. Gallstones and hepatic failure are treated as previously described. Results of experimental treatment with immunosuppressive agents such as cyclosporine and methotrexate are inconclusive thus far.[34]

Prognosis and Outcome. Prognosis is variable. Asymptomatic persons have the same life expectancy as those without the disease. However, those who are symptomatic at the time of diagnosis have an average life expectancy of 5 to 10 years.[35] Prognosis relates to the severity of concurrent autoimmune disorders as well as response to treatment of hepatic failure. PBC is a common indication for hepatic transplantation. Five-year survival after surgery is 69%, and 25% of patients will require retransplantation because of subsequent development of the disease in the graft.[34]

Primary Sclerosing Cholangitis

Definition. Primary sclerosing cholangitis (PSC) is a chronic cholestatic liver disease characterized by inflammation and fibrosis of intrahepatic and extrahepatic bile ducts.

Epidemiology. Prevalence of PSC in the United States has been estimated at 7 per 100,000.[36] Most adult patients are between the ages of 27 to 55 years, and 70% to 80% have inflammatory bowel disease, usually ulcerative colitis (see Chapter 24). Individuals with specific HLA subtypes (HLA-B8 and HLA-DR3) are at higher risk.[37] Males outnumber females 3:1.[35] In children, PSC may present during the neonatal period and is usually idiopathic.[38]

Etiology. The precise etiology is unknown, but, similarly to PBC, an immunologic cause is likely. A cross-reaction between an antibody to an intestinal virus or bacterium may trigger an autoimmune response in genetically susceptible persons.[37]

Pathophysiology. Over a 10- to 15-year period, a chronic inflammatory process leads to twisting, dilations, and strictures within the entire biliary ductal system. Bile ducts eventually become nonfunctional, and hepatic failure ensues.[36]

Clinical Manifestations. Patients may be asymptomatic for a variable period after initiation of the process. The initial manifestations typically are fatigue, pruritus, and jaundice. Steatorrhea and deficiency of fat-soluble vitamins develops later, and sludging and obstruction of the biliary tree may lead to inflammatory pain. Onset of hepatic failure may be sudden, with associated bleeding esophageal varices, ascites, and hepatic encephalopathy. Hepatic enzymes are elevated in a cholestatic pattern (see Table 26–5). Up to 30% of patients develop cholelithiasis.

Prevention and Treatment. Individuals with ulcerative colitis should be closely monitored for development of PSC. Symptomatic treatment of pruritus and malabsorption is indicated. Definitive treatment of gallstones is also warranted. The treatment of choice for end-stage primary sclerosing cholangitis is liver transplantation.

Prognosis and Outcome. Patients with PSC who undergo liver transplantation have a 1-year survival rate of 85% and a 5-year survival rate of 75%. The disease recurs in the grafts of a significant number of patients. Ten to 15% of patients with PSC develop cholangiocarcinoma (cancer of the bile ducts), which has a 2-year survival rate of less than 10%.[36]

Extrahepatic Biliary Atresia

Definition. Extrahepatic biliary atresia is congenital obstruction or absence of all or part of the extrahepatic bile ducts, leading to cholestasis and progressive biliary cirrhosis.[38] Biliary atresia is the most common congenital structural anomaly associated with hepatic failure. Other disorders are summarized in Table 26–14.

Epidemiology. One in 10,000 to 15,000 infants is born with extrahepatic atresia, and the condition is more prevalent in females than in males. Risk factors are unknown, although prenatal viral infection with reovirus type 3, rubella, Epstein-Barr virus, or cytomegalovirus may be implicated.[38]

Etiology. The precise etiology of biliary atresia is unknown. In most cases, the hepatic damage occurs postnatally, ruling out failure of morphogenesis during embryonic development.

Pathophysiology. Retention of bile within the liver leads to chronic inflammation, with fibrosis, edema, and sloughing of the biliary epithelium into the duct lumen. Inflammatory cells infiltrate liver tissue, and hepatocytes may be transformed into giant cells. Bile ducts are gradually destroyed, and hepatic fibrosis and possibly cirrhosis are evident during the first year of life.

Clinical Manifestations. Most infants are full term and of normal birth weight.[38] Jaundice persists beyond the time attributable to physiologic jaundice (about 14 days). Stools gradually become pale as ductal obstruction progresses. Hyperbilirubinemia results from an approximate 50:50 mixture of unconjugated and conjugated types, reflecting biliary obstruction and hepatocyte dysfunction. Liver enzymes are moderately elevated. The infant eventu-

TABLE 26-14
CONGENITAL ANOMALIES OF HEPATIC STRUCTURE

DISORDER	DESCRIPTION
Extrahepatic biliary atresia	Obstruction or absence of biliary ducts below the porta hepatis (15%) or above the porta hepatis (85%), leading to cholestasis, obstructive jaundice, and potentially hepatic fibrosis
Choledochal cysts	Cystic dilation of the common bile duct, permitting reflux of pancreatic secretions into the biliary tree; associated with fibrosis and increased risk of cholangiocarcinoma
Congenital biliary ectasia (Caroli's disease)	Cystic dilation of the intrahepatic bile ducts; associated with liver abscesses, sepsis, biliary cirrhosis, and increased risk of cholangiocarcinoma
von-Meyenburg complexes	Small clusters of dilated bile ducts embedded in fibrous tissue; usually of no clinical significance
Polycystic liver disease	Multiple diffuse cystic lesions containing serous fluid (not bile); often associated with polycystic kidney disease, which dominates the clinical picture
Congenital hepatic fibrosis	Enlargement of portal tracts by broad bands of collagenous tissue, dividing the liver into irregular islands; may result in portal hypertension

Data from Cotran, R.S., Kumar, V., and Robbins, S.L. (1994). *Robbins Pathologic Basis of Disease.* (5th Ed.). Philadelphia: W.B. Saunders. (pp. 870–871).

ally demonstrates "failure to thrive," with poor weight gain and development. Signs of hepatic failure are soon apparent. An estimated 10% to 25% of affected infants have other congenital anomalies, such as cardiac defects, bowel malrotation or atresia, and multiple spleens.

Prevention and Treatment. Specific preventive measures are unknown. Extrahepatic biliary atresia is potentially treatable with surgical repair of ducts or with bypass procedures (e.g., the Kasai procedure) that shunt bile from the liver to the common bile duct or duodenum. Surgical outcomes are most successful if surgery is performed within the first 2 months of life, before extensive liver damage occurs. Liver transplantation is indicated for those infants in whom surgical repair or bypass fails to restore bile flow. Because infants require smaller amounts of hepatic tissue, living relatives may serve as graft donors, donating a portion of their livers.

Prognosis and Outcome. Prognosis is increasingly positive for those whose atresia is treatable with shunting or transplantation. Without treatment, biliary atresia is usually fatal within 2 years. The Kasai procedure is successful in 80% to 90% of infants referred for surgery within 60 days of birth. One-year survival after liver transplantation exceeds 90%.[38]

Gallbladder Cancer

Definition. Gallbladder cancer refers to malignant tumors originating in the gallbladder.

Epidemiology. Carcinomas of the gallbladder occur in 1 in 100,000 males and twice as many females in the United States.[39] Peak incidence is in the eighth decade of life, and more than 70% have coexisting gallstones.

Etiology. The precise etiology is unknown.

Pathophysiology. More than 90% of gallbladder cancers are adenocarcinomas. Less common types are lymphomas, sarcomas, large cell carcinomas, and small cell (oat cell) carcinomas. Local infiltration leads to cholecystitis and contributes to cholelithiasis. Metastasis to the liver, regional lymph nodes, and lungs commonly occurs. Tumors occasionally secrete hormones, resulting in a paraneoplastic syndrome resembling Cushing's syndrome.

Clinical Manifestations. The presentation is similar to that of cholelithiasis, with progressive, severe right upper quadrant pain and possibly jaundice. Abdominal distention usually develops, and low-grade fever is commonly seen. Gallstones are frequently detected with ultrasonography or other testing. Surgical intervention and tissue biopsy establishes the diagnosis of cancer. With progressive metastasis, pain becomes increasingly severe and jaundice worsens. Hepatic failure eventually occurs.

Prevention and Treatment. Specific preventive measures are unknown. Surgical excision of the gallbladder (cholecystectomy) is the treatment of choice. Chemotherapeutic agents such as etoposide (VP-16) may be used adjunctively to reduce the tumor burden if complete excision is not possible.

Prognosis and Outcome. Prognosis in gallbladder cancer is poor, with an overall 5-year survival of 5%. Prognosis in oat cell cancer is even worse, with a mean survival time of 7 months after diagnosis.[39]

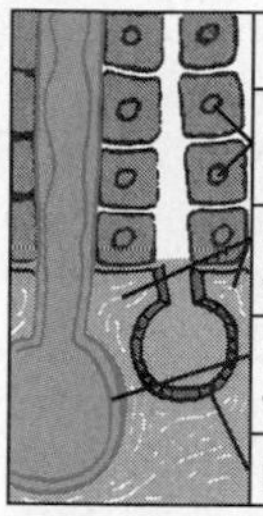

ORIGIN	BENIGN	MALIGNANT
Hepatocytes	Adenoma	Hepatocellular carcinoma
Connective tissue	Fibroma	Sarcoma
Blood vessels	Hemangioma	Hemangioendothelioma
Bile ducts	Cholangioma	Carcinoma

FIGURE 26–11

Classification of primary liver neoplasms. Benign and malignant tumors may arise from hepatocytes, connective tissue, blood vessels, or bile ducts. (From Black, J.M., and Matassarin-Jacobs, E. [1997]. *Medical-Surgical Nursing: Clinical Management for Continuity of Care.* [5th Ed.]. Philadelphia: W.B. Saunders. [p. 1896].)

Hepatocellular Carcinoma

Definition. Hepatocellular carcinoma is a malignant neoplasm originating from hepatocytes. Primary tumors, arising from the liver, may also develop from connective tissue cells, blood vessels, or bile ducts (Fig. 26–11). Benign and malignant tumors originating from liver tissues are summarized in Table 26–15. Metastatic tumors of the liver are very common. They most often originate in the skin (malignant melanoma), GI tract (gastric and gallbladder tumors), lung, and breast and metastasize to the liver via direct extension, blood, or lymph.

Epidemiology. Primary hepatocellular carcinoma is relatively rare in the United States but very common worldwide. It is more common in men than women. Risk factors include history of chronic hepatitis from HBV or HCV infections, cirrhosis, hemochromatosis, abuse of anabolic steroids, long-term androgen therapy, and exposure to carcinogenic agents such as aflatoxin B, a toxin found in some inappropriately stored grain. HBV carriers have a 100-fold risk of hepatocellular carcinoma after 30 years, and the concurrent presence of cirrhosis increases risk another 10-fold. Primary hepatic cancers are more common in immigrants from Africa and Asia and in Alaskan natives.[40] In children, malignant tumors of the liver are uncommon.

Etiology. The precise etiology of hepatocellular carcinoma is unknown. In patients with chronic HBV infection, predisposition probably originates from incorporation of viral DNA into the hepatocyte DNA. This mechanism does not occur in chronic HCV infection, however. Aflatoxin B appar-

TABLE 26–15
BENIGN AND MALIGNANT NEOPLASMS OF THE LIVER

TUMOR	DESCRIPTION
Benign Tumors	
Liver cell adenoma	Originates from hepatocytes; tends to occur in young women on oral contraceptives and to regress on discontinuance of use; may rupture during pregnancy, resulting in hemorrhage
Bile duct adenoma (cholangioma)	Originates from bile duct epithelium; usually found incidentally
Focal nodular hyperplasia	Well-demarcated nodule composed of normal hepatocytes, lymphocytic infiltrates, and bile ducts; usually occurs in young to middle-aged adults
Cavernous hemangioma	Red-blue, spongy mass filled with blood separated by scant connective tissue stroma
Fibroma	Small, firm, encapsulated tumor composed of spindled fibroblasts and collagen
Malignant Tumors	
Hepatoblastoma	Childhood tumor composed of fetal or embryonic epithelial cells or a mixture of epithelial cells and other cells of mesenchymal origin; most common in boys; presence of family history, Wilms' tumor, or fetal alcohol syndrome imposes increased risk
Angiosarcoma (hemangioendothelioma)	Originates from blood vessels; composed of mass of atypical endothelial cells; increased risk with exposure to polyvinylchloride, widely used in plastics
Hepatocellular carcinoma	Accounts for 90% of all primary liver cancers; originates from hepatocytes; most prevalent cancer worldwide; cirrhosis imposes increased risk
Cholangiocarcinoma	Originates from bile duct epithelium; early blood-borne metastasis is common; usually no risk factors are apparent

Data from Cotran, R.S., Kumar, V., and Robbins, S.L. (1994). *Robbins Pathologic Basis of Disease.* (5th Ed.). Philadelphia: W.B. Saunders. (pp. 510, 878–882).

ently induces mutation of *p53,* a tumor suppressor gene.[41]

Pathophysiology. In many cases, growth of tumors within the liver is insidious until as much as 90% of normal hepatic tissue is involved.[12] All hepatic functions are potentially affected, leading to metabolic and nutritional abnormalities, alteration of biotransformation, bleeding tendencies, and other manifestations of hepatic failure. Enlargement of the liver leads to tenderness and potential infringement on the thoracic space and other abdominal organs. The neoplastic process may invade or rupture blood vessels, leading to hemorrhage.

Clinical Manifestations. Clinical signs of hepatic cancer are usually vague or absent until the disease is well advanced. Abdominal tenderness is present, and a palpable abdominal mass may be detected. Weight loss, vomiting, and paraneoplastic syndromes may be present. Serum levels of α-fetoprotein, a tumor cytokine, are often elevated in patients with primary, but not metastatic, hepatic tumors. Signs of hepatic failure are apparent with advanced hepatic cancers.

Prevention and Treatment. Prevention of cancer is discussed in Chapter 7. Surgical resection (wedge resection or lobectomy) is the treatment of choice. In those with unresectable tumors, hepatic arterial embolization, chemotherapy, or radiation may be used in an effort to reduce tumor mass, slow the progression of the neoplastic process, and enhance patient comfort. Chemotherapy is most effective if administered via direct infusion into the hepatic artery.

Prognosis and Outcome. Most individuals with primary liver cancer have a poor prognosis. If the tumor is not resectable, mean survival time is about 2 years. Five-year survival after surgical resection is approximately 68%.[40] Prognosis in secondary liver cancer is variable depending on the nature of the primary neoplasm and the degree of metastasis, but it is generally unfavorable.

CLINICAL SIGNIFICANCE OF HEPATIC AND BILIARY DISORDERS

As illustrated by the conditions discussed in this chapter, hepatobiliary disorders are clinically significant by virtue of their commonality and prevalence within individuals of all age groups (see Developmental Perspective). Given the hundreds of functions served by the liver, it is not surprising that morbidity and mortality are significant in biliary tract disease. Liver transplantation has improved prognosis for many with congenital and acquired disorders of the liver, and research continues toward the goal of refining this procedure. Basic and pharmacologic research are ongoing in an effort to develop therapeutic agents with reduced hepatotoxicity.

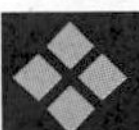

Summary of Key Points

- Functional liver cells (hepatocytes) are surrounded by outlets to the biliary ducts and the vascular system. When bilirubin is prevented from entering the bile, increased amounts enter the blood instead, promoting hyperbilirubinemia caused by cholestasis. Phagocytic Kupffer cells lining the hepatic sinusoids clear bacteria from portal venous blood. In liver disease, failure of this function may promote septicemia. Loss of hepatocyte functions in hepatic failure manifests as disruption of metabolism, storage, synthesis, and biotransformation.

- Most bilirubin is produced when RBCs are hemolyzed, either because of normal turnover or pathology. Plasma enzymes catalyze the formation of bilirubin from heme proteins. In the hepatocytes, bilirubin is conjugated (rendered more water soluble) for excretion in the bile. Failure of hepatocytes to conjugate bilirubin because of an increased bilirubin load or enzymatic dysfunction, or obstruction of biliary drainage from the liver, may lead to clinically evident hyperbilirubinemia.

- Bile is synthesized by hepatocytes from bilirubin, bile salts, electrolytes, proteins, cholesterol, and water. It is excreted from the liver via the hepatic duct, and enters the gallbladder for concentration and storage. Gallbladder stimulation with entry of food into the duodenum results in gallbladder contraction and release of bile into the common bile duct, from which it enters the duodenum.

- Because of the position of the liver with respect to the venous circulation, rising pressure in the vena cava (as in congestive heart failure) results in storage of 300 to 400 mL of blood. Liver enlargement (hepatomegaly) results. This stored blood may be shunted back into the central circulation when the liver contracts under sympathetic nervous system stimulation in hypovolemic shock.

Summary continued on next page

- Hepatic function is central to the metabolism of all major nutrients. Carbohydrate metabolism by hepatic enzyme systems is essential in glucose buffering (maintenance of stable serum glucose levels). The processes of glycogenesis, glycogenolysis, and gluconeogenesis are balanced to achieve glucose homeostasis. Dysruption of lipid metabolism by hepatocytes may lead to accumulation of lipid within lobules, contributing to the early changes leading to cirrhosis. Hepatocytes also convert ammonia, a product of protein metabolism, to urea for renal excretion. Ammonia may accumulate to toxic levels in hepatic failure. Many genetic disorders are associated with abnormality of one or more metabolic functions of the liver.
- The liver normally stores a variety of substances other than blood. These include minerals such as iron and copper and vitamins A, B_{12}, and D. Excessive accumulation of stored material may be toxic to the liver. This abnormal storage may result from excessive intake or from inborn errors of metabolism.
- Failure of the liver to synthesize protein clotting factors may lead to bleeding disorders. Lack of synthesis of transport proteins such as albumin and transferrin may result in abnormal serum osmolarity and fluid imbalance as well as in toxicity caused by an increase in the unbound fraction of circulating drugs or hormones. Abnormal apoprotein synthesis may contribute to dyslipidemia.
- Most circulating drugs and hormones are inactivated by enzymatic reactions as they pass through the liver. Failure of this biotransformation in hepatic disease may contribute to exaggerated or toxic effects of these agents.
- When hepatic reserve is exceeded, disorders of hepatobiliary function manifest as altered synthetic, metabolic, synthetic, or storage processes or as failure of biotransformation. In addition to loss of hepatocyte function, normal biliary excretion may be impaired. The function of nearly all organ systems is affected. Systemic toxicity may result from hepatic failure or may contribute to its development. In many hepatobiliary disorders, treatment is essentially supportive after removal of the hepatotoxic agent. Hepatic transplantation is the treatment of choice in end-stage liver disease.

REFERENCES

1. Lasker, M.R., and Holzman, I.R. (1996). Neonatal jaundice: When to treat, when to watch and wait. *Postgraduate Medicine* 99(3), 187–198.
2. Reishtein, J. (1993). Liver failure: Case study of a complex problem. *Critical Care Nurse* October 1993, 36–44.
3. Lee, W.M. (1993). Acute liver failure. *New England Journal of Medicine* 329(25), 1862–1872.
4. Lee, W.M. (1994). Acute liver failure. *American Journal of Medicine* 96(1A suppl.), 1A-3S–1A-9S.
5. Lee, W.M. (1995). Drug-induced hepatotoxicity. *New England Journal of Medicine* 333(17), 1118–1127.
6. Jaffe, D.L., Chung, R.T., and Friedman, L.S. (1996). Management of portal hypertension and its complications. *Medical Clinics of North America* 80(5), 1021–1034.
7. Bhuva, M., Ganger, D., and Jensen, D. (1994). Spontaneous bacterial peritonitis: An update on evaluation, management, and prevention. *American Journal of Medicine* 97, 169–175.
8. Lange, P.A., and Stoller, J.K. (1995). The hepatopulmonary syndrome. *Annals of Internal Medicine* 122, 521–529.
9. Laine, L., and Cook, D. (1995). Endoscopic ligation compared with sclerotherapy for treatment of esophageal variceal bleeding: A meta-analysis. *Annals of Internal Medicine* 123, 280–287.
10. Runyon, B.A. (1994). Care of patients with ascites. *New England Journal of Medicine* 330(5), 337–342.
11. Trevillyan, J., and Carroll, P.J. (1997). Management of portal hypertension and esophageal varices in alcoholic cirrhosis. *American Family Physician* 55(5), 1851–1858.
12. Black, J.M., and Matassarin-Jacobs, E. (1997). *Medical-Surgical Nursing: Clinical Management for Continuity of Care.* (5th ed.). Philadelphia: W.B. Saunders. (pp. 1872, 1896–1898).
13. Friedman, S.L. (1993). The cellular basis of hepatic fibrosis: Mechanisms and treatment strategies. *New England Journal of Medicine* 328(25), 1828–1835.
14. Cotran, R.S., Kumar, V., and Robbins, S.L. (1994). *Robbins Pathologic Basis of Disease.* (5th ed.). Philadelphia: W.B. Saunders. (pp. 834–835, 838).
15. Hicks, B.A., and Altman, R.P. (1993). The jaundiced newborn. *Pediatric Clinics of North America* 40(6), 1161–1175.
16. Ghiloni, B.W. (1993). Cholelithiasis: Current treatment options. *American Family Physician* 48(5), 762–768.
17. Jaffe, Philip E. (1993). Gallstones: Who are good candidates for nonsurgical treatment? *Postgraduate Medicine* 94(6), 45–57.
18. Johnston, D.E., and Kaplan, M.M. (1993). Pathogenesis and treatment of gallstones. *New England Journal of Medicine* 328(6), 412–421.
19. Goldschmid, S., and Brady, P.G. (1993). Approaches to the management of cholelithiasis for the medical consultant. *Medical Clinics of North America* 77(2), 413–426.
20. Soper, N.J., Brunt, L.M., and Kerbl, K. (1994). Laparoscopic general surgery. *New England Journal of Medicine* 330(6), 409–419.
21. Ransohoff, D.F., and Gracie, W.A. (1993). Treatment of gallstones. *Annals of Internal Medicine* 119, 606–619.
22. Scully, R.E., Mark, E.J., McNeely, W.F., *et al.* (Eds). (1997). Weekly clinicophatological exercises—Case 10-1997. *New England Journal of Medicine* 336(13), 939–947.
23. Becherer, P.R. (1995). Viral hepatitis: What have we learned about risk factors and transmission? *Postgraduate Medicine* 98(1), 65–74.
24. Moyer, L., Warwick, M., and Mahoney, F.J. (1996). Prevention of hepatitis A virus infection. *American Family Physician* 54(1), 107–114.
25. Frymoyer, C.L. (1993). Preventing the spread of viral hepatitis. *American Family Physician* 48(8), 1479–1486.
26. Regenstein, F. (1994). New approaches to the treatment of chronic viral hepatitis B and C. *American Journal of Medicine* 96(1A suppl.), 1A-47S–1A-51S.
27. Antai-Otong, D. (1995). Helping the alcoholic patient to recovery. *American Journal of Nursing* August 1995, 22–30.
28. Lieber, C.S. (1995). Medical disorders of alcoholism. *New England Journal of Medicine* 333(16), 1058–1065.

29. Morrison, S.F., Rogers, P.D., and Thomas, M.H. (1995). Alcohol and adolescents. *Pediatric Clinics of North America* 42(2), 371–387.
30. Council on Scientific Affairs, American Medical Association. (1996). Alcoholism in the elderly. *Journal of the American Medical Association* 275(10), 797–801.
31. Gejman, P.V., Ram, A., Gelernter, J., *et al.* (1994). No structural mutation in the dopamine D_2 receptor gene in alcoholism or schizophrenia. *Journal of the American Medical Association* 271(3), 204–208.
32. Blondell, R.D., Frierson, R.L., and Lippmann, S.B. (1996). Alcoholism: Taking a preventive public health approach. *Postgraduate Medicine* 100(1), 69–80.
33. Woods, S.E., Hitchcock, M., and Meyer, A. (1993). Alcoholic hepatitis. *American Family Physician* 47(5), 1171–1178.
34. Sherlock, S. (1994). Primary biliary cirrhosis: Clarifying the issues. *American Journal of Medicine* 96(1A suppl.), 1A-27S–1A-33S.
35. Buckley, S.E., and Dipalma, J.A. (1996). Recognizing primary biliary cirrhosis and primary sclerosing cholangitis. *American Family Physician* 53(1), 195–200.
36. Wiesner, R.H. (1994). Current concepts in primary sclerosing cholangitis. *Mayo Clinic Proceedings* 69, 969–982.
37. Bhutani, M.S., Rostami, G., and Gopalswamy, N. (1995). Hepatobiliary complications of inflammatory bowel disease. *American Family Physician* 52(5), 1440–1444.
38. McEvoy, C.F., and Suchy, F.J. (1996). Biliary tract disease in children. *Pediatric Clinics of North America* 43(1), 75–98.
39. Johnstone, A.K., Zuch, R.H., and Anders, K.H. (1993). Oat cell carcinoma of the gallbladder. *Archives of Pathology and Laboratory Medicine* 117, 1009–1012.
40. Smith, C.S., and Paauw, D.S. (1993). Hepatocellular carcinoma: Identifying and screening populations at increased risk. *Postgraduate Medicine* 94(8), 71–74.
41. Khakoo, S.I., Grellier, L.F.L., Soni, P.N., *et al.* (1996). Etiology, screening, and treatment of hepatocellular carcinoma. *Medical Clinics of North America* 80(5), 1121–1145.

SELECTED BIBLIOGRAPHY

Baird, R.E., Foley, C., Bresee, J., *et al.* (1994). Reye's syndrome: Lessons for family physicians. *American Family Physician* (Editorial). 50(7), 1454–1461.

Besson, I., Ingrand, P., Person, B., *et al.* (1995). Sclerotherapy with or without octreotide for acute variceal bleeding. *New England Journal of Medicine* 333(9), 555–560.

Blackburn, S.T., and Loper, D.L. (1992). *Maternal, Fetal, and Neonatal Physiology: A Clinical Perspective.* Philadelphia: W.B. Saunders.

Caty, M.G., and Shamberger, R.C. (1993). Abdominal tumors in infancy and childhood. *Pediatric Clinics of North America* 40(6), 1253–1271.

Chari, R.S., Collins, B.H., Magee, J.C., *et al.* (1994). Brief report: Treatment of hepatic failure with ex vivo pig-liver perfusion followed by liver transplantation. *New England Journal of Medicine* 331(4), 234–237.

Czaja, A.J. (1996). Diagnosis and therapy of autoimmune liver disease. *Medical Clinics of North America* 80(5), 973–994.

Czaja, A.J. (1996). The variant forms of autoimmune hepatitis. *Annals of Internal Medicine* 125, 588–598.

Dana, F., Becherer, P.R., and Bacon, B.R. (1994). *Postgraduate Medicine* 95(6), 121–130.

DiBisceglie, A.M. (1995). Chronic hepatitis B: Hope for decreasing its impact. *Postgraduate Medicine* 98(1), 99–106.

Everhart, J.E. (1993). Contributions of obesity and weight loss to gallstone disease. *Annals of Internal Medicine* 119(10), 1029–1035.

Figueredo, V.M. (1997). The effects of alcohol on the heart: Detrimental or beneficial? *Postgraduate Medicine* 101(2), 165–176.

Fishman, L.N., Jonas, M.M., and Lavine, J.E. (1996). Update on viral hepatitis in children. *Pediatric Clinics of North America* 43(1), 57–74.

Fried, M.W. (1996). Therapy of chronic viral hepatitis. *Medical Clinics of North America* 80(5), 957–972.

Ganne, E.J., Portmann, B.C., Naoumov, N.V., *et al.* (1996). Long-term outcome of hepatitis C infection after liver transplantation. *New England Journal of Medicine* 334(13), 815–820.

Gholson, C.F., McDonald, J., and McMillan, R. (1995). Liver transplantation: When is it indicated and what can be expected afterwards? *Postgraduate Medicine* 97(2), 101–114.

Herrera, J.L. (1993). Abnormal liver enzyme levels: The spectrum of causes. *Postgraduate Medicine* 93(2), 113–116.

Jackson, G.H., Meyer, A., and Lippmann, S. (1994). Wilson's disease: Psychiatric manifestations may be the clinical presentation. *Postgraduate Medicine* 95(8), 135–138.

Jutabha, R., and Jenson, D.M. (1996). Management of upper gastrointestinal bleeding in the patient with chronic liver disease. *Medical Clinics of North America* 80(5), 1035–1068.

Kadakia, S.C. (1993). Biliary tract emergencies: Acute cholecystitis, acute cholangitis, and acute pancreatitis. *Medical Clinics of North America* 77(5), 1015–1036.

Knox, T.A., and Olans, L.B. (1996). Liver disease in pregnancy. *New England Journal of Medicine* 335(8), 569–576.

Lieber, C.S. (1994). Mechanisms of ethanol-drug-nutrition interactions. *Clinical Toxicology* 32(6), 631–681.

Lindsay, K.L. (1994). Management of chronic hepatitis in special populations. *American Journal of Medicine* 96 (1A suppl.), 1A-57S–1A-60S.

Lisanti, P., and Talotta, D. (1994). An overview of viral hepatitis. *AORN Journal* 59(5), 997–1005.

Lohr, R.H. (1995). Treatment of alcohol withdrawal in hospitalized patients. *Mayo Clinic Proceedings* 70, 777–782.

Mammen, E.F. (1994). Coagulation defects in liver disease. *Medical Clinics of North America* 78(3), 545–554.

Miller, M., and Hutchins, G.M. (1994). Hemochromatosis, multiorgan hemosiderosis, and coronary artery disease. *Journal of the American Medical Association* 272(3), 231–233.

Moore, K.L., and Persaud, T.V.N. (1993). *The Developing Human: Clinically Oriented Embryology.* (5th ed.). Philadelphia: W.B. Saunders.

Naylor, C.D. (1994). Physical examination of the liver. *Journal of the American Medical Association* 271(23), 1859–1865.

Nemes, J., and Donahue, M.C. (1994). Solid tumors in children. *Nursing Clinics of North America* 29(4), 585–598.

Neuschwander-Tetri, B.A. (1995). Common blood tests for liver disease: Which ones are most useful? *Postgraduate Medicine* 98(1), 49–63.

Neuschwander-Tetri, B.A., and Bacon, B.R. (1996). Nonalcoholic steatohepatitis. *Medical Clinics of North America* 80(5), 1147–1166.

NIH Consensus Development Panel on Gallstones and Laparoscopic Cholecystectomy. (1993). Gallstones and laparoscopic cholecystectomy. *Journal of the American Medical Association* 269(8), 1018–1024.

Nunes, F.A., and Raper, S.E. (1996). Liver-directed gene therapy. *Medical Clinics of North America* 80(5), 1201–1213.

Olynyk, J.K., and Bacon, B.R. (1995). Hepatitis C: Recent advances in understanding and management. *Postgraduate Medicine* 98(1), 79–94.

Quam, D.A. (1994). Recognizing a case of Reye's syndrome. *American Family Physician* 50(7), 1491–1496.

Reily, C.A. (1994). Hepatic disease in pregnancy. *American Journal of Medicine* 96 (1A suppl.), 1A-18S–1A-22S.

Rubin, R.A., Kowalski, T.E., Khandelwal, M., *et al.* (1994). Ursodiol for hepatobiliary disorders. *Annals of Internal Medicine* 121(3), 207–218.

Sackier, J.M. (1996). New applications of laparoscopy in gastrointestinal surgery. *American Family Physician* 53(1), 237–242.

Schiffmann, R. (1996). Niemann-Pick disease type C: From bench to bedside. *Journal of the American Medical Association* 276(7), 561–564.

Schwarzenberg, S.J., and Sharp, H.L. (1996). Update on metabolic liver disease. *Pediatric Clinics of North America* 43(1), 27–56.

Sempos, C.T., Looker, A.C., Gillum, R.F., *et al.* (1994). Body iron stores and the risk of coronary heart disease. *New England Journal of Medicine* 330(16), 1119–1124.

Sharara, A.I., Hunt, C.M., and Hamilton, J.D. (1996). Hepatitis C. *Annals of Internal Medicine* 125, 658–668.

Sheth, S.G., Gordon, F.D., and Chopra, S. (1997). Nonalcoholic steatohepatitis. *Annals of Internal Medicine* 126(2), 137–145.

Tanaka, E., Alter, H.J., Nakatsuji, Y., *et al.* (1996). Effect of hepatitis G virus infection on chronic hepatitis C. *Annals of Internal Medicine* 125(9), 740–743.

Theal, R.M., and Scott, K. (1996). Evaluating asymptomatic patients with abnormal liver function test results. *American Family Physician* 53(6), 2111–2119.

Zein, N.N., Rakela, J., Krawitt, E.L., *et al.* (1996). Hepatitis C virus genotypes in the United States: Epidemiology, pathogenicity, and response to interferon therapy. *Annals of Internal Medicine* 125(8), 634–639.

Zetterman, R.K. (1994). Primary care management of the liver transplant patient. *American Journal of Medicine* 96(1A suppl.), 1A-10S–1A-17S.

Unit X

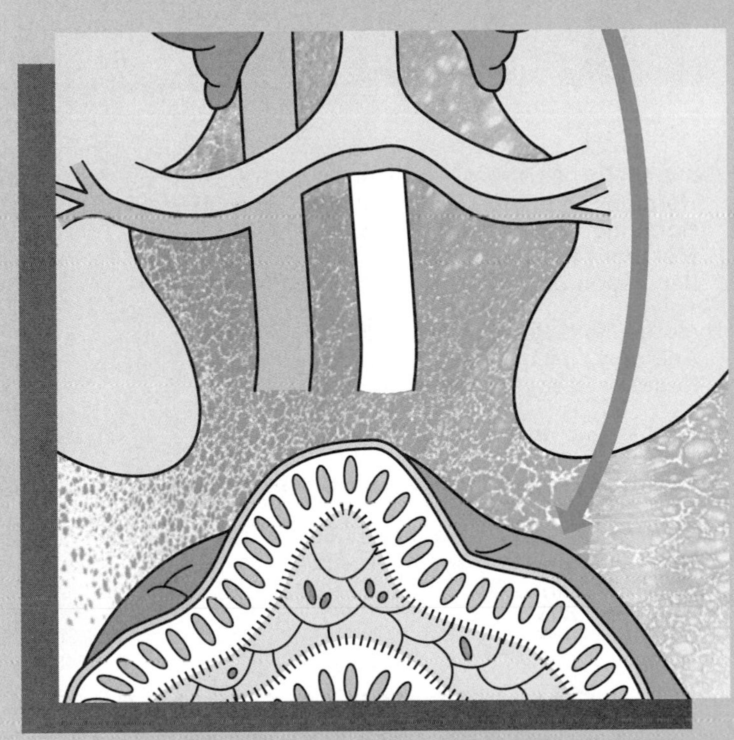

ENDOCRINE SYSTEM

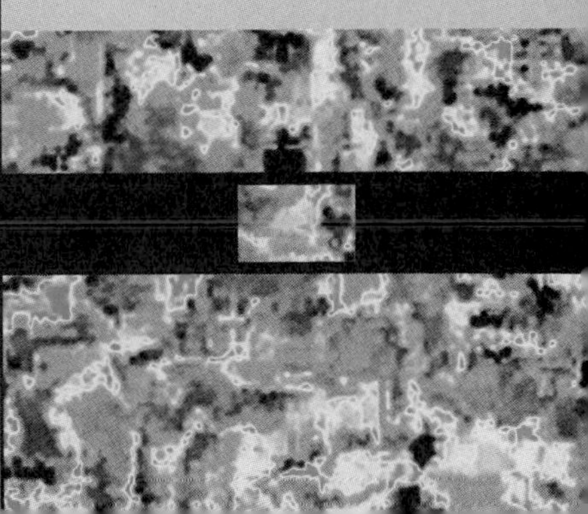

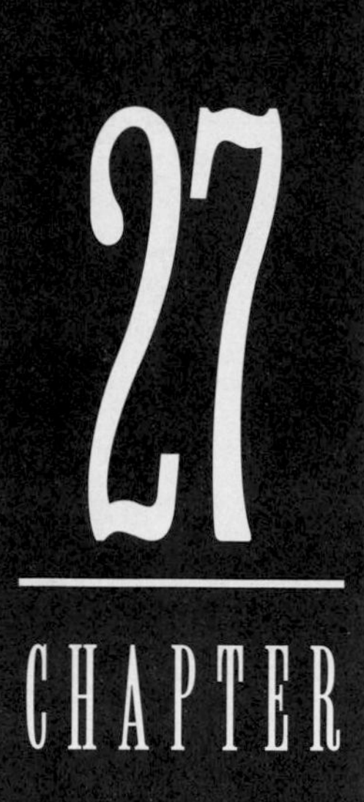

Hypothalamic and Pituitary Disorders

LEARNING OBJECTIVES

1. Differentiate between neural and endocrine mechanisms of regulation.
2. Classify the most important hormones with respect to structure, synthesis, transport, receptor-mediated actions, and inactivation.
3. Describe the structure and function of the hypothalamic–pituitary axis.
4. Discuss the principal hormones and endocrine functions of the hypothalamus, pituitary gland, and pineal gland.
5. Comprehend the pathophysiologic mechanisms that underlie the clinical manifestations and rationalize the treatment of selected disorders of the endocrine hypothalamus and pituitary gland.

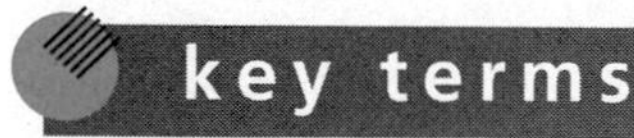

key terms

acromegaly
adrenocorticotropic hormone (ACTH)
aldosterone
androgen
antidiuretic hormone (ADH)
β-endorphin
classic endocrine system
cortisol
diabetes insipidus
diffuse endocrine system
empty sella syndrome
estrogen
follicle-stimulating hormone
glucagon
gonadotropin-releasing hormone
growth hormone (GH)
growth hormone deficiency
growth hormone release–inhibiting hormone
growth hormone–releasing hormone
hormone
hypopituitarism

hypothalamic–pituitary axis (HPA)
insulin
insulin-like growth factor (IGF)
luteinizing hormone
melanocyte-stimulating hormone
melatonin
oxytocin
panhypopituitarism
parathyroid hormone
pituitary dwarfism
pituitary giantism
prolactin
seasonal affective disorder
Sheehan's syndrome
syndrome of inappropriate antidiuretic hormone secretion (SIADH)
thyroid-stimulating hormone (TSH)
thyrotropin-releasing hormone

Together, the nervous system and the endocrine system regulate all of human function. These two systems have much in common. As discussed in Chapter 21, many of the chemicals that mediate neurotransmission also serve as **hormones**, signaling molecules that are transported in the bloodstream to distant organs on which they exert slower-onset, longer-duration effects than those mediated by the nervous system. Epinephrine, norepinephrine, and dopamine are examples of major *neurotransmitters* that also act as hormones. Among the growing list of *neuromodulators* (chemicals that influence neurotransmission but are not essential to it) are several peptides, which are also classified as components of the **diffuse endocrine system** (Table 27–1). This system consists of a wide variety of cell types that secrete mediators with predominantly local (autocrine and paracrine) effects. To the extent that these chemicals travel in the bloodstream to more distant targets, they function as hormones.

The emphasis in this and the succeeding chapters is on the **classic endocrine system**, composed of several organs that have as their *primary* function the secretion of hormones (Fig. 27–1). The major organs of the classic endocrine system are the hypothalamus, pituitary gland, pineal gland, thyroid gland, parathyroids, adrenal cortex, endocrine pancreas, and gonads (ovaries and testes).

A number of organ systems have *secondary* endocrine functions. Specialized cells of the liver secrete **insulin-like growth factors (IGFs)**, which mediate **growth hormone** (GH) action, and hepatic enzymes are involved in the activation of vitamin D, a steroid hormone important in the regulation of calcium and phosphate metabolism. The kidneys are also involved in vitamin D activation and secrete the hormones erythropoietin and renin. Erythropoietin is critical to the regulation of erythrocyte proliferation and maturation in the bone marrow, whereas renin secretion mediates fluid and electrolyte homeostasis. The endocrine functions of the corpus luteum and placenta are essential to the maintenance of pregnancy. During childhood and adolescence, the thymus gland secretes hormones that direct the maturation of lymphocytes and the development of normal immune function.

This chapter presents an overview of endocrine function, with emphasis on cellular mechanisms of activity and regulation. The interdependent functions of the endocrine hypothalamus and pituitary

TABLE 27–1
EXAMPLES OF HORMONES OF THE DIFFUSE ENDOCRINE SYSTEM

HORMONE	EFFECTS
Acetylcholine	Stimulates gastric secretion of HCl, pepsinogen, and mucus Stimulates pancreatic secretion of digestive enzymes
Gastrin	Stimulates gastric secretion of HCl
Histamine	Stimulates gastric secretion of HCl
Secretin	Decreases gastrointestinal motility (weak effect) Increases pancreatic secretion of digestive juice (water and bicarbonate)
Cholecystokinin (CCK)	Blocks increased gastric motility induced by gastrin Stimulates gallbladder contraction Stimulates secretion of pancreatic enzymes
Gastric inhibitory peptide (GIP)	Stimulates insulin secretion by the pancreas Inhibits gastric secretion
Vasoactive intestinal polypeptide	Inhibits gastric secretion
Endothelin	Constricts vascular smooth muscle
Serotonin	Either constricts or dilates vascular smooth muscle
Angiotensin II	Constricts vascular smooth muscle Stimulates release of aldosterone from adrenal cortex
Atrial natriuretic peptide	Inhibits renal tubular reabsorption of sodium and water
Pancreatic polypeptide	Uncertain pancreatic effect

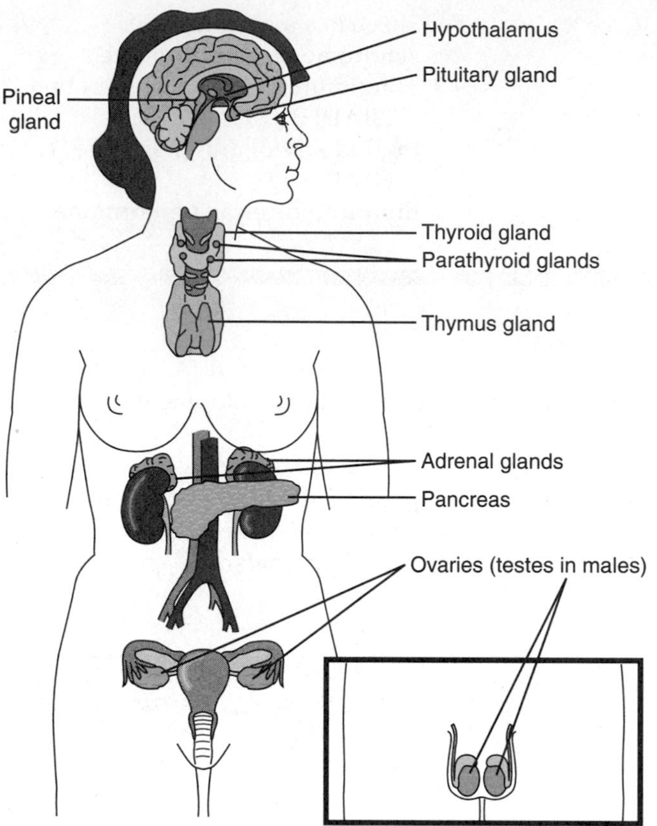

FIGURE 27–1

Organs of the classic endocrine system. Organs that have as their primary function the secretion of hormones include the hypothalamus; the pituitary, pineal, thyroid, parathyroid, and adrenal glands; the gonads (ovaries and testes); and the endocrine pancreas. The thymus gland, which secretes hormones critical to the maturation and differentiation of lymphocytes, normally atrophies after puberty.

gland are detailed, along with postulated contributions of the pineal gland to hypothalamic function. Thyroid and parathyroid function are discussed in Chapter 28, and the adrenal cortex and endocrine pancreas are examined in Chapter 29. The male and female reproductive systems and their endocrine regulation are covered in Chapters 30 and 31. The function of the adrenal medulla, which secretes catecholamine hormones in response to sympathetic nervous system stimulation, is detailed in Chapter 22.

GENERAL MECHANISMS OF ENDOCRINE ACTIVITY

Hormone Structure, Synthesis, and Transport

Hormones are either protein derivatives (glycoproteins, polypeptides, or amines) or cholesterol derivatives (steroid hormones). Table 27–2 categorizes the major hormones according to their biochemical structure. Most protein derivatives (except thyroid hormones) are water soluble, whereas the steroids are lipid soluble. As is true of all cellular protein synthesis, the protein hormones are synthesized in the rough endoplasmic reticulum and processed by the Golgi complexes. Protein hormones are then stored in vesicles within the cells until their release is stimulated. Steroid hormones, in contrast, are not stored, but are instead synthesized as needed from

TABLE 27–2
BIOCHEMICAL CLASSIFICATION OF THE MAJOR HORMONES

Classification	Examples	Source
Steroids	Cortisol	Adrenal cortex
	Aldosterone	Adrenal cortex
	Estrogen	Ovary, adrenal cortex, placenta
	Progesterone	Ovary, adrenal cortex, placenta
	Testosterone	Testis
Proteins	Thyroxine	Thyroid
	Tri-iodothyronine	Thyroid
	Calcitonin	Thyroid
	Parathyroid hormone	Parathyroid
	Epinephrine	Adrenal medulla
	Norepinephrine	Adrenal medulla
	Releasing hormones	Hypothalamus
	Release-inhibiting hormones	Hypothalamus
	Oxytocin	Hypothalamus and posterior pituitary
	Antidiuretic hormone	Hypothalamus and posterior pituitary, pineal
	Melatonin	Pineal
	Insulin	Pancreatic islets
	Glucagon	Pancreatic islets
	Trophic hormones	Anterior pituitary

cholesterol precursors in the smooth endoplasmic reticulum.

Because most water-soluble hormones circulate in free (unbound) form in the plasma, they have a more rapid onset of action. They are also more accessible to metabolic inactivation by the liver and excretion by the kidneys, however, and thus have relatively short half-lives. Lipid-soluble hormones circulate in both free form and bound to albumin and other plasma proteins. Only the free portion is active. The bound fraction serves as a reservoir for hormone: as free hormone is metabolized, more is released from protein binding. Because protein binding also protects the hormone from excretion, the greater the percentage of protein binding, the longer the half-life of the hormone.

Hormone–Receptor Interactions

Water-soluble hormones bind to fixed receptors on the target cell plasma membrane, activating second-messenger systems that culminate in activation of enzymes affecting intracellular activity (see Chapter 2). Lipid-soluble hormones pass freely through membrane lipids and bind either to mobile cytoplasmic receptors, with the complex then entering the nucleus (in the case of steroid hormones), or to nuclear receptors (in the case of thyroid hormones). The hormone–receptor complexes influence transcription factors that direct the synthesis of structural proteins and enzymes, thus affecting target organ growth and function.

At the cellular level, endocrine activity depends on the number and the affinity of receptors for hormones. Both of these factors can vary under physiologic and pathologic conditions. The number of receptors may be down-regulated as part of an adaptive negative feedback loop, or receptor proteins may be targeted by autoantibodies. Down-regulation of insulin receptors is believed to play a role in the pathophysiology of type 2 diabetes mellitus, for example (see Chapter 29).

The affinity of receptor for hormone is often variable with changes in extracellular pH, osmolarity, or concentration of hormone, or it may be altered by the presence of competitive ligands (e.g., other hormones or drugs). Binding of a water-soluble hormone to its receptor on the plasma membrane may enhance the affinity of another hormone receptor, resulting in a *permissive effect*. For example, GH in normal concentrations is permissive for **insulin**, although when present in excess, GH inhibits insulin effects. Hormones administered exogenously, in very high (nonphysiologic) doses, may produce *pharmacologic effects* that differ from the usual hormonal effect. For example, **antidiuretic hormone (ADH)**, which opposes the loss of excess water in the urine when present at physiologic levels, acts as a powerful vasoconstrictor when administered in high doses.

Metabolic Inactivation of Hormones

Like drugs, hormones must be inactivated and cleared from the plasma to prevent "overdose" effects. Protein hormones are inactivated when enzymes in the liver and kidneys cleave the peptide bonds, whereas steroid hormones are first conjugated in the liver, then excreted in bile or urine. Clinical manifestations of renal failure and hepatic failure thus include effects due to altered biotransformation and excretion of hormones (see Chapters 20 and 26).

Regulation of Endocrine Function

Some hormones (notably insulin, **glucagon**, ADH, **aldosterone**, and **parathyroid hormone**) are released in direct response to levels of one or more serum constituents. Many hormones (e.g., sex hormones, **melatonin**, and **cortisol**) demonstrate a predictable rhythmic fluctuation in their serum levels. For most endocrine glands, however, regulation of hormone secretion involves the **hypothalamic–pituitary axis (HPA)**.

HYPOTHALAMIC–PITUITARY AXIS

Anatomy

Regulation of hormone secretion from all major endocrine organs except the pancreas and parathyroids depends on the coordinated function of the hypothalamus and the pituitary gland. Anatomic proximity and the presence of both neural and vascular connections between these two organs facilitates this function. The pineal gland functions within this system as well, although the precise functions and clinical importance of this gland are still incompletely understood.

As illustrated in Figure 27–2, the pituitary gland is located centrally in the cranial vault, near the optic chiasm. Projecting below the hypothalamic nuclei, the pituitary has two major subdivisions. The anterior pituitary (adenohypophysis), the larger por-

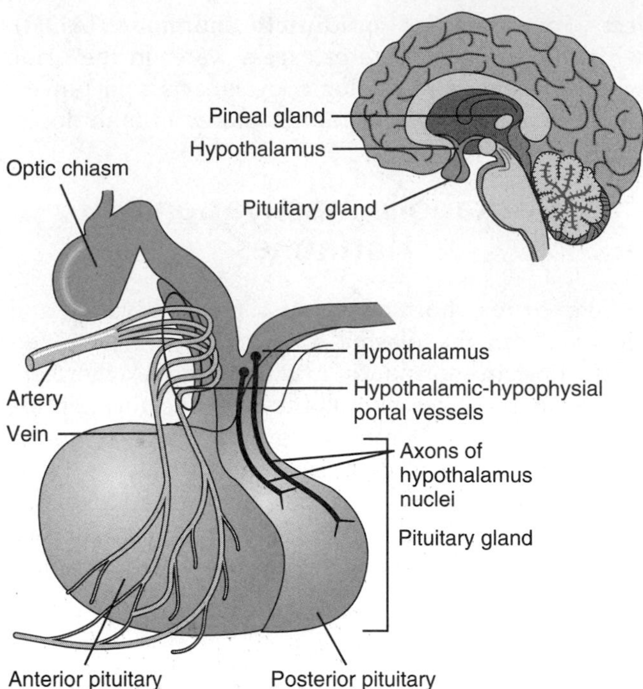

FIGURE 27–2

Relationships among the hypothalamus, pituitary, and pineal glands. The pituitary gland is located centrally within the cranial vault, projecting below the hypothalamic nuclei. The hypothalamus signals the anterior pituitary by the release of hormones into the vascular portal system. Other hypothalamic hormones are stored within the posterior pituitary gland and are released in response to neural stimuli. The pineal gland lies above and behind the hypothalamus, from which it receives neural signals. Binding of the pineal hormone, melatonin, to hypothalamic receptors may influence rhythmic biologic functions.

tion, consists of several distinct cell types, each secreting a different hormone. The vascular connection (portal system) between the hypothalamus and the anterior pituitary permits the release of anterior pituitary hormones in response to endocrine signals from hypothalamic releasing or inhibiting hormones. The posterior pituitary (neurohypophysis) does not synthesize any hormones of its own but does receive and store two hypothalamic hormones through its axonal connections to the hypothalamus.

The pineal gland, a small organ lying in the center of the brain behind the third ventricle, receives neural signals from the suprachiasmatic nucleus of the hypothalamus. This gland, like the hypothalamus, functions as a *neuroendocrine transducer*, receiving neural stimuli and responding with hormone secretion.

Negative Feedback Regulation

The HPA is a negative feedback system that regulates the release of many major hormones. Shown schematically in Figure 27–3, the system begins with the hypothalamus, which in response to certain exogenous and endogenous stimuli, secretes stimulatory or inhibitory hormones that bind to specific receptors on cells of the anterior pituitary gland. In response, the anterior pituitary gland releases trophic hormones, which in turn bind to receptors on endocrine target organs, stimulating growth, metabolism, and release of their hormones. Table 27–3 summarizes the functions of hypothalamic releasing hormones and release-inhibiting hormones. Under physiologic conditions, the releasing hormones usually predominate.

Functions of the anterior pituitary trophic hormones are summarized in Table 27–4. Most of these hormones are discussed in other chapters related to the function of their target endocrine glands. GH and related disorders are detailed later in this chap-

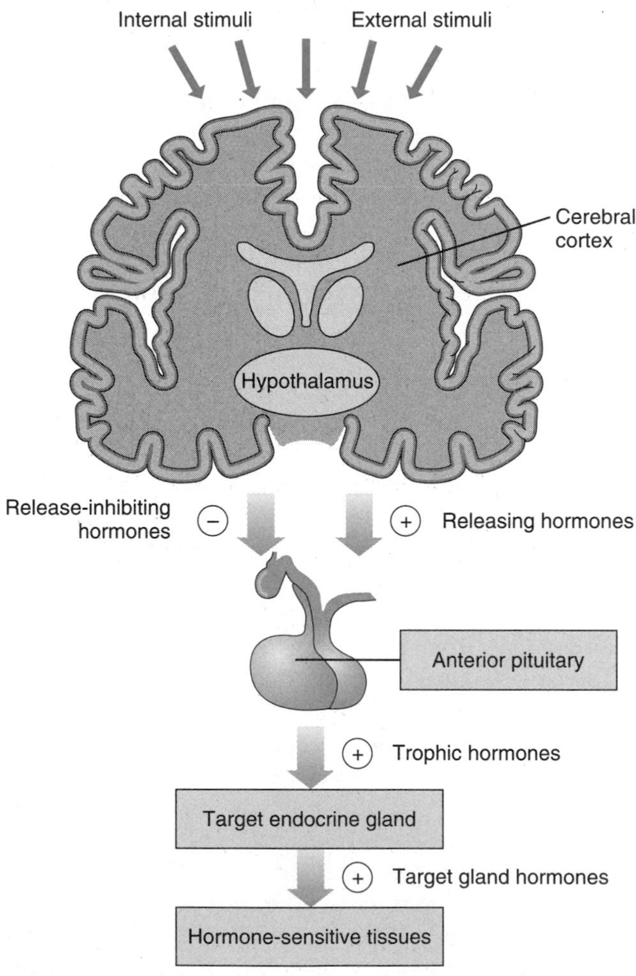

FIGURE 27–3

Hypothalamic–pituitary axis. The hypothalamic–pituitary axis is a negative feedback system that regulates the secretion of most classic hormones. The system begins with hypothalamic secretion of releasing hormones or, less commonly, release-inhibiting hormones into the portal system. These influence the secretion of specific trophic (growth and function-promoting) hormones from the anterior pituitary gland. The trophic hormones regulate the growth and secretion of target endocrine organs.

TABLE 27-3
HYPOTHALAMIC REGULATION OF PITUITARY SECRETION

Hypothalamic Hormone	Pituitary Effect
Growth hormone–releasing hormone (GHRH, or somatocrinin)	Stimulates release of growth hormone (GH, or somatotropin)
Growth hormone release–inhibiting hormone (GHRIH, or somatostatin)	Inhibits release of growth hormone
Thyrotropin-releasing hormone (TRH)	Stimulates release of thyroid-stimulating hormone (TSH, or thyrotropin) Stimulates release of prolactin
Prolactin-inhibitory hormone (PIH, or dopamine)	Inhibits release of prolactin
Gonadotropin-releasing hormone (GnRH)	Stimulates release of luteinizing hormone (LH) and follicle-stimulating hormone (FSH)
Corticotropin-releasing hormone (CRH)	Stimulates release of adrenocorticotropic hormone (ACTH, or corticotropin)

ter. Within the HPA system, negative feedback tightly regulates the rate of hormone secretion. Potentially, three levels of feedback are possible (Fig. 27–4): (1) *long-loop feedback*, in which the level of target endocrine gland hormone signals the hypothalamus to alter its rate of secretion of releasers or release inhibitors; (2) *short-loop feedback*, in which the target gland hormone feeds back to the anterior pituitary, altering trophic hormone release, or in which the trophic hormone level feeds back to the hypothalamus; and (3) *ultrashort-loop feedback*, in which the hormone released at any of the three levels feeds back to the gland that released it. The relative importance of these three forms of feedback is variable among the endocrine glands regulated by the hypothalamus–pituitary axis.

Endocrine disorders involving these glands are classified as primary, secondary, or tertiary, depending on the site of the defect within the HPA. In primary disorders, the target endocrine gland is defective. A destructive thyroid tumor could produce primary hypothyroidism, for example. In secondary disorders, the defect lies within the anterior pituitary, and in tertiary disorders the defect is at the level of the hypothalamus. Secondary hypothyroid-

TABLE 27-4
ACTIONS OF THE PITUITARY HORMONES

Hormone	Effects
Anterior Pituitary Hormones	
Growth hormone	Enhances growth and maturation of bone, cartilage, and skeletal muscle Stimulates lipolysis and protein metabolism (decreases fat deposition and increases lean body mass) Stimulates insulin release and glucose oxidation at physiologic levels; antagonizes insulin effects if present in excess Sensitizes the ovary to the effects of gonadotropins
Adrenocorticotropic hormone	Stimulates secretion and growth of the zona fasciculata and zona reticularis of the adrenal cortex Stimulates melanin production by skin cells (melanocytes)
Thyroid-stimulating hormone	Stimulates secretion and growth of the thyroid gland
Luteinizing hormone	Stimulates ovulation and corpus luteum formation in females Stimulates testosterone secretion in males
Follicle-stimulating hormone	Stimulates growth of the ovarian follicle in females Stimulates spermatogenesis in males
Prolactin	Stimulates breast development and lactation in pregnant females Enhances lymphocyte function Enhances libido and reproductive function
Posterior Pituitary Hormones	
Antidiuretic hormone	Enhances permeability of the distal tubular and collecting duct cells to water and urea Stimulates contraction of vascular smooth muscle (at pharmacologic levels) Stimulates contraction of smooth muscle within spermatic cord during ejaculation Releases clotting factor VIII from von Willebrand factor
Oxytocin	Stimulates letdown of milk from the lactating mammary gland Stimulates contraction of uterine smooth muscle May contribute to male orgasm

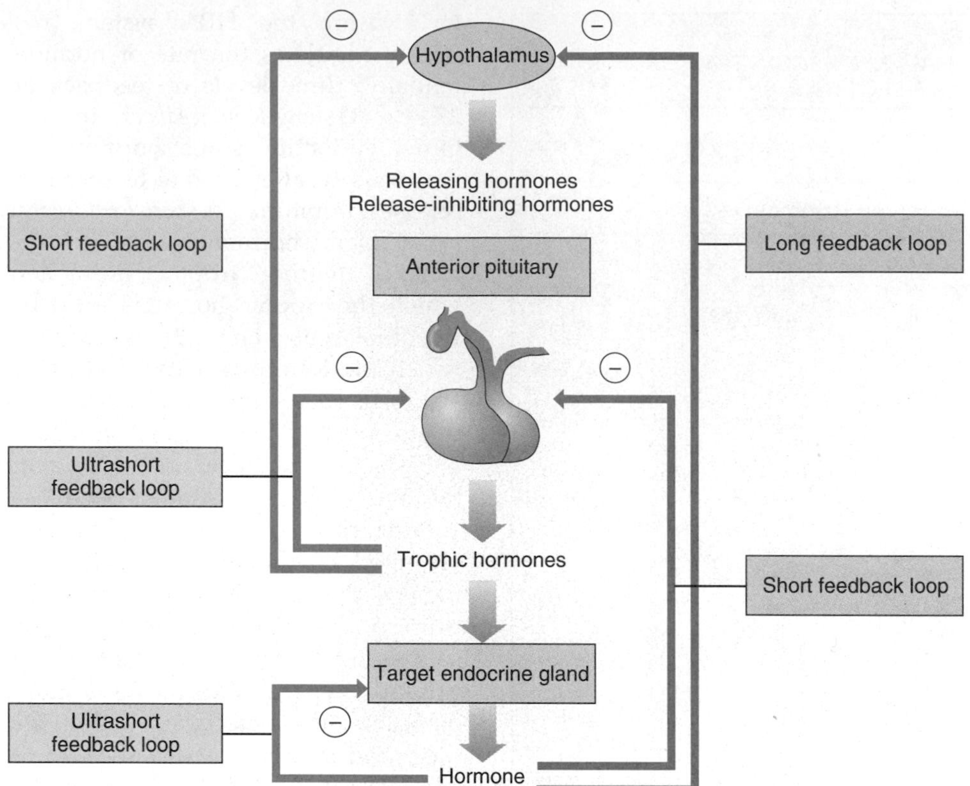

FIGURE 27–4

Negative feedback within the hypothalamic–pituitary axis. Three levels of negative feedback regulate secretion within the hypothalamic–pituitary axis. In *long loop feedback,* circulating levels of the target endocrine gland hormone influence hypothalamic secretion of releasing and release-inhibiting hormones. In *short loop feedback,* levels of target gland hormone or trophic hormones feed back to the anterior pituitary or hypothalamus, respectively. In *ultrashort loop feedback,* hormone levels signal the gland from which they were secreted.

ism could result from a tumor destroying cells of the anterior pituitary that produce **thyroid-stimulating hormone (TSH),** whereas tertiary hypothyroidism may occur due to a defect in the cells of the hypothalamus that produce **thyrotropin-releasing hormone**.

HYPOTHALAMIC HORMONES AND FUNCTIONS

Nonendocrine functions of the hypothalamus include integration of autonomic reflexes (see Chapter 22), function as a component of the limbic system (see Chapter 21), and thermoregulation (see Chapter 11). As discussed later, the hypothalamus, in conjunction with the pineal gland, also functions in regulation of the body's circadian rhythms, or "biologic clock." Endocrine functions of the hypothalamus include the regulation of anterior pituitary secretion by the HPA. Functions of the hypothalamic releasing and release-inhibiting hormones are summarized in Table 27–3.

The hypothalamus also synthesizes two other hormones, **oxytocin** and ADH. These hormones, released in response to neural stimuli, are synthesized in the cell bodies of the supraoptic and paraventricular nuclei of the hypothalamus, then transported by axoplasmic flow to the axon terminals located in the posterior pituitary gland. Actions of oxytocin and ADH are discussed later in this chapter within the context of posterior pituitary functions.

ANTERIOR PITUITARY HORMONES AND FUNCTIONS

A critical component of endocrine regulation by the HPA, the anterior pituitary gland secretes six trophic hormones that affect nearly all tissues of the body (see Table 27–4).

Growth Hormone

GH (or somatotropin) is a water-soluble polypeptide secreted by somatotrope cells, which constitute 30% to 40% of the anterior pituitary gland.[1] Basal secretion of GH is pulsatile and episodic and is regulated in response to hypothalamic **growth hormone–releasing hormone** (or somatocrinin) or **growth hormone release–inhibiting hormone** (or somatostatin). Illustrated in Figure 27–5, HPA regulation of GH secretion involves the liver as a target endocrine organ and many other tissues as end organs for GH effects. GH induces the secretion of small peptides that are structurally similar to proinsulin, the precursor of insulin. These IGFs (or somatomedins) are, in many cases, essential to the anabolic (tissue-building) effects of GH. Binding of GH to hepatic cells stimulates the production of most of the circulating IGF-I. Both IGF-I and IGF-II may be synthesized by many tissue types in response to numerous stimuli, including GH and other trophic hormones. These tissue IGFs serve primarily autocrine and paracrine functions.

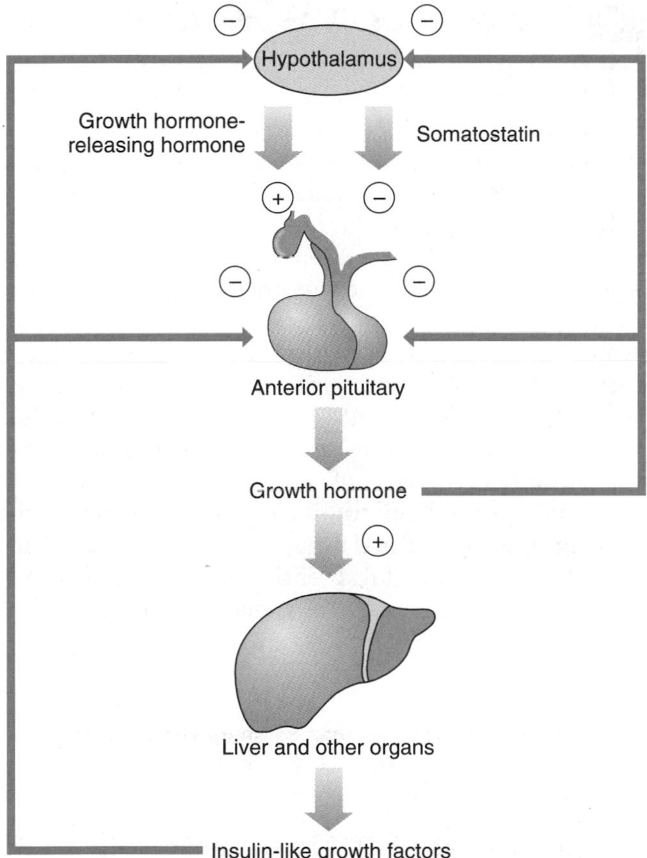

FIGURE 27–5
Hypothalamic–pituitary regulation of growth hormone activity. In response to multiple stimuli, the hypothalamus may release growth hormone–releasing hormone, which promotes secretion of growth hormone from the anterior pituitary. Alternatively, hypothalamic secretion of growth hormone release-inhibiting hormone (somatostatin) may inhibit pituitary secretion of growth hormone. Growth hormone binds to receptors in liver and other tissues, initiating its effects either directly or by stimulation of the release of insulin-like growth factors. Three levels of negative feedback may modulate growth hormone effects.

GH may exert its effects directly, by binding to GH receptors on target tissues, or indirectly, through the induction of IGF mediators. Both IGF-I and IGF-II act primarily through binding with the IGF-I receptor, although a unique IGF-II receptor also exists.[2] Furthermore, IGFs may bind to insulin receptors. IGF levels are determined not only by the rate of secretion but also by their interaction with *IGF-binding proteins*. Whether binding of IGFs to these proteins is inhibitory or stimulatory to their actions is still uncertain.

The effects of GH and the IGFs include stimulation of linear growth of bone by actions on epiphyseal cartilage and activation of vitamin D, and stimulation of visceral hypertrophy and hyperplasia, resulting in increased functional capacity of internal organs. Metabolic effects of GH are consistent with facilitation of growth but depend on the serum levels of the hormone. At physiologic levels, GH is permissive for insulin secretion, augmenting insulin effects and enhancing glucose uptake. GH deficiency results in hypoglycemia, whereas GH excess promotes hyperglycemia and lipolysis, owing to insulin resistance. Elevated GH levels also stimulate the renin–angiotensin–aldosterone system, contributing to an increase in extracellular fluid volume.

Elevated GH levels are seen in stress, in fasting states, during puberty, and during non-REM sleep, especially during childhood. Decreasing GH levels with aging may account for some of the characteristic physiologic and cognitive changes seen in older people (see Developmental Perspective). Many obese people (particularly those with visceral or central obesity) have decreased levels of GH, possibly secondary to increased levels of cortisol, which generates negative feedback to the HPA.[3] Disorders related to GH excess and deficiency are detailed later in this chapter.

Adrenocorticotropic Hormone

Adrenocorticotropic hormone (ACTH, or corticotropin) is a polypeptide hormone, cleaved from a precursor protein that also gives rise to the endogenous opiate **β-endorphin** (see Chapter 23) and to **melanocyte-stimulating hormone**, which regulates production of the skin pigment *melanin* (see Chapter

Developmental Perspective

Embryonic and Fetal Periods

GH synthesis begins in the fetal pituitary as early as 12 weeks' gestation, but normal or near-normal linear growth of the fetus may occur in the absence of GH. (It is believed that fetal growth is primarily determined by human placental somatomammotropin.) Placental production of GH occurs but is not regulated by the HPA. Fetal GH levels peak at about 22 ng/mL at 22 weeks' gestation and decline to about 10 ng/mL at term. Intrauterine growth retardation due to placental insufficiency or other factors is associated with growth delay and reduced adult height.

Infancy and Childhood

Children with genetic defects leading to pituitary dwarfism or giantism are usually normal in size at birth, but altered growth rates soon become apparent. Short stature and delayed bone age in children may be due to true GH deficiency or to genetic defects, normal genetic variation, constitutional short stature, neurosecretory disorder, or nutritional and metabolic factors. Serum melatonin levels are low at birth but increase and become circadian in older infants. Melatonin levels are highest in children 1 to 3 years of age, after which they gradually decline.

Adolescence and Young Adulthood

Melatonin production drops sharply before puberty. During normal development, a marked elevation in the amplitude of pulses of GH secretion occurs at puberty, leading to rapid linear growth in 10- to 13-year-old girls and 12- to 15-year-old boys. Growth stimulation during puberty is interrelated with the effects of elevated sex hormone levels. Estrogens and androgens stimulate GH secretion and enhance the responsiveness of target organs to GH effects. Anorexia nervosa is associated with reduced IGF levels. GH excess occurring before epiphyseal plate closure results in giantism, whereas that occurring after epiphyseal fusion results in acromegaly. Serum GH levels are elevated during pregnancy, which may adaptively stimulate the production of insulin.

Middle and Older Adulthood

The pituitary content of GH increases with aging, whereas circulating GH levels decrease. This decline is more marked in women than in men, owing to the association with declining estrogen levels at menopause. IGF-I levels are also reduced. Obesity is common in this age group and is associated with decreased GH or IGF levels. In diabetes, also prevalent among older people, GH levels are increased, but IGF-I levels are reduced. Probable effects of GH reduction with aging include decreased lean body mass, increased central obesity, decreased muscle strength, reduced aerobic exercise capacity, reduced bone mineral density, and increased atherogenicity of the serum lipid profile. Melatonin production continues to decline with advancing age. Serum melatonin levels are reduced in patients with colorectal, breast, and prostate cancer. A reduction in the ratio of melatonin to serotonin may contribute to the effects of aging.

36). ACTH secretion is regulated by the HPA and displays a diurnal pattern, with a peak in serum levels seen 2 to 4 hours before awakening. Stress and daylight exposure stimulate ACTH secretion, whereas therapy with opiates and cortisol decreases secretion. The principal function of ACTH is to regulate the growth and function of the adrenal cortex, primarily the secretion of the hormone cortisol, which promotes mobilization of energy stores. Because ACTH contains an amino acid sequence that is identical to that of melanocyte-stimulating hormone, and because ACTH levels are normally much higher than melanocyte-stimulating hormone levels, ACTH is also important in the stimulation of skin pigmentation. Disorders of adrenocortical function are discussed in Chapter 29.

Thyroid-Stimulating Hormone

TSH, also known as thyrotropin, is a glycoprotein that regulates the growth and metabolism of the thyroid gland as well as the secretion of thyroid hormones. TSH release is regulated by the HPA, as discussed in Chapter 28.

Gonadotropins

The gonadotropins **luteinizing hormone** and **follicle-stimulating hormone** are glycoproteins that regulate the development and function of the female ovaries and male testes. Although the HPA is critical to regulation of secretion of these hormones, regulation of reproductive function, especially in females, is complex, involving limited periods of positive feedback (see Chapters 30 and 31).

Prolactin

Prolactin, a polypeptide similar in structure to GH, is now known to have more comprehensive functions than its name suggests and has been found to be present in males as well as females. Regulated by the HPA, prolactin secretion is normally inhibited by hypothalamic PIH (dopamine). Functions of prolactin include the stimulation of breast development during pregnancy and production of milk (lactogenesis) in lactating females (see Chapter 32). Prolactin levels also affect sexual desire (libido) and reproductive function in both males and females by the inhibition of **gonadotropin-releasing hormone**. T lymphocytes are known to have receptors for prolactin, and binding of hormone to these receptors may play a regulatory role in immune function.[4]

Prolactin, like GH, is believed to act through the production of intermediary substances rather than by directly binding to target tissues. Prolactin secretion is stimulated by suckling of the infant in lactating females, by oxytocin, and by opiates. Secretion is inhibited by norepinephrine (during stress) and by exogenous dopamine administration. Nonphysiologic prolactin excess (*hyperprolactinemia*) is most evident in females, manifesting as menstrual irregularity and milk production (galactorrhea) independent of childbirth (see Chapter 31).

POSTERIOR PITUITARY HORMONES AND FUNCTIONS

The posterior pituitary gland releases two polypeptide hormones that are similar in structure. These hormones, synthesized by the hypothalamus, are not regulated by the HPA, but rather are regulated in direct linear response to stimulation of the hypothalamus by a variety of agents.

Antidiuretic Hormone

As discussed in detail in Chapter 8, ADH (also known as arginine vasopressin) is integral to the regulation of the osmolarity and volume of body fluids. In pharmacologic doses, ADH also has a potent vasoconstrictor effect and releases clotting factor VIII from its carrier protein, von Willebrand factor (see Chapter 14). ADH has been postulated to serve as a neuromodulator in facilitating memory and may stimulate smooth muscle contraction within the spermatic cord during ejaculation. ADH secretion is stimulated primarily by increased osmolarity of extracellular fluids (as sensed by osmoreceptors in the hypothalamus and other tissues) and secondarily by decreased extracellular fluid volume (as sensed by baroreceptors). Disorders associated with ADH excess and deficiency are detailed later in this chapter.

Oxytocin

Oxytocin has as its primary function the stimulation of ejection of milk from the lactating mammary gland. Because oxytocin also stimulates rhythmic contraction of uterine smooth muscle, it is frequently administered exogenously to induce labor. At physiologic levels, however, other hormones are probably more critical to labor and delivery than oxytocin (see Chapter 32). Oxytocin is present in males as well as females and has been postulated to contribute to male orgasm. Suckling of the infant at the breast is the major stimulus for oxytocin secretion, initiating hypothalamic stimulation by afferent neural pathways. **Estrogen** also stimulates oxytocin release, whereas catecholamines, endorphins, and opiate drugs inhibit release. The role of oxytocin in lactation is discussed further in Chapter 32.

PINEAL GLAND HORMONES AND FUNCTIONS

The importance of pineal gland function in humans is poorly understood. This small gland consists of two types of cells: pinealocytes, which secrete melatonin and other peptides (including ADH), and neuroglial cells. Melatonin, the primary pineal hormone, is synthesized from serotonin in response to the level of light received by retinal photoreceptors.[5] During daylight hours, photoreceptor cells are hyperpolarized, inhibiting release of the neurotransmitter norepinephrine. During darkness, norepinephrine is released, activating a neural signaling pathway that includes the suprachiasmatic and

TABLE 27–5
BIOLOGIC FUNCTIONS POSSIBLY MEDIATED BY MELATONIN

FUNCTION	MECHANISM
Promotion of sleep	Hypothermic effect at pharmacologic doses Receptor-mediated effect on limbic system
Regulation of circadian rhythms	Secretion of melatonin in response to stimulation of retinal photoreceptors by light and dark Receptor-mediated effects on neural and peripheral tissues
Mood elevation	Unknown
Inhibition of reproduction	Inhibition of hypothalamic–pituitary–gonadal axis Effects on ovarian steroid production
Antineoplastic effect	Direct antiproliferative effect Enhanced immune response Scavenging of reactive oxygen species
Stimulation of immune response	Increased interleukin production by helper T cells
Anti-aging effect	Scavenging of reactive oxygen species

Adapted with permission from Brzezinski, A. (1997). Melatonin in humans. *New England Journal of Medicine* 336(3), 187.

paraventricular nuclei of the hypothalamus and the superior cervical ganglion of the sympathetic nervous system. Norepinephrine binds to α_1- and β_1-adrenergic receptors in the pineal gland, and the numbers of these receptors are also up-regulated by darkness. Norepinephrine binding induces the synthesis and release of melatonin.

Melatonin binds to at least two types of receptors, which are present in the hypothalamus and other regions of the brain as well as in the gastrointestinal tract, ovaries, and blood vessels.[5] Proposed functions of melatonin, as well as possible mechanisms of these effects, are summarized in Table 27–5. Many of these mechanisms are unproved, as is the purported association of melatonin imbalance with **seasonal affective disorder**, a depressive illness that has been linked to lack of light exposure.[6]

DISORDERS OF HYPOTHALAMIC AND PITUITARY FUNCTION

The general syndrome of **hypopituitarism** is detailed next, along with specific disorders resulting from excess or deficiency of GH and ADH. Disorders of thyroid function, adrenocortical function, and reproductive system function may also relate to dysfunction of the HPA. These are discussed in subsequent chapters.

Hypopituitarism

Definition. Hypopituitarism is a deficiency of pituitary hormones. It may be partial, affecting one or a few trophic hormones, or complete (**panhypopituitarism**), affecting all trophic hormones and their target endocrine organs.

Epidemiology. The annual incidence of pituitary tumor, the most common cause of acquired hypopituitarism, has been estimated at 2.0 to 2.8 per 100,000 of the U.S. population.[7] Risk factors for the syndrome of hypopituitarism are related to the specific underlying causes. The most common factors are diabetes mellitus, pregnancy, radiation therapy, anticoagulation therapy, bleeding disorders, head injury, and carotid artery instrumentation.

Etiology. Primary pituitary tumors (usually benign adenomas) that destroy hormone-synthesizing cells are the most common cause of hypopituitarism. Tumors of the breast, lung, colon, or prostate may metastasize to the pituitary. The pituitary gland may also be damaged by radiation, trauma, hemorrhage, stroke, or inflammatory diseases such as tuberculosis. Less common causes of hypopituitarism include **Sheehan's syndrome,** in which pituitary necrosis follows postpartum hemorrhage and hypovolemia, and **empty sella syndrome**, which refers to an enlarged space surrounding the pituitary gland, caused by herniation of the arachnoid membrane into the area. The pituitary gland is usually flattened against the floor of the sella in this disorder. During pregnancy, the pituitary gland is hypertrophied and highly vascular, rendering it more vulnerable to ischemia and hemorrhage. Empty sella syndrome may result from a congenital defect in the diaphragm surrounding the space, or from an acquired defect secondary to trauma or to a tumor. Surgical resection of pituitary tumors results in iatrogenic hypopituitarism.

Pathophysiology. Deficiency of one or more trophic hormones results in lack of stimulation of target endocrine organs. Some degree of deficiency of target organ hormone results, which may be noted as a baseline state or may be uncovered by stress states in which increased secretion would be expected.

Clinical Manifestations. Manifestations of dysfunction affect most body systems, depending on which trophic hormones are deficient and the degree of deficiency (Table 27–6). ACTH deficiency may lead to signs of cortisol deficiency, including weakness, fatigue, weight loss, and altered cognitive function (see Chapter 29). Deficiency of the adrenocortical hormone aldosterone may lead to orthostatic hypotension and hyponatremia, and lack of adrenal **androgens** may cause loss of axillary and pubic hair in females. TSH deficiency may cause fatigue, weight gain, constipation, intolerance of cold, and other signs of hypothyroidism (see Chapter 28). Gonadotropin deficiency leads to sexual dysfunction and infertility (see Chapters 30 to 32). GH deficiency usually manifests as fatigue, decreased exercise tolerance, higher percentage of body fat, and increased serum lipids in adults. In children, GH deficiency leads to some degree of growth retardation, as discussed later in this chapter. Because prolactin is normally inhibited, deficiency is apparent only in lactating females. ADH deficiency leads to **diabetes insipidus (DI)**, discussed later in this chapter. Oxytocin deficiency results in decreased milk ejection during lactation (see Chapter 32).

TABLE 27–6
MANIFESTATIONS OF HYPOPITUITARISM

Deficient Hormone	Clinical Manifestations
Adrenocorticotropic hormone	Fatigue, weakness, headache, anorexia, weight loss, nausea, vomiting, abdominal pain, altered mental activity, orthostatic hypotension, loss of axillary and pubic hair in females, anemia, eosinophilia
Thyroid-stimulating hormone	Fatigue, weakness, weight gain or inability to lose weight, puffiness, constipation, cold intolerance, impaired memory, altered mental activity, bradycardia, delayed relaxation of deep-tendon reflexes, hyponatremia, anemia
Gonadotropins	In males: decreased libido, erectile dysfunction, decreased volume of ejaculate, hot flashes, decreased facial and body hair, fine facial wrinkles, gynecomastia, soft testes In females: alteration of the menstrual cycle, hot flashes, decreased libido, vaginal dryness, dyspareunia
Growth hormone	In children: growth failure In adults: lack of vigor, decreased exercise tolerance, decreased social functioning, increased body fat percentage, fine facial wrinkles
Prolactin	Failure of lactation
Antidiuretic hormone	Diabetes insipidus
Oxytocin	Decreased milk ejection during lactation

Data from Vance, M.L. (1994). Hypopituitarism. *New England Journal of Medicine* 330(23), 1651–1662.

Prevention and Treatment. Prevention of hypopituitarism is possible in cases in which risk factors may be eliminated or minimized. Pituitary adenomas are not known to be preventable, but early diagnosis based on assay of serum levels of pituitary hormones and on radiologic imaging is associated with a favorable prognosis. The treatment of choice is surgical excision of the tumor through either a trans-sphenoidal approach (through the sphenoidal sinus, with an incision though the upper gum line) or a traditional craniotomy approach. Hypopituitarism is treated with hormone replacement therapy, including exogenous hydrocortisone, thyroxine, estrogen, progesterone, or testosterone to restore normal levels. GH, now produced by recombinant DNA technology, is approved for use only in children.

Prognosis and Outcome. Prognosis depends on the underlying disorder. Most pituitary tumors are surgically resectable. As long as appropriate replacement therapy is continued, the patient is usually able to lead a normal life. Careful monitoring of serum hormone levels is essential. Although hydrocortisone doses may require adjustment in the case of unusual stressors (e.g., serious illness), replacement doses of other hormones generally remain stable.

Growth Hormone Deficiency

Definition. Growth hormone deficiency includes a group of disorders of children characterized by subnormal growth velocity, a delayed bone age, and, on provocative testing, a subnormal GH response to at least two stimuli for release of the hormone.[8] A GH deficiency syndrome has also been described in adults and is characterized by general debility and increased mortality, owing to altered metabolism, strength, and body composition.[9] Controversy exists regarding the definition of a subnormal GH response. The most rigorous criterion is a maximum serum GH level of less than 7 ng/mL, but many clinicians argue that current methods of provocative testing are not adequate to detect more subtle forms of GH deficiency, such as secretory failure, GH resistance, or structurally abnormal (bioin-

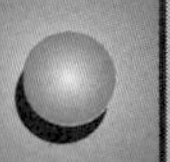

TABLE 27–7
CLINICAL SYNDROMES OF GROWTH HORMONE DEFICIENCY IN CHILDREN

SYNDROME	DESCRIPTION
Isolated growth hormone deficiency	Genetic disorder leading to dwarfism if not treated with growth hormone (GH) replacement
Neurosecretory failure	Idiopathic disorder in which growth velocity is subnormal and bone age is delayed, but growth hormone levels exceed the limits for deficiency; variable response to GH replacement
Panhypopituitarism	Growth hormone and other trophic hormones deficient, requiring replacement
Turner's syndrome	Chromosomal defect leading to multiple abnormalities, including decreased GH response to provocative stimuli and possibly increased target organ resistance to GH or insulin-like growth factors; administration of GH in high doses produces modest increases in height
Down syndrome	Chromosomal defect leading to multiple abnormalities, including short stature; GH replacement stimulates growth but does not result in improved quality of life
Intrauterine growth retardation	Birth weight is low; children who do not exhibit catch-up growth during the first year have short adult stature; GH therapy may stimulate catch-up growth in those who do not experience it spontaneously
Normal variant short stature	Children are short but have normal growth velocity and bone age; predicted adult heights are at least 10 cm less than expected on the basis of parental heights; response to GH therapy is modest and inconsistent
Familial short stature	Children are short but have normal growth velocity and bone age; predicted adult heights are within the range expected on the basis of parental heights; response to GH therapy is modest and inconsistent
Constitutional delay of growth and development	Children are short and have delayed bone ages, but their growth velocities and rates of bone age advancement are normal; pubertal development is also delayed; adult heights are normal; androgen therapy is as effective as GH in increasing the rate of development
Chronic renal failure and renal transplantation	Children grow slowly, although GH response and insulin-like growth factor I levels are normal; GH therapy may increase height but is associated with increased risk of malignancy in patients taking immunosuppressive drugs

Data from Drug and Therapeutics Committee of the Lawson Wilkins Pediatric Endocrine Society. (1995). Guidelines for the use of growth hormone in children with short stature. *Journal of Pediatrics* 127(6), 857–867; and Strobl, J.S., and Thomas, M.J. (1994). Human growth hormone. *Pharmacological Reviews* 46(1), 1–34.

active) GH.[8] Table 27–7 summarizes features of clinical syndromes of GH deficiency in children.

Epidemiology. Given the lack of agreement on the criteria for GH deficiency, the overall prevalence of the disorder is uncertain. The prevalence in children has been estimated at 1 in 4000 to 10,000 in various studies.[10] Risk factors include cerebral defects or insults, radiation, anorexia nervosa, cortisol therapy, and family history. Aging and obesity are risk factors for adult GH deficiency syndrome.

Etiology. Isolated GH deficiency in children may be inherited as an autosomal recessive, autosomal dominant, or X-linked trait. **Pituitary dwarfism** (discussed later) is usually due to a de novo genetic defect but may also be inherited. Chromosomal defects such as Turner's syndrome and Down syndrome are characterized by short stature, although not all of these children have documented GH deficiency. GH deficiency may be a component of panhypopituitarism, as has been discussed.

Children who are well-nourished but whose growth curves are below the fifth percentile for height may be diagnosed with *idiopathic growth deficiency* if testing does not establish diminished serum GH levels or GH response. This category includes those with normal variant short stature, familial short stature, or constitutional delay of growth (see Table 27–7). Intrauterine growth retardation, cortisol therapy, and chronic renal failure have also been associated with growth failure, although GH levels are variable. Increased hypothalamic secretion of somatostatin occurs when cortisol levels are high.[11] Elevated somatostatin levels and a blunted response to stimuli for GH release have been implicated in GH deficiency in obese people. The etiology of GH deficiency in most adults is the decreased activity of the

GH–IGF axis associated with normal aging, termed the *somatopause*.[9]

Pathophysiology. In children, growth failure results from absence or deficiency of GH synthesis, secretory failure, or resistance to the effects of GH or IGFs. In adults, metabolic derangements predominate, owing to decreased GH response to stimuli.

Clinical Manifestations. In children, isolated GH deficiency is manifested by height at least 2 standard deviations below the predicted mean for age and gender. Bone age, determined from x-ray evaluation of the number, size, and fusion of epiphyseal centers, is less than normal for chronologic age. If untreated, these children also demonstrate increased body fat and decreased muscle strength. Adults with GH deficiency report nonspecific symptoms, such as fatigue, inability to lose weight, and a diminished sense of well-being.[9] Muscle strength, bone density, and exercise capacity are reduced. An atherogenic serum lipid profile is common, with elevation of low-density lipoprotein cholesterol and triglycerides and reduction of high-density lipoprotein cholesterol (see Chapter 25).

Prevention and Treatment. Early detection and treatment of documented GH deficiency in children has been shown to improve growth velocity and final adult height (see Focus of Current Research). Recombinant GH has been available since 1985. Treatment is expensive and may involve multiple weekly injections for years. Use of GH replacement in idiopathic growth deficiency in children is controversial. A short-term increase in growth velocity is usually seen, but the increase in final adult height is unimpressive.[12] GH replacement for idiopathic growth deficiency has not been approved in the United States. GH replacement in adult GH deficiency syndrome is investigational.[9]

Prognosis and Outcome. In children with isolated GH deficiency, replacement therapy results in doubling or tripling of height velocity, peaking after 1 to 2 years of treatment.[11] In idiopathic growth deficiency, treatment with GH results in accelerated growth in 75% to 80% of children. Short-term improvement of metabolic abnormalities may be achieved with GH replacement in adults, but effects on mortality and functional status have not been demonstrated.[9] The risks associated with GH replacement have not been thoroughly investigated. In children, increased risk of leukemia has been associated with GH replacement, particularly in those also immunosuppressed.[12] Other reported adverse effects include hypothyroidism, slipping of the femoral epiphyseal plate, insulin resistance, and sodium and water retention. Some patients also develop features of **acromegaly**.

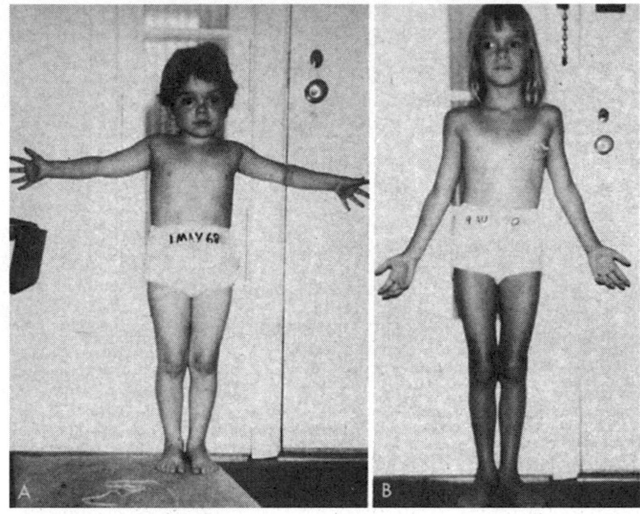

FIGURE 27–6

Pituitary dwarfism. A young girl with pituitary dwarfism is shown before (*A*) and after (*B*) treatment with growth hormone replacement. (From Wilson, J.D., and Foster, D.W. [1985]. *Williams' Textbook of Endocrinology*. [7th ed.]. Philadelphia: W.B. Saunders. [p. 599].)

Pituitary Dwarfism

Definition. Pituitary dwarfism is a markedly abnormal small stature due to deficiency of GH or somatomedins (Fig. 27–6).

Epidemiology. Pituitary dwarfism is uncommon. Because most cases are idiopathic, risk factors are uncertain. A high incidence of breech delivery has been reported among these patients.[13] Pituitary dwarfism may be due to an isolated deficiency or may occur as a component of panhypopituitarism.

Etiology. The cause of most cases of pituitary dwarfism is an idiopathic deficiency in hypothalamic growth hormone–releasing hormone secretion. In some cases, there is congenital agenesis of the pituitary, or hypopituitarism due to a destructive tumor. A rare form, Laron's dwarfism, results from an idiopathic deficiency in somatomedin production despite normal GH levels.

Pathophysiology. The abnormality within the HPA regulating synthesis of GH and somatomedins results in inadequate stimulation of tissue growth as well as metabolic abnormalities due to impaired interaction between GH and insulin.

Clinical Manifestations. The affected infant may be small for gestational age or of normal length and weight at birth, but delayed growth becomes apparent during the first year of life. Hypoglycemia is common, resulting in increased feeding demands, irritability, shakiness, and possibly seizures. Visceral

Focus of Current Research

Study	Objective and Findings
Blethen, et al. (1996) Overview of the National Cooperative Growth Study substudy of serial growth hormone measurements.	*Objective:* To evaluate spontaneous growth hormone (GH) secretion in children with idiopathic short stature compared with children classified as GH-deficient on the basis of pharmacologic testing *Findings:* Children who were classified as having GH deficiency had lower spontaneous GH secretion than those classified as having idiopathic short stature, but considerable overlap existed between groups.
Fazio, et al. (1996) A preliminary study of growth hormone in the treatment of dilated cardiomyopathy.	*Objective:* To determine the effect of inducing cardiac hypertrophy with growth hormone treatment on patients with idiopathic dilated cardiomyopathy, a condition in which compensatory hypertrophy is believed to be deficient *Findings:* GH therapy increased myocardial mass and reduced the size of the left ventricular chamber, resulting in improvement in hemodynamics, myocardial energy metabolism, and clinical status.
Kaplowitz (1995) Effect of growth hormone therapy on final versus predicted height in short twelve- to sixteen-year-old boys without growth hormone deficiency.	*Objective:* To determine whether adult height in these children exceeded that predicted from bone age at the start of therapy *Findings:* After 2 years of treatment, final height was close to that predicted from pretherapy bone age, although the rate of bone growth increased.
Albanese & Stanhope (1995) Predictive factors in the determination of final height in boys with constitutional delay of growth and puberty.	*Objective:* To identify predictive factors of final height outcome in order to select patients who may benefit from alternative therapeutic approaches *Findings:* A late onset in the timing of puberty appears to be deleterious to spinal growth and final height attainment. Treatment with androgens did not affect outcomes.
Malozowski & Stadel (1995) Prepubertal gynecomastia during growth hormone therapy.	*Objective:* To describe the cases of gynecomastia (breast enlargement) developing before puberty in boys treated with growth hormone *Findings:* Gynecomastia developed in 22 boys treated with GH, usually between 0.5 and 7 months after treatment was begun. The condition appears to be self-limited and benign.

Continued

Continued

Golden, et al. (1994) Disturbances in growth hormone secretion and action in adolescents with anorexia nervosa.	*Objectives:* To compare serum levels of GH and insulin-like growth factors (IGFs) in patients with anorexia versus controls; to correlate findings with measures of body composition, energy expenditure, and hypothalamic–pituitary function; and to evaluate the effects of nutritional rehabilitation on GH and IGF levels *Findings:* GH levels did not differ between groups, but levels of IGF and IGF-binding proteins were lower in subjects with anorexia, correlating with body mass index. Refeeding normalized IGF levels.

obesity may result from altered lipid metabolism. Linear growth is proportionately deficient (unlike *achondroplastic dwarfism*, a hereditary skeletal disorder in which the growth deficiency disproportionately affects the limbs). The bones of the skull demonstrate variable growth rates, with protrusion of the frontal bones and flattening of the bridge of the nose. In many affected children, puberty is delayed or absent. Intellectual development is normal unless there is brain damage associated with prolonged hypoglycemia and seizures. If a pituitary tumor is present, signs of increased intracranial pressure may be evident, and alterations in the levels of other pituitary hormones may produce specific manifestations.

Prevention and Treatment. Early diagnosis of GH deficiency is optimal. Surgical removal of any pituitary tumor is indicated. Subsequent replacement of GH may modulate short stature and metabolic abnormalities.

Prognosis and Outcome. The earlier the diagnosis and onset of treatment, the more favorable the outcome. Social development is critical to outcome and requires treating the child according to age instead of size.

Pituitary Giantism

Definition. Pituitary giantism (or gigantism) is objectively defined as height and weight greater than 3 standard deviations above the mean for age and sex.[14]

Epidemiology. Pituitary giantism is rare. Risk factors are the general factors associated with neoplasia.

Etiology. Pituitary giantism is caused by a GH-producing pituitary adenoma in which GH excess is present before closure of the epiphyseal growth plates of long bones.

Pathophysiology. Excess GH stimulates linear growth, increased bulk of bones and joints, enlargement of internal organs, and metabolic abnormalities. The pituitary tumor constitutes a space-occupying intracranial mass. Secretion of other pituitary hormones may also be altered by the tumor.

Clinical Manifestations. If untreated, the patient may grow to a height of 7 to 9 feet. Joints are painful, and bones may be osteoporotic. Enlargement of intracranial tissues may lead to headache and other signs of increased intracranial pressure. Cardiomegaly may lead to hypertension and heart failure. Excessive GH opposes insulin, leading to hyperglycemia and related metabolic abnormalities.

Prevention and Treatment. Routine monitoring of infant growth and development nearly always results in early detection of the condition. Treatment requires surgical removal of the pituitary tumor, with postoperative replacement of hormones as necessary.

Prognosis and Outcome. With early diagnosis and treatment, prognosis is excellent. If untreated, the condition leads to shortened life expectancy, owing to hypertension and heart failure.

Acromegaly

Definition. Acromegaly is accelerated growth and metabolism due to GH excess arising in adults, following epiphyseal closure.

Epidemiology. Acromegaly is uncommon, occurring in an estimated 50 to 70 people per 1 million in the United States.[15] The disorder is diagnosed with equal frequency in both sexes, with most cases diagnosed in patients in their 30s, 40s or 50s.[16]

Etiology. In 98% of cases, acromegaly is caused by a GH-secreting pituitary adenoma.[17]

Pathophysiology. Because epiphyseal plates have

fused, GH excess does not increase linear growth of bone. Bone density and width do increase, and there is proliferation of the connective tissue matrix of soft tissues. Excess GH opposes the effects of insulin, promoting hyperglycemia and, ultimately, diabetes mellitus (see Chapter 29). Altered levels of other pituitary hormones may be present concurrently.

Clinical Manifestations. Increased nonlinear bone growth manifests as large hands and feet, protruding jaw, enlarged joints, and splayed teeth (Fig. 27–7). Soft tissue enlargement is evident in broadening of the nose, enlargement of the lips, and deep voice due to enlargement of the larynx. The heart is enlarged, and hypertension is common. Diabetes mellitus due to insulin resistance is common, and atherosclerosis is accelerated, owing to the combined effects of the cardiac and metabolic abnormalities. The growing intracranial tumor may cause increased intracranial pressure.

Prevention and Treatment. Surgical excision of the tumor is the treatment of choice. Administration of a somatostatin analog (octreotide) and radiation therapy have been employed to shrink unresectable tumors or as an adjunct to surgery if the tumor cannot be completely removed. Replacement of pituitary hormones (other than GH) may be used postoperatively to restore normal levels. GH replacement is not used in the treatment of adults.

Prognosis and Outcome. Prognosis is most favorable with early diagnosis and treatment. Morbidity and mortality are associated with the presence and severity of diabetes and atherosclerosis. Acromegaly is associated with a two- to three-fold increase in mortality rates.[15]

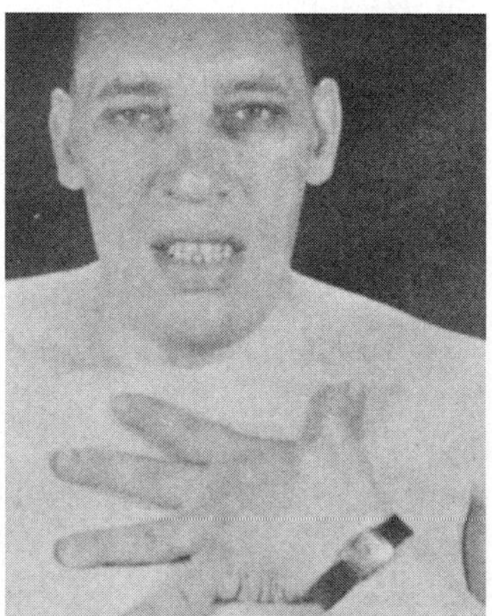

FIGURE 27–7
Acromegaly. Note the enlarged hands, protruding jaw, broad nose, thick lips, and splayed teeth. (From Wilson, J.D., and Foster, D.W. [1985]. *Williams' Textbook of Endocrinology*. [7th ed.]. Philadelphia: W.B. Saunders. [p. 602].)

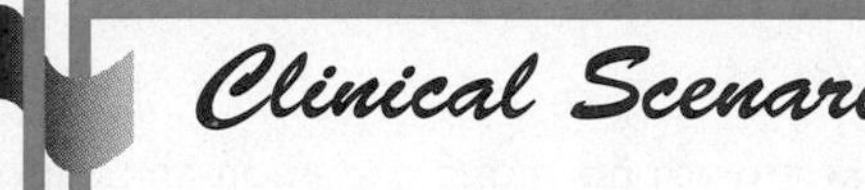

During a routine physical examination, T.M., 45 years of age, reports enlargement of his hands, weight gain, deepening of his voice, and increases in his clothing and shoe sizes. His dentist had recently noted widening of the spaces between his teeth. Serum testing reveals elevated levels of GH and IGF-I. Magnetic resonance imaging demonstrates the presence of a pituitary tumor.

1. What process is causing T.M.'s clinical manifestations? Would T.M.'s height be expected to increase? Explain.
2. What additional disorders might arise as a consequence of GH excess? How might this risk be minimized?

Syndrome of Inappropriate Antidiuretic Hormone Secretion

Definition. The **syndrome of inappropriate antidiuretic hormone secretion (SIADH)** is the disorder resulting from excess ADH secretion triggered by stimuli other than increased extracellular fluid osmolarity and decreased extracellular fluid volume.

Epidemiology. SIADH is a relatively common complication of critical illness and surgery. The conditions most frequently associated with the syndrome are cancers, including oat cell carcinoma of the lung, carcinomas of the duodenum or pancreas, leukemias, and lymphomas. Craniotomy and other surgeries may precipitate increased ADH release. Respiratory infections, psychiatric disease, extreme stress and pain, and certain drugs have also been linked to SIADH (Table 27–8).

Etiology. Cancers result in increased ADH release, owing to ectopic hormone production as a paraneoplastic syndrome (see Chapter 7). With craniotomy, particularly pituitary surgery, stored ADH may be mechanically released by manipulation. After most major surgeries, ADH secretion and release are increased for several days, probably secondary to iatrogenic and adaptive alterations in fluid volume and osmolarity. The mechanisms by which other diseases, stress, and drugs increase ADH secretion are uncertain and probably variable. Iatrogenic ADH excess may result from overtreatment of diabetes insipidus.

Pathophysiology. In the presence of excess ADH, excessive water is reabsorbed from the distal convoluted tubule and collecting ducts of the renal neph-

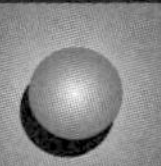

TABLE 27–8
CONDITIONS ASSOCIATED WITH SIADH SECRETION

Ectopic antidiuretic hormone
Malignancies
Lung (oat cell)
Lymphoma
Pancreas and duodenum
Endogenous causes
Central nervous system disorders
Brain tumors
Hemorrhagic states (subdural hematoma, cerebral vascular accident)
Head trauma
Infections: meningitis, encephalitis, brain abscesses
Guillain-Barré syndrome
Lupus erythematosus
Pulmonary conditions
Positive-pressure mechanical ventilation
Acute respiratory failure (↓ Po_2, ↑ Pco_2)
Infection
Viral pneumonia
Tuberculosis
Chronic obstructive pulmonary disease
Lung abscesses
Postoperative period
Drugs
Nicotine
Carbamazepine (Tegretol)
Chlorpropamide
Barbiturates
Analgesics (morphine)
Antineoplastic drugs
Anesthetics
Tricyclic antidepressants

Po_2, partial pressure of oxygen; Pco_2, partial pressure of carbon dioxide; SIADH, syndrome of inappropriate antidiuretic hormone. From Batcheller, J. (1994). Syndrome of inappropriate antidiuretic hormone secretion. *Critical Care Nursing Clinics of North America* 6(4), 687–692.

rons, leading to dilution of the extracellular fluid compartment. Clinical manifestations are due to hypervolemia (see Chapter 8) and hyponatremia (see Chapter 9).

Clinical Manifestations. Serum osmolarity is low, whereas urine osmolarity is disproportionately elevated. Serum sodium levels are low, and the degree of hyponatremia determines the severity of the condition. The earliest signs include thirst, anorexia, fatigue, and lethargy; these are followed by vomiting and intestinal cramping as Na^+ levels drop further. At serum levels of 115 MEq/L or less, more severe central nervous system manifestations, including seizures and coma, may occur, owing to osmotic swelling of cells.

Prevention and Treatment. Prevention requires careful monitoring of serum osmolarity and electrolytes in patients at risk. Optimal treatment of the underlying disorder is warranted. Drug therapy that may contribute to the condition is discontinued. Hyponatremia and hypervolemia are usually correctable with water restriction alone. Intravenous hypertonic (3%) sodium chloride may be used for patients with acute hypernatremia. Loop diuretics (e.g., furosemide) may be used in treatment of those who are severely hypervolemic.[18]

Prognosis and Outcome. Prognosis depends on both the degree of ADH excess and the rate at which it develops. SIADH usually resolves within 2 to 3 days of effective intervention.

Diabetes Insipidus

Definition. DI is a disorder characterized by excessive output of dilute urine due to lack of ADH secretion by the posterior pituitary gland (*neurogenic* or *central DI*) or lack of renal response to normal ADH levels (*nephrogenic DI*).

Epidemiology. Neurogenic DI may be associated with stroke, hypothalamic or pituitary tumors, and cranial trauma or surgery (see Chapter 21). Nephrogenic DI is less common but may occur in patients with end-stage renal failure (see Chapter 20). One form of nephrogenic DI is familial, and certain drugs, including lithium, demeclocycline, and methoxyflurane, may result in transient DI.

Etiology. Neoplastic, traumatic, or ischemic destruction of the paraventricular and supraoptic nuclei of the hypothalamus results in neurogenic DI. The disorder is permanent when more than 80% of the supraoptic and paraventricular nuclei are affected or when the proximal end of the pituitary stalk is destroyed.[19] If damage is lower on the pituitary stalk, ADH release is decreased, but other pituitary sites may compensate to some extent. In nephrogenic DI, damage to renal tubular cells interferes with the normal ADH effect, in which protein channels are inserted in the tubular membrane to enhance the permeability of the distal nephron to water and urea.

Pathophysiology. Lack of ADH, or lack of renal ADH effect, leads to large outputs of dilute urine. If the thirst reflex is intact, the patient drinks large volumes of fluids to compensate. If fluid intake is not increased, hypovolemic shock ensues.

Clinical Manifestations. Polydipsia (excessive thirst) and polyuria (excessive urination) are the cardinal symptoms of DI. (These are also characteristic of diabetes mellitus, discussed in Chapter 29). Nocturia (frequent urination at night) disturbs sleep and leads to fatigue. Urine volumes approach 15 liters per 24 hours.[19] Patients may drink nearly continuously to compensate, with resulting abdominal fullness, anorexia, and weight loss. Serum osmolarity is high, whereas urine osmolarity is low. If dehydration is severe, manifestations of shock and renal failure are evident.

Prevention and Treatment. Reduction of risk factors for stroke, head injury, and conditions leading to renal failure are relevant to the prevention of DI. Underlying conditions should be optimally managed. Maintenance of adequate hydration is essential in patients with DI. Free water is replaced, and hypernatremia is corrected. Neurogenic DI is treated with replacement of ADH, usually in the form of a synthetic analog, desmopressin (DDAVP). In patients who retain some degree of ADH synthesis, drugs that enhance its release may be used. These include clofibrate (Atromid-S) and carbamazepine (Tegretol). ADH replacement is not effective in treatment of nephrogenic DI. Water replacement is indicated, and restriction of dietary protein and sodium may assist in reducing urine excretion. Drug therapy is aimed at reduction of the delivery of fluid to the distal tubules of the nephron and may include thiazide diuretics, chlorpropamide, and nonsteroidal anti-inflammatory drugs.[19]

Prognosis and Outcome. Prognosis relates to the severity of the underlying intracranial disorder in neurogenic DI. Hypothalamic and pituitary tumors can often be successfully excised or controlled with adjunctive therapy. Nephrogenic DI is associated with end-stage renal failure, in which the prognosis is poor.

CLINICAL SIGNIFICANCE OF HYPOTHALAMIC AND PITUITARY DISORDERS

The significance of hypothalamic and pituitary disorders does not reside with their commonality because they are relatively rare. Rather, their significance lies in their illustration of mechanisms of endocrine control by the HPA. Clinical understanding of the regulation of hormone synthesis and release is still limited, although research is ongoing in an effort to illuminate the mechanisms. The importance of the multiple hormones of the diffuse endocrine system is under intensive study, as are the cellular mechanisms of hormone action. As illustrated by the disorders detailed in this chapter, hypothalamic and pituitary disorders affect children as well as adults. HPA regulation of thyroid, adrenocortical, and reproductive function is detailed in Chapters 28 to 32.

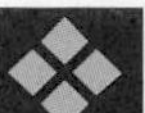

Summary of Key Points

- Endocrine mechanisms of regulation differ from neural regulation in that their effects are of slower onset and longer duration. Both systems use signaling molecules, and to the extent that these molecules travel in the bloodstream to more distant targets, they serve as hormones.
- Hormones are either protein derivatives (glycoproteins, polypeptides, or amines) or cholesterol derivatives (steroids). Proteins are synthesized at basal rates and stored within vesicles until their release is stimulated. Steroids are not stored but rather are synthesized on demand. Protein hormones (except thyroid hormones) circulate primarily in unbound form, whereas steroids may bind to albumin and other plasma proteins. Protein hormones (except thyroid hormones) exert their actions through binding to cell surface receptors. Steroids and thyroid hormones pass through membrane lipids and bind to intracellular or, in the case of thyroid hormones, nuclear receptors. Protein hormones are metabolized to amino acids by renal and hepatic enzymes, then excreted in the urine. Steroid hormones are conjugated in the liver, then excreted in the bile or urine.
- The hypothalamus, a group of nuclei serving varied neuroendocrine functions, is located above the pituitary gland. Vascular (portal) connections exist between the hypothalamus and the anterior pituitary gland. In response to varied stimuli, the hypothalamus releases protein releasing hormones or release-inhibiting hormones into the portal system. These hormones influence the secretion of trophic hormones by the anterior pituitary gland. Trophic hormones stimulate the secretion of hormones from target endocrine organs, including the thyroid, adrenal cortex, gonads, mammary glands, and liver. Negative feedback loops act at each level of this HPA to modulate fluctuations in serum levels of hormones.
- In addition to releasing hormones and release-inhibiting hormones, the hypothalamus secretes oxytocin and ADH. In response to neural stimuli, these hormones are released from storage in the posterior pituitary gland to influence lactation and fluid balance, re-

Continued

spectively. The pineal gland responds to stimulation of photoreceptors in the retina by a pathway that involves the hypothalamus and sympathetic nervous system. Darkness stimulates the release of the pineal hormone melatonin, which binds to hypothalamic receptors to influence biologic rhythms, such as sleep–wake cycles.

◆ Hypothalamic and pituitary disorders may be the result of hypofunction (hormone deficiency) or hyperfunction (hormone excess). Primary disorders of endocrine organs regulated by the HPA are due to a defect of the target endocrine gland; secondary disorders are due to a defect in anterior pituitary function; and tertiary disorders are due to a defect in hypothalamic function. Clinical manifestations of deficiency syndromes reflect absence of hormonal action (lack of principal hormone effect or permissive effects on other hormones). Manifestations of excess reflect exaggerated hormonal actions or pharmacologic effects. Intervention is aimed at early detection of abnormalities and at normalization of hormone levels.

REFERENCES

1. Guyton, A.C., and Hall, J.E. (1996). *Textbook of Medical Physiology*. (9th ed.). Philadelphia: W.B. Saunders. (pp. 933–944).
2. Jones, J.J., and Clemmons, D.R. (1995). Insulin-like growth factors and their binding proteins: Biological actions. *Endocrine Reviews* 16(1), 3–34.
3. Bjorntorp, P. (1995). Endocrine abnormalities of obesity. *Metabolism* 44(9 suppl. 3), 21–23.
4. Reber, P.M. (1993). Prolactin and immunomodulation. *American Journal of Medicine* 95, 637–644.
5. Brzezinski, A. (1997). Melatonin in humans. *New England Journal of Medicine* 336(3), 186–195.
6. Rosenthal, N.E. (1993). Diagnosis and treatment of seasonal affective disorder. *Journal of the American Medical Association* 270(22), 2717–2720.
7. Vance, M.L. (1994). Hypopituitarism. *New England Journal of Medicine* 330(23), 1651–1662.
8. Drug and Therapeutics Committee of the Lawson Wilkins Pediatric Endocrine Society. (1995). Guidelines for the use of growth hormone in children with short stature. *Journal of Pediatrics* 127(6), 857–867.
9. Lieberman, S.A., and Hoffman, A.R. (1996). Growth hormone deficiency in adults: Characteristics and response to growth hormone replacement. *Journal of Pediatrics* 128(5 Pt. 2), S58–S60.
10. Phillips, J.A., and Cogan, J.D. (1994). Molecular basis of familial human growth hormone deficiency. *Journal of Clinical Endocrinology and Metabolism* 78(1), 11–16.
11. Strobl, J.S., and Thomas, M.J. (1994). Human growth hormone. *Pharmacological Reviews* 46(1), 1–34.
12. Neely, E.K., and Rosenfeld, R.G. (1994). Use and abuse of human growth hormone. *Annual Review of Medicine* 45, 407–420.
13. Triulzi, F., Scotti, G., di Natale, B., *et al.* (1994). Evidence of a congenital midline brain anomaly in pituitary dwarfs: A magnetic resonance imaging study in 101 patients. *Pediatrics* 93(3), 409–416.
14. Job, J.C., and Pierson, M. (Eds.). (1981). *Pediatric Endocrinology*. New York: John Wiley & Sons. As cited in: Foster, R.L.R., Hunsberger, M.M., and Anderson, J.J.T. (1989). *Family-Centered Nursing Care of Children*. Philadelphia: W.B. Saunders. (p. 1909).
15. Acromegaly Therapy Consensus Development Panel. (1994). Consensus statement: Benefits versus risks of medical therapy for acromegaly. *American Journal of Medicine* 97, 468–473.
16. Maugans, T.A., and Coates, M.L. (1995). Diagnosis and treatment of acromegaly. *American Family Physician* 52(1), 207–213.
17. Melmed, S., Ho, K., Klibanski, A., *et al.* (1995). Recent advances in pathogenesis, diagnosis, and management of acromegaly. *Journal of Clinical Endocrinology and Metabolism* 80(12), 3395–3402.
18. Batcheller, J. (1994). Syndrome of inappropriate antidiuretic hormone secretion. *Critical Care Nursing Clinics of North America* 6(4), 687–692.
19. Bell, T.N. (1994). Diabetes insipidus. *Critical Care Nursing Clinics of North America* 6(4), 675–685.

SELECTED BIBLIOGRAPHY

Albanese, A., and Stanhope, R. (1995). Predictive factors in the determination of final height in boys with constitutional delay of growth and puberty. *Journal of Pediatrics* 126(4), 545–550.

Allen, D.B. (1996). Safety of human growth hormone therapy: Current topics. *Journal of Pediatrics* 128(5 Pt 2), S8–S13.

Blethen, S.L., Breen, T.J., and Attie, K.M. (1996). Overview of the National Cooperative Growth Study substudy of serial growth hormone measurements. *Journal of Pediatrics* 128(5 Pt. 2), S38–S41.

Blondell, R.D. (1991). Hypopituitarism. *American Family Physician* 43(6), 2029–2036.

Buyalos, R.P. (1995). Insulin-like growth factors: Clinical experience in ovarian function. *American Journal of Medicine* 98(suppl. 1A), 55S–66S.

Cavallo, A. (1993). The pineal gland in human beings: Relevance to pediatrics. *Journal of Pediatrics* 123(6), 843–851.

Chrousos, G.P. (1995). The hypothalamic-pituitary-adrenal axis and immune-mediated inflammation. *New England Journal of Medicine* 332(20), 1351–1362.

Conn, P.M. (1994). Gonadotropin-releasing hormone and its analogs. *Annual Review of Medicine* 45, 391–405.

Edge, D.S., and Segatore, M. (1993). Assessment and management of galactorrhea. *Nurse Practitioner* 18(6), 35–49.

Fazio, S., Sabatini, D., Capaldo, B., *et al.* (1996). A preliminary study of growth hormone in the treatment of dilated cardiomyopathy. *New England Journal of Medicine* 334(13), 809–814.

Francomano, C.A. (1995). The genetic basis of dwarfism. *New England Journal of Medicine* 332(1), 58–59.

Gelber, S.J., Heffez, D.S., and Donohoue, P.A. (1992). Pituitary gigantism caused by growth hormone excess from infancy. *Journal of Pediatrics* 120(6), 931–934.

Giudice, L. (1995). The insulin-like growth factor system in normal and abnormal human ovarian follicle development. *American Journal of Medicine* 98(suppl. 1A), 48S–54S.

Golden, N.H., Kreitzer, P., Jacobson, M.S., *et al.* (1994). Disturbances in growth hormone secretion and action in adolescents with anorexia nervosa. *Journal of Pediatrics* 125(4), 655–660.

Hughes, J.M., Ellsworth, C.A., and Harris, B.S. (1995). Clinical case seminar: A 33-year-old woman with a pituitary mass and panhypopituitarism. *Journal of Clinical Endocrinology and Metabolism* 80(5), 1521–1525.

Kaplowitz, P.B. (1995). Effect of growth hormone therapy on final versus predicted height in short twelve- to sixteen-year-old boys without growth hormone deficiency. *Journal of Pediatrics* 126(3), 478–480.

Kaye, T.B. (1996). Hyperprolactinemia: Causes, consequences, and treatment options. *Postgraduate Medicine* 99(5), 265–268.

Kendler, B.S. (1997). Melatonin: Media hype or therapeutic breakthrough. *Nurse Practitioner* 22(2), 66–77.

Korte, C., Styne, D., Merritt, A., *et al.* (1996). Adrenocortical function in the very low birth weight infant: Improved testing sensitivity and association with neonatal outcome. *Journal of Pediatrics* 128(2), 257–263.

Lamberts, S.W.J., van der Lely, A-J., de Herder, W.W., *et al.* (1996). Octreotide. *New England Journal of Medicine* 334(4), 246–254.

LeRoith, D. (Moderator). (1995). NIH Conference: Insulin-like growth factors and cancer. *Annals of Internal Medicine* 122(1), 54–59.

Loriaux, T.C. (1996). Endocrine assessment: Red flags for those on the front lines. *Nursing Clinics of North America* 31(4), 695–713.

Malozowski, S., and Stadel, B.V. (1995). Prepubertal gynecomastia during growth hormone therapy. *Journal of Pediatrics* 126(4), 659–661.

Miller, M. (1996). Endocrine disorders: New technology allows quick, accurate diagnosis. *Geriatrics* 51(1), 52–58.

Moffatt, M.E.K., Harlos, S., Kirshen, A.J., *et al.* (1993). Desmopressin acetate and nocturnal enuresis: How much do we know? *Pediatrics* 92(3), 420–425.

Nachtigall, L.B., Boepple, P.A., Pralong, F.P., *et al.* (1997). Adult-onset idiopathic hypogonadotropic hypogonadism: A treatable form of male infertility. *New England Journal of Medicine* 336(6), 410–415.

Romero, J.H. (1996). Hyperfunction and hypofunction in the anterior pituitary. *Nursing Clinics of North America* 31(4), 769–778.

Rusterholtz, A. (1996). Interpretation of diagnostic laboratory tests in selected endocrine disorders. *Nursing Clinics of North America* 31(4), 715–724.

Schachter, S.C. (1994). Neuroendocrine aspects of epilepsy. *Neurologic Clinics* 12(1), 31–37.

Seeman, T.E., and Robbins, R.J. (1994). Aging and hypothalamic-pituitary-adrenal response to challenge in humans. *Endocrine Reviews* 15(2), 233–260.

Spagnoli, A., Spadoni, G.L., Cianfarani, S., *et al.* (1995). Prediction of the outcome of growth hormone therapy in children with idiopathic short stature. *Journal of Pediatrics* 126(6), 905–909.

Takahashi, T., Shoji, Yu., Shoji, Ya., *et al.* (1997). Active hypothalamic-pituitary-gonadal axis in an infant with X-linked adrenal hypoplasia congenita. *Journal of Pediatrics* 130(3), 485–488.

Van Cauter, E., and Plat, L. (1996). Physiology of growth hormone secretion during sleep. *Journal of Pediatrics* 128(5 Pt. 2), S32–S37.

Winger, J.M., and Hornick, T. (1996). Age-associated changes in the endocrine system. *Nursing Clinics of North America* 31(4), 827–844.

Yanovski, J.A., Yanovski, S.Z., Cutler, G.B., *et al.* (1996). Differences in the hypothalamic-pituitary-adrenal axis of black girls and white girls. *Journal of Pediatrics* 129(1), 130–135.

Zadik, A., Zung, A., Sarel, R., *et al.* (1997). Evolving growth hormone deficiency in children with a subnormal secretion of growth hormone. *Journal of Pediatrics* 130(3), 481–484.

Thyroid and Parathyroid Disorders

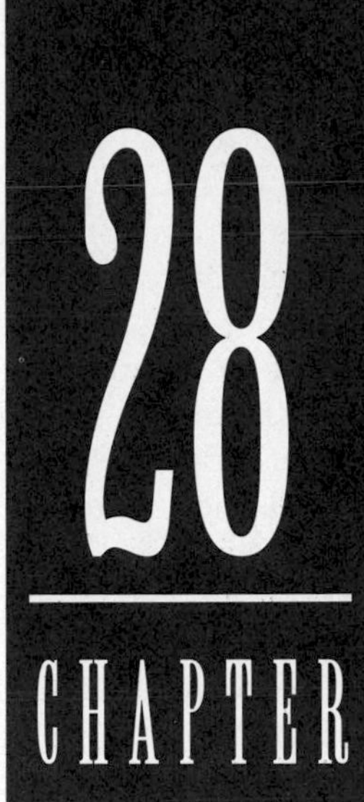

LEARNING OBJECTIVES

1. Discuss the clinical importance of the anatomic relationship of the thyroid and parathyroid glands.
2. Describe the processes of thyroid hormone synthesis, transport, and storage.
3. Discuss the cellular mechanism and target organ effects of thyroid hormone.
4. Characterize the relationship between parathyroid hormone and serum calcium.
5. Discuss the pathophysiologic mechanisms that predict clinical manifestations and rationalize treatment of the more prevalent thyroid and parathyroid disorders.

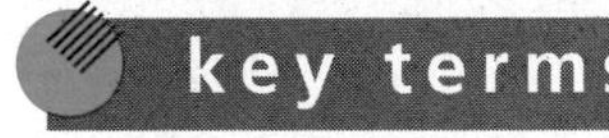

calcitonin
euthyroid sick syndrome
exophthalmos
goiter
Graves' disease
Hashimoto's thyroiditis
hyperparathyroidism
hyperthyroidism
hypoparathyroidism
hypothyroidism
multiple endocrine neoplasia
myxedema
parathyroid hormone (PTH)
parathyroid hormone–related protein
thyroid cancer
thyroiditis
thyroid-stimulating hormone (TSH)
thyroid storm
thyroglobulin
thyrotoxicosis
thyrotropin-releasing hormone (TRH)
thyroxine (T_4)
thyroxine-binding globulin (TBG)
toxic nodular goiter
tri-iodothyronine (T_3)
Wolff-Chaikoff effect

Thyroid disorders are among the most common endocrine diseases. Although the mechanism is still uncertain, thyroid hormones are known to be essential to normal cognitive and physiologic development in infants and children. In adults, thyroid hormones influence the growth and metabolism of nearly all tissues. The importance of parathyroid function is inherent in the role of **parathyroid hormone (PTH)** in the regulation of serum calcium levels. Calcium, in turn, is critical to the cellular regulation of action potentials, muscle contraction, and the secretory processes that underlie neurotransmission and hormone function, as discussed in Chapter 9. In this chapter, the normal anatomy and function of the thyroid and parathyroid glands are reviewed, along with the processes involved in the regulation of synthesis and release of thyroid hormones and PTH. The widespread effects of excess or deficiency of these hormones are illustrated through discussion of the clinical syndromes of **hypothyroidism, hyperthyroidism, hypoparathyroidism,** and **hyperparathyroidism**. **Thyroid cancer** is also described.

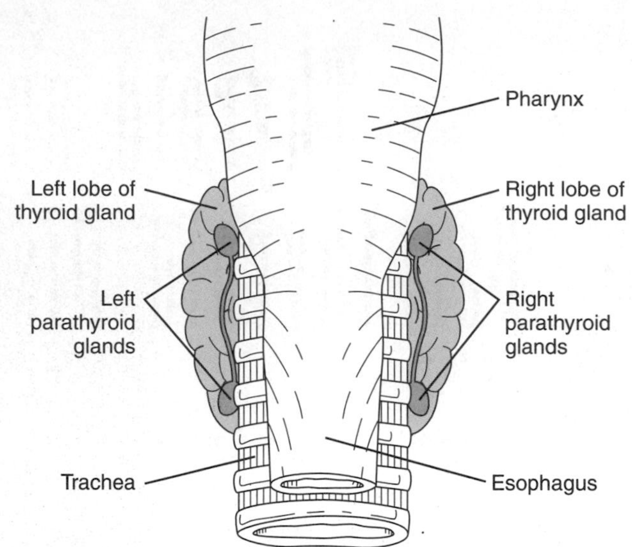

FIGURE 28–2
Parathyroid glands. The four parathyroid glands are located posterior to the thyroid. Two parathyroids are associated with each thyroid lobe.

FUNCTIONAL ANATOMY OF THE THYROID AND PARATHYROID GLANDS

Gross Anatomy

The thyroid gland is a butterfly-shaped organ located anteriorly to the trachea, just below the cricoid cartilage (Fig. 28–1). The right and left lobes of the gland lie deep to the sternocleidomastoid muscles, and the narrow middle portion (*isthmus*) extends across the trachea at midline. In about half of the population, a slender third lobe (*pyramidal lobe*) extends upward from the isthmus and attaches to the hyoid bone. The pyramidal lobe represents persistence of an embryonic structure and may or may not contain functional thyroid tissue.

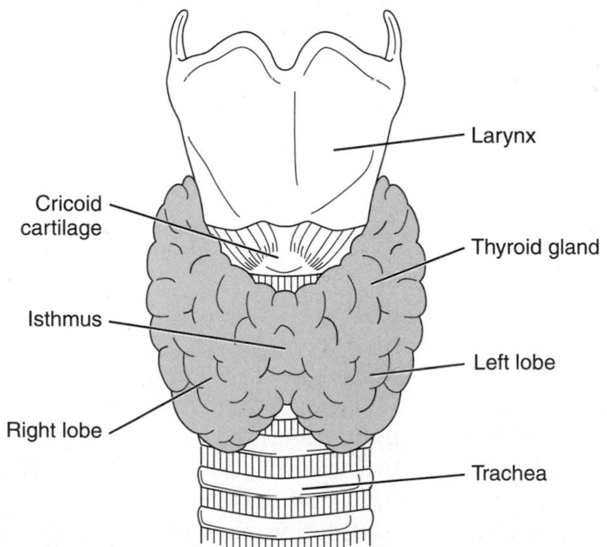

FIGURE 28–1
Thyroid gland. The butterfly-shaped thyroid is located anterior to the trachea, below the cricoid cartilage and larynx. The gland consists of two lobes, which lie deep to the sternocleidomastoid muscles of the neck, connected by a narrow isthmus, which is normally palpable.

The four parathyroid glands are located posteriorly to the thyroid; two are associated with each of the lobes of the thyroid (Fig. 28–2). The precise location of these glands is variable, and in rare cases, there are more than four. The parathyroid glands develop within the embryonic thymus gland and normally separate from it before its descent from the neck region to the mediastinum. If thymic descent occurs before separation of the parathyroids, the glands are carried with the thymus to positions below the thyroid in the neck or thorax. Because of their anatomic proximity to thyroid tissue, surgical excision of thyroid nodules may inadvertently result in disruption of parathyroid function. The recurrent laryngeal nerve may also be damaged by thyroid or parathyroid lesions or surgery, leading to monotony of the voice.

Microscopic Anatomy

The thyroid gland is composed of functional units known as *follicles*, each formed by an encircling layer of epithelial cells that secrete **thyroglobulin** into the interior of the follicle (Fig. 28–3). Thyroglobulin is a glycoprotein that binds and stores thy-

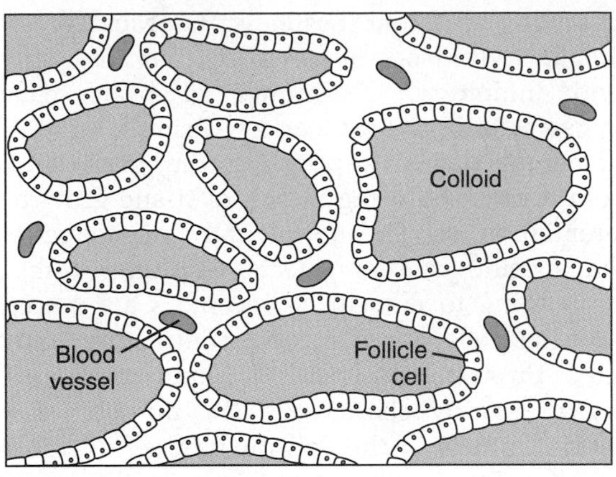

FIGURE 28–3

Thyroid follicles. The functional unit of the thyroid gland is the follicle, consisting of a layer of epithelial cells that secrete a colloid substance, thyroglobulin, into the interior. Rich perfusion facilitates follicular uptake of iodine and secretion of thyroid hormones into the blood.

roid hormones and their substrates. Follicular epithelial cells are richly perfused, facilitating exchange between the blood and the follicles. Parafollicular cells secrete the minor thyroid hormone **calcitonin.** The functional units of the parathyroid gland are the *chief cells,* which synthesize and release PTH (Fig. 28–4).

THYROID FUNCTION

Synthesis of Thyroid Hormones

The three thyroid hormones are **thyroxine (T_4)**, **tri-iodothyronine (T_3)**, and calcitonin. T_4 and T_3 are synthesized through a three-step process (Fig. 28–5). In the first step, known as *iodine trapping,* the trace mineral iodine is reduced to iodide (I^-), then actively transported against a steep concentration gradient from the blood into the thyroid follicles. Within the follicles, the oxidation of iodide and its subsequent binding to the amino acid tyrosine occur (*iodination*). Tyrosine, a component of follicular thyroglobulin, has an aromatic (ring) structure, which confers lipid solubility. Binding of a single iodine to tyrosine produces monoiodotyrosine (MIT); binding of two iodines produces di-iodotyrosine (DIT). In the final step, *coupling* of MIT and DIT molecules occurs, with linking of MIT and DIT producing T_3, and combination of two DIT molecules producing T_4. Iodination and coupling are catalyzed by the enzyme *thyroid peroxidase.*

Calcitonin, a water-soluble polypeptide produced by parafollicular C cells, is considered to be a minor hormone in humans. It binds with high affinity to receptors on osteoclasts (bone-resorbing cells), inhibiting the release of calcium and phosphate from bone. Calcitonin is important only when present in excess, as in the case of a calcitonin-producing tumor or pharmacologic use of the hormone. In common clinical usage, and throughout this chapter, the term *thyroid hormones* refers to T_4 and T_3.

Hormone Transport and Tissue Storage

Thyroid hormone synthesis occurs while tyrosine is still attached to thyroglobulin within the follicle. The hormones may be stored in this form or may be cleaved from thyroglobulin and secreted into the blood by follicular cells. In the baseline state, 90% of the hormone released is T_4.

After their release into the blood, thyroid hormones bind to plasma proteins for transport. Eighty per cent bind to a specific transport protein, **thyroxine-binding globulin (TBG)**, whereas some binds to thyroxine-binding prealbumin (transthyretin) and albumin. A small amount of hormone circulates in the unbound (free) form, which is biologically active. Protein-bound hormone serves as a reservoir for inactive hormone. Because thyroid hormones have particularly high affinity for TBG, release from binding sites is slow, with T_4 having a half-life of 6 days and T_3, 1 day.

Circulating T_4 is believed to be essentially inactive, serving as a precursor for the active hormone T_3. T_4 is converted to T_3 by the removal of one of its iodines, as catalyzed by the enzyme *monodeiodinase.* Because little T_3 is released directly from the thyroid gland, peripheral conversion of T_4 serves as the

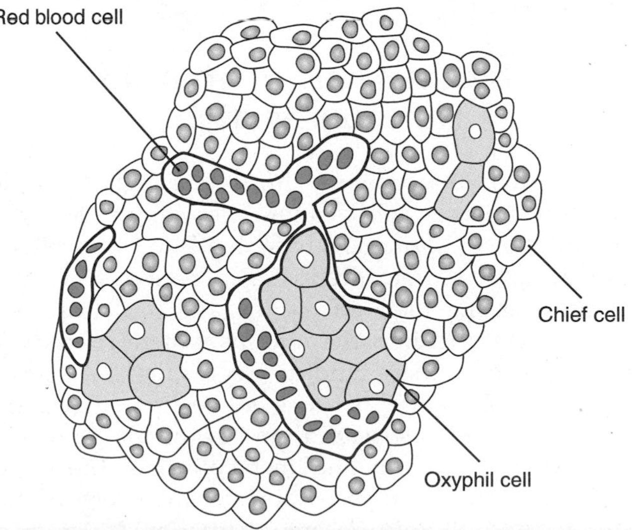

FIGURE 28–4

Parathyroid chief cells. Parathyroid hormone is synthesized and secreted by chief cells, which make up the bulk of each gland. Oxyphil cells probably represent quiescent chief cells.

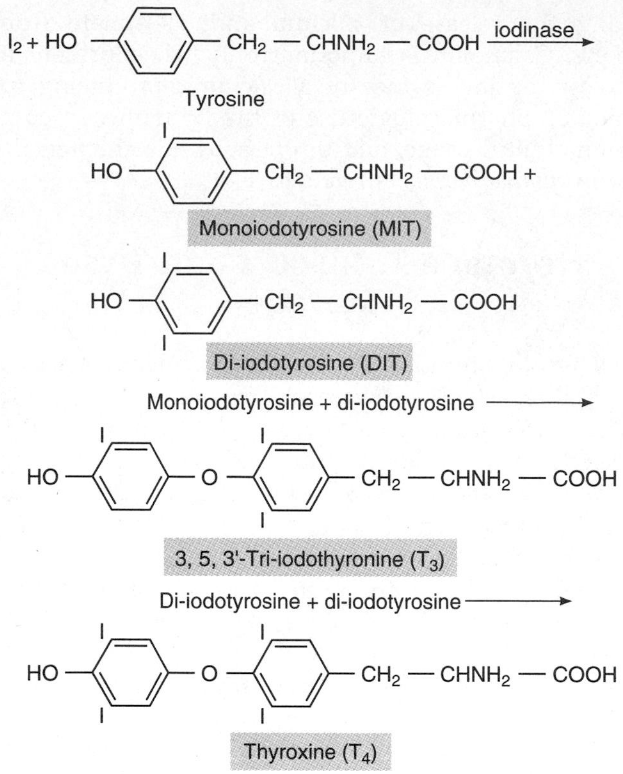

I_2 + HO—C₆H₄—CH_2—$CHNH_2$—COOH —iodinase→

Tyrosine

HO—C₆H₃(I)—CH_2—$CHNH_2$—COOH +

Monoiodotyrosine (MIT)

HO—C₆H₂(I)₂—CH_2—$CHNH_2$—COOH

Di-iodotyrosine (DIT)

Monoiodotyrosine + di-iodotyrosine ⟶

HO—C₆H₃(I)—O—C₆H₂(I)₂—CH_2—$CHNH_2$—COOH

3, 5, 3'-Tri-iodothyronine (T_3)

Di-iodotyrosine + di-iodotyrosine ⟶

HO—C₆H₂(I)₂—O—C₆H₂(I)₂—CH_2—$CHNH_2$—COOH

Thyroxine (T_4)

FIGURE 28–5

Synthesis of thyroid hormones. Thyroxine (T_4) and tri-iodothyronine (T_3) are synthesized within follicular epithelial cells from iodine and the amino acid tyrosine. Iodination of tyrosine produces monoiodotyrosine (MIT) or di-iodotyrosine (DIT); these are then coupled to form T_4 (DIT + DIT) or T_3 (DIT + MIT).

principal source of active thyroid hormone. Some of the T_3 produced by peripheral conversion is an inactive isomer, *reverse* T_3. Most peripheral conversion occurs in the liver and kidneys.

Mechanisms of Thyroid Hormone Activity

Free thyroid hormones diffuse through the lipid bilayer of target cell membranes. Within the cytoplasm, these hormones may bind to intracellular proteins for a time, producing a period of latency before exerting their effects. T_3 (and to a lesser extent T_4) diffuses into the nucleus, where it binds to receptors that then bind to regulatory regions of genes. Modification of gene expression affects the synthesis of new structural and regulatory proteins, thus altering growth and metabolism of the target tissues. Nuclear T_3 receptors are members of the steroid and thyroid receptor superfamily of transcription factors (see Chapter 6). Several T_3 receptor subtypes exist, and these are differentially distributed among different tissue types. Most receptors stimulate thyroid hormone effects, but some are apparently inhibitory.[1] The number of specific receptor subtypes within tissues varies during different developmental stages, supporting the importance of thyroid hormones in regulation of tissue growth and differentiation (see Developmental Perspective).

The specific cellular effects resulting from hormone binding to nuclear T_3 receptors are varied. In myocardial cells, for example, contractility may be affected through synthesis of a particular myosin isoenzyme or by changes in the number of slow calcium channels in the cell membrane.[2] Nuclear receptors for T_3 are present not only in the heart but also in the anterior pituitary, liver, kidney, brain, skeletal muscle, skin, and bone.[3] Lymphatic tissues and the gonads have few, if any, receptors.

T_3 receptors are believed to exist outside the nucleus as well. Increased mitochondrial oxygen consumption may result as a direct effect of binding to mitochondrial DNA, which influences synthesis of cytochromes (see Chapter 3). Up-regulation of Na^+-K^+-ATPase pumps also occurs with increased levels of T_3, but this effect is believed to be due a post-transcriptional mechanism. Increased ATP use by this active transport protein may contribute to the hyperthermic effects of thyroid hormones.[2]

Regulation of Thyroid Growth and Secretion

The synthesis and release of thyroid hormones is regulated in two ways: (1) by the hypothalamic–pituitary axis (see Chapter 27), and (2) by an autoregulatory mechanism. The hypothalamic–pituitary–thyroid axis is illustrated in Figure 28–6. In response to a variety of factors, discussed subsequently, the hypothalamus synthesizes **thyrotropin-releasing hormone (TRH)**. TRH is transported to the anterior pituitary by the portal system, stimulating release of stored **thyroid-stimulating hormone (TSH)** and inducing accelerated synthesis of TSH by pituitary thyrotroph cells.

TSH binds to follicular cells of the thyroid gland, accelerating the cleavage and secretion of stored thyroid hormones. TSH also accelerates all three stages of thyroid hormone synthesis and results in hypertrophy of follicular cells. TSH stimulates release of other iodinated tyrosines from thyroglobulin for the purpose of recycling of their iodine into accelerated synthesis of T_3 and T_4. Multiple levels of negative feedback are possible along the hypothalamic–pituitary–thyroid axis. Elevation of circulating T_3 and T_4 suppresses the release of TRH and TSH, whereas

Developmental Perspective

Embryonic and Fetal Periods

Thyroglobulin is produced by the 8th week of gestation, iodine trapping occurs by the 10th week, and TSH secretion occurs by the 12th week. Fetal T_4 production is first detectable at 8 to 10 weeks, then rises until 35 to 37 weeks, when it plateaus. The role of thyroid hormones in later fetal growth and development is uncertain because in infants with congenital hypothyroidism, replacement of thyroid hormones beginning at birth promotes nearly normal physical and intellectual development. Fetal thyroid development is independent of the mother's hypothalamic–pituitary axis because little T_4 crosses the placenta. The parathyroid glands develop within the thymus gland.

Infancy and Childhood

Until the age of 1 to 2 years, appropriate thyroid hormone levels are essential to normal brain development. Thyroid diseases occurring during childhood include congenital hypothyroidism (cretinism), autoimmune thyroiditis, and neonatal Graves' disease (due to maternal transfer of thyroid-stimulating antibodies). Thyroid nodules are uncommon in children. Thyroid deficiency leads to delayed bone growth, whereas thyroid excess leads to advanced bone age in children. Familial hyperparathyroidism and, rarely, congenital hypoparathyroidism may be evident during infancy as calcium imbalances.

Adolescence and Young Adulthood

Attainment of normal adult height requires normal levels of thyroid hormones. Menstrual irregularity is a common manifestation of thyroid disease, but it is uncertain whether fertility is significantly impaired. Hyperthyroidism during pregnancy is associated with low birth weight and increased neonatal mortality. Human chorionic gonadotropin, a hormone of pregnancy, shares a common amino acid sequence with TSH and is capable of stimulating thyroid function. More than half of pregnant women with hyperemesis gravidarum have elevated serum T_4 concentrations. Pregnancy increases maternal requirements for T_4 by 25% to 50%. Hyperthyroidism most commonly manifests in young women between the ages of 20 and 40 years. Hypothyroidism is most common among women aged 30 to 50 years.

Middle and Older Adulthood

Thyroid function decreases with normal aging, as evidenced by decreased TRH, TSH, and T_4 levels. The sensitivity of the hypothalamic–pituitary–thyroid axis diminishes with age. Systemic diseases, most common in the elderly, are associated with increased frequency of euthyroid sick syndrome in patients without thyroid disease, and with thyroid storm in those with hyperthyroidism. Inappropriate empiric therapy of weight gain and fatigue may result in iatrogenic hyperthyroidism, particularly in middle-aged women. The incidence of Graves' disease declines after 60 years of age. Hyperthyroidism presents atypically in the elderly, with eye signs usually absent and with weakness and apathy seen more often than nervousness and tremors. Subclinical hyperthyroidism may precipitate atrial fibrillation. Elderly women are at highest risk of myxedema coma. Half of the population older than 50 years have thyroid nodules.

---

low levels of circulating thyroid hormones stimulate release of TRH and TSH.

The autoregulatory mechanism resides within the thyroid gland and serves to maintain a constant level of thyroid hormones and their precursors (MIT and DIT) within the follicles despite alterations in the availability of iodine. A large increase in circulating iodine inhibits synthesis of thyroid hormones by blocking the peroxidase enzyme (**Wolff-Chaikoff effect**). If the iodine excess is chronic, decreased thyroid hormone output results in increased TSH release and thyroid stimulation, producing thyroid enlargement (**goiter**).

Because of its multiple levels of regulation, protein binding, and storage within follicles and target cells, thyroid activity is normally stable. Factors po-

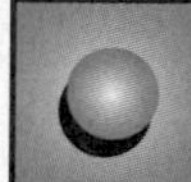

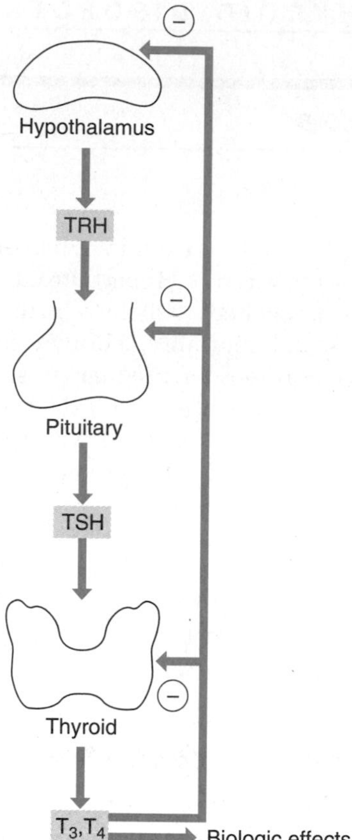

FIGURE 28–6

Hypothalamic–pituitary–thyroid axis. In response to multiple stimuli, the hypothalamus secretes thyrotropin-releasing hormone (TRH), which stimulates the release of thyroid-stimulating hormone (TSH, or thyrotropin) from the anterior pituitary. TSH stimulates thyroid growth and function, enhancing the release of the thyroid hormones. Multiple levels of negative feedback regulation are possible.

tentially affecting thyroid function relate to the availability of iodine and the status of metabolic energy balance, although tight autoregulation of these processes usually maintains thyroid homeostasis within narrow limits. The normal iodine requirement is about 1 mg/wk, obtained principally from seafood or iodized table salt. Excess iodine intake results in inhibition of iodine trapping and an increase in its excretion by the urine and feces. The Wolff-Chaikoff effect inhibits thyroid hormone synthesis in cases of chronic iodine excess, but the thyroid gland eventually "escapes" from this effect. When iodine intake is low and storage forms are depleted, thyroid hormone synthesis is reduced. TSH release is then stimulated, augmenting iodine trapping and influencing the preferential synthesis and release of T_3 rather than T_4.[4] Direct synthesis of T_3 is presumably more efficient with respect to iodine use. Goiter due to TSH stimulation could also result from this state of thyroid hormone deficiency.

Thyroid function also varies with caloric intake; a

TABLE 28–1
DRUGS AFFECTING THYROID FUNCTION

DRUGS THAT DECREASE TSH SECRETION
Dopamine
Glucocorticoids
Octreotide
DRUGS THAT ALTER THYROID HORMONE SECRETION
Decreased thyroid hormone secretion
Lithium
Iodide
Amiodarone
Aminoglutethimide
Increased thyroid hormone secretion
Iodide
Amiodarone
DRUGS THAT DECREASE T_4 ABSORPTION
Colestipol
Cholestyramine
Aluminum hydroxide
Ferrous sulfate
Sucralfate
DRUGS THAT ALTER T_4 AND T_3 TRANSPORT IN SERUM
Increased serum TBG concentration
Estrogens
Tamoxifen
Heroin
Methadone
Mitotane
Fluorouracil
Decreased serum TBG concentration
Androgens
Anabolic steroids (e.g., danazol)
Slow-release nicotinic acid
Glucocorticoids
Displacement from protein-binding sites
Furosemide
Fenclofenac
Mefenamic acid
Salicylates
DRUGS THAT ALTER T_4 AND T_3 METABOLISM
Increased hepatic metabolism
Phenobarbital
Rifampin
Phenytoin
Carbamazepine
Decreased T_4 5′-deiodinase activity
Propylthiouracil
Amiodarone
β-Adrenergic antagonist drugs
Glucocorticoids
CYTOKINES
Interferon-α
Interleukin-2

TSH, thyrotropin; T_4, thyroxine; T_3, tri-iodothyronine; TBG, thyroxine-binding globulin.

From Surks, M.I., and Sievert, R. (1995). Drugs and thyroid function. *New England Journal of Medicine* 333(25), 1691.

long-term increase in intake results in increased thyroid output of T_3 and a concurrent increase in basal metabolic rate. Notably, however, increased caloric intake does *not* increase T_4 output (recall that T_4 is the most important source of the active hormone, T_3, by peripheral conversion). The opposite effect occurs with decreased caloric intake, whether intentional or disease related. Thyroid function thus acts to modulate the effects of variable caloric intake but cannot prevent obesity with excess, nor weight loss with caloric deficiency. Metabolic alterations during prolonged stress and catabolic diseases affect the rate of peripheral conversion of T_4 to T_3, thus adaptively altering thyroid function. The altered metabolic state of pregnancy also influences thyroid hormone effects. Human chorionic gonadotropin produced during pregnancy has a thyrotropic effect, resulting in slightly increased levels of free hormones. The importance of thyroid function in thermoregulation is discussed in Chapter 11. Prolonged exposure to a cold environment stimulates hypothalamic release of TRH, stimulating thyroid function. A number of drugs affect thyroid function by inhibiting the enzymes involved in thyroid hormone synthesis or peripheral conversion (Table 28–1).

Hormonal Effects on Target Tissues

T_3 increases the metabolic rate (up to 100% above normal) of all body tissues except the retina, spleen, testes, and lungs. Specific thyroid-induced alterations in metabolism are detailed in Table 28–2. During the embryonic and fetal periods, and in infants and young children, T_3 is critical to normal development of the nervous system and other tissues.

TABLE 28–2
EFFECTS OF THYROID HORMONES

FUNCTION	EFFECTS
Oxidative metabolism	Increases size and number of mitochondria Increases rate of adenosine triphosphate production, but uncoupling of oxidative phosphorylation at higher thyroid hormone levels produces more heat than adenosine triphosphate Regulates basal metabolic rate
Growth and development	Increases skeletal growth during childhood Promotes development of the brain during late fetal life and early childhood
Carbohydrate metabolism	Stimulates uptake of glucose by cells Enhances glycolysis and gluconeogenesis Increases glucose absorption from the gastrointestinal tract Increases insulin secretion
Lipid metabolism	Mobilizes lipids from adipose tissue Accelerates β-oxidation of free fatty acids for energy Decreases serum cholesterol and triglycerides Enhances biliary excretion of cholesterol Up-regulates low-density lipoprotein receptors on liver cells
Appetite	Stimulates appetite
Cardiovascular function	Enhances perfusion Increases cardiac output Increases heart rate Increases cardiac contractility
Respiratory function	Increases rate and depth of ventilation
Central nervous system function	Increases rapidity of cerebration May promote nervousness and anxiety at higher levels
Muscle contraction	Increases vigor of contraction Causes fine tremors at higher levels
Sleep	Promotes normal sleep Difficulty sleeping is typical of excess, whereas somnolence is seen with hormone deficiency
Endocrine function	Promotes secretion from other endocrine organs while increasing tissue requirements for hormones (e.g., insulin, parathyroid hormone) Increases the rate of hepatic inactivation of cortisol
Sexual function	Maintains normal libido Maintains normal menstrual cycle

Data from Guyton, A.C., and Hall, J.E. (1996). *Textbook of Medical Physiology*. (9th ed.). Philadelphia: W.B. Saunders. (pp. 949–951).

PARATHYROID FUNCTION

Synthesis and Secretion of Parathyroid Hormone

PTH secretion from parathyroid chief cells is governed by an inverse linear relationship to serum calcium levels. PTH is the major endocrine regulator of calcium metabolism. When serum calcium is low, PTH secretion increases until Ca^{2+} rises to about 7 mg/dL; it then levels off to a basal secretion rate. Serum magnesium levels are known to exert a similar, but weaker, effect on PTH secretion.

Parathyroid hormone–related protein has a structure similar enough to PTH to bind to its receptor and mimic most of its actions. It is secreted by tumor cells as well as by many normal tissues.[5]

Effects of Parathyroid Hormone

PTH increases serum calcium and, reciprocally, decreases serum phosphate through its effects on bone and on the kidneys. PTH increases the resorption (mobilization) of calcium and phosphate from the crystalline matrix of bone, returning these ions to the blood. Through its actions on the proximal tubular cells of renal nephrons, PTH inhibits the excretion of calcium while increasing the excretion of phosphate in the urine. PTH also increases the activation of vitamin D_3 by the kidneys, thus indirectly enhancing the absorption of calcium from the gastrointestinal tract. Calcium metabolism is discussed in detail in Chapter 9. Metabolism of bone is discussed further in Chapter 34.

The thyroid hormone calcitonin weakly opposes PTH effects. As stated previously, the effects of this hormone are insignificant unless it is present in excess, owing to a calcitonin-secreting tumor or to exogenous administration.

DISORDERS OF THYROID AND PARATHYROID FUNCTION

Hypothyroidism

Definition. Hypothyroidism is the syndrome resulting from a deficiency of thyroid hormone or, much less commonly, resistance to thyroid hormone effect. Hypothyroidism may be congenital or acquired. *Primary hypothyroidism*, due to a disorder of the thyroid gland, is the usual form. *Secondary hypothyroidism* results from deficiency of pituitary TSH, whereas *tertiary hypothyroidism* is due to lack of hypothalamic TRH. True hypothyroidism must be distinguished from **euthyroid sick syndrome**, in which thyroid hormone levels may be low as a consequence of impaired peripheral conversion due to nonthyroidal illness (e.g., severe infection). In this transient syndrome, T_3 and T_4 are low; however, contrary to true hypothyroidism, TSH is low or normal, and reverse T_3 is elevated.

Epidemiology. The overall prevalence of hypothyroidism within the U.S. population has been estimated at 3%.[6] Females receive thyroid hormone replacement 10 times more often than males, but it is uncertain whether this finding represents differential incidence or diagnosis rates. Risk factors relate to the specific etiology (Table 28–3). Worldwide, the most common risk factor for hypothyroidism is iodine deficiency, but this is uncommon in the United States. Family history, presence of systemic inflammatory conditions (infectious or autoimmune), and specific human leukocyte antigen subtypes are associated with higher risk. Therapy with certain drugs (e.g., amiodarone, lithium) may also increase risk (see Table 28–1), and the disorder may be induced iatrogenically with surgical or other ablative treatment of hyperthyroidism.

Etiology. Congenital hypothyroidism usually results from thyroid agenesis (failure of the gland to develop in utero). Congenital hypothyroidism (also known as *cretinism*) is endemic in areas of iodine deficiency, but maternal ingestion of goiter-inducing substances in foods is often implicated as well. These *goitrogens*, which inhibit iodine uptake by the thyroid, are found in cassava, maize, sweet potatoes, lima beans, pearl millet, and cruciferous vegetables such as cabbage and broccoli. Genetic and teratogenic mechanisms may also produce thyroid agenesis. Premature infants are particularly susceptible to iodine-induced hypothyroidism as a consequence of exposure to iodine-containing agents during intensive care.[7]

The most common cause of primary hypothyroidism is **Hashimoto's thyroiditis**, which is believed to be an autoimmune condition resulting from a genetic defect in the function of thyroid-specific suppressor T cells. The patient develops cytotoxic T cells directed against normal thyroid antigens, leading to activation of B cells and the production of antibodies that target thyroid cell membranes and thyroid peroxidase enzyme.

Pathophysiology. Lack of thyroid hormone leads to insufficient stimulation of metabolism and tissue development in infants and children. In adult-onset

TABLE 28–3
ETIOLOGY OF HYPOTHYROIDISM

MECHANISM	EXAMPLES	RISK FACTORS
Autoimmune destruction of thyroid tissue	Hashimoto's thyroiditis Chronic autoimmune thyroiditis Subacute thyroiditis Silent thyroiditis Postpartum thyroiditis	Family history Female sex Middle age White or Asian race Presence of other autoimmune disease Pregnancy Turner's or Down syndrome
Infection of thyroid tissue	Acute (suppurative) thyroiditis Subacute granulomatous thyroiditis	Bacterial, fungal, or parasitic infection (acute) Viral infection (subacute)
Fibrous invasion of thyroid tissue	Riedel's thyroiditis	Middle age or older Female sex
Iatrogenic destruction of thyroid tissue	Thyroidectomy Radioactive iodine ablation Neck irradiation	Thyroid tumors Hyperthyroidism
Iodine deficiency	Endemic cretinism Goiter	Geographic and cultural factors Ingestion of goitrogens
Inhibition of thyroid hormone biosynthesis, release, or peripheral conversion of thyroxine (T_4) to tri-iodothyronine (T_3)	Autosomal recessive dyshormonogenesis Secondary hypothyroidism Tertiary hypothyroidism Iatrogenic hypothyroidism Euthyroid sick syndrome Transient neonatal hypothyroidism	Family history Pituitary tumor Hypothalamic disorder Iatrogenic iodine excess Iodinated contrast media Antithyroid drug therapy Amiodarone therapy for dysrhythmias Lithium therapy for psychiatric illness Surgery or acute systemic illness
Peripheral resistance to thyroid hormones	Hereditary resistance syndromes	Autosomal dominant inheritance

hypothyroidism, a hypometabolic state is present. Due to an unknown mechanism, edema (**myxedema**) develops gradually as a result of accumulation of a mucopolysaccharide-rich fluid in connective tissues. Swelling and loss of striation of skeletal and cardiac muscle fibers are sometimes seen.

Clinical Manifestations. Clinical manifestations affect virtually all body systems. In congenital hypothyroidism, evidence of impaired physical and mental growth becomes apparent weeks to months after birth. Stunted physical growth, mental retardation, squinting, deafness, joint deformity, and gait disorder are commonly seen.

Clinical manifestations of acquired hypothyroidism are similar regardless of specific cause and are listed in Table 28–4. Goiter is often seen early as the thyroid hyperfunctions adaptively. There may be periods of transient hyperthyroidism due to leakage of thyroid hormones from the damaged gland. Myxedema manifests as puffiness of the face (Fig. 28–7), cardiomegaly, and edematous effusions (possibly pleural or pericardial). The hypometabolic state is evidenced by fatigue, weight gain, hyperlipidemia, intolerance of cold, decreased gastrointestinal motility, mental dullness, dry skin, brittle hair, and loss of the outer third of the eyebrows.

Tests of thyroid function usually demonstrate the presence of hypothyroidism and may delineate the cause (Table 28–5). Except in the unusual case of isolated TSH excess, elevation of serum TSH indicates an adaptive response to hypothyroidism. Patients with *subclinical hypothyroidism* have increased TSH levels but have adequate thyroid hormone levels and no overt symptoms.

Myxedema coma, a rare syndrome that is the most serious manifestation of hypothyroidism, may present with hypothermia and unresponsiveness and progress to multiple-system organ failure. This medical emergency may be precipitated by concurrent acute illness (e.g., pneumonia, stroke, cardiac failure)

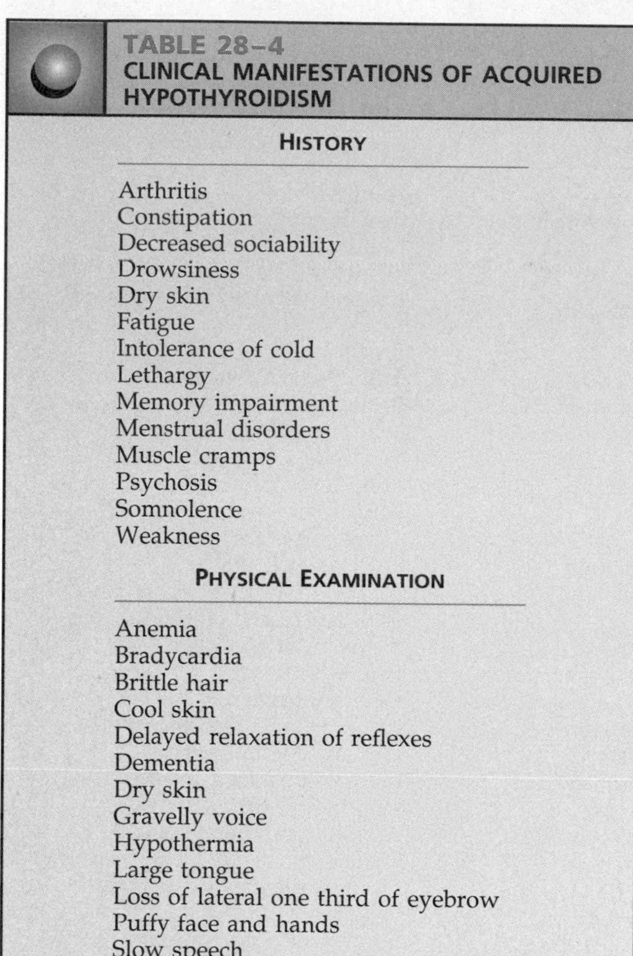

TABLE 28–4
CLINICAL MANIFESTATIONS OF ACQUIRED HYPOTHYROIDISM

History
Arthritis
Constipation
Decreased sociability
Drowsiness
Dry skin
Fatigue
Intolerance of cold
Lethargy
Memory impairment
Menstrual disorders
Muscle cramps
Psychosis
Somnolence
Weakness
Physical Examination
Anemia
Bradycardia
Brittle hair
Cool skin
Delayed relaxation of reflexes
Dementia
Dry skin
Gravelly voice
Hypothermia
Large tongue
Loss of lateral one third of eyebrow
Puffy face and hands
Slow speech
Weight changes

From Martinez, M., Derksen, D., and Kapsner, P. (1993). Making sense of hypothyroidism: An approach to testing and treatment. *Postgraduate Medicine* 93(6), 143.

in a patient (usually an elderly female) with hypothyroidism. All organ systems become infiltrated with mucopolysaccharides, and blunting of the ventilatory response to hypoxia or CO_2 retention is seen.

Prevention and Treatment. Optimal iodine intake should be ensured. Concurrent inflammatory or autoimmune disorders should be appropriately managed. Neonates are routinely screened for thyroid hormone deficiency at birth. Early replacement of thyroid hormone does not always prevent developmental impairment, however. Acquired hypothyroidism is usually treated with synthetic levothyroxine (T_4); the rate of conversion to T_3 is then physiologically regulated. If T_3 is administered directly, hyperthyroid effects, such as tachycardia and palpitations, are more common. In postmenopausal women receiving thyroid replacement therapy, estrogen replacement is also recommended to reduce the risk of osteoporosis. Myxedema coma is treated with large doses of T_4, usually administered intravenously. Slow, passive rewarming and support of system function are also indicated, with careful monitoring in a critical care setting. Treatment of pituitary or hypothalamic disorders is warranted in cases of secondary and tertiary hypothyroidism (see Chapter 27).

Prognosis and Outcome. Treatment of hypothyroidism results in symptomatic improvement in most patients. The unfavorable serum lipid profile typical of hypothyroidism does not always improve with treatment, however. Congenital hypothyroidism, if untreated, results in loss of 3 to 5 intelligence quotient points monthly during the first year of life.[8] Untreated subclinical hypothyroidism progresses to overt hypothyroidism at a rate of 5% to 20% per year. With early recognition and appropriate intensive care, the mortality rate in myxedema coma has dropped to 15% to 20%.[9] The need for monitoring and therapy of hypothyroidism is lifelong.

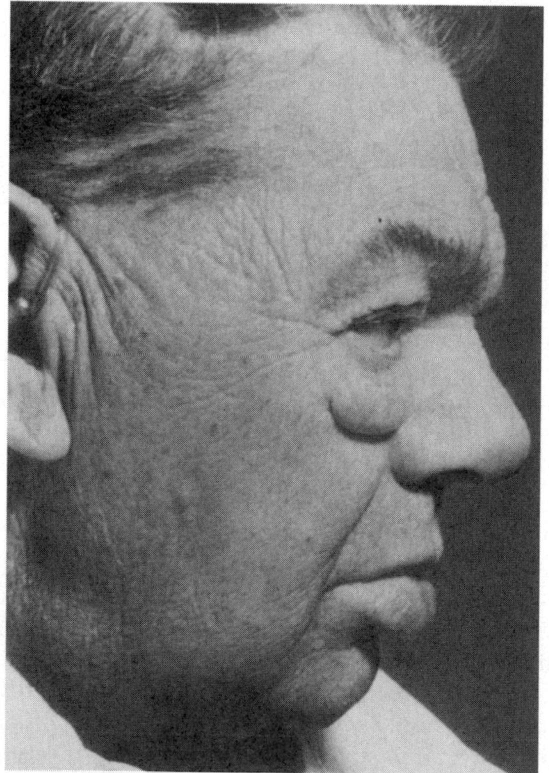

FIGURE 28–7
Myxedema. In hypothyroidism, a mucopolysaccharide-rich fluid accumulates in connective tissues. Note the facial puffiness, especially around the eyes, as well as the coarse facial features, dry skin, and dry, coarse hair and eyebrows. (From Jacob, S.W., Francone, C.A., and Lossow, W.J. [1982]. *Structure and Function in Man.* [5th ed.]. Philadelphia: W.B. Saunders. [p. 555].)

TABLE 28–5
THYROID FUNCTION TESTS

Test	Description	Significance of Abnormality
Thyroxine (T_4)	Measurement of bound T_4 in serum	Elevated in hyperthyroidism, reduced in hypothyroidism False high or low levels possible in disorders that alter the amount of available binding proteins (thyroxine-binding globulin [TBG], or albumin)
Tri-iodothyronine (T_3)	Measurement of bound T_3 in serum	Usually elevated in hyperthyroidism; usually reduced in hypothyroidism Minimally bound by proteins, so may be normal in some patients with T_4 elevation Reduced in conditions in which peripheral conversion of T_4 is impaired
Reverse T_3 (rT_3)	Measurement of serum rT_3	Increased in hyperthyroidism and in nonthyroidal illnesses that reduce T_3, and in conditions in which peripheral conversion is blocked Decreased in hypothyroidism
T_3 resin uptake (T_3RU)	Measurement of amount of T_3 remaining after unbound TBG sites have been filled	Elevated (indicating few unbound sites) in states of hyperthyroidism or low TBG levels Reduced (indicating many unbound sites) in states of hypothyroidism or high TBG levels
Free T_4 index ($T_4 \times T_3RU$)	Approximation of the amount of free T_4	Elevated in hyperthyroidism; reduced in hypothyroidism Usually normal in conditions causing false alterations in T_4 or T_3RU
Free T_4	Measurement of free T_4 in serum	Elevated in hyperthyroidism; reduced in hypothyroidism Most accurate assessment of thyroid status, especially in conjunction with thyroid-stimulating hormone (TSH) level
TSH	Measurement of serum TSH, with "sensitive" assay more accurate than "conventional" assay	Elevated in primary hypothyroidism, reduced in hyperthyroidism Usually normal in nonthyroid disease
Thyroid-releasing hormone (TRH)	Measurement of responsiveness of pituitary to intravenously administered TRH	Low baseline TSH and suppressed TSH release in hyperthyroidism High baseline TSH and exaggerated TSH release in hypothyroidism
Thyroglobulin	Measurement of serum thyroglobulin	Increased in hyperthyroidism and thyroiditis Reduced or undetectable in suppression of thyroid function by inappropriate ingestion of thyroid hormone (thyrotoxicosis factitia)
TSH receptor antibodies (TRAb)	Measurement of antibodies to TSH receptor	Presence of stimulating TRAb in early Graves' disease Presence of blocking TRAb in hypothyroidism due to treatment of Graves' disease, in Hashimoto's thyroiditis, or in transient neonatal hypothyroidism

Data from Costa, A.J. (1995). Interpreting thyroid tests. *American Family Physician* 52(8), 2325–2330.

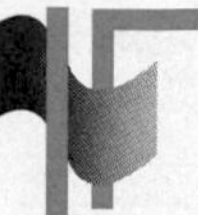

Clinical Scenario

R.M., age 74 years, is seen by her family doctor for evaluation of symptoms of fatigue and constipation. She appears lethargic and has a mask-like facial expression. R.M. reports increasing difficulty with memory during the past 2 years. On examination, her blood pressure is 170/96 mm Hg, pulse is 56 beats/minute, and oral temperature is 96.6°F. Her skin is dry and scaly, and her hair is coarse and brittle. She has noticeable puffiness around her eyes, and her deep tendon reflexes are diminished. Her serum total T_4 is 1.2 μg/dL (normal is 5.0 to 12.5), and her TSH is 85 μU/L (normal is 0.5 to 5.0).

1. Are R.M.'s physical examination findings suggestive of hypothyroidism? Do they mimic other disorders of the elderly? Explain.

2. For what complications is R.M. at risk? How might this risk be minimized?

Hyperthyroidism

Definition. Hyperthyroidism is a hypermetabolic state induced by elevated levels of thyroid hormones in the blood, usually due to hyperfunction of the thyroid gland (**thyrotoxicosis**). Less commonly, hyperthyroidism results from nonthyrotoxic mechanisms, such as inflammation-induced release of hormones, ectopic hormone production, or ingestion of foods or drugs containing thyroid hormones.

Epidemiology. Hyperthyroidism affects an estimated 2% of women and 0.2% of men.[10] In **Graves' disease**, which accounts for 85% of cases of hyperthyroidism, the risk is highest in females, with onset between the ages of 20 and 40 years. Inappropriate diagnosis or therapy of hypothyroidism imposes risk for iatrogenic hyperthyroidism.

Etiology. Specific disorders that may manifest as hyperthyroidism are summarized in Table 28–6. In Graves' disease, the development of immunoglobulin G antibodies to the TSH receptor occurs due to an unknown mechanism. These thyroid-stimulating immunoglobulins bind to TSH receptors and inappropriately stimulate the thyroid gland. In **toxic nodular goiter**, parts of the gland do not respond to normal negative feedback regulation by the hypothalamic–pituitary–thyroid axis. In inflammatory conditions such as **thyroiditis**, inflammatory mediators may release thyroid hormones. Excessive therapy of hypothyroidism or inappropriate empiric therapy of chronic fatigue and obesity may also result in increased circulating levels of thyroid hormone.

Pathophysiology. Elevation of T_3 results in a hypermetabolic state, with increased oxygen consumption by body tissues. Goiter, if present, is secondary to inflammation. The enlarged thyroid may compress the trachea, esophagus, and superior vena cava. Thyroid hormones in excess act as pseudocatecholamines, inducing a sympathetic nervous system–like response. Tonic contraction of extraocular muscles is usually present due to an unknown mechanism. Negative feedback induced by elevated thyroid hormones may result in deficiencies of other hypothalamic and pituitary hormones. When untreated hyperthyroidism is present as a baseline state, imposition of the additional stress of trauma, serious illness, or thyroid manipulation may produce a sudden, massive output of thyroid hormones known as **thyroid storm.**

Clinical Manifestations. Clinical manifestations of hyperthyroidism are summarized in Table 28–7. Thyroid function tests reveal elevated levels of T_3 and T_4, whereas TSH (and possibly TBG) levels are reduced. Typical clinical findings include goiter, **exophthalmos** (a characteristic bulging of the eyes), and a stimulated expression (Fig. 28–8). Other endocrine effects commonly seen are menstrual irregularities in females, hyperglycemia, decreases in serum lipids, excessive sweating, flushing, and heat intolerance. Obstructive goiter may result in dysphagia, airway obstruction, or superior vena cava syndrome, in which headache, jugular venous distention, and upper extremity edema are seen as a result of impaired venous return. Hair loss and changes in hair texture result from altered perfusion of the integument. Tachycardia at rest and increased stroke volume result in palpitations. Emotional lability, restlessness, tremors, and insomnia are common central nervous system manifestations.

Subclinical hyperthyroidism, which is much less common than subclinical hypothyroidism, is characterized only by decreased serum TSH. The patient does not have symptoms, and T_3 and T_4 levels are normal. Thyroid storm is manifested by a high temperature; extreme increase in heart rate and cardiac output, leading to high-output cardiac failure and angina; and central nervous system effects, including delirium and agitation.

Prevention and Treatment. Iatrogenic hyperthyroidism is preventable with appropriate diagnostic testing and monitoring of therapy. Thyroid storm is nearly always preventable with appropriate treatment of baseline hyperthyroidism. Hyperthyroidism due to Graves' disease or toxic nodular goiter may be treated with antithyroid drugs, radioactive iodine

TABLE 28–6
ETIOLOGY OF HYPERTHYROIDISM

Cause	Pathogenesis	Comment
Common		
Graves' disease	Production of thyroid-stimulating antibodies	Most frequent cause
Toxic nodular goiter		
Multiple nodules	Thyroid autonomy*	Causes 10% of cases of hyperthyroidism among middle-aged and elderly patients (outside the United States)
Single toxic adenoma		Causes less than 5% of cases of toxic nodular goiter
Thyroiditis	Inflammation-induced release of thyroxine and tri-iodothyronine	Confirmed by low uptake or absence of uptake of radioiodine into the thyroid
Subacute		
Silent		
Postpartum		
Iatrogenic illness	Administration of thyroxine or tri-iodothyronine	Second most common cause
Rare		
Neonatal hyperthyroidism	Transplacental passage of thyroid-stimulating antibodies	Occurs transiently in infants of mothers with Graves' disease
Inappropriate secretion of thyrotropin	Pituitary tumor	
	Pituitary resistance to thyroxine and tri-iodothyronine	
Exogenous iodide	Augmented thyroid secretion in patients with underlying thyroid autonomy	Sources of iodine include health-food preparations, kelp, amiodarone, and radiographic contrast agents
Factitious illness		
Very rare		
Thyroid cancer		
Choriocarcinoma, hydatidiform mole, embryonal testicular carcinoma	Tumor production of chorionic gonadotropin, stimulating the thyroid	
Struma ovarii	Ovarian teratoma containing thyroid tissue	

* Nodules functioning independently of normal feedback regulation.
From: Franklyn, J.A. (1994). The management of hyperthyroidism. *New England Journal of Medicine* 330(24), 1732.

(for radioactive ablation of the gland), or thyroidectomy (Table 28–8). In some cases, T_4 replacement is administered concurrently with antithyroid drugs to suppress TSH activity. Use of antithyroid drugs is favored in Europe and Japan, whereas radioactive iodine ablation is most often used in the United States.[11] Total or subtotal thyroidectomy is indicated in patients with large, compressive goiters. The decision to treat subclinical hyperthyroidism must be individualized. Patients at risk for atrial fibrillation or osteoporosis are most likely to benefit from treatment.[12] Hyperthyroidism due to thyroiditis is usually transient, requiring only symptomatic treatment (e.g., β-adrenergic blocking agents to suppress tachycardia).

Prognosis and Outcome. In patients older than 40 years, antithyroid drugs may not permit achievement of complete remission, and relapse rates are high.[13] Hepatitis, arthritis, rash, or agranulocytosis may occur as a complication of this therapy. Radioactive iodine is usually effective in inducing remission but may lead to a transient thyrotoxic state as stored hormone is released from the damaged gland. About half of patients treated with radioactive iodine or subtotal thyroidectomy demonstrate hypothyroidism after 25 years, requiring thyroid hormone replacement.

Thyroid Cancer

Definition. Thyroid cancers are malignant neoplasms of the thyroid gland. About 75% to 85% of these are classified on the basis of tissue appearance as papillary carcinomas, whereas 10% to 20% are classified as follicular.[14] Medullary and anaplastic carcinomas, which are rare, are the other two histologic classifications.

Epidemiology. The prevalence of occult thyroid cancer in the United States has been estimated at

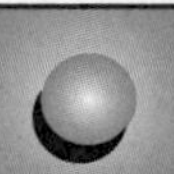

TABLE 28-7
CLINICAL MANIFESTATIONS OF HYPERTHYROIDISM

History
Amenorrhea or oligomenorrhea
Difficulty concentrating
Difficulty sleeping
Dyspnea
Eye complaints (dry, scratchy eyes, photophobia, eye pressure, double vision)
Fatigue
Frequent bowel movements
Heat intolerance
Irritability
Nervousness
Palpitations
Weight loss or stable weight with increased appetite
Physical Examination
Decreased visual acuity
Exophthalmos
Fine hair
Goiter
Gynecomastia in males
Hyper-reflexia
Irregular pulse
Proximal muscle weakness
Systolic ejection murmur
Thyroid nodules
Stimulated appearance
Systolic hypertension
Tachycardia
Tremors
Warm, smooth, moist skin
Widened pulse pressure

Data from Streff, M.M., and Pachucki-Hyde, L.C. (1996). Management of the patient with thyroid disease. *Nursing Clinics of North America* 31(4), 779–796; Tietgens, S.T., and Leinung, M.C. (1995). Thyroid storm. *Medical Clinics of North America* 79(1), 169–184; and McGuinness, M.E., and Talbert, R.L. (1994). Management of thyroid disorders. *American Pharmacy* NS34(12), 36–47.

3.9% to 4.1%.[15] The incidence of thyroid cancers in the United States has been steadily increasing, although they still account for fewer than 1% of all cancer deaths (about 1000 per year).[14] Although thyroid cancer can occur in both sexes, with onset at any age, two thirds of patients with thyroid cancer are women, with usual onset in middle age. Radiation to the head and neck, particularly during the first two decades of life, constitutes a significant risk factor for thyroid cancer. Hashimoto's thyroiditis has also been associated with increased risk. Medullary carcinomas have a familial incidence. Benign thyroid adenomas and nonpalpable nodules discovered on ultrasonography ("incidentalomas") rarely become cancerous. Patients with a chronic autoimmune form of thyroiditis are at increased risk for development of non-Hodgkin's lymphoma, which is usually confined to the thyroid gland[16] (see Chapter 13).

Etiology. The precise etiology of thyroid cancer is generally unknown, although a specific oncogene has been identified in some cases of papillary carcinoma, and a familial syndrome has been implicated in medullary thyroid carcinoma. Mechanisms of neoplastic transformation are discussed in detail in Chapter 7.

Pathophysiology. Thyroid tumors usually begin as single nodular lesions that grow slowly. Thyroid tumors may or may not take up iodine. Papillary tumors may cause a mild degree of thyrotoxicosis, and metastasis to cervical lymph nodes is common. Distant metastasis is unusual with this type. Follicular carcinomas also present as painless, slow-growing lesions, with direct invasion and lymphatic metastasis more likely than in papillary tumors. Many follicular tumors secrete thyroglobulin. Medullary tumors arise from calcitonin-secreting parafollicular cells and tend to metastasize early. Medullary thyroid carcinoma may be a component of the rare familial syndrome of **multiple endocrine neoplasia.** Anaplastic tumors have the highest rate of malignancy, spreading by both the bloodstream and the lymphatics.

Clinical Manifestations. Specific manifestations depend on tumor size, growth rate, tumor secretion, and metastasis. In most cases, the initial manifestations of the growing thyroid nodule lead to early diagnosis and treatment. Untreated disease results in local obstructive manifestations of dysphagia and airway obstruction. Systemic effects depend on the site and degree of metastasis. Manifestations of thyrotoxicosis, if present, are usually mild.

Prevention and Treatment. Reduction of radiation

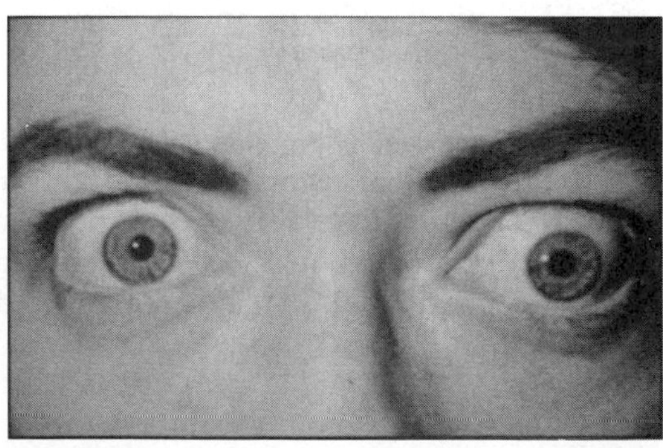

FIGURE 28–8
Exophthalmos. Protrusion of the eyes, a common sign of hyperthyroidism, is probably due to tonic contraction of extraocular muscles. Note the visible white sclera above the iris. (From Scheie, H.G., and Albert, D.M. [1977]. *Textbook of Ophthalmology.* [9th ed.]. Philadelphia: W.B. Saunders. [p. 427].)

TABLE 28–8
TREATMENT OF HYPERTHYROIDISM

Treatment	Mechanism of Action	Comments
Antithyroid Drugs (ATDs)		
Methimazole (Tapazole) Propylthiouracil (PTU)	Inhibits thyroid peroxidase Inhibits thyroid peroxidase Inhibits peripheral conversion of thyroxine (T_4)	Relieves symptoms within a few days Remission may occur within 6 mo to 2 y Relapse may occur after discontinuation of therapy Adverse effects include skin rashes, leukopenia, and (rarely) agranulocytosis Most common form of therapy in Japan and Europe
Lithium carbonate Stable iodine (saturated solution of potassium iodide [SSKI], Lugol's solution)	Blocks release of thyroid hormone from the gland	Used in patients who are intolerant of other ATDs Use is uncommon
Radiation		
Radioactive iodine (RAI, or ^{131}I)	Taken up by the thyroid and used in hormone synthesis; β-emission radioactivity destroys follicles over time	Renders patient permanently hypothyroid within 3–6 mo; lifelong thyroxine replacement is then required Most common form of therapy in the United States
Adjunctive Therapy		
β-blockers (propranolol [Inderal], nadolol [Corgard]) Calcium-channel blockers (diltiazem [Cardizem])	Provides symptomatic improvement until euthyroid state can be achieved	Contraindicated in patients with low-output cardiac failure, asthma, diabetes mellitus, bradycardia
Surgery		
Thyroidectomy (total or subtotal)	Surgical removal of thyroid tissue	Use is uncommon except for in patients with large goiters

Data from Singer, P.A., Cooper, D.S., Levy, E.G., *et al.* (1995). Treatment guidelines for patients with hyperthyroidism and hypothyroidism. *Journal of the American Medical Association* 273(10), 808–812.

risk is warranted. Radiation to the head and neck, particularly in the young, should be avoided. (Such treatment was once common for acne and other dermatologic conditions.) Thyroid cancer is optimally treated with total or subtotal thyroidectomy, with radioactive iodine uptake or external radiation used as adjunctive treatments. TSH may be administered to suppress thyroglobulin secretion. Thyroid hormone replacement is often required after initial treatment.

Prognosis and Outcome. Anaplastic thyroid carcinoma is nearly always fatal within months, regardless of mode of therapy. Prognosis in medullary cancer depends on its extent and resectability at the time of diagnosis. Papillary and follicular carcinomas are effectively treated with a combination of near-total thyroidectomy, radioactive iodine, and thyroid hormone replacement. A 30-year mortality rate of 8% was recently demonstrated in long-term follow-up study of 1355 patients.[17] The same study found that 36% of patients did show recurrence of the cancer, indicating a need for careful lifelong monitoring after initial diagnosis and treatment (see Focus of Current Research).

Hypoparathyroidism

Definition. Hypoparathyroidism is the syndrome resulting from the effects of PTH deficiency or PTH resistance on calcium homeostasis.

Epidemiology. Hypoparathyroidism due to primary disorder of the parathyroid glands is an uncommon disorder. Rarely, it is congenital. Transient hypoparathyroidism during infancy is a component of *DiGeorge syndrome* and *velocardiofacial syndrome*, both of which result from a deletion on chromosome 22.[18] A rare idiopathic form of hypoparathyroidism may be associated with an autosomal recessive disorder in which multiple autoimmune disorders are concurrently present (*autoimmune polyglandular syndrome type I*).[19] *Pseudohypoparathyroidism* is a rare in-

Focus of Current Research

Study	Objective and Findings
Sherman, et al. (1996) Clinical and socioeconomic predispositions to complicated thyrotoxicosis: A predictable and preventable syndrome?	*Objective:* To identify the clinical, demographic, and hormonal features that characterize and place patients at greater risk for complicated thyrotoxicosis *Findings:* There was a high correlation between organ systems with pre-existing dysfunction and those with a complication of thyrotoxicosis. Patients with serum T_4 concentrations greater than twice the upper limit of normal were at highest risk.
Kohler, et al. (1996) Transient congenital hypothyroidism and hyperthyrotropinemia: Normal thyroid function and physical development at the ages of 6–14 years.	*Objective:* To re-evaluate the thyroid function and physical development of 61 children with transient thyroid disorders *Findings:* Thyroid function and growth were normal in all except two children, who had elevated thyroid-stimulating hormone levels.
Skuza, et al. (1996) Prediction of neonatal hyperthyroidism in infants born to mothers with Graves' disease.	*Objective:* To determine whether thyrotropin-receptor antibody levels in newborn infants of women with Graves' disease would predict which infants will have hyperthyroidism *Findings:* Seven infants with antibody levels of more than 0.25 binding inhibition developed signs of hyperthyroidism.
Kremer, et al. (1996) Parathyroid-hormone-related peptide in hematologic malignancies.	*Objective:* To determine whether parathyroid hormone–related peptide is an important mediator of hypercalcemia in patients with hematologic malignancies *Findings:* Significant elevations in parathyroid hormone–related peptide were noted in most patients with hypercalcemia and malignancy (usually non-Hodgkin's lymphoma).
Winer, et al. (1996) Synthetic human parathyroid hormone 1-34 vs calcitriol and calcium in the treatment of hypoparathyroidism.	*Objective:* To test the hypothesis that treatment with human parathyroid hormone 1-34 can maintain normal serum calcium levels in patients with hypoparathyroidism *Findings:* Treatment with parathyroid hormone 1-34 maintained normal serum calcium levels, with reduced urinary calcium excretion compared with calcitriol treatment.

Box continued on following page

Study	*Objective and Findings*
Massaferri & Jhiang (1994) Long-term impact of initial surgical and medical therapy on papillary and follicular thyroid cancer.	*Objective:* To determine the long-term impact of medical and surgical treatment of well-differentiated papillary and follicular thyroid cancer *Findings:* For tumors of 1.5 cm or greater diameter that are not initially metastatic, near-total thyroidectomy followed by radioactive iodine and thyroid hormone therapy confers a distinct outcome advantage.
Erickson, et al. (1994) The prevalence of hypothyroidism in gout.	*Objective:* To examine the potential relationship between gout and hypothyroidism *Findings:* The prevalence of hypothyroidism is significantly increased in patients with gout.
Schneider, et al. (1994) Thyroid hormone use and bone mineral density in elderly women.	*Objective:* To determine the effect of long-term use of thyroid hormone on bone mineral density and the potential effects of estrogen replacement therapy *Findings:* Long-term thyroid use was associated with significant bone loss. This effect was negated with estrogen use.

herited disorder of PTH resistance, in which hormone levels are normal but the renal response to PTH is impaired. Secondary hypoparathyroidism is much more common and may be associated with neck surgery, sepsis, pancreatitis, major burns, magnesium imbalance, hypothyroidism, and primary bone diseases.

Etiology. Hypoparathyroidism is nearly always iatrogenic. With neck surgery, particularly thyroidectomy, inadvertant mechanical or ischemic damage to the parathyroids may result in deficiency. In sepsis, pancreatitis, and burns, circulating mediators of inflammation apparently suppress PTH secretion. The relationship between magnesium imbalance and PTH activity is poorly understood. A decrease in PTH secretion may result from either hypermagnesemia or hypomagnesemia. Several drugs may also suppress PTH secretion; these include aluminum, ethanol, cimetidine, and several antineoplastic agents.

Pathophysiology. PTH deficiency results in a reduction of serum calcium as a consequence of a reduction in bone resorption and renal conservation of calcium. Deficiency in activation of vitamin D_3 results in impaired intestinal absorption of calcium.

Clinical Manifestations. Hypoparathyroidism results in hypocalcemia and reciprocal hyperphosphatemia, with clinical manifestations usually apparent when serum calcium levels fall below 3.2 mg/dL. The congenital forms also manifest skeletal abnormalities, and some degree of developmental disability is usually present. The manifestations of hypocalcemia are particularly evident in cardiac and skeletal muscle and in the nervous system, as detailed in Chapter 9.

Prevention and Treatment. Iatrogenic hypoparathyroidism is potentially preventable. Treatment of hypocalcemia consists of replacement of calcium and vitamin D, as discussed in Chapter 9. A synthetic form of PTH has been developed, and its use is under study.[20]

Prognosis and Outcome. Without treatment, hypoparathyroidism may cause life-threatening tetany and seizures. Treatment of congenital forms results in resolution of hypocalcemia and hyperphosphatemia within a few weeks to months, but these manifestations are likely to recur later in life. Prognosis in iatrogenic hypoparathyroidism depends on early recognition and response to hypocalcemia and on the severity of the underlying disorder.

Hyperparathyroidism

Definition. Hyperparathyroidism is the clinical syndrome resulting from excessive secretion of PTH.

Epidemiology. About 100,000 new cases of primary hyperparathyroidism are diagnosed each year in the United States.[21] Incidence is higher in women than men and increases with age. Risk factors include a family history of hyperparathyroidism or multiple endocrine neoplasia, history of radiation to the head or neck during childhood, or use of thiazide diuretics. Secondary hyperparathyroidism is seen in renal failure, vitamin D deficiency, and osteomalacia (see Chapter 34).

Etiology. More than 80% of cases of primary hyperparathyroidism are caused by PTH-secreting parathyroid adenomas (benign tumors). Parathyroid carcinoma accounts for less than 1% of all cases.[21] Parathyroid hyperplasia accounts for the remainder of cases. In secondary hyperparathyroidism, persistent hypocalcemia triggers excess secretion of PTH.

Pathophysiology. PTH levels are elevated in 90% of patients with hyperparathyroidism. In the remaining 10%, PTH levels are within the high-normal range but are elevated beyond what would be expected given their serum calcium levels. In renal failure, phosphate retention and hypocalcemia result in an adaptive increase in PTH secretion. Vitamin D deficiency may directly increase PTH secretion, although the mechanism is uncertain. When PTH levels are elevated, excessive bone resorption and renal reabsorption of calcium result in hypercalcemia.

Clinical Manifestations. Seventy-five per cent of patients are asymptomatic except for elevated serum PTH and calcium levels. When present, the effects of elevated serum calcium are primarily manifested in excitable tissues, producing muscle weakness, cardiac dysrhythmias, and neurologic effects (see Chapter 9). Increased resorption leaves bones weak and prone to fracture (see Chapter 34). Renal calculi and calcium deposition into soft tissues may be seen.

Prevention and Treatment. Asymptomatic patients require only careful monitoring, unless serum calcium levels exceed 14 mg/dL. These patients should avoid dehydration, immobilization, excessive dietary intake of calcium and vitamin D, and use of loop or thiazide diuretics.[21] Surgery is the treatment of choice for patients with symptoms, who may be cured with partial or complete parathyroidectomy. If apparently normal parathyroidal tissue can be salvaged, it may be transplanted to an accessible area, usually the muscle of the forearm. Such autotransplantation preserves some PTH secretion while eliminating the risks associated with recurrent surgical dissection of the neck (e.g., airway obstruction, laryngeal nerve injury). Hypercalcemic emergencies are treated with fluids to dilute serum calcium, diuretics to increase calcium excretion, and biphosphonates drug to inhibit resorption of calcium from bone. Calcitonin has also been administered in pharmacologic doses for treatment of hyperparathyroidism. Its rapid onset of action in opposing PTH is beneficial in emergencies, but calcitonin has not been shown to be as effective as the biphosphonates for long-term use.[22] General interventions in hypercalcemia are detailed in Chapter 9.

Prognosis and Outcome. Surgery is curative in some cases of primary hyperparathyroidism, but most patients have a high probability of recurrence. Long-term monitoring is essential. Parathyroid carcinoma has a 5-year survival rate of 50%.[21]

CLINICAL SIGNIFICANCE OF THYROID AND PARATHYROID DISORDERS

The impact of thyroid disorders on human function is considerable in view of the fact that thyroid hormones influence the function of nearly all tissues. The extent of this influence is probably underappreciated at this time. The developmental effects of lack of thyroid hormone are deleterious to both cognitive and physiologic function (see Developmental Perspective). Much progress has been made in clarifying the cellular mechanisms underlying thyroid hormone actions, and research in this area is ongoing. Parathyroid disorders are less common; however, their clinical effects may be life-threatening if serum calcium levels are severely deranged.

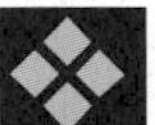

Summary of Key Points

- The thyroid gland is located anterior to the trachea, below the cricoid cartilage. The four parathyroid glands are associated with the thyroid lobes and may be inadvertently damaged due to direct trauma or ischemia during thyroid surgery.
- Thyroid hormone synthesis is regulated by the hypothalamic–pituitary–thyroid axis. Synthesis begins with active uptake of iodine from the blood. Iodination of tyrosine produces the hormone precursors, which then couple to form the thyroid hormones T_4 and T_3. Nearly all circulating thyroid hormones are transported in complex with TBG or other plasma proteins. T_4 is deiodinated in the liver and kidney to form T_3. Thyroid hormones may be stored within the gland, in association with the protein thyroglobulin, then released on stimulation by pituitary TSH.

Summary continued on following page

- The lipophilic quality of free thyroid hormones permits their diffusion through membrane lipids and into the nucleus. T_3, the active hormone, binds to specific receptors that serve as transcription factors, influencing the expression of genes encoding structural and regulatory proteins. Target organ effects of thyroid hormones reflect enhancement of tissue metabolism and growth. During the embryonic, fetal, neonatal, and early childhood stages, thyroid hormone is critical to growth and to normal development of the nervous system.
- PTH is released in response to decreased serum calcium levels. Its release is inhibited when serum calcium levels are elevated. PTH increases serum calcium through several mechanisms. It induces the resorption of calcium and phosphate from bone matrix, inhibits the renal excretion of calcium, and increases the activation of vitamin D_3 by the kidneys. Vitamin D_3 enhances the absorption of dietary calcium.
- Disorders of thyroid and parathyroid function are usually due to hyperfunction or hypofunction of the glands. Less commonly, disorders of hypothalamic or pituitary stimulation may result in secondary or tertiary thyroid disorders, and primary excess or deficiency of calcium may precipitate abnormality of PTH secretion. Resistance syndromes rarely produce disorders of thyroid or parathyroid function. Treatment is aimed at normalizing circulating levels of hormones through suppressive or ablative measures or, in the case of hypothyroidism, through exogenous hormone replacement.

REFERENCES

1. McNabb, F.M.A. (1995). Thyroid hormones, their activation, degradation and effects on metabolism. *Journal of Nutrition* 125, 1773S–1776S.
2. Tietgens, S.T., and Leinung, M.C. (1995). Thyroid storm. *Medical Clinics of North America* 79(1), 169–184.
3. Ridgway, E.C. (1996). Modern concepts of primary thyroid gland failure. *Clinical Chemistry* 42(1), 179–182.
4. Boyages, S.C. (1993). Iodine deficiency disorders. *Journal of Clinical Endocrinology and Metabolism* 77(3), 587–591.
5. Deftos, L.J. (1996). Hypercalcemia: Mechanisms, differential diagnosis, and remedies. *Postgraduate Medicine* 100(6), 119–126.
6. McGuinness, M.E., and Talbert, R.L. (1994). Management of thyroid disorders. *American Pharmacy* NS34(12), 36–47.
7. Kohler, B., Schnabel, D., Biebermann, H., *et al.* (1996). Transient congenital hypothyroidism and hyperthyrotropinemia: Normal thyroid function and physical development at the ages of 6–14 years. *Journal of Clinical Endocrinology and Metabolism* 81(4), 1563–1567.
8. Toft, A.D. (1994). Thyroxine therapy. *New England Journal of Medicine* 331(3), 174–179.
9. Jordan, R.M. (1995). Myxedema coma: Pathophysiology, therapy, and factors affecting prognosis. *Medical Clinics of North America* 79(1), 185–194.
10. Franklyn, J.A. (1994). The management of hyperthyroidism. *New England Journal of Medicine* 330(24), 1731–1738.
11. Feldt-Rasmussen, U., Glinoer, D., and Orgiazzi, J. (1993). Reassessment of antithyroid drug therapy of Graves' disease. *Annual Review of Medicine* 44, 323–334.
12. Surks, M.I., and Ocampo, E. (1996). Subclinical thyroid disease. *American Journal of Medicine* 100, 217–223.
13. Kennedy, J.W., and Caro, J.F. (1996). The ABCs of managing hyperthyroidism in the older patient. *Geriatrics* 51(5), 22–32.
14. Cotran, R.S., Kumar, V., and Robbins, S.L. (1994). *Robbins Pathologic Basis of Disease.* (5th ed.). Philadelphia: W.B. Saunders. (pp. 1136–1142).
15. Tan, G.H., and Gharib, H. (1997). Thyroid incidentalomas: Management approaches to nonpalpable nodules discovered incidentally on thyroid imaging. *Annals of Internal Medicine* 126(3), 226–231.
16. Dayan, C.M., and Daniels, G.H. (1996). Chronic autoimmune thyroiditis. *New England Journal of Medicine* 335(2), 99–107.
17. Massaferri, E.L., and Jhiang, S.M. (1994). Long-term impact of initial surgical and medical therapy on papillary and follicular thyroid cancer. *American Journal of Medicine* 97, 418–428.
18. Greig, F., Paul, E., DiMartino-Nardi, J., *et al.* (1996). Transient congenital hypoparathyroidism: Resolution and recurrence in chromosome 22q11 deletion. *Journal of Pediatrics* 128(4), 563–567.
19. Reber, P.M., and Heath III, H. (1995). Hypocalcemic emergencies. *Medical Clinics of North America* 79(1), 93–106.
20. Winer, K.K., Yanovski, J.A., and Cutler, Jr., G.B. (1996). Synthetic human parathyroid hormone 1-34 vs calcitriol and calcium in the treatment of hypoparathyroidism. *Journal of the American Medical Association* 276(8), 631–636.
21. Deftos, L.J., Parthemore, J.G., and Stabile, B.E. (1993). Management of primary hyperparathyroidism. *Annual Review of Medicine* 44, 19–26.
22. Kaye, T.B. (1995). Hypercalcemia: How to pinpoint the cause and customize treatment. *Postgraduate Medicine* 97(1), 153–160.

SELECTED BIBLIOGRAPHY

Bishnoi, A., and Sachmechi, I. (1996). Thyroid disease during pregnancy. *American Family Physician* 53(1), 215–220.

Burrow, G.N. (1993). Thyroid function and hyperfunction during gestation. *Endocrine Reviews* 14(2), 194–202.

Burrow, G.N., Fisher, D.A., and Larsen, P.R. (1994). Maternal and fetal thyroid function. *New England Journal of Medicine* 331(16), 1072–1078.

Costa, A.J. (1995). Interpreting thyroid tests. *American Family Physician* 52(8), 2325–2330.

Cushing, G.W. (1993). Subclinical hypothyroidism: Understanding is the key to decision making. *Postgraduate Medicine* 94(1), 95–107.

Edelson, G.W., and Kleerekoper, M. (1995). Hypercalcemic crisis. *Medical Clinics of North America* 79(1), 79–92.

Erickson, A.R., Enzenauer, R.J., Nordstrom, D.M., *et al.* (1994). The prevalence of hypothyroidism in gout. *American Journal of Medicine* 97, 231–234.

Fisher, D.A. (1996). Physiological variations in thyroid hormones: Physiological and pathophysiological considerations. *Clinical Chemistry* 42(1), 135–139.

Guyton, A.C., and Hall, J.E. (1996). *Textbook of Medical Physiology.* (9th ed.). Philadelphia: W.B. Saunders.

Haggerty, Jr., J.J., and Prange, Jr., A.J. (1995). Borderline hypothyroidism and depression. *Annual Review of Medicine* 46, 37–46.

Hall, T.G., and Schaiff, R.A.B. (1993). Update on the medical treatment of hypercalcemia of malignancy. *Clinical Pharmacy* 12, 117–125.

Heitman, B., and Irizarry, A. (1995). Hypothyroidism: Common complaints, perplexing diagnosis. *Nurse Practitioner* 20(3), 54–60.

Hennessey, J.V. (1996). Diagnosis and management of thyrotoxicosis. *American Family Physician* 54(4), 1315–1324.

Hurley, D.L., and Gharib, H. (1995). Detection and treatment of hypothyroidism and Graves' disease. *Geriatrics* 50(4), 41–44.

Isley, W.L. (1993). Thyroid dysfunction in the severely ill and elderly: Forget the classic signs and symptoms. *Postgraduate Medicine* 94(3), 111–128.

Kremer, R., Shustik, C., Tabak, T., *et al.* (1996). Parathyroid-hormone-related peptide in hematologic malignancies. *American Journal of Medicine* 100, 406–411.

Loriaux, T.C. (1996). Endocrine assessment: Red flags for those on the front lines. *Nursing Clinics of North America* 31(4), 695–713.

Maberly, G.F. (1994). Iodine deficiency disorders: Contemporary scientific issues. *Journal of Nutrition* 124, 1437S–1478S.

Mandel, S.J., Brent, G.A., and Larsen, P.R. (1993). Levothyroxine therapy in patients with thyroid disease. *Annals of Internal Medicine* 119(6), 492–502.

Martinez, M., Derksen, D., and Kapsner, P. (1993). Making sense of hypothyroidism: An approach to testing and treatment. *Postgraduate Medicine* 93(6), 135–145.

McDermott, M.T., and Ridgway, E.C. (1993). Thyroid hormone resistance syndromes. *American Journal of Medicine* 94, 424–432.

Miller, M. (1996). Endocrine disorders: New technology allows quick, accurate diagnosis. *Geriatrics* 51(1), 52–58.

Moruzzi, P., Doria, E., and Agostoni, P.G. (1996). Medium-term effectiveness of L-thyroxine treatment in idiopathic dilated cardiomyopathy. *American Journal of Medicine* 101, 461–467.

Pittman, J.G. (1996). Evaluation of patients with mildly abnormal thyroid function tests. *American Family Physician* 54(3), 961–966.

Porterfield, S.P., and Hendrich, C.E. (1993). The role of thyroid hormones in prenatal and neonatal neurological development: Current perspectives. *Endocrine Reviews* 14(1), 94–106.

Pronovost, P.H., and Parris, K.H. (1995). Perioperative management of thyroid disease: Prevention of complications related to hyperthyroidism and hypothyroidism. *Postgraduate Medicine* 98(2), 83–98.

Reginster, J.Y., Deroisy, R., Lecart, M.P., *et al.* (1995). A double-blind, placebo-controlled, dose-finding trial of intermittent nasal salmon calcitonin for prevention of postmenopausal lumbar spine bone loss. *American Journal of Medicine* 98, 452–458.

Rogers, D.G. (1994). Thyroid disease in children. *American Family Physician* 50(2), 344–350.

Rusterholtz, A. (1996). Interpretation of diagnostic laboratory tests in selected endocrine disorders. *Nursing Clinics of North America* 31(4), 715–724.

Sakiyama, R. (1993). Thyroiditis: A clinical review. *American Family Physician* 48(4), 615–621.

Schneider, D.L., Barrett-Connor, E.L., and Morton, D.J. (1994). Thyroid hormone use and bone mineral density in elderly women. *Journal of the American Medical Association* 271(16), 1245–1249.

Schubert, M.F., and Kountz, D.S. (1995). Thyroiditis: A disease with many faces. *Postgraduate Medicine* 98(2), 101–112.

Sherman, S.I., Simonson, L., and Ladenson, P.W. (1996). Clinical and socioeconomic predispositions to complicated thyrotoxicosis: A predictable and preventable syndrome? *American Journal of Medicine* 101, 192–198.

Siminoski, K. (1995). Does this patient have a goiter? *Journal of the American Medical Association* 273(10), 813–817.

Singer, P.A., Cooper, D.S., Levy, E.G., *et al.* (1995). Treatment guidelines for patients with hyperthyroidism and hypothyroidism. *Journal of the American Medical Association* 273(10), 808–812.

Skuza, K.A., Sills, I.N., Stene, M., *et al.* (1996). Prediction of neonatal hyperthyroidism in infants born to mothers with Graves' disease. *Journal of Pediatrics* 128(2), 264–268.

Smith, S.A. (1995). Commonly asked questions about thyroid function. *Mayo Clinic Proceedings* 70, 573–577.

Streff, M.M., and Pachucki-Hyde, L.C. (1996). Management of the patient with thyroid disease. *Nursing Clinics of North America* 31(4), 779–796.

Surks, M.I., and Sievert, R. (1995). Drugs and thyroid function. *New England Journal of Medicine* 333(25), 1688–1694.

Tonner, D.R., and Schlechte, J.A. (1993). Neurologic complications of thyroid and parathyroid disease. *Medical Clinics of North America* 77(1), 251–263.

Winger, J.M., and Hornick, T. (1996). Age-associated changes in the endocrine system. *Nursing Clinics of North America* 31(4), 827–844.

Woeber, K.A. (1991). Iodine and thyroid disease. *Medical Clinics of North America* 75(1), 169–178.

Wysolmerski, J.J., and Broadus, A.E. (1994). Hypercalcemia of malignancy: The central role of parathyroid hormone-related protein. *Annual Review of Medicine* 45, 189–200.

Disorders of the Adrenal Cortex and Endocrine Pancreas

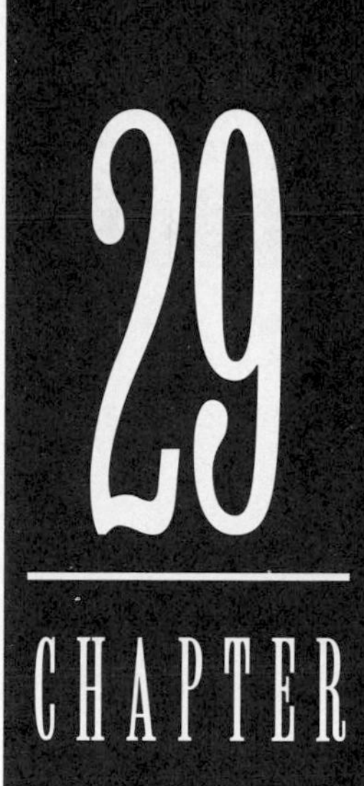

LEARNING OBJECTIVES

1. Discuss the importance of the adrenocortical and pancreatic islet cell hormones in glucose homeostasis during stressed and unstressed states.
2. Identify the hormones produced by each zone of the adrenal cortex and by each cell type of the pancreatic islets of Langerhans.
3. Compare and contrast the principal functions of the adrenal mineralocorticoids, glucocorticoids, and androgens.
4. Discuss the pathophysiologic basis and clinical importance of the phenomenon of insulin resistance.
5. Explain the pathophysiologic mechanisms underlying disorders of adrenocortical hyperfunction and hypofunction.
6. Compare and contrast the etiologies and clinical manifestations of type 1 versus type 2 diabetes mellitus.
7. Identify the rationales for the primary modes of clinical intervention in diabetes mellitus.
8. Discuss the pathophysiologic mechanisms that result in the clinical manifestations of hypoglycemia.

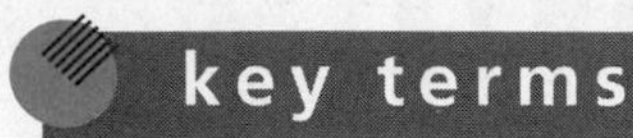

Addison's disease
adrenal insufficiency
adrenocorticotropic hormone (ACTH)
aldosterone
androgen
congenital adrenal hyperplasia (CAH)
corticotropin-releasing hormone (CRH)
cortisol
Cushing's syndrome
diabetes mellitus
diabetic ketoacidosis (DKA)
glucagon
glucocorticoid
gluconeogenesis
glycogenolysis
gonadocorticoid
hyperglycemia
hyperinsulinemia
hyperosmolar nonketotic state
hypoglycemia
impaired glucose tolerance
insulin
insulin resistance
macrovascular disease
microvascular disease
mineralocorticoid
nephropathy
neuropathy
pancreatic polypeptide hormone
primary aldosteronism
retinopathy
somatostatin
syndrome X

Under physiologic conditions, the brain requires a steady supply of glucose for normal function. Maintenance of stable levels of serum glucose despite normal variations in nutrient intake and metabolic demands requires coordination of processes of hepatic glucose production, secretion of **insulin** and **glucagon** by the endocrine pancreas, and cellular actions of insulin in muscle and adipose tissues. Under extraordinary circumstances, such as stress, illness, or starvation states, the actions of the adrenal hormones and autonomic nervous system are also critical to glucose homeostasis. In this chapter, the anatomy and normal functions of the adrenal cortex and endocrine pancreas are examined, along with the functions of the most important adrenocortical and pancreatic hormones. The endocrine regulation of glucose homeostasis under physiologic and nonphysiologic circumstances is detailed.

Primary disorders of the adrenal cortex are uncommon; however, the more prevalent conditions resulting in hyperfunction and hypofunction are discussed to illustrate the endocrine regulatory mechanisms. The role of the principal adrenocortical hormone, **cortisol**, is of particular clinical importance in that its pharmacologic equivalent is frequently (and often inappropriately) used in the treatment of inflammatory disorders. Iatrogenic **Cushing's syndrome**, which may result from excessive or prolonged administration of exogenous corticosteroid therapy, is commonly encountered in clinical situations.

Diabetes mellitus, which results from lack of insulin or lack of insulin effect, afflicts more than 16 million people in the United States.[1] The various forms of diabetes are discussed in detail, along with the potential acute and chronic complications of this disease. **Hypoglycemia,** which most often results from inappropriate insulin therapy, also is addressed.

ADRENOCORTICAL ANATOMY AND FUNCTION

Cortical Zones

Composed of several distinct zones, each producing different hormones, the adrenal glands have important functions in the regulation of fluid and electrolyte balance, metabolic adaptation during stress, and inflammatory and immune responses. Adrenal hormones also have a minor role in the regulation of sexual development and function. The central portion of the gland, the adrenal medulla, is functionally integrated with the sympathetic nervous system, as discussed in Chapter 22.

Figure 29–1 illustrates the gross anatomy and position of the adrenals atop the kidneys in the retroperitoneal space. The adrenal zones are shown in cross-section in Figure 29–2. The inner medulla secretes the catecholamine hormones epinephrine and norepinephrine in response to sympathetic stimulation. The adrenal cortex consists of three zones: the inner *zona reticularis* and *zona fasciculata* and the outer *zona glomerulosa.*

Adrenocortical Hormones

Classification

Three categories of hormones are produced by the adrenal cortex: the **mineralocorticoids**, of which **al-**

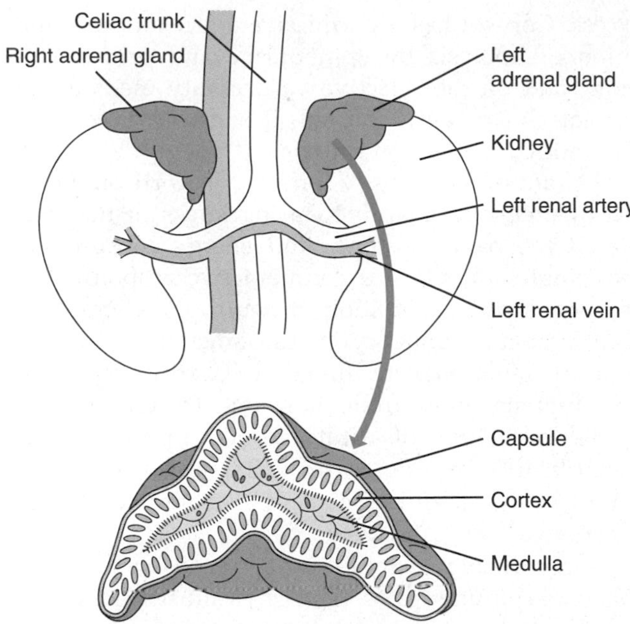

FIGURE 29–1
Adrenal anatomy. The adrenal glands lie atop the kidneys in the retroperitoneal space. Each gland is composed of an outer capsule and two functionally distinct endocrine glands: the outer adrenal cortex and the inner adrenal medulla.

dosterone is most important; the **glucocorticoids**, of which cortisol is most important; and the **gonadocorticoids** (adrenal sex hormones), of which **androgens** are most important. Table 29–1 lists the principal hormones in each category.

Synthesis

In contrast to the peptide catecholamines, the adrenocortical hormones are steroids, are lipid soluble, and are dependent on the availability of cholesterol as a substrate for their synthesis (Fig. 29–3). Specific enzymes are essential to each step of hormone synthesis. Deficiency of any of these enzymes may lead to a lack of production of one or more adrenocortical hormones and overproduction of others, as discussed later in this chapter.

Hormone Transport and Cellular Mechanism of Action

The adrenocortical hormones are primarily transported bound to *transcortin* (also known as *corticosteroid-binding globulin*) and other plasma proteins. Aldosterone precursors are almost completely protein bound, whereas aldosterone is only 50% to 70% protein bound. Cortisol is 90% to 95% protein bound. As discussed in Chapter 27, the free (unbound) fraction is biologically active. Free hormone is also accessible for hepatic and renal metabolism and excretion. Aldosterone thus has a much more rapid onset of action, but also a shorter half-life, than cortisol (35 minutes for aldosterone versus 120 minutes for cortisol).[2]

As described in Chapter 27, steroid hormones exert their actions by entering target cells, binding to intracellular receptors, and influencing transcription of genes within the nucleus. Because receptors for the different steroid hormones are structurally similar, there is a considerable degree of cross-reactivity; that is, mineralocorticoids may bind to glucocorticoid receptors, and vice versa. Actions of the adrenocortical steroids thus overlap to some degree.

Mineralocorticoid Actions

The mineralocorticoids are so named because they affect the homeostasis of *minerals*, primarily sodium and potassium. The importance of the mineralocorticoid aldosterone in sodium and potassium regulation, as well as its secondary effects on fluid balance and acid-base balance, are detailed in Chapters 8, 9, and 10. Briefly, aldosterone stimulates the synthesis of the Na^+-K^+-ATPase membrane pump, which reabsorbs sodium from renal tubules into the blood while secreting potassium into the distal nephron for potential excretion in the urine. Aldosterone also stimulates similar pumps in other tissues (e.g., the gastrointestinal tract and salivary glands), with lesser effect.

Associated with this primary function is the reabsorption of water along the osmotic gradient created by active reabsorption of sodium. This action of aldosterone makes it an important component of the renin–angiotensin–aldosterone system (RAAS), a critical regulator of fluid balance. The role of aldosterone in acid-base balance lies in the potential excretion of hydrogen instead of potassium by the Na^+-K^+-ATPase pump. Although potassium is the principal cation exchanged for sodium, some H^+ is

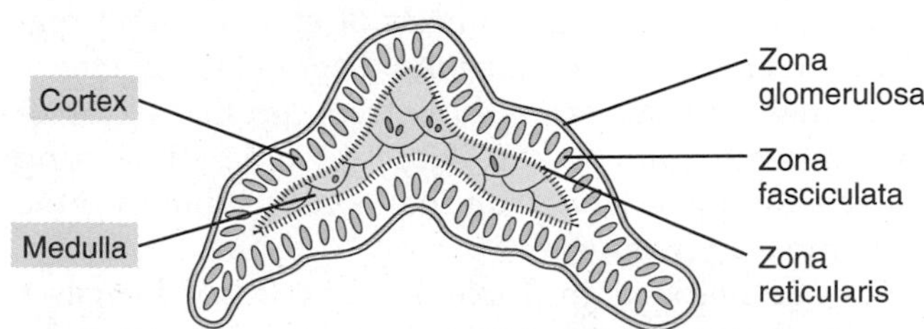

FIGURE 29–2
Adrenal zones. The adrenal cortex is composed of the outer zona glomerulosa, which secretes aldosterone and other mineralocorticoids, and the zona fasciculata and zona reticularis, which secrete the glucocorticoids and adrenal sex hormones. The adrenal medulla, which is functionally integrated with the sympathetic nervous system, secretes the catecholamines epinephrine and norephinephrine.

TABLE 29–1
CLASSIFICATION OF THE ADRENOCORTICAL HORMONES

CLASSIFICATION	EXAMPLES
Mineralocorticoids	Aldosterone (90% of mineralocorticoid activity) Desoxycorticosterone (DOC) Corticosterone
Glucocorticoids	Cortisol (95% of glucocorticoid activity) 11-Deoxycortisol Corticosterone
Gonadocorticoids	Dehydroepiandrosterone (DHEA) Androstenedione Androstenediol Testosterone Estrone Estradiol

also exchanged, particularly if serum H^+ is elevated or if serum K^+ is low.

Regulation of aldosterone secretion by the RAAS is discussed in detail in Chapter 8. This negative feedback system begins with the renal secretion of renin, triggered by decreased blood volume or by decreased serum Na^+. Elevated serum K^+ also stimulates aldosterone secretion independently of the RAAS. Circulating K^+ apparently depolarizes membranes of zona glomerulosa cells, opening calcium channels and subsequently increasing aldosterone secretion.

Glucocorticoid Actions

Cortisol is the most important of the glucocorticoid hormones, named for their effects on glucose. Glucocorticoid effects extend beyond glucose homeostasis, however, affecting metabolism of other nutrients and also modulating the effects of a number of other hormones and neurotransmitters. Secreted by cells of the zona reticularis and zona fasciculata, cortisol stimulates the synthesis of enzymes that regulate diverse cellular functions. The metabolic effects of cortisol during stress have the common goal of maximizing glucose availability and stimulating muscle strength while simultaneously inhibiting the inflammatory response.

As summarized in Table 29–2, cortisol increases serum glucose and hepatic glycogen deposition by stimulating protein catabolism and **gluconeogenesis**. Furthermore, cortisol antagonizes insulin and vitamin D, inhibiting glucose uptake and bone formation. Collagen synthesis is also inhibited, producing thin skin and capillary fragility in cases of cortisol excess. Cortisol has a permissive effect on the stimulation of lipolysis by epinephrine and growth hormone and on the selective vasoactivity mediated by the catecholamines. Cortisol also has a direct positive inotropic effect on muscle.

The anti-inflammatory effects of cortisol, which are theoretically adaptive during stress in that they inhibit the pain, swelling, and energy consumption that might impede the counteractive response to a stressor, include inhibition of neutrophil chemotaxis, stabilization of phagocytic lysosomes, and suppression of T-lymphocyte function. Cortisol in excess also inhibits antidiuretic hormone (resulting in an increased output of dilute urine), increases emotional lability, and decreases REM sleep and sensory acuity by its modulation of central nervous system function.

Glucocorticoid secretion is regulated by the hypothalamic–pituitary axis (HPA), as illustrated in Figure 29–4. In response to a variety of neural and hormonal signals, the paraventricular nuclei of the hypothalamus release **corticotropin-releasing hormone (CRH),** which then stimulates the anterior pituitary to release **adrenocorticotropic hormone** (ACTH, or corticotropin). In addition to this major endocrine effect, CRH also stimulates the secretion of the neurotransmitter norepinephrine, enhancing the stress response (see Chapter 1), as well as endorphins and other peptides that mediate the inflammatory response and the endogenous analgesia system (see Chapters 13 and 23).

Inflammatory cytokines, including tumor necrosis factor, interleukin-1, and interleukin-6, are known to activate the hypothalamic–pituitary–adrenal axis.[3] Baseline CRH secretion follows a predictable circa-

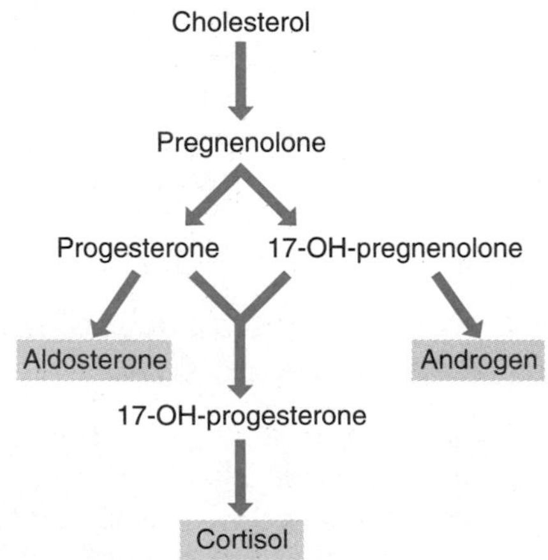

FIGURE 29–3
Synthesis of the adrenocortical hormones. The adrenocortical hormones are steroids synthesized from cholesterol under regulation by specific enzymes. Deficiency of any of these enzymes may lead to lack of certain hormones and overproduction of others.

TABLE 29–2
ACTIONS OF CORTISOL

Primary Action	Mechanisms
Mobilization of energy stores (increasing serum glucose)	Stimulation of hepatic gluconeogenesis Induction of appropriate enzymes Mobilization of amino acids from nonhepatic tissues Increased hepatic glycogen stores Decreased cellular glucose use Decreased protein synthesis (except in liver) Increased protein catabolism (except in liver) Mobilization of fatty acids from adipose tissue Increased β-oxidation of fatty acids for energy
Suppression of inflammatory and immune responses	Stabilization of lysosomal membranes Blockade of prostaglandin and leukotriene synthesis Decreased capillary permeability Decreased neutrophil migration Decreased phagocytic activity Suppression of eosinophil production Suppression of lymphocyte proliferation and immunoglobulin secretion Reduction of fever by decreased production of interleukin-1 by leukocytes
Enhancement of erythrocyte production	Unknown

Data from Guyton, A.C., and Hall, J.E. (1996). *Textbook of Medical Physiology.* (9th ed.). Philadelphia: W.B. Saunders. (pp. 962–965).

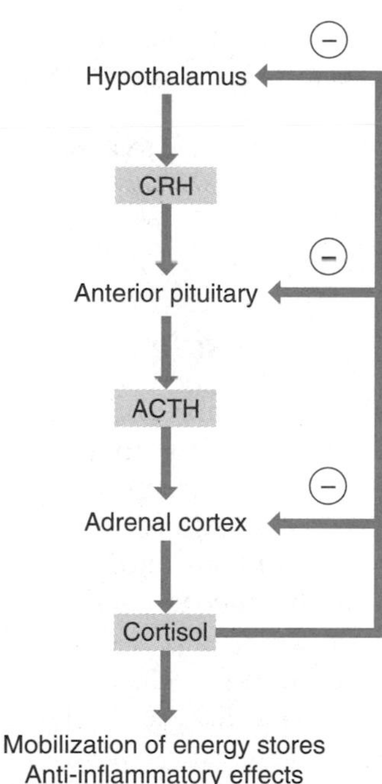

FIGURE 29–4
Hypothalamic–pituitary–adrenal axis. Secretion of cortisol and other glucocorticoids is regulated in response to hypothalamic corticotropin-releasing hormone (CRH), which stimulates the release of adrenocorticotropic hormone (ACTH, or corticotropin) from the anterior pituitary. ACTH stimulates the secretion of cortisol and, to a lesser extent, other adrenocortical hormones. Negative feedback to this system is primarily modulated by circulating cortisol levels.

dian rhythm, with peak output during the early morning. CRH is known to be produced by cells outside the hypothalamus, including thymus and spleen, and the hormone is found within circulating white blood cells and in inflammatory exudate. This "peripheral" CRH is proinflammatory. The term *tissue CRH* has been used to describe a number of other proinflammatory cytokines released into sites of inflammation, but these substances have no structural similarity to CRH.

Within the HPA, CRH stimulates the anterior pituitary to produce ACTH and β-endorphin (both cleaved from the same peptide prohormone), which trigger the release of cortisol and, to a lesser extent, other adrenocortical hormones. The systemic *anti*-inflammatory effects of ACTH and cortisol are derived in part from their negative feedback to the HPA, which suppresses the secretion of CRH.

Gonadocorticoid Actions

A subset of cells located in the inner adrenocortical layers secrete the gonadocorticoids, which include some estrogens and progesterone but which are mainly androgens. Estrogens and progesterone, which confer "female" characteristics, and androgens, which confer "male" characteristics, are present in both sexes. The adrenals normally supply about 25% of circulating sex hormones, a physiologically insignificant amount when compared with ovarian and testicular hormone production.

In females, adrenal androgens sustain the normal growth of pubic and axillary hair, and in males, these hormones contribute to a minor extent to the development of masculine characteristics. The clinical importance of adrenal androgens is evident only when they are present in excess, in which case pronounced masculinization of females and precocious puberty in males may result (see later discussion of **congenital adrenal hyperplasia [CAH]).**

Adrenal androgens have been postulated to enhance immune function by a receptor that is present in T lymphocytes. The mechanisms by which sex hormones (whether from adrenal or gonadal sources) influence immune function are unknown. Autoimmune disorders are known to affect females more often than males (see Chapter 13).

Regulation of adrenal sex hormone secretion is poorly understood. ACTH stimulates the secretion of gonadocorticoids as well as glucocorticoids and mineralocorticoids, but only cortisol appears to feed back negatively to the HPA.

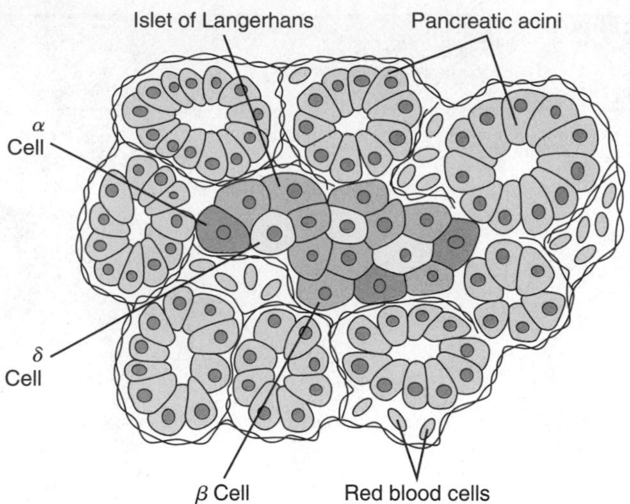

FIGURE 29–5

Endocrine pancreas. The endocrine function of the pancreas originates from the 1% of the gland composed of the islets of Langerhans. Principal cell types within the islets include (1) α cells, which secrete glucagon, (2) β cells, which secrete insulin, and (3) δ cells, which secrete somatostatin. The bulk of the pancreas is composed of acini, which serve an exocrine function.

ANATOMY AND FUNCTION OF THE ENDOCRINE PANCREAS

Cells of the Islets of Langerhans

The mass of the pancreas is largely composed of the acinar cells and ducts, which secrete pancreatic enzymes, bicarbonate, and water into the duodenum. This exocrine function of the pancreas, essential to the digestion and absorption of nutrients, is discussed in Chapter 25. The endocrine function of the pancreas resides in the *islets of Langerhans*, integrated groups of endocrine cells distributed among the exocrine cells. Although the islets make up only 1% of pancreatic mass, the endocrine function of the pancreas is critical to glucose homeostasis, which is, in turn, essential to energy metabolism (see Chapter 3).

Figure 29–5 illustrates the cellular structure of the islets of Langerhans. Each islet contains four types of cells, each producing a different peptide hormone: (1) α cells, which produce glucagon, (2) β cells, which produce insulin, (3) δ cells, which produce **somatostatin**, and (4) *PP cells*, which produce **pancreatic polypeptide hormone**. The islets are innervated by the autonomic nervous system, and gap junctions between cells facilitate exchange of molecules as a basis for local regulation of secretion. As is true of all endocrine glands, the islets are richly perfused, facilitating secretion of hormones into the bloodstream.

Pancreatic Hormones

The pancreatic hormones are essential to the regulation of: (1) serum glucose levels, which comprise the body's readily available energy fuel, and (2) the uptake of glucose by selected body cells.

Insulin

Insulin is the *only* hormone that acts to lower blood glucose. The hypoglycemic effects of insulin are the result of its enhancement of glucose uptake by skeletal muscle and adipose tissue, enhancement of hepatic glucose uptake and glycogen synthesis, and inhibition of gluconeogenesis, lipolysis, and proteolysis (Table 29–3). As directed by a gene on chromosome 11, insulin is synthesized by β cells via cleavage of a large peptide prohormone (Fig. 29–6), producing the active hormone as well as an inactive *C-protein* fragment. The C-protein level in the blood serves as a clinical marker of β-cell activity.

Insulin reduces serum glucose by altering the metabolism of carbohydrates, fats, and proteins to achieve the homeostatic goal of enhancing peripheral uptake of glucose for energy metabolism and storage, thus sparing lipids and proteins for anabolic processes. In support of anabolism, insulin also af-

TABLE 29–3
ACTIONS OF INSULIN

Primary Action	Mechanisms
Promotion of glucose uptake, storage, and use (decreasing serum glucose)	Promotion of rapid uptake and preferential use of glucose by skeletal muscle after meals Promotion of muscle glycogenesis after meals Promotion of hepatic glycogenesis after meals Inactivation of enzymes that catalyze glycogenolysis Activation of enzymes that enhance hepatic glucose uptake (e.g., glucokinase) and glycogenesis (e.g., glycogen synthase) Promotion of triglyceride synthesis from excess glucose Promotion of glucose uptake by most other body cells (except brain cells)
Suppression of lipolysis (sparing fat from metabolism and reducing serum glucose)	Inhibition of the hormone-sensitive lipase enzyme that causes splitting of fatty acids from stored triglycerides in adipose tissue
Promotion of fat storage in adipose cells	Promotion of hepatic uptake of glucose, making excess glucose available to form acetyl–coenzyme A, from which fatty acids are synthesized Activation of the enzyme lipoprotein lipase, which cleaves fatty acids from circulating triglycerides, permitting their uptake into adipose cells Promotion of glucose uptake into adipose cells for use in synthesis of the glycerol backbone of triglycerides
Suppression of proteolysis	Inhibition of catabolism of muscle cell proteins Inhibition of the use of plasma amino acids for gluconeogenesis
Promotion of protein synthesis and growth	Increased uptake of the amino acids valine, leucine, isoleucine, tyrosine, and phenylalanine into cells Increased translation of mRNA by ribosomes Increased rate of transcription of selected DNA genetic sequences in the nucleus

Data from Guyton, A.C., and Hall, J.E. (1996). *Textbook of Medical Physiology.* (9th ed.). Philadelphia: W.B. Saunders. (pp. 973–976).

fects electrolyte balance by stimulating cellular uptake of potassium, phosphate, and magnesium into muscle and liver cells and by promoting reabsorption of potassium, phosphate, and sodium by renal tubular cells.

Although the synthesis and release of insulin may be stimulated or inhibited by a number of agents and conditions, the most important factor is the serum glucose level. Amino acids in the blood have a significant synergistic effect with glucose on insulin secretion, whereas triglycerides and fatty acids have only minor effects. Sympathetic stimulation and catecholamines produce a net inhibition of insulin secretion (mediated by β-adrenergic receptors), whereas parasympathetic stimulation increases insulin release. At physiologic levels, cortisol, growth hormone, thyroid hormones, and sex hormones stimulate hyperplasia of β cells in response to the increased peripheral uptake of glucose mediated by these hormones, thus chronically increasing insulin output. Insulin secretion also varies with nutrient intake, stress, and exercise, as discussed later.

Glucagon

Glucagon is the most important of the *counter-regulatory* hormones that mobilize energy stores, raising serum glucose. Glucagon is synthesized by α cells under the direction of a gene located on chromosome 2. The actions of glucagon directly oppose those of insulin; and the *ratio* of insulin to glucagon is more important than the absolute amounts of either hormone in determining net effects.

Glucagon increases blood glucose by promoting the mobilization of stored nutrients (Table 29–4). The major effects of glucagon are on the liver, where it stimulates **glycogenolysis** and gluconeogenesis by activating selected enzymes. Glucagon has little effect on muscle and adipose tissue except in cases of complete or near-complete lack of insulin, when unopposed glucagon promotes lipolysis. Glucagon also decreases hepatic cholesterol synthesis by inhibiting the enzyme hydroxymethylglutaryl–coenzyme A reductase (HMG–CoA reductase). Other actions of glucagon include inhibition of renal sodium reabsorp-

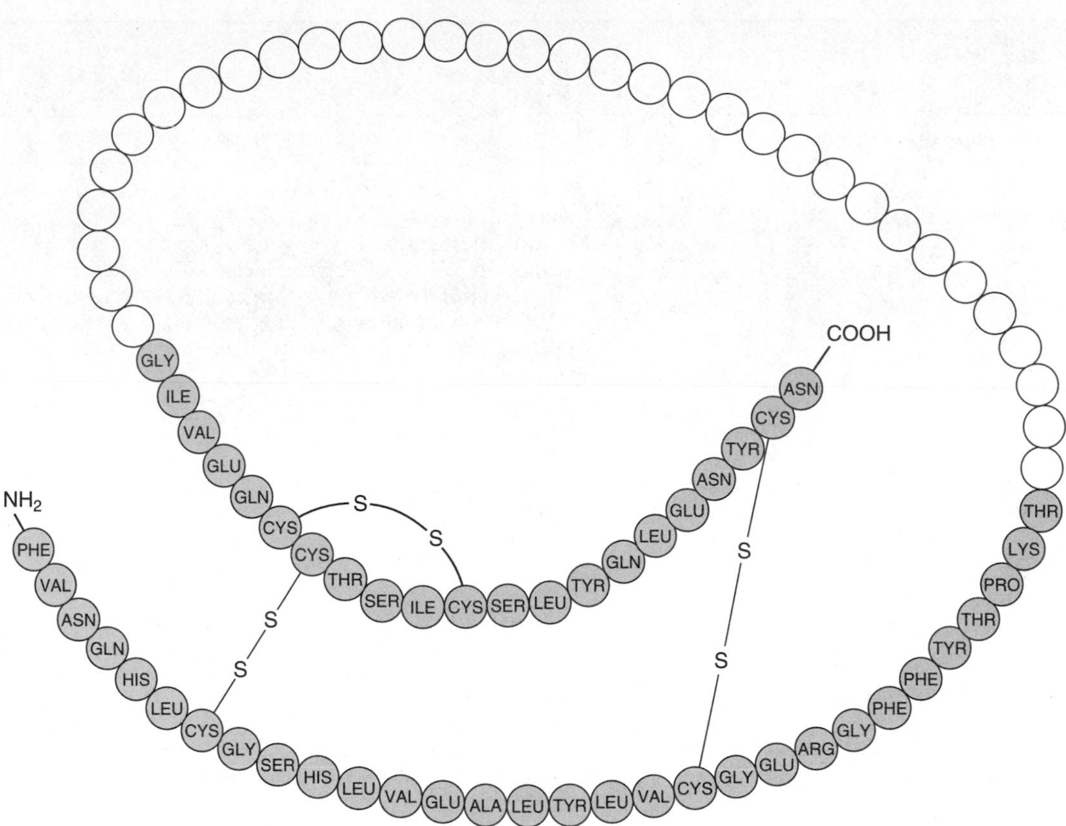

FIGURE 29–6

Structure of insulin. Cleavage of a large peptide prohormone yields the active hormone, insulin (illustrated in color), and an inactive C-protein fragment (illustrated in white). Assay of serum C-protein serves as a clinical marker of β-cell activity.

tion and activation of the cyclic adenosine monophosphate mechanism, mediating enhanced contraction of cardiac muscle. Glucagon may also act as a neuromodulator in central nervous system regulation of appetite.

Glucagon synthesis is enhanced by low serum glucose and insulin levels as well as by protein intake in the absence of glucose. Sympathetic stimulation in stress and exercise (by α-adrenergic receptors) enhances glucagon secretion, as does parasympathetic stimulation.

TABLE 29–4
ACTIONS OF GLUCAGON

PRIMARY ACTION	MECHANISMS
Promotion of glycogenolysis (increasing serum glucose)	Activation of the glycolytic enzyme cascade in hepatic cells
Promotion of gluconeogenesis (increasing serum glucose)	Promotion of amino acid uptake by hepatic cells Activation of enzyme systems for gluconeogenesis

Data from Guyton, A.C., and Hall, J.E. (1996). *Textbook of Medical Physiology*. (9th ed.). Philadelphia: W.B. Saunders. (pp. 978–979).

Somatostatin

Somatostatin, also known as *growth hormone release–inhibiting hormone*, is produced not only by pancreatic δ cells but also by hypothalamic nuclei (see Chapter 27) and by intestinal cells. Somatostatins from these different sources are structurally similar, but not identical. In addition to its best-known effect of inhibiting secretion of growth hormone from the pituitary, somatostatin decreases the intestinal absorption and cellular uptake of all nutrients, apparently serving to modulate the metabolic responses to both insulin and glucagon.

Somatostatin secretion is enhanced by elevated serum glucose, amino acids, and free fatty acids as well as by several hormones (including glucagon)

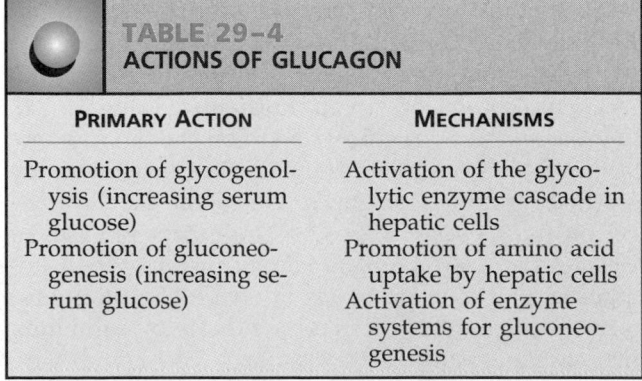

and neurotransmitters. Insulin inhibits somatostatin release.

Pancreatic Polypeptide Hormone

Pancreatic polypeptide hormone is secreted by PP cells in response to hypoglycemia and to food ingestion. Its effect is to decrease pancreatic exocrine secretion by inhibiting the uptake of enzyme precursors by acinar cells (see Chapter 25). The physiologic importance of this function is unknown.

ENDOCRINE REGULATION OF GLUCOSE HOMEOSTASIS

Cellular Mechanisms

Because the hydrophobic interior of the cell membrane prevents the simple diffusion of polar molecules such as glucose, carrier proteins are essential to glucose uptake into cells. A glucose–sodium cotransporter actively transports glucose into the cells of the small intestine and the proximal convoluted tubule of the kidney. Glucose uptake also occurs by a saturable system in which a carrier protein binds to glucose, rendering it more lipid soluble and capable of concentration-driven passive transport through the membrane.

Several subclasses of glucose transporter proteins (GLUTs) have been identified, and differences among tissue types are evident. GLUT1 has the highest affinity for glucose and is most widely distributed in tissues, including the brain, placenta, liver, kidney, small intestine, and pancreatic β cells. It mediates basal glucose uptake, that is, the uptake of glucose without insulin, even when serum glucose is low. GLUT2 mediates transport of glucose into and out of hepatocytes and may also be involved in glucose-stimulated insulin secretion by pancreatic β cells. GLUT4 is found only in tissues in which glucose uptake is mediated by insulin, namely skeletal muscle, cardiac muscle, liver, and adipose tissue.

Although the cellular mechanism by which insulin facilitates glucose uptake is still uncertain, it has been postulated that the binding of insulin to cell membrane receptors stimulates the migration of GLUT4 carrier proteins from the cytoplasm to the cell membrane.[4] Insulin may also increase the intrinsic activity of these proteins. In contrast, glucagon may antagonize the actions of insulin by decreasing this intrinsic activity.

Adaptation to Stress or Starvation

Whether glucose uptake is insulin-mediated depends not only on tissue type but also on physiologic conditions (e.g., fed versus fasted state, stressed versus nonstressed state, muscle rest versus exercise). In the resting, nonstressed, fed (absorptive) state, 80% of cellular glucose uptake is not insulin mediated, and most uptake is by the central nervous system. About 20% of peripheral glucose uptake from the blood is accounted for by skeletal muscle, and about half of that is insulin mediated. The higher the serum glucose, the greater the uptake by non–insulin-mediated carriers.

The increase in serum glucose that results from intestinal absorption stimulates insulin secretion, with insulin levels normally peaking about 30 minutes after a meal (Fig. 29–7). Insulin stimulates the peripheral use of glucose for fuel, sparing amino acids for anabolic activities (synthesis, tissue growth, and repair). Glucose uptake that exceeds immediate cellular needs for energy is diverted to storage forms: glycogen in liver and muscle, and triglycerides in liver and adipose tissue.

In the fasted (postabsorptive) state, peripheral use of glucose for energy quickly consumes available serum glucose, which suppresses further insulin secretion and stimulates glucagon secretion. Lack of insulin removes the stimulus for insulin-mediated glucose uptake and storage and disinhibits glycogenolysis, gluconeogenesis, lipolysis, and proteolysis. Glucagon promotes glycogenolysis and gluconeogenesis in the liver, increasing serum glucose, and also stimulates the use of fatty acids for energy by β-oxidation (see Chapter 3). β-Oxidation of fatty acids provides energy fuel in the absence of glucose,

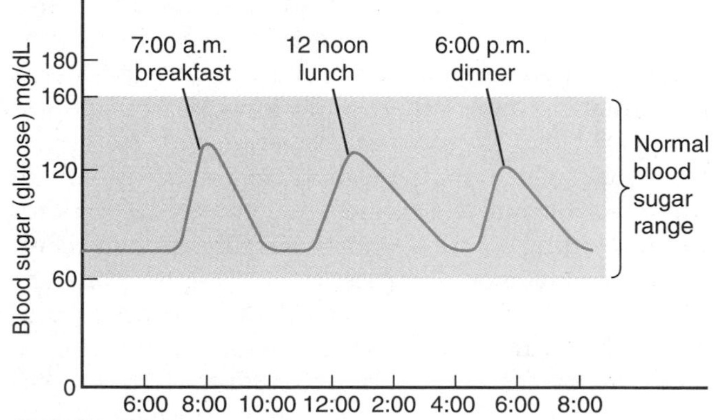

FIGURE 29–7

Pattern of insulin secretion. A relatively stable basal secretion occurs, with superimposed surges (postprandial peaks) about 30 minutes after meals.

but also produces the organic ketoacids acetoacetate and β-hydroxybutyric acid. In diabetes mellitus, excessive production of these acids may promote a form of metabolic acidosis known as **diabetic ketoacidosis (DKA),** discussed later in this chapter.

In the stressed state, peripheral glucose uptake is increased even if serum glucose is low. This increased uptake is apparently due primarily to enhanced glucose use by tissues rich in macrophages, particularly the spleen, ileum, liver, and lung.[4] A unique form of non–insulin-mediated glucose transport, this enhanced uptake is associated with the cellular immune response and is mediated by a number of cytokines released from stressed or injured cells. Gluconeogenesis is enhanced during stress and is mediated not only by glucagon but also by the "stress hormones" epinephrine and cortisol. It is notable, however, that in the absence of glucagon, these hormones have little effect on glucose homeostasis.

Insulin Resistance

Insulin resistance refers to decreased sensitivity to insulin, that is, a lack of insulin effect at the cellular level despite elevated levels of circulating insulin. Sensitivity to insulin is known to vary about three-fold in lean, healthy people. Those with less sensitivity are usually able to secrete enough additional insulin to overcome resistance and maintain normal serum glucose levels. Others, particularly those who have visceral obesity (fat distributed primarily in the trunk and abdomen), cannot secrete sufficient insulin. Serum glucose levels rise above normal, and the individual demonstrates **impaired glucose tolerance,** or type 2 diabetes mellitus.

Insulin resistance not only affects glucose homeostasis but also is associated with the following disorders: (1) coronary heart disease; (2) an atherosclerotic pattern of dyslipidemia (increased triglycerides, reduced high-density lipoprotein cholesterol, and smaller, more atherogenic low-density lipoprotein particles); (3) essential hypertension; (4) hyperuricemia (which may promote gouty arthritis); (5) impaired fibrinolysis (which may promote inappropriate clotting); and (6) microvascular angina (chest pain despite normal patency of larger coronary arteries). Many of these disorders may occur concurrently within the same person, producing a constellation of clinical manifestations termed **syndrome X.**[5]

The precise mechanism of insulin resistance is unknown. Initially, it primarily affects glucose use by skeletal muscle. Because 75% of glucose use normally occurs in skeletal muscle, serum glucose levels remain elevated, and β cells are stimulated to secrete more insulin. Binding of insulin to membrane receptors may be impaired under certain conditions, and chronic exposure to high levels of insulin may down-regulate the number of receptors on skeletal muscle, hepatic, and adipose cells. Alternatively, a postreceptor effect on glucose transport or use may account for lack of cellular response to insulin. The cellular defect may have both acquired and genetic components. People who consume excess calories and increase their body weight as little as 15% may develop some degree of insulin resistance, and physical inactivity also promotes the syndrome.[6] The importance of insulin resistance syndrome and compensatory **hyperinsulinemia** in the pathophysiology of type 2 diabetes is discussed further later in this chapter.

DISORDERS OF THE ADRENAL CORTEX AND ENDOCRINE PANCREAS

The more prevalent disorders resulting from excess or deficiency of adrenocortical hormones are discussed next. Disorders of the adrenal medulla are associated with altered function of the sympathetic nervous system and are detailed in Chapter 22. The principal forms of diabetes mellitus and the syndrome of hypoglycemia are also reviewed.

Cushing's Syndrome

Definition. Cushing's syndrome (hypercortisolism) is the constellation of clinical manifestations resulting from long-term glucocorticoid excess. The term *Cushing's disease* is more narrowly applied when the cause is excessive secretion of ACTH by a pituitary tumor.

Epidemiology. Cushing's disease and other disorders of endogenous cortisol excess are rare, with an approximate incidence of two to four cases per 1 million people per year.[7] The incidence of Cushing's syndrome resulting from exogenous administration of cortisol is uncertain, but it is known to be much greater than that of the endogenous types. Specific risk factors for development of tumors that secrete excess CRH, ACTH, or cortisol are unknown. Pituitary tumors are associated with excessive ACTH production, whereas adrenocortical tumors may produce cortisol in excess. Ectopic production of these hormones is rare and is most commonly seen with lung cancer, particularly small cell carcinoma, and with tumors of other endocrine glands. The risk factor for iatrogenic Cushing's syndrome is prolonged use of exogenous cortisol in the treatment of inflammatory conditions. Clinical depression and alcoholism are associated with a secondary *pseudo-Cushing's syndrome,* in which transient hyperactivity of the HPA or impaired hepatic inactivation of hormones produces a similar clinical picture.

Etiology. Two mechanisms may result in Cushing's syndrome: (1) an ACTH-dependent mechanism, in which elevated plasma ACTH levels stimulate the adrenal cortex to produce excess cortisol; and (2) an ACTH-independent mechanism, in which excess cortisol is either produced by the adrenal cortex or administered exogenously, suppressing the secretion of both CRH and ACTH. The first mechanism is operative in Cushing's disease, in which an ACTH-producing pituitary tumor (usually a micro adenoma) induces bilateral adrenocortical hyperplasia. Ectopic production of ACTH or, more rarely, CRH stimulates the HPA independently of normal feedback inhibition by cortisol. Excessive cortisol production is most often seen with adrenal adenomas, whereas adrenal carcinomas tend to stimulate androgen production to a greater extent than cortisol. Iatrogenic cortisol excess may result from prolonged cortisol therapy for chronic inflammatory conditions such as arthritis.

Pathophysiology. Cortisol excess results in anti-inflammatory effects, but also in excessive catabolism of protein and peripheral fat to support hepatic glucose production. Chronic cortisol excess also suppresses the HPA.

Clinical Manifestations. The most immediately apparent sign is weight gain, which may be generalized but more often occurs in a typical pattern of truncal obesity, "moon" face, and increased fat pads above the clavicles (Fig. 29–8). Metabolic abnormalities seen include glucose intolerance (with diabetes in 20% of cases), hypertension, muscle wasting, and weakness. Thin skin and fragile capillaries result in a reddened complexion, frequent bruising, gastrointestinal bleeding, and striae (stretch marks).

If ACTH excess is present, hyperpigmentation of the skin may be seen due to elevated levels of the melanocyte-stimulating hormone segment of the peptide (see Chapter 27). With long-term Cushing's syndrome in older people, osteoporosis is prevalent, manifesting as low back pain and possible pathologic fractures (see Chapter 34). Cushing's syndrome in children is rare, but manifests as impairment of linear growth and excessive weight gain (see Focus of Current Research). Derangement of HPA regulation of adrenal androgen secretion may result in masculinization signs in females, including acne and hirsutism. Laboratory evidence of Cushing's syndrome includes elevation of urinary cortisol excretion and failure of exogenous cortisol (dexamethasone) to suppress cortisol secretion.

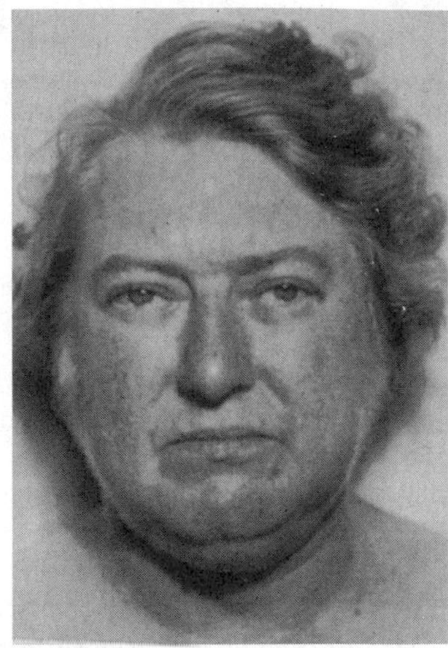

FIGURE 29–8
Cushing's syndrome. Note the plethoric, rounded, moon-like face, prominent jowels, and hirsutism on the upper lip, lower cheeks, and chin. (From Williams, R.H. [1968]. *Textbook of Endocrinology.* [4th ed.]. Philadelphia: W.B. Saunders. [p. 352].)

Prevention and Treatment. Patients receiving excessive or inappropriate steroid therapy should be gradually weaned off the drugs if at all possible. (After long-term suppression of the HPA by cortisol, sudden withdrawal of steroids may precipitate acute **adrenal insufficiency**.) ACTH-secreting pituitary tumors are optimally treated with surgical excision if tumors are well-circumscribed. If surgery is not possible or desirable, pituitary irradiation may be used. If radiation also fails to contain the pituitary tumor, bilateral total adrenalectomy is done, with lifelong replacement of glucocorticoids and mineralocorticoids. Adrenalectomy is the treatment of choice for adrenal tumors. Ectopic hormone secretion is usually not curable by surgical excision. Medical therapy may be used as an adjunctive treatment to minimize hypercortisolism in patients with mild disease or in cases of disease recurrence after surgery. Antiadrenal drugs include adrenal enzyme inhibitors, such as ketoconazole (Nizoral) or aminoglutethimide (Cytadren), and the adrenocorticolytic agent mitotane (Lysodren).

Prognosis and Outcome. Surgery is curative in 80% of cases of Cushing's disease.[8] The incidence of recurrence after surgery increases over time, however. Eighty-five per cent of children are cured with irradiation of the pituitary gland. The process of weaning patients from chronic glucocorticoid therapy may be difficult in many cases, owing to exacerbation of the underlying problems (e.g., arthritis) or

Focus of Current Research

Study	Objective and Findings
Diabetes Control and Complications Trial Research Group (1996) Lifetime benefits and costs of intensive therapy as practiced in the Diabetes Control and Complications Trial.	*Objective:* To examine the cost-effectiveness of alternative approaches to the management of insulin-dependent diabetes *Findings:* Over a lifetime, intensive therapy reduces complications, improves quality of life, and can be expected to increase longevity.
Westphal (1996) The occurrence of diabetic ketoacidosis in non-insulin-dependent diabetes and newly diagnosed diabetic adults.	*Objective:* To examine the occurrence of diabetic ketoacidosis (DKA) in adults without a prior history of type I diabetes *Findings:* DKA occurs in patients with type 2 diabetes. Older patients may present with clinically apparent type I diabetes. Some adults who present with DKA do not remain insulin-dependent.
Carter, *et al.* (1996) Non-insulin-dependent diabetes mellitus in minorities in the United States.	*Objective:* To review the data on prevalence, complications, and mortality of non-insulin-dependent diabetes among nonwhites in the United States *Findings:* All minorities except Alaskan natives have a two- to six-fold increased incidence of type 2 diabetes as compared with whites.
Colditz, *et al.* (1995) Weight gain as a risk factor for clinical diabetes mellitus in women.	*Objective:* To examine the relation between adult weight change and the risk for clinical diabetes among middle-aged women *Findings:* The excess risk for diabetes with even modest and typical adult weight gain is substantial.
Lazarevic, *et al.* (1995) Reduction of cortisol levels after single intra-articular and intramuscular steroid injection.	*Objective:* To determine the influence of a single injection of methylprednisolone on the hypothalamic–pituitary–adrenal axis *Findings:* Decreased adrenocortical secretion can result from a single low-dose injection of depot corticosteroids.
Garg, *et al.* (1994) Effects of varying carbohydrate content of diet in patients with non-insulin-dependent diabetes mellitus.	*Objective:* To study effects of variation in carbohydrate content of diet on glycemia and plasma lipoproteins in patients with type 2 diabetes *Findings:* High carbohydrate diets, compared with high monounsaturated fat diets, caused persistent deterioration in glycemic control, accentuation of hyperinsulinemia, and increased plasma triglycerides and very-low-density lipoprotein cholesterol.

Box continued on following page

Study	*Objective and Findings*
Berlin, *et al.* (1994) Suspected postprandial hypoglycemia is associated with β-adrenergic hypersensitivity and emotional distress.	*Objective:* To study physiologic responses in patients with suspected postprandial hypoglycemia versus control subjects *Findings:* Patients with suspected hypoglycemia have normal glucose tolerance, increased β-adrenergic sensitivity, and emotional distress.
Magiakou, *et al.* (1994) Cushing's syndrome in children and adolescents: Presentation, diagnosis, and therapy.	*Objective:* To analyze the clinical presentation, diagnostic evaluation, and treatment of 59 patients, aged 4 to 20 years, with Cushing's syndrome *Findings:* Weight gain and growth retardation are common characteristics. Diagnostic evaluation is accurate, and therapy is usually successful.

presence of withdrawal symptoms, such as hypotension, fatigue, and abdominal pain.[9]

Adrenal Insufficiency

Definition. Adrenal insufficiency is a clinical syndrome associated with deficient production of adrenocortical hormones. **Addison's disease**, the most common form of *primary adrenal insufficiency*, is a chronic disorder resulting from autoimmune destruction of all three zones of the adrenal cortex. *Secondary adrenal insufficiency*, which is due to suppression of CRH or ACTH secretion, differs from Addison's disease in that it results in deficiency of cortisol and androgens but not aldosterone.

Epidemiology. Adrenal insufficiency is uncommon but can occur at any age. The prevalence of Addison's disease has been estimated at 39 to 60 cases per 1 million population.[10] Most cases of Addison's disease are seen in adult white females, and a genetic predisposition is probable in these cases. Tuberculosis, acquired immunodeficiency syndrome, systemic fungal infections, and metastatic cancers (especially lymphomas, malignant melanomas of the skin, and cancers of the lung, breast, and gastrointestinal tract) also constitute risk factors because these diseases may involve the adrenals.

Etiology. Disorders associated with primary and secondary adrenal insufficiency are listed in Table 29–5. Most cases (80%) are caused by autoimmune destruction of the adrenal glands, either exclusively or as part of a syndrome in which other endocrine glands (e.g., thyroid, endocrine pancreas) are also damaged.[11] Infections cause 15% of cases, with a variety of disorders accounting for the remainder.

Pathophysiology. Adrenal cells are destroyed by immune-mediated inflammation or, less commonly, by ischemic necrosis. Manifestations of adrenocortical hormone deficiency become apparent when 90%

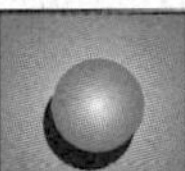

TABLE 29–5
ETIOLOGY OF ADRENAL INSUFFICIENCY

PRIMARY ADRENAL INSUFFICIENCY
Autoimmune adrenalitis (e.g., Addison's disease)
Tuberculosis
Adrenomyeloneuropathy
Systemic fungal infections (e.g., histoplasmosis, cryptococcosis, blastomycosis)
Acquired immunodeficiency syndrome (associated with opportunistic infections or Kaposi's sarcoma)
Metastatic carcinoma (usually of lung, breast, or kidney origin)
Lymphoma
Isolated glucocorticoid deficiency (often familial)
Adrenal hemorrhage or necrosis (due to sepsis, coagulation disorders, or antiphospholipid syndrome)
SECONDARY ADRENAL INSUFFICIENCY
Pituitary tumor
Craniopharyngioma
Pituitary surgery or radiation
Lymphocytic hypophysitis
Sarcoidosis
Histiocytosis
Empty sella syndrome
Hypothalamic tumor
Long-term glucocorticoid therapy
Sheehan's syndrome
Pituitary trauma
Pituitary or adrenal surgery

Adapted from Oelkers, W. (1996). Adrenal insufficiency. *New England Journal of Medicine* 335(16), 1207.

of functional cells in both glands are lost. In most cases, cellular atrophy is limited to the cortex, although in some cases, the medulla is involved also, resulting in catecholamine deficiency. Adrenocortical hormone levels are low, and in primary adrenal insufficiency, ACTH excess develops as a result of lack of negative feedback to the HPA. ACTH excess does not occur in secondary adrenal insufficiency.

Clinical Manifestations. The altered metabolic state induced by cortisol deficiency may manifest as hypoglycemia, weakness, fatigue, and low resistance to stress and infection. Emotional lability may be noted. Mineralocorticoid deficiency (in primary adrenal insufficiency) may result in hyponatremia ("salt-wasting"), hyperkalemia, nausea and vomiting, abdominal pain, dehydration, and hypotension. Lack of adrenal androgens may cause loss of axillary and pubic hair in females. ACTH excess manifests as hyperpigmentation of the skin. Except in cases of acute adrenal insufficiency, however, symptoms are mild and may go undetected. *Addisonian crisis* (or adrenal crisis), in which hypoglycemia, hypotension, and electrolyte depletion are severe enough to produce seizures or coma, may occur in untreated patients who are subjected to additional stress, such as trauma or intercurrent acute illness.

Prevention and Treatment. Adrenal insufficiency is not preventable in most cases. Addisonian crises may be anticipated in those at risk, and usual steroid doses may need to be increased during periods of increased stress. Optimal treatment of tuberculosis, fungal infections, and cancers may reduce the risk of adrenal involvement in the minority of cases with these etiologies. Treatment of adrenal insufficiency involves addressing the underlying cause, if possible, and replacing cortisol and, usually, mineralocorticoid hormones.[12]

Prognosis and Outcome. Steroid therapy is successful in the management of most cases. Therapy is lifelong in Addison's disease patients and must be accompanied by close monitoring to minimize adverse effects of either cortisol deficiency or iatrogenic excess.

Primary Aldosteronism

Definition. Primary aldosteronism (also known as *primary hyperaldosteronism* or *Conn's syndrome*) is an adrenocortical hyperfunction disorder manifested primarily by mineralocorticoid excess. Secondary aldosteronism results from renin excess and is usually due to decreased renal perfusion, as discussed in Chapter 20.

Epidemiology. Primary aldosteronism is uncommon but accounts for an estimated 1% of cases of hypertension.[13] It is more common in women and demonstrates a peak onset during the third to fifth decades of life.

Etiology. The usual cause of primary aldosteronism is an aldosterone-producing adenoma (benign *aldosteronoma*), but primary aldosteronism may also result from bilateral adrenal hyperplasia or adrenocortical carcinoma.

Pathophysiology. Excessive secretion of aldosterone results in inappropriate renal reabsorption of sodium and water and increased renal excretion of potassium. Plasma renin activity is suppressed, but cortisol production is usually normal. Secondary hypertension results from volume expansion.

Clinical Manifestations. Hypertension is usually moderate to severe and is not seen in all patients.[13] Electrolyte imbalances may affect excitable cells, resulting in weakness, paresthesias, muscle cramping, tetany, fatigue, or cardiac failure. Volume expansion may lead to frequent urination (*polyuria*).

Prevention and Treatment. Although secondary aldosteronism may be prevented with optimal therapy of cardiac failure and other disorders that can reduce renal perfusion, there is no known prevention for primary aldosteronism. Surgical resection of adrenal tumors is the treatment of choice. Bilateral adrenal hyperplasia is treated with sodium restriction, potassium replacement, and spironolactone (Aldactone), an aldosterone antagonist.

Prognosis and Outcome. Hypertension may be cured with surgery but frequently recurs. Management of hypertension then requires treatment with spironolactone. Conventional antihypertensive drugs are usually ineffective in cases of secondary hypertension (see Chapter 15).

Congenital Adrenal Hyperplasia

Definition. Congenital adrenal hyperplasia (CAH) encompasses a group of genetic disorders resulting in deficiency or absence of an enzyme necessary for synthesis of glucocorticoids or mineralocorticoids. Cortisol synthesis is most commonly impaired. Manifestations are usually apparent at birth or during early childhood, but symptoms may manifest later in life in the case of *nonclassic CAH*.[14]

Epidemiology. These conditions are uncommon. Specific risk factors other than family history are unknown.

Etiology. The disorder is inherited as an autosomal recessive trait. In 95% of cases, there is deficiency of the enzyme 21-hydroxylase.[15] Rarely, a genetic defect results in glucocorticoid resistance, with compensatory hyperstimulation of the HPA.[16]

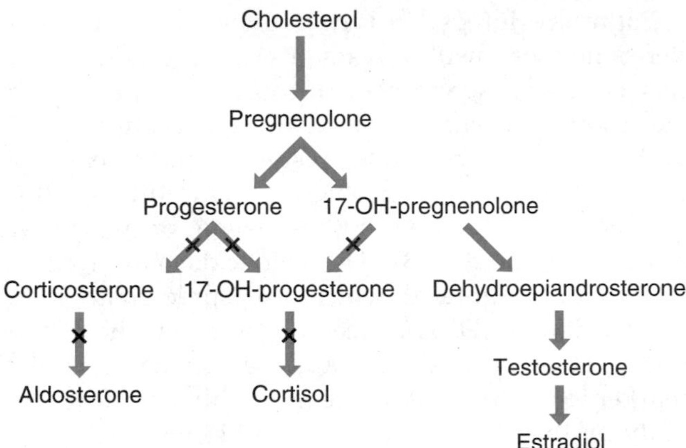

FIGURE 29–9
Androgen excess in 21-hydroxylase deficiency. Blockade of the enzymatic pathways leading to synthesis of mineralocorticoids and glucocorticoids diverts more substrate to androgen production.

Pathophysiology. Figure 29–9 illustrates the metabolic alterations induced by 21-hydroxylase deficiency. Blockade of mineralocorticoid and glucocorticoid synthesis diverts more substrate into androgen production. Lack of negative feedback to the HPA leads to ACTH excess and adrenal hyperplasia.

In glucocorticoid resistance syndromes, all adrenocortical hormones are present in excess. Because cells are resistant to cortisol effects, however, clinical manifestations are primarily those of androgen excess and, to a lesser degree, hyperaldosteronism.

Clinical Manifestations. Although manifestations vary depending on degree of enzyme deficiency, lack of mineralocorticoid may produce salt wasting, manifested as hyponatremia, hyperkalemia, and hypotension. Clinical signs become apparent soon after birth. Androgen excess is detectable in female infants as virilization, with some degree of ambiguity of the genitalia (Fig. 29–10). The clitoris is enlarged, and the labia may be fused. The condition may go undetected in males unless signs of salt wasting are evident. Lack of cortisol (or cortisol effect, in resistance syndromes) is manifested as decreased resistance to stress and infection and may not be apparent until the child contracts an intercurrent illness. Nonclassic CAH may manifest at the time of puberty in females, and hirsutism and menstrual abnormalities are commonly seen.

Prevention and Treatment. Genetic counseling may be indicated in those with a positive family history. Oral dexamethasone may be given to pregnant women who are carrying a female fetus at risk for the disorder.[15] Routine newborn screening for CAH is done in some states. Prevention of severe hypotension and shock due to salt wasting requires early diagnosis and intervention. CAH is treated with lifelong replacement of cortisol and mineralocorticoids and with surgical correction of abnormalities of the sexual organs.

Prognosis and Outcome. With early diagnosis and hormone replacement, metabolic abnormalities are usually successfully managed. If untreated, 21-hydroxylase deficiency results in advancement of bone age (see Chapter 27). Adult stature is short, however, because of early epiphyseal closure. Psychosocial factors significantly affect outcome if sexual ambiguity is present, and early detection and surgical intervention promote a positive outcome.

Diabetes Mellitus

Definition. Diabetes mellitus is a metabolic disorder characterized by **hyperglycemia** (elevated serum glucose) resulting from lack of insulin, lack of insulin effect, or both. Three general classifications are recognized: (1) type 1, formerly known as insulin-dependent or juvenile-onset diabetes, (2) type 2, formerly known as noninsulin-dependent or maturity-onset diabetes, and (3) gestational diabetes (diabetes that emerges during pregnancy).

Epidemiology. More than 6% of all adults in the United States have diabetes,[17] and 90% of cases are type 2. About half of people with type 2 diabetes are never diagnosed. A genetic predisposition (specific HLA subtype) is known to impose risk in type 1 disease, and family history is an even stronger risk factor in type 2 diabetes. People of northern European descent are at highest risk for type 1 disease, which most frequently manifests in children and

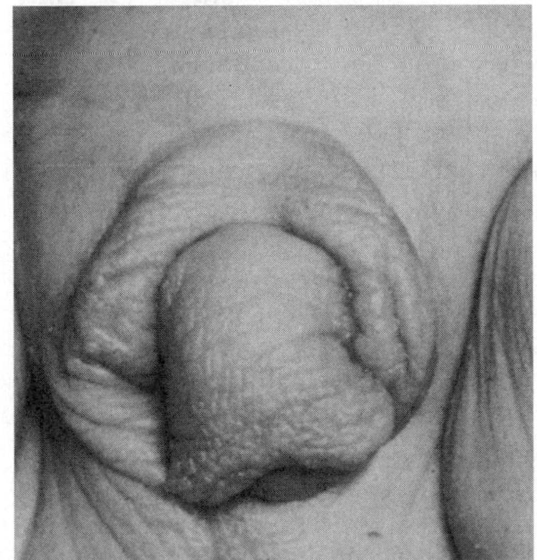

FIGURE 29–10
Ambiguous female genitalia in congential adrenal hyperplasia. Note that the clitoris is enlarged, simulating a penis, and the labia are partially fused to form a scrotum-like structure. (From Moore, K.L., and Persaud, T.V.N. [1993]. *Before We Are Born*. Philadelphia: W.B. Saunders. [p. 222].)

young adults. Both major forms of diabetes are prevalent among Hispanics, blacks, and some Native American populations. Aging and obesity are significant risk factors in type 2 diabetes.

Disorders that predispose to diabetes include Cushing's syndrome, pancreatitis and pancreatic cancer (see Chapter 25), and acromegaly (see Chapter 27). Pregnancy increases the risk of diabetes in women who have baseline impaired glucose tolerance, manifested as inadequate insulin secretion in response to ingestion of a measured glucose load. Many of these women have a history of obesity and evidence of insulin resistance.

Etiology

Type 1 Diabetes Mellitus. Type 1 diabetes results from a chronic autoimmune process that usually exists in a preclinical phase for years before the onset of clinical manifestations. Two major hypotheses have been advanced regarding the initiation of the autoimmune response: (1) infection with a virus that has an amino acid sequence similar to that of a β-cell protein, and (2) an environmental insult that generates inflammatory mediators that induce the expression of adhesion molecules in the vascular endothelium of the pancreatic islets.[18]

Type 2 Diabetes Mellitus. In type 2 diabetes, insulin resistance and genetically programmed β-cell dysfunction probably interact to cause diabetes in vulnerable patients. Insulin resistance, which is often related to visceral obesity, is initially overcome by increased secretion of insulin. Insulin resistance progresses to hyperglycemia and clinical diabetes mellitus when β-cell secretion of insulin can no longer compensate for insulin resistance.[19] The elevation in circulating glucose is believed to contribute to β-cell dysfunction, although the precise mechanism of this "glucose toxicity" is unknown.

Destruction of islet cells by pancreatitis or pancreatic cancer may produce insulin deficiency that is sufficient to cause diabetes in some people. Cortisol excess in Cushing's syndrome may elevate serum glucose to the point at which a relative lack of insulin is created, and growth hormone excess in acromegaly may inhibit insulin activity.

Gestational Diabetes Mellitus. Many of the hormones of pregnancy mediate increased glucose mobilization to supply the growing fetus. Hormones with diabetogenic potential include luteinizing hormone, human chorionic gonadotropin, estrogen, cortisol, progesterone, prolactin, and human chorionic somatomammotropin.[20] In an estimated 1% to 3% of pregnant women, diabetes mellitus results from the unmasking of insulin resistance or a pre-existing defect in insulin secretion. Gestational diabetes is discussed in detail in Chapter 32.

Pathophysiology. In type 1 diabetes, the absolute deficiency of insulin leads to hyperglycemia, enhanced lipolysis, and protein catabolism. Ketosis, the elevation of acetoacetic acid, β-hydroxybutyric acid, and acetone in the blood, results from increased β-oxidation of lipids for energy, with the resulting production of ketone bodies, some of which are acidic (see Chapter 3). The ketoacids may accumulate to the degree at which they precipitate metabolic acidosis (DKA). Acetone, a nonacidic ketone body, is also produced and serves as a clinical marker of ketosis. Acetone is eliminated from the body by the respiratory tract and kidneys.

Patients with type 2 diabetes usually produce enough insulin to suppress lipolysis and protein catabolism. As previously discussed, the presence of insulin resistance may contribute to the development of disorders associated with syndrome X.

In all forms of diabetes, hyperglycemia increases serum osmolarity, and increased renal filtration of glucose leads to osmotic diuresis when the renal glucose reabsorption threshold is exceeded. Increased glucose in intraocular fluid may cause altered light refraction and blurred vision. Infection risk is enhanced by the presence of increased serum glucose, which may provides a rich medium for organism growth and which also impairs neutrophil chemotaxis in the inflammatory response.

Chronically elevated blood glucose is known to contribute to long-term vascular and neural complications of diabetes, although the precise mechanism is unknown. Three mechanisms are postulated: (1) nonenzymatic binding of glucose to structural and regulatory proteins (glycosylation or glycation); (2) intracellular accumulation of sugar alcohols, such as sorbitol, produced by a secondary (aldose reductase) pathway of glucose metabolism; and (3) alteration in the function of protein kinase C, an enzyme important to intracellular signal transduction pathways.[21]

In tissues such as blood vessels and nerves, which do not require insulin for glucose uptake, elevated intracellular levels of glucose and its metabolites may lead to glycosylation of proteins, impairing their function. In the microcirculation, glycosylation of hemoglobin shifts the oxyhemoglobin dissociation curve to the left, decreasing oxygen release to tissues (see Chapter 19). Intracellular metabolism of glucose is typically altered as well. The enzyme aldose reductase catalyzes the reduction of glucose to sorbitol, which inhibits Na^+-K^+-ATPase activity in retinal, neural, and renal tissues. Sorbitol accumulation in the lenses of the eyes may contribute to cataract formation. Alteration of protein kinase C activity may manifest as impaired contractility of vascular smooth muscle or as increased permeability of vascular endothelial cells.

Clinical Manifestations. The clinical manifestations of diabetes may be considered to represent one of three aspects of the pathophysiology: onset, acute complications, or chronic complications.

Clinical Signs of Diabetes Onset. Type 1 diabetes demonstrates a relatively rapid onset of clinical manifestations, whereas the onset of type 2 diabetes is usually more gradual. Onset is typically marked by the presence of the classic "three Ps": polyuria (frequent urination), polydipsia (thirst), and polyphagia (hunger). Dehydration, hyponatremia, weight loss, blurred vision, fatigue, and weakness may occur secondary to hyperglycemia and impaired energy metabolism. Laboratory evidence of hyperglycemia is present (Table 29–6). In type 1 diabetes, islet cell antibodies are usually demonstrated in the serum. Insulin levels are low or, more commonly, undetectable. Polyphagia and weight loss are less evident in type 2 diabetes, and insulin levels may be normal or elevated. (Reduction in circulating insulin levels usually occurs late in type 2 diabetes.)

Acute Complications. The acute complications of diabetes include DKA and **hyperosmolar nonketotic state**, two decompensation syndromes resulting from extreme hyperglycemia. A third complication, hypoglycemia, demonstrates the opposite extreme.

Some patients demonstrate DKA as a presenting sign of diabetes, but this syndrome is more often encountered in patients known to have type 1 diabetes who are poorly compliant with insulin therapy or who experience an intercurrent illness, trauma, or other stressor. In DKA, which may develop in 1 or 2 days, the patient's level of consciousness is gradually impaired by acidosis until, if untreated, the patient goes into *diabetic coma*. Fasting serum glucose is elevated well above the normal range of about 80 mg/dL, possibly approaching 1000 mg/dL. Serum ketones are also elevated, and clinical signs are of hypovolemia and shock due to osmotic diuresis. High anion gap metabolic acidosis, due to accumulation of organic ketoacids, is accompanied by potassium imbalance (see Chapter 10). Potassium may be elevated initially as a consequence of cellular shifts and renal exchange for hydrogen in acidosis but is eventually decreased as a consequence of osmotic diuresis. An acetone (fruity) odor to the breath is apparent.

A significant percentage of patients with DKA have abdominal pain, possibly due to disinhibition of prostaglandin production in adipose tissue in the insulin-deficient state.[22] Patients are usually warm and flushed despite their hypovolemic state, and this finding has also been attributed to altered prostaglandin synthesis. Most patients demonstrate rapid

TABLE 29–6
LABORATORY EVIDENCE OF ALTERED GLUCOSE HOMEOSTASIS

Test	Normal Value	Comments
Fasting plasma glucose (FPG)	80–115 mg/dL*	Low values indicate hypoglycemia; values of ≥126 mg/dL on two separate occasions confirm diagnosis of diabetes mellitus. Values exceed 250 mg/dL in diabetic ketoacidosis and usually exceed 400 mg/dL in the hyperosmolar nonketotic state.
Postprandial oral glucose tolerance test (OGTT)	<140 mg/dL	May be used after an abnormally high fasting plasma glucose to diagnose diabetes in patients without symptoms. A measured dose of glucose is given after a fast, followed by serum glucose testing after 2 h. Values between 140 and 200 mg/dL indicate impaired glucose tolerance; values of >200 mg/dL indicate diabetes mellitus.
Glycosylated hemoglobin (HbA_{1c})	<6%	High values indicate persistent hyperglycemia during previous 2–3 mo.
C-peptide suppression test	C-peptide of <1.2 ng/mL when glucose is 40 mg/dL or less	High values indicate an insulin-producing tumor (insulinoma).
Serum insulin	2–25 μU/mL	High values indicate insulin resistance or insulinoma. Undetectable levels indicate type 1 diabetes mellitus.
Serum glucagon	<250 pg/mL	Very high values indicate glucagon-producing tumor (glucagonoma). Values may be low in idiopathic glucagon deficiency or pancreatitis.

*To convert mg/dL to mmol/L, multiply by 0.05551.

FPG and OGTT values confirming diagnosis from the Report of the Expert Committee on the Diagnosis and Classification of Diabetes Care, American Diabetes Association, 1997.

breathing (tachypnea), and Kussmaul's respirations (deep, gasping ventilation or air hunger) may be present in respiratory compensation for metabolic acidosis (see Chapter 10). When the serum pH falls below 7.0, respirations are typically shallow.[22] DKA is rare in patients with type 2 diabetes, presumably because these patients have enough circulating insulin to suppress lipolysis and ketosis.

The hyperosmolar nonketotic state, usually seen in elderly patients with type 2 diabetes, resembles DKA in that the patient is severely dehydrated, owing to osmotic diuresis. This syndrome evolves gradually over days to weeks, however, and is characterized by absence of ketosis. If acidosis is present, it is not DKA but rather lactic acidosis secondary to hypovolemia and decreased tissue perfusion (see Chapter 10).

Clinical signs of the hyperosmolar nonketotic state are similar to those of DKA except that acidosis and Kussmaul's respirations are uncommon and there is no fruity acetone odor to the breath. Serum glucose levels may rise to a greater degree than in DKA, possibly as high as 2000 mg/dL.[23]

Hypoglycemia, the third acute complication of diabetes, is now seen much more frequently in diabetic patients as a consequence of intensive therapy aimed at achievement of tighter glucose control. Hypoglycemia is discussed in detail later in this chapter.

Chronic Complications. Chronic complications of both type 1 and type 2 diabetes manifest as damage to tissues that are freely permeable to glucose: the retinas (**retinopathy**), kidneys (**nephropathy**), and nerves (**neuropathy**). Damage to small-diameter vessels (**microvascular disease**) accounts for the manifestations of retinopathy and nephropathy and, along with metabolic derangement, may play a role in neuropathy. Disorders of larger blood vessels (**macrovascular disease**) may manifest as coronary heart disease, cerebrovascular disease, or peripheral vascular disease. Insulin resistance, hyperinsulinemia, hypertension, visceral obesity, and impaired fibrinolysis, which may also contribute to macrovascular disorders, cause more problems in patients with type 2 diabetes.

The general syndrome of retinopathy is discussed in Chapter 23 (see also Color Fig. 23–4). Some degree of retinopathy is found in nearly all patients with type 1 diabetes and in more than 60% of those with type 2 diabetes within 20 years of diagnosis.[24] Diabetic retinopathy is classified as *nonproliferative* or *proliferative*. Nonproliferative (background) retinopathy initially manifests as microaneurysms and increased permeability of retinal capillaries, leading to retinal edema, fluid exudation, and leaking of blood ("dot-and-blot" hemorrhages). Retinal veins may become twisted and may demonstrate variable lumen sizes ("beading"). Occlusion of some retinal capillaries ("capillary dropout") may promote visual loss if it occurs near the macula, the area of the most acute central vision. Proliferative retinopathy occurs later in the disease and is characterized primarily by ischemia-induced growth of new vessels and proliferation of preretinal fibrous tissue. Contraction of this fibrous tissue may cause hemorrhage into the vitreous humor or retinal detachment.

Diabetic nephropathy manifests as nodular lesions and thickening of the glomerular basement membrane (Kimmelstiel-Wilson syndrome). Glomerular foot processes are blunted and surface proteins lose their capacity to repel plasma proteins. Mesangial tissue proliferates, encroaching on the glomerular capillary wall to decrease the available surface area for filtration (see Chapter 20). Intraglomerular pressure is markedly elevated due to: (1) dilation of the afferent arteriole, which increases renal blood flow, and (2) increased responsiveness of the efferent arteriole to endogenous vasoconstrictors, such as angiotensin II and endothelin. Concurrent presence of hypertension speeds the progression of nephropathy. Loss of protein in the urine (microalbuminuria) is common early in diabetic nephropathy, with eventual chronic renal failure occurring in about 35% of all patients with diabetes.[25]

Diabetic neuropathy results from neural hypoxia and demyelination secondary to microvascular disease and to hyperglycemia-induced metabolic derangement. Neuropathy most commonly affects peripheral sensory and motor nerves, although isolated motor neuropathy and autonomic neuropathy may also occur. Loss of peripheral sensation may contribute to *diabetic foot disease* because the patient may be unaware of injury to the foot due to normal wear and tear, hot bath water, or ill-fitting footwear. Ischemic ulcers of the feet may result from impaired perfusion due to peripheral vascular disease, and infection is enhanced by hyperglycemia. Peripheral sensorimotor neuropathy may also manifest as paresthesias, decreased deep tendon reflexes, or muscle weakness, whereas autonomic neuropathy may cause postural hypotension, decreased gastrointestinal motility (*diabetic gastroparesis*), decreased bladder tone, and erectile dysfunction. The general syndrome of peripheral neuropathy is discussed in Chapter 23.

Microvascular disease in diabetes contributes to hypertension, which worsens nephropathy and retinopathy and promotes macrovascular disease. In diabetic patients, larger vessels become atherosclerotic earlier, and atherosclerosis progresses more rapidly, owing to hypertension, possible glycosylation of vessel proteins, and dyslipidemia resulting from insulin resistance. Atherosclerosis is detailed in Chapter 15.

Prevention and Treatment

Prevention. Prevention of type 1 diabetes may be possible in the near future. Immune markers (islet cell antibodies) are present in the serum of patients long before they develop insulin deficiency, and research is ongoing to develop immunotherapy that may prevent or interrupt the autoimmune process.[18] People at risk for diabetes because of family history or visceral obesity should be closely monitored for the development of insulin resistance or abnormal glucose tolerance. Dietary and exercise interventions are warranted in treatment of obesity, and pharmacologic treatment may be used in some cases (see Chapter 25).

Glycemic Control. Prevention of acute and chronic complications depends on tight control of serum glucose. Glucose control in type 1 diabetes requires the administration of insulin, augmented with diet and exercise. Insulin is usually required in gestational diabetes as well. Type 2 diabetes may be treated with diet and exercise alone, with oral hypoglycemic agents, or with insulin. Table 29–7 describes the forms of insulin in common use. A longer-acting insulin is used to simulate the normal basal secretion of insulin, and a short-acting insulin is used to mimic postprandial peaks (i.e., increases in insulin secretion stimulated by increased blood glucose after eating). Intensive therapy mandates frequent injection of insulin (at least four injections each day or continuous subcutaneous infusion by an insulin pump), with the dosage determined by concurrent testing of blood glucose.

Because the mechanisms of action of the oral agents used in the treatment of type 2 diabetes are varied, these agents might be used in combination (Table 29–8). When oral agents are insufficient to maintain normoglycemia in type 2 diabetes, insulin may be added to the regimen. Often, high insulin doses may be required to overcome insulin resistance.

The ideal diabetic diet is a matter of some controversy, and may differ depending on the needs of individual patients. The American Diabetes Association has revised its dietary recommendations to permit the consumption of modest amounts of simple sugars, as long as adequate control of serum glucose can be maintained.[26] In general, dietary recommendations for people with diabetes are the same as those advocated for prevention of or intervention in dyslipidemia (see Chapter 25). Increased dietary fiber and decreased dietary fat, particularly saturated and *trans*-polyunsaturated fats, are recommended. Obese patients clearly benefit from caloric restriction. Whether the nonprotein calories in the diabetic diet should come primarily from increased complex carbohydrates (as is usually advocated) or from unsaturated fats is uncertain. A recent study has demonstrated a detrimental effect on glucose control as well as an elevation of very-low-density lipoprotein cholesterol with the former approach.[27]

Moderate, consistent exercise promotes weight control and circulatory function and enhances glucose uptake by muscle, reducing the need for insulin. Beneficial effects of exercise are detailed in Chapter 35.

Pancreatic transplantation has been used in selected cases since 1983. Islet cell transplantation, from fetal tissue or from living donors, is in limited experimental use.[28]

Management of Acute Complications. DKA is treated with fluid resuscitation, intravenous insulin, and potassium replacement. The hyperosmolar nonketotic state is treated supportively with fluid and electrolyte replacement in addition to treatment of the precipitating condition. Insulin replacement, if necessary, is usually by continuous low-dose infusion. Hypoglycemia is treated with glucose replacement, as detailed subsequently.

Management of Chronic Complications. The pro-

TABLE 29–7
FORMS OF EXOGENOUS HUMAN INSULIN

Category	Examples	Peak Action (h)	Duration of Action (h)
Short-acting	Lispro	0.5–1.5	2–4
	Regular	2–3	3–6
Intermediate-acting	NPH	4–10	10–16
	Lente	4–12	12–18
Long-acting	Ultralente	None	18–20

Adapted from Black, J.M., and Matassarin-Jacobs, E. (1997). *Medical-Surgical Nursing: Clinical Management for Continuity of Care.* (5th ed.). Philadelphia: W.B. Saunders. (p. 1969).

TABLE 29–8
ORAL HYPOGLYCEMIC AGENTS

Category	Examples	Duration of Action (h)	Mechanism of Action
Sulfonylureas	First generation		Stimulates insulin secretion from pancreas
	Tolbutamide (Orinase)	6–12	
	Chlorpropamide (Diabinese)	60	
	Tolazamide (Tolinase)	12–24	
	Second generation		
	Glipizide (Glucotrol)	16–24	
	Glyburide (DiaBeta, Micronase, Glynase)	18–24	
	Glimepiride (Amaryl)	24	
Biguanides	Metformin (Glucophage)	12	Decreases hepatic glucose production; enhances peripheral glucose uptake; decreases intestinal absorption of glucose
	Precose (Acarbose)	4–6	Slows carbohydrate digestion and glucose absorption
Thiazolidinediones	Troglitazone (Rezulin)	—	Directly improves action of insulin in liver, skeletal muscle, and adipose tissue

gression of nonproliferative diabetic retinopathy may be slowed by tight glucose control. Patients should be screened frequently to detect retinal changes as early as possible. Antiplatelet agents, such as aspirin and dipyridamole (Persantine), may reduce the number of microaneurysms.[29] Use of photocoagulation by argon laser or xenon arc light has been shown to reduce visual loss in patients with proliferative retinopathy and macular edema. Vitrectomy, in which vitreous humor is removed and replaced with a physiologic solution to maintain intraocular pressure, may be beneficial in patients with vitreous hemorrhage or traction on the retina.

Diabetic nephropathy is also lessened with tight glucose control, and the use of angiotensin-converting enzyme inhibitors such as enalapril (Vasotec) at the first sign of microalbuminuria has been shown to slow its progression. These agents not only decrease intraglomerular pressure but also help to manage the systemic hypertension that is frequently present.[30] Restriction of dietary protein and avoidance of nephrotoxic agents is also warranted. End-stage chronic renal failure may be treated conservatively, with dialysis, or with renal transplantation (see Chapter 20).

The incidence of diabetic neuropathy may be significantly reduced with intensive management of serum glucose. Treatment of neuropathy is supportive and symptomatic. Pain may be managed with topical capsaicin or antidepressant drugs[29] (see Chapter 23). The use of nonsteroidal anti-inflammatory drugs should be avoided because of the risk of nephrotoxicity. Diabetic gastroparesis may be treated with metoclopramide (Reglan), which enhances gastrointestinal motility. Gastroparesis and other autonomic manifestations are frequently resistant to treatment, however. Meticulous foot care is warranted to reduce the risk of diabetic foot disease. In severe cases, however, amputation of toes, or even the lower limb, may be necessitated by ischemic necrosis.

Prognosis and Outcome. The large Diabetes Control and Complications Trial, completed in 1993, demonstrated that intensive therapy achieves tighter glucose control and significantly reduces the chronic complications of type 1 diabetes.[31] In this study, the risk of progression of retinopathy was reduced by 50%, the risk of nephropathy was reduced by 43%, and the risk of neuropathy was reduced by 60%. However, target goals for serum glucose and glycosylated hemoglobin (Hb A_{1c}) were not achieved with either intensive or conventional therapy, weight gain was enhanced, and the risk for hypoglycemia was increased two- to three-fold with intensive treatment. Large studies are underway to determine whether the study findings may be applied to treatment of type 2 diabetes as well.[32] The complication of weight gain, which may exacerbate insulin resistance, might prove detrimental to many with this form of diabetes.

Diabetes mellitus is a contributor to at least 7% of

all deaths in the United States, primarily owing to its association with coronary heart disease.[1] The incidence of diabetes (particularly type 2) has been increasing steadily. Morbidity is also high, and the health care costs related to diabetes and its complications have been estimated at greater than $92 billion per year.

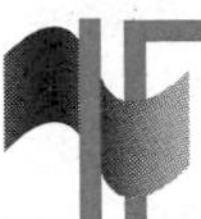

Clinical Scenario

C.K., a 67-year-old widow, suffers from diabetes mellitus, asthma, and rheumatoid arthritis. C.K. lives alone in a subsidized housing unit for senior citizens. During a monthly home visit, the community health checks C.K.'s blood glucose level and finds it to be 259 mg/dL. C.K. reports that she has "not been feeling well." Her daily medications include a nonsteroidal anti-inflammatory drug for her arthritis, an inhaled bronchodilator for her asthma, the oral hypoglycemic agent glipizide (Glucotrol), and Humulin N insulin, 40 units each morning and 34 units each evening.

1. What type of diabetes does C.K. have? For what complications is she at risk?
2. Would C.K. be likely to benefit from more intensive therapy of her diabetes? What measures might be taken?
3. What obstacles to optimal outcomes are evident in this situation?

Hypoglycemia

Definition. Hypoglycemia is the syndrome resulting from serum glucose levels below 60 mg/dL.

Epidemiology. Hypoglycemia is the most common endocrine medical emergency.[33] Many conditions either cause or predispose to hypoglycemia (Table 29–9). The most common cause is the excessive administration of insulin in treatment of diabetes, and the risk of hypoglycemic episodes ("insulin reactions") is increased with intensive therapy, as has been discussed. Stress or illness, as well as alterations in diet or exercise regimen, may promote hypoglycemia in diabetics. Hypoglycemic disorders are uncommon in nondiabetic patients but may be triggered by a number of drugs and underlying disorders.

Elderly people with long-standing diabetes are at particular risk of hypoglycemia because they frequently have diminished awareness of hypoglycemic symptoms. Decreased sensory and autonomic function associated with aging and neuropathy may contribute to more severe hypoglycemia in these patients (see Developmental Perspective). Use of alcohol may also contribute to decreased awareness of symptoms, leading to more severe episodes of hypoglycemia.

TABLE 29–9
CONDITIONS ASSOCIATED WITH HYPOGLYCEMIA

ETIOLOGY	EXAMPLES
Insulin-producing tumor	Insulinoma
Elevated levels of insulin-like growth factor II	Non–β-cell tumor
Cortisol deficiency	Adrenal insufficiency
Abnormal hepatic response to glucagon	Glycogen storage disease
Systemic disease	Sepsis Congestive heart failure Shock Malnutrition Hepatic failure Renal failure Autoimmune disease
Iatrogenic	Excess or inappropriate administration of insulin in treatment of diabetes Abrupt termination of glucocorticoid therapy Drug-induced (e.g., ethanol, salicylates, quinine, haloperidol, disopyramide)

Data from Service, F.J. (1995). Hypoglycemic disorders. *New England Journal of Medicine* 332(17), 1144–1152.

Etiology. Hypoglycemia results from excess insulin (or insulin-like activity) or from impaired counter-regulation.

Pathophysiology. Glucose homeostasis is disrupted by insufficient glucose counter-regulation, that is, by relatively inadequate activity of glucagon and epinephrine in the presence of declining serum glucose levels. Deficiencies of cortisol or growth hormone apparently do not play a significant role in hypoglycemia.[34] Lack of glucose in cells of the central nervous system results in defective central nervous system function (*neuroglycopenic symptoms*) and triggers the stress response (*autonomic symptoms*).

Clinical Manifestations. Neuroglycopenic symptoms include hunger, blurred vision, drowsiness, weakness, shaking, dizziness, confusion, difficulty speaking, and headache. In severe hypoglycemia, coma and seizures may be present. Autonomic manifestations include palpitations, nervousness, anxiety, and sweating. (NOTE: The syndrome once referred

Developmental Perspective

Embryonic and Fetal Periods

Unlike the adrenal medulla, which develops from the neuroectoderm, the adrenal cortex develops from the mesodermal germ layer. The adrenal cortex is first detectable during the sixth week of gestation and grows rapidly, equaling the kidneys in size by mid-gestation. The fetal cortex secretes large quantities of adrenal androgens and preferentially converts progesterone to corticosteroids. The fetal pancreas appears at about 5 weeks' gestation. Insulin, which acts as a fetal growth hormone, is present in fetal islet cells at about 9 weeks' gestation. Glucagon is produced by 15 weeks. Fetal liver and other tissues have proportionately more receptors for insulin than glucagon, thus promoting anabolic processes rather than catabolism. Acute changes in maternal glucose levels do not significantly affect fetal secretion of insulin or glucagon, but chronic maternal hyperglycemia (e.g., diabetes mellitus) increases fetal insulin secretion, depresses glucagon secretion, and leads to macrosomia. Chronic maternal malnutrition has the opposite effect. Inadequate nutrition during fetal life and early infancy may lead to inadequate development of islet cells, increasing the risk of diabetes mellitus later in life.

Infancy and Childhood

Preterm infants have diminished ability to secrete cortisol in response to stress, and this deficiency may contribute to chronic lung disease. The adrenal glands continue to secrete androgens during the first year of life, but the glands involute, or decrease in size, during this period. At about 6 to 8 years of age, the zona reticularis again becomes active, and this developmental event has been termed *adrenarche*. Excess weight, early acne, hirsutism, or precocious puberty during childhood may signify abnormality of adrenocortical function. Removal of the maternal glucose source at birth results in glycogenolysis and mobilization of fat stores. Gluconeogenic enzymes develop soon after birth, and regulation of metabolism approaches adult patterns. Neonatal diabetes mellitus is a rare disorder that may be transient or permanent. Because of ongoing brain development, young children have proportionately higher requirements for glucose and are thus at higher risk of adverse consequences of hypoglycemia. A number of inborn errors of metabolism, including glycogen storage diseases and mitochondrial defects, may result in abnormal glucose homeostasis. Children with cystic fibrosis have a higher prevalence of diabetes mellitus. Onset of type 1 diabetes

---

to as *functional* or *reactive* hypoglycemia and manifested only by autonomic symptoms after the ingestion of food is no longer considered to be a true hypoglycemia.[34])

Prevention and Treatment. Iatrogenic hypoglycemia is preventable with careful monitoring of serum glucose and management of diabetes therapy, diet, and exercise. Treatment of acute episodes consists of glucose administration, with the route depending on the patient's level of consciousness. Glucagon may also be administered to evaluate the plasma glucose response, serving both diagnostic and therapeutic purposes. Drug therapy contributing to the condition is discontinued, and underlying disorders are managed appropriately.

Prognosis and Outcome. Hypoglycemia that is promptly recognized and treated is not associated with adverse outcomes in most cases. Recurrent episodes of severe hypoglycemia in children may increase the risk of cognitive impairment.[33] The elderly may be at higher risk of injury related to falls. Seizures impose risk of musculoskeletal injuries and aspiration (see Chapter 21).

CLINICAL SIGNIFICANCE OF ADRENOCORTICAL AND PANCREATIC ENDOCRINE DISORDERS

Adrenocortical disorders are relatively uncommon but are clinically important in view of the systemic effects of cortisol and aldosterone on the stress response, inflammation, energy metabolism, and fluid and electrolyte homeostasis. Indiscriminate administration of steroids for their anti-inflammatory effects is of concern because of the concomitant effects on metabolism. Clinical research has shown little or no benefit (and sometimes adverse effects) of steroid therapy in a number of conditions (see Focus of

in childhood is common, whereas childhood onset of type 2 diabetes is rare. Inadequate nutrition during early childhood may limit adipocyte development and promote hypertrophy of visceral adipocytes later in life. This pattern of obesity is associated with insulin resistance. The hyperosmolar nonketotic state occurs rarely in childhood and is usually due to dehydrating conditions such as diarrhea rather than to diabetes.

Adolescence and Young Adulthood

Adrenal androgen production peaks at puberty and then progressively declines. Type 1 diabetes mellitus usually has its onset during adolescence or young adulthood. Despite the challenges imposed by physiologic and psychosocial changes, adolescents with type 1 diabetes benefit from intensive therapy to the same extent as adults. Intensive therapy of diabetes increases body mass index in adolescents but does not affect linear growth. Greater irregularities in diet and exercise occur in younger people with diabetes, and these impose higher risk of hypoglycemic episodes. The hormones of pregnancy induce maternal insulin resistance and may precipitate gestational diabetes mellitus in childbearing women who cannot mount a compensatory increase in insulin secretion. The associations among obesity, insulin resistance, and dyslipidemia are evident during adolescence and young adulthood.

Middle and Older Adulthood

Aging, per se, does not alter serum adrenal hormone levels or function of the hypothalamic–pituitary–adrenal axis. There are differences among individual patients, however, and those who have had more lifetime cumulative exposure to episodes of stress may demonstrate more prolonged cortisol exposure after challenge. Type 2 diabetes mellitus typically presents in middle or older age, although the underlying insulin resistance and β-cell dysfunction are usually present for decades before the disease becomes clinically evident. Weight gain and sedentary lifestyle may accompany aging, and these factors contribute to higher risk of type 2 diabetes. Elderly people with diabetes are particularly prone to diabetic foot disease, infections, and poor wound healing. Diminished awareness of neuroglycopenic and autonomic symptoms in older people with diabetes increases the frequency and severity of hypoglycemic episodes.

Current Research). The complexity of the relationships between mediators of the hypothalamic–pituitary–adrenal axis and immune function is becoming increasingly apparent, and the importance of peripheral production of these mediators remains to be clarified. In addition, the neuroendocrine interactions that regulate local inflammation and the generalized stress response associated with disorders of all body systems warrant continued investigation through basic research.

The impact of diabetes mellitus on the health of people of all ages cannot be overstated. Diabetes is the most prevalent chronic disease of childhood, and its incidence rises throughout the life span (see Developmental Perspective). The contribution of diabetes to morbidity of multiple systems and to mortality from cardiovascular and renal diseases is clear. The cost of these diseases, in terms of both human impact and stress on the health care system, is staggering. Significant progress has been made in clarifying the genetic basis of diabetic predisposition as well as the environmental factors that promote the development of diabetes. The Diabetes Control and Complications Trial has provided new evidence of the efficacy of intensive treatment of type 1 diabetes, and research is ongoing in an effort to document the most effective approaches to management of type 2 diabetes, the most common form. Many clinicians and investigators believe that a cure for diabetes is on the horizon.

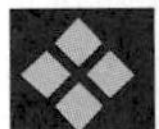

Summary of Key Points

- Maintenance of glucose homeostasis during basal metabolism and during stressed states depends on the complex interplay among the effects of insulin and glucagon produced by the pancreatic islets of Langerhans and on the anabolic and catabolic effects of numerous other hormones, particularly the adrenal hormones (cortisol and the catecholamines), growth hormone, and thyroid hormones.

Summary continued on following page

- Each zone of the adrenal cortex produces different hormones. The outer zona glomerulosa secretes aldosterone and other mineralocorticoids, whereas the inner zona reticularis and zona fasciculata produce the glucocorticoids (e.g., cortisol) and the gonadocorticoids (e.g., adrenal androgens).

- The adrenal mineralocorticoids are so named because they exert their effects on minerals. Aldosterone, for example, stimulates sodium reabsorption and potassium secretion in the distal nephron. Cortisol and other glucocorticoids act primarily on glucose, mobilizing the body's energy stores by promoting lipolysis and proteolysis and thus antagonizing the anabolic effects of insulin. The glucocorticoids also exert an anti-inflammatory effect. The gonadocorticoids (adrenal androgens) are normally of minor importance in promotion of sexual characteristics but may become clinically important in states of excess.

- Insulin resistance, a state of decreased cellular sensitivity to insulin despite normal or increased circulating levels, underlies the most prevalent form of diabetes (type 2 diabetes mellitus). The precise molecular mechanism of this phenomenon is unknown, but both genetic and environmental factors are believed to play a role. Insulin resistance is associated with visceral obesity in many people and also contributes to hypertension, dyslipidemia, and other syndrome X disorders, which greatly increase the risk of coronary heart disease, stroke, and peripheral vascular disease.

- Primary disorders of adrenal hypofunction or hyperfunction are rare. Hypofunction of the adrenal cortex is usually due to chronic autoimmune destruction of the gland (e.g., Addison's disease). Destructive tumors may induce hypofunction, whereas functional tumors (of the adrenal gland, the pituitary, or the hypothalamus) may result in hyperfunction syndromes such as Cushing's disease or primary aldosteronism. Ectopic production of these hormones is rare. Iatrogenic Cushing's syndrome, due to exogenous administration of cortisol, is common. Congenital adrenal hyperplasia results from deficiency of an enzyme, usually within the synthetic pathway for cortisol and aldosterone. Lack of cortisol results in reduction of negative feedback inhibition to the hypothalamic–pituitary–adrenal axis. Overstimulation of the gland then yields hyperplasia and excess of the adrenal androgens.

- Type 1 diabetes mellitus is due to an absolute lack of insulin resulting from autoimmune destruction of the β cells of the islets of Langerhans. Type 2 diabetes is a result of lack of insulin effect, initially due to insulin resistance, but later due to lack of insulin secretion as well. Clinical manifestations of the two types are similar in that hyperglycemia induces osmotic diuresis and predisposes to the development of long-term complications (e.g., retinopathy, nephropathy, and neuropathy) within tissues that are freely permeable to glucose. Patients with type 1 diabetes are dependent on insulin for life, and their absolute lack of insulin places them at risk for DKA due to increased lipolysis and β-oxidation of lipids for energy. Type 2 diabetic patients may have low, normal, or high levels of circulating insulin, but usually have enough to suppress lipolysis. Macrovascular disease (e.g., coronary heart disease) is more prevalent in type 2 diabetes because other risk factors associated with insulin resistance may independently promote damage to larger vessels.

- Tight control of serum glucose has been shown to reduce greatly the incidence of morbidity due to chronic complications of diabetes. Patients with type 1 diabetes require insulin therapy aimed at reproducing normal baseline insulin secretion as well as postprandial peaks. Intensive treatment of type 1 diabetes involves self-monitoring of serum glucose at least four times a day, with adjustment of insulin dosage based on the results. Treatment of type 2 diabetes is aimed at glycemic control and reduction of insulin resistance. This type may respond to diet and exercise alone, to oral hypoglycemic agents, or to insulin therapy. Normalization of weight, particularly in patients with visceral obesity, is a worthy goal but is difficult to achieve. Exercise promotes weight reduction as well as non–insulin-mediated glucose uptake by muscle cells. Oral agents are varied in their mechanisms of action. The newest agent, troglitazone, is believed to enhance cellular sensitivity to insulin. Many type 2 diabetic patients require high doses of insulin to overcome insulin resistance.

Summary continued on following page

◆ Hypoglycemia usually results from excessive administration of insulin in treatment of diabetes. Failure to monitor serum glucose adequately or to adjust the insulin dosage on the basis of changing dietary intake or metabolic demands may precipitate the disorder. Less commonly, insulin-producing tumors (insulinomas), glycogen storage diseases, or other inborn errors of metabolism result in hypoglycemia. Clinical manifestations result from neuroglycopenia (insufficient glucose supply to the central nervous system) and autonomic activation during the stress response induced by the glucose-deficient state.

REFERENCES

1. Cefalu, W.T. (1996). Treatment of type II diabetes: What options have been added to traditional methods? *Postgraduate Medicine* 99(3), 109–122.
2. Agarwal, M.K. (1994). Perspectives in receptor-mediated mineralocorticoid hormone action. *Pharmacological Reviews* 46(1), 67–87.
3. Chrousos, G.P. (1995). The hypothalamic-pituitary-adrenal axis and immune-mediated inflammation. *New England Journal of Medicine* 332(20), 1351–1362.
4. Mizock, B.A. (1995). Alterations in carbohydrate metabolism during stress: A review of the literature. *American Journal of Medicine* 98, 75–84.
5. Davidson, M.B. (1995). Clinical implications of insulin resistance syndromes. *American Journal of Medicine* 99, 420–426.
6. Arrants, J. (1994). Hyperinsulinemia and cardiovascular risk. *Heart & Lung* 23(2), 118–124.
7. Tsigos, C., and Chrousos, G.P. (1996). Differential diagnosis and management of Cushing's syndrome. *Annual Review of Medicine* 47, 443–461.
8. Orth, D.N. (1995). Cushing's syndrome. *New England Journal of Medicine* 332(12), 791–803.
9. Kountz, D.S., and Clark, C.L. (1997). Safely withdrawing patients from chronic glucocorticoid therapy. *American Family Physician* 55(2), 521–525.
10. Oelkers, W. (1996). Adrenal insufficiency. *New England Journal of Medicine* 335(16), 1206–1212.
11. Reasner, C.A., and Isley, W.L. (1997). Endocrine emergencies: Recognizing clues to classic problems. *Postgraduate Medicine* 101(3), 231–242.
12. Ackerman, R.J. (1994). Adrenal disorders: Know when to act and what tests to give. *Geriatrics* 49(7), 32–37.
13. Gumowski, J., and Loughran, M. (1996). Diseases of the adrenal gland. *Nursing Clinics of North America* 31(4), 747–768.
14. Azzi, R., Dewailly, D., and Owerback, D. (1994). Nonclassic adrenal hyperplasia: Current concepts. *Journal of Clinical Endocrinology and Metabolism* 78(4), 810–815.
15. New, M.I. (1995). Steroid 21-hydroxylase deficiency (congenital adrenal hyperplasia). *American Journal of Medicine* 98(suppl. 1A), 2S–8S.
16. Chrousos, G.P., moderator. (1993). Syndromes of glucocorticoid resistance. *Annals of Internal Medicine* 119(11), 1113–1124.
17. Laine, C., and Caro, J.F. (1996). Preventing complications in diabetes mellitus. *Medical Clinics of North America* 80(2), 457–474.
18. Atkinson, M.A., and Maclaren, N.K. (1994). The pathogenesis of insulin-dependent diabetes mellitus. *New England Journal of Medicine* 331(21), 1428–1436.
19. Polonsky, K.S., Sturis, J., and Bell, G.I. (1996). Non-insulin-dependent diabetes mellitus: A genetically programmed failure of the beta cell to compensate for insulin resistance. *New England Journal of Medicine* 334(12), 777–783.
20. Davidson, J.A., and Roberts, V.L. (1996). Gestational diabetes: Ensuring a successful outcome. *Postgraduate Medicine* 99(3), 165–172.
21. Porte, D., Jr., and Schwartz, M.W. (1996). Diabetes complications: Why is glucose potentially toxic? *Science* 272, 699–700.
22. Fish, L.H. (1994). Diabetic ketoacidosis: Treatment strategies to avoid complications. *Postgraduate Medicine* 96(3), 75–96.
23. O'Hanlon-Nichols, T. (1996). Hyperglycemic hyperosmolar nonketotic syndrome. *American Journal of Nursing* 96(3), 38–39.
24. Hirsch, I.B. (1996). Surveillance for complications of diabetes: Don't wait for symptoms before intervening. *Postgraduate Medicine* 99(3), 147–162.
25. Bakris, G.L. (1993). Diabetic nephropathy: What you need to know to preserve kidney function. *Postgraduate Medicine* 93(5), 89–100.
26. Wolever, T.M.S., and Miller, J.B. (1995). Sugars and glucose control. *American Journal of Clinical Nutrition* 62(suppl.), 212S–227S.
27. Garg, A.G., Bantle, J.P., Henry, R.R., *et al.* (1994). Effects of varying carbohydrate content of diet in patients with non-insulin-dependent diabetes mellitus. *Journal of the American Medical Association* 271(18), 1421–1427.
28. Lacy, P.E. (1995). Treating diabetes with transplanted cells. *Scientific American* 273(1), 50–58.
29. Clark, Jr., C.M., and Lee, D.A. (1995). Prevention and treatment of the complications of diabetes mellitus. *New England Journal of Medicine* 332(18), 1210–1217.
30. Adler, S., Nast, C., and Artishevsky, A. (1993). Diabetic nephropathy: Pathogenesis and treatment. *Annual Review of Medicine* 44, 303–315.
31. Diabetes Control and Complications Trial Research Group. (1996). Lifetime benefits and costs of intensive therapy as practiced in the Diabetes Control and Complications Trial. *Journal of the American Medical Association* 276(17), 1409–1415.
32. Pritchard, C.E. (1996). Update in diabetes: Applications for clinical practice from the diabetes control and complications trial. *Nursing Clinics of North America* 31(4), 725–735.
33. Service, F.J. (1995). Hypoglycemia. *Medical Clinics of North America* 79(1), 1–8.
34. Service, F.J. (1995). Hypoglycemic disorders. *New England Journal of Medicine* 332(17), 1144–1152.

SELECTED BIBLIOGRAPHY

Baliga, B.S., and Fonseca, V.A. (1997). Recent advances in the treatment of type II diabetes mellitus. *American Family Physician* 55(3), 817–824.

Bell, D.S.H. (1993). Insulin resistance: An often unrecognized problem accompanying chronic medical disorders. *Postgraduate Medicine* 93(7), 99–107.

Berlin, I., Grimaldi, A., Landault, C., *et al.* (1994). Suspected postprandial hypoglycemia is associated with β-adrenergic hypersensitivity and emotional distress. *Journal of Clinical Endocrinology and Metabolism* 79(5), 1428–1433.

Bienkowski, J. (1994). An overview of the progression of diabetic retinopathy with treatment recommendations. *Nurse Practitioner* 19(7), 50–58.

Blackburn, S.T., and Loper, D.L. (1992). *Maternal, Fetal, and Neonatal Physiology: A Clinical Perspective.* Philadelphia: W.B. Saunders.

Bochicchio, D., Losa, M., Buchfelder, M., and the European Cushing's Disease Survey Study Group. (1995). Factors influencing the immediate and late outcome of Cushing's disease treated by transsphenoidal surgery: A retrospective study by the European Cushing's Disease Survey Group. *Journal of Clinical Endocrinology and Metabolism* 80(11), 3114–3120.

Bohannon, N.J.V. (1997). Benefits of lispro insulin: Control of postprandial glucose levels is within reach. *Postgraduate Medicine* 101(2), 73–80.

Bohannon, N.J.V. (1994). Effective use of insulin: A balancing act. *Postgraduate Medicine* 95(8), 52–67.
Bose, H.S., Sugawara, T., Strauss III, J.F., *et al.*, for the International Congenital Lipoid Adrenal Hyperplasia Consortium. (1996). The pathophysiology and genetics of congenital lipoid adrenal hyperplasia. *New England Journal of Medicine* 335(25), 1870–1878.
Boumpas, D.T., moderator. (1993). Glucocorticoid therapy for immune-mediated diseases: Basic and clinical correlates. *Annals of Internal Medicine* 119(12), 1198–1208.

Caputo, G.M., Cavanagh, P.R., Ulbrecht, J.S., *et al.* (1994). Assessment and management of foot disease in patients with diabetes. *New England Journal of Medicine* 331(13), 854–860.
Carter, J.S., Pugh, J.A., and Monterrosa, A. (1996). Non-insulin-dependent diabetes mellitus in minorities in the United States. *Annals of Internal Medicine* 125(3), 221–232.
Charles, M.A., Pettitt, D.J., McCance, D.R., *et al.* (1994). Gravidity, obesity, and non-insulin-dependent diabetes among Pima Indian women. *American Journal of Medicine* 97, 250–255.
Colditz, G.A., Willett, W.C., Rotnitzky, A., *et al.* (1995). Weight gain as a risk factor for clinical diabetes mellitus in women. *Annals of Internal Medicine* 122(7), 481–486.
Cook, D.M., and Loriaux, D.L. (1996). The incidental adrenal mass. *American Journal of Medicine* 101, 88–94.
Cotran, R.S., Kumar, V., and Robbins, S.L. (1994). *Robbins Pathologic Basis of Disease.* (5th ed.). Philadelphia: W.B. Saunders. (pp. 907–925).

DeFronzo, R.A., Goodman, A.M., and the Multicenter Metformin Study Group. (1995). Efficacy of metformin in patients with non-insulin-dependent diabetes mellitus. *New England Journal of Medicine* 333(9), 541–549.
Despres, J-P., Lamarche, B., Mauriege, P., *et al.* (1996). Hyperinsulinemia as an independent risk factor for ischemic heart disease. *New England Journal of Medicine* 334(15), 952–957.
Diabetes Control and Complications Trial Research Group. (1994). Effect of intensive diabetes treatment on the development and progression of long-term complications in adolescents with insulin-dependent diabetes mellitus: Diabetes Control and Complications Trial. *Journal of Pediatrics* 125(2), 177–188.
Diabetes Control and Complications Trial Research Group. (1995). The effect of intensive diabetes therapy on the development and progression of neuropathy. *Annals of Internal Medicine* 122(8), 561–568.

Expert Committee on the Diagnosis and Classification of Diabetes Mellitus. (1997). Report of the Expert Committee on the Diagnosis and Clarification of Diabetes Mellitus. *Diabetes Care* 20(7), 1183–1197.

Fava, G.A. (1994). Affective disorders and endocrine disease: New insights from psychosomatic studies. *Psychosomatics* 35(4), 341–353.
Field, A.E., Colditz, G.A., Willett, W.A., *et al.* (1994). The relation of smoking, age, relative weight, and dietary intake to serum adrenal steroids, sex hormones, and sex hormone-binding globulin in middle-aged men. *Journal of Clinical Endocrinology and Metabolism* 79(5), 1310–1316.
Freckmann, M-L., Thorburn, D.R., Kirby, D.M., *et al.* (1997). Mitochondrial electron transport chain defect presenting as hypoglycemia. *Journal of Pediatrics* 130(3), 431–436.

Gonzalez-Campoy, J.M., and Robertson, R.P. (1996). Diabetic ketoacidosis and hyperosmolar nonketotic state: Gaining control over extreme hyperglycemic complications. *Postgraduate Medicine* 99(6), 143–152.
Grossman, E., and Messerli, F.H. (1996). Diabetic and hypertensive heart disease. *Annals of Internal Medicine* 125(4), 304–310.
Guyton, A.C., and Hall, J.E. (1996). *Textbook of Medical Physiology.* (9th ed.). Philadelphia: W.B. Saunders. (pp. 957–983).

Henry, R.R. (1996). Glucose control and insulin resistance in non-insulin-dependent diabetes mellitus. *Annals of Internal Medicine* 124(1 Pt. 2), 97–103.
Hoeldtke, R.D., and Boden, G. (1994). Epinephrine secretion, hypoglycemia unawareness, and diabetic autonomic neuropathy. *Annals of Internal Medicine* 120(6), 512–517.

Jabbar, M., Pugliese, M., Recker, B., *et al.* (1991). Excess weight and precocious pubarche in children: Alterations of the adrenocortical hormones. *Journal of the American College of Nutrition* 10(4), 289–296.
Jackson, P., and Bash, D.M. (1994). Management of the uncomplicated pregnant diabetic client in the ambulatory setting. *Nurse Practitioner* 19(12), 64–73.

Kochar, M.S., and Kalluru, V.B. (1994). Hypertension in the diabetic patient: Controlling its harmful effects. *Postgraduate Medicine* 96(6), 101–110.
Korte, C., Styne, D., Merritt, A., *et al.* (1996). Adrenocortical function in the very low birth weight infant: Improved testing sensitivity and association with neonatal outcome. *Journal of Pediatrics* 128(2), 257–263.
Krolewski, A., Laffel, L.M.B., Krolewski, M., *et al.* (1995). Glycosylated hemoglobin and the risk of microalbuminuria in patients with insulin-dependent diabetes mellitus. *New England Journal of Medicine* 332(19), 1251–1255.

Laffel, L.M.B., McGill, J.B., and Gans, D.J., on behalf of the North American Microalbuminuria Study Group. (1995). The beneficial effect of angiotensin-converting enzyme inhibition with captopril on diabetic nephropathy in normotensive IDDM patients with microalbuminuria. *American Journal of Medicine* 99, 497–504.
LaRochelle, G.E., LaRochelle, A.G., Ratner, R.E., *et al.* (1993). Recovery of the hypothalamic-pituitary-adrenal (HPA) axis in patients with rheumatic diseases receiving low-dose prednisone. *American Journal of Medicine* 95, 258–264.
Lazarevic, M.B., Skosey, J.L., Djordjevic-Denic, G., *et al.* (1995). Reduction of cortisol levels after single intra-articular and intramuscular steroid injection. *American Journal of Medicine* 99, 370–373.
Levy, J., Gavin III, J.R., and Sowers, J.R. (1994). Diabetes mellitus: A disease of abnormal cellular calcium metabolism? *American Journal of Medicine* 96, 260–273.
Lillioja, S., Mott, D.M., Spraul, M., *et al.* (1993). Insulin resistance and insulin secretory dysfunction as precursors of non-insulin-dependent diabetes mellitus. *New England Journal of Medicine* 329(27), 1988–1992.
Loriaux, T.C. (1996). Endocrine assessment: Red flags for those on the front lines. *Nursing Clinics of North America* 31(4), 695–713.

Magiakou, M.A., Mastorakos, G., Oldfield, E.H., *et al.* (1994). Cushing's syndrome in children and adolescents: Presentation, diagnosis, and therapy. *New England Journal of Medicine* 331(10), 629–636.
Marcus, A.O., and Fernandez, M.P. (1996). Insulin pump therapy: Acceptable alternative to injection therapy. *Postgraduate Medicine* 99(3), 125–144.
McMahon, M.M., and Rizza, R.A. (1996). Nutrition support in hospitalized patients with diabetes mellitus. *Mayo Clinic Proceedings* 71, 587–594.
Merke, D.P., and Cutler, Jr., G.B. (1997). New approaches to the treatment of congenital adrenal hyperplasia. *Journal of the American Medical Association* 277(13), 1073–1076.
Meyer, J.S. (1996). Diabetes and wound healing. *Critical Care Nursing Clinics of North America* 8(2), 195–201.
Miller, M. (1996). Type II diabetes: A treatment approach for the older patient. *Geriatrics* 51(8), 43–50.
Mitamura, R., Kimura, H., Murakami, Y., *et al.* (1996). Ultralente insulin treatment of transient neonatal diabetes mellitus. *Journal of Pediatrics* 128(2), 268–270.
Moore, K.L., and Persaud, T.V.N. (1993). *The Developing Human: Clinically Oriented Embryology.* (5th ed.). Philadelphia: W.B. Saunders.
Murphy, R.P. (1995). Management of diabetic retinopathy. *American Family Physician* 51(4), 785–796.

Nathan, D.M. (1996). The pathophysiology of diabetic complications: How much does the glucose hypothesis explain? *Annals of Internal Medicine* 124(1 Pt. 2), 86–89.

Nathan, D.M., McKitrick, C., Larkin, M., *et al.* (1996). Glycemic control in diabetes mellitus: Have changes in therapy made a difference? *American Journal of Medicine* 100, 157–163.

Nolan, J.J., Ludvik, B., Beerdsen, P., *et al.* (1994). Improvement in glucose tolerance and insulin resistance in obese subjects treated with troglitazone. *New England Journal of Medicine* 331(18), 1188–1193.

Pandit, M.K., Burke, J., Gustafson, A.B., *et al.* (1993). Drug-induced disorders of glucose tolerance. *Annals of Internal Medicine* 118(7), 529–539.

Partanen, J., Niskanen, L., Lehtinen, J., *et al.* (1995). Natural history of peripheral neuropathy in patients with non-insulin-dependent diabetes mellitus. *New England Journal of Medicine* 333(2), 89–94.

Patterson, J.E., and Andriole, V.T. (1995). Bacterial urinary tract infections in diabetes. *Infectious Disease Clinics of North America* 9(1), 25–51.

Pimenta, W., Korytkowski, M., Mitrakou, A., *et al.* (1995). Pancreatic beta-cell dysfunction as the primary genetic lesion in NIDDM. *Journal of the American Medical Association* 273(23), 1855 1861.

Pugliese, A., Bugawan, T., Moromisato, R., *et al.* (1994). Two subsets of HLA-DQA1 alleles mark phenotypic variation in levels of insulin autoantibodies in first degree relatives at risk for insulin-dependent diabetes. *Journal of Clinical Investigation* 93, 2447–2452.

Reaven, G.M., Lithell, H., and Landsberg, L. (1996). Hypertension and associated metabolic abnormalities: The role of insulin resistance and the sympathoadrenal system. *New England Journal of Medicine* 334(6), 374–381.

Ritz, E. (1993). Hypertension in diabetic nephropathy: Prevention and treatment. *American Heart Journal* 125(5 Pt. 2), 1514–1519.

Rosenecker, J., Eichler, I., Kuhn, L., *et al.* (1995). Genetic determination of diabetes mellitus in patients with cystic fibrosis. *Journal of Pediatrics* 127(3), 441–443.

Rother, K.I., and Schwenk II, F. (1995). An unusual case of the nonketotic hyperglycemic syndrome during childhood. *Mayo Clinic Proceedings* 70(1), 62–65.

Rusterholtz, A. (1996). Interpretation of diagnostic laboratory tests in selected endocrine disorders. *Nursing Clinics of North America* 31(4), 715 724.

Seeman, T.E., and Robbins, R.J. (1994). Aging and hypothalamic-pituitary-adrenal response to challenge in humans. *Endocrine Reviews* 15(2), 233–260.

Skyler, J.S. (1997). Insulin therapy in type II diabetes: Who needs it, how much of it, and for how long? *Postgraduate Medicine* 101(2), 85–96.

Smith, U. (1994). Carbohydrates, fat, and insulin action. *American Journal of Clinical Nutrition* 59(suppl.), 686S–689S.

Steinberger, J., Moorehead, C., Katch, V., *et al.* (1995). Relationship between insulin resistance and abnormal lipid profile in obese adolescents. *Journal of Pediatrics* 126(5 Pt. 1), 690–695.

Stern, M.P. (1996). Do non-insulin-dependent diabetes mellitus and cardiovascular disease share common antecedents? *Annals of Internal Medicine* 124(1 Pt. 2), 110–116.

Stoffer, S.S. (1993). Addison's disease: How to improve patients' quality of life. *Postgraduate Medicine* 93(4), 265–278.

Stumvoll, M., Nurjhan, N., Perriello, G., *et al.* (1995). Metabolic effects of metformin in non-insulin-dependent diabetes mellitus. *New England Journal of Medicine* 333(9), 550–554.

Talente, G.M., Coleman, R.A., Alter, C., *et al.* (1994). Glycogen storage disease in adults. *Annals of Internal Medicine* 120(3), 218–226.

Tan, G.H., and Nelson, R.L. (1996). Pharmacologic treatment options for non-insulin-dependent diabetes mellitus. *Mayo Clinic Proceedings* 71, 763–768.

Trevisan, R., and Viberti, G. (1995). Genetic factors in the development of diabetic nephropathy. *Journal of Laboratory and Clinical Medicine* 126(4), 342–349.

von Muhlendahl, K.E., and Herkenhoff, H. (1995). Long-term course of neonatal diabetes. *New England Journal of Medicine* 333(11), 704–708.

Walston, J., Silver, K., Bogardus, C., *et al.* (1995). Time of onset of non-insulin-dependent diabetes mellitus and genetic variation in the β_3-adrenergic receptor gene. *New England Journal of Medicine* 333(6), 343–347.

Watkins, J.B., III, and Sanders, R.A. (1995). Diabetes mellitus-induced alterations of hepatobiliary function. *Pharmacological Reviews* 47(1), 1–23.

Weber, K.T., and Villarreal, D. (1993). Role of aldosterone in congestive heart failure. *Postgraduate Medicine* 93(5), 203–221.

Westphal, S.A. (1996). The occurrance of diabetic ketoacidosis in non-insulin-dependent diabetes and newly diagnosed diabetic adults. *American Journal of Medicine* 101, 19–24.

White, J.R., Jr., Campbell, R.K., and Hirsch, I. (1997). Insulin analogues: New agents for improving glycemic control. *Postgradute Medicine* 101(2), 58–70.

White, J.R., Jr., Hartman, J., and Campbell, R.K. (1993). Drug interactions in diabetic patients: The risk of losing glycemic control. *Postgraduate Medicine* 93(3), 131–139.

Wing, R.R., Blair, E., Marcus, M., *et al.* (1994). Year-long weight loss treatment for obese patients with type II diabetes: Does including an intermittent very-low-calorie diet improve outcome? *American Journal of Medicine* 97, 354–362.

Winger, J.M., and Hornick, T. (1996). Age-associated changes in the endocrine system. *Nursing Clinics of North America* 31(4), 827–844.

Yanovski, J.A., Yanovski, S.Z., Cutler, Jr., G.B., *et al.* (1996). Differences in the hypothalamic-pituitary-adrenal axis of black girls and white girls. *Journal of Pediatrics* 129(1), 130–135.

Unit XI

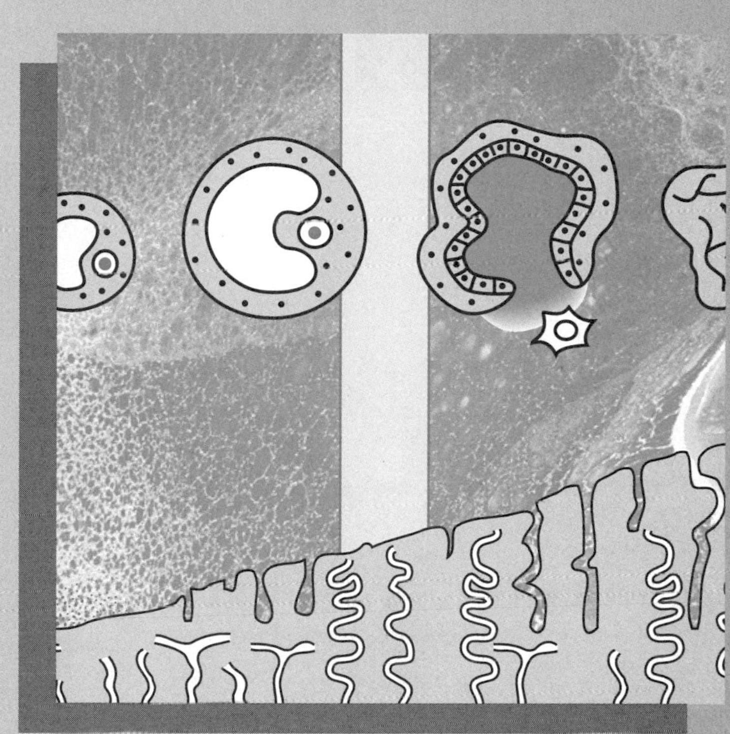

REPRODUCTIVE SYSTEM

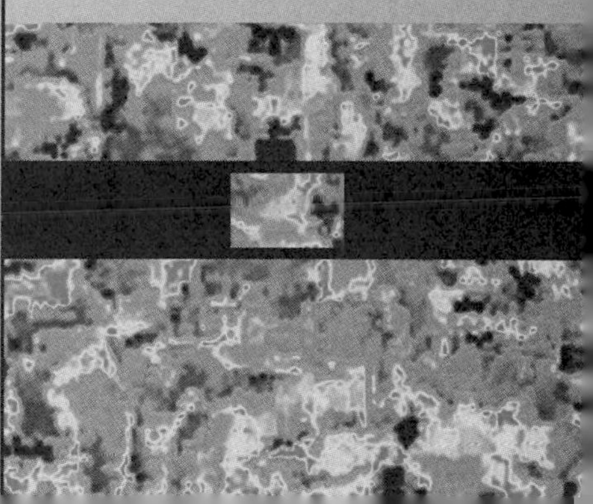

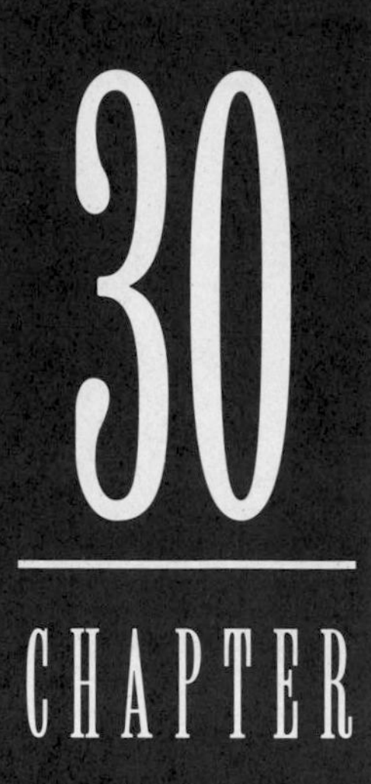

Disorders of the Male Reproductive System

LEARNING OBJECTIVES

1. Discuss the anatomic relationships underlying reproductive and urinary disorders in males.
2. Describe the process of spermatogenesis with reference to fertility and potential neoplasia.
3. Discuss pathologic processes and iatrogenic factors that may impair neuroendocrine regulation of male sexual function.
4. Relate clinical manifestations of selected disorders of male reproductive function to congenital or acquired structural defects.
5. Discuss the impact of sexually transmitted disease on reproductive function in males.
6. Compare and contrast the pathophysiologic processes, clinical manifestations, and treatment of benign prostatic hyperplasia and prostate cancer.

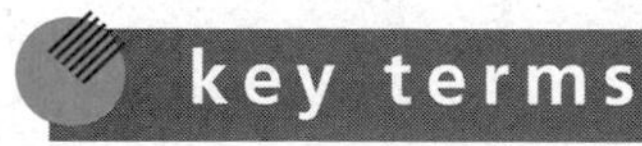

key terms

activin
azoospermia
balanitis
benign prostatic hyperplasia (BPH)
chlamydial infection
circumcision
cryptorchidism
dihydrotestosterone (DHT)
ejaculation
emission
epididymitis
epispadias
erectile dysfunction
erection
estradiol
genital herpes
genital warts
gonorrhea
hematocele
hydrocele
hypogonadism
hypospadias
infertility
inguinal hernia
inhibin
micropenis
oligospermia
orchitis
paraphimosis
Peyronie's disease
phimosis
posthitis
priapism
prostate cancer
prostate-specific antigen (PSA)

prostatitis
sexually transmitted disease (STD)
spermatogenesis
syphilis
testicular cancer
testicular torsion
testosterone
trichomoniasis
varicocele
vasectomy

A growing body of epidemiologic evidence suggests that the incidence of reproductive disorders in males has increased during the past 50 years.[1] **Testicular cancer**, **hypospadias**, and **cryptorchidism** have increased in incidence, and semen quality (volume and sperm density) has declined. Lifestyle factors (e.g., abuse of alcohol or tobacco, sexual behavior) and environmental exposures (to estrogen-like products, ionizing radiation, or toxic agents) have been implicated as possible causes of this trend. **Prostate cancer** is now the second-leading cause of cancer death in males, and **benign prostatic hyperplasia (BPH)** causes significant morbidity for many older men. **Sexually transmitted diseases (STDs)** remain a major public health concern. Because sexual function and reproductive capacity are integral to self-esteem, quality of life may be greatly affected by disorders of the male reproductive system.

Because the reproductive and urinary systems are structurally and functionally integrated in males, most disorders adversely affect both systems (see Chapter 20). In this chapter, the anatomy of the male reproductive system is reviewed, and the physiologic processes underlying sexual and reproductive function are detailed. Selected disorders of the male reproductive system are discussed in detail, including those mentioned earlier. Clinical features of less common disorders are briefly summarized.

ANATOMY OF THE MALE REPRODUCTIVE SYSTEM

The male reproductive system, illustrated in Figure 30–1, consists of: (1) the male gonads (*testes*), contained within the *scrotum*; (2) a number of accessory organs and ducts, including the *epididymis*, *seminal vesicles*, *prostate gland*, and *Cowper's glands*; and (3) the penetrating organ of sexual intercourse, the *penis*. Within the penis, the urethra transports both urine and semen, consistent with its function as a component of both the urinary and reproductive systems.

Testes and Scrotum

The bilateral testes (or testicles) are smooth, oval organs, suspended in the scrotum by the *spermatic cord*. Contained within the spermatic cord are arteries, veins, lymphatics, excretory ducts, and the *cremaster muscle*, which elevates the scrotum. The scrotal sac surrounds each testis. Within the scrotum, a serosa-lined sac, the *tunica vaginalis*, contains a small amount of clear fluid. This potential fluid space may be the site of accumulation of clear fluid (**hydrocele**) or blood (**hematocele**) in traumatic, structural, or inflammatory disorders of the testis. **Varicocele** refers to scrotal swelling due to dilation of veins within the spermatic cord. This idiopathic

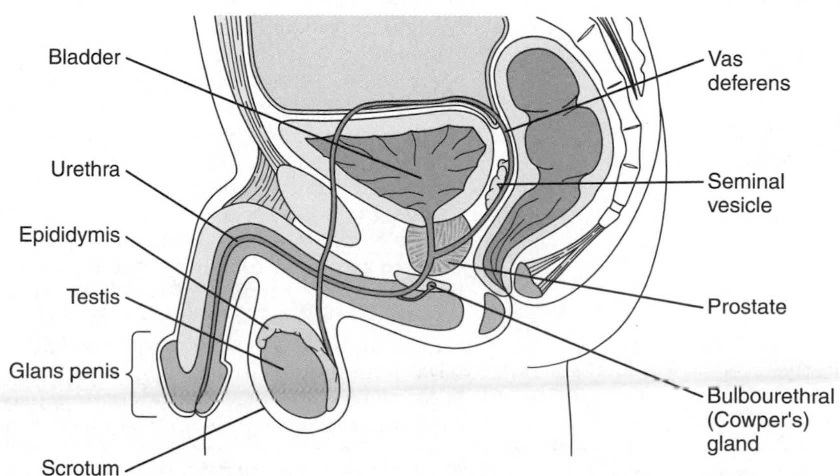

FIGURE 30–1
Male reproductive system. The reproductive organs of the male include (1) the male gonads (*testis*), contained within the *scrotum* and serving as sites of spermatogenesis and testosterone synthesis; (2) the ductal system, which transports, nourishes, and releases sperm and which includes the *epididymis*, *vas deferens*, and *seminal vesicle*; (3) accessory organs, such as the *Cowper's glands* and *prostate gland*, which contract to add components to the sperm-containing fluid, or semen; and (4) the *penis*, which serves as the penetrating organ of intercourse.

disorder may contribute to **infertility** in some men (see Chapter 32).

Suspension of the testes maintains scrotal temperature at about 2° to 3°F below core body temperature, a range that is optimal for **spermatogenesis** (sperm production). When testicular temperature falls below optimum, contraction of the cremaster muscle elevates the scrotum, bringing it closer to the abdominal wall.

The testes initially develop within the abdominal cavity (see Developmental Perspective). During the third trimester, under the influence of the male hormone **testosterone**, the testes normally descend through an opening in the peritoneum, the *inguinal canal*, into the scrotum. The inguinal canal usually closes just before birth, but this area remains relatively weak in a number of males, increasing the risk of **inguinal hernia,** as discussed later.

Accessory Organs and Ducts

Epididymis

Located posteriorly and superiorly to each testis is the epididymis. Each of these comma-shaped glands consists of a tightly coiled duct (*vas deferens*) that receives sperm from the testis. As sperm are slowly conducted (over about 12 days) through the duct, their maturation is facilitated by testosterone and nutrients. At the end of each vas deferens is an *ampulla* (pouch) that stores the mature sperm until they are released during sexual activity. Mature sperm remain fertile within the ampulla for up to 42 days. Surgical sterilization of the male is accomplished with **vasectomy**, in which the vas deferens is interrupted with clipping, ligation, or cautery, preventing ascent of sperm from the testes. Vasectomy is a safe and effective procedure, although not absolutely free of complications[2] (Table 30–1). Contraceptive practices are further detailed in Chapter 32.

Seminal Vesicles

During sexual activity, sperm are released from the ampulla into the seminal vesicles, a process known as **emission**. The seminal vesicles secrete a fluid containing nourishing fructose as well as prostaglandins, which assist with breakdown of the protective cervical mucus of the female, facilitating its

TABLE 30–1
EFFECTS OF VASECTOMY

Effects	Comments
Expected Effects	
Contraception	Vasectomy is equal to tubal ligation in efficacy and has a better safety profile and lower cost. The potential reversibility of the procedure varies with the technique but is similar to that for tubal ligation.
Anatomic changes	Back pressure may induce damage to the epididymis and vas deferens. Blow-outs and extravasation (leakage) of sperm may occur at the body and tail of the epididymis. Sperm granulomas may form at blow-out sites (in ligation procedures) or at cut sites (in open-ended procedures). There is no significant anatomic change in testis, prostate, or seminal vesicles, and testicular volume does not change. Pressure effects usually arrest spermatogenesis initially, but normal sperm production usually returns.
Hormonal changes	The testis may have decreased responsiveness to follicle-stimulating hormone and luteinizing hormone because of pressure effects.
Immunologic changes	Antisperm antibodies are detected in 70% of men and are more likely to be present if sperm extravasation occurs. This change is not associated with increased incidence of autoimmune disease.
Complications	
Contraceptive failure	Failure of vasectomy occurs in 1 in 250 to 400 procedures and is usually due to unprotected intercourse too soon after vasectomy. Absence of sperm must be demonstrated by two sperm counts 6 weeks apart. Late vasectomy failure may be due to failure to cut both vas deferens, presence of an accessory duct, or insufficient ejaculations to clear out remaining sperm. Spontaneous recanalization (reconnection) of the vas may occur in cases in which sperm granulomas are present at the cut site or in which less than 1 cm of vas is removed.
Surgical complications	Bleeding and hematoma formation rarely occur. Incisional infections are also uncommon. Pain may be associated with sperm granulomas. Erectile dysfunction, if present, is psychogenic in origin. Epididymitis may occur in patients who had a genitourinary tract infection before the procedure. Vasourinary fistulas are rare.

Data from Raspa, R.F. (1993). Complications of vasectomy. *American Family Physician* 48(7), 1264–1268.

penetration by sperm. The outlet from each seminal vesicle is the ejaculatory duct, through which the sperm-containing fluid, or semen, traverses the prostate gland and enters the urethra for **ejaculation**, or release to the exterior. Injury (e.g., surgical trauma) to the prostatic urethra or its innervation may result in *retrograde ejaculation*, in which semen from the ejaculatory ducts enters the bladder rather than being ejected to the exterior.

Prostate Gland

The prostate gland is normally chestnut-sized in adults, encircling the urethra at the neck of the bladder. The prostatic portion of the urethra is entered by the paired ejaculatory ducts. The prostate is divided functionally into three zones (Fig. 30–2), each of which has a ductal system draining into a specific part of the prostatic urethra. The inner transitional zone, which immediately surrounds the urethra, is the site of BPH, whereas the outer peripheral zone is the usual site of origin of prostate cancer. The prostate contracts during ejaculation, adding a milky, alkaline fluid to the semen. The fluid aids in transport and nourishment of sperm. Because vaginal secretions are acidic, the alkalinity of the seminal fluid normalizes pH to facilitate fertilization. (The process of fertilization is detailed in Chapter 32.)

Cowper's Glands

Located near the base of the penis, the Cowper's glands, also known as bulbourethral glands, secrete mucus into the urethra. This last addition to the semen provides lubrication for sexual function.

Penis

The *glans* or tip of the penis contains the urethral meatus, through which urine and semen pass to the exterior. The glans contains many nerve endings for sexual sensation. The meatus is normally centrally located, although malposition may occur as a congenital defect. As discussed in Chapter 20, these disorders, **hypospadias** and **epispadias**, may result in urinary problems that require surgical correction during childhood. The *foreskin* (prepuce) is a retractable cuff of loose skin covering the glans. Surgical removal of the foreskin (**circumcision**) is performed on more than 60% of male newborns in the United States, but this procedure is increasingly controversial.[3] There is disagreement about whether a medical indication for the procedure exists, and its performance may be painful for the neonate. Circumcision has significant social significance for some groups and is a religious ritual within the Jewish culture. Table 30–2 summarizes the major points of contention regarding the circumcision procedure.

The penis may be affected by infections (often sexually transmitted), congenital abnormalities, or cancer. STDs are discussed later in this chapter. Inflammation of the glans (**balanitis**) or foreskin (**posthitis**) may result in swelling, redness, and pain. In uncircumcised males, inflammation may lead to **phimosis**, in which the constricted foreskin cannot be retracted over the glans. **Paraphimosis** is the inability to replace the foreskin, once retracted. If severe, phimosis and paraphimosis may obstruct the flow of blood or urine, requiring surgical intervention.

Peyronie's disease, an idiopathic disorder in which fibrous plaques develop on the dorsal surface of the shaft, is common among older men. This disorder leads to curvature of the penis during **erection**

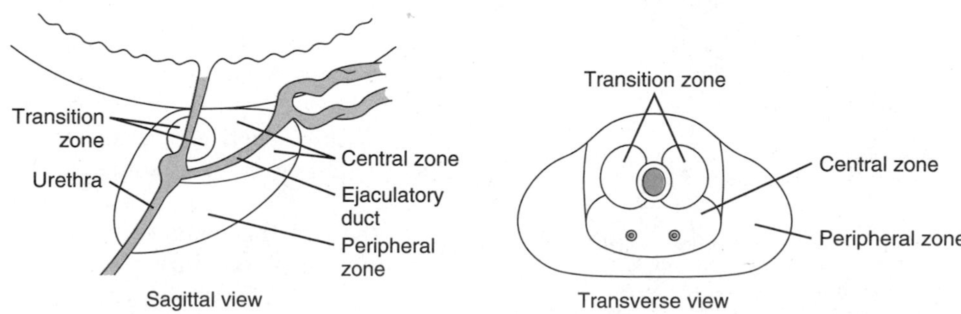

FIGURE 30–2

Zonal anatomy of the prostate gland. The prostate gland is depicted here in cross-section, from sagittal (side) and transverse (horizontal) views. The inner transitional zone is the area affected by benign prostatic hyperplasia, whereas prostate cancer most frequently arises from the peripheral zone. (Redrawn from Maxwell, M.B. [1993]. Cancer of the prostate. *Seminars in Oncology Nursing* 9[4], 238.)

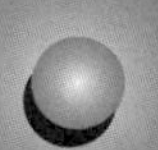

TABLE 30–2
BENEFITS AND RISKS RELATED TO CIRCUMCISION

Possible Benefits	Comments
Protection against penile cancer	Penile cancer occurs almost exclusively in uncircumcised men; however, the difference may relate to hygienic factors rather than to intrinsic protection by circumcision.
Protection of partner from cervical cancer	Some strains of human papillomavirus, found more commonly in uncircumcised men, have been linked to squamous cell carcinoma of the cervix.
Protection against sexually transmitted disease	Nearly all sexually transmitted diseases occur more frequently among uncircumcised men.
Protection against urinary tract infection	Circumcised boys are less likely to have urinary tract infections during infancy.
Cultural acceptability	Jewish men report the largest proportion circumcised. Whites are much more likely to be circumcised than blacks or Hispanics in the United States.
Facilitation of hygiene	Lack of the foreskin simplifies hygiene, and this may be the source of protective effects.
Possible Risks	**Comments**
Pain	Neonates do experience pain during the procedure. Use of dorsal block and local anesthetic infiltration is indicated.
Psychological trauma	Restraint during the procedure may be stressful. Maternal–infant bonding during the neonatal period may be impaired.
Bleeding and infection	These complications are rare.
Disfigurement	Poor surgical technique may rarely result in deformation of the penis. Excessive tissue removal may cause denudation of the penile shaft or trauma to the glan or meatus. Inadequate removal of foreskin may lead to adhesions or phimosis.
Reduction in sensitivity of the glans	Little consensus exists regarding the role of the foreskin in sexual performance and satisfaction.

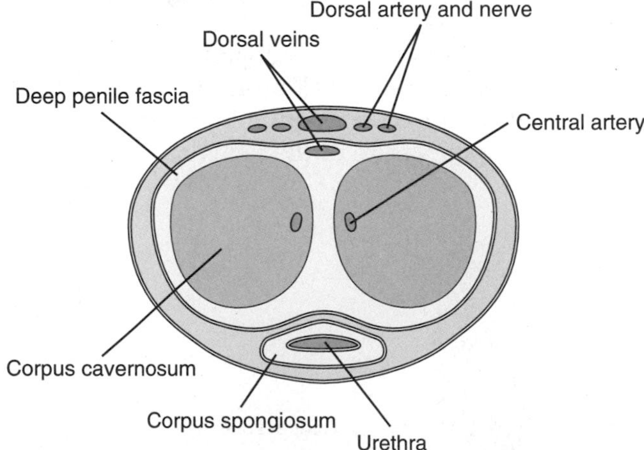

FIGURE 30–3
Vascular structures of the penis. The erectile tissues *(corpus cavernosum* and *corpus spongiosum)* within the shaft of the penis are seen in cross-section, along with the principal blood vessels. Sinusoids of the erectile tissue are relatively empty at baseline, and the penis is flaccid. With sexual stimulation, these tissues distend with blood, owing to rapid arterial inflow and partial obstruction of venous outflow, leading to penile erection. (Redrawn from Guyton, A.C., and Hall, J.E. [1996]. *Textbook of Medical Physiology.* [9th ed.]. Philadelphia: W.B. Saunders. [p. 1009].)

and may cause unsatisfactory sexual function or urinary obstruction. Peyronie's disease may resolve spontaneously in some cases or may require surgical correction. With the exceptions of hypospadias and epispadias, congenital defects of the penis are rare. A congenitally small penis (**micropenis**) may be associated with other structural anomalies (e.g., exstrophy of the bladder, epispadias, neural tube defects) or with **hypogonadism** due to chromosomal abnormalities. Surgical correction may be possible in some cases. Genetically male infants may be assigned female gender in some cases of genital ambiguity.[4]

The shaft of the penis contains erectile tissue that distends with blood during sexual arousal (Fig. 30–3). As detailed later in this chapter, impaired arousal (**erectile dysfunction**) may be a consequence of systemic disorders that affect peripheral perfusion or innervation, notably cardiovascular disease, diabetes mellitus, and spinal cord injury.

MALE REPRODUCTIVE FUNCTION

Reproductive function in males depends on the production of sperm and the capability of sexual intercourse.

Spermatogenesis

Testicular Microstructure

The functional unit of the testis is the *lobule*, illustrated in Figure 30–4. Production of sperm begins at puberty in males, at about 13 years of age, and continues throughout life. Each lobule contains *seminiferous tubules*, smooth muscle tubes (totaling 750 feet in length) that are lined with *spermatogonia* and *Sertoli cells*. Spermatogonia are the primary germ cells from which spermatozoa develop during a series of divisions, as discussed later. Sertoli cells secrete nutrients to sustain spermatogenesis, digestive enzymes essential to the final maturation of sperm, and several hormones necessary for normal testicular development and spermatogenesis. In the interstitial spaces between seminiferous tubules are the *Leydig cells*, which produce testosterone.

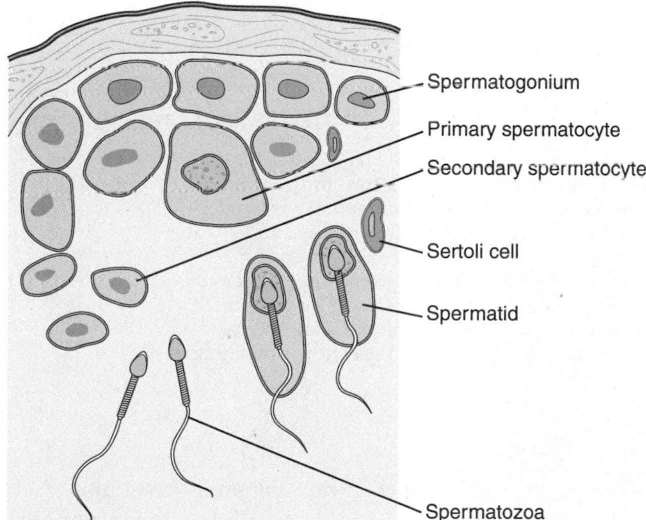

FIGURE 30–4
Testicular microstructure. Each lobule, or functional unit of the testis, contains seminiferous tubules lined with spermatogonia, the primitive germ cells from which spermatozoa develop. A seminiferous tubule is shown in cross-section, along with spermatogonia and spermatozoa in progressive stages of development. *Sertoli cells* contained within the lobules support the process of spermatogenesis by secreting nutrients, digestive enzymes, and hormones.

Mitotic and Meiotic Processes

Spermatogenesis involves a series of cell divisions, illustrated in Figure 30–5. During the first stage, the most mature spermatogonia divide mitotically to form two daughter cells known as *primary spermatocytes*. During the second stage, each primary spermatocyte undergoes meiotic division to form two smaller *secondary spermatocytes*, each having the haploid number of chromosomes (see Chapter 6). During the third stage, each secondary spermatocyte divides by mitosis to form two *spermatids*. The fourth and final stage consists of the maturation of spermatids into *spermatozoa*, or *sperm*, under the influence of testosterone and Sertoli cell enzymes.

Alterations in Spermatogenesis

Reduction in the quantity or motility of the sperm may be a factor in infertility (see Chapter 32). **Azoospermia** (absence of sperm in the semen) and **oligospermia** (deficient numbers of sperm) may occur idiopathically or in association with known disorders (Table 30–3). An estimated 15% of couples attempting pregnancy have less-than-normal fertility, and in half of these cases, the abnormality resides completely or partially with the male.[5] Clinical interventions designed to stimulate spermatogenesis, enhance sperm motility, remove serum antisperm antibodies, and increase sperm counts are being investigated.[6]

Decreased sperm motility is typical of aging, although the degree and pattern of this decrease are not universal. Although the term "male menopause" has been applied to alterations in spermatogenesis, sexual function, and androgen levels that occur in males at midlife, an identifiable cessation in the production of sex cells does not normally occur.[7] Reproductive function potentially remains intact throughout the lifetime of the male.

Endocrine Regulation of Male Reproductive Function

The primary male hormone is the androgen testosterone, a steroid synthesized from cholesterol. Ninety-five per cent of testosterone is secreted by the Leydig cells of the testes, with the remaining 5% secreted by the adrenal cortex (see Chapter 29). Testosterone may act directly on target cells or may be converted to **dihydrotestosterone (DHT)** by the 5α-reductase enzyme, or to the estrogen **estradiol** by the aromatase enzyme. Testosterone and DHT bind

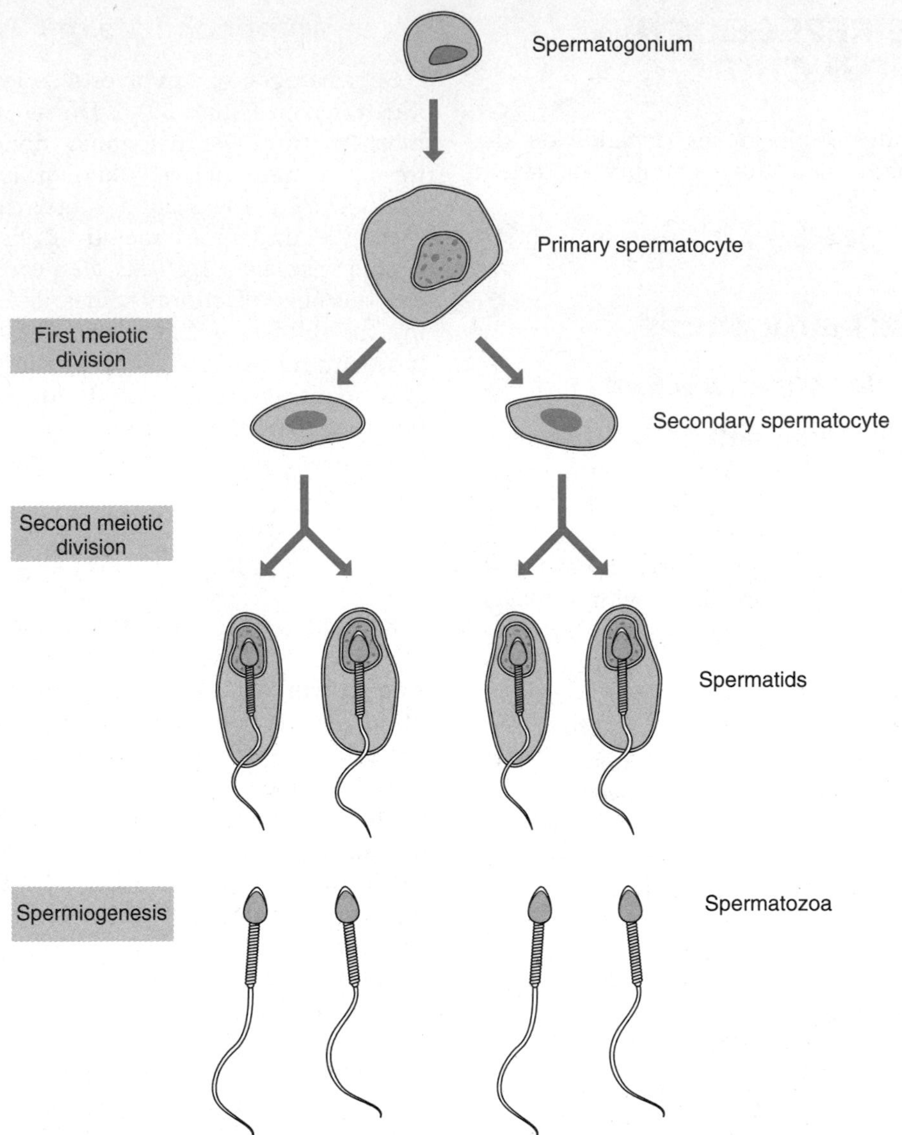

FIGURE 30–5

Spermatogenesis. Spermatogenesis occurs by a series of cell divisions culminating in the production of spermatozoa from primary germ cells, or spermatogonia. Each spermatogonium first undergoes two cycles of mitosis, resulting in four primary spermatocytes (one is shown, for simplicity). Each primary spermatocyte then undergoes the first of two meiotic divisions, producing two secondary spermatocytes, each with 23 duplicated but attached (bivalent) chromosomes. Meiotic division of each secondary spermatocyte produces two spermatids, each containing 23 unreplicated chromosomes (the haplid number). Spermatids then undergo maturation to functional spermatozoa, ejecting much of their cytoplasm and developing a flagellum (tail), a midsection containing mitochondria, and an acrosome (head).

to the same receptor in target cells, but DHT is more potent because of its higher affinity. The 5α-reductase enzyme is found primarily in prostate, skin, and reproductive system tissues, whereas the aromatase enzyme predominates in adipose tissue, liver, and the central nervous system.

Similarly to other steroid hormones, testosterone circulates primarily in bound form, with this form serving as a reservoir for release of free (active) hormone. Testosterone binds to sex hormone–binding globulin (SHBG) and other plasma proteins. Free testosterone binds to an intracellular receptor, and this complex then enters the nucleus to influence protein synthesis (see Chapter 27). Secretion of testosterone by the Leydig cells is regulated by the hypothalamic–pituitary axis, as illustrated in Figure 30–6. Hypothalamic gonadotropin-releasing hormone, also known as luteinizing hormone–releasing hormone (LHRH), induces the release of the gonadotropins luteinizing hormone (LH) and follicle-

TABLE 30-3
FACTORS ASSOCIATED WITH INFERTILITY IN MALES

CATEGORY	EXAMPLES
Medical history	Mumps orchitis Thyroid disease Erectile dysfunction Testicular trauma Chromosomal defect Hypogonadism Retrograde ejaculation
Structural defects	Cryptorchidism Testicular torsion Hypospadias Agenesis of testis or vas deferens Varicocele
Lifestyle factors	Excessive alcohol intake Cigarette smoking Marijuana use Abuse of anabolic steroids Hot tub use
Iatrogenic factors	Cytotoxic chemotherapy Hormonal therapy Radiation therapy

Data from Trantham, P. (1996). The infertile couple. *American Family Physician* 54(3), 1001–1010.

stimulating hormone (FSH) from the anterior pituitary gland. In males, LH stimulates testosterone production by Leydig cells, whereas FSH induces Sertoli cells to initiate spermatogenesis.

A number of peptides, of which **activin** and **inhibin** are best known, participate in the regulation of gonadal, adrenal, and placental hormone production, both within the hypothalamic–pituitary axis and by local autocrine or paracrine effects.[8] These peptides are produced not only by the ovary and testis but also by extragonadal tissues. As their names suggest, activin simulates gonadotropin release from the pituitary, whereas inhibin inhibits this release. Rising gonadotropin levels stimulate inhibin release in a negative feedback mechanism. Activin stimulates ovarian progesterone secretion and aromatase enzyme activity.

Effects of Testosterone and Estradiol

The effects of testosterone, summarized in Table 30–4, include promotion of spermatogenesis, promotion of prostate growth, and regulation of the development of male physical characteristics of the genitalia, body hair and skin, voice, and muscle. The role of testosterone in sexual function is uncertain, but it is probable that there is a threshold level below which lack of testosterone impairs the frequency and quality of erections.[9] The role of estradiol in males is also uncertain but may involve regulation of spermatogenesis and maintenance of bone density (see Chapter 34). Because of their negative feedback effect on the hypothalamic–pituitary axis, estrogens have been administered therapeutically in treatment of benign prostatic hyperplasia and prostatic cancer. As discussed subsequently, more effective means of reducing testosterone levels have been developed, and estrogen therapy is no longer considered as first-line intervention in these disorders.

Testosterone Deficiency (Hypogonadism)

Testosterone deficiency (hypogonadism) may occur as a primary disorder or secondary to systemic disorders or constitutional delay of puberty (Table 30–5). Males with primary hypogonadism have low serum testosterone concentrations despite elevated levels of the gonadotropins LH and FSH. Exogenous hormone replacement maintains secondary sex characteristics in these patients, but they remain infertile. In secondary hypogonadism, both testosterone and gonadotropin levels are low. Treatment with gonadotropin replacement often stimulates both spermatogenesis and endogenous release of testosterone.[8]

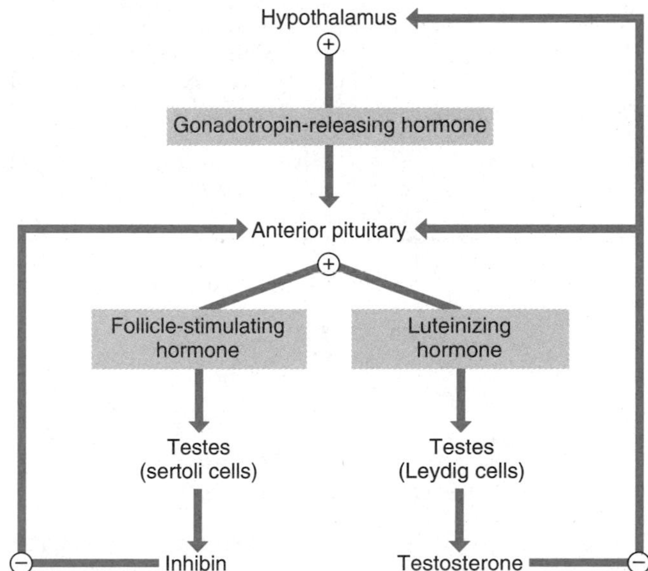

FIGURE 30–6
Hypothalamic–pituitary axis regulation of testosterone secretion. Release of gonadotropin-releasing hormone from the hypothalamus stimulates gonadotrope cells of the anterior pituitary to produce follicle-stimulating hormone and luteinizing hormone. These gonadotropins then stimulate the testes, with follicle-stimulating hormone inducing Sertoli cell secretion and luteinizing hormone stimulating testosterone systhesis. Rising testosterone levels provide negative feedback to this regulatory axis.

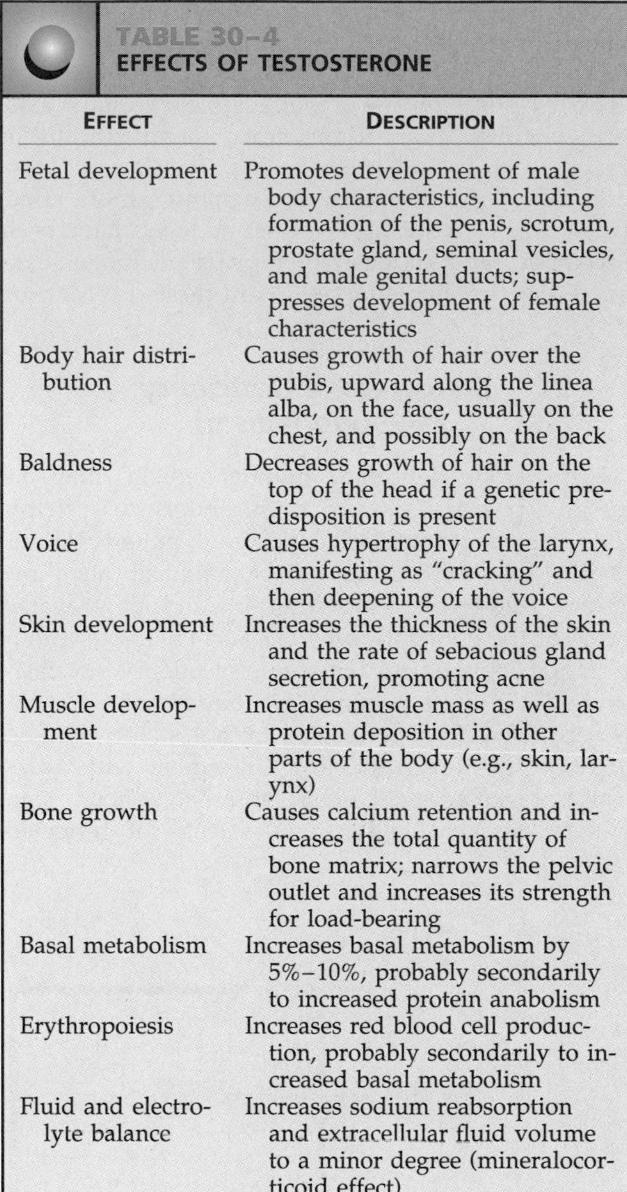

TABLE 30–4
EFFECTS OF TESTOSTERONE

Effect	Description
Fetal development	Promotes development of male body characteristics, including formation of the penis, scrotum, prostate gland, seminal vesicles, and male genital ducts; suppresses development of female characteristics
Body hair distribution	Causes growth of hair over the pubis, upward along the linea alba, on the face, usually on the chest, and possibly on the back
Baldness	Decreases growth of hair on the top of the head if a genetic predisposition is present
Voice	Causes hypertrophy of the larynx, manifesting as "cracking" and then deepening of the voice
Skin development	Increases the thickness of the skin and the rate of sebaceous gland secretion, promoting acne
Muscle development	Increases muscle mass as well as protein deposition in other parts of the body (e.g., skin, larynx)
Bone growth	Causes calcium retention and increases the total quantity of bone matrix; narrows the pelvic outlet and increases its strength for load-bearing
Basal metabolism	Increases basal metabolism by 5%–10%, probably secondarily to increased protein anabolism
Erythropoiesis	Increases red blood cell production, probably secondarily to increased basal metabolism
Fluid and electrolyte balance	Increases sodium reabsorption and extracellular fluid volume to a minor degree (mineralocorticoid effect)

Data from Guyton, A.C., and Hall, J.E. (1996). *Textbook of Medical Physiology*. (9th ed.). Philadelphia: W.B. Saunders. (pp. 1011–1012).

Abuse of Anabolic Steroids

The androgenic effect of testosterone derivatives on muscle development has led to widespread illicit use of these agents to enhance athletic performance.[9] Usually, these androgens are taken in amounts up to 100 times the doses used for replacement therapy in hypogonadism. Complications of such use include acne, gynecomastia (breast enlargement), reduction of serum high-density lipoprotein and increase in low-density lipoprotein cholesterol (with inherent risk of cardiovascular disease), obstructive sleep apnea, polycythemia, platelet abnormalities, hepatic failure, decreased testicular size, and azoospermia. Behavioral effects, such as increased aggression, altered libido, and psychosis ("'roid rage") have been reported, along with signs of physiologic and psychological withdrawal.

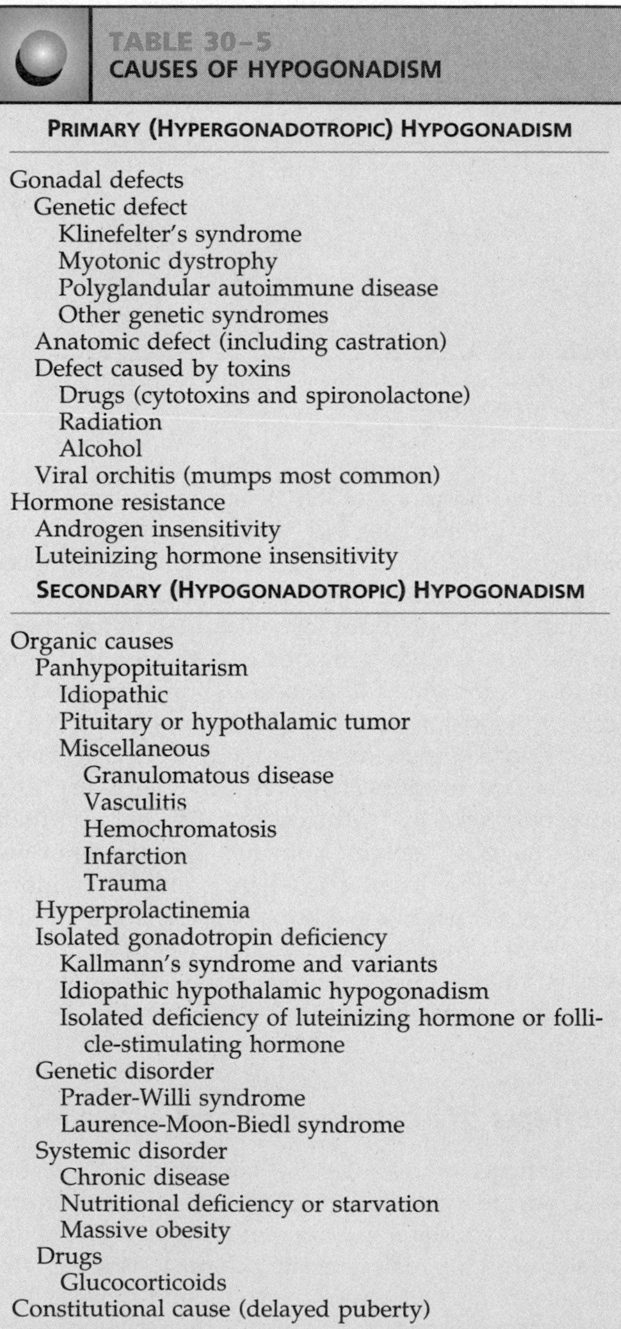

TABLE 30–5
CAUSES OF HYPOGONADISM

Primary (Hypergonadotropic) Hypogonadism

- Gonadal defects
  - Genetic defect
    - Klinefelter's syndrome
    - Myotonic dystrophy
    - Polyglandular autoimmune disease
    - Other genetic syndromes
  - Anatomic defect (including castration)
  - Defect caused by toxins
    - Drugs (cytotoxins and spironolactone)
    - Radiation
    - Alcohol
  - Viral orchitis (mumps most common)
- Hormone resistance
  - Androgen insensitivity
  - Luteinizing hormone insensitivity

Secondary (Hypogonadotropic) Hypogonadism

- Organic causes
  - Panhypopituitarism
    - Idiopathic
    - Pituitary or hypothalamic tumor
    - Miscellaneous
      - Granulomatous disease
      - Vasculitis
      - Hemochromatosis
      - Infarction
      - Trauma
  - Hyperprolactinemia
  - Isolated gonadotropin deficiency
    - Kallmann's syndrome and variants
    - Idiopathic hypothalamic hypogonadism
    - Isolated deficiency of luteinizing hormone or follicle-stimulating hormone
  - Genetic disorder
    - Prader-Willi syndrome
    - Laurence-Moon-Biedl syndrome
  - Systemic disorder
    - Chronic disease
    - Nutritional deficiency or starvation
    - Massive obesity
  - Drugs
    - Glucocorticoids
- Constitutional cause (delayed puberty)

From Bagatell, C.J., and Bremner, W.J. (1996). Androgens in men: Uses and abuses. *New England Journal of Medicine* 334(11), 711.

Role of the Y Chromosome

Presence of the Y chromosome is the genetic determinant of male sex (see Chapter 6). Embryonic development of the testes and male genital pattern requires genetic direction from DNA codes on the Y chromosome as well as presence of androgen hormone receptors, which are encoded by genetic material on the X chromosome. Autosomal DNA may also participate in directing the development of male characteristics. Genes on the long arm of the Y chromosome have been associated with regulation of spermatogenesis.[10] Microdeletions of genetic material in this region have been associated with infertility in some men.

Sexual Function

Sexual function in males has three components: erection, emission, and ejaculation. Erection occurs as a result of dilation of arterioles in the corpus cavernosum of the penis. Rapid inflow of blood results in a local increase in vascular pressure, which occludes small veins, decreasing outflow and trapping blood within the corpus. Emission, which immediately precedes ejaculation, occurs when rhythmic contraction of accessory organs and ducts fills the urethra with semen. Emission and ejaculation, the propulsion of semen to the exterior, constitute the male orgasm.

Erection, emission, and ejaculation are mediated by the autonomic nervous system and by endothelial factors. A parasympathetic neural impulse carried by pudendal nerve fibers initiates the arteriolar dilation of early erection. Relaxation of the cavernosal tissues is mediated by locally produced nitric oxide. Erection is sustained until a sympathetic reflex signals emission and ejaculation. Signals from higher centers are not essential but usually contribute to sexual function. Inputs from the limbic system, the seat of innate libido (sex drive), are of particular importance and may, in turn, be affected by higher cortical stimuli.

Priapism, which is prolonged, often painful erection in the absence of sexual stimulation, results from sludging of blood or arteriovenous shunting within the corpus cavernosum, leading to inefficient or obstructed venous outflow from the penis. Priapism is usually idiopathic or due to trauma in adults but may be associated with sickle cell disease in children. Priapism must be resolved quickly to prevent ischemic fibrosis and infertility. Treatment may involve aspiration of blood or injection of vasoactive agents. Failure to achieve satisfactory erection (erectile dysfunction) is much more common and is detailed next.

DISORDERS OF MALE REPRODUCTIVE FUNCTION

Erectile Dysfunction

Definition. Erectile dysfunction (formerly referred to as *impotence*) is the consistent inability to attain and maintain a penile erection sufficient to permit satisfactory sexual intercourse.[11]

Epidemiology. Because many men may not report sexual problems, estimation of the number affected by erectile dysfunction is imprecise. As many as 30 million men in the United States may be affected.[11] Risk factors are summarized in Table 30–6. After 40 years of age, increased time and more stimulation may be needed to achieve erection, and the refractory period between successive erections is usually longer. These are considered to be normal developmental changes.

Etiology. The etiology of erectile dysfunction may be hormonal, neurologic, vascular, or psychogenic.[12] Most men with erectile dysfunction have a physiologic cause, although psychological problems may contribute.[11]

Hormonal causes include hypogonadism, drug therapy with steroids or lipid-lowering agents, and hormonal drug treatment of prostatic disorders (e.g., LHRH agonists, estrogens, and 5α-reductase inhibitors). Metoclopramide (Reglan), used in treatment of decreased gastrointestinal motility, can cause erectile dysfunction by raising prolactin levels, thus suppressing pituitary output of gonadotropins. Patients with cirrhosis of the liver often have increased levels of circulating estrogen because of reduced hepatic inactivation (see Chapter 26).

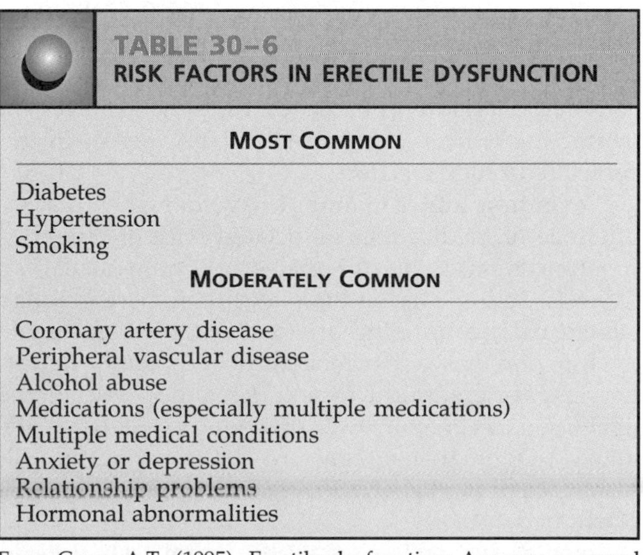

TABLE 30–6
RISK FACTORS IN ERECTILE DYSFUNCTION

MOST COMMON
Diabetes
Hypertension
Smoking
MODERATELY COMMON
Coronary artery disease
Peripheral vascular disease
Alcohol abuse
Medications (especially multiple medications)
Multiple medical conditions
Anxiety or depression
Relationship problems
Hormonal abnormalities

From Guay, A.T. (1995). Erectile dysfunction: Are you prepared to discuss it? *Postgraduate Medicine* 97(4), 130.

Neurologic impairment may result from spinal cord injury, diabetic neuropathy, multiple sclerosis, pelvic nerve injury (e.g., surgical trauma), or drug therapy with antidepressants, antihypertensives, tranquilizers, antipsychotic agents, and H_2-receptor antagonists.

Vascular causes include peripheral vascular disease, diabetic microvascular disease, and the vasoactive effects of nicotine, α-adrenergic and β-adrenergic antagonists, thiazide diuretics, sympatholytic agents, and vasodilators. Many of the older antihypertensive drugs are commonly associated with erectile dysfunction, whereas the newer agents (e.g., calcium-channel blockers and angiotensin-converting enzyme inhibitors) carry a low risk.[13]

Psychogenic causes may include anxiety, depression, or relationship problems. Erectile dysfunction in this setting can further exacerbate emotional problems in a positive feedback loop.

Pathophysiology. Lack of the autonomic signal, impairment of perfusion, or both may interfere with arteriolar dilation. Inappropriate adrenergic stimulation due to anxiety or with use of certain medications may mimic the effect of ejaculation, causing premature collapse of the sacs of the corpus cavernosum. Venous incompetence or decreased inflow pressure of blood may result in shunting of blood around the sacs into medium-sized veins, preventing the sacs from filling completely. *Pelvic steal syndrome* may result in loss of erection before ejaculation in cases in which increased blood flow to pelvic muscles during intercourse (with penile thrusting) "steals" perfusion from the corpus cavernosum. Typically, this perfusion was initially compromised by partial obstruction of small arteries.[13]

Clinical Manifestations. Erectile dysfunction usually presents as difficulty obtaining the initial erection or achieving adequate rigidity.[13] Early detumescence, or loss of erection, is also common. Interruption of the autonomic reflex arc may result in complete flaccidity of the penis, whereas lack of neural input from higher centers may result in uncontrolled reflex erection.

Prevention and Treatment. Avoidance or discontinuance of medications associated with erectile dysfunction is advisable for males in whom sexual activity is desired. Individuals and their partners may benefit from counseling or sex therapy when erectile dysfunction has a psychogenic component. Newer, nerve-sparing surgical techniques aim to reduce the likelihood of erectile dysfunction due to traumatic injury. Optimal management of contributing illnesses, such as diabetes or cardiovascular disease, is warranted.

Erectile dysfunction may be definitively treated with drug therapy, vacuum constriction devices, self-injection therapy, or penile prostheses. The α_2-adrenergic antagonist yohimbine (Yocon) may enhance parasympathetic neurotransmission, resulting in more satisfactory erections in some men. Testosterone supplementation is indicated only for men who are hypogonadal and is avoided in men with prostate cancer. The vacuum constriction device consists of a hollow cylinder placed over the penis and a pump mechanism that applies negative pressure to pull blood into the corpus cavernosum. A constricting ring is then placed at the base of the penis, trapping blood and sustaining the erection. Injection of vasoactive agents, such as prostaglandin E, directly into the corpus cavernosum with a fine-gauge needle may induce an erection for 30 to 60 minutes in some men. Surgical implantation of a malleable or inflatable penile prosthesis is a less common but permanent intervention in erectile dysfunction.

Prognosis and Outcome. Yohimbine has resulted in subjective improvement in 40% of men taking the drug.[12] Half of hypogonadal men achieve erections with testosterone supplementation. Sixty-eight per cent of men using vacuum constriction and 79% of men using self-injection report satisfaction with this therapy, as do 90% of men with penile implants.

Cryptorchidism

Definition. Cryptorchidism is the failure of one or both testes to descend into the scrotum during the fetal period. The testis may remain within the abdominal cavity or inguinal canal, or may be located ectopically, outside the normal pathway of descent (Fig. 30–7). A testis that has been fully descended at one time but that later becomes cryptorchid is known as a *retractile testis*.

Epidemiology. An estimated 5.9% of male infants have cryptorchidism at birth, and 1.6% of infants demonstrate the condition at 3 months of age.[14] Major risk factors are prematurity and deficiency of testosterone. A genetic predisposition may be involved in a minority of cases, and the incidence increases in infants with neural tube defects and in a number of rare, inherited metabolic disorders.

Etiology. The precise cause of cryptorchidism is unknown. The most prevalent hypothesis is one of hormonal imbalance. Deficiency of testosterone, owing to a defect at some point on the hypothalamic–pituitary–gonadal axis, may result in failure of gonadal differentiation and descent, usually affecting both testes. Maternal antibodies against fetal gonadotropins have been found to be elevated in some studies, and affected infants have demonstrated decreased levels of LH. Mechanical obstruction due to structural abnormality (such as ectopic location of

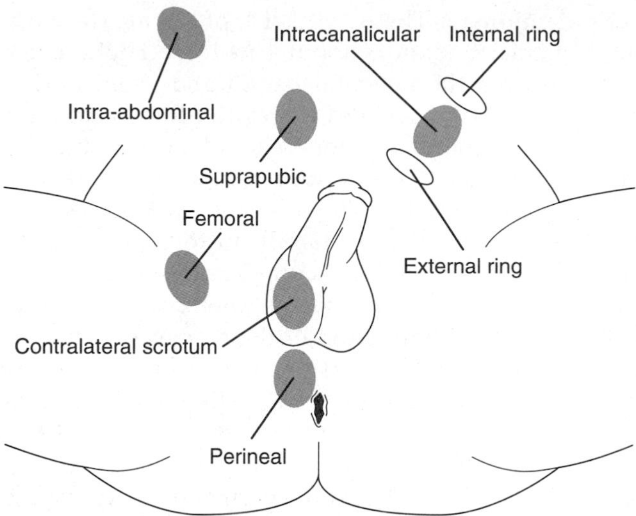

FIGURE 30–7

Cryptorchid and ectopic testes. One or both testes may fail to descend normally from their intra-abdominal sites of embyronic development. *Cryptorchidism* refers to retention of the testis within the abdomen or within the normal pathway of descent (the inguinal canal), whereas *ectopic testis* refers to a location of the testis outside the normal pathway of descent (e.g., suprapubic area, perineal area, femoral area, or contralateral scrotum).

the testis or short spermatic cord) may also impede descent, usually of one testis.

Pathophysiology. The undescended testis is maintained at higher temperature than is optimum for spermatogenesis. Faulty spermatogenesis leads to reduced fertility. The significantly increased risk of neoplasia in undescended testes may be due to inherent abnormality of the testis or to abnormal division of germ cells due to higher testicular temperature.

Clinical Manifestations. Lack of testicular mass within the scrotum is apparent. Infertility may manifest after maturity in untreated males. By the age of 2 years, 40% of undescended testes demonstrate azoospermia.[14]

Prevention and Treatment. Early intervention is advisable to prevent the complication of infertility and to reduce the risk of subsequent testicular cancer. Medical treatment consists of hormone replacement with exogenous testosterone or with human chorionic gonadotropin, which consists mainly of LH and thus stimulates endogenous testosterone production. Surgical correction of cryptorchidism (orchiopexy) is most often recommended and should be done between the ages of 6 and 18 months.

Prognosis and Outcome. Hormonal therapy is most effective in retractile testes but may induce descent of a cryptorchid testis if it is in a low position. Surgical therapy is successful in 90% to 95% of cases.[14] Fertility is greatly reduced in untreated males, and their risk of testicular cancer is increased by 10-fold to 40-fold.[15] Early treatment reduces, but does not remove, these risks.

Testicular Cancer

Definition. Testicular cancers are malignant neoplasms of testicular tissue or germ cells.

Epidemiology. Testicular cancers constitute 1% of all cancers in males and are the leading cause of death due to illness in males aged 15 to 35 years.[16] A lesser peak in incidence is seen after 75 years of age. As previously mentioned, the incidence of testicular cancer has been increasing at a rate of about 2.8% per year, for reasons that are uncertain. The incidence in white men is four times that in blacks. Cryptorchidism is the most significant risk factor. Males with chromosomal abnormalities, such as Klinefelter's syndrome, are also at higher risk, and there is a six-fold increase in incidence among first-degree relatives of men with testicular cancer.

Etiology. The precise etiology of testicular cancer is unknown.

Pathophysiology. Ninety-five per cent of testicular cancers arise from germ cells associated with some stage of spermatogenesis, whereas 5% are derived from stromal or sex cord cells.[17] The most common and least malignant form of testicular cancer is the *seminoma,* which originates within the seminiferous tubules. Some testicular cancers secrete sex hormones, resulting in paraneoplastic syndromes of virilization or feminization. Testicular cancers are classified in Table 30–7.

Clinical Manifestations. A painless scrotal mass is evident early as a small nodule at the front or side of the testis. Pain and obstructive signs and symptoms may occur later as the cancer extends locally and metastasizes through the lymphatic system. Signs of ectopic hormone production include changes in skin texture, hair distribution, and muscle mass consistent with feminization or virilization; gynecomastia is common in non–germ cell tumors.

Prevention and Treatment. Early treatment of cryptorchidism reduces the risk of testicular cancer. Testicular self-examination, involving systematic palpation, promotes early detection of testicular masses. Treatment of testicular cancer is based on the cell type of origin and on the stage of the disease (Fig. 30–8). Surgical removal of the affected testis (orchiectomy) is the initial treatment. Retroperitoneal lymph node dissection (RPLND), the exploration and removal of affected regional lymph nodes, is often performed as well, although the extent of the procedure varies depending on the stage. In some cases, chemotherapy is used instead of, or in addition to, RPLND. Seminomas are particularly respon-

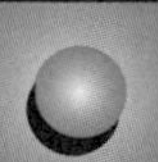

TABLE 30–7
CLASSIFICATION OF TESTICULAR CANCERS

Germ Cell Tumors
Tumors of one histologic pattern
Seminoma
Spermatocytic seminoma
Embryonal carcinoma
Yolk sac tumor (embryonal carcinoma, infantile type)
Polyembryoma
Choriocarcinoma
Teratomas
Mature
Immature
With malignant transformation
Tumors showing more than one histologic pattern
Embryonal carcinoma plus teratoma (teratocarcinoma)
Choriocarcinoma and any other types (specify types)
Other combinations (specify)
Sex Cord–Stromal Tumors
Well-differentiated forms
Leydig cell tumor
Sertoli cell tumor
Granulosa cell tumor
Mixed forms (specify)
Incompletely differentiated forms

From Cotran, R.S., Kumar, V., and Robbins, S.L. (1994). *Robbins Pathologic Basis of Disease.* (5th ed.). Philadelphia: W.B. Saunders. (p. 1015.)

sive to radiation therapy, which may be substituted for RPLND in many cases. Cisplatin-based chemotherapy has shown significant cure rates even in advanced seminoma. Treatment of testicular cancer with high-dose chemotherapy may be supported with autologous bone marrow transplantation as "rescue" therapy (see Chapter 12).

Prognosis and Outcome. Prognosis depends on tumor classification and stage but is generally good. For seminomas limited to the testis, more than 95% of patients experience long-term disease-free survival with appropriate treatment.[15] Nearly 85% of those with non–germ cells tumors achieve complete remission.[17] The least favorable prognosis is found with highly malignant cancers of embryonic origin (*choriocarcinomas*). These tumors more often affect the female genital tract and are discussed in Chapter 32.

Testicular Torsion

Definition. Testicular torsion is an acute ischemic injury of the testis due to its rotation around the vascular pedicle of the spermatic cord.

Epidemiology. The overall risk of a male developing testicular torsion is about 1 in 160.[14] Highest risk occurs during the neonatal period and again during puberty. The risk declines thereafter. Risk factors for neonatal torsion have not been identified, but infants with torsion of one testis are at increased risk of developing torsion of the other. Risk factors for pubertal torsion include family history and a horizontal lie of the testis. Acute torsion occurs more frequently during the winter months, apparently owing to reflex contraction of the cremaster muscle.

Etiology. Testicular torsion in neonates is caused by a maldeveloped tunica vaginalis membrane that nearly surrounds the entire spermatic cord and testis[18] (Fig. 30–9). In pubertal torsion, incomplete attachment of the testis and spermatic fascia to the scrotal wall leaves the testis free to rotate around its vascular pedicle.

Pathophysiology. Twisting of the spermatic cord causes venous occlusion, resulting in acute ischemia, scrotal edema, and possible third spacing of fluid (hydrocele). Irreversible testicular damage occurs within a matter of hours. In 80% of cases, the testis is no longer viable after 12 hours of torsion.[14]

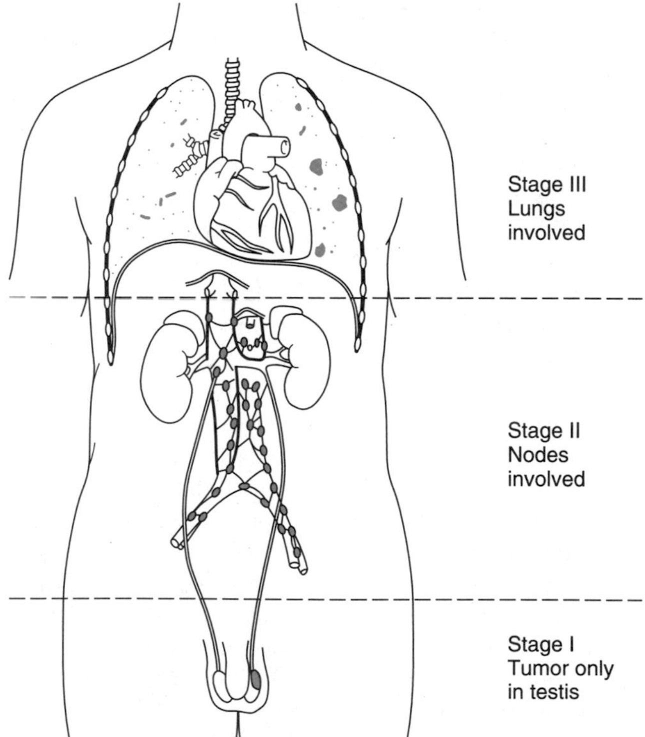

FIGURE 30–8
Staging of testicular cancer. A common staging system for seminoma is pictured. Stage I cancer is confined to the testis, stage II extends to regional lymph nodes, and stage III demonstrates dissemination beyond regional nodes to distant organs such as the lungs, bones, or other viscera. (Redrawn from Brock, D., Fox, S., Goslin, G., *et al.* [1993]. Testicular cancer. *Seminars in Oncology Nursing* 9[4], 226.)

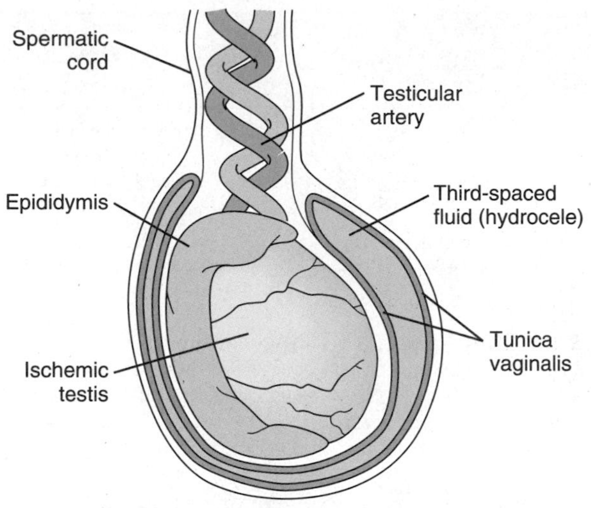

FIGURE 30–9
Testicular torsion. As a consequence of abnormal development of the tunica vaginalis or incomplete attachment of the testis to the scrotal wall, the testis may rotate about its vascular pedicle. The resulting venous occlusion causes acute ischemia, scrotal edema, and possibly third spacing of fluid (hydrocele).

Clinical Manifestations. On the affected side, the scrotum is edematous, ecchymotic, and elevated ("bell-clapper" deformity).[18] In pubertal torsion, the patient usually experiences acute onset of severe testicular pain, abdominal pain, nausea, and vomiting. Twisting of the spermatic cord may be palpable.

Prevention and Treatment. In neonates, surgical fixation of the contralateral testis may prevent its subsequent torsion and preserve gonadal function. Surgical removal of a nonviable testis decreases the risk of antisperm antibody formation and subsequent infertility. Treatment of acute testicular torsion is done on an emergent basis. Manual detorsion, in which the testis is twisted counterclockwise, may be attempted in an effort to improve blood flow before surgery. Surgical fixation (orchiopexy) is the treatment of choice. If the testis is nonviable, orchiectomy is performed.

Prognosis and Outcome. When surgery is performed within 6 hours of the onset of pain, the rate of testicular salvage approaches 100%.[18] Surgical fixation preserves Leydig cell function and testosterone production. Spermatogenesis is usually reduced, possibly owing to the formation of antisperm antibodies in response to testicular antigens released during the ischemic episode.[14]

Inguinal Hernia

Definition. Inguinal hernia is the protrusion of abdominal viscera, usually a loop of bowel, through a weakened area of the abdominal wall in the inguinal or groin region. In *indirect* inguinal hernia, protrusion is through the inguinal canal. In males, the herniated bowel often descends into the scrotal sac. In *direct* inguinal hernia, protrusion is through a weakened area other than the inguinal canal.

Epidemiology. Inguinal hernias may be congenital or acquired and are the most common of several types of herniation of viscera through the abdominal wall (Fig. 30–10). Congenital hernias are the most common of all congenital anomalies, occurring in an estimated 10 to 20 infants per 1000 live births.[19] Inguinal hernias are much more common in males but may occur in females as well, with herniation into the labia. Prematurity is a significant risk factor for congenital hernia. General risk factors include the following: (1) factors that weaken the abdominal wall, such as congenital weakness, lack of exercise, aging, and poorly healed surgical incisions; and (2) factors that increase intra-abdominal pressure, such as obesity, pregnancy, heavy lifting or straining, violent coughing, and in infants, vigorous crying.

Etiology. Herniation results from the combination of abdominal wall weakness and increased intra-abdominal pressure.

Pathophysiology. Protrusion of abdominal viscera through the abdominal wall creates a bulge in the scrotal sac or in an area of the abdominal wall. Visceral function is not adversely affected unless the contents of the sac become obstructed or ischemic. If the sac contents can be manipulated back into normal position, the hernia is said to be *reducible*. If not

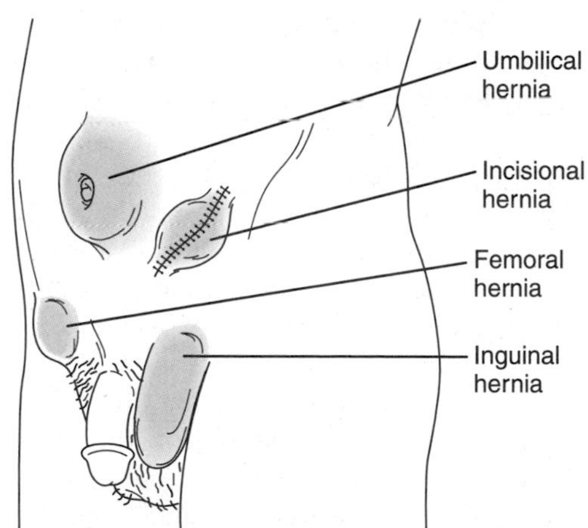

FIGURE 30–10
Types of hernias. Hernias result from congenital or acquired weakness of the abdominal wall, which bulges outward from intra-abdominal pressure. Obstruction of perfusion to abdominal viscera in the area of the bulge may occur with strangulation or incarceration of the hernia. The umbilical region, femoral ring, and inguinal canal are often congenitally weak. The inguinal canal is an especially common site of muscular wall weakness in males and may permit herniation of a loop of bowel into the scrotum. Inadequately healed abdominal incisions may also give rise to hernias.

easily reducible, the hernia is said to be *incarcerated* and may become *strangulated* if blood flow to the bowel or other visceral contents is obstructed.

Clinical Manifestations. In reducible hernias, the only clinical evidence may be the bulge within the scrotal sac or on the abdominal wall. If scrotal swelling persists after reduction of the hernia, hydrocele may be present. Strangulation is a surgical emergency, potentially leading to scrotal edema, ischemic pain, bowel obstruction, peritonitis, and septic shock.

Prevention and Treatment. Many hernias in adults are preventable with weight control, maintenance of muscle strength with exercise, and appropriate technique during lifting. Most hernias are treated with manual reduction, aided by positioning and sedation. In adults, a truss may be used to provide external support to the weakened area. Nonreducible hernias are surgically repaired with herniorrhaphy. Scrotal edema is managed supportively with elevation and ice packs.

Prognosis and Outcome. Incarcerated hernias that are not strangulated can be manually reduced in 80% of cases. Herniorrhaphy is a relatively benign procedure with few complications.

Sexually Transmitted Diseases

Definition. STDs (formerly referred to as venereal diseases) are infections affecting both males and females that are communicated primarily through sexual contact. In the United States, the most prevalent STDs are **syphilis, gonorrhea, chlamydia, genital herpes, genital warts, trichomoniasis**, and acquired immunodeficiency syndrome (AIDS). AIDS is discussed in detail in Chapter 13.

Epidemiology. The annual incidence of STD has been estimated at 12 million in the United States.[20] Risk factors are primarily behavioral, derived from frequent, unprotected sexual activity. Risk rises exponentially with the number of sexual partners. Presence of genital lesions due to one STD may predispose to superinfection with another STD organism. Immunosuppressed people are at higher risk for all types of infections (see Chapter 13). Syphilis and AIDS may be acquired in utero by the fetus, and infants may be infected with other STDs during vaginal delivery by infected mothers.

Etiology. The infectious agent is a bacterium in syphilis, gonorrhea, and chlamydia. AIDS, genital herpes, and genital warts are viral infections. Trichomoniasis is caused by a protozoan parasite. Table 30–8 lists causative organisms implicated in STDs.

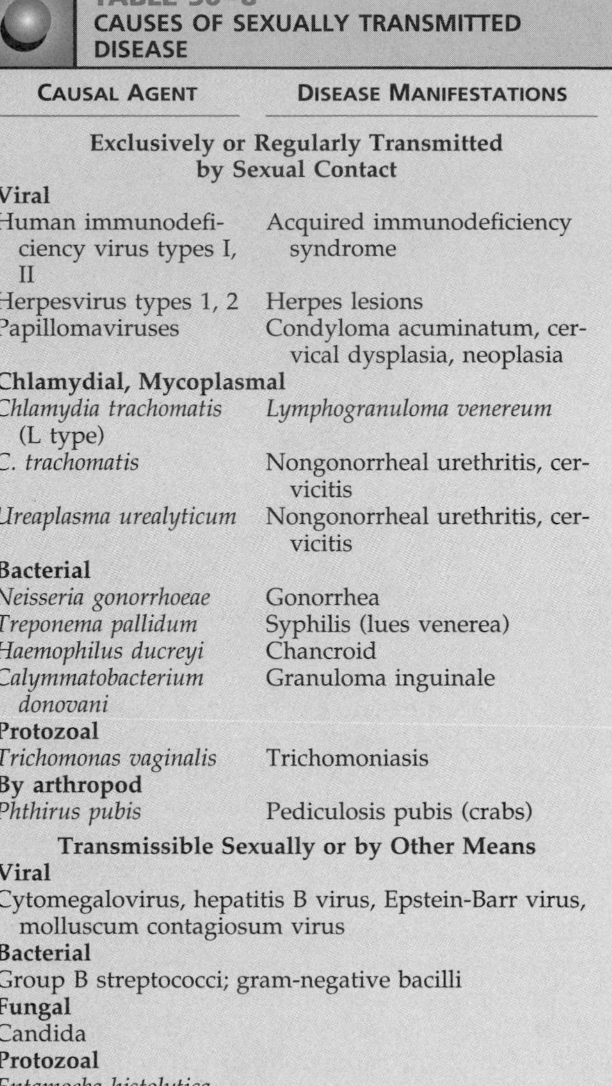

TABLE 30–8
CAUSES OF SEXUALLY TRANSMITTED DISEASE

CAUSAL AGENT	DISEASE MANIFESTATIONS
Exclusively or Regularly Transmitted by Sexual Contact	
Viral	
Human immunodeficiency virus types I, II	Acquired immunodeficiency syndrome
Herpesvirus types 1, 2	Herpes lesions
Papillomaviruses	Condyloma acuminatum, cervical dysplasia, neoplasia
Chlamydial, Mycoplasmal	
Chlamydia trachomatis (L type)	*Lymphogranuloma venereum*
C. trachomatis	Nongonorrheal urethritis, cervicitis
Ureaplasma urealyticum	Nongonorrheal urethritis, cervicitis
Bacterial	
Neisseria gonorrhoeae	Gonorrhea
Treponema pallidum	Syphilis (lues venerea)
Haemophilus ducreyi	Chancroid
Calymmatobacterium donovani	Granuloma inguinale
Protozoal	
Trichomonas vaginalis	Trichomoniasis
By arthropod	
Phthirus pubis	Pediculosis pubis (crabs)
Transmissible Sexually or by Other Means	
Viral	
Cytomegalovirus, hepatitis B virus, Epstein-Barr virus, molluscum contagiosum virus	
Bacterial	
Group B streptococci; gram-negative bacilli	
Fungal	
Candida	
Protozoal	
Entamoeba histolytica	

From Cotran, R.S., Kumar, V., and Robbins, S.L. (1994). *Robbins Pathologic Basis of Disease.* (5th ed.). Philadelphia: W.B. Saunders. (p. 340).

Pathophysiology. After exposure to the causative organism, there is a variable incubation period during which the patient is usually symptom free. Skin lesions then become apparent in most cases, and discharge (urethral or vaginal) may be noted. The causative organism is present in lesions or discharge and may be transmitted by sexual activity unless barriers are employed. Untreated infections may disseminate to other organ systems, causing signs of systemic inflammation and specific organ dysfunction. Although rare in the United States, untreated syphilis may lead to death due to infiltration of the aorta and aortic valve.

Clinical Manifestations. Clinical manifestations of the more prevalent STDs are summarized in Table 30–9. Systemic signs of inflammation are generally vague and may not be present at all. Characteristics of the discharge and skin lesions (Color Figs. 30–1

TABLE 30–9
CLINICAL MANIFESTATIONS OF PREVALENT SEXUALLY TRANSMITTED DISEASES

Disease	Clinical Manifestations
Syphilis	*Incubation period:* 10–90 d (average, 3 wk) *Primary stage:* Painless chancre at site of infection, possible phimosis due to edema, enlarged inguinal lymph nodes *Secondary stage:* Early macular or roseolar rash, generalized lymphadenopathy, influenza-like syndrome, late papular rash *Tertiary stage:* Mucocutaneous lesions; cardiovascular, neural, and visceral infiltration
Gonorrhea	*Incubation period:* 3–8 d *Manifestations in males:* May be asymptomatic; purulent discharge from anterior urethra, dysuria, urinary frequency *Manifestations in females:* May be asymptomatic; purulent discharge (heavy, yellow-green), cervical erythema, vulvar inflammation, menstrual abnormalities, dysuria, urinary frequency
Chlamydia	*Incubation period:* 7–21 d *Manifestations in males:* May be asymptomatic; white or clear urethral discharge, mild dysuria, possible epididymitis *Manifestations in females:* May be asymptomatic; vaginal discharge (yellow, mucopurulent), midcycle bleeding, dysuria, Bartholin's duct obstruction, possible pelvic inflammatory disease
Genital herpes	*Incubation period:* 3–7 d *First-episode primary disease:* Prodrome of malaise, fever, headache, myalgias, and genital paresthesias; multiple, painful, bilateral vesicles that become ulcerated *First-episode nonprimary disease* (patient with previous unrecognized exposure and antibody development): Fewer lesions, less pain, fewer systemic symptoms, faster healing *Recurrent disease* (follows an identified first episode): Prodrome of pruritus, tingling or dysesthesias; eruption of a single lesion, vaginal discharge, dysuria
Genital warts	*Incubation period:* 1–2 m *Manifestations in males:* Clusters of painless warts on the glans, urethral meatus, or anorectal area; may bleed with friction *Manifestations in females:* Clusters of painless warts on the vulva, vagina, cervix, perineum, urethral meatus, or anorectal area; may bleed with friction
Trichomoniasis	*Manifestations in males:* May be asymptomatic; urethritis, prostatitis *Manifestations in females:* Persistent vaginitis, vaginal discharge (thin, gray or yellow, frothy, odorous), vulvar itching, dyspareunia, dysuria

through 30–6) provide presumptive diagnosis of specific disorders, with confirmation by detection of the causative organism in serum or by culture of lesions or discharge.

Prevention and Treatment. Prevention of STDs depends on behavioral interventions to reduce high-risk sexual activity and on the use of barrier methods such as condoms to protect against transmission of organisms. Identification and treatment of partners of infected people, whether they do or do not have symptoms, is central to public health programs aimed at eradicating STD. Syphilis, gonorrhea, and chlamydia are treated with appropriate antibiotic therapy. Genital herpes may be treated with the antiviral agent acyclovir (Zovirax) to reduce the severity and recurrence rate of infection. There is no curative therapy for herpes, however. Trichomoniasis is treated with the antibiotic metronidazole (Flagyl). Warts are treated with local eradication of lesions by cryotherapy (freezing), laser treatment, or surgical excision. Treatment of AIDS is discussed in Chapter 13.

Prognosis and Outcome. With the notable exception of AIDS, STDs may be cured or effectively controlled with therapy. In females, infertility is a significant long-term complication of an STD that has extended locally into the reproductive system (see Chapter 32). Although the prevalence of specific types of STDs has varied during the past several decades, the overall incidence of STDs has continued to rise despite medical and behavioral intervention.

Epididymitis

Definition. Epididymitis is inflammation of the epididymis and its ducts.

Epidemiology. Epididymitis is a relatively common infection in patients prone to STD or urinary tract infection; thus risk factors for those conditions apply (see Chapter 20). Rarely, the epididymis is infected secondarily to a systemic infection such as tuberculosis.

Etiology. Most cases result from ascending infection with sexually transmitted gonorrhea or chlamydia, or from urinary tract infection with *Escherichia coli*, streptococci, or staphylococci.

Pathophysiology. Organisms ascend the vas deferens or lymphatics to the epididymis, initiating inflammation. Other reproductive organs may also be involved, including the testes (**orchitis**) and prostate (**prostatitis**). Chronic inflammation with recurrent episodes may result in scarring and obstruction of the ducts.

Clinical Manifestations. Local inflammation results in scrotal swelling, which is often severe and painful. Dysuria, pyuria, and urethral discharge are common with epididymitis, and systemic signs of inflammation, including fever and malaise, are often present. Infertility may result from prolonged obstruction.

Prevention and Treatment. Measures for prevention of STDs and urinary tract infections are applicable. Appropriate antibiotic therapy is administered, and supportive measures such as bed rest and scrotal elevation are employed. Chronically affected males in whom sterility is acceptable may consider vasectomy to interrupt the pathway for ascent of organisms.

Prognosis and Outcome. Treatment of acute epididymitis with antibiotics is generally effective. Recurrent episodes may respond to treatment, but the risk of infertility is greater in these men.

Benign Prostatic Hyperplasia

Definition. BPH is the nonmalignant enlargement of the prostate gland due to excessive growth of both the glandular and stromal elements of the gland.[21]

Epidemiology. BPH is common, and its prevalence increases in a direct linear relationship to age, affecting up to 50% of men older than 50 years and 75% of men older than 80 years.[22] Aging is therefore the most significant risk factor.

Etiology. The precise etiology is unknown. Because growth of the prostate is under endocrine control, the cause of hyperplasia has been hypothesized to be an age-related imbalance in androgenic stimulation of the gland. DHT, the androgen that exerts the most potent growth-promoting effect on prostatic tissue, accumulates in the gland and binds to receptors in the transitional zone surrounding the urethra.

Pathophysiology. The clinical effects of BPH result from both static and dynamic components of the disease. The static component is prostatic enlargement, with resulting compression of the bladder neck and obstruction of urine flow. The dynamic component relates to periodic increases in sympathetic stimulation of the smooth muscle of the prostatic urethra and bladder neck.

Clinical Manifestations. The prostate is palpably enlarged on digital rectal examination. Static (obstructive) signs include hesitancy and intermittency in voiding, weak urinary stream, straining to void, and dribbling. Dynamic (irritative) signs and symptoms include urgency, feeling of incomplete emptying of the bladder, and possible overflow incontinence (see Chapter 20). Dynamic symptoms are often worse with stress. Increased force of bladder contraction compensates for obstruction at first, but urinary stasis eventually occurs, evidenced by a palpable suprapubic bulge due to distention of the bladder. Urinary stasis increases the risk of urinary tract infection and urolithiasis, as discussed in Chapter 20. BPH can result in an elevated serum level of **prostate-specific antigen (PSA)**, although usually not to the same degree as that due to prostate cancer (see later discussion).

Prevention and Treatment. There is no known prevention for BPH. Medical and surgical treatments are available, with the decision depending on severity of the condition and patient preference. Those with mild to moderate symptoms are often treated initially with "watchful waiting" to determine if obstructive manifestations worsen. If clinical manifestations are distressing, the patient may be treated medically with α-adrenergic blocking agents, such as terazosin hydrochloride (Hytrin), to reduce the dynamic symptoms. The drug finasteride (Proscar) may be used to block the 5α-reductase enzyme, which converts testosterone to DHT, resulting in some shrinkage of the prostate and modest relief of obstructive symptoms in many cases.

Several surgical procedures are used in treatment of more severe BPH. Surgical resection of the prostate may be accomplished with either a transurethral approach (transurethral resection of the prostate) or an open approach (suprapubic prostatectomy). A less extensive approach, transurethral incision of the prostate, may be sufficient in some cases. In this procedure, incisions are made to relieve bladder outlet obstruction, with no removal of prostatic tissue. Balloon dilation of the urethra and insertion of prostatic stents may be used to maintain urethral patency, and laser excision techniques and microwave therapy are in experimental use for relief of prostatic enlargement.

Prognosis and Outcome. In some studies, treatment with finasteride has been reported to result in a 20% to 30% reduction in prostate size.[23] α-Adrenergic blocking agents, such as terazosin, are effective in relieving dynamic symptoms in most cases (see Focus of Current Research). Transurethral resec-

Focus of Current Research

Study	Objective and Findings
Laumann, et al. (1997) Circumcision in the United States: Prevalence, prophylactic effects, and sexual practice.	*Objective:* To assess the prevalence of circumcision across various social groups and to examine the health and sexual outcomes of circumcision *Findings:* No significant differences were found between circumcised and uncircumcised men in their likelihood of contracting sexually transmitted diseases. Uncircumcised men were slightly more likely to experience sexual dysfunction, especially later in life.
Natchigall, et al. (1997) Adult-onset idiopathic hypogonadotropic hypogonadism: A treatable form of male infertility.	*Objective:* To characterize the clinical and biochemical features of men developing gonadotropin-releasing hormone (GnRH) deficiency after puberty, without an identifiable cause *Findings:* Compared with men with classic GnRH deficiency, men with the adult-onset form had higher testicular volumes, serum testosterone levels, and serum inhibin B concentrations. Treatment with GnRH reversed the hypogonadism and restored fertility in men with the adult-onset form.
Linet, et al. (1996) Efficacy and safety of intracavernosal alprostadil in men with erectile dysfunction.	*Objective:* To investigate the efficacy and safety of intracavernosal injection of a vasodilator agent in erectile dysfunction *Findings:* The therapy was 94% successful, with tolerable side effects of pain, bruising, or prolonged erection.
Lepor, et al. (1996) The efficacy of terazosin, finasteride, or both in benign prostatic hyperplasia.	*Objective:* To compare the efficacy of these drugs, singly and in combination, with placebo *Findings:* Terazosin was effective, whereas finasteride was not. The combination of the two drugs was no more effective than terazosin alone.
Potosky, et al. (1995) The role of increasing detection in the rising incidence of prostate cancer.	*Objective:* To assess the reasons for the dramatic surge in prostate cancer incidence from 1986 to 1991 *Findings:* The recent increase is due to increased intensity of medical surveillance for the disorder.
Krahn, et al. (1994) Screening for prostate cancer: A decision analytic view.	*Objective:* To determine the clinical and economic effects of screening for prostate cancer *Findings:* Screening may result in poorer health outcomes and will increase costs dramatically.

Continued on following page

continued

Epstein, et al. (1994) Pathologic and clinical findings to predict tumor extent of nonpalpable (stage T1c) prostate cancer.	*Objective:* To examine preoperative clinical and pathologic parameters in men with early prostate cancer and to correlate these findings with the pathologic extent of disease in the surgical specimen in an attempt to identify a subset of patients who might be followed with watchful waiting *Findings:* 84% of tumors were higher grade, warranting immediate treatment. 16% were insignificant and could have been followed with watchful waiting.
Field, et al. (1994) The relation of smoking, age, relative weight, and dietary intake to serum adrenal steroids, sex hormones, and sex hormone–binding globulin in middle-aged men.	*Objective:* To examine the relationships of a variety of potential risk factors with serum levels of adrenal steroids, sex hormones, and sex hormone–binding globulin *Findings:* Adrenal steroid and sex hormone concentrations are more influenced by cigarette smoking and obesity than by dietary intake.

tion of the prostate may cause considerable blood loss, urethral stricture, and nerve damage, leading to erectile dysfunction or incontinence. Newer, nerve-sparing surgical therapies are associated with fewer complications.

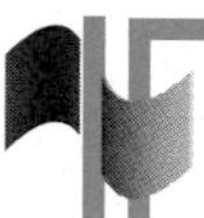

Clinical Scenario

C.P., aged 65 years, sees his family physician at the insistence of his wife, who is distressed by his need to get up three or four times a night to urinate. C.P. reports difficulty starting his urinary stream and a decreased, slow stream. He has also been embarrassed by slight incontinence after urinating, and has avoided playing golf because of this. Rectal examination reveals a moderately enlarged prostate gland, without any nodularity or hardness. The remainder of C.P.'s physical examination is normal.

1. Could C.P.'s urinary symptoms be caused by enlargement of the prostate? Explain.
2. Do these clinical findings represent normal developmental changes? Do they warrant further evaluation? What tests might be done?

Prostate Cancer

Definition. Prostate cancer is a malignant neoplasm of the prostate gland.

Epidemiology. An estimated 318,000 men in the United States were diagnosed with prostate cancer in 1996, nearly double the rate of 1993.[24] Prostate cancer is now the second-leading cause of cancer death (behind lung cancer) in males. The dramatic increase in the incidence of prostate cancer in recent years has been attributed to more aggressive screening and detection procedures. Aging is the most significant risk factor for prostate cancer, with most cases diagnosed in men older than 65 years. The death rate due to prostatic cancer is twice as high in black males as in whites. A familial predisposition is also evident. Several other risk factors have been suggested by epidemiologic studies but remain unproved. These include increased consumption of red meat and dairy products, excessive intake of essential fatty acids (especially the combination of high α-linoleic acid and low linoleic acid), and history of vasectomy.[25]

Etiology. The precise etiology of prostate cancer is unknown.

Pathophysiology. Ninety-five per cent of prostate cancers are adenocarcinomas, arising in the peripheral zone of the prostate.[26] Sarcomas, transitional cell carcinomas (associated with bladder cancer), small

Developmental Perspective

Embryonic and Fetal Periods

Early embryos exhibit indifferent gonads, capable of development either as males or females. During the seventh week of gestation, the testes begin to develop under the influence of the testis-determining factor (TDF) gene on the Y chromosome. The epididymis, vas deferens, and ejaculatory ducts develop from the mesonephric (wolffian) ducts of the male embryo. Testosterone production by the fetal testis begins during the eighth week, stimulating further development of the male genitalia. The testes develop within the abdominal cavity and normally descend through the inguinal canals into the scrotum by 32 weeks' gestation. Cryptorchidism, or undescended testis, occurs in about 30% of premature males and in about 3% of full-term males. Weakness of the inguinal canal may cause congenital inguinal hernia. Rarely, chromosomal defects may result in various degrees of indeterminate sex (hermaphroditism or intersexuality). Malposition of the urethral meatus is common, whereas other penile abnormalities are rare.

Infancy and Childhood

Neonatal circumcision is common in the United States, although its medical indication is questionable. The infant's prostate gland is about the size of an almond, and it changes little in size until puberty. In many cases of cryptorchidism, the undescended testis descends spontaneously within 3 months. Neonates are one of the at-risk groups for testicular torsion, which is likely to affect both testes in sequence.

Adolescence and Young Adulthood

Normal puberty in boys begins before the age of 15 years. Maturation of the genitalia and development of secondary sex characteristics becomes evident, and spermatogenesis begins. Boys who do not manifest signs of puberty by this time may have primary hypogonadism or a constitutional delay of puberty. The prostate gland grows rapidly, soon doubling in size. Young men are normally easily able to achieve an erection by fantasizing. STDs, abuse of anabolic steroids, infertility, testicular torsion, and testicular cancer are prevalent in this age group.

Middle and Older Adulthood

There is no "male menopause," or specific cessation of male reproductive function with aging. Although testosterone levels decline, spermatogenesis may continue throughout the life of the male. Fertility may be reduced, owing to decreased motility of sperm. About two thirds of men older than 55 years have some manifestations of prostatic enlargement due to BPH, leading to manifestations of urinary obstruction. Expected developmental changes in sexual function include the need for more time and stimulation to achieve erection, and a longer refractory period between erections. The incidence of erectile dysfunction increases with aging, often due to neuropathy, vascular disease, or the effects of medications. Eighty per cent of cases of prostate cancer are diagnosed in men older than 65 years.

---

cell carcinomas, and squamous cell carcinomas are much less common. The prostate may be a site of metastasis from cancers of the lung, colon, and bladder. Under the influence of androgens, prostatic enlargement occurs, giving rise to manifestations of urinary obstruction and possibly erectile dysfunction. As the tumor spreads throughout most of the gland, the prostate becomes hard and extends through its outer capsule into the seminal vesicles, bladder neck, and pelvic lymph nodes. Metastasis to the liver and to bone may occur by the hematogenous route. Uncontrolled growth leads to increased serum levels of PSA, a glycoprotein secreted by prostate cells, and prostate-specific membrane antigen, a protein bound to the membranes of prostate cells.

Clinical Manifestations. Digital rectal examination reveals a prostatic mass or hardness, nodularity, and fixation of the prostate. Transrectal ultrasonography may detect some nonpalpable tumors. Signs of urinary obstruction are identical to those of BPH but usually progress more rapidly. Elevated PSA levels are suggestive of, but not always specific for, prostate cancer. PSA production increases proportionately to the volume of the gland, which typically increases with age-associated BPH. Cancer cells produce more PSA per gram of tissue than do normal prostate cells or those present in BPH. Age-specific norms have been used as reference points for PSA elevation, and additional tests, such as the more specific prostate-specific membrane antigen, have been used in screening for prostate cancer and in monitoring of response to therapy. The rate of change in PSA value over time (PSA velocity) and the PSA density (PSA value divided by the volume of the prostate gland) may also provide more meaningful data than PSA values alone. Bony metastasis in advanced prostate cancer may result in low back pain and pathogenic fractures.

Prevention and Treatment. There is no known prevention. The value of mass screening for prostate cancer is controversial because the choice of subsequent treatment is also uncertain. The early detection of small tumors may lead to aggressive treatment and a reduction in *quality* of life with no assurance that the cancer would have otherwise progressed. Surgery and radiation both impose risk of postoperative incontinence and erectile dysfunction. Chemotherapy, including hormone therapy, is not curative, but may be used palliatively in advanced disease.

The choice of treatment is usually made on the basis of staging of the disease as well as the patient's age, presence of comorbid conditions, and personal preference. The American Urological System designates four stages of the disease. Stage A disease is not clinically detectable but is found incidentally during removal of prostate tissue for BPH. Stage B disease is clinically detectable but confined to the gland. Stage C disease is locally advanced, and stage D disease demonstrates distant metastasis.[27]

Stage A disease may be treated with watchful waiting (frequent clinical assessment and monitoring of PSA and other indexes). If PSA values are significantly elevated, transurethral resection of the prostate, radical prostatectomy, or radiation therapy may be recommended. Stage B disease is usually treated with radical prostatectomy or radiation therapy. State C disease is treated with radiation therapy, whereas stage D disease may be treated with watchful waiting or with hormonal therapy. Hormonal therapy usually consists of an LHRH agonist (leuprolide or goserelin) in combination with an antiandrogen (flutamide). LHRH initially stimulates the hypothalamic–pituitary axis, increasing testosterone levels transiently. Rising testosterone soon suppresses the hypothalamic–pituitary axis, however, and testosterone production declines. Antiandrogens act by blocking androgen receptors. Cytotoxic chemotherapy is minimally effective in treatment of prostate cancer.

Prognosis and Outcome. The likelihood of disease progression has traditionally been predicted on the basis of the PSA level and the Gleason score, the most commonly used histologic grading system for prostate cancer. In this scale, the two most prominent cell patterns within the tumor are each assigned a score of 1 to 5, and the two numbers are added.[27] Slow-growing, well-differentiated tumors are graded 2 to 4; moderately differentiated tumors are graded 5 to 7; and poorly differentiated, aggressive tumors are graded 8 to 10. A PSA level of less than 10 ng/mL and a Gleason score of less than 4 confer low risk, whereas a PSA level of more than 20 ng/mL and a Gleason score of 8 or greater confer high risk and poor prognosis.[28]

Median survival in prostate cancer is more than 5 years, with or without treatment.[26] When it is confined to the prostate gland, the cancer is often curable with surgery or radiation therapy. Median survival in men with metastatic disease is 1 to 3 years, but the disease has a prolonged course in many patients. Despite the significant incidence and death rate, most men die *with*, not *of*, prostate cancer.

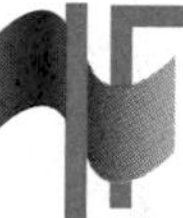

Clinical Scenario

F.W., a 70-year-old retired plumber, is found to have a serum PSA level of 8.5 ng/mL during a routine checkup. Rectal examination of his prostate reveals slight asymmetric enlargement but no nodularity. F.W. is referred for evaluation by a urologist and undergoes a biopsy, which is positive for adenocarcinoma of the left peripheral zone of the prostate. The tumor is given a Gleason score of 6.

1. What treatment options are available to F.W.?
2. What factors should be considered in the choice of treatment?

CLINICAL SIGNIFICANCE OF DISORDERS OF THE MALE REPRODUCTIVE SYSTEM

Sexual and reproductive capacity are integral to the physical and emotional health of the male. The disorders discussed in this chapter illustrate the potential impact on males of all ages. Although much current research is focused on prostate cancer, this condition is still relatively understudied (and research underfunded) in comparison to breast cancer in females.[29] Because the appropriateness of aggressive treatment of early prostate cancer is uncertain, the potential value of mass screening programs is questionable. Epidemiologic research is ongoing in an effort to clarify this issue. Clinical trials are underway to determine the relative efficacy of a variety of approaches to treatment of prostatic cancer and BPH. STDs have assumed more critical importance in the era of AIDS, and research into the prevention and cure of these conditions continues to be a national health care priority. The effects of STDs on the female reproductive system are discussed further in the next chapter, along with prevalent gynecologic and breast disorders.

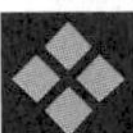

Summary of Key Points

- Because the reproductive and urinary systems are structurally integrated in males, most disorders adversely affect both systems. The prostate gland encircles the urethra at the bladder neck, and the urethra carries both urine and semen. Congenital abnormalities or prostatic enlargement may impair both urinary and sexual functions.
- Spermatogenesis begins at puberty and normally persists throughout the lifetime of the male. Male infertility is frequently idiopathic but may be related to ischemic disorders affecting the seminiferous tubules or to abnormal hormonal regulation. Because spermatogenesis involves the frequent division and differentiation of germ cells, testicular cancer is more likely to arise from these cells than from cells with lower rates of division.
- The process of spermatogenesis, the maturation and development of the male reproductive system and secondary sex characteristics, and male sexual function are under regulation by androgens produced primarily by the Leydig cells of the testis. Testosterone production by the testis is regulated by the hypothalamic–pituitary axis. Erectile function is regulated by parasympathetic and sympathetic signals to vascular structures within the penis as well as to accessory organs and ducts. Hormonal disorders, vascular disorders, surgical or radiation trauma, or drug therapy may impede regulatory signals or tissue responses, resulting in disorders of male sexual and reproductive function.
- Structural defects of the male reproductive system may be congenital or acquired. Testicular disorders, such as cryptorchidism or torsion, may culminate in testicular loss or infertility.
- STDs are increasing in incidence in the United States despite the availability of public education and preventive measures. The skin lesions of STDs may expose the male and his partner to superinfection with other STDs, including AIDS. Untreated infections may become disseminated to other organ systems, causing systemic inflammation and specific organ dysfunction. Infertility and the risk of ectopic pregnancy are increased as a consequence of STDs. Condom use reduces the risk of communication of STDs but is far from universal. Behavioral risk factors, such as early and frequent sexual activity and multiple sex partners, also contribute to the rising incidence of STDs.
- BPH and prostate cancer are both disorders of prostatic enlargement due to androgen-induced growth of prostate cells. Both are more prevalent with aging, and both result in urinary obstructive symptoms and rising PSA levels. Surgical treatment is similar for both disorders. BPH and prostate cancer arise from different regions within the gland. BPH is confined to the prostate gland, whereas prostate cancer is potentially locally invasive, metastatic, and lethal.

REFERENCES

1. Giwercman, A., Carlsen, E., Keiding, N., *et al.* (1993). *Environmental Health Perspectives Supplements* 101(suppl. 2), 65–71.
2. Raspa, R.F. (1993). Complications of vasectomy. *American Family Physician* 48(7), 1264–1268.
3. Holman, J.R., Lewis, E.L., and Ringler, R.L. (1995). Neonatal circumcision techniques. *American Family Physician* 52(2), 511–518.
4. Woodhouse, C.R.J. (1994). The sexual and reproductive consequences of congenital genitourinary anomalies. *Journal of Urology* 152, 645–651.
5. Howards, S.S. (1995). Treatment of male infertility. *New England Journal of Medicine* 332(5), 312–317.
6. Jones, H.W., and Toner, J.P. (1993). The infertile couple. *New England Journal of Medicine* 329(23), 1710–1715.
7. Schow, D.A., Redmon, B., and Pryor, J.L. (1997). Male menopause: How to define it, how to treat it. *Postgraduate Medicine* 101(3), 62–79.
8. Jaffe, R.B., Spencer, S.J., and Rabinovici, J. (1993). Activins and inhibins: Gonadal peptides during prenatal development and adult life. *Annals of the New York Academy of Sciences* 687, 1–9.

9. Bagatell, C.J., and Bremner, W.J. (1996). Androgens in men: Uses and abuses. *New England Journal of Medicine* 334(11), 707–714.
10. de Kretser, D.M. (1997). The Y chromosome and spermatogenesis. *New England Journal of Medicine* 336(8), 576–577.
11. Linet, O.I., and Ogring, F.G., for the Alprostadil Study Group. (1996). Efficacy and safety of intracavernosal alprostadil in men with erectile dysfunction. *New England Journal of Medicine* 334(14), 873–877.
12. Dewire, D.M. (1996). Evaluation and treatment of erectile dysfunction. *American Family Physician* 53(6), 2101–2106.
13. Guay, A.T. (1995). Erectile dysfunction: Are you prepared to discuss it? *Postgraduate Medicine* 97(4), 127–143.
14. Cilento, B.G., Najjar, S.S., and Atala, A. (1993). Cryptorchidism and testicular torsion. *Pediatric Clinics of North America* 40(6), 1133–1149.
15. Brock, D., Fox, S., Gosling, G., *et al.* (1993). Testicular cancer. *Seminars in Oncology Nursing* 9(4), 224–236.
16. Peck, R. (1993). Descriptive epidemiology of genitourinary cancers. *Seminars in Oncology Nursing* 9(4), 218–223.
17. Cotran, R.S., Kumar, V., and Robbins, S.L. (1994). *Robbins Pathologic Basis of Disease.* (5th ed.). Philadelphia: W.B. Saunders. (pp. 1015–1023).
18. Samm, B.J., and Dmochowski, R.R. (1996). Urologic emergencies: Trauma injuries and conditions affecting the penis, scrotum, and testicles. *Postgraduate Medicine* 100(4), 187–200.
19. Scherer, L.R., III, and Grosfeld, J.L. (1993). Inguinal hernia and umbilical anomalies. *Pediatric Clinics of North America* 40(6), 1121–1131.
20. Black, J.M., and Matassarin-Jacobs, E. (1997). *Medical-Surgical Nursing: Clinical Management for Continuity of Care.* Philadelphia: W.B. Saunders. (pp. 2459–2476).
21. Oesterling, J.E. (1995). Benign prostatic hyperplasia: Medical and minimally invasive treatment options. *New England Journal of Medicine* 332(2), 99–109.
22. Moul, J.W. (1993). Benign prostatic hyperplasia: New concepts in the 1990s. *Postgraduate Medicine* 94(6), 141–152.
23. Geller, J., Kirschenbaum, A., Lepor, H., *et al.* (1995). Therapeutic controversies: Clinical treatment of benign prostatic hyperplasia. *Journal of Clinical Endocrinology and Metabolism* 80(3), 745–747.
24. Garnick, M.B., and Fair, W.R. (1996). Prostate cancer: Emerging concepts, part I. *Annals of Internal Medicine* 125(2), 118–125.
25. Hostetler, R.M., Mandel, I.G., and Marshburn, J. (1996). Prostate cancer screening. *Medical Clinics of North America* 80(1), 83–98.
26. Maxwell, M.B. (1993). Cancer of the prostate. *Seminars in Oncology Nursing* 9(4), 237–251.
27. Cersosimo, R.J., and Carr, D. (1996). Prostate cancer: Current and evolving strategies. *American Journal of Health-System Pharmacy* 53, 381–396.
28. Garnick, M.B., and Fair, W.R. (1996). Prostate cancer: Emerging concepts, part II. *Annals of Internal Medicine* 125(3), 205–212.
29. Garnick, M.B. (1994). The dilemmas of prostate cancer. *Scientific American* 270(4), 72–81.

SELECTED BIBLIOGRAPHY

American Academy of Family Physicians. (1995). Fact sheet for physicians regarding neonatal circumcision. *American Family Physician* 52(2), 523–526.

Burnett, A.L. (1995). Nitric oxide control of lower genitourinary tract functions: A review. *Urology* 45(6), 1071–1083.

Catalona, W.J. (1994). Management of cancer of the prostate. *New England Journal of Medicine* 996–1004.

Clark, J.L., and Tatum, N.O. (1995). Management of genital herpes. *American Family Physician* 51(1), 175–182.

Epstein, J.I., Walsh, P.C., Carmichael, M., *et al.* (1994). Pathologic and clinical findings to predict tumor extent of nonpalpable (stage T1c) prostate cancer. *Journal of the American Medical Association* 271(5), 368–374.

Field, A.E., Colditz, G.A., Willett, W.C., *et al.* (1994). The relation of smoking, age, relative weight, and dietary intake to serum adrenal steroids, sex hormones, and sex hormone-binding globulin in middle-aged men. *Journal of Clinical Endocrinology and Metabolism* 79(5), 1310–1316.

Freedman, A., Hahn, G., and Love, N. (1996). Follow-up after therapy for prostate cancer: Treating the problems and caring for the man. *Postgraduate Medicine* 100(3), 125–136.

Guisti, R.M., Iwamoto, K., and Hatch, E.E. (1995). Diethylstilbestrol revisited: A review of the long-term health effects. *Annals of Internal Medicine* 122(10), 778–788.

Guyton, A.C., and Hall, J.E. (1996). *Textbook of Medical Physiology.* (9th ed.). Philadelphia: W.B. Saunders. (pp. 1003–1015).

Hess, R.A., Bunick, D., and Bahr, J.M. (1995). Sperm, a source of estrogen. *Environmental Health Perspectives* 103(suppl. 7), 59–62.

Hicks, R.J., and Cook, J.B. (1995). Managing patients with benign prostatic hyperplasia. *American Family Physician* 52(1), 135–142.

Holmes, K.K. (1994). Human ecology and behavior and sexually transmitted bacterial infections. *Proceedings of the National Academy of Sciences U.S.A.* 91, 2448–2455.

Hutchinson, K.A. (1995). Androgens and sexuality. *American Journal of Medicine* 98(suppl. 1A), 111S–115S.

Koeppel, K.M. (1995). Sperm banking and patients with cancer: Issues concerning patients and healthcare professionals. *Cancer Nursing* 18(4), 306–312.

Krahn M.D., Mahoney, J.E., Eckman, M.H., *et al.* (1994). Screening for prostate cancer: A decision analytic view. *Journal of the American Medical Association* 272(10), 773–780.

L'Archevesque, C.I., and Goldstein-Lohman, H. (1996). Ritual circumcision: Educating parents. *Pediatric Nursing* 22(3), 228–234.

Laumann, E.O., Masi, C.M., and Zuckerman, E.W. (1997). Circumcision in the United States: Prevalence, prophylactic effects, and sexual practice. *Journal of the American Medical Association* 277(13), 1052–1057.

Lepor, H., Williford, W.O., Barry, M.J., *et al.* (1996). The efficacy of terazosin, finasteride, or both in benign prostatic hyperplasia. *New England Journal of Medicine* 335(8), 533–539.

Martin, D.H., and Mroczkowski, T.F. (1994). Dermatologic manifestations of sexually transmitted diseases other than HIV. *Infectious Disease Clinics of North America* 8(3), 533–582.

Miller, D.M., and Brodell, R.T. (1996). Human papillomavirus infection: Treatment options for warts. *American Family Physician* 53(1), 135–143.

Moore, K.L., and Persaud, T.V.N. (1993). *The Developing Human: Clinically Oriented Embryology.* (5th ed.). Philadelphia: W.B. Saunders.

Moul, J.W. (1993). Prostatitis: Sorting out the different causes. *Postgraduate Medicine* 94(5), 191–194.

Nachtigall, L.B., Boepple, P.A., Pralong, F.P., *et al.* (1997). Adult-onset idiopathic hypogonadotropic hypogonadism: A treatable form of male infertility. *New England Journal of Medicine* 336(6), 410–415.

O'Reilly, K.R., and Piot, P. (1996). International perspectives on individual and community approaches to the prevention of sexually transmitted disease and human immunodeficiency virus infection. *Journal of Infectious Diseases* 174(suppl. 2), S214–S222.

Potosky, A.L., Miller, B.A., Albertsen, P.C., *et al.* (1995). The role of increasing detection in the rising incidence of prostate cancer. *Journal of the American Medical Association* 273(7), 548–552.

Taub, M., Begas, A., and Love, N. (1996). Advanced prostate cancer: Endocrine therapies and palliative measures. *Postgraduate Medicine* 100(3), 139–154.

Trantham, P. (1996). The infertile couple. *American Family Physician* 54(3), 1001–1010.

Williams, T.R., and Love, N. (1996). Treatment of localized prostate cancer: Choosing the best alternative. *Postgraduate Medicine* 100(3), 105–120.

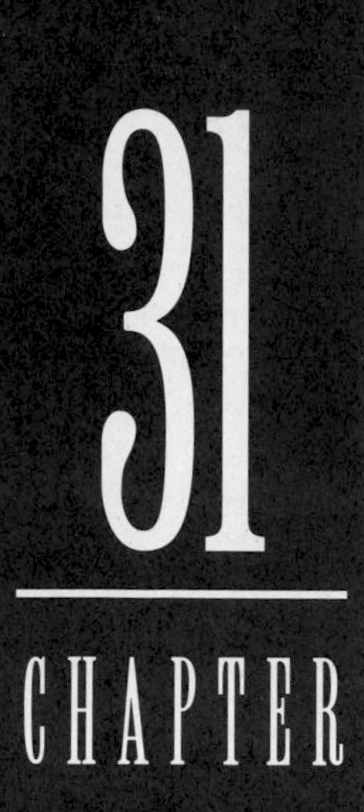

Gynecologic and Breast Disorders

LEARNING OBJECTIVES

1. Discuss the anatomic features of the external and internal reproductive organs that may predispose to gynecologic disorders.
2. Describe the processes of oogenesis and ovulation with reference to fertility and potential gynecologic disorders.
3. Discuss the endocrine regulation of the menstrual cycle, including the endocrine changes occurring at menarche and menopause.
4. Relate alterations in sexual function, fertility, and uterine bleeding to specific gynecologic disorders.
5. Identify the pathophysiologic mechanisms that predict clinical manifestations and rationalize intervention in selected gynecologic disorders.
6. Compare and contrast the pathophysiologic processes, clinical manifestations, and treatment of fibrocystic change of the breast and breast cancer.

key terms

abnormal uterine bleeding
adenomyosis
amenorrhea
androgen
atrophic vaginitis
bacterial vaginosis
breast cancer
cervical cancer
coitus
dyspareunia
endometrial cancer
endometriosis
endometritis
estrogen
fibrocystic change of the breast
follicle-stimulating hormone (FSH)
galactorrhea
gonadotropin-releasing hormone (GnRH)
hyperandrogenism
inhibin
insulin-like growth factor (IGF)
intromission
luteinizing hormone (LH)
menarche
menopause

menstrual cycle
menstruation
oligomenorrhea
oogenesis
ovarian cancer
ovarian cyst
ovulation
pelvic inflammatory disease (PID)
pelvic support disorder
perimenopause
polycystic ovary syndrome (PCOS)
premenstrual syndrome (PMS)
progesterone
uterine fibroid tumor
vaginal candidiasis
vulvovaginitis

Gynecology is the medical specialty that focuses on disorders associated with reproductive function in nonpregnant females. In most clinical settings, gynecology is integrated with obstetrics, which encompasses the process of childbearing. From the time women enter their reproductive years until their 60s and beyond, gynecologic and obstetrical issues are central to their health care. Gynecologic problems are a significant source of morbidity, and their impact on health care costs and quality of life is considerable. Cessation of **menstruation (menopause),** a normal developmental transition, is nevertheless attended by discomfort and imposes significant risk of cardiovascular disease and osteoporosis. More than 30 million women in the United States are postmenopausal, and this number is expected to increase by 6 million during the next decade.[1] **Breast cancer** is second only to lung cancer as a cause of cancer death in women. One in eight women will develop breast cancer during their lifetimes.[2] Until recent years, women's health was relatively understudied; however, this situation is now changing, with several major studies in progress (see Focus of Current Research).

In this chapter, the anatomy of the female reproductive system and breast will be reviewed. The menstrual cycle and its regulation will be detailed. Developmental changes in reproductive function, including the onset and cessation of menstruation, will be described. The more prevalent gynecologic and breast disorders affecting nonpregnant women will be described in detail. Less common gynecologic and breast disorders will be briefly summarized. Disorders associated with pregnancy and lactation are reviewed in Chapter 32.

ANATOMY OF THE FEMALE REPRODUCTIVE SYSTEM

In contrast to the male reproductive system, the female reproductive organs are anatomically separate from the urinary structures. Still, the structures are in close enough proximity that disorders such as infections frequently affect sexual-reproductive and urinary function.

External Genitalia

The external genitalia of the female, illustrated in Figure 31-1, include the *labia, clitoris, introitus,* and *perineum.* The external opening from the bladder, the urethral meatus, is located just anteriorly to the introitus. The outer labia majora and inner labia minora are folds of tissue homologous to the scrotum of the male in their protective function. The labia contain *sebaceous glands,* which secrete the oily sebum that nourishes hair follicles, and *Bartholin's glands,* which secrete mucus for lubrication during sexual activity. Inflammation and obstructive cysts affecting these glands are common. The *clitoris* is a small erectile organ homologous to the male penis. It contains many nerve endings for sexual stimulation. The introitus, which leads to the internal genital tract, is partially or completely covered by a connective tissue membrane, the *hymen,* which is normally stretched or torn with initial sexual intercourse. In a small number of women, the hymen is congenitally imperforate, requiring surgical excision to permit menstruation and sexual function.

Internal Organs

The internal reproductive organs of the female, illustrated in Figure 31-2, include the *vagina, uterus, ovaries,* and *fallopian tubes.* The vagina is a tube of smooth muscle that extends upward and backward between the bladder and the rectum. The vagina serves as the route of menstrual flow to the exterior, the receptive organ of intercourse, and the birth canal. The lower end of the uterus, the *cervix,* projects into the upper end of the vagina.

The uterus is a small, hollow, pear-shaped organ with thick walls of smooth muscle. It consists of three regions: the upper fundus, middle body, and lower cervix. Uterine walls have three layers: the outer serosa, which is continuous with the peritoneum; the middle myometrium or smooth muscle

Focus of Current Research

Study	*Objective and Findings*
Olson, et al. (1996) Relation between sodium balance and menstrual cycle symptoms in normal women.	*Objective:* To determine whether sodium balance affects expression of menstrual symptoms *Findings:* Breast tenderness and bloating did not result from sodium retention during the luteal phase. Women actually had sodium loss during this phase.
Writing Group for the PEPI Trial (1996) Effects of hormone replacement therapy on endometrial histology in postmenopausal women.	*Objective:* To report the histologic findings of the endometrium of postmenopausal women receiving placebo, estrogen only, or a combination of estrogen and progesterone *Findings:* Treatment with estrogen only enhanced the development of endometrial hyperplasia. Combination therapy protected the endometrium from these changes.
Grodstein, et al. (1996) Postmenopausal estrogen and progestin use and the risk of cardiovascular disease.	*Objective:* To examine the relation between cardiovascular disease and hormone therapy during 16 years of follow-up *Findings:* Addition of progestin to hormone therapy does not reduce the cardioprotective effects of hormone replacement.
Sanchez-Guerrero, et al. (1995) Silicone breast implants and the risk of connective-tissue diseases and symptoms.	*Objective:* To study the relation between silicone breast implants and connective tissue diseases and symptoms *Findings:* No association was found.
Jacobson, et al. (1995) Ten-year results of a comparison of conservation with mastectomy in the treatment of stage I and II breast cancer.	*Objective:* To compare lumpectomy with mastectomy for stage I and II breast cancer *Findings:* Lumpectomy and radiation offer equivalent results to mastectomy.
Colditz, et al. (1995) The use of estrogens and progestins and the risk of breast cancer in postmenopausal women.	*Objective:* To quantify the relation between the use of hormones and the risk of breast cancer *Findings:* The risk of breast cancer is increased with both forms of treatment, especially among older women.
Newcomb, et al. (1994) Lactation and a reduced risk of premenopausal breast cancer.	*Objective:* To describe the association between lactation and the risk of breast cancer *Findings:* There is a reduction in breast cancer risk among premenopausal women who have lactated. No risk reduction was seen in postmenopausal women with a history of lactation.

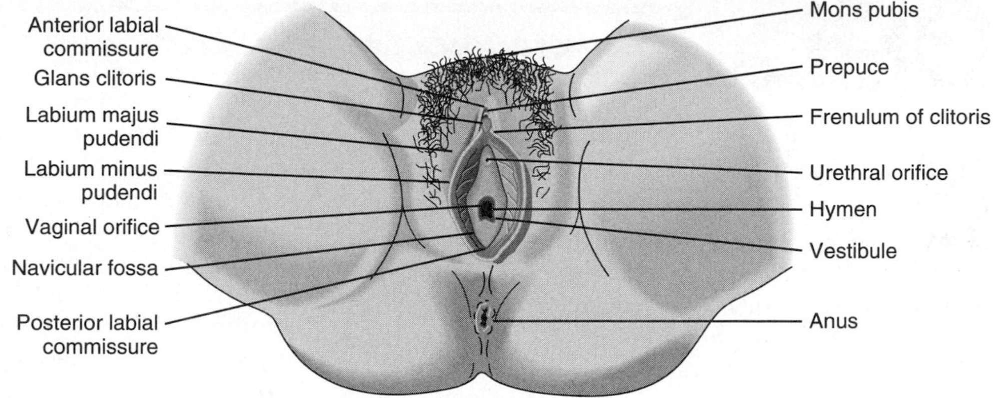

FIGURE 31–1

Female genitalia. The external reproductive organs of the female are functionally separate from the urinary system. The *labia* are folds of tissue that protect the vaginal opening (*introitus*) and provide lubrication via Bartholin's glands. The introitus is partially or completely covered by a connective tissue membrane, the *hymen,* which is stretched or torn with initial intercourse. The *clitoris* is a small erectile organ homologous to the male penis.

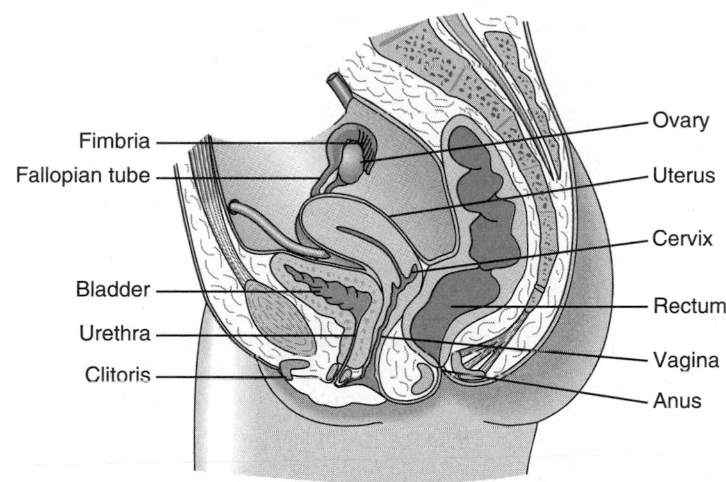

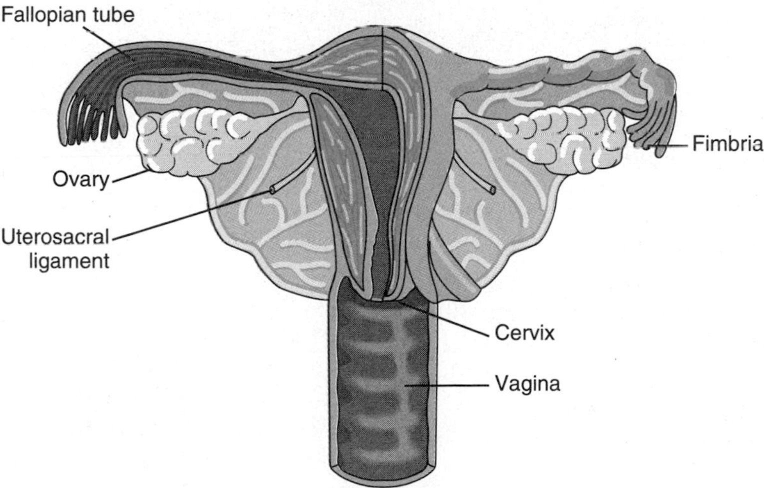

FIGURE 31–2

Internal reproductive organs. The *vagina* is a tube of smooth muscle that extends upward between the bladder and the rectum. The *uterus* is a pear-shaped organ composed of smooth muscle. Its lower portion, the *cervix,* protrudes slightly into the upper vaginal vault. The *ovaries,* or female gonads, are suspended by ligaments on either side of the uterus. The *fallopian tubes,* which emerge from the upper portion of the uterus, are open at their distal fringed (fimbriated) ends to receive the ovum released during each menstrual cycle.

Developmental Perspective

Embryonic and Fetal Periods

Under the influence of the X chromosome and an autosome, the ovaries develop from the initially indifferent gonad. The ovaries are identifiable by the 10th week of gestation. Primitive ovarian follicles are apparent at 16 weeks. Active mitosis of oocytes occurs during fetal life, although many degenerate before birth. An estimated 1 to 2 million ovarian follicles are present at birth. The fallopian tubes, uterus, and vagina develop from the paired paramesonephric (müllerian) ducts. Fusion of the lower portion of the ducts is essential to uterine and vaginal development, and abnormal fusion may give rise to congenital anomalies such as bicornuate (heart-shaped) uterus. Abnormal separation of structures may result in obstruction (e.g., cervical atresia or imperforate hymen). In the absence of androgens, feminization of the neutral external genitalia occurs, and definitive characteristics are apparent by the 9th to 12th weeks. The breasts develop at about 4 to 6 weeks of gestation, when ectoderm thickens to form mammary ridges ("milk lines") on the ventral surface of the embryo. Normally, the ridges regress except in the pectoral regions, but failure of this regression may lead to congenital abnormalities such as ectopic breast tissue or additional (supernumerary) breasts or nipples along the milk lines.

Infancy and Childhood

The hypothalamic–pituitary–gonadal axis is normally quiescent during infancy and childhood. Early onset (precocious) puberty in females, evidenced by breast development, pubic and axillary hair, and onset of menstrual cycles, is often idiopathic, and is termed *constitutional* if no other abnormalities are found. Serum levels of FSH, LH, and estrogen may be normal or elevated in these cases. Central nervous system lesions, ovarian tumors, and exogenous sources of estrogen are uncommon causes of this syndrome.

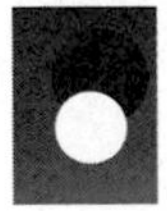

Adolescence and Young Adulthood

Secretion of GnRH increases to adult levels at puberty, inducing menarche in the presence of adequate body fat. Delayed menarche may be associated with lack of body fat, hormonal imbalance, or congenital defects of the outlet tract such as imperforate hymen. Amenorrhea and oligomenorrhea associated with anovulatory cycles are common during adolescence. Sexual function and orgasm in females are apparently influenced by psychosocial factors to a greater degree than in males. Hyperandrogenism is commonly associated with amenorrhea and anovulation and may also manifest as hirsutism, acne, and PCOS. Adolescents and young women are at particular risk for sexually transmitted diseases that may progress to PID, with its inherent risks of infertility and ectopic pregnancy. Premenstrual syndrome, endometriosis, benign ovarian cysts, and fibrocystic change of the breast are common throughout the reproductive years.

Middle and Older Adulthood

Uterine fibroid tumors, endometriosis, and premenstrual syndrome are very common among middle-aged women and lead (perhaps inappropriately) to a high incidence of hysterectomies and surgical menopause in the United States. More rigorous screening for gynecologic cancers has resulted in earlier diagnosis and lower mortality rates in these tumors. Multiparous women are prone to pelvic support disorders because of the additive effects of aging and the trauma of childbirth on the pelvic musculature. Discomforts of the perimenopause often include hot flashes, genitourinary tract dysfunction, and psychological distress; and removal of estrogen imposes a gradually increasing risk of osteoporosis and cardiovascular disease. The use of hormone replacement therapy may reduce these discomforts and risks, but it imposes increased risk of endometrial and breast cancer. The risk of breast cancer is particularly high in middle-aged and older women, even if they have no risk factors other than age and sex.

layer; and the inner endometrium, the lining cells that undergo predictable changes during the menstrual cycle. Cells of the cervix produce mucus that varies in thickness during the cycle, serving to protect the internal organs from ascending infection. Cervical mucus forms a thick barrier during pregnancy to protect the growing fetus. The cervical os, or opening, is normally less than 1 cm in diameter, except during late pregnancy. Congenital anomalies of the uterus are uncommon, but may occur when normal fusion of the müllerian ducts does not occur during embryogenesis (see Developmental Perspective). Examples include septate (divided) uterus and bicornuate (heart-shaped) uterus (Fig. 31–3).

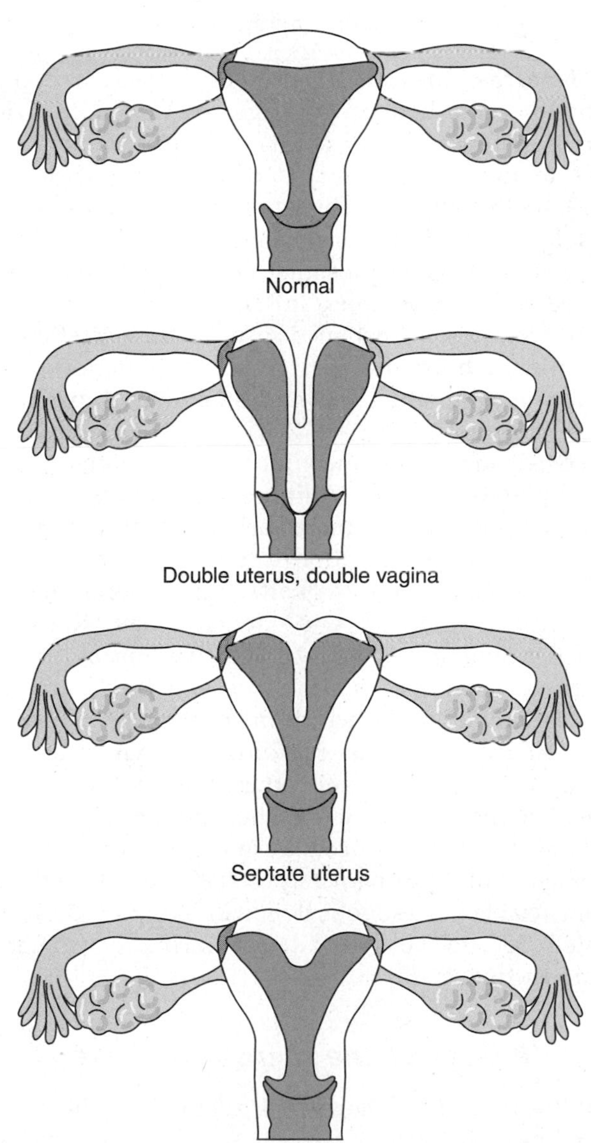

FIGURE 31–3
Congenital abnormalities of the uterus. Failure of normal fusion during embryonic development may result in doubling or division of the uterus, vagina, or both.

The ovaries are the female gonads, serving as the principal source of the female sex hormones **estrogen** and **progesterone** as well as the site of storage, maturation, and release of *ova,* or eggs. The bilateral ovaries are small oval organs, suspended by ligaments in the *adnexae* on either side of the uterus. **Oogenesis,** the development of ova within the ovaries, begins at about 6 weeks' gestation in the female embryo. By the time of birth, the ovaries of the female fetus have produced 1 to 2 million *oocytes* (germ cells from which ova may develop), at which time oogenesis is complete. The meiotic cell division, which results in oocyte formation, was described in Chapter 6.

The fallopian tubes, slender tubes of smooth muscle, serve to conduct ova to the uterus. The tubes have open, fimbriated (fringed) distal ends that receive the ovum after its release into the peritoneal cavity from one ovary. Connected to the uterus at their proximal ends, the fallopian tubes are lined with ciliated epithelium and mucus that sweep the ovum into the uterus. If spermatozoa are present, fertilization of the ovum usually occurs while the ovum is still within the fallopian tube.

The perineum, the tissue between the introitus and the anus, is notable in that it may easily tear during childbirth. *Episiotomy,* surgical incision to enlarge the introitus, is frequently done to facilitate vaginal delivery (see Chapter 32).

Breast

The female breast, illustrated in Figure 31–4, is composed of the *mammary glands,* which produce milk during lactation, along with supportive tissues including smooth muscle, ligaments, adipose tissue, blood vessels, and lymphatics. A system of ducts connects and drains the functional units of the mammary glands, known as alveoli or lobules. The milk-conducting lactiferous ducts converge at the nipple, from which milk may be ejected. Breast cancer most frequently arises from the epithelial lining of these glands and ducts. Lactation and its regulation are discussed in Chapter 32.

FEMALE REPRODUCTIVE FUNCTION

Female reproductive function includes sexual function to permit access of spermatozoa as well as cyclic changes associated with **ovulation** (release of

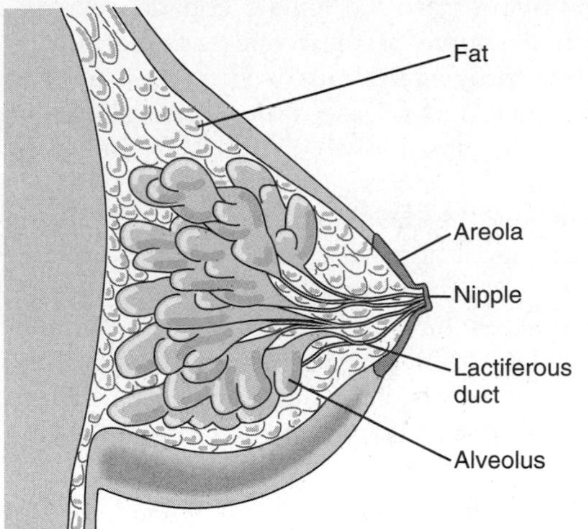

FIGURE 31–4
Female breast. The breast is composed of the *mammary alveoli,* which synthesize and secrete milk into *lactiferous ducts* under stimulation by prolactin during lactation. Ducts converge at the *nipple,* which is surrounded by an area of pigmentation, the *areola.* Supportive tissues within the breast include smooth muscle, ligaments, fatty tissue, blood vessels, and lymphatics.

an ovum from the ovary) and support of a potential pregnancy.

Sexual Function

The phases of female sexual activity parallel those of the male, although they are not as readily observed because of anatomic differences. With physical or psychological stimulation before intercourse, the clitoris becomes distended and erect, and the labia become engorged with blood. Vaginal walls secrete lubricating fluid, in preparation for **intromission,** or entry of the penis. Vaginal smooth muscle relaxes, and the vaginal canal is extended by elevation of the uterus. Female orgasm usually requires clitoral stimulation, either directly or secondarily to movement of the labia during intercourse or **coitus.** During orgasm, smooth muscle of the outer third of the vagina contracts rhythmically, and the uterus also contracts in a top-to-bottom pattern similar to its contraction during labor. Orgasm, which is not achieved with all sexual intercourse, apparently serves the physiologic purpose of enhancing retention of semen in the vagina, facilitating conception. Pelvic blood flow and muscle tone return to the baseline state relatively quickly after orgasm, or more slowly if orgasm does not occur.

Menstrual Cycle

Definitions and Normal Parameters

Menstruation is the cyclic shedding of cells of the endometrial lining, evidenced as uterine contraction (with crampy pain) and vaginal bleeding. The usual length of the **menstrual cycle,** the time between menstrual periods, is 21 to 35 days (average, 28 days).[3] The duration of menstrual flow is 2 to 6 days, and the expected blood loss with each cycle is approximately 30 mL, although up to 80 mL may be normal for some women. Any pattern outside this range is termed **abnormal uterine bleeding.** This syndrome is detailed subsequently.

Menarche

Menarche, the initial onset of menstrual cycles, usually occurs between the ages of 11 and 15, with variation depending primarily on genetic factors and the amount of body fat. Under genetic regulation, the hypothalamic-pituitary axis, which regulates gonadal release of sex hormones, slowly matures. At puberty, increasing pulsatile secretion of **gonadotropin-releasing hormone (GnRH)** from the hypothalamus produces a sustained rise in the secretion of **luteinizing hormone (LH)** from the anterior pituitary gland, initiating the first ovulation. A body fat percentage of 22% to 24% must generally be achieved and maintained for a few months before menarche will occur. Adipose cells produce some estrogen and may promote earlier sexual maturation and onset of menstruation in girls with more body fat. Other factors that may affect the onset of menarche include physical and mental stress. Rigorous athletic training may reduce body fat and induce an energy drain. Stress is also associated with increased catecholamine levels, which may interrupt LH secretion. Abnormal uterine bleeding is common among adolescents for these and other reasons, as detailed later. At the time of menarche, most of the 1 to 2 million oocytes produced during gestation have atrophied, but approximately 300,000 to 400,000 remain viable. These oocytes will support an estimated 350 to 400 ovulations during a woman's reproductive years.

Phases of the Menstrual Cycle

With respect to hormonal regulation, the menstrual cycle consists of two phases, illustrated in Figure 31–5. During each *follicular phase,* the pituitary hormone **follicle-stimulating hormone (FSH)** stimulates the development of 6 to 12 ovarian follicles,

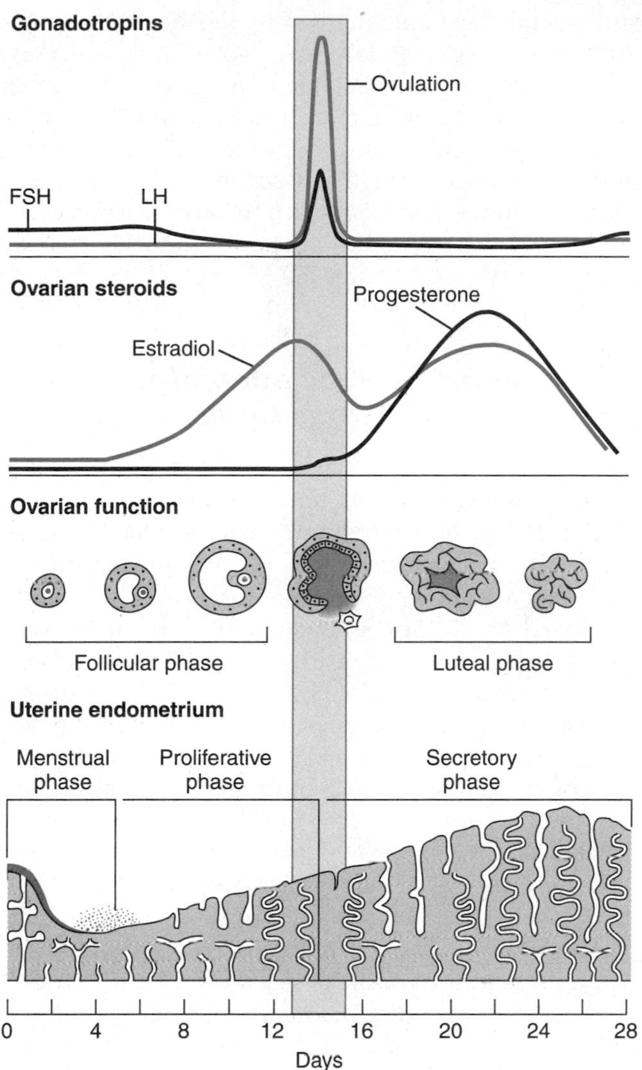

FIGURE 31–5

Phases of the menstrual cycle. The menstrual cycle consists of two phases: the *follicular phase,* during which one ovarian follicle develops under the influence of follicle-stimulating hormone (FSH) and estrogen and is released with ovulation at midcycle; and the *luteal phase,* during which the remaining follicular coat (corpus luteum) secretes progesterone to maintain the uterine lining (endometrium) to sustain a possible pregnancy. In the absence of pregnancy, the progesterone level falls and the endometrial lining is shed during menstruation. LH, luteinizing hormone.

each consisting of an ovum surrounded by fluid and two layers of supporting cells, the inner granulosa and outer thecal cells (Fig. 31–6). As they enlarge, the granulosa cells of these primary follicles begin to synthesize estrogen. Typically, one follicle secretes more estrogen than the others, and, in a limited positive feedback loop, stimulates its own development to a greater degree. This dominant follicle then continues to develop and produce estrogen while the others atrophy. FSH secretion, which is under regulation by the hypothalamic–pituitary–gonadal axis, is eventually suppressed by rising estrogen levels near midcycle. When LH secretion exceeds FSH secretion, LH stimulates rupture of the follicle at the ovarian surface, and ovulation occurs, marking the end of the follicular phase and the beginning of the *luteal phase* of the menstrual cycle. Minimal bleeding from the ovarian surface into the peritoneal cavity at the time of rupture may irritate pain receptors and cause *mittelschmerz,* or crampy pain of ovulation.

The empty follicle that remains on the ovarian surface after ovulation collapses to form the *corpus luteum,* which produces the hormone progesterone for regulation of the luteal phase. Progesterone maintains the growth and function of the endome-

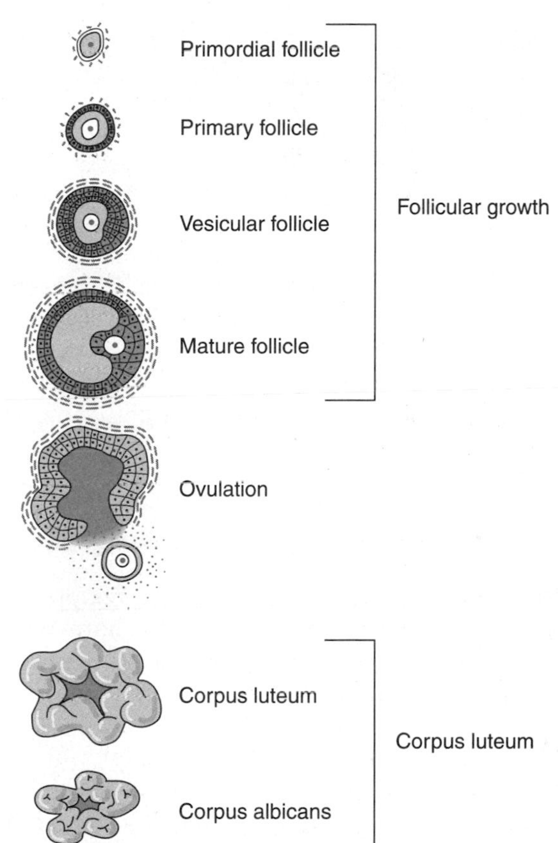

FIGURE 31–6

Follicular development. Oogenesis, the formation of oocytes (ova or eggs) via meiosis, is complete at birth in females. Many oocytes then degenerate, and the ovaries at puberty contain 300,000 or more oocytes, surrounded by a layer of supportive cells, to sustain the reproductive years. During the follicular phase of each menstrual cycle, 6 to 12 of these follicles begin to develop and secrete estrogen; however, 1 follicle dominates and the others soon atrophy. This primary follicle continues to grow until ovulation, when its ovum is released from the ovarian surface. The follicular coat remaining in the ovary forms the corpus luteum, which secretes progesterone during the luteal phase. After menstruation, the corpus luteum involutes to form a white scar, the corpus albicans.

trium to support a potential pregnancy. If pregnancy does not occur, the corpus luteum atrophies and becomes a white scar (*corpus albicans*) on the ovarian surface. Removal of progesterone then allows menstruation to occur. If fertilization does take place, the corpus luteum persists, secreting progesterone for about 3 months. At that time, the placenta has developed to the point where it becomes the primary source of progesterone secretion during pregnancy. Inadequate secretion of progesterone by the corpus luteum (luteal phase deficiency) may contribute to recurrent spontaneous abortion in some women (see Chapter 32). Anovulatory cycles, with phase disruption and lack of ovulation, are common during adolescence and during **perimenopause,** the period preceding menopause, discussed later.

Endometrial Changes During the Menstrual Cycle

Endometrial cells evolve through three sequential phases during the cycle. During the *proliferative phase* (days 6 to 14 preceding ovulation), these cells, along with uterine glands and vessels, grow rapidly under the influence of estrogen. After ovulation, during the *secretory phase,* progesterone stimulates increased secretory function, vascularity, and edema of the endometrium. The *menstrual phase* occurs with the removal of progesterone, when the inner layer of endometrium degenerates and sloughs, producing the menstrual flow.

Changes in Cervical Mucus

Mucus production by glands in the region of the cervical os also varies cyclically under hormonal influences. Before ovulation, when estrogen levels are high, increased amounts of thin, watery mucus are produced. This mucus is easily penetrated by sperm, facilitating fertilization. After ovulation, increased progesterone levels result in production of thick mucus, which serves as a protective barrier (mucus plug) in the event of pregnancy. Consistency of the cervical mucus is one parameter by which the ovulatory cycle of the female may be monitored as a basis for "natural" family planning methods (see Chapter 32).

Changes in the Breasts

During the follicular phase, estrogen promotes an increase in adipose deposition, fluid accumulation, and ductal development within the breasts. Nipple growth and pigmentation are also influenced by estrogen. Progesterone sustains these effects during the luteal phase until menstruation, when selective programmed cell death (apoptosis) reduces the proliferative changes and the tissue returns to baseline state. Lactation, the production and secretion of breast milk, requires the presence of the hormones of pregnancy (see Chapter 32).

Hormonal Regulation of the Menstrual Cycle

Endocrine regulation of menstrual function is complex, depending not only on absolute amounts of circulating hormones but also on the ratios of hormones. The effects of the sex hormones on tissues other than reproductive organs, particularly vascular smooth muscle, bone, and brain, are incompletely understood. Table 31–1 details known effects of the gonadotropins (FSH and LH), the estrogens, progesterone, and androgens. In males and females, the pituitary hormones FSH and LH are a component of the hypothalamic–pituitary–gonadal regulatory axis. Figure 31–7 depicts this regulatory system in females.

Gonadotropin-releasing hormone secretion from the hypothalamus is pulsatile, released in a predictable pattern during the menstrual cycle but potentially influenced by multiple neuroendocrine stimuli. The neurotransmitter norepinephrine stimulates GnRh release, and dopamine inhibits it. The secretion of FSH and LH is mediated not only by GnRH but also by serotonin and melatonin, which stimulate release, and by γ-aminobutyric acid (GABA), acetylcholine, β-endorphins, and the ovarian peptide **inhibin,** which inhibit secretion. FSH and LH stimulate ovarian growth. FSH stimulates estrogen production by follicle cells, and LH stimulates progesterone production by the corpus luteum.

The ovaries produce steroid hormones (estrogens, progesterone, and **androgens**) as well as a number of peptides (notably inhibin and insulin-like growth factors [IGFs]). Of the three forms of estrogen synthesized, *estradiol, estrone,* and *estriol,* estradiol is most abundant and most potent. Adipose tissue also secretes estrogen, and a marked decrease in body fat (as in anorectic conditions, starvation, or elite athletes) may alter menstrual cycles or cause them to cease. Estrogen synthesis also results from conversion of adrenal androgens.

Estrogen (named for its function of "generation of the estrus," or female cycle) is essential to ovulation

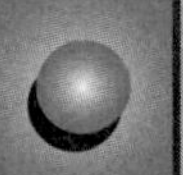

TABLE 31–1
EFFECTS OF THE GONADOTROPINS AND SEX STEROID HORMONES IN FEMALES

Hormone	Principal Effects
Follicle-stimulating hormone (FSH)	Stimulates development of 6 to 12 primary ovarian follicles each month, including proliferation of granulosa cells, generation of thecal cells, and stimulation of secretion of estrogen-rich fluid from granulosa cells that accumulates to form an antrum
	Stimulates expression of luteinizing hormone (LH) and FSH receptors on granulosa cells
	With LH, causes rapid swelling of the follicle just before ovulation
Luteinizing hormone (LH)	Stimulates secretion by granulosa and thecal cells in follicles beyond the antral stage
	Stimulates final follicular development and swelling before ovulation
	Converts granulosa cells and thecal cells to favor progesterone secretion just before ovulation
	Stimulates ovulation via promotion of follicular swelling and release of proteolytic enzymes from thecal cells to dissolve the capsular wall
	Promotes luteinization (yellowing) of the postovulatory follicle, forming the corpus luteum
Estrogens	Promote development of the uterus, fallopian tubes, ovaries, external genitalia, and breasts at puberty
	Promote increased osteoblastic activity, resulting in linear growth and closure of the epiphyseal plates
	Promote deposition of fat in the subcutaneous tissues in the female (gynoid) pattern
	Weakly promote protein deposition and increased metabolic rate
	Promote soft, smooth texture and increased vascularity of the skin
	Weakly promote sodium and water retention (mineralocorticoid effect)
	Stimulate endometrial proliferation during the follicular phase of the menstrual cycle
	Promote systemic and reproductive tissue changes in support of pregnancy
	Increase HDL cholesterol and decrease LDL cholesterol
	Promote vasomotor stability and relaxation of vascular smooth muscle
Progesterone	Stimulates secretory changes in the endometrium during the luteal phase of the menstrual cycle in preparation for potential implantation
	Stimulates increased secretion by the mucosal lining of the fallopian tubes, facilitating nutrition and transport of the fertilized ovum
	Promotes lobular and alveolar development of the breasts during the luteal phase or during pregnancy
	Weakly promotes sodium and water excretion via competitive inhibition of aldosterone
	Promotes smooth muscle relaxation and other systemic changes during pregnancy
Androgens	Promote growth of pubic and axillary hair
	Stimulate sebum production by the pilosebaceous unit of the skin
	May promote libido

Data from Guyton, A.C., and Hall, J.E. (1996). *Textbook of Medical Physiology*. (9th ed.). Philadelphia: W.B. Saunders. (pp. 1017–1026).

and pregnancy and promotes the development of the female reproductive organs and breasts. Estrogens derived from adrenal androgens may be most important in the development of the female skin characteristics and the female distribution of hair and body fat. Estrogens exert a favorable effect on blood vessels, promoting their resiliance, and on serum lipids, promoting increased high-density lipoprotein (HDL) and decreased low-density lipoprotein (LDL) cholesterol levels (see Chapter 25). The increases in very-low-density lipoprotein (VLDL) and coagulability of the blood mediated by estrogen may be less favorable to some. Estrogen also promotes cyclic fluid retention. The role of estrogen in protecting against increased bone resorption and osteoporosis is well established (see Chapter 34).

Progesterone (named for its function of "promotion of gestation," or pregnancy) is essential in preparation of the endometrium for the support of pregnancy. This hormone also mediates a cyclic elevation in body temperature at the time of ovulation. The physiologic purpose of this elevation is uncertain. Although most progesterone is produced by the corpus luteum, as has been discussed, some is pro-

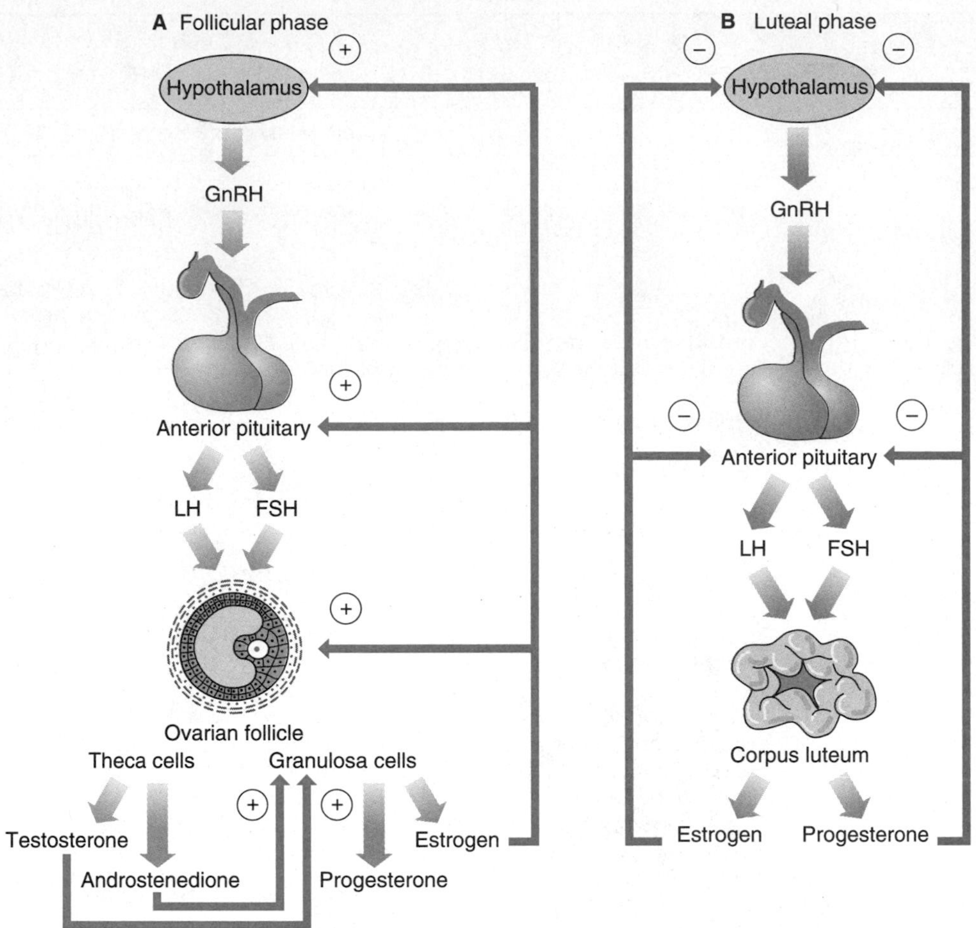

FIGURE 31–7

Hormonal regulation of the menstrual cycle. Endocrine regulation of the menstrual cycle is a function of the *hypothalamic-pituitary-gonadal axis.* The hypothalamus secretes a basal amount of gonadotropin-releasing hormone (GnRH), which then stimulates the release of the gonadotropins follicle-stimulating hormone (FSH) and luteinizing hormone (LH). FSH and LH stimulate follicular growth and estrogen secretion. Estrogen augments the FSH effect on the follicle and stimulates its own increased secretion in a limited positive feedback loop. Estrogen also induces increased pituitary secretion of LH, and LH stimulates follicular release of progesterone and the androgens testosterone and androstenedione, which serve as estrogen precursors. A surge in LH at midcycle produces follicular changes that result in ovulation. During the luteal phase, LH is of particular importance in stimulating the secretion of progesterone and a smaller amount of estrogen by the corpus luteum. These hormones then exert negative feedback (indicated by minus signs) to the hormonal axis, reducing the secretion of GnRH, FSH, and LH.

duced by the adrenal cortex along with the adrenal androgens.

The ovaries produce 25% of the circulating androgens, or "male hormones," in females. Androgens of ovarian and adrenal sources serve as estrogen precursors and are known to play a role in muscle development, hair growth, and function of the pilosebaceous units of the skin. Testosterone, the major circulating androgen in females, may also mediate sex drive, or *libido.* **Hyperandrogenism,** a syndrome of excess androgen secretion or enhanced androgen effect in females, may be idiopathic, associated with reproductive or other endocrine disorders, or caused by the androgenic effects of a number of drugs (Table 31–2). Hyperandrogenism manifests as variable degrees of anovulation, hirsutism, cystic acne, and male-pattern hair loss.

Insulin-like growth factors (IGFs) are produced by a variety of tissues, including the ovaries. As detailed in Chapter 27, these peptides are structurally and functionally similar to proinsulin and are essential to most effects of growth hormone. The ovarian IGF system seems to act synergistically with the FSH and LH in regulation of the menstrual cycle. The dominant follicle has been shown to have up to three times the amount of IGF-I in comparison

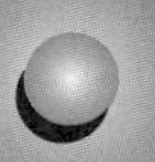

TABLE 31–2
CONDITIONS ASSOCIATED WITH HYPERANDROGENISM

Endogenous
Ovarian origin
- Primary tumors
- Metastatic tumors
- Polycystic ovary syndrome (including idiopathic hirsutism)
- Ovarian stromal hyperthecosis
- Androgen excess in pregnancy
- Abnormal gonadal or sexual development

Adrenal Origin
- Cushing's syndrome/disease
- Late-onset (attenuated) congenital adrenal hyperplasia
- Tumors

Exogenous [Iatrogenic]
- Danazol*
- Phenytoin*
- Diazoxide*
- Hexachlorobenzene*
- Hexachlorophene*
- Minoxidil*
- Cyclosporine*
- Testosterone and other androgens
- Anabolic steroids
- Synthetic progestins (OCs)
- Metapyrone

*Hirsutism without significant virilization.
OCs, oral contraceptives.
Reprinted from Derman, R.J. (1995). Effects of sex steroids on women's health: Implications for practitioners. *American Journal of Medicine* 98 (1A suppl.), 138S. Copyright 1995, with permission from Excerpta Medica Inc.

with the nondominant follicles that atrophy.[4] Ovarian tissue has receptors that bind insulin and IGF-I. Binding of either peptide to these receptors enhances gonadotropin effects and stimulates androgen production. Abnormal function of the ovarian IGF system has been linked to **polycystic ovary syndrome (PCOS),** characterized by menstrual abnormalities, hyperandrogenism, and insulin resistance. PCOS is detailed later in this chapter.

In clinical settings, endogenous administration of hormones and blockade of hormone receptors are used in treatment of reproductive system disorders. This *hormonal therapy* is of particular importance in treatment of prostate cancer in males (see Chapter 30), infertility (see Chapter 32), and many of the gynecologic and breast disorders detailed in this chapter. *Hormone replacement therapy* is the foundation of intervention for the discomforts associated with menopause, but imposes some iatrogenic risk, as discussed next.

Menopause and the Perimenopause

Menopause, the cessation of menstrual cycles that accompanies the depletion of oocytes, occurs physiologically at an average age of 51 years. Surgical menopause is iatrogenically induced with removal of the ovaries (*oophorectomy*). As previously stated, the number of postmenopausal women is increasingly rapidly. This trend is because of the increased longevity of American women as well as the arrival of the postwar "baby boom" generation into the menopausal transition.

It is unknown whether menopause, also known as the *climacteric*, occurs because of depletion of ovarian follicles, with resulting alteration of feedback to the hypothalamic–pituitary–adrenocortical (HPA) axis, or whether it occurs because of genetically programmed changes in neural input to the HPA axis, resulting in altered signaling to the ovaries. It is possible that both events serve a "pacemaker" function.[5] Years before the follicular reserve is exhausted, manifestations of reduced fertility and irregularity of menstrual cycles become apparent. The frequency of GnRH pulses decreases, and circulating GnRH declines. FSH levels rise and inhibin levels fall in perimenopausal women who are still menstruating. Progesterone is depleted first, followed by estradiol, and finally ovarian androgens. Follicular development ceases, and menstrual cycles stop, sometimes suddenly, but usually during a time period of 1 to 5 years. Adipose and adrenal production of estrone, a weak estrogen, continues for a time (see Chapter 29).

Menstrual irregularity resulting from occasional anovulatory cycles is often the first manifestation of the perimenopause. Cycle length becomes more variable, and bleeding may be prolonged or heavy. Scanty bleeding between periods may also be seen. Instability of vascular smooth muscle, manifested as headaches, dizziness, and palpitations, occurs in many women. The precise mechanism responsible for these symptoms is uncertain, but they may relate to increased FSH or wide fluctuations in circulating estradiol levels.

Temperature lability is believed to result from inappropriate inputs to the hypothalamus during altered HPA regulation. Hot flashes are recurrent periods of flushing, sweating, and chills, reflecting a downward resetting of the hypothalamic thermostat (see Chapter 11).[6] To achieve the lower set point, the hypothalamus initiates cooling mechanisms (peripheral dilation and sweating). When the set point is reset to normal, heat production mechanisms (chills) are triggered. Hot flashes may occur frequently during the day, causing psychological distress in social and occupational settings. External factors such as anxiety, caffeine, sugar, spicy foods, hot drinks, and high environmental temperature may trigger some hot flashes, but others occur with no apparent stimuli. Hot flashes at night (night sweats) may interrupt sleep.

With declining levels of estrogen, progesterone, and androgens, gradual atrophy is seen in glandular breast tissue, and in the ovaries, uterus, cervix, and vagina. Female-patterned body hair and fat distribution, as well as elasticity of the skin, are gradually lost. Vaginal walls become thinner and dryer, possibly resulting in **atrophic vaginitis** or in difficult, painful sexual intercourse (**dyspareunia**).

Psychological manifestations such as anxiety, depression, irritability, and decreased libido are common but not universal during the perimenopause. Cognitive disturbances and decreased short-term memory are often reported as well. Hormonal fluctuations and sleep disturbances certainly underlie some of these symptoms. Situational factors associated with midlife roles and cultural factors related to aging may increase the risk of emotional distress.

Loss of the protective effects of estrogen on serum lipids and blood vessels permits acceleration of atherosclerosis in postmenopausal women. By age 65, their risk of cardiovascular disease is equal to that of men.[7] Removal of estrogen also promotes osteoporosis, especially in women with intrinsically higher rates of bone loss, inadequate calcium intake, and inactive lifestyles (see Chapter 34).

Because some estrogen is produced by adipose tissue, women who are obese may have more constant estrogen levels and milder perimenopausal symptoms. Typically, women who smoke cigarettes have more severe symptoms because of thinner body habitus as well as more rapid degeneration of the ovarian follicles.[6]

Although menopause is a natural transition, the increased life expectancy beyond the reproductive years results in a sustained estrogen deficiency state that clearly has adverse effects. Hormone replacement therapy is used by many women to alleviate menopausal symptoms and decrease the risks of cardiovascular disease and osteoporosis. Conjugated equine estrogen (Premarin) is the most frequently prescribed drug in the United States.[8] Unfortunately, therapy with estrogen alone is known to increase the risk of gallbladder disease, **endometrial cancer,** and probably breast cancer. Controversy exists as to whether combination regimens in which progesterone is also administered are safer or as effective as unopposed estrogen in reducing cardiovascular risk (see Focus of Current Research). Risks and benefits of therapy vary with different hormone preparations and routes of administration, as detailed in Table 31–3.

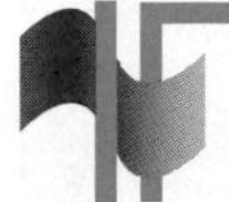

Clinical Scenario

During her yearly check-up, S.M., age 48, tells her gynecologist that she has been having "terrible headaches" and often wakes during the night in a "cold sweat." She also notes that she is "impossible to live with most of the time" and often snaps at her husband and teenage children. S.M. is still having menstrual periods, but her cycles have become increasingly irregular, and the bleeding may vary from very scanty periods to "gushing of blood." S.M.'s physical examination is normal, although lab studies reveal a mild microcytic, hypochromic anemia and increased serum FSH.

1. What is the probable physiologic basis of S.M.'s symptoms?
2. Should S.M. begin hormone replacement therapy? What factors should be considered?

DISORDERS OF THE FEMALE REPRODUCTIVE SYSTEM AND BREAST

Amenorrhea

Definition. Amenorrhea is the absence of menstruation in a woman of reproductive age. *Primary amenorrhea* is defined as the lack of spontaneous uterine bleeding by the age of 14 in the absence of development of secondary sex characteristics or by age 16 if development is otherwise normal.[9] *Secondary amenorrhea* is the absence of menstrual bleeding for 6 months in a woman with previously regular cycles or for 12 months in a woman with previous **oligomenorrhea** (irregular, prolonged periods between bleeding episodes).

Epidemiology. Primary amenorrhea has a demonstrated prevalence of 0.3%, and secondary amenorrhea is seen in 1 to 3% of women.[9] Primary amenorrhea is usually caused by an endocrine disorder or structural abnormality of the reproductive tract. Risk factors for specific conditions are discussed subsequently with etiology. Secondary amenorrhea is seen

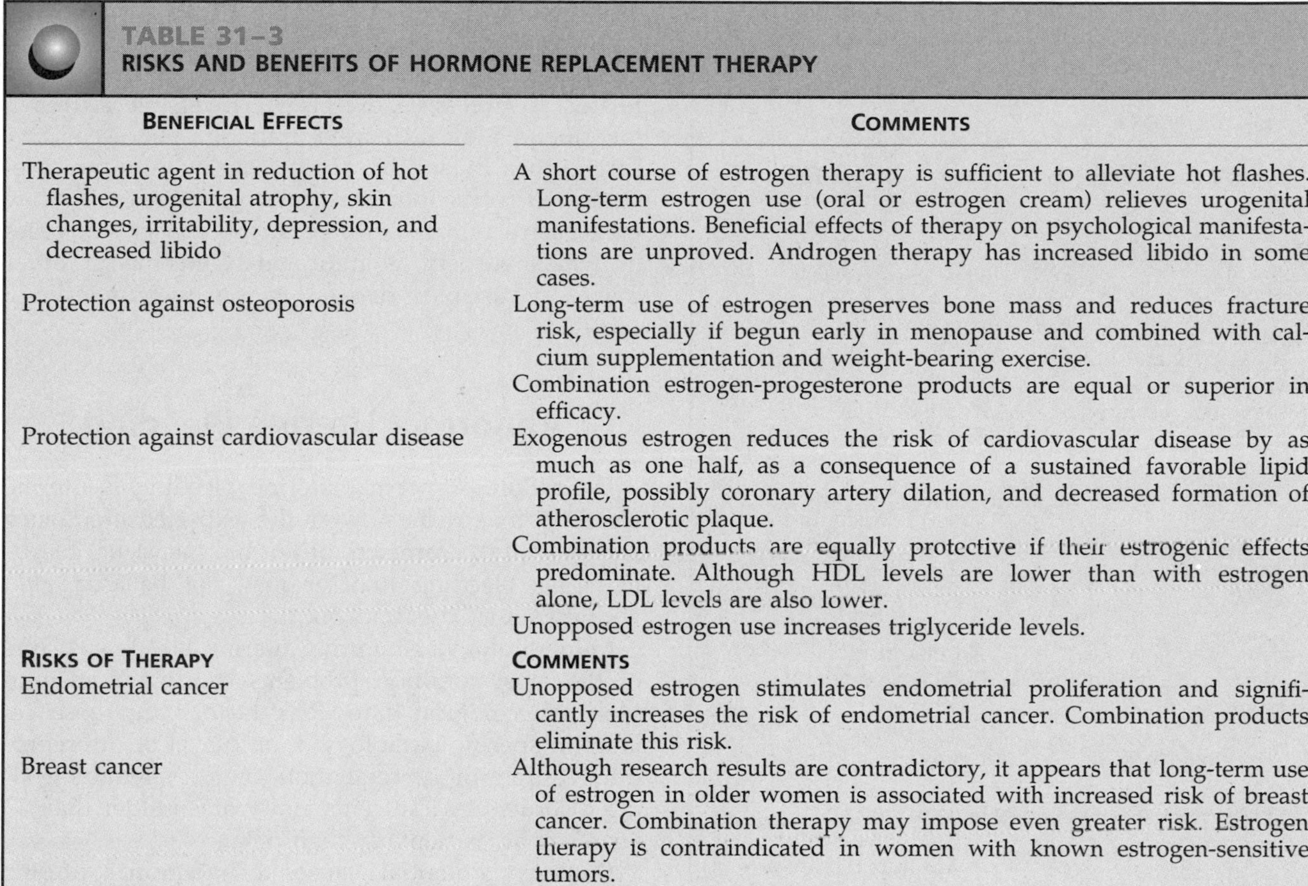

TABLE 31–3
RISKS AND BENEFITS OF HORMONE REPLACEMENT THERAPY

BENEFICIAL EFFECTS	COMMENTS
Therapeutic agent in reduction of hot flashes, urogenital atrophy, skin changes, irritability, depression, and decreased libido	A short course of estrogen therapy is sufficient to alleviate hot flashes. Long-term estrogen use (oral or estrogen cream) relieves urogenital manifestations. Beneficial effects of therapy on psychological manifestations are unproved. Androgen therapy has increased libido in some cases.
Protection against osteoporosis	Long-term use of estrogen preserves bone mass and reduces fracture risk, especially if begun early in menopause and combined with calcium supplementation and weight-bearing exercise. Combination estrogen-progesterone products are equal or superior in efficacy.
Protection against cardiovascular disease	Exogenous estrogen reduces the risk of cardiovascular disease by as much as one half, as a consequence of a sustained favorable lipid profile, possibly coronary artery dilation, and decreased formation of atherosclerotic plaque. Combination products are equally protective if their estrogenic effects predominate. Although HDL levels are lower than with estrogen alone, LDL levels are also lower. Unopposed estrogen use increases triglyceride levels.
RISKS OF THERAPY	**COMMENTS**
Endometrial cancer	Unopposed estrogen stimulates endometrial proliferation and significantly increases the risk of endometrial cancer. Combination products eliminate this risk.
Breast cancer	Although research results are contradictory, it appears that long-term use of estrogen in older women is associated with increased risk of breast cancer. Combination therapy may impose even greater risk. Estrogen therapy is contraindicated in women with known estrogen-sensitive tumors.
Thromboembolism	Research data are inconclusive.
Gallbladder disease	Research data are inconclusive.

HDL, high-density lipoprotein; LDL, low-density lipoprotein.

most often in college students (associated with anorexia nervosa) and in competitive athletes and ballet dancers (associated with low body fat and intense physical exertion). Drug therapy with agents that have estrogen-like activity, increase prolactin levels, or cause ovarian toxicity may also induce secondary amenorrhea.

Etiology. Table 31–4 lists the more common causes of amenorrhea. The most common cause is pregnancy, which must be initially ruled out before proceeding with further clinical evaluation. Menstruation requires a functional HPA, hormonally responsive reproductive organs, and an intact outflow tract. Dysfunction of any of these elements may result in amenorrhea. Inadequate release of hypothalamic GnRh may result from stress, depression, severe weight loss, anorexia nervosa, or strenuous exercise.[9] Hyperandrogenism is present in 37% of amenorrheic women, many of whom also have polycystic ovary syndrome.[10] *Premature ovarian failure,* defined as the depletion of ovarian follicles before the age of 35, may be idiopathic, associated with autoimmune disease, or caused by a chromosomal defect (mosaicism with predominant XX karyotype but some XO or XY cells). Prolactin-secreting pituitary tumors, which may impair secretion of gonadotropins, are a less common cause of amenorrhea. Imperforate hymen may obstruct menstrual outflow in primary amenorrhea, and intrauterine adhesions and endometrial ablation (*endometrial failure* or *Asherman's syndrome*) may be the cause in women who have previously undergone *dilatation and curettage* (scraping) of the endometrial lining of the uterus.

Pathophysiology. The mechanism of amenorrhea varies depending on whether the cause is hypothalamic failure, pituitary failure, ovarian failure, endometrial failure, or outflow tract obstruction. Other variables include ovulatory status and circulating levels of reproductive hormones. Amenorrheic women who have adequate estrogen levels but deficiency of progesterone do not ovulate and are thus infertile.[9] These women are at increased risk of endometrial cancer and possibly breast cancer because of unopposed estrogen. Others have estrogen defi-

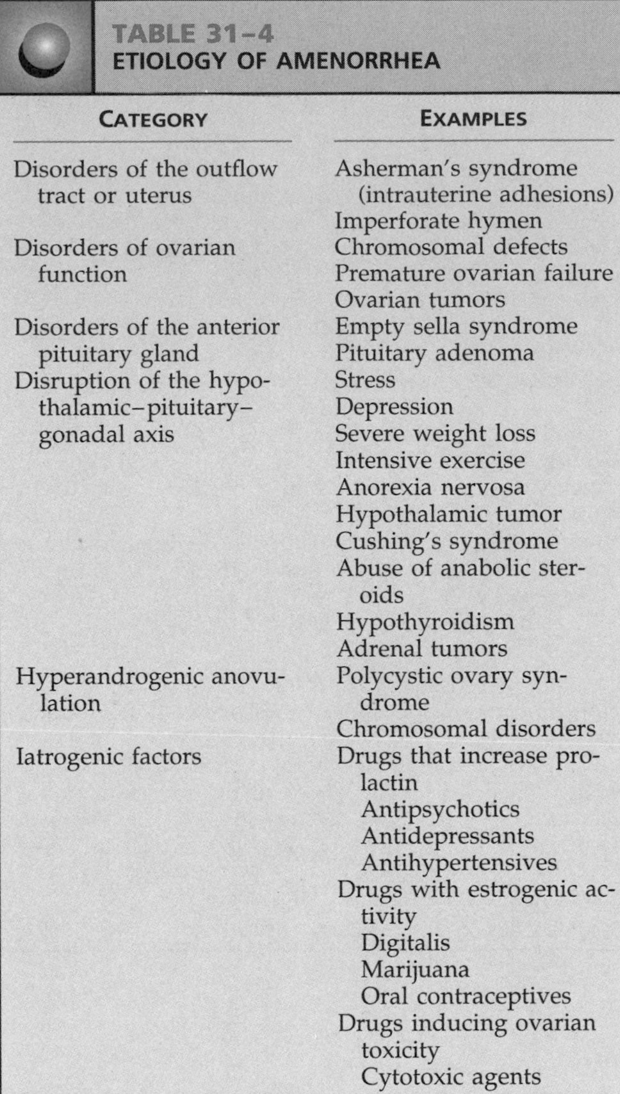

TABLE 31–4
ETIOLOGY OF AMENORRHEA

Category	Examples
Disorders of the outflow tract or uterus	Asherman's syndrome (intrauterine adhesions) Imperforate hymen
Disorders of ovarian function	Chromosomal defects Premature ovarian failure Ovarian tumors
Disorders of the anterior pituitary gland	Empty sella syndrome Pituitary adenoma
Disruption of the hypothalamic–pituitary–gonadal axis	Stress Depression Severe weight loss Intensive exercise Anorexia nervosa Hypothalamic tumor Cushing's syndrome Abuse of anabolic steroids Hypothyroidism Adrenal tumors
Hyperandrogenic anovulation	Polycystic ovary syndrome Chromosomal disorders
Iatrogenic factors	Drugs that increase prolactin Antipsychotics Antidepressants Antihypertensives Drugs with estrogenic activity Digitalis Marijuana Oral contraceptives Drugs inducing ovarian toxicity Cytotoxic agents

ciency, and are at risk for osteoporosis and cardiovascular disease. Presence of a Y chromosome may give rise to malignancy in undeveloped testicular tissue. Pituitary tumors may cause panhypopituitarism with widespread organ effects (see Chapter 27).

Clinical Manifestations. Amenorrhea is the common denominator among the many associated disorders. Additional manifestations depend on the specific cause.

Prevention and Treatment. Many factors associated with secondary amenorrhea are amenable to intervention, e.g., nutritional counseling, modification of exercise regimens, and discontinuation of offending drugs. Surgical treatment is warranted in the presence of testicular tissue, pituitary tumors, or outflow tract abnormalities. Chronic anovulation is usually treated with oral contraceptives or cyclic progesterone. Hormone replacement therapy with a combination of estrogen and progesterone is usually indicated in those with premature ovarian failure or hypothalamic failure.

Prognosis and Outcome. Secondary amenorrhea related to excessive exercise is reversible within a few months of decreased training, but secondary amenorrhea caused by anorexia nervosa is more resistant to correction. Surgical correction or outflow tract obstruction is curative in the majority of cases in which surgery is indicated. Outcome in other cases is variable, depending on the underlying cause.

Abnormal Uterine Bleeding

Definition. Abnormal uterine bleeding is uterine bleeding that differs from the expected frequency and quantity parameters of normal menstrual bleeding. This bleeding may or may not be associated with ovulatory dysfunction.

Epidemiology. Abnormal uterine bleeding is one of the most common problems causing women to seek gynecological care. Risk factors are those related to specific pathology at any level of the reproductive tract or its regulation, or to systemic bleeding disorders. Adolescents and women older than 40 years are at particularly high risk.

Etiology. Potential causes of abnormal uterine bleeding may be related to trauma, pregnancy, anatomic abnormality, inflammation, coagulopathy, systemic disease, or hormonal imbalance. Examples of disorders in each category are listed in Table 31–5. Bleeding associated with pregnancy is discussed in Chapter 32.

Pathophysiology. If the bleeding is regular and cyclic, the patient is presumed to be ovulating. Irregular bleeding is associated with anovulation and hormonal imbalance.[10] Increased estrogenic stimulation of the endometrium may cause endometrial proliferation and increased risk of endometrial cancer in some cases. Excessive bleeding may result in iron-deficiency anemia or, rarely, in hemorrhagic shock.

Clinical Manifestations. The pattern of abnormal uterine bleeding relates to the underlying cause (Table 31–6). Manifestations of anemia include fatigue, dyspnea, and palpitations (see Chapter 12). Anovulation manifests as infertility and hormonal imbalance.

Prevention and Treatment. Intervention is aimed at the underlying disorder. Iron replacement may be warranted in severe anemia. Acute bleeding leading to hemodynamic compromise of the patient may require dilatation and curettage of the endometrium or surgical evacuation of blood clots. Estrogen excess in anovulation is treated with cyclic progester-

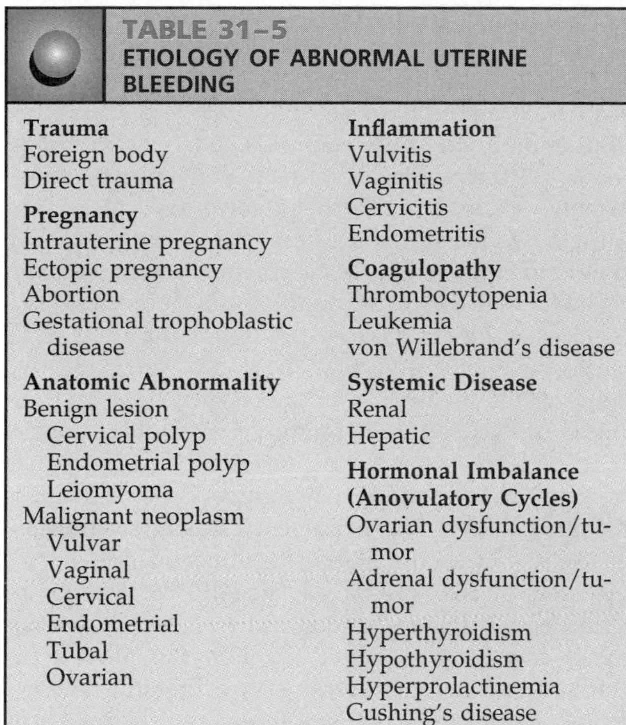

TABLE 31–5
ETIOLOGY OF ABNORMAL UTERINE BLEEDING

Trauma	**Inflammation**
Foreign body	Vulvitis
Direct trauma	Vaginitis
Pregnancy	Cervicitis
Intrauterine pregnancy	Endometritis
Ectopic pregnancy	**Coagulopathy**
Abortion	Thrombocytopenia
Gestational trophoblastic disease	Leukemia
	von Willebrand's disease
Anatomic Abnormality	**Systemic Disease**
Benign lesion	Renal
Cervical polyp	Hepatic
Endometrial polyp	**Hormonal Imbalance (Anovulatory Cycles)**
Leiomyoma	Ovarian dysfunction/tumor
Malignant neoplasm	Adrenal dysfunction/tumor
Vulvar	Hyperthyroidism
Vaginal	Hypothyroidism
Cervical	Hyperprolactinemia
Endometrial	Cushing's disease
Tubal	
Ovarian	

From Galle, P.C., and McRae, M.A. (1993). Abnormal uterine bleeding: Finding and treating the cause. *Postgraduate Medicine* 93(2), 76.

one administration to induce normal sloughing of the endometrium.

Prognosis and Outcome. Correction of hormonal imbalance or structural disorder yields a good prognosis in most cases. Prognosis in reproductive tract cancers or systemic diseases is variable depending on the severity of the underlying disorder.

Premenstrual Syndrome

Definition. Premenstrual syndrome (PMS) is the predictable occurrence of distressing physical and psychological manifestations during the luteal phase of the menstrual cycle. Controversy exists as to whether PMS represents a physiologic disorder, a psychiatric disorder, or enhanced sensitivity of some individuals to normal cyclic changes.

Epidemiology. An estimated 70% to 90% of women report some symptoms associated with menstruation, and about 10% have symptoms severe enough to disrupt their lives.[11] When formal diagnostic criteria are applied, fewer than 50% of women who self-diagnose with PMS have the diagnosis confirmed.[10]

Etiology. No definitive cause has been found for PMS. Emotional and situational factors may play a role in heightened sensitivity to physiologic changes during the menstrual cycle.

Pathophysiology. Hormone levels and patterns are not significantly different from those of women who do not complain of PMS symptoms, and physical examination findings are normal.

Clinical Manifestations. Common symptoms of PMS are listed in Table 31–7. Manifestations such as abdominal bloating, breast tenderness, headache, anxiety, tension, and irritability are perceived as stressful or even disabling. To support the diagnosis

TABLE 31–6
TERMINOLOGY ASSOCIATED WITH ABNORMAL UTERINE BLEEDING

Term	Description	Common Etiologies
Menorrhagia	Excessive menstrual bleeding at normal intervals	Excessive endometrial proliferation resulting from high estrogen state
Metrorrhagia	Bleeding that is not excessive but occurs at irregular, frequent intervals	Breakthrough bleeding with oral contraceptive use; endometrial polyps; use of an intrauterine device; chlamydial endometritis
Intermenstrual bleeding	Bleeding that is not excessive but occurs between regular menstrual cycles	May be a precursor for more ominous types of abnormal uterine bleeding; often idiopathic
Metromenorrhagia	Either prolonged or excessive bleeding occurring at irregular intervals	Anovulation; uterine fibroids; uterine polyps; gynecologic cancers
Polymenorrhea	Regular bleeding at intervals of less than 21 days	Associated with ovulation and reduced length of the follicular phase
Oligomenorrhea	Uterine bleeding at intervals of 35 days to 6 months	Hypothalamic disorder
Amenorrhea	Absence of bleeding for at least 6 months	Pregnancy; menopause; anovulation

Data from Jennings, J.C. (1995). Abnormal uterine bleeding. *Medical Clinics of North America* 79(6), 1358–1359.

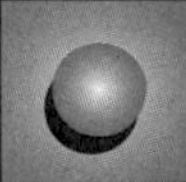

TABLE 31–7
COMMON MANIFESTATIONS OF PREMENSTRUAL SYNDROME

Emotional/Behavioral	Physical
Aggression	Abdominal bloating
Altered libido	Acne, cold sores, styes
Anger	Breast swelling, tenderness
Anxiety	Constipation
Decreased motivation	Dizziness
Depression	Fatigue
Food cravings	Fluid retention
Forgetfulness	Headaches, migraines
Hostility	Hot flashes
Insomnia	Muscle aches and pains
Irritability	Palpitations
Mood lability	Weight gain
Panic attacks	
Poor concentration	
Reduced coping skills	
Suicidal tendencies	
Tearfulness	
Tension	

Reprinted with permission from Parker, P.D. (1994). Premenstrual syndrome. *American Family Physician* 50(6), 1310, published by the American Academy of Family Physicians.

of PMS, the patient is asked to document the presence and severity of her emotional/behavioral and physical symptoms for at least two consecutive cycles. Consistent with PMS, symptoms should be at least three times worse during the luteal phase than the follicular phase.[10]

Prevention and Treatment. Intervention in PMS is usually symptomatic and supportive, including emotional support, dietary modification (reduction of salt and refined sugar), ensuring sufficient sleep, and a prescribed exercise routine. Diuretics have not been shown to be superior to placebo in treating symptoms of bloating and breast tenderness.[10] Modest improvement in symptoms has been reported with supplementation of vitamin B_6, calcium, and magnesium.[11] Anxiety and irritability may be treated with anxiolytic agents such as alprazolam (Xanax) and antidepressants such as fluoxetine (Prozac). In more severe cases, suppression of ovulation with oral contraceptives, progesterone, estrogen, androgen derivatives, and GnRH agonists has been used, but these agents have not proved superior to placebo. A few patients have undergone bilateral oophorectomy in treatment of PMS.

Prognosis and Outcome. A wide range of interventions has been reported to be effective in treatment of PMS, on the basis of subjective improvement in symptoms. Patients with PMS have been shown to have an extremely high response to placebo, however, so the true efficacy of any therapy is uncertain.[11]

Vulvovaginitis

Definition. Vulvovaginitis is inflammation of the vulva and vaginal tissues.

Epidemiology. Vulvovaginitis is very common among postmenopausal women and among young, sexually active women. Behavioral risk factors in younger women are those associated with sexually transmitted diseases (see Chapter 30). Women who are metabolically or immunologically compromised are also at higher risk. Conditions imposing such compromise include pregnancy, oral contraceptive use, diabetes mellitus, immunosuppression, and antibiotic or corticosteroid therapy.[12] Atrophic changes caused by the removal of estrogen at menopause result in tissue changes that reduce the effectiveness of epithelial and pH barriers of the vagina, increasing the risk of local irritation or infection.

Etiology. Vulvovaginitis is usually caused by infection or atrophic changes induced by postmenopausal estrogen deficiency. Among the most common vulvovaginal infections are genital herpes, genital warts, and trichomoniasis, which are sexually transmitted. Vaginitis may also be caused by **bacterial vaginosis,** associated with polymicrobial infection with agents such as *Gardnerella vaginalis, Corynebacterium, Bacteroides, Peptococcus, Eubacterium,* and *Mycoplasma hominis.*[12] **Vaginal candidiasis** (yeast infection) is also common. The *Candida* fungus is a component of the normal vaginal flora in many women, and it may induce inflammation in response to immunologic or metabolic compromise.

Removal of estrogen at menopause leads to atrophic effects predisposing to urinary incontinence (see Chapter 20), **pelvic support disorders** (discussed later in this chapter), and atrophic vaginitis. Thinning of the vaginal epithelium, decreased blood supply, and increased vaginal pH lead to decreased lubrication and protection and increase the risk of local irritation.[13]

Rarely, lesions of the vulva or vagina are caused by neoplasia (Table 31–8). Occurrence of a rare clear-cell cancer of the vagina in a cohort of young women whose mothers had taken the steroid diethylstilbestrol (DES) to reduce the risk of spontaneous abortion led to banning of the use of this agent in the United States in 1971.[14]

Pathophysiology. Vulvovaginitis is an inflammatory disorder (see Chapter 13). Release of local mediators by infectious agents or local irritation induces erythema, irritation, itching, and altered vaginal discharge. (Normal lubricatory vaginal secretions are odorless, clear or white, and viscous.) Sexual and urinary function may be impaired. Some strains of human papillomavirus (HPV) have been associated with the development of **cervical cancer;** how-

TABLE 31–8
NEOPLASTIC LESIONS OF THE VULVA AND VAGINA

LESION	DESCRIPTION
Tumors of the Vulva	
BENIGN TUMORS	
Papillary hidradenoma	Arises from modified apocrine sweat glands
Condyloma acuminatum	Sexually transmitted warts, polyps, or other raised lesions
MALIGNANT TUMORS	
Carcinoma of the vulva	Eighty-five per cent are squamous cell carcinomas, associated with human papillomaviruses and precancerous changes (vulvar intraepithelial neoplasia)
Paget's disease	Arises from primitive epithelial progenitor cells; manifests as pruritic, red, crusted, map-like area on labia majora
Malignant melanoma	Arises from melanocytes; capable of widespread metastasis
Tumors of the Vagina	
BENIGN TUMORS	
Rhabdomyoma	Arises from skeletal muscle
Stromal polyps	Arise from stromal cells; may be precancerous
MALIGNANT TUMORS	
Squamous cell carcinoma	Usually follows a previous cervical carcinoma
Adenocarcinoma	Clear cell type is associated with intrauterine exposure to diethylstilbestrol
Embryonal rhabdomyosarcoma	Arises from embryonic cells; seen in infants and young children

Data from Cotran, R.S., Kumar, V., and Robbins, S.L. (1994). *Robbins Pathologic Basis of Disease.* Philadelphia: W.B. Saunders. (pp. 1041–1045).

ever, these are not the same strains that usually cause genital warts.

Clinical Manifestations. Common manifestations include irritation, itching, dysuria, dyspareunia, and possibly skin lesions or altered vaginal discharge. Genital herpes presents as painful, tender vesicles that may be preceded by burning, paresthesias, or pain radiating to the back, hips, or legs.[10] Genital warts are apparent as painless, clustered "cauliflower-like" lesions that may involve the cervix and well as the vulva. Trichomoniasis may produce copious, foul-smelling, frothy, yellow-green drainage. Vulvovaginal erythema is mild, and the vaginal mucosa and cervix may have a "strawberry" appearance (red with petechiae). Bacterial vaginosis usually produces a thin, white, yellow, or gray creamy discharge with minimal irritation and itching.[13] The discharge has a fishy or musty odor. Patients with candidiasis have intense vulvar itching and irritation, and thick, white, curd-like discharge. Atrophic vaginitis is characterized by vaginal dryness, burning, watery or blood-tinged vaginal discharge, erythema, and possible petechiae.

Prevention and Treatment. Preventive measures for sexually transmitted diseases were discussed in Chapter 30. Optimal management of pregnancy and diabetes mellitus and discontinuation of antibiotic or steroid therapy may reduce the risk of vaginal infections. The patient should be advised to wear loose clothing and cotton underwear and should avoid use of local creams or sprays that might alter the vaginal flora or pH. Genital herpes is treated with antiviral agents such as acyclovir (Zovirax). Genital warts may be treated with local application of antimitotic agents such as podophyllum (Podocon), topical cytotoxic agents (e.g., 5-fluorouracil), acyclovir, or systemic or intralesional interferon therapy.[10] Antibiotic therapy with metronidazole (Flagyl) is the treatment of choice for trichomoniasis and bacterial vaginosis, and candidiasis is treated with an antifungal agent such as miconazole (Monistat).[13] Use of estrogen vaginal cream may relieve symptoms of atrophic vaginitis, and consideration should be given to hormone replacement therapy in some cases.

Prognosis and Outcome. Most forms of vulvovaginitis respond to symptomatic treatment, but tend to persist as recurrent conditions.

Pelvic Inflammatory Disease

Definition. Pelvic inflammatory disease (PID) is infection of the uterus, fallopian tubes, and adjacent pelvic structures that is not associated with surgery or pregnancy.[15]

Epidemiology. Pelvic inflammatory disease is diagnosed in approximately 1 million women each year in the United States.[15] Risk factors for sexually transmitted diseases and bacterial vaginosis apply to PID, because ascending infection is usually implicated. Other risk factors are use of intrauterine contraceptive devices (IUDs), cigarette smoking, and vaginal douching.

Etiology. Pelvic inflammatory disease results from ascending infection with *Chlamydia trachomatis, Neisseria gonorrheae,* or other organisms that have colonized the cervix. More than one third of women with untreated chlamydia or gonorrhea develop PID.[16] Although sexually transmitted organisms may initiate the process, other organisms (including the normal flora) have been implicated in its development as well. The precise mechanisms by which host factors interact with the infecting organism are unknown.

Pathophysiology. Organisms ascend from the cervical region, triggering an inflammatory response within the upper genital tract. Chronic inflammation frequently results in scarring and obstruction of fallopian tubes, increasing the risk of tubal pregnancy or infertility (see Chapter 32). Each episode of PID impairs host defenses, increasing the likelihood of subsequent attacks and long-term effects.

Clinical Manifestations. Local signs and symptoms of inflammation include lower abdominal pain, abnormal vaginal discharge or bleeding, dysuria, and dyspareunia. Systemic manifestations may also be present, including nausea, vomiting, fever, and leukocytosis, as well as an increase in the erythrocyte sedimentation rate and other acute phase reactants (see Chapter 13). Either infertility or tubal pregnancy may be the presenting sign in some women who have had clinically silent PID. The diagnosis may be confirmed with laparoscopic visualization of inflamed pelvic organs.

Prevention and Treatment. Reduction of risk factors for sexually transmitted diseases is essential (see Chapter 30). Treatment consists of appropriate antibiotic therapy, usually administered on an outpatient basis. The male sexual partners of women with PID must also be assessed and treated if necessary to prevent reinfection. Surgical treatment, including drainage of pelvic abscesses or resection of damaged organs, is rarely required. Treatment of infertility is discussed in Chapter 32.

Prognosis and Outcome. Acute episodes of PID are usually successfully managed with medical therapy. Chronic pelvic pain persists in about 18%, and the risk of tubal pregnancy is increased sixfold.[15] Infertility remains a long-term problem in 25% of women after one or more episodes of PID.

Endometriosis

Definition. Endometriosis is a non-neoplastic condition in which functioning endometrial tissue is found in ectopic sites, outside the uterus (Fig. 31–8).

Epidemiology. Endometriosis is relatively common, with a prevalence of 5% to 10% among premenopausal women.[17] As many as 50% of infertile women have endometriosis. The highest incidence is among women whose mothers also had the condition. Women who have postponed childbearing are at particularly high risk, with whites at higher risk than women of other races.

Etiology. The precise etiology of endometriosis is unknown. Three theories have been advanced: (1) retrograde menstruation with coelomic metaplasia; (2) embryonic implantation; and (3) endometrial metastasis. Retrograde menstruation refers to the regurgitation of menstrual flow through the fallopian tubes into the abdominal cavity. Endometrial tissue then implants on pelvic organs and reproduces itself. However, because not all women with retro-

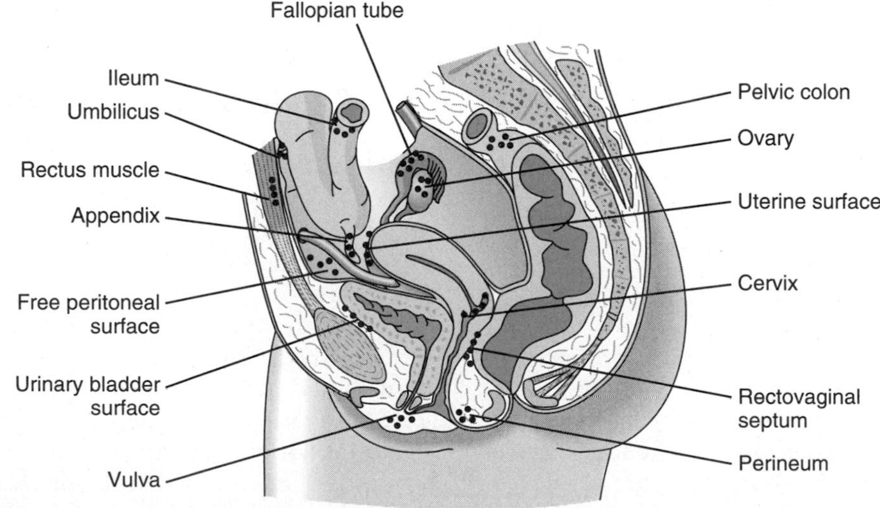

FIGURE 31–8

Common sites of endometriosis. Ectopic endometrial tissue is most commonly found on the ovaries and in dependent areas of the peritoneum, but it may be located throughout the peritoneal cavity and at distant sites such as the lungs.

grade menstruation develop endometriosis, other factors must also be involved. Immunologic alteration is often present in these women and may contribute to progression of the disease. In addition, irritants within menstrual fluid may induce coelomic metaplasia, or transformation of peritoneal mesothelium to endometrium. (Mesothelium and endometrium both originate from the same embryonic tissue.)

The embryonic implantation theory holds that some embryonic müllerian cells (which give rise to endometrial tissue) remain in pelvic tissues and may be induced to differentiate into endometrial tissue with later estrogenic stimulation. The endometrial metastasis theory proposes that endometrial cells are transported to extrauterine sites via the bloodstream or lymphatics, similarly to neoplastic metastasis.

Pathophysiology. Ectopic endometrial tissue responds to cyclic hormonal changes with proliferation, secretion, and sloughing, but in a more unpredictable way than does normal endometrial tissue. Bleeding chronically triggers the inflammatory response, resulting in formation of scar tissue adhesions that may be obstructive. Endometrial tissue developing on the ovary produces an ovarian cyst known as an endometrioma or "chocolate" cyst because of the brown blood it contains. Endometriosis regresses with the hormonal alterations of pregnancy and subsides completely with menopause.

Clinical Manifestations. Although many women are asymptomatic, some suffer excessive pain (dysmenorrhea) before, during, and after menstruation. Dyspareunia and irregularity of the menstrual cycle are common. The incidence of infertility is high, whether or not tubal obstruction is present. Tender, nodular masses are often palpable along thickened uterosacral ligaments or in the region of the posterior uterus or cul-de-sac. Ovarian implants (chocolate cysts) may manifest as adnexal tenderness. Signs of urinary or gastrointestinal obstruction may be apparent as bleeding into the urine or stool, ureteral colic, or bowel obstruction. Rarely, hemoptysis or pneumothorax is present because of dissemination of endometrial tissue to the lungs. Laparoscopic evaluation reveals the endometrial implants, which may appear as bluish black "powder burn" lesions; white, red, or clear vesicles; white or yellow papules; flame-shaped hemorrhages; nodules; or fibroses.[17]

Prevention and Treatment. There is no known prevention for the disorder. Staging is done during diagnostic laparoscopy. Treatment depends on severity, the woman's age, and whether she desires pregnancy. In patients with stage I (minimal) or stage II (mild) endometriosis who wish to attain or retain fertility, the disorder may be treated expectantly with analgesics during periods of pain or with conservative surgery. Hormone therapy with oral contraceptives, progesterone, or antigonadotropins is designed to induce pseudopregnancy, pseudomenopause, or chronic anovulation, and it may result in regression of endometrial tissue. Hormone therapy is often used in patients with extensive endometriosis (stage III or IV disease) manifested by severe pain and infertility.

Surgical treatment of endometriosis is conservative (limited to laser excision of isolated adhesions and ectopic endometrial implants) in women who wish to conceive, and it may be done at the time of diagnostic laparoscopy. In severe endometriosis, definitive treatment consists of radical resection of the uterus, ovaries, fallopian tubes, and as many ectopic sites as possible. Surgery may also be used to free any obstructions of fallopian tubes, ureters, or bowel. Treatment of infertility is discussed in Chapter 32.

Prognosis and Outcome. Hormonal treatment of endometriosis is generally very effective in relieving discomfort. Assisted reproductive techniques have been successful in many cases of endometriosis-associated infertility. Ovarian hyperstimulation with gonadotropins has resulted in pregnancy in up to 18% of affected women, and up to 25% of women have successful pregnancies after in vitro fertilization or gamete intrafallopian transfer.[18] Women with advanced stages of endometriosis are usually not successfully treated with assisted reproductive techniques because of impaired follicle development.

Adenomyosis

Definition. Adenomyosis, sometimes referred to as "internal endometriosis," is a benign disorder in which endometrial tissue invades the uterine myometrium.

Epidemiology. Adenomyosis is a common disorder, occurring in up to 80% of women with other pelvic diseases such as uterine fibroid tumors, endometriosis, PID, and endometrial cancer. In most cases, the diagnosis is made incidentally in women undergoing surgical removal of the uterus (*hysterectomy*) in treatment of endometriosis or uterine fibroid tumors. Most women with adenomyosis are between 30 and 50 years of age and usually have borne several children.[19]

Etiology. The etiology of adenomyosis is unknown. Hypothetical causes include heredity, trauma by cesarean section or uterine infection, viral infection, excessive estrogen stimulation of the endometrium, or hyperprolactinemia. No controlled studies have confirmed these associations, however.[19]

The link between multiparity (history of more than one pregnancy) and adenomyosis may relate to the presence of chronic postpartum inflammation (**endometritis**) that breaks down the barrier between the endometrial and myometrial layers of the uterus.

Pathophysiology. Endometrial tissue invades much of the myometrium and bleeds in response to hormonal stimulation. The uterus enlarges as a result of compensatory hypertrophy and hyperplasia of myometrial muscle fibers. Disruption of the uterine wall prevents normal muscle contraction and predisposes to abnormal uterine bleeding. Fertility is usually not affected.

Clinical Manifestations. Uterine enlargement nearly always occurs, to a maximum size equivalent to that seen at 8 to 14 weeks of pregnancy. Pelvic pain and menorrhagia are present in most cases. Childbearing imposes risk of postpartum hemorrhage, uterine atony, and uterine rupture in women with adenomyosis.

Prevention and Treatment. There is no known prevention or medical therapy for adenomyosis. For severely symptomatic patients in whom loss of reproductive capacity is acceptable, hysterectomy is the treatment of choice.

Prognosis and Outcome. It has been proposed that adenomyosis may predispose patients to the development of endometrial cancer, but this association is unproved.[19] Symptoms of adenomyosis subside at menopause. Hysterectomy is curative.

Uterine Fibroid Tumors

Definition. Uterine fibroid tumors (leiomyomas) are benign tumors composed of myometrial smooth muscle and fibrous connective tissue.

Epidemiology. Uterine fibroids are present in 25% of all women during their fertile years.[20] Black women are at higher risk than whites.

Etiology. The precise etiology of uterine fibroids is unknown. The tumors are known to be estrogen responsive.

Pathophysiology. The tumors develop as twisted bundles of smooth muscle cells that may be very small or may fill the pelvic cavity. They usually involve the body and fundus of the uterus, sparing the cervix and the ligaments that suspend the uterus. Individual muscle cells are normal in appearance and function and rarely undergo malignant transformation. Mechanical effects of tumor growth may produce abnormal uterine bleeding, compression of the bladder, and impaired fertility.

Clinical Manifestations. Uterine fibroids are often asymptomatic, but they may cause abnormal uterine bleeding if submucosal vessels are disrupted, urinary frequency if the bladder is compressed, ischemic pelvic pain if blood vessels are obstructed, and infertility if tumors impair intrauterine transport of sperm or implantation of the conceptus. If pregnancy does occur, the frequency of complications is increased, including spontaneous abortion, malposition of the fetus, uterine dystocia during labor, and hemorrhage after delivery (see Chapter 32).

Prevention and Treatment. Asymptomatic leiomyomas do not require treatment and usually regress spontaneously with removal of estrogen at menopause. Symptomatic leiomyomas may be managed with hormonal therapy or nonsteroidal anti-inflammatory drugs (NSAIDs) for relief of menorrhagia, dysmenorrhea, or pelvic discomfort.[21] Myomectomy (removal of the tumor) may be done laparoscopically in those who wish to preserve reproductive function. Hysterectomy may be indicated for women who have finished childbearing and who have severe discomfort, anemia unresponsive to iron replacement, or menorrhagia caused by large fibroids. Uterine fibroids are the most common indication for hysterectomy, a procedure that has been criticized as unjustified and unnecessary by many.[21] More than 90% of hysterectomies are done electively in women with nonmalignant conditions for which conservative treatment is available.

Prognosis and Outcome. Uterine fibroid tumors are usually effectively managed with conservative treatment or surgery. Laparoscopic myomectomy is associated with a 15% to 30% risk of tumor recurrence.[21]

Ovarian Cysts

Definition. Ovarian cysts are fluid-filled, non-neoplastic lesions within the ovary. The cysts may be single or multiple, involving one or both ovaries. Ovarian cysts are classified as *functional cysts* if they arise from some variation of the ovulatory process. Presence of numerous functional cysts is a component of polycystic ovary syndrome, discussed next.

Epidemiology. Ovarian cysts are very common. Specific risk factors other than age within the reproductive years are unknown. Endometriosis is a risk factor for chocolate cysts of the ovaries, as discussed in the section on endometriosis.

Etiology. The precise etiology of most functional cysts is unknown. It is possible that they may not represent pathology at all, but rather are physiologic variants within the sequence of ovarian follicle development.[20]

Pathophysiology. *Follicular cysts* originate from unruptured primary follicles or from follicles that have ruptured but resealed before their fluid contents have been reabsorbed. *Luteal cysts* arise from the corpus luteum and are believed to be physiologic. Older cysts may incorporate old blood and fibrous tissue, and, if they rupture into the peritoneal cavity, an inflammatory reaction occurs.

Clinical Manifestations. The majority of functional cysts are less than 2 cm in diameter and are asymptomatic. Larger cysts may cause pelvic pain because of peritoneal inflammation, and an adnexal mass may be palpable. Irregular menstrual cycles and dysmenorrhea may be present. Rupture of a large cyst may be acutely painful and result in manifestations of intra-abdominal hemorrhage or peritonitis.

Prevention and Treatment. Use of oral contraceptives to regulate the menstrual cycle may prevent the formation of functional cysts in women who are prone to them. Follicular cysts may regress or rupture spontaneously. Symptomatic cysts that do not regress are treated surgically with laparoscopic removal of the cyst only or with open excision of the entire ovary.

Prognosis and Outcome. Ovarian cysts are successfully managed in most cases. Functional ovarian cysts do not increase the risk of **ovarian cancer.**

Polycystic Ovary Syndrome

Definition. Polycystic ovary syndrome (PCOS) is a metabolic disorder characterized by multiple ovarian cysts, insulin resistance, hyperandrogenism, and chronic anovulation in women without specific disease of the adrenal or pituitary glands.[22]

Epidemiology. The overall prevalence of PCOS has been estimated at 22% in the United States.[22] Among women who seek treatment for infertility associated with anovulation, more than 75% have polycystic ovaries and 90% have elevated serum LH, androgens, or both. A genetic predisposition is apparent, and in some families the disorder demonstrates autosomal dominant inheritance. Central (visceral) obesity is present in 50% to 80% of women with PCOS.[23]

Etiology. The precise etiology of PCOS is unknown. Excess androgen secretion from the ovaries and possibly the adrenal glands is believed to trigger the endocrine and metabolic abnormalities that characterize PCOS, which may result from abnormal enzymatic activity. Abnormal function of the ovarian IGF system has also been postulated.[24]

Pathophysiology. Ovarian follicle development is initially normal, but selection of a dominant follicle does not occur. Many small follicles accumulate, and these may respond abnormally to stimulation by steroid hormones (estrogens, progesterone, and androgens) and peptides (gonadotropins and IGFs). Endocrine abnormalities in PCOS may be the cause or the result of the cystic abnormalities. These include elevation of LH, testosterone, and androstenedione and an abnormal pattern of estrogen secretion during the menstrual cycle. Sustained estrogenic stimulation of the endometrium may impose increased risk of endometrial cancer. Abnormalities in the secretion of prolactin and growth hormone are less commonly seen. Insulin resistance in women with PCOS differs from that seen in type 2 diabetes mellitus (see Chapter 29). In PCOS, muscle and adipose tissue, but not hepatic tissue, are resistant to the effects of insulin.

Clinical Manifestations. Hyperandrogenism manifests as hirsutism, acne, and male-pattern hair loss. Polycystic ovaries are evident on ultrasonography, and ovarian dysfunction manifests as anovulation with associated infertility, amenorrhea, oligomenorrhea, or other abnormal uterine bleeding. The history of menstrual disturbance usually dates back to menarche.[22] Insulin resistance is associated with dyslipidemia and increased risk of cardiovascular disease and type 2 diabetes mellitus.

Prevention and Treatment. There is no specific prevention for PCOS. Achievement and maintenance of a body mass index within the optimal range are indicated to reduce the risks associated with insulin resistance and may result in spontaneous ovulation in some women.[22] Anovulation is usually treated with an antiandrogen such as clomiphene (Clomid). Abnormal uterine bleeding may be treated with low-dose oral contraceptives or cyclic progesterone administration. Antiandrogen therapy also improves hirsutism, male-pattern hair loss, and acne, and more specific modes of intervention such as hair removal and retinoic acid derivatives may also be used (see Chapter 36).

Prognosis and Outcome. Ovulation and fertility can be restored with antiandrogen therapy in 77% to 80% of women with PCOS. Symptomatic treatment of hirsutism and acne is usually effective. Patients should be carefully monitored for the development of cardiovascular disease, type 2 diabetes mellitus, or endometrial cancer.

Cervical Cancer

Definition. Cervical cancer is a malignant neoplasm of the cervix. Eighty-five per cent of cervical cancer is squamous cell carcinoma; the remaining cancers are adenocarcinomas.

Epidemiology. The incidence of cervical cancer is increasing, but overall mortality is declining. Both of these trends are the result of improved detection by cytologic testing using the Papanicolaou (Pap) smear. About 16,000 cases are diagnosed each year in the U.S.[25] Once the leading cause of cancer deaths in women, cervical cancer now ranks eighth, causing an estimated 4500 deaths per year.

Risk factors suggest a sexually transmitted etiologic basis in many cases, and include early age of first intercourse and multiple sexual partners. HPV has been strongly linked to cervical cancer, particularly in those in whom other factors such as immunosuppression coexist. Cervical cancer is common among women with HPV who are also positive for human immunodeficiency virus (HIV), and it has been designated as an acquired immunodeficiency syndrome (AIDS)–defining illness (see Chapter 13). Other risk factors implicated with less certainty are oral contraceptive use, cigarette smoking, parity (pregnancy history), family history, other genital infections, and lack of circumcision of the male partner.

Etiology. Although the precise cause of cervical cancer is unknown, nearly 90% of cervical specimens with dysplasia contain DNA from HPV.[25] Immunosuppression enhances the risk of virally induced neoplastic transformation.

Pathophysiology. Most cervical cancers are preceded by precancerous changes that are noninvasive for as long as 20 years. The progression of these cellular alterations to cancer does not always occur; however, the risk of progression increases with the degree of cellular dysplasia. Squamous cell carcinoma usually arises from cells at the transition zone between squamous and columnar epithelium near the external cervical os.

Table 31–9 compares the three histology-based grading systems for cervical cancer, representing progression of the disease from atypical changes to dysplasia to localized carcinoma (carcinoma in situ) to invasive cancer. Cervical cancer may extend locally to pelvic organs and ultimately metastasize to the liver, lungs, bone marrow, and other tissues. The most severe clinical manifestations usually result from urinary tract obstruction.

Clinical Manifestations. Early cervical cancer is asymptomatic, often for several years, with the only clinical evidence being cellular abnormality detected by the Pap smear. Later, with local extension and invasion, cervical cancer may manifest as cervical lesions, vaginal bleeding, painful coitus, and dysuria.

Prevention and Treatment. Many of the risk factors for cervical cancer are controllable with behavioral and lifestyle modification. Women aged 18 or older who are or have been sexually active should undergo annual Pap smear screening. After three consecutive negative smears, the frequency of screening may be reduced at the discretion of the woman and her physician.[25] A low-power magnification device (colposcope) permits screening for intraepithelial lesions during cervical examination.

The majority of atypical cervical lesions resolve spontaneously and require no intervention beyond frequent monitoring. Early cervical cancer may be treated with cryotherapy (freezing of abnormal cells with nitrous oxide or other volatile gas), conization (removal of a cone of tissue from the cervical os), or laser surgery directed at abnormal tissues only. More advanced cancer is treated with simple hysterectomy. Radical hysterectomy, in which surrounding ligaments, part of the vagina, and regional pelvic lymph nodes are also resected, may be done in more advanced cases. Pelvic radiation therapy may

TABLE 31–9
HISTOLOGIC GRADING SYSTEMS IN CERVICAL CANCER

Bethesda	World Health Organization	Papanicolaou
Within normal limits	Normal	Class I
Benign epithelial cell change	Atypia	Class II
Epithelial cell abnormalities	Atypia	Class II
Atypical squamous cells of unknown significance (ASCUS)		
Atypical glandular cells of unknown significance (AGUS)	Atypia	Class II
Low-grade squamous intraepithelial lesion (LGSIL)	Mild dysplasia (CIN I)	Class III
High-grade squamous intraepithelial lesion (HGSIL)	Moderate dysplasia (CIN II)	Class III
	Severe dysplasia, carcinoma in situ (CIN III)	Class IV
Invasive carcinoma	Invasive carcinoma	Class V

CIN, cervical intraepithelial neoplasia.
From Stack, P.S. (1997). Pap smears: Still a reliable screening tool for cervical cancer. *Postgraduate Medicine* 101(4), 212.

be used after surgery or instead of surgery in extensive disease with distant metastasis. Cervical cancer that recurs after initial therapy may be treated with chemotherapy (e.g., cisplatin), radiation therapy, or pelvic exenteration (surgical removal of the bladder, uterus, vagina, and possibly the rectum followed by reconstructive procedures).

Prognosis and Outcome. Survival rates depend on stage at the time of diagnosis and treatment, ranging from 95% 5-year survival for localized disease to 20% for those with extension beyond the pelvis.[26]

Endometrial Cancer

Definition. Endometrial cancer is a malignant neoplasm arising from the endometrial glands of the uterus. Ninety-seven per cent of uterine cancers are endometrial in origin; the remaining 3% are sarcomas.[27]

Epidemiology. Endometrial carcinoma is diagnosed in an estimated 34,000 women each year, and the median age at diagnosis is 63 years.[27] Risk factors other than age include early menarche, nulliparity (never having borne children), infertility, obesity, and estrogen replacement therapy without opposing progesterone. Use of the antiestrogen tamoxifen in treatment of breast cancer is also associated with increased risk, because this drug acts as an estrogen agonist on the endometrium. Women from families affected by hereditary nonpolyposis colorectal cancer syndrome demonstrate a 4% to 11% incidence of endometrial cancer, at a younger age than that seen among the general population (see Chapter 24).[27]

Etiology. Endometrial cancers usually develop in women with a history of endometrial hyperplasia related to excessive or prolonged estrogen stimulation.

Pathophysiology. The tumor may develop as a localized polyp, or may involve virtually the entire surface of the endometrium. Endometrial cancer spreads by local invasion to pelvic structures at first, then metastasizes via lymphatic and hematogenous routes to the lungs, liver, bones, and other tissues.

Clinical Manifestations. Endometrial cancer is often asymptomatic at first, but it may cause abnormal uterine bleeding. The uterus may or may not be enlarged. Cytologic diagnosis may be established with the Pap smear, but more often biopsy of the endometrial tissue is required.[28]

Prevention and Treatment. In recent years, the administration of unopposed estrogen for treatment of menopausal symptoms has largely been replaced by the use of combined estrogen-progesterone preparations. The incidence of endometrial cancer has decreased proportionately. Surgical removal of the uterus, ovaries, and fallopian tubes (total abdominal hysterectomy with bilateral salpingo-oophorectomy) is the treatment of choice for endometrial cancer. Radiation therapy, hormonal therapy, and chemotherapy are often used adjunctively when a high risk of recurrence is present. In a small number of younger women with early cancer, treatment with hormonal therapy alone has resulted in complete remission with preservation of fertility. Very elderly women may be treated with radiation therapy alone.

Prognosis and Outcome. Prognosis in endometrial cancer depends on the stage of the tumor at diagnosis (Table 31–10). Fortunately, most cases are diagnosed at stage I, which demonstrates a 5-year survival rate of 83%.

Ovarian Cancer

Definition. Ovarian cancer is a malignant neoplasm arising from ovarian surface epithelial cells, germ cells, and sex cord or stromal cells. The ovary is an uncommon site of metastatic cancer.

Epidemiology. Malignant tumors of the ovaries account for 6% of cancers in females, and they tend to occur in women between 40 and 65 years of age.[20] (About 80% of ovarian tumors are benign, and these tend to occur in younger women, aged 20 to 45 years). Ovarian cancer displays a familial predisposition, and a specific genetic locus for neoplastic alteration in ovarian and breast cancer (BRCA1) has recently been identified.[29] Other risk factors in-

TABLE 31–10
CLINICAL STAGING OF ENDOMETRIAL CANCER

Stage	Description	5-Year Survival
IA	Tumor limited to endometrium	83%
IB	Invasion of less than half the myometrium	
IC	Invasion of more than half the myometrium	
IIA	Involves endocervical glands	73%
IIB	Invasion of cervical stroma	
IIIA	Invasion of serosa or adnexa, or malignant peritoneal cytology	52%
IIIB	Vaginal metastasis	
IIIC	Metastasis to pelvic or para-aortic lymph nodes	
IVA	Invasion of bladder or bowel mucosa	27%
IVB	Distant metastasis	

Adapted with permission from Rose, P.G. (1996). Endometrial carcinoma. *New England Journal of Medicine* 335(9), 642–643.

clude advancing age, nulliparity, North American or Northern European descent, and history of congenital abnormalities of sex organ development (*gonadal dysgenesis*). Protective factors (anti–risk factors) associated with lower risk include more than one full-term pregnancy, use of oral contraceptives, and breast feeding.[30]

Etiology. The precise cause of ovarian cancer is unknown. Known genetic syndromes account for fewer than 0.05% of cases.[30] Abnormalities associated with ovulation are apparently significant, because factors that reduce the frequency of ovulation protect against the disorder.

Pathophysiology. Ovarian cancers may be unilateral or bilateral. The tumors may produce hormones in excess, resulting in paraneoplastic syndromes, but in most cases they are nonfunctional. Clinical manifestations caused by invasion and obstruction become evident with enlargement of the tumor.

Clinical Manifestations. Ovarian cancer is often asymptomatic, although local invasion and compression may result in vague abdominal pain, distention, urinary tract obstruction, and abnormal uterine bleeding. An adnexal mass may be palpable on physical examination.

Prevention and Treatment. Annual gynecologic examination is recommended for most women, and bimanual rectovaginal pelvic examination might detect ovarian masses at an earlier stage. Women who are known to be at risk for ovarian cancer because of genetic factors might also undergo transvaginal ultrasonography or serum testing for the tumor marker CA-125. Some women with the *BRCA1* gene elect to have prophylactic surgical removal of the ovaries.

Definitive treatment depends on the stage of the cancer and the cell type of origin. Early-stage epithelial tumors, found in 25% of cases, are treated with total abdominal hysterectomy (removal of the uterus) and bilateral salpingo-oophorectomy (removal of both ovaries and fallopian tubes). Younger women with unilateral tumors who wish to retain fertility might elect to undergo resection of only the involved ovary and fallopian tube. Adjuvant therapy with chemotherapy (e.g., cisplatin and paclitaxel) is also used except in very early tumors. Any finding other than stage I disease represents advanced ovarian cancer, found in 75% of cases. Total abdominal hysterectomy and bilateral salpingo-oophorectomy are indicated, with optimal tumor debulking and lymph node resection. Systemic chemotherapy is instituted after surgery. For patients who relapse, systemic chemotherapy is reinstituted. Clinical trials of high-dose chemotherapy followed by bone marrow transplantation or stem cell infusions to rescue the marrow are ongoing (see Chapter 12).

Prognosis and Outcome. Prognosis in ovarian cancer depends on the cell type of origin and degree of advancement at time of diagnosis. Most ovarian carcinomas are not diagnosed until they extend beyond the ovary, and 5-year survival rates in these women are just 10% to 20%.[30]

Pelvic Support Disorders

Definition. Pelvic support disorders include a number of conditions characterized by abnormal position or instability of pelvic organs caused by decreased ligament support or weakness of pelvic outlet muscles.

Epidemiology. Pelvic support disorders are very common in women, especially in middle age. An estimated 20% of postmenopausal women may be affected, although the precise incidence is uncertain.[31] Many women may not report the problem because of embarrassment or belief that it is an unavoidable consequence of aging. Risk factors for pelvic support disorders are female sex, removal of estrogen (with natural or surgical menopause), history of childbearing (with increased risk proportionate to parity), and pelvic floor muscle weakness associated with aging or deconditioning.

Etiology. Repeated pregnancy and vaginal delivery result in stretching and weakening of pelvic ligaments and muscles. Trauma of childbearing and degenerative changes with aging may also weaken or damage connective tissue in the walls of the vagina, bladder, and rectum.

Pathophysiology. With uterine *prolapse,* the poorly supported uterus descends downward into the vagina and may exert pressure on the adjacent bladder and rectum (Fig. 31–9). With severe prolapse, the cervix extends to the exterior, through the vaginal opening (introitus). Herniation of the bladder (*cystocele*) or rectum (*rectocele*) into the weakened vagina are also associated with structural alterations. In cases where there is associated inflammation, openings (*fistulas*) may develop between the vagina and the bladder or bowel.

Clinical Manifestations. Mild pelvic discomfort may be present in some cases, but the most distressing manifestation is stress or urge incontinence (see Chapter 20). Incontinence and fistulas constitute infection risks.

Prevention and Treatment. Exercises that strengthen the pelvic floor musculature and the external urinary sphincter (Kegel exercises) are usually taught to women after childbearing. These may aid in preventing or minimizing subsequent development of support disorders and may also decrease severity of incontinence in middle-aged women. An

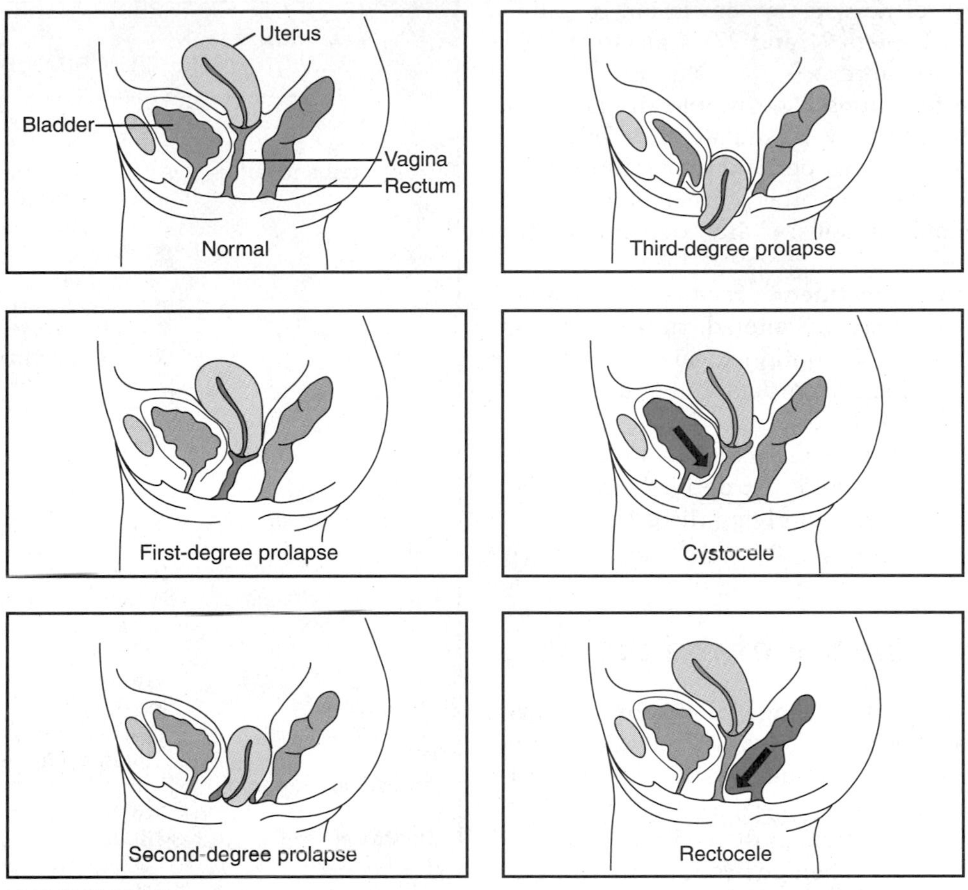

FIGURE 31–9

Pelvic support disorders. Relaxation of pelvic floor muscles and ligaments may result in herniation of the uterus into the vagina (*uterine prolapse*), herniation of the bladder into the vagina (*cystocele*), or herniation of the rectum into the vagina (*rectocele*).

internal fixation device (pessary) may be used to support a mildly prolapsed uterus. Many women elect to tolerate mild incontinence, using absorbent pads or undergarments to protect clothing. Surgical repair is the treatment of choice for more severe pelvic support disorders.

Prognosis and Outcome. Pelvic support disorders are potentially well managed with optimal physical conditioning and, when necessary, surgical repair of structural abnormalities. Untreated fistulas and urinary tract infections may impose significant risk of sepsis.

Galactorrhea

Definition. Galactorrhea is breast milk production independent of the normal stimuli for lactation.

Epidemiology. Isolated galactorrhea, in which prolactin levels and menstruation are normal, is estimated to occur in 2% to 20% of normal women.[32] Up to 25% of patients with secondary amenorrhea have hyperprolactinemia because of a pituitary abnormality (see Chapter 27), and many of these women also have galactorrhea.[33]

Etiology. Many different etiologies may result in galactorrhea. Stimulation of the neural reflex arc mediating lactation and milk letdown may occur with herpes zoster lesions, hypothalamic plaques (in multiple sclerosis), breast prosthesis implantation, thoracotomy, fondling of the breasts, or a poorly fitting brassiere. Endocrine disorders, pituitary tumors, or pituitary compression by other intracranial lesions may disrupt the regulation of prolactin secretion via the HPA. Other tumors may secrete prolactin or estrogen ectopically, producing galactorrhea as a paraneoplastic syndrome (see Chapter 7). Galactorrhea is an expected side effect of therapy with a number of drugs affecting neurotransmission (e.g., opiates, amphetamines, benzodiazepines, haloperidol, phenothiazines, tricyclic antidepressants). These agents affect the function of hypothalamic neurons (see Chapter 21).

Pathophysiology. Galactorrhea is significant if it is

caused by a central nervous system lesion or pituitary tumor (see Chapters 21 and 27). Galactorrhea is not a sign of breast cancer.

Clinical Manifestations. The nipple discharge is thin and off-white. It may be unilateral or bilateral, expressed or spontaneous, persistent or intermittent. Serum prolactin levels may be normal or elevated. Other clinical manifestations, if any, depend on the underlying cause.

Prevention and Treatment. Factors stimulating the letdown reflex may be altered, and offending medications may be discontinued in some cases. Treatment of neurologic disorders and pituitary tumors is discussed elsewhere.

Prognosis and Outcome. Galactorrhea in itself is a benign condition. Prognosis is derived from the presence and severity of underlying disorders.

Fibrocystic Change of the Breast

Definition. Fibrocystic change of the breast, formerly known as fibrocystic disease, includes three forms of benign breast tissue alterations: (1) cyst formation; (2) ductal hyperplasia; and (3) fibrosis.[34] Fibrocystic change is the most common benign breast disorder. Other benign conditions of the breast are described in Table 31–11.

Epidemiology. Fibrocystic change is seen in an estimated 10% of women younger than 21 years of age, 25% of women during their reproductive years, and 50% of postmenopausal women.[34] Specific risk factors are unknown.

Etiology. The precise etiology of fibrocystic change is unknown, and controversy exists as to whether it represents pathology or an expected developmental transition in some women. Several etiologic theories have been advanced, including an imbalance between estrogen and progesterone levels, altered prolactin levels, and enzymatic alteration caused by increased intake of methylxanthines. Methylxanthines, found in tea, coffee, chocolate, and some soft drinks, inhibit cyclic adenosine monophosphate and cyclic guanosine monophosphate phosphodiesterase enzymes.[34]

Pathophysiology. Cysts may form within lobular or subareolar areas. Those smaller than 1 mm, termed *microcysts,* are asymptomatic and nonpalpable. In 20% to 40% of women, these cysts dilate to 3 mm or more, becoming *macrocysts.* Cysts are usually bilateral. *Ductal ectasia* refers to dilations of the ductal system below the areola and nipple. These dilations may fill with yellowish lipid material. In ductal hyperplasia, the normally cuboidal or cylindrical ductal epithelium may undergo a metaplastic

TABLE 31–11
BENIGN DISORDERS OF THE BREAST

Disorder	Description
Congenital anomalies	Amastia (absence of one or both breasts) Delayed thelarche (absence of breast development by age 15 years) Juvenile hypertrophy (excessively large breasts) Poland's syndrome (lack of development of breast, pectoral muscle, shoulder girdle, and upper arm) Polymastia (supernumerary breasts) Symmastia (webbing between breasts) Asymmetry
Fibrocystic change	Benign alterations of breast tissue including cyst formation, ductal hyperplasia, and fibrosis
Fat necrosis	Spontaneous or post-traumatic; irregular mass that often becomes calcified
Fibroadenoma	Benign breast neoplasm; may calcify after menopause
Galactocele	Milk-filled cyst in the retroalveolar area; associated with lactation
Intraductal papilloma	Benign neoplasm that may be nonpalpable but causes spontaneous serosanguinous discharge from the nipple; presence of multiple papillomas is a precancerous condition
Lipoma	Soft, painless mass composed of fat and connective tissue; usually self-limited in size with no malignant potential
Mammary duct ectasia	Tender, dilated subareolar ducts producing dark green nipple discharge
Mastitis	Breast inflammation, usually related to pregnancy or lactation (puerperal mastitis); nonpuerperal mastitis is caused by bacterial infection
Mondor's disease	Thrombophlebitis of the superficial thoracoepigastric breast vein
Phyllodes tumors	Larger than fibroadenomas; may be benign, premalignant, or malignant
Sclerosing adenosis	Benign lesions presenting as a painless mass or discovered incidentally on mammography; weakly associated with risk of malignant transformation

Data from Hindle, W.H. (1994). Other benign breast problems. *Clinical Obstetrics and Gynecology* 37(4), 910–924.

transformation, either without disrupting the lobular architecture or by forming intraductal papillomas that may be palpable and induce nipple discharge that contains fat, proteins, sloughed ductal cells, macrophage-derived foam cells, and erythrocytes. Fibrosis may occur as a result of an inflammatory response to cystic changes or ductal hyperplasia. Fibrotic areas are palpable, immobile, firm, irregular masses up to 5 cm in diameter. Inflammatory edema and nerve root irritation stimulate pain receptors in breast tissue.

Clinical Manifestations. Breast pain (*mastalgia*) is the most universal symptom of fibrocystic change, and it typically begins 4 to 7 days into the luteal phase of the menstrual cycle and continues until the onset of menstruation.[34] The pain is usually located in the upper outer quadrant of both breasts. Tender, firm masses may be apparent, usually in the upper outer quadrant, and these may noticeably increase in size during the luteal phase. Nipple discharge, if present, is usually greenish brown to black. Ultrasound usually differentiates between cystic and solid masses. Tissue biopsy, obtained with fine-needle aspiration or surgical excision, differentiates between benign and malignant changes.

Prevention and Treatment. Simple reassurance is sufficient in cases in which discomfort is mild. The patient is advised to wear a comfortable, supporting brassiere. A mild diuretic may be prescribed for 2 to 3 days before menstruation to reduce breast edema. Restriction of dietary methylxanthines has not been shown to be superior to placebo in management of fibrocystic change; however, many women report symptomatic improvement. Hormonal therapy, including oral contraceptives, and antiestrogens have been beneficial to some. The dopamine agonist bromocriptine (Parlodel) has also been used to inhibit the secretion of prolactin, but this drug has significant toxic effects. Large cysts may be surgically excised for diagnostic purposes, and it has been proposed that their removal may preclude neoplastic transformation.

Prognosis and Outcome. Fibrocystic change may regress spontaneously in some women and may be managed successfully in most. The association of fibrocystic change with subsequent development of breast cancer is a matter of controversy; study results have been inconsistent. In ductal hyperplasia, certain metaplastic changes (termed *atypica*) are considered to be premalignant, and women with these changes *and* a family history of breast cancer have been shown to have a 20% chance of developing breast cancer within 15 years.[34] A small number of women with premalignant fibrocystic change elect to undergo prophylactic breast removal (mastectomy).

Breast Cancer

Definition. Breast cancer (carcinoma of the breast) is a malignant neoplasm arising from one of several tissue types within the breast (Table 31–12).

Epidemiology. The incidence of breast cancer in the United States has increased significantly in recent years in part because of better screening procedures and because of the aging of the population. In 1995, 182,000 new cases were diagnosed.[2] Nearly all (99%) of cases occur in females. Breast cancer is rare

TABLE 31–12
HISTOLOGIC CLASSIFICATION OF BREAST CANCER

Classification	Description
Intraductal carcinoma in situ	Malignant population of ductal epithelial cells that are incapable of invasion through the basement membrane (20% to 30% of breast carcinomas)
Lobular carcinoma in situ	Proliferation of loosely cohesive cells within terminal ducts or acini; commonly develops into invasive carcinoma
Invasive ductal carcinoma, not otherwise specified	Rock-hard growths (1–2 cm) of mixed cell types attached to surrounding and underlying tissues (65% to 80% of breast carcinomas)
Medullary carcinoma	Larger, fleshy tumor masses (5 cm or greater) with foci of hemorrhage and necrosis (1% to 5% of breast carcinomas)
Colloid (mucinous) carcinoma	Rare, slow-growing tumor having the consistency and appearance of pale gray-blue gelatin
Paget's disease of the breast	Associated with intraductal carcinoma (in situ or invasive) in which cells have migrated up a main duct to the skin of the nipple
Invasive lobular carcinoma	Rubbery, poorly circumscribed tumor arising from terminal ductules of breast lobule (5% to 10% of breast carcinomas)

Data from Cotran, R.S., Kumar, V., and Robbins, S.L. (1994). *Robbins Pathologic Basis of Disease.* (5th ed.). Philadelphia: W.B. Saunders. (pp. 1101–1106).

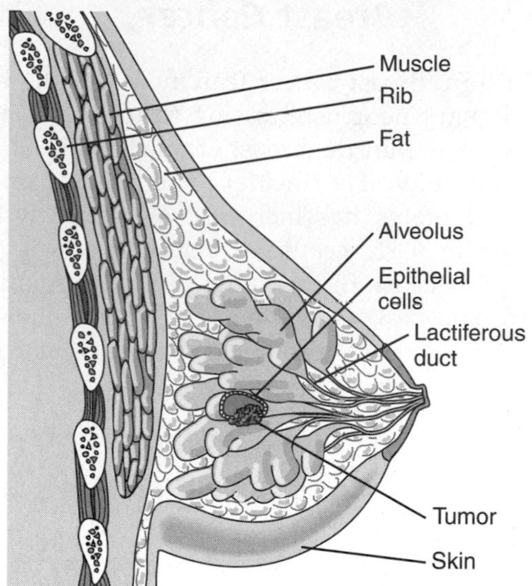

FIGURE 31–10
Origin of breast cancer. Breast tumors are most likely to arise from epithelial cells lining the mammary alveoli or ducts.

in those younger than age 25 years, but risk then increases proportionately with age.

The most well-defined risk factor is family history. Presence of the *BRCA1* gene is now known to confer greatly increased risk of breast and ovarian cancers in a small number of families, with the trait demonstrating autosomal dominant inheritance. Women with *BRCA1* mutations have an 85% lifetime risk of developing breast cancer. This mutation is believed to be present in 30% of women who develop breast cancer before age 45 years.[35]

Other risk factors that are less certain include early menarche, late menopause, nulliparity, giving birth to one's first child after age 30, obesity, radiation of the chest, hormone replacement therapy, fibrocystic change with atypia, or exposure to environmental substances with estrogen activity (*xenoestrogens*). Xenoestrogens include a number of pesticides and herbicides, hydrocarbons in petroleum-based fuels, and plastics.[36] It should be noted, however, that 80% of those in whom breast cancer is diagnosed have no risk factors except female sex and age older than 50 years.[37]

Etiology. The precise etiologic mechanism of breast cancer is unknown. Susceptibility is conveyed by presence of the *BRCA1* gene, which results in abnormal protein synthesis. In many, but not all, breast cancers, tumor cells have receptors for estrogen. Estrogen may promote secretion of growth-promoting cytokines by these cells, which then promote their own growth in an autocrine positive feedback loop.

Excessive or prolonged exposure to estrogen (associated with many of the risk factors) or an abnormality in the metabolism of estrogen are the best-accepted etiologic theories in breast cancer. Estradiol may be metabolized to either of two metabolites: 16-alpha-hydroxyestrone ("bad" estrogen) or 2-hydroxyestrone ("good" estrogen).[36] The 16-alpha-hydroxyestrone is known to strongly increase the interaction of estrogen receptors with growth-promoting genes. Progesterone is also believed to be involved in the pathogenesis of breast cancer. Activation of oncogenes expressing tumor growth–promoting factors and mutation of tumor suppressor genes have been implicated in some studies.

Pathophysiology. Approximately 50% of breast cancers arise in the upper outer quadrant of the breast. The majority of breast cancers arise from the ductal epithelium (Fig. 31–10). About 30% of breast cancers are noninvasive, proliferating within the ductal system or lobules as solid tumors or necrotic areas. Invasive carcinomas are most common and result in hard, infiltrative tumors that fix breast tissue to the underlying pectoral muscle and chest wall. Involvement of adjacent lymph nodes has often occurred by the time of diagnosis, and distant metastasis may result from lymphatic or hematogenous spread (Fig. 31–11). Inflammatory breast cancer, an uncommon type, differs in that it mimics breast infection (mastitis) or fibrocystic change, causing rapidly worsening erythema and edema involving at least a third of the breast.[2]

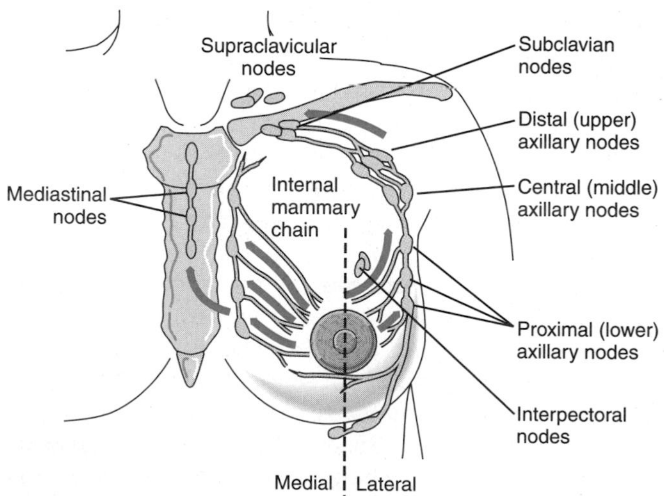

FIGURE 31–11
Lymphatic metastasis of breast cancer. Lateral lesions of the breast usually metastasize to axillary and supraclavicular lymph nodes, and medial tumors tend to metastasize to the internal mammary, mediastinal, and supraclavicular nodes. (Redrawn from Shapiro, T.J., and Clark, P.M. [1995]. Breast cancer: What the primary care provider needs to know. *Nurse Practitioner* 20[3], 45. © 1995 Springhouse Corporation.)

Clinical Manifestations. Cancers confined to the ducts may not be manifested as a mass, but spontaneous, often bloody, discharge from the nipple of the affected side is likely. When of sufficient size, tumors are detectable with mammography or with palpation. Unilateral edema, "orange peel" texture of overlying skin (*peau d'orange*), fixation of the breast with position change, prominent venous pattern, retraction of the nipple, or dimpling of the skin may demonstrate the underlying lesion. Clinical manifestations associated with metastasis depend on the tissues involved. Bony metastasis is common, with resulting bone pain and pathogenic fractures.

Prevention and Treatment. Breast self-examination (BSE) and routine mammography have long been advocated for the early detection of breast cancer. Their efficacy with regard to improving outcomes is uncertain, however, and controversy exists with respect to recommended frequency of mammography before age 50 years.[36] Dietary measures (e.g., low fat, high fiber) and weight reduction are also unproved in reducing risk. The antiestrogen drug tamoxifen (Nolvadex) is currently being tested as a chemopreventative measure in a cohort of women who are at high risk of breast cancer.[38] A small number of women with high familial risk have elected to undergo mastectomy as a preventive measure.

Recommended treatment of breast cancer depends on tumor stage (Table 31–13), patient age, and treatment preference. For stage I and II disease, breast-conserving surgery followed by radiation therapy (plus tamoxifen or cytotoxic chemotherapy in those with lymph node involvement) has been shown to be as effective as more radical surgery. Breast-conserving surgery involves removal of the mass (lumpectomy) or the affected quadrant of the breast (segmental mastectomy or quadrantectomy), with minimal disfigurement. Radical mastectomy includes removal of the entire breast, along with pectoral muscle tissue and axillary nodes.

For stage III disease, systemic chemotherapy is often used before tumor debulking with surgery or radiation therapy. Chemotherapy and hormonal therapy are first-line treatment of stage IV disease. In premenopausal women, tamoxifen and luteinizing hormone–releasing hormone analogs are used to achieve "chemical oophorectomy" or "total estrogen blockade," depriving estrogen-sensitive tumors of their hormonal stimulus. In postmenopausal women, tamoxifen, progesterone, and the cytotoxic agent aminoglutethimide (Cytadren) are most often used.[39] High-dose chemotherapy followed by rescue of the bone marrow has been used in some women with metastatic breast cancer and has induced remission in 30%.[39]

TABLE 31–13
STAGING OF BREAST CANCER

Stage	Description
0	TIS (carcinoma in situ) N0 (no lymph node metastasis) M0 (no distant metastasis)
I	T1 (tumor diameter <2 cm) N0 M0
IIA	T0 (no evidence of primary tumor) N1 (metastasis to movable ipsilateral axillary lymph nodes) M0
IIB	T2 (tumor 2–5 cm diameter) N1 M0 or T3 (tumor diameter >5 cm) N0 M0
IIIA	T0, T1, or T2 N2 (metastasis to ipsilateral fixed axillary lymph nodes) M0 or T3 N1 or N2 M0
IIIB	T4 (tumor of any size with extension into chest wall or skin) any N M0 or any inflammatory breast cancer
IV	any T any N M1 (distant metastasis)

Adapted with permission from Phillips, D.M., and Balducci, L. (1996). Current management of breast cancer. *American Family Physician* 53(2), 658, published by the American Academy of Family Physicians.

Breast cancer in men is treated similarly, except that orchiectomy may be indicated for those who do not respond to tamoxifen. In women, surgery may be followed by a breast reconstruction procedure to effect a satisfactory cosmetic outcome. Reconstruction may involve the use of saline-filled implants. Silicone implants are no longer used because of their unproved association with connective tissue diseases (see Focus of Current Research).

Prognosis and Outcome. Five-year survival statistics for breast cancer are increasingly favorable. In women with early cancer and no lymph node involvement, a 70% to 80% cure rate has been observed.[40] When primary tumor size is less than 1 cm, this rate rises to 90%. The 5-year rate of recurrence of cancer in women with 10 or more tumor-positive nodes is 75%, and the mortality rate in this group is 22% within 5 years. Overall mortality rates have been stable as a result of concurrent increases in detection and survival. In the United States, breast cancer is still the leading cause of death for women between ages 35 and 54 years.[41]

CLINICAL SIGNIFICANCE OF GYNECOLOGIC AND BREAST DISORDERS

The disorders discussed in this chapter represent significant sources of morbidity across the life span (see Developmental Perspective). Sexually transmitted diseases affect many young women and may leave them with lifelong deficiencies in reproductive function. The human distress inherent in the inability to bear children is inestimable. With the "baby boom" generation of women now entering the perimenopausal and menopausal years, management of the manifestations of this period may be expected to consume considerable health care resources. An increasing emphasis has been placed on women's health in recent years, with establishment of research priorities in the areas of breast cancer prevention and treatment as well as risks versus benefits of hormone replacement therapy (see Focus of Current Research).

Issues related to pregnancy and childbearing are also a significant component of women's health. Although pregnancy is certainly not a disease, it represents a major stressor to the human system. The physiology of pregnancy and the processes of delivery and lactation will be described in Chapter 32, along with disorders related to pregnancy, labor, and delivery.

Summary of Key Points

- Although the female reproductive and urinary systems are anatomically separate, they are in close enough proximity that infections, structural disorders, and neoplasias may affect both systems. Because the upper genital tract is an open system, retrograde menstruation is possible and may induce endometriosis.
- In females, oogenesis is complete at birth. At puberty, an estimated 300,000 to 400,000 ovarian follicles remain, constituting the pool from which ovulation occurs during the reproductive years. During each menstrual cycle, one dominant follicle develops and releases its ovum from the ovarian surface. The empty follicle (corpus luteum) secretes progesterone for maintenance of the endometrium in support of a potential pregnancy. Anovulation, usually associated with hormonal imbalance, leads to infertility and abnormal uterine bleeding. Luteal phase abnormalities increase the risk of spontaneous abortion. Benign ovarian cysts commonly arise from some stage of follicle development.
- The menstrual cycle is regulated by estrogen and progesterone, steroid hormones released by the ovaries in a complex process mediated by the hypothalamic–pituitary–gonadal axis. Hypothalamic GnRH release is pulsatile and potentially influenced by numerous factors. The pituitary gonadotropins LH and FSH act in concert with ovarian IGFs in the regulation of ovarian function. Menarche occurs at puberty as the hypothalamic–pituitary–gonadal axis matures. Increased GnRH secretion produces a sustained rise in LH, initiating the first ovulation and menstrual cycle if adequate body fat is present. Menopause, the cessation of ovulation and menstrual cycles, occurs when the follicular pool is depleted. Estrogen levels fall, and decreased negative feedback to the HPA causes a transient rise in FSH, and later LH.
- Hormonal changes associated with menopause or gynecologic disorders may impair sexual function by reducing libido, as a consequence of lesions or atrophy of the external genitalia or of prolapse of the uterus. Fertility may be adversely affected by gynecologic disorders in which ovulation, fertilization, or implantation are impaired. Treatment of many gynecologic disorders may induce infertility because of hormonal or anatomic alterations. Abnormal uterine bleeding is a primary manifestation of gynecologic disorders, and it may range from absence of bleeding (amenorrhea) to excessive menstrual bleeding or intermenstrual bleeding.
- Gynecologic disorders may arise from inflammatory, neoplastic, traumatic, degenerative, or idiopathic mechanisms. Intervention is aimed at alleviating the underlying cause, when possible, or at manipulating the hormonal environment or correcting anatomic abnormalities. Most gynecologic infections are preventable with behavioral methods and

are responsive to treatment. Earlier detection has resulted in greatly improved survival rates in gynecologic cancers, with the exception of ovarian cancer.

- Fibrocystic change of the breast is very common and may represent normal developmental processes rather than pathology in many cases. In contrast to the lesions of breast cancer, the formation of cysts, ductal hyperplasia, and fibroses in fibrocystic change is a benign process. Both disorders may manifest as lumps or nodularity of the breast, but fibrocystic change is usually associated with breast pain and lump enlargement during the luteal phase of the menstrual cycle. Development of atypical cells with fibrocystic change represents a precancerous state that warrants careful monitoring and, in a few women, prophylactic mastectomy. Breast cancer is also common, affecting one in eight women in the United States. More rigorous screening and more effective treatment has resulted in improving outcomes, but breast cancer is still the leading cause of death among women 35 to 54 years of age.

REFERENCES

1. Hammond, C.B. (1997). Management of menopause. *American Family Physician* 55(5), 1667–1674.
2. Dahlbeck, S.W., Donnelly, J.F., and Theriault, R.L. (1995). Differentiating inflammatory breast cancer from acute mastitis. *American Family Physician* 52(3), 929–934.
3. Jennings, J.C. (1995). Abnormal uterine bleeding. *Medical Clinics of North America* 79(6), 1357–1376.
4. Buyalos, R.P. (1995). Insulin-like growth factors: Clinical experience in ovarian function. *American Journal of Medicine* 98(1A suppl.) 55S–66S.
5. Wise, P.M., Krajnak, K.M., and Kashon, M.L. (1996). Menopause: The aging of multiple pacemakers. *Science* 273, 67–70.
6. Shaw, C.R. (1997). The perimenopausal hot flash: Epidemiology, physiology, and treatment. *Nurse Practitioner* 22(3), 55–66.
7. LeBoeuf, F.J., and Carter, S.G. (1996). Discomforts of the perimenopause. *Journal of Obstetric, Gynecologic, and Neonatal Nursing* 25(2), 173–180.
8. Thomas, D.J. (1996). Benefits and risks of hormone/estrogen replacement. *Nursing Clinics of North America* 31(4), 815–825.
9. Kiningham, R.B., Apgar, B.S., and Schwenk, T.L. (1996). Evaluation of amenorrhea. *American Family Physician* 53(4), 1185–1194.
10. Klein, T.A. (1996). Office gynecology for the primary physician, part II. *Medical Clinics of North America* 80(2), 321–336.
11. Parker, P.D. (1994). Premenstrual syndrome. *American Family Physician* 50(6), 1309–1317.
12. Reife, C.M. (1996). Office gynecology for the primary physician, part I. *Medical Clinics of North America* 80(2), 299–319.
13. Kvale, J.N., and Kvale, J.K. (1993). Common gynecologic problems after age 75. *Postgraduate Medicine* 93(5), 263–273.
14. Giusti, R.M., Iwamoto, K., and Hatch, E.E. (1995). Diethylstilbestrol revisited: A review of the long-term health effects. *Annals of Internal Medicine* 122(10), 778–788.
15. McCormack, W.M. (1994). Pelvic inflammatory disease. *New England Journal of Medicine* 330(2), 115–119.
16. Newkirk, G.R. (1996). Pelvic inflammatory disease: A contemporary approach. *American Family Physician* 53(4), 1127–1135.
17. Lu, P.Y., and Ory, S.J. (1995). Endometriosis: Current management. *Mayo Clinic Proceedings* 70, 453–463.
18. Olive, D.L., and Schwartz, L.B. (1993). Endometriosis. *New England Journal of Medicine* 328(24), 1759–1769.
19. Pavlik, R.M. (1995). Adenomyosis—An ignored uterine disease. *Nurse Practitioner* 20(4), 32–41.
20. Cotran, R.S., Kumar, V., and Robbins, S.L. (1994). *Robbins Pathologic Basis of Disease.* (5th ed.). Philadelphia: W.B. Saunders. (pp. 1058–1067, 1099–1109).
21. Kramer, M.G., and Reiter, R.C. (1997). Hysterectomy: Indications, alternatives and predictors. *American Family Physician* 55(3), 827–834.
22. Franks, S. (1995). Polycystic ovary syndrome. *New England Journal of Medicine* 333(13), 853–861.
23. Wild, R.A. (1995). Obesity, lipids, cardiovascular risk, and androgen excess. *American Journal of Medicine* 98(1A suppl.), 27S–32S.
24. Giudice, L.C. (1995). The insulin-like growth factor system in normal and abnormal human ovarian follicle development. *American Journal of Medicine* 98(1A suppl.), 48S–54S.
25. Warner, E.A., and Parsons, A.K. (1996). Screening and early diagnosis of gynecologic cancers. *Medical Clinics of North America* 80(1), 45–61.
26. Cannistra, S.A., and Niloff, J.M. (1996). Cancer of the uterine cervix. *New England Journal of Medicine* 334(16), 1030–1038.
27. Rose, P.G. (1996). Endometrial carcinoma. *New England Journal of Medicine* 335(9), 640–649.
28. Shelly, M.S. (1997). Endometrial biopsy. *American Family Physician* 55(5), 1731–1736.
29. Shattuck-Eidens, D., McClure, M., Simard, J., *et al.* (1995). A collaborative survey of 80 mutations in the BRCA1 breast and ovarian cancer susceptibility gene. *Journal of the American Medical Association* 273(7), 535–541.
30. NIH Consensus Development Panel on Ovarian Cancer. (1995). Ovarian cancer: Screening, treatment, and follow-up. *Journal of the American Medical Association* 273(6), 491–497.
31. Davila, G.W. (1996). Vaginal prolapse: Management with nonsurgical techniques. *Postgraduate Medicine* 99(4), 171–185.
32. Edge, D.S., and Segatore, M. (1993). Assessment and management of galactorrhea. *Nurse Practitioner* 18(6), 35–49.
33. Kaye, T.B. (1996). Hyperprolactinemia: Causes, consequences, and treatment options. *Postgraduate Medicine* 99(5), 265–268.
34. Drukker, B.H. (1994). Fibrocystic change of the breast. *Clinical Obstetrics and Gynecology* 37(4), 903–915.
35. Miki, Y., Swenson, J., Shattuck-Eidens, D., *et al.* (1994). A strong candidate for the breast and ovarian cancer susceptibility gene BRCA1. *Science* 266, 66–71.
36. Davis, D.L. (1995). Can environmental estrogens cause breast cancer? *Scientific American* 273(4), 166–172.
37. Buyske, J., Mackarem, G., Ulmer, B.C., *et al.* (1996). Breast cancer in the nineties. *AORN Journal* 64(1), 64–72.
38. O'Schaughnessy, J.A. (1996). Chemoprevention of breast cancer. *Journal of the American Medical Association* 275(17), 1349–1353.
39. Phillips, D.M., and Balducci, L. (1996). Current management of breast cancer. *American Family Physician* 53(2), 657–665.
40. Berkowitz, L.D., and Love, N. (1995). Adjuvant systemic therapy for breast cancer: Issues for primary care physicians. *Postgraduate Medicine* 98(4), 85–94.
41. Porterfield, L.A., and Love, N. (1995). Local and regional therapy for primary breast tumors: Answers to major questions. *Postgraduate Medicine* 98(4), 65–80.

SELECTED BIBLIOGRAPHY

Adimora, A.A., and Quinlivan, E.B. (1995). Human papillomavirus infection: Recent findings on progression to cervical cancer. *Postgraduate Medicine* 98(3), 109–120.

Ambrosone, C.B., Freudenheim, J.L., Graham, S., *et al.* (1996). Cigarette smoking, N-acetyltransferase 2 genetic polymorphisms, and breast cancer risk. *Journal of the American Medical Association* 276(18), 1494–1501.

Appleby, J. (1995). Management of the abnormal Papanicolaou smear. *Medical Clinics of North America* 79(2), 345–361.

Ault, K.A., and Faro, S. (1993). Pelvic inflammatory disease: Current diagnostic criteria and treatment guidelines. *Postgraduate Medicine* 93(2), 85–91.

Bachmann, G.A. (1994). The changes before "the change": Strategies for the transition to the menopause. *Postgraduate Medicine* 95(4), 113–124.

Barrett-Connor, E. (1993). Estrogen and estrogen-progestogen replacement: Therapy and cardiovascular diseases. *American Journal of Medicine* 95(1A suppl.), 40S–43S.

Bayer, S.R., and DeCherney, A.H. (1993). Clinical manifestations and treatment of dysfunctional uterine bleeding. *Journal of the American Medical Association* 269(14), 1823–1828.

Belchetz, P.E. (1994). Hormonal treatment of postmenopausal women. *New England Journal of Medicine* 330(15), 1062–1071.

Bonadonna, G., Valagussa, P., Moliterni, A., *et al.* (1995). Adjuvant cyclophosphamide, methotrexate, and fluorouracil in node-positive breast cancer. *New England Journal of Medicine* 332(14), 901–906.

Carlson, K.J., Nichols, D.H., and Schiff, I. (1993). Indications for hysterectomy. *New England Journal of Medicine* 328(12), 856–860.

Carmichael, J.M. (1995). Understanding infertility treatment plans. *American Pharmacy* NS35(11), 41–54.

Cauley, J.A., Lucas, F.L., Kuller, L.H., *et al.* (1996). Bone mineral density and risk of breast cancer in older women: The study of osteoporotic fractures. *Journal of the American Medical Association* 276(17), 1404–1408.

Cobleigh, M.A., Berris, R.F., Bush, T., *et al.* (1994). Estrogen replacement therapy in breast cancer survivors. *Journal of the American Medical Association* 272(7), 540–545.

Colditz, G.A., Hankinson, S.E., Hunter, D.J., *et al.* (1995). The use of estrogens and progestins and the risk of breast cancer in postmenopausal women. *New England Journal of Medicine* 332(24), 1589–1593.

DeLancey, J.O.L. (1993). Anatomy and biomechanics of genital prolapse. *Clinical Obstetrics and Gynecology* 36(4), 897–909.

Derman, R.J. (1995). Effects of sex steroids on women's health: Implications for practitioners. *American Journal of Medicine* 98(1A suppl.), 137S–143S.

DiFiori, J.P. (1995). Menstrual dysfunction in athletes: How to identify and treat patients at risk for skeletal injury. *Postgraduate Medicine* 97(3), 143–156.

Ernster, V.L., Barclay, J., Kerlikowske, K., *et al.* (1996). Incidence of and treatment for ductal carcinoma in situ of the breast. *Journal of the American Medical Association* 275(12), 913–918.

Freeman, E.W., Rickels, K., Sondheimer, S.J., *et al.* (1995). A double-blind trial of oral progesterone, alprazolam, and placebo in treatment of severe premenstrual syndrome. *Journal of the American Medical Association* 274(1), 51–57.

Gabriel, S.E., Woods, J.E., O'Fallon, M., *et al.* (1997). Complications leading to surgery after breast implantation. *New England Journal of Medicine* 336(10), 677–682.

Galle, P.C., and McRae, M.A. (1993). Abnormal uterine bleeding: Finding and treating the cause. *Postgraduate Medicine* 93(2), 73–81.

Gibson, M. (1995). Reproductive health and polycystic ovary syndrome. *American Journal of Medicine* 98(1A suppl.), 67S–75S.

Ginsburg, E.S., Mello, N.K., Mendelson, J.H., *et al.* (1996). Effects of alcohol ingestion on estrogens in postmenopausal women. *Journal of the American Medical Association* 276(21), 1747–1751.

Grodstein, F., Stampfer, M.J., Manson, J.E., *et al.* (1996). Postmenopausal estrogen and progestin use and the risk of cardiovascular disease. *New England Journal of Medicine* 335(7), 453–461.

Guyton, A.C., and Hall, J.E. (1996). *Textbook of Medical Physiology.* (9th ed.). Philadelphia: W.B. Saunders.

Hadjiathanasiou, C.G., Brauner, R., Lortat-Jacob, S., *et al.* (1994). True hermaphroditism: Genetic variants and clinical management. *Journal of Pediatrics* 125(5 pt. 1), 738–744.

Hargrove, J.T., and Eisenberg, E. (1995). Menopause. *Medical Clinics of North America* 79(6), 1337–1356.

Hindle, W.H. (1994). Other benign breast problems. *Clinical Obstetrics and Gynecology* 37(4), 916–924.

Hutchinson, K.A. (1995). Androgens and sexuality. *American Journal of Medicine* 98(1A suppl.), 111S–115S.

Jacobson, J.A., Danforth, D.N., Cowan, K.H., *et al.* (1995). Ten-year results of a comparison of conservation with mastectomy in the treatment of stage I and II breast cancer. *New England Journal of Medicine* 332(14), 907–911.

Kottmann, L.M. (1995). Pelvic inflammatory disease: Clinical overview. *Journal of Obstetric, Gynecologic, and Neonatal Nursing* 24(8), 759–767.

Kushi, L.H., Folsom, A.R., Prineas, R.J., *et al.* (1996). Dietary antioxidant vitamins and death from coronary heart disease in postmenopausal women. *New England Journal of Medicine* 334(18), 1156–1162.

Lafferty, F.W., and Fiske, M.E. (1994). Postmenopausal estrogen replacement: A long-term cohort study. *American Journal of Medicine* 97, 66–77.

Lee-Feldstein, A., Anton-Culver, H., and Feldstein, P.J. (1994). Treatment differences and other prognostic factors related to breast cancer survival. *Journal of the American Medical Association* 271(15), 1163–1168.

Lindfors, K.K., and Rosenquist, J. (1995). The cost-effectiveness of mammographic screening strategies. *Journal of the American Medical Association* 274(11), 881–884.

Moore, A.A., and Noonan, M.D. (1996). A nurse's guide to hormone replacement therapy. *Journal of Obstetric, Gynecologic, and Neonatal Nursing* 25(1), 24–31.

Moore, K.L., and Persaud, T.V.N. (1993). *The Developing Human: Clinically Oriented Embryology.* Philadelphia: W.B. Saunders.

Moormeier, J. (1996). Breast cancer in black women. *Annals of Internal Medicine* 124(10), 897–905.

Newcomb, P.A., Storer, B.E., Longnecker, M.P., *et al.* (1994). Lactation and a reduced risk of premenopausal breast cancer. *New England Journal of Medicine* 330(2), 81–87.

Olson, B.R., Forman, M.R., Lanza, E., *et al.* (1996). Relation between sodium balance and menstrual cycle symptoms in normal women. *Annals of Internal Medicine* 125(7), 564–567.

Phelps, W.C., and Alexander, K.A. (1995). Antiviral therapy for human papillomaviruses: Rationale and prospects. *Annals of Internal Medicine* 123(5), 368–382.

Poehlman, E.T., Toth, M.J., and Gardner, A.W. (1995). Changes in energy balance and body composition at menopause: A controlled longitudinal study. *Annals of Internal Medicine* 123(9), 673–675.

Redmond, G.P. (1995). Androgenic disorders of women: Diagnostic and therapeutic decision making. *American Journal of Medicine* 98(1A suppl.), 120S–129S.

Rittmaster, R.S. (1995). Clinical relevance of testosterone and dihydrotestosterone metabolism in women. *American Journal of Medicine* 98(1A suppl.), 17S–21S.

Rush, C.B., and Entman, S.S. (1995). Pelvic organ prolapse and stress urinary incontinence. *Medical Clinics of North America* 79(6), 1473–1479.

Sanchez-Guerrero, J., Colditz, G.A., Karlson, E.W., *et al.* (1995). Silicone breast implants and the risk of connective tissue diseases and symptoms. *New England Journal of Medicine* 332(25), 1666–1670.

Sanchez-Guerrero, J., Liang, M.H., Karlson, E.W., *et al.* (1995). Postmenopausal estrogen therapy and the risk for developing systemic lupus erythematosus. *Annals of Internal Medicine* 122(6), 430–433.
Scharbo-Dehaan, M. (1994). Management strategies for hormonal replacement therapy. *Nurse Practitioner* 19(12), 47–57.
Schrott, H.G., Bittner, V., Vittinghoff, E., *et al.* (1997). Adherence to National Cholesterol Education Program Treatment goals in postmenopausal women with heart disease: The Heart and Estrogen/Progestin Replacement Study (HERS). *Journal of the American Medical Association* 277(16), 1281–1286.
Shapiro, T.J., and Clark, P.M. (1995). Breast cancer: What the primary care provider needs to know. *Nurse Practitioner* 20(3), 36–53.
Shepherd, J.C., and Fried, R.A. (1995). Preventing cervical cancer: The role of the Bethesda system. *American Family Physician* 51(2), 434–440.
Silverman, B.G., Brown, S.L., Bright, R.A., *et al.* (1996). Reported complications of silicone gel breast implants: An epidemiologic review. *Annals of Internal Medicine* 124(8), 744–756.
Soper, D.E. (1994). Pelvic inflammatory disease. *Infectious Disease Clinics of North America* 8(4), 821–840.
Speroff, L., Rowan, J., Symons, J., *et al.* (1996). The comparative effect on bone density, endometrium, and lipids of continuous hormones as replacement therapy (CHART study): A randomized controlled trial. *Journal of the American Medical Association* 276(17), 1397–1403.
Stack, P.S. (1997). Pap smears: Still a reliable screening tool for cervical cancer. *Postgraduate Medicine* 101(4), 207–214.
Stanford, J.L., Weiss, N.S., Voigt, L.F., *et al.* (1995). Combined estrogen and progestin hormone replacement therapy in relation to risk of breast cancer in middle-aged women. *Journal of the American Medical Association* 274(2), 137–142.

Thune, I., Brenn, T., Lund, E., *et al.* (1997). Physical activity and the risk of breast cancer. *New England Journal of Medicine* 336(18), 1269–1275.

Velanovich, V. (1995). Ectopic breast tissue, supernumerary breasts, and supernumerary nipples. *Southern Medical Journal* 88(9), 903–906.

Walker, L.O., and Tinkle, M.B. (1996). Toward an integrative science of women's health. *Journal of Obstetric, Gynecologic, and Neonatal Nursing* 25(5), 379–382.
Wall, L.L. (1993). The muscles of the pelvic floor. *Clinical Obstetrics and Gynecology* 36(4), 910–925.
Weber, B.L. (1994). Susceptibility genes for breast cancer. *New England Journal of Medicine* 331(22), 1523–1524.
Writing Group for the PEPI Trial. (1995). Effects of estrogen or estrogen/progestin regimens on heart disease risk factors in postmenopausal women. *Journal of the American Medical Association* 273(2), 199–208.
Writing Group for the PEPI Trial. (1996). Effects of hormone therapy on bone mineral density: Results from the Postmenopausal Estrogen/Progestin Interventions (PEPI) Trial. *Journal of the American Medical Association* 276(17), 1389–1396.
Writing Group for the PEPI Trial. (1996). Effects of hormone replacement therapy on endometrial histology in postmenopausal women: The Postmenopausal Estrogen/Progestin Interventions (PEPI) Trial. *Journal of the American Medical Association* 275(5), 370–375.

Unit XII

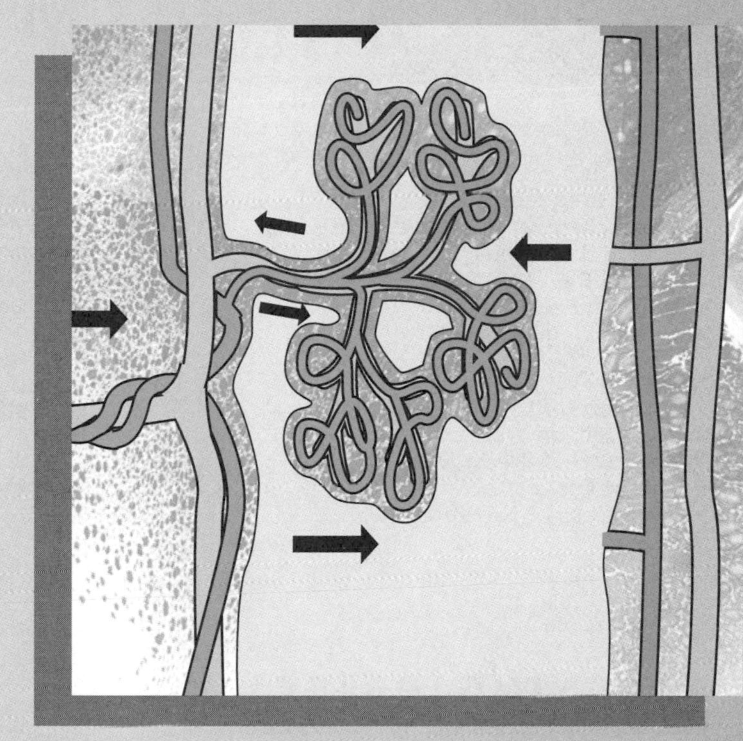

Chapter 32
Disorders Related to Pregnancy and Lactation

Chapter 33
Neonatal Disorders

PREGNANCY AND THE NEONATAL PERIOD

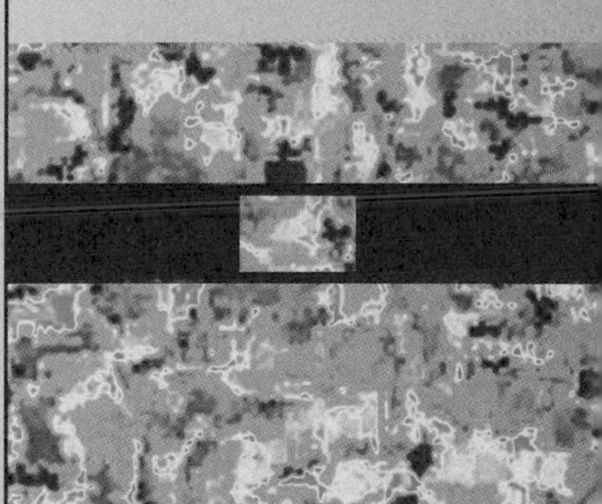

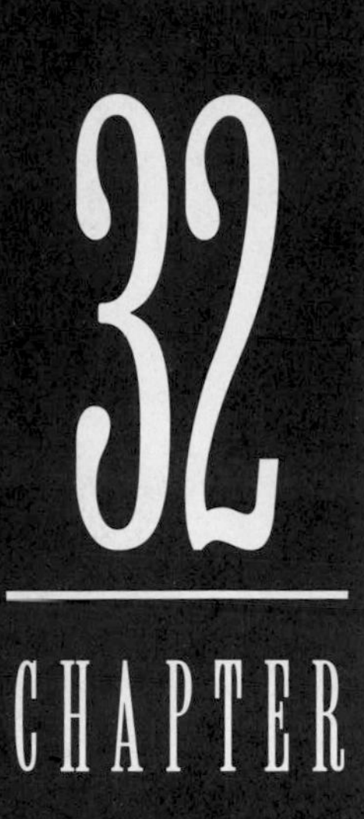

32 CHAPTER Disorders Related to Pregnancy and Lactation

LEARNING OBJECTIVES

1. Identify developmental landmarks occurring at each stage of pregnancy.
2. Describe the endocrine regulation of pregnancy.
3. Differentiate between normal and pathologic changes induced in each body system during pregnancy.
4. Describe the critical events that differentiate the stages of labor and delivery.
5. Identify risks associated with multifetal pregnancy.
6. Discuss the physiologic processes underlying breast tissue changes and regulation of lactation.
7. Comprehend the pathophysiologic processes that explain clinical manifestations and rationalize intervention in maternal disorders related to pregnancy.
8. Discuss the clinical significance of pregnancy-related disorders for mother and infant.

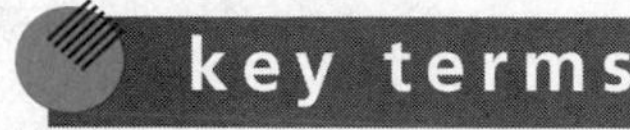

key terms

abruptio placentae
acute fatty liver of pregnancy (AFLP)
amniotic fluid embolism
anemia of pregnancy
cesarean section
choriocarcinoma
contraception
dilatation and curettage (D&C)
dystocia
eclampsia
ectopic pregnancy
endometritis
engorgement
fibromata molle
gestational diabetes mellitus
gestational trophoblastic disease
HELLP syndrome
hydatidiform mole
hyperemesis gravidarum
incompetent cervix
infertility
lactogenesis
letdown reflex

mastitis
melasma
multifetal pregnancy
obstetrics
oligohydramnios
parity
peripartum hemorrhage
placenta accreta
placental insufficiency
placenta previa
polyhydramnios
preeclampsia
pregnancy-induced hypertension
premature rupture of the membranes (PROM)
preterm labor
retraction ring
spontaneous abortion
striae gravidarum
subinvolution
TORCH infections
tubal ligation

Pregnancy and lactation are normal physiologic processes. Nevertheless, complications of pregnancy still result in an overall maternal mortality rate of 10 per 100,000 live births in the United States.[1] Causes of maternal death are indicated in Figure 32–1. Highest maternal risk is associated with age older than 40 years, black race, poor nutrition, lack of prenatal care, and abuse of drugs. The biomedical specialty of **obstetrics** is concerned with support of normal pregnancy and with prevention and treatment of associated disorders. Significant morbidity for mother and infant may result from the conditions discussed in this chapter. Pregnancy is a major stressor on all body systems of the mother, with inherent adaptive processes and clinical risks.

In this chapter, the processes of fertilization and implantation, introduced in Chapter 6, are described in more detail. Mechanisms of **infertility** and methods of **contraception** are discussed within this context. The anatomic and physiologic adaptations of pregnancy that occur within the maternal systems are detailed, along with potential disorders, including **spontaneous abortion**, **preterm labor**, **ectopic pregnancy**, **gestational diabetes mellitus**, **preeclampsia**, and **hydatidiform mole**. Processes and complications related to labor and delivery (parturition) are described, including **dystocia** and **peripartum hemorrhage**. Normal lactation and associated problems are also examined. In Chapter 33, fetal physiology is reviewed, and abnormalities of the newborn related to intrauterine development, labor and delivery, and the neonatal period are described.

PREGNANCY

Stages of Pregnancy

Figure 32–2 illustrates the typical anatomic changes that occur during the approximate 40 weeks of the pregnancy, or gestation period. Most obvious are the enlargement of the uterus by hypertrophy and hyperplasia, which increases its weight from about 60 g to 1000 g, and the changes in the breasts, which typically enlarge to at least twice their prepregnant size. Pregnancy begins with fertilization and implantation of the ovum, followed by the gestation period, which is divided into three 3-month periods (trimesters), during which maternal adaptations designed to support the growing fetus take place. Birth of the infant after a complete gestation period is said to occur at full-term (or simply "term").

Fertilization of the Ovum

After ovulation, there is an approximate 24-hour window of opportunity during which the ovum is available for penetration by spermatozoa. Even under optimal conditions, only a small fraction of the sperm deposited during ejaculation ever reaches the ovum; most die along the way to the fallopian tubes, where fertilization normally takes place. Ciliary movement and rhythmic contraction of fallopian tube smooth muscle assist with conduction of ovum and sperm toward each other. The ovum also releases a peptide that attracts sperm. As they near the ovum, sperm must undergo two final developmental changes: *capacitation*, in which surface glycoproteins are removed, and *activation*, in which sperm motility is altered to facilitate penetration.

The process of fertilization is illustrated in Figure 32–3. Several sperm are able to attach to the surface of the ovum through binding between molecules on the sperm head (acrosome) and the outer layers of the ovum (corona radiata and zona pellucida). This binding triggers the *acrosomal reaction*, in which the acrosome releases enzymes that break down the ovum's outer cell layers, fusing the two germ cells. When one spermatozoon is able to penetrate to the nucleus of the ovum, the *cortical reaction* occurs within the ovum. Cytoplasmic (cortical) vesicles adjacent to the cell membrane fuse with the membrane in a calcium-dependent process, forming a *fertilization membrane*. Enzymes released from the vesicles alter the receptors on the ovum surface, preventing penetration by more than one spermatozoon, except in rare cases.

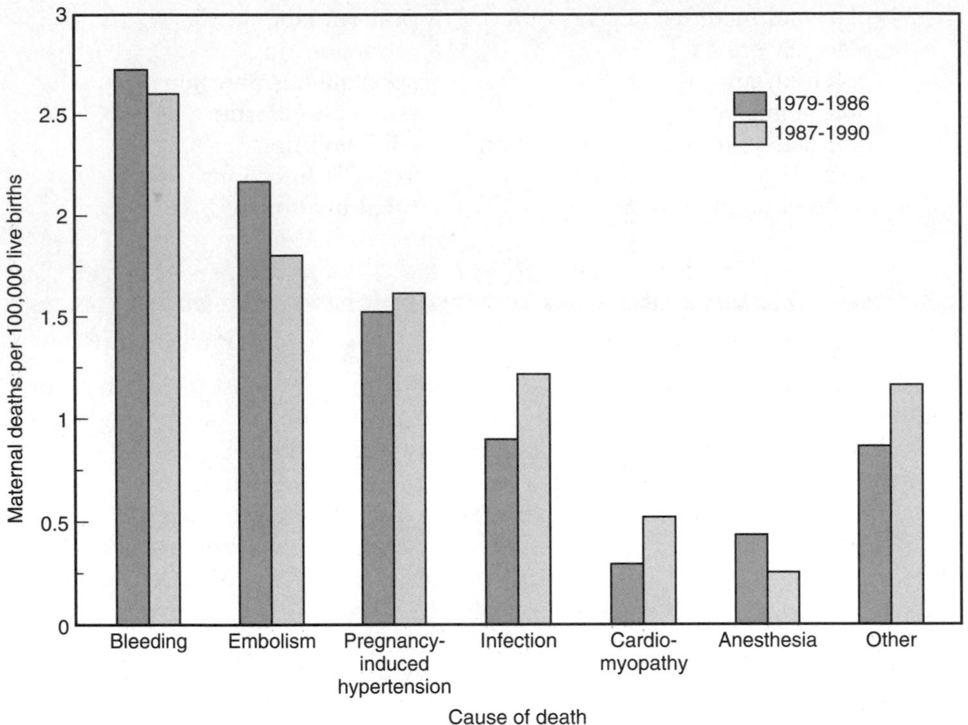

FIGURE 32–1

Causes of maternal mortality. Cardiovascular complications, including intrapartum bleeding, thromboembolism, and pregnancy-induced hypertension, account for most maternal deaths. (From Berg, C.J., Atrash, H.K., Doonin, L.M., *et al.* [1996]. Pregnancy-related mortality in the United States, 1987–1990. *Obstetrics and Gynecology* 88[2], 164. Reprinted by permission from the American College of Obstetricians and Gynecologists.)

As detailed in Chapter 6, fertilization triggers a series of cell divisions within the fertilized ovum (zygote), creating multiple smaller cells within the original outer layer of the ovum. As this cell mass, or *morula*, continues its transit through the fallopian tube to the uterus, it evolves into the *blastocyst* stage, when a fluid-filled cavity divides the mass into two cell layers (Fig. 32–4). The inner cell mass will become the embryo, and the outer cell mass or *trophoblast* will become the *chorion*, a membrane that covers the embryo and provides the fetal component of the placenta.

Disorders that may occur during this stage include some mechanisms of infertility, such as failure to ovulate (anovulation) or impairment of sperm numbers, motility, or response to chemical attraction by the ovum. Blockage or impaired motility of the fallopian tube caused by scar tissue or other factors may result in infertility or in ectopic pregnancy. **Multifetal pregnancy** results from penetration of more than one ovum by sperm (e.g., fraternal or nonidentical twins) or from initial division of the zygote into daughter cells that then undergo separate development (e.g., monozygotic or identical twins).

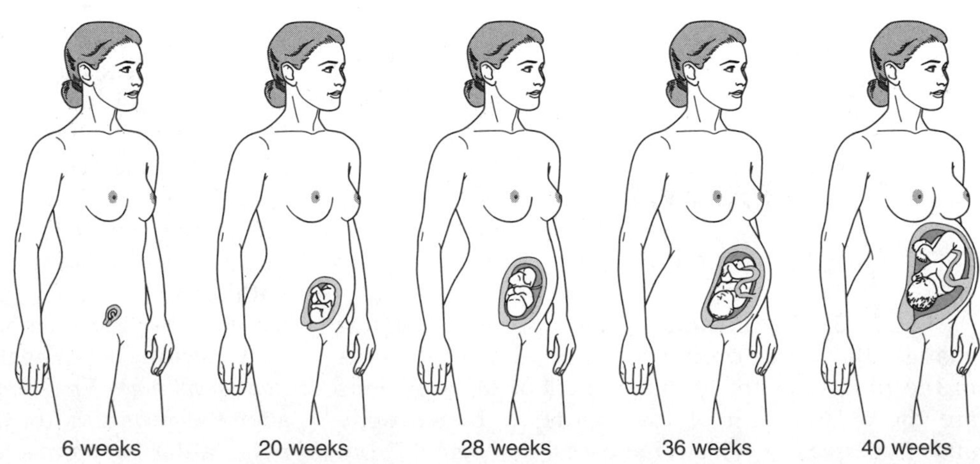

FIGURE 32–2

Anatomic stages of pregnancy. Uterine and breast enlargement occurs proportionately to fetal growth. Uterine weight increases from 60 to 1000 g, and the breasts may enlarge to more than double their prepregnant mass.

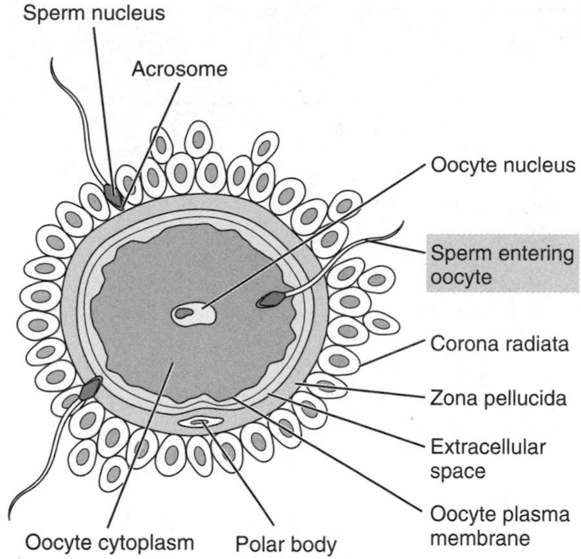

FIGURE 32–3

Fertilization. Several sperm attach to the ovum via binding of the sperm head *(acrosome)* to receptors on the outer layers of the ovum *(corona radiata* and *zona pellucida).* When one sperm is able to penetrate these layers, cytoplasmic vesicles fuse with the oocyte membrane, altering membrane receptors and preventing penetration by other sperm.

Implantation

Within the uterus, the blastocyst floats freely for 7 to 9 days, receiving nutrients from endometrial secretions. It then selects a site for attachment to the endometrium (implantation). Implantation normally occurs in the upper, posterior portion of the uterus. Enzymes secreted by the trophoblast erode the endometrium, embedding the blastocyst. Expression of adhesion molecules is also involved in this process. In addition, adequate levels of the hormone progesterone must be maintained to enhance the receptivity of the uterus to implantation. Abnormalities of these molecular processes may underlie spontaneous abortions (miscarriages).

The placenta develops from trophoblast and endometrial cells at the point of implantation. Hydatidiform mole is a condition in which initial trophoblastic cell division is abnormal and uncontrolled, resulting in rapid, neoplastic-like growth within the uterus. Should the blastocyst implant low in the uterus, at a site near to or covering the cervical os, the developing fetus may eventually obstruct its own placental blood supply. This disorder, **placenta previa**, may also result in peripartum hemorrhage.

Methods of **contraception**, the voluntary prevention of pregnancy, are based on prevention of ovulation, fertilization, or implantation (Table 32–1).

Development and Function of the Placenta

Immediately after implantation, the blastocyst receives nutrients and oxygen and eliminates carbon dioxide and metabolic wastes via simple diffusion between endometrial and trophoblastic cells. Fingerlike projections of the trophoblast (chorionic villi)

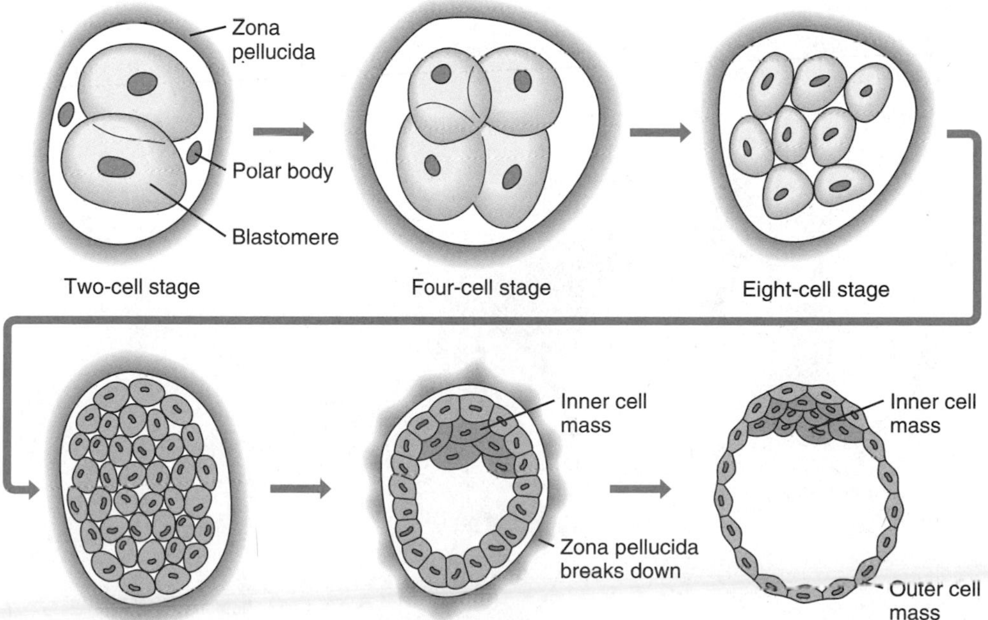

FIGURE 32–4

Blastocyst development. Fertilization initiates division of the oocyte, creating multiple smaller cells within the outer layer of the ovum. This cell mass *(morula)* evolves into a *blastocyst,* with a fluid cavity separating the cells into two layers. The inner cell mass will become the embryo, and the outer cell mass *(trophoblast)* will form a fetal membrane, the chorion, as well as the fetal component of the placenta.

TABLE 32–1
METHODS OF CONTRACEPTION

Method	Efficacy	Comments
Vasectomy	99.9%	Surgical sterilization of male by interruption of the vas deferens, preventing access of sperm to seminal fluid
Tubal ligation	99.6%	Surgical sterilization of female by blockage of the fallopian tube, preventing the ovum from entering the uterus or contacting sperm
Hormonal methods Oral contraceptives Injectable progestogen Hormonal implants	97%–99%	Alteration of the hormonal environment (estrogen or progesterone levels), suppressing ovulation and disrupting cyclic endometrial changes
Intrauterine devices (IUDs) Copper T Progestasert	97%	Uncertain mechanism; may induce a sterile inflammatory response or hormonal effects that alter the endometrial environment, inhibiting implantation; may alter cervical mucus or sperm function
Barrier methods Male condom Female condom Diaphragm Vaginal sponge Cervical cap Spermicides	72%–88%	Inhibit contact of sperm and ovum; spermicides also kill sperm; protect against sexually transmitted disease
Natural family planning (periodic abstinence) Calendar rhythm Ovulation method Symptothermal method Postovulation method	80%	Based on identification of the female's fertile period by assessment of basal body temperature, cervical mucus, and other symptoms indicating ovulation

grow into the endometrium and are functional as exchange vessels between the maternal and fetal blood at 4 weeks' gestation (Fig. 32–5). Fetal blood flows from the descending aorta through two umbilical arteries into the villi of the placenta and returns to the fetal vena cava via the ductus venosus near the fetal liver (see Chapter 33). Maternal blood flows via uterine arteries into the intervillous spaces surrounding the villi and returns via uterine veins.

Exchange across the walls of the villi occurs by active and passive transport processes. Because most fetal venous blood bypasses the collapsed fetal

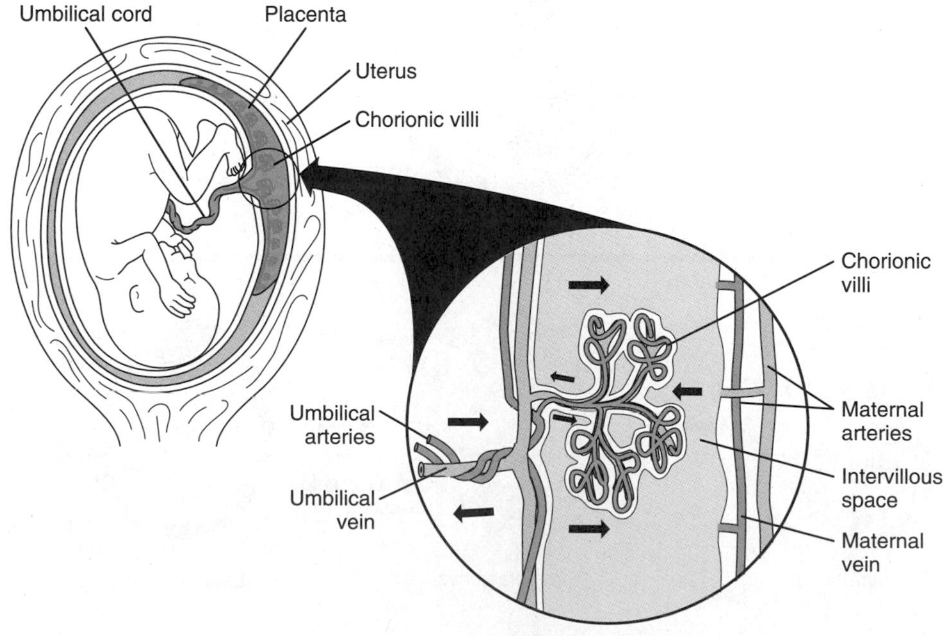

FIGURE 32–5
Placental exchange vessels. Finger-like projections of the trophoblast *(chorionic villi)* grow into the maternal endometrium and are functional as exchange vessels by 4 weeks' gestation.

lungs, the partial pressure of oxygen in the fetal arterial blood is low in comparison with the maternal blood, facilitating exchange along this gradient. Fetal hemoglobin (Hb F) has a slightly different structure from that of adult hemoglobin (Hb A), conferring higher affinity for oxygen and facilitating fetal uptake of oxygen (see Chapter 12).

Water, electrolytes, blood gases, some nutrients, and most drugs readily cross the placenta by simple diffusion (Table 32–2). Glucose uptake occurs by facilitated diffusion and active transport. Amino acids are exchanged by active transport, and proteins such as albumin and γ-globulin are taken up by pinocytosis (see Chapter 2). Selective transport processes of the placenta normally act as a barrier between fetal antigenic proteins and the maternal circulation, preventing the production of antifetal antibodies that could damage or destroy the fetus.

The placenta expands to cover half the endometrial surface during the first 20 weeks of gestation. As discussed later, the placenta gradually assumes importance as an endocrine organ as well as an exchange structure. Structural and functional abnormalities of the placenta may lead to significant complications of pregnancy. **Abruptio placentae** (placental abruption) is a disorder in which the placenta separates prematurely from the uterine wall, leading to life-threatening maternal hemorrhage and abrupt loss of fetal support. **Placental insufficiency**, a general term for inadequate placental function, may lead to deficient development of the fetus, and has also been implicated in the etiology of preeclampsia.

TABLE 32–2
PLACENTAL TRANSPORT OF SELECTED SUBSTANCES

Mechanism	Substance
Simple (passive) diffusion	Water, electrolytes, oxygen, carbon dioxide, urea, simple amines, creatinine, fatty acids, steroids, fat-soluble vitamins, narcotics, antibiotics, barbiturates, and anesthetics
Facilitated diffusion	Glucose, oxygen
Active transport	Amino acids, water-soluble vitamins, calcium, iron, iodine
Pinocytosis and endocytosis	Globulins, phospholipids, lipoproteins, antibodies, viruses
Bulk flow/solvent drag	Water, electrolytes
Accidental capillary breaks	Intact blood cells
Independent movement	Maternal leukocytes, organisms such as *Treponema pallidum*

From Blackburn, S.T., and Loper, D.L. (1992). *Maternal, Fetal, and Neonatal Physiology: A Clinical Perspective.* Philadelphia: W.B. Saunders. (p. 79). Used with permission.

Endocrine Regulation of Pregnancy

Pregnancy is under endocrine regulation by several hormones (Fig. 32–6). During early pregnancy (the *luteal phase*), hormonal support originates from the trophoblast, which secretes human chorionic gonadotropin (hCG) and human chorionic somatomammotropin (hCS), also known as human placental lactogen (hPL), and from the corpus luteum, which secretes those hormones as well as progesterone, estrogen, and relaxin. During the second and third trimesters (the *placental phase* of pregnancy), placental secretion of hCG, estrogen, and progesterone overtakes luteal secretion. The placenta also secretes antidiuretic hormone (ADH), aldosterone, and renin.

The anterior pituitary hormone prolactin and the posterior pituitary hormone oxytocin are of particular importance in the regulation of lactation.

Human Chorionic Gonadotropin

Human chorionic gonadotropin, which is similar in structure to luteinizing hormone (LH), prevents the degeneration of the corpus luteum, extending its hormone production throughout the first trimester. hCG also maintains the endometrium and stimulates secretion of testosterone by the testes in male fetuses. Detection of hCG in the maternal urine allows early confirmation of pregnancy.

Human Chorionic Somatomammotropin

Human chorionic somatomammotropin is structurally similar to growth hormone (GH) and prolactin (see Chapter 27). Its GH-like effects favor fetal growth and inhibit maternal nutrient storage. Fetal bone growth is enhanced directly, and maternal insulin resistance is induced, reducing glucose uptake and elevating serum glucose levels for use by the fetus. Maternal use of lipids for energy is thus favored, and insulin resistance may precipitate gestational diabetes mellitus in some women. The prolactin-like effects of hCS may promote development of the breast in preparation for milk production (lactation).

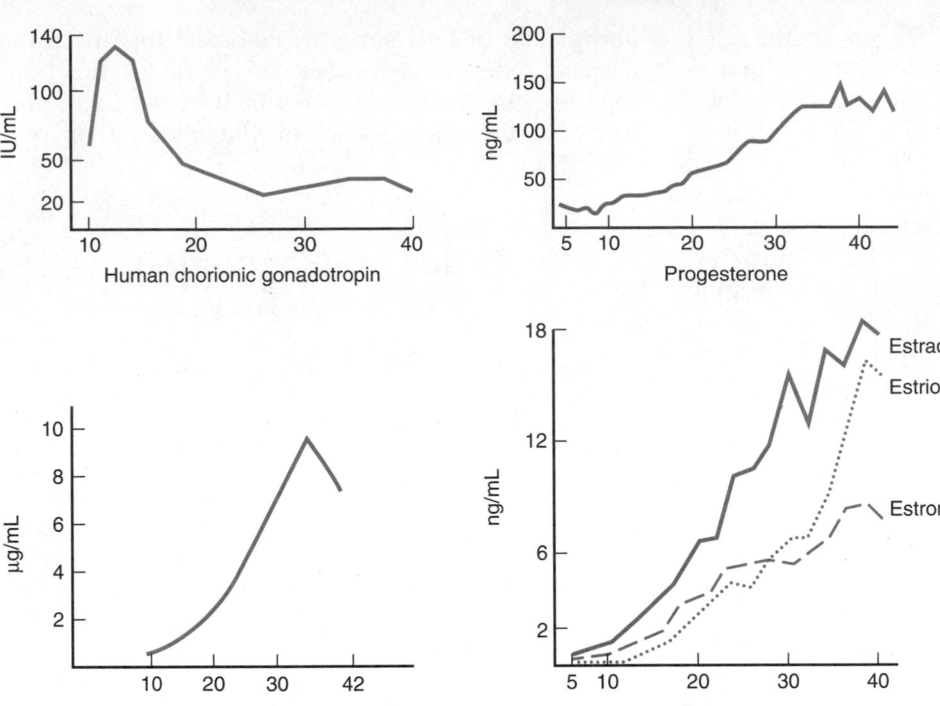

FIGURE 32–6
Hormone levels during pregnancy. The serum level of human chorionic gonadotropin (hCG) rises sharply during early pregnancy, as a consequence of trophoblastic secretion. Later in pregnancy, hCG secretion by the placenta is stabilized at a lower level. Levels of human chorionic somatomammotropin (hCS), estrogen (particularly estradiol), and progesterone continue to rise until term. (Redrawn from Freinkle, N. [1980]. Pregnancy and progeny: Banting lecture, 1980. *Diabetes* 29, 1023–1035.)

Relaxin

Relaxin initially softens the cervix and uterus, facilitating uterine enlargement, and later softens ligaments of the pelvis, enlarging the pelvic aperture in anticipation of delivery. Relaxin also promotes expression of oxytocin receptors on uterine smooth muscle. Withdrawal of relaxin at term may enhance the uterine smooth-muscle contraction of labor.

Estrogen

Estrogen synthesis by the placenta requires the assistance of the fetal and maternal adrenal glands for intermediate steps (see Chapter 29). Placental estrogen is mostly estriol, which is lower in potency than the estradiol that mediates the menstrual cycle (see Chapter 31). However, because of its elevated levels during pregnancy, estriol assumes major importance in stimulating enlargement of the uterus and development of the breasts.

Progesterone

Placental cells contain the enzymes for complete synthesis of progesterone from cholesterol. Progesterone levels are very high during pregnancy, mediating endometrial and breast development and decreasing contractility of uterine smooth muscle to prevent spontaneous abortion or preterm labor.

Antidiuretic Hormone, Aldosterone, and Renin

Antidiuretic hormone, aldosterone, and renin (from placental, posterior pituitary, or renal sources) promote maternal fluid retention and enhanced blood volume during pregnancy to perfuse the growing fetus (see Chapter 8). The vasoconstricting effects of ADH and angiotensin II, produced with stimulation of the renin–angiotensin–aldosterone system, increase resistance of the circulation in the lower body of the fetus, thereby promoting increased oxygen delivery to the vital structures of the head and chest. Maternal alteration in sensitivity to angiotensin II may play a role in hypertension associated with preeclampsia.

Prolactin

The secretion of prolactin by the anterior pituitary is increased 10-fold during pregnancy, but its effect of stimulating **lactogenesis** (milk production by mammary glands) is inhibited by the concurrently high levels of estrogen and progesterone. Removal of estrogen and progesterone with delivery of the placenta permits lactogenesis.

Oxytocin

The hypothalamic hormone oxytocin, released from the posterior pituitary, is of particular importance to the processes of labor and lactation. Oxytocin receptors on uterine cells are expressed in increasing numbers throughout pregnancy. Binding of oxytocin induces smooth-muscle contraction directly and also triggers the synthesis of prostaglandins by endometrial macrophages and other tissues. Local mediators (prostaglandins) further induce uterine contraction and mediate softening ("ripening") of the cervix. Before term, oxytocin and prostaglandin effects are normally inhibited by high progesterone levels. Oxytocin also mediates the milk **letdown reflex** during lactation by inducing contraction of smooth muscle surrounding milk-filled alveoli in the breasts.

Additional effects of the hormones of pregnancy are described in the next section.

Systemic Adaptations During Pregnancy

The extreme physiologic changes of pregnancy affect every body system and must be appreciated so that they are not misinterpreted as pathology.

Cardiovascular System

The mother's circulating blood volume increases by an average of 45% to adequately perfuse the enlarged uterus, breasts, and fetus and to accommodate the expected blood loss that occurs during delivery. This *hypervolemia of pregnancy* is primarily caused by increases in plasma volume mediated by placental ADH, renin, and aldosterone, although red blood cell volume also increases.

Cardiac output increases 30% to 50% by 24 weeks' gestation, a level that is maintained throughout the remainder of the pregnancy. The heart rate typically increases 10 to 15 beats/min, and stroke volume increases 30%, leading to increased myocardial oxygen demand. The increased cardiac workload is well-tolerated unless the mother has underlying cardiac disease such as valve disease or cardiomyopathy, in which case pregnancy may precipitate cardiac failure (see Chapter 16).

Progesterone relaxes venous smooth muscle, enlarging circulatory capacity but also contributing to the development of superficial varicosities and hemorrhoids. Hemorrhoids also result from increased venous pressure caused by obstruction of venous return from the legs by the enlarged uterus. Reduced vascular resistance contributes to lower blood pressure early in pregnancy, and hypotension may worsen when the woman lies supine, permitting the gravid uterus to obstruct venous return. Increased vascularization of the uterus, cervix, and vagina changes their color to bluish purple, a presumptive sign of pregnancy (Chadwick's sign).

Hematopoietic System

The disproportionate increase in plasma volume results in a dilutional reduction in hemoglobin, hematocrit, and erythrocyte count during pregnancy. Erythropoietin release is stimulated by hCS, progesterone, and prolactin during the second and third trimesters, leading to increased erythropoiesis (see Chapter 12). Iron supplementation is often necessary to support increased red blood cell (RBC) synthesis during pregnancy.

In the case of an Rh-negative mother bearing an Rh-positive fetus, the possibility of Rho(D) isoimmunization exists (see Chapter 13). Normally, the placenta effectively separates fetal RBCs from the maternal circulation, so that anti-Rh antibodies do not develop during pregnancy. In disorders of placental function, such as preeclampsia, contact may occur and antibodies may develop during pregnancy. Antibody-induced lysis of fetal RBCs induces anemia and hyperbilirubinemia (hemolytic disease of the newborn). The first Rh-positive infant born to an Rh-negative mother is usually not affected, because sensitizing contact of maternal blood with fetal RBCs does not occur until the time of delivery. This contact would then induce the formation of anti-Rh antibodies that would attack the RBCs of the Rh-positive fetus in a subsequent pregnancy. Pregnant women are routinely assessed for Rh type and sensitization status. At the time of delivery, or after any potentially sensitizing event (e.g., abortion, ectopic pregnancy), the mother is given anti-Rh antibody by injection. This agent (RhoGAM or RhIGIV) lyses any fetal Rh-positive RBCs in the maternal circulation, preventing development of anti-Rh antibody.

Under the influence of estrogen and progesterone, serum levels of several protein clotting factors are elevated (see Chapter 14). The resulting hypercoagulable state serves to limit blood loss during delivery, but also increases the risk of deep vein thrombosis and pulmonary emboli. Thrombotic events are among the more common complications of pregnancy. Anemia and a low platelet count (thrombocytopenia) are components of the **HELLP syndrome** (*h*emolysis, *e*levated *l*iver enzymes, and *l*ow *p*latelet count) that may accompany preeclampsia.

Respiratory System

The growing uterus displaces the diaphragm upward and causes the lower rib cage to expand outward. Despite this infringement on the thoracic space, alveolar ventilation actually increases during pregnancy, exceeding the increased oxygen demands. Increased ventilation is primarily caused by an increase in tidal volume, although a slight increase in resting respiratory rate is often seen as well. Expiratory reserve volume and residual volume decrease adaptively; thus, the pregnant woman maintains normal ventilation above a decreased functional residual capacity (see Chapter 18).

Arterial blood gases usually reveal a mild, compensated respiratory alkalosis (see Chapter 10). Progesterone-mediated relaxation of bronchial smooth muscle decreases airway resistance, facilitating ventilation. Progesterone may also cause heightened sensitivity of the chemoreceptors to carbon dioxide, promoting the hyperventilation and dyspnea often associated with pregnancy. Nasal stuffiness is common during pregnancy, and it is believed to result from estrogen-induced vasomotor instability.

Renal-Urinary System

Increased blood volume, progesterone-mediated relaxation of ureteral smooth muscle, and outflow obstruction by the growing uterus lead to a physiologic hydroureter and hydronephrosis in the majority of pregnant women (see Chapter 20). Bladder tone is decreased, and bladder capacity is increased. Renal blood flow increases by 50% during the first trimester, caused by increased cardiac output, increased blood volume, and decreased renal vascular resistance. Glomerular filtration rate (GFR) rises proportionately. Urine volumes are typically increased 25%.

Tubular reabsorption rates of filtered substances increase adaptively up to their maximum capacities, but increased urinary excretion of glucose, amino acids, urea, and protein are common during pregnancy. Potassium reabsorption is increased during pregnancy to supply the demands of fetal synthesis. The mechanism of this increase may be inhibition of the aldosterone-driven Na^+,K^+-ATPase in the distal tubule (see Chapter 9). The kidneys retain hydrogen ions and excrete bicarbonate in compensation for respiratory alkalosis. Urinary loss of calcium and water-soluble vitamins is increased because of "washout" with increased tubular flow rates. Most pregnant women require supplementation of vitamins and minerals to offset these losses. Increases in ADH and activity of the renin–angiotensin–aldosterone system mediate sodium reabsorption proportionate to fluid retention, thus maintaining osmolar balance.

An estimated 5% to 8% of pregnant women develop asymptomatic bacteriuria during pregnancy, and 25% of these cases will progress to renal infection (pyelonephritis) if untreated.[2] Screening urinalysis is indicated during prenatal care, and antibiotic therapy may be required for treatment of urinary tract infection.

Gastrointestinal System

The effects of pregnancy on the alimentary canal are caused mainly by estrogen-mediated vascular changes, progesterone-mediated relaxation of intestinal smooth muscle, and external pressure by the growing uterus. Estrogen increases blood flow to the gingivae (gums) of the oral cavity and enhances turnover of cells, leading to gingivitis in many pregnant women. Decreased tone of the lower esophageal sphincter accompanied by increased intra-abdominal pressure leads to an increased incidence of gastroesophageal reflux of acid (see Chapter 24). Gastric motility is decreased, leading to slowed digestion and a tendency toward reverse peristalsis. Intestinal motility is also decreased, leading to prolonged transit time. Digestive enzyme activity is increased, however, and intestinal villi elongate, increasing the absorptive surface. These changes facilitate increased absorption of nutrients from the gut, but also increase the risk of constipation and flatulence.

Nausea and vomiting (morning sickness) occur in the majority of pregnant women, most frequently between the 5th and 12th weeks of gestation. The precise etiology is unknown, and research results have been conflicting. Hormonal theories implicate high levels of estrogen, hCG, or both, but correlations between levels of these hormones and severity of symptoms have been inconsistent across several studies. Psychogenic factors, such as ambivalence about the pregnancy, or heightened sensitivity to hormonal changes have also been implicated but remain unproved. **Hyperemesis gravidarum** is extensive and prolonged vomiting leading to severe alteration in nutritional status and fluid-electrolyte balance.[3] The cause of this disorder, seen in 1% to 2% of pregnant women, is unknown. More than 50% of women with hyperemesis have elevated levels of thyroxine (see Chapter 28).

Hepatobiliary System

Gallbladder tone is decreased during pregnancy, leading to retention of bile after contraction. Reabsorption of water from stored bile is decreased, and the resulting dilute bile does not solubilize cholesterol optimally. Formation of cholesterol-based gallstones is more common during pregnancy, and retention of bile salts may cause pruritus (see Chapter 26). The liver is displaced from its normal position by the growing uterus, and its fraction of the cardiac output is reduced by the demands of the placenta. Liver function is usually within normal limits during pregnancy, but changes in hepatic synthesis of plasma proteins, bilirubin, and serum lipids are evident. Albumin synthesis is decreased, but protein clotting factors are increased. Bilirubin synthesis may be increased slightly, and cholesterol synthesis may be doubled.

Acute fatty liver of pregnancy (AFLP) is a serious complication in 1 in 13,000 pregnancies.[4] This idiopathic disorder, usually associated with preeclampsia, arises later in pregnancy and typically progresses to acute hepatic failure (see Chapter 26). Immediate termination of pregnancy is warranted in AFLP. The HELLP syndrome, characterized by elevated liver enzymes and coagulopathy, may also accompany preeclampsia.

Integumentary System

The skin and its associated blood vessels, glands, and hair follicles are greatly affected by pregnancy, and many of the manifestations persist after delivery of the infant. Hyperpigmentation, caused by increased production of the pigment *melanin*, manifests as darkening of the areolae of the breasts, genital skin, and the *linea alba* that extends from the xiphoid process to the symphysis pubis at the abdominal midline. Existing freckles, nevi (moles), and scars may enlarge and darken during pregnancy. **Melasma** (chloasma or "mask of pregnancy") occurs in 50% to 75% of pregnant women. Melasma manifests as brownish pigmentation over the cheeks, forehead, upper lip, nose, or chin. There is an apparent genetic predisposition to development of melasma. The pigmentation fades in most women during the year after pregnancy, but it may persist longer in dark-haired women. Pigmentation demarcation lines, abrupt transitions between lighter and darker skin areas, are most common in Japanese, black, and Hispanic women. Hyperpigmentation of pregnancy is believed to be caused by the effects of estrogen and progesterone on melanin production. No increase in melanocyte-stimulating hormone activity is seen (see Chapter 27).

Striae gravidarum or "stretch marks" are caused by tearing of dermal collagen in the skin of the enlarging breasts and abdomen. Striae typically appear at 6 to 7 months' gestation and are apparently caused by the combined effects of hormonally mediated changes in the skin structure and mechanical stretching by growth of underlying tissues. Striae appear as pink or purple wavy lines that eventually become silvery white, fading with time, but usually not disappearing completely. Estrogen-induced vasomotor instability may result in the appearance of superficial vascular lesions, including angiomata, palmar erythema, purpura, and varicosities. Existing moles and freckles usually darken, and skin tags (**fibromata molle**) are common during the second and third trimesters.

Increased activity of the sebaceous glands results in oiliness of the skin. Enlargement of sebaceous glands of the areolae of the breasts produces the characteristic tiny bumps of *Montgomery's tubercles*. Activity of apocrine sweat glands (which empty into the hair follicles of selected areas such as the axillae and groin) is decreased, whereas that of eccrine sweat glands (which empty onto the skin surface over the entire body) is increased. Eccrine gland activity is of particular importance to thermoregulation, and evaporative cooling assists in dissipating the excess heat produced by the increased metabolic rate of pregnancy.

Hair growth is commonly altered during pregnancy, with mild hirsutism often seen early because of hormonal alterations. Although this effect is greatly lessened during the weeks after delivery, a few coarse hairs may remain on the face and in the midline of the suprapubic area. After delivery, a period of increased hair loss is often seen, resulting from estrogen-induced lengthening of the follicular growth phase during pregnancy. Cyclic hair growth usually returns to normal within 6 to 15 months after pregnancy, although hair may be permanently thinner in some women.

Nervous System

The neurologic manifestations of pregnancy are believed to be hormonally mediated, but most are incompletely understood. Sleep patterns are altered during pregnancy as well as after delivery. During the first trimester, total sleep time is typically increased. Later in pregnancy, sleep time decreases, with increased night awakenings possibly associated with nocturia, dyspnea, or other physiologic manifestations. Sleep alteration usually persists until about 2 weeks after delivery.

Early pregnancy is often characterized by emotional lability (mood swings). A period of mild depression (postpartum blues) is experienced by many women during the first 2 weeks after delivery. In a few women, this phenomenon manifests as severe depression or psychosis. The specific causes of these manifestations are unknown.[5]

Seizure activity arising in a woman with preeclampsia indicates that the condition has degenerated to **eclampsia**.

Musculoskeletal System

The characteristic "waddling" gait of advanced pregnancy is caused by relaxation of pelvic ligaments and by the functional lordosis that compensates for the shifted center of gravity. It is widely believed that calcium loss from maternal bones and teeth occurs during pregnancy, but there is no research evidence of such demineralization. Carpal tunnel syndrome is common during pregnancy, probably secondary to hypervolemia, but usually resolves spontaneously after delivery (see Chapter 23).

Endocrine System

Many effects of the hormones of pregnancy have been detailed in the preceding discussion. Increased estrogen and progesterone levels also suppress the hypothalamic–pituitary–gonadal axis, and ovulation ceases during pregnancy (see Chapter 31). The pituitary gland is hypertrophied and highly vascular during pregnancy, increasing the risk of hypopituitarism secondary to Sheehan's syndrome (see Chapter 27). Output of thyroid hormones increases due to the thyrotropic effect of hCG, mediating a 25% increase in basal metabolic rate. Thyroid disorders are associated with increased risk of spontaneous abortion. Parathyroid hormone, cortisol, and insulin output are also increased in support of the altered metabolism of pregnancy.

Inflammatory and Immune Responses

Adaptations in host defenses during pregnancy serve the physiologic purpose of increasing tolerance of the "foreign" fetus, but they may also increase maternal susceptibility to infection and to autoimmune disorders, as evidenced by the commonality of intrapartum infections and the significantly higher incidence of autoimmune disorders in females. White blood cell (WBC) counts are usually slightly increased during pregnancy, but neutrophil chemotaxis is decreased, possibly delaying onset of inflammation (see Chapter 13). Numbers of natural killer cells are decreased, reducing the nonspecific immune response. Numbers of T helper cells are reduced during pregnancy, and T suppressor cell activity may increase during late pregnancy. These changes reduce the efficiency of the cell-mediated immune response and may suppress humoral immunity as well. Significant alterations in immunoglobulin (antibody) levels are usually not seen.

Most pregnant women are not significantly compromised by changes in host defense. However, an increase in viral infections and those caused by opportunistic organisms is seen, particularly during the second and third trimesters. These infections often take longer to resolve in pregnant women. Urinary tract infections are particularly common because of urine stasis induced by the pressure of the growing uterus. Infections are associated with increased incidence of preterm labor, possibly because of disruption of fetal membranes or stimulation of prostaglandin synthesis by maternal lymphokines. Although it has been suspected as a contributing factor, consistent correlations have not been found between maternal infection and spontaneous abortion. Maternal infections may significantly affect fetal development, however. The **TORCH infections** (*t*oxoplasmosis, *o*ther agents, *r*ubella, *c*ytomegalovirus, and *h*erpes simplex virus) may be directly teratogenic or may induce placental lesions (see Chapter 7). The risk of vertical transmission of the human immunodeficiency virus (HIV) from mother to infant is significant. HIV-infected mothers and their newborns are routinely treated with the antiretroviral drug zidovudine (see Chapter 13). An autoimmune mechanism has recently been implicated in the etiology of preeclampsia.

Human breast milk contains many substances of importance to fetal immunologic defense, including phagocytic WBCs, complement proteins, B and T lymphocytes, and their products of immunoglobulin (Ig) A, IgG, IgM, interferons, and other lymphokines. The early breast secretion, colostrum, is especially rich in these substances. IgA is the predominant immunoglobulin in breast milk, serving as a protective barrier against mucosal invasion by viruses, bacterial toxins, and antigenic proteins.[6] Because the HIV virus may be transmitted in breast milk, HIV-infected mothers are encouraged to bottle-feed their infants.

Energy Metabolism and Nutrition

Optimal weight gain during pregnancy has been the subject of controversy for many years. Recent guidelines issued by the Institute of Medicine recommend a gain of 25 to 35 pounds for women of normal weight, with less for those who are overweight before pregnancy and more for those who are underweight.[7] To ensure optimal growth of fetal and maternal tissues, a gain of 8 pounds during the first trimester is recommended, followed by a gain of 1 pound per week during the remainder of the pregnancy. The early gain is constituted primarily as maternal fat stores and blood volume, and later gains represent growth of the fetus, uterus, and breasts.

Pregnancy is an anabolic state, characterized by increased demands for energy fuel to meet the needs of the stressed maternal system and the growing fetus. Basal metabolic rate (BMR) increases by an average of 30%. The most notable changes in carbohydrate metabolism result from increasing maternal resistance to insulin, which has been referred to as the "diabetogenic effect" of pregnancy. Insulin resistance is believed to result from the hormonal effects of hCS, cortisol, progesterone, and estrogen. Maternal use of glucose decreases, making more available to the fetus. Gestational diabetes may develop as a result of insulin resistance in susceptible women. These women, as well as those whose diabetes predates pregnancy, are at increased risk for a number of complications. Infants of diabetic mothers are also vulnerable, as detailed in Chapter 33.

Protein metabolism displays a biphasic pattern. In early pregnancy, maternal protein synthesis is enhanced; in late pregnancy, an "accelerated starvation" state develops in which some protein is catabolized to supply maternal energy fuel and amino acid substrates for fetal protein synthesis.[8] Triglyceride synthesis and adipose storage increase during the first and second trimesters. During third trimester "starvation," there is increased lipolysis, apparently to serve as a source of maternal energy fuel during a period of increased uptake of glucose and amino acids by the fetus. Ketosis is common during this period, but it is not harmful to mother or infant. Ketone bodies cross the placenta and may be used by the fetus as energy fuel (see Chapter 3).

To optimize outcomes of pregnancy, supplemental vitamins and minerals are indicated for most pregnant women and possibly for women of childbearing age who are contemplating pregnancy. Supplements are intended to enhance, not to replace, an adequate diet. Iron, calcium, folate, vitamins B_6, B_{12}, C, and D, and possibly some trace elements are needed for tissue synthesis. Supplementation of these nutrients before and during pregnancy has been shown to enhance the health of mother and fetus and possibly to reduce the incidence of certain congenital defects.[9] Folate deficiency, for example, is strongly associated with neural tube defects such as spina bifida (see Chapter 21). **Anemia of pregnancy** is usually caused by relative deficiency of iron or folate that develops as a consequence of increased erythropoiesis.[10]

Labor and Delivery

Onset of Labor

The factors that initiate labor are incompletely understood. Those factors believed to play an active or permissive role include (1) genetic programming; (2) hormones of pregnancy; (3) prostaglandins; and (4) mechanical factors such as myometrial stretch or membrane disruption. Neurologic input to uterine smooth muscle is not essential to contraction.

Genetic Programming. Evidence for genetic programming lies in the observed consistency of length of gestation within species. The precise mechanisms of this regulation have not been identified.

Hormones of Pregnancy. The ratio of estrogen to progesterone near term may also be important. Progesterone suppresses uterine contraction throughout pregnancy, and administration of progesterone inhibitors has been used to terminate premature labor. Increased estrogen levels near term may trigger synthesis of a progesterone-binding protein, exerting a permissive effect on labor onset. Estrogen levels in amniotic fluid increase 2 to 3 weeks before onset of labor (whether term, preterm, or post-term). Estrogens facilitate labor by promoting formation of gap junctions between myometrial cells, inducing expression of oxytocin and estrogen receptors on myometrial cells, stimulating prostaglandin synthesis via the arachidonic acid pathway (see Chapter 13), increasing intracellular calcium binding, and increasing phosphorylation of the contractile protein myosin.

Oxytocin binding to its receptors on the myometrium enhances ion flux, increasing the frequency of pacemaker potentials and lowering the depolarization threshold for uterine smooth-muscle contraction (see Chapter 4). Exogenous oxytocin (Pitocin) has long been used to induce or augment labor. Before term, estrogen inhibits the sensitivity of the myometrium to oxytocin. In the absence of prostaglandins, oxytocin is ineffective in stimulation of labor.

Prostaglandins. Local levels of two prostaglandins, PGE_2 and PGF_{2a}, increase before and during labor. These are apparently important in facilitating the molecular mechanism of smooth-muscle contraction, similarly to estrogen, and are directly involved in softening of the cervix to permit dilation. The sources of these prostaglandins may include cells of the placenta, uterus, and fetal membranes, which are known to contain the enzymes of the arachidonic acid pathway. Prostaglandin inhibitors may be used to inhibit preterm labor, and prostaglandin gel applied to the cervix may enhance ripening and facilitate labor.

Mechanical Factors. Release of lysosomal enzymes

by mechanical stressors such as uterine contraction or manual stripping of the fetal membranes may promote labor by initiating prostaglandin synthesis. The uterine myometrium contracts via the sliding filament mechanism for smooth muscle, discussed in detail in Chapter 5. Much is still unknown regarding regulation of this contraction at the molecular level. The hormonal factors discussed previously may apply. The mechanical stretch reflex may play a role, as may availability of calcium and adenosine triphosphate.

Stages of Labor

Labor proceeds in three discernible stages (Fig. 32–7).

First Stage. During the first stage, rhythmic, top-to-bottom contractions of the myometrium begin. Contractions are typically mild at first and approximately 30 minutes apart. The regularity and increasing intensity of these contractions distinguish them from the irregular, usually painless contractions (Braxton Hicks' contractions), which occur throughout the second and third trimesters. The length of the first stage may vary from less than 1 hour to more than 24 hours depending on **parity** (number of previous deliveries) and other factors. Contractions gradually become more frequent and intense (every 2 to 3 minutes) and of longer duration (approximately 60 seconds). Uterine contractions serve to push the baby downward toward the cervix and also assist in thinning (*effacement*) and dilation of the ripened (softened) cervix.

The fluid-filled amniotic sac usually ruptures spontaneously during this stage (the "water breaks"). Although its use is controversial, intentional rupture of the membranes may be done as a component of labor induction or facilitation. In approximately 10% of women, the amnion ruptures unexpectedly, before the onset of labor.[11] **Premature rupture of the membranes (PROM)** constitutes a high risk of ascending infection and accounts for one third of all cases of preterm labor. The first stage of labor is complete when the cervix is fully dilated, to about 10 cm diameter.

Second Stage. The second stage of labor includes the time from full dilation to delivery. The mother feels the urge to push, and the presenting part of the fetus (usually the back of the head, the *vertex* presentation) crowns, or is visible at the cervix during contractions. An *episiotomy* (surgical incision of the perineum) may be done at this point to enlarge the introitus and prevent laceration of the perineum. Uterine contraction, upright maternal position, and maternal pushing (contraction of abdominal muscles to increase intra-abdominal pressure) are usually sufficient to deliver the baby with minimal assist-

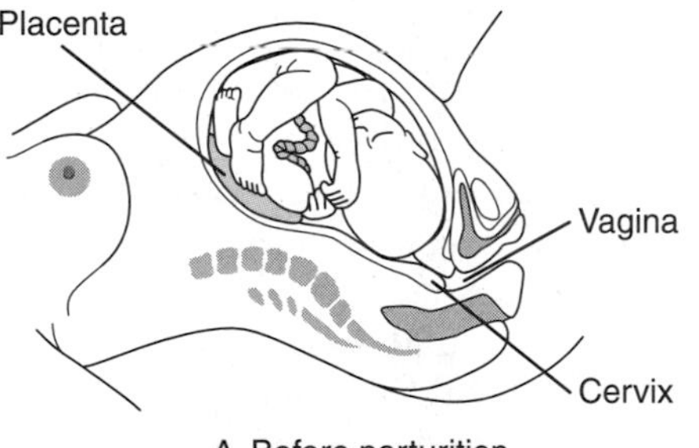

A. Before parturition

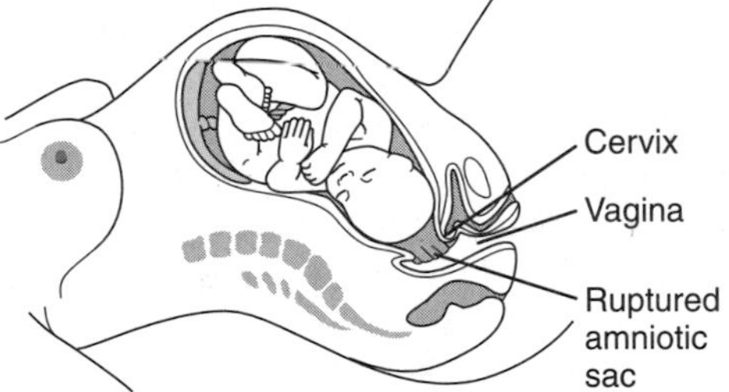

B. Dilation of cervix, rupture of amniotic sac

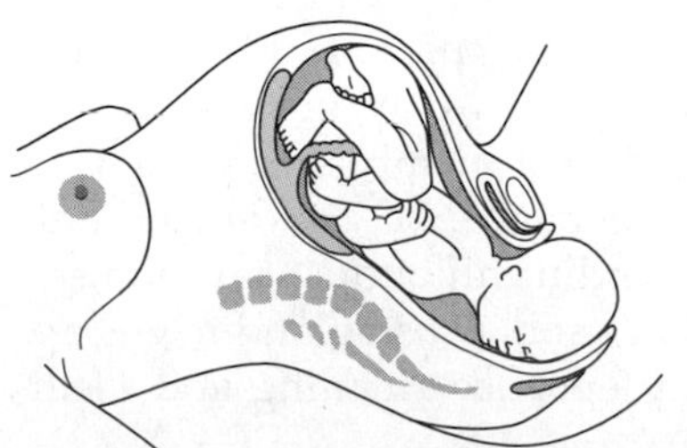

C. Fetus moving through the birth canal

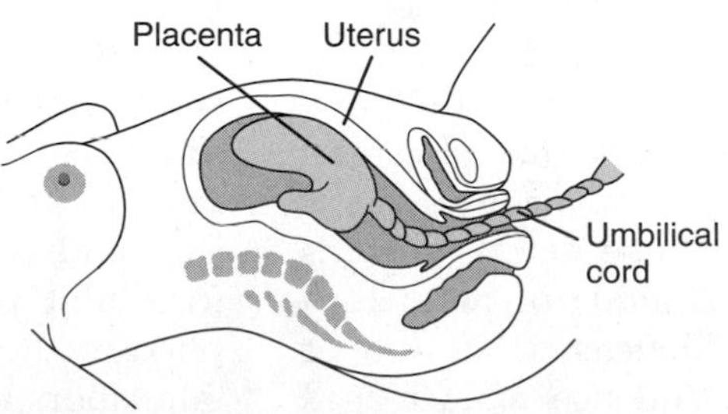

D. Placenta separates from wall of the uterus

FIGURE 32–7

Stages of labor. *A,* Just before labor, the cervix is closed but soft ("ripened"). *B,* During the *first stage of labor,* uterine contractions serve to push the baby downward and to thin (efface) and dilate the cervix. The amniotic sac usually ruptures during this stage. *C,* The *second stage of labor* begins when the cervix is fully dilated and the mother feels the urge to contract her abdominal muscles to push the baby through the birth canal. The back of the baby's head (occiput) usually presents (vertex presentation). *D,* the *third stage of labor* results in separation and delivery of the placenta.

ance or manipulation. Pushing is most beneficial if it is involuntary (reflex) rather than directed, and the mother should be cautioned against straining against a closed glottis, to avoid triggering vagal stimulation via the Valsalva maneuver (see Chapter 15).

Manual rotation of the baby (*version*) may be required in cases of *breech* presentation (buttocks or feet first), and forceps may assist delivery when the mother is too weak to push effectively. Some fetal positions and presentations, such as transverse (sideways) or footling breech (one foot extending through the cervix), may be undeliverable (see later discussion of dystocia).

Fetal malposition, ineffective labor (dystocia), or fetal distress during labor may necessitate surgical delivery of the infant through an abdominal incision (**cesarean section**). The most frequent indications for cesarean birth are listed in Table 32–3. The rate of cesarean delivery in the United States is nearly 1 in 4—much higher than that in other developed countries.[12] Concern about this "epidemic" is often expressed, and it is based on increased maternal and fetal morbidity and mortality as well as the high costs associated with potentially unnecessary surgical procedures (see Focus of Current Research).

Third Stage. The third stage of labor results in separation and delivery of the placenta. Separation normally occurs as a consequence of decreased endometrial surface area after delivery of the infant. Uterine contractions then continue to expel the placenta. Blood loss during this stage is usually estimated at less than 500 cc. In **placenta accreta**, the chorionic villi penetrate beyond the endometrium into the myometrium. Placental detachment is impaired with this complication, and hemorrhage is likely.

TABLE 32–3
INDICATIONS FOR CESAREAN BIRTH

CAUSE	PERCENTAGE
Previous cesarean	39
Dystocia	28
Fetal distress	14
Breech presentation	9
Other	10

United States data for the years 1970 to 1978 and 1980 to 1985.
Data from Porreco, R.P., and Thorp, J.A. (1996). The cesarean birth epidemic: Trends, causes, and solutions. *American Journal of Obstetrics and Gynecology* 175(2), 369–374.

Postpartum Period

The postpartum period, or puerperium, begins with delivery of the placenta and lasts approximately 6 weeks. Unless suppressed, lactation begins during this time, and the maternal organ systems gradually approach their prepregnant state. The uterus involutes, or returns nearly to its original size, within about 10 days. Involution involves contraction of the myometrium, which limits bleeding, and lysis of some intracellular proteins to decrease cell size. Regeneration of the endometrium also occurs. The placental site normally heals without scarring in 6 to 7 weeks. Vaginal discharge (*lochia*) varies in a manner reflecting these events. Initially, it is darkly bloody (*lochia rubra*), then pink (*lochia serosa*), then whitish yellow (*lochia alba*) in decreasing amounts during a period of 3 to 6 weeks. **Subinvolution** (late postpartum hemorrhage) is characterized by persistent lochia and failure of the uterus to decrease in size. Transient bleeding may occur with normal sloughing of the placental eschar at 7 to 10 days postpartum. Retention of placental fragments or endometrial infection (**endometritis**) may also promote postpartum hemorrhage.

After 4 weeks, the cervix has shortened and the os has closed, appearing as a small transverse slit. The vagina gradually heals and regains most, but not all, of its prepregnancy tone. Regeneration of the vaginal epithelium usually takes 6 to 10 weeks, and decreased lubrication during this time may cause *dyspareunia* (discomfort during intercourse). Pelvic joints may remain lax for a time, especially in women who have had several children. Weakening of pelvic floor muscles and ligaments associated with childbirth, compounded by age-related changes, may give rise to pelvic support disorders, as discussed in Chapter 31.

Removal of the hormones of pregnancy initiates return of maternal organ systems to their prepregnancy functional state. Nonlactating women are infertile for about 5 weeks, and lactating women are infertile for about 8 weeks after delivery. Elevated prolactin levels may constitute negative feedback to the hypothalamic–pituitary–gonadal axis, decreasing pituitary output of LH and follicle-stimulating hormone (FSH) to levels insufficient to stimulate follicular development and ovulation.

Multifetal Pregnancy

Multiple fetuses produce proportionately greater maternal systemic changes during pregnancy. Physical effects related to the oversized uterus and increased levels of placental hormones may account

Focus of Current Research

Study	Objective and Findings
Peterson, et al. (1997) The risk of ectopic pregnancy after tubal sterilization	*Objective:* To estimate the risk of ectopic pregnancy in women who had undergone the common types of tubal sterilization *Findings:* The 10-year cumulative probability of ectopic pregnancy for all methods combined was 7.3 per 1000 procedures.
Naylor, et al. (1996) Cesarean delivery in relation to birth weight and gestational glucose tolerance	*Objective:* To examine the relationship between birth weight and mode of delivery among women with borderline and overt gestational diabetes and normoglycemic women *Findings:* Untreated borderline gestational diabetes was associated with macrosomia and cesarean delivery. Those with treated gestational diabetes and without macrosomia also had high rates of cesarean delivery, possibly because of a lower threshold for surgical delivery resulting from recognition of the disorder.
McMahon, et al. (1996) Comparison of a trial of labor with an elective second cesarean section.	*Objective:* To explore maternal and perinatal morbidity and mortality associated with this method of delivery *Findings:* Major maternal complications are almost twice as likely among those managed with a trial of labor as among those who undergo a second cesarean section.
Hannah, et al. (1996) Induction of labor compared with expectant management for prelabor rupture of the membranes at term.	*Objective:* To determine whether inducing labor decreases the risk of fetal and maternal infection in those with prelabor rupture of the membranes at term *Findings:* Both methods of management were asociated with similar rates of neonatal infection and cesarean section. Risk of maternal infection was lower with induction of labor.
Ananth, et al. (1996) Effect of maternal age and parity on the risk of uteroplacental bleeding disorders in pregnancy.	*Objective:* To examine the risk of placental abruption, placenta previa, and uterine bleeding of unknown etiology in relation to advanced maternal age and parity *Findings:* Placenta previa is linked to aging of the uterus and the effects of repeated pregnancies.

continued

Frigoletto, et al. (1995) A clinical trial of active management of labor.	*Objective:* To evaluate whether active management of labor (childbirth classes, manual rupture of the membranes, high-dose oxytocin, and one-to-one nursing) would lower the rate of cesarean section among women delivering their first babies. *Findings:* Active management did not reduce the cesarean section rate but was associated with shorter duration of labor.
Fraser, et al. (1995) Association of young maternal age with adverse reproductive outcomes.	*Objective:* To determine whether young age confers intrinsic risk when socioeconomic and environmental factors are removed *Findings:* Younger age confers an increased risk attributed to biologic immaturity.
Mahon, et al. (1994) Short labor: Characteristics and outcome.	*Objective:* To determine the characteristics and consequences of labors of 3 hours or less *Findings:* Short labors are strongly associated with placental abruption, but were otherwise not major contributors to maternal and fetal morbidity.

for the higher risk state associated with multiple gestations. Preterm delivery is usual. Risks associated with multifetal pregnancy are summarized in Table 32–4.

LACTATION

Preparation for Lactogenesis

During pregnancy, elevated levels of estrogen and progesterone stimulate development of the mammary alveoli (secretory cells) and ducts. Prolactin and hCLS further stimulate alveolar growth. Actual production of milk (lactogenesis) is inhibited by estrogen and progesterone during pregnancy, but removal of these hormones with delivery of the placenta allows prolactin to induce alveolar secretion and milk production. Prolactin levels remain high as long as lactation continues. Figure 32–8 illustrates the anatomic changes in breast tissue that occur in preparation for lactation.

Milk Production and Letdown

Suckling by the infant triggers sensory signals to the hypothalamus, resulting in secretion of prolactin-releasing factor and inhibition of prolactin-inhibiting factor (structurally identical to dopamine). Prolactin-releasing factor then stimulates prolactin release from the anterior pituitary (see Chapter 27). Prolactin is aided by the permissive effects of insulin, cortisol, and thyrotropin-releasing hormone in stimulating synthesis of milk by mammary alveoli. A second reflex, mediated by oxytocin, allows milk letdown, or conduction of milk through the ducts to the nipple. Letdown is normally stimulated by suckling of the infant, but reflex letdown may also occur with cortical stimulation of the hypothalamus when the infant cries or with maternal thoughts of the infant. Milk is secreted into alveolar ducts by exocytosis.

Composition of Breast Milk

Breast milk is composed of fat, protein, and lactose synthesized within alveolar cells as well as water, vitamins, and minerals obtained from maternal plasma (Table 32–5). The composition of the initial colostrum differs in that it is higher in protein (including immunoglobulins) and lower in fat, carbohydrates, and calories. Colostrum is yellow because of its high content of carotene, a vitamin A derivative.

TABLE 32–4
RISKS ASSOCIATED WITH MULTIFETAL PREGNANCY

DISORDER	COMMENTS
Spontaneous abortion	May affect one or all fetuses
Perinatal mortality	Often caused by intertwining umbilical cords
Low birth weight	Caused by intrauterine growth retardation or preterm birth
Fetal malformations	Twice as common as in single fetuses; associated with polyhydramnios
Fetal hemorrhage	
Pregnancy-induced hypertension	More severe and earlier onset than in single pregnancies
Maternal anemia	Caused by acute blood loss at delivery, iron deficiency, or folate deficiency
Placental accidents	Placenta previa and placental abruption are more likely
Uterine atony	May contribute to hemorrhage
Cord prolapse	Caused by polyhydramnios
Preterm labor	
Dystocia	
Abnormal fetal presentation	May contribute to dystocia

Data from Cunningham, F.G., MacDonald, P.C., and Gant, N.F. (1989). *Williams Obstetrics.* (18th ed.). Norwalk, CT: Appleton & Lange. (pp. 629–652).

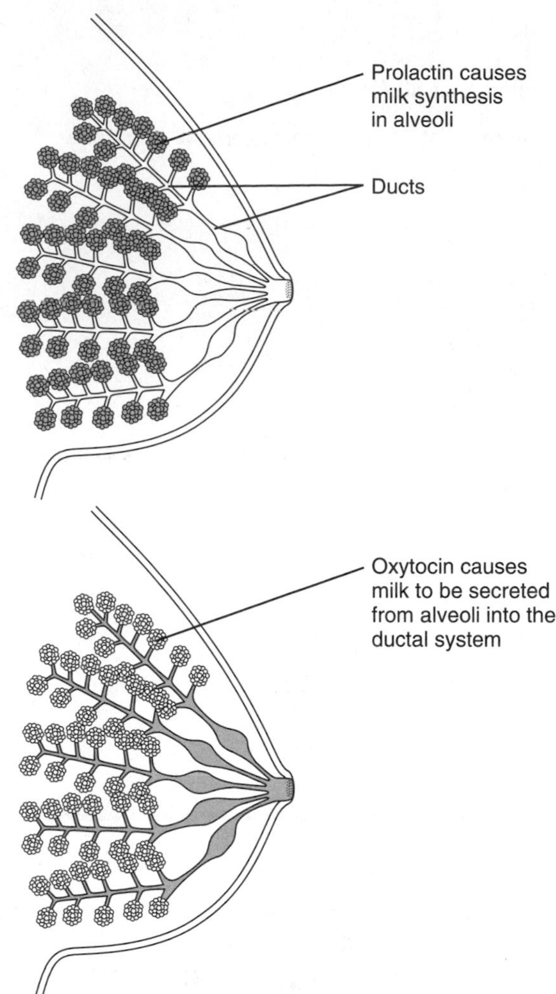

FIGURE 32–8
Process of lactation. Reduction of estrogen and progesterone levels at delivery permits the effects of elevated prolactin levels to be expressed. Prolactin induces synthesis of milk by mammary alveoli. The oxytocin-mediated milk letdown reflex causes secretion of milk from alveoli into the ductal system.

TABLE 32–5
COMPOSITION OF BREAST MILK

FUNCTION	COMPONENT
Nutrition	Protein (whey, casein)
	Carbohydrate (lactose)
	Fat
	Minerals
	Vitamins
	Water
Immune/antibacterial	B and T lymphocytes
	Macrophages
	Neutrophils
	Immunoglobulin A
	γ-Interferon
	Lysozyme
	Fibronectin
	Lactoferrin
	Mucins
Regulation of growth and maturation	Hormones
	Growth factors

Uptake of constituents of maternal plasma across the *blood-milk barrier*, composed of the alveolar cell membrane, interstitial space, and maternal capillary membrane, is selective, depending on the size and polarity of the transported particles as well as the transport mechanism. Nearly all drugs cross this barrier, with resulting pharmacologic effects on the infant. Some drugs directly affect lactation; for example, alcohol blocks milk ejection, and oral contraceptives suppress lactogenesis.[13]

Metabolic Cost of Lactation

The process of lactation demands a 60% increase in the mother's basal metabolic rate, compounding the energy requirements of postpartum healing and involutional processes. During the first few months, fat stores acquired during the first trimester may be used for this purpose, but prolonged lactation requires increased caloric intake. Lactating women experience a decrease in bone density because of rapid mobilization of calcium, which is apparently mediated by a peptide synthesized by mammary tissue.[14] This *parathyroid hormone–related peptide* is expressed when prolactin levels are high and estradiol levels are low (see Chapter 28).

Complications of Lactation

Complications of lactation are few, although inflammation of the mammary glands (**mastitis**) may result from organisms that ascend through cracks or erosions in the nipple. **Engorgement,** painful distention of the alveoli with milk, may occur 2 to 4 days after delivery. Removal of milk with suckling of the infant relieves distention in women who breast feed, and local application of heat may also promote comfort and milk flow. In women who do not wish to breast feed, suckling is withheld and cold compresses may be used to reduce milk production. Other complications associated with breast feeding are summarized in Table 32–6.

TABLE 32–6
COMPLICATIONS ASSOCIATED WITH BREAST FEEDING

Complication	Comments
Engorgement (milk stasis)	Provides rich culure medium for bacteria entering via nipple
Sore nipples	May be associated with infection, poor position of the infant's mouth, prolonged feeding periods
Inhibited letdown reflex	Often caused by maternal pain, cold, or anxiety; may lead to prolongation of feeding and sore nipples
Blocked milk ducts (galactocele)	Noted as smooth, tender lump; may be caused by incomplete emptying of breast or failure to vary the position of the infant on the breast
Mastitis	Infection of lactating breast caused by *Staphylococcus aureus*, *Escherichia coli*, or streptococcus species; may lead to systemic manifestations of inflammation
Breast abscess	Pus-filled cyst associated with mastitis

MATERNAL DISORDERS ASSOCIATED WITH PREGNANCY

The most common maternal disorders related to pregnancy, detailed in the subsequent section, are (1) those associated with achieving and maintaining pregnancy (infertility, spontaneous abortion, preterm labor, and ectopic pregnancy); (2) those associated with the prenatal period (gestational diabetes, preeclampsia, and hydatidiform mole); and (3) those occurring during or after labor and delivery (dystocia and peripartum hemorrhage). Thromboembolism, discussed in Chapter 14, may also complicate any phase of pregnancy, with clinical disorders ranging from asymptomatic deep vein thrombosis to life-threatening pulmonary embolism or stroke. Table 32–7 describes risk factors for thromboembolitic complications of pregnancy. Maternal infections may also complicate pregnancy. Common examples are summarized in Table 32–8.

Infertility

Definition. Infertility is the failure to conceive after 1 year of unprotected intercourse.[15] *Primary* infertility is present in couples who have not achieved pregnancy. *Secondary* infertility refers to couples who are unable to conceive within a year after having previously achieved pregnancy.[16]

Epidemiology. An estimated 15% of couples have subnormal fertility, and the incidence is increasing.[17]

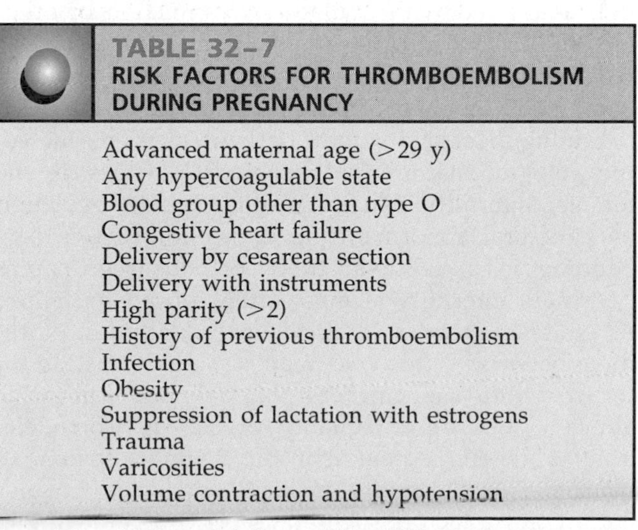

TABLE 32–7
RISK FACTORS FOR THROMBOEMBOLISM DURING PREGNANCY

Advanced maternal age (>29 y)
Any hypercoagulable state
Blood group other than type O
Congestive heart failure
Delivery by cesarean section
Delivery with instruments
High parity (>2)
History of previous thromboembolism
Infection
Obesity
Suppression of lactation with estrogens
Trauma
Varicosities
Volume contraction and hypotension

From Ritter, D.C., and deShazo, R.D. (1994). Peripartum complications: Hemorrhage, embolism, hypertension, and infection. *Postgraduate Medicine* 95(2), 182.

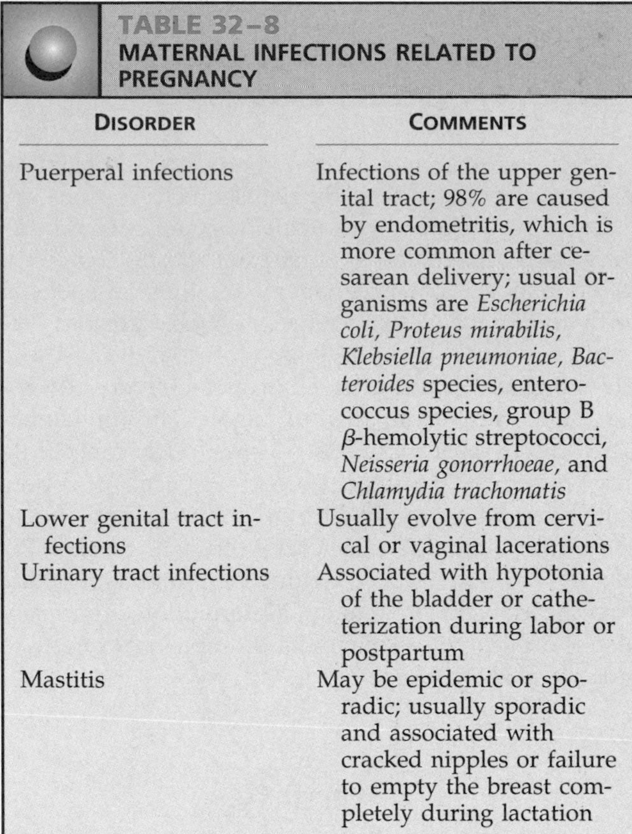

TABLE 32–8
MATERNAL INFECTIONS RELATED TO PREGNANCY

Disorder	Comments
Puerperal infections	Infections of the upper genital tract; 98% are caused by endometritis, which is more common after cesarean delivery; usual organisms are *Escherichia coli, Proteus mirabilis, Klebsiella pneumoniae, Bacteroides* species, enterococcus species, group B β-hemolytic streptococci, *Neisseria gonorrhoeae*, and *Chlamydia trachomatis*
Lower genital tract infections	Usually evolve from cervical or vaginal lacerations
Urinary tract infections	Associated with hypotonia of the bladder or catheterization during labor or postpartum
Mastitis	May be epidemic or sporadic; usually sporadic and associated with cracked nipples or failure to empty the breast completely during lactation

In 50%, the causative defect is in the female; in 30%, the problem is in the male; and in 20% there are abnormalities in both partners. The incidence of infertility is rising as a consequence of sexually transmitted diseases, resulting in pelvic adhesions and tubal dysfunction, and because of delayed childbearing, associated with ovulatory dysfunction or other factors. Advanced ovarian age, demonstrated by elevated serum FSH levels, indicates that remaining oocytes are few and of poor quality.

Etiology. Infertility may be caused by hormonal, physiologic, anatomic, or behavioral factors. In the female, infertility usually results from anovulation or structural abnormality of the endometrium (e.g., endometriosis), fallopian tubes, or both (see Chapter 31). Male infertility is most often caused by failure of emission, *retrograde ejaculation* (deposition of semen backward into the man's bladder instead of forward into the partner's vagina), and idiopathic abnormalities in the quality of semen. Microdeletions of genetic sequences in the Y chromosome may contribute to infertility in some men (see Chapter 30). Lifestyle factors such as use of drugs (including tobacco) that inhibit spermatogenesis and exposure of the testes to excessive heat (as with frequent hot tub use) may also be contributing factors. Table 32–9 summarizes causes of infertility.

Pathophysiology. Mechanisms of infertility include: (1) failure of the female to ovulate; (2) mechanical or functional obstruction of the fallopian tubes; (3) impenetrability or other adverse qualities of the cervical mucus; (4) deficient numbers or abnormality of responsiveness or motility of sperm; (5) abnormal liquefaction or viscosity of semen; (5) failure of implantation because of endometrial abnormalities.

Clinical Manifestations. Infertility is manifested by the inability to conceive. Specific manifestations of the underlying disorders, such as pelvic inflammatory disease in females or failure of emission or ejaculation in males, may also be apparent on clinical examination. Analysis of semen may reveal abnormalities in quantity or quality of sperm and seminal fluid. *Oligospermia* is a total sperm count of less than 50 million per ejaculate, and *asthenospermia* is less than 50% motility.

Prevention and Treatment. Reduction of controllable risk factors such as drug and tobacco use is warranted. Prevention of sexually transmitted disease is of particular importance (see Chapter 30). Consideration should be given to the risks inherent in delayed childbearing. Hormonal therapy with fertility drugs such as the antiestrogen clomiphene

TABLE 32–9
CAUSES OF INFERTILITY

Factors	Incidence (%)
Male	20–40
Ovulation	15–30
Anovulation	
Hyperprolactinemia	
Hypothalamic dysfunction	
Thyroid dysfunction	
Adrenal dysfunction	
Primary ovarian failure	
Polycystic ovary disease	
Multifactorial	15–30
Peritoneal abnormality, including endometriosis	6–25
Unexplained	10–20
Tubal	12–20
Uterine	2–10
Coital	5–6
Cervical	3–5
Luteal phase defects	3–4
Immunologic	Unknown
"Reluctant ovum" syndrome	Unknown

Reprinted with permission from Trantham, P. (1996). The infertile couple. *American Family Physician* 54(3), 1003, published by the American Academy of Family Physicians.

(Clomid) or the gonadotropin preparations Pergonal or Humegon may induce ovulation in anovulatory women, but their use also increases the risk of multifetal pregnancies. Fallopian tube obstructions may be amenable to surgical restoration of patency.

Assisted reproduction techniques such as in vitro fertilization (IVF), gamete intrafallopian transfer (GIFT), zygote intrafallopian transfer (ZIFT), donor sperm or oocytes, donor embryos, and gestational carriers (surrogate uteri) may be appropriate in some cases. These procedures are described in Table 32–10.

For male infertility, hormonal therapy (testosterone and antiestrogens) has been used with limited success. Semen processing (washing and extracting the best-quality sperm from the ejaculate) followed by intrauterine insemination has achieved variable results. Failure of emission, often related to spinal cord injury, diabetic neuropathy, multiple sclerosis, or psychogenic factors, may be treated with α-adrenergic agonists or external vibratory stimulation to induce peristalsis in the vas deferens. Spinal cord injury patients may achieve ejaculation with electrical stimulation of the sacral reflex arc (electroejaculation).

Prognosis and Outcome. The efficacy of conventional treatment for infertility varies from 20% to 90%, depending on the method and the nature and severity of the underlying abnormality.[16]

TABLE 32–10
ASSISTED REPRODUCTION TECHNIQUES

METHOD	DESCRIPTION
Artificial insemination	Donor sperm is deposited directly into the uterus, at the cervical os, or inside the cervical canal; donor sperm is frozen until negative human immunodeficiency virus status is certain
In vitro fertilization	Fertilization is accomplished in a test tube or petri dish after retrieval of mature ova from the ovary; fertilized ova are then implanted in the uterus
Gamete intrafallopian transfer	Transfer of ova and sperm directly into the fallopian tube via a catheter
Zygote intrafallopian transfer	Transfer of zygote (from in vitro fertilization) directly into the fallopian tube

Spontaneous Abortion

Definition. Spontaneous abortion (miscarriage) is unintended termination of pregnancy before fetal viability (usually 20 weeks, or fetal weight less than 500 g).[18] *Habitual* or *recurrent* spontaneous abortion refers to three or more consecutive spontaneous abortions conceived with the same partner.

Epidemiology. The reported incidence of spontaneous abortion has been estimated at 31% of all pregnancies, with 22% of these occurring before the pregnancy was clinically evident.[19] Most spontaneous abortions (80%) occur during the first trimester. Risk factors associated with habitual abortion include uterine abnormalities (e.g., leiomyomas, double or bicornuate uterus), cervical abnormalities (e.g., **incompetent cervix** [short or funneled cervix that thins or dilates prematurely] or history of surgical abortion or cervical conization), genetic abnormality of one or both partners, and maternal hormone imbalance or subclinical autoimmune disease. When the pregnancy is terminated in the first few weeks after conception, chromosomal abnormalities are almost always present in the aborted fetus.

Etiology. The specific etiology of isolated spontaneous abortion is usually unknown, and sporadic miscarriage usually occurs in the absence of any known risk factors. In habitual abortion, structural or functional disorders of the reproductive system, lethal genetic defects, or immunologic mechanisms are possible. Genetic abnormalities of the fetus may preclude normal cell division and precipitate early abortion, as discussed in Chapter 7. Table 32–11 summarizes known etiologic factors for spontaneous abortion.

Pathophysiology. With *threatened abortion*, uterine bleeding and cramping pose a risk to the developing fetus. The cervical os remains closed, however. Abortion is classified as *imminent* when bleeding and cramping increase, and the cervical os dilates. Fetal membranes may rupture. With *complete* abortion, all products of the conception are expelled from the uterus. With *incomplete* abortion, parts of the fetus or placenta are retained. *Missed* abortion results in fetal demise but the products of pregnancy are not expelled. In this case, the cervix remains closed, uterine growth stops, and other signs of pregnancy regress. Retention of the fetus beyond 6 weeks results in autolysis of fetal tissue with release of tissue thromboplastin, possibly triggering disseminated intravascular coagulation (see Chapter 14).

Clinical Manifestations. Vaginal bleeding in combination with uterine cramping or backache are the characteristic manifestations of spontaneous abor-

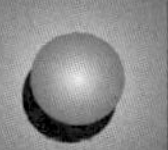

TABLE 32–11
ETIOLOGY OF SPONTANEOUS ABORTION

Chromosomal Abnormalities (from either the Maternal or Paternal Gonadocytes)
The earlier the abortion, the higher the proportion of chromosomal abnormalities.

Abortions with Normal Chromosomes (Euploidy)
Many investigators reported the occurrence of malformed or blighted embryos as a cause of abortion. These embryonic losses may occur later in the first trimester and have been shown to have normal karyotypes. The causes of these abortions include:
- Genetic abnormalities (i.e., dominant mutations [lethals], polygenic genetic abnormalities, recessive disease [from the maternal gonadocytes, the paternal gonadocytes, or both]). In rare instances, these conditions may account for repetitive abortion, but in most cases, they will occur sporadically.
- Maternal disease states
  - Maternal diabetes
  - Maternal hypothyroidism
  - Corpus luteum or placental progesterone deficiency (luteal phase deficiency)
  - Maternal genital infection: The consensus is that herpes simplex type 2 and maternal syphilis increase the risk of abortion. Controversy surrounds the relationship of the following organisms to the incidence of abortion: *Chlamydia trachomatis, Mycoplasma hominis, Listeria monocytogenes, Toxoplasma gondii,* and *Ureaplasma urealyticum.*
  - Severe, debilitating maternal diseases, such as hepatitis, collagen diseases, or untreated hyperthyroidism; or severe malnutrition
- Antiphospholipid antibodies (lupus anticoagulant, anticardiolipin antibodies)
- Maternal-fetal histocompatibility
- Overmature gametes
- Mechanical or physical problems related to uterine abnormalities, multiple pregnancies, or, very rarely, trauma
- Cervical incompetence
- Abnormal placentation (hypoplastic trophoblast, circumvallate implantation)
- Some environmental teratogens

From Brent, R.L., and Beckman, D.A. (1994). The contribution of environmental teratogens to embryonic and fetal loss. *Clinical Obstetrics and Gynecology* 37(3), 648.

tion. Expulsion of identifiable products of conception is diagnostic.

Prevention and Treatment. Most cases are not associated with known risk and are therefore not preventable. Structural abnormalities of the uterus or cervix may be corrected with surgical intervention in some cases. An incompetent cervix may be sutured closed during pregnancy, with the *cerclage* (encircling) suture released at term or, in some cases, retained while the infant is delivered by cesarean birth.

After miscarriage, the woman is treated with supportive care. Intravenous fluids may be given, but blood transfusion is not usually necessary. If the products of pregnancy are not completely expelled, surgical methods such as suction evacuation or **dilatation and curettage (D&C)** are used to ensure removal of the fetus and placenta. In unusual cases of missed abortion in the second trimester, labor may be induced with oxytocin and prostaglandin gel.

Prognosis and Outcome. Physiologic complications of spontaneous abortion are uncommon if the products of conception are completely expelled, either spontaneously or surgically. After one spontaneous abortion, a couple's chances of achieving a term pregnancy are not reduced. Each sequential abortion confers increased risk of another, however.

Preterm Labor

Definition. Preterm labor is defined as labor occurring before 37 completed weeks of gestation, and it is characterized by regular uterine contractions with progressive cervical dilation or effacement.[20]

Epidemiology. Despite efforts aimed at prevention and despite improved management of preterm labor, the incidence of preterm birth has remained constant at 7% to 9% in the United States during the past 20 years.[21] Increased risk is associated with behavioral and medical factors, including inadequate prenatal care, history of preterm labor or spontaneous abortion, abuse of alcohol or other addictive drugs, nonwhite race, low socioeconomic status, and age younger than 17 years or older than 35 years.[22] Medical conditions associated with preterm labor include cigarette smoking, preeclampsia, infection, incompetent cervix, uterine structural anomalies, multifetal pregnancy, excessive amniotic fluid (**polyhydramnios**), deficient amniotic fluid (**oligohydramnios**), placenta previa, and abruptio placentae. Women who undergo prenatal diagnostic testing (e.g., amniocentesis in the second trimester or chorionic villus sampling late in the first trimester) are at increased risk of premature rupture of the membranes (PROM), which often precedes preterm labor (see Chapter 33).

Etiology. In 50% of cases, the etiology of preterm labor is unknown. About 30% of cases begin with PROM. The remaining cases are medically induced, as a result of an adverse maternal or fetal condition.

Pathophysiology. If preterm labor begins before 20 weeks of gestation, the cause is often a genetic abnormality of the fetus (spontaneous abortion), and intervention to stop labor may not be indicated. Similarly, if the fetus is known to have died, to be severely compromised, or to have anomalies incompatible with life, preterm labor is viewed as adaptive. PROM occurring near term is usually followed by the spontaneous onset of labor within 48 hours and has a benign course.[11] PROM occurring before 35 weeks or lasting longer than 24 hours is associated with increased neonatal mortality and morbidity because of the possibility of ascending infection. Spontaneous preterm labor, occurring when the membranes are intact and the fetus is viable, is associated with high risk of preterm birth, which in turn imposes high risk of neonatal morbidity and mortality (see Chapter 33).

Clinical Manifestations. Subtle signs such as vaginal or lower abdominal pressure, discharge, or frequent urination may warn of incompetent cervix. Preterm cervical dilation may be evident on examination. PROM is noted as a gush or leakage of fluid from the vagina, occasionally experienced as a "popping" sensation.[11] The frequency of uterine contractions during late pregnancy is specific to gestational age and increases significantly in the 24-hour period preceding the onset of preterm labor.[23]

Prevention and Treatment. Optimal management of underlying maternal disorders is indicated. Cerclage may be used in treatment of incompetent cervix, for example, and maternal infections should be appropriately treated. Intervention to delay labor and delivery is warranted in spontaneous preterm labor not associated with PROM or significant fetal abnormality, as indicated earlier. Patient education and home monitoring (tocodynamometry) of uterine contractions may permit earlier detection of preterm labor in those at risk. Bedrest is usually advised to relieve cervical pressure, and optimal fluid status is ensured with hydration as necessary. Early detection improves the efficacy of drug therapy (tocolytic therapy) aimed at halting uterine contraction. Tocolytic drugs include the β-adrenergic agents ritodrine hydrochloride and terbutaline sulfate, and magnesium sulfate, which is believe to relax smooth muscle by blocking the influx of calcium. Ritodrine and terbutaline can be given orally or intravenously. Terbutaline may also be administered subcutaneously or by continuous pump infusion, and thus may be used long-term on an outpatient basis. Magnesium sulfate is administered intravenously in the hospital setting, often in combination with a β-agonist. The use of corticosteroids (e.g., betamethasone) during preterm labor to hasten fetal lung maturity is controversial (see Chapter 33).

Treatment of preterm labor associated with PROM is controversial. Bedrest and hydration are usually warranted. Antibiotics may be used in an effort to prevent ascending infection, but the value of this treatment is unproved.[21] Tocolytic therapy and corticosteroids are usually not indicated. Delivery of the infant is indicated when infection is known to be present. In these cases, labor is induced or a cesarean section is performed.

Prognosis and Outcome. An estimated 40% to 50% of patients "break through" tocolytic therapy and resume preterm labor, giving birth prematurely.[21] After 35 to 37 weeks' gestation, therapy is usually discontinued and the patient is allowed to begin labor. As stated earlier, the overall incidence of preterm birth has not changed despite efforts at improved prevention, monitoring, and therapy.

Ectopic Pregnancy

Definition. Ectopic pregnancy is implantation of the blastocyst at a site outside the body of the uterus, e.g., fallopian tube, cervix, ovary, or bowel. Implantation within the fallopian tube (tubal pregnancy) accounts for 95% of ectopic pregnancies.[24]

Epidemiology. The incidence of ectopic pregnancy in the United States has been estimated at 16.8 per 1000 pregnancies.[25] Quadrupling of the incidence of ectopic pregnancy since 1970 has been attributed to the increased number of cases of sexually transmitted disease and resultant pelvic inflammatory disease (see Chapter 31). Hemorrhage associated with ruptured tubal pregnancy is the most common cause of maternal death during the first 20 weeks of pregnancy. A history of sexually transmitted disease is the major risk factor, but risk is also increased with the use of the intrauterine device (IUD) for contraception, previous ectopic pregnancy, previous surgical abortion, previous pelvic or tubal surgery (including **tubal ligation** for sterilization), previous in vitro fertilization, cigarette smoking, congenital malformations of the reproductive tract, or hormonal changes (as during perimenopause). In some cases, ectopic pregnancy is the first sign of pelvic inflammatory disease. Ectopic pregnancy also occurs in a significant number of women with no known risk factors.

Etiology. When fallopian tubes have been damaged by inflammation, cilia may be lost, impairing conduction of the fertilized ovum to the uterus. Alteration in the local hormonal environment may also play a role in impeding ovum transport.

Pathophysiology. With delayed transport to the uterus, the blastocyst implants at another available vascularized site, usually the lining of the fallopian tube. The hormones of pregnancy are released normally from the corpus luteum, and the normal signs of pregnancy are usually present at first. Some uterine enlargement occurs in one fourth of ectopic pregnancies. The hCG-based test for pregnancy is

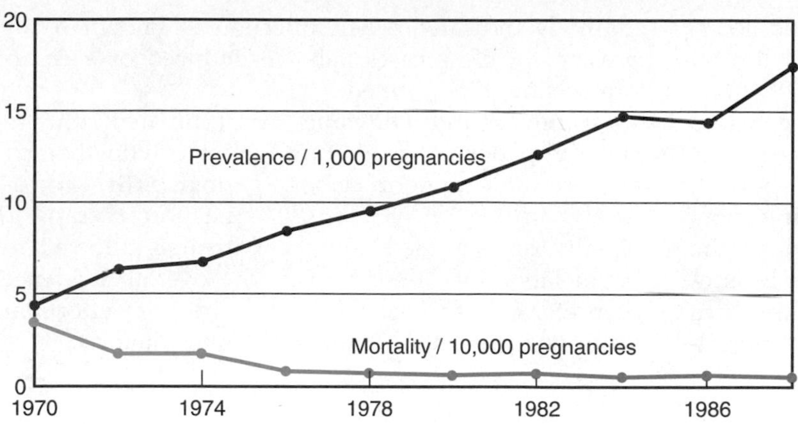

FIGURE 32–9

Trends in ectopic pregnancy. Since 1970, the prevalence of ectopic pregnancy has increased, but mortality has declined. These trends suggest that although preventive efforts have been unsuccessful, treatment has improved. (From Nederlof, K., Lawson, H., Saftlas, A., *et al.* [1990]. Ectopic pregnancy surveillance, U.S. 1970–1987. *Morbidity and Mortality Weekly Report* 39[SS-4], 9–17.)

positive, but amounts of the hormone are usually lower than in uterine pregnancies. Chorionic villi grow into the wall of the tube or other implantation site, establishing a vascular connection. Very few ectopic pregnancies are carried to term, with the infant delivered through an abdominal incision. In most cases of uninterrupted ectopic pregnancy, internal hemorrhage occurs when the tube ruptures, terminating the pregnancy and jeopardizing the life of the mother.

Clinical Manifestations. Symptoms are usually evident at 6 to 12 weeks' gestation. Signs of bleeding may be subtle, including irregular spotting, vague abdominal discomfort, and dizziness caused by low hemoglobin. An adnexal mass or adnexal tenderness may be apparent on palpation. Measurement of serum progesterone and hCG may reveal low levels consistent with a nonviable pregnancy. Ultrasound imaging may demonstrate the ectopic pregnancy. Occasionally, laparoscopic investigation of the fallopian tube is necessary for diagnosis. As the ectopic pregnancy continues, slow hemorrhage eventually results in abdominal rigidity and more severe discomfort. Profuse hemorrhage leads to sharp abdominal pain, often referred to the shoulder, and signs of hypovolemic shock (see Chapter 15).

Prevention and Treatment. Prevention involves reduction of risk for sexually transmitted disease. Early detection is facilitated with optimal prenatal care. Tubal pregnancy may be treated surgically, with laparoscopic removal of the fetus and placenta. The affected tube is repaired and spared, if possible. Medical intervention with the cytotoxic drug methotrexate (Folex) has been used effectively to destroy the pregnancy if it is detected while the cell mass is less than 4 cm in diameter. Ruptured ectopic pregnancies require laparotomy. Surgical resection of fallopian tubes or other pelvic organs is done only when massive infection or scarring are present, in an effort to preserve fertility if at all possible. Shock is treated as discussed in Chapter 15.

Prognosis and Outcome. Paradoxically, maternal mortality from ectopic pregnancy has fallen while incidence has increased, indicating that treatment has improved while prevention has failed (Fig. 32–9). Mortality is now estimated at 30 per 10,000.[25]

Gestational Diabetes Mellitus

Definition. Gestational diabetes mellitus is carbohydrate intolerance that has its onset or first recognition during pregnancy.[26]

Epidemiology. Gestational diabetes is the most common medical complication of pregnancy in the United States, affecting an estimated 3% to 6% of pregnancies.[26] Among black, Hispanic, and Native American populations, the incidence is as high as 12%.[27] Risk factors are listed in Table 32–12.

Etiology. In a minority of cases, gestational diabetes results when the diabetogenic effect (insulin resistance) of pregnancy "uncovers" a previously unrecognized type 2 diabetes. In most cases, however, the hyperglycemia of gestational diabetes is caused

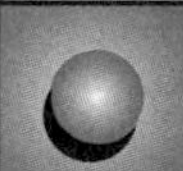

TABLE 32–12
RISK FACTORS FOR GESTATIONAL DIABETES MELLITUS

Age older than 30 years
Family history of diabetes
Problems with infant in previous pregnancy; macrosomia, malformation, stillborn
Obesity
Hypertension
Glucosuria
Previous gestational diabetes

Reprinted with permission from Weller, K.A. (1996). Diagnosis and management of gestational diabetes. *American Family Physician* 53(6), 2054, published by the American Academy of Family Physicians.

by insulin resistance *and* compromised insulin secretion.[8] The precise etiology of these defects is unknown.

Pathophysiology. The pathophysiology of diabetes mellitus was discussed in detail in Chapter 29. During pregnancy, diabetes imposes risks on mother and fetus. Diabetic mothers are at increased risk for the development of preeclampsia, dystocia, and postpartum hemorrhage. They are also more likely to require cesarean section.

Elevated serum glucose induces excessive insulin secretion by the fetus, and this hyperinsulinemia accelerates fat deposition in insulin-sensitive tissues, promoting increased and asymmetric fetal growth (*macrosomia*). The trunk, shoulders, and upper arms are particularly large, contributing to potentially difficult labor (shoulder dystocia). Hyperinsulinemia also raises the fetal metabolic rate, increasing oxygen demand, while shifting the oxyhemoglobin-dissociation curve to the left, decreasing oxygen release to tissues (see Chapter 19). Fetal hypoxia induces a secondary polycythemia, which may contribute to hyperbilirubinemia and toxicity, and increases the risk of infant respiratory distress syndrome. The infant of the diabetic mother is discussed in further detail in Chapter 33.

Clinical Manifestations. Abnormal glucose tolerance testing establishes the presence of gestational diabetes (see Chapter 29). Signs and symptoms of diabetes during pregnancy include polyuria, nocturia, polydipsia, recurrent vaginal infections, and failure to gain weight to the degree expected.[27] Fasting plasma glucose is greater than 105 mg/dL.[28] Most women with gestational diabetes (75%) have type A-1, which means that their postprandial glucose level (measured after ingestion of a standard test dose) is less than 120 mg/dL. The remaining women are type A-2; that is, their postprandial glucose is greater than 120 mg/dL.

Prevention and Treatment. Ideally, women having a history of gestational diabetes or risk factors for the disorder should undergo screening glucose tolerance testing *before* conception. Intervention is warranted in modifiable risk factors, i.e., obesity and hypertension. Half of all women with gestational diabetes have no risk factors.[28] Identification of these individuals early in pregnancy facilitates tight regulation of blood glucose levels, which reduces the risk of maternal and fetal complications. Frequent monitoring of serum glucose and diet and exercise modification are prudent, as discussed in Chapter 29. Oral hypoglycemic agents are not used during pregnancy because of the associated risks of fetal malformation or fetal hyperinsulinemia. Insulin is required in treatment of type A-2 gestational diabetes.

Prognosis and Outcome. With adequate control of serum glucose throughout pregnancy, outcomes are comparable to nondiabetic pregnancies.[28] When gestational diabetes is inadequately treated, the risk of maternal, fetal, and neonatal complications is increased. Delivery of the infant removes the hormones of pregnancy and decreases insulin resistance. Glucose homeostasis is re-established over days to weeks, and women who did not require insulin before pregnancy do not require it after pregnancy. Women with gestational diabetes have a 50% chance of developing type 2 diabetes mellitus within 20 years.[26]

Preeclampsia

Definition. Preeclampsia, formerly known as toxemia of pregnancy, is defined by the American College of Obstetricians and Gynecologists as (1) an elevation of greater than 30 mm Hg in systolic or 15 mm Hg in diastolic blood pressure; (2) blood pressure greater than 140/90 after 20 weeks' gestation; (3) proteinuria of greater than 300 mg per 24 hours; and (4) clinically evident edema, especially of the face and hands.[29]

Preeclampsia is the most common form of **pregnancy-induced hypertension (PIH)**, a more inclusive term that refers to high blood pressure in pregnant women. PIH also includes pregnancy-induced exacerbation of pre-existing *chronic hypertension* and *transient hypertension*, which develop late in pregnancy and are not associated with edema or proteinuria. Transient hypertension is usually present with each pregnancy and predicts the development of essential hypertension later in life.[30] Eclampsia is defined as seizure activity in a patient with preeclampsia, if other causes of seizures are excluded.

Epidemiology. An estimated 5% to 7% of pregnancies in otherwise healthy women are complicated by preeclampsia.[30] Risk factors are summarized in Table 32–13.

Etiology. The causative mechanism of preeclampsia is uncertain, but the best-accepted theory relates to abnormal synthesis of prostaglandins and thromboxanes. As discussed earlier, certain prostaglandins are normally elevated in pregnancy, serving as mediators of uterine and cervical changes. In women with preeclampsia, levels of these lipid mediators are altered. As discussed in Chapter 13, prostaglandins and thromboxanes produced by the arachidonic acid pathway have multiple effects on vascular function. Some act as vasoconstrictors, and others act as vasodilators. Some agents promote platelet aggregation, facilitating the hemostatic response. Increased synthesis of the prostaglandin prostacyclin (PGI_2)

TABLE 32–13
RISK FACTORS FOR PREECLAMPSIA

Risk Factor	Relative Risk	Comments
Nulliparity	6–8	Two thirds of cases of preeclampsia occur in nulliparous patients
Extremes of maternal age*	Not quantified	Preeclampsia does not appear to be more common among young women after controlling for parity
Family history of preeclampsia	Not quantified	The risk of preeclampsia is three to four times greater in women whose mothers and sisters had preeclampsia
History of preeclampsia in a previous pregnancy	Not quantified	The risk of overt toxemia in subsequent pregnancies is 10 to 15%; among women with chronic hypertension, the risk of recurrence may be as high as 70%
Preexisting hypertension or renal disease	Not quantified	Superimposed toxemia is common but difficult to diagnose in this group
Diabetes mellitus	Not quantified	The precise relative risk is confounded by coexisting hypertension
Multiple gestation	Not quantified	Relative risk is 5 for twins
Hydatidiform mole	10	May cause early preeclampsia
Hydrops fetalis	10	May cause early preeclampsia

*Whether the apparent association of young maternal age and preeclampsia is the result of confounding by nulliparity is controversial.
Published with permission from Zamorski, M.A., and Green, L.A. (1996). Preeclampsia and hypertensive disorders of pregnancy. *American Family Physician* 53(5), 1596, published by the American Academy of Family Physicians.

and thromboxane A_2 presumably leads to a tendency toward systemic vasoconstriction and hypercoagulability in preeclampsia.[31] Sympathetic nervous system overactivity has also been implicated in the pathogenesis of this disorder.[32]

Pathophysiology. The blood vessels of women with preeclampsia are hyper-responsive to vasoconstrictor substances. Decreased vessel caliber leads to hypertension as a consequence of increased vessel resistance (see Chapter 15). Vasoconstriction also results in decreased perfusion of maternal organ systems, fetus, and placenta. An immune reaction similar to organ rejection is believed to impair trophoblastic invasion during implantation, and the arterial connection is underdeveloped, resulting in further reduction of placental perfusion. The hypoperfused placenta releases local mediators that induce abnormal endothelial regulation of vessel caliber.

High vascular pressure directly damages the endothelium and may initiate clotting or even a mild form of disseminated intravascular coagulation, which consumes platelets and further impairs perfusion (see Chapter 14). The HELLP syndrome may complicate preeclampsia during the third trimester, with the worst manifestations occurring just after delivery. HELLP differs from disseminated intravascular coagulation in that prothrombin times, partial thromboplastin times, and fibrinogen levels are normal. In HELLP, hepatic damage and fibrin deposition in small vessels are characteristic. Bleeding may result from thrombocytopenia secondary to aggregation of platelets at sites of fibrin deposition and vessel injury.

Proteinuria results from increased glomerular permeability caused by renal hypoxia, and loss of protein from the vascular space (decreased colloid osmotic pressure) promotes edema because of shift of intravascular fluid to the extracellular space (see Chapter 8). The GFR is decreased as a result of decreased renal perfusion (see Chapter 20). Seizure activity in eclampsia may be caused by cerebral vasospasm.

Clinical Manifestations. With severe elevation of blood pressure, signs and symptoms may include headache, visual disturbances, confusion, pulmonary edema, and abdominal pain. Renal effects include oliguria and proteinuria. Edema and excessive weight gain demonstrate the fluid shift. Disseminated intravascular coagulation manifests as bleeding in some women, but in most cases only laboratory evidence of the disorder is present (see Chapter 14). HELLP may manifest as abdominal pain, nausea, and vomiting as a result of hepatic effects (see Chapter 26). Generalized seizure activity characterizes eclampsia (see Chapter 21). Potentially fatal manifestations include hepatic rupture and cerebral hemorrhage. Signs of intrauterine growth retardation are apparent because of placental hypoperfusion, and fetal demise is possible (see Chapter 33).

Prevention and Treatment. Optimal prenatal monitoring facilitates early detection, appropriate treatment, and favorable outcomes in preeclampsia. Early detection and treatment may prevent advancement of preeclampsia to eclampsia, HELLP, or disseminated intravascular coagulation. Preeclampsia is treated with bedrest to reduce metabolic demands and improve renal perfusion. Antihypertensive medications may be used if diastolic pressure exceeds 110 mm Hg. In eclampsia, seizures are prevented or treated with magnesium sulfate, which opposes calcium uptake by neurons without producing generalized central nervous system depression in the mother or the fetus. Organ system failure (e.g., acute renal failure, hepatic failure, encephalopathy) is treated supportively. HELLP may be treated with plasmapheresis to remove endogenous toxins and with fresh frozen plasma to supply clotting factors. Treatment of disseminated intravascular coagulation is discussed in Chapter 14. Induction of labor and delivery of the infant is mandated in situations in which the life of the mother or the fetus is in imminent danger.

Prognosis and Outcome. Outcome depends on the severity of the manifestations and the degree of end-organ damage. Extreme elevations in blood pressure impose high risk of mortality from cerebral hemorrhage. Preeclampsia complicated by HELLP syndrome has a very high mortality rate.

Hydatidiform Mole

Definition. Hydatidiform mole is the most common form of **gestational trophoblastic disease,** in which there is abnormal proliferation of trophoblast cells. With hydatidiform mole (molar pregnancy), cells derived from the chorionic villi divide uncontrollably producing grape-like clusters of clear, fluid-filled vesicles (Fig. 32–10).

Epidemiology. The incidence of hydatidiform mole is approximately 1 in 2000 in the United States.[33] The condition is much more common in Asia, Mexico, and among native Alaskans. Women older than 45 years have a 10-fold risk of having a molar pregnancy.

Etiology. Hydatidiform mole is believed to result from a genetic defect in one of the germ cells comprising the zygote. With *complete mole,* in which vesicles completely fill the uterus, the defect is in the sperm, which always carries an X chromosome. With *incomplete mole,* only part of the uterus is involved with vesicular development, and the remains of a degenerating fetus or amniotic sac may be present. Incomplete mole may result from fertilization of a normal ovum with two sperm or with one diploid sperm, or from fertilization of an "empty" ovum with two haploid sperm.

Pathophysiology. Proliferation of trophoblastic cells leads to rapid, disproportionate enlargement of

Clinical Scenario

J.M., a 20-year-old who is in the 30th week of her first pregnancy, is found to have a blood pressure of 170/102 and significant proteinuria during a routine prenatal visit. She is hospitalized for monitoring. During the first 2 days of hospitalization, J.M.'s blood pressure remained elevated, and blood tests revealed elevated hepatic enzymes, increased creatinine and blood urea nitrogen, and a decreased platelet count. The decision was made to induce labor.

1. What disorder is suggested by the presence of hypertension and proteinuria?
2. What complications are evident from the results of blood testing? What clinical manifestations might be expected?
3. What are the risks and benefits of induction of labor at this time?

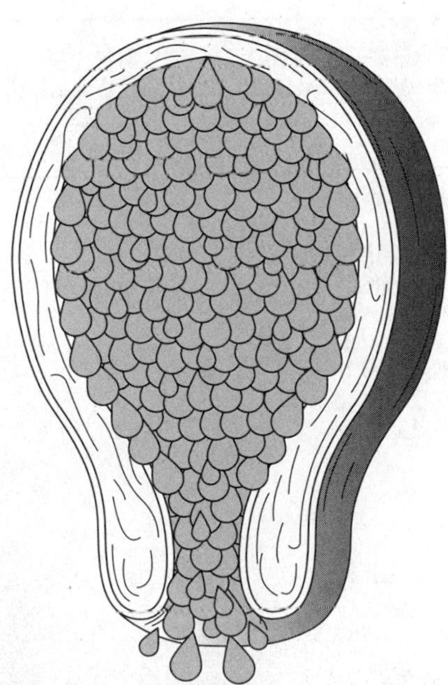

FIGURE 32–10
Hydatidiform mole. A complete mole is shown here, in which no embryonic or fetal tissue is identifiable. This gestational trophoblastic disease results from uncontrolled proliferation of trophoblast cells.

the uterus. By the end of the first trimester, intermittent vaginal bleeding begins, caused by abnormal vascularization. Vesicles may also be passed vaginally or into the venous system, imposing risk of pulmonary embolism (see Chapter 19). Serum hCG levels are significantly higher than normal because of the excessive trophoblastic growth, possibly contributing to the preeclampsia and hyperemesis that are common in molar pregnancy.

Clinical Manifestations. Vaginal bleeding is usually the first sign of molar pregnancy. In many patients with partial moles, the initial diagnosis is of missed abortion. Uterine size in excess of duration of pregnancy, severe nausea and vomiting, manifestations of preeclampsia, and elevation of hCG levels are usually noted as well. Pulmonary emboli, if present, are usually small, and cardiac and respiratory manifestations, if any, are minor. About 2% of cases are complicated by hyperthyroidism, apparently the result of the thyrotropic hormone–like effect of hCG. Fetal heart tones are absent, and no fetal movement is felt.

Prevention and Treatment. There are no known means of prevention. In partial moles, the pregnancy usually spontaneously aborts. In most cases, however, intervention is required to completely empty the uterus. Vacuum aspiration is used to evacuate the bulk of the mole, with additional curettage if necessary. Induction of uterine contraction with oxytocin and prostaglandins may be useful in evacuation of larger moles. In older women and those with high parity, the risk of malignant transformation may indicate the need for prophylactic hysterectomy or chemotherapy.

Prognosis and Outcome. With early detection and treatment, immediate mortality is essentially zero.[33] Levels of hCG are monitored for at least a year after termination of the pregnancy to ensure that malignant transformation of trophoblastic cells has not occurred. **Choriocarcinoma** develops in nearly 20% of hydatidiform moles in older, multiparous women, and this cancer is associated with a high mortality rate. If hCG levels remain normal after a year, the probability of another molar pregnancy is low.

Dystocia

Definition. Dystocia includes all conditions that result in dysfunctional labor, that is, labor which is suboptimal in achieving cervical effacement and dilation as well as descent and delivery of the infant. Dystocia imposes risk for laboring mother and fetus. Criteria for dysfunctional labor are quantified in Table 32–14.

Epidemiology. Dystocia is the leading indication for a first cesarean delivery among U.S. women.[34] Nulliparous women are at highest risk for pro-

TABLE 32–14
CRITERIA FOR DYSFUNCTIONAL LABOR

Labor Pattern	Diagnostic Criterion: Nulliparas	Diagnostic Criterion: Multiparas	Preferred Treatment	Exceptional Treatment
Prolongation disorder				
Prolonged latent phase	>20 hr	>14 hr	Therapeutic rest	Oxytocin or cesarean section for urgent problems
Protraction disorders				
Protracted active phase dilatation	<1.2 cm/hr	<1.5 cm/hr		
Protracted descent	<1.0 cm/hr	<2 cm/hr	Expectant and supportive	Cesarean section for CPD
Arrest disorders				
Prolonged deceleration phase	>3 hr	>1 hr	Without CPD: oxytocin	Rest if exhausted
Secondary arrest of dilatation	>2 hr	>2 hr		
Arrest of descent	>1 hr	>1 hr	With CPD: cesarean section	Cesarean section
Failure of descent	No descent in deceleration phase or second stage of labor			

CPD, cephalopelvic disproportion.
From Cohen, W., and Friedman, E.A. (eds.). (1983). *Management of Labor*. Baltimore: University Park Press.

longed (longer than 24 hours) or inefficient labor. Iatrogenic risk factors associated with dysfunctional labor include injudicious use of sedatives or analgesics, which may prolong labor, and overdosage of oxytocin (Pitocin) for labor induction.

Etiology. The numerous conditions that may result in dystocia are summarized in Table 32–15. Four types of mechanisms may be involved. These are classically referred to as problems of the *psyche* (maternal stress and anxiety), *powers* (abnormalities of uterine structure or regulation of contraction), *passage* (pelvic outlet abnormalities), and *passenger* (fetal malposition, enlargement of the fetal head).

Pathophysiology. Neuroendocrine alterations with stress may alter the hormonal environment and divert energy substrates from the uterine muscle. The catecholamine hormones of stress may induce uncoordinated, ineffective uterine contraction or hyperactive contraction, depending on whether epinephrine (inhibitory) or norepinephrine (excitatory) dominates.

The molecular mechanism of smooth-muscle contraction may be impaired by any factor that reduces available energy, impedes availability or transport of calcium, alters the contractile proteins, or alters the local hormonal environment. Dysfunctional uterine contractions may be *hypertonic* (high frequency but poor quality contractions present from the onset of labor) or *hypotonic* (effective contractions early in labor, degenerating to weak or absent contractions later). Either pattern is likely to prolong labor.

With hypertonic contractions, the refractory period between depolarizations is shortened, and resting uterine muscle tone is increased. Uterine vessels are compressed at baseline, leading to uterine muscle hypoxia and ischemic pain with contractions as well as impairment of placental exchange. Fetal distress is evident. Because hypertonic contractions often occur early, before the cervix is capable of rapid dilation and effacement, labor is ineffective and exhausting, and maternal stress is enhanced in a positive feedback loop. Hypertonic contractions may also result in precipitous delivery (labor less than 3 hours), especially if they occur in cases of multiparity, large maternal pelvis, or small fetus in a favorable position.

Hypotonic contractions may ensue in women who have progressed normally during the early part of labor. Hypotonic contractions may subside entirely, and labor may stop. Factors contributing to this pattern include (1) overstretching of uterine muscle fibers because of multiple gestations, large infant size, polyhydramnios, or multiparity; (2) maternal sedation; or (3) reflex decline in neural stimulation as a result of bladder or bowel distention. Prolonged la-

TABLE 32–15
CONDITIONS ASSOCIATED WITH DYSTOCIA

CATEGORY	EXAMPLES
Uterine dysfunction	Hypotonic, hypertonic, or incoordinate uterine contraction caused by pelvic contraction or fetal malposition
Inadequate voluntary expulsive force	Failure to bear down or push as a result of abdominal muscle weakness, conduction anesthesia, heavy sedation, extreme pain, or pre-existing neuromuscular disease
Localized uterine muscle abnormality	Development of pathologic retraction rings that obstruct fetal descent, associated with prolonged rupture of the membranes, protracted labor, or delivery of the first of twins
Precipitate labor and delivery	Extremely rapid labor and delivery caused by low resistance of the birth canal or from abnormally strong uterine contractions; may be associated with multiparity
Fetal malpresentation	Breech, face, brow, transverse, compound (extremity prolapse in addition to presenting part), persistent occiput posterior, or persistent occiput transverse presentations
Fetal macrosomia	Large fetus, hydrocephalus, large trunk leading to shoulder dystocia, large abdomen secondary to ascites or organ enlargement (kidneys or liver)
Pelvic contraction	Small pelvic inlet, midpelvis, or pelvis outlet; pelvic fractures
Soft tissue abnormalities	Atresia of the vulva, vagina, or cervix secondary to scarring or congenital anomaly
Uterine displacement	Anteflexion or retroflexion of the uterus
Tumors or masses	Uterine myomas, ovarian tumors, distended bladder, or polycystic kidney

Data from Cunningham, F.G., MacDonald, P.C., and Gant, N.F. (1989). *Williams Obstetrics*. (18th ed.). Norwalk, CT: Appleton & Lange. (pp. 341–392).

bor is associated with increased risk of intrapartum infection. After delivery, the hypotonic or atonic uterus is prone to bleed excessively.

Retraction rings between the upper uterus, which thickens as the fetus descends, and the lower uterus, which thins with dilation by the descending fetus, form and release physiologically during labor. A retraction ring may become obstructive to labor if uterine muscle becomes tetanic (see Chapter 5). The fetus, or part of the fetus, is located above the constriction and cannot descend. The sustained contraction must be released with general anesthesia, and the infant delivered via cesarean birth. In rare cases, a pathologic retraction ring results in rupture of the uterus and severe maternal hemorrhage.

Fetal malposition or malpresentation (Fig. 32–11) may result in prolonged labor, necessitating manual repositioning of the fetus or instrument-assisted delivery. Cesarean section may be necessary in some cases to prevent uterine rupture and fetal demise. Macrosomia, as in the case of the infant of a diabetic mother, imposes risk of shoulder dystocia, which complicates 0.15% to 0.6% of vaginal deliveries.[35] Prolapse of the umbilical cord is more likely with malposition, imposing risk of fetal hypoxia. Multifetal pregnancies are often complicated by hypotonic contractions, fetal malposition, and preterm labor.

Clinical Manifestations. The most obvious manifestation of prolonged dysfunctional labor is maternal exhaustion. Vaginal examination reveals deficiency in cervical effacement or dilation. Monitoring of the frequency and duration of uterine contractions may demonstrate a hypertonic or hypotonic pattern. Fetal monitoring reveals alterations in heart rate indicative of fetal distress (see Chapter 33). Uterine rupture may occur in rare cases, resulting in massive bleeding.

Prevention and Treatment. Optimal prenatal care may identify many risk factors for dysfunctional labor, and careful monitoring during the labor process should allow early detection of problems. The laboring mother must be supported physiologically and emotionally during the natural process of labor, with provision of fluids and nutrition and facilitation of as much rest as possible. Oxytocin is commonly used to enhance hypotonic labor contractions, and forceps-aided delivery may be indicated. Hypertonic labor usually requires no intervention other than supporting the delivery of the infant. Fetal malposition or macrosomia may necessitate rotational maneuvers (version), forceps-aided delivery, or intentional fracture of a fetal part (controlled destructive procedures). General anesthesia and emergent surgical delivery of the infant are mandated in cases of hemorrhage or significant fetal distress.

Prognosis and Outcome. Dysfunctional labor imposes increased risk to mother and fetus. Highest maternal mortality is associated with hemorrhagic complications, discussed further in the next section. Fetal manifestations of dysfunctional labor and delivery are discussed in Chapter 33.

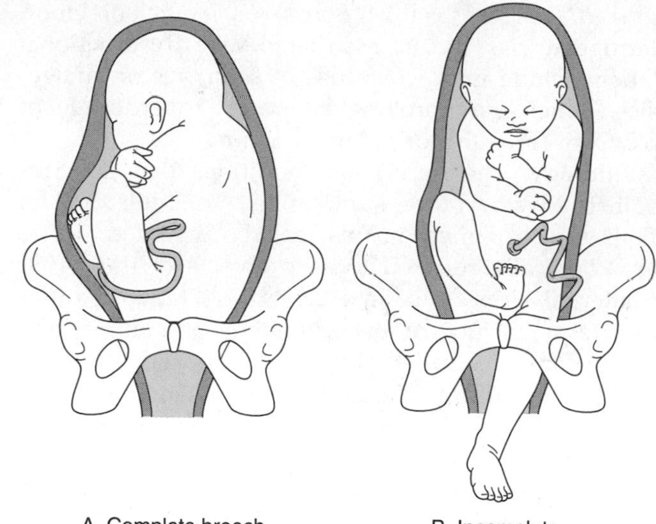

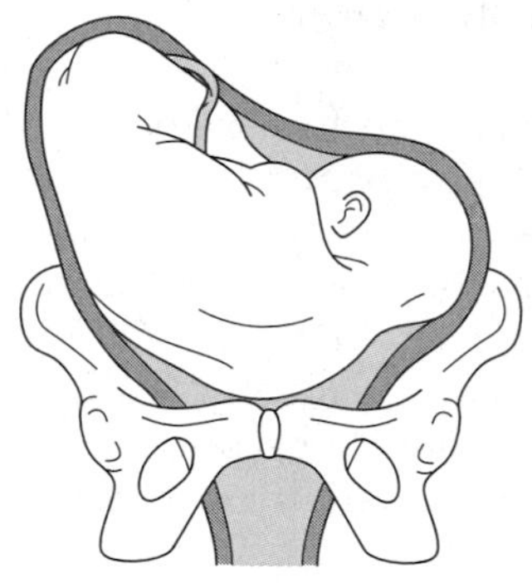

FIGURE 32–11
Fetal presentation associated with dystocia. *A,* In a *complete breech* presentation, the fetal buttocks present. *B,* In an *incomplete (footling) breech* presentation, one foot protrudes through the introitus. *C,* In a *transverse* lie, one shoulder presents.

Peripartum Hemorrhage

Definition. Peripartum hemorrhage is excessive blood loss (>500 mL for a vaginal delivery) during the prenatal period, labor and delivery, or the postpartum period.

Epidemiology. Hemorrhage is the leading cause of maternal mortality in the United States, causing 30% of all maternal deaths.[36] Risk factors are associated with the specific causative disorders, as discussed in this section.

Etiology. During the antepartum period (before labor), the most frequent causes of hemorrhage are abortion (spontaneous or induced), ruptured ectopic (tubal) pregnancy, and abruptio placentae. Spontaneous abortion and tubal pregnancy have been previously discussed. Abruptio placentae (placental abruption), responsible for 17% of cases of fatal maternal hemorrhage, is the premature separation of the placenta from its site of implantation before delivery.[36] Risk factors for abruption include eclampsia, trauma, abnormally short umbilical cord, polyhydramnios, and maternal abuse of alcohol or cocaine.

During the intrapartum period (labor and delivery), hemorrhage may result from a hypotonic or atonic uterus or, uncommonly, uterine rupture. Risk factors for these conditions were discussed in the previous section on dysfunctional labor. Postpartum hemorrhage usually results from subinvolution, retained placental fragments, placenta accreta, or placenta previa. Placenta previa may also present as bleeding in the second or third trimesters. The lower segment of the uterus is less contractile than the upper segment and is less able to constrict to minimize bleeding after placental separation. Risk factors for subinvolution are the same as those for uterine hypotonicity or atony. Risk factors for retention of placental fragments, placenta accreta, and placenta previa are unknown.

Extrauterine factors such as trauma (accidental or surgical), maternal bleeding disorders unrelated to pregnancy (see Chapter 14), disseminated intravascular coagulation, or HELLP syndrome may also promote hemorrhage. An uncommon event that may trigger disseminated intravascular coagulation during pregnancy (typically during labor and the postpartum period) is **amniotic fluid embolism**. During the period when the placenta has begun to separate, uterine contraction may force a bolus of amniotic fluid into the mother's bloodstream. Amniotic fluid is rich in tissue thromboplastin, which may trigger disseminated intravascular coagulation and resultant hemorrhage. Amniotic fluid embolism may predispose to the development of adult respiratory distress syndrome (ARDS) (see Chapter 19).

Pathophysiology. Maternal hemorrhage may lead to hypovolemic shock, with potentially fatal complications of hypoxic organ failure, disseminated intravascular coagulation, and ARDS. With hemorrhage before delivery, fetal hypoxia also results.

Clinical Manifestations. General manifestations of shock and disseminated intravascular coagulation are detailed in Chapters 14 and 15. ARDS is discussed in Chapter 19. Excessive vaginal bleeding and a "boggy" uterus (i.e., one that fails to involute after delivery, remaining palpable above the umbilicus) are apparent. Signs of fetal distress occur with hemorrhage before delivery, and the infant may demonstrate varying degrees of hypoxia. Fetal demise is common with severe antepartum or intrapartum hemorrhage.

Prevention and Treatment. Optimal prenatal care facilitates the early recognition and potential removal of risk factors. Treatment is aimed at restoration of hemodynamic balance (see Chapter 15) and removal of the underlying cause of bleeding. Treatment of ectopic pregnancy, hypotonic uterine contraction, shock, disseminated intravascular coagulation, and ARDS are discussed in the indicated chapters. The fetus and placenta are delivered (often surgically) as soon as is feasible to preserve viability of the infant and to access the bleeding source. Oxytocin may be given to enhance involution of the uterus. Ligation of major bleeding sources may be possible. Uterine rupture usually necessitates hysterectomy.

Prognosis and Outcome. Maternal mortality is uncommon in the United States, but when it does occur, hemorrhage is the usual cause. Most incidents of maternal hemorrhage are not fatal, but are successfully managed with appropriate monitoring and support of pregnancy, labor, delivery, and postpartum recovery.

CLINICAL SIGNIFICANCE OF DISORDERS RELATED TO PREGNANCY AND LACTATION

Although childbearing is a physiologic process, it is a major stressor even when uncomplicated. Disorders related to pregnancy impose additional physiologic (and psychological) stress on women who are in a vulnerable state. Although maternal mortality has declined significantly in recent decades, childbearing is not without risk, as illustrated by the disorders discussed in this chapter. The factors involved in the regulation of pregnancy and lactation are still not completely understood. Research is ongoing in an effort to identify the interdependent roles of the many hormones, cytokines, and lipid mediators that direct the maternal systemic changes of pregnancy and the processes of labor, delivery, and lactation. Effects of very young maternal age or advanced maternal age are also under study. Fetal abnormalities may adversely affect the mother during pregnancy, and maternal disorders of pregnancy invariably affect development of the fetus. Chapter

33 reviews fetal and neonatal physiology and describes common disorders affecting neonates.

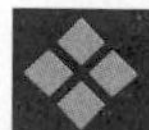

Summary of Key Points

- Pregnancy begins with fertilization of the ovum, which normally takes place in the fallopian tube. Fertilization initiates a series of cell divisions within the fertilized ovum (zygote), forming the blastocyst. The two cell layers of the blastocyst become the embryo and the trophoblast. Implantation of the blastocyst normally occurs in the upper portion of the uterus, and the placenta forms from trophoblastic and endometrial tissues. Placental exchange begins at 4 weeks' gestation, and placental growth parallels fetal growth until near term (40 weeks' gestation).
- Uterine growth supportive of pregnancy is under endocrine regulation by the hormones human chorionic gonadotropin (hCG), human chorionic somatomammotropin (hCS), progesterone, estrogen, and relaxin, secreted by the corpus luteum during the luteal phase of pregnancy. The placental phase is regulated by these same hormones, secreted by the placenta. Labor onset and progression depend on the additional influence of the hypothalamic hormone oxytocin, secreted by the posterior pituitary gland.
- Blood volume and cardiac output increase significantly during pregnancy; however, hypertension is abnormal. Dilutional effects on hemoglobin and hematocrit are expected, but significant anemia is preventable. Hypercoagulability is normal, but thrombosis is pathologic. Although hyperventilation and dyspnea may occur, alveolar ventilation normally increases during pregnancy. Hydroureter and hydronephrosis are physiologic, but increased tubular flow rates may lead to washout of electrolytes and water-soluble vitamins. Hormonally mediated relaxation of gastrointestinal smooth muscle promotes acid reflux and constipation. Nausea and vomiting are common; however, extreme cases (hyperemesis gravidarum) may lead to significant fluid and electrolyte imbalance. Hepatobiliary function is altered during pregnancy, with increased incidence of gallbladder disease and infrequent liver failure. Hyperpigmentation and striae of the skin are common. Emotional lability and mild depression are common during pregnancy and the postpartum period; psychosis and seizures indicate significant pathology.
- The first stage of labor is variable in length and serves to push the baby downward and assist in effacement and dilation of the cervix. The amniotic sac usually ruptures spontaneously during this stage. The second stage includes the time from full cervical dilation and effacement to delivery. During the third stage, the placenta separates and is delivered.
- Multifetal pregnancy is associated with proportionately greater maternal systemic changes and higher risk. Preterm labor and delivery is usual.
- Development of the mammary alveoli and ducts is stimulated by estrogen, progesterone, prolactin, and hCS during pregnancy. Removal of progesterone and estrogen with delivery of the placenta allows prolactin to induce alveolar secretion and milk production. Prolactin levels remain high as long as lactation continues. Milk letdown is mediated by oxytocin, released in response to suckling.
- Maternal disorders related to pregnancy include (1) those associated with achieving and maintaining pregnancy (infertility, spontaneous abortion, preterm labor, and ectopic pregnancy); (2) those associated with the prenatal period (gestational diabetes, preeclampsia, and hydatidiform mole); and (3) those occurring during labor and delivery (dystocia and peripartum hemorrhage).
- Although maternal mortality has declined significantly in recent decades, childbearing is not without risk, particularly for those of nonwhite race, age younger than 20 years or older than 40 years, or those not receiving optimal prenatal care. Fetal abnormalities may adversely affect the mother during pregnancy, and maternal disorders of pregnancy invariably affect development of the fetus.

REFERENCES

1. Berg, C.J., Atrash, H.K., Koonin, L.M., *et al.* (1996). Pregnancy-related mortality in the United States, 1987–1990. *Obstetrics and Gynecology* 88(2), 161–167.
2. Prevost, R.R. (1995). Treatment of pregnancy-related illnesses. *American Pharmacy* NS35(10), 25–32.
3. Hod, M., Orvieto, R., Kaplan, B., *et al.* (1994). Hyperemesis gravidarum: A review. *Journal of Reproductive Medicine* 39(8), 605–612.

4. Knox, T.A., and Olans, L.B. (1996). Liver disease in pregnancy. *New England Journal of Medicine* 335(8), 569–576.
5. Jermain, D.M. (1995). Treatment of postpartum depression. *American Pharmacy* NS35(1), 33–38.
6. Newman, J. (1995). How breast milk protects newborns. *Scientific American* 273(6), 76–79.
7. King, J.C., Butte, N.F., Bronstein, M.N., *et al.* (1994). Energy metabolism during pregnancy: Influence of maternal energy status. *American Journal of Clinical Nutrition* 59(suppl.), 439S–445S.
8. Boden, G. (1996). Fuel metabolism in pregnancy and in gestational diabetes mellitus. *Obstetrics and Gynecology Clinics of North America* 23(1), 1–10.
9. Keen, C.L., and Zidenberg-Cherr, S. (1994). Should vitamin-mineral supplements be recommended for all women with childbearing potential? *American Journal of Clinical Nutrition* 59(suppl.), 532S–539S.
10. Lops, V.R., Hunter, L.P., and Dixon, L.R. (1995). Anemia in pregnancy. *American Family Physician* 51(5), 1189–1197.
11. Greenwald, J.L. (1993). Premature rupture of the membranes: Diagnostic and management strategies. *American Family Physician* 48(2), 293–306.
12. Porreco, R.P., and Thorp, J.A. (1996). The cesarian birth epidemic: Trends, causes, and solutions. *American Journal of Obstetrics and Gynecology* 175(2), 369–374.
13. Karew, S. (1993). Adverse effects of drugs and chemicals in breast milk on the nursing infant. *Journal of Clinical Pharmacology* 33, 213–221.
14. Sowers, M.F., Hollis, B.W., Shapiro, B., *et al.* (1996). Elevated parathyroid hormone-related peptide associated with lactation and bone density loss. *Journal of the American Medical Association* 276(7), 549–554.
15. Pryor, J.L., Kent-First, M., Muallem, A., *et al.* (1997). Microdeletions in the Y chromosome of infertile men. *New England Journal of Medicine* 336(8), 534–539.
16. Trantham, P. (1996). The infertile couple. *American Family Physician* 54(3), 1001–1010.
17. Howards, S.S. (1995). Treatment of male infertility. *New England Journal of Medicine* 332(5), 312–317.
18. Brent, R.L., and Beckman, D.A. (1994). The contribution of environmental teratogens to embryonic and fetal loss. *Clinical Obstetrics and Gynecology* 37(3), 646–670.
19. Rand, S.E. (1993). Recurrent spontaneous abortion: Evaluation and management. *American Family Physician* 48(8), 1451–1457.
20. McCombs, J. (1995). Update on tocolytic therapy. *Annals of Pharmacotherapy* 29, 515–522.
21. Papke, K.R. (1993). Management of preterm labor and prevention of premature delivery. *Nursing Clinics of North America* 28(2), 279–288.
22. Travis, B.E., and McCullough, J.M. (1993). Pharmacotherapy of preterm labor. *Pharmacotherapy* 13(1), 28–36.
23. U.S. Preventive Services Task Force. (1993). Home uterine activity monitoring for preterm labor. *Journal of the American Medical Association* 270(3), 371–376.
24. Maiolatesi, C.R., and Peddicord, K. (1996). Methotrexate for nonsurgical treatment of ectopic pregnancy: Nursing implications. *Journal of Obstetric, Gynecologic, and Neonatal Nursing* 25(3), 205–208.
25. Bernstein, J. (1995). Ectopic pregnancy: A nursing approach to excess risk among minority women. *Journal of Obstetric, Gynecologic, and Neonatal Nursing* 24(9), 803–810.
26. Weller, K.A. (1996). Diagnosis and management of gestational diabetes. *American Family Physician* 53(6), 2053–2057.
27. Davidson, J.A., and Roberts, V.L. (1996). Gestational diabetes: Ensuring a successful outcome. *Postgraduate Medicine* 99(3), 165–172.
28. Jackson, P., and Bash, D.M. (1994). Management of the uncomplicated pregnant diabetic client in the ambulatory setting. *Nurse Practitioner* 19(12), 64–73.
29. Zamorski, M.A., and Green, L.A. (1996). Preeclampsia and hypertensive disorders of pregnancy. *American Family Physician* 53(5), 1595–1604.
30. Fadigan, A.B., Sealy, D.P., and Schneider, E.F. (1994). Preeclampsia: Progress and puzzle. *American Family Physician* 49(4), 849–856.
31. Meagher, E.A., and FitzGerald, G.A. (1993). Disordered eicosanoid formation in pregnancy-induced hypertension. *Circulation* 88(3), 1324–1333.
32. Schobel, H.P., Fischer, T., Heuszer, K., *et al.* (1996). Preeclampsia: A state of sympathetic overactivity. *New England Journal of Medicine* 335(20), 1480–1485.
33. Cunningham, F.G., MacDonald, P.C., and Gant, N.F. (1989). *Williams Obstetrics*. (18th ed.). Norwalk, CT: Appleton & Lange. (pp. 541–549).
34. Peaceman, A.M., and Socol, M.L. (1996). Active management of labor. *American Journal of Obstetrics and Gynecology* 175(2), 363–368.
35. Gianoppoulos, J.G. (1994). Emergency complications of labor and delivery. *Emergency Medicine Clinics of North America* 12(1), 201–217.
36. Ritter, D.C., and deShazo, R.D. (1994). Peripartum complications: Hemorrhage, embolism, hypertension, and infection. *Postgraduate Medicine* 95(2), 178–192.

SELECTED BIBLIOGRAPHY

Aldous, M.B., and Edmonson, B. (1993). Maternal age at first childbirth and risk of low birth weight and preterm delivery in Washington State. *Journal of the American Medical Association* 270(21), 2574–2577.

Ananth, C.V., Wilcox, A.J., Savitz, D.A., *et al.* (1996). Effect of maternal age and parity on the risk of uteroplacental bleeding disorders in pregnancy. *Obstetrics and Gynecology* 88(4 pt. 1), 511–516.

Barth, W.H. (1994). Cervical incompetence and cerclage: Unresolved controversies. *Clinical Obstetrics and Gynecology* 37(4), 831–841.

Berkowitz, R.S., and Goldstein, D.P. (1996). Chorionic tumors. *New England Journal of Medicine* 335(23), 1740–1748.

Blackburn, S.T., and Loper, D.L. (1992). *Maternal, Fetal, and Neonatal Physiology: A Clinical Perspective.* Philadelphia: W.B. Saunders.

Bright, D.A. (1994). Postpartum mental disorders. *American Family Physician* 50(3), 595–598.

Bucher, H.C., Guyatt, G.H., Cook, R.J., *et al.* (1996). Effect of calcium supplementation on pregnancy-induced hypertension and preeclampsia. *Journal of the American Medical Association* 275(14), 1113–1117.

Carmichael, J.M. (1995). Understanding infertility treatment plans. *American Pharmacy* NS35(11), 41–52.

Carpenter, C.C.J., Fischl, M.A., Hammer, S.M., *et al.* (1996). Antiretroviral therapy for HIV infection in 1996: Recommendations of an international panel. *Journal of the American Medical Association* 276(2), 146–154.

Carson, S.A., and Buster, J.E. (1993). Ectopic pregnancy. *New England Journal of Medicine* 329(6), 1174–1181.

Charles, M.A., Pettitt, D.J., and McCance, D.R. (1994). Gravidity, obesity, and non–insulin-dependent diabetes among Pima Indian women. *American Journal of Medicine* 97, 250–255.

Clark, R.A. (1995). Infections during the postpartum period. *Journal of Obstetric, Gynecologic, and Neonatal Nursing* 24(6), 542–548.

Coulam, C.B., and Stern, J.J. (1994). Endocrine factors associated with recurrent spontaneous abortion. *Clinical Obstetrics and Gynecology* 37(3), 730–744.

Dawood, M.Y. (1993). Nonsteroidal antiinflammatory drugs and reproduction. *American Journal of Obstetrics and Gynecology* 169(5), 1255–1265.

Errickson, C.V., and Matus, N.R. (1994). Skin disorders of pregnancy. *American Family Physician* 49(3), 605–610.

Fraser, A.M., Brockert, J.E., and Ward, R.H. (1995). Association of young maternal age with adverse reproductive outcomes. *New England Journal of Medicine* 332(17), 1113–1117.

Fretts, R.C., Schmittdiel, J., McLean, F.H., *et al.* (1995). Increased maternal age and the risk of fetal death. *New England Journal of Medicine* 333(15), 953–957.

Fretts, R.C., and Usher, R.H. (1997). Causes of fetal death in women of advanced maternal age. *Obstetrics and Gynecology* 89, 40–45.

Frigoletto, F.D., Lieberman, E., Lang, J.M., *et al.* (1995). A clinical trial of active management of labor. *New England Journal of Medicine* 333(12), 745–750.

Geerling, J.H. (1995). Natural family planning. *American Family Physician* 52(6), 1749–1756.

Hannah, M.E., Ohlsson, A., Farine, D., *et al.* (1996). Induction of labor compared with expectant management for prelabor rupture of the membranes at term. *New England Journal of Medicine* 334(16), 1006–1010.

Hill, J.A., Polgar, K., and Anderson, D.J. (1995). T-helper 1-type immunity to trophoblast in women with recurrent spontaneous abortion. *Journal of the American Medical Association* 273(24), 1933–1936.

Iams, J.D., Goldenberg, R.L., and Meis, P.J., *et al.* (1996). The length of the cervix and the risk of spontaneous premature delivery. *New England Journal of Medicine* 334(9), 567–572.

Infante-Rivard, C., Fernandez, A., Gauthier, R., *et al.* (1993). Fetal loss associated with caffeine intake before and during pregnancy. *Journal of the American Medical Association* 270(24), 2940–2943.

Jones, H.W., and Toner, J.P. (1993). The infertile couple. *New England Journal of Medicine* 329(23), 1710–1715.

Kaunitz, A.M., Illions, E.H., Jones, J.L., *et al.* (1995). Contraception: A clinical review for the internist. *Medical Clinics of North America* 79(6), 1377–1409.

Kinningham, R.B. (1993). Asymptomatic bacteriuria in pregnancy. *American Family Physician* 47(5), 1232–1238.

Kittner, S.J., Stern, B.J., and Feeser, B.R. (1996). Pregnancy and the risk of stroke. *New England Journal of Medicine* 335(11), 768–774.

Koenigseder, L.A., Crane, P.B., and Lucy, P.W. (1993). HELLP: A collaborative challenge for critical care and obstetric nurses. *American Journal of Critical Care* 2(5), 385–392.

Kousen, M. (1993). Treatment of nausea and vomiting in pregnancy. *American Family Physician* 48(7), 1279–1283.

Lowe, N.K. (1996). The pain and discomfort of labor and birth. *Journal of Obstetric, Gynecologic, and Neonatal Nursing* 25(1), 82–92.

Mahon, T.R., Chazotte, C., and Cohen, W.R. (1994). Short labor: Characteristics and outcome. *Obstetrics and Gynecology* 84(1), 47–51.

Major, C.A., de Veciana, M., Lewis, D.F., *et al.* (1995). Preterm premature rupture of membranes and abruptio placentae: Is there an association between these pregnancy complications? *American Journal of Obstetrics and Gynecology* 172(2 pt. 1), 672–676.

Mazor, M., Furman, B., Wiznitzer, A., *et al.* (1995). Maternal and perinatal outcome of patients with preterm labor and meconium-stained amniotic fluid. *Obstetrics and Gynecology* 86(5), 830–833.

McKennett, M., and Fullerton, J.T. (1995). Vaginal bleeding in pregnancy. *American Family Physician* 51(3), 639–646.

McMahon, M.J., Luther, E.R., Bowes, W.A., *et al.* (1996). Comparison of a trial of labor with an elective second cesarean section. *New England Journal of Medicine* 335(10), 689–695.

Melnikow, J., and Bedinghaus, J.M. (1994). Management of common breast-feeding problems. *Journal of Family Practice* 39(1), 56–64.

Minakami, H., and Sato, I. (1996). Reestimating date of delivery in multifetal pregnancies. *Journal of the American Medical Association* 275(18), 1432–1434.

Moore, T.R. (1995). Assessment of amniotic fluid volume in at-risk pregnancies. *Clinical Obstetrics and Gynecology* 38(1), 78–90.

Naylor, C.D., Sermer, M., Chen, E., *et al.* (1996). Cesarean delivery in relation to birth weight and gestational glucose tolerance: Pathophysiology or practice style? *Journal of the American Medical Association* 275(15), 1165–1170.

Newcomb, P.A., Storer, B.E., Longnecker, M.P., *et al.* (1994). Lactation and a reduced risk of premenopausal breast cancer. *New England Journal of Medicine* 330(2), 81–86.

Newman, V., Fullerton, J.T., and Anderson, P.O. (1993). Clinical advances in the management of severe nausea and vomiting during pregnancy. *Journal of Obstetric, Gynecologic, and Neonatal Nursing* 22(6), 483–490.

Norris, T.C. (1997). Management of postpartum hemorrhage. *American Family Physician* 55(2), 635–640.

Paul, R.H., and Miller, D.A. (1994). Cesarean birth: How to reduce the rate. *American Journal of Obstetrics and Gynecology* 172(6), 1903–1911.

Peterson, H.B., Xia, Z., Hughes, J.M., *et al.* (1997). The risk of ectopic pregnancy after tubal sterilization. *New England Journal of Medicine* 336(11), 762–767.

Reife, C.M. (1996). Office gynecology for the primary care physician, part I. *Medical Clinics of North America* 80(2), 299–319.

Riely, C.A. (1994). Hepatic disease in pregnancy. *American Journal of Medicine* 96(1A suppl.), 18S–22S.

Sabai, B.M., Ramadan, M.K., Chari, R.S., *et al.* (1995). Pregnancies complicated by HELLP syndrome (hemolysis, elevated liver enzymes, and low platelets): Subsequent pregnancy outcome and long-term prognosis. *American Journal of Obstetrics and Gynecology* 172(1 pt. 1), 125–129.

Schoener, C.J., and Krysa, L.W. (1996). The comfort and discomfort of infertility. *Journal of Obstetric, Gynecologic, and Neonatal Nursing* 25(2), 167–172.

Scott-Conner, C.E.H., and Schorr, S.J. (1995). The diagnosis and management of breast problems during pregnancy and lactation. *American Journal of Surgery* 170, 401–405.

Sibai, B.M., Caritis, S.N., Thom, E., *et al.* (1993). Prevention of preeclampsia with low-dose aspirin in healthy, nulliparous pregnant women. *New England Journal of Medicine* 329(17), 1213–1218.

Silver, R.M., and Branch, D.W. (1994). Recurrent miscarriage: Autoimmune considerations. *Clinical Obstetrics and Gynecology* 37(3), 745–760.

Stover, A.M., and Marnejon, J.G. (1995). Postpartum care. *American Family Physician* 52(5), 1465–1472.

Sulik, S.M., and Greenwald, J.L. (1994). Evaluation and management of postdate pregnancy. *American Family Physician* 49(5), 1177–1186.

Summers, P.R. (1994). Microbiology relevant to recurrent miscarriage. *Clinical Obstetrics and Gynecology* 37(3), 722–729.

Surratt, N. (1993). Severe preeclampsia: Implications for critical-care obstetric nursing. *Journal of Obstetric, Gynecologic, and Neonatal Nursing* 22(6), 500–507.

Surratt, N., and Troiano, N.H. (1994). Adult respiratory distress in pregnancy: Critical care issues. *Journal of Obstetric, Gynecologic, and Neonatal Nursing* 23(9), 773–780.

Tagg, P.I. (1995). The diaphragm: Barrier contraception has a new social role. *Nurse Practitioner* 20(12), 36–42.

Toohey, J.S., Keegan, K.A., Morgan, M.A., *et al.* (1995). The "dangerous multipara": Fact or fiction? *American Journal of Obstetrics and Gynecology* 172(2 pt. 1), 683–686.

Neonatal Disorders

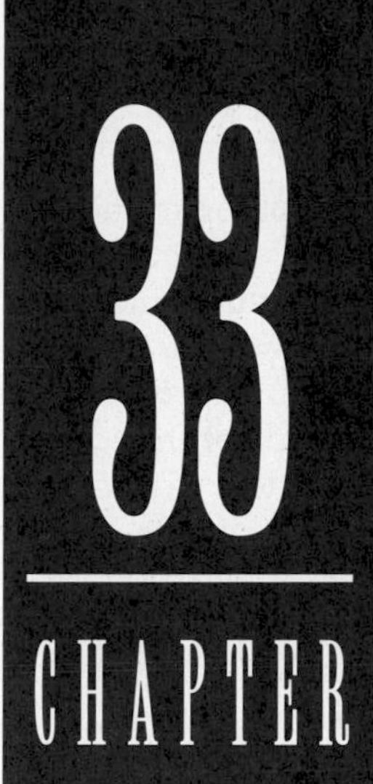

LEARNING OBJECTIVES

1. Identify anatomic differences between term and preterm neonates.
2. Discuss aspects of fetal and neonatal systemic physiology that may induce vulnerability to disease or dysfunction.
3. Compare and contrast clinical manifestations and pathophysiologic processes associated with prematurity and postmaturity.
4. Comprehend maternal, fetal, uterine, and placental factors that may result in intrauterine growth retardation.
5. Identify the pathophysiologic processes that predict clinical manifestations and rationalize prevention and treatment of common congenital disorders affecting multiple body systems.

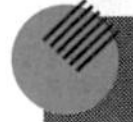

key terms

acrocyanosis
anemia of prematurity
apnea
asphyxia
bronchopulmonary dysplasia (BPD)
diving reflex
Down syndrome
fetal alcohol syndrome
hemolytic disease of the newborn
infant of a diabetic mother (IDM)
infant respiratory distress syndrome (IRDS)
intrauterine growth retardation (IUGR)
intraventricular hemorrhage
macrosomia
meconium aspiration syndrome
necrotizing enterocolitis (NEC)
ophthalmia neonatorum
patent ductus arteriosus (PDA)
periventricular hemorrhage
periventricular leukomalacia
persistent pulmonary hypertension of the newborn (PPHN)
phenylketonuria
physiologic jaundice
postmaturity
prematurity
retinopathy of prematurity (ROP)

The physiologic and potentially pathologic effects of pregnancy on the maternal system were detailed in Chapter 32. In this chapter, pregnancy is viewed from the other side of the placenta, with emphasis on fetal-neonatal physiology and potential disorders developing during gestation, delivery, or the *neonatal period,* usually defined as the first month of life. The physiologic changes that occur during this period of transition to extrauterine life are proportionately greater than will ever again be experienced during the lifetime of the individual.

Overall infant mortality (death within the first year of life) is now at an all-time low in the United States, reported in 1994 at 8.3 deaths per 1000 live births.[1] Mortality continues to decline slowly, but the risk of first-year mortality is still about 2.5 times greater for black infants than white infants, and the leading causes of death differ between races. Congenital anomalies are the leading cause of mortality in white infants, whereas black infants most often die of conditions related to preterm delivery or low birth weight.

Many congenital defects have been detailed previously in chapters related to the major organ systems. Processes underlying defective organ system development were discussed in Chapter 6. In this chapter, the structure and function of the fetal-neonatal systems and the processes of adaptation to extrauterine life are discussed. The most significant neonatal disorders relate to abnormal length of gestation (**prematurity** and **postmaturity**) or to insufficient fetal development during gestation (**intrauterine growth retardation**). These conditions and their related disorders are discussed in this chapter. Three congenital disorders that affect multiple body systems and that are usually evident during the neonatal period are also detailed: **phenylketonuria**, **fetal alcohol syndrome**, and **Down syndrome.**

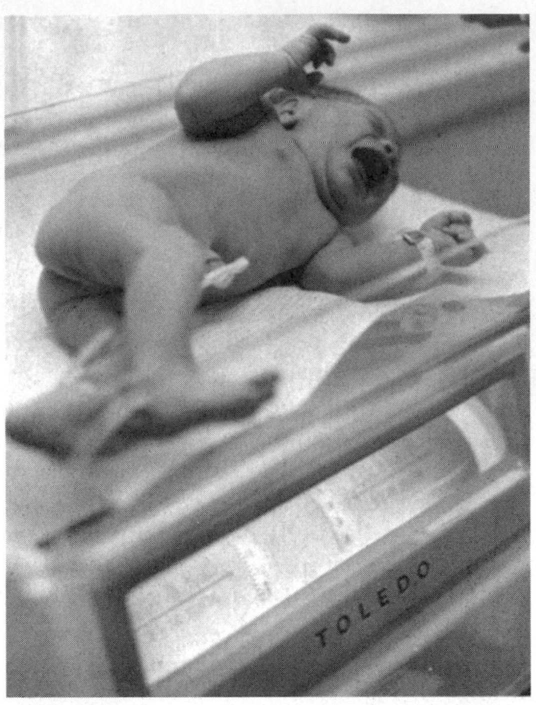

FIGURE 33–1
Full-term infant. At term, the newborn has apparent subcutaneous fat stores. The neck and extremities are short and flexed. The skin is slightly reddened, with some lanugo (fine hair) on the shoulders and arms. The head is slightly large in proportion to the body and may appear elongated because of molding during labor and delivery. (From Thompson, E.D. [1995]. *Introduction to Maternity and Pediatric Nursing.* [2nd ed.]. Philadelphia: W.B. Saunders. [p. 304].)

ANATOMY OF THE NEONATE

Term Infant

Figures 33–1 and 33–2, which contrast the general appearances of the term infant and the premature infant, illustrate the final developmental changes that normally occur late in gestation. The size of the term infant, born after 38 to 42 weeks' gestation, is deemed appropriate for gestational age (AGA) if the infant weighs about 3200 g (7 pounds) and is about 49 cm (19 inches) long. Much normal variation is possible as a result of characteristics inherited from the infant's parents.

Length of gestation as determined by the mother's recollection of the date of the last menstrual period is often inaccurate, because of faulty memory and because of possible confusion related to the slight vaginal bleeding that may occur with implantation of the blastocyst. Weight and length assume more importance in determining the possible presence of abnormality if they are correlated with an accurate estimation of the infant's gestational age, which may be obtained from standardized assessment of the infant's physical and behavioral characteristics (Fig. 33–3).

Infants are classified as small for gestational age (SGA) if they fall below the 10th percentile for height and weight at a given gestational age, and as large for gestational age (LGA) if they are above the 90th percentile. Low birth weight (LBW), regardless of gestational age, is highly correlated with neonatal morbidity and mortality. Low birth weight is defined as 500 to 2499 g and contains the subclasses of very low birth weight (VLBW), defined as less than 1500 g, and extremely low birth weight (ELBW), defined as less than 1000 g. During the past decade, survival of VLBW infants has increased markedly as a result of the introduction of exogenous surfactant therapy for the treatment of the **infant respiratory**

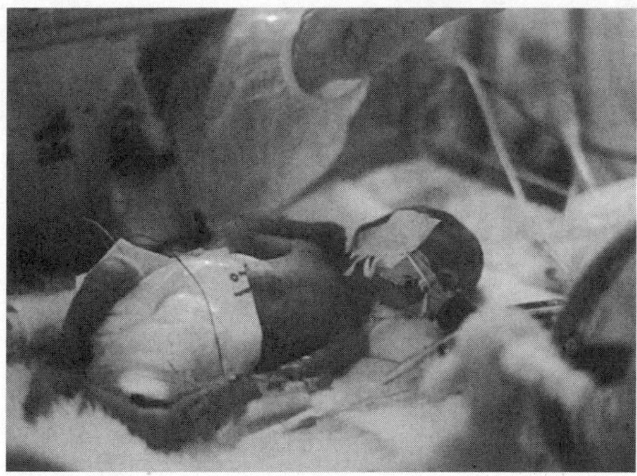

FIGURE 33–2
Premature infant. The premature infant appears very lean, with underdeveloped flexor muscles and diminished muscle tone. The extremities are extended. The skin is thin and friable, with clearly visible vessels. Lanugo covers most of the skin. The head appears very large in proportion to the body. (From Mahan, K., and Escott-Stump, S. [1996]. *Krause's Food, Nutrition, and Diet Therapy: A Textbook of Nutritional Care.* [9th ed.]. Philadelphia: W.B. Saunders. [p. 235].)

distress syndrome (IRDS) associated with immaturity of the lungs. Prematurity and IRDS are discussed later in this chapter.

The head of the neonate is proportionately large in comparison with the body and may transiently appear elongated because of molding during labor and delivery. The face may appear edematous for a time because of the trauma of delivery, and some asymmetry may be apparent as a result of the infant's position in utero. Subcutaneous fat stores are evident. The baby's abdomen protrudes slightly, and the stump of the umbilical cord sloughs off by the 10th day. The neck and extremities are short and flexed, approximating the intrauterine position. Skin appears reddened the first few days after birth, and some **acrocyanosis** is common, especially with crying, as a result of incomplete circulatory adaptation. Lanugo (fine, downy hair) may cover the shoulders and arms. Vernix caseosa, a cheesy-white secretion, is apparent in skin folds of the axilla, genitalia, and neck. A yellow tinge to the skin and sclerae (**physiologic jaundice**) may become apparent during the first few days because of lysis of fetal red blood cells and hepatic immaturity. The testes of the male infant are normally fully descended, but they may retract upward through the inguinal canal during periods of cold stress. The female genitalia are engorged with blood for a short time after birth because of the influence of maternal hormones that have crossed the placenta. These hormones may also cause some enlargement and discharge from the breasts of male and female infants.

Preterm Infant

The infant born prematurely demonstrates fetal anatomy consistent with shortened gestation. Because the current limit of viability is estimated at 23 weeks,[2] fetal development from that period to term is relevant to prematurity. At 26 weeks, some body fat is apparent, but the infant still appears very lean. The flexor muscles are underdeveloped and muscle tone is somewhat diminished. Little cartilage is evident, and plantar creases are absent. The skin is thin and transparent, with visible blood vessels. Lanugo and vernix caseosa are more extensive than in the term neonate. The baby's head is significantly larger than the body until 36 weeks. During the last 2 months of gestation, about 14 g of body fat are gained each day.

FETAL AND NEONATAL PHYSIOLOGY

In contrast to the embryonic period, the fetal period (which begins at the 9th week of gestation) is characterized by very little organ system differentiation. Most organ systems are therefore less vulnerable to teratogens during the fetal period (see Chapter 6). Through processes of hypertrophy and hyperplasia, fetal organ systems grow in size and attain functional capacity. Some anatomic differences and functional immaturity are still evident at term, however, as discussed in the following sections.

Cardiovascular System

The transition between fetal circulation and neonatal circulation is critical to independent existence of the newborn. The fetal circulation, illustrated in Figure 33–4, demonstrates the dependence of the fetus on maternal systems and placental exchange of oxygen and carbon dioxide, nutrients, and metabolic wastes.

Placental blood enters the fetal circulation via the umbilical vein, which enters the hepatic portal microcirculation and then the fetal vena cava either directly or via the *ductus venosus*. The ductus venosus is a specialized fetal vascular channel that shunts 40% to 60% of fetal venous flow past the immature liver to the heart. Half of the blood entering the right atrium is shunted directly to the left atrium through an opening in the septum, the *foramen ovale*, bypassing the collapsed fetal lungs. The remaining blood in the right atrium passes through the right ventricle into the pulmonary artery. Be-

Estimation of Gestational Age

NEUROMUSCULAR MATURITY

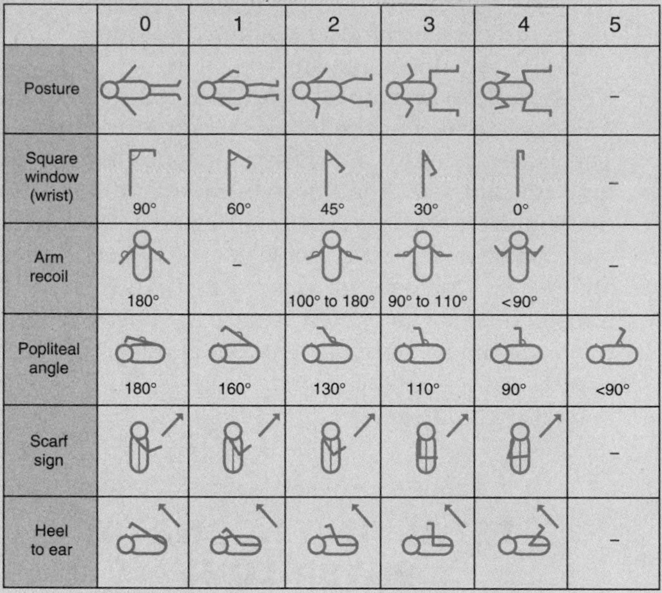

	0	1	2	3	4	5
Posture						–
Square window (wrist)	90°	60°	45°	30°	0°	–
Arm recoil	180°	–	100° to 180°	90° to 110°	<90°	–
Popliteal angle	180°	160°	130°	110°	90°	<90°
Scarf sign						–
Heel to ear						–

Gestation by dates ______

Birth date ______ Hour ______

APGAR ______ 1 min ______

MATURITY RATING

Score	Wks
5	26
10	28
15	30
20	32
25	34
30	36
35	38
40	40
45	42
50	44

PHYSICAL MATURITY

	0	1	2	3	4	5
Skin	Gelatinous, red, transparent	Smooth, pink visible veins	Superficial peeling and /or rash; few veins	Cracking pale areas, rare veins	Parchment, deep cracking, no veins	Leathery, cracked, wrinkled
Lanugo	None	Abundant	Thinning	Bald areas	Mostly bald	–
Plantar creases	No crease	Faint red marks	Anterior transverse crease only	Creases anterior 2/3	Creases over entire sole	–
Breast	Barely perceptible	Flat areola; no bud	Stippled areola; 1–2 mm bud	Raised areola; 3–4 mm bud	Full areola; 5–10 mm bud	–
Ear	Pinna flat, stays folded	Slightly curved pinna; soft, slow recoil	Well-curved pinna; soft but ready recoil	Formed and firm with instant recoil	Thick cartilage, ear stiff	–
Genitals male	Scrotum empty, no rugae	–	Testes descending, few rugae	Testes down, good rugae	Testes pendulous, deep rugae	–
Genitals female	Prominent clitoris & labia minora	–	Majora & minora equally prominent	Majora large, minora small	Clitoris & minora completely covered	–

SCORING SECTION

	1st Exam = X	2nd Exam = O
Estimating gestational age by maturity rating	______ Weeks	______ Weeks
Time of exam	Dates ______ Hours ______ am pm	Dates ______ Hours ______ am pm
Age at exam	______ Hours	______ Hours
Signature of examiner	______ ______ M.D.	______ ______ M.D.

FIGURE 33–3

Assessment of gestational age. A simplified scoring system for estimating gestational age on the basis of physical signs and neuromuscular maturity is illustrated. (Redrawn from Ballard, J.L., *et al.* [1977]. A simplified assessment of gestational age. *Pediatric Research* 11, 374. Figures adapted from Sweet, A.Y. [1977]. Classification of the low-birth-weight infant. In: Klaus, M.H., and Fanaroff, A.A. *Care of the High-Risk Infant*. Philadelphia: W.B. Saunders.)

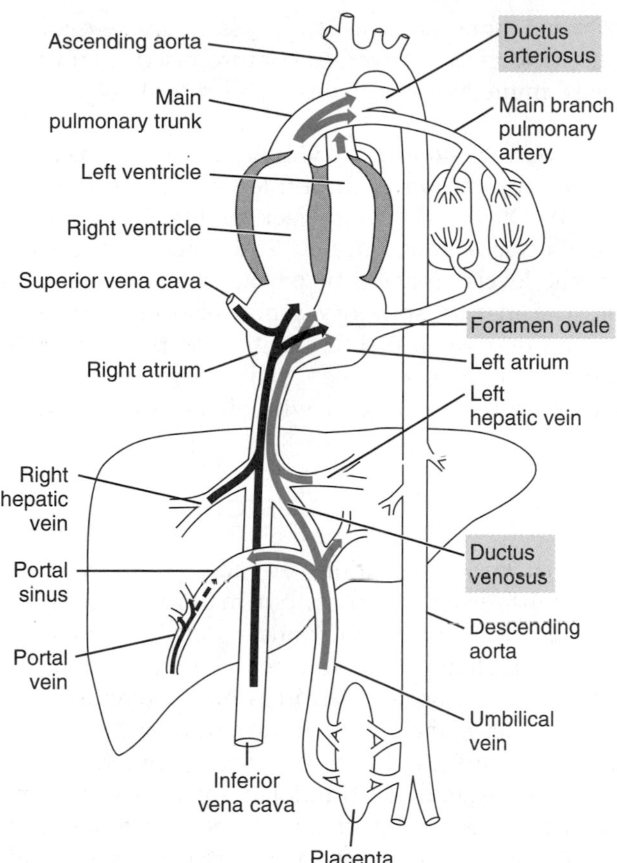

FIGURE 33–4

Fetal circulation. Placental blood enters the fetal circulation via the umbilical vein, which enters the hepatic portal micrcocirculation and then the vena cava either directly or through the *ductus venosus,* which shunts about half of the fetal venous blood past the immature liver to the heart. Half of the blood entering the right atrium is shunted into the left atrium through the *foramen ovale,* an opening in the atrial septum. The remaining right atrial blood enters the right ventricle and the pulmonary artery, where more than 90% of it is shunted across the *ductus arteriosus* to the descending aorta. From the aorta, fetal blood enters the placenta via the two umbilical arteries. Structures are illustrated schematically, not anatomically.

cause of the high pulmonary vascular resistance (PVR) within the collapsed lungs, only about 5% to 10% of the right ventricular output perfuses the lungs. Most pulmonary arterial blood follows the path of least resistance across the *ductus arteriosus* to the descending aorta. From the descending aorta, fetal blood enters the placenta via the two umbilical arteries. In 0.25% to 1% of deliveries, the umbilical cord has only a single umbilical artery. This anomaly is associated with other malformations in 25% to 50% of cases, such as renal defects, tracheoesophageal fistula, and central nervous (CNS) abnormalities.[2]

At delivery, the low-resistance placenta is removed from the circulation and the infant initiates respiratory efforts that expand the lungs, lowering PVR (see Chapter 15). The gradients that mediated flow through the three fetal shunts are thus reduced, decreasing flow and facilitating closure of these structures. When left atrial pressure exceeds right, an overriding flap of tissue closes the foramen ovale, separating the atria. The ductus venosus closes when the umbilical vein is clamped, effectively stopping blood flow. Functional closure resulting from altered pressure gradients is soon followed by anatomic closure caused by fibrosis.

The circular smooth muscle of the ductus arteriosus constricts after birth in response to the higher oxygen content of the blood flowing through it. Responsiveness of the ductal smooth muscle to oxygen increases throughout fetal life, creating a tendency toward constriction that is opposed by the action of prostaglandin E_2, produced by cells of the ductus itself as well as by the placenta and umbilical vessels. Removal of these prostaglandin sources at delivery is also important to functional closure of the ductus, which normally occurs within 24 hours. Delayed closure of the ductus arteriosus is very common in neonatal conditions in which PVR is elevated, such as IRDS and **persistent pulmonary hypertension of the newborn (PPHN).** Prolonged **patent ductus arteriosus (PDA)** is one of a number of congenital heart defects that may precipitate congestive heart failure. PDA and pulmonary hypertension are discussed in detail in Chapters 16 and 19, respectively.

The fetal circulation is characterized by a lower partial pressure of oxygen (PO_2) than the maternal circulation, as discussed in Chapter 32. Fetal tissues are normally well oxygenated, however, because the structure of fetal hemoglobin confers a higher affinity for oxygen, shifting the oxyhemoglobin-dissociation curve to the left and facilitating oxygen uptake by fetal blood (see Chapter 19). Fetal hemoglobin concentration is also significantly higher than adult hemoglobin, and increased erythropoiesis occurs in response to any intrauterine hypoxic condition.

During the first week of life, neonatal hemoglobin concentration falls to a level that is lower than adult norms, because of increased hemolysis of red blood cells containing fetal hemoglobin. Potentially fatal hemolysis (**hemolytic disease of the newborn**) may occur in utero or soon after birth in cases of Rh incompatibility (see Chapter 13). The newborn is more prone to bleed during the first few days of life because of the lack of intestinal colonization with bacteria that synthesize vitamin K (see Chapter 14). Routine administration of vitamin K at birth counteracts this risk.

Respiratory System

The precise stimulus for initial ventilatory efforts at birth is uncertain. At term, the fetal lungs contain a volume of fluid approximately equal to the functional residual capacity, or the volume of air normally retained in the lungs at the end of a passive expiration (see Chapter 18). Much of this fluid is cleared during labor, although not as a consequence of mechanical compression of the fetal chest, as once believed.[4] Rather, lung fluid is apparently reabsorbed into the pulmonary blood because of changes in the pulmonary epithelium. Active sodium reabsorption pulls water along an osmotic gradient, and the action of this "sodium pump" is increased during labor and the early neonatal period. Persistent lung fluid is seen more often in infants delivered prematurely or by cesarean section.

Gravitational drainage or suctioning of fluid from the upper airways is done to clear airways, but both inspiration and expiration require muscular effort at first. Exposure to cold, physical stress of delivery, the catecholamine surge occurring at birth, and manual stimulation may have excitatory effects on neurons of the medullary respiratory center. Initial ventilatory efforts are inadequate in fully exchanging oxygen and carbon dioxide, resulting in falling Po_2, rising partial pressure of carbon dioxide (Pco_2), and falling pH (acidosis). Chemoreceptor-mediated stimulation of the respiratory center thus occurs. Each breath meets with less resistance as the lungs continue to expand, increasing pulmonary compliance and functional residual capacity (see Chapter 18).

At 1 minute and again at 5 minutes after birth, an *Apgar score* is determined based on observation of the infant's heart rate, respiratory effort, reflex irritability, muscle tone, and color (Table 33–1).[5] Each observation area is scored from 0 to 2, and the five scores added. An Apgar score of 7 to 10 indicates that the infant is vigorous and will need no further resuscitation. A score of 3 to 6 indicates mild-to-moderate respiratory depression and a possible need for intubation and ventilatory assistance. A score of 0 to 2 indicates a severely compromised infant who needs immediate intubation and ventilatory assistance.

Presence of *surfactant* normally assists in overcoming surface tension in fluid-filled airways (see Chapter 18). During the first week of life, lung compliance increases and airway resistance decreases to normal levels. Sensitivity of the chemoreceptors of the medullary respiratory center also increases during the first week of life. Ventilation-perfusion relationships normalize when pulmonary vascular resistance falls concurrently with airway expansion.

Renal System

By 34 weeks' gestation, the adult number of nephrons has been achieved, but nephrons are neither full-sized nor fully functional. Renal vascular resistance is high, reducing fetal circulation to the kidneys. The placenta performs most excretory functions in utero, and the fetal kidneys mainly produce amniotic fluid. At birth, the renin–angiotensin–aldosterone system is stimulated by decreased renal blood flow. Secretion of antidiuretic hormone is increased, possibly in response to release of catecholamines, prostaglandins, or other mediators of stress. Fluid retention, increased blood volume, and selective distribution of blood to vital organs occurs. Withdrawal of maternal hormones may also account for some of the increase in extracellular fluid seen in newborns during the first few days.

Renal vascular resistance decreases rapidly, the glomerular filtration rate (GFR) increases, and a period of diuresis follows, contributing to the loss of 5% to 10% of the birth weight that commonly occurs during the first week of life. Urine output increases to 250 to 400 mL/24 hours by 1 month of age, with

TABLE 33–1
APGAR SCORING SYSTEM

Observation	Score 0	Score 1	Score 2
Heart rate	Absent	Slow (<100)	>100
Respiratory effort	Absent	Slow, irregular, shallow	Good, sustained cry; regular respirations
Reflex irritability	No response	Grimace, frown	Sneeze, cough, cry
Muscle tone	Limp, completely flaccid	Some flexion of extremities; some resistance to extension of extremities	Active motion, good muscle tone, spontaneous flexion
Color	Cyanotic, pale	Body pink, extremities pale	Completely pink

From Apgar, V. (1953). A proposal for a new method of evaluating the newborn infant. *Current Research in Anesthesia and Analgesia.* Jul/Aug, 260.

a maximum urine osmolarity of 600 to 800 mOsm/L (about half that of maximum adult levels). The newborn has a higher ratio of body water to body mass than older children and adults, increasing risk of significant dehydration with vomiting, diarrhea, or fever. During the period when GFR is decreased, infants are at increased risk of toxicity caused by drugs that must be cleared by the kidneys.

Gastrointestinal System

Fetal gastrointestinal (GI) function is essentially limited to swallowing of amniotic fluid and formation of the first stool *(meconium)*. Digestion and absorption of nutrients and elimination of wastes are accomplished by the maternal system. At birth, the immature gut wall is more permeable to antigenic proteins, bacteria, and bilirubin, conferring increased risk of allergy, infection, and physiologic jaundice. Initiation of feeding induces the increased secretion of a number of peptide hormones that increase the motility and secretion of the alimentary canal.

Passage of meconium is also essential to establishment of GI function, and usually occurs within 24 hours of birth. Failure to pass meconium may indicate presence of congenital bowel obstruction (see Chapter 24) or cystic fibrosis (see Chapter 18). Fetal hypoxia or other factors may lead to passage of meconium into the amniotic fluid, with subsequent aspiration in utero or during delivery. Meconium aspiration is one of several mechanisms of **asphyxia** discussed later in this chapter.

Neural pathways for reflex coordination of sucking, swallowing, and breathing are not completely developed until about 38 weeks' gestation, which may increase the risk of aspiration in preterm infants. However, the oropharynx of the term infant is small because of elevation of the larynx, facilitating nipple feeding and ingestion of liquids without aspiration (see Chapter 25). Decreased tone and location of the lower esophageal sphincter above the diaphragm contribute to the reflux (spitting up) that is common in neonates. Immaturity of the smooth muscle of the GI tract results in slower, more disorganized contraction and decreased motility. Surface cells are also immature, with fewer villi and epithelial cells than adults, decreasing surface area for absorption. Enteral feeding induces maturation of these tissues.

Hepatobiliary System

The fetal liver is largely bypassed in utero, because the maternal liver fulfills the synthetic and conjugation functions required by the fetus. After birth, the liver is very active in hematopoiesis for a few weeks. If maternal iron intake was adequate, hepatic iron stores should be sufficient to support hematopoiesis for several months, after which supplementation may be required. Increased glycogen storage begins at birth, and liver enzyme systems for biotransformation of drugs and hormones gradually mature as the smooth endoplasmic reticulum develops.

Metabolism of bilirubin is depressed during the last month of gestation to route bilirubin across the placenta for metabolism by the maternal liver and excretion in the bile. Depressed conjugation enzymes and increased bilirubin load caused by hemolysis result in physiologic jaundice (*icterus neonatorum*) in 50% of full-term and 80% of preterm infants (see Chapter 26). Physiologic jaundice is usually evident *after* the first 24 hours and may be prolonged in infants who are breast fed.

Hepatic synthesis of protein clotting factors XI, XII, and XIII is reduced at birth. Platelet counts are normal, but platelets are functionally immature. Phototherapy for treatment of physiologic jaundice worsens platelet dysfunction, contributing to bleeding tendencies.

Inflammatory and Immune Responses

The neonate is at increased risk of sepsis because of immaturity of host defense systems. The inflammatory response is relatively ineffective in walling off infections because of reduced activity of neutrophils (see Chapter 13). Neonatal neutrophils are less flexible and less mobile. Deficiency of serum chemotactic factors also contributes to reduction of the inflammatory response. Phagocytic activity may or may not be affected, but complement proteins are reduced by at least 50%. The hypothalamic thermal response to pyrogenic organisms is also reduced (see Chapter 11). Decreased local and systemic signs of inflammation complicate clinical detection of sepsis in newborns.

Both B-cell and T-cell activity are reduced in neonates. Immunoglobulin G (IgG) crosses the placenta beginning in the third month and accounts almost entirely for immunoglobulin levels, which are 55% to 80% of adult values. The other immunoglobulins, IgA, IgM, IgD, and IgE, do not cross the placenta in clinically significant amounts, although the fetus may produce IgM in response to intrauterine infection after about 20 weeks. Breast-fed infants receive maternal IgA. Numbers of T cells are consistent with adult levels, but lymphokine secretion and cytotoxic activity are significantly reduced. Activity of T suppressors exceeds that of T helpers. Immaturity of physical barriers such as the gut wall, skin, and mucous membranes increases the risk of sepsis in the newborn, as do maternal infections and vaginal delivery. Clinical features of the more significant neonatal infections are summarized in Table 33–2.

Integumentary System

Epidermal thickness increases with gestational and postnatal age. Cohesion between the epidermis and dermis is decreased in neonates, and dermal collagen and elastin are immature, increasing the risk of skin injury caused by shearing (frictional) forces as well as the risk of absorption of toxic substances through the skin. Preterm infants have markedly increased skin permeability, epidermal water content, and transepidermal water loss until about 2 weeks after delivery, when their skin function is similar to that of a term infant. Skin pH at birth is relatively alkaline, but pH declines within a few days. This protective "acid mantle" apparently results from eccrine gland activity and alterations in surface lipids. Colonization of skin with normal flora bacteria begins at birth and conveys protection against invasive pathogens.

Nervous System

Neonatal sensory function is immature, but more functional than was once believed. The sense of touch develops earliest during gestation, followed by smell, proprioception, taste, hearing, and vision. Also contrary to earlier belief, neonates *do* perceive pain, demonstrating a stress response to painful stimuli. Vision is relatively acute at birth, particularly within close range, and improves rapidly during the first few months of life. In the United States, antibiotic prophylaxis against **ophthalmia neonatorum**, infection of the conjunctiva of the neonate caused by organisms acquired during vaginal delivery, is legally mandated. Auditory acuity in neonates is best for lower frequencies. Vestibular system function is well developed, as evidenced by infants' responsiveness to rocking and other rhythmic movements.

Neonates spend much of their time sleeping, with sleep–wake cycles independent of light-dark exposures. Coordination of sleep–wake cycles is especially chaotic for a few days after birth, with increased alertness typical. Infants then establish their own, highly individual patterns as their neurologic development continues. *State modulation* is the ability of the infant to make smooth transitions between sleep and wake states. Lack of this ability (*state oscillation*) is characteristic of prematurity or infant discomfort caused by pain or stress.

Motor activity in neonates is largely reflexive. The *primitive reflexes* exhibited by neonates gradually disappear with motor system maturation, reappearing later in life only in cases of motor system pathology (see Chapter 22).

Immaturity of systems for regulation of cerebral blood flow increases the risk of **intraventricular hemorrhage** or **periventricular hemorrhage**, particularly in preterm infants. The *subependymal germinal matrix*, a structure located near the ventricles, is richly perfused with very fragile capillaries. This vascular structure is largest at about 28 weeks' gestation, after which it begins to decrease in size (involute). Involution, which decreases the risk of hemorrhage, continues throughout the third trimester and the neonatal period. Any condition that increases cerebral blood flow, such as hypoxemia, hypercapnia, acidosis, pain, or stress, may precipitate hemorrhage from the matrix.

Hypoxic conditions may also damage neural cells directly. Ischemic episodes early in gestation often lead to necrosis of white matter surrounding the ventricles (**periventricular leukomalacia**) or elsewhere in the brain. Periventricular leukomalacia is often seen in children with cerebral palsy (see Chapter 22). Later in gestation (after 34 weeks), most cerebral blood flow is directed to the cerebral cortex. Hypoxic conditions during this period may contribute to later cortical dysfunction. Neonatal seizures may result from hypoxia, electrolyte imbalance, or hypoglycemia, and repeated seizure activity may further damage the developing nervous system.

Thermoregulation

Because of their increased ratio of body surface area to body mass, decreased amounts of insulating subcutaneous fat, and increased skin permeability to water, neonates readily lose heat to the environment. Term infants rely heavily on nonshivering thermogenesis via brown fat metabolism for heat production (see Chapter 11). Brown fat develops in tissues of the neck, thorax, and abdomen, beginning at 26 to 30 weeks' gestation and continuing through the neonatal period. Lack of brown fat contributes to hypothermia in preterm infants. Sweat gland activity in infants is about one third that of adults, but this is easily offset by increased transepidermal water loss.

TABLE 33–2
COMMON INFECTIONS DURING THE NEONATAL PERIOD

Disorder	Usual Pathogens	Comments
Ophthalmia neonatorum	*Chlamydia trachomatis*	Conjunctival infection caused by maternal STD; newborn prophylaxis is mandatory although incidence is low in U.S. (8.2/1000 live births)
Neonatal sepsis	Group B streptococci *Escherichia coli* *Listeria monocytogenes* *Pseudomonas*	Mothers colonized with group B streptococci may infect healthy infants VLBW infants may develop sepsis caused by normal flora organisms Meningitis and septicemia are the usual presentations
HIV infection	Human immunodeficiency virus type I	May be transmitted antepartally, intrapartally, or postpartally; may be transmitted via breast milk Premature rupture of the membranes enhances risk of transmission 15% to 20% develop AIDS in the first year of life
Hepatitis B	Hepatitis B virus	May be acquired from mother via infected vaginal secretions, amniotic fluid, blood, saliva, or breast milk Infant may or may not develop fulminant liver failure
Candidiasis	*Candida albicans*	Normal vaginal flora in 10% to 30% of healthy women Usually affects mouth (thrush) and skinfold areas
Omphalitis	*Staphylococcus aureus* *E. coli*	Infection of the umbilical stump Umbilical artery catheters may contribute to subsequent sepsis
Necrotizing enterocolitis	*E. coli* *Clostridium* species	Normal bowel flora may contribute to pathogenesis
TORCH infections	*Toxoplasma gondii* Other infections (syphilis, varicella, parvovirus B19) Rubella Cytomegalovirus Herpes simplex	Cytomegalovirus is the most common cause of congenital infection in the U.S.; occurs in 1% of all newborns; infection occurs via transplacental passage of virus from mother; may cause sensorineural deafness and mental retardation Congenital toxoplasmosis may occur with initial maternal infection during pregnancy; cats serve as host for parasite; may cause severe CNS defects Herpes simplex and syphilis are STDs increasing in incidence and associated with intrauterine (syphilis) or intrapartum (herpes) infection of newborns; may cause severe CNS defects Risk of dissemination of maternal varicella to fetus is low Parvovirus B19 (which causes fifth disease) is usually not associated with adverse outcomes Congenital rubella is highly teratogenic, but incidence is low since advent of MMR vaccine

STD, sexually transmitted disease; HIV, human immunodeficiency virus; AIDS, acquired immunodeficiency syndrome; CNS, central nervous system; MMR, measles, mumps, rubella.

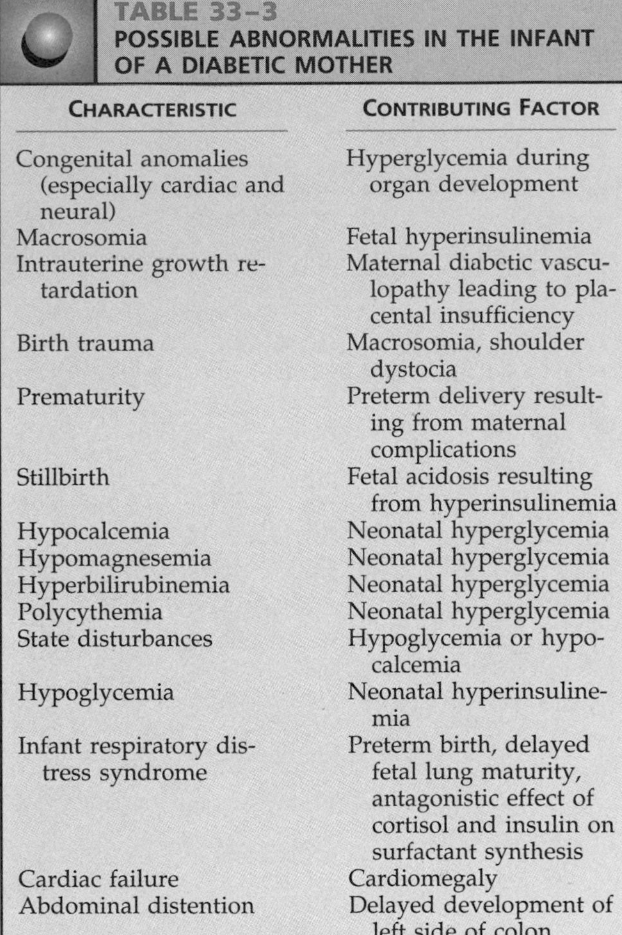

TABLE 33–3
POSSIBLE ABNORMALITIES IN THE INFANT OF A DIABETIC MOTHER

Characteristic	Contributing Factor
Congenital anomalies (especially cardiac and neural)	Hyperglycemia during organ development
Macrosomia	Fetal hyperinsulinemia
Intrauterine growth retardation	Maternal diabetic vasculopathy leading to placental insufficiency
Birth trauma	Macrosomia, shoulder dystocia
Prematurity	Preterm delivery resulting from maternal complications
Stillbirth	Fetal acidosis resulting from hyperinsulinemia
Hypocalcemia	Neonatal hyperglycemia
Hypomagnesemia	Neonatal hyperglycemia
Hyperbilirubinemia	Neonatal hyperglycemia
Polycythemia	Neonatal hyperglycemia
State disturbances	Hypoglycemia or hypocalcemia
Hypoglycemia	Neonatal hyperinsulinemia
Infant respiratory distress syndrome	Preterm birth, delayed fetal lung maturity, antagonistic effect of cortisol and insulin on surfactant synthesis
Cardiac failure	Cardiomegaly
Abdominal distention	Delayed development of left side of colon

Nutrition and Metabolism

Sudden removal of the maternal source of glucose at birth, together with the low level of glycogen storage by the fetal liver, may lead to mild hypoglycemia. The neonate relies on adipose and protein stores for some energy metabolism, which may contribute to early weight loss until breast or bottle feeding is well established. The term neonate has sufficient pancreatic and intestinal enzyme activity to digest most simple carbohydrates, proteins, and fats, but these may not be well absorbed in preterm infants. Calcium needed for ossification of bones is provided with breast or formula feeding, and other minerals and vitamins needed for tissue growth may be supplemented as necessary.

The **infant of a diabetic mother (IDM)** is often LGA and at higher risk for asphyxia and birth trauma at delivery. Increased levels of glucose during gestation trigger a resulting hyperplasia of fetal islet cells to increase insulin secretion. Fetal insulin permits increased systemic growth and fat deposition. After delivery, removal of maternal glucose may trigger a more severe hypoglycemia in these infants because of high levels of circulating insulin. IDMs are at higher risk for congenital anomalies and neonatal complications, as summarized in Table 33–3.

NEONATAL DISORDERS

Major congenital defects affecting specific organ systems are listed in Table 33–4, with reference to the chapters in which they are discussed. Three systemic congenital disorders are detailed in this section. The primary emphasis of *neonatology* is on the care of infants who are born too soon or too small. That emphasis is also apparent in the section that follows. The clinical syndromes seen in these infants

TABLE 33–4
SELECTED CONGENITAL DISORDERS

Body System	Disorders	Chapter
Hematopoietic	Sickle cell anemia	12
	Hereditary spherocytosis	12
	Polycythemia vera	12
	Porphyria	12
	Severe combined immunodeficiency	13
	Hemophilia	14
	von Willebrand disease	14
Cardiovascular	Congenital heart defects	16
	Wolff-Parkinson-White syndrome	17
Respiratory	Cystic fibrosis	18
Renal-urinary	Polycystic kidney disease	20
Nervous	Neural tube defects	21
	Epilepsy	21
	Hydrocephalus	21
	Cerebral palsy	22
	Cataracts	23
Gastrointestinal	Hirschsprung's disease	24
	Hypertrophic pyloric stenosis	24
	Esophageal atresia	24
	Cleft lip and palate	25
	Biliary atresia	26
Endocrine	Pituitary dwarfism	27
	Congenital hypothyroidism	28
	Congenital adrenal hyperplasia	29
Reproductive	Cryptorchidism	30
Multisystemic	Phenylketonuria	33
	Fetal alcohol syndrome	33
	Down syndrome	33
Musculoskeletal	Scoliosis	34
	Muscular dystrophy	35

may also occur in term infants, although that is less often the case.

Prematurity

Definition. Prematurity is delivery of a viable infant before the 37th week of gestation.

Epidemiology. Approximately 9% of infants in the United States are born prematurely.[6] Risk factors for premature labor include maternal factors such as infection, systemic illness, trauma, or uterine abnormalities; fetal factors such as multiple gestation or polyhydramnios; and iatrogenic factors such as premature elective induction of labor or cesarean section resulting from inaccurate assessment of gestational age (see Chapter 32). The increased risk of preterm labor in nonwhites and in those with lower socioeconomic status has been attributed to lifestyle factors such as substance abuse and lack of prenatal care.

Etiology. The precise etiology of preterm labor is unknown in most cases (see Chapter 32). About 30% of preterm labors begin with premature rupture of the membranes.

Pathophysiology. The stress of labor and delivery superimposed on immaturity of the fetal organ systems results in the pathophysiologic effects of prematurity. Mechanisms underlying specific clinical manifestations are discussed in the next section.

Clinical Manifestations. The most significant manifestations of prematurity are respiratory failure, hypothermia, cardiac failure, anemia, renal insufficiency, necrotizing enterocolitis, intracranial hemorrhage, and retinopathy.

Respiratory Failure. Respiratory failure accounts for most morbidity and mortality in premature infants. Infant respiratory distress syndrome (IRDS), also known as hyaline membrane disease, may occur in term infants, but is much more common in prematurity. With birth before the onset of sufficient surfactant production (at 28 to 30 weeks), alveoli and terminal airways are difficult to inflate and collapse easily because of increased surface tension (see Chapter 18). Fetal lung maturity may be evaluated clinically by the ratio of the surface-active phospholipids lecithin and sphingomyelin (L/S ratio). Fetal lung maturity is demonstrated by a ratio greater than 2 : 1, and IRDS rarely occurs in these infants.[7]

Decreased lung compliance and poor inspiratory muscle development further impair ventilation, and immaturity of the the medullary respiratory control center leads to periods of **apnea**, or absence of ventilatory efforts. Hypoxic damage to the alveolar-capillary membrane results in "cartilage-like" (hyaline) changes within these tissues and severely impairs gas exchange, similarly to adult respiratory distress syndrome (ARDS) (see Chapter 19). The precise mechanism of membrane damage in IRDS is unknown, but it may relate to generation of reactive oxygen species with reperfusion of ischemic areas and with toxicity of oxygen therapy (see Chapters 3 and 18).[8]

Meconium aspiration syndrome may be present in premature, postmature, or other high-risk infants who are meconium-stained at birth. Meconium passage in utero is probably a maturational event in fetuses after 37 weeks' gestation, but it may indicate fetal hypoxia or acidosis in others. Gasping activity induced by hypoxia may lead to aspiration of meconium into the airways in utero or during labor and delivery. About 10% of all fetuses pass meconium in utero, mandating careful suctioning of the upper airways before the first breath at delivery to minimize aspiration risk. Meconium aspiration produces respiratory distress caused by mechanical obstruction of airways and an inflammatory response induced by locally irritating components of meconium.

Meconium aspiration is commonly associated with persistent pulmonary hypertension of the newborn (PPHN), although surfactant deficiency, lung hypoplasia, and neonatal pneumonia may also contribute to PPHN.[9] In many cases, no etiology is apparent.[10] In PPHN, pulmonary vasoconstriction results in sustained elevation of pulmonary vascular resistance, probably because of local imbalance in vasodilator and vasoconstrictor substances. The normal left-to-right pressure gradient between the systemic and pulmonary vascular systems is not established, and closure of the foramen ovale and ductus arteriosus is inhibited. Hypoxemic respiratory failure and potential cardiac failure ensue because of right-to-left shunting (see Chapter 16).

Bronchopulmonary dysplasia (BPD), also known as chronic lung disease of the newborn, is one of the most significant iatrogenic disorders of neonates. More than 75% of cases occur in premature infants weighing less than 1000 g.[11] BPD follows ventilator and oxygen therapy for neonatal respiratory failure. It is characterized by chronic respiratory distress, persistent hypoxemia when breathing room air, and abnormal chest radiograph ("cobblestone" appearance of lungs caused by scarring and areas of atelectasis or hyperinflation) at 1 month of age. BPD is caused by high airway pressures (barotrauma) and oxygen toxicity, both of which directly injure the lung and induce an inflammatory response (see Chapter 18).

Hypothermia. Cold stress in premature infants may result from immaturity of hypothalamic control, lack of brown fat and adipose insulation, evaporative cooling with increased transepidermal water loss, and inefficient energy metabolism (see Chapter 11). Hypothermia may worsen respiratory status as the infant's basal metabolic rate increases to produce heat, resulting in increased oxygen demand. Failure to gain weight is common, because oxygen and nutrients are diverted to heat production rather than tissue synthesis. Metabolic acidosis and hypoglycemia may also result from the increased metabolic demands of cold stress.

Cardiac Failure. Congestive heart failure (CHF), with resultant pulmonary edema, may also compromise respiratory status (see Chapter 16). CHF may be caused by immaturity of the left ventricle or by high right ventricular afterload resulting from increased pulmonary vascular resistance. Patent ductus arteriosus (PDA) occurs in the majority of LBW infants because of persistent high pressure in the pulmonary circulation, and it may also contribute to cardiac failure.

Anemia. Many premature infants develop a normocytic, normochromic anemia (**anemia of prematurity**) between 6 and 10 weeks of age, resulting from a blunted erythropoietin response to tissue hypoxemia (see Chapter 12).[12] This condition is usually self-limited, but some infants may require transfusion.

Renal Insufficiency. Renal insufficiency is common in preterm infants because of immaturity of nephron function. If the infant has suffered asphyxia (oxygen deprivation during labor and delivery), the primitive **diving reflex** may be elicited. This reflex results in vasoconstriction to the kidneys and GI tract to preserve perfusion of the head and heart, and it is stimulated by lack of oxygen to the medullary vasomotor center. Decreased renal perfusion under these circumstances may precipitate renal failure (see Chapter 20).

Necrotizing Enterocolitis. Ischemia of the bowel secondary to the diving reflex may be a contributing factor in the development of **necrotizing enterocolitis (NEC),** with ischemic injury potentially resulting in bowel perforation and peritonitis (see Chapter 24). NEC is characterized by abdominal distention, trapping of gas in the bowel wall, lower GI bleeding, and possible sepsis and shock.[13] Any portion of the bowel from the stomach to the rectum may be involved, but most lesions are located in the terminal ileum or proximal colon. Immaturity of the mucosal barrier and immune responses are believed to increase the susceptibility of premature infants to NEC, and aggressive enteral feeding may trigger the inflammatory process. The involvement of bacterial toxins in causing NEC has also been hypothesized.

Intracranial Hemorrhage. Rupture of vessels of the subependymal germinal matrix is common in infants born before 28 weeks' gestation, leading to intraventricular or periventricular hemorrhage with increased intracranial pressure (see Chapter 21). Immaturity, possibly complicated by birth trauma or asphyxia, may produce CNS dysfunction manifested by jitteriness, state oscillations, and possible seizures.

Retinopathy of Prematurity. **Retinopathy of prematurity (ROP),** formerly known as retrolental fibroplasia, includes a spectrum of disorders of the retina ranging from mild myopia (nearsightedness) to blindness resulting from retinal detachment (see Chapter 23). Developing retinal vessels in premature infants are vulnerable to injury occurring either in utero or soon after birth. Retinal injury may be induced by prolonged oxygen therapy (oxygen toxicity), shock, sepsis, asphyxia, or other stressors during the perinatal or neonatal periods.[14] Developing capillaries are destroyed by the injuring agent or process, and their regrowth is delayed, excessive, and disorganized. Tortuous vessels, retinal hemorrhages, scarring, and detachment are possible (see Color Fig. 23–6). Retinopathy is usually not evident until 4 to 6 weeks after birth and may display either a regressive (stabilizing) or progressive (worsening) course.

Prevention and Treatment. Prevention of preterm labor requires reduction of risks. Healthy maternal lifestyle and optimal prenatal care are advocated in risk reduction. Surgical intervention may correct maternal reproductive system anomalies contributing to spontaneous abortion and preterm labor (see Chapter 32). When appropriate, preterm labor may be arrested with tocolytic therapy. Treatment of the mother with corticosteroids may be done to stimulate maturation of the fetal cardiovascular, respiratory, nervous, and GI systems, reducing morbidity and mortality.[15]

Treatment of the preterm infant is based on support of immature organ system function while minimizing iatrogenic risks. Exogenous surfactant is administered in definitive therapy of IRDS.[7] Oxygen therapy is often required, and mechanical ventilation or extracorporeal membrane oxygenation may be indicated (see Chapter 18). *Amnioinfusion,* the introduction of warm normal saline into the amniotic cavity during labor, has been shown to reduce the incidence of meconium aspiration syndrome.[16] Closure of a PDA is accomplished pharmacologically or surgically as soon as possible to reduce cardiac workload and pulmonary vascular resistance.

Fluid and electrolyte status are carefully monitored, with replacement as necessary. The premature infant is not fed enterally until the risk of NEC is ruled out. If NEC is present, total parenteral nutrition is administered intravenously. If the risk of aspiration is high because of poor sucking-swallowing coordination, the baby is fed through a feeding tube. The thermal environment is carefully controlled with use of isolettes, warmers, or other means. In view of the immaturity of renal and hepatic systems, drug therapy in support of system function is administered cautiously, with careful monitoring of physiologic responses.

Prognosis and Outcome. Morbidity and mortality associated with prematurity depend on the related factors of gestational age and birth weight, with the lower ranges being strongly associated with life-threatening respiratory failure and intracranial hemorrhage. Intracranial hemorrhage is usually fatal. Increased survival rates in VLBW infants have resulted from the introduction of exogenous surfactant therapy for IRDS. These children have a high incidence of chronic respiratory problems, visual defects, and neurodevelopmental disorders (see Focus of Current Research).

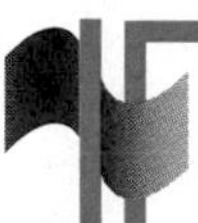

Clinical Scenario

S.A., a male infant weighing 2 lb, 8 oz, was delivered by cesarean section at 30 weeks' gestation after 5 hours of preterm labor. His spontaneous respiratory efforts were ineffective, and S.A. required intubation and mechanical ventilation in the delivery room. Surfactant was also administered. At 48 hours, S.A. demonstrated a PDA and continued to require ventilation with 60% oxygen at high inspiratory pressure. Chest radiography showed bilateral pneumonia, and blood cultures were positive for group B streptococcus. S.A. required mechanical ventilation for 40 days and was discharged on supplemental oxygen therapy.

1. What factors probably contributed to S.A.'s respiratory insufficiency?
2. Are there any iatrogenic risks in this situation?

Postmaturity

Definition. The postmature infant is one delivered after a postdate pregnancy extending beyond 42 weeks' gestation.

Epidemiology. Post-term labor occurs in an estimated 10% of all pregnancies.[17] *Primigravidas* (women pregnant for the first time), women who have given birth more than four times, and women with a history of postdate pregnancy are at higher risk. Presence of fetal anomalies or maternal disorders that reduce secretion of estrogen or cortisol may contribute to failure of initiation of spontaneous labor.

Etiology. The precise etiology of postdate pregnancy is often unknown. A severe abnormality of the fetus (e.g., anencephaly or congenital adrenal hypoplasia) (see Chapters 21 and 29) may result in lack of fetal cortisol, which normally reduces adrenal production of progesterone and increases production of estrogen precursors, tipping the balance in favor of uterine contraction. Maternal hormone imbalance may result in delayed ovulation, confounding determination of the precise onset of pregnancy and leading to misdiagnosis of postdate pregnancy.

Pathophysiology. With prolonged gestation, the placenta often begins to degenerate before delivery of the infant. Placental insufficiency may lead to intrauterine growth retardation (IUGR—discussed in the next section), meconium aspiration syndrome related to fetal stress, fetal hypoxia, and possible fetal demise.

Large fetal size (**macrosomia**) may result in dystocia during labor as well as asphyxia or birth trauma to the infant during delivery. The postmature infant is usually long and thin rather than fat, however, because body stores of fat have been used to compensate for decreased placental delivery of nutrients. With prolonged placental deficiency, the infant is small and underdeveloped.

Clinical Manifestations. Many of the clinical manifestations of postmaturity resemble those of prematurity, although organ system failure is caused by placental insufficiency or birth trauma rather than by immaturity. Signs of asphyxia and respiratory distress may be evident because of meconium aspiration or difficult delivery. Persistence of fetal shunts may result in a heart murmur and possibly CHF. Polycythemia is common if placental deficiency and hypoxia have been prolonged. The vernix is absent because of prolonged gestation, and the skin is dry and cracked because of prolonged exposure to amniotic fluid. Skin and nails are often stained with meconium. Depletion of glycogen stores predisposes the infant to hypoglycemia, whereas loss of subcutaneous fat predisposes to hypothermia. Seizure activity is common if hypoxic insults have occurred. If there has been no hypoxia, the infant is usually more alert than most term infants. Birth trauma may result in skull fracture or subdural hematomas with increased intracranial pressure or in impaired mobility caused by peripheral nerve injury, fractures, or dislocations.

Prevention and Treatment. Prevention of post-term delivery requires careful prenatal monitoring of mother and fetus, with induction of labor at the first

Focus of Current Research

Study	Objective and Findings
Bauer, et al. (1997) Body temperatures and oxygen consumption during skin-to-skin (kangaroo) care in stable preterm infants weighing less than 1500 grams.	*Objective:* To test the hypothesis that skin-to-skin care is a cold stress for preterm infants weighing less than 1500 g *Findings:* For stable preterm infants younger than 1 week of age, 1 hour of skin-to-skin care is not a cold stress.
McEvoy, et al. (1997) Prone positioning decreases episodes of hypoxemia in extremely low birth weight infants (1000 grams or less) with chronic lung disease.	*Objective:* To compare average oxygenation and episodes of hypoxemia in the supine versus prone position with the use of pulse oximetry *Findings:* Prone positioning increased oxygen saturation and significantly decreased episodes of hypoxemia.
Tyson, et al. (1996) Viability, morbidity, and resource use among newborns of 501- to 800-g birth weight.	*Objective:* To assess risk factors affecting viability and analyze the effects of mechanical ventilation on neonatal outcome and resource use among extremely premature infants *Findings:* Overall mortality was 43%. Mortality in infants without mechanical ventilation was 93%. Females, small-for-gestational age infants, and those whose mothers received steroids antenatally had a survival advantage.

sign of placental insufficiency. Cesarean delivery may be required because of fetal macrosomia. Treatment of the postmature infant is symptomatic and supportive, similar to that of the premature infant. Birth injuries are treated appropriately, with reduction and fixation of fractures and dislocations (see Chapter 34).

Prognosis and Outcome. Although neonatal morbidity is increased, the mortality rate of postmature infants is only slightly higher than that of term infants, with most deaths caused by asphyxia during labor. When the postdate pregnancy is complicated by maternal diabetes or hypertension, however, the neonatal mortality rate is greater than 50%.[17] Such pregnancies are usually not allowed to proceed beyond the 41st week.

Intrauterine Growth Retardation

Definition. Intrauterine growth retardation is deficient support of fetal growth in utero, resulting in birth of an infant who is SGA.

Epidemiology. The precise incidence of IUGR is unknown. The National Institutes of Health has estimated that approximately 40,000 infants of low birth weight at term are growth restricted and that two thirds of preterm infants were small as a consequence of prematurity and growth restriction.[18] Risk factors, detailed in Figure 33–5, include maternal, uterine, placental, and fetal abnormalities.

Etiology. Although the precise etiology is uncertain in some cases, IUGR is usually the result of (1) a chromosomal or genetic defect in the fetus that impairs intrauterine development or (2) insufficient delivery of oxygen and nutrients to the fetus caused by maternal, uterine, or placental factors. Defective production of insulin-like growth factor I (IGF-I) has been implicated in reduction of fetal growth.[19] Deficiency of other hormones (e.g., growth hormone or human chorionic somatomammotropin) may also play a role in the development of IUGR. The degree of IUGR resulting from placental abnormality is proportionate to the number and severity of placental lesions.[20]

Pathophysiology. Two patterns of IUGR may be

Rojas, et al. (1995) Changing trends in the epidemiology and pathogenesis of neonatal chronic lung disease.	*Objective:* To assess the role of specific risk factors that may predispose preterm infants with mild or no initial respiratory distress syndrome to the development of chronic lung disease *Findings:* Chronic lung disease is a frequent sequela in very low birth weight infants with mild or no respiratory distress syndrome. Late patent ductus arteriosus and nosocomial infection play a role.
Spinillo, et al. (1995) Epidemiologic association between maternal smoking during pregnancy and intracranial hemorrhage in preterm infants.	*Objective:* To evaluate the effect of maternal smoking during pregnancy on the risk of intracranial hemorrhage in preterm infants born at 24 to 33 weeks of gestation *Findings:* The risk of hemorrhage was three times higher in infants of heavy smokers.
Philip (1995) Neonatal mortality rate: Is further improvement possible?	*Objective:* To determine whether improvement in neonatal and infant mortality rates is possible or likely *Findings:* During the decade of 1982 to 1991, the gestational age at which there was a 50% survival rate fell from 26 weeks to 24 weeks. A marked increase in survival of infants with birth weights less than 1500 g occurred after the introduction of exogenous surfactant therapy.

seen, depending on the timing of the insult to the developing fetus. *Symmetric* IUGR is demonstrated by a proportionate decrease in the size of all body organs, including head circumference. Symmetric IUGR results from abnormality of the fetus from the beginning of pregnancy, such as that caused by genetic defect or long-term adverse maternal conditions. *Asymmetric* IUGR results from compromise of fetal blood supply later in gestation, usually during the third trimester, caused by acute maternal illness or trauma or by late-developing fetal or placental abnormality. Asymmetric IUGR is characterized by normal length and head circumference, but decreased subcutaneous fat and muscle tissue and loose skin folds. Organ size is small, but development is physiologically normal for gestational age.

Clinical Manifestations. The infant is SGA, with a general appearance consistent with symmetric or asymmetric IUGR. Compromise during gestation leaves the infant less able to tolerate the stress of labor and delivery, increasing the likelihood of asphyxia and intracranial bleeding. Intrauterine hypoxia may lead to meconium aspiration syndrome, with resulting respiratory failure and persistent pulmonary hypertension. Hypothermia risk is high because of lack of insulating subcutaneous fat. Hypoglycemia is common in IUGR infants, caused by poor glycogen stores and possibly a cold stress–induced increase in metabolic rate. The skin is dry and cracked and often stained with meconium because of fetal distress. Asymmetric IUGR infants often have poor brain development later in childhood, with hyperactivity, attention deficit, poor motor coordination, and possibly speech disorders or hearing loss.

Prevention and Treatment. Maternal risk factors must be reduced if possible. Careful monitoring and appropriate intervention in any critical events during the pregnancy are warranted. The high-risk infant may be delivered via cesarean section to avoid the stress of labor and vaginal delivery. Treatment of the infant after delivery is symptomatic and supportive, similar to the care of premature infants.

Prognosis and Outcome. Prognosis in asymmetric IUGR infants, especially those born before 37 weeks' gestation, is poor, primarily because of the detri-

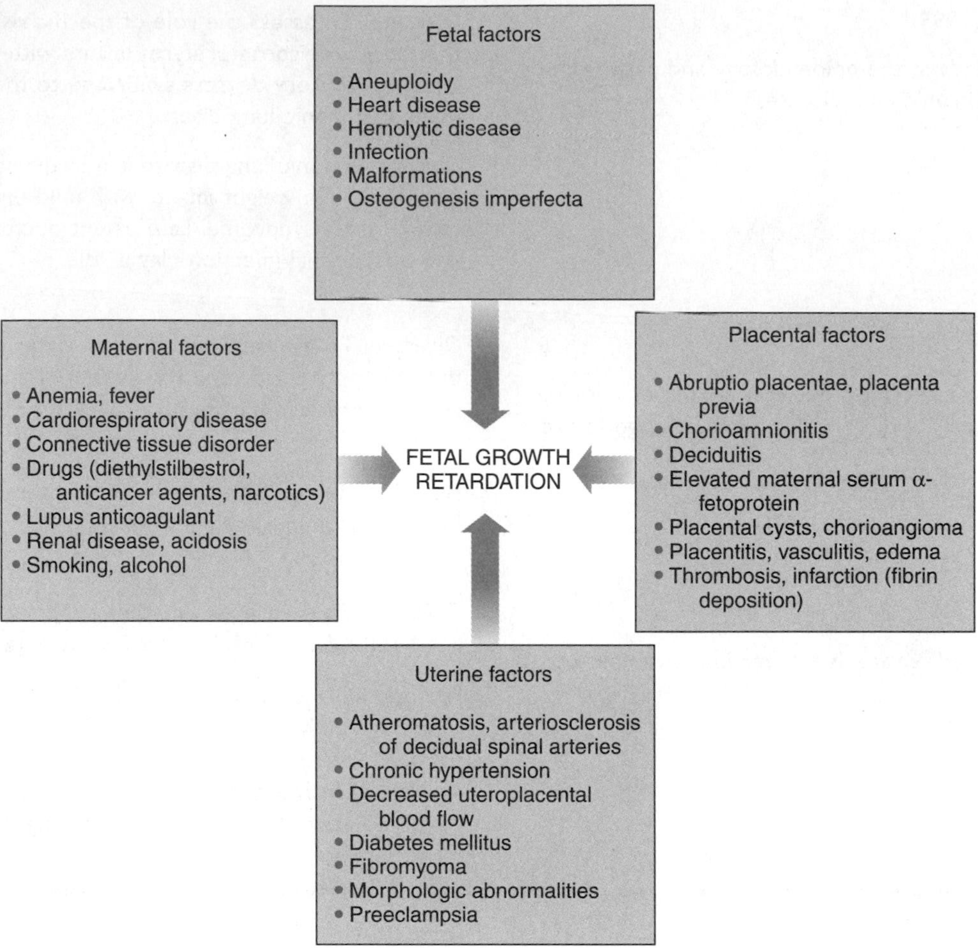

Fetal factors
• Aneuploidy
• Heart disease
• Hemolytic disease
• Infection
• Malformations
• Osteogenesis imperfecta
Maternal factors
• Anemia, fever
• Cardiorespiratory disease
• Connective tissue disorder
• Drugs (diethylstilbestrol, anticancer agents, narcotics)
• Lupus anticoagulant
• Renal disease, acidosis
• Smoking, alcohol
FETAL GROWTH RETARDATION
Placental factors
• Abruptio placentae, placenta previa
• Chorioamnionitis
• Deciduitis
• Elevated maternal serum α-fetoprotein
• Placental cysts, chorioangioma
• Placentitis, vasculitis, edema
• Thrombosis, infarction (fibrin deposition)
Uterine factors
• Atheromatosis, arteriosclerosis of decidual spinal arteries
• Chronic hypertension
• Decreased uteroplacental blood flow
• Diabetes mellitus
• Fibromyoma
• Morphologic abnormalities
• Preeclampsia

FIGURE 33–5

Factors associated with intrauterine growth retardation. Fetal, maternal, placental, and uterine factors may impose risk of retardation of fetal growth. (Redrawn from Weiner, C.P. [1989]. Pathogenesis, evaluation, and potential treatments for severe, early onset growth retardation. *Seminars in Perinatology* 13, 321.)

mental effects on neural development. Outcomes in other infants vary depending on the duration and severity of insufficient fetal blood flow or on any direct fetal effects, for example, congenital anomalies, meconium aspiration, or intrauterine infections. Delayed growth and reduced adult height are common.

Phenylketonuria

Definition. Phenylketonuria (PKU) is an inborn error of metabolism in which the amino acid phenylalanine accumulates as a result of inadequate conversion of phenylalanine to tyrosine.

Epidemiology. The incidence of PKU in the United States is approximately 1 in 12,000 live births.[21] Because the disorder is inherited as an autosomal recessive trait, risk is derived from the parental genotype.

Etiology. In classic PKU, a deficiency of the enzyme phenylalanine hydrolase prevents the hydroxylation of phenylalanine to tyrosine, the precursor of epinephrine, norepinephrine, and thyroid hormones. The gene for this enzyme is located on the long arm of chromosome 12. Deficiency of a cofactor for phenylalanine hydrolase may also result in persistent elevation of serum phenylalanine.

Pathophysiology. Excess phenylalanine is metabolized to products that are toxic to the developing brain and other tissues.

Clinical Manifestations. Phenylketonuria is one of a number of disorders for which neonatal screening is routine (Table 33–5). The diagnosis is established when serum phenylalanine levels exceed 20 mg/dL, with normal or decreased tyrosine levels.[21] The affected infant may appear normal at birth, but developmental delay and potentially severe mental retardation eventually manifest. Vomiting is an early symptom, and the child has a characteristic odor

TABLE 33–5
ROUTINE METABOLIC SCREENING IN NEONATES

DISORDER	DESCRIPTION
Phenylketonuria	Deficiency of enzyme for conversion of phenylalanine to tyrosine (see text); may cause mental retardation
Congenital hypothyroidism	Deficiency of thyroxine; may cause growth deficiency and mental retardation
Galactosemia	Deficiency of one of three enzymes for metabolism of galactose; may cause feeding intolerance, liver dysfunction, and coagulopathy during the neonatal period; and mental retardation, cataracts, and cirrhosis later
Maple syrup urine disease	Deficiency of enzyme resulting in accumulation of certain branched-chain amino acids and their ketoacids; urine smells like maple syrup or curry; leads to severe mental retardation and neurologic impairment
Homocystinuria	Deficiency of enzyme converting homocysteine to cystathionine; elevated homocysteine and methionine result in mental retardation, lens dislocation, osteoporosis, and thromboembolism
Biotinidase deficiency	Deficiency of this enzyme; prevents the activation of four mitochondrial enzymes; may lead to alopecia, skin infections, and neurologic impairment
Sickle cell disease	Genetic disorder of hemoglobin synthesis; leads to vascular occlusion and hemolytic anemia

Data from Irons, M. (1993). Screening for metabolic disorders: How are we doing? *Pediatric Clinics of North America* 40(5), 1073–1085.

that has been described as barn-like or mousy. Infants with PKU have fair skin and blue eyes and usually manifest a seborrheic or eczematous skin rash. Microcephaly, jaw prominence, widely spaced teeth, hypoplasia of dental enamel, and growth retardation are common in untreated children. In addition to retardation, neural signs include seizures, autism, hyperactivity, and aggressive behavior.

Infants of women with untreated PKU often have IUGR and severe congenital heart defects. Spontaneous abortion is also common.

Prevention and Treatment. Primary prevention requires identification and treatment of PKU in potentially childbearing women. Neonatal screening should identify infants with the condition and permit early intervention. Treatment should begin no later than 3 weeks of age and consists of a phenylalanine-restricted diet. Special phenylalanine-free formulations are available to supply protein and vitamins, and nitrogen-free foods (sugars and fats) are used to supply remaining calories. Adequate dietary intake of tyrosine must be ensured. It is now recommended that monitoring of phenylalanine levels and dietary restriction be continued indefinitely to prevent adverse effects on nervous system development and function. Replacement of the cofactor tetrahydrobiopterin (BH_4) and administration of precursors for tyrosine-derived neurotransmitters may be required in some cases.

Prognosis and Outcome. Early treatment may prevent mental retardation and other complications of classic PKU. Learning disabilities are sometimes seen even in those who are optimally treated, however. Treatment is less successful for those with cofactor deficiency. These patients are more likely to have mental retardation or other neurologic manifestations despite treatment.

Fetal Alcohol Syndrome

Definition. Fetal alcohol syndrome (FAS) is a constellation of clinical manifestations that are typically seen in children born to mothers who consume alcohol in excess during pregnancy.

Epidemiology. The incidence of FAS has been estimated at between 1 in 600 and 1 in 3000 live births.[22] It is the third most common cause of birth defects in the United States (after Down syndrome and spina bifida). Risk is highest among blacks and Native Americans, but all racial groups are affected. It is apparent that risk factors other than alcohol consumption are also important, because equivalent patterns of alcohol abuse may produce severe FAS in some infants and no apparent effects in others. Additional risk factors may include genetic differences in the maternal metabolism of alcohol or in fetal sensitivity to alcohol, multiple drug use, and nutritional deficiency.

Etiology. Alcohol is a weak teratogen, but it has significant detrimental effects on the developing CNS if blood alcohol levels are consistently high during gestation. Exposure to alcohol during the first trimester is thought to be responsible for craniofacial anomalies in FAS, and exposure during the second and third trimesters produces most neuronal loss.[23]

Pathophysiology. Alcohol easily crosses the placental and blood–brain barriers. Fetal alcohol exposure disrupts many aspects of CNS development. Alterations in embryonic division and differentiation of neural tissues are seen, and significant death of neurons is also apparent. Development of appropriate connections between neurons is impaired. Specific mechanisms of CNS damage are uncertain, but may involve alcohol-impaired protein synthesis, reduction in oxygen supply, free radical toxicity, stimulation of prostaglandin synthesis, methylation of DNA, fluidization of biologic membranes, impairment of vitamin and mineral functions, or impairment of synaptic transmission.[23]

Clinical Manifestations. Fetal alcohol syndrome manifests as prenatal and postnatal growth deficiency, developmental delay, microcephaly, and characteristic malformations of the face, including short palpebral fissures and epicanthal folds ("almond" eyes), short nose and flat nasal bridge, and thin upper lip with lack of a distinct indentation (Fig. 33–6). Altered palmar creases are also typical, and congenital heart defects are frequently seen. Behavioral manifestations are of learning disability, poor motor development, and hyperactivity.

Prevention and Treatment. Because the amount of alcohol that can be safely consumed during pregnancy is unknown, and because its teratogenic effects are seen throughout the gestation period, prevention of FAS requires abstinence from alcohol use throughout pregnancy. Treatment of the child with FAS is symptomatic and supportive.

Prognosis and Outcome. Follow-up studies of FAS infants reveal that most remain small in stature but achieve normal weight. Head size remains small in most, and facial features become coarser. Problems with cognitive and social function persist throughout life.

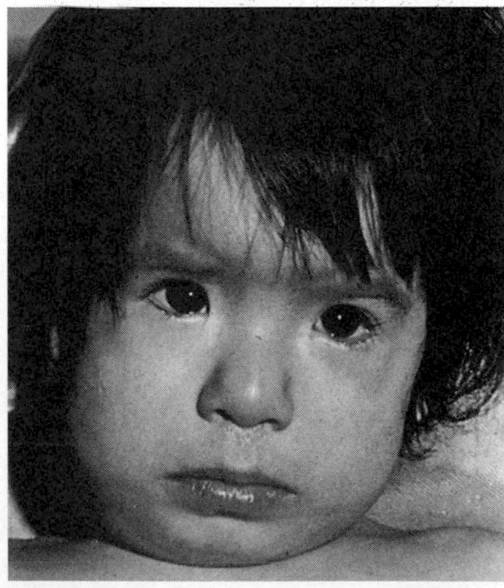

FIGURE 33–6
Infant with fetal alcohol syndrome. Characteristic facial features include almond-shaped eyes, short nose, flat nasal bridge, and thin upper lip with lack of distinct indentation. (From Jones, K.L., *et al.* [1973]. Pattern of malformation in offspring of chronic alcoholic mothers. *Lancet* 1, 1267.)

Down Syndrome

Definition. Down syndrome is the phenotype resulting from trisomy of chromosome 21.

Epidemiology. Down syndrome is the most common chromosomal disorder in humans, occurring in 1 in 700 live births.[24] Trisomy 21 is also present in a similar number of spontaneously aborted conceptuses. The primary risk factor is maternal age. The risk of giving birth to an infant with Down syndrome is approximately 3% at age 35, and this risk rises exponentially to 41% at age 46.[25] Although mothers older than age 35 years account for just 7% of all pregnancies, 20% to 25% of all fetuses with Down syndrome are detected with prenatal diagnosis in this group.[24] Techniques for prenatal diagnosis of Down syndrome and other chromosomal anomalies are summarized in Table 33–6.

Etiology. Trisomy 21 is almost always the result of nondisjunction, usually during a meiotic division (see Chapter 7). Abnormality of the chromosome provided by the mother is implicated in nearly all cases, and it is widely believed that aging of the ovum induces the defect. In a few cases, a de novo translocation is the mechanism of Down syndrome.

Pathophysiology. Except in the 2% to 4% of individuals with Down syndrome who are mosaics, trisomy 21 is evident in all body cells. Triplication of gene products of chromosome 21 apparently induces arrested development of some organs and as well as features suggestive of a premature aging process.[24]

Clinical Manifestations. Major clinical manifestations of Down syndrome include mental retardation, short stature, hypotonia, characteristic facial features (Fig. 33–7), abnormal palmar creases, conductive hearing loss, ocular defects, thyroid dysfunction, cardiac defects, and GI disorders (e.g., tracheoesophageal fistula, volvulus, or Hirschsprung's disease). In the neonatal period, congenital heart defects and GI malformations account for most morbidity and may require surgical correction. Acute leukemia occurs with greater frequency in individuals with Down syndrome, and certain biochemical abnormalities, such as increased levels of superoxide dismutase enzyme, interferon receptors, and amyloid protein deposition, have been noted.

Prevention and Treatment. Genetic counseling and prenatal diagnosis are recommended for women older than age 35 years. Prenatal diagnostic procedures permit analysis of fetal products such as α-fetoprotein (AFP) and DNA analysis for detection of abnormalities. Parents may then elect to terminate the pregnancy. The individual with Down syndrome is treated symptomatically and supportively, with early intervention and special education systems being of primary importance.

Prognosis and Outcome. The presence of congenital heart disease is the most significant factor influencing survival. Those without heart disease may survive well into their 60s.[24] Cognitive impairment is usually moderate (intelligence quotient, 40 to 54). About 20% of individuals with Down syndrome have psychiatric disorders, requiring behavioral or pharmacologic intervention. Alzheimer's disease is evident in 15% of individuals in their 50s, and it is rapidly progressive over 5 years. Most persons with Down syndrome are able to function fairly well in a structured, protected environment and can live full and rewarding lives.

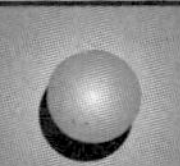

TABLE 33–6
PRENATAL DIAGNOSTIC TESTING

METHOD	CLINICAL USE
Noninvasive Imaging Techniques	
High resolution sonography (passing of ultrasound waves through structures, with reflection back to the source proportional to different tissue densities)	Documentation of fetal measurements, level of amniotic fluid, fetal position, placental location, structural abnormality of organs
Invasive Genetic Evaluation	
Amniocentesis (sampling of amniotic fluid)	Performed after 14 weeks' gestation; provides fetal cells for karyotyping for chromosomal defects; can provide information about fetal lung maturity
Chorionic villus sampling (sampling of developing placental tissue)	Performed after 8 to 12 weeks' gestation; cells obtained via needle with transabdominal or via catheter with transcervical approach; karyotyping done for detection of chromosomal defects
Percutaneous umbilical blood sampling	Performed using ultrasound guidance to insert needle transabdominally into the umbilical cord; permits rapid karyotyping and detection of infection
Maternal Serum Screening	
Triple screen (measurement of maternal unconjugated estriol, α-fetoprotein [AFP], and human chorionic gonadotropin [hCG])	Assay of proteins from fetus or placenta; elevation of AFP in neural tube defect; low AFP in Down syndrome; hCG elevated in Down syndrome; estriol low in Down syndrome; does not detect sex chromosome abnormalities
Fetal cell isolation from maternal blood	Fetal trophoblastic remnants, lymphocytes, granulocytes, and nucleated erythrocytes isolated from maternal blood for karyotyping

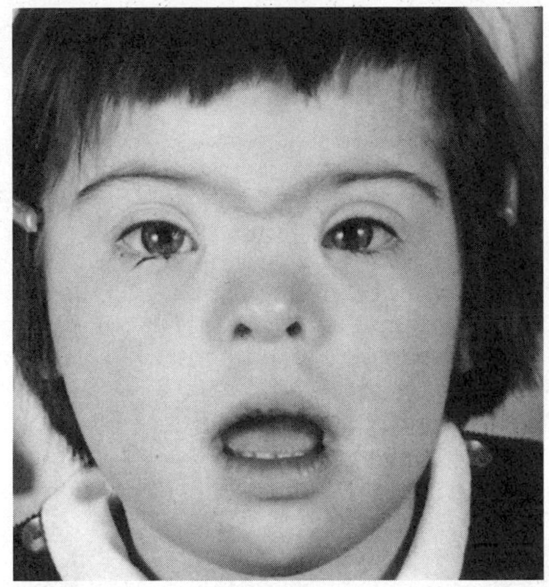

FIGURE 33–7
Child with Down syndrome. Typical facial characteristics include upslanted eyes with epicanthal folds, short nose with flat bridge, and protruding tongue resulting from small oral cavity. The head is short and flat. (From Bartalos, M., and Baramki, T.A. [1967]. *Medical Cytogenes.* Baltimore: Williams & Wilkins.)

CLINICAL SIGNIFICANCE OF NEONATAL DISORDERS

The illness, developmental abnormality, or death of an infant is arguably the greatest crisis faced by parents. Loss or threat of loss of the infant is often compounded by parental feelings of guilt. With improved prenatal care and clinical intervention, survival rates for high-risk infants are improving, and overall neonatal mortality is decreasing. Many infants who survive are left with lifelong developmental disability, however, and their consumption of health care resources and educational support services is disproportional. Research is ongoing in an effort to clarify etiologic mechanisms of preterm and post-term labor and to develop clinical interventions that support physiologic function without imposing concurrent risk of iatrogenic disorders.

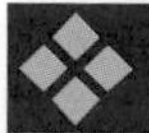

Summary of Key Points

- The organ systems of the term neonate are fully differentiated at birth, although functional maturation is incomplete. The head is large in proportion to the body, and physiologic jaundice and acrocyanosis are common. The preterm infant is smaller, as reflective of shortened gestation, and the head is disproportionately large. Little body fat is present, and the skin is covered with lanugo and vernix caseosa.

- At birth, all neonatal body systems must adapt to extrauterine life. Fetal shunts close, establishing the normal left-to-right gradient in arterial pressure. Red blood cells containing fetal hemoglobin are lysed. Lung fluid is cleared and airways expand, reducing pulmonary vascular resistance. Renal nephrons are normal in number but decreased in size and function at birth. Body water–to–body mass ratio is high. GI motility is uncoordinated and intestinal surface cells are immature, decreasing absorptive capacity. Hepatobiliary function is also reduced, potentiating physiologic jaundice, bleeding tendencies, and deficient biotransformation of drugs. Host defense systems are immature, predisposing to neonatal infection. Sensory function is more complete than widely believed. Patterns of behavior become apparent and are individual to each infant. Primitive reflexes are evident. Thermoregulation is inefficient, and metabolic regulation is not fully developed.

- Clinical manifestations of prematurity are the result of developmental immaturity of organ systems and any insults occurring as a consequence of preterm labor and delivery. Manifestations of postmaturity are similar; however, the mechanism of impaired organ function is not immaturity but rather placental insufficiency. Birth trauma caused by macrosomia may impose further problems.

- Maternal factors such as toxins or systemic disease, fetal factors such as infections or congenital anomalies, uterine factors such as preeclampsia or structural abnormalities, and placental factors such as thrombosis, infection, or premature separation may result in IUGR.

- Congenital disorders may result from genetic or chromosomal defects, as in PKU and Down syndrome, or from preventable environmental teratogens, as in fetal alcohol syndrome. Arrested or abnormal development is evident in utero and during the neonatal period, and effects persist for the life of the individual.

REFERENCES

1. Centers for Disease Control and Prevention. (1994). Infant mortality: United States, 1991. *Journal of the American Medical Association* 271(1), 15–16.
2. Allen, M.C., Donohue, P.K., and Dusman, A.E. (1993). The limit of viability: Neonatal outcome of infants born at 22 to 25 weeks' gestation. *New England Journal of Medicine* 329(22), 1597–1601.
3. Altshuler, G. (1987). Abnormalities of the placenta, membranes, and umbilical cord. In: Danforth, D.N., and Scott, J.R.(Eds.). *Obstetrics and Gynecology*. (5th ed.). Philadelphia: J.B. Lippincott. (p. 830).
4. Lowe, N.K., and Reiss, R. (1996). Parturition and fetal adaptation. *Journal of Obstetric, Gynecologic, and Neonatal Nursing* 25(4), 339–349.
5. Foster, R.L.R., Hunsberger, M.M., and Anderson, J.J.T. (1989). *Family-Centered Nursing Care of Children*. Philadelphia: W.B. Saunders. (pp. 181–182).
6. Travis, B.E., and McCullough, J.M. (1993). Pharmacotherapy of preterm labor. *Pharmacotherapy* 13(1), 28–36.
7. Ishisaka, D.Y. (1996). Exogenous surfactant use in neonates. *Annals of Pharmacotherapy* 30, 389–398.
8. Wiswell, T.E., and Mendiola Jr., J. (1993). Respiratory distress syndrome in the newborn: Innovative therapies. *American Family Physician* 47(2), 407–414.
9. Kinsella, J.P., and Abman, S.H. (1995). Recent developments in the pathophysiology and treatment of persistent pulmonary hypertension of the newborn. *Journal of Pediatrics* 126(6), 853–864.
10. Roberts, J.D., and Shaul, P.W. (1993). Advances in the treatment of persistent pulmonary hypertension of the newborn. *Pediatric Clinics of North America* 40(5), 983–1004.
11. Abman, S.H., and Groothius, J.R. (1994). Pathophysiology and treatment of bronchopulmonary dysplasia: Current issues. *Pediatric Clinics of North America* 41(2), 277–315.
12. Walters, M.C., and Abelson, H.T. (1996). Interpretation of the complete blood count. *Pediatric Clinics of North America* 43(3), 599–622.
13. Neu, J. (1996). Necrotizing enterocolitis: The search for a unifying pathogenic theory leading to prevention. *Pediatric Clinics of North America* 43(2), 409–432.
14. Phelps, D.L. (1993). Retinopathy of prematurity. *Pediatric Clinics of North America* 40(4), 705–714.
15. NIH Consensus Development Panel on the Effect of Corticosteroids for Fetal Maturation on Perinatal Outcomes. (1995). Effect of corticosteroids for fetal maturation on perinatal outcomes. *Journal of the American Medical Association* 273(5), 413–417.
16. Wallerstedt, C., Higgins, P., Kasnic, T., *et al.* (1993). Amnioinfusion: An update. *Journal of Obstetric, Gynecologic, and Neonatal Nursing* 23(7), 573–578.
17. Sulik, S.M., and Greenwald, J.L. (1994). Evaluation and managment of postdate pregnancy. *American Family Physician* 49(5), 1177–1186.
18. Cunningham, F.G., MacDonald, P.C., and Gant, N.F. (1989). *Williams Obstetrics*. (18th ed.). Norwalk, CT: Appleton & Lange. (p. 764).

19. Gluckman, P.D. (1995). The endocrine regulation of fetal growth in late gestation: The role of insulin-like growth factors. *Journal of Clinical Endocrinology and Metabolism* 80(4), 1047–1050.
20. Salafia, C.M., Minior, V.K., Pezzullo, J.C., *et al.* (1995). Intrauterine growth restriction in infants of less than thirty-two weeks' gestation: Associated placental pathologic features. *American Journal of Obstetrics and Gynecology* 173(4), 1049–1057.
21. Irons, M. (1993). Metabolic disorders: How are we doing? *Pediatric Clinics of North America* 40(5), 1073–1085.
22. Bratton, R.L. (1995). Fetal alcohol syndrome: How you can help prevent it. *Postgraduate Medicine* 98(5), 197–200.
23. West, J.R., Chen, W-J.A., and Pantazis, N.J. (1994). Fetal alcohol syndrome: The vulnerability of the developing brain and possible mechanisms of damage. *Metabolic Brain Disease* 9(4), 291–321.
24. Hayes, A., and Batshaw, M.L. (1993). Down syndrome. *Pediatric Clinics of North America* 40(3), 523–535.
25. Epstein, C.J. (1995). Down syndrome (trisomy 21). In: Scriver, C.R., Beaudet, A.L., Sly, W.S. (Eds.). *The Metabolic and Molecular Bases of Inherited Disease.* (7th ed.). Volume 1. New York: McGraw-Hill. (pp. 749–794).

SELECTED BIBLIOGRAPHY

Acosta, P.B., and Wright, L. (1992). Nurses' role in preventing birth defects in offspring of women with phenylketonuria. *Journal of Obstetric, Gynecologic, and Neonatal Nursing* 21(4), 270–352.

Akinbi, H., Abbasi, S., and Hilpert, P.L. (1994). Gastrointestinal and renal blood flow velocity profile in neonates with birth asphyxia. *Journal of Pediatrics* 125(4), 625–627.

Allen, M.C. (1993). The high-risk infant. *Pediatric Clinics of North America* 40(3), 479–491.

Alyn, I.B., and Baker, L.K. (1992). Cardiovascular anatomy and physiology of the fetus, neonate, infant, child, and adolescent. *Journal of Cardiovascular Nursing* 6(3), 1–11.

Bauer, K., Uhrig, C., Sperling, P., *et al.* (1997). Body temperature and oxygen consumption during skin-to-skin (kangaroo) care in stable preterm infants weighing less than 1500 grams. *Journal of Pediatrics* 130(2), 240–244.

Behnke, M., Eyler, F.D., Conlon, M., *et al.* (1993). The relationship between umbilical cord and infant blood gases and developmental outcome in very low birth weight infants. *Clinical Obstetrics and Gynecology* 36(1), 73–81.

Behrman, R.E. (Ed.). (1992). *Nelson Textbook of Pediatrics.* (14th ed.). Philadelphia: W.B. Saunders.

Bianchi, D.W. (1995). Prenatal diagnosis by analysis of fetal cells in maternal blood. *Journal of Pediatrics* 127(6), 847–856.

Blackburn, S.T., and Loper, D.L. (1992). *Maternal, Fetal, and Neonatal Physiology: A Clinical Perspective.* Philadelphia: W.B. Saunders.

Carey, B.E., and Trotter, C. (1996). Bronchopulmonary dysplasia. *Neonatal Network* 15(4), 73–77.

Charlton, A. (1994). Children and passive smoking: A review. *Journal of Family Practice* 38(3), 267–277.

Crawford, D., and Morris, M. (Eds.). (1994). *Neonatal Nursing.* London: Chapman & Hall.

Darby, M.K., and Loughead, J.L. (1996). Neonatal nutritional requirements and formula composition: A review. *Journal of Obstetric, Gynecologic, and Neonatal Nursing* 25(3), 209–217.

Davidson, J.A., and Roberts, V.L. (1996). Gestational diabetes: Ensuring a successful outcome. *Postgraduate Medicine* 99(3), 165–172.

Davis, S.F., Byers, Jr., R.H., Lindegren, M.L., *et al.* (1995). Prevalence and incidence of vertically acquired HIV infection in the United States. *Journal of the American Medical Association* 274(12), 952–955.

Doran, L. (1992). Periventricular leukomalacia. *Neonatal Network* 11(4), 7–13.

Ferrara, T.B., Hoekstra, R.E., Couser, R.J., *et al.* (1994). Survival and follow-up of infants born at 23 to 26 weeks of gestational age: Effects of surfactant therapy. *Journal of Pediatrics* 124(1), 119–124.

Hack, M., Taylor, H.G., Klein, N., *et al.* (1994). School-age outcomes in children with birth weights under 750 g. *New England Journal of Medicine* 331(12), 753–759.

Hicks, B.A., and Altman, R.P. (1993). The jaundiced newborn. *Pediatric Clinics of North America* 40(6), 1161–1175.

Howell, L.J. (1994). The unborn surgical patient: A nursing frontier. *Nursing Clinics of North America* 29(4), 681–694.

Jackson, P., and Bash, D.M. (1994). Management of the uncomplicated pregnant diabetic client in the ambulatory setting. *Nurse Practitioner* 19(12), 64–73.

Jacobson, J.L., Jacobson, S.W., Sokol, R.J., *et al.* (1994). Effects of alcohol use, smoking, and illicit drug use on fetal growth in black infants. *Journal of Pediatrics* 124(5 pt. 1), 757–764.

Johnson, L., Quinn, G.E., Abbasi, S., *et al.* (1995). Severe retinopathy of prematurity in infants with birth weights less than 1250 grams: Incidence and outcome of treatment with pharmacologic serum levels of vitamin E in addition to cryotherapy from 1985 to 1991. *Journal of Pediatrics* 127(4), 632–639.

Klonoff-Cohen, H.S., Edelstein, S.L., Lefkowitz, E.S., *et al.* (1995). The effect of passive smoking and tobacco exposure through breast milk on sudden infant death syndrome. *Journal of the American Medical Association* 273(10), 795–798.

Lachance, C., Chessex, P., Fouron, J-C., *et al.* (1994). Myocardial, erythropoietic, and metabolic adaptations to anemia of prematurity. *Journal of Pediatrics* 125(2), 278–282.

Landesman, S.H., Kalish, L.A., Burns, D.N., *et al.* (1996). Obstetrical factors and the transmission of human immunodeficiency virus type 1 from mother to child. *New England Journal of Medicine* 334(25), 1617–1623.

Lasker, M.R., and Holzman, I.R. (1996). Neonatal jaundice: When to treat, when to watch and wait. *Postgraduate Medicine* 99(3), 187–198.

Leuther, S.R., Jansen, R.D., and Hageman, J.R. (1994). Cardiopulmonary resuscitation of the newborn: An update. *Pediatric Clinics of North America* 41(5), 893–907.

MacKendrick, W., and Caplan, M. (1993). Necrotizing enterocolitis: New thoughts about pathogenesis and potential treatments. *Pediatric Clinics of North America* 40(5), 1047–1059.

May, K.A., and Mahlmeister, L.R. (1990). *Comprehensive Maternity Nursing: Nursing Process and the Childbearing Family.* (2nd ed.). Philadelphia: J.B. Lippincott.

McEvoy, C., Mendoza, M.E., Bowling, S., *et al.* (1997). Prone positioning decreases episodes of hypoxemia in extremely low birth weight infants (1000 grams or less) with chronic lung disease. *Journal of Pediatrics* 130(2), 305–309.

Metcoff, J. (1994). Clinical assessment of nutritional status at birth: Fetal malnutrition and SGZ are not synonymous. *Pediatric Clinics of North America* 41(5), 875–891.

Moffatt, M.E.K., Longstaffe, S., Besant, J., *et al.* (1994). Prevention of iron deficiency and psychomotor decline in high-risk infants through use of iron-fortified infant formula: A randomized clinical trial. *Journal of Pediatrics* 125(4), 527–534.

Moore, K.L., and Persaud, T.V.N. (1993). *The Developing Human: Clinically Oriented Embryology.* (5th ed.). Philadelphia: W.B. Saunders.

O'Hara, M.A. (1993). Ophthalmia neonatorum. *Pediatric Clinics of North America* 40(4), 715–725.

Page, J.M., Schneeweiss, S., Whyte, H.E.A., *et al.* (1993). Ocular sequelae in premature infants. *Pediatrics* 92(6), 787–790.

Peckham, C., and Gibb, D. (1995). Mother-to-child transmission of the human immunodeficiency virus. *New England Journal of Medicine* 333(5), 298–302.

Philip, A.G.S. (1995). Neonatal mortality rate: Is further improvement possible? *Journal of Pediatrics* 126(3), 427–433.

Pisacane, A., DeVizia, B., Valiante, A., *et al.* (1995). Iron status in breast-fed infants. *Journal of Pediatrics* 127(3), 429–431.

Platt, M.W., and Gilson, G.J. (1994). Group B streptococcal disease in the perinatal period. *American Family Physician* 49(2), 434–442.

Rojas, M.A., Gonzalez, A., Bancalari, E., *et al.* (1995). Changing trends in the epidemiology and pathogenesis of neonatal chronic lung disease. *Journal of Pediatrics* 126(4), 605–610.

Spinillo, A., Ometto, A., Stronati, M., *et al.* (1995). Epidemiologic association between maternal smoking during pregnancy and intracranial hemorrhage in preterm infants. *Journal of Pediatrics* 127(3), 472–478.

Stamos, J.K., and Rowley, A.H. (1994). Timely diagnosis of congenital infections. *Pediatric Clinics of North America* 41(5), 1017–1033.

Tan, K.L. (1994). Comparison of the efficacy of fiberoptic and conventional phototherapy for neonatal hyperbilirubinemia. *Journal of Pediatrics* 125(4), 607–612.

Tyson, J.E., Younes, J., Verter, J., *et al.* (1996). Viability, morbidity, and resource use among newborns of 501- to 800-g birth weight. *Journal of the American Medical Association* 276(20), 1645–1651.

Walsh-Sukys, M.C., Bauer, R.E., Cornell, D.J., *et al.* (1994). Severe respiratory failure in neonates: Mortality and morbidity rates and neurodevelopmental outcomes. *Journal of Pediatrics* 125(1), 104–110.

Wandstrat, T.L., and Kaplan, B. (1995). Use of erythropoietin in premature neonates: Controversies and the future. *Annals of Pharmacotherapy* 29, 166–173.

White, C.W., Stabler, S.P., Allen, R.H., *et al.* (1994). Plasma cysteine concentrations in infants with respiratory distress. *Journal of Pediatrics* 125(5 pt. 1), 769–777.

Wiswell, T.E., and Bent, R.C. (1993). Meconium staining and the meconium aspiration syndrome. *Pediatric Clinics of North America* 40(5), 955–981.

Witek-Janusek, L., and Cusack, C. (1994). Neonatal sepsis: Confronting the challenge. *Critical Care Nursing Clinics of North America* 6(2), 405–419.

Woods, K.A., Camaco-Hubner, C., Savage, M.O., *et al.* (1996). Intrauterine growth retardation and postnatal growth failure associated with deletion of the insulin-like growth factor I gene. *New England Journal of Medicine* 335(18), 1363–1367.

Unit XIII

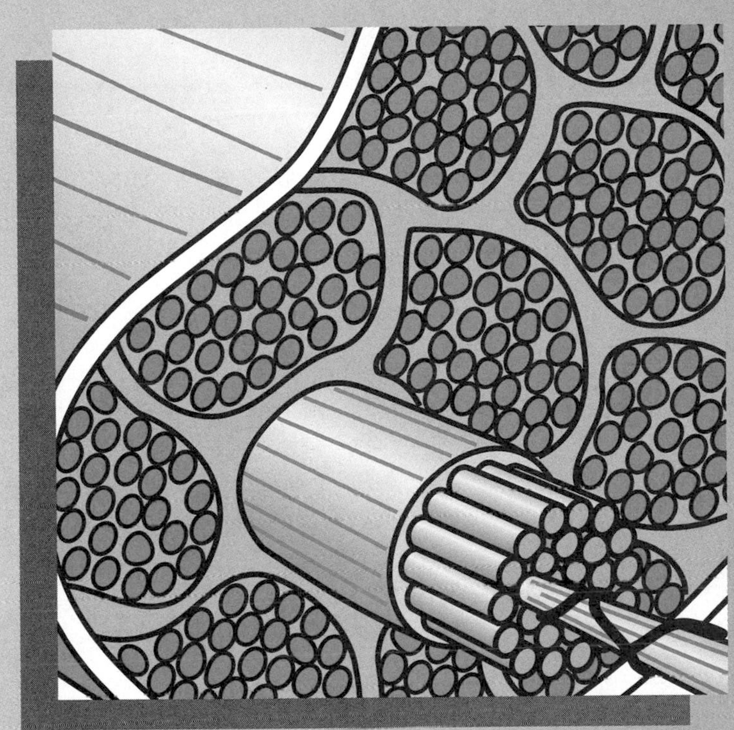

MUSCULOSKELETAL SYSTEM

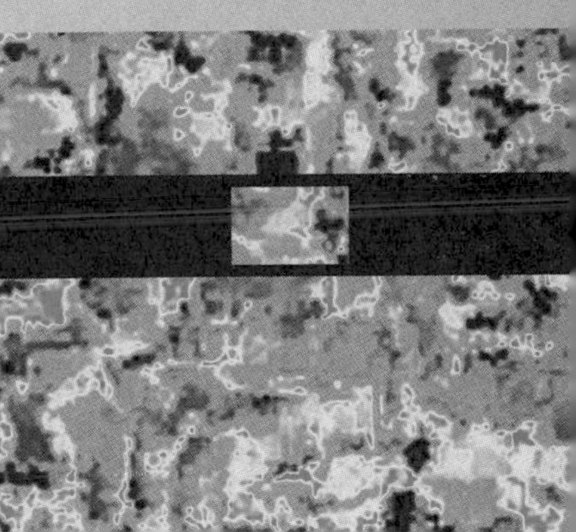

CHAPTER 34

Disorders of the Bones and Joints

LEARNING OBJECTIVES

1. Discuss the relationships among musculoskeletal disorders, hematopoietic disorders, connective tissue diseases, and rheumatic diseases.
2. Describe the mechanisms of bone growth and remodeling with reference to bone disorders and bone healing.
3. Relate structural and functional characteristics of diarthrotic joints to the manifestations of arthritis.
4. Differentiate among the prevalent bone disorders that may result in decreased bone density.
5. Identify risk factors associated with traumatic injury to bones and joints.
6. Differentiate among the prevalent forms of arthritis with respect to the mechanism of joint damage.
7. Discuss the pathophysiologic processes underlying the systemic manifestations of systemic lupus erythematosus.

key terms

ankylosing spondylitis
ankylosis
antinuclear antibody (ANA)
arthritis
bursitis
chondrosarcoma
compartmental syndrome
developmental hip dysplasia (DHD)
discoid lupus erythematosus
dislocation
Ewing's sarcoma
Felty's syndrome
fracture
gout
hypercalcemia of malignancy
hyperuricemia
kyphosis
Legg-Calvé-Perthes disease
lordosis
multiple myeloma
Osgood-Schlatter disease
osteoarthritis (OA)
osteochondrosis
osteomalacia
osteomyelitis
osteoporosis
osteosarcoma
Paget's disease
renal osteodystrophy

rheumatoid arthritis (RA)
rheumatoid factor (RF)
rickets
scoliosis
Sjögren's syndrome
sprain
subluxation
synovitis
systemic lupus erythematosus (SLE)
tendinitis

The musculoskeletal system includes the bones of the body's skeletal chassis, the skeletal muscles that effect voluntary movement, and the joints that permit that movement. The skeletal system (bones and teeth) serves as an essential reservoir for calcium, phosphate, and other minerals and as a principal site of hematopoiesis (see Chapters 9 and 12), and the skeletal muscles are a significant source of energy metabolism and body heat generation (see Chapter 3). This chapter focuses on the support and mobility functions served by the bones and joints and on disorders that may impede those functions. Chapter 35 examines the structure and function of skeletal muscles as well as clinical features of selected muscle disorders.

Traumatic and degenerative disorders of the bones and joints are a major source of morbidity in the United States. **Fractures** of bones and **dislocations** of joints are exceedingly common outcomes of motor vehicle accidents, falls, and sports injuries. **Arthritis**, in its many forms, significantly reduces quality of life for many individuals of all ages and both sexes. **Rheumatoid arthritis (RA)** is the prototypical disorder within a category of immune-mediated systemic disorders affecting the joints and other tissues, known variously as *rheumatic diseases, connective tissue diseases,* or *collagen diseases*. **Osteoporosis** is of particular importance in view of its prevalence in postmenopausal women and its potential prevention with hormone replacement, calcium supplementation, and exercise. These and other disorders are discussed in detail later in this chapter. The structure and function of the bones and joints are also reviewed as a basis for understanding clinical manifestations and rationalizing treatment of these disorders.

STRUCTURE AND FUNCTION OF THE BONES AND JOINTS

Classification and General Structure of Skeletal Tissues

Figure 34–1 depicts the skeletal system, with its axial (truncal) and appendicular (extremity) components and its 206 articulating bones. Bone tissue consists of two structural types: *cancellous (trabecular)* and *compact (cortical) bone* (Fig. 34–2). Cancellous bone is light and spongy in appearance because of marrow spaces dispersed throughout its matrix; compact bone is much more dense because of a high degree of calcification. Bones are composed of combinations of these two tissue types. The long bones of the extremities have a surface of compact bone, with cancellous bone in the interior *marrow cavity* and at the *epiphyseal growth plates* at each end. Flat bones, such as those of the skull, sternum, ribs, scapulae, vertebrae, and iliac crests, consist of a layer of cancellous bone sandwiched between two layers of compact bone.

Bone marrow, the fluid found in cancellous spaces, is of two types: red marrow, which is hematopoietically active, and yellow marrow, which is hematopoietically inert and consists primarily of fat cells. In response to biochemical stimuli during severe anemia, yellow marrow may revert to red marrow, increasing the body's hematopoietic capacity (see Chapter 12). With extremity fractures, yellow marrow may enter the bloodstream, and the resulting fat emboli may cause potentially fatal cardiac dysrhythmias and respiratory dysfunction. Cell lines in the marrow differentiate not only into hematopoietic cells, but also into bone cells (*osteoblasts* and *osteoclasts*).

The exterior surface of bones is covered by the *periosteum*, a membrane that also extends across joints to lend stability. The outer layer of the periosteum is tough and fibrous, and the inner layer contains osteogenic cells (immature, inactive osteoblasts), blood vessels, and nerve endings. A second type of bone membrane, the *endosteum*, lines cancellous spaces and *haversian canals* (see next section). Endosteum also contains osteogenic cells.

Microstructure of Skeletal Tissues

Skeletal tissues include bone, cartilage, tendons, and ligaments, all classified as connective tissues. These tissues consist of an organic matrix composed of fibrous collagen proteins embedded within an adhesive ground substance of fluid and complex protein-carbohydrate molecules (proteoglycans).

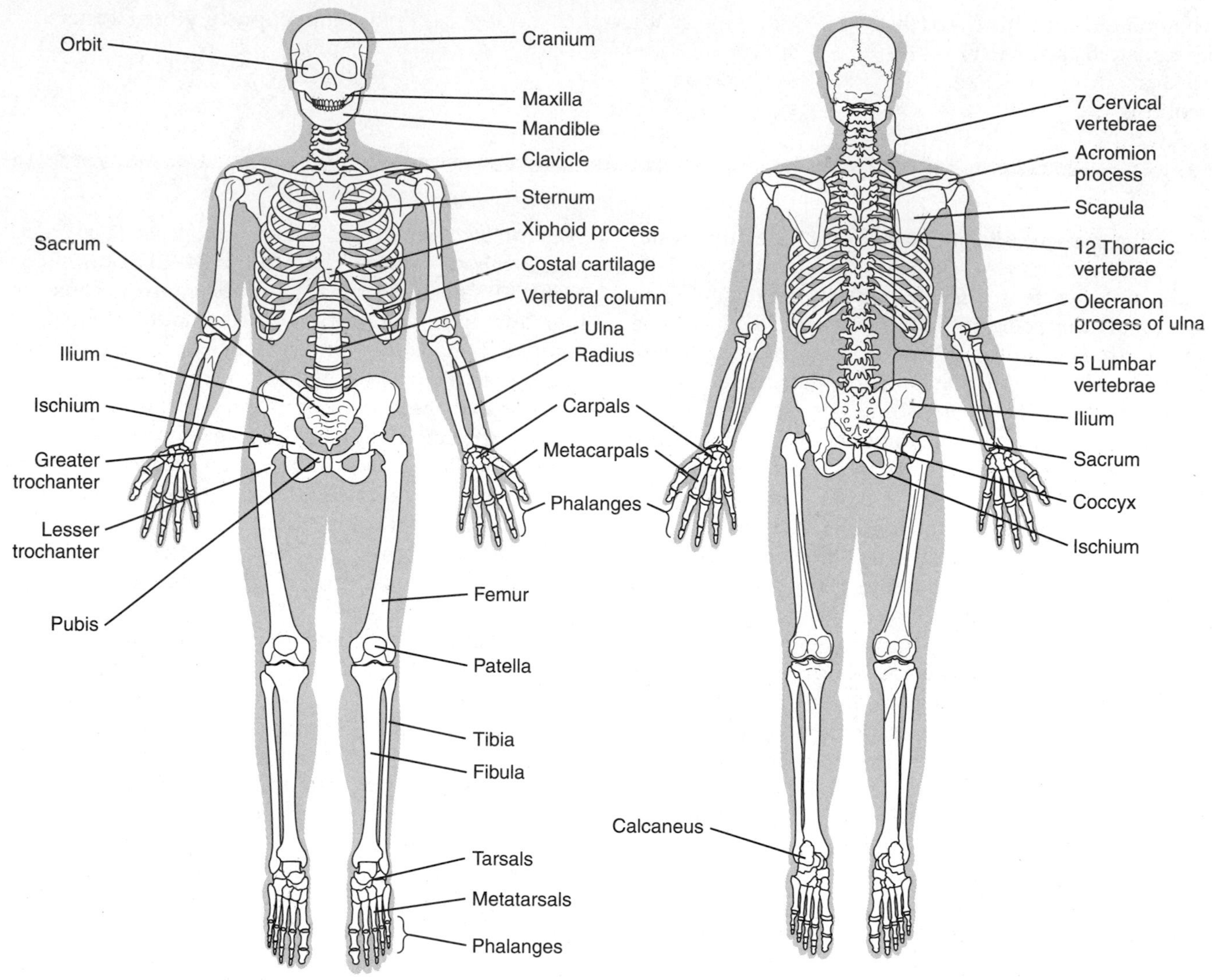

FIGURE 34–1

Skeletal system. The *axial skeleton* includes the cranium, the vertebral column, and bony thorax (ribs and sternum). The *appendicular skeleton* includes the bones of the pelvic girdle and extremities.

Bone

In bone, minerals such as calcium and phosphate are deposited into the organic matrix to confer structural rigidity and strength. The cell types found within this matrix include osteogenic cells (which become osteoblasts when activated), osteoblasts (bone-forming cells), osteoclasts (which phagocytize bone), and osteocytes (mature bone cells or "trapped" osteoblasts).

The functional unit of compact bone is the haversian system or osteon, illustrated in Figure 34–3. Each osteocyte is immediately surrounded by a lacuna (lake) of fluid, then by a calcified matrix through which canaliculi (small channels) permit access of blood vessels and nerves. These bony matrices are arranged in concentric layers around a central haversian canal that also carries blood vessels and nerve fibers. Because of this innervation, disorders of bone may be exquisitely painful.

Cartilage

The structure of cartilage, tendons, and ligaments differs from bone in that calcium and phosphate crystals do not precipitate into the matrix (except under pathologic conditions). The strength of these tissues derives from the collagen fibers in the matrix, and the lack of crystallization permits increased flexibility. Cartilage is higher in fluid content than bone and contains no blood vessels, being nourished instead by diffusion of nutrients into its fluid matrix.

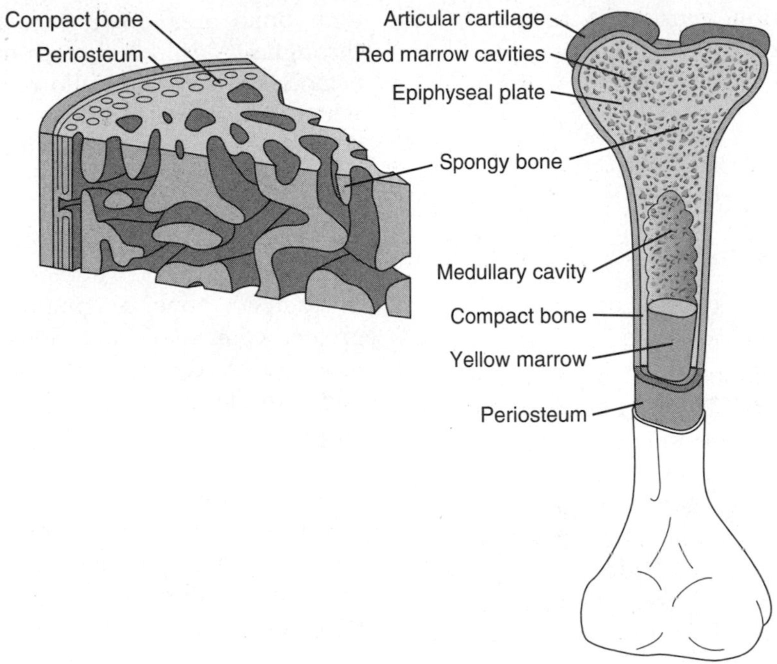

FIGURE 34–2
Cancellous and compact bone. Bone tissue consists of two structural types. *Cancellous bone* (spongy bone) is light and spongy in appearance because of dispersed marrow spaces, whereas *compact bone* is much more dense because of a high degree of calcification.

Cartilage also lacks nerve endings, permitting extensive injury or degeneration that is nonpainful unless adjoining innervated tissues are affected.

Hyaline cartilage is the most abundant form of cartilage in the body, forming the fetal skeleton as well as the cartilage within most joints and epiphyseal plates. *Fibrocartilage*, the most rigid form, is found in the intervertebral disks, the pubic joints, and at points of attachment of tendons to bone. In the knee, fibrocartilage forms shock-absorbing pads (menisci) that are prone to damage with acute trauma or arthritis.

Tendons and Ligaments

Tendons and ligaments are fibrous bands composed mainly of bundled collagen fibers, although they do contain a few blood vessels. Tendons, which connect muscle to bone, are enclosed by sheaths consisting of two membranes separated by a thin layer of fluid for lubrication during movement. With **tendinitis**, inflammatory exudation into this potential fluid space may occur. Ligaments are critical structures within most joints, connecting the articulating bones. Ligament tears and **sprains,** commonly

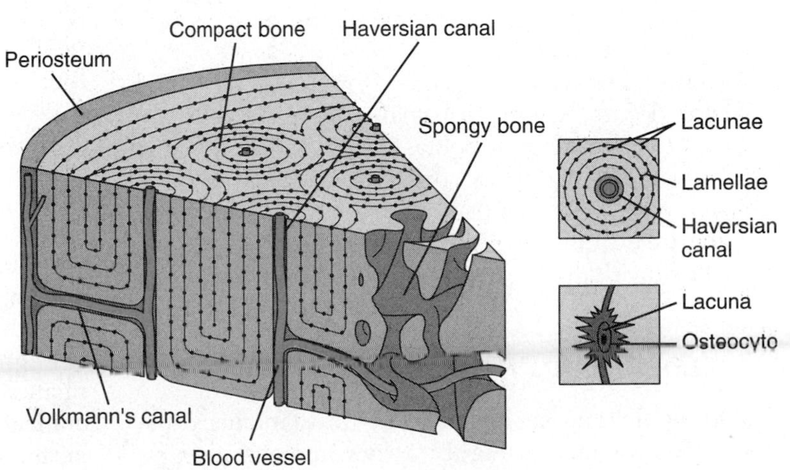

FIGURE 34–3
Haversian system. The functional unit of compact bone is the *haversian system* or osteon. Each bone cell (osteocyte) is surrounded by a lacuna (lake) of fluid, then by a calcified matrix through which small channels (Volkmann's canals) permit access of blood vessels and nerves. The bony matrix is arranged in concentric circles around a central haversian canal, which carries larger blood vessels and nerve fibers.

seen with hyperextension injuries of the joints, are discussed later in this chapter.

Bone Formation and Remodeling

Bone Growth

In most individuals, linear bone growth is complete by age 18 in women and age 22 in men, with a particularly rapid period of bone growth during puberty (see Developmental Perspective).[1] Bones continue to accumulate more mineral deposits, however, and *peak bone mass* is typically attained during the third decade of life. Depending on genetic, nutritional, and mechanical factors, bone mass is normally constant until the 4th decade in women and then declines fairly rapidly after menopause. This decline in bone mass occurs about two decades later in men.

Linear bone growth occurs at the epiphyseal plates located at the cartilaginous ends (epiphyses) of long bones (Fig. 34–4). Activity at the epiphysis progresses from outside in. The outermost layer of epiphyseal cartilage cells (chondrocytes) is a resting cell layer, awaiting activation by hormones (growth hormone, thyroid hormone, and sex hormones). The next layer (*zone of proliferation*) consists of actively dividing cells that are pushed toward the shaft (diaphysis) of the bone into the *zone of hypertrophy*. The cells in this area enlarge in size, but become structurally weaker in doing so. Children may suffer epiphyseal fractures at this vulnerable site, resulting in impairment or arrest of bone growth. From the zone of hypertrophy, cells push inward to the *zone of provisional calcification*, where they begin to undergo ossification, which is deposition of organic matrix and inorganic salts resulting in formation of mature bone. When linear growth is completed, the inner epiphyseal layers ossify (i.e., the epiphyseal plate "fuses"), and the outer layer differentiates into mature articular cartilage.

Growth in bone diameter (appositional bone growth) occurs when periosteal osteogenic cells are activated, increasing osteoblastic deposition of bone on the outside of the existing bone. Increased bone density and bone deposition associated with bone healing or continuous remodeling also occurs by this mechanism.

Continuous Remodeling of Bone

Although bone seems more static than many tissues, it is, in fact, a highly active homeostatic system. Bone breakdown (*resorption*) occurs in cycles throughout adulthood, with each period of increased osteoclastic activity followed by a period during which osteoblasts deposit new bone. After completion of growth and acquisition of peak bone mass, osteoblastic and osteoclastic processes are normally in equilibrium, so that total bone mass and density are relatively stable until late adulthood. The rate of remodeling is much higher in cancellous bone than in compact bone, as might be expected given the greater contact of cancellous bone with bone marrow, which contains the precursors of osteoblasts and osteoclasts.

Regulation of Osteoblastic and Osteoclastic Activity

The activity of osteogenic stem cells, osteoblasts, and osteoclasts is under a complex system of regulation that is still being clarified. Several hormones are known to enhance or inhibit bone growth and remodeling, including growth hormone (GH), parathyroid hormone (PTH), calcitonin, vitamin D_3, estrogen, and testosterone. In addition, the importance of a number of locally produced cytokines and lipid mediators (e.g., prostaglandins, interleukins, tumor necrosis factor-α, insulin-like growth factors, and transforming growth factor-β) is increasingly appreciated.[2] Table 34–1 summarizes the effects of these hormones and mediators on bone homeostasis. New bone formation occurs in areas of bone strain, such as that caused by weight-bearing, whereas bone resorption is accelerated when this stress is removed for extended lengths of time (e.g., during prolonged bedrest). The mechanisms underlying this mechanical regulation of bone metabolism are unknown, but presumably involve local regulation by cytokines and tissue matrix signaling (see Chapter 2).

Energy and substrate must be available for new bone formation, requiring sufficient dietary intake and normal serum levels of calcium and phosphate. As discussed in Chapter 9, the ratio of calcium to phosphate is also important. A low calcium-to-phosphate ratio, whether caused by inadequate calcium intake or excessive phosphate intake or retention, promotes decreased levels of ionized calcium and persistent elevation of PTH. The actions of PTH increase serum levels of ionized calcium at the expense of bone mass (see Chapter 28).

Although PTH is the central regulator of bone mass, the steroid hormone vitamin D_3 is also important in calcium homeostasis and stimulation of bone growth (see Chapter 9). Physiologic levels of vitamin D augment the effects of PTH on calcium and phosphate absorption from the gut and enhance mineralization of bone. At the same time, vitamin D permits PTH-mediated bone resorption. Lack of acti-

Developmental Perspective

Embryonic and Fetal Periods

The skeletal system and other connective tissues develop from embryonic mesenchyme, derived from mesoderm and neural crest cells. Cartilage first appears at 5 weeks' gestation. Bone develops in mesenchyme and from some cartilaginous models through osteoblastic deposition of protein matrix. Bone mineral deposition into the limb bones begins at the end of the embryonic period and requires an adequate supply of calcium and phosphate. At birth, the ends of the long bones (epiphyses) are still cartilaginous, although the rest of the skeleton is well mineralized. Joints begin to develop by the sixth week of gestation, resembling adult joints by 8 weeks. Fibrous joints (sutures) between the bones of the skull permit molding of the head during delivery. The most significant congenital abnormalities of the bones and joints are spina bifida, accessory ribs, microcephaly, and achondroplastic dwarfism. Some primary bone tumors have their origin in embryonic mesenchymal tissues.

Infancy and Childhood

Before puberty, adequate dietary intake of protein, energy, and calcium results in robust gains in bone mass. Pediatric musculoskeletal injuries are a common reason for emergency-department treatment and hospitalization in children. Although most injuries occur accidentally while the child is at play, intentional abuse is also a source of injury. Growth plate injuries with fractures or severe sprains may result in significant deformity. The periosteum is thicker in children's bones, reducing displacement during fractures and speeding bone healing. Pediatric bone is less dense than normal adult bone and tends to bend in response to the same amount of force that would fracture bone in older individuals. Fracture of the clavicle is the most common childhood fracture. Osteochondroses are also common in growing children. Juvenile RA and systemic lupus erythematosus (SLE) may have their onset during childhood or adolescence.

Adolescence and Young Adulthood

Bone growth during adolescence and young adulthood is largely driven by growth hormone and sex hormones. Linear bone growth ceases at about age 18 in women and age 22 in men, but bone mass continues to increase during young adulthood. Physical activity during this period is associated with modeling of bone for function. Participation in sports and other activities imposes risk of musculoskeletal injury. Scoliosis is commonly detected during school screening, and juvenile RA commonly manifests in adolescents. Primary bone tumors are often diagnosed in this age group. SLE is most frequently diagnosed in young women during their childbearing years.

Middle and Older Adulthood

Although osteoporosis and osteoarthritis are not inevitable with aging, they are exceedingly common among the elderly, particularly elderly women. Removal of estrogen at menopause imposes significant risk of osteoporosis, especially among those who demonstrate a genetically determined rapid rate of loss of bone mass. Osteoarthritis affects about 80% of individuals older than 65 years, leading to a significant decline in quality of life for many. RA, gout, and less common forms of arthritis also have their highest incidence among the elderly. Fractures in the elderly may be traumatic (associated with falls), but they are more often pathologic, associated with normal weight-bearing, movement, or coughing and occurring in bones weakened by osteoporosis or bony metastasis.

vated vitamin D_3 may result from dietary deficiency, lack of sunlight exposure, malabsorption, liver disease, or kidney disease, promoting **rickets** in children or **osteomalacia** in adults. These disorders are discussed later in this chapter.

Deposition of Bone by Osteoblasts

Osteoblasts first secrete collagen and ground substance to form *osteon,* a matrix that is receptive to precipitation of calcium and phosphate. About 75% of the calcium and phosphate precipitated forms

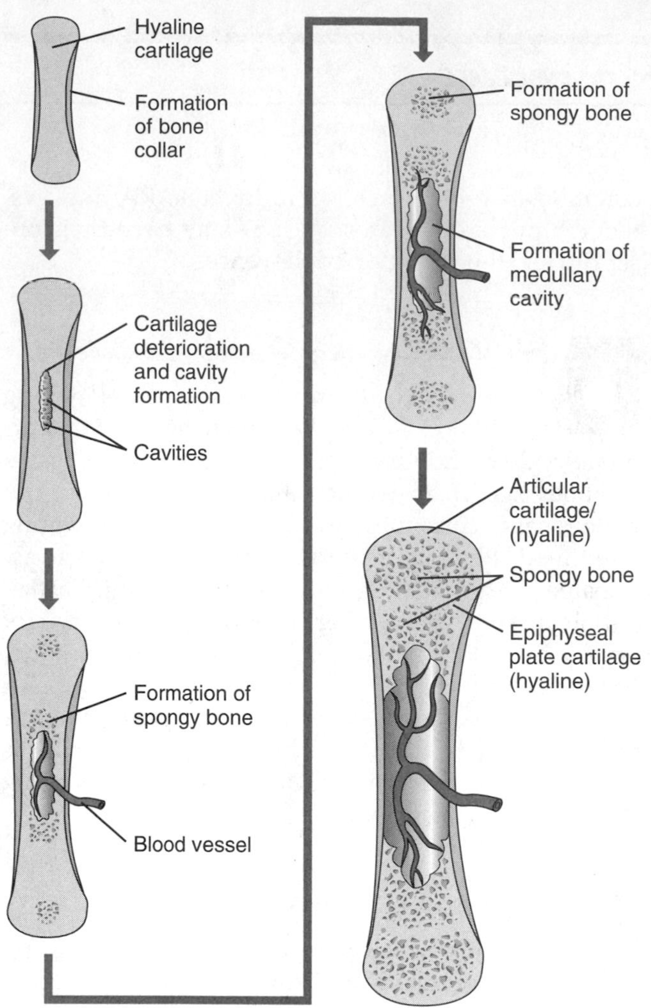

FIGURE 34–4
Bone growth and ossification. Embryonic development of most bones occurs by a process that uses hyaline cartilage structures as models for bone formation. Linear bone growth occurs at the epiphyseal plates located at the cartilaginous ends of long bones.

crystalline plates that are rigid, and 25% (at the bone surface) remains in a more disorganized form, constituting an exchangeable pool of these ions between bone and blood. Any osteoblasts trapped by calcium and phosphate deposition become osteocytes.

Resorption of Bone by Osteoclasts

Osteoclasts, derived from the same hematopoietic stem cells as monocyte-macrophages, are characterized by the same phagocytic activity. These cells digest the organic matrix, releasing the calcium and phosphate salts from bone. Osteoclasts are responsive to a number of cytokines, including several interleukins. Interleukin-6 is known to be particularly important in pathologic conditions in which osteoclastic activity occurs in excess of bone formation, such as **multiple myeloma, Paget's disease** of bone, and RA.[3]

Structure and Function of the Joints

Definition and Classification

Joints are points where two or more bones join, or articulate. The term *articular cartilage* refers to cartilage within joints, and the dynamic function of this cartilage is essential to withstand weight-bearing and the shearing forces inflicted with movement. Three types of joints are found within the human body: *synarthroses*, which are normally immovable; *amphiarthroses*, which are slightly movable; and *diarthroses*, which are freely movable within their normal range of motion. The sutures of the skull, which are normally fused with new bone formation after 18 months of age, are examples of synarthroses. Fibrocartilage, with its very limited flexibility, is found in the amphiarthroses of the symphysis pubis and intervertebral joints.

Structure of Diarthrotic Joints

Most joints in the body are diarthroses, also known as *synovial joints* (Fig. 34–5). Within these joints, the bones are covered with articular cartilages that distribute the weight load on the joint and that slide over each other during movement. A capsule of periosteum encloses the joint, and ligaments con-

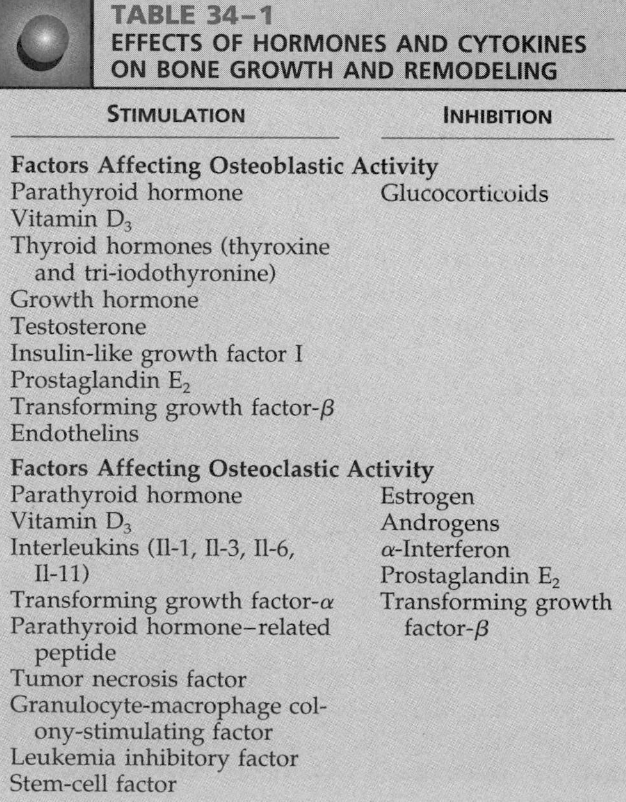

TABLE 34–1
EFFECTS OF HORMONES AND CYTOKINES ON BONE GROWTH AND REMODELING

STIMULATION	INHIBITION
Factors Affecting Osteoblastic Activity	
Parathyroid hormone	Glucocorticoids
Vitamin D_3	
Thyroid hormones (thyroxine and tri-iodothyronine)	
Growth hormone	
Testosterone	
Insulin-like growth factor I	
Prostaglandin E_2	
Transforming growth factor-β	
Endothelins	
Factors Affecting Osteoclastic Activity	
Parathyroid hormone	Estrogen
Vitamin D_3	Androgens
Interleukins (Il-1, Il-3, Il-6, Il-11)	α-Interferon
Transforming growth factor-α	Prostaglandin E_2
Parathyroid hormone–related peptide	Transforming growth factor-β
Tumor necrosis factor	
Granulocyte-macrophage colony-stimulating factor	
Leukemia inhibitory factor	
Stem-cell factor	

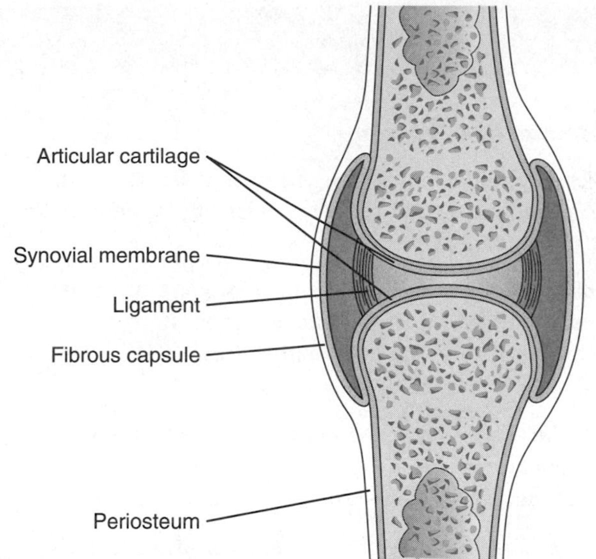

FIGURE 34–5
Synovial joint structure. Most joints of the body are synovial (diarthrotic) joints. The articulating surfaces of the bones are covered with weight-bearing *articular cartilage.* A capsule of *periosteum* encloses the joint, and *ligaments* connect the bones. The *synovial membrane* lines the joint cavity and secretes synovial fluid, which lubricates the joint and serves as a diffusion medium for nutrients.

nect the bones. The *synovial membrane* that lines the joint capsule secretes *synovial fluid,* a viscous fluid that transudes from the plasma. Synovial fluid lubricates the joint and serves as a diffusion medium for nutrients. Hydrostatic movement of fluid between the matrix of the articular cartilage and the joint space normally prevents damage to the cartilage with repeated weight-bearing and movement.

In some diarthroses, the synovial membrane separates in places to form fluid-filled sacs (*bursae*), which serve to cushion tendons. In **bursitis** caused by joint injury, these areas may become acutely inflamed. Membranes associated with joints, tendons, and ligaments contain pain receptors and proprioceptors that relay sensory information and are served by the same spinal nerves as the associated muscles. The synovial membrane is richly perfused, and its vessels are surrounded by mast cells, facilitating the inflammatory response.

Microstructure and Function of the Articular Cartilage

Articular cartilage is hyaline cartilage, composed of collagen fibers, water, proteoglycans, and chondrocytes. The collagen fibers are arranged in arches at the articular surface, allowing them to deform with weight-bearing and distribute the load across a greater area. The proteoglycans play an important role in regulation of water flux between the cartilage matrix and the synovial space. Water that is squeezed out with weight-bearing is attracted back into the matrix by proteoglycans when weight is released.

Chondrocytes contain enzymes regulating synthesis of the cartilage matrix as well as its digestion. Because cartilage is without blood supply, these processes are under regulation by local cytokines rather than by circulating hormones. Similarly to bone formation and resorption, collagen deposition and digestion are normally in equilibrium, permitting continuous renewal and remodeling of articular cartilage.

DISORDERS OF THE BONES AND JOINTS

Osteoporosis

Definition. Osteoporosis is a multifactorial disorder in which decreased bone mass and increased bone fragility result from disequilibrium of osteoblastic and osteoclastic activity.

Epidemiology. Osteoporosis is very common, affecting an estimated 25 million Americans.[4] It is primarily a disease of postmenopausal females, causing painful and debilitating fractures in one of two women, but it also affects one in eight men. Aging and loss of gonadal function are the two most important risk factors for its development. Premenopausal women who are amenorrheic or oligomenorrheic are also at increased risk, presumably because of estrogen deficiency, as are women who take antiestrogen drugs (e.g., tamoxifen) for therapy or prophylaxis of breast cancer or other gynecologic disorders (see Chapter 31). Blacks, who have denser bones as a baseline state, are at much lower risk than whites.

There is clearly a genetic predisposition toward the disease, related to inherent bone density and rate of bone loss. Women whose mothers had an osteoporosis-related fracture are at very high risk of developing the condition. Cortisol excess, whether caused by an endocrine disorder affecting the hypothalamic–pituitary–adrenal axis or caused by prolonged glucocorticoid therapy, contributes to osteoporosis by mobilizing bone proteins for energy (see Chapter 29). Hyperthyroidism may also promote demineralization of bone (see Chapter 28). Lack of exercise deprives bone of normal mechanical stresses, and dietary deficiencies of calcium and vitamin D also contribute to low bone mass. A high intake of caffeine has been shown to enhance bone loss in

Focus of Current Research

Study	Objective and Findings
Ettinger, et al. (1997) A randomized trial comparing aerobic exercise and resistance exercise with a health education program in older adults with knee osteoarthritis: The Fitness Arthritis and Seniors Trial (FAST).	*Objective:* To determine the effect of structured exercise programs on self-reported disability in older adults with knee osteoarthritis *Findings:* Older disabled persons with knee osteoarthritis had modest improvements in disability, physical performance, and pain with either form of exercise.
Karpf, et al. (1997) Prevention of nonvertebral fractures by alendronate.	*Objective:* To evaluate the effect of treatment with alendronate on the incidence of nonvertebral fractures in postmenopausal women with osteoporosis *Findings:* Treatment with alendronate reduces the risk of nonvertebral fractures for at least 3 years.
O'Dell, et al. (1996) Treatment of rheumatoid arthritis with methotrexate alone, sulfasalazine, and hydroxychloroquine, or a combination of all three medications.	*Objective:* To determine whether disease-modifying agents were effective as combination therapy for rheumatoid arthritis and whether the combinations studied had better efficacy than methotrexate alone *Findings:* Combination therapy is more effective than methotrexate alone. The combination of methotrexate, sulfasalazine, and hydroxychloroquine was more effective than sulfasalazine and hydroxychloroquine.
To, et al. (1995) Regulation of adhesion molecule expression by human synovial microvascular endothelial cells in vitro.	*Objective:* To examine the expression of adhesion molecules by synovial microvascular endothelial cells in comparison with similar cells in neonatal foreskin and umbilical vein *Findings:* Regulation is different in synovial cells. Augmented expression of adhesion molecules in rheumatoid arthritis may facilitate recruitment of leukocytes to this site.
Kirwan, et al. (1995) The effect of glucocorticoids on joint destruction in rheumatoid arthritis.	*Objective:* To compare oral prednisolone with placebo in adults with active rheumatoid arthritis of less than 2 years' duration *Findings:* Prednisolone substantially reduced the rate of progression of the disease.
Cummings, et al. (1995) Risk factors for hip fracture in white women.	*Objective:* To assess potential risk factors for hip fracture in white women 65 years of age or older *Findings:* Women with multiple risk factors and low bone density have an especially high risk of hip fracture. Maintaining body weight, walking for exercise, avoiding long-acting benzodiazepines, minimizing caffeine intake, and treating impaired visual function may decrease risk.

continued

Barrett-Connor, et al. (1994) Coffee-associated osteoporosis offset by daily milk consumption: The Rancho Bernardo Study	*Objective:* To describe the association of lifetime intake of caffeinated coffee to bone mineral density in postmenopausal women, and to determine the effect of regular milk intake on this association *Findings:* Coffee intake equivalent to 2 cups per day is associated with decreased bone density in older women who do not drink milk on a daily basis.
Henderson and Specter (1994) Kyphosis and fractures in children and young adults with cystic fibrosis.	*Objective:* To examine children and adolescents with cystic fibrosis for increased frequency of fractures or kyphosis. *Findings:* Females 6 to 16 years of age had higher-than-normal rates of fracture. Seventy-seven per cent of females and 36% of males older than 15 years had kyphosis exceeding 40 degrees. Decreased bone density was probably a contributing factor.

those who are also calcium-deficient (see Focus of Current Research).[5] Cigarette smoking, alcohol abuse, and sedentary lifestyle are other factors that promote loss of bone mass.

Etiology. The combination of low bone density (caused by developmental, genetic, hormonal, and lifestyle factors) and genetically determined rapid rate of bone loss results in the development of osteoporosis in older individuals.

Pathophysiology. Estrogen and, to a lesser extent, testosterone, protect against excessive osteoclastic activity, apparently by interfering with transcription of the gene for interleukin-6. Gonadal deficiency thus enhances osteoclastic activity. In addition, aging has a depressant effect on the bone marrow, reducing the availability of osteoblastic cells. Dietary and lifestyle factors may contribute to low bone density as a baseline state on which the imbalance in bone remodeling is superimposed.

Cancellous (trabecular) bone is most greatly affected, because its remodeling rate is much greater than that of cortical bone. Osteoporosis results in significant weakening and loss of the normal architecture of cancellous bone, as shown in Figure 34–6. The risk of fractures is greatly increased, particularly in areas where cancellous bone is predominant (e.g., vertebrae, the distal radius, and the femoral neck).

Clinical Manifestations. Initially, bone loss is asymptomatic. Conventional radiography does not detect osteoporosis until about 30% of bone mass has been lost. Diagnosis may be established earlier with the use of dual energy x ray absorptiometry (DXA), which provides a measure of bone mineral content in the spine, hip, and wrist.[6]

A fracture of the spine or hip is often the first clinical sign of osteoporosis. Compression fractures of the vertebrae alter their architecture from a cylindrical to a wedge shape, which forces a forward bending curvature and results in loss of height and **kyphosis** (dowager's hump) (Fig. 34–7). Back pain is common because of pressure and inflammation associated with vertebral fractures. Hip fractures are particularly common with falls and involve the femoral neck or intertrochanteric region in 90% of cases (Fig. 34–8).[7]

Prevention and Treatment. Optimal dietary intake of calcium and vitamin D and regular weight-bearing exercise promote maintenance of bone density. Screening of at-risk populations with DXA is controversial; although it may detect early bone loss, the procedure is costly and does not predict the rate of progression of the disease. Hormone replacement therapy (HRT) has been shown to reduce bone resorption to premenopausal levels, particularly if begun soon after menopause. All forms of estrogen and estrogen-progesterone combination therapy are effective if sufficient doses are used, but extended treatment is required. The increased risk of endometrial cancer and possibly breast cancer with HRT must be considered in the decision to advocate HRT in postmenopausal women (see Chapter 31). Testosterone replacement prevents bone loss in men with documented gonadal deficiency, but it may exacerbate prostatic hyperplasia and dyslipidemia (see Chapter 30).

In addition to HRT, pharmacologic treatment of osteoporosis includes biphosphonates such as alendronate (Fosamax), calcitonin, and slow-release so-

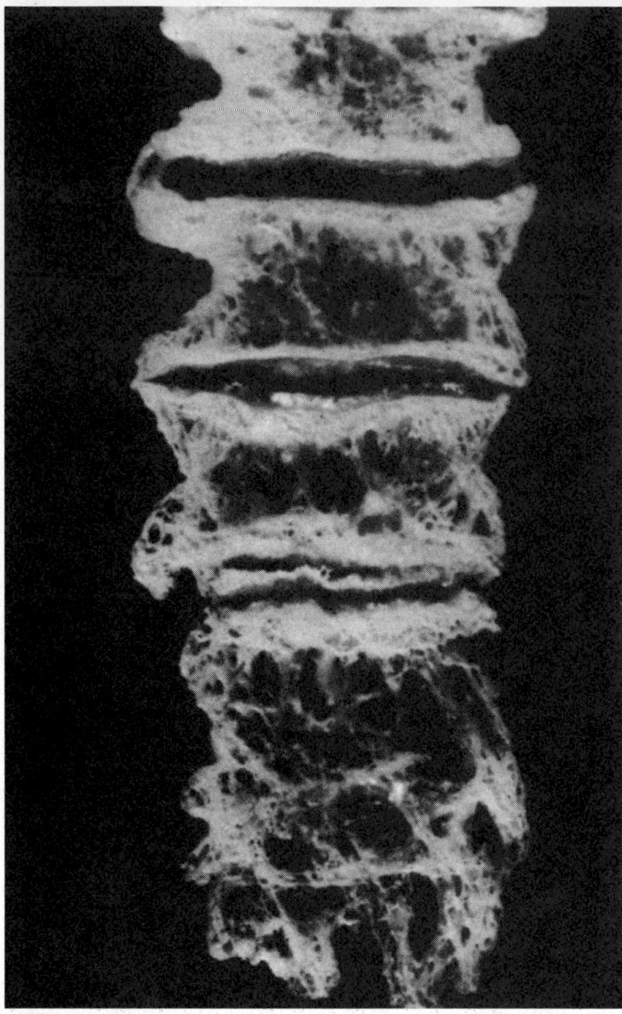

FIGURE 34–6
Osteoporosis. In this section of vertebrae, marked loss of bone matrix is apparent, caused by an excess of osteoclastic activity. (From Cotran, R.S., Kumar, V., and Robbins, S.L. [1994]. *Robbins' Pathologic Basis of Disease.* [5th ed.]. Philadelphia: W.B. Saunders. [p. 1221].)

dium fluoride. The biphosphonates bind to calcium-phosphate (hydroxyapatite) crystals that, when deposited into newly synthesized bone matrix, inhibit osteoclastic activity. At physiologic levels, the thyroid hormone calcitonin weakly opposes the effects of PTH, thus inhibiting bone resorption (see Chapter 28). Therapeutic use of calcitonin is generally reserved for those who cannot take HRT or alendronate. At pharmacologic doses, calcitonin inhibits bone resorption and has an analgesic effect on the pain of osteoporotic fractures. Calcitonin must be administered parenterally or intranasally, however, and its use is accompanied by side effects such as nausea and vomiting. Sodium fluoride has the advantage of lower cost, and it has been shown to increase the number of osteoblasts, stimulating bone formation. However, some studies have demonstrated an *increased* incidence of fractures with fluoride use, as a consequence of the formation of weaker, more brittle bone under fluoride stimulation.[6]

Prognosis and Outcome. The protective effects of HRT can only be maintained with continuous therapy. Loss of bone density is apparently inevitable with aging, although the rate of loss may be markedly slowed with hormonal, dietary, and activity-based interventions. Osteoporosis-related fractures result in significant morbidity and mortality. Spinal fractures occur in 25% of white women by age 65 years, resulting in considerable pain, deformity, and disability.[8] More than 200,000 hip fractures occur annually, and nearly one in four of these patients dies within a year of the injury.[9] Twenty per cent of women sustaining hip fractures require institutional care within a skilled nursing facility, and the average length of stay is 7 years.

Osteomyelitis

Definition. Osteomyelitis is an infectious disorder of bone characterized by progressive inflammatory destruction after new formation of bone.

Epidemiology. Osteomyelitis is becoming more prevalent, possibly because of greater numbers of immunosuppressed individuals, the emergence of new organisms and resistant strains, and frequent

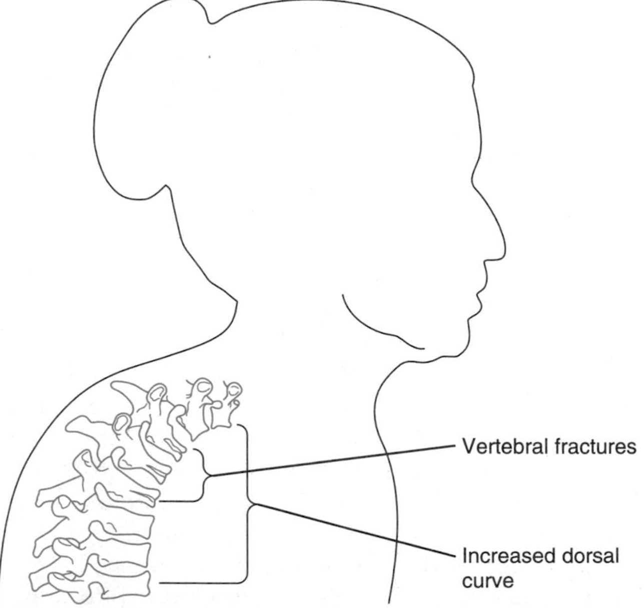

FIGURE 34–7
Kyphosis and vertebral fracture in osteoporosis. Compression fractures of the vertebrae are common with osteoporosis. Fractured vertebrae flatten and assume a wedge shape, resulting in concave curvature of the thoracic spine (kyphosis or dowager's hump) and loss of height.

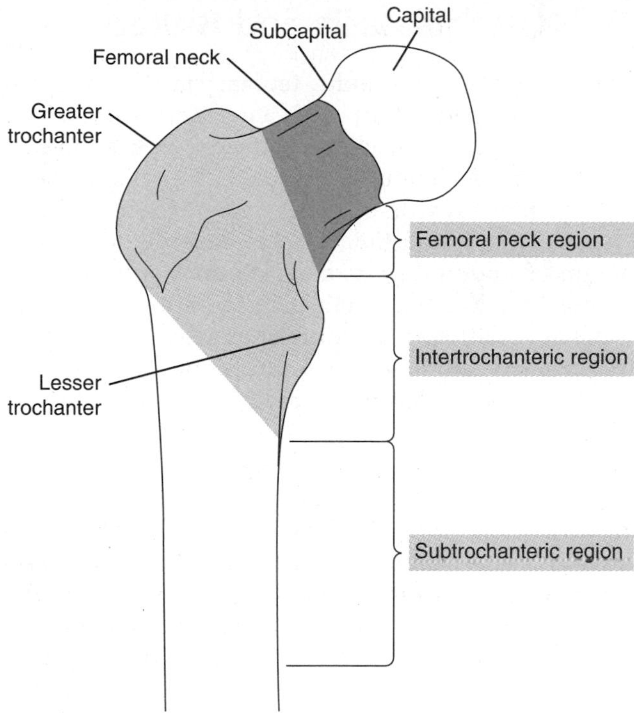

FIGURE 34–8

Usual sites of hip fracture. Ninety per cent of hip fractures associated with osteoporosis and falls involve the femoral neck or intertrochanteric region.

use of prosthetic devices in fracture fixation and joint replacement. General risk factors for systemic infection, attributable to exposure to organisms and host vulnerability, thus apply (see Chapter 13). Risk is highest among the elderly and among children. Individuals with sickle cell anemia are at increased risk because of impaired circulation to epiphyseal areas with sickling crises (see Chapter 12). Rapidly growing children are at increased risk because increased vascularity of epiphyseal tissues facilitates access of organisms. Each year in the United States, 1 in 5000 children under the age of 13 is diagnosed with osteomyelitis.[10] Boys are affected 2.5 times as often as girls.

Etiology. Although a wide variety of organisms may cause osteomyelitis, *Staphylococcus aureus* is the cause in 85% to 90% of cases (Table 34–2). Organisms may access bone endogenously, traveling through the bloodstream from primary sites in the upper respiratory tract, middle ear, gastrointestinal (GI) tract, or urinary system. Less commonly, organisms gain exogenous access via compound fractures, surgery, injection sites (especially with intravenous drug abuse), or the bites of humans or animals.

Pathophysiology. Organisms such as *S. aureus* adhere to bone by expressing adhesion molecules that bind components of the bone matrix. In this adherent state, microorganisms are highly resistant to antibiotics. After invading the vascular supply in bone, the organism triggers an inflammatory response within this enclosed space. Inflammatory exudate infiltrates the canaliculi and the bone marrow, and, particularly in children, may extend beneath the periosteum, forming abscesses. Stripping of the periosteum disrupts the blood supply to underlying bone, infarcting the endosteum and resulting in the development of a necrotic area known as a *sequestrum.* Osteogenic cells in the periosteum are also activated with stripping, resulting in formation of a layer of new bone that surrounds the sequestrum. Inflammation continues within the sequestrum, and inflammatory mediators released by phagocytic cells may generate reactive oxygen species and activate proteolytic enzymes that injure bone and surrounding soft tissues.

Clinical Manifestations. The bacteremia that precedes the development of endogenous osteomyelitis

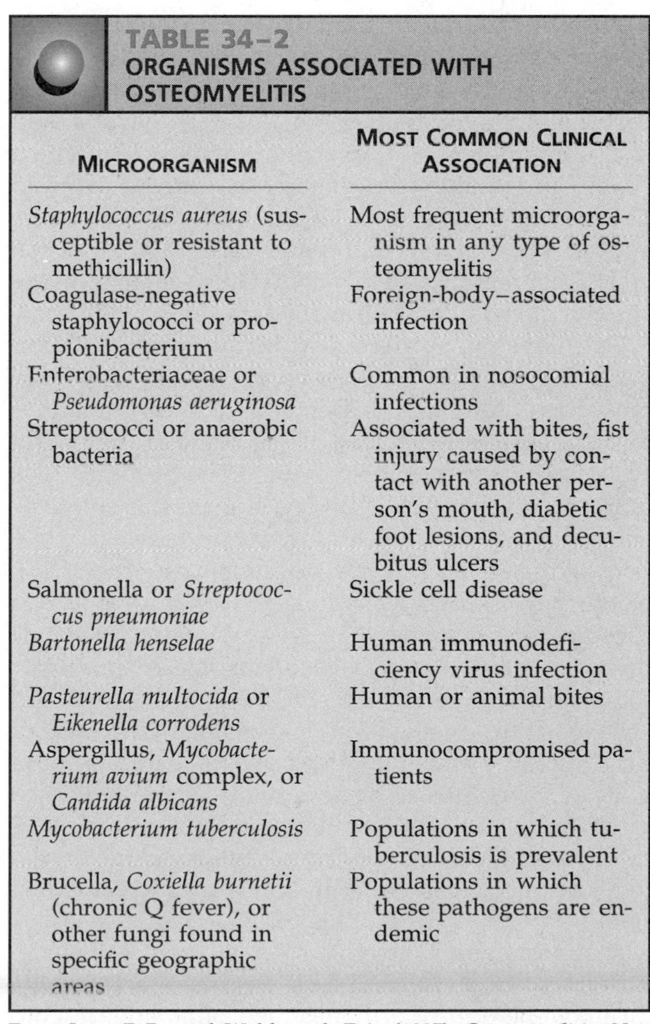

TABLE 34–2
ORGANISMS ASSOCIATED WITH OSTEOMYELITIS

MICROORGANISM	MOST COMMON CLINICAL ASSOCIATION
Staphylococcus aureus (susceptible or resistant to methicillin)	Most frequent microorganism in any type of osteomyelitis
Coagulase-negative staphylococci or propionibacterium	Foreign-body–associated infection
Enterobacteriaceae or *Pseudomonas aeruginosa*	Common in nosocomial infections
Streptococci or anaerobic bacteria	Associated with bites, fist injury caused by contact with another person's mouth, diabetic foot lesions, and decubitus ulcers
Salmonella or *Streptococcus pneumoniae*	Sickle cell disease
Bartonella henselae	Human immunodeficiency virus infection
Pasteurella multocida or *Eikenella corrodens*	Human or animal bites
Aspergillus, *Mycobacterium avium* complex, or *Candida albicans*	Immunocompromised patients
Mycobacterium tuberculosis	Populations in which tuberculosis is prevalent
Brucella, *Coxiella burnetii* (chronic Q fever), or other fungi found in specific geographic areas	Populations in which these pathogens are endemic

From Lew, D.P., and Waldvogel, F.A. (1997). Osteomyelitis. *New England Journal of Medicine* 336(14), 1001.

may be asymptomatic in some cases, but systemic signs of inflammation, including fever and malaise, are usually present. The location of the bone lesion (or lesions) depends on the cause. Needle aspiration of the affected area of bone may reveal the presence of the organism. In children, the infection is usually localized to a single focus, commonly in the metaphyseal area of the tibia or femur where blood flow is sluggish. In adults, the vertebrae and the sternoclavicular, sacroiliac, and symphysis pubis joints are commonly affected. Osteomyelitis in individuals with diabetes or vascular insufficiency usually affects the feet. Lesions associated with prostheses are located at the insertion or implantation site.

Bone pain may range from vague to excruciating. Inflammatory mediators often trigger muscle spasm in the affected area, which further contributes to pain and may dislocate affected joints. Pathologic fractures are also possible. Redness, warmth, and edema of overlying soft tissue are common, and lymph nodes proximal to the infected site are enlarged.

Prevention and Treatment. Preventive measures for common infections should be undertaken. Meticulous aseptic technique must be used in care of invasive lines, surgical incisions, fixation devices, and any other potential exogenous source of infection. Prophylactic antibiotic therapy is commonly used before bone surgery as well as during the procedure and for a short time postoperatively. Early detection and intervention of osteomyelitis may prevent chronic infection and ultimate deformity.

Osteomyelitis is treated with appropriate antibiotic therapy as well as symptomatic and supportive measures. Although parenteral administration is most often used, delivery of the drug to the poorly vascularized area of the lesion may be limited. A number of innovative delivery systems are currently being investigated, including closed suction-irrigation of the lesion and direct implantation of pellets or other substances impregnated with antibiotic.[12] In chronic osteomyelitis that is resistant to antibiotic therapy, surgery may be done to release pus from the lesion and to débride all devitalized bone and soft tissue in preparation for healing. The wound may then be covered and revascularized with a graft of bone, muscle, or skin.[11] Osteomyelitis associated with a prosthetic device usually requires surgical removal of the device.[12] Osteomyelitis of the foot may necessitate amputation if necrosis is extensive.

Prognosis and Outcome. The course of osteomyelitis is often prolonged, but outcomes are usually positive. Deformity of bones and joints and, in children, arrest of growth of an extremity may occur with severe cases.

Osteomalacia and Rickets

Definition. Rickets and osteomalacia are bone disorders characterized by deficient mineralization of the bone matrix caused by deficiency or abnormal metabolism of vitamin D. In children, rickets results in abnormal growth of cartilage and bone, and in adults, osteomalacia (adult rickets) results in the formation of undermineralized bone during cyclic bone remodeling. **Renal osteodystrophy**, commonly seen in patients with end-stage renal disease, is a form of osteomalacia, although factors other than vitamin D deficiency also contribute to bone weakness (see Chapter 20).

Epidemiology. In developing countries, rickets and osteomalacia commonly occur as a result of dietary deficiency. In the United States, these nutritional deficiencies are uncommon, but they may occur in pregnant women, children or the elderly who do not ingest dairy products fortified with vitamin D, or others with restricted or bizarre diets. Lack of sunlight exposure during long winters in the Northern hemisphere may also contribute, because the second source of vitamin D is through conversion of a precursor, 7-dehydrocholesterol, by skin cells exposed to ultraviolet light. Individuals with malabsorption syndromes, hepatic failure, or renal disease are also at increased risk, as discussed next.

Etiology. Although dietary deficiency and lack of sunlight exposure may contribute to the etiology, most cases of rickets and osteomalacia in the United States are caused by (1) impaired absorption of fat-soluble vitamins (including vitamin D) or (2) impaired hepatic or renal activation of dietary or skin-produced vitamin D, which are inert forms, to the active hormone, 1,25-dihydroxycholecalciferol (vitamin D_3).[13] Malabsorption of fat is characteristic of cholestatic liver disease, pancreatic insufficiency, gluten-sensitive enteropathy, and inflammatory bowel disease (see Chapter 25). Impaired activation of vitamin D is common with chronic renal failure and hepatic failure (see Chapters 20 and 26).

Pathophysiology. In adults and children, delayed or inadequate mineralization of bone matrix results in formation of bone that is disorganized in its structure and lacks density. Unlike osteoporosis, in which bone matrix is mineralized but deficient in quantity, osteomalacia and rickets are characterized by an adequate quantity of matrix but deficient mineralization. In children, there is also lack of provisional calcification of epiphyseal cartilage, leading to deformation during skeletal growth.

Clinical Manifestations. Skeletal abnormalities seen in children include short stature, squaring of the head, pigeon-breast deformity of the chest, lumbar **lordosis** (swayback), and bowing of the legs.

Clinical manifestations in adults are similar to those of osteoporosis. Serum levels of calcium, phosphorus, and vitamin D are low. Fractures of the vertebrae, hips, wrists, and ribs are common, and bone cysts may occur.

Prevention and Treatment. In dietary deficiency states, rickets and osteomalacia may be prevented with supplementation of the vitamin, along with calcium, phosphorus, and protein as necessary. Vitamin D supplementation is also used in treatment of the disorder. Optimal management of malabsorption syndromes, renal failure, and hepatic failure is also indicated.

Prognosis and Outcome. Mineralization of bone is usually evident on radiographs within 2 to 4 weeks of treatment. Depending on the age at which treatment of rickets is instituted, the skeletal deformities may improve or disappear over months to years. Failure of the individual to respond to vitamin D supplementation suggests an inherited defect in bone metabolism. Prognosis in malabsorption syndromes, renal failure, or hepatic failure is associated with the underlying cause. The osteomalacia of renal osteodystrophy usually does not respond to treatment with vitamin D supplementation.[14]

Osteochondroses

Definition. The **osteochondroses** are a group of disorders characterized by avascular necrosis of the epiphyseal growth plates in growing children and adolescents. The two best known osteochondroses are **Legg-Calvé-Perthes disease** (osteochondrosis of the femoral head) and **Osgood-Schlatter disease** (osteochondrosis of the tibial tubercle, just below the knee).

Epidemiology. The osteochondroses are relatively common. Legg-Calvé-Perthes disease usually affects children between 4 and 8 years of age and is four times more common in boys than in girls.[15] Osgood-Schlatter disease is most common in adolescents, particularly males who participate in sports.

Etiology. Although these disorders are related to bone growth, the precise etiology of the avascular necrosis is unknown. In Osgood-Schlatter disease, repetitive stress on the tibial tubercle with running or biking may contribute, especially if the quadriceps muscles are tight.[16]

Pathophysiology. Legg-Calvé-Perthes disease follows a predictable, self-limited course during a 12- to 36-month period. Lack of blood supply to the femoral head leads to septic necrosis, with softening and resorption of bone. Revascularization then results in reossification (new bone deposition) in the femoral head. Without treatment, the femoral head may become permanently flattened. The pattern is similar in Osgood-Schlatter disease, and new bone growth causes enlargement of the tibial tubercle.

Clinical Manifestations. Symptoms of Legg-Calvé-Perthes disease usually become apparent during the revascularization stage. Pain is present in the affected leg during activity, and the child may limp noticeably. Decreased range of motion and atrophy of buttock or thigh muscles may also be apparent. Osgood-Schlatter disease manifests as pain and swelling in the area of the tibial tubercle.

Prevention and Treatment. There is no known prevention. Early detection and treatment may prevent significant deformity. The goal of treatment in Legg-Calvé-Perthes disease is to prevent stress on the femoral head and to keep it within the joint capsule so that it regains its normal configuration with reossification. Bedrest may be indicated during acute pain. A non–weight-bearing brace and crutches may be used to permit some mobility. Surgery may also be required to keep the femoral head in position. Osgood-Schlatter disease is usually treated with activity restriction and possibly with immobilization in a long-leg cast to reduce pain and swelling. Activity is gradually resumed.

Prognosis and Outcome. With appropriate therapy, Legg-Calvé-Perthes disease usually resolves with little deformity of the hip. These children do have a higher risk of degenerative arthritis of the hip as adults, however.[16] The pain and swelling of Osgood-Schlatter disease disappear when growth stops, but enlargement of the tibial tubercle is permanent.

Sprains

Definition. A sprain is a traumatic injury of one or more ligaments within a joint.

Epidemiology. Although believed to be very common, the precise incidence of these injuries is unknown, because mild sprains are usually self-treated. The ankle is most frequently sprained. Collateral ligament sprains of the knee are also common. Risk factors are related to lack of physical conditioning or to any conditions (e.g., excessive or abnormal movements, environmental hazards) under which injury is more likely.

Etiology. The injury occurs as a result of direct trauma that induces movement of the joint outside its normal range of motion, such as turning an ankle, a football tackle to the knee, or whiplash sprain of cervical ligaments.

Pathophysiology. Sprain injury is classified in four grades (Fig. 34–9). A grade I sprain is a stretch injury of the ligament, resulting in a relatively mild inflammatory response. Grade II is a more severe

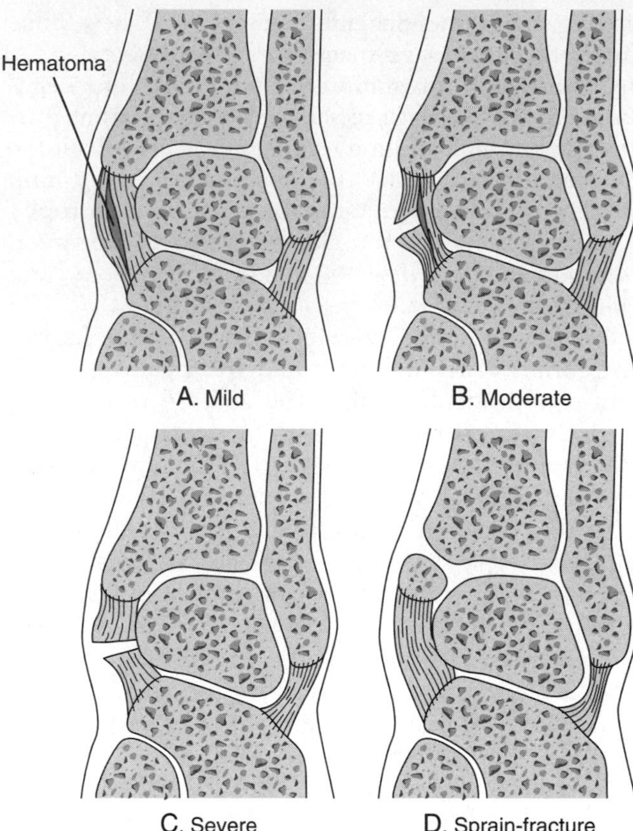

FIGURE 34–9

Classification of sprains. With mild (grade I) sprain, there is a stretch injury of the ligament, resulting in a mild inflammatory response. Hematoma may be present. With moderate (grade II) sprain, inflammation and hematoma result from more severe ligament stretch and tearing of some collagen fibers. In severe sprain (grade III), the ligament is completely torn, and in sprain-fracture (grade IV), the bony fragment to which the ligament is attached is broken away. (Redrawn from Black, J.M., and Matassarin-Jacobs, E. [1997]. *Medical-Surgical Nursing: Clinical Management for Continuity of Care.* [5th ed.]. Philadelphia: W.B. Saunders. [p. 2164].)

stretch with some tearing of collagen fibers and damage to blood vessels, resulting in inflammation and hematoma. In grade III, the ligament is completely torn, and in grade IV (sprain fracture), the bony fragment to which the ligament attaches is also broken away.

Clinical Manifestations. Clinical manifestations of some degree of inflammation are apparent, including pain, heat, and swelling. Ecchymosis (bruising) may be evident with hematoma formation. Mobility is impaired by pain in grades I and II and also by loss of joint integrity in grades III and IV.

Prevention and Treatment. Prevention requires that appropriate measures be taken to ensure optimal safety during risk-related activities, such as protective support of joints during sports, use of automobile headrests, and environmental lighting to prevent missteps. Immediate intervention consists of elevating the extremity and applying ice to limit inflammation. Limitation of the inflammatory response is adaptive in this case, because the joint constitutes an enclosed space (see Chapter 13). The joint is supported with a compression bandage, brace, or cast to provide support during healing and to limit further damage. Early protected mobilization and resistive exercises are encouraged to increase the tensile strength of the affected ligaments.[17] Severe sprains may require surgical intervention to evacuate hematomas, reduce fractures, or reconstruct the joint.

Prognosis and Outcome. Although prognosis varies with severity of the sprain, the outcome is positive in most cases, with complete or near-complete restoration of joint function.

Fractures

Definition. A fracture is a break in the continuity of bone. Fractures are described as *closed* if bone fragments do not penetrate the overlying skin and soft tissues or *open* if there is associated damage to overlying tissues. With a *complete* fracture, bone fragments are completely separated; with a *partial* fracture, the integrity of part of the bone has been retained. Figure 34–10 illustrates common patterns of fracture.

Epidemiology. An estimated 25% of the population suffers traumatic musculoskeletal injury each year, and a significant portion of these involve fractures.[18] Risk factors are those associated with the application of force to bone, such as falls, sports activities, motor vehicle accidents, or use of drugs that impair mobility or judgment, as well as those factors that decrease the ability of bone to withstand a deforming force, such as immaturity, osteoporosis, and metastatic or primary bone tumors.

Etiology. Fractures are caused by the application of a deforming force to bone, with the magnitude of the force being greater than the bone can withstand. Traumatic forces of great magnitude are required to fracture dense, mature bone, whereas much less force, such as that attributable to normal weight-bearing, may fracture weaker bone. *Pathologic (pathogenic) fractures* may occur with normal movement (such as coughing or changing position in bed) in persons with bone demineralization resulting from immobility, osteoporosis, or bone tumors. Because the bones of children are less dense, they are more likely to bend or buckle than more dense adult bones, which would probably fracture completely in response to the same force.[19] Table 34–3 lists the

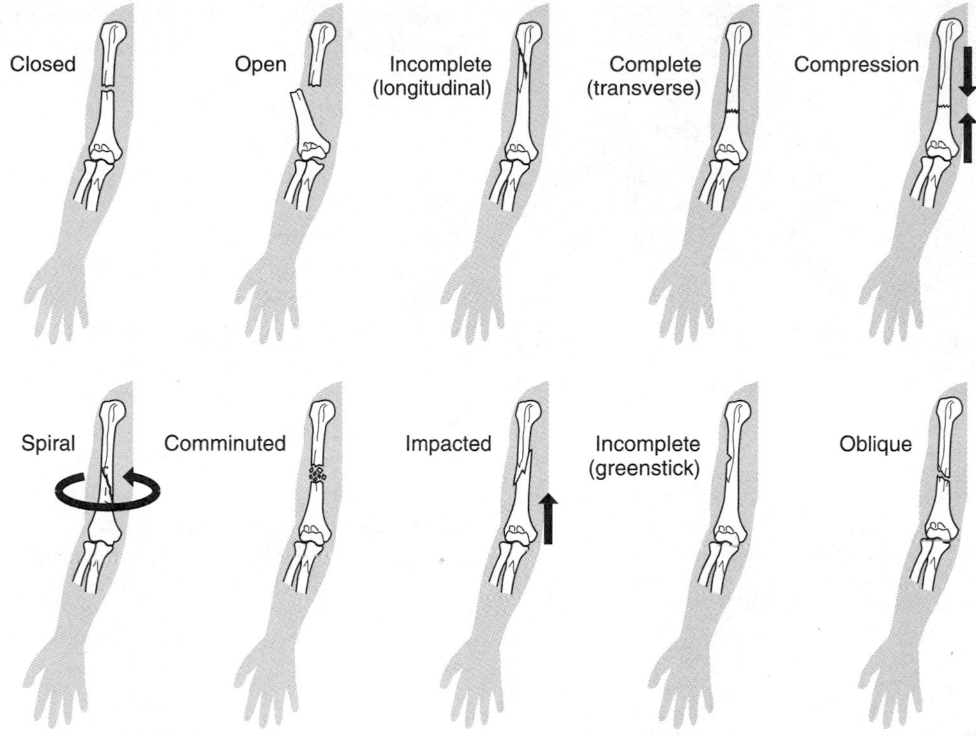

FIGURE 34–10

Patterns of fracture. Fractures may be classified on the basis of relative fragment position, integrity of the skin and soft tissues, or mechanism of injury. Common types of fracture are illustrated.

more common fractures along with the mechanism of injury.

Pathophysiology. Fractures in which bone ends are displaced not only disrupt the continuity of the bone but also damage the bone membranes, nerves, and blood vessels in the area. Surrounding soft tissues (muscle, nerves, connective tissue, and skin) may also be traumatized to some degree, triggering an inflammatory response. Loss of function of the affected skeletal area results. With long bone fractures in adults, the risk of fat emboli is present (see Chapter 14). **Compartmental syndrome** may complicate soft tissue damage if the anatomic configuration of the wound restricts the inflammatory response to a compartment enclosed by fascia (membranes) that surround muscle groups (Fig. 34–11). Edema within this enclosed tissue space compresses blood vessels, resulting in ischemic injury.

Clinical Manifestations. Severity of manifestations varies with the location and extent of the fracture and soft tissue damage. Typical findings are of deformity or abnormal mobility (if the fracture ends are displaced), surface bleeding (with possible severe hemorrhage) in compound fractures or ecchymosis and hematoma formation in simple fractures, possible *crepitus* with attempted movement (crunching sound caused by small fragments), and severe pain resulting from mechanical stimulation of pain receptors. Inflammation results in redness, warmth, edema, further pain, and loss of function. Fat emboli, a life-threatening complication, may result in acute respiratory failure or cardiac arrest. Compartmental syndrome is evidenced by increasingly severe pain caused by ischemia, followed by loss of sensation and mobility in the affected area as nerves are deprived of blood supply.

When the bone ends are realigned, bone healing begins (Fig. 34–12). A number of local cytokines, referred to as *osteogenic proteins* or *bone morphogenic proteins*, apparently direct healing in a process that mimics the embryologic development of bone.[20] Initially, angiogenic factors induce capillaries from the bone ends to grow into the hematoma site. Phagocytic cells, attracted during the inflammatory response, clear the area of dead bone cells and debris. Fibroblasts then migrate in, wall off the inflammatory process, and produce the fibrin meshwork for wound healing (see Chapter 13). Some fibroblasts differentiate into chondroblasts and begin secreting cartilage. Osteoblasts migrate into this *fibrocartilage callus* from adjacent viable bone and begin forming cancellous bone. The outer part of this callus is more highly calcified and extends beyond the bone edges. Osteoblastic activity gradually converts the fibrocartilage callus to a *bony callus*.

When mechanical stress can again be applied to

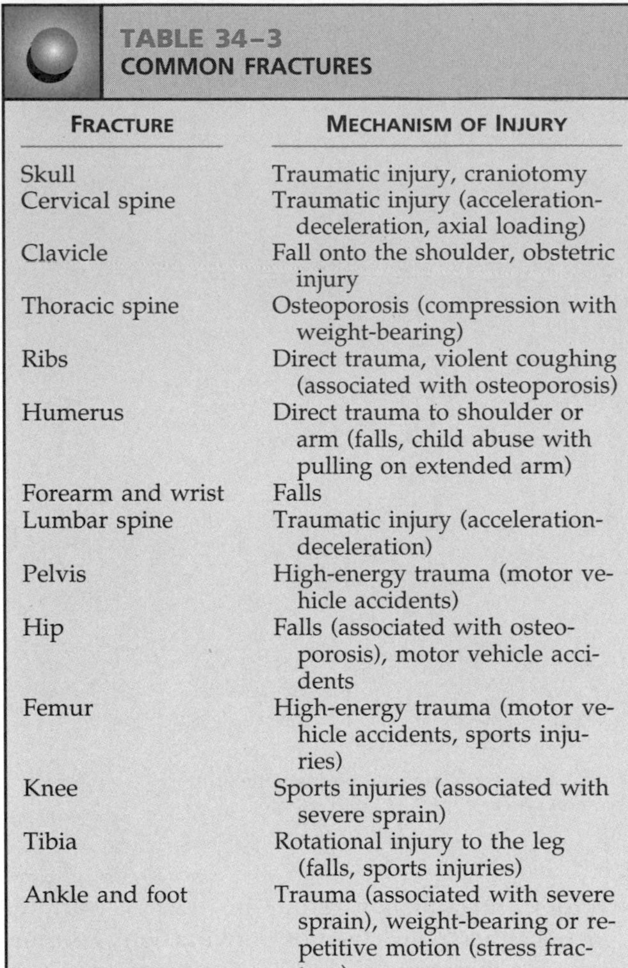

TABLE 34–3
COMMON FRACTURES

Fracture	Mechanism of Injury
Skull	Traumatic injury, craniotomy
Cervical spine	Traumatic injury (acceleration-deceleration, axial loading)
Clavicle	Fall onto the shoulder, obstetric injury
Thoracic spine	Osteoporosis (compression with weight-bearing)
Ribs	Direct trauma, violent coughing (associated with osteoporosis)
Humerus	Direct trauma to shoulder or arm (falls, child abuse with pulling on extended arm)
Forearm and wrist	Falls
Lumbar spine	Traumatic injury (acceleration-deceleration)
Pelvis	High-energy trauma (motor vehicle accidents)
Hip	Falls (associated with osteoporosis), motor vehicle accidents
Femur	High-energy trauma (motor vehicle accidents, sports injuries)
Knee	Sports injuries (associated with severe sprain)
Tibia	Rotational injury to the leg (falls, sports injuries)
Ankle and foot	Trauma (associated with severe sprain), weight-bearing or repetitive motion (stress fracture)

the bone, the equilibrium of osteoblastic and osteoclastic activity is reestablished, and the bony callus is remodeled, nearly resuming its original configuration. Bone healing is typically more rapid in young children and slower in the elderly or in anyone with limited blood supply to the affected bone.

Prevention and Treatment. Implementation of measures that enhance safety during high-risk activities is warranted. Maximizing the safety of children and vulnerable adults (e.g., the cognitively impaired or the physically frail or disabled) through personal assistance or supervision and environmental design measures is of particular importance. Optimal prevention and treatment of osteoporosis is critical to the prevention of fractures of the spine and hip, as discussed previously.

Fractures are treated with reduction (realignment of bone ends) followed by immobilization until the bone heals. Closed reduction is accomplished with manual manipulation, and open reduction is done directly through a surgical incision. Traction may be necessary to pull bone fragments into position before surgical fixation or to maintain their position during healing. Traction involves the use of suspended weights attached to the affected bone via screws or pins or to overlying skin via adhesive straps. Fixation involves surgical access to the bone and the use of pins, wires, screws, rods, or plates to fuse bone fragments.

Prognosis and Outcome. With appropriate intervention, the integrity of most fractured bones may be successfully restored. Fixation and healing of fractures are usually possible even in cases of severe osteoporosis or neoplastic involvement of bone, and they should be undertaken to minimize pain and permit optimal mobility. Growth plate fractures in children are associated with more severe deformity. Healing of fractures may also be less than satisfactory in the elderly or in others with underlying systemic illnesses.

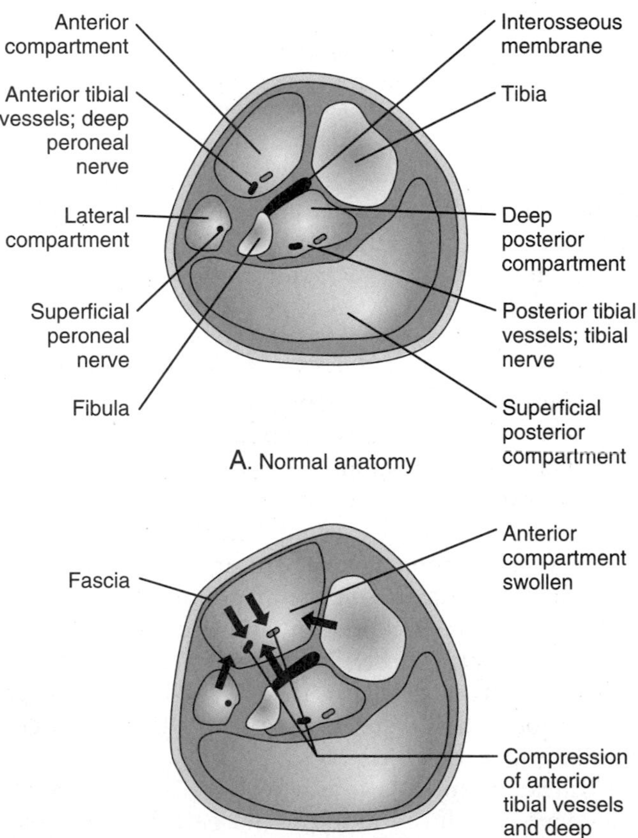

FIGURE 34–11

Compartmental syndrome. A cross-section of the lower leg, with its four fascial compartments, is illustrated. In anterior compartmental syndrome, edema exerts pressure on the blood vessels and nerves contained within the compartment. (Redrawn from Black, J.M., and Matassarin-Jacobs, E. [1997]. *Medical-Surgical Nursing: Clinical Management for Continuity of Care.* [5th ed.]. Philadelphia: W.B. Saunders. [p. 2140].)

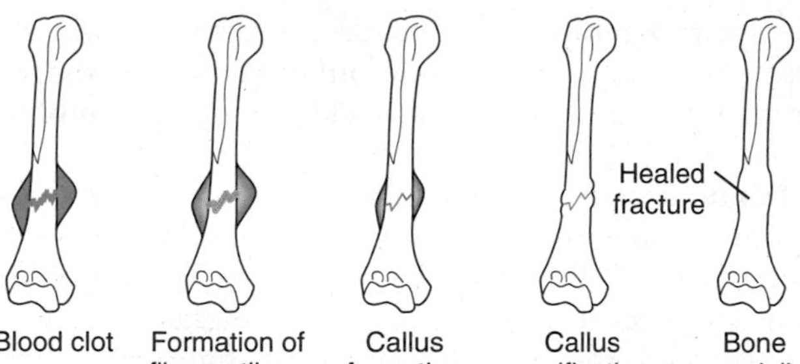

FIGURE 34–12

Process of bone healing. Local cytokines direct bone healing in a process that mimics embryonic bone development. Angiogenic factors induce bone capillaries to grow into the blood clot that forms at the time of injury. Fibroblasts also migrate in, producing a meshwork foundation for healing. Some fibroblasts differentiate into chondroblasts that secrete cartilage, forming a *fibrocartilage callus*. Osteoblasts then migrate into this tissue and secrete protein matrix. Deposition of bone minerals into this matrix forms the *bony callus*, which is remodeled by mechanical stress and other regulatory factors.

Bone Tumors

Definition. Bone tumors are benign or malignant neoplasms of skeletal tissue. Primary bone tumors, which originate in skeletal tissues, are more common in children and young adults, whereas the majority of bone tumors in older adults represent metastatic lesions. Technically, cancers arising from bone marrow could also be classified as bone tumors. Usually only multiple myeloma, which is characterized by extensive infiltration of bone tissue, is discussed in this context; leukemias and lymphomas are considered to be hematopoietic cancers. Multiple myeloma is detailed in the next section; leukemias and lymphomas were examined in Chapters 12 and 13. Table 34–4 classifies the more common bone tumors.

Epidemiology. Most bone tumors are benign, although the precise incidence of these is unknown. Of the malignant neoplasms, the most common are **osteosarcoma, chondrosarcoma,** and **Ewing's sarcoma**. Osteosarcoma (also known as osteogenic sarcoma), the most common malignant bone tumor of children, is diagnosed in 600 to 800 individuals each year in the United States, with males affected more often than females.[20] Most affected individuals are between the ages of 10 and 20 years, but the tumor can affect any age group. Rapid growth constitutes a risk factor for osteosarcoma and other tumors that favor epiphyseal sites. Other risk factors include bone infarcts, chronic osteomyelitis, Paget's disease, radiation exposure, and use of metal in fixation of fractures. Primary cancers of the breast, lung, prostate, and kidney impose the greatest risk of metastasis to bone.[13]

Etiology. The precise etiology of primary bone tumors is unknown. A genetic alteration apparently triggers neoplastic transformation, but no specific gene locus is identifiable in most cases.

Pathophysiology. Tumors of skeletal tissue are typically composed of cells that demonstrate uncontrolled proliferation and increased production of abnormal bone, cartilage, or fibrous tissue, depending on the cell of origin. Bone tumors disrupt the structural integrity of bone in varying patterns and degrees, depending on tumor classification. Benign bone tumors are usually well demarcated and limited in extent. Their growth compresses, but does not invade, surrounding normal bone. Malignant tumors are invasive and destructive to adjacent normal cells, weakening the bone. Destruction may be

TABLE 34–4
CLASSIFICATION OF PRIMARY BONE TUMORS

Tissue of Origin	Benign Tumors	Malignant Tumors
Hematopoietic		Malignant myeloma, lymphoma
Cartilage	Osteochrondroma, chondroma, chondroblastoma, chondromyxoid fibroma	Chondrosarcoma
Bone	Osteoid osteoma, osteoblastoma	Osteosarcoma
Unknown	Giant cell tumor	Ewing's sarcoma, malignant giant cell tumor, adamantinoma
Histiocytes	Fibrous histiocytoma	Malignant histiocytoma
Fibrous tissue	Fibroma	Desmoplastic fibroma, fibrosarcoma
Notochord		Chordoma
Blood vessels	Hemangioma	Hemangioendothelioma, hemangiopericytoma
Adipose tissue	Lipoma	Liposarcoma
Nervous tissue	Neurilemoma	

Adapted from Cotran, R.S., Kumar, V., and Robbins, S.L. (1994). *Robbins Pathologic Basis of Disease.* (5th ed.). Philadelphia: W.B. Saunders. (p. 1233). By permission of the Mayo Foundation.

localized or may extensively permeate the bone. Primary bone tumors are considered to be systemic diseases, with micrometastasis assumed at the time of diagnosis.[21]

In osteosarcoma, affected bone appears "moth-eaten." When tumors invade the outer cortical bone and periosteum, osteogenic activity is stimulated at the bone surface, producing disorderly thickening caused by abnormal bone surrounding the neoplastic area. Some bone tumors extend to adjacent soft tissue, and metastasis to the lung is possible. Calcium homeostasis may be disrupted; hypercalcemia caused by increased bone resorption is more common than hypocalcemia. **Hypercalcemia of malignancy** may result from two mechanisms: (1) increased resorption (local osteolysis) resulting from factors secreted at the site of metastasis or (2) release of factors such as PTH-related peptide from tumor sites remote from bone (see Chapter 28).[22]

Clinical Manifestations. Depending on the size and location of the tumor, the patient may be asymptomatic at first or may have vague manifestations (aches and pains) that mimic arthritis or muscle strains. Pain and swelling increase until deformity is apparent and mobility is severely limited. In some patients, pathologic fracture is the presenting sign. Lysis of bone cells results in elevated serum levels of the intracellular enzyme alkaline phosphatase.

Prevention and Treatment. Specific preventive measures for bone tumors are unknown. Avoidance of radiation exposure and repeated trauma to bone is warranted. The treatment of choice for localized tumors is surgical excision, which may necessitate amputation. Limb salvage surgery is possible in some cases and may involve joint reconstruction or the use of grafts or expandable prostheses. Systemic chemotherapy with multiple agents is used before and after surgery in an effort to eradicate micrometastases. Because bone pain may be very severe, adequate analgesia is a priority in the care of patients with bone tumors. Treatment of hypercalcemia is discussed in Chapter 9.

Prognosis and Outcome. Benign tumors of bone and many malignant tumors are successfully treated with surgical excision. Adjunctive chemotherapy has produced increasingly positive outcomes in localized malignant tumors and in those with limited metastasis. Five-year survival rates for patients with localized primary tumors now exceeds 60%.[21]

Multiple Myeloma

Definition. Multiple myeloma is a malignant neoplasm of bone marrow origin characterized by abnormal proliferation of a single clone of plasma cells that produce an immunoglobulin known as the M protein. Multiple myeloma is classified as a lymphoproliferative disorder (see Chapter 13).

Epidemiology. Multiple myeloma affects an estimated 14,000 individuals each year in the United States, with 10,000 deaths.[23] Most patients are older than 60 years of age. Blacks are at higher risk than whites, and men are at slightly higher risk than women. Risk factors other than aging include exposure to ionizing radiation, herbicides, pesticides, benzene, wood, metal, rubber, textiles, and petroleum products. A history of recurrent infections and drug allergies is also associated with increased risk.

Etiology. The precise etiology is unknown. Chronic antigenic stimulation of the immune system is thought to play a role.

Pathophysiology. The transformed cell in multiple myeloma is the plasma cell, which is the mature, immunoglobulin-secreting B-lymphocyte mediating humoral immunity (see Chapter 13). The malignant plasma cell secretes large quantities of M protein, which is not functional in antigen-antibody reactions. Cytokines such as interleukin-6 have been implicated in promoting the growth and differentiation of the plasma cell clone by an autocrine or paracrine mechanism. The tumor may produce other cytokines such as interleukin-1β, which is thought to act as an osteoclast-activating factor promoting invasive bone lesions.

The kidney is affected by M protein proliferation in 50% of cases. *Myeloma kidney* may be caused by deposition of the light chain component of the M protein within renal tubules, causing obstruction, dilation, inflammation, and fibrosis.[23] In addition, amyloid material (a waxy, protein substance) may infiltrate renal blood vessels, glomeruli, and the interstitium. Hypercalcemia is often present because of lytic bone lesions, and calcium deposition may also play a role in renal insufficiency. Increased blood viscosity caused by the presence of excess protein may promote sludging of blood flow and inappropriate bleeding or clotting within the kidney.

The direct effects of multiple myeloma on the bone marrow are confined to the erythrocyte line. Erythrocyte progenitor cells are replaced by plasma cells, and erythrocyte production is reduced. The rate of erythrocyte destruction is increased because of coating of red blood cells (RBCs) with M protein, causing them to undergo rouleau formation (stacking like a roll of coins). In this form, they are trapped and lysed by phagocytic cells. Reduction in platelets (thrombocytopenia) and leukocytes (leukopenia) is usually caused by chemotherapy or radiation therapy rather than by the disease process.

Multiple myeloma usually begins with a slowly

progressive (indolent) phase, and about 20% of patients are diagnosed by chance when laboratory studies reveal the increased serum M-protein concentration or presence of Bence Jones protein in the urine.[24] Most asymptomatic patients will remain stable for more than 5 years. Patients who have one or more lytic bone lesions at diagnosis usually demonstrate progression of the disease within 1 year.

Clinical Manifestations. Most patients (75% to 80%) with multiple myeloma develop bone disease, characterized by bone pain and pathologic fractures.[23] Radiographic imaging studies may reveal single or multiple, discrete osteolytic lesions, giving the bone a "punched out" appearance, or they may show a generalized depletion of bone mass similar to that of osteoporosis. Myeloma kidney manifests as varying degrees of azotemia, leading to renal failure. Anemia, bleeding disorders, and infections are common because of the hematopoietic effects of the disease and its therapy.

Prevention and Treatment. There is no specific prevention for multiple myeloma, other than reduction of exposures associated with increased risk. Standard chemotherapy of multiple myeloma consists of intermittent courses of melphalan and prednisone, although other combinations are being evaluated in clinical trials.[24] Destruction of the bone marrow (myoablative therapy) with high-dose chemotherapy, followed by rescue bone marrow transplantation, has been used in a small number of patients younger than 50 years who have an HLA-matched sibling. Bone pain, hypercalcemia, anemia, renal failure, and infection are treated appropriately if present.

Prognosis and Outcome. Multiple myeloma is a fatal disease. Initial chemotherapy induces remission in about 40% of cases.[24] Remission typically lasts about 2 years, and median survival after diagnosis is 3 years. Fewer than 10% of patients survive longer than 10 years, and relapse is apparently inevitable unless patients die earlier of infection or leukemia caused by chemotherapy.

Dislocations and Subluxations

Definition. Dislocation is the complete separation of the bones within a joint. **Subluxation** is partial separation of the articulating surfaces of the bones. These disorders may be congenital or acquired (traumatic).

Epidemiology. Traumatic dislocations and subluxations are very common. Risk factors for traumatic dislocation are the same as those for sprains and traumatic fractures, such as participation in athletics or other strenuous activity, especially by those who lack fitness or knowledge of appropriate technique. The most common type of congenital dislocation is **developmental hip dysplasia (DHD),** with an estimated incidence of 0.1% to 1.0% in white neonates.[25] Breech position in utero is a risk factor for congenital hip dislocation, and firstborn infants are also at higher risk. There is an apparent genetic predisposition promoting dysplasia of the hip joint capsule (acetabulum), and elevated maternal relaxin levels may promote relaxation of the ligaments within the joint, predisposing to dislocation or subluxation. Large infants may have shoulder dislocation or subluxation during delivery.

Etiology. Trauma associated with excessive or abnormal movement of the joint is the usual cause of dislocation or subluxation. Except in the case of birth trauma, the precise etiology of congenital dislocations is unknown. Mechanical, genetic, and hormonal factors have been implicated.

Pathophysiology. Displacement of bones within the joint may damage joint structures, including blood vessels, ligaments, tendons, and nerves. Fractures may occur at the articulating surfaces. Ischemic necrosis is possible because of disruption of the blood supply to the joint.

Clinical Manifestations. With traumatic dislocations, the joint is visibly deformed and the affected extremity appears shortened. Local pain, swelling, and limitation of function result from inflammation. Ischemic pain is particularly severe and may be followed by numbness. With DHD, unequal skinfolds are apparent on the thighs and buttocks, and unequal knee height and limitation of abduction on the affected side are usually apparent (Fig. 34–13).

Prevention and Treatment. Measures for reduction of risk in other musculoskeletal injuries, such as sprains and fractures, apply to dislocations as well. Newborns are routinely screened for the presence of hip dysplasia with the Barlow provocative test and the Ortolani maneuver, tests that detect abnormal movement between the femoral head and the acetabulum. Treatment of dislocations usually consists of closed reduction, often done under anesthesia. Open reduction may be required in severe dislocations. For congenital hip dislocation, a period of traction may be required to pull the hip into position. Once reduced, joints are immobilized for a time (typically 3 to 6 weeks) while tissues heal. The congenitally dislocated hip is maintained in abduction by a Pavlik harness (which permits some movement) or hip spica cast (which immobilizes the joint). After healing is complete, active exercise of the joint is encouraged to restore mobility.

Prognosis and Outcome. With appropriate intervention, full function is usually restored.

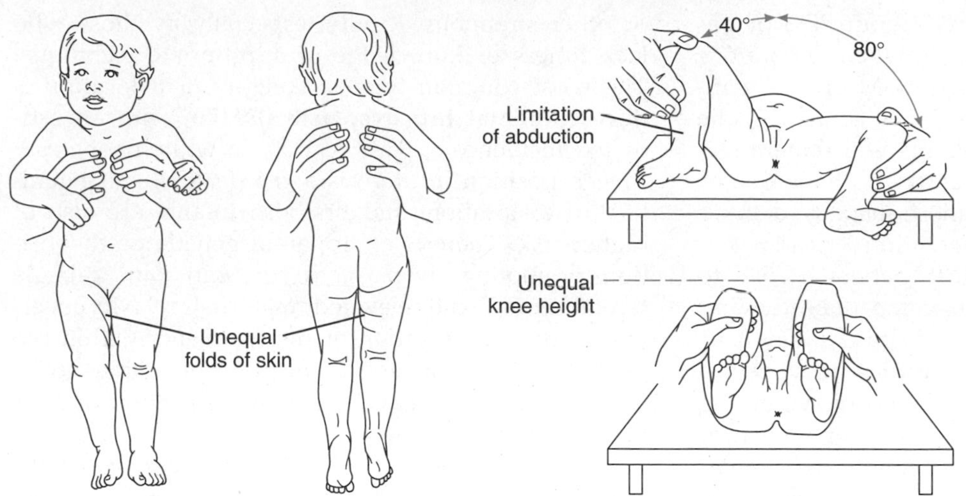

FIGURE 34–13
Developmental hip dysplasia. The three classic signs of developmental hip dysplasia are shown: unequal skinfolds, limitation of abduction, and unequal knee height. (Redrawn from Tachdjian, M. [1972]. *Pediatric Orthopedics*. Philadelphia: W.B. Saunders.)

Scoliosis

Definition. Scoliosis is a lateral, sigmoid (S-shaped) spinal curvature greater than 10 degrees, as determined by the Cobb angle (Fig. 34–14). Scoliosis is classified as *nonstructural* (compensatory) if there is no anatomic abnormality, and *structural* if there are associated abnormalities of vertebral joints, bones, muscles, or ligaments.

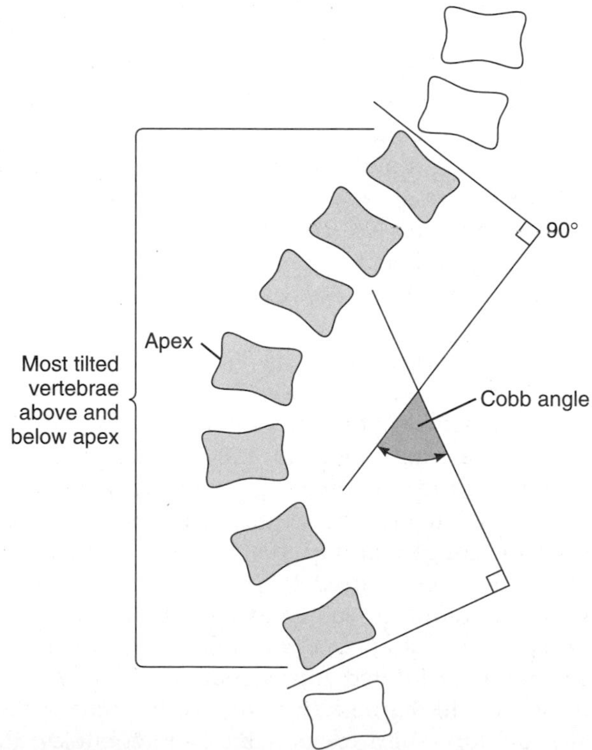

FIGURE 34–14
Cobb angle in scoliosis. This method of measuring the degree of curvature draws lines perpendicular to the plane of the most tilted vertebrae at the top and bottom of the curve. The angle formed by the intersection of these lines is the Cobb angle.

Epidemiology. Scoliosis is usually diagnosed in adolescents between ages 10 and 14, during routine school screening. About 2% to 3% of adolescents have scoliosis. Most forms are more common in girls. Scoliosis diagnosed in infancy is more common in boys. Specific risk factors for nonstructural scoliosis include malnutrition, chronic fatigue, lack of exercise, poor posture, or muscle spasm related to injury. Structural scoliosis is associated with a genetic predisposition in most cases. Teratogenic factors, intrauterine position, and neuromuscular diseases may also predispose to scoliosis.

Etiology. Nonstructural scoliosis is the result of postural or functional factors, in which habitual assumption of poor spinal posture produces spinal curvature. Over time, anatomic changes result. With structural scoliosis, several etiologies are possible. Anatomic abnormalities (e.g., vertebral rotation or deformity, rib fusion) that are present at birth may result in spinal curvature that becomes pronounced during the period of adolescent growth. Congenital abnormality of proprioceptive function of the dorsal column–medial lemniscus system may also contribute to compensatory changes in spinal structures. Primary neuromuscular disease (e.g., poliomyelitis, muscular dystrophy, myelomeningocele, cerebral palsy) results in muscle imbalance that may pull the spine out of alignment. Because specific genetic or teratogenic factors often cannot be identified, 65% of cases are usually classified as idiopathic.[26] Table 34–5 further describes subtypes of structural scoliosis and other congenital spinal deformities.

Pathophysiology. The curve may be evident in any area of the spine, but the most common pattern is that of a right thoracic and left lumbar curve (Fig. 34–15). The earliest signs of misalignment result from shortening of the muscles and ligaments on the concave side of the curve, followed by compression of vertebral joints. Differential stresses on vertebral

TABLE 34–5
CLASSIFICATION OF CONGENITAL DISORDERS OF SPINAL ALIGNMENT

DEFORMITY	DESCRIPTION
Scoliosis	Lateral, sigmoid curvature of spine
Congenital scoliosis	Caused by embryonic malformation of vertebrae, often coexists with other anomalies
Neuromuscular (paralytic) scoliosis	Results from muscle imbalance (e.g., in muscular dystrophy, polio, cerebral palsy, spina bifida)
Infantile idiopathic scoliosis	Often associated with intrauterine position; occurs in children younger than 4 years; usually left thoracic curve
Juvenile idiopathic scoliosis	Occurs between ages 4 and 10 years; usually progressive right thoracic curve
Adolescent idiopathic scoliosis	Occurs after age 10 years; most prevalent form in U.S.: 7:1 female predominance; may or may not progress
Kyphosis	Exaggerated convexity of thoracic spine (humpback or hunchback)
Congenital kyphosis	Caused by abnormal embryonic development of vertebrae; may become apparent at birth or during pubertal growth spurt
Postural kyphosis (roundback)	Caused by indifferent posture; no structural impairment
Scheuermann's kyphosis	An osteochondrosis affecting thoracic vertebrae; more common in males
Pott's curvature	Caused by tuberculosis of the spine
Lordosis	Exaggerated concavity of the lumbar spine (swayback); nearly always compensatory; associated with scoliosis or kyphosis

Adapted from Betz, C.L., Hunsberger, M.M., and Wright, S. (1994). *Family-Centered Nursing Care of Children,* (2nd ed.). Philadelphia: W.B. Saunders. (pp. 1854–1855).

bone result in imbalance of osteoblastic activity, which causes rapid progression of the curve during adolescence. If not corrected, this imbalance continues into adulthood, with curves greater than 50 degrees likely to progress at an average rate of 1 degree per year. Curves greater than 60 degrees impair ventilatory function.

Clinical Manifestation. Mild scoliosis is noted on careful inspection as prominence of one hip, shoulder, scapula, or rib cage area, especially with spinal flexion. Asymmetry of the spaces between the arms and trunk may be seen when the patient stands upright. Leg length may differ by more than ½ inch on measurement, or uneven skirt hems may be evident in girls. Back pain may be reported, although this manifestation does not differ from that of the general population.[26] Greater curves result in obvious asymmetry and may be associated with severe back pain, respiratory distress, and neurologic impairment.

Prevention and Treatment. Nonstructural scoliosis is preventable with voluntary reduction of contributing factors. When structural changes have occurred, however, exercise and posture alone are not sufficient to correct the deformity. Early detection of scoliosis may be facilitated through routine spinal screening programs during junior high school, but studies have not shown a definite benefit of this practice. As many as two thirds of adolescents identified as having scoliosis are found to have no spinal abnormality with more careful evaluation.[27] In general, the younger the child at diagnosis and the greater the magnitude of the curve, the greater the risk of progression of the spinal abnormality. For curves less than 30 degrees, observation alone may be sufficient, because these curves often do not progress. If the curve progresses by 5 degrees, bracing is indicated. Use of a rigid underarm brace for 23 hours a day is usually prescribed, but many patients do not fully comply with this regimen. Bracing is about 40% effective in preventing curve progression.

In growing children and adolescents, curves of greater than 40 degrees are treated with surgical fusion (arthrodesis) of the spine, which may involve bone grafts or use of metal instrumentation (e.g., Harrington rods, Dwyer instrumentation, or Luque wires). Bracing and surgery are augmented with appropriate exercise programs to restore balance in muscle support. Differential electrostimulation of muscles on either side of the curve has also been used in treatment of scoliosis, but has not been shown to be effective.[26]

Prognosis and Outcome. Curves of less than 40 degrees at skeletal maturity remain stable without treatment. Although the treatment period is often long, tedious, and socially stressful, favorable outcomes are usually achieved with optimal treatment of scoliosis. Without treatment, curves greater than 40 degrees progress, potentially impairing respiratory and neurologic function if the spinal cord becomes compressed.

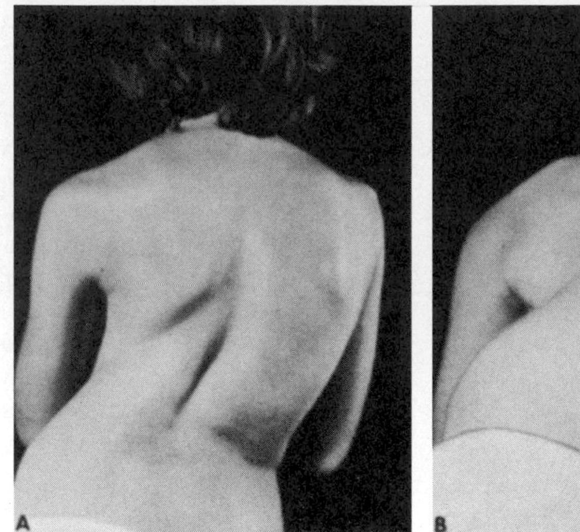
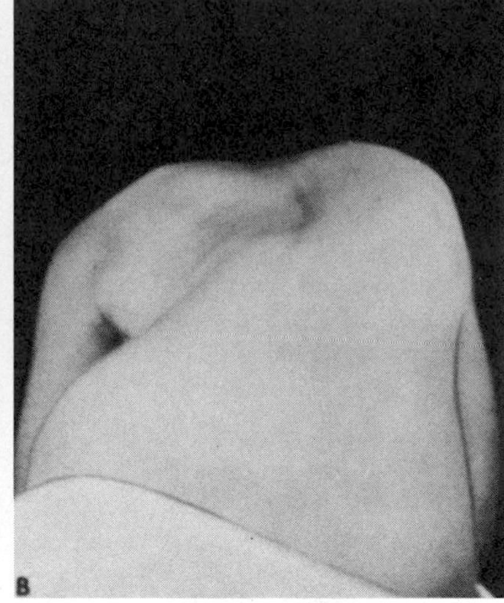

FIGURE 34–15
Scoliosis. A severe right thoracic curve is shown here. Note the scapular elevation and asymmetry of the spaces between the arms and trunk. (From Gartland, M. [1979]. *Fundamentals of Orthopedics.* Philadelphia: W.B. Saunders. [p. 307].)

Ankylosing Spondylitis

Definition. Ankylosing spondylitis, also known as Marie-Strümpell disease, is a chronic, progressive disorder characterized by inflammation of the spine and sacroiliac joints. Ankylosing spondylitis is the most prevalent of the *seronegative spondyloarthropathies*, joint disorders of apparent immunologic origin in which the **rheumatoid factor (RF)** autoantibody is absent from the serum (Table 34–6).

Epidemiology. Ankylosing spondylitis has been diagnosed in about 400,000 people in the United States.[28] The diagnosis is usually made between the ages of 20 and 40 years, and men are affected nine times more frequently than women. A genetic predisposition is evident, with 90% of patients demonstrating a specific genetic marker, HLA-B27.

Etiology. The precise etiology is unknown, but presence of the specific HLA subtype suggests an immunologic basis for the disease.

Pathophysiology. Inflammation typically begins in the sacroiliac joints and moves progressively up the spine. The inflammatory process destroys the articular cartilage, which is then replaced by deposition of new bone. This process eventually fuses the entire spine.

Clinical Manifestations. Early symptoms include morning backache and stiffness in the lumbar area. Pain and stiffness progress upward, and symptoms are typically worse at rest than with activity. Systemic signs of inflammation are often present and may include iritis, arthritis, weight loss, and malaise.[18]

Prevention and Treatment. There is no effective intervention to prevent or slow the progress of ankylosing spondylitis. Treatment is symptomatic and supportive, with use of nonsteroidal anti-inflammatory drugs (NSAIDs); application of heat, splinting or bracing; and occasionally surgical reconstruction.

Prognosis and Outcome. After 10 to 20 years, the patient's spine is fused into a bent-forward position (kyphosis), and the patient's knees are flexed in an effort to hold the head upright.

Osteoarthritis

Definition. Osteoarthritis (OA), formerly known as degenerative joint disease, is joint damage and inflammation caused by biochemical alteration of the articular cartilage in one or a few joints. OA is the most prevalent form of arthritis. Table 34–7 lists and classifies the more common forms of arthritis. Two of these, RA and gout, are detailed after this section.

Epidemiology. Eighty per cent of all individuals older than age 65 years are known to have some degree of OA.[29] Postmenopausal women are at highest risk. OA may also occur in younger persons, as a result of repeated trauma to a joint (as in athletes), rare hereditary syndromes (e.g., familial chondrocalcinosis and Stickler syndrome), inflammatory arthritis (e.g., RA or psoriatic arthritis), metabolic disorders (e.g., Wilson's disease or hemochromatosis), congenital joint deformity, or Legg-Calvé-Perthes disease. Obesity is correlated with OA affecting the knees and hips. Most older individuals with OA have no apparent risk factors other than aging. In

TABLE 34–6
AUTOANTIBODY TESTING IN RHEUMATOLOGIC DISORDERS

AUTOANTIBODY	CLINICAL SIGNIFICANCE
Antinuclear antibody (ANA)	Detects serum antibodies that bind to various nuclear antigens; positive in more than 95% of patients with systemic lupus erythematosus (SLE), but may also be detectable in other connective tissue disorders, infections, malignancies, and in some healthy persons
Anti-dsDNA antibodies	Detects serum antibodies that bind double-stranded DNA; more specific for SLE but less sensitive; also elevated in renal disease and immune-mediated hepatitis
Anti–Scl 70 and anti-centromere tests	Derivatives of the ANA test; specific staining patterns confirm the diagnosis of CREST syndrome, a variant of the connective tissue disease scleroderma
Extractable nuclear antibodies	Detects antibodies against RNA; associated with SLE, autoimmune liver disease, scleroderma, Sjögren's syndrome, and other connective tissue diseases
Rheumatoid factor	Immunoglobulin antibodies directed against the Fc portion of IgG; often detected in rheumatoid arthritis and Sjögren's syndrome; less commonly elevated in other connective tissue disorders, chronic infections, or gammopathies
Antineutrophil cytoplasmic antibodies	Antibodies directed against components of neutrophil cytoplasm; positive in Wegener's granulomatosus
Jo1	Antibody directed against the enzyme transfer-RNA histydyl synthetase; detected in idiopathic inflammatory myopathy

Data from Moder, K.G. (1996). Use and interpretation of rheumatologic tests: A guide for clinicians. *Mayo Clinic Proceedings* 71, 391–396.

women, the knees and hands are more commonly affected; in men, the hips are more often involved.

Etiology. OA results from progressive breakdown in the articular cartilage. In a minority of cases, this breakdown is initiated by repetitive trauma, disease, or deformity, as indicated above; however, most OA is idiopathic. The secretion of regulatory cytokines is apparently altered, although the mechanisms of this alteration are unknown. In response, chondrocytes secrete an excess of digestive enzymes that initiate breakdown of the matrix of the articular cartilage.

Pathophysiology. Typical joint changes in OA are illustrated in Figure 34–16. Initially, chondrocytes in the articular cartilage proliferate, and the water content of the matrix increases in proportion to the proteoglycans. Cracks appear in the matrix, and superficial layers of cartilage are degraded. As the disease progresses, the articular cartilage is completely destroyed in places, exposing the underlying bone. Stress on this bone results in disordered bone growth. Bone spurs (*osteophytes*) may develop, and microscopic fractures may free bone fragments within the joint. Synovial fluid may be forced into defects in the bone, forming cysts. The synovial membrane is not usually affected until late in the disease, when it may become mechanically irritated by bone spurs and fracture fragments. Repeated inflammation results in formation of a fibrous *pannus* over parts of the synovial membrane and articular surface, and effusion into the joint space may occur.

Uncommon variants of OA include *diffuse idiopathic skeletal hyperostosis (DISH)*, also called Forestier's disease, and *neuropathic (Charcot's) arthropathy*.[30] DISH is seen in older men and is often associated with diabetes mellitus. Calcifications of at least four adjacent vertebral bodies are present in DISH. Neuropathic arthropathy is a severe, progressive form of OA that follows loss of normal sensation within a joint. This form is associated with diabetic neuropathy and other neurologic disorders.

Clinical Manifestations. Joint pain, morning stiffness, crepitus, and limitation of movement are the usual signs. In most cases, only one or two joints are involved. The degree of joint pain does not correlate well with the degree of apparent deformity seen with radiography.[30] The joint appears enlarged because of abnormal bone growth, and subluxation is possible. OA involving the hands may manifest as *Heberden's nodes* or *Bouchard's nodes* caused by bone spurs in the joints (Fig. 34–17). Involvement of intervertebral joints may compress spinal nerve roots, resulting in pain and radiculopathy similar to that of a herniated lumbar disk (see Chapter 23).

Prevention and Treatment. Weight reduction and termination or modification of activities associated with repetitive joint trauma are reasonable preven-

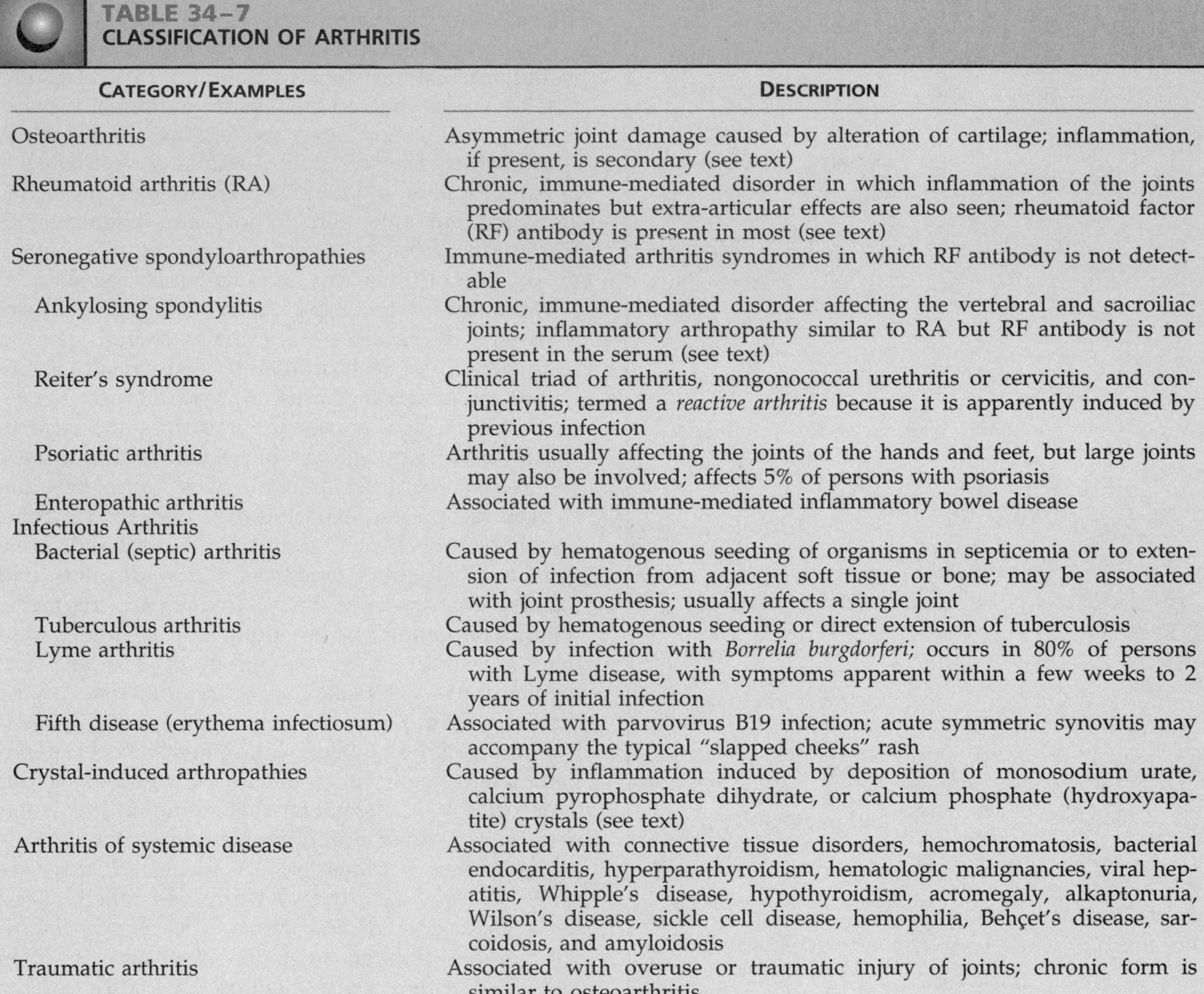

TABLE 34–7
CLASSIFICATION OF ARTHRITIS

Category/Examples	Description
Osteoarthritis	Asymmetric joint damage caused by alteration of cartilage; inflammation, if present, is secondary (see text)
Rheumatoid arthritis (RA)	Chronic, immune-mediated disorder in which inflammation of the joints predominates but extra-articular effects are also seen; rheumatoid factor (RF) antibody is present in most (see text)
Seronegative spondyloarthropathies	Immune-mediated arthritis syndromes in which RF antibody is not detectable
Ankylosing spondylitis	Chronic, immune-mediated disorder affecting the vertebral and sacroiliac joints; inflammatory arthropathy similar to RA but RF antibody is not present in the serum (see text)
Reiter's syndrome	Clinical triad of arthritis, nongonococcal urethritis or cervicitis, and conjunctivitis; termed a *reactive arthritis* because it is apparently induced by previous infection
Psoriatic arthritis	Arthritis usually affecting the joints of the hands and feet, but large joints may also be involved; affects 5% of persons with psoriasis
Enteropathic arthritis	Associated with immune-mediated inflammatory bowel disease
Infectious Arthritis	
Bacterial (septic) arthritis	Caused by hematogenous seeding of organisms in septicemia or to extension of infection from adjacent soft tissue or bone; may be associated with joint prosthesis; usually affects a single joint
Tuberculous arthritis	Caused by hematogenous seeding or direct extension of tuberculosis
Lyme arthritis	Caused by infection with *Borrelia burgdorferi;* occurs in 80% of persons with Lyme disease, with symptoms apparent within a few weeks to 2 years of initial infection
Fifth disease (erythema infectiosum)	Associated with parvovirus B19 infection; acute symmetric synovitis may accompany the typical "slapped cheeks" rash
Crystal-induced arthropathies	Caused by inflammation induced by deposition of monosodium urate, calcium pyrophosphate dihydrate, or calcium phosphate (hydroxyapatite) crystals (see text)
Arthritis of systemic disease	Associated with connective tissue disorders, hemochromatosis, bacterial endocarditis, hyperparathyroidism, hematologic malignancies, viral hepatitis, Whipple's disease, hypothyroidism, acromegaly, alkaptonuria, Wilson's disease, sickle cell disease, hemophilia, Behçet's disease, sarcoidosis, and amyloidosis
Traumatic arthritis	Associated with overuse or traumatic injury of joints; chronic form is similar to osteoarthritis

tive measures. There are no known preventive measures for most individuals with idiopathic OA. Treatment depends on severity of the condition as well as the patient's age and lifestyle. Conservative measures include rest, analgesics (usually acetaminophen), range of motion and isometric exercises, and use of an adjunctive device such as a cane or walker to decrease stress on the joint. If symptoms are not controlled with this regimen, an NSAID may be used, although this is controversial because synovial inflammation is usually only a minor component of the disease process. Surgical interventions range from removal of bone spurs to replacement of the affected joint with an artificial prosthesis.

Prognosis and Outcome. Although it may stabilize without treatment, OA is usually chronically progressive, leading to permanent disability. Joint replacement surgery is usually well tolerated and significantly improves mobility and quality of life for many.[30]

Rheumatoid Arthritis

Definition. RA is a chronic systemic disorder in which connective tissues throughout the body (principally the joints) are damaged, probably by an autoimmune mechanism.

Epidemiology. RA affects about 1% of the U.S. population.[31] Females outnumber males 3 : 1 for most types. Peak onset is in middle adulthood, but RA afflicts individuals of all ages. With onset before the age of 16, the disease is known as *juvenile rheumatoid arthritis*. A genetic predisposition is evident, with two HLA subtypes (DR4 and DR1) known to confer higher risk.

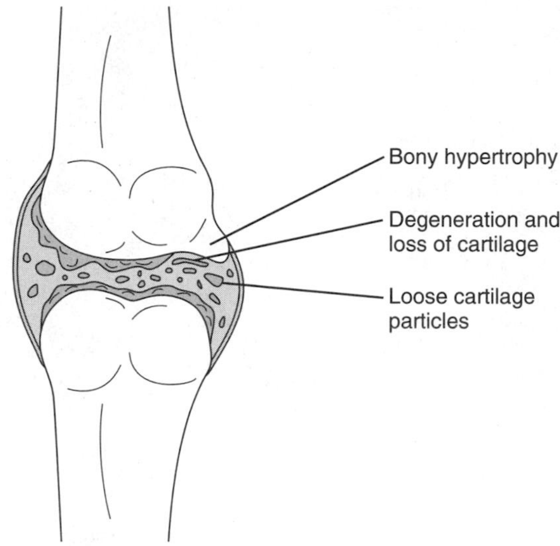

FIGURE 34–16
Joint pathology in osteoarthritis. Cracks appear in the articular cartilage, and its superficial layers are degraded. Eventually, areas of cartilage may be completely destroyed, exposing underlying bone. Stress on this bone causes disordered bony overgrowth, with formation of bone spurs, microscopic fractures, and cysts.

Etiology. The precise mechanism of RA is unknown, but there is significant indirect evidence of autoimmune involvement. The principal theory is that specific HLA subtypes provide a binding site for an initiating (arthritogenic) agent.[13] This agent is probably a microorganism, with Epstein-Barr virus most frequently implicated. An initial, self-limited infection may thus trigger an autoimmune attack against synovial membranes and other tissues.

Pathophysiology. The initial infection induces inflammation of the synovial membrane (**synovitis**). T lymphocytes (mainly CD4+) migrate to the inflamed area, activating monocyte-macrophages and B lymphocytes (see Chapter 13). In most RA patients, antibodies produced during this activation are autoantibodies of the immunoglobulin (Ig) M class, directed against the Fc portion of the individual's native IgG. Binding of these RF autoantibodies produces immune complexes that perpetuate local inflammation and may also circulate to tissues outside the joints, producing the systemic or extra-articular manifestations of RA. A number of antibodies directed at other cellular components may contribute to RA and other connective tissue diseases (see Table 34–6).

The process of joint destruction in RA begins with edema and hyperplasia of the inflamed synovial membrane (Fig. 34–18). Inflammatory fluid seeps between the articular cartilages, forming a fibrous pannus that causes **ankylosis** (fusion of the joint), and contributes to destruction of the underlying bone by erosion and cyst formation. Osteoclastic activity, triggered by mediators of inflammation, is involved in this process. Ultimately, osteoblastic activity is also initiated, and the fibrous ankylosis is replaced by bony ankylosis that totally immobilizes the joint.

Clinical Manifestations. The onset of RA is variable. In the majority of patients, there are initial vague systemic signs of inflammation, including malaise, fatigue, and generalized musculoskeletal pain. After several weeks, joint inflammation, manifested by pain, warmth, redness, swelling, and stiffness, is evident. Joint involvement may begin in one, a few, or several joints. If multiple joints are affected, the pattern is usually symmetric. The joints of the hands and feet are typically affected first, followed by the wrists, ankles, elbows, and knees. Involvement of the spine and hips is unusual. Deformities of the hand that are characteristic of RA include *ulnar deviation, boutonniere deformity,* and *swan-neck deformity* (Fig. 34–19).

The most common extra-articular manifestations

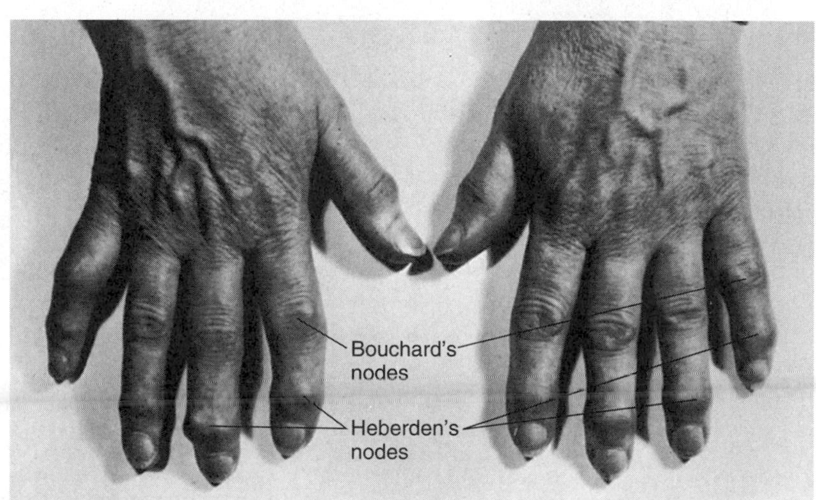

FIGURE 34–17
Heberden's and Bouchard's nodes. Enlargement of the interphalangeal joints caused by bony overgrowth is a typical manifestation of osteoarthritis. Heberden's nodes involve the distal joints, and Bouchard's nodes involve the proximal joints. (From Polley, H.F., and Hunder, G.G. [1978]. *Physical Examination of the Joints.* [2nd ed.]. Philadelphia: W.B. Saunders. [p. 120].)

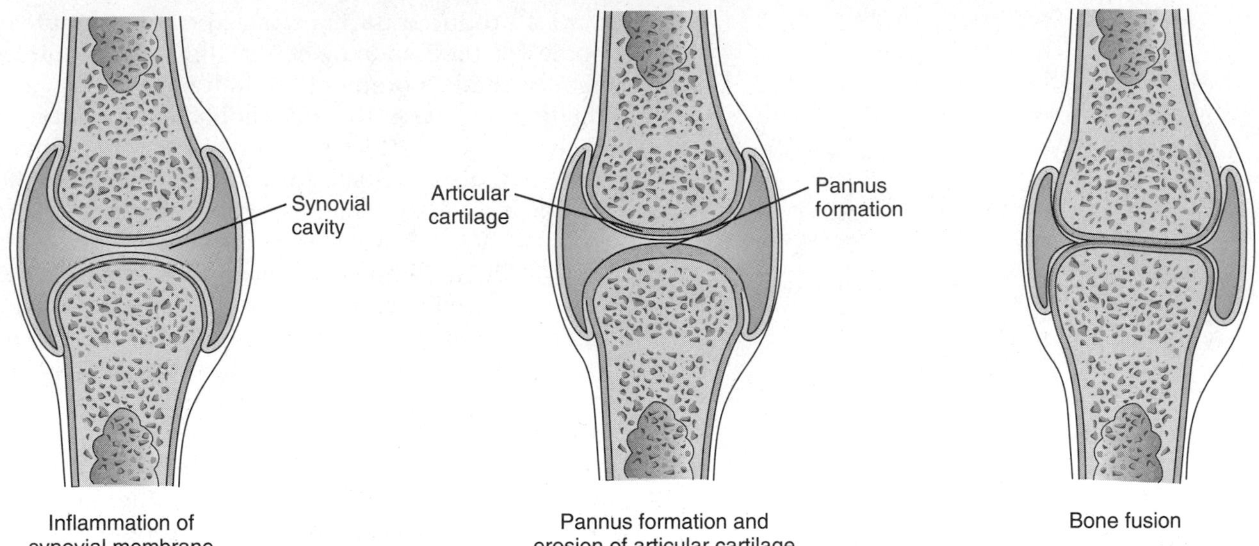

FIGURE 34–18

Joint pathology in rheumatoid arthritis. The synovial membrane is initially inflamed. Inflammatory fluid seeps between the articular cartilages, forming a fibrous *pannus.* Osteoclastic activity contributes to erosion of bone and cartilage. Osteoblastic activity eventually results in bony *ankylosis* (fusion) of the joint.

of RA are *rheumatoid nodules* composed of immune complexes and inflammatory cells. Nodules are most often present in areas of skin overlying pressure points and occur less commonly in tissues of the lungs, retina, spleen, dura, and heart. In a small percentage of patients, RA has an acute systemic onset, manifested by high fever and extra-articular manifestations such as splenomegaly, lymphadenopathy, pericarditis, myocarditis, or amyloidosis. Inflammation of small blood vessels (*rheumatoid vasculitis*) may contribute to nodule formation and may also result in vascular skin lesions (purpura), peripheral neuropathy, and ischemic ulcers of the skin. **Felty's syndrome** refers to the combined manifestations of RA, splenomegaly, and neutropenia. **Sjögren's syndrome**, in which immune-mediated destruction of the lacrimal and salivary glands leads to dry eyes and mouth, commonly occurs in association with RA. (Sjögren's syndrome may also present as an isolated condition or in association with other connective tissue disorders such as **systemic lupus erythematosus [SLE]**.)

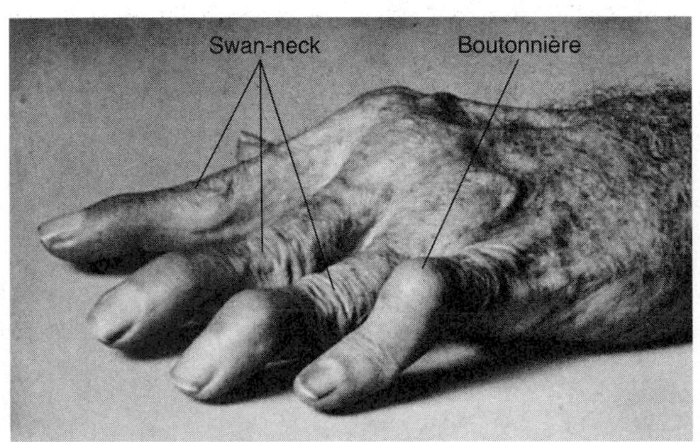

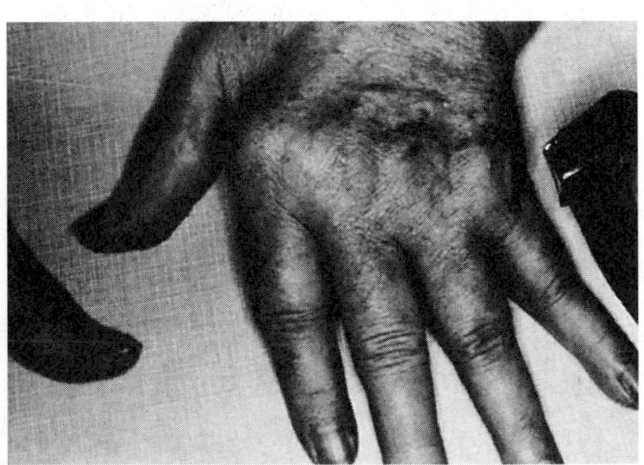

FIGURE 34–19

Hand deformities in rheumatoid arthritis. Swan-neck deformity and boutonniere deformity (left), and ulnar deviation (right) result from joint contractures and stretching of joint capsules. (From Polley, H.F., and Hunder, G.G. [1978]. *Physical Examination of the Joints.* [2nd ed.]. Philadelphia: W.B. Saunders. [p. 118].)

Prevention and Treatment. There are no known preventive measures for RA. Nonpharmacologic measures such as rest and physical therapy may optimize mobility, but definitive treatment requires drug therapy to decrease joint inflammation and slow disease progression. Four classes of drugs are used: NSAIDS, corticosteroids, cytotoxic (immunosuppressive) agents, and a fourth category known variously as slow-acting antirheumatoid drugs (SAARDs) or disease-modifying antirheumatic drugs (DMARDs). Currently, controversy exists with respect to the best sequence and combination of therapy. In the traditional "therapeutic pyramid" approach, NSAIDs are used first, followed by corticosteroids, DMARDs, and cytotoxic drugs, particularly methotrexate. Based on the finding that major joint damage occurs during the first 2 years of the disease, there is currently a trend toward reversing the therapeutic pyramid, using more aggressive pharmacotherapy early in the disease.[32] The early use of methotrexate, possibly in combination with cyclosporine, is advocated by many, but these drugs have significant toxicity. Table 34–8 lists examples of drugs used in treatment of RA, their probable mechanisms of action, and potential toxicity associated with therapy.

Prognosis and Outcome. More aggressive drug therapy has resulted in some preservation of function, particularly during the early years of the disease. Longer-term outcome is often poor, however, characterized by progressive joint destruction and loss of function. In its most severe stage (involving more than 30 joints), RA has a 5-year survival rate of less than 50%.[32] Death may be caused by vascular, pulmonary, or cardiac complications or may be related to adverse effects of therapy such as GI bleeding or lowered resistance to infection.

TABLE 34–8
DRUG THERAPY OF RHEUMATOID ARTHRITIS

CATEGORY/EXAMPLES	MECHANISM	POSSIBLE TOXICITY
Nonsteroidal anti-inflammatory drugs Aspirin Fenoprofen (Nalfon) Ibuprofen (Motrin) Naproxen (Naprosyn) Indomethacin (Indocin) Etodolac (Lodine) Sulindac (Clinoril) Meclofenamate (Meclomen) Piroxicam (Feldene)	Inhibition of cyclooxygenase enzyme within arachidonic acid pathway, reducing production of inflammatory mediators (e.g., prostaglandins)	Gastrointestinal bleeding; interstitial nephritis; fluid retention; dizziness; anemia; thrombocytopenia; alterations in vision, taste, or hearing
Corticosteroids (Glucocorticoids) Prednisone Prednisolone	Inhibition of synthesis of inflammatory mediators; suppression of phagocyte infiltration and leukocytosis	Decreased calcium absorption and bone mass; avascular necrosis with large doses; potential Cushing's syndrome with prolonged systemic use
Slow-acting or disease-modifying agents Gold compounds, e.g., aurothioglucose (Solganal), auranofin (Ridaura) Penicillamine (Cuprimine) Hydroxychloroquine (Plaquenil) Sulfasalazine (Azulfidine)	Altered production of cytokines such as interleukin-1 and tumor necrosis factor; some have weak immunosuppressive effects	Gastrointestinal irritation; rash; flushing and dizziness (with gold); nephritis; bone marrow depression
Cytotoxic agents (immunosuppressants) Methotrexate (Rheumatrex) Azathioprine (Imuran) Cyclosporine (Sandimmune, Neoral)	Inhibition of immune-mediated inflammation	Nausea; mucosal ulcers; cytopenias and anemia; hepatotoxicity; pulmonary fibrosis; nephrotoxicity

Data from Blackburn, W.D. Jr. (1996). Management of osteoarthritis and rheumatoid arthritis: Prospects and possibilities. *American Journal of Medicine* 100 (2A suppl.), 24S–30S; and Flynn, B.L. (1994). Rheumatoid arthritis and osteoarthritis: Current and future therapies. *American Pharmacy* NS34(11), 31–42.

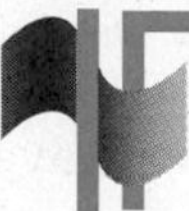

Clinical Scenario

L.R., a 61-year-old dairy farmer, is admitted to the orthopedic unit for treatment of inflammation of his left knee. L.R. has a 40-year history of RA, for which he underwent joint replacement (left total knee arthroplasty) 2 years ago. He is complaining of chills, generalized stiffness, and marked pain in his knee. Fine-needle aspiration of the swollen joint reveals the presence of β-hemolytic streptococcus.

1. What are the possible mechanisms of L.R.'s inflammation?
2. What modes of intervention are indicated in this case?

Gout

Definition. Gout includes a group of metabolic disorders characterized by elevation of uric acid in the blood. *Gouty arthritis* results when uric acid precipitates into joints, forming needle-like monosodium urate crystals. Uric acid, a product of the metabolism of purines in nucleic acids, may have either endogenous or exogenous sources. Table 34–9 compares features of gout and other crystal-induced forms of arthritis.

Epidemiology. The incidence of gout in the United States has been estimated at 2.7 cases per 1000 persons.[33] It is the most common form of inflammatory joint disease in men older than 40 years. Removal of estrogen at menopause also confers a slight risk for females, because estrogen promotes uric acid excretion. Risk factors for **hyperuricemia**, the elevation in serum uric acid that precedes gout, include a high-purine diet (Table 34–10), genetic errors in purine metabolism, hematologic cancers, alcohol abuse, diabetes, renal disorders, obesity, and use of drugs that decrease urinary excretion of uric acid (e.g., thiazide diuretics, levodopa, nicotinic acid).

Etiology. Gout is etiologically classified as either *primary* or *secondary*. Primary gout is most common by far and results from an intrinsic (often idiopathic) mechanism by which uric acid is overproduced or underexcreted. Secondary gout is caused by the effects of another disease or medication use. In either

TABLE 34–9
COMMON FORMS OF CRYSTAL-INDUCED ARTHRITIS

Disorder	Etiology	Clinical Features	Treatment
Gout (gouty arthritis)	Deposition of monosodium urate crystals, usually associated with hyperuricemia in males	Typically affects one joint (big toe); intermittent flare ups occur suddenly, often at night; raised lesions (tophi) may develop after many years	NSAIDs for acute attacks; urate-lowering drugs; low-purine diet
Pseudogout (CPPD disease)	Deposition of calcium pyrophosphate dihydrate (CPPD) crystals; usually associated with aging; metabolic diseases; and previous joint trauma	Typically affects knees, wrists, or hands	NSAIDs for acute attacks; management of underlying disease
Hydroxyapatite-associated arthritis	Deposition of calcium hydroxyapatite, a normal crystalline component of bone; may be associated with calcium or phosphate imbalance, as in renal failure; also seen in some connective tissue disorders and after tissue injury or corticosteroid injections	Usually causes inflammation of tendons or bursae, but may affect joints of shoulders, hips, elbows, wrists, and digits; may be asymptomatic	NSAIDs; surgical aspiration

NSAID, nonsteroidal anti-inflammatory drug.
Data from Schumacher, H.R. Jr. (1996). Crystal-induced arthritis: An overview. *American Journal of Medicine* 100 (2A suppl.), 46S–52S; and Joseph, J., and McGrath, H. (1995). Gout or "pseudogout": How to differentiate crystal-induced arthropathies. *Geriatrics* 50(4), 33–39.

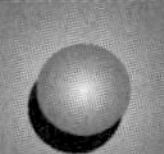

TABLE 34–10
DIETARY SOURCES OF PURINES*

Low-Purine Foods
Refined cereals and cereal products, cornflakes, white bread, pasta, flour, arrowroot, sago, tapioca, cakes
Milk, milk products, and eggs
Sugar, sweets, and gelatin
Butter, polyunsaturated margarine, and all other fats
Fruit, nuts, and peanut butter
Lettuce, tomatoes, and green vegetables (except those listed below)
Cream soups made with low-purine vegetables but without meat or meat stock
Water, fruit juice, cordials, and carbonated drinks

High-Purine Foods
All meats, including organ meats, and seafood
Meat extracts and gravies
Yeast and yeast extracts, beer, and other alcoholic beverages
Beans, peas, lentils, oatmeal, spinach, asparagus, cauliflower, and mushrooms

*The purine content of a food reflects its nucleoprotein content and turnover. Foods containing many nuclei (e.g., liver) have many purines, as do rapidly growing foods such as asparagus. The consumption of large amounts of a food containing a small concentration of purines may provide a greater purine load than consumption of a small amount of a food containing a large concentration of purines.

From Emmerson, B.T. (1996). The management of gout. *New England Journal of Medicine* 334(7), 448.

case, hyperuricemia is a necessary antecedent of gouty arthritis. Supersaturation of extracellular fluid with uric acid promotes deposition of crystals in joints and other connective tissues. Although hyperuricemia is essential to the development of gout, it results in gout in only a small percentage of individuals with elevated uric acid levels.

Overproduction of uric acid may be caused by genetic deficiency of an enzyme that normally promotes purine synthesis by a "salvage" pathway with recycling of uric acid. Enzyme deficiency leads to increased purine synthesis by an alternative de novo pathway. Increased cell turnover in cancers or trauma releases endogenous nucleic acids, whereas a high-purine diet provides more exogenous sources. Underexcretion of uric acid may occur with diabetic nephropathy, renal failure, or use of certain drugs. Alcohol excess also promotes uric acid retention, because metabolism of alcohol produces increased amounts of lactate, which blocks renal excretion of uric acid.

Pathophysiology. The first stage of gout is a period of asymptomatic hyperuricemia, in which serum uric acid levels rise to about double the normal level. About 20% of these individuals progress to the second stage, in which hyperuricemia leads to an acute attack of gouty arthritis caused by precipitation of crystals in joints. Synovial fluid does not solubilize uric acid as well as serum, and this may be a contributing factor to precipitation in joints. The first metatarsophalangeal joint of the big toe is most often involved, probably because of its lower temperature and its tendency to be traumatized.[34] Deposits of monosodium urate in other tissues are also seen, forming raised lesions (*tophi*). Uric acid stones may also form within the urinary tract (see Chapter 20). In joints, crystals trigger an inflammatory response. Phagocytosis of crystals may release mediators that induce further precipitation from the serum. The initial attack usually subsides spontaneously within 3 to 10 days.[35]

The third stage is a period of alternating acute attacks and remissions, often referred to as *intercritical periods*. Intercritical periods rarely last longer than a few months without treatment. The fourth stage, which develops over a period of about 10 years, is one of chronic tophaceous gout, during which acute attacks may be superimposed. Without treatment, tophi enlarge and proliferate because of increasing deposition of uric acid. Tophi in joints are associated with erosion of articular cartilage and underlying bone, resulting in permanent deformity of the affected joints.

Clinical Manifestations. Serum uric acid levels are elevated to 9 to 10 mg/dL or more. An acute attack, often precipitated by stress, trauma, or increased alcohol intake, is manifested by sudden onset of severe pain and swelling of one joint, usually of the big toe. Inflammation of surrounding soft tissues is also evident. Aspiration of monosodium urate crystals from synovial fluid or tophi confirms the diagnosis.

Prevention and Treatment. The risk of acute attacks may be reduced with avoidance of precipitating factors such as alcohol use, high-purine diet, stress, and use of drugs that impair renal excretion of uric acid. Hyperuricemia exceeding 12 mg/dL is usually treated prophylactically. Treatment of acute attacks of gout consists of resting, elevating, and icing the affected joint. NSAIDs such as indomethacin (Indocin), or naproxen (Naprosyn), or corticosteroids are used to relieve inflammation.

Colchicine, the mainstay of treatment in the past, is now less commonly used because of its toxic effects (e.g., nausea, vomiting, diarrhea) and its potential interaction with many other drugs.[36] Colchicine, which inhibits the phagocytosis of uric acid crystals by neutrophils, is particularly effective in aborting an acute attack when administered at the onset of the first signs of the episode. Drugs that lower uric acid levels, such as allopurinol (Zyloprim) or probenecid (Benemid) may be used to decrease the risk of precipitation and promote dissolution of tophi. Allopurinol blocks the synthesis of uric acid, and probenecid blocks renal tubular reabsorption of uric acid. Adequacy of fluid intake must be ensured to decrease the risk of urolithiasis with this therapy.

Prognosis and Outcome. Gout is successfully managed with risk reduction and drug therapy. Tophi are largely preventable with early diagnosis and treatment and are rarely seen in clinical practice.

Systemic Lupus Erythematosus

Definition. SLE is a chronic multisystem disorder characterized by arthritis, dermatitis, and other systemic manifestations and by the presence in the blood of autoantibodies directed at one or more components of cell nuclei.[37] SLE is generally considered to be a connective tissue disorder, but it may also be classified as an autoimmune disorder, a collagen vascular disorder, or a rheumatic (joint-involving) disease. The connective tissue diseases also include RA and other forms of arthritis (see Table 34–7); ankylosing spondylitis and Sjögren's syndrome (described earlier in this chapter); vasculitis (see Chapter 15); fibromyalgia (see Chapter 35); and dermatomyositis and progressive systemic sclerosis (see Chapter 36). The coexistence of more than one of these disorders in the same individual is quite common and is termed *mixed connective tissue disease.*

Epidemiology. The overall incidence of SLE in the United States is about 40 cases per 100,000 population.[37] More than 80% of cases occur in women during their childbearing years, with incidence in this group estimated at 1 in 1000. SLE may also affect children and the elderly, however, and female prevalence is higher in these groups as well. There is some evidence that SLE is more prevalent and more severe in blacks and Hispanics than in whites. A genetic predisposition is apparent, and certain HLA subtypes (DR2 and DR3) and complement deficiencies (C4a and C4b) are more prevalent among individuals with SLE.

Etiology. High levels of **antinuclear antibodies (ANAs)** in the serum of SLE patients support the diagnosis, but have not been shown to be directly involved in causing manifestations (see Table 34–6). In the strictest sense, SLE is not an autoimmune disease, that is, significant immune attack against self-antigens does not occur. Rather, the pathology originates from persistent nonspecific activation of multiple clones of B lymphocytes, resulting in widespread tissue deposition of immune complexes.[38] Normally, such B-cell activation is stimulated during overwhelming infection, but subsides when the infection resolves. In SLE, for unknown reasons, the B-cell activation persists and excessive immune complex formation continues. Certain drugs, notably procainamide (Pronestyl), may cause a lupus-like syndrome that subsides within 4 to 6 weeks after the drug is discontinued (Table 34–11).

Pathophysiology. Connective tissue damage in SLE is the result of deposition of immune complexes, most of which do not contain antibodies against self tissues. Damage results from organ-specific inflammatory responses to excessive deposition of these immune complexes. Toxic effects of concurrent, long-term corticosteroid therapy also contribute to pathology in SLE, promoting premature atherosclerosis, avascular necrosis of bone, hypertension, and weight gain (see Chapter 29).

Clinical Manifestations. Nearly every organ system is potentially affected by SLE, and the presence of at least four typical manifestations must be present to confirm the diagnosis (Table 34–12). Arthritis is the most common manifestation, occurring in a pattern similar to RA except that joint involvement is migratory (passing from one joint to another), nondeforming, and much more painful than would be expected given the degree of synovitis. Tendinitis is also common, and may cause rupture of tendons. Dermatitis is also characteristic of SLE, although the type and distribution of skin rash is variable. The classic malar or "butterfly" rash over the nose and cheeks that is unique to SLE is present in only a third of patients. More commonly, a reddened (erythematous) rash caused by hypersensitivity to ultraviolet light (*photosensitivity*) is distributed in patches over all sun-exposed areas. **Discoid lupus erythematosus** is a syndrome of erythematous rash accompanied by scaling, plugging of hair follicles, and atrophic scarring.

Painful ischemic lesions of the distal fingers result from the vasculitis-induced vasospasm of Raynaud's

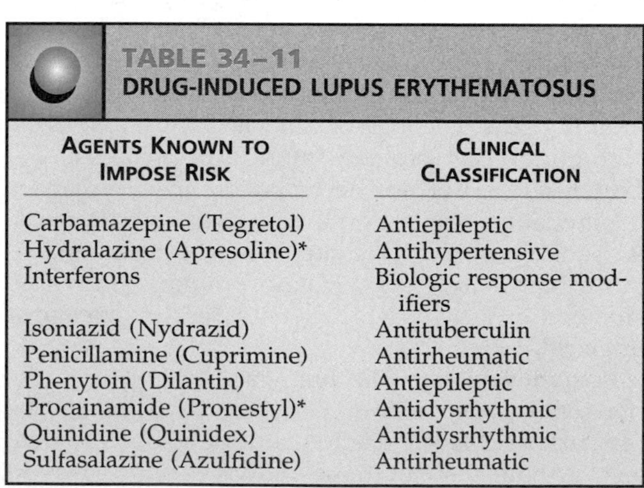

TABLE 34–11
DRUG-INDUCED LUPUS ERYTHEMATOSUS

Agents Known to Impose Risk	Clinical Classification
Carbamazepine (Tegretol)	Antiepileptic
Hydralazine (Apresoline)*	Antihypertensive
Interferons	Biologic response modifiers
Isoniazid (Nydrazid)	Antituberculin
Penicillamine (Cuprimine)	Antirheumatic
Phenytoin (Dilantin)	Antiepileptic
Procainamide (Pronestyl)*	Antidysrhythmic
Quinidine (Quinidex)	Antidysrhythmic
Sulfasalazine (Azulfidine)	Antirheumatic

*Most commonly implicated in drug-induced lupus.

TABLE 34–12
MANIFESTATIONS OF SYSTEMIC LUPUS ERYTHEMATOSUS

System	Typical Manifestations
Integumentary	Malar (butterfly) rash
	Photosensitivity
	Discoid lupus erythematosus
	Alopecia
	Mucosal ulcerations
Musculoskeletal	Acute arthritis of the hands, wrists, and knees, usually episodic and symmetric, nonerosive
	Jaccoud's arthritis (hand deformity caused by ligament relaxation)
	Avascular necrosis of hip (associated with steroid therapy)
	Fatigue
Cardiovascular	Pericarditis
	Myocarditis
	Endocarditis
	Premature atherosclerosis
	Hypertension (associated with steroid therapy and atherosclerosis)
Renal	Glomerulonephritis
Pulmonary	Pneumonitis
	Pulmonary alveolar hemorrhage
	Chronic interstitial lung disease
	Pulmonary hypertension
	Shrinking lung syndrome
	Pulmonary embolism
	Pleuritis
	Pulmonary infiltrates
Gastrointestinal	Serositis
	Mesenteric vasculitis
	Acute pancreatitis
	Weight loss
Central nervous system	Seizures
	Psychosis
	Depression
	Dementia
	Stroke
	Movement disorders
	Transverse myelitis
	Headache
	Fever
Hematologic	Anemia
	Leukopenia
	Lymphopenia
	Thrombocytopenia
	Lupus anticoagulant syndrome (prolonged partial thromboplastin time)
	Antiphospholipid antibody syndrome (immune thrombocytopenia, recurrent fetal loss, and thrombosis)
	Positive ANA in more than 95% of patients
	Positive LE cell prep (for ANA), anti-dsDNA, ENA, or false-positive VDRL test for syphilis
	Complement deficiency

ANA, antinuclear antibody; LE, lupus erythematosus; dsDNA, double-stranded DNA; ENA, extractable antinuclear antibodies; VDRL, Veneral Disease Research Laboratory.

Data from Von Feldt, J.M. (1995). Systemic lupus erythematosus: Recognizing its various presentations. *Postgraduate Medicine* 97(4), 79–94.

phenomenon (see Chapter 15). Mucous membrane manifestations include GI symptoms caused by inflammation of the serosa (*serositis*), noninfectious pharyngitis, and ulcers of the oral, vaginal or nasal mucosa. The more serious manifestations of SLE are renal (*lupus glomerulonephritis*), neurologic (*lupus encephalopathy*), or pulmonary (*lupus pneumonitis*), resulting from vasculitis. Small pericardial effusions and acute pericarditis, myocarditis, or endocarditis may also occur. Valve lesions are common, but do not usually precipitate cardiac failure. Patients with SLE are prone to infection, even if they are not receiving immunosuppressive or glucocorticoid therapy. Pregnancy exacerbates manifestations of SLE and is associated with a high rate of second-trimester abortion.[37]

Prevention and Treatment. There are no known means of preventing SLE, nor is there any definitive treatment. Acute exacerbations (SLE flares) may be precipitated by sun exposure and possibly by ingestion of alfalfa sprouts, which should be avoided.[39] Pregnancy in patients with active SLE may also induce a flare and is associated with adverse outcomes for the fetus.[37] However, women whose disease has been in remission for at least 4 to 6 months have normal outcomes of pregnancy. Treatment is supportive and symptomatic, directed at organ-specific manifestations. Glucocorticoids are the most widely used agents for treatment of acute inflammation in SLE; however, prolonged use of steroids is associated with increased morbidity, as has been stated. NSAIDs may be used to treat more minor inflammatory manifestations such as serositis, synovitis, fever, soft-tissue pain, and headache.[40] Sunscreens are advocated to block ultraviolet light exposure.

Skin manifestations may be treated with antimalarial drugs, retinoids, or azathioprine (see Chapter 36). There is recent evidence that low-dose therapy with azathioprine or cyclophosphamide (Cytoxan) and prednisone may reduce the need for corticosteroid therapy for many of the manifestations of SLE.[40] In selected patients, plasmapheresis has been used to reduce the number of circulating immune complexes, but this regimen has not shown any beneficial effects beyond those of the standard pharmacologic regimen.

Prognosis and Outcome. The 10-year survival rate for patients with SLE is nearly 90%.[37] Women and those whose disease onset is after the age of 60 have the most positive prognosis, and men and children have a poorer prognosis. Death is commonly caused by renal failure or by coronary atherosclerosis, possibly exacerbated by vasculitis-associated hypertension and long-term glucocorticoid therapy.

CLINICAL SIGNIFICANCE OF DISORDERS OF THE BONES AND JOINTS

The disorders discussed in this chapter are of clinical importance primarily because of their commonality and, in the case of arthritis, their impact on quality of life for so many individuals of all ages. The pathophysiologic mechanisms that underlie the development of bone tumors, most forms of arthritis, and most connective tissue disorders, including SLE, are still obscure, and treatment is still empiric in many cases. Active research is continuing in an effort to clarify etiologic mechanisms and develop rational therapies. Many of the connective tissue disorders introduced in this chapter affect not only the bones or joints but also the muscles and skin, as detailed in the remaining chapters.

Summary of Key Points

- Musculoskeletal disorders may represent localized trauma, neoplasia, inflammation, or congenital defects. In their roles as connective tissues, bones, muscles, and joints are a significant source of morbidity in a number of systemic disorders as well.
- Despite its static appearance, bone tissue is highly homeostatic. Linear bone growth early in life and remodeling of bone throughout life depend on a balance of osteoblastic (bone-forming) and osteoclastic (bone-resorbing) processes. Imbalance of these processes underlies many disorders of bone. The process of bone healing is also mediated by osteoblastic and osteoclastic processes and simulates the embryonic development of bone.
- Most joints in the body are diarthroses, in which articulating bones are covered with weight-distributing cartilage and connected by ligaments that allow movement within the range of motion. A capsule of periosteum encloses the joint, and a vascular, innervated synovial membrane lines the capsule. Synovial fluid, secreted by the synovial membrane, lubricates and nourishes joint structures. Traumatic and inflammatory conditions affecting diarthrotic joints may result in damage to cartilage, ligaments, and bones within the joint. Impaired mobility, disordered bone and cartilage remodeling, pain and third spacing of fluid are characteristic of disorders involving these joints.
- Many bone disorders are characterized by decreased bone density as a result of imbalance of osteoblastic and osteoclastic activity, although the pattern and degree of impairment is variable. Osteoporosis is characterized by decreased matrix and mineralization, and

osteomalacia presents as decreased mineralization of normal amounts of bone matrix. Other disorders such as bone tumors, osteomyelitis, and osteochondrosis are limited to specific areas of the skeleton.

- Traumatic injuries to the bones and joints include sprains, fractures, dislocations, and subluxations. Risk of these injuries is highest among those who engage in sports or other activities that stress these tissues, particularly by those who are not in optimal physical condition or have not been trained in proper technique. Children, whose play activities and lack of inhibition or judgment may place them at risk, are prone to traumatic fractures. The elderly, whose bones may be weakened by osteoporosis, frequently suffer hip fractures caused by falls.
- The most prevalent forms of arthritis are OA, RA, and gouty arthritis. Joint damage in OA is characterized by progressive degeneration of articular cartilage. Disordered bone growth and inflammation are caused by this degenerative process. Joint damage in RA and gout is induced by inflammation, triggered by an immune-mediated process in RA and by deposition of needle-like monosodium urate crystals in gout.
- SLE is a systemic disorder in which excessive production of antibody-secreting B lymphocytes results in deposition of immune complexes in joints, skin, and other tissues throughout the body. Because most of the antibody in the immune complexes is not directed against self antigens, SLE is not a true *auto*immune disease, although it certainly represents a disordered immune response.

REFERENCES

1. Anderson, J.J.B. (1996). Calcium, phosphorus, and human bone development. *Journal of Nutrition* 126, 1153S–1158S.
2. Stern, P.H., Tatrai, A., Semler, D.E., *et al.* (1995). Endothelin receptors, second messengers, and actions in bone. *Journal of Nutrition* 125, 2028S–2032S.
3. Manolagas, S.C., and Jilka, R.L. (1995). Bone marrow, cytokines, and bone remodeling. *New England Journal of Medicine* 332(5), 305–311.
4. Ybarra, J., Ade, R., and Romeo, J.H. (1996). Osteoporosis in men: A review. *Nursing Clinics of North America* 31(4), 805–813.
5. Barrett-Connor, E., Chang, J.C., and Edelstein, S.L. (1994). Coffee-associated osteoporosis offset by daily milk consumption: The Rancho Bernardo Study. *Journal of the American Medical Association* 271(4), 280–283.
6. Kessenich, C.R. (1996). Update on pharmacologic therapies for osteoporosis. *Nurse Practitioner* 21(8), 19–24.
7. Zuckermann, J.D. (1996). Hip fracture. *New England Journal of Medicine* 334(23), 1519–1525.
8. Bellantoni, M.F. (1996). Osteoporosis prevention and treatment. *American Family Physician* 54(3), 986–992.
9. Galsworthy, T.D., and Wilson, P.L. (1996). Osteoporosis: It steals more than bone. *American Journal of Nursing* 96(6), 27–33.
10. Sonnen, G.M., and Henry, N.K. (1996). Pediatric bone and joint infections: Diagnosis and antimicrobial management. *Pediatric Clinics of North America* 43(4), 933–947.
11. Lew, D.P., and Waldvogel, F.A. (1997). Osteomyelitis. *New England Journal of Medicine* 336(14), 999–1007.
12. Haas, D.W., and McAndrew, M.P. (1996). Bacterial osteomyelitis in adults: Evolving considerations in diagnosis and treatment. *American Journal of Medicine* 101, 550–561.
13. Cotran, R.S., Kumar, V., and Robbins, S.L. (1994). *Robbins Pathologic Basis of Disease.* (5th ed.). Philadelphia: W.B. Saunders. (pp. 414–418, 1232–1246, and 1249–1253).
14. Hruska, K.A., and Teitelbaum, S.L. (1995). Renal osteodystrophy. *New England Journal of Medicine* 333(3), 166–174.
15. Gartland, J.J. (1979). *Fundamentals of Orthopedics.* Philadelphia: W.B. Saunders. As cited in: Foster, R.L.R., Hunsberger, M.M., and Anderson, J.J.T. (1989). *Family-Centered Nursing Care of Children.* Philadelphia: W.B. Saunders. (p. 1831).
16. Foster, R.L.R., Hunsberger, M.M., and Anderson, J.J.T. (1989). *Family-Centered Nursing Care of Children.* Philadelphia: W.B. Saunders. (pp. 1831–1834).
17. Swain, R.A., and Holt, W.S., Jr. (1993). Ankle injuries: Tips from sports medicine physicians. *Postgraduate Medicine* 93(3), 91–100.
18. Black, J.M., and Matassarin-Jacobs, E. (1997). *Medical-Surgical Nursing: Clinical Management for Continuity of Care.* (5th ed.). Philadelphia: W.B. Saunders. (pp. 678, 2129).
19. Englund, S.P., and Sundberg, S. (1996). Management of common pediatric fractures. *Pediatric Clinics of North America* 43(5), 991–1012.
20. Alper, J. (1994). Boning up: Newly isolated proteins heal bad breaks. *Science* 263, 324–325.
21. Himelstein, B.P., and Dormans, J.P. (1996). Malignant bone tumors of childhood. *Pediatric Clinics of North America* 43(4), 967–984.
22. Hall, T.G., and Schaiff, R.A.B. (1993). Update on the medical treatment of hypercalcemia of malignancy. *Clinical Pharmacy* 12, 117–125.
23. Sheridan, C.A. (1996). Multiple myeloma. *Seminars in Oncology Nursing* 12(1), 59–69.
24. Alexanian, R., and Dimopoulos, M. (1994). The treatment of multiple myeloma. *New England Journal of Medicine* 484–489.
25. Novacheck, T.F. (1996). Developmental dysplasia of the hip. *Pediatric Clinics of North America* 43(4), 829–848.
26. U.S. Preventive Services Task Force. (1993). Screening for adolescent idiopathic scoliosis. *Journal of the American Medical Association* 269(20), 2667–2672.
27. Skaggs, D.L., and Bassett, G.S. (1996). Adolescent idiopathic scoliosis: An update. *American Family Physician* 53(7), 2327–2334.
28. Schumacher, H.R. (1988). *Primer on the Rheumatic Diseases.* (9th ed.). Atlanta: Arthritis Foundation. As cited in Long, B.C., Phipps, W.J., and Cassemeyer, V.L. (1993). *Medical-Surgical Nursing: A Nursing Process Approach.* St. Louis: Mosby–Year Book. (p. 1378).
29. Oddis, C.V. (1996). New perspectives on osteoarthritis. *American Journal of Medicine* 100(2A suppl.), 10S–15S.
30. Harris, C. (1993). Osteoarthritis: How to diagnose and treat the painful joint. *Geriatrics* 48(8), 39–46.
31. Lyssy, K.J., and Ascalante, A. (1996). Perioperative management of rheumatoid arthritis: Areas of concern for primary care physicians. *Postgraduate Medicine* 99(2), 191–206.
32. Blackburn, W.D. (1996). Management of osteoarthritis and rheumatoid arthritis: Prospects and possibilities. *American Journal of Medicine* 100(2A suppl.), 24S–30S.
33. Schumacher, H.R. (1996). Crystal-induced arthritis: An overview. *American Journal of Medicine* 100(2A suppl.), 46S–52S.

34. Joseph, J., and McGrath, H. (1995). Gout or 'pseudogout': How to differentiate crystal-induced arthropathies. *Geriatrics* 50(4), 33–39.
35. Beutler, A., and Schumacher, H.R. (1994). Gout and 'pseudogout': When are arthritis symptoms caused by crystal deposition? *Postgraduate Medicine* 95(2), 103–120.
36. Emmerson, B.T. (1996). The management of gout. *New England Journal of Medicine* 334(7), 445–451.
37. Mills, J.A. (1994). Systemic lupus erythrmatosus. *New England Journal of Medicine* 330(26), 1871–1879.
38. Lehman, T.J.A. (1995). A practical guide to systemic lupus erythematosus. *Pediatric Clinics of North America* 42(5), 1223–1238.
39. Von Feldt, J.M. (1995). Systemic lupus erythematosus: Recognizing its various presentations. *Postgraduate Medicine* 97(4), 79–94.
40. Redford, T.W., and Small, R.E. (1995). Update on pharmacotherapy of systemic lupus erythematosus. *American Journal of Health-System Pharmacy* 52, 2686–2695.

SELECTED BIBLIOGRAPHY

Aaron, A.D. (1994). The management of cancer metastatic to bone. *Journal of the American Medical Association* 272(15), 1206–1209.

Attal, M., Harousseau, J-L., Stoppa, A-M., *et al.* (1996). A prospective, randomized trial of autologous bone marrow transplantation and chemotherapy in multiple myeloma. *New England Journal of Medicine* 335(2), 91–97.

Bamberger, D.M. (1993). Osteomyelitis: A commonsense approach to antibiotic and surgical treatment. *Postgraduate Medicine* 94(5), 177–184.

Boachie-Adjei, O., and Lonner, B. (1996). Spinal deformity. *Pediatric Clinics of North America* 43(4), 883–897.

Boumpas, D.T., Austin, H.A. III, Fessler, B.J., *et al.* (1995). Systemic lupus erythematosus: Emerging concepts. Part 1: Renal, neuropsychiatric, cardiovascular, pulmonary, and hematologic disease. *Annals of Internal Medicine* 122(12), 940–950.

Boumpas, D.T., Fessler, B.J., Austin, H.A. III, *et al.* (1995). Systemic lupus erythematosus: Emerging concepts. Part 2: Dermatologic and joint disease, the antiphospholipid antibody syndrome, pregnancy and hormonal therapy, morbidity and mortality, and pathogenesis. *Annals of Internal Medicine* 123(1), 42–53.

Brechtelsbauer, D.A. (1994). Managing rheumatologic disease in nursing home patients. *Postgraduate Medicine* 96(2), 91–96.

Buckley, T.J. (1996). Radiologic features of gout. *American Family Physician* 54(4), 1232–1238.

Bulbul, R., Williams, W.V., and Schumacher, H.R. Jr. (1995). Psoriatic arthritis: Diverse and sometimes highly destructive. *Postgraduate Medicine* 97(4), 97–108.

Cummings, S.R., Nevitt, M.C., Browner, W.S., *et al.* (1995). Risk factors for hip fracture in white women. *New England Journal of Medicine* 332(12), 767–773.

Eiff, M.P. (1997). Management of clavicle fractures. *American Family Physician* 55(1), 121–128.

Erickson, A.R., Enzenauer, R.J., Nordstrom, D.M., *et al.* (1994). The prevalence of hypothyroidism in gout. *American Journal of Medicine* 97, 231–234.

Ettinger, W.H., Burns, R., Messier, S.P., *et al.* (1997). A randomized trial comparing aerobic exercise and resistance exercise with a health education program in older adults with knee osteoarthritis: The Fitness Arthritis and Seniors Trial (FAST). *Journal of the American Medical Association* 277(1), 25–31.

Felson, D.T. (1996). Weight and osteoarthritis. *American Journal of Clinical Nutrition* 63(suppl.), 430S–432S.

Fish, D. (1995). Environmental risk and prevention of Lyme disease. *American Journal of Medicine* 98(4A suppl.), 2S–9S.

Flynn, B.L. (1994). Rheumatoid arthritis and osteoarthritis: Current and future therapies. *American Pharmacy* NS34(11), 31–42.

Greenspan, S.L., Myers, E.R., Maitland, L.A., *et al.* (1994). Fall severity and bone mineral density as risk factors for hip fracture in ambulatory elderly. *Journal of the American Medical Association* 271(2), 128–133.

Guyton, A.C., and Hall, J.E. (1996). *Textbook of Medical Physiology.* (9th ed.). Philadelphia: W.B. Saunders. (pp. 985–996).

Henderson, R.C., and Specter, B.B. (1994). Kyphosis and fractures in children and young adults with cystic fibrosis. *Journal of Pediatrics* 125(2), 208–212.

Johnston, C.C., and Slemenda, C.W. (1993). Risk assessment: Theoretical considerations. *American Journal of Medicine* 95(5A suppl.), 2S–5S.

Karpf, D.B., Shapiro, D.R., Seeman, E., *et al.* (1997). Prevention of nonvertebral fractures by alendronate: A meta-analysis. *Journal of the American Medical Association* 277(14), 1159–1164.

Kirchner, J.T. (1995). Reiter's syndrome: A possibility in patients with reactive arthritis. *Postgraduate Medicine* 97(3), 111–122.

Kirwan, J.R., and the Arthritis and Rheumatism Council Low-Dose Glucocorticoid Study Group. (1995). The effect of glucocorticoids on joint destruction in rheumatoid arthritis. *New England Journal of Medicine* 333(3), 142–146.

Kremer, R., Shustik, C., Tabak, T., *et al.* (1996). Parathyroid-hormone-related peptide in hematologic malignancies. *American Journal of Medicine* 100, 406–411.

Kyle, R.A. (1994). The monoclonal gammopathies. *Clinical Chemistry* 40(11B), 2154–2161.

LaRochelle, G.E., LaRochelle, A.G., Ratner, R.E., *et al.* (1993). Recovery of the hypothalamic-pituitary adrenal (HPA) axis in patients with rheumatic diseases receiving low-dose prednisone. *American Journal of Medicine* 95, 258–264.

Liberman, U.A., Weiss, S.R., Broll, J., *et al.* (1995). Effect of oral alendronate on bone mineral density and the incidence of fractures in postmenopausal osteoporosis. *New England Journal of Medicine* 333(22), 1437–1443.

Lindsay, R. (1993). Hormone replacement therapy for prevention and treatment of osteoporosis. *American Journal of Medicine* 95(5A suppl.), 37S–39S.

Marchall, J.B., and McMurray, R. (1994). Acute polyarthritis: Fifth disease passed from adult to child. *Postgraduate Medicine* 95(8), 165–168.

Michelson, D., Stratakis, C., Hill, L., *et al.* (1996). Bone mineral density in women with depression. *New England Journal of Medicine* 335(16), 1176–1181.

Moder, K.G. (1996). Use and interpretation of rheumatologic tests: A guide for clinicians. *Mayo Clinic Proceedings* 71, 391–396.

Moore, K.L., and Persaud, T.V.N. (1993). *The Developing Human: Clinically Oriented Embryology.* Philadelphia: W.B. Saunders. (pp. 354–368).

Nietfeld, J.J. (1993). Cytokines and proteoglycans. *Experientia* 49, 456–469.

O'Dell, J.R., Haire, C.E., Erikson, N., *et al.* (1996). Treatment of rheumatoid arthritis with methotrexate alone, sulfasalazine, and hydroxychloroquine, or a combination of all three medications. *New England Journal of Medicine* 334(20), 1287–1291.

Oken, M.M. (1994). Standard treatment of multiple myeloma. *Mayo Clinic Proceedings* 69, 781–786.

Ostezan, L.B., and Callen, J.P. (1996). Cutaneous manifestations of selected rheumatologic diseases. *American Family Physician* 53(5), 1625–1633.

Pak, C.Y.C., Sakhaee, K., Adams-Huet, B., *et al.* (1995). Treatment of postmenopausal osteoporosis with slow-release sodium fluoride. *Annals of Internal Medicine* 123(6), 401–408.

Pope, R.M. (1996). Rheumatoid arthritis: Pathogenesis and early recognition. *American Journal of Medicine* 100(suppl 2A), 3S–9S.

Rahn, D.W. (1994). Lyme disease—Where's the bug? *New England Journal of Medicine* 330(4), 282–283.

Raisz, L.G. (1997). The osteoporosis revolution. *Annals of Internal Medicine* 126(6), 458–462.

Reginster, J.Y., Deroisy, R., Lecart, M.P., *et al.* (1995). A double-blind, placebo-controlled, dose-finding trial of intermittent nasal salmon calcitonin for prevention of postmenopausal lumbar spine bone loss. *American Journal of Medicine* 98, 452–458.

Reid, I.R., Ames, R.W., Evans, M.C., *et al.* (1995). Long-term effects in calcium supplementation on bone loss and fractures in postmenopausal women: A randomized controlled trial. *American Journal of Medicine* 98, 331–335.

Ribot, C., Tremollieres, F., and Pouilles, J-M. (1995). Can we detect women with low bone mass using clinical risk factors? *American Journal of Medicine* 98(2A suppl.), 52S–55S.

Rich, M.W. (1996). Drug-induced lupus. *Postgraduate Medicine* 100(3), 299–308.

Riis, B.J. (1995). The role of bone loss. *American Journal of Medicine* 98(2A suppl.), 29S–32S.

Saag, K.G., Koehnke, R., Caldwell, J.R., *et al.* (1994). Low dose long-term corticosteroid therapy in rheumatoid arthritis: An analysis of serious adverse events. *American Journal of Medicine* 96, 115–123.

Schneider, D.L., Barrett-Connor, E.L., and Morton, D.J. (1994). Thyroid hormone use and bone mineral density in elderly women: Effects of estrogen. *Journal of the American Medical Association* 271(16), 1245–1249.

Schumacher, H.R. Jr. (1995). Arthritis of recent onset: A guide to evaluation and initial therapy for primary care physicians. *Postgraduate Medicine* 97(4), 52–63.

Smith, B.W., and Green, G.A. (1995). Acute knee injuries: Part II. Diagnosis and management. *American Family Physician* 51(4), 799–806.

Tibbitts, G.M. (1994). Juvenile rheumatoid arthritis: Old challenges, new insights. *Postgraduate Medicine* 96(2), 75–87.

To, S.S.T., Newman, P.M., Hyland, V.J., *et al.* (1996). Regulation of adhesion molecule expression by human synovial microvascular endothelial cells in vitro. *Arthritis and Rheumatism* 39(3), 467–477.

Totemchokchyakarn, K., and Ball, G.V. (1996). Arthritis of systemic disease. *American Journal of Medicine* 101, 642–647.

Towheed, T.E., and Hochberg, M.C. (1996). Acute monoarthritis: A practical approach to assessment and treatment. *American Family Physician* 54(7), 2239–2243.

Tugwell, P., Pincus, T., Yocum, D., *et al.* (1995). Combination therapy with cyclosporine and methotrexate in severe rheumatoid arthritis. *New England Journal of Medicine* 333(3), 137–141.

Uy, J.P., Nuwayhid, N., and Saadeh, C. (1996). Unusual presentations of gout: Tips for accurate diagnosis. *Postgraduate Medicine* 100(1), 253–268.

van der Heide, A., Jacobs, J.W.G., Bijlsma, W.J., *et al.* (1996). The effectiveness of early treatment with "second-line" antirheumatic drugs: A randomized, controlled trial. *Annals of Internal Medicine* 124(8), 699–707.

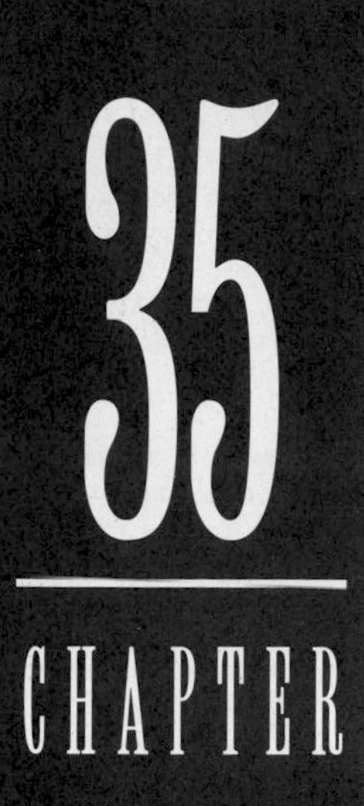

Muscle Disorders and Effects of Exercise

LEARNING OBJECTIVES

1. Differentiate among the normal and pathophysiologic mechanisms that may result in muscle fatigue.
2. Discuss the effects of gender, physical conditioning, and exercise on type I and type II muscle fibers.
3. Identify normal and pathophysiologic mechanisms of muscle atrophy and hypertrophy.
4. Discuss the interdependence of the skeletal muscles, bones, and joints with respect to the mechanics of mobility.
5. Differentiate between neural and muscular causes of abnormally increased muscle contraction.
6. Discuss the adaptive responses of the skeletal muscles and other body systems to strength and resistance training.
7. Identify the relationship between physical fitness and risk of disease.
8. Comprehend the pathophysiologic mechanisms that predict clinical manifestations and rationalize intervention in selected muscle disorders.

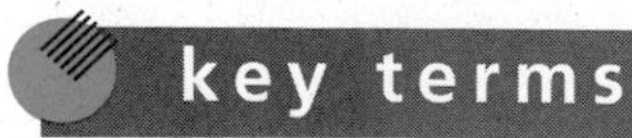

key terms

athlete's heart
atrophy
Becker's muscular dystrophy (BMD)
chronic fatigue syndrome
dermatomyositis
Duchenne's muscular dystrophy (DMD)
dynamic exercise
fibromyalgia
hyperplasia
hypertrophy
hypoplasia
inclusion-body myositis
inflammatory myopathy

muscular dystrophy
myalgia
myoglobinuria
myotonia
myotonia congenita
oxygen debt
polymyositis
rhabdomyolysis
rhabdomyosarcoma
spasticity
static exercise
strain

Skeletal muscle is, by mass, is the most abundant tissue in the body. Skeletal muscles are the effectors of voluntary movement, which is the essence of interaction between individuals and the environment. Contraction of skeletal muscle is absolutely dependent on neural stimulation, and each muscle cell (fiber) is served by its own axonal connection (neuromuscular junction). Muscle contraction is energy dependent; any contraction longer than a few seconds' duration requires a continuous supply of oxygen and glucose to drive the molecular mechanism of contraction. Neural, vascular, and metabolic factors have great influence on the process of skeletal muscle contraction. The energy consumed by muscle contraction generates not only work (movement or resistance against gravity or other forces), but also heat. Muscle contraction is the major contributor to the generation of core body temperature (see Chapter 11).

Primary muscle disorders are relatively uncommon, but the skeletal muscles are secondarily affected by disease of other major systems. Motor system disorders such as spinal cord injury are a classic model of the interdependence of neural and muscular function (see Chapter 22). The muscle fatigue and wasting that are manifestations of many systemic disorders result from deficiency of oxygen and nutrients caused by problems with source (respiratory or metabolic function) or delivery (cardiovascular function).

The functional interdependence of the major body systems and skeletal muscle has beneficial as well as detrimental aspects. Endurance and resistance types of exercise have been shown to significantly reduce morbidity and mortality caused by coronary heart disease, hypertension, obesity, diabetes, osteoporosis, cancer, and depression. In this chapter, the most significant primary muscle disorders are discussed, including muscle trauma (**strains**), the common idiopathic disorders **fibromyalgia** and **chronic fatigue syndrome**, the syndrome of **rhabdomyolysis, muscular dystrophies, inflammatory myopathies,** and the most common muscle tumor (**rhabdomyosarcoma**). The adaptive responses of skeletal muscle and other body systems to exercise are also discussed, along with the mechanisms by which these responses may protect against specific disorders.

ANATOMY OF SKELETAL MUSCLE

Organization and Connective Tissue Support

The microscopic anatomy of skeletal muscle fibers was described in Chapter 5. Figure 35–1 illustrates and names the major skeletal muscles. Each muscle is composed of thousands of individually innervated and perfused fibers, bundled together in a functional configuration by several layers of supportive connective tissue. As shown in Figure 35–2, a layer of *endomysium* surrounds each muscle fiber. Several fibers are bundled together into *fascicles* by a wrapping of *perimysium*, and several fascicles are bundled into an individual muscle by *epimysium*, also referred to as *fascia*. In most muscles, the epimysium extends beyond the body of the muscle to become a flat, fibrous *tendon* that attaches the muscle to bone (indirect attachment). In a few muscles, the epimysium covering the body of the muscle is fused to adjacent bone or cartilage (direct attachment). This multilayered connective tissue support enables muscle to withstand the deforming forces associated with contraction. Connective tissue diseases, discussed in Chapter 34 within the context of joint dysfunction, may also manifest as skeletal muscle dysfunction (Table 35–1).

Fascicular Arrangement

Fascicular arrangement determines the shape and functional capacity of a given muscle (Fig. 35–3). Muscles of the extremities are in *parallel* arrangement, aligned parallel to the long axis of the muscle and giving the muscle a strap-like or spindle shape (e.g., the biceps). In a *pennate* arrangement, fascicles are arranged obliquely to a central tendon, similarly to a feather (e.g., the quadriceps). A *convergent* arrangement is demonstrated by the pectoral and deltoid muscles, in which fascicles converge toward a single tendon in a fan-like pattern. A *circular* arrangement of fascicles, found in the external anal and urinary sphincters and in the muscles surrounding the mouth and eyes, facilitates opening or clo-

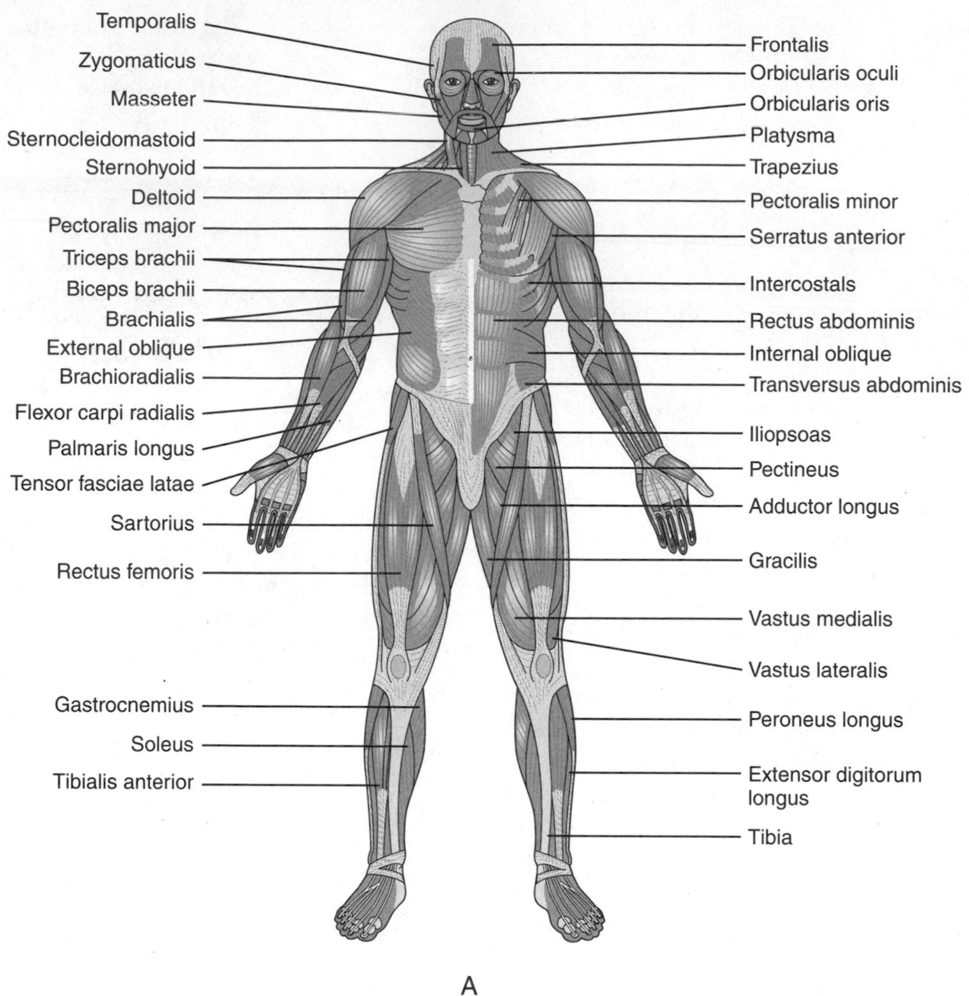

FIGURE 35–1
Major muscle groups. *A*, Anterior view.

sure of orifices. Muscles with parallel arrangement typically effect more movement, and pennate and convergent muscles generate more power because of the greater number of fibers exerting force on a given point.

CONTRACTION OF SKELETAL MUSCLE

The molecular mechanism of muscle contraction (the sliding filament mechanism) was discussed in detail in Chapter 5. Factors that affect contraction of whole muscle are emphasized in this section and include: (1) predominant fiber type and energetics; (2) neural stimulation; (3) hormonal regulation of muscle growth and development; and (4) muscle mechanics. Mechanisms of abnormal muscle contraction are derived from these factors.

Fiber Types and Energy Metabolism

Muscle contraction requires the expenditure of energy, released within the cell with the cleavage of high-energy phosphate bonds in adenosine triphosphate (ATP) molecules (see Chapter 3). Four sources of ATP are potentially available to muscle: stored ATP, phosphocreatine, anaerobic glycolysis, and oxidative (aerobic) metabolism. The first three sources do not require oxygen. Muscle cells store enough ATP to sustain contraction for approximately 6 seconds. Phosphocreatine, a high-energy compound unique to muscle, may then transfer energy and a phosphate group to adenosine diphosphate (ADP) to regenerate ATP, sustaining muscle work for another 5 or 10 seconds. These short-term energy stores are replenished during periods of muscle rest, when more ATP is generated than expended.

Anaerobic glycolysis can generate small amounts

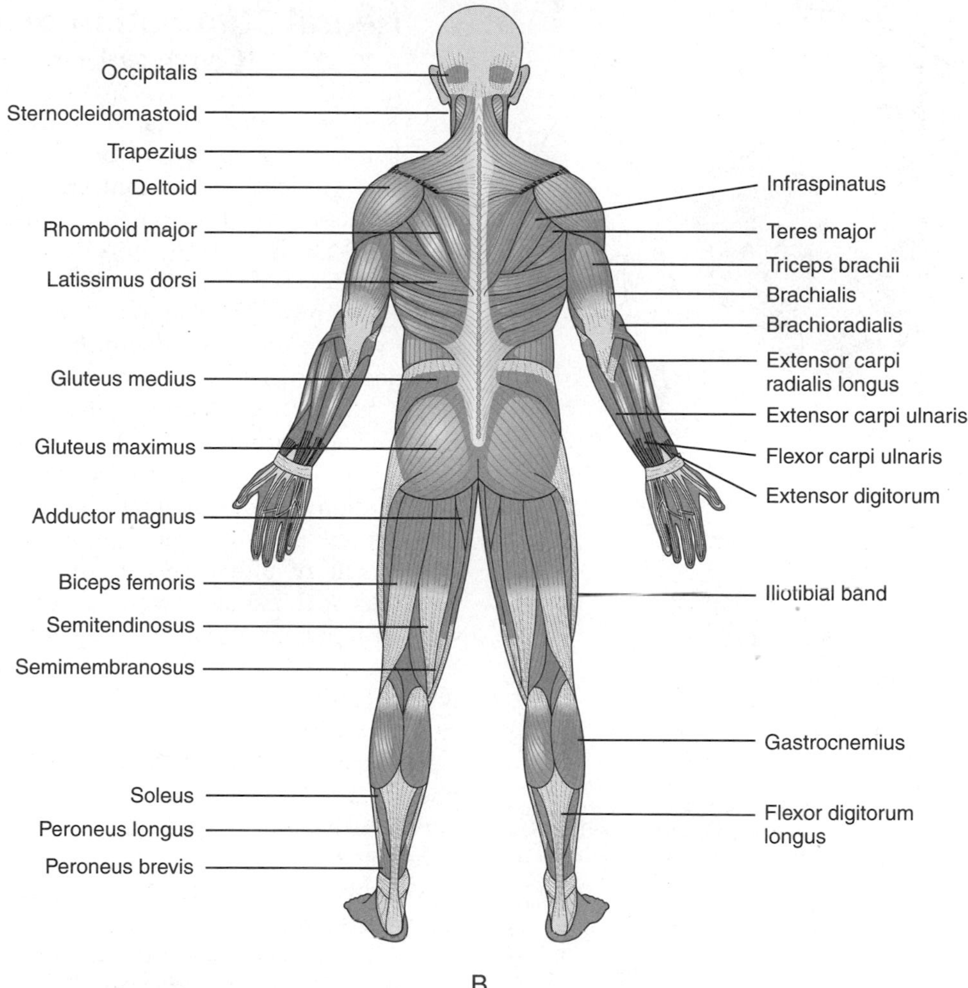

FIGURE 35–1 *Continued*
B, Posterior view.

of ATP from stored muscle glycogen, but this metabolic pathway also produces lactic acid, contributing to a local acidosis that is believed to induce muscle aching and fatigue. In the presence of oxygen, the pyruvic acid produced during glycolysis is not converted to lactic acid, but rather enters the Krebs cycle and, ultimately, mitochondrial oxidative phosphorylation. Oxidative metabolism produces much more ATP than does anaerobic glycolysis, but does not produce it as quickly. When insufficient ATP is available, muscle contraction is impaired because of (1) inability of actin-myosin cross-bridges to detach and recycle (see Chapter 5) and (2) lack of energy to drive the Na^+,K^+-ATPase pump during the repolarization phase of the action potential (see Chapter 4). Table 35–2 lists congenital and nutritional disorders in which abnormal energy metabolism manifests as defective skeletal muscle function.

As discussed briefly in Chapter 5, specific muscles are specialized for greater efficiency in either anaerobic glycolysis or oxidative metabolism, depending on their predominant fiber type. Skeletal muscle fibers are classified as slow oxidative (type I or "slow twitch"), fast oxidative (type IIA "fast twitch") or fast glycolytic (type IIB "fast twitch"). Table 35–3 classifies major muscles on the basis of these types. Type I fibers are found primarily in antigravity muscles that must maintain contraction for long periods of time. Oxidative metabolism, which provides a slow, continuous supply of oxygen, is more efficient under such circumstances, and these fibers thus contain large numbers of mitochondria and are richly perfused. Type I fibers appear red because of the presence of *myoglobin*, an iron-containing molecule that facilitates diffusion of oxygen within the fiber in a manner similar to that of hemoglobin in the blood.

Type IIA fibers are a mixed type, containing mito-

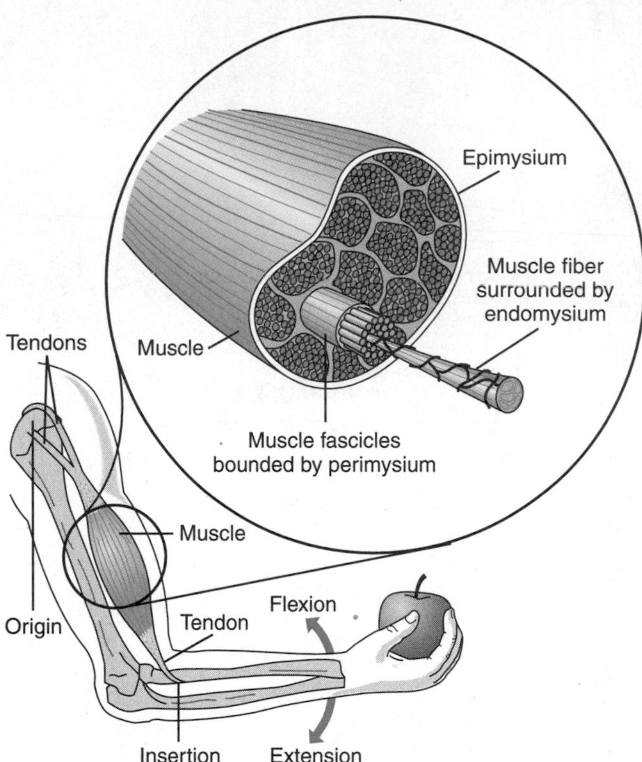

FIGURE 35–2

Organization of skeletal muscle. Each muscle fiber is surrounded by a layer of *endomysium.* Several fibers are bundled together by a layer of *perimysium,* forming muscle fascicles, and several fascicles are bundled together by a layer of *epimysium (fascia)* to form the body of the muscle. In most muscles, the epimysium extends beyond the muscle to form the tendon that attaches muscle to bone. (Redrawn from Moffett, D.F., Moffett, S.B., and Schauf, C.L. [1993]. *Human Physiology: Foundations & Frontiers.* [2nd ed.]. St. Louis: Mosby–Year Book. [pp. 292–293]. Reproduced with permission of The McGraw-Hill Companies.)

chondria and myoglobin, but also glycogen, which can be quickly converted to ATP via glycolysis. Type IIA fibers fatigue more quickly than type I, but not as quickly as type IIB. Type IIB fibers appear white because of the absence of myoglobin. They have few mitochondria and large glycogen stores, relying almost exclusively on anaerobic glycolysis for ATP production. Energy can be generated quickly, but glycogen and phosphocreatine stores are quickly depleted. These fibers are thus specialized for brief, powerful contraction.

Within individuals, the distribution of fiber types is genetically limited, but may be influenced within these limits by physical conditioning, as discussed later. A shift in the proportion of small type I and larger type II fibers probably contributes to the decline in muscle mass seen with aging. Type IIA fibers seem to be preferentially lost, and this may be because of degeneration of these fibers or their conversion to type I fibers (see Developmental Perspective).[1]

Neural Stimulation of Muscle Contraction

As discussed in Chapter 5, contraction of a muscle fiber is initiated by an action potential from a motor nerve fiber, which contacts the muscle fiber at the myoneural junction. The neurotransmitter acetylcholine (ACh) is released into this synapse, inducing voltage-gated sodium channels to open in the muscle cell membrane. The resultant change in membrane voltage releases calcium from the sarcoplasmic reticulum into the cytoplasm. Calcium then triggers contraction by the sliding filament mechanism. Variation in the frequency of action potentials caused by local alterations in electrolyte concentrations results in variation in the characteristics of the resulting contraction. Contractions may be weak or enhanced as a result of alterations in the resting membrane potential or threshold potential of muscle fibers, and they are potentially altered by summation mechanisms (see Chapter 5). Altered contraction of all types of muscle is characteristic of electrolyte imbalance (see Chapter 9).

Innervation ratios, that is, the numbers of muscle fibers served by axonal branches of single motor nerves, are also variable among muscles and influence the nature of the resulting contractions. Muscles involved in very fine motor activity receive neural inputs from a greater number of nerves, and muscles involved in limb motion and posture are served by fewer motor nerves.

Regulation of Muscle Growth and Development

The functional capacity of muscle is greatly affected by its structural mass, that is, the *size* of its component cells. An increase in muscle size because of structural enlargement of muscle cells is termed **hypertrophy**, and a decrease in size because of loss of structural components of cells is known as **atrophy**. Hypertrophy increases the functional capacity of muscle, whereas atrophy decreases it. Hypertrophy occurs only in muscle tissue and is distinct from other mechanisms of organ enlargement (organomegaly) such as edema, engorgement of blood vessels, or **hyperplasia** (increased *numbers* of cells because of normal or abnormal mitotic activity). Atrophy is different from organ shrinkage caused by dehydration, death of cells caused by apoptosis or necrosis, or **hypoplasia** (decreased numbers of cells caused by arrest or impairment of mitosis). The stimuli that result in hypertrophy or atrophy may trigger hyperplasia or hypoplasia at the same time.

TABLE 35–1
CONNECTIVE TISSUE DISEASES INVOLVING SKELETAL MUSCLE

Category	Examples	Clinical Features
Nutritional	Scurvy	Dietary deficiency of ascorbic acid (vitamin C); results in fragility of collagen-containing tissues in blood vessels and skeletal muscles
	Protein-energy malnutrition	Continued synthesis of connective tissue proteins but significant proteolysis of muscle in severe deficiency; invasion of muscle fibers by non–muscle cells containing hydrolytic enzymes
Genetic	Ehlers-Danlos syndrome	Group of at least 10 disorders of collagen metabolism; joints affected most severely
	Osteogenesis imperfecta	Maldistribution of collagen types of connective tissues; bone fractures especially common
	Marfan syndrome	Defect in cross-linking of collagen; primarily affects eye, blood vessels, and skeleton
	Homocystinuria	Deficiency of enzyme cystathionine β-synthase; defective collagen cross-linking caused by accumulation of homocysteine secondary to blockade of cystathionine synthesis from serine and homocysteine; mainly affects lens of eye, bones, medium-sized arteries and veins, cognitive function
	Alkaptonuria	Deficiency of enzyme homogentisic acid oxidase, leading to pigment deposition in connective tissues; associated with degenerative joint disease
Immunologic	Rheumatoid arthritis	Inflammatory destruction of cartilage in joints; affects connective tissues throughout the body
	Systemic lupus erythematosus	Acute necrotic and dystrophic changes caused by immune complexes in connective tissues and other tissues throughout the body
Idiopathic	Abnormal calcification	Deposition of calcium in collagen and elastin in soft tissue, muscle, and ligaments; associated with hypercalcemia and tissue trauma
	Scleroderma	Excessive collagen deposition; mainly in skin and subcutaneous tissue; may result in fibrosis of deep subcutaneous tissue and fascia

Data from Pearson, A.M., and Young, R.B. (1993). Diseases and disorders of muscle. *Advances in Food and Nutrition Research* 37, 339–423.

Muscle tissue is incapable of true hyperplasia, although hypertrophied fibers will ultimately split longitudinally. Only one of the resulting fibers retains the original innervation, however, and the other will not survive unless it is reinnervated by another axon branch.

Alterations in muscle mass result from variation in mechanical, neural, hormonal, and local chemical stimulation of muscle cells, although the precise cellular regulation of these changes is incompletely understood. At birth, muscle fibers measure about 10 μm in cross-sectional diameter, but reach adult size (approximately 40 to 60 μm) by puberty.[2] During normal development, muscle growth is regulated primarily through the anabolic effects of growth hormone, insulin, and sex hormones and is coordinated with the regulation of linear bone growth. In males, increased testosterone mediates sex differences in muscle bulk, preferentially enlarging type II fibers and increasing performance in brief but intense activities such as weight-lifting and sprinting. Under the influence of estrogen, muscle fibers in females incorporate more lipids, enhancing performance in aerobic and endurance activities such as long-distance running.

Muscle atrophy resulting from breakdown of muscle proteins occurs under conditions of immobility or denervation of muscle and in fasting, acidosis, sepsis, acquired immunodeficiency syndrome (AIDS wasting syndrome), and neoplasia (cancer cachexia). Proteins in all body cells are continuously being degraded and replaced to inactivate enzymes and other regulatory proteins and to eliminate any abnormally folded or damaged proteins. This adaptive proteolysis is regulated at the cellular level by the *ubiquitin-proteasome pathway*, an energy-dependent process that is itself regulated by nuclear transcription factors.[3] The protein ubiquitin binds to cellular proteins destined for destruction, marking them as targets for proteolytic enzymes.

Normally, synthesis of new proteins keeps pace or, during growth or resistance training, exceeds the

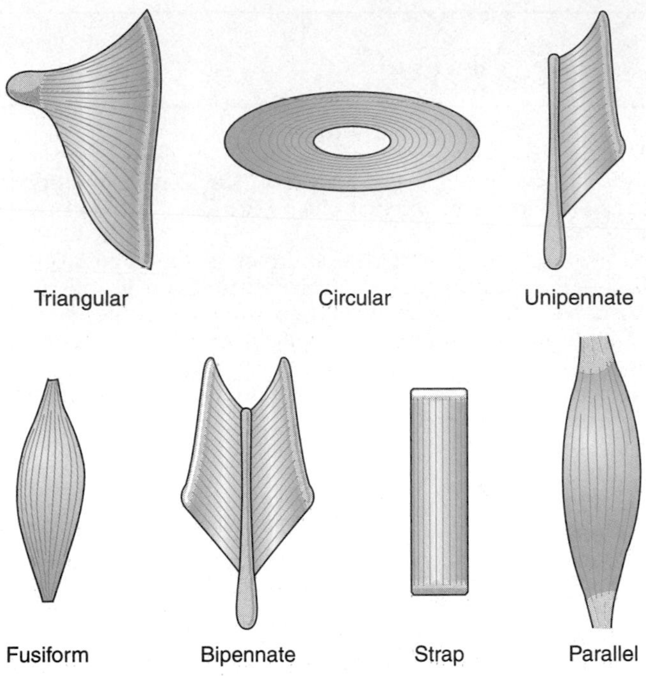

FIGURE 35–3

Fascicular arrangement of muscles. Fascicular arrangement determines the shape and specialized function of a muscle.

rate of proteolysis. In immobilized or denervated muscle cells, enhanced proteolysis results from inappropriate or increased activation of the ubiquitin-proteasome pathway by an intracellular signal. In fasting or wasting syndromes associated with systemic disease or trauma, the signal is extracellular, mediated primarily by glucocorticoids (unopposed by insulin) and cytokines such as interleukins 1 and 6 and tumor necrosis factor. Excess thyroid hormone (thyrotoxicosis) also promotes proteolysis in skeletal muscle.

In response to increased neural stimulation and mechanical stress (resistance or workload), muscle fibers synthesize more proteins and filaments to "share the load." The level of metabolic activity per unit volume of each muscle cell remains fairly stable. Increased muscle size is thus an adaptive response to heavy work or weight training.

Muscle Mechanics

Lever Dynamics

Nearly all movement of the musculoskeletal system is accomplished with the use of leverage to modify speed of movement, range of movement, or capacity to oppose a force or lift a weight. Bones act as levers, moving on fixed points or fulcrums (the joints) in response to an applied force (muscle contraction) to move a load or oppose a resisting force. The relative positions of the lever, fulcrum, and force determine the nature of the leverage. Three classes of leverage are illustrated with musculoskele-

TABLE 35–2

METABOLIC DISORDERS AFFECTING SKELETAL MUSCLE

Category	Examples	Clinical Features
Glycolytic disorders	Von Gierke's disease (glycogen storage disease—several types)	Genetic deficiency of enzymes required for glycolysis, glyconeogenesis, or glycogenesis; affects liver, skeletal muscle, kidney, erythrocytes, and other tissues as a result of accumulation of abnormal forms of glycogen
	Alcoholism	Muscle weakness associated with reduced glycolysis and impaired lactate metabolism
	Hypothyroidism	Impairment in glycolysis caused by predominance of slow oxidative fibers; reversible with thyroid hormone replacement
Disorders of mitochondrial oxidation	Myoclonus epilepsy and ragged red fibers syndrome	Reduced activity of first and fourth cytochromal enzyme complexes for oxidative phosphorylation; muscle wasting and neural manifestations predominant
	Mitochondrial myopathy, encephalopathy, lactic acidosis, stroke-like episodes	Reduced activity of first complex and cytochrome *c*-oxidase enzyme for oxidative phosphorylation; myopathy, short stature, and neural manifestations predominant
Disorders of lipid metabolism	Carnitine deficiency	Failure of carnitine synthesis in liver or failure of carnitine uptake by muscle; impairment of fatty acid uptake into mitochondria for β-oxidation; muscle weakness
	Carnitine palmityltransferase (CPT) deficiency	Lack of CPT resulting in lipid accumulation within muscle; recurrent muscle pain and myoglobinuria; exacerbated by fasting or exercise; improved with high carbohydrate–low fat diet

Data from Pearson, A.M., and Young, R.B. (1993). Diseases and disorders of muscle. *Advances in Food and Nutrition Research* 37, 339–423; and Luft, R. (1994). The development of mitochondrial medicine. *Proceedings of the National Academy of Sciences* USA 91(9), 8731–8738.

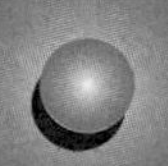

TABLE 35–3
CHARACTERISTICS OF MUSCLE FIBER TYPES

	Muscle Fiber Type		
Characteristic	**Type I**	**Type IIA**	**Type IIB**
Color	Red	White	White
Fiber size	Small	Large (boys>girls)	Large (boys>girls)
Alkaline myofibrillar ATPase histochemistry	Light	Dark	Dark
Cellular organelles	Numerous mitochondria, rich in sarcoplasmic reticulum, rich in myoglobin	Some mitochondria, poor in sarcoplasmic reticulum, some myoglobin	Few mitochondria, poor in sarcoplasmic reticulum, poor in myoglobin
Fuel stores	Lipid rich, glycogen poor	Lipid rich, glycogen rich	Lipid poor, glycogen rich
Energy metabolism	High oxidative (aerobic), low glycolytic (anaerobic)	High oxidative (aerobic), high glycolytic (anaerobic)	Low oxidative (aerobic), high glycolytic (anaerobic)
Energy stores	High intracellular resting levels of phosphocreatine	Moderate intracellular resting levels of phosphocreatine	Low intracellular resting levels of phosphocreatine
Vascularity	Prominent surrounding capillaries, good blood flow	Some surrounding capillaries, moderate blood flow	Few capillaries, blood flow rapidly insufficient
Twitch (contraction) speed	Slow	Fast	Fast
Twitch tension (force, strength)	Low (weak)	High (strong)	High (strong)
Fatigue	Resistant (fatigues slowly)	Resistant (fatigues slowly)	Sensitive (fatigues quickly)
Functional role	Postural and prolonged (sustained) contractions	Rapid, repeated or prolonged voluntary movements	Rapid strong voluntary contractions of short duration ("quick burst")
Motor unit characteristics	Small motor neuron cell body, small diameter slow-conducting axon, fewer muscle fibers in motor unit, low recruitment threshold, low firing frequency	Large motor neuron cell body, large diameter fast-conducting axon, many muscle fibers in motor unit, high recruitment threshold, high firing frequency	Large motor neuron cell body, large diameter fast-conducting axon, many muscle fibers in motor unit, high recruitment threshold, high firing frequency

From Brumback, R.A., Feeback, D.L., and Leech, R.W. (1992). Rhabdomyolysis in childhood: A primer on normal muscle function and selected metabolic myopathies characterized by disordered energy production. *Pediatric Clinics of North America* 39(4), 826.

tal function (Fig. 35–4). With a *first-class lever,* the force is applied at one end of the lever, and the load is at the other, with the fulcrum in between. Contraction of the triceps to extend the forearm against resistance is an example of this type of leverage. First-class levers are often inefficient, requiring the application of greater force than that to be resisted. With a *second-class lever,* the force is applied at one end of the lever, the fulcrum is at the other end, and the load or resisting force is in between (like a wheelbarrow). An example of this type of leverage is contraction of the gastrocnemius muscle of the calf to pull one's weight up on one's toes. Second-class leverage facilitates lifting of greater weight, but speed and range of movement are limited.

Most muscle contraction occurs within *third-class lever* systems, in which the fulcrum is at one end, and the load at the other. The force is applied in the middle of the lever. This system permits rapid movement and extended range of motion, but requires greater force of contraction. Lever dynamics illustrate the interdependence of the bones, joints, and muscles in effecting movement and in resisting deforming forces.

Loss of integrity of any component of this lever system impairs mobility and work capacity. In addi-

Developmental Perspective

Embryonic and Fetal Periods

Skeletal muscle is derived from the embryonic mesoderm. Most muscles are developed before birth, with the remaining ones formed by the end of the first year of life. Injury to the sternocleidomastoid muscle at birth may lead to tilting and twisting of the head (torticollis or wryneck). Embryonic muscle cells may give rise to rhabdomyosarcoma.

Infancy and Early Childhood

After birth, muscles increase in length and width to keep pace with skeletal growth. Some embryonic muscle fibers normally degenerate, but may persist as vestigial anomalies. Absence of single muscles is also common. Congenital anomalies of the limbs originate from concurrently abnormal development of muscles, joints, and bones and may include congenital hip dislocation, talipes equinovarus (clubfoot), syndactyly (webbing of digits), polydactyly (supernumerary digits), and other, less common deformities. Duchenne's muscular dystrophy manifests during early childhood, when the child begins to walk. Lack of physical activity in childhood may predispose to obesity and dyslipidemias, increasing the risk of cardiovascular disease later in life.

Adolescence and Young Adulthood

Before puberty, type I and type II muscle fibers are the same size in boys and girls. After puberty, type II fibers are larger in boys, as a consequence of stimulation by testosterone. Peak performances in sports are seen during the late teens to early 30s. Participation in sports enhances fitness in this age group, but also imposes risk of sports injuries. Females may manifest addiction to exercise in conjunction with eating disorders. Excessive exercise may delay onset of menarche or induce amenorrhea. Fibromyalgia and chronic fatigue syndrome most commonly affect young and middle-aged women.

Middle and Older Adulthood

Exercise may slow the rate of decline in cardiac reserve to 5% per decade, as opposed to the 10% seen in sedentary individuals. By 60 to 70 years of age, muscle mass decreases by 25% to 30%. A decrease in large type II fibers accompanied by an increase in small type I fibers contributes to muscle atrophy with aging. Muscle strength declines by 30% to 40% between ages 30 and 80, in association with loss of muscle mass. Muscle tissue retains its capacity to regenerate if injured, but impairment of reinnervation, revascularization, nutrition, or hormonal stimulation may limit tissue recovery in older persons.

---

tion to primary muscle pathology, altered muscle contraction may result from fracture of a bone, joint fusion or painful arthropathy, or stretching or tearing of ligaments or tendons (see Chapter 34). Maladaptive healing of the skin overlying joints (*contractures*), as is common with burn wounds, may also impede leverage and mobility (see Chapter 36).

Interactions Among Muscle Groups

Complex body movements require the coordinated actions of multiple muscle groups. This coordination originates from interneuronal connections between motor reflex arcs (see Chapter 22). Reciprocal innervation normally results in reflex relaxation of muscle groups opposing those that are contracting, although partial contraction of the opposing group may allow "fine-tuning" or grading of movement. A muscle whose shortening is primarily responsible for a given movement is referred to as an *agonist*, and a muscle that contracts to oppose or to reverse the original movement is an *antagonist*. Muscle groups that act together to strengthen or stabilize a movement are known as *synergists*. Muscles that facilitate efficiency of movement by minimizing movement of bones that are the insertion points of the other muscles are known as *fixators*. Coordinated contraction of several muscle groups is essential to directionally accurate, graded, smooth and efficient movement. Pathology affecting one or a few muscle groups thus influences the function of others.

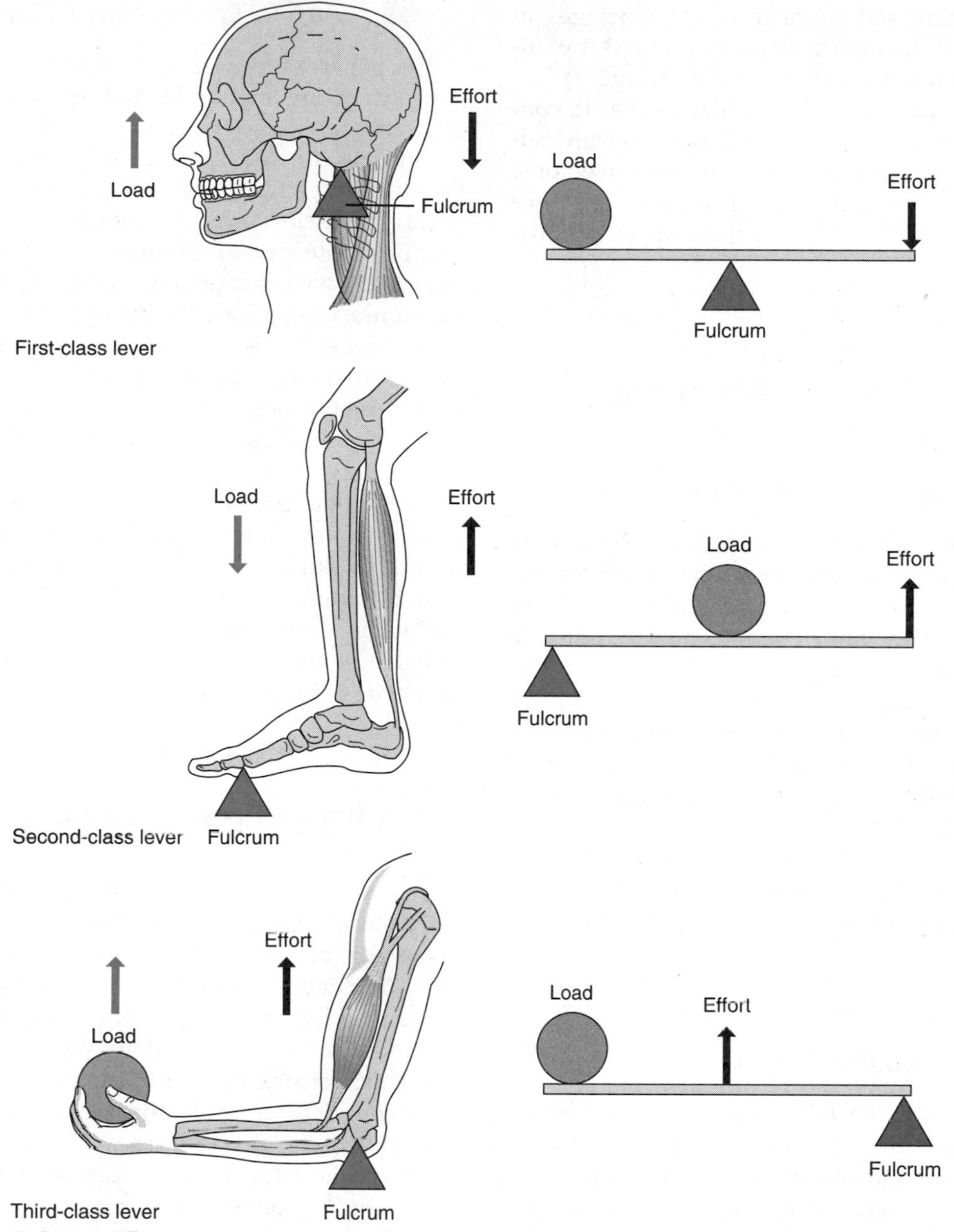

FIGURE 35–4

Leverage in muscle movement. Leverage is used to modify the speed, range of movement, or load-bearing capacity of a muscle. *First-class levers* have the fulcrum between the effort (contractile force) and the load (resistance). *Second-class levers* have the fulcrum at one end, the effort at the opposite end, and the load between them. *Third-class levers* have the fulcrum at one end, the load at the opposite end, and the effort between them.

Length-Tension Relationships

Not all skeletal muscle contraction results in muscle fiber shortening. For fiber shortening to occur, the amount of force or tension generated by cross-bridge formation must exceed the weight or resistance to be overcome. With *isotonic contraction* (**dynamic exercise**), force generated within the muscle fiber overcomes the resisting force and movement occurs: tension within the muscle fiber is constant, and fiber length shortens. With *isometric contraction* (**static exercise**), the resisting force is greater, and fiber shortening does not occur. Cross-bridge formation generates increasing force or tension, but fiber length remains constant. With *lengthening contraction*, the resisting force or load is greater than the force developed by the muscle, and the muscle fiber lengthens. Lengthening contraction is characterized by a slightly increased number of cross-bridges in comparison with isometric contraction and by increased tension development per cross-bridge.[1]

Most activities consist of an initial isometric contraction as force is generated, followed by an isotonic contraction as the resisting force is overcome and movement occurs. Exercise programs are usually designed to include both of these types of muscle contraction.

Mechanisms of Abnormal Muscle Contraction

Muscle Weakness

Because the amount of force developed by a muscle is proportional to its cross-sectional diameter (reflecting the quantity of contractile proteins, sarcoplasmic reticulum, and mitochondria), muscle atrophy decreases the force generation of muscle. As indicated previously, atrophy may result from disuse, denervation, or systemic wasting disorders, and some degree of atrophy is apparently inevitable with aging. Most of the primary muscle disorders detailed later in this chapter are also characterized by muscle weakness resulting from destruction or damage to contractile tissue or from replacement of contractile elements by fat and connective tissue.

Muscle Fatigue

Muscle fatigue is the failure to achieve or maintain the expected force or power output of a muscle.[4] Fatigue after vigorous exercise is a natural phenomenon, as discussed later, but abnormal fatigue may result from pathology. The mechanisms of fatigue may involve conduction of action potentials within the nervous system or the process of transduction of the electrical impulses into mechanical force production by the muscle itself.[5] At the cellular level, fatigue may originate from intracellular acidosis, lack of energy production, or disruption in calcium flux. Atrophic conditions manifest as more rapid tiring in addition to weakness. Disorders in which defective energy metabolism rapidly depletes glycogen stores are primarily characterized by fatigue. In myasthenia gravis, depletion of ACh activity at the neuromuscular junction leads to progressive muscle fatigue (see Chapter 22). Chronic fatigue may have a psychogenic component, as discussed later.

Muscle Spasms and Cramps

The general types of abnormally increased muscle contraction are **myotonia** and **spasticity**. Myotonia, an intrinsic characteristic of muscle, is the inability of muscle to relax completely after contraction.[4] Spasticity describes involuntary, intense, and often painful muscle contraction that is associated with inappropriate neural stimulation. Myotonia may be associated with congenital muscle disorders such as **myotonia congenita** or with some muscular dystrophies. Spasticity is a major component of neuromotor disorders such as spinal cord injury and cerebral palsy (see Chapter 22).

Myoclonus (tics, tremors, and fasciculations) and clonus (e.g., ankle clonus, decerebrate or decorticate posturing, seizures) are other forms of abnormal muscle contraction resulting from impaired neural input. Involuntary contraction (cramping) of muscles is a common form of spasticity that is often idiopathic but may also be associated with electrolyte imbalance, systemic toxicity, muscle overuse, or certain drugs (Table 35–4).[6]

EXERCISE PHYSIOLOGY

The recent development of the fields of exercise physiology and sports medicine reflects a growing awareness of the potential benefits and risks of exercise. Technically, exercise is any skeletal muscle movement resulting in energy expenditure, which includes activities of daily living as well as "planned, structured, and repetitive bodily movement done to improve or maintain one or more components of physical fitness."[7] This discussion focuses on the latter type of exercise, with its goals of improving or maintaining performance capacity and reducing the risk of morbidity and mortality from a number of disorders.

Systemic Effects of Exercise

In addition to their adaptive effects on muscle fibers, exercise programs alter cardiovascular, respiratory, endocrine, metabolic, and thermoregulatory systems.

Effects of Exercise on Skeletal Muscle

Exercise programs are of two basic types: strength (resistance) training and endurance (aerobic) train-

TABLE 35-4
CONDITIONS ASSOCIATED WITH MUSCLE CRAMPING

Classification	Etiology	Examples
True cramps	Motor unit hyperactivity	Ordinary muscle cramps Cramps associated with lower motor neuron disease (e.g., spinal cord injury) Cramps caused by medications (e.g., calcium-channel blockers, β-blockers, diuretics, alcohol, nicotinic acid) Cramps caused by fluid and electrolyte imbalance (e.g., heat cramps, hemodialysis cramps, hypoglycemia, hyponatremia, hypocalcemia, hypomagnesemia, hyperkalemia, or hypokalemia)
Contractures	Electrically silent, caused by metabolic abnormality	Glycogen storage disease Thyroid disease
Tetany	Sensory and motor unit hyperactivity	Hypocalcemia Hypomagnesemia Hypokalemia Hyperkalemia
Dystonia	Simultaneous contraction of agonist and antagonist muscles	Occupational cramps (e.g., writer's cramp, musician's cramp) Cramps caused by antipsychotic medications such as phenothiazines

Data from Riley, J.D., and Antony, S.J. (1995). Leg cramps: Differential diagnosis and management. *American Family Physician* 52(6), 1794–1798.

ing. Resistance training, consisting mainly of weight-lifting, has a greater isometric component, generating greater force within the muscle and triggering more muscle hypertrophy. Fast-twitch (glycolytic) fibers are affected by resistance training, with increased muscle size and strength resulting from increased numbers of myofibrils and increased capacity for storage of glycogen. Although its basis is poorly understood, weight training also has a neurologic component, enhancing the individual's ability to voluntarily "recruit" more muscle fibers during activity, increasing strength through this synergism.

Endurance training affects slow-twitch (oxidative) muscle fibers as well as respiratory and cardiovascular capacity, increasing maximum oxygen uptake and, as a result, increasing the threshold at which energy expenditure during exercise exceeds oxygen supply. Changes in slow-twitch fibers seen with endurance training include increased size and number of mitochondria, increased capillary perfusion of each muscle fiber, increased capacity for oxidation of fat for energy, and increased myoglobin concentration. As previously stated, proportionate numbers of fast- and slow-twitch fibers are genetically determined to a significant degree, imposing a limitation on the degree of adaptation possible with exercise training. The elite athletes of the world have apparently been genetically endowed with exceptional capacity for such adaptation.

Cardiovascular Responses to Exercise

When untrained individuals exercise, cardiac output increases within the limits of cardiac reserve, as a result of increases in heart rate and stroke volume (see Chapter 16). With endurance training, cardiac reserve is greatly enhanced as a result of myocardial hypertrophy and dilation in response to increased oxygen demand. These changes result in cardiomegaly (**athlete's heart**) and in reduction of the resting heart rate, presumably because of changes in baseline parasympathetic stimulation. Particularly in males, the ventricular chamber size and wall thickness of athlete's heart may approach those seen in dilated cardiomyopathy (see Focus of Current Research).[8]

The oxygen-carrying capacity of the blood remains relatively stable, unless the individual trains in high altitude to induce a secondary polycythemia. Oxygen extraction by exercising muscle increases as much as 20-fold, however, because of tissue level changes (increased temperature, increased pH, decreased partial pressure of oxygen [PO_2], and increased partial pressure of carbon dioxide [PCO_2]) that shift the oxyhemoglobin dissociation curve to the right, decreasing affinity of hemoglobin for oxygen and favoring its release to tissues (see Chapter 19). Within capillary beds, these local changes favor

Focus of Current Research

Study	Objective and Findings
Kushi, et al. (1997) Physical activity and mortality in postmenopausal women	*Objective:* To evaluate the association between physical activity and all-cause mortality in postmenopausal women *Findings:* A graded, inverse association exists between physical activity and all-cause mortality in these women.
Thune, et al. (1997) Physical activity and the risk of breast cancer.	*Objective:* To investigate whether everyday exercise is related to risk of breast cancer *Findings:* Physical activity during leisure time and at work is associated with a reduced risk of breast cancer.
Pelliccia, et al. (1996) Athlete's heart in women.	*Objective:* To determine the alterations in cardiac dimensions associated with long-term intense conditioning in elite female athletes *Findings:* Left ventricular cavity size exceeding normal limits was evident in 8% of women, and was within the range of dilated cardiomyopathy in 1%.
MacDonald, et al. (1996) A case-control study to assess possible triggers and cofactors in chronic fatigue syndrome.	*Objective:* To assess possible triggers and cofactors in chronic fatigue syndrome and to compare levels of selected cytokines between cases and controls *Findings:* Cases were more likely to have exercised regularly before illness, to be nulliparous, and to have a history of depression. Cytokine levels were similar between groups.
Luepker, et al. (1996) Outcomes of a field trial to improve children's dietary patterns and physical activity (CATCH Trial).	*Objective:* To assess the outcomes of health behavior interventions, focusing on the elementary school environment, classroom curricula, and home programs for the primary prevention of cardiovascular disease *Findings:* The CATCH intervention was able to modify the fat content of school lunches, increase moderate-to-vigorous activity in physical education, and improve eating and physical activity behaviors in children during 3 school years.

continued

Zeni, et al. (1996) Energy expenditure with indoor exercise machines.	*Objective:* To compare the rates of energy expenditure at given rating of performance exertion levels among six different indoor exercise machines *Findings:* The treadmill is the most effective indoor exercise machine for enhancing energy expenditure when perceived exertion is used to establish exercise intensity.
Ginsburg, et al. (1996) Effects of a single bout of ultraendurance exercise on lipid levels and susceptibility of lipids to peroxidation in triathletes.	*Objective:* To determine the effects of a single bout of ultraendurance exercise, as a model for physiologic stress, on lipid and lipoprotein levels and oxidative susceptibility in highly trained athletes *Findings:* A single bout of exercise can reduce lipid risk factors for developing cardiovascular disease.
Mendell, et al. (1995) Myoblast transfer in the treatment of Duchenne's muscular dystrophy.	*Objective:* To evaluate the effectiveness of injection of donor myoblasts into muscles of patients with muscular dystrophy *Findings:* Myoblasts transferred once a month for 6 months failed to improve strength in patients with Duchenne's muscular dystrophy.
Blair, et al. (1995) Changes in physical fitness and all-cause mortality: A prospective study of healthy and unhealthy men.	*Objective:* To evaluate the relationship between changes in physical fitness and risk of mortality in men *Findings:* Improvement in fitness was associated with lower death rates after adjusting for age, health status, and other risk factors for premature mortality.

closure of arteriovenous shunts (thoroughfare channels), increasing flow through true capillaries, or exchange vessels (see Chapter 15). The proportional distribution of blood flow to specific tissues is altered during exercise, as regulated by the sympathetic nervous system (see stress response, Chapter 1) and local factors. Exercising muscle receives the greater share of the cardiac output, and nonexercising muscle, gastrointestinal (GI), and renal systems receive less. Blood flow to the skin is also decreased early in exercise, but as core temperature rises as a consequence of muscle activity, cutaneous vessels dilate to enhance heat loss to the environment.

The effects of exercise on systemic vascular resistance (SVR) and, consequently, on blood pressure depend on the type of program. Isotonic exercise (which predominates in endurance programs) decreases SVR as peripheral flow to exercising muscle is enhanced, decreasing blood pressure as well. In contrast, isometric exercise (typical of bodybuilding and some weight-training regimens) tends to increase SVR because high tension in the muscle fibers promotes collapse of adjacent capillaries. Isometric exercise thus tends to increase blood pressure. Care must also be taken during such exercise to "breathe through" the activity so that the Valsalva maneuver is not initiated (see Chapter 15).

Respiratory Function During Exercise

The intensity of exercise may be quantified on the basis of the degree of increase in energy expenditure (and resulting oxygen uptake) induced by the exercise state as compared with the resting state. One *metabolic unit (MET)* represents an energy expenditure of 1 kcal/kg body weight per hour, or an oxygen uptake of 3.5 mL/kg/min, which is typical of the seated adult at rest.[9] Table 35–5 categorizes vari-

TABLE 35–5
METABOLIC UNIT EQUIVALENTS IN COMMON PHYSICAL ACTIVITIES*

LIGHT (<3.0 METs or <4 kcal · min⁻¹)	MODERATE (3.0–6.0 METs or 4–7 kcal · min⁻¹)	HARD/VIGOROUS (>6.0 METs or >7 kcal · min⁻¹)
Walking, slowly (strolling) (1–2 mph)	Walking, briskly (3–4 mph)	Walking, briskly uphill or with a load
Cycling, stationary (<50 W)	Cycling for pleasure or transportation (≤10 mph)	Cycling, fast or racing (>10 mph)
Swimming, slow treading	Swimming, moderate effort	Swimming, fast treading or crawl
Conditioning exercise, light stretching	Conditioning exercise, general calisthenics	Conditioning exercise, stair ergometer, ski machine
—	Racket sports, table tennis	Racket sports, singles tennis, racketball
Golf, power cart	Golf, pulling cart or carrying clubs	—
Bowling	—	—
Fishing, sitting	Fishing, standing/casting	Fishing in stream
Boating, power	Canoeing, leisurely (2.0–3.9 mph)	Canoeing, rapidly (≥4 mph)
Home care, carpet sweeping	Home care, general cleaning	Moving furniture
Mowing lawn, riding mower	Mowing lawn, power mower	Mowing lawn, hand mower
Home repair, carpentry	Home repair, painting	—

*The METs (work metabolic rate/resting metabolic rate) are multiples of the resting rate of oxygen consumption during physical activity. One MET represents the approximate rate of oxygen consumption of a seated adult at rest, or about 3.5 mL · min^{-1} · kg^{-1}. The equivalent energy cost of 1 MET in kilocalories · min^{-1} is about 1.2 for a 70-kg person, or approximately 1 kcal · kg^{-1} · hr^{-1}.

From Pate, R.R., Pratt, M., Blair, S.N., *et al.* (1995). Physical activity and public health: A recommendation from the Centers for Disease Control and Prevention and the American College of Sports Medicine. *Journal of the American Medical Association* 273(5), 404. Copyright 1995, American Medical Association.

ous types of activities in terms of their MET equivalents.

Oxygen uptake during exercise typically increases to 8 to 20 times the resting rate. The highest rates of oxygen uptake are associated with exercises involving both the arms and legs, because a greater proportion of muscle mass is active. Pulmonary ventilation increases to meet this demand through increases in rate and use of inspiratory reserve volume to increase tidal volume (see Chapter 18). The regulatory mechanism that mediates this increase is uncertain, because blood gas values do not change significantly during moderate exercise. Increased cardiac output during exercise also increases pulmonary blood flow, and more areas of the lung approach ideal ventilation-perfusion (V/Q) ratios, enhancing oxygen uptake in pulmonary capillaries. Maximum oxygen uptake is genetically limited, but with aerobic training it increases proportionately to lean body mass.

Endocrine and Metabolic Responses to Exercise

Exercise is a stressor, resulting in elevated catecholamine levels caused by increased sympathetic stimulation and adrenal medullary secretion (see Chapter 1). Activation of the hypothalamic–pituitary–adrenal axis results in enhanced secretion of cortisol. Catecholamines mediate some of the selective perfusion during exercise, and, along with cortisol, mobilize energy stores (e.g., lipids in adipose tissue, glycogen in liver and muscle). Consistent with mobilizing energy stores, exercise inhibits insulin secretion and enhances glucagon secretion, probably in response to increased sympathetic stimulation of the pancreas. It should be recalled that exercising muscle does not require insulin for uptake of glucose (see Chapter 29).

Depletion of glycogen stores is a limiting factor in fast-twitch fibers, which use anaerobic glycolysis almost exclusively. Glycogen depletion is also a factor in slow-twitch fibers during high-intensity exercise, because the cardiovascular system cannot deliver glucose at an adequate rate to sustain maximal performance. The technique of *carbohydrate loading* is often used by athletes to enhance their glycogen stores before a competitive event. The athlete first depletes glycogen stores with a period of low intake of carbohydrates, and then begins a high-carbohydrate diet a few days before the event. Intensive training is also stopped during these last few days.

Lactic acid levels rise rapidly with short-duration, high-intensity exercise involving primarily fast-twitch glycolytic fibers (such as weight-lifting and sprints). As detailed in Chapter 3, some of this lactate may be reconverted to pyruvate and used in oxidative metabolism by slow-twitch muscle fibers or oxidative tissues of the heart, brain, liver, or kidney. Lactate released into the blood may also be taken up by the liver or kidneys and converted to pyruvate and then to glucose via energy-dependent gluconeogenesis (the Cori cycle). Accumulation of lactate and exhaustion of glucose supplies may contribute to the related but poorly understood states of fatigue and **oxygen debt**. Oxygen debt refers to the period after strenuous exercise during which oxygen uptake remains elevated to restore pre-exercise levels of lactate and glycogen.

Thermoregulatory Responses to Exercise

The increased contraction of skeletal muscle generates heat at greatly increased rates (see Chapter 11). Muscle temperature rises immediately, and core body temperature rises more slowly, attaining a steady state temperature as high as 40°C (104°F) with sustained high-intensity activity. This temperature increase is beneficial in enhancing oxygen uptake to tissues, as has been discussed, but represents a risk for heat exhaustion or heat stroke if excess heat cannot be dissipated. If environmental temperature and humidity are low enough, heat is lost to the environment by radiation and evaporative cooling. Increased sweating results in fluid losses as high as 2 to 5 L per hour. Electrolytes are also lost in the sweat, but at a much lower rate than fluid (see Chapter 8). Under most conditions, fluid losses during exercise are optimally replaced with plain water or other hypotonic fluids to enhance gastric emptying and absorption.

Exercise and the Prevention of Disease

A growing number of epidemiologic studies have demonstrated protective effects of exercise with regard to several chronic and life-threatening diseases (see Focus of Current Research). It has been estimated that up to 250,000 deaths per year in the United States could be prevented with programs of regular exercise.[9] Exercise training has been shown to improve several risk factors for coronary heart disease, including the serum lipid profile (increased high-density lipoprotein and decreased low-density lipoprotein and triglycerides). Enhanced fibrinolytic activity also reduces the risk of thrombosis, which contributes to myocardial infarction. Venous compression during skeletal muscle contraction (the skeletal muscle pump) reduces venous pooling, lowering the risk of deep vein thrombosis. Reduction in weight, as a result of increased caloric expenditure, and reduction in blood pressure, as a result of decreased SVR, are also related to decreased coronary risk. Weight reduction also reduces insulin resistance, associated with type 2 diabetes mellitus, hypertension, and atherosclerosis.

The increased stress on bone with exercise reduces demineralization and aids in the prevention of osteoporosis. Exercise may reduce, but not eliminate entirely, the muscle atrophy associated with aging.[1] Aerobic exercise has been shown to improve mood, apparently by inducing release of enkephalins and endorphins. An active lifestyle has been associated with reduction in mortality from colon cancer, but the mechanism of this protection is unknown.[10] The risk of breast cancer is also reduced, possibly because of suppression of gonadotropin-releasing hormone and estrogen release.[11] The Centers for Disease Control and Prevention and the American College of Sports Medicine recently issued a consensus statement recommending that every adult in the United States accumulate 30 minutes or more of moderate-intensity physical activity (3 to 6 METs) on most, or preferably all, days of the week.[9]

Risks Associated with Exercise

Although the risks associated with exercise are insignificant in comparison with the benefits in most cases, there are potential adverse effects. Exercise-associated musculoskeletal trauma is common, particularly in those who lack fitness, appropriate equipment, or knowledge of proper technique. Table 35–6 lists common types of injuries. As discussed in Chapter 31, exercise-induced amenorrhea is common in elite female athletes, as a result of suppression of the hypothalamic–pituitary–gonadal axis. Decreased estrogen levels in these women may lead to infertility and increased risk of stress fractures caused by decreased bone density.[12] GI tract problems, including diarrhea, gastroesophageal reflux, and abdominal pain ("side stitch") are common in runners and may be the result of electrolyte imbalance, altered GI blood flow, autonomic nervous system effects, or mechanical factors.[13] Individuals with athlete's heart may be prone to atrial dysrhythmias. Of serious concern is the possibility of sudden cardiac death, associated with congenital anomalies or drug abuse in young competitive athletes, and with myocardial infarction triggered by unusual physical exertion in older, untrained individuals.[14, 15]

TABLE 35–6
COMMON EXERCISE-INDUCED INJURIES

INJURY	DESCRIPTION
Knee injury	Torn ligaments or cartilage; "runner's knee" (irritation of patellar tendon); patellar displacement
Ankle sprain	Overstretched or torn ligament; avulsion fracture or growth plate fracture
Shinsplints	Strain of muscles and tendons on medial shin
Muscle strains	Usually hamstring, calf, or groin
Back pain	Usually strain of muscles and ligaments; less commonly back spasms or herniated intervertebral disk
Rotator cuff injury	Sprain, strain, or dislocation of shoulder caused by injury of muscles and tendons surrounding joint
Tennis elbow (golf elbow)	Strain of muscles on lateral side of elbow

MUSCLE DISORDERS

Muscle Strains

Definition. A muscle strain is a localized injury of muscle or tendon fibers ranging from excessive stretch (a muscle "pull") to tearing or rupture of a muscle. In the case of rupture, the body of the muscle protrudes through the fascia.

Epidemiology. Muscle strains are very common. Engaging in a physical activity (recreational or occupational) for which one is not physically fit nor properly trained constitutes the major risk factor for muscle strain.

Etiology. Muscle strains are usually caused by sudden mechanical overloading of the muscle (generation of excessive force), especially when the muscle is not adequately stretched before the activity. Penetrating trauma such as gunshot wounds and stab wounds may also result in muscle rupture.

Pathophysiology. Bleeding into the muscle and surrounding tissue occurs if vessels are torn. An inflammatory response ensues, after which healing by regeneration normally occurs. Calcium may deposit into muscle that is chronically strained.

Clinical Manifestations. Muscle pain (**myalgia**), swelling, and limitation of function result from inflammation. Swelling may continue for as long as 72 hours.[16] Bruising (ecchymosis) is often evident.

Prevention and Treatment. Physical conditioning and appropriate stretching and warm-up before strenuous activity may prevent most strains. Frequent relaxation breaks and optimal technique may reduce the risk of injury caused by overuse. Strains are usually treated with the RICE technique, with *r*est (cessation of the activity), application of *i*ce and a *c*ompression wrap, and *e*levation of the injured part to reduce pain and swelling. After signs of acute inflammation have subsided, heat and ultrasound may be applied to enhance blood flow, reduce cramping, and promote healing. Topical anti-inflammatory or analgesic medications may be transferred to underlying tissues when used with ultrasound or electrically induced ion flux through the skin (iontophoresis). Nonsteroidal anti-inflammatory drugs (NSAIDs) or corticosteroids may also be used, but are associated with toxic effects if their use is prolonged or excessive (see Chapters 13 and 29). Exercise is gradually resumed as healing progresses. Treatment of ruptures requires surgical repair, followed by a longer period of rehabilitation.

Prognosis and Outcome. Most muscle strains heal without complications.

Fibromyalgia

Definition. Fibromyalgia is a syndrome of diffuse pain and specific tender points in muscles, accompanied by sleep disturbance, fatigue, depression, and anxiety.

Epidemiology. The estimated prevalence of fibromyalgia in the general population is 2%. The condition usually occurs in young women. Risk may be associated with a hypersensitive or prolonged stress response, as seen in such disorders as chronic fatigue syndrome, irritable bowel syndrome, multiple-chemical sensitivity, and manifestations that follow silicone breast-implant surgery.[17]

Etiology. The etiology of fibromyalgia is unknown. Inflammation is not involved, because serum markers of inflammation and muscle damage (e.g., erythrocyte sedimentation rate, creatine kinase) are not increased. Hypothetical mechanisms include neurotransmitter imbalance associated with affective disorder (anxiety or depression) or sleep disturbance (disordered non-REM sleep), endocrine imbalance caused by enhanced reactivity of the hypothalamic–pituitary–adrenal axis,[17] and muscle ischemia caused by sleep-induced reduction of arterial oxygen saturation.[18]

Pathophysiology. Biopsy of skeletal muscles in tender areas reveals microstructural changes (ragged red fibers and mitochondrial changes) similar to those in some disorders of mitochondrial DNA function (see Chapter 3). Muscle fibers are also deficient in ATP and phosphocreatine. These changes are suggestive of hypoxia.[18] Sleep disruption may be a cause or an effect in fibromyalgia. Low levels of serotonin, normally produced during non-REM sleep by the raphe nuclei of the brain stem, may influence the affective aspects of fibromyalgia, particularly depression. The clinical course of fibromyalgia is typically waxing and waning, with little ultimate improvement.

Clinical Manifestations. Patients report generalized muscle aching and acute pain with palpation of specific tender points (Fig. 35–5). Sleep disturbance manifests as difficulty falling asleep, frequent awakening, early awakening, and morning fatigue and stiffness. Fibromyalgia patients demonstrate a high level of anxiety and depression on psychological testing.

Prevention and Treatment. Because the the etiology is uncertain, specific preventive measures are unknown. Reduction in exposure to stressors or modulation of the individual's coping methods is generally advised but difficult to achieve. Tricyclic antidepressant drugs, which enhance non-REM sleep and reduce the metabolic clearance of serotonin, are the most effective treatment.[17] Aerobic exercise, which has a mood-enhancing effect because of endorphin release as well as beneficial effects on muscle, may also be helpful.

Prognosis and Outcome. Fibromyalgia does not result in serious, long-term organ damage, but it has a significant negative impact on quality of life for many. Response to treatment is often less than satisfactory. On the basis of patient-reported improvement of symptoms, the rate of favorable response has ranged from 11% to 46%.[17]

Chronic Fatigue Syndrome

Definition. Chronic fatigue syndrome is an idiopathic disorder characterized by fatigue, muscle and joint pain, neuropsychiatric symptoms, and various other manifestations. The Centers for Disease Control and Prevention has established clinical criteria for diagnosis of the disorder (Table 35–7).[19]

Epidemiology. Given the lack of specificity in definition of the disorder, the precise incidence of

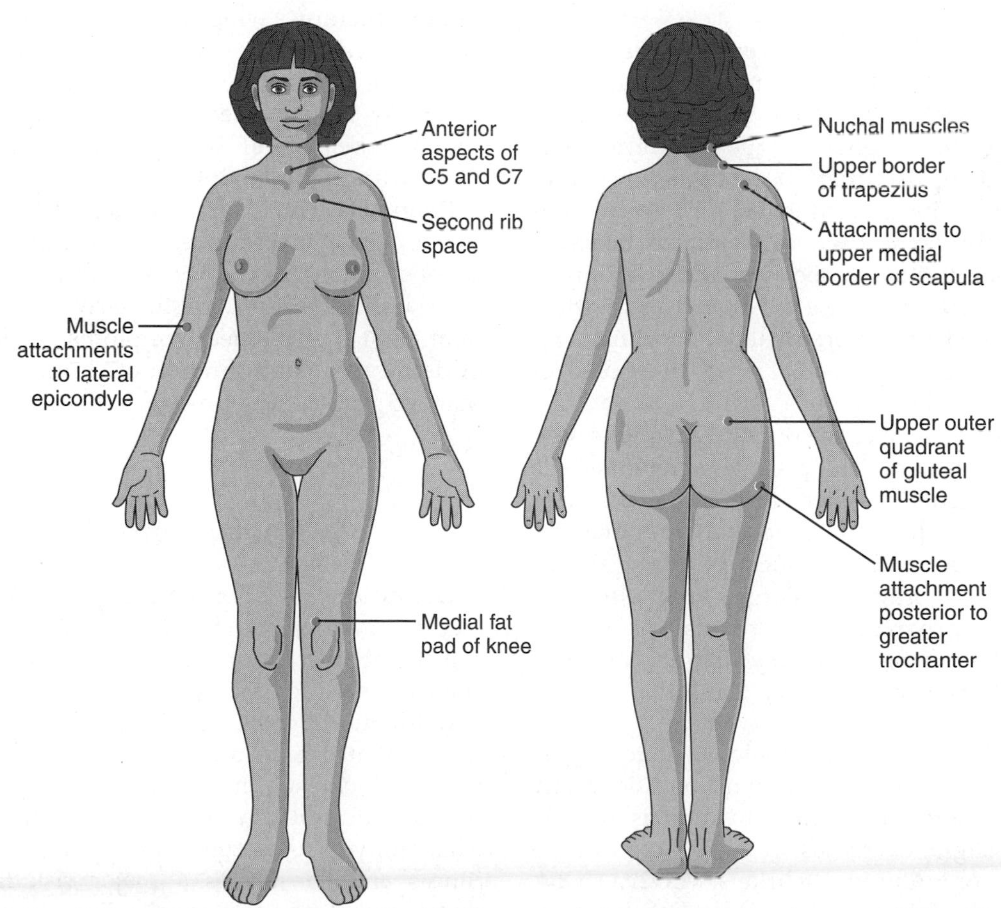

FIGURE 35–5

Tender points in fibromyalgia. According to the American College of Rheumatology, nine paired tender points establish the diagnosis of fibromyalgia.

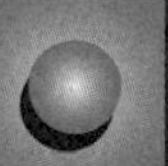

TABLE 35–7
CRITERIA FOR DIAGNOSIS OF CHRONIC FATIGUE SYNDROME

1. New onset of disabling fatigue for 6 months with at least 50% reduction in activity
2. Exclusion of other diagnostic possibilities
3. Six or more of the following symptoms:
    - Mild fever
    - Sore throat
    - Painful lymph nodes
    - Muscle weakness
    - Myalgia
    - Prolonged fatigue after exercise
    - Headaches
    - Migratory arthralgias
    - Neuropsychological complaints
    - Sleep disturbance
    - Acute onset of symptom complex

    plus

    Two or more of the following signs:
    - Low-grade fever
    - Nonexudative pharyngitis
    - Palpable or tender lymph nodes

From Bell, D.S. (1994). Chronic fatigue syndrome update: Findings now point to CNS involvement. *Postgraduate Medicine* 96(6), 74.

chronic fatigue syndrome is uncertain. The prevalence of unexplained fatigue as a presenting symptom in clinical practice has been estimated at 20%.[20] The prevalence of chronic fatigue syndrome has been reported at up to 3 per 1000 population.[21] Median age of onset in one study was 37 years.[22] Patients are usually females with a characteristic stress response similar to that associated with fibromyalgia. If their primary response to stress is pain, they may be diagnosed with fibromyalgia; a primary response of fatigue may result in a diagnosis of chronic fatigue syndrome.[17]

Etiology. The specific cause of chronic fatigue syndrome remains obscure. The prevalent hypothesis is that infectious agents or other environmental factors serve as triggers for an abnormal immune response.[22] Individual cofactors such as stress, history of depression, and previous allergies may also play a role in disease progression. There is also considerable debate whether the neuropsychiatric manifestations of the disorder are primary (causative) or secondary (reactive).

Pathophysiology. The immunologic state of the individual with chronic fatigue syndrome is subtly but measurably altered. T-cell activation is usually evidenced by slight decreases in CD4+ cells or increased levels of adhesion markers (CD29, CD54, CD 58) on T cells (see Chapter 13).[19] High levels of interleukin-1 and tumor necrosis factor are found in the most disabled individuals. Hormonal alterations are also common and include prolactin elevation, erratic secretion of antidiuretic hormone, decreased cortisol, and increased adrenocorticotropin levels. Many patients have increased levels of angiotensin-converting enzyme. Increased activity of the sympathetic nervous system is indicated by lower levels of the norepinephrine metabolite 3-methoxy-4-hydroxyphenylglycol. Cerebral blood flow, particularly in the right temporal area, is reduced in many patients. Whether these manifestations are primary or secondary to an unidentified stimulus (e.g., a viral infection) is unknown.

Clinical Manifestations. Profound fatigue of at least 6 months' duration is the characteristic symptom. Patients often report that the fatigue began abruptly after an acute viral infection and that it is worse after levels of physical exertion that had been easily tolerated in the past.[21] Other common symptoms include light-headedness, difficulty concentrating, headache, sore throat, lymph node pain, abdominal pain, muscle and joint pain, temperature instability, emotional problems, and sleep disturbance.

Prevention and Treatment. Specific preventive measures are unknown, and there is no rational basis for therapy, which is essentially symptomatic and supportive. Tricyclic antidepressants such as desipramine (Norpramin) and imipramine (Tofranil) are most widely used. Psychotherapy, particularly cognitive-behavioral therapy, may be indicated in those with predominant neuropsychiatric symptoms.

Prognosis and Outcome. An estimated 70% to 80% of patients improve with antidepressant medications.[20] Persistent illness is likely in older women with less education, particularly those with more than eight unexplained symptoms, a lifetime history of depression, and duration of chronic fatigue longer than 1.5 years at the time of initial diagnosis.[23]

Rhabdomyolysis

Definition. Rhabdomyolysis is a syndrome associated with excessive breakdown of skeletal muscle cell membranes, releasing large quantities of muscle cell contents such as myoglobin into the blood.

Epidemiology. Because rhabdomyolysis is a syndrome that complicates other primary disorders, its precise incidence has not been reported. Milder forms are probably undiagnosed in many cases. Rhabdomyolysis is common in the setting of critical illness and constitutes a major risk factor for the development of acute renal failure (see Chapter 20). Risk factors for the development of rhabdomyolysis include crush injuries, excessive exercise, heat stroke, malignant hyperthermia, compartmental syndrome, viral infections, status epilepticus, electrical shock, and alcohol or drug abuse (with overdose followed by prolonged immobility).

Etiology. Extensive damage to the muscle cell membrane (sarcolemma) usually results from direct physical trauma or ischemia, although a number of less common conditions may also cause rhabdomyolysis (Table 35–8). The inflammatory response to infection or trauma may lead to ischemia as edema builds in muscle compartments bounded by fascia. In the case of prolonged immobility, gravitational fluid shifts may contribute to edema. Crush injuries or excessive muscle contraction with extreme exertion, malignant hyperthermia, or status epilepticus may directly traumatize muscle cells. Thermal injury is the mechanism of injury with heat stroke and electrical shock.

Pathophysiology. Loss of integrity of the sarcolemma permits myoglobin, normally found only within muscle cells, to enter the blood. Other intracellular components, such as enzymes (particularly creatine kinase), uric acid, and potassium, also spill into the blood. Myoglobin normally binds to plasma proteins, then is gradually released, filtered into the glomerulus, and excreted in the urine. When 100 to 200 g of muscle has been injured, the binding capacity of plasma proteins is exceeded, and sufficient free myoglobin is released into the urine to change its color (*pigmenturia*).[24] The mechanism of renal damage in rhabdomyolysis is uncertain. The potential nephrotoxicity of myoglobin apparently requires a renal tubular pH of less than 5.6, common in the setting of dehydration and acidosis.[24] Nearly all patients with acute rhabdomyolysis also develop some degree of disseminated intravascular coagulation (DIC) (see Chapter 14).[25]

Clinical Manifestations. The most serious effects of rhabdomyolysis are on the urinary system. Myoglobin in the urine (**myoglobinuria**) is detectable on microscopic urinalysis and turns the urine a dark reddish brown color if present in sufficient quantities. Myoglobinuria also causes a false-positive response to urine testing for occult blood. Serum creatine kinase is greater than 10 times normal,[25] with nearly 100% the result of the skeletal muscle isozyme (CK-MM).[24] Hyperkalemia, hyperphosphatemia, and proteinuria are also present. The patient often is acutely ill with fever, weakness, malaise, nausea and vomiting, and pain and swelling of the involved muscles.[24] Manifestations of acute renal failure may include oliguria, azotemia, electrolyte imbalance, and fluid overload (see Chapter 20). DIC is usually moderate but may manifest as severe hemorrhage. Manifestations of the underlying disorder are also apparent.

Prevention and Treatment. Risk factors related to the underlying disorders should be reduced if possible. Prolonged, lower-intensity training (as opposed to more intense exercise over a shorter period) reduces the risk for exertional rhabdomyolysis.[25] Optimal treatment of the underlying condition and careful monitoring for signs of myoglobinuria may prevent renal failure. Administration of intravenous fluids and diuretics to increase tubular flow rates may reduce nephrotoxicity. Hyperkalemia may be treated with glucose and insulin to drive potassium intracellularly or with cation exchange resins (see Chapter 9). Short-term dialysis is usually indicated in the treatment of acute renal failure (see Chapter 20). DIC usually resolves spontaneously within 2 weeks, but severe hemorrhage may require transfusion of clotting factors in fresh frozen plasma.

Prognosis and Outcome. If recognized early and treated appropriately, rhabdomyolysis usually resolves completely. Longer-term morbidity and mortality are related to the severity of the underlying disorder.

TABLE 35–8
CONDITIONS ASSOCIATED WITH RHABDOMYOLYSIS

Etiology	Examples
Muscle necrosis	Physical trauma (e.g., crush injury) Extreme exertion (recreational or occupational) Ischemia (shock, vascular disease, arterial thrombosis, sickle cell crisis)
Inflammation	Dermatomyositis Polymyositis Inclusion-body myositis Systemic infections
Toxicity	Snake or insect venoms Alcohol or cocaine abuse Drugs (e.g., clofibrate, aminocaproic acid, anticholinergics, aspirin, phenothiazines)
Metabolic disorder	Glycogen storage disease Disorder of mitochondrial oxidative phosphorylation Carnitine palmityltransferase deficiency Malignant hyperthermia Heat stroke

Data from Brumback, R.A., Feeback, D.L., and Leech, R.W. (1992). Rhabdomyolysis in childhood: A primer on normal muscle function and selected metabolic myopathies characterized by disordered energy production. *Pediatric Clinics of North America* 39(4), 821–858; and Line, R.L., and Rust, G.S. (1995). Acute exertional rhabdomyolysis. *American Family Physician* 52(2), 502–506.

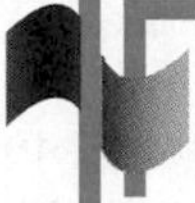

Clinical Scenario

M.L., a 24-year-old track athlete, is seen in the walk-in clinic complaining of pain and swelling in his arms and chest. Two days earlier, he had completed an intense, 2-hour weight-lifting session. Tenderness and edema of the pectoralis, biceps, and triceps muscles is evident on physical examination. Urinalysis is positive for heme protein, and serum creatine kinase is elevated to over 13,000 IU/L with nearly 100% CK-MM fraction.

1. What is the pathophysiologic basis of M.L.'s laboratory findings? Does he have blood in his urine? Explain.
2. For what life-threatening complications is M.L. at risk?

Muscular Dystrophies

Definition. The muscular dystrophies are a group of familial disorders characterized by progressive degeneration of skeletal muscle fibers. The major types of muscular dystrophy, **Duchenne's muscular dystrophy (DMD)** and **Becker's muscular dystrophy (BMD)**, are detailed here. Table 35–9 compares clinical features of less common muscular dystrophies.

Epidemiology. Duchenne's muscular dystrophy, the most severe form of muscular dystrophy, occurs in about 1 in 3500 males.[4] A small number of females have also had the disease. DMD and BMD may be inherited as X-linked recessive disorders; however, about one third of DMD cases are caused by de novo mutations. BMD is much less common than DMD.[26] Female carriers of the defective gene may have elevated serum levels of the muscle cell enzyme creatine kinase, histologic changes on muscle biopsy, and higher risk of development of cardiomyopathy.[27]

Etiology. Although DMD and BMD are caused by defects in different genes, the defective trait in both forms is located on the short arm of the X chromosome. The diseases are thus ordinarily expressed in males because they have no opposing normal allele. In the few females with the disorder, the normal X chromosome that would otherwise confer carrier status is preferentially inactivated for unknown reasons. Factors that lead to de novo mutation are also unknown.

Pathophysiology. The mechanisms by which the genetic defect results in increasing structural abnormality and loss of muscle function are uncertain. The defective gene normally encodes a protein, *dystrophin,* which is completely absent from muscle cells in most patients with DMD. Those with BMD demonstrate variable deficiencies of dystrophin. The defect is present from fetal life onward, but the progressive muscle wasting that characterizes the disease manifests later, suggesting that other factors

TABLE 35–9
LESS COMMON MUSCULAR DYSTROPHIES

DISEASE	INHERITANCE	CLINICAL FINDINGS	PATHOLOGIC FINDINGS
Fascioscapulohumeral (FSH) muscular dystrophy	Autosomal dominant	Variable age at onset (most commonly 10–30 years); weakness of muscles of face, neck, and shoulder girdle (gene localized to 4q35)	Dystrophic myopathy, but also often including inflammatory infiltrate of muscle
Oculopharyngeal muscular dystrophy	Autosomal dominant	Onset in midadult life; ptosis and weakness of extraocular muscles; difficulty in swallowing	Dystrophic myopathy, but often including rimmed vacuoles in type 1 fibers
Limb-girdle dystrophy (heterogeneous group)	Autosomal recessive and sporadic cases are common	Onset often 10–30 years; weakness of proximal muscles of upper and lower extremities; usually slowly progressive but prognosis extremely variable	Variable findings of dystrophic myopathy
Emery-Dreifuss muscular dystrophy	X-linked	Variable onset (most common 10–20 years); prominent contractures, especially of elbows and ankles	Mild myopathic changes

From Cotran, R.S., Kumar, V., and Robbins, S.L. (1994). *Robbins Pathologic Basis of Disease.* (5th ed.). Philadelphia: W.B. Saunders. (p. 1287).

compound the initiating effect of dystrophin deficiency. Dystrophin is located on the internal surface of the muscle cell membrane and may serve a stabilizing structural role or as a component of tissue matrix signaling (see Chapter 2).

On histologic examination early in the disease, muscle tissue shows abnormally large as well as abnormally small fibers; splitting, degeneration, and phagocytosis of fibers; regenerating fibers; increased numbers of nuclei; and excessive endomysium. As the disease progresses, skeletal muscle becomes almost totally replaced by fat and connective tissue. Cardiac muscle often becomes fibrotic late in the disease, and similar changes may occur in the smooth muscle of the GI tract. Functional neurologic impairment is common, although no consistent structural abnormalities are seen.

Clinical Manifestations. The infant appears normal at birth. In DMD, walking is delayed and muscle weakness becomes apparent by age 5 years. Characteristic signs include a waddling gait; *Gowers' maneuver*, in which the child compensates for lower extremity weakness by using his arms to "climb his legs" when attempting to stand (Fig. 35–6); and *pseudohypertrophy*, in which enlargement of calf muscles is caused first by dystrophic enlargement of muscle fibers and then by replacement of muscle with fat and connective tissue.

A wheelchair is usually required by age 10 to 12 years. Respiratory muscle weakness and severe scoliosis caused by spinal muscle weakness eventually predispose to respiratory failure. Cardiac involvement may manifest as heart failure or dysrhythmias, and GI involvement may be seen as bowel obstruction or malabsorption. Variable degrees of cognitive impairment develop, with some children manifesting mental retardation.

Becker's muscular dystrophy manifests as a milder form. The onset of clinical manifestations in patients with BMD is typically during later childhood or adolescence, and the rate of progression is slower and more variable.[26]

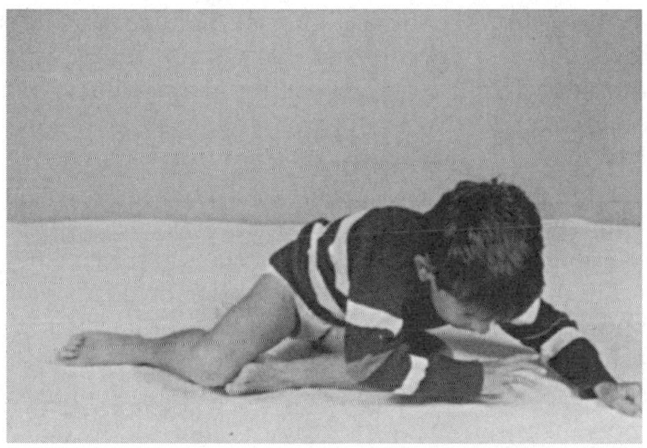
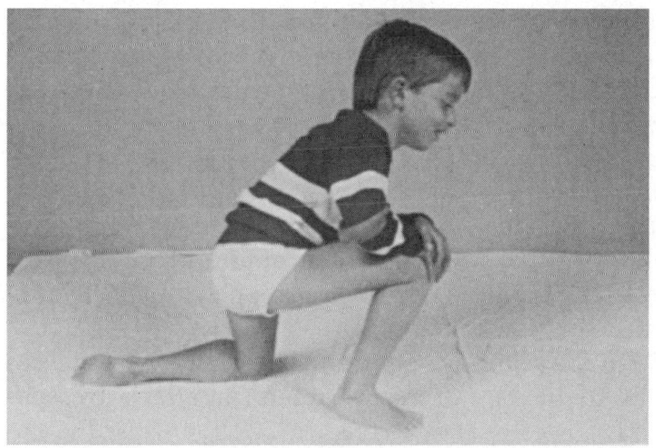
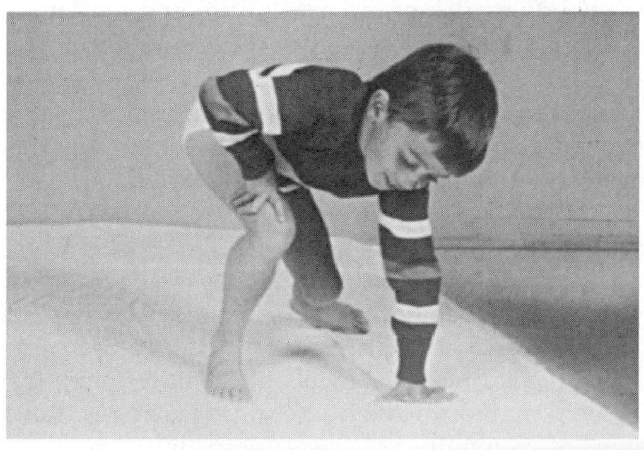
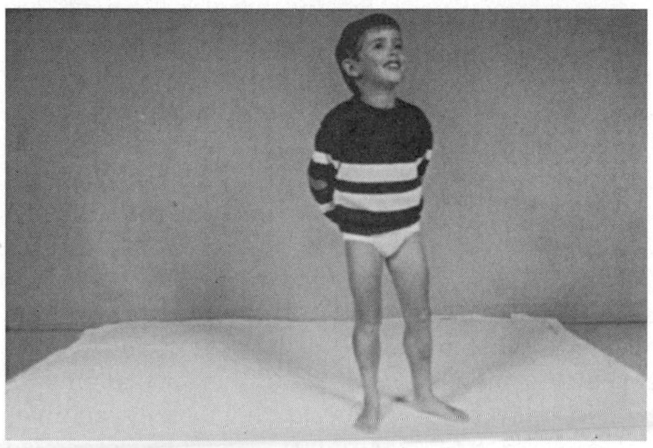

FIGURE 35–6
Gowers' maneuver in a child with muscular dystrophy. The child compensates for lower extremity weakness by using his arms to "climb his legs" when attempting to stand. (From Behrman, R.E., *et al.* [1996]. *Nelson Textbook of Pediatrics.* Philadelphia: W.B. Saunders. [p. 1672].)

Prevention and Treatment. There is no known prevention of muscular dystrophy. In cases where carriers can be identified or intrauterine diagnosis can be made, subsequent counseling is provided. Treatment of DMD and BMD is symptomatic and supportive. Gene replacement therapy and transplantation of muscle-forming (myoblast) cells are in early experimental phases.[4]

Prognosis and Outcome. Death usually occurs in the early 20s in DMD because of respiratory or cardiac failure. Patients with BMD may have a nearly normal life span.[26]

Inflammatory Myopathies

Definition. The inflammatory myopathies are a group of disorders characterized by immune-mediated inflammation of skeletal muscle. This category includes **dermatomyositis**, named because of its involvement of skin as well as muscle, **polymyositis**, and **inclusion-body myositis**.

Epidemiology. The incidence of the inflammatory myopathies has been estimated at 5 per million, but this estimate is believed to be low.[28] Presence of another connective tissue disease such as rheumatoid arthritis, systemic lupus erythematosus, or scleroderma is associated with increased risk, as is the presence of malignancy. Females are more commonly afflicted than males, but the age and sex distribution varies with the specific disorder.

Etiology. The precise etiology of these disorders is unknown, although an autoimmune process, possibly triggered by a virus or tumor cytokine, is suggested by the clinical picture.

Pathophysiology. In dermatomyositis, capillaries seem to be the primary targets of attack by self-reactive B cells and T cells. In polymyositis, the endomysium is the apparent target. In inclusion-body myositis, rimmed vacuoles and tubular filaments are seen within muscle cells. An inflammatory response underlies muscle tissue injury in each case.

Clinical Manifestations. Muscle weakness is the principal characteristic of all three forms, accompanied by a violet-colored skin rash around the eyes and over distal bony prominences in dermatomyositis. In dermatomyositis and polymyositis, muscle weakness is slow in onset and symmetric, affecting the proximal muscles first. Late in the disease, fine movements are impaired by distal muscle involvement. Inclusion-body myositis differs in that muscle weakness may be asymmetric and usually involves distal muscles first. Laboratory evidence associated with the inflammatory myopathies includes the presence of antinuclear or Jo-1 antibodies (see Chapter 34) and elevation of serum creatine kinase. Electromyography and muscle biopsy establish the diagnosis.[26]

Prevention and Treatment. There is no known prevention of these disorders. Corticosteroids are the mainstay of treatment, although cytotoxic agents such as azathioprine, cyclophosphamide, and methotrexate may be used in severe cases.

Prognosis and Outcome. Most patients improve with treatment, but are subject to relapse at any time. Five-year survival in inflammatory myopathies is about 75%, with death usually caused by pulmonary, renal, or cardiac complications.[28]

Rhabdomyosarcoma

Definition. Rhabdomyosarcoma is a malignant neoplasm arising from embryonic mesenchymal cells that differentiate into skeletal muscle.

Epidemiology. Rhabdomyosarcoma is the most common soft tissue tumor occurring during childhood and adolescence. Incidence has been estimated at 8.4 per million in white children and about half that incidence in black children.[29] Incidence peaks are seen at age 5 years and younger and again at 15 to 19 years. The tumor affects slightly more males than females. Specific risk factors are unknown, although a familial predisposition is apparent. Embryonic exposure to teratogenic chemicals and viruses has induced the tumor in laboratory animals, and the tumor may be associated with other cancers and with congenital anomalies.

Etiology. The specific etiology is unknown.

Pathophysiology. Rhabdomyosarcoma may arise in any skeletal muscle tissue, with certain histologic subtypes more likely to be found in specific regions of the body. The most common type in children is more likely to arise in the head and neck, and the most common type in adolescents usually begins in the deep muscles of the extremities and may involve the genital tract. The early childhood form is the least differentiated and thus the most aggressive. The tumor spreads first by local infiltration, replacing muscle tissue with a grayish white mass. Metastasis is by hematogenous and lymphatic spread. In young children, the disease is often metastatic at the time of diagnosis.

Clinical Manifestations. The soft tissue mass is visible or palpable and may cause local edema and signs of obstruction or bleeding (e.g., of the sinuses, airway, middle ear, bowel, or genitourinary tract). Tumors may also invade neural tissues, resulting in signs of meningitis or sensorimotor impairment.

Prevention and Treatment. Specific means of prevention are unknown. Treatment depends on the stage of the disease, with stage I disease representing localized, completely resectable disease, stage II disease manifested by involvement of regional lymph nodes and micrometastasis, stage III disease indicating gross residual disease, and stage IV disease demonstrating distant metastasis at the time of diagnosis.[29] Rhabdomyosarcoma is ideally treated with surgical excision, but complete tumor removal is often not possible, and surgery may result in permanent disfigurement. Radiation therapy in combination with chemotherapy may be used as an adjunct to surgery in stages II and III. Stage IV disease is treated with systemic chemotherapy.

Prognosis and Outcome. Prognosis depends on the location of the tumor, clinical stage of the disease at diagnosis, and the histologic subtype. Approximately 65% of patients are cured of their disease.[26]

CLINICAL SIGNIFICANCE OF MUSCLE DISORDERS AND EXERCISE

Skeletal muscle is the most abundant tissue in the body, and its function is interdependent with that of the other major body systems. Although life-threatening primary disorders of muscle are rare, clinical manifestations of muscle pain and fatigue are exceedingly common. Impairment of mobility may significantly reduce quality of life as well as predispose to development of major systemic disorders, including cardiovascular disease, hypertension, diabetes, and osteoporosis. The disorders discussed in this chapter demonstrate the impact of muscle disorders on individuals of all ages. Despite widespread publication of the health benefits of exercise and the risks of inactivity, a significant segment of the U.S. population is sedentary. The impact of inactivity on subsequent development of major illness constitutes a major public health concern. Research is ongoing in an effort to illuminate mechanisms underlying the common but obscure disorders manifesting as muscle pain and fatigue and to further define the type and duration of activity that is of most benefit in prevention of the major causes of morbidity and mortality.

Summary of Key Points

- Muscle fatigue after exercise is a normal phenomenon, possibly associated with depletion of glycogen stores and accumulation of lactic acid. Failure to achieve or maintain the expected force or power of a muscle is typical of pathology and may be the result of impairment of neural stimulation of muscle, energy metabolism, or disruption in calcium flux. Primary muscle disorders, such as atrophy and dystrophy, result in more rapid fatigue as well as weakness because of actual loss of cross-sectional area of muscle.
- Skeletal muscles are composed of mixed fibers classified as either type I (slow oxidative) or type II (fast glycolytic) fibers. Smaller type I fibers are specialized for endurance, and larger type II fibers are specialized for brief, powerful contraction. In adult males, type II fibers occupy the larger volume of muscle mass, accounting for greater muscle bulk; in females, type I fibers predominate. Endurance training (e.g., aerobics) primarily affects type I fibers, increasing the size and number of mitochondria, myoglobin concentration, capillary perfusion, and capacity for utilization of lipids for energy. Resistance training (e.g., weight-lifting) primarily affects type II fibers, increasing the number of myofibrils and storage of glycogen. Type II fibers are preferentially lost with aging, contributing to atrophy.
- Some degree of muscle atrophy is normal with aging. Pathologic atrophy occurs with denervation, immobility, or enhanced proteolysis caused by altered regulation by hormones or cytokines. Muscle hypertrophy occurs adaptively in response to increased neural stimulation and mechanical stress.
- Nearly all movement is accomplished with the use of leverage to modify its speed, strength, and range. Normal function of lever systems depends on the integrity of muscle, joints, bones, ligaments, and tendons as well as flexibility of overlying skin. The two general types of abnormally increased muscle contraction are myotonia, a property of muscle itself, and spasticity, a function of the neural stimulation of muscle. Myotonia is the inability of muscle to relax completely after contraction and may be seen in muscular dystrophies and other primary muscle disorders. Spasticity is much more common and is associated with electrolyte imbalance, muscle overuse, systemic toxicity, epilepsy, neuromuscular diseases, and neurotrauma.
- The function of type I and type II muscle fi-

Summary continued on following page

bers is enhanced by endurance and resistance training, respectively. With endurance training, cardiac reserve may be greatly enhanced as a result of cardiac hypertrophy and dilation and increased efficiency of peripheral oxygen utilization. Systemic vascular resistance decreases with endurance training and increases with resistance training. Pulmonary ventilation increases to meet the demands of exercise, and maximum oxygen uptake increases adaptively with endurance training. Exercise activates the stress response, mobilizing energy stores. Core body temperature rises during exercise, imposing risk of hyperthermia and dehydration in adverse environmental conditions.

- Exercise protects against many chronic and life-threatening diseases, including coronary heart disease, dyslipidemia, thrombosis, obesity, hypertension, type 2 diabetes, osteoporosis, depression, and some cancers.

- Primary muscle disorders are relatively uncommon, but may arise from trauma, inherited or de novo genetic defects, immune-mediated inflammation, or neoplasia. The underlying mechanisms in the common disorders of fibromyalgia and chronic fatigue syndrome remain obscure.

REFERENCES

1. Brooks, S.V., and Faulkner, J.A. (1994). Skeletal muscle weakness in old age: Underlying mechanisms. *Medicine and Science in Sports and Exercise* 26(4), 432–439.
2. Brumback, R.A., Feeback, D.L., and Leech, R.W. (1992). Rhabdomyolysis in childhood: A primer on normal muscle function and selected metabolic myopathies characterized by disordered energy production. *Pediatric Clinics of North America* 39(4), 821–858.
3. Mitch, W.E., and Goldberg, A.L. (1996). Mechanisms of muscle wasting: The role of the ubiquitin-proteasome pathway. *New England Journal of Medicine* 335(25), 1897–1905.
4. Pearson, A.M., and Young, R.B. (1993). Diseases and disorders of muscle. *Advances in Food and Nutrition Research* 37, 339–423.
5. Luckin, K.A., Biedermann, M.C., Jubrias, S.A., *et al.* (1991). Muscle fatigue: Conduction or mechanical failure? *Biochemical Medicine and Metabolic Biology* 46, 299–316.
6. Riley, J.D., and Antony, S.J. (1995). Leg cramps: Differential diagnosis and management. *American Family Physician* 52(6), 1794–1798.
7. NIH Consensus Development Panel on Physical Activity and Cardiovascular Health. *Journal of the American Medical Association* 276(3), 241–246.
8. Pelliccia, A., Maron, B.J., Culasso, F., *et al.* (1996). Athlete's heart in women: Echocardiographic characterization of highly trained elite female athletes. *Journal of the American Medical Association* 276(3), 211–215.
9. Pate, R.R., Pratt, M., Blair, S.N., *et al.* (1995). *Journal of the American Medical Association* 273(5), 402–407.
10. Giovannucci, E., Ascherio, A., Rimm, E.B., *et al.* (1995). Physical activity, obesity, and risk for colon cancer and adenoma in men. *Annals of Internal Medicine* 122(5), 327–334.
11. Thune, I., Brenn, T., Lund, E., *et al.* (1997). Physical activity and the risk of breast cancer. *New England Journal of Medicine* 336(18), 1269–1275.
12. DiFiori, J.P. (1995). Menstrual dysfunction in athletes: How to identify and treat patients at risk for skeletal injury. *Postgraduate Medicine* 97(3), 143–156.
13. Butcher, J.D. (1993). Runner's diarrhea and other intestinal problems of athletes. *American Family Physician* 48(4), 623–627.
14. Maron, B.J., Shirani, J., Poliac, L.C., *et al.* (1996). Sudden death in young competitive athletes: Clinical, demographic, and pathological profiles. *Journal of the American Medical Association* 276(3), 199–204.
15. Willich, S.N., Lewis, M., Lowel, H., *et al.* (1993). Physical exertion as a trigger of acute myocardial infarction. *New England Journal of Medicine* 329(23), 1684–1690.
16. Baumert, P.W. Acute inflammation after injury: Quick control speeds rehabilitation. *Postgraduate Medicine* 97(2), 35–49.
17. Wilke, W.S. (1996). Fibromyalgia: Recognizing and addressing the multiple interrelated factors. *Postgraduate Medicine* 100(1), 153–170.
18. Lario, B.A., Valdivielso, J.L.A., Lopez, J.A., *et al.* (1996). Fibromyalgia syndrome: Overnight falls in arterial oxygen saturation. *American Journal of Medicine* 101, 54–60.
19. Bell, D.S. (1994). Chronic fatigue syndrome update: Findings now point to CNS involvement. *Postgraduate Medicine* 96(6), 73–81.
20. Wilson, A., Hickie, I., Lloyd, A., *et al.* (1994). The treatment of chronic fatigue syndrome: Science and speculation. *American Journal of Medicine* 96, 544–550.
21. Bou-Holaigah, I., Rowe, P.C., Kan, J., *et al.* (1995). The relationship between neurally mediated hypotension and the chronic fatigue syndrome. *Journal of the American Medical Association* 274(12), 961–967.
22. MacDonald, K.L., Osterholm, M.T., LeDell, K.H., *et al.* (1996). A case-control study to assess possible triggers and cofactors in chronic fatigue syndrome. *American Journal of Medicine* 100, 548–554.
23. Clark, M.R., Katon, W., Russo, J., *et al.* (1995). Chronic fatigue: Risk factors for symptom persistence in a 2½-year follow-up study. *American Journal of Medicine* 98, 187–195.
24. Dayer-Berenson, L. (1994). Rhabdomyolysis: A comprehensive guide. *American Nephrology Nurses Association Journal* 21(1), 15–18.
25. Line, R.L., and Rust, G.S. (1995). Acute exertional rhabdomyolysis. *American Family Physician* 52(2), 502–506.
26. Cotran, R.S., Kumar, V., and Robbins, S.L. (1994). *Robbins Pathologic Basis of Disease.* (5th ed.). Philadelphia: W.B. Saunders. (pp. 213–214, 1267–1268, 1285–1288).
27. Politano, L., Nigro, V., Nigro, G., *et al.* (1996). Development of cardiomyopathy in female carriers of Duchenne and Becker muscular dystrophies. *Journal of the American Medical Association* 275(17), 1335–1338.
28. Braunwald, E., Isselbacher, K.J., Petersdorf, R.G., *et al.* (Eds.). (1987). *Harrison's Principles of Internal Medicine.* (11th ed.). New York: McGraw-Hill. (pp. 2069–2072).
29. Behrman, R.E., Kliegman, R.M., Arvin, A.M. (1996). *Nelson Textbook of Pediatrics.* (15th ed.). Philadelphia: W.B. Saunders.

SELECTED BIBLIOGRAPHY

Bernadet, P. (1995). Benefits of physical activity in the prevention of cardiovascular diseases. *Journal of Cardiovascular Pharmacology* 25(1 suppl.), S3–S8.

Blair, S.N., Kohl, H.W., III, Barlow, C.E., *et al.* (1995). Changes in physical fitness and all-cause mortality: A prospective study of healthy and unhealthy men. *Journal of the American Medical Association* 273(14), 1093–1098.

Brooks, G.A. (1991). Current concepts in lactate exchange. *Medicine and Science in Sports and Exercise* 23(8), 895–906.

Catlin, D.H., and Murray, T.H. (1996). Performance-enhancing drugs, fair competition, and Olympic sport. *Journal of the American Medical Association* 276(3), 231–237.

Chati, Z., Zannad, F., Jeandel, C., *et al.* (1996). Physical deconditioning may be the mechanism for the skeletal muscle energy phosphate metabolism abnormalities in chronic heart failure. *American Heart Journal* 131(3), 560–566.

Clark, M.G., Colquhoun, E.Q., Rattigan, S., *et al.* (1995). Vascular and endocrine control of muscle metabolism. *American Journal of Physiology* 268, E797–E812.

Fiatarone, M.A., O'Neill, E.F., Ryan, N.D., *et al.* (1994). Exercise training and nutritional supplementation for physical frailty in very elderly people. *New England Journal of Medicine* 330(25), 1769–1775.

Ginsburg, G.S., Agil, A., O'Toole, M., *et al.* (1996). Effects of a single bout of ultraendurance exercise on lipid levels and susceptibility of lipids to peroxidation in triathletes. *Journal of the American Medical Association* 276(3), 221–225.

Glockner, S.M. (1995). Shoulder pain: A diagnostic dillemma. *American Family Physician* 51(7), 1677–1687.

Guyton, A.C., and Hall, J.E. (1996). *Textbook of Medical Physiology*. (9th ed.). Philadelphia: W.B. Saunders. (pp. 1059–1070).

Klesges, R.C., Ward, K.D., Shelton, M.L., *et al.* (1996). Changes in bone mineral content in male athletes: Mechanisms of action and intervention effects. *Journal of the American Medical Association* 276(3), 226–230.

Kushi, L.H., Fee, R.M., Folsom A.R., *et al.* (1997). Physical activity and mortality in postmenopausal women. *Journal of the American Medical Association* 277(16), 1287–1292.

Lakka, T.A., Venalainen, J.M., Rauramaa, R., *et al.* (1994). Relation of leisure-time physical activity and cardiorespiratory fitness to the risk of acute myocardial infarction in men. *New England Journal of Medicine* 330(22), 1549–1554.

Leonard, J.C., and Townsend, H.E. (1996). Ready, set, go! Sports medicine on and off the field. *Postgraduate Medicine* 99(5), 237–244.

Luepker, R.V., Perry, C.L., McKinlay, S.M., *et al.* (1996). Outcomes of a field trial to improve children's dietary patterns and physical activity: The Child and Adolescent Trial for Cardiovascular Health (CATCH). *Journal of the American Medical Association* 275(10), 768–776.

Luft, R. (1994). The development of mitochondrial medicine. *Proceedings of the National Academy of Sciences USA* 91(9), 8731–8738.

Mendell, J.R., Kissel, J.T., Amato, A.A., *et al.* (1995). Myoblast transfer in the treatment of Duchenne's muscular dystrophy. *New England Journal of Medicine* 333(13), 832–838.

Mittleman, M.A., Maclure, M., Tofler, G.H., *et al.* (1993). Triggering of acute myocardial infarction by heavy physical exertion. *New England Journal of Medicine* 329(23), 1677–1683.

Moffett, D.R., Moffett, S.B., and Schauf, C.L. (1993). *Human Physiology: Foundations and Frontiers*. St. Louis: Mosby–Year Book. (pp. 290–312).

Moore, K.L., and Persaud, T.V.N. (1993). *The Developing Human: Clinically Oriented Embryology*. (5th ed.). Philadelphia: W.B. Saunders. (pp. 370–374).

Ostezan, L.B., and Callen, J.P. (1996). Cutaneous manifestations of selected rheumatologic diseases. *American Family Physician* 53(5), 1625–1633.

Pahor, M., Guralnik, J.M., Salive, M.E., *et al.* (1994). Physical activity and risk of severe gastrointestinal hemorrhage in older persons. *Journal of the American Medical Association* 272(8), 595–599.

Sharma, K.R., Mynhier, M.A., and Miller, R.G. (1995). Muscular fatigue in Duchenne muscular dystrophy. *Neurology* 45, 306–310.

Schlicker, S.A., Borra, S.T., and Regan, C. (1994). The weight and fitness status of United States children. *Nutrition Reviews* 52(1), 11–17.

Sherman, S.E., D'Agostino, R.B., Cobb, J.L., *et al.* (1994). Does exercise reduce mortality rates in the elderly? Experience from the Framingham Heart Study. *American Heart Journal* 128(5), 965–972.

Sherman, S.E., D'Agostino, R.B., Cobb, J.L., *et al.* (1994). Physical activity and mortality in women in the Framingham Heart Study. *American Heart Journal* 128(5), 879–884.

Wilson, D.F. (1995). Energy metabolism in muscle approaching maximal rates of oxygen utilization. *Medicine and Science in Sports and Exercise* 27(1), 54–59.

Worton, R. (1995). Muscular dystrophies: Diseases of the dystrophin-glycoprotein complex. *Science* 270, 755–756.

Zeni, A.I., Hoffman, M.D., and Clifford, P.S. (1996). Energy expenditure with indoor exercise machines. *Journal of the American Medical Association* 275(18), 1424–1427.

Unit XIV

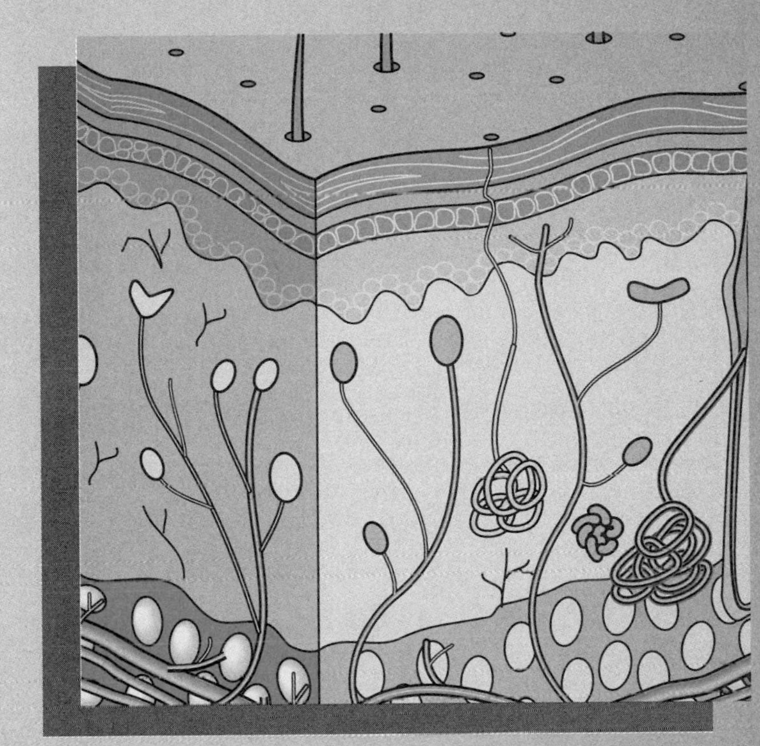

Chapter 36
Integumentary Disorders

INTEGUMENTARY SYSTEM

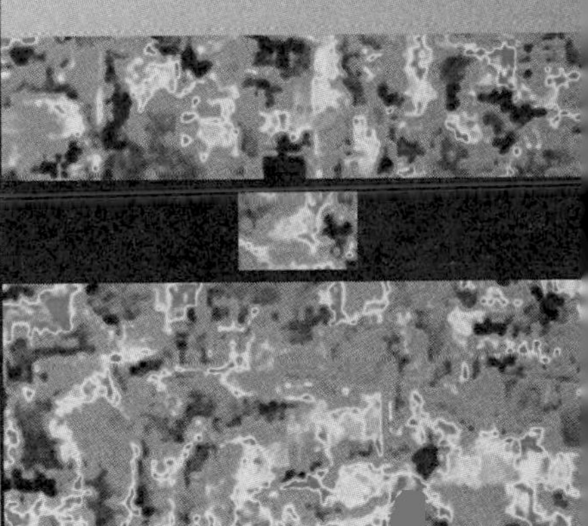

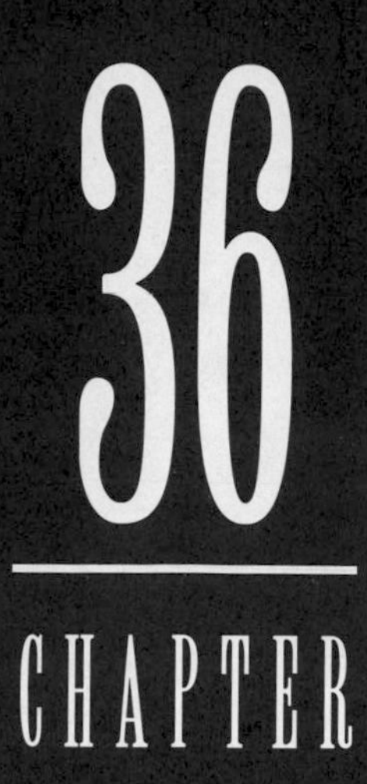

Integumentary Disorders

LEARNING OBJECTIVES

1. Identify the anatomic features of the skin, hair, and nails that underlie their physiologic functions.
2. Discuss the principal neural, hormonal, and local mechanisms by which integumentary function is regulated, with reference to manifestations of altered regulation.
3. Compare and contrast primary and secondary skin lesions on the basis of morphology and mechanism.
4. Differentiate between primary integumentary disorders and systemic disorders with integumentary manifestations.
5. Discuss the pathophysiologic mechanisms that predict clinical manifestations and rationalize intervention in infectious, allergic, immune-mediated, and idiopathic disorders of the skin.
6. Compare and contrast the major forms of skin cancer on the basis of etiology and risk factors, lesion morphology, and metastatic potential.
7. Discuss the pathophysiologic mechanisms resulting in the multisystemic manifestations of major burn injury.

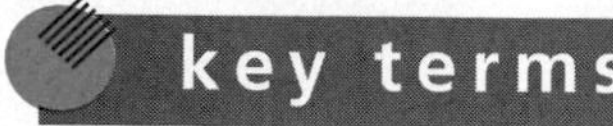

key terms

acne vulgaris
actinic keratosis
alopecia
angioedema
atopic dermatitis
basal cell carcinoma
burn shock
candidiasis
cellulitis
contact dermatitis
CREST syndrome
Curling's ulcer
eczema
eschar
exanthem
folliculitis
furunculosis
gangrene
herpes simplex
herpes zoster
impetigo
Kaposi's sarcoma
leukoplakia
malignant melanoma
nevus
pediculosis
photodermatitis

photosensitivity
primary skin lesion
pruritus
psoriasis
rubella
rubeola
scabies
scalded skin syndrome
scarlet fever
scleroderma
seborrheic dermatitis
secondary skin lesion
squamous cell carcinoma
tinea
urticaria
varicella
verrucae
xerosis

The skin and its related structures, the hair and nails, comprise the integument or "covering" of the body. The most important function of the integument, protection, is inherent in this term. The intact skin and mucous membranes, with their acid pH, enzymatic secretions, and normal flora of microorganisms, constitute the first line of defense of human beings against invasion by environmental toxins and pathogens (see Chapter 13). The skin is far more than a physicochemical barrier, however. The high vascularity and dense innervation of the skin are evidence of the dynamic nature of the integument that enables it to reflect, and to some degree direct, the function of the underlying organ systems.

Skin turgor (texture and resilience) is a manifestation of the general state of fluid balance, and the skin participates in that balance through sweating (see Chapter 8). Skin temperature reflects core body temperature, and the skin participates in thermoregulation by radiation, conduction, convection, and evaporative cooling (see Chapter 11). Skin color varies with changes in oxygenation and perfusion, and skin vessels represent a high-volume, variable-resistance reservoir of blood, the status of which (under autonomic regulation) impacts perfusion of all other systems (see Chapter 15). Skin cells also contain enzymes that activate Vitamin D_3, a steroid hormone of importance to calcium and phosphate homeostasis and bone metabolism (see Chapters 9 and 34).

With the notable exceptions of **malignant melanoma** and major burn injuries, disorders of the integument are rarely life-threatening. Skin disorders are common, however, and the resulting physical discomfort is often magnified by the psychological discomfort associated with disfigurement. In this chapter, the structure and function of the skin and its appendages are reviewed, and the skin manifestations resulting from disorders of other body systems are discussed. The most common inflammatory, idiopathic, and neoplastic disorders of the skin are detailed. Burns are also discussed, illustrating the multisystem dysfunction that may result from traumatic loss of the integument. Structure, function, and disorders of the hair and nails are briefly summarized.

ANATOMY AND FUNCTION OF THE INTEGUMENT

Skin

Figure 36–1 illustrates the cross-sectional anatomy of the skin, revealing its two principal interactive layers, the outer *epidermis* and inner *dermis*, which are separated by a basement membrane zone and supported by subcutaneous tissue composed of fibrous connective tissue and adipose tissue. The thickness of the skin varies in different regions of the body and also with age, as a function of external pressure and friction, hormonal stimuli (notably androgens and estrogens), and genetic makeup.

Epidermis

The epidermis consists of four cell types. Several layers of squamous epithelial cells (called *keratinocytes* because of their production of the protein keratin) provide the epidermis with its basic structure (Fig. 36–2). The innermost layer of epidermis consists of a single layer of *basal cells* attached to the basement membrane zone. In the process of keratinization, these cells actively divide (at different rates under different stimuli), forming daughter cells that migrate outward while accumulating keratin and changing in shape, function, and viability. The outermost layer of epidermis, the *stratum corneum*, consists of dead cells that are continuously sloughed. Epidermal cells normally turn over every 15 to 30 days, a rate that varies with normal stimuli as well as with exfoliative (skin-sloughing) disorders such as **psoriasis**.

Three other cell types are interspersed among the epithelial cells of the epidermis: *Langerhans cells*, *Merkel cells*, and *melanocytes*. Langerhans cells migrate into the epidermis from the bone marrow and

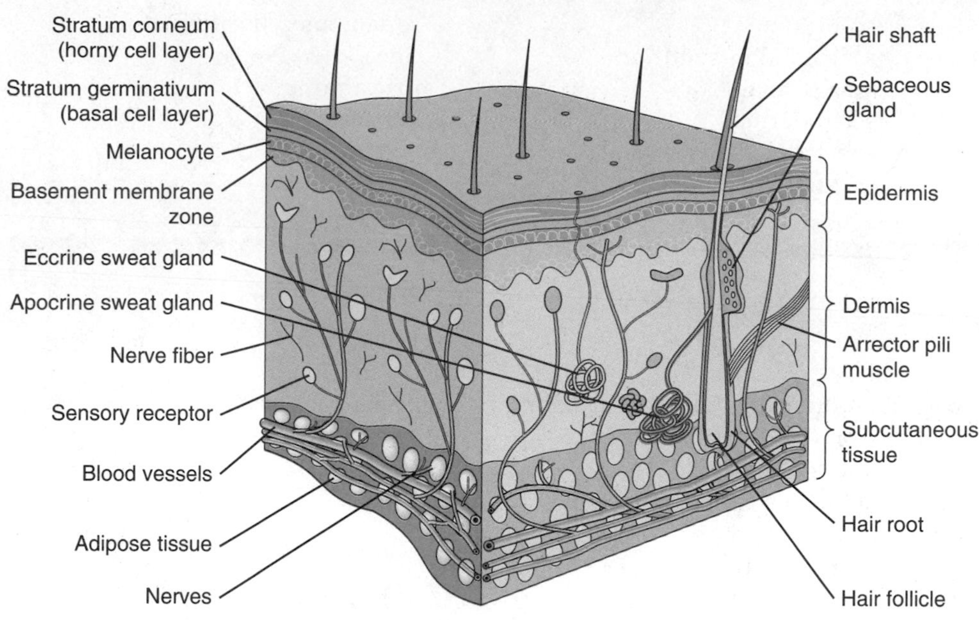

FIGURE 36–1
Three-dimensional view of the skin. The layers of the skin are the outer *epidermis,* the *basement membrane zone,* the *dermis,* and the *subcutaneous layer.* The epidermis is composed primarily of epithelial cells that are continuously sloughed from the outer layer and regenerated by division of the basal cells, or inner layer. The basement membrane zone anchors the epidermis to the dermis. The dermis is a connective tissue layer that supports the appendages (hair follicles, sebaceous glands, and sweat glands) as well as blood vessels, pilomotor muscles, and nerves. The subcutaneous layer of fat and connective tissue provides support, insulation, and energy fuel storage.

are believed to serve as antigen-presenting cells in the immune response (see Chapter 13). Merkel cells are mechanoreceptors, mediating the sense of touch (see Chapter 23). Melanocytes, located within the basal cell layer, synthesize the brown pigment *melanin,* which is taken up by the keratinocytes. Genetically determined variations in amount and color of melanin produced determine baseline skin color and response to ultraviolet (UV) light (Table 36–1). Disorders characterized primarily by abnormal skin pigmentation are briefly described in Table 36–2.

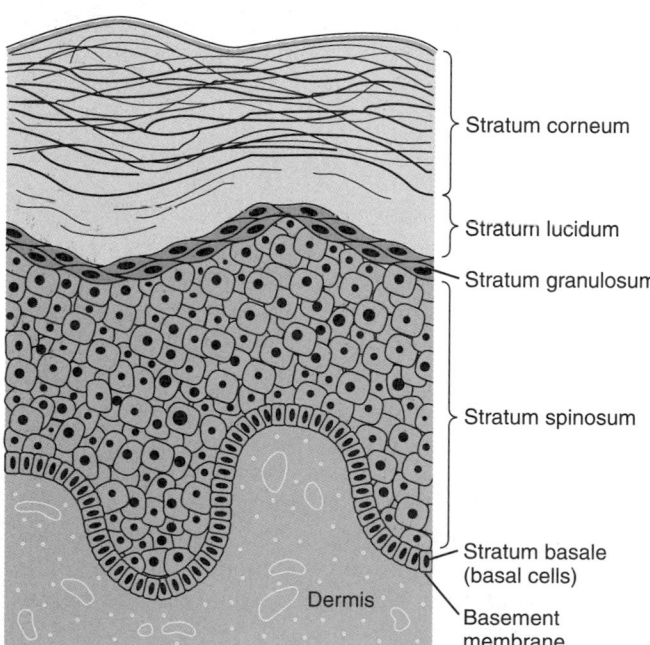

FIGURE 36–2
Layers of the epidermis. The epidermis consists of layers of epithelial cells known as *keratinocytes* because they contain the protein keratin. A single layer of basal cells, attached to the basement membrane, divides to form daughter cells that migrate upward while accumulating keratin and becoming flatter. The outer layer, the *stratum corneum,* consists of dead cells that are continuously sloughed. Epidermal cells normally turn over every 15 to 30 days.

Exposure to UV light stimulates increased melanin production, producing the "tan" that, in addition to its cosmetic effect, affords some protection against UV damage. Squamous cells, basal cells, and melanocytes are the cells of origin of the significant types of skin cancer. As discussed later, cumulative exposure to UV light and baseline skin color are the significant risk factors for these cancers.

Basement Membrane Zone

The basement membrane zone between the epidermis and the dermis contains collagen fibers that anchor the two layers, providing strength, cohesion, and elasticity. In neonates (especially premature infants), incomplete development of this adhesive layer predisposes to ease of injury and increased permeability of the skin. Degeneration of collagen with chronologic aging and photoaging (cumulative, sunlight-induced damage) contributes to thinning and wrinkling of the skin (see Developmental Perspective).

Dermis

The dermis is a connective tissue layer, containing fibroblasts that secrete collagen fibers and mucopolysaccharide ground substance as well as tissue

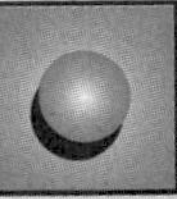

TABLE 36–1
CLASSIFICATION OF SKIN TYPES WITH RESPECT TO INTRINSIC PIGMENTATION AND SUN SENSITIVITY

CATEGORY	DESCRIPTION
Type I	Individuals who never tan and always sunburn if exposed to any amount of sunlight (primarily red-haired individuals and light-complexioned blondes)
Type II	Individuals who frequently sunburn but are able to tan to a small degree after extended sun exposure
Type III	Individuals who burn infrequently and tan readily
Type IV	Individuals who rarely burn and tan heavily with moderate sun exposure (primarily individuals of Asian, Native American, Mediterranean, and Latin American descent)
Type V	Individuals with intrinsic dark pigmentation who become noticeably darker with sun exposure (primarily light-complexioned African-American persons and those of east Indian descent)
Type VI	Individuals with very dark intrinsic pigmentation (dark-skinned African-Americans)

Data from Farmer, K.C., and Naylor, M.F. (1996). Sun exposure, sunscreens, and skin cancer prevention: A year-round concern. *Annals of Pharmacotherapy* 30, 662–673.

macrophages and mast cells that mediate the inflammatory and immune responses. The dermis supports the *dermal appendages* (hair follicles, sebaceous glands, and sweat glands) as well as pilomotor muscles, blood vessels, lymphatics, and nerves. Sebaceous glands secrete the oily *sebum* that lubricates the skin and nourishes hair follicles. Sweat glands are of two types: eccrine glands, which secrete sweat through pores on most of the body surface, and apocrine glands, located in the axillae, groin, abdomen, face, and scalp, which secrete a more viscous sweat into hair follicles. Modified apocrine glands in

TABLE 36–2
SELECTED DISORDERS OF SKIN PIGMENTATION

DISORDER	DESCRIPTION
Vitiligo	Idiopathic, possibly autoimmune disorder characterized by partial or complete loss of melanocytes; flat, asymptomatic, well-demarcated zones of pigment loss of variable size; usual distribution to wrists, axillae, periorbital and perioral regions of face, and anogenital regions; most noticeable in dark-skinned persons
Freckles (ephelides)	Tan-red or light brown macules 1 to 10 mm in diameter; most noticeable during childhood in light-skinned whites after sun exposure; fade and reappear cyclically during winter and summer; caused by increased melanin in basal cells
Melasma (mask of pregnancy)	Blotchy macules over the cheeks, temples, and forehead during pregnancy; enhanced by sunlight exposure; usually resolves spontaneously after pregnancy; caused by increased pigment transfer to basal cells and dermal macrophages in hormonal environment of pregnancy; may also occur with oral contraceptive use
Senile (solar) lentigines (liver spots)	Small, flat brown macules on the forearms and hands of older persons; caused by benign hyperplasia of melanocytes induced by extensive sun exposure
Café-au-lait spots	Tan or light brown, irregularly shaped patches with well-defined borders; may be normal variant or associated with neurofibromatosis
Mongolian spots	Blue-black or purple area at sacrum or buttocks caused by deep dermal melanocytes; present in many blacks, Asians, and Native Americans and in a few whites; fades during the first year of life
Acanthosis nigricans	Thickened areas of hyperpigmentation in skinfold areas of the axillae, neck, groin, or anogenital region; may be congenital or associated with endocrine disorders (e.g., type 2 diabetes mellitus, pituitary and pineal disorders); may signal an underlying adenocarcinoma if arising in older individuals

Data from Cotran, R.S., Kumar, V., and Robbins, S.L. (1994). *Robbins Pathologic Basis of Disease.* (5th ed.). Philadelphia: W.B. Saunders. (pp. 1175–1176); and Jarvis, C. (1992). *Physical Examination and Health Assessment.* Philadelphia: W.B. Saunders. (pp. 223–273).

Developmental Perspective

Embryonic and Fetal Periods

The two principal skin layers develop from different embryonic tissues: the epidermis from the ectoderm and the dermis from the mesoderm. The epidermis grows in thickness during the first and second trimesters. Exfoliated cells and sebum form part of the vernix caseosa, which protects fetal skin from exposure to amniotic fluid. Neural crest cells migrate into the dermoepidermal junction during the early fetal period, differentiating into melanocytes. Melanocytes begin producing melanin at birth. Fine, colorless hairs (lanugo) are apparent by the end of the 12th week. Melanin stimulates the development of hair color several weeks before birth. Nail development is apparent at about 10 weeks of gestation. Fingernails reach the tips of the fingers by 32 weeks, and toenails reach the tips of the toes by 36 weeks, providing a marker of gestational age in premature infants. Significant congenital anomalies of the skin are uncommon. Congenital ectodermal dysplasia is characterized by lack of body hair and presence of dental anomalies. Albinism is a rare autosomal recessive disorder in which the skin, hair, and retina lack melanin pigment. Mongolian spots are areas of hyperpigmentation in the sacrum or buttocks caused by deep dermal melanocytes, found as a normal variant in black, Native American, Latin, and Asian newborns.

Infancy and Childhood

Physiologic jaundice is present in about half of all newborns, imparting a yellow cast to the skin. Infants are first able to sweat at about 1 month of age. The epidermis of newborns is thin, predisposing to injury, dermatitis, and absorption of toxins in soaps and lotions. Eczematous dermatitis first manifests during the first year of life in most cases, then gradually subsides. Infectious disorders of the skin such as impetigo and pediculosis are common among school-age children. Young children are an at-risk group for burn injury related to neglect or abuse.

Adolescence and Young Adulthood

The adrenal and gonadal hormone surges at puberty stimulate increased production of sebum, promoting the development of acne vulgaris. Individuals with more severe acne probably have sebaceous glands that are hyper-responsive to androgens. Areas of skin hyperpigmentation may be seen during pregnancy as a result of the effects of the altered hormonal environment. Skin tags, nevi, and hemangiomas may become more numerous or prominent during pregnancy. Stretch marks are caused by stretching of collagen with pregnancy or weight gain. Malignant melanoma commonly presents in young adults.

Middle and Older Adulthood

Both photoaging (cumulative effects of sun exposure) and chronologic aging affect the skin. The epidermis and dermis become thinner, sweat glands decrease in number and function, and sebum production declines. Growth of body hair decreases as a consequence of fewer hair follicles and arrest of many follicles in the telogen, or resting phase. Skin becomes increasingly dry, wrinkled, and furrowed, and turgor is decreased. Nonmalignant lesions common to aging include senile (solar) lentigines (liver spots), telangiectases, purpura, and actinic keratoses. Nonmelanoma skin cancers have their highest incidence in this age group. The elderly are prone to hyperthermia because of decreased ability to sweat. The elderly constitute a high-risk group for burn injury, and their mortality rates are higher because of diminished adaptive responses and possible underlying systemic illnesses.

the external auditory canal secrete protective cerumen (ear wax).

Subcutaneous Tissue

The subcutaneous tissue layer of fat and connective tissue (also known as the *hypodermis*) lends support and texture to the skin layers, insulates against heat loss, and serves as a storage depot for energy fuel. Some hair follicles and eccrine sweat glands extend into this layer. Deposition of lipophilic bilirubin in the subcutaneous fat produces the yellow color of jaundice in hemolytic disorders and biliary tract pathology (see hyperbilirubinemia, Chapter 26).

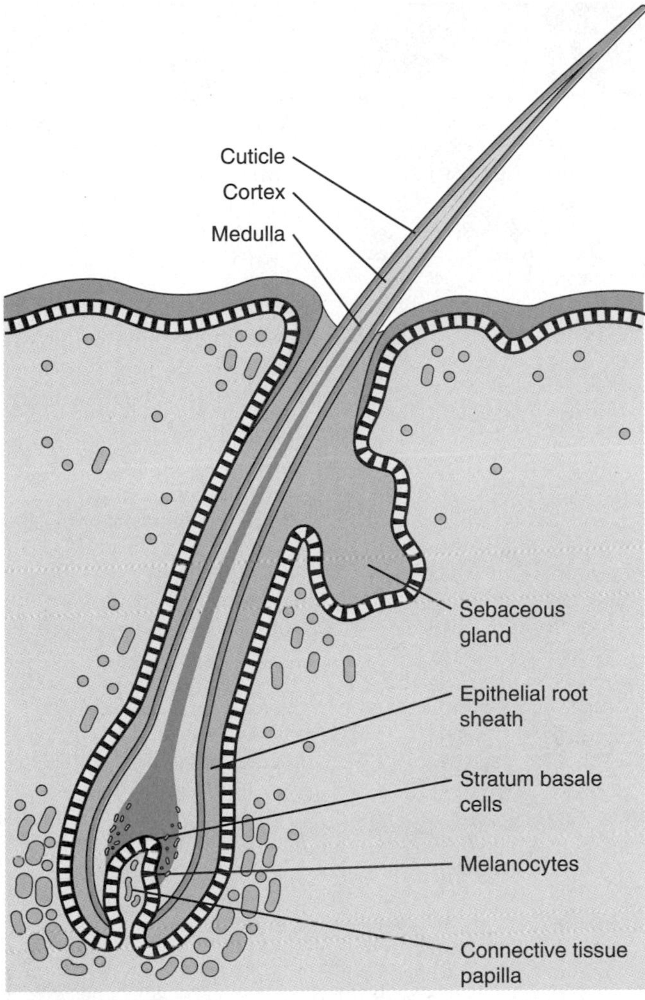

FIGURE 36–3
Hair follicle structure. Hair, like epidermis, is composed of keratinocytes. Hair follicle walls are composed of cells derived from the dermis and epidermis. Melanocytes within the basal layer contribute pigment to the hair.

Hair

Figure 36–3 depicts a typical hair follicle. Hair, like epidermis, is composed of keratinocytes. Hair follicle walls consist of an outer sheath derived from the dermis and an inner sheath formed from an invagination of the epidermis. The epithelial lining of hair follicles may serve as a source of regeneration of epidermis in healing of partial thickness burns, as discussed later in this chapter.

Hair growth results from active division of epithelial cells at the base of the follicle, which is normally richly perfused. In a process similar to epidermal keratinization, new cells formed at the base grow outward and differentiate, overlapping each other in concentric layers. Melanocytes within the basal layer contribute pigment in varying proportions of brown, black, and yellow. With aging, or in some cases extreme stress or systemic illness, melanin production ceases, resulting in gray, then white hair. The pilomotor muscles (arrector pili) are composed of smooth muscle fibers under sympathetic innervation. Their contraction pulls the hair follicle upward, resulting in piloerection, or "goose bumps," a primitive reflex response to fright or environmental cold (see Chapter 11).

Body hair is of two types: *vellus hair*, the fine, silky hair that covers most of the body surface, and *terminal hair*, the coarser, longer hair of the scalp, eyebrows, and, beginning at puberty, the axillary and pubic hair of both sexes and the facial hair and increased body hair of males. Hair growth occurs in repeated cycles throughout the lifetime of the individual, proceeding through *telogen* (resting), *anagen* (growth), and *catagen* (shortening and sloughing) phases. The duration of anagen determines the ultimate length of the hair, and varies in different parts of the body. The rate of hair growth is relatively stable within an individual, with slight spurts typical in the summer, possibly caused by increased stimulation by androgens. Sebaceous secretion is also increased with androgenic stimulation, provid-

TABLE 36–3
DISORDERS AFFECTING HAIR GROWTH AND TEXTURE

Disorder	Associated Conditions
Alopecia (sporadic loss of scalp hair)	Cancer chemotherapy Thyroid disorder Tinea capitis Traumatic hair care practices Alopecia areata (idiopathic) Trichotillomania (habitual rubbing or twisting of hair)
Male pattern baldness (receding hairline or loss of hair at top of head)	Genetic pattern in males Androgen excess in females
Hirsutism (excess facial and body hair in females)	Androgen excess
Abnormal onset, amount, or pattern of pubic hair	Adrenogenital deficiency Precocious puberty
Sudden-onset loss of hair or hair pigment	Extreme stress Severe illness Chemotherapy
Asymmetric loss of hair on extremity	Peripheral arterial disease
Brittle, dry texture of hair	Thyroid disorder Nutritional disorder Normal aging
Dandruff, cradle cap	Seborrheic dermatitis Pediculosis

ing oily protection and nourishment for the skin as well as the hair. The hair follicle with its sebaceous gland is known as the *pilosebaceous unit*. Among the integumentary disorders affecting this unit is **acne vulgaris,** discussed later in this chapter. Many chemotherapeutic agents used in treatment of cancer reversibly arrest hair growth as a consequence of their effects on DNA. Table 36–3 describes common disorders affecting hair growth and texture.

Nails

Nails protect the dorsal surfaces of the fingers and toes. Like hairs, nails consist of modified epidermis (Fig. 36–4). Just as in the skin and hair, keratinocytes divide within a basal layer (in the nail root in this case), and migrate outward over a supportive layer (the nailbed). The nail is enclosed by skin folds (paronychium) except at its distal end, with the eponychium or cuticle extending from the proximal nail fold. Nail growth is regulated by the same factors as skin and is dependent on adequate perfusion and oxygenation. Systemic disorders and local trauma are thus reflected in the characteristics of the nail. Transverse ridges (*Beau's lines*) may reflect altered growth during periods of systemic illness. Superficial vessels below the nail surface permit monitoring of oxygenation and perfusion. Delayed capillary refill after pressure is released from the nailbed reflects lack of distal perfusion, and cyanosis caused by deoxygenated hemoglobin is readily seen with inspection of the nailbeds (see Chapter 15). Table 36–4 summarizes clinical features of selected disorders of the nails.

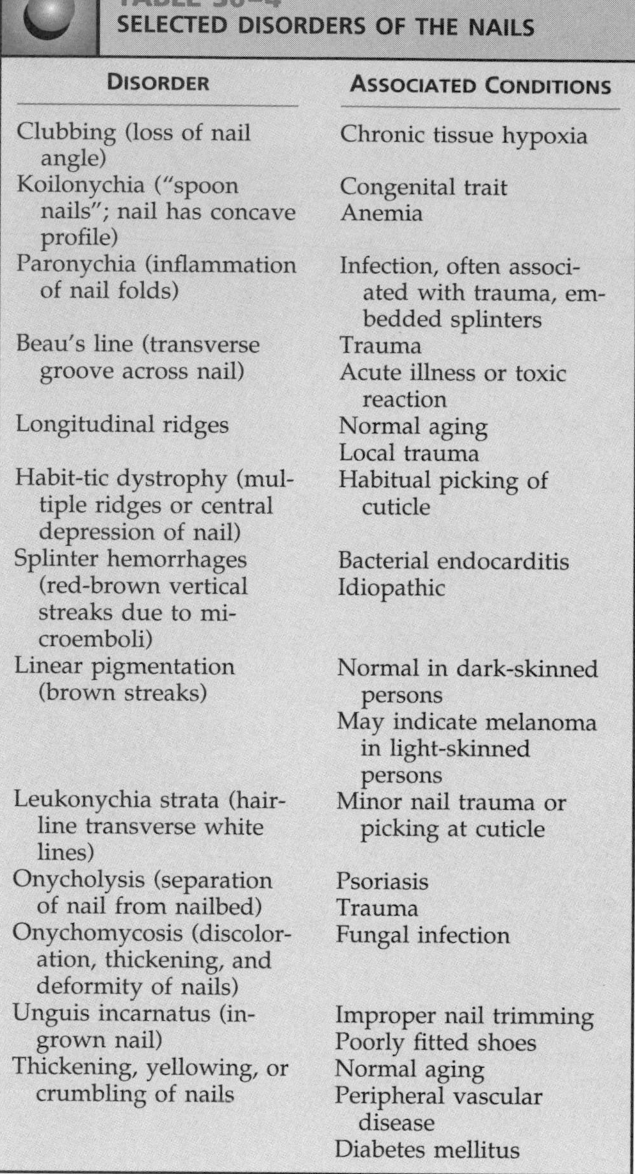

TABLE 36–4
SELECTED DISORDERS OF THE NAILS

Disorder	Associated Conditions
Clubbing (loss of nail angle)	Chronic tissue hypoxia
Koilonychia ("spoon nails"; nail has concave profile)	Congenital trait Anemia
Paronychia (inflammation of nail folds)	Infection, often associated with trauma, embedded splinters
Beau's line (transverse groove across nail)	Trauma Acute illness or toxic reaction
Longitudinal ridges	Normal aging Local trauma
Habit-tic dystrophy (multiple ridges or central depression of nail)	Habitual picking of cuticle
Splinter hemorrhages (red-brown vertical streaks due to microemboli)	Bacterial endocarditis Idiopathic
Linear pigmentation (brown streaks)	Normal in dark-skinned persons May indicate melanoma in light-skinned persons
Leukonychia strata (hairline transverse white lines)	Minor nail trauma or picking at cuticle
Onycholysis (separation of nail from nailbed)	Psoriasis Trauma
Onychomycosis (discoloration, thickening, and deformity of nails)	Fungal infection
Unguis incarnatus (ingrown nail)	Improper nail trimming Poorly fitted shoes
Thickening, yellowing, or crumbling of nails	Normal aging Peripheral vascular disease Diabetes mellitus

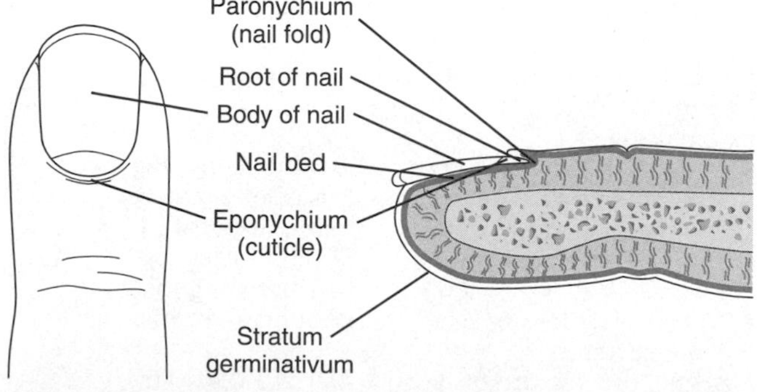

FIGURE 36–4
Nail structure. Keratinocytes divide at the root of the nail and migrate outward over a supportive layer, the nail bed. The nail is enclosed by nail folds (paronychium) except at the distal end. The cuticle (eponychium) protects the nail root.

REGULATION OF INTEGUMENTARY FUNCTION

As is true of other organ systems, the integument is subject to regulation by neural, endocrine, and local stimuli.

Neural Regulation

As the primary interface between the human being and the environment, the skin is replete with sensory receptors for pain, touch, and temperature.

These specialized structures receive and transmit sensory information to the central nervous system, initiating reflex and voluntary motor responses as well as autonomic responses. Sensitivity of these receptors varies physiologically, as discussed in Chapter 23.

The complex sensations of tickle and itch are also readily perceived, although the mechanisms are incompletely understood. Itching, or **pruritus**, is a common manifestation of skin disorders. Pruritic sensations arise from stimulation of sensory receptors (free nerve endings) in the junction between the dermis and epidermis and are transmitted along unmyelinated C fibers of the lateral spinothalamic tract to the cerebral cortex.[1] This pathway also carries pain impulses, and the neuromodulators involved in transmission of itch sensation are the same as those for pain (substance P, calcitonin gene-related peptide, somatostatin, and neurokinins). Histamine, released by mast cells near the free nerve endings, is one of several chemicals capable of initiating the sensation of pruritus.

Skin blood vessels are subject to regulation by autonomic innervation via α-adrenergic receptors. Neurally mediated alterations in skin perfusion are critical to thermoregulation (see Chapter 11) and to the selective vasoconstriction that characterizes the stress response (see Chapter 1) and the compensatory stage of shock (see Chapter 15).

Regulation by Hormones and Local Mediators

Local mediators (endothelial cytokines and mechanical factors) are also essential to regulation of all peripheral perfusion, including that of the skin, hair, and nails. Regulation of cellular growth and glandular secretion by the integument is genetically programmed, but clearly subject to other regulatory factors as well.

Integumentary cells in men and women have receptors for androgens, which are known to stimulate hair growth and sebaceous secretion. The integumentary response to a given androgen level is highly variable in different areas of the body and between individuals, demonstrating that other regulatory factors are also involved. Recently, estrogen replacement therapy has been shown to decrease the degeneration of collagen that was once believed to be a genetically programmed consequence of aging.[2] Estrogen and other hormones of pregnancy are believed to mediate the changes in skin and hair that commonly occur in pregnant women (see Chapter 32). Oral contraceptives may have similar effects.

Glucocorticoid excess in Cushing's syndrome is associated with dysfunction of the pilosebaceous unit, predisposing to acne and hirsutism (see Chapter 29). Melanocyte-stimulating hormone (MSH), produced by the anterior pituitary gland, mediates baseline melanin production. Excess adrenocorticotropic hormone (ACTH) (as in Addison's disease) results in hyperpigmentation of the skin because of melanocyte stimulation by the MSH subunit of ACTH (see Chapter 27). Hyperprolactinemia is associated with hirsutism and increased sebum production, and thyroid disorders manifest as altered hair quality and growth. Growth hormone may sensitize receptors in the pilosebaceous units to the effects of androgens.

Nutritional factors, including vitamins A and C, are essential to keratinization. Nutritional deficiencies, whether dietary or caused by lack of perfusion, are often evidenced by dry, scaly skin; brittle hair and nails; and delayed wound healing. Exposure of the skin to UV rays provokes physiologic (melanin production and vitamin D_3 activation) and pathologic (degenerative and neoplastic changes) responses. Keratinocytes are known to synthesize a number of cytokines that influence keratinization as well as the function of dermal appendages, although the mechanisms of this regulation are poorly understood. Interestingly, the epidermis contains levels of interleukin-1 (IL-1) up to 100 times higher than in other tissues (see Focus of Current Research).[3]

SKIN LESIONS

Classification of Skin Lesions

The language of *dermatology*, the medical specialty that focuses on integumentary disorders, classifies skin lesions on the bases of primary or secondary origin, morphology, and distribution.

Primary Skin Lesions

Primary skin lesions are those that arise from previously normal skin. These are classified morphologically as *macules, papules, plaques, patches, nodules, tumors, wheals, cysts, vesicles, bullae,* or *pustules* (Fig. 36–5). Table 36–5 lists examples of disorders characterized by each of these types of lesions.

Secondary Skin Lesions

Secondary skin lesions are those that arise as a consequence of rupture, mechanical irritation, extension, invasion, normal healing, or abnormal healing of primary lesions. These include *erosions, ulcers, fissures, crusts, scales, lichenification* (thickening and hardening with exaggeration of normal markings),

Focus of Current Research

Study	Objective and Findings
Stern, et al. (1997) Malignant melanoma in patients treated for psoriasis with methoxsalen (psoralen) and ultraviolet A radiation (PUVA).	*Objective:* To study the occurrence of melanoma among patients treated with PUVA *Findings:* About 15 years after the first treatment with PUVA, the risk of melanoma increases, especially among patients who receive 250 treatments or more.
Rabkin, et al. (1997) Monoclonal origin of multicentric Kaposi's sarcoma lesions.	*Objective:* To test the hypothesis that the spindle cells in Kaposi's sarcoma lesions originate from a single clone of precursor cells *Findings:* Kaposi's sarcoma is a disseminated monoclonal cancer.
Lucky, et al. (1997) Predictors of severity of acne vulgaris in young adolescent girls: Results of a five-year longitudinal study.	*Objective:* To determine which factors in early pubertal girls are predictive of later, severe facial acne *Findings:* The early development of comedonal acne is one of the best predictors of later, more severe disease. Androgens play a role in the perpetuation of severe acne.
Clark, et al. (1996) Effects of selenium supplementation for cancer prevention in patients with carcinoma of the skin: A randomized controlled trial.	*Objective:* To determine whether a nutritional supplement of selenium will decrease the incidence of cancer *Findings:* Selenium treatment did not protect against development of basal cell or squamous cell carcinomas of the skin.
Schwartz, et al. (1996) Current and future management of serious skin and skin-structure infections.	*Objective:* To compare the efficacy and safety of cefepime with that of ceftazidime in patients with serious skin and skin-structure infections *Findings:* Cefepime, a new parenteral cephalosporin administered every 12 hours, is an effective alternative to ceftazidime given every 8 hours.
Eller, et al. (1995) A role for interleukin-1 in epidermal differentiation: Regulation by expression of functional versus decoy receptors.	*Objective:* To determine the role of interleukin-1 (IL-1) in epidermal biology *Findings:* Epidermal IL-1 probably functions to promote keratinocyte differentiation.
Meinking, et al. (1995) The treatment of scabies with ivermectin.	*Objective:* To determine whether the antihelmintic agent ivermectin is effective treatment in scabies *Findings:* Ivermectin is an effective agent for treatment of scabies in otherwise healthy patients and in many patients with HIV infection.

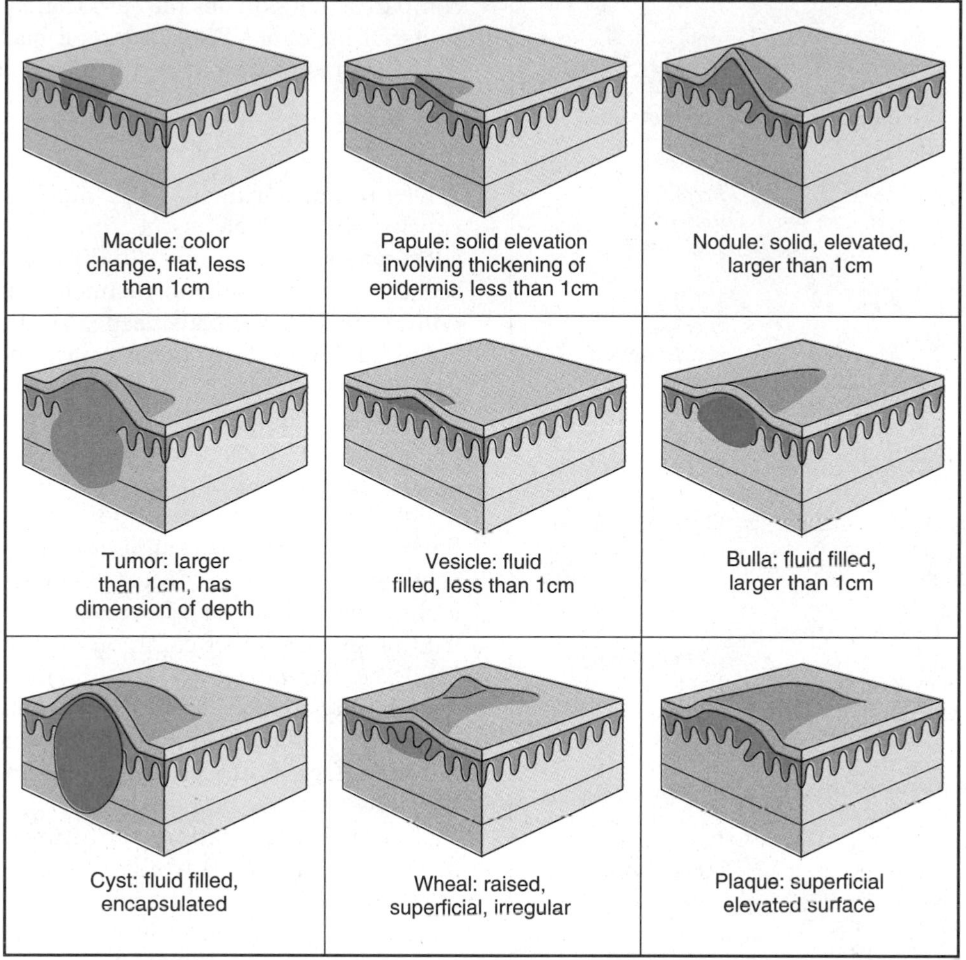

FIGURE 36–5
Primary skin lesions. Primary skin lesions arise from previously normal skin.

excoriations (scratches), *scars,* and *keloids* (hypertrophic scars) (Fig. 36–6).

Distribution of Skin Lesions

The configuration of lesions and their relationship to each other, that is, the nature of the rash or **exanthem**, is often important in determining the underlying cause (Fig. 36–7). Examples of disorders characterized by different configurations or distributions of skin lesions are listed in Table 36–6.

Lesions Associated with Systemic Diseases

In addition to signaling the presence of primary integumentary disorders, skin manifestations may often be clues to the presence of underlying systemic disease. Genetic disorders (inborn errors of metabolism), connective tissue diseases, hematopoietic disorders, sepsis, and neoplasia are commonly characterized by integumentary changes. Table 36–7 lists examples of skin lesions associated with each of these etiologies.

Cutaneous Reactions to Drugs

Adverse cutaneous drug reactions affect 2% to 3% of hospitalized patients[4] and certainly many more outpatients. In most cases, these reactions are not severe, but approximately 1 in 1000 patients has a life-threatening reaction. Common skin reactions to drugs, along with the usual initiating agents, are described in Table 36–8.

TABLE 36–5
EXAMPLES OF PRIMARY SKIN LESIONS

Lesion	Description	Examples
Pigment Changes		
Macule	Flat, circumscribed, <1 cm diameter; tan, brown, or red	Freckles Flat nevi Petechiae Liver spots Vitiligo Measles Scarlet fever
Patch	Coalescence of macules; >1 cm diameter	Mongolian spot Mask of pregnancy Measles
Solid Lesions		
Papule	Solid, elevated, circumscribed; <1 cm diameter	Elevated nevus Lichen planus Molluscum Warts
Plaque	Coalescence of papules; >1 cm diameter	Psoriasis Lichen planus
Nodule	Solid, elevated, lesion >1 cm diameter; deeper than plaque	Xanthoma Fibroma Intradermal nevus
Tumor	Larger and deeper than nodule	Lipoma Hemangioma Carcinoma
Wheal	Superficial, raised erythematous lesion; irregular shape; often associated with angioedema	Urticaria Mosquito bite
Fluid-Filled Lesions		
Vesicle	Elevated lesion with cavity containing clear fluid; <1 cm diameter	Herpes simplex Herpes zoster Varicella Contact dermatitis
Bulla	Similar to vesicle but >1 cm diameter	Pemphigus Burns Contact dermatitis Friction blister
Pustule	Similar to vesicle but filled with pus	Acne vulgaris Impetigo
Cyst	Similar to pustule but larger and deeper	Acne vulgaris Sebaceous cyst Epidermal cyst (wen)

Adapted from Jarvis, C. (1992). *Physical Examination and Health Assessment*. Philadelphia: W.B. Saunders. (pp. 257–258).

PRIMARY DISORDERS OF THE INTEGUMENT

Bacterial Infections

The most common bacterial infections of the skin are **furunculosis, folliculitis, impetigo,** and **cellulitis**. These disorders are detailed below. Figure 36–8 compares the skin lesions associated with common bacterial infections. Less common bacterial infections of the skin are summarized in Table 36–9.

Furunculosis

Definition. Furunculosis is the formation of a furuncle (boil), which is an abscess of the skin and subcutaneous tissue surrounding a hair follicle or sebaceous gland. Several furuncles may interconnect within the subcutaneous tissue, forming a *carbuncle*.

Epidemiology. The precise incidence is unknown, because many cases are probably self-treated. Furuncles are seen in individuals of all ages. Risk factors include poor hygiene, occupational exposure to grease or oil, infection of pre-existing skin lesions, malnutrition, alcoholism, and immunosuppression.[5] For unknown reasons, athletes are particularly susceptible to furuncles. Most patients do not have identifiable risk factors, however.

Etiology. The most common causative organism is *Staphylococcus aureus*.

Pathophysiology. Infection results in inflammation of perifollicular tissues of hairy skin, usually of the neck, face, buttocks, thighs, perineum, breast, or axillae.

Clinical Manifestations. A furuncle appears as an indurated (hardened), dull red nodule with a pus-filled core. Carbuncles are similar in appearance, but larger, and usually drain pus through several points in the skin surface. Systemic signs of inflammation, including fever and enlargement of adjacent lymph nodes, may be present with severe cases.

Prevention and Treatment. If known risk factors are present, they should be minimized, although such intervention has often been unsuccessful.[5] Furuncles and carbuncles are treated with good hygiene and warm compresses to support the inflammatory response. Oral antibiotic therapy (usually penicillin) is administered for at least a 2-week course. Surgical drainage and débridement may speed resolution of lesions.

Prognosis and Outcome. Acute inflammation usually resolves within 2 weeks; however, the overlying skin may remain reddened for several weeks. Drainage of large carbuncles leaves an ulcer that may heal with scarring.

Folliculitis

Definition. Folliculitis is inflammation within the hair follicle, resulting in the formation of pustules.

Epidemiology. The precise incidence is unknown, because many individuals do not seek treatment. Risk factors include poor hygiene, maceration (softening) of the skin with water because of prolonged

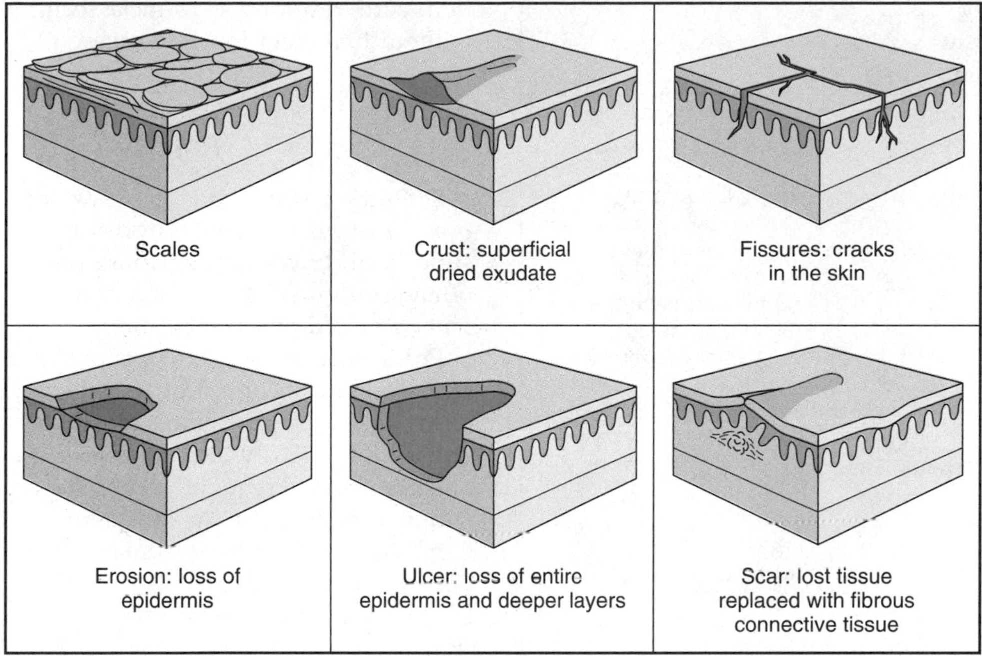

FIGURE 36–6

Secondary skin lesions. Secondary skin lesions arise as a consequence of rupture, mechanical irritation, extension, invasion, or healing of primary skin lesions.

soaking or occlusive dressings, occupational exposure to solvents, and immunosuppression.[5] Impairment of the normal skin flora with long-term antibiotic therapy also constitutes a risk.

Etiology. The usual cause of superficial folliculitis is *S. aureus*. Gram-negative folliculitis is more common with long-term antibiotic therapy (often for treatment of acne) and usually results from *Kleb-*

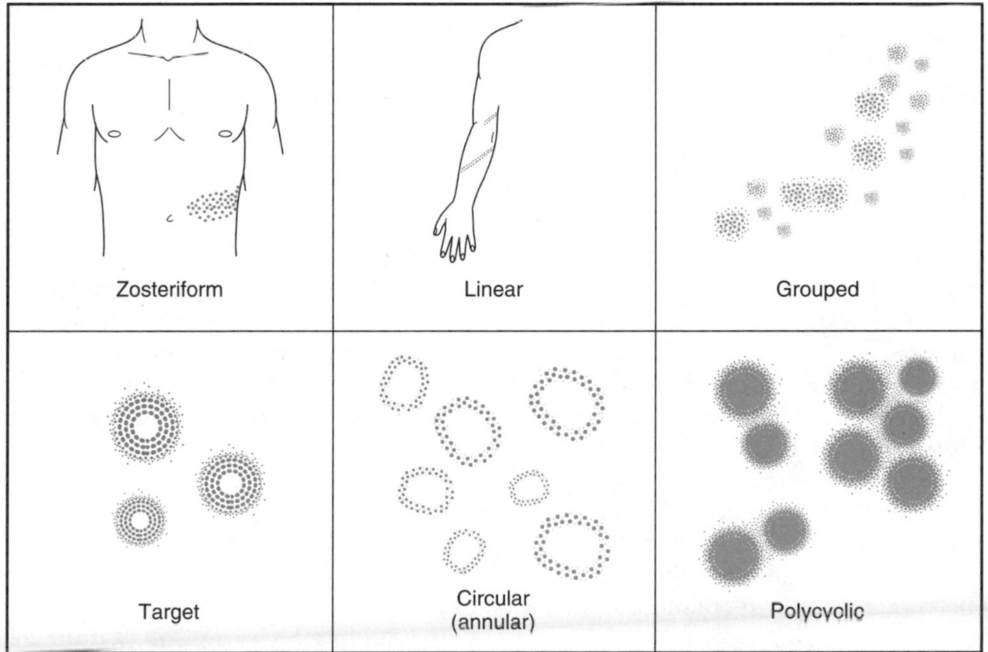

FIGURE 36–7

Configuration and distribution of lesions. Superficial characteristics of lesions and the relationship of multiple lesions to each other may provide clues to the underlying cause.

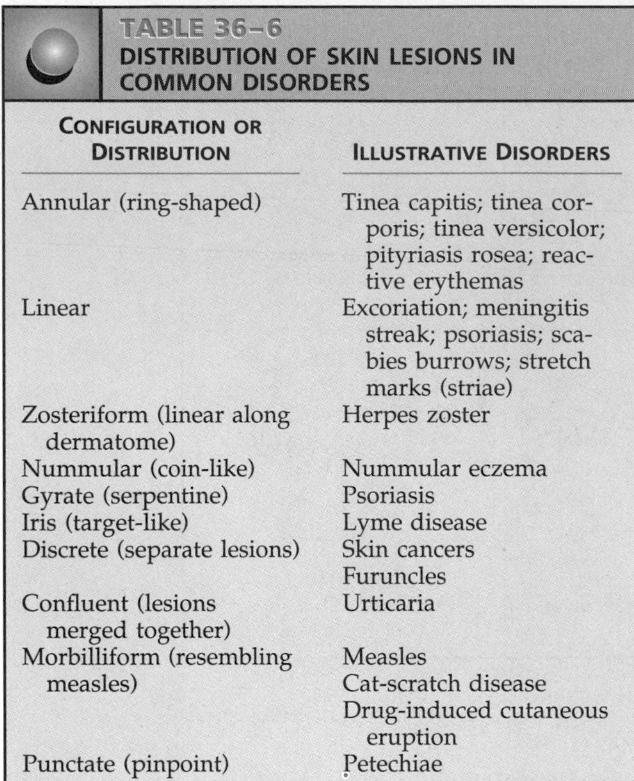

TABLE 36–6
DISTRIBUTION OF SKIN LESIONS IN COMMON DISORDERS

Configuration or Distribution	Illustrative Disorders
Annular (ring-shaped)	Tinea capitis; tinea corporis; tinea versicolor; pityriasis rosea; reactive erythemas
Linear	Excoriation; meningitis streak; psoriasis; scabies burrows; stretch marks (striae)
Zosteriform (linear along dermatome)	Herpes zoster
Nummular (coin-like)	Nummular eczema
Gyrate (serpentine)	Psoriasis
Iris (target-like)	Lyme disease
Discrete (separate lesions)	Skin cancers Furuncles
Confluent (lesions merged together)	Urticaria
Morbilliform (resembling measles)	Measles Cat-scratch disease Drug-induced cutaneous eruption
Punctate (pinpoint)	Petechiae

siella, Enterobacter, or *Proteus*. A newer variant, "hot-tub folliculitis," is caused by *Pseudomonas aeruginosa*, an organism that thrives in the low chlorine, high pH, warm environment of hot tubs and whirlpools.[5]

Pathophysiology. Organisms gain access, possibly assisted by skin barrier breakdown, and initiate inflammation within hair follicles.

Clinical Manifestations. Superficial folliculitis manifests as small pustules at the openings of hair follicles. Lesions may be single or multiple and typically appear on the scalp, back, and extremities. Pruritus is often quite severe. Gram-negative folliculitis is usually deeper and more nodular, typically involving the skin around the nose. Hot-tub folliculitis affects areas exposed to water. There are usually no systemic manifestations.

Prevention and Treatment. Known risk factors should be avoided. Treatment consists of topical antibiotics (i.e., solutions applied directly to the skin) in the case of superficial folliculitis. Erythromycin (E-Mycin) is the usual drug of choice. Oral antibiotics such as amoxicillin-claviculanate (Augmentin) are used in treatment of gram-negative folliculitis. Hot-tub folliculitis usually resolves spontaneously with avoidance of tub use.

Prognosis and Outcome. Folliculitis usually resolves within 2 to 3 weeks. Extension of inflammation with resulting carbuncle formation may occur without treatment in some cases.

Impetigo

Definition. Impetigo, the most prevalent type of *pyoderma* (pus-forming skin disease), is a contagious, superficial, crust-forming infection of the skin, most often seen in children. There are two forms: *impetigo contagiosa* and *impetigo bullosa*.

Epidemiology. Impetigo is the most common pediatric skin infection, but it may occur in people of all ages. Exposure to causative organisms increases risk of impetigo, which is endemic in the southern United States. Frequent outbreaks occur during the summer months in the northern United States. Insect bites and minor trauma that disrupt the skin barrier may increase risk. Individuals who are chronic carriers of *S. aureus* in their oropharyngeal tissues are also at higher risk.

Etiology. Impetigo contagiosa is usually caused by either *S. aureus* or group A β-hemolytic streptococci.[6] Impetigo bullosa is usually caused by a toxin produced by *S. aureus*.

Pathophysiology. Impetigo contagiosa results from entry of the organism through traumatized skin and triggers superficial infection. Impetigo bullosa inflames nontraumatized skin via chemical trauma produced by the bacterial toxin. Inflammation results in pus formation in impetigo contagiosa, and impetigo bullosa is nonpurulent. Impetigo contagiosa caused by streptococci results in subsequent acute glomerulonephritis in 2% to 6% of cases, most often in children younger than 6 years. This form of acute glomerulonephritis is caused by a delayed hypersensitivity reaction and is associated with particular nephritogenic strains of streptococcus (see Chapter 20). Unlike "strep throat," streptococcal impetigo does not give rise to rheumatic fever and subsequent cardiac complications.[7] Rare complications of impetigo bullosa result from systemic extension of the staph infection and include **scarlet fever**, **scalded skin syndrome**, pneumonia, and meningitis.

Clinical Manifestations. Impetigo contagiosa usually affects exposed surfaces, beginning with small vesicles that later become pustules. Distribution is usually *annular* (in the shape of a circle or arc). Drainage from these vesicles forms a honey-colored crust that sticks to the lesions. Impetigo bullosa begins with small vesicles on nonexposed skin. Vesicles develop into bullae, larger lesions filled with clear fluid, which rupture within 24 to 48 hours, leaving a thin, "varnish-like" crust. Lesions are nonpainful, but itching is usually present.

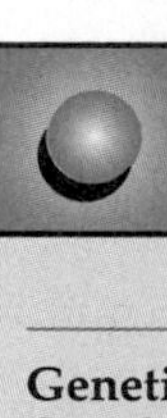

TABLE 36–7
SKIN LESIONS ASSOCIATED WITH SYSTEMIC DISEASE

Systemic Disorder	Associated Skin Lesions
Genetic Disorders	
Cowden's disease (multiple hamartoma syndrome)	Multiple papules of the face, oral cavity, palms of hands and soles of feet
Connective Tissue Diseases	
Dermatomyositis	Gottron's papules over knuckles or other bony prominences; heliotrope (violet or red) rash in periorbital region; poikiloderma (erythema, scaling, telangiectasia, and atrophy) on sun-exposed areas
Eosinophilia myalgia syndrome (caused by ingestion of L-tryptophan)	Urticaria, macules, papules, or hyperpigmented lesions; severe pruritus; alopecia
Amyloidosis	Purpura, oral papules
Systemic lupus erythematosus	Malar rash, discoid lupus erythematosus, photosensitivity
Systemic sclerosis	Scleroderma, CREST syndrome
Hematopoietic Disorders	
Anticoagulant therapy	Skin necrosis
Chronic myelogenous leukemia, polycythemia vera	Atypical or bullous pyoderma
Acute myelogenous leukemia	Sweet's syndrome (painful, erythematous plaques on arms, head, and neck)
Hemophilias and thrombocytopenias	Petechiae, purpura, ecchymoses
Sepsis	
Lyme disease	Erythema migrans (expanding red plaque) or target-like lesion
AIDS	Bacillary angiomatosis (subcutaneous vascular lesions caused by infection with *Bartonella bacilliformis*); eosinophilic folliculitis; pruritic papules
Toxic shock syndrome	Erythema, bullae, exfoliation
Cat-scratch disease	Papules or pustules at site of inoculation; morbilliform rash with macules, papules, erythema nodosum, erythema multiforme, erythema marginatum, or petechiae
Neoplasia	
Widespread metastatic carcinoma	Sister Mary Joseph's nodule (red, white, bluish violet, and brownish red nodule or hardened area near the umbilicus); may signify underlying adenocarcinoma
Leukemia or lymphoma	Paraneoplastic pemphigus; dermatitis herpetiformis (pruritic papulovesicular rash); leukemia cutis (papules and nodules caused by infiltration of leukemic cells into the skin)
Intra-abdominal cancer	Acanthosis nigricans
Paget's disease	Erythematous, exudative plaque of nipple area, vulva, perianal area, penis, scrotum, groin
Hodgkin's disease	Ichthyosis (dry scaliness), exfoliation, pruritus, papules, nodules

Prevention and Treatment. Prevention involves good hygiene and avoidance of minor trauma and insect bites whenever possible. Topical antibiotic therapy is effective if there are only a few lesions, but oral therapy is also required in most cases. Topical mupirocin (Bactroban) is particularly effective against staphylococcus species.[5] Dicloxacillin (Dynapen) may be used for treatment of resistant strains. Antibiotic therapy does not prevent acute glomerulonephritis in susceptible persons.

Prognosis and Outcome. Most cases of impetigo respond to antibiotic therapy with no complications, but recurrences are common.

Cellulitis

Definition. Cellulitis is diffuse, pus-forming inflammation of the dermis and subcutaneous tissue (Color Fig. 36–1).

Epidemiology. Any existing break in the integrity of skin imposes risk for cellulitis. Skin trauma and superficial skin infections are the usual predisposing factors.

TABLE 36–8
ADVERSE CUTANEOUS REACTIONS TO DRUGS

DRUG ERUPTION	ASSOCIATED MEDICATIONS
Erythema	Bismuth, barbiturates, sulfonamides, antihistamines, penicillins
Lichenoid or eczematous	Gold, quinidine, methyldopa, antituberculin agents, antidysrhythmics, antiepileptics
Acneiform lesions	Corticosteroids, bromides, iodides
Urticaria	Penicillins, antibiotics, vaccines
Bullae	Iodides, penicillamine, bleomycin
Exfoliation	Gold
Nodules	Sulfathiazole, salicylates, oral contraceptives
Photodermatitis	Phenothiazines, chlorothiazide, dimeclocycline, griseofulvin, oral hypoglycemics
Erythema multiforme (macules, papules, vesicles, bullae, and "target" lesions); Variants: (1) severe, febrile form known as Stevens-Johnson syndrome; (2) diffuse exfoliative form known as toxic epidermal necrolysis	Allopurinol, barbiturates, dapsone, digitalis, phenytoin, gold, hydralazine, salicylates, sulfonamides, tetracycline, trimethoprim-sulfamethoxazole; aminopenicillins, carbamazepine, phenylbutazone, piroxicam, chlormezanone, amithiozone
Necrosis	Warfarin, heparin
Angioedema	Penicillin, cephalosporins, contrast media, anesthetics, nonsteroidal anti-inflammatory drugs, angiotensin-converting enzyme inhibitors

Adapted with permission from Beacham, B.E. (1993). Common dermatoses in the elderly. *American Family Physician* 47(6), 1447. Published by the American Academy of Family Physicians.

Etiology. The usual causative organisms are *S. aureus* and β-hemolytic streptococci.

Pathophysiology. Cellulitis represents failure of the inflammatory response to adequately contain the infecting organism, permitting wider and deeper extension. The potential for hematogenous or lymphatic dissemination of infection exists, especially in young children and the elderly.[6] Systemic manifestations of inflammation may precede the development of skin lesions.

Clinical Manifestations. The individual may or may not be aware of the initial skin trauma or infection site. Malaise and fever often precede the appearance of skin lesions, which begin as isolated, solid red lesions that coalesce to form a larger red, raised, warm plaque. Vesicles may also develop within the area, often at the edges. The inflamed area is usually tender and pruritic. Bacteremia may be present, potentially leading to septic shock.

Prevention and Treatment. Optimal care of minor skin trauma and infections may prevent the development of cellulitis in some cases. Systemic antibiotic therapy, appropriate to the causative organism, is the definitive treatment. Cold compresses, bedrest, and elevation of the affected area may provide some symptomatic relief.

Prognosis and Outcome. Except in immunosuppressed individuals, cellulitis is usually successfully resolved with antibiotic therapy. **Gangrene** (tissue necrosis) and toxic shock syndrome (systemic sepsis) are rare complications.

Fungal Infections

Superficial fungal infections of the skin are common in clinical practice. Fungi that can infect and survive on the keratin in hair, nails, and the dead top layer of skin are known as *dermatophytes*. The most common of the fungal disorders, **tinea** and

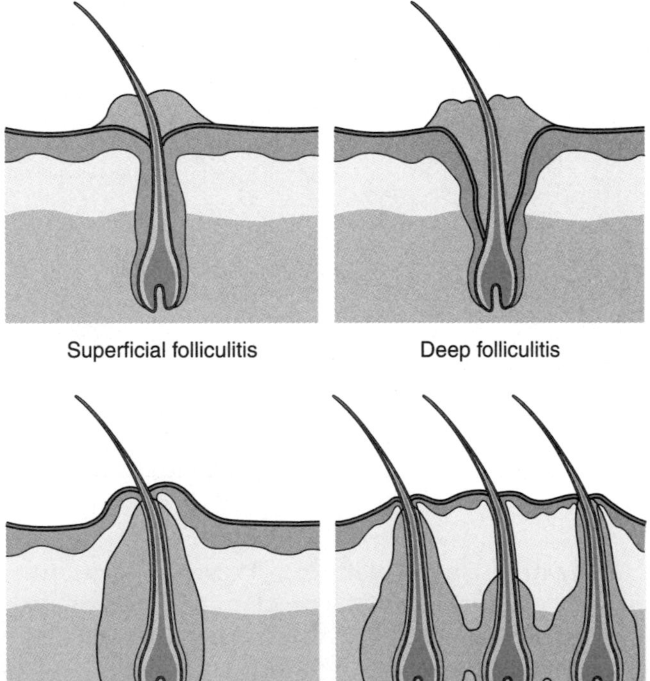

FIGURE 36–8
Comparison of bacterial skin infections. Bacterial infection of the skin, often caused by *Staphylococcus aureus*, may form pustules within the hair follicle (folliculitis) or an abscess of the skin and subcutaneous tissue surrounding a hair follicle or sweat gland (furunculosis). A carbuncle is formed when several adjacent follicles and their subcutaneous tissues are affected.

TABLE 36–9
LESS COMMON BACTERIAL INFECTIONS OF THE SKIN

Disorder	Description
Leprosy (Hansen's disease)	Slowly progressive infection of the skin and peripheral nerves leading to deformity and disability; caused by *Mycobacterium leprae,* which is endemic in poor tropical countries
Erysipelas	Streptococcal infection of the superficial layers of the skin and cutaneous lymphatics; characterized by raised, erythematous areas that are well-demarcated; usually affecting the face
Necrotizing fasciitis	Streptococcal infection of deep tissues resulting in progressive destruction of fascia and fat; may complicate primary trauma of the skin or other skin infections; may precede toxic shock syndrome
Gas gangrene	Clostridial infection complicating trauma, crush injuries, neoplasia, or chemotherapy
Secondary syphilis	Macular or papular disseminated rash caused by *Treponema pallidum;* follows primary venereal infection in 6 to 8 weeks
Scarlet fever	Associated with group A streptococcal pharyngitis and tonsillitis; rash is punctate and erythematous, involving the face, trunk, and inner aspects of the arms and legs
Scalded skin syndrome	Generalized exfoliative dermatitis caused by infection with certain strains of *Staphylococcus aureus;* typically occurs in newborns and children under the age of 5; rash similar to that of scarlet fever progressing to large bullae that ulcerate, leaving a wound similar to a major burn

candidiasis, are detailed below, and others are summarized in Table 36–10.

Tinea

Definition. Tinea infections are fungal infections of superficial skin layers, classified according to their body location. *Tinea corporis* ("body ringworm") is found on the skin of the trunk and extremities, excluding the head, hands, feet, and groin. *Tinea capitis* ("scalp ringworm") is found on the scalp (Color Fig. 36–2). *Tinea cruris* ("jock itch") is located in the groin of males, and *tinea pedis* ("athlete's foot") is found on the feet. *Tinea manuum* affects the hands, and *tinea unguium* affects the toenails or fingernails.[8] *Tinea versicolor* is usually located on the upper trunk and is so named because of the varied pigmentation associated with the lesions.[9]

Epidemiology. Tinea infections are very common, especially among children and athletes. The fungus is acquired through contact with contaminated objects or surfaces (*fomites*) or from direct person-to-person or animal-to-person transmission. Risk factors include activities where contact with the fungus is likely, suppression of normal flora organisms (as with antibiotic therapy), and obesity, in which skin fold (intertriginous) areas may provide the ideal conditions for fungal growth. Maceration of the skin with water sports or sweating in poorly ventilated shoes or clothing may also contribute to risk.

Etiology. Tinea infections are usually caused by *Microsporum, Trichophyton,* or *Epidermophyton* species. These organisms are not highly infectious, and infection does not confer immunity.[8]

Pathophysiology. The fungi feed on the dead cells

TABLE 36–10
LESS COMMON FUNGAL INFECTIONS OF THE SKIN

Disorder	Description
Cryptococcosis	Caused by inhalation of *Cryptococcus neoformans,* found in the soil and in bird droppings; may be caused by disseminated infection including skin manifestations in immunosuppressed persons
Aspergillosis	Caused by infection with *Aspergillus* species; disseminated to skin in less than 5% of patients; increased risk in immunosuppressed persons; single or multiple papules that become pustular
Fusariosis	Caused by *Fusarium* species found in contaminated grain; may cause disseminated infection in immunosuppressed patients; skin and soft tissue lesions are small, rounded, grayish lesions that ulcerate and become covered with a black eschar

of the outer skin layers, preferring dark, warm, moist areas. Deep invasion and systemic dissemination are rare, but may occur in immunosuppressed individuals.[8]

Clinical Manifestations. The classic "ringworm" or annular distribution is not always seen, but is characteristic of tinea corporis and tinea capitis (see Color Fig. 36–2). Pustules are surrounded by redness (erythema) and associated with scaling. Itching is often severe. With tinea capitis, oval patches of hair loss (**alopecia**) also result. Tinea cruris causes similar lesions in the groin, possibly extending to the inner thighs but not involving the scrotum. Tinea pedis often begins in the intertriginous area between the fourth and fifth toes, then extends to the plantar surface (bottom) of the foot. Tinea versicolor usually presents as small, scaly, hyperpigmented or hypopigmented patches.[9] The term *tinea incognito* refers to an inflamed, scaling rash that is mistaken for eczematous dermatitis.[8]

Prevention and Treatment. Reduction of risk factors is warranted. In concentrated outbreaks, efforts are made to locate and treat the source. Tinea is treated with topical antifungal sprays, ointments, lotions, gels, or powders, such as undecylenic acid (Cruex, Desenex), tolnaftate (Aftate, Tinactin), ciclopirox (Loprox), or imidazoles (Monistat, Nizoral). Oral antifungal drugs such as griseofulvin (Fulvicin) or ketoconazole (Nizoral) are used for extensive infections and for tinea capitis and tinea unguium, in which topical medication cannot reach the source of infection.[8]

Prognosis and Outcome. Tinea usually resolves with appropriate drug therapy and risk reduction.

Candidiasis

Definition. Candidiasis (*moniliasis*) is superficial fungal infection of the skin or mucous membranes caused by *Candida albicans*. Candidiasis of the oral mucosa is known as *thrush*. Candidiasis of the vagina (vaginitis) and penis (balanitis) may be sexually transmitted (see Chapter 30).

Epidemiology. Candidiasis is common, especially in children; in immunosuppressed individuals, including those with acquired immunodeficiency syndrome (AIDS) or those on glucocorticoid therapy; in individuals receiving long-term antibiotic therapy; and as a sexually transmitted infection or perinatal infection. Pregnancy and diabetes mellitus are also associated with higher rates of candidiasis, as are other endocrine disorders and presence of indwelling catheters and intravenous lines.[10] Warm, moist skin areas best support the infection.

Etiology. *Candida* species (usually *Candida albicans*) are normal flora organisms of the skin, mouth, gastrointestinal (GI) tract, and genitalia in many individuals. Candida overgrowth and infection may occur as a result of depletion of competing organisms in the normal flora with antibiotic therapy. The fungus may be transmitted sexually, and infants may become infected via a nipple infection or vaginal infection in the mother. A severe, disseminated form of candidiasis may occur in those with neutropenia (deficiency of neutrophils) caused by bone marrow suppression (see Chapter 12).[11]

Pathophysiology. The organism penetrates the epidermis after first binding to integrin receptors and other adhesion molecules. Secretion of proteolytic enzymes then facilitates tissue invasion. Inflammation results from attraction of neutrophils to the area and from activation of the complement cascade by the alternative pathway (see Chapter 13).

Clinical Manifestations. Superficial papules and pustules are seen on a red, swollen area of epidermis or mucous membrane. As inflammation continues, a whitish yellow, curd-like crust soon covers the infected area. Lesions are painful and pruritic and may ulcerate with chronic infection.

Prevention and Treatment. Risk factors should be minimized as much as possible, including indiscriminate use of antibiotics and glucocorticoids. Treatment of the underlying disorder in immunosuppression or neutropenia is warranted. Superficial candidiasis is treated similarly to tinea, with antifungal agents such as miconazole, nystatin (Mycostatin), or ketoconazole. Disseminated candidiasis is treated with intravenous or oral antifungal agents such as amphotericin B (Fungizone), fluconazole (Diflucan), or flucytosine (Ancobon).[11]

Prognosis and Outcome. Candidiasis usually responds to antifungal therapy, but may recur chronically if risk factors persist.

Viral Infections

Viral infections affecting the skin are of two types: (1) those in which the skin is the principal site of viral replication and (2) those in which the skin rash is one of several manifestations of systemic viral infection. The most common examples of the former are **verrucae** (warts), **herpes simplex** (cold sores and genital herpes), and **herpes zoster** (shingles) (Color Fig. 36–3). **Rubeola** ("hard" measles), **rubella** (German measles), and **varicella** (chickenpox) (Color Fig. 36–4) are the most common examples of the latter. These disorders are detailed in the following section. Clinical features of other viral infections affecting the skin are summarized in Table 36–11.

TABLE 36–11
LESS COMMON VIRAL INFECTIONS AFFECTING THE SKIN

Disorder	Description
Molluscum contagiosum	Superficial cutaneous infection of children caused by a Poxviridae virus; lesions are smooth, firm, shiny, hemispherical papules with depressed centers; may be solitary or grouped; usually affect lower abdomen, genitalia, palms, soles, eyelids, conjunctivae; may be widely disseminated in AIDS patients
Roseola infantum	May be caused by numerous viruses; usually seen in children 6 to 18 months of age; macular or maculopapular rash over trunk associated with high fever; rash spreads to other parts of the body and fades within 24 hours
Fifth disease (erythema infectiosum)	Caused by human parvovirus; flu-like prodrome followed by bright red rash over cheeks ("slapped cheeks" rash); more generalized maculopapular rash follows; rash fades from center in lacy pattern

Verrucae

Definition. Warts are benign hyperplastic lesions of the skin or mucous membranes caused by human papillomavirus (HPV). *Verrucae vulgaris* (common warts) are found most often on the hands, but also on the face, trunk, arms, or legs. Those on the plantar surface of the foot are called *plantar warts*. *Condylomata acuminata* (genital warts) are located in the genitalia and perianal areas. Genital warts, a sexually transmitted disease, is discussed in Chapter 30.

Epidemiology. Warts are very common and are communicated by direct contact with the virus, either between individuals or via site-to-site autoinoculation within the same individual. Transmission via fomites has also been postulated.[12] Occupations associated with warm, moist environments and repeated trauma to the skin facilitate transmission of the virus, and immunosuppression confers increased risk of infection.

Etiology. The causative organism is HPV, a DNA virus that replicates within the nuclei of epithelial cells of the skin or mucous membranes. More than 63 types of the virus have been identified.[12]

Pathophysiology. The incubation period is not clearly defined. Uncontrolled replication of the virus causes irregular thickening of the stratum corneum in the infected areas. The lesions resolve spontaneously when immunity to the virus develops, but this process may take several years in some cases.

Clinical Manifestations. Skin lesions are typically rough and nodular. Plantar warts (on the sole or plantar surface of the foot) may be particularly large, with black dots within them representing sclerosed capillaries. Mucosal warts are more moist and usually occur in multiples. Lesions are usually nonpainful, but frictional stress or pressure may cause pain in some cases. Bleeding and secondary infection may also be associated with frictional stress.

Prevention and Treatment. Contact with infected lesions should be avoided, and known risk factors should be avoided if possible. Warts may resolve on their own without treatment, but this approach may lead to the development of more lesions due to autoinoculation.[12] Common warts may be removed with application of the keratolytic agent podophyllum (Podocon), cryosurgery ("freezing" with liquid nitrogen or nitrous oxide gas), laser excision, or electrocautery ("burning"). Plantar warts are often treated with application of mild salicylic acid solutions (Compound W, Sal-Acid, Trans-Ver-Sal) to induce keratinolysis.

Prognosis and Outcome. Common warts and plantar warts resolve spontaneously or are easily managed with treatment. Infection with some strains of HPV imposes increased risk of malignancy, however. The association of HPV infection with cervical cancer is discussed in Chapter 31. HPV infection is less commonly associated with skin cancer (squamous cell carcinoma) and cancers of the prostate, larynx, and conjunctivae.[12]

Herpes Simplex

Definition. Herpes simplex infections include those of the lips, mouth, nose, eyes, and skin, usually caused by herpes simplex virus type 1 (HSV-1), and those of the genital areas, usually caused by herpes simplex virus type 2 (HSV-2). Genital herpes is a common sexually transmitted disease (see Chapter 30).

Epidemiology. Herpes simplex infection is very common. By age 5 years, an estimated 90% of the population has experienced this infection.[13] HSV-1 is acquired through direct contact with the virus, such as with kissing, touching, sharing of glasses or towels, etc. Immunosuppressed individuals are more susceptible to recurrence of this viral infection.

Etiology. Herpes simplex virus is the causative organism. Individuals vary widely in their susceptibility to infection.

Pathophysiology. The virus penetrates the skin and is sequestered in the sensory nerve ganglion that innervates the site of entry. After an incubation period of up to 2 weeks, inflammation is initiated. Virus continues to be shed over several weeks, after which the virus remains dormant in the ganglion. Acute inflammation may recur at any time, sometimes years later, usually in response to sunlight, fever, trauma, or emotional stress.

Clinical Manifestations. The initial viral infection may be asymptomatic or very mild, but recurrent episodes are more severe. Lesions are multiple, grouped vesicles (e.g., fever blisters or canker sores) that may be very painful. Vesicles eventually rupture, forming a crust over the inflamed area. Ocular infection may lead to corneal scarring.[14] Lesions usually persist for about 2 weeks. Ulceration occurs with recurrent infections, and in rare cases systemic dissemination and encephalitis may occur.

Prevention and Treatment. Infections with HSV-1 may be prevented with avoidance of contact with persons known to be infected. Towels and clothing should not be shared. Treatment of uncomplicated HSV is essentially supportive and symptomatic, with topical analgesics. Immunosuppressed individuals or others at particular risk may be treated with antiviral agents such as acyclovir (Zovirax) or foscarnet (Foscavir). This therapy is not curative, but it may slow disease progression, inhibit recurrence, or lessen severity of manifestations in some cases.[14]

Prognosis and Outcome. Lesions usually resolve within 2 to 6 weeks, but recurrent outbreaks are common.

Herpes Zoster and Varicella

Definition. Herpes zoster (shingles) and varicella (chickenpox) are manifestations of infection with a highly contagious herpesvirus known as the varicella-zoster virus (VSV). Varicella is the initial infection, which usually occurs during childhood. Herpes zoster represents recurrence of infection caused by activation of dormant virus that has been sequestered in dorsal root ganglia.

Epidemiology. Varicella is among the most common communicable childhood diseases in the United States. An estimated 4 million cases occur each year.[15] The VSV vaccine introduced in 1995 is now recommended for routine use in children 12 to 18 months of age, a practice that should markedly affect the incidence of the disease and the age of the affected population in coming years. Currently, most cases occur before the age of 11 years. The rate of infection is highest in the winter and spring months, probably because of high contact rates during the school year. Herpes zoster is also very common. Incidence increases with advancing age and declining immune function. Annual incidence is 0.4 to 1.6 per 1000 among healthy individuals younger than age 20 years, and 4.5 to 11 cases per 1000 among those older than age 80 years.[16] Acute eruptions are usually triggered by stress, intercurrent illness, or immunosuppression. Children with leukemia and adults with AIDS are at much higher risk than others of their age groups.

Etiology. The VSV, a DNA virus, is the etiological agent in these disorders.

Pathophysiology. The initial viral infection produces the systemic illness of chickenpox, which is soon followed by the characteristic skin rash. Acute inflammation usually resolves in about a week, but the virus may not be cleared from the body. Instead, it may persist in a dormant state within the dorsal root ganglia of the sensory system, usually those of the thoracic or lumbar spine, or the cranial nerves. Cell-mediated immunity keeps the virus inactive during this time, but waning immunocompetence with aging or systemic disease may permit clinical reactivation. Herpes zoster lesions usually persist for about 3 weeks. Histologic examination of affected nerve roots shows inflammation, hemorrhagic necrosis, and neuronal loss, resulting in altered central processing of pain impulses.[16] Dissemination of the reactivated virus throughout the body is rare. Some axonal regrowth occurs after acute episodes, usually leading to hypersensitivity of the affected area.

Clinical Manifestations. Varicella is usually a mild illness in children, although older adolescents and adults may have more systemic manifestations. Malaise, fever, and occasionally upper respiratory symptoms precede the development of multiple small erythematous macules and papules. Lesions then develop into vesicles, which rupture, crust over, and heal spontaneously, usually within a week (see Color Fig. 36–4). The trunk and face are the initial sites of the rash, which then usually spreads to the extremities. In immunosuppressed children, and in adult-onset varicella, dissemination of the virus may result in pneumonia or encephalitis, manifested as respiratory failure and increased intracranial pressure. Fortunately, these complications are rare.

Herpes zoster manifests as multiple vesicles distributed along one or two adjacent dermatomes (see Color Fig. 36–3). Edema and superficial hemorrhage of adjacent skin are also seen. Intense, burning pain in the dermatomal area is characteristic of herpes zoster and may persist for months or years after resolution of the skin lesions. This *postherpetic neuralgia* is more common in elderly patients. Some patients have lack of pain sensation or abnormal sensation of light touch or temperature in the affected area. Rarely, involvement of the trigeminal nerve results in visual impairment as a result of infection and perforation of the cornea. Dissemination is more likely in immunosuppressed individuals.

Prevention and Treatment. Immunization with live attenuated VSV vaccine is now recommended for young children, and "catch-up" immunization may also be warranted for susceptible older children and adults. Isolation of infected individuals may be warranted to prevent varicella in those who are not immune, either as a result of having had the disease or having been immunized. Treatment of varicella is usually symptomatic and supportive. The American Pediatric Association has not recommended routine antiviral treatment of varicella in otherwise healthy children. Adolescents and adults with varicella are usually treated with oral acyclovir (Zovirax) and may require hospitalization for fluid support in some cases. Treatment of varicella does not influence the sequestration of the virus in nerve roots. Herpes zoster is treated with antiviral agents (acyclovir or famciclovir) to shorten the duration and lessen the severity of acute outbreaks and with systemic steroids to reduce the severity of postherpetic neuralgia.[14]

Prognois and Outcome. Most varicella is experienced as a mild, self-limiting illness. Herpes zoster is often recurrent and severe despite treatment, especially in the elderly.

Rubeola

Definition. Rubeola ("red," "hard," or "7-day" measles) is a systemic viral infection characterized by upper respiratory, ophthalmic, and integumentary manifestations.

Epidemiology. Rubeola was once a very common contagious disease of childhood, but introduction of the measles-mumps-rubella (MMR) vaccine has significantly reduced the incidence of the disease in recent years. Transmission is through inhalation of virus in droplet nuclei or hand-to-nose transmission after direct contact with the virus.

Etiology. The *Morbillivirus* (paramyxovirus), an RNA virus, is the cause of measles.

Pathophysiology. Manifestations of the disorder are caused by viral replication and resultant inflammation (see Chapter 13).

Clinical Manifestations. An incubation period of 8 to 10 days follows the initial exposure. A prodromal phase characterized by malaise, fever, cough, headache, light-induced sensitivity of the skin (**photosensitivity**), and eyes (photophobia) is then seen. Koplik's spots (white spots circumscribed in red) may be seen on the buccal mucosa opposite the lower molars. The prodrome is followed by the appearance of lesions on the skin and mucous membranes of the mouth. Skin lesions are dark red macules that usually become confluent, first over the face and then the trunk and extremities. Fever subsides as the rash erupts. The rash turns brown and scaly after about 5 to 6 days and disappears after about 2 weeks.[17] Rare complications include hemorrhage from lesions or dissemination resulting in otitis media, pneumonia, or encephalitis.

Prevention and Treatment. The MMR vaccine prevents the disorder and is now a required immunization for children 15 months of age or older. Treatment is symptomatic and supportive.

Prognosis and Outcome. Except in immunosuppressed or otherwise debilitated children and adults, measles resolves spontaneously with no adverse outcomes.

Rubella

Definition. Rubella ("German" or "3-day" measles) is a communicable systemic viral infection characterized by mild systemic signs and a skin rash.

Epidemiology. Like rubeola, rubella was once a very common contagious childhood disease, but its incidence has been greatly reduced since the advent of the MMR vaccine. Airborne transmission is usual. Transplacental exposure of the fetus to rubella virus imposes risk of significant teratogenic effects.

Etiology. The cause of the disorder is the rubella virus (rubivirus).

Pathophysiology. Viral replication triggers mild inflammatory illness and skin eruption. The virus is known to be highly teratogenic. Transmission of the virus to a pregnant woman during the first trimester may result in congenital cataracts, microcephaly, deafness, or other serious malformations in the fetus (see Chapter 7).

Clinical Manifestations. The incubation period for rubella is 14 to 21 days.[17] Lymph node enlargement or upper respiratory symptoms may precede the development of the rash. A pinpoint macular rash begins on the face and trunk and soon spreads to the arms and legs. The rash lasts about 3 days. Rare complications include encephalitis, arthritis, and thrombocytopenia.

Prevention and Treatment. MMR vaccination prevents the disease in children, greatly reducing the likelihood of transmission to a pregnant woman. Antirubella antibody titer is routinely assessed during pregnancy, but immunization against rubella is contraindicated *during* pregnancy. Pregnant women should be isolated from infected persons. Treatment of the illness is symptomatic and supportive.

Prognosis and Outcome. The initial rubella infection nearly always resolves within a few days without complications. Teratogenic complications are potentially significant adverse outcomes in pregnancy.

Bites, Stings, and Parasitic Infestations

Humans are subject to cutaneous and systemic disorders resulting from bites, stings, and infestations of a large number of insects and animals. Three common disorders, **scabies, pediculosis**, and insect stings are discussed below. Clinical features of other parasitic infestations, bites, and stings are summarized in Table 36–12.

Scabies

Definition. Scabies is a communicable inflammatory disorder of the skin caused by infestation with mites.

Epidemiology. Scabies is common among those subject to close human contact, particularly children and and sexually active adults. Its estimated worldwide incidence is 300 million.[18] Scabies is most commonly spread by sexual contact, but may also be communicated by fomites (e.g., clothing).

Etiology. The human itch mite *Sarcoptes scabiei* is the causative agent.

Pathophysiology. The male mite remains on the skin surface, but the impregnated female releases a proteolytic secretion that allows her to penetrate to inner epidermal layers. The mite survives in the skin for up to 30 days, laying 2 to 3 eggs per day. Eggs hatch and mature within 2 months. Skin regions between the fingers and in areas often constricted by clothing, such as the wrists, breasts, waist, and groin, are the usual sites of penetration. Dead mites, eggs, larvae, and their excrement trigger an inflammatory eruption of the skin in infested areas.

Clinical Manifestations. Linear burrows may be evident. Skin lesions are small erythematous papules and vesicles that may rupture, resulting in secondary crusts and scales (Color Fig. 36–5). The rash is intensely pruritic, especially at night. Mites may or may not be seen with microscopic examination of the skin. A variant of scabies, Norwegian (crusted) scabies, is common among those with AIDS and may lead to life-threatening septicemia.

Prevention and Treatment. Prevention involves avoidance of contact with infested persons. Prophylaxis with application of gamma benzene hexachloride or lindane (Kwell) is indicated for family members or other close contacts of known infested persons. Gamma benzene hexachloride, permethrin (Elimite), and crotamiton (Eurax) are principal antiparasitic agents used in treatment of scabies. These agents penetrate the exoskeletons of the mites, stimulating their nervous systems and causing seizures and death. Mild topical glucocorticoids and systemic antihistamines may also be used to manage itching. (Clinical use of glucocorticoids and antihistamines is detailed in Chapters 13, 18, and 29.) An antihelmintic (worm-eradicating) agent, ivermectin, has recently been shown to be effective in treating scabies in AIDS patients.[19]

Prognosis and Outcome. Treatment is usually effective in eradicating the mites. Most pruritus will resolve, but some may persist for weeks until dead mite parts are sloughed. Systemic sepsis in Norwegian scabies may be fatal.

TABLE 36–12
LESS COMMON DISORDERS ASSOCIATED WITH BITES, STINGS, AND PARASITIC INFESTATIONS

Disorder	Description
Rocky Mountain spotted fever	Caused by an intracellular bacterium (*Rickettsiae* species) transmitted by tick bites; eschar forms at bite site, followed by hemorrhagic rash extending over entire body
Lyme disease	Caused by spirochete *Borrelia burgdorferi,* transmitted from rodents to humans via deer tick bite; skin lesion at bite site is target-like; disseminated erythematous, "onion-skin" lesions associated with arteritis
Strongyloidiasis	Infection by the nematode *Strongyloides stercoralis* (threadworm); endemic in southern United States and tropical countries; causes a linear, pruritic lesion caused by larvae burrowing through the skin; petechiae and purpura may also be seen
Seabather's eruption	Caused by stings of jellyfish, Portuguese man-of-war, coral, sea urchins; pruritic rash and neurotoxicity are possible

Pediculosis

Definition. Pediculosis is cutaneous inflammation of the scalp, body, or groin caused by infestation with lice.

Epidemiology. An estimated 6 to 12 million persons are affected by pediculosis each year in the United States.[20] Outbreaks of head lice (*pediculosis capitis*) are very common among children in schools and day care centers. Pubic lice or "crabs" (*pediculosis pubis*) is a sexually transmitted infestation. Infestation with body lice (*pediculosis corporis*) is associated with close human contact or sharing of contaminated clothing or linens. Head lice affect only humans and are not transmitted by pets or other animals. The shape of the hair shaft in African-American individuals protects them from infestation.

Etiology. The causative agents are the lice *Phthirus pubis* and *Pediculosis humanus.*

Pathophysiology. Lice do not burrow, but rather crawl and attach superficially to the epidermis and hair, laying their eggs (nits). During her 30-day life span, the female louse attaches a total of 60 to 150 nits to hair shafts near the body surface. Nits survive by ingesting blood from the human host for up to 10 days, then hatch and mature into adults in about 2 weeks.[20] Lice inject their saliva into the scalp and skin, causing pruritus. Scratching the area may predispose the individual to secondary bacterial infections.

Clinical Manifestations. Lice and nits are visible with careful inspection (Fig. 36–9). Pruritus is also present and may be intense.

Prevention and Treatment. Avoidance of contact with infested persons or contaminated objects is warranted. The drug of choice for treatment of head lice is a 1.0% solution of permethrin (Nix), used as a creme rinse after shampoo.[20] Nits must be removed with a fine-toothed comb to prevent reinfestation. Body and pubic lice are treated similarly to scabies with antiparasitic agents in lotion, cream, or gel form.

Prognosis and Outcome. Pediculosis is readily eradicated with short-term treatment.

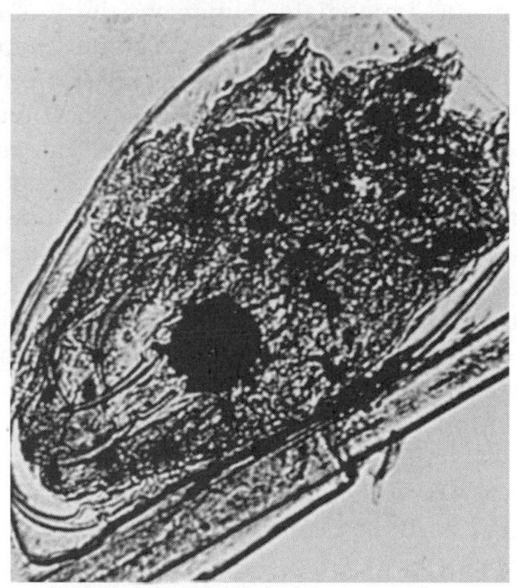

FIGURE 36–9

Pediculosis. The eggs (nits) of the female louse are attached to hair shafts near the body surface and are visible with careful inspection. Here, a nit is illustrated under magnification. (From Behrman, R.E., Kliegman, R.M., and Arvin, A.M. [1996]. *Nelson Textbook of Pediatrics.* [15th ed.]. Philadelphia: W.B. Saunders. [p. 1907].)

Insect Stings

Definition. The category of insect stings is inclusive of all injuries caused by the injection of insect venom into the skin.

Epidemiology. Insect stings are very common and may be a serious medical problem for some individuals. Potentially fatal allergic reactions (anaphylaxis) induced by stings occur in 0.3% to 3% of the general population each year in the United States.[21] Individuals engaged in outdoor activities such as lawn-mowing, gardening, or other recreational or occupational activities in areas where insects are plentiful are at highest risk. The risk of an anaphylactic response to an insect sting is highest among people younger than 20 years of age, with males affected twice as commonly as females. About one third have a history of allergy.

Etiology. Stinging insects include members of the order Hymenoptera, class Insecta. There are two major subgroups: vespids (yellow jackets, hornets, and wasps), and apids (honeybees and bumblebees).[21] Yellow jacket stings are most common because these insects nest near the ground and are frequently disturbed by human activity. Bees are normally docile and sting only when provoked. Africanized honeybees ("killer bees"), which are spreading northward and have been found in Texas, California, and Arizona, are more aggressive than honeybees, but their venom is no more toxic. Biting insects such as mosquitoes, deerflies, and bedbugs inject saliva rather than venom, and, with rare exceptions, the reaction is one of local inflammation rather than anaphylaxis.

Pathophysiology. The major allergens in venom are phospholipase A_2, hyaluronidase, melittin, and a protein known as antigen 5.[21] The humoral immune response to these allergens is mediated by venom-specific immunoglobulin (Ig) E and IgG and either sensitizes the individual or elicits a clinical immune response (see Chapter 13). The reaction may be limited to a local inflammatory reaction, or may take the form of immediate hypersensitivity (anaphylaxis). Complications such as vasculitis, nephrosis, neuritis, encephalitis, and serum sickness are rare.

Clinical Manifestations. The local reaction to an insect sting is manifested by pain, swelling, and erythema at the sting site. Swelling may extend over a large area, but usually peaks within 48 hours.[21] Anaphylaxis usually manifests within 20 minutes of the sting as generalized **urticaria** (hives), flushing, and **angioedema**. Life-threatening manifestations include laryngeal edema, bronchospasm, and circulatory collapse (see anaphylactic shock, Chapter 15).

Prevention and Treatment. Wearing dark-colored protective clothing and avoiding high-risk exposures may be of some benefit in preventing insect stings. Cosmetics, perfumes, and hair sprays that attract insects should be avoided. Because food odors attract yellow jackets, care should be taken when cooking or eating outdoors.[21] Individuals known to be at risk for anaphylaxis should carry a preloaded cartridge of epinephrine (e.g., Ana-Kit, EpiPen), which may be self-administered in the event of a sting. Immunotherapy with venom-specific IgG and IgE has also been shown to be effective.

Local reactions to insect stings require symptomatic and supportive care. With honeybee and bumblebee stings, the insect leaves the stinger in the skin. It should be gently removed, with care to not squeeze more venom from the attached sac. Aspirin and antihistamines may alleviate pain and itching. Use of glucocorticoids is warranted in some cases of extensive swelling. Tetanus prophylaxis is not necessary.[21] Anaphylaxis is treated with epinephrine and antihistamines, as discussed in Chapter 13. Anaphylactic shock may require intubation to maintain the airway and extensive fluid resuscitation, as detailed in Chapter 15.

Prognosis and Outcome. Local reactions to stings normally subside within 7 days. The risk of anaphylaxis is less than 5% per sting episode and can be nearly eliminated with immunotherapy.[21] With appropriate treatment, the acute symptoms of anaphylaxis usually subside within 15 to 30 minutes. Untreated episodes may be fatal.

Dermatitis

Dermatitis, also known as **eczema** (literally, "to boil out") is a general term inclusive of a variety of noninfectious, often immune-mediated, conditions characterized by erythematous, blistering, weeping lesions of skin areas. The three most common forms, **atopic dermatitis, contact dermatitis,** and **seborrheic dermatitis**, are discussed below. Table 36–13 describes less common forms of dermatitis.

TABLE 36–13
LESS COMMON FORMS OF DERMATITIS

Disorder	Description
Stasis dermatitis	Erythematous, edematous, sometimes oozing eruption on the lower legs caused by chronic venous insufficiency
Neurodermatitis (lichen simplex chronicus)	Hypertrophic lichenification caused by idiopathic pruritus and chronic scratching; associated with stress and psychiatric disorders; hereditary predisposition
Dyshidrotic dermatitis	Related to emotional distress; may magnify effects of contact dermatitis
Dermatitis medicamentosa	Adverse cutaneous drug eruptions; may be allergic, irritative, multifactorial, or idiopathic
Photodermatitis	Caused by photoallergic (cell-mediated delayed hypersensitivity) or phototoxic (irritant) reaction to ultraviolet light; drug-induced photosensitivity may enhance response; usually classified as a form of contact dermatitis
Exfoliative dermatitis	Erythematous, scaling eruption involving the entire skin surface; may be associated with lymphoma or leukemia, psoriasis, eczematous dermatitis, or drug allergy

Atopic Dermatitis

Definition. Atopic dermatitis is a systemic inflammatory response to an allergen that manifests primarily as a skin eruption.

Epidemiology. Atopic dermatitis is common, occurring in allergy-prone (atopic) individuals who often demonstrate a family history as well as other forms of allergy (e.g., asthma, hay fever). The disorder usually manifests first in infants between 2 and 6 months of age.[22] Allergens in the home and workplace may trigger or worsen atopic dermatitis later in life. The lifetime incidence has been estimated at 15% to 20%, with an equal distribution between males and females.[23]

Etiology. The combination of inherited genetic susceptibility and exposure to environmental irritants causes atopic dermatitis. Disordered cell-mediated immunity is demonstrated in many individuals, with underactivity of Il-2 and overactivity of Il-4 and Il-5.[23] It is uncertain whether these findings represent a cause or an effect of the disease, however. The inflammatory response results from an IgE-mediated immediate hypersensitivity reaction (a "true" allergy). Although the specific precipitating allergen may never be identified, agents such as moisture, wool, deodorants, solvents, plants, latex rubber, and lanolin are commonly implicated. Cutaneous reactions to drugs may also take the form of atopic dermatitis (see Table 36–8). Food allergies probably play a limited role.[23] Emotional stress may exacerbate the reaction.

Pathophysiology. The allergic mechanism of immediate hypersensitivity, detailed in Chapter 13, results in release of inflammatory mediators via sensitized antibodies of the IgE class. Histamine and other cytokines induce an inflammatory response that is excessive, resulting in edema and breakdown of the skin as well as intense pruritus.

Clinical Manifestations. The skin lesions of atopic dermatitis are typically red, blistering, weeping, scaly, and thickened (Color Fig. 36–6). They are intensely pruritic, with the patient's scratching possibly exacerbating the condition and promoting secondary lesions and bacterial infection. Distribution of the rash is variable, limited to skinfold areas in some cases and more generalized in others.

Prevention and Treatment. If possible, triggering agents should be identified and avoided. Topical steroids such as hydrocortisone are the mainstay of treatment, used for their anti-inflammatory effect. Systemic corticosteroids may be indicated in exceptionally severe cases. Antihistamines may reduce the intensity of inflammation and itching for selected patients, but are of limited benefit in most cases.[23] Hyposensitization therapy is rarely beneficial in atopic dermatitis.

Prognosis and Outcome. Most patients gain significant relief with avoidance of triggers and use of topical steroids, but no cure exists for the condition. Many children with atopic dermatitis improve significantly as they grow older, but may manifest other allergies in adulthood. Atopic dermatitis may persist as a lifelong condition in some adults.

Contact Dermatitis

Definition. Contact dermatitis is a localized inflammatory response of the skin caused by contact with an irritant.

Epidemiology. The condition is by far the most common form of eczema, occurring to some extent in nearly everyone. Table 36–14 lists common contact irritants. The severity of response to a given agent varies among individuals; however, children and the elderly are more vulnerable because of their lower thresholds for skin irritation.[24]

Etiology. Contact dermatitis may be classified according to its etiologic mechanism as allergic contact dermatitis, irritant contact dermatitis, **photodermatitis**, or contact urticaria.[25] Allergic contact dermatitis is caused by a cell-mediated delayed hypersensitivity reaction (see Chapter 13). Irritant contact dermatitis is an appropriate inflammatory response to skin cell damage by a toxic effect of an irritant.

Photodermatitis is caused by a *photoallergic reaction* (delayed hypersensitivity reaction to UV light) or a *phototoxic reaction* (irritant-induced inflammation) in which UV light activates some agent that then produces the response. In photoallergy, an allergen is formed by this reaction, whereas in phototoxicity, the agent formed apparently binds to DNA or leads to oxidation of skin cellular components.[24]

Contact urticaria is a wheal-and-flare reaction (hives) that occurs on contact with irritants. It may

TABLE 36–14
EXAMPLES OF CONTACT IRRITANTS

Substance	Source
Contact Allergens	
Rhus (urushiol)	Poison ivy, poison oak, mango
Nickel sulfate	Hairpins, jewelry, zippers, hair dyes, bleaches, insecticides
Potassium dichromate	Cement, leather, household cleansers, bleaches
Formaldehyde	Cosmetics, fabrics, cigarettes, newsprint and newspaper, preservatives
Ethylenediamine	Hair dyes, fungicides, topical medications
Mercaptobenzothiazole	Rubber products
Thiuram	Fungicides, insecticides, rubber products
Paraphenylenediamine	Hair dyes, fur dyes, photographic chemicals
Chemical irritants	Acids, alkali, solvents, enzymes, surfactants, oxidants, enzymes (in household and occupational products)
Photoirritants	Ultraviolet B and, to a lesser degree, ultraviolet A spectra of sunlight

Adapted with permission from Klaus, M.V., and Wieselthier, J.S. (1993). Contact dermatitis. *American Family Physician* 48(4), 629–632. Published by the American Academy of Family Physicians.

have an allergic mechanism (IgE-mediated hypersensitivity) or a nonallergic mechanism (induced by physical pressure, moisture, scratching or rubbing, or cold exposure). In a significant number of cases, urticaria is idiopathic, occurring without an identifiable cause.[26]

Pathophysiology. An adaptive response designed to clear the irritant usually results in mild inflammation limited to the area of contact. With cell-mediated hypersensitivity, the inflammatory response becomes progressively worse with each contact and may extend to adjacent regions of the skin. Anaphylaxis is also possible. Cell-mediated hypersensitivity and anaphylaxis are discussed in Chapter 13.

Clinical Manifestations. The characteristics of the rash vary with severity and mechanism, but usually clearly delineate the area of contact with the irritant. Erythematous, weeping, scaly lesions are most typical, with development of vesicles in some cases (Color Fig. 36–7). Drying (**xerosis**) and cracking of the skin are common, and epidermal necrosis, in which the epidermis is separated from the dermis by vesicles, may occur in some cases. With chronic exposure, hyperpigmentation and lichenification may occur. Photoallergic or phototoxic reactions are limited to sun-exposed areas. Urticarial lesions (hives) are small wheals caused by fluid exudation into the upper dermis and are associated with erythema and intense itching. Hives usually appear in clusters that persist for 2 or 3 hours, then disappear to flare up elsewhere on the body surface.[27] Angioedema, a painful but nonpruritic swelling of loose connective tissues, may accompany urticaria in many cases. Angioedema usually manifests as swelling of the lips or eyelids, but may impose risk of airway obstruction if it involves the tongue or larynx.

Prevention and Treatment. Prevention requires identification and avoidance of offending agents. Symptomatic treatment of pruritus and crusting may involve baths (tap water, with the possible addition of oilated oatmeal [Aveeno] powder, or application of wet compresses with astringent or anesthetic agents [e.g., Burow's solution]).[22] Antihistamines such as chlorpheniramine (Chlor-Trimeton) and loratadine (Claritin) may also be used in an effort to alleviate pruritus. Corticosteroid creams and ointments (e.g., hydrocortisone) are most frequently used in the treatment of contact dermatitis. Topical or systemic antibiotics may be indicated if secondary infection is present.

Prognosis and Outcome. The skin rash usually resolves spontaneously within 1 to 3 weeks after contact with the offending agent is discontinued.[24] Most cases of chronic contact dermatitis are successfully managed with behavioral and symptomatic interventions.

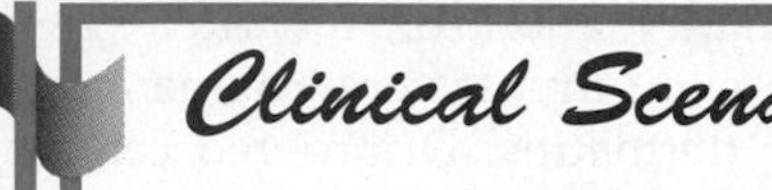

A.F., a 38-year-old elementary teacher, consults her family physician about a skin rash that has developed in recent weeks as she has been working on renovation of some antique furniture. The red, blistering rash is confined to her hands and wrists, and painful fissures have begun to form on her fingertips. She has been wearing rubber gloves while using a commercial paint stripping chemical; however, some of the solution may have seeped through small holes in the gloves or leaked around the wrist area. A.F. denies any systemic symptoms.

1. What additional information would be helpful in determining the probable cause of A.F.'s dermatitis? Is A.F.'s medical history relevant? Explain.
2. What is the first priority in intervention in this case?

Seborrheic Dermatitis

Definition. Seborrheic dermatitis is a noninfectious, scaling inflammation of the skin appearing in areas of increased sebaceous gland activity.

Epidemiology. Seborrheic dermatitis is very common, affecting individuals of all ages. Infants younger than 3 months of age and adults 30 to 60 years of age are at highest risk. A severe form may be associated with AIDS.[28] Increased risk is also seen among those with Parkinson's disease and with neuroleptic drug therapy.

Etiology. The precise cause of sebaceous overactivity is unknown. Several theories of causation have been advanced.[28] It may be a hormonally dependent disorder, which would explain its presence in childhood and disappearance at puberty. Seborrheic dermatitis in AIDS is associated with overgrowth of the fungus *Pityrosporum ovale*, a component of the normal skin flora. Pooling of sebum in areas of altered innervation has been proposed as a mechanism in neurologic disorders, but no specific neurotransmitter imbalances have been implicated. Deficiency of certain vitamins (e.g., riboflavin, biotin, or pyridoxine) has also been proposed as an etiologic mechanism.

Pathophysiology. Increased sebum production is associated with an oily complexion and is particularly evident in the scalp, nasolabial folds and other skinfold areas, eyebrows, eyelid margins, external ear, and trunk. Secreted sebum induces erythema and scaling, but, except in AIDS, does not cause acute dermatitis.

Clinical Manifestations. In infants, the disorder may manifest as dry, patchy scaling overlying erythematous scalp (cradle cap) or as diaper dermatitis. In adolescents and adults, seborrheic dermatitis usually manifests as dandruff or as erythema of the nasolabial folds. Blepharitis (inflammation of the eyelid margins) and external ear inflammation (otitis externa) are also common. Truncal lesions may manifest as small, reddish brown papules and greasy scaling near hair follicles or as generalized macules and patches. In most cases, scaling in seborrheic dermatitis is of fine texture and white or yellow in color.

Prevention and Treatment. Antidandruff shampoos are widely available for the control of seborrheic dermatitis involving the scalp. More severe cases of seborrheic dermatitis in adolescents and adults are treated with topical corticosteroid lotions.

Prognosis and Outcome. The disorder is usually mild and responsive to treatment. Severe, persistent seborrheic dermatitis may suggest an underlying disorder, warranting further diagnostic testing.[28]

Idiopathic and Immune-Mediated Disorders

Some of the most common disorders seen in dermatologic practice have unknown or multifactorial etiology, involving possible immune mechanisms in many cases. Three significant disorders in this category, acne vulgaris, psoriasis, and **scleroderma**, are detailed in this section. Table 36–15 summarizes clinical features of other idiopathic disorders and immune-mediated disorders of the skin.

Acne Vulgaris

Definition. Acne vulgaris is a multifactorial skin disorder characterized by chronic inflammation and obstruction of the pilosebaceous unit.

Epidemiology. Acne is very common, affecting an estimated 80% of the population between the ages of 11 and 30 years.[29] Persistent or sporadic recurrence into the middle years is also common. As many as 40% to 50% of adult women are affected by a low-grade, persistent form of acne.[30] Risk factors for acne are uncertain. A familial predisposition is apparent. Hormonal stimulation of the pilosebaceous unit with the androgen surge at puberty plays a role in the development of acne, and reduction in estrogen levels may contribute to worsening of acne during perimenopause. Stress hormones may play a role, because exacerbations are apparently stress-induced in

TABLE 36–15
IDIOPATHIC AND IMMUNE-MEDIATED DISORDERS OF THE SKIN

Disorder	Description
Erythema nodosum	Inflammation of subcutaneous fat, producing skin manifestations of tender, erythematous nodules that gradually become bruise-like; usually affects lower legs
Erythema induratum	Inflammation of subcutaneous fat, possibly caused by an underlying vasculitis; presents as tender, erythematous nodules that eventually ulcerate; most common in adolescents and postmenopausal women
Lichen planus	Self-limited disorder of skin and mucous membranes; skin lesions are itchy, purple, flat-topped papules that may coalesce to form plaques; wrists and elbows involved symmetrically, also glans penis of males; oral lesions are white and net-like
Pemphigus	Rare autoimmune blistering disorder resulting from loss of attachment of epidermis and mucosal epithelium; bullous lesions of oral mucosa and skin of scalp, face, axilla, trunk, groin, and pressure points
Dermatitis herpetiformis	Urticarial plaques and vesicles grouped symmetrically on extensor surfaces, elbows, knees, upper back, and buttocks; extremely pruritic; associated with gluten-sensitive enteropathy
Rosacea	Erythema on cheeks, nose, chin, or forehead; waxes and wanes at first; telangiectasia and acne-like lesions eventually develop; nose may become edematous; highest risk in fair-skinned persons; usually affects those in their 30s and 40s

Data from Cotran, R.S., Kumar, V., and Robbins, S.L. (1994). *Robbins Pathologic Basis of Disease.* (5th ed.). Philadelphia: W.B. Saunders. (pp. 1196–1205).

many individuals. Corticosteroid therapy is notoriously acnegenic.

Several foods and food additives have been implicated, including oils, chocolate, and iodide, but dietary restriction does not usually result in noticeable benefit. Obstruction of pilosebaceous units by cosmetics or poor hygiene may worsen inflammation, but is not believed to be causative. Mechanical trauma to the skin, such as that caused by manipulation of lesions or abrasion by hatbands and collars, may also contribute, as evidenced by the frequency of lesions in these areas. Very humid environments, heavy sweating, and exposure to polluted air may aggravate the disorder.

Etiology. The precise etiology of acne is unknown, but probably involves a combination of genetic, hormonal, environmental, and lifestyle factors.

Pathophysiology. The acne-prone areas of the body are the face, upper chest, and back, where pilosebaceous units are larger, containing vellus hairs and opening onto the skin surface via a visible pore. Obstruction of these units results from a combination of factors, including possible increased amount or viscosity of sebum or increased sloughing of follicular cells. Obstructed units are prone to secondary bacterial infections, usually with *Propionibacterium acnes*, a constituent of the normal skin flora.

Clinical Manifestations. Noninflammatory lesions (comedones) and inflammatory lesions (pustules, papules, nodules, and cysts) are characteristic of acne (Fig. 36–10). The microcomedo forms first as a result of plugging of the pilosebaceous unit with sebum. A visible closed comedo (whitehead) is apparent when enough sebum accumulates. Continuing distention of the follicle causes protrusion of follicular contents from the orifice, forming an open comedo (blackhead). The dark color is caused by the presence of oxidized lipids, melanin, and densely packed keratinocytes, not dirt.

Pustules develop when the compacted follicle ruptures near the skin surface, releasing bacteria and bacterial toxins (e.g., free fatty acids) into the dermis. Papules, nodules, and cysts may result from deeper and more extensive follicular rupture and subsequent inflammation. Inflammatory lesions are painful and pruritic.

Prevention and Treatment. There is no known prevention nor cure. Reduction of possible contributing factors is warranted. Vigorous scrubbing of the skin is not advised; the skin should instead be gently washed with mild, unscented soap and water. Treatment of acne depends on its severity (Table 36–16). Milder forms are treated with topical antibacterial agents such as benzoyl peroxide, erythromycin, clindamycin (Cleocin T), or meclocycline

Three major pathophysiologic processes occur in the development of acne vulgaris.

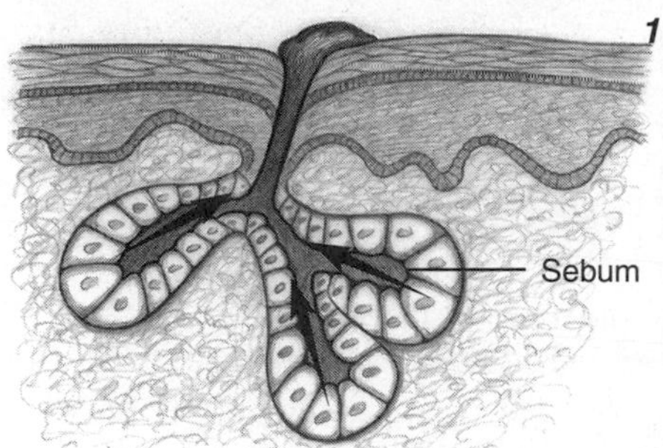

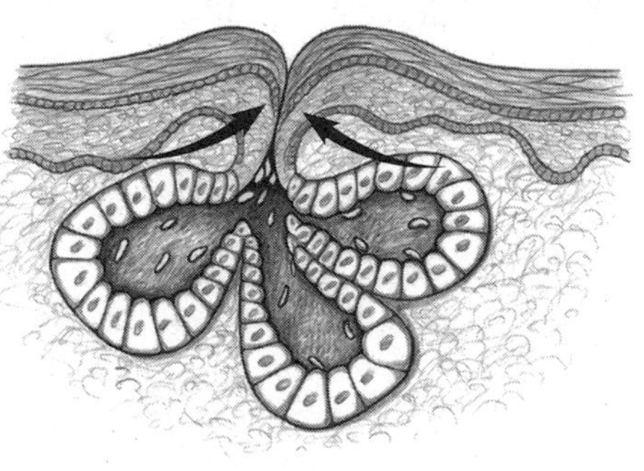

1 Sebum production is excessive and occurs with the onset of adrenal and gonadal androgen production.

2 There is an increased shedding of epithelial cells lining the *sebaceous follicles* (hair follicles with oil-producing glands). This process expands and blocks the follicle.

3 The cutaneous flora, *Propionibacterium acnes*, multiplies in this anaerobic environment and initiates an inflammatory response in the follicle. Open or closed comedones are then formed, and the follicle may rupture.

FIGURE 36–10

Pathogenesis of acne vulgaris. (From Luckmann, J. [1997]. *Saunders Manual of Nursing Care.* Philadelphia: W.B. Saunders. [p. 1645].)

(Meclan). Azelaic acid (Azelex), a naturally occurring substance derived from cereal grains, has recently been approved for topical use in treatment of mild to moderate acne as well.[31] Its mechanism of action is unknown. Keratinolytic agents such as salicylic acid or the retinoic acid derivative tretinoin (Retin-A) are commonly used to clear superficially plugged follicles. More severe forms of acne are treated with oral antibiotics such as tetracycline or erythromycin in addition to topical tretinoin. In very

TABLE 36–16
SEVERITY GRADES IN ACNE VULGARIS

GRADE	CHARACTERISTICS
I	Comedonal, fewer than 10 lesions on face only, no scarring
II	Papular, 10–25 lesions on face and trunk, mild scarring
III	Pustular, more than 25 lesions, moderate scarring
IV	Nodulocystic, extensive scarring

Data from Nguyen, Q.H., Kim, Y.A., and Schwartz, R.A. (1994). Management of acne vulgaris. *American Family Physician* 50(1), 89–96.

severe nodulocystic acne a potent keratolytic agent, isotretinoin (Accutane) may be prescribed. Use of this retinoic acid derivative is limited to short courses of therapy because of its potential detrimental effects on serum lipids and on liver function, kidney function, and hematopoiesis. Isotretinoin is a known teratogen, and must never be used by pregnant women or by those contemplating pregnancy. Surgical intervention may also be indicated in severe acne for drainage of cystic lesions and smoothing (dermabrasion) of acne-scarred skin.

Prognosis and Outcome. In most individuals, acne remains mild, and acute flare-ups resolve spontaneously or with topical therapy. Ninety per cent of patients with severe acne achieve a satisfactory response to 4 to 5 months of therapy with isotretinoin.[30] Some severe cases result in permanent scarring. Episodes of recurrent acne are common later in life because of hormonal changes, stress, or other factors.

Psoriasis

Definition. Psoriasis is a chronic inflammatory disorder of the skin characterized by episodes of excessively rapid turnover of keratinocytes.

Epidemiology. An estimated 1% to 2% of individuals in the United States are afflicted with the disorder.[10] Onset is usually before age 20 years, but individuals of any age may be affected. Genetic and environmental factors apparently increase the risk of psoriasis. Certain HLA subtypes are associated with increased incidence. Areas of skin trauma are frequent sites of lesions.

Etiology. The specific etiology of psoriasis is unknown. Two principal theories have been advanced.[10] According to one, damage to the stratum corneum "unmasks" antigenic proteins that trigger an autoimmune response limited to the epidermis. As a consequence of the resulting inflammation, factors that promote keratogenesis are released. A second hypothesis holds that capillary endothelial cell sensitivity to certain cytokines is genetically enhanced in the epidermis of psoriasis patients, leading to increased neutrophil chemotaxis and promoting inflammation.

Pathophysiology. Lesions most often develop on the elbows, knees, scalp, lumbosacral area, gluteal cleft, and penis. Lesions result from structural disorder of the epidermis and dermis as a result of greatly accelerated turnover of keratinocytes (3 to 4 days rather than the normal 15 to 30). Basal cell activity is increased, as is the rate of transit from the inner to the outer layers of the epidermis. Production of keratin is abnormal, resulting in thick, poorly adhesive cells that appear as silvery scales. An adaptive increase in vascular growth in the involved areas produces an erythematous base beneath the scales. The course of the disorder is usually one of spontaneous exacerbations and remissions.

Clinical Manifestations. Lesions initially appear as small red papules that enlarge and coalesce into large plaques that become covered with scales (Fig. 36–11). Up to 15% to 20% of patients also develop an associated psoriatic arthritis, which usually affects the distal interphalangeal joints of the hands but may be more generalized. Psoriatic changes in the nails affect 30% to 50% of patients.[13]

Prevention and Treatment. There are no known

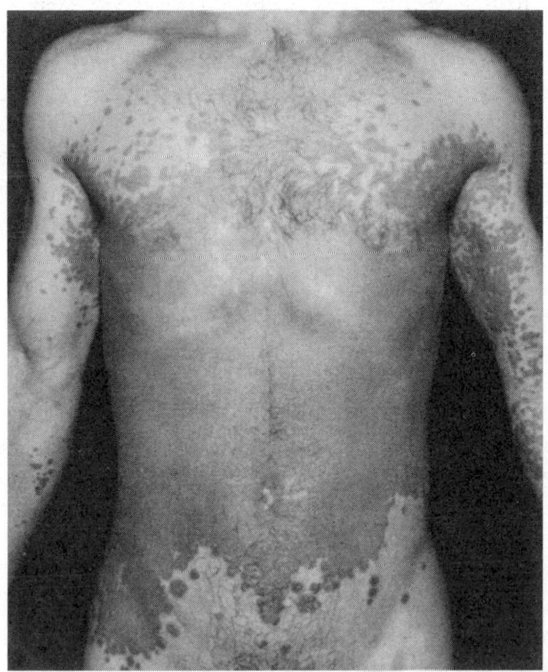

FIGURE 36–11
Psoriasis. Lesions initially appear as small, red papules that enlarge and coalesce into large, scale-covered plaques. (From Moschella, S.L., and Hurley, H.J. [1992.] *Dermatology.* [3rd ed.]. Philadelphia: W.B. Saunders. [p. 614].)

means of prevention of the disorder. Many interventions have been used in treatment, although none have been entirely successful. Topical or systemic corticosteroids are most commonly used for their anti-inflammatory effects. Agents that decrease the rate of cell proliferation may also be used; these include the topical antipsoriatic agent anthralin (Anthra-Derm), antineoplastic drugs such as methotrexate (Rheumatrex), and the combination of a photosensitizing drug (psoralen) with UV light (PUVA). An oral retinoid, etretinate (Tegison) has resulted in improvement in some cases, although its precise mechanism of action in psoriasis is uncertain. Treatment with PUVA, although effective for many patients, is controversial because of the associated risk of squamous cell carcinoma and possibly malignant melanoma of the skin.[32]

Prognosis and Outcome. Psoriasis is a chronic, recurrent disorder for which there is no known cure. Severity and extent of the lesions and presence of systemic manifestations such as arthritis vary widely among individuals. In immunosuppressed individuals, psoriasis may become generalized to most of the skin surface. This condition (*pustular psoriasis*) may be fatal because of fluid and electrolyte loss through the skin.

Scleroderma (Systemic Sclerosis)

Definition. Scleroderma ("hardening of the skin"), also known as systemic sclerosis, is a connective tissue disorder characterized by fibrosis and degenerative changes in multiple organs. Although the skin is primarily affected, changes also occur in the GI tract, kidneys, heart, muscles, and lungs.[10] The term *scleroderma* best applies during the phase where involvement is limited to the skin, whereas *systemic sclerosis* reflects the progression to other organ systems that nearly always occurs.

Epidemiology. Scleroderma is an uncommon disorder, affecting women three to four times as often as men, with peak incidence during the fifth and sixth decades.[10] Specific risk factors are not apparent in most cases; however, systemic sclerosis may be associated with occupational exposure to silica dust or polyvinyl chloride or with use of the anticancer agent bleomycin (Blenoxane) or the non-narcotic analgesic pentazocine (Talwin).[33]

Etiology. The precise etiology is unknown. Two major hypotheses have been proposed to explain the pathogenesis of scleroderma. The *immunologic hypothesis* holds that fibrosis occurs as a result of abnormal activation of the immune system. Alterations in humoral and cell-mediated immunity may induce inflammation with release of mediators that up-regulate collagen synthesis. Nearly all patients demonstrate antinuclear antibodies (ANA) in the serum (see Chapter 34). The *vascular hypothesis* is derived from the observation that microvascular disease with intimal fibrosis, capillary dilation, and platelet activation is present in distal arteries early in systemic sclerosis. Persistent perfusion deficit could then trigger tissue changes.

Pathophysiology. In scleroderma, diffuse, sclerotic atrophy of the skin occurs, usually beginning in the fingers and extending proximally to the upper arms, shoulders, neck, and face.[10] Edema and infiltrates containing CD4+ T cells surround blood vessels, and collagen fibers are swollen and degenerative. Fibrosis binds the dermis tightly to underlying subcutaneous structures, and dermal appendages atrophy. With progressive systemic sclerosis, similar changes occur in other organs. The mucosal layer of the GI tract (esophagus and lower bowel) may be replaced with fibrous tissue, leading to impaired motility, ulceration, and malabsorption. Muscles and joints may become fibrotic in a small number of patients. Renal vessels are affected in most patients, leading to hypertension and renal failure. Pulmonary fibrosis may lead to respiratory failure. Pericarditis with effusion is also common and may lead to cardiac failure as a result of decreased preload.

Clinical Manifestations. The skin is initially edematous, and Raynaud's phenomenon of digital vascular spasm is frequently present (see Chapter 15). Calcium deposition into subcutaneous tissue then occurs, resulting in small white lumps that may rupture and drain.[13] Spidery vascular lesions (*telangiectases*) result from permanent dilation of capillaries, arterioles, and venules. With increasing collagen deposition and fibrosis, the fingers demonstrate a tapered and claw-like appearance (*sclerodactyly*) (Fig. 36–12), and the face becomes mask-like.[10] The term **CREST syndrome** is often applied to the syndrome of *c*alcinosis, *R*aynaud's phenomenon, *e*sophageal dysfunction, *s*clerodactyly, and *t*elangiectasia. In systemic sclerosis, symptoms of multiple organ failure are progressive.

Prevention and Treatment. Avoidance of occupational exposures or use of drugs associated with the disorder may benefit a small number of persons. Treatment of scleroderma is symptomatic and supportive. High-dose corticosteroids and immunosuppressive agents are usually used.

Prognosis and Outcome. Scleroderma and systemic sclerosis manifest a slowly progressive course, usually for 10 to 20 years or more. Prognosis is favorable when the disorder is limited to the skin; however, systemic involvement signals a fatal course, with death usually caused by infection, renal failure, or cardiac failure.[13]

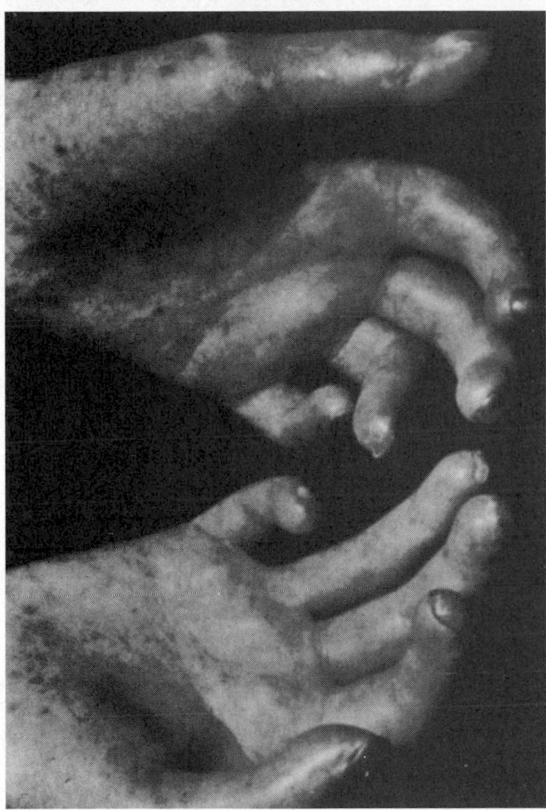

FIGURE 36–12
Scleroderma. Extensive subcutaneous fibrosis has immobilized the fingers, creating a claw-like flexion deformity. (From Cotran, R.S., Kumar, V., and Robbins, S.L. [1994]. *Robbins Pathologic Basis of Disease.* [5th ed.]. Philadelphia: W.B. Saunders. [p. 212].)

Skin Cancers

The most common skin cancers are **basal cell carcinoma** (Color Fig. 36–8) and **squamous cell carcinoma** (Color Fig. 36–9), both of which are highly curable. The most deadly form of skin cancer is malignant melanoma (Color Fig. 36–10). These disorders are detailed below. **Kaposi's sarcoma (KS)**, a cancer of the vascular endothelium in skin and other tissues that was once uncommon, has emerged as an opportunistic cancer in AIDS (see Chapter 13). Table 36–17 summarizes clinical characteristics of KS and several other benign, premalignant, and malignant skin tumors.

Nonmelanoma Skin Cancer (Basal Cell Carcinoma and Squamous Cell Carcinoma)

Definition. Basal cell carcinoma and squamous cell carcinoma are malignant lesions arising from epidermal epithelial cells.

Epidemiology. Nonmelanoma skin cancer is the most common cancer in the United States, with an annual incidence of about 900,000 cases.[34] The most important risk factors are sunlight exposure and aging. Aging, of course, is associated with longer duration of exposure to solar radiation, but may also be an independent risk factor for cancer. Because they produce less protective melanin, light-skinned persons (types I to III) are more susceptible to harmful effects of sunlight than dark-skinned individuals. A genetic predisposition may play a minor role in basal cell carcinoma. Skin cancers may be opportunistic in immunosuppressed individuals.

Etiology. The precise etiologic mechanism in these skin cancers is unknown, but the primary role of UV light exposure is well accepted. UV light (particularly within the spectrum referred to as UVB) is known to create mutations at points on DNA where pyrimidine bases lie adjacent to each other.[35] In most cases of nonmelanoma skin cancer, these mutations are found in the *p53* gene, a tumor suppressor gene. Normally, the *p53* gene either prevents a DNA-damaged cell from reproducing until its repair systems have had time to work or induces apoptosis (programmed cell death) in the damaged cell, preventing its reproduction.

Pathophysiology. Basal cell carcinoma originates from basal cells in the deepest layer of the epidermis. Tumors occur in sun-exposed areas (usually the head and neck) and extend locally but do not metastasize. Squamous cell carcinoma also develops in sun-exposed areas (usually the head, neck, extremities, or back), often arising from a premalignant lesion such as an area of **actinic keratosis, leukoplakia,** scarring, or ulceration. The in situ type tumor extends within the epidermis and dermis, whereas the invasive type may spread to regional lymph nodes.

Clinical Manifestations. Growth of basal cell carcinoma is slow, beginning as a light-colored nodule and often developing into a lesion with a characteristic central depression and rolled border (see Color Fig. 36–8). Several different types of clinical lesions are possible, however. As the tumor grows, it often ulcerates and crusts over. Local tissue destruction may be extensive. Squamous cell carcinomas are usually firm, elevated, granular-appearing tumors that bleed easily (see Color Fig. 36–9). Lymphadenopathy is associated with the invasive type.

Prevention and Treatment. Prevention requires minimization of sun exposure with appropriate use of protective clothing and sun block preparations with a skin protection factor (SPF) of 15 or greater, depending on skin type. Protection of children is particularly important, because it is the cumulative dose of UV light exposure that is implicated in

TABLE 36–17
BENIGN, PREMALIGNANT, AND LESS COMMON MALIGNANT TUMORS OF THE SKIN

Tumor	Description
Benign Tumors	
Seborrheic keratoses (senile keratoses)	Common epidermal tumor occurring most frequently in middle-aged and older individuals; round, flat plaques that are tan to dark brown; cells of origin are basal cells that produce excess keratin
Fibroepithelial polyp (skin tag)	Soft, flesh-colored bag-like tumor connected to the skin by a slender stalk; most common in middle-aged and older persons; consist of fibrovascular core covered by squamous epithelium; may become more numerous during pregnancy
Keratoacanthoma	Rapidly developing neoplasm similar to well-differentiated squamous cell carcinoma, but heals spontaneously; most common in middle-aged white men; appears as flesh-colored, dome-shaped nodules with central, keratin-filled plug
Benign fibrous histiocytoma	Dermal neoplasm originating from fibroblasts and histiocytes (tissue macrophages); often occurs on legs of young and middle-aged women; lesions are tan to brown, firm papules that may flatten and grow to several centimeters in diameter
Dermatofibrosarcoma protuberans	Well-differentiated benign tumor originating from dermal fibroblasts; may extend deeply into subcutaneous fat; tumor is a firm, solid nodule that may ulcerate; usually located on the trunk
Xanthoma	Collection of foamy histiocytes within the dermis; associated with dyslipidemias and lymphomas or may occur in the absence of underlying disorder
Premalignant Tumors	
Actinic keratosis	Lesion developing as a result of excess keratin production in response to sunlight exposure; usually less than 1 cm in diameter, tan, brown, red, and flesh-colored; may develop cutaneous "horns"; highest prevalence in light-skinned individuals; located in sun-exposed areas
Malignant Tumors	
Merkel's cell carcinoma	Rare neoplasm originating from Merkel's cells of the epidermis; closely resembles small-cell tumors of the lung
Mycosis fungoides (cutaneous T-cell lymphoma)	Scaly, red-brown patches and nodules that may remain localized to the skin for many years or may disseminate systemically; cell of origin is a CD4+ T-helper cell that forms band-like clusters within the superficial dermis and invades the epidermis; may be virally induced
Kaposi's sarcoma	Most common malignant lesion in patients with AIDS; transformed cell is a spindle-shaped cell of probable vascular origin; skin and oral mucosa most frequently affected with discrete, irregular, red, purple, or brown nodules, macules, patches, or plaques in symmetric distribution; systemic dissemination is common

Data from Cotran, R.S., Kumar, V., and Robbins, S.L. (1994). *Robbins Pathologic Basis of Disease.* (5th ed.). Philadelphia: W.B. Saunders. (pp. 1185–1192).

DNA damage. Individuals who have disorders or are taking drugs that may induce photosensitivity should also be particularly vigilant. Surgical removal of premalignant lesions is advocated. Malignant tumors are treated with surgical removal or destruction with heat (electrocautery), freezing with liquid nitrogen or nitrous oxide (cryosurgery), or radiation.

Prognosis and Outcome. Basal cell carcinoma and squamous cell carcinoma are highly curable. Squamous cell carcinoma may metastasize in some cases, and it causes an estimated 1200 deaths per year.[34] Disfigurement is also possible because of the destructive effects of the tumor or its excision.

Malignant Melanoma

Definition. Malignant melanoma is a malignant neoplasm originating from melanocytes.

Epidemiology. The incidence of malignant melanoma is rising more rapidly than that of any other cancer. The expected annual incidence is now about 34,000 cases.[34] Fair-skinned individuals between 20 and 40 years of age who live in sunbelt states are at highest risk. Melanoma is uncommon in children and adolescents, with only 1% to 4% occurring in these age groups.[36] Both sexes are equally affected. Risk factors include sunlight exposure, genetic predisposition, immunosuppression, radiation therapy, PUVA light therapy, and chemotherapy. Although melanomas may arise from normal skin, they are much more likely to develop from transformation of an existing **nevus** (benign mole). Nevi that are most likely to undergo malignant transformation are those that are: (1) large and present at birth (congenital melanocytic nevi); (2) atypical or dysplastic (larger and more irregular in color, texture, and contour than typical nevi); or (3) caused by an autosomal dominant syndrome of multiple moles (familial atypical mole/melanoma syndrome [FAMM]).[36]

Etiology. The precise etiology of malignant melanoma is unknown. Mutation of the *p53* gene is apparently not involved.[35]

Pathophysiology. Malignant transformation occurs within melanocytes in the basal layer of the epidermis, or, more commonly, within the aggregated melanocytes of an existing nevus. The initial appearance and pattern of tumor growth and metastasis differ among tumor subtypes. *Superficial spreading melanoma* and *lentigo malignant melanoma* tend to extend horizontally within the epidermal and superficial dermal layers, whereas *nodular melanoma* extends vertically into deeper tissues and demonstrates a high potential for metastasis. Local invasion, regional lymph node metastasis, and distant metastasis are possible with all subtypes, however.

Clinical Manifestations. Appearance of a new nevus or changes in a pre-existing nevus are characteristic of malignant melanoma. Nevi that are suspicious meet the "ABCD" criteria: they are *a*symmetric, with irregular *b*orders and deep brown, blue, black or variable *c*olor, and a *d*iameter greater than 6 mm (see Color Fig. 36–10).[34] Any itching or nontraumatic bleeding of a nevus is also characteristic of melanoma. Regional lymph node enlargement may be evident, and signs of distant metastasis depend on metastatic site.

Prevention and Treatment. Protection from sunlight exposure is warranted. Surgical excision and biopsy should be done for any suspicious nevi. For known malignant melanoma, surgical excision is the treatment of choice. Dissection of regional lymph nodes may also be required. Treatment of metastatic disease may include immunotherapy and combination chemotherapy. The most effective chemotherapeutic agent is dacarbazine (DTIC), especially in combination with α-interferon.

Prognosis and Outcome. Prognosis depends on the site and depth of the initial lesions as well as the extent of metastasis. Lesions of the extremities have the most favorable prognosis, and trunk lesions have the poorest. Five-year survival in early, nonmetastatic disease is approximately 75%. The survival rate drops to about 35% with metastatic disease.[37] About 7200 deaths occur each year because of melanoma.[34]

Burns

Definition. A burn is an injury to skin and possibly deeper tissues resulting from direct contact with excessive heat, corrosive chemicals, electricity, or radiation.

Epidemiology. Each year in the United States, an estimated 1.25 million individuals are burned severely enough to seek treatment.[38] The incidence has been steadily declining in recent years. Those at highest risk are the elderly, whose risk relates to impairment of mobility or sensation, and children, whose risk often relates to neglect or abuse. Occupational exposure (e.g., in laboratory workers, farm laborers, or rural electrical lineworkers) often plays a role in chemical or electrical burns. Lightning is also a significant source of electrical burns and may be associated with recreational exposure (e.g., golfers). In the absence of nuclear war, radiation burns are the least common, but may occur with accidental occupational exposure or as an unavoidable consequence of radiation therapy. Sunburn is technically a radiation burn, but it is more commonly considered to be a form of photodermatitis.

Etiology. Thermal burns result from exposure of the skin or mucous membranes to direct flame, hot liquids, or radiant energy. Chemical burns result from direct contact with the skin (chemical spills) or mucous membranes (inhalation of toxic gases such as smoke or ammonia or ingestion of corrosive agents such as lye). Electrical burns result from passage of current from a high-voltage source through the body to the ground.

Pathophysiology. Cellular proteins are denatured by the injuring agent. Death of some cells occurs because of traumatic or ischemic necrosis. Loss of collagen cross-linking also occurs with denaturation, creating abnormal osmotic and hydrostatic pressure gradients for movement of intravascular fluid to the interstitial space. Cellular injury triggers the release of mediators of inflammation, contributing to local and, in the case of major burns, systemic increases in capillary permeability. Specific pathophysiologic events depend on the cause and classification of the burn.

Classification of Burn Wounds. In *first-degree (superficial) burns,* cellular damage is limited to the epidermis, and the barrier function of the skin remains intact. *Second-degree (partial-thickness) burns* include two categories: superficial second degree, in which there is destruction of the epidermis and some of the dermis, and deep second degree, in which the epidermis and dermis are destroyed but some dermal appendages remain intact. Barrier function is lost in both types of second-degree burns. A *third-degree (full-thickness) burn* is one in which the entire epidermis and dermis are destroyed, along with some subcutaneous tissue. The designation of *fourth-degree burn* is sometimes used to denote burns extending to muscle and bone or in reference to electrical burns, which may burn deeper tissues while leaving surface cells intact.

Burn severity criteria are used in clinical practice to determine the nature of treatment. Generally, *major burns* include partial-thickness burns involving more than 20% of the body surface, full-thickness burns involving more than 10%, any burns associated with inhalation injury or major trauma to other systems, and electrical burns complicated by dysrhythmias. Either of two methods may be used to estimate the total burn surface area (TBSA): the rule of nines (Fig. 36–13) or the Lund and Browder Chart (Fig. 36–14).

The site of the injury and the degree of pretraumatic disability of the individual are also relevant to classifications of burn severity. Edema associated with the inflammatory response may lead to airway obstruction with burns of the face and neck, for example. Circumferential burns could result in ischemia of underlying and distal tissues related to edema and later contraction of scar tissue. In individuals with limited functional reserve because of pre-existing cardiovascular, respiratory, or renal disease, less severe burns could precipitate system failure.

Local and Systemic Responses to Major Burns. Minor burns trigger an appropriate inflammatory response, which leads to healing by regeneration if the wound is relatively small, adequately perfused and nourished, and uncomplicated by infection. Larger wounds or suboptimal conditions lead to healing with scar tissue.

The pathophysiology of major burns includes not only the inflammatory response designed to restore integrity of the wound, but the profound systemic responses resulting from (1) loss of normal skin functions, (2) the stress response, and (3) release of massive amounts of cytokines and other local mediators associated with large-scale inflammation. With electrical burns, dysrhythmias such as ventricular fibrillation may result from depolarization of myocardial cells (see Chapter 17). With inhalation injury, direct thermal injury (above the larynx) and chemical injury from toxins in inhaled gases or smoke may damage the alveolar-capillary membrane, leading to adult respiratory distress syndrome (ARDS), and carbon monoxide intoxication may also occur (see Chapter 19). Even in the absence of direct trauma to the cardiac or respiratory systems, major burns induce significant functional alterations in all body systems. These are discussed in the next section with their resulting clinical manifestations.

Clinical Manifestations

Appearance and Sensation of the Burn Wound. First-degree burns are red (erythematous) and painful, and blisters may form after 24 hours. Superficial

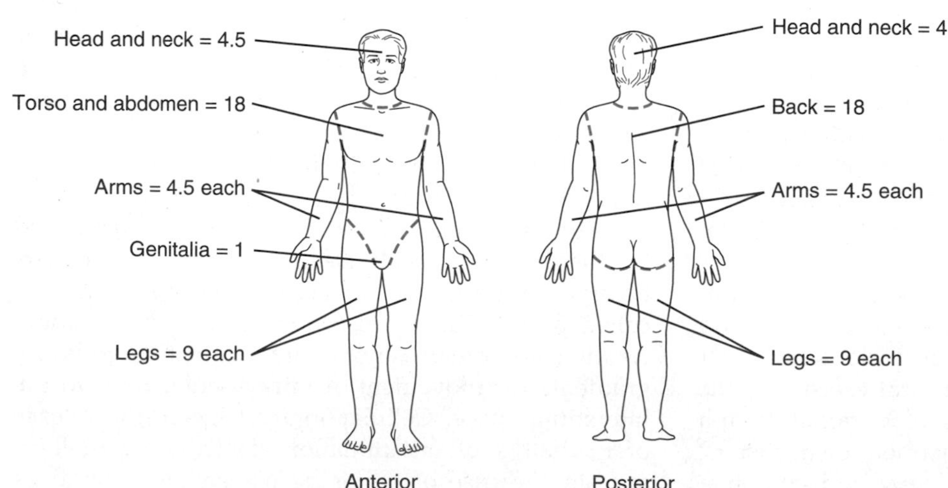

FIGURE 36–13
Rule of nines. Total burn surface area may be quickly estimated with this method, in which the body parts are assigned percentages based on the number nine. The anterior and posterior legs are each 9%, the head 4.5%, anterior and posterior arms 4.5% each, the torso and abdomen 18%, and the back 18%. The remaining 1% is assigned to the genitalia.

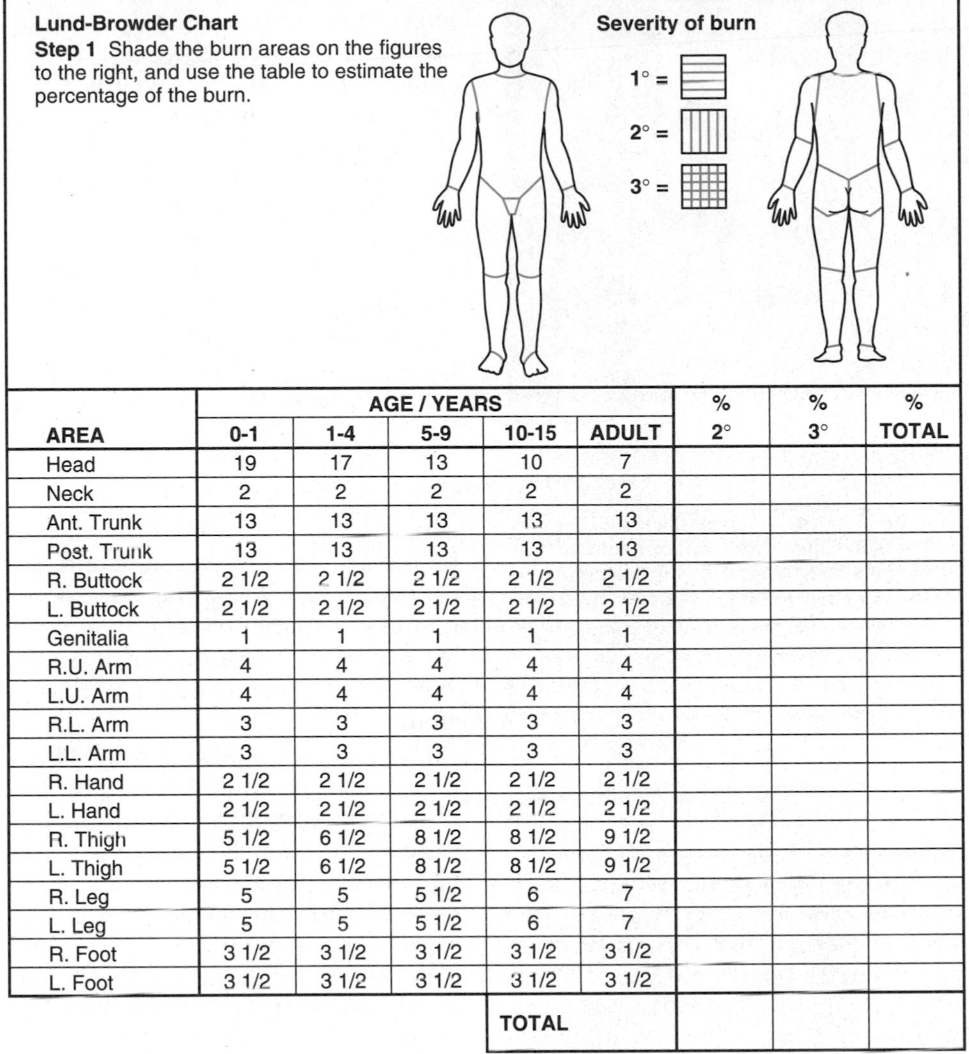
Lund-Browder Chart
Step 1 Shade the burn areas on the figures to the right, and use the table to estimate the percentage of the burn.
Severity of burn
1° =
2° =
3° =

AREA	AGE / YEARS 0-1	1-4	5-9	10-15	ADULT	% 2°	% 3°	% TOTAL
Head	19	17	13	10	7			
Neck	2	2	2	2	2			
Ant. Trunk	13	13	13	13	13			
Post. Trunk	13	13	13	13	13			
R. Buttock	2 1/2	2 1/2	2 1/2	2 1/2	2 1/2			
L. Buttock	2 1/2	2 1/2	2 1/2	2 1/2	2 1/2			
Genitalia	1	1	1	1	1			
R.U. Arm	4	4	4	4	4			
L.U. Arm	4	4	4	4	4			
R.L. Arm	3	3	3	3	3			
L.L. Arm	3	3	3	3	3			
R. Hand	2 1/2	2 1/2	2 1/2	2 1/2	2 1/2			
L. Hand	2 1/2	2 1/2	2 1/2	2 1/2	2 1/2			
R. Thigh	5 1/2	6 1/2	8 1/2	8 1/2	9 1/2			
L. Thigh	5 1/2	6 1/2	8 1/2	8 1/2	9 1/2			
R. Leg	5	5	5 1/2	6	7			
L. Leg	5	5	5 1/2	6	7			
R. Foot	3 1/2	3 1/2	3 1/2	3 1/2	3 1/2			
L. Foot	3 1/2	3 1/2	3 1/2	3 1/2	3 1/2			
				TOTAL				

FIGURE 36–14

Lund-Browder chart. Total burn surface area may be more precisely assessed using this chart, which assigns specific percentages to each body part and accounts for burn thickness and developmental differences.

second-degree burns are characterized by redness and blisters that develop soon after the injury. The wound is especially painful when blisters rupture, exposing nerve endings. Deep second-degree and third-degree wounds are similar in appearance (Fig. 36–15). They are typically waxy-white and surrounded by areas of partial-thickness injury. In deep second-degree burns, hair follicles are intact and hair regrowth is evident after 7 to 10 days. Deep second-degree and third-degree burns are essentially nonpainful, because pain receptors have been destroyed. Pain may be present as a result of a lesser depth of burn at the wound edges, however.

Fluid Imbalances and Shifts. During the immediate postburn period, capillaries throughout the body "unseal," or attain maximal dilation and permeability. The precise mechanism of this response is uncertain, but it is probably related to massive release of inflammatory mediators such as histamine, prostaglandins, and kinins from the injured area. Intravascular fluid then shifts into interstitial space, and insensible (evaporative) fluid loss to the environment is increased to about 10 times the normal rate.[39] Hypovolemic shock (**burn shock**) results, manifesting as decreased cardiac output, hypotension, tachycardia, and decreased urine output (see Chapter 15). Burn shock necessitates intravenous infusion of large volumes of isotonic fluid to restore intravascular volume and perfuse vital organs; however, a significant portion of the infused volume shifts immedi-

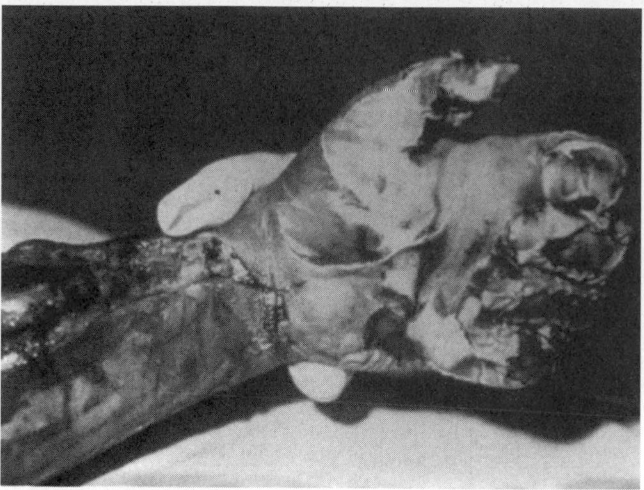

FIGURE 36–15

Third-degree (full-thickness) burn. This full-thickness burn injury to the hand and arm resulted from direct flame contact. Natural débridement of the skin is visible in the palmar aspect and digits. Escharotomy has been done on the forearm. (From Kitt, S., *et al.* [1995]. *Emergency Nursing.* [2nd ed.]. Philadelphia: W.B. Saunders. [p. 586].)

ately to the interstitial space, manifesting as massive edema. Myocardial contractility is decreased in patients with major burns, possibly because of hypothermia, right ventricular dysfunction, acidosis, poor myocardial perfusion, or release of cytokines that have a myocardial depressant effect.[40] Cardiac output remains lower than normal, even when intravascular volume is restored. Hypovolemic shock, along with possible rhabdomyolysis related to sepsis or muscle injury, may result in acute renal failure. Disseminated intravascular coagulation (DIC) is a common complication of major burns, resulting from release of massive amounts of tissue thromboplastin from burn-injured or ischemic tissues.

About 24 hours after the injury, capillary beds (except those suffering direct burn injury) return to their preburn diameter and permeability, or are said to "reseal." This response, apparently mediated by cytokines, restores normal capillary dynamics, halting the plasma-to-interstitial shift and favoring reabsorption of edema fluid because of the high interstitial fluid pressure. If the kidneys are functional, a period of increased urine output (diuresis) follows. Hypokalemia often results from potassium washout with increased tubular flow rates, placing the individual at risk for cardiac dysrhythmias (see Chapter 9).

Impairment of Barrier Function and Defense. Loss of the skin barrier not only permits increased evaporative water loss, but also allows access of pathogenic microorganisms to the wound. Infection of major burns is probably inevitable, despite meticulous aseptic technique and a limited access environment in burn care centers. Translocation of microorganisms across the gut wall is a consequence of the stress response in major trauma, because selective vasoconstriction mediated by the sympathetic nervous system decreases perfusion of the GI system (see Chapter 15). Stress ulceration of the intestinal wall is very common and is known as **Curling's ulcer** when it occurs in burn patients. Bacterial translocation and disruption of the skin barrier by the burn wound and invasive lines and tubes places the burn victim at high risk for septic shock, which may contribute to prolongation of peripheral vasodilation and edema, ARDS, DIC, rhabdomyolysis and renal failure, as well as hypermetabolism and hyperthermia (discussed later).

In addition to impairment of barrier defense, immunologic defense is also suppressed. The functions of phagocytic cells, the complement system, and lymphocytes are less effective in burn patients, for reasons that are incompletely understood. Presumably, local cytokines mediate these apparently maladaptive effects.

Hypermetabolism and Hyperthermia. Initially, the patient's body temperature may be low because of increased evaporative fluid loss. Body temperature is soon elevated, however, as a consequence of inflammatory mediators (interleukins) that reset the hypothalamic thermostat upward (see Chapter 11). This high set point can only be sustained with an increase in the basal metabolic rate. Other mechanisms contributing to hyperthermia in burn patients include the profound stress response and the demands of injured tissues for substrate for wound healing. The patient with major burns may need up to 3500 to 5000 calories a day to support the hypermetabolic state.

Prevention and Treatment. Prevention of burn injuries is the focus of many public education efforts and legislative campaigns. School children are taught to "stop, drop, and roll" if their clothing is on fire. Smoke detectors are in widespread use in homes and public buildings. Safety measures and employee education are mandated in industries where the risk of fire, chemical exposure, and electrical injury exist. Fire-retardant materials are used in the manufacturing of clothing, and appliance manufacturers are incorporating safer design (e.g., placing stove burner controls at the front).

Minor burns without systemic manifestations usually heal spontaneously within a few days to weeks. Fluid resuscitation is the immediate priority in major burns, with the amount usually determined by standard protocols based on the patient's weight and the total burn surface area. Crystalloid solutions such as lactated Ringer's solution are infused in very large volumes, because only 20% to 30% of the fluid administered remains in the vascular system. When capillaries reseal, fluid administration is titrated against cardiac output and urine output. Renal function may require support with diuretics or dialysis. Inhalation injury may require intubation and mechanical ventilation of the patient. Carbon monoxide intoxication is treated with 100% oxygen.

The burn wound must be cleaned and débrided to remove dead tissue, reduce infection risk, and promote healing. In some centers, this procedure is done while the patient is in a water-filled tank or whirlpool (hydrotherapy). Débridement is very painful in tissues where pain receptors and sensory nerves are intact, and provision of adequate analgesia may be difficult because pain originates from superficial tissues that are poorly perfused. The crust of drainage and sloughed cells (**eschar**) that forms over the burn surface may restrict underlying circulation, requiring surgical incision (escharotomy) to relieve or prevent pressure. Incision of the fascia (fasciotomy) may be necessary to relieve pressure in deeper wounds.

Topical antibiotics are applied to the wound, and it is covered with a light dressing to provide a barrier against microorganism access. Skin grafts are usually applied as early as possible to restore the barrier. Grafts may be temporary allografts or permanent autografts (see Chapter 13). The use of cultured and artifical skin products is a recent innovation in the treatment of burn injury. Major burns may require repeated skin graft surgeries over months or years. Scarring associated with burn healing is disfiguring, and excessive scarring (keloid formation) is common (see Chapter 13). Burned joint areas must be splinted in positions of function so that contractures do not develop. Compression masks and garments are used to minimize scarring. Because nutritional needs are very great during wound healing as well as during the hypermetabolic state, a high-calorie diet and supplementation of vitamins and minerals are provided.

Prognosis and Outcome. Deaths caused by burns have declined from 12,000 to 6000 per year since 1990, in part the result of improved care of major burns.[39] Present alternatives for minimization of scarring are not very effective, however, and major burns are associated with unsightly, restrictive, and uncomfortable hypertrophic scars.[38] Optimal recovery from major burns requires not only physical rehabilitation, but often emotional support and vocational rehabilitation as well.

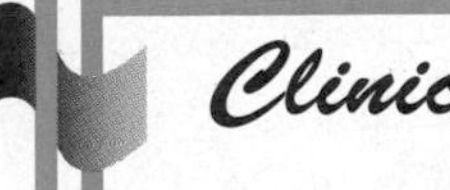

Clinical Scenario

J.L., an 86-year-old widower, suffers a burn injury while attempting to put out a kitchen grease fire. On arrival at the emergency department he is semiconscious and is found to have partial-thickness and full-thickness burns of his face, both arms and hands, and the upper third of his anterior chest. J.L. appears to have difficulty breathing and is moaning as if in pain. He has a cough that is productive of black, soot-like material.

1. What is the estimated extent of body surface area involved with J.L.'s burn? Is this a major burn?
2. What is the probable cause of J.L.'s respiratory distress?

CLINICAL SIGNIFICANCE OF INTEGUMENTARY DISORDERS

The integumentary system not only encloses, but interacts functionally with all body systems. Disorders of the integument affect individuals of all ages. Although few integumentary disorders are life threatening, the visibility of manifestations and the chronicity of many dermatologic diseases is often emotionally traumatic and financially stressful. Much has yet to be learned about the etiology of acne vulgaris and psoriasis, two very common integumentary disorders. The cellular mechanisms of burn injury are also obscure. The incidence of malignant melanoma is increasing epidemically, and means must be found of reducing the risk of this and other skin cancers. Development of definitive therapy for many disorders that are now treated empirically is an ongoing priority.

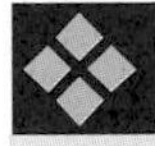

Summary of Key Points

- The skin is composed of two principal layers, the outer epidermis, composed of layers of epithelial cells, and the inner dermis, composed of connective tissue supporting appendages (hair follicles, sebaceous glands, and sweat glands), blood vessels, and nerves.

Summary continued on following page

The skin is replete with sensory receptors, as required for its function in interacting with the external environment. The vascular supply to the skin serves as a high-volume reservoir that responds to the need to shunt blood to more critical organs during stress or shock or to retain or dissipate core body temperature.

- Skin receptors transmit sensory information to the central nervous system, initiating reflex and voluntary motor responses and autonomic responses. Tickle and itch are complex sensations initiated from skin structures and are apparently mediated by the same pathways and neuromodulators as pain sensation. Skin growth and secretion are mediated by numerous hormones, notably androgens, estrogen, cortisol, growth hormone, and melanocyte-stimulating hormone. Alteration in hormone levels with developmental changes or with endocrine disease manifests as changes in integumentary function.

- Primary skin lesions are those arising from previously normal skin as a consequence of disease and include a number of solid and fluid-filled lesions of variable depth and diameter. Secondary skin lesions arise as a consequence of rupture, mechanical irritation, extension, invasion, normal healing, or abnormal healing of primary lesions.

- In addition to signaling the presence of primary integumentary disorders, skin manifestations may often be clues to the presence of underlying systemic disease. Genetic disorders, connective tissue diseases, hematopoietic disorders, sepsis, and neoplasia commonly produce integumentary manifestations.

- Infection often causes inflammatory disorders of the skin. Skin infections may be bacterial, viral, fungal, or parasitic. Inflammation of the skin may also occur in response to allergic or irritative processes and as a component of immune-mediated or idiopathic disorders.

- Nonmelanoma skin cancers, the most common form of cancer, include squamous cell carcinoma and basal cell carcinoma. Malignant melanoma is the other major type of skin cancer. Nonmelanoma skin cancers arise from basal cells and keratinocytes of the epidermal layer, whereas malignant melanoma arises from pigment-producing melanocytes. Risk in all three types is associated with cumulative dose of sunlight exposure, a risk that is magnified in fair-skinned individuals. Squamous cell carcinoma remains superficial. Basal cell carcinoma may metastasize in a minority of cases and has caused some deaths. Malignant melanoma is highly metastatic unless discovered and treated in an early stage.

- A major burn is an extreme stressor that initiates a cascade of physiologic responses extending beyond the burned area to affect all body systems. The inflammatory response to this injury is profound, and the associated release of inflammatory mediators as well as the injury-induced loss of normal skin functions results in significant alteration of fluid and electrolyte balance, metabolism, thermoregulation, and function of the cardiovascular, respiratory, renal, and GI systems.

REFERENCES

1. Millikan, L.E. (1996). Treating pruritus: What's new in safe relief of symptoms? *Postgraduate Medicine* 99(1), 173–184.
2. Bologna, J.L. (1995). Aging skin. *American Journal of Medicine* 98(1A suppl.), 99S–103S.
3. Eller, M.S., Yaar, M., Ostrom, K., *et al.* (1995). A role for interleukin-1 in epidermal differentiation: Regulation by expression of functional versus decoy receptors. *Journal of Cell Science* 108, 2741–2746.
4. Roujeau, J.C., and Stern, R.S. (1994). Severe adverse cutaneous reactions to drugs. *New England Journal of Medicine* 331(19), 1272–1285.
5. Hacker, S.M. (1994). Common infections of the skin: Characteristics, causes, and cures. *Postgraduate Medicine* 96(2), 43–52.
6. Kahn, R.M., and Goldstein, E.J.C. (1993). Common bacterial skin infections: Diagnostic clues and therapeutic options. *Postgraduate Medicine* 93(6), 175–182.
7. Bisno, A.L., and Stevens, D.L. (1996). Streptococcal infections of skin and soft tissues. *New England Journal of Medicine* 334(4), 240–245.
8. Bergus, G.R., and Johnson, J.S. (1993). Superficial tinea infections. *American Family Physician* 48(2), 259–268.
9. Brodell, R.T., and Elewski, B. (1997). Superficial fungal infections: Errors to avoid in diagnosis and treatment. *Postgraduate Medicine* 101(4), 279–287.
10. Cotran, R.S., Kumar, V., and Robbins, S.L. (1994). *Robbins Pathologic Basis of Disease*. Philadelphia: W.B. Saunders. (pp. 210–213, 354–355, 1197–1198).
11. Bodey, G.P. (1994). Dermatologic manifestations of infections in neutropenic patients. *Infectious Disease Clinics of North America* 8(3), 655–675.
12. Miller, D.M., and Brodell, R.T. (1996). Human papillomavirus infection: Treatment options for warts. *American Family Physician* 53(1), 135–143.
13. Black, J.M., and Matassarin-Jacobs, E. (1997). *Medical-Surgical Nursing: Clinical Management for Continuity of Care*. (5th ed.). Philadelphia: W.B. Saunders. (pp. 677–678, 1724, 2210–2211).
14. Dudley, M.N. (1995). Management of herpesvirus infections in the healthy host. *Pharmacotherapy* 15(5 pt. 2), 43S–48S.

15. Wharton, M. (1996). The epidemiology of varicella-zoster virus infections. *Infectious Disease Clinics of North America* 10(3), 571–581.
16. Kost, R.G., and Straus, S.E. (1996). Postherpetic neuralgia—Pathogenesis, treatment, and prevention. *New England Journal of Medicine* 335(1), 32–42.
17. Foster, R.L.R., Hunsberger, M.M., and Anderson, J.J.T. (1989). *Family-Centered Nursing Care of Children*. Philadelphia: W.B. Saunders. (pp. 1640–1641).
18. Mackey, S.L., and Wagner, K.F. (1994). Dermatologic manifestations of parasitic diseases. *Infectious Disease Clinics of North America* 8(3), 713–743.
19. Meinking, T.L., Taplin, D., Hermida, J.L., *et al.* (1995). The treatment of scabies with ivermectin. *New England Journal of Medicine* 333(1), 26–30.
20. Sokoloff, F. (1994). Identification and management of pediculosis. *Nurse Practitioner* 19(8), 62–64.
21. Reisman, R.E. (1994). Insect stings. *New England Journal of Medicine* 331(8), 523–527.
22. Zug, K.A., and McKay, M. (1996). Eczematous dermatitis: A practical review. *American Family Physician* 54(4), 1243–1250.
23. Landow, K. (1997). Atopic dermatitis: Current concepts support old therapies and spur new ones. *Postgraduate Medicine* 101(3), 101–118.
24. Agency for Toxic Substances and Disease Registry. (1993). Contact dermatitis and urticaria from environmental exposures. *American Family Physician* 48(5), 773–780.
25. Klaus, M.V., and Wieselthier, J.S. (1993). Contact dermatitis. *American Family Physician* 48(4), 629–632.
26. Greaves, M.W. (1995). Chronic urticaria. *New England Journal of Medicine* 332(26), 1767–1772.
27. Sveum, R.J. (1996). Urticaria: The diagnostic challenge of hives. *Postgraduate Medicine* 100(2), 77–84.
28. Janniger, C.K., and Schwartz, R.A. (1995). Seborrheic dermatitis. *American Family Physician* 52(1), 149–155.
29. Leyden, J.J. (1997). Therapy for acne vulgaris. *New England Journal of Medicine* 336(16), 1156–1162.
30. Nguyen, Q.H., Kim, Y.A., and Schwartz, R.A. (1994). Management of acne vulgaris. *American Family Physician* 50(1), 89–96.
31. Mackrides, P.S., and Shaughnessy, A.F. (1996). Azelaic acid therapy for acne. *American Family Physician* 54(8), 2457–2459.
32. Wolff, K. (1997). Should PUVA be abandoned? *New England Journal of Medicine* 336(15), 1090–1091.
33. Braunwald, E., Isselbacher, K.J., Petersdorf, R.G., *et al.* (Eds). (1987). *Harrison's Principles of Internal Medicine*. (11th ed.). New York: McGraw-Hill. (pp. 1428–1433).
34. Brandt, T.P. (1996). Skin cancer screening. *Medical Clinics of North America* 80(1), 99–114.
35. Leffell, D.J., and Brash, D.E. (1996). Sunlight and skin cancer. *Scientific American* 275(1), 52–59.
36. Williams, M.L., and Pennella, R. (1994). Melanoma, melanocytic nevi, and other melanoma risk factors in children. *Journal of Pediatrics* 124(6), 833–845.
37. Ceballos, P.I., Ruiz-Maldonado, R., and Mihm, M.C., Jr. (1995). Melanoma in children. *New England Journal of Medicine* 332(10), 656–662.
38. Monafo, W.W. (1996). Initial management of burns. *New England Journal of Medicine* 335(21), 1581–1586.
39. Allwood, J.S. (1995). The primary care management of burns. *Nurse Practitioner* 20(8), 76–87.
40. Byers, J.F., and Flynn, M.B. (1996). Acute burn injury: A trauma case report. *Critical Care Nurse* 16(4), 55–66.
41. Greenfield, E., and Jordan, B. (1996). Advances in burn wound care. *Critical Care Nursing Clinics of North America* 8(2), 203–215.

SELECTED BIBLIOGRAPHY

Beacham, B.E. (1993). Common dermatoses in the elderly. *American Family Physician* 47(6), 1445–1450.

Bulbul, R., Williams, W.V., and Shumacher, H.R. Jr. (1995). Psoriatic arthritis: Diverse and sometimes highly destructive. *Postgraduate Medicine* 97(4), 97–108.

Caldwell, S.H., and Popenoe, R. (1995). Perceptions and misperceptions of skin color. *Annals of Internal Medicine* 122(8), 614–617.

Clark, L.C., Combs, G.F. Jr., Turnbull, B.W., *et al.* (1996). Effects of selenium supplementation for cancer prevention in patients with carcinoma of the skin: A randomized controlled trial. *Journal of the American Medical Association* 276(24), 1957–1963.

Cohen, P.R. (1994). Cutaneous paraneoplastic syndromes. *American Family Physician* 50(6), 1273–1282.

Cohen, P.R. (1995). Skin cues to primary and metastatic malignancy. *American Family Physician* 51(5), 1199–1204.

Farmer, K.C., and Naylor, M.F. (1996). Sun exposure, sunscreens, and skin cancer prevention: A year-round concern. *Annals of Pharmacotherapy* 30, 662–673.

Hocutt, J.E. Jr. (1993). Skin cryosurgery for the family physician. *American Family Physician* 48(3), 445–452.

Holmes, C.E., and Massa, M.C. (1994). Skin signs of systemic disease: When the problem is more than skin-deep. *Postgraduate Medicine* 96(8), 93–102.

Jarvis, C. (1992). *Physical Examination and Health Assessment*. Philadelphia: W.B. Saunders. (pp. 223–273).

Juckett, G. (1996). Plant dermatitis: Possible culprits go far beyond poison ivy. *Postgraduate Medicine* 100(3), 159–171.

Khorenian, S.D., and Lebwohl, M. (1995). New cutaneous manifestations of systemic diseases. *American Family Physician* 51(3), 625–630.

Kuflik, A.S., and Janniger, C.K. (1993). Basal cell carcinoma. *American Family Physician* 48(7), 1273–1276.

Levin, M.J., and Hayward, A.R. (1996). Prevention of herpes zoster. *Infectious Disease Clinics of North America* 10(3), 657–675.

Lucky, A.W. (1995). Hormonal correlates of acne and hirsutism. *American Journal of Medicine* 98(1A suppl.), 89S–94S.

Lucky, A.W., Biro, F.M., Simbarti, L.A., *et al.* (1997). Predictors of severity of acne vulgaris in young adolescent girls: Results of a five-year longitudinal study. *Journal of Pediatrics* 130(1), 30–39.

Martin, D.H., and Mroczkowski, T.F. (1994). Dermatologic manifestations of sexually transmitted diseases other than HIV. *Infectious Disease Clinics of North America* 8(3), 533–582.

Moore, K.L., and Persaud, T.V.N. (1993). *The Developing Human: Clinically Oriented Embryology*. (5th ed.). Philadelphia: W.B. Saunders. (pp. 443–448).

Ostezan, L.B., and Callen, J.P. (1996). Cutaneous manifestations of selected rheumatologic diseases. *American Family Physician* 53(5), 1625–1633.

Rabkin, C.S., Janz, S., Lash, A., *et al.* (1997). Monoclonal origin of multicentric Kaposi's sarcoma lesions. *New England Journal of Medicine* 336(14), 988–993.

Rosenfield, R.L., and Deplewski, D. (1995). Role of androgens in the developmental biology of the pilosebaceous unit. *American Journal of Medicine* 98(1A suppl.), 80S–88S.

Ruddy, R.M. (1994). Smoke inhalation injury. *Pediatric Clinics of North America* 41(2), 317–336.

Schwartz, R., Das-Young, L.R., and Frank, E. (1996). Current and future management of serious skin and skin-structure infections. *American Journal of Medicine* 100(6A suppl.), 90S–95S.

Stern, R.S., Nichols, K.T., and Vakeva, L.H., for the PUVA Follow-Up Study. (1997). Malignant melanoma in patients treated for psoriasis with methoxsalen (psoralen) and ultraviolet A radiation (PUVA). *New England Journal of Medicine* 336(15), 1041–1045.

Sussman, G.L., and Beezhold, D.H. (1995). Allergy to latex rubber. *Annals of Internal Medicine* 122(1), 43–46.

Walter, J.B. (1992). *An Introduction to the Principles of Disease.* (3rd ed.). Philadelphia: W.B. Saunders. (pp. 142–204).

Wang, C-Y.E., Schroeter, A.L., and Su, W.P.D. (1995). Acquired immunodeficiency syndrome–related Kaposi's sarcoma. *Mayo Clinic Proceedings* 70, 869–879.

Wang, C-Y., Brodlund, D.G., and Su, W.P.D. (1995). Skin cancers associated with acquired immunodeficiency syndrome. *Mayo Clinic Proceedings* 70, 766–772.

APPENDIX A: Glossary

α_2-antiplasmin—plasma protein that inactivates circulating plasmin.

abdominal aortic aneurysm—aneurysm occurring within the lower abdominal aorta, commonly at the point of bifurcation into the iliac arteries.

abnormal uterine bleeding—uterine bleeding that differs from the expected frequency and quantity parameters of normal menstrual bleeding; it may or may not be associated with ovulatory dysfunction.

ABO incompatibility—clinical syndrome resulting from transfusion of blood with erythrocytes bearing an incompatible antigen of the ABO group. Antibodies in the recipient's blood then attack antigen on the donor cells, resulting in agglutination and lysis and a generalized inflammatory response to the tissue injury.

abruptio placentae—disorder in which the placenta separates prematurely from the uterine wall, leading to life-threatening maternal hemorrhage and abrupt loss of fetal support.

abscess—localized collection of pus in a cavity formed by tissue necrosis.

absolute refractory period—time immediately after depolarization to just above threshold, when an excitable cell cannot depolarize in response to a stimulus.

absorptive state—period during and approximately 4 hours after eating.

acclimation—long-term adaptation to changes in environmental temperature, mediated by the hypothalamic-pituitary axis.

acetyl CoA—biochemical intermediate in the Krebs cycle; formed by the attachment to coenzyme A of acetic acid during oxidation of pyruvate; it can also be synthesized from lipid and protein metabolites.

achalasia—motor disorder of the esophagus characterized by the absence of esophageal peristalsis and impaired relaxation of the lower esophageal sphincter during swallowing.

achlorhydria—lack of hydrochloric acid secretion.

acid—substance capable of releasing hydrogen ions into a solution, contributing to a lower pH.

acidemia—serum pH less than 7.35.

acidosis—pathologic condition resulting from accumulation of acid or depletion of base in the blood and body tissues and characterized by a pH lower than the normal range (i.e., below 7.35).

acne vulgaris—multifactorial skin disorder characterized by chronic inflammation and obstruction of the pilosebaceous unit.

acquired immunodeficiency syndrome—epidemic disorder caused by human immunodeficiency virus type 1 (HIV-1), characterized by destruction of immune cells (primarily CD4+ helper T cells). The resulting immunodeficiency predisposes to opportunistic infections and neoplasms.

acrocyanosis—persistent cyanosis of the of the fingers and hands or the toes and feet, with mottled blue or red discoloration, coldness, and profuse sweating of the digits.

acromegaly—accelerated growth and metabolism due to growth hormone excess arising in adults after epiphyseal closure.

actin—intracellular protein that, along with myosin, is essential to muscle contraction.

actinic keratosis—sharply outlined wart-like or keratotic growth caused by excessive exposure to the sun that may develop into a cutaneous horn and may become malignant.

action potential—maximal discharge of the membrane potential in an excitable cell, occurring when membrane potential rises from the resting level to threshold.

active transport—energy-consuming transport in opposition to a natural gradient; "pumping."

activin—peptide that participates in the regulation of gonadal, adrenal, and placental hormone production; stimulates gonadotropin release from the pituitary, ovarian progesterone secretion, and aromatase enzyme activity; and is produced by the ovary, testis, and extragonadal tissues.

acute bronchitis—inflammation of one or more bronchi, often as an extension of a viral infection of the upper respiratory tract.

acute fatty liver of pregnancy—idiopathic disorder, usually associated with preeclampsia, that arises late in pregnancy and typically progresses to acute hepatic failure; immediate termination of pregnancy is warranted.

acute interstitial nephritis—disorder of sudden onset of inflammation of kidney tissue caused by proliferation of microorganisms or, more commonly, by the toxic effects of antibiotics, nonsteroidal anti-inflammatory drugs, or diuretics; it may also be idiopathic.

acute lymphoblastic leukemia (ALL)—malignant neoplasm of lymphocyte precursors that originates in the bone marrow; the transformed cell is usually a B lymphocyte.

acute myeloid leukemia (AML)—malignant neoplasm of immature hematopoietic cells of the myeloid line that originates in the bone marrow. The transformed cell may be any of several in the myeloid line. Patients with severe polycythemia vera are at high risk for acute myeloid leukemia.

acute renal failure (ARF)—sudden onset of decreased or absent urine output, leading to accumulation of metabolic waste products as well as fluid and electrolyte imbalance.

acute tubular necrosis—syndrome associated with inflammatory destruction of renal tubular cells, especially in the proximal tubule and thick ascending limb of the loop of Henle. Epithelial cells are denuded and tubular lumens are occluded by cellular debris and casts. In acute tubular necrosis due to rhabdomyolysis or hemolysis, heme pigments also occlude the lumens.

adaptation—processes by which a system seeks to restore or maintain homeostasis.

Addison's disease—chronic disorder resulting from autoimmune destruction of all three zones of the adrenal cortex; it is the most common form of primary adrenal insufficiency.

adenomyosis—benign disorder in which endometrial tissue invades the uterine myometrium; it is also called internal endometriosis.

adenosine triphosphate (ATP)—nucleotide containing two high-energy phosphate bonds serving as an energy storage molecule in all living cells.

adhesion molecule—cell surface protein that acts as ligand or receptor in mediating stable or transient contact between cells.

adhesive junction—membrane junction that serves to hold cells together in the face of deforming forces; it is also called a desmosome.

adipose tissue—connective tissue containing fat cells; long-term form of energy fuel storage.

adrenal insufficiency—clinical syndrome associated with deficient production of adrenocortical hormones.

adrenocorticotropic hormone (ACTH)—hormone secreted by the anterior lobe of the pituitary gland that stimulates the cortex of the adrenal gland to secrete its hormones, including cortisol; it is also called corticotropin.

adult respiratory distress syndrome (ARDS)—acute respiratory failure syndrome resulting from ischemic or toxic injury of the alveolar-capillary membrane; it is characterized by impaired gas diffusion, with low PaO_2 despite oxygen therapy.

aerobic metabolism—conversion of glucose to pyruvate in the presence of oxygen, yielding small amounts of adenosine triphosphate, substrate for the Krebs cycle, and reduced coenzymes for oxidative phosphorylation.

afterdrop—untoward effect of active external rewarming measures used in treatment of hypothermia, in which peripheral vasodilation permits cold blood to return to the core organs, decreasing core temperature and potentially causing acidosis and dysrhythmias.

afterload—force or pressure opposing ventricular ejection, originating primarily from pressure or vascular resistance in the systemic circulation for the left ventricle and the pulmonary circulation for the left ventricle.

agonist—substance other than the natural ligand that may bind to a receptor and initiate its normal activity.

akinesia—muscle paralysis.

alcoholism—excessive or prolonged abuse of alcohol resulting in dependence and impairment of biologic, interpersonal, or occupational function.

aldosterone—principal mineralocorticoid hormone produced by the adrenal cortex; it regulates electrolytic and water balance by promoting the retention of sodium and the excretion of potassium.

alkalemia—serum pH greater than 7.45.

alkalosis—pathologic condition resulting from accumulation of base, or from loss of acid from body fluids and tissues, and characterized by a pH higher than the normal range (i.e., above 7.45).

all or none law—commitment of an excitable cell to a full action potential if threshold is reached and absence of an action potential if depolarization does not reach threshold.

allele—alternative form of a gene at a particular locus on homologous chromosomes.

allergen—substance, usually a protein, capable of inducing allergy.

allergy—IgE-mediated immediate hypersensitivity initiated by exposure to an allergen.

allodynia—production of pain by low-intensity stimuli.

alopecia—hair loss.

alveolar hypoventilation—decrease in the rate of delivery of fresh atmospheric air to the alveoli for exchange.

alveolar-capillary membrane—collective term for the tissues through which gases must diffuse from the alveolar air to the blood, or vice versa; the alveolar wall, pulmonary interstitium, and capillary wall.

Alzheimer's disease (AD)—a primary degenerative dementia diagnosed after other causes of dementia have been ruled out. It may be confirmed at autopsy by the presence of cortical atrophy, ventricular dilation, neuritic plaques, neurofibrillary tangles, and amyloid deposition.

amenorrhea—absence of menstruation in a woman of reproductive age.

amnesia—loss of memory.

amniotic fluid embolism—bolus of amniotic fluid forced into the maternal bloodstream by strong uterine contractions during the period of pregnancy when the placenta has begun to separate.

amyotrophic lateral sclerosis (ALS)—motor disorder resulting from progressive degeneration of the anterior horn cells and the corticospinal tracts; also called Lou Gehrig's disease.

anabolism—synthetic reactions resulting in formation of new cells and tissues; opposite of catabolism.

anaerobic metabolism—energy processing reactions occurring in conditions of absence or deficit of oxygen (i.e., anaerobic glycolysis).

analgesia—reduction of pain.

anaphase lag—mechanism leading to a numeric chromosomal abnormality; occurs when one chromosome (in meiosis) or one chromatid (in mitosis) lags behind and is left out of the nucleus of the daughter cell or gamete.

anaphylactic shock—distributive shock resulting from a severe hypersensitivity reaction to an allergen.

anaphylactoid reaction—syndome resembling allergic hypersensitivity but that results from mast cell degranulation induced by mechanisms other than IgE cross-linking.

anaphylaxis—unusual or exaggerated allergic reaction.

androgen—steroid hormone that promotes male characteristics; produced in the testes, ovaries, and adrenal cortex; serves as estrogen precursor.

anemia—reduction below normal in the number or volume of erythrocytes or in the quantity of hemoglobin in the blood.

anemia of pregnancy—anemia due to relative deficiency of iron or folate, which develops as a consequence of increased erythropoiesis.

anemia of prematurity—normocytic, normochromic anemia occurring in premature infants between 6 and 10 weeks of age.

anencephaly—absence of brain tissue above a rudimentary brain stem and basal ganglia.

anesthesia—reduction of all sensation.

aneuploid—referring to a number of chromosomes other than 46 (the diploid number) or 23 (the haploid number).

aneurysm—sac formed by the localized dilation of the wall of an artery, vein, or the heart.

angina pectoris—acute pain in the chest resulting from decreased blood supply to the heart muscle.
angioedema—third spacing of fluid due to excess of capillary forces favoring outward fluid movement (filtration).
angiogenesis—development of blood vessels.
angiotensin I (AGT I)—a relatively inactive peptide formed by the action of renin on a serum globulin, angiotensinogen. AGT I is converted to active AGT II by angiotensin-converting enzyme (ACE).
angiotensin II (AGT II)—peptide formed from activation of AGT I by angiotensin-converting enzyme (ACE). AGT II is a potent vasoconstrictor and stimulates the secretion of aldosterone by the adrenal cortex.
angiotensin-converting enzyme (ACE)—enzyme synthesized primarily by pulmonary cells that catalyzes the conversion of angiotensin I to angiotensin II and that mediates vasoconstriction and stimulation of aldosterone release from the adrenal cortex.
angiotensinogen—serum α-globulin synthesized and released by the liver that gives rise to angiotensin I when hydrolyzed by renin.
anhydrosis—decreased sweating.
anion—negatively charged ion.
anion gap (A^-)—concentration of unmeasured anions in the plasma, normally 12 to 14 mEq/L, usually calculated by subtracting the sum of the bicarbonate and chloride concentrations from the sodium concentration.
ankylosing spondylitis—chronic, progressive disorder characterized by inflammation of the spine and sacroiliac joints; a joint disorder of apparent immunologic origin in which the rheumatoid factor autoantibody is absent from the serum.
ankylosis—immobility and consolidation of a joint due to injury, disease, or surgical procedure; caused by inflammatory fluid seeping between the articular cartilages, forming a fibrous pannus.
anorexia—loss of appetite.
anorexia nervosa—psychological and physiologic disorder of self-starvation defined by four criteria: failure to maintain a minimal weight for height and age, fear of fatness, distorted body image, and absence of menstruation in females.
antagonist—substance similar enough to a natural ligand to bind to its receptor but that does not induce the receptor-mediated response; a receptor-blocking agent.
antibody—a protein molecule capable of adhering and interacting with the antigen that induced its synthesis; an immunoglobulin.
anticoagulant—substance that inhibits blood clotting.
antidiuretic hormone (ADH)—hypothalamic hormone, released from the posterior pituitary, that opposes the loss of excess water in the urine when present at physiologic levels, resulting in concentration of urine; acts as a powerful vasoconstrictor when administered in high doses; possibly serves as a neuromodulator in facilitating memory; may stimulate smooth muscle contraction in the spermatic cord during ejaculation; also called vasopressin.
antigen—substance, usually a protein or large carbohydrate, that is capable of inducing a specific immune response by interaction with antibodies or sensitized T lymphocytes.
antinuclear antibodies (ANA)—antibodies directed against components of the cell nucleus, such as DNA, RNA, and histones; a positive ANA test is characteristic of systemic lupus erythematosus, rheumatoid arthritis, Sjögren's syndrome, and scleroderma.
antioxidant—substance that in small amounts will inhibit oxidation by converting radicals to stable forms.
antipyretic—category of drugs that reduce fever by blocking prostaglandin synthesis, preventing upward resetting of the hypothalamic thermostat. Aspirin and other nonsteroidal anti-inflammatory drugs are commonly used for this purpose.
antithrombin III—plasma protein that inactivates thrombin and acts as a heparin cofactor in anticoagulation.
aortic insufficiency—incomplete closure of the aortic valve during diastole.
aortic stenosis—incomplete opening of the aortic valve during systole.
aphakia—absence of the lens of the eye.
aphasia—impairment of language expression by speech, writing, or signs or impairment of comprehension of such language.
aplasia—complete absence or defective development of an organ.
apnea—absence of ventilatory efforts, often seen in infants younger than 40 weeks' conceptual age.
apoptosis—noninflammatory, orderly process leading to DNA fragmentation and cell death; genetically programmed or induced cell suicide.
appendicitis—inflammation of the vermiform appendix.
arachidonic acid—fatty acid derived from membrane lipids; the products of its degradation are among the most important of the lipid mediators of inflammation and other biologic processes.
arginine vasopressin (AVP)—vasoconstrictor peptide hormone synthesized by the hypothalamus and released from the posterior pituitary. It is also known as antidiuretic hormone (ADH) because of its principal effect of rendering the distal tubule and collecting duct of the kidney permeable to water, permitting its reabsorption.
arterial blood gases (ABGs)—laboratory measurement of the pH and partial pressures of carbon dioxide and oxygen in a sample of arterial blood. The bicarbonate concentration is calculated from the measured parameters and is also reported in this analysis.
arteriosclerosis—group of diseases characterized by thickening and loss of elasticity of the arterial walls; "hardening of the arteries."
arteriosclerosis obliterans—peripheral vascular disorder characterized by chronic, progressive hardening and occlusion of arteries due to lesions consisting primarily of atherosclerotic plaque.
arteriovenous malformation (AVM)—tangle of dilated blood vessels that form an abnormal communication between the arterial and venous systems.
arthritis—inflammation of a joint.
ascites—third spacing of vascular fluid into the peritoneal cavity.
asphyxia—condition in which there is a deficiency of oxygen in the blood and an increase in carbon dioxide in the blood and tissues; it can occur in newborns during labor and delivery owing to oxygen deprivation.
aspiration—unintended entry of a substance other than inspired air (e.g., a foreign body, gastric contents) into the airways of the pulmonary system.
aspiration pneumonia—inflammation of respiratory unit tissues secondary to pathologic inhalation of infectious or toxic substances.
asterixis—motor disturbance of the upper extremity often referred to as liver flap because of its occurrence in coma associated with liver disease.
asthma—inflammatory airway disease characterized by

increased airway responsiveness to a variety of stimuli that results in airway obstruction, which is at least partially reversible.

astigmatism—nonuniform curvature of the cornea or lens.

asystole—absence of detectable electrical activity on the electrocardiogram (i.e., a straight line); form of cardiac arrest.

atelectasis—alveolar collapse.

atherosclerosis—form of arteriosclerosis in which deposits of plaque composed of cholesterol and other materials occlude arteries.

athlete's heart—cardiac hypertrophy and dilation occurring as an adaptive response to habitual endurance exercise.

atonia—absence of muscle tone; atony.

atony—absence of muscle tone; atonia.

atopic dermatitis—systemic inflammatory response to an allergen that manifests primarily as a skin eruption.

atrial fibrillation—totally irregular rhythm generated by disorganized atrial depolarization at a rate of 400 to 600 beats per minute, with random conduction of some impulses through the atrioventricular junction to the ventricles. Atrial activity is represented on the electrocardiogram by a wavy baseline (f waves).

atrial flutter—rapid, usually regular rhythm of atrial origin in which the atrial rate is 250 to 350 beats per minute and the ventricular rate varies according to the degree of atrioventricular block. Atrial activity is represented on the electrocardiogram by characteristic "sawtooth" F waves.

atrial natriuretic peptide (ANP)—one of a family of peptide hormones released by the atrial myocardium and other tissues, particularly the brain. It is a weak endogenous antagonist of the renin-angiotensin-aldosterone system and antidiuretic hormone in that it promotes sodium excretion and diuresis, protecting the body from hypervolemia.

atrial septal defect (ASD)—acyanotic heart defect in which there is a hole in the septum between the atria.

atrial tachycardia—rapid rhythm originating from atrial myocardium, outside the sinus node.

atrioventricular (AV) block—conduction disturbance in which one or more atrial impulses are delayed or prevented from being transmitted throughout the atrioventricular junction to the ventricles.

atrophic vaginitis—inflammation of the vagina occurring in postmenopausal women, associated with estrogen deficiency.

atrophy—decrease in muscle size due to loss of structural components of muscle cells.

atypical pneumonia—type of lower respiratory tract infection in which inflammation is patchy and diffuse, involving the alveolar ducts and interstitial spaces but sparing the alveoli; it commonly results from infection with influenza virus or *Mycoplasma or Legionella* bacteria.

autoantibody—antibody formed in response to, and reacting against, an antigenic component of the individual's own tissues.

autoantigen—tissue constituent that stimulates production of autoantibodies in the organism in which it occurs.

autocrine—form of signaling that occurs when the target cell is the same cell that released the signaling molecule (typically a growth factor).

autoimmunity—humoral or cell-mediated immune attack against the body's own tissues.

automaticity—capacity of an excitable cell to initiate an action potential without external stimulation.

autonomic hyperreflexia—exaggeration of reflexes, sometimes due to excessive activity of the sympathetic nervous system; life-threatening complication of many cases of spinal cord injury involving a triggering stimulus, intact autonomic reflex arcs, and impaired communication with higher integrative centers.

autonomic neuropathy—clinical syndrome resulting from hypofunction or hyperfunction of the autonomic nervous system; usually a component of polyneuropathy.

autosomal dominant—referring to an inherited genetic disorder in which the defect is located on an autosome and is expressed in heterozygous individuals.

autosomal recessive—referring to an inherited genetic disorder in which the defect is located on an autosome and is fully expressed only in homozygous individuals.

autosome—any of the 22 pairs of chromosomes in humans not concerned with determination of sex.

axis deviation—abnormal direction of the mean current vector within the heart, due to abnormal position of the heart in the chest or disruption of the cardiac conduction system.

azoospermia—absence of spermatozoa in the semen or failure of formation of spermatozoa.

azotemia—presence of nitrogen-containing compounds (e.g., creatinine, blood urea nitrogen) in the blood, characteristic of renal insufficiency.

β-endorphin—one of a group of opiate-like peptides produced at neural synapses at various points in the central nervous system pathways, where they modulate the transmission of pain perceptions.

β-oxidation—metabolic pathway by which fatty acids are converted to acetyl CoA and reduced coenzymes, ultimately yielding energy via the Krebs cycle and oxidative phosphorylation.

bacterial vaginosis—nonspecific vaginitis associated with polymicrobial infection with agents such as *Gardnerella vaginalis, Corynebacterium, Bacteroides, Peptococcus, Eubacterium,* and *Mycoplasma hominis.*

balanitis—inflammation of the glans penis.

baroreceptor—sensory nerve terminal that is stimulated by changes in pressure.

baroreceptor reflex—autonomic regulatory mechanism whereby specialized mechanoreceptors sense changes in vessel wall stretch or intraluminal pressure, initiating sensory input to the vasomotor centers and cardioregulatory centers in the medulla, which results in alteration in the degree of autonomic stimulation of heart rate, contractility, and vessel caliber.

Barrett's metaplasia—premalignant condition of the esophagus in which chronic epithelial injury induces metaplastic transformation of the native squamous epithelium into columnar epithelium; the risk of developing adenocarcinoma of the esophagus is much higher in people with Barrett's metaplasia than in the general population.

basal cell carcinoma—malignant tumor that arises from epidermal epithelial cells and seldom metastasizes.

basal metabolic rate (BMR)—lowest possible level of energy expenditure, obtained with measurement in a well-rested, fasted, and quietly awake individual.

base—substance that may combine with acid to form a salt, contributing to a rise in the pH of a solution.

basophil—granulocyte that is the circulating equivalent of a tissue mast cell. Basophils and mast cells synthesize and release histamine and other mediators of inflammation.

Becker's muscular dystrophy—form of muscular dystrophy closely resembling Duchenne's but having a later onset and milder course; the defective trait is located on the short arm of the X chromosome; thus the disease is usually expressed in males.

Bell's palsy—peripheral facial nerve paralysis in which an inflammatory process leads to dysfunction of cranial nerve VII.

benign—nonmalignant; favorable in terms of course and recovery.

benign positional vertigo—peripheral vestibular disorder affecting the posterior semicircular canal and resulting in episodic vertigo with assumption of certain head positions.

benign prostatic hyperplasia—nonmalignant enlargement of the prostate gland due to excessive growth of both the glandular and stromal elements of the gland.

bicarbonate (HCO_3^-)—anion important in the regulation of the pH of body fluids.

bicarbonate reclamation—process by which bicarbonate anions are regenerated within renal tubular cells and reabsorbed into the blood. The process begins with the generation of CO_2 from a dehydration reaction in the tubules. CO_2 then diffuses into the tubular cells, and bicarbonate is regenerated via its hydrolysis.

bicarbonate regeneration—buffering process in which for every hydrogen ion secreted, one bicarbonate ion is regenerated from the tubular cell and returned to the blood; identical to bicarbonate reclamation, except that the hydrogen ion is excreted in the urine.

body mass index (BMI)—preferred epidemiologic means of quantifying obesity-related risk; correlates with body fat. BMI is calculated from height in meters and weight in kilograms: BMI = w/h^2. A BMI of less than 25 is desirable; a BMI of 30 or more places a person at major health risk due to obesity.

Bohr effect—reduction in the affinity of hemoglobin for oxygen as a result of local acidosis.

bone marrow transplantation—a procedure in which bone marrow is aspirated and reinfused into another human or into the donor after treatment of the marrow; used in the treatment of many hematopoietic and neoplastic disorders.

bowel obstruction—blockade of chyme transport along the alimentary canal, hindering the passage of feces; commonly caused by adhesions on the serosa. An obstruction may be congenital or acquired, complete or partial, mechanical (due to an obstructive mass, constriction, or lesion) or functional (due to impaired neural stimulation of motility).

bradycardia—heart rate below 60 beats per minute.

bradykinesia—abnormal slowness of movement.

brain death—irreversible coma.

breast cancer—malignant neoplasm arising from one of several tissue types within the breast.

bronchiectasis—permanent dilation and distortion of the bronchi and bronchioles due to breakdown of airway smooth muscle and connective tissue support.

bronchiolitis—lower respiratory illness of primarily viral etiology that typically occurs in infants younger than 2 years of age.

bronchogenic carcinoma (lung cancer)—malignant neoplasm originating in lung tissue.

bronchopneumonia—most common pattern of lower respiratory tract inflammation, in which inflammation starts simultaneously in several areas, producing patchy, diffuse consolidations.

bronchopulmonary dysplasia (BPD)—injury of airways secondary to barotrauma with high ventilation pressures or oxygen toxicity associated with prolonged administration of oxygen at a high FIO_2. It produces fluid exudation, airway scarring, and decreased surfactant production and leads to permanent impairment of pulmonary function.

brown fat—specialized adipose tissue that develops in the fetus late in gestation and atrophies after the first month of life. Brown fat is highly vascular and contains large numbers of mitochondria, and its metabolism produces large quantities of heat.

buffer—system that consists of a weak acid and a corresponding base.

bulimia nervosa—eating disorder characterized by periods of excessive consumption of high-calorie foods followed by purging behaviors, including self-induced vomiting and abuse of diuretics and laxatives.

bulk flow—a flow of water carrying dissolved and suspended particles that is transported through pores between cells composing multicellular membranes.

bundle branch block (BBB)—delayed or blocked conduction through the right bundle branch or through either or both fascicles of the left bundle branch.

burn shock—form of hypovolemic shock that occurs when blood or plasma is lost in such quantities that the remaining blood cannot fill the circulatory system despite constriction of the blood vessels. The blood may be lost into spaces inside the body where it is no longer accessible to the circulatory system, as in major burns that attract large quantities of blood fluids to the burn site outside blood vessels and capillaries.

bursitis—inflammation of a bursa; often caused by excessive use of the joint.

cachexia—profound and marked state of constitutional disorder; general ill health and malnutrition.

cadherin—one of the four major categories of adhesion molecules.

calcitonin—peptide hormone secreted by parafollicular (C) cells of the thyroid. Calcitonin weakly opposes the effects of parathyroid hormone (PTH), lowering serum calcium levels.

calcium (Ca^{2+})—most abundant mineral in the body, forming bones and teeth and participating in many critical regulatory functions, including blood clotting, muscle contraction, neurotransmission, and energy metabolism.

caldesmon—protein associated with actin in smooth muscle; it may play a role in latch-bridge formation.

calmodulin—regulatory protein that serves a calcium-binding function in smooth muscle.

calponin—protein associated with actin in smooth muscle; it may play a role in latch-bridge formation.

cancer—malignant neoplasm.

candidiasis—fungal infection of the superficial skin or mucous membranes, usually due to *Candida albicans.*

capillary hydrostatic pressure (CHP)—hemodynamic force favoring outward movement of fluid from capillaries.

carbamino compound—compound formed from the combination of carbon dioxide with hemoglobin.

carbon monoxide intoxication—syndrome resulting from the inhalation of carbon monoxide gas in amounts sufficient to induce cerebral hypoxia.

carbonic acid (H_2CO_3)—weak acid formed from the chemical combination of CO_2 and H_2O.

carbonic acid–bicarbonate buffer system—chemical buffer system in body fluids, consisting of the weak acid carbonic acid and the base bicarbonate; the most clinically important and closely monitored of the extracellular fluid buffers.

carbonic anhydrase (CA)—enzyme that catalyzes the hydrolysis of carbon dioxide to form carbonic acid, which immediately dissociates into H^+ and HCO_3^-.

carcinogen—substance capable of initiating or promoting neoplasia.

carcinoma—term applied to many malignant neoplasms of epithelial origin.

cardiac axis—mean direction or vector of current flow within the heart; the geometric average of the multiple current vectors present in the heart at any given time.

cardiac cirrhosis—uncommon complication of chronic hepatomegaly associated with cardiac failure.

cardiac cycle—series of events occurring during one complete heart beat or contraction-relaxation sequence.

cardiac failure—inability of the heart to contract with sufficient rate and force to satisfy the metabolic demands of tissues.

cardiac index (CI)—cardiac output divided by the body surface area; means of quantifying cardiac contractile function.

cardiac output (CO)—volume of blood pumped by the left ventricle per minute; the product of the heart rate and the stroke volume.

cardiac reserve—degree to which the heart can increase cardiac output in response to increased metabolic demands.

cardiac tamponade—limitation of ventricular filling due to external pressure exerted on the heart when the pericardial sac or mediastinal space fills with blood or exudate.

cardiogenic shock—state of generalized deficit in tissue perfusion resulting from inadequate pumping force of the heart.

cardiomyopathy—impairment of cardiac contraction due to primary disease of the myocardium, unrelated to the effects of hypertension or coronary heart disease.

cardiopulmonary resuscitation (CPR)—technique of basic life support performed after sudden cardiac death in an effort to maintain some ventilation through mouth-to-mouth or bag breathing and some perfusion through external cardiac compression.

carpal tunnel syndrome—neuropathy syndrome resulting from entrapment of the median nerve within a narrowed carpal tunnel.

catabolism—conversion of complex substances into simpler compounds, liberating energy; opposite of anabolism.

cataract—opacity of the lens; may be congenital or acquired.

catecholamine—hormone containing an amine and a catechol group in its chemical structure; includes norepinephrine, epinephrine, and dopamine

cation—positively charged ion.

cauda equina syndrome—dull, aching pain of the saddle region (areas served by sacral nerves) accompanied by urinary retention and radiculopathy; due to compression of the spinal nerve roots.

celiac disease—gluten-sensitive enteropathy; also called nontropical sprue.

cell cycle—sequence of events during which a cell divides.

cell-mediated immunity—immune response dependent on T lymphocytes, exemplified by graft rejection, response against intracellular infections, delayed hypersensitivity reactions, some autoimmune disorders, and surveillance for neoplastic cells.

cellular respiration—utilization of oxygen and production of carbon dioxide during cellular energy metabolism.

cellulitis—diffuse, pus-forming inflammation of the dermis and subcutaneous tissue; a bacterial infection.

central venous pressure—blood pressure measured at the right atrium or at the vena cava proximal to the right atrium.

cerebral palsy—symptom complex covering a group of nonprogressive motor impairment syndromes that may result from lesions or anomalies of the brain in the early stages of its development.

cervical cancer—malignant neoplasm of the cervix. Eighty-five percent of cervical cancer is squamous cell carcinoma; the remaining cancers are adenocarcinomas.

cervical radiculopathy—disease of the cervical nerve roots; occurs with herniation of disks in the lower cervical region of the spine and manifests as neck pain and upper extremity paresthesias.

cesarean section—delivery of an infant through an abdominal and uterine incision.

chemomechanical coupling—modulation of muscle contraction by cytokines, hormones, neurotransmitters, or drugs via a variety of receptor-mediated processes.

chemotaxis—stimulation of the movement of neutrophils and monocytes toward the site of inflammation, probably in response to complement proteins, leukotrienes, and lymphokines at the site.

chest trauma—physical injury of the thorax by either a blunt or sharp force.

chlamydia infection—sexually transmitted disease caused by the bacterium *Chlamydia trachomatis* and treated with an antibiotic such as tetracycline or doxycycline.

chloride (Cl^-)—principal anion in extracellular fluid.

chloride shift—exchange of chloride for bicarbonate across the erythrocyte membrane. In the tissues, chloride leaves the red blood cell as bicarbonate enters. The process is reversed in the lungs, as bicarbonate undergoes reverse hydrolysis and is exhaled as CO_2.

cholecystitis—inflammation of the gallbladder.

cholelithiasis—disorder resulting from formation of obstructive stones in the gallbladder, cystic duct, or common bile duct.

cholestasis—obstruction of bile flow due to factors in the liver (intrahepatic) or outside the liver (extrahepatic).

cholesteatoma—cystic lesion occurring most commonly in the middle ear and mastoid region.

chondrosarcoma—malignant neoplasm of skeletal tissue derived from cartilage cells or their precursors.

choriocarcinoma—malignant neoplasm of trophoblastic cells formed by abnormal proliferation of the placental epithelium, without production of chorionic villi.

chromosomal defect—abnormality of DNA affecting one or more chromosomes and, consequently, multiple genes (e.g., a translocation, monosomy, or trisomy); cytogenetic disorder.

chromosome—nuclear structure composed of genetic material (DNA) coiled around a protein (histone) core.

chronic bronchitis—inflammation of bronchi with increased mucus production and chronic productive cough, persisting for at least 3 months of the year for 2 successive years.

chronic fatigue syndrome—idiopathic disorder characterized by fatigue, muscle and joint pain, neuropsychiatric symptoms, and other manifestations.

chronic lymphocytic leukemia (CLL)—slowly progressive

malignant neoplasm of bone marrow origin in which the transformed cell is a mature B lymphocyte expressing the CD5 antigen.

chronic myeloid leukemia (CML)—malignant neoplasm of bone marrow origin in which the transformed cell is the committed progenitor cell of the myeloid line.

chronic obstructive pulmonary disease (COPD)—functional category designating a condition of persistent obstruction of bronchial air flow (e.g., emphysema, chronic bronchitis, asthma, bronchiectasis, and cystic fibrosis); also referred to as chronic obstructive lung disease (COLD) and chronic airflow limitation (CAL).

chronic renal failure (CRF)—progressive, irreversible loss of renal function due to replacement of functional nephrons with fibrous scar tissue, also known as end-stage renal disease (ESRD). In CRF, the patient's glomerular filtration rate is consistently less than 10 ml/min, a level insufficient to fulfill the homeostatic functions of the kidney.

chronic venous insufficiency—includes a spectrum of disorders resulting from elevated venous pressure in the legs; ranges in severity from varicose veins to lipodermatosclerosis and venous stasis ulcers.

Chvostek's sign—classic indication of impending tetany, in which twitching of facial muscles is elicited by tapping over the facial nerve.

circumcision—surgical removal of the foreskin of the penis.

cirrhosis—progressive tissue response to chronic (not acute) liver injury resulting in extensive hepatic fibrosis and regenerative nodules disrupting the parenchymal architecture of the entire liver.

classic endocrine system—comprises several organs having as their primary function the secretion of hormones; the major organs are the hypothalamus, pituitary gland, pineal gland, thyroid gland, parathyroids, adrenal cortex, endocrine pancreas, and gonads.

cleavage—initial mitotic division of the zygote.

cleft lip and palate—congenital splitting or defect in the lip or roof of the mouth (palate), sometimes concurrently.

clinical intervention—action by health professionals designed to prevent disease, relieve signs and symptoms, or support the body's efforts to overcome disease; prevention and treatment

clinical manifestation—physical or verbal evidence of disease; sign or symptom

clotting cascade—stepwise series of enzymatic activations of serum clotting factors, culminating in formation and dissolution of a fibrin blood clot.

clotting factor—plasma substance, usually a protein synthesized by the liver, that circulates in inactive form as part of the procoagulant fraction. Clotting factors are sequentially activated during the clotting cascade, culminating in formation of a fibrin blood clot.

CNS ischemic response—limited period of intense sympathetic stimulation of the heart and blood vessels that is initiated by vasomotor center neurons in response to a very low mean arterial pressure.

coarctation of the aorta—acyanotic congenital heart defect in which there is a stricture in the aorta, usually within the aortic arch.

coitus—sexual union by vagina between male and female.

colloid—medium consisting of small particles that do not settle out of solution under the influence of gravity, nor pass through a semipermeable membrane under physiologic conditions.

color blindness—inherited disorder in which a person lacks one or more of the cone types and therefore is unable to distinguish between certain colors.

colorectal cancer—primary malignant neoplasm of the colon or rectum.

coma—state of being neither awake nor aware.

common cold—acute and highly contagious viral infection of the upper respiratory tract; also referred to as acute viral rhinitis.

compartmental syndrome—condition in which increased tissue pressure in a confined anatomic space causes decreased blood flow leading to ischemia and dysfunction of contained myoneural elements, marked by pain, muscle weakness, sensory loss, and palpable tenseness in the involved compartment; ischemia can lead to necrosis, resulting in permanent impairment of function.

complement—series of enzymes present in serum that when activated (either directly by bacterial products or by antigen-antibody binding) produce widespread inflammatory effects and lysis of bacteria.

concentration gradient—force driving net thermal movement of particles from an area of higher density to that of lower density of particles.

conceptus—term for the developing human during the preembryonic period.

concussion—injury resulting from a violent jar or shock; concussion of the brain results in transient loss of consciousness as well as other manifestations of cortical dysfunction. Structural injury is usually minimal.

conduction—heat transfer between two objects or media having different temperatures.

conduction disturbance—dysrhythmia resulting from absence of normal impulse generation, excessive slowing of the impulse, or blockage of conduction of some or all impulses within the cardiac conduction system.

conductive hearing loss—hearing loss due to defects in sound transmission through the auditory canal or middle ear.

congenital—present at and existing from the time of birth.

congenital adrenal hyperplasia—encompasses a group of genetic disorders resulting in deficiency or absence of an enzyme necessary for synthesis of glucocorticoids or mineralocorticoids.

congenital heart defect—structural abnormality of the heart that is present at birth.

congestive heart failure (CHF)—syndrome in which cardiac output is not adequate to meet tissue metabolic demands, usually accompanied by rising pressure and volume in the pulmonary or systemic venous systems.

conjunctivitis—inflammation of the palpebral conjunctiva and the bulbar conjunctiva due to chemical irritation, bacterial or viral infection, or allergy.

connectin (titin)—cytoskeletal protein associated with actin in striated muscle that lends structural stability and resistance to passive stretch.

constipation—two or more of the following for at least 12 months: fewer than three bowel movements per week, excessive straining with at least 25% of bowel movements, a feeling of incomplete evacuation at least 25% of the time, and bowel movements that produce hard or pellet-like stools at least 25% of the time.

constrictive pericarditis—type of pericardial inflammation in which scarring of pericardial layers causes them to fuse and thicken, restricting diastolic filling.

contact dermatitis—localized inflammatory response of the skin due to contact with an irritant.

contraception—prevention of conception or impregnation.

convection—currents created by wind, fans, or moving water, which accelerate heat loss by continuously carrying transferred heat away from a warm object.

cor pulmonale—congestive heart failure resulting from increased right ventricular afterload.

Cori cycle—metabolic pathway by which lactic acid, produced during muscle glycolysis, is converted to glucose by the liver and returned to the circulation.

corneal opacity—loss of transparency of the cornea; can occur as a result of traumatic abrasion, toxic injury of the cornea, or, rarely, congenital disorders.

corneal reflex—reflex closure of the eyelids on irritation of the cornea; mediated by cranial nerves V and VII.

coronary heart disease—condition of decreased perfusion of the myocardium due to occlusion of one or more coronary arteries by atherosclerosis, thrombosis, or spasm; also known as coronary artery disease, ischemic heart disease, and atherosclerotic cardiovascular disease.

coronary steal syndrome—complication of coronary artery bypass graft surgery using an internal mammary artery graft. Pressure gradients created by atherosclerotic stenosis of the left subclavian artery proximal to the graft origin induce retrograde flow through the graft, "stealing" myocardial perfusion and inducing ischemia.

corticotropin-releasing hormone (CRH)—neuropeptide secreted by the hypothalamus that stimulates the anterior pituitary to release adrenocorticotropic hormone (ACTH or corticotropin); also stimulates the secretion of the neurotransmitter norepinephrine, enhancing the stress response, and endorphins and other peptides that mediate the inflammatory response and the endogenous analgesia system.

cortisol—hormone from the adrenal cortex; the principal glucocorticoid; stimulates synthesis of enzymes that regulate diverse cellular functions.

cotransport—transport mechanism utilizing symport proteins.

countertransport—transport mechanism utilizing antiport proteins.

crackle—abnormal discontinuous nonmusical sound heard on auscultation of the lungs, primarily during inhalation.

creatine phosphate—compound of creatine and phosphoric acid that serves as the primary energy buffer in muscle, potentially forming adenosine triphosphate by transferring energy from its single phosphate bond to adenosine diphosphate; also known as phosphocreatine.

CREST syndrome—form of systemic scleroderma consisting of calcinosis, Raynaud's phenomenon, esophageal dysfunction, sclerodactyly, and telangiectasia.

Crohn's disease—granulomatous, transmural inflammation of discontinuous segments of bowel, usually confined to the terminal ileum and proximal colon but potentially affecting any portion of the gastrointestinal tract.

cross-bridge—binding between actin and myosin that underlies the sliding filament theory of muscle contraction.

croup (laryngotracheobronchitis)—inflammatory condition of the upper airways in children, characterized by acute laryngeal obstruction and stridor.

cryogen—agent that causes low temperatures.

cryptorchidism—failure of one or both testes to descend into the scrotum during the fetal period. The testis may stay in the abdominal cavity or inguinal canal or may be located ectopically, outside the normal pathway of descent.

cure—complete eradication of disease.

Curling's ulcer—stress ulceration of the stomach or intestinal wall in burn patients.

Cushing's syndrome—group of symptoms produced by an excess of free circulating cortisol from the adrenal cortex; may result from excessive or prolonged administration of exogenous corticosteroid therapy.

cutaneous reflex—superficial muscle contraction in response to stroking of the skin of the umbilical or anogenital areas.

cystic fibrosis—inherited abnormality of exocrine gland function that affects the secretory surfaces of the respiratory, gastrointestinal, and genitourinary systems as well as the sweat glands. Respiratory function is most severely impaired due to the presence of thick, obstructive mucus in airways.

cystitis—inflammation of the bladder.

cytokine—regulatory substance (usually a protein) secreted by a cell.

de novo—referring to a defect that arises within the affected individual, as opposed to being inherited.

dead space—the volume of air in the lungs that does not participate in gas exchange; "wasted" ventilation that increases the work of breathing. Dead space includes anatomic dead space (the volume of the conducting airways) and physiologic dead space (the volume of any nonperfused alveoli).

decompression disorder—any of a group of related disorders resulting from the entry of bubbles of nitrogen into body tissues as a result of exposure to an abnormal gas pressure environment.

deep tendon reflex—automatic contraction of a muscle elicited by a sharp tap on a tendon to induce brief stretch of the muscle.

deep vein thrombosis—state of excessive or inappropriate clotting in one or more deep veins, typically of the legs or pelvis.

defervescence—clinical manifestations associated with activation of heat loss mechanisms (vasodilation, sweating) following return of the hypothalamic set point to normal after a pyrogen-induced fever; "breaking" of fever.

definitive therapy—clinical interventions designed to achieve cure or remission.

dementia—one of a group of syndromes characterized by progressive decline in memory, judgment, intellectual function, and adaptive ability.

deoxyribonucleic acid (DNA)—double-stranded nucleic acid that constitutes the genetic code.

depolarization—discharge of the membrane potential; phase 0 of the action potential.

depression—morbid sadness, dejection, or melancholy; distinguishable from grief, which is an appropriate reaction to personal loss.

dermatomyositis—acute, subacute, or chronic disease marked by nonsuppurative inflammation of the skin, subcutaneous tissue, and muscles, with necrosis of muscle fibers; a type of inflammatory myopathy.

developmental hip dysplasia—congenital defect promoting subluxation or dislocation of the hip; the most common type of congenital dislocation; breech position in utero is a risk factor.

diabetes insipidus—disorder characterized by excessive

e (ESRD)—period in which serum
l urea nitrogen levels continue to
pairment of all body systems; mani-
ılar filtration rate consistently less
evel inadequate to serve the homeo-
kidney.

gnaling that occurs when signaling
) travel in the blood to distant tar-
bind and exert their effects.

ependent process by which large
into cells (e.g., phagocytosis, pino-
ediated endocytosis).

tissue layer that gives rise to epi-

alignant neoplasm arising from the
f the uterus. Ninety-seven percent
endometrial in origin; the rest are

oplastic condition in which func-
issue is found in ectopic sites, out-

ation of the endometrium; may
hemorrhage.

distention of the mammary alveoli

ntinence in a child older than 3
manifesting as bedwetting.

upational lung disease—includes
tory conditions of the lower respi-
riggered by inhaled toxins associ-
environment or occupation.

ermia—elevation of body tempera-
diant heat gain from a warm envi-
elms the body's heat loss mecha-

granulocyte that targets antigenic
antibody complexes.

f the cause and distribution of dis-

tion of the epididymis and its
es secondary to sexually transmit-
tract infection.

calized collection of clotted blood
between the dura and the skull.

on of the flap of tissue that reflex-
ance into the trachea during swal-

acterized by recurrent seizure ac-
e cause.

echolamine hormone and neuro-
rimarily by the adrenal medulla
the sympathetic nervous system.

malformation with absence of the
thra, occurring in both sexes but
male, the urethral opening being
e dorsum of the penis.

nsport across the skin, the intesti-
iologic membranes composed of

g region on an antigen; antigenic

nsistent inability to attain and
on.

igidity that occur in the penis as
arterioles in the corpus caver-
ient rapid inflow of blood during
stimulation.

ımation of a diverticulum, an area in
l layer of the colon wall herniates
the muscular layers, creating bal-

ence, but not inflammation, of diverti-

itive reflex initiated by facial contact
impulses carried by the trigeminal
ain-stem centers to slow the heart rate
ctive vasoconstriction, which shunts
s of the skin and abdominal organs to
rt.

ıagnification of the plasma colloid
by sodium and other cations that
the negative charges on serum albu-

-congenital condition characterized by
ıations and some degree of mental re-
ienotype results from trisomy of chro-

ular dystrophy—childhood type of
phy characterized by progressive degen-
al muscle fibers. The defective trait is
ıort arm of the X chromosome; thus the
rily expressed in males.

ne—rapid emptying of gastric contents
ntestine, which creates a high osmotic
umen of the bowel, resulting in hypovo-
uid shifts from the surrounding vessels
ıtestinal tract.

—isotonic contraction; force generated
ıcle fiber overcomes the resisting force,
rtens, and movement occurs.

ımation of the intestine, especially the
by bacteria, chemical irritants, protozoa,
sitic worms.

ormal muscle movement.

ment of reading ability.

clusive term for abnormality (excess or
erum lipids.

is—abnormal physical development; de-
onormality of structure.

fficult or painful sexual intercourse in

aired swallowing.

lessness, malaise, or disquiet.

ormality of size, shape, or development of

ed or difficult breathing.

ıbnormal origin, rate, and/or direction of
the electrical impulse within the heart;

onditions that result in dysfunctional labor
at is suboptimal in achieving cervical ef-
dilation as well as descent and delivery of
mposes risk for both laboring mother and

rder of muscle tone; includes atonia, hypo-
pertonia.

normal cellular growth and development.

r—psychological and physiologic disorder
tion or excessive consumption of high-calo-

ıemorrhagic lesion in the skin or mucous
forming a nonelevated blue or purplish
se.

eclampsia—seizure activity in a patient with preeclampsia, if other causes of seizures are excluded.

ectoderm—embryonic tissue layer that differentiates into the surface ectoderm, which gives rise to the epidermis and other tissues, and the neuroectoderm, which gives rise to the nervous system.

ectopic pregnancy—implantation of the blastocyst at a site outside the body of the uterus, such as the fallopian tube, cervix, ovary, or bowel.

eczema—general term inclusive of a variety of noninfectious, often immune-mediated conditions characterized by erythematous, blistering, weeping, crusting, and scaling lesions of skin areas.

edema—accumulation of excess fluid in the interstitial space.

effusion—shift of excess fluid from the plasma into a potential fluid space (e.g., the peritoneal, pleural, pericardial, alveolar, or synovial spaces).

ejaculation—expulsion of semen from the male urethra, a reflex action that occurs as a result of sexual stimulation.

ejection fraction—percentage of end-diastolic ventricular volume expelled during each systole.

electrical gradient—driving force for movement of particles based on the attraction of particles of unlike charge and the repulsion of particles of like charge.

electrocardiogram (ECG)—record produced by electrocardiography; a tracing representing the heart's electrical action derived by amplification of the minutely small electrical impulses generated by the heart.

electrolyte—chemical substance that dissociates into electrically charged particles (ions) when dissolved in water and is able to conduct an electrical current.

electromechanical coupling—conversion of an electrical stimulus (an action potential) to mechanical activity (muscle contraction).

electrotonic potential—short-distance current flow induced by subthreshold depolarization or by a single action potential.

embolus—substance, usually a blood clot but possibly fat, air, bacterial vegetation, amniotic fluid, or a foreign body, brought by the blood from one vessel and forced into a smaller one, obstructing circulation.

embryo—term applied to the developing human between the third and eighth weeks of gestation.

embryonic period—weeks 3 through 8 of gestation.

emesis—the act of vomiting.

emission—release of sperm from the ampulla into the seminal vesicles; immediately precedes ejaculation.

emphysema—abnormal, permanent enlargement of alveoli and alveolar ducts, with destruction of alveolar walls and breakdown of connective tissue support of lower airways.

empty sella syndrome—refers to an enlarged space surrounding the pituitary gland caused by herniation of the arachnoid membrane into the area; results in flattening of the pituitary gland against the floor of the sella.

empyema—accumulation of pus in a body cavity, usually the pleural cavity.

encephalitis—inflammation of brain tissue.

encephalocele—external sac or mass that may occur at any point over the vertex or base of the skull and may be covered either with scalp or a transparent membrane.

encephalopathy—general term for degenerative disease of the brain, usually secondary to disease of another system.

end-stage renal diseas
creatinine and bloo
rise and there is im
fested by a glomer
than 10 mL/min, a l
static functions of th

endocrine—form of si
molecules (hormones
get cells, where they

endocytosis—energy-d
molecules are taken
cytosis, or receptor-m

endoderm—embryonic
thelial tissues.

endometrial cancer—m
endometrial glands
of uterine cancers ar
sarcomas.

endometriosis—non-ne
tioning endometrial
side the uterus.

endometritis—inflamm
promote postpartum

engorgement—painful
with milk.

enuresis—urinary inco
years of age, usually

environmental and occ
a variety of inflamma
ratory tract that are
ated with a particular

environmental hyperth
ture resulting from ra
ronment that overwh
nisms.

eosinophil—phagocytic
proteins and antigen–

epidemiology—study o
ease in populations

epididymitis—inflamma
ducts; common in ma
ted disease or urinary

epidural hematoma—lo
in the epidural space,

epiglottitis—inflammati
ively occludes the entr
lowing.

epilepsy—disorder char
tivity without reversib

epinephrine—major cat
transmitter; secreted
but also by neurons of

epispadias—congenital
upper wall of the ure
more commonly in the
located anywhere on t

epithelial transport—tra
nal wall, and other
adjacent epithelial cells

epitope—specific bindin
determinant.

erectile dysfunction—c
maintain a penile erect

erection—swelling and
a result of dilation o
nosum and the subseq
sexual or other types

eructation—belching.
erythrocyte—red blood cell.
erythroplasia—red mucosal plaques having no inflammatory cause; often precancerous.
erythropoiesis—red blood cell formation.
erythropoietin—glycoprotein hormone, secreted by the adult kidney and the fetal liver, that acts on the bone marrow to stimulate erythropoiesis, the production of red blood cells.
eschar—slough produced by a thermal burn or a corrosive application, or by gangrene.
esophageal atresia—congenital obstruction of the esophagus that is usually associated with concurrent abnormality of the trachea.
esophageal cancer—includes two types of malignant tumors of the esophagus: squamous cell carcinoma and adenocarcinoma.
esophageal varices—elevated pressure in the portal venous system that causes engorgement of the vessels of the esophagus and increases the risk of hemorrhage.
essential hypertension—most common form of chronically high blood pressure. The cause of essential hypertension is unknown.
essential thrombocythemia—myeloproliferative disorder resulting from proliferation of the myeloid stem cell.
estradiol—most potent naturally occurring estrogen in humans; can be formed from the conversion of testosterone by the aromatase enzyme.
estrogen—generic term for female sex hormones, including estradiol, estriol, and estrone; produced at a high rate during maturation of the ovum.
etiology—identified cause of a disease.
euthyroid sick syndrome—transient syndrome characterized by low thyroid hormone levels as a consequence of impaired peripheral conversion due to nonthyroidal illness; triiodothyronine and thyroxine levels are low but, contrary to true hypothyroidism, the level of thyroid-stimulating hormone is low or normal and that of reverse triiodothyronine is elevated.
evaporation—conversion of a liquid to a gaseous state, consuming heat and cooling the surface from which the evaporation occurs. Evaporation is the body's only means of heat loss when ambient temperature exceeds body temperature.
Ewing's sarcoma—malignant tumor of the bone that always arises in medullary tissue; usually occurs in cylindrical bones, with pain, fever, and leukocytosis as symptoms.
exanthem—skin eruption or rash.
exchange transfusion—procedure by which an individual's blood is removed by means of phlebotomy while simultaneously being replaced by transfused blood. Exchange transfusion removes an undesirable element such as sickled cells, abnormal hemoglobin, antibody-coated cells, or bilirubin while providing normal blood elements.
exocytosis—vesicular mechanism by which movement of particles occurs from the interior to the exterior of the cell. Exocytosis consumes energy and involves formation of vesicles that first fuse with, then are released from, the cell membrane.
exophthalmos—abnormal protrusion of the eye; usually due to hyperthyroidism.
expressivity—degree of expression, or severity of manifestations, seen in an inherited disorder.
extracellular fluid—compartment comprising one third of the body's fluid volume; includes intravascular, interstitial, and transcellular fluids.
extrahepatic biliary atresia—congenital obstruction or absence of all or part of the extrahepatic bile ducts, leading to cholestasis and progressive biliary cirrhosis.
extrapyramidal symptoms—effects of neuroleptic drugs on the accessory motor systems, or clinical disorders affecting major motor pathways, including parkinsonism, chorea, and athetosis.
exudate—third-space fluid containing protein, associated with conditions such as inflammation in which increased capillary permeability is an etiologic factor.
exudation—transport of fluid, cells, or cellular debris from blood vessels into tissues.
facilitated diffusion—movement of particles with the assistance of membrane transporter proteins; mediated transport.
familial hypercholesterolemia—type II hyperlipoproteinemia; autosomal dominant single gene defect resulting in dysfunction of low density lipoprotein receptors and decreased cellular uptake of low density lipoproteins; associated with the highest risk of atherosclerosis.
fatigue—subjective feeling of tiredness or exhaustion; in muscle, lack of capacity to perform active work.
febrile seizure—generalized seizure triggered by high body temperature in children. Febrile seizures are usually benign but may predispose to epilepsy in a small number of cases.
fecal incontinence—deficient control of defecation in a mature person.
feedback—return of system output to the system as a means of regulation.
Felty's syndrome—combined manifestations of rheumatoid arthritis, splenomegaly, and neutropenia.
fetal alcohol syndrome—constellation of symptoms characterized by mental and physical abnormalities of the infant, linked to maternal consumption of excessive alcohol during pregnancy.
fetal period—time between the ninth week of gestation and birth.
fetor hepaticus—acetone-like, "old wine" odor of the breath characteristic of hepatic disease.
fetus—term applied to the developing human being from the ninth week of gestation to the time of delivery.
fever—pyrogenic hyperthermia.
fever of unknown origin (FUO)—temperature of 101°F (38.3°C) or higher for 3 weeks or longer, the cause of which is not diagnosed after a week of intensive investigation.
fibrin—insoluble protein essential to blood clotting; formed from fibrinogen by action of thrombin.
fibrinogen—plasma protein precursor of fibrin; also known as clotting factor I.
fibrinolysis—dissolution of fibrin by enzymatic action.
fibrocystic change of the breast—disorder characterized by single or multiple benign tumors in the breast; the most common breast disorder of premenopausal women; usually abates after menopause.
fibromata molle—acrochordon, usually occurring on the neck, upper chest, and axillae of middle-aged women, that commonly appears during the second and third trimesters of pregnancy; also called skin tag.
fibromyalgia—muscle disorder in which deconditioning or repeated microtrauma causes diffuse pain and specific tender points in muscles; accompanied by sleep disturbance, fatigue, depression, and anxiety.
filtration—outward movement of fluid across a capillary membrane.

first-degree atrioventricular (AV) block—conduction disturbance in which the atrial impulse is slowed but eventually conducted through the atrioventricular node to the ventricles.

first-pass effect—effect of orally ingested drugs passing through the liver before being delivered to their target sites; can either inactivate much of the drug (the usual case) or activate the drug through hepatic metabolism.

flail chest—thoracic injury in which rib fractures separate a section of ribs from the sternum and spine, creating a free-floating segment that moves paradoxically inward with inspiration and outward with expiration.

flatulence—excessive formation of gases in the stomach or intestine.

follicle-stimulating hormone (FSH)—gonadotropic hormone of the anterior pituitary gland that stimulates the growth and maturity of graafian follicles in the female ovary and spermatogenesis in the male seminiferous tubules.

folliculitis—inflammation within the hair follicle, resulting in the formation of pustules; a bacterial infection.

fracture—break in the continuity of bone.

frame shift—genetic defect in which insertion or deletion of a base results in misreading of the genetic code.

Frank-Starling mechanism—relationship between the degree of tension generated within myocardial fibers and the contractile force generated during their subsequent contraction. Up to a maximal point, the greater the myocardial fiber stretch or tension, the greater will be the force of contraction that ejects that volume.

fulminant hepatitis—acute hepatitis with coma; results from extensive hepatic necrosis.

functional incontinence—involuntary urination associated with lack of voluntary control of micturition due to developmental or environmental factors.

furunculosis—bacterial infection of the skin characterized by formation of a furuncle, which is an abscess of the skin and subcutaneous tissue surrounding a hair follicle or sebaceous gland.

G protein—signal-transducing protein associated with a transmembrane receptor and a guanine nucleotide (guanosine diphosphate [GDP]); prevalent signal transduction mechanism in human cells.

galactorrhea—breast milk production independent of the normal stimuli for lactation.

gallbladder cancer—malignant tumors originating in the gallbladder.

gallop rhythm—disordered rhythm of the heart produced by a third heart sound, fourth heart sound, or both.

gamete—germ cell within sex organs; an oocyte or a spermatocyte.

gangrene—death of body tissue, generally in considerable mass, usually associated with loss of vascular supply and followed by bacterial invasion and putrefaction.

gap junction—area in which the membranes of adjacent cells are close together and connected by protein channels that traverse both membranes, facilitating communication and syncytial function.

gastric cancer—primary malignant neoplasm of the stomach; ninety percent are adenocarcinomas, and most of the remainder are non-Hodgkin's lymphomas or leiomyosarcomas.

gastritis—acute or chronic inflammation of the gastric mucosa.

gastroenteritis—inflammation of the stomach or intestines due to viruses, toxins, or bacteria.

gastroesophageal reflux disease—includes a group of disorders in which reflux of gastric contents into the lower esophagus results in either clinical symptoms or structural alterations in the tissue of the esophagus or other organs.

gene—segment of genetic material (DNA) that encodes the synthesis of a specific protein or that regulates that synthesis.

gene therapy—delivery of corrective genes to genetically abnormal cells, giving rise to production of normal or therapeutic gene products.

general adaptation syndrome—Selye's concept of a three-phase stress response. The initial stage is the *alarm reaction,* which is a brief fight-or-flight response mediated primarily by catecholamines. The second stage is the *stage of resistance,* in which there is mobilization of energy stores and suppression of immune and inflammatory responses, mediated primarily by cortisol. The third stage is the *stage of exhaustion,* which gives rise to disease and even death as adaptive resources are depleted.

general resistance equation—statement of the relationships between factors determining blood flow, derived from Ohm's law, where F = flow, P_a = pressure generated by the heart at the beginning of the systemic circuit (arterial pressure), P_v = pressure at the end of the circuit (venous pressure), and R = the resistance in the circuit: $F = (P_a - P_v)/R$.

genetic polymorphism—normal variation; presence within a population of multiple alleles at specific genetic loci.

genital herpes—herpes simplex virus infection of the genitalia, usually caused by the type 2 strain of herpes simplex virus; there is no cure.

genital warts—sexually transmitted papillomatous lesions caused by the human papillomavirus; treated with local eradication by cryotherapy, surgical excision, or laser.

genogram—family tree diagram that provides a pictorial representation of patterns of inheritance.

genomic imprinting—condition of inheritance in which the nature and degree of expression of a trait depend on whether it originates from maternal or paternal genes.

genotype—genetic constitution of an individual; also the alleles present at one or more specific loci.

gestational diabetes mellitus—carbohydrate intolerance beginning or first recognized during pregnancy.

gestational trophoblastic disease—group of disorders characterized by abnormal proliferation of trophoblast cells in the placenta; most common form is hydatidiform mole.

gingivitis—superficial inflammation of the gums; can lead to periodontal disease.

glaucoma—progressive damage to the optic nerve characterized by increased intraocular pressure, resulting in loss of vision.

glioblastoma multiforme—grade III or IV malignant astrocytoma; a rapidly growing tumor, usually of the cerebral hemispheres, in which the transformed cell is an astrocyte.

glomerular filtration rate (GFR)—rate at which water is transported from the plasma into the renal tubules by means of glomerular capillaries.

glomerulonephritis—general category that includes a number of primary and secondary disorders characterized by inflammation of the glomerular capillaries.

glucagon—polypeptide hormone secreted by the α cells of the islets of Langerhans in response to hypoglycemia or to stimulation by growth hormone; the most important of the counter-regulatory hormones that mobilize energy stores, raising serum glucose. The actions of glucagon directly oppose those of insulin, with the ratio of insulin to glucagon being more important than the absolute amounts of either hormone.

glucocorticoid—corticoid substance, released from the adrenal cortex, that increases gluconeogenesis, raising the concentration of liver glycogen and blood glucose. The principal glucocorticoid hormone is cortisol.

gluconeogenesis—synthesis of glucose from noncarbohydrate sources such as amino acids and glycerol; stimulated by cortisol and other glucocorticoids and by thyroxine.

gluten-sensitive enteropathy—malabsorption syndrome characterized by abnormal small bowel structure and intolerance of gluten (found in wheat, barley, rye, malt, and possibly oats).

glycogen—polysaccharide (starch) that is synthesized by liver and muscle and serves as a short-term storage form of energy fuel.

glycogenesis—the process by which excess nutrients are converted in the liver to glycogen for short-term storage.

glycogenolysis—splitting of glycogen in the liver, yielding glucose; stimulated by glucagon.

glycolysis—conversion of glucose to lactate or pyruvate, yielding energy (adenosine triphosphate [ATP]) and substrate for further oxidative energy metabolism; also known as preliminary metabolism (if oxygen is present) and as the Embden-Meyerhof pathway (if oxygen is absent).

goiter—thyroid enlargement; usually caused by chronic excessive iodine, which leads to decreased thyroid hormone output resulting in increased thyroid-stimulating hormone release and thyroid stimulation; may also be present in states of normal or increased thyroid hormone production.

gonadocorticoid—corticoid substance released from the adrenal cortex; gonadocorticoid hormones are mainly androgens, which confer male characteristics, but also include estrogens and progesterone, which confer female characteristics.

gonadotropin-releasing hormone—decapeptide hormone released in a pulsatile manner from the hypothalamus; stimulates the release of follicle-stimulating hormone and luteinizing hormone from the pituitary gland.

gonorrhea—highly contagious bacterial infection of the genitourinary system caused by *Neisseria gonorrhoeae;* a common sexually transmitted disease.

gout—group of metabolic disorders characterized by elevation of uric acid in the blood; gouty arthritis results when uric acid precipitates into joints, forming needle-like monosodium urate crystals.

graded potential—subtheshold potential. Its amplitude depends on the intensity of the stimulus that initiates it.

graft rejection—immune attack against a transplanted organ or tissue, involving both humoral and cell-mediated immunity and resulting in failure of the transplanted organ and a generalized inflammatory response.

graft-versus-host disease (GVHD)—isoimmune response to infused or surgically implanted tissues, typically bone marrow transplantation or blood transfusions, from a human donor; may occur when transplanted tissue contains viable T cells. The T cells recognize the host tissue antigens as foreign and mount an immune response against them. Removal of T cells from the graft decreases the risk of GVHD but also increases the risk of graft failure.

granulocyte—nonlymphocytic white blood cell that develops in bone marrow from the myeloid progenitor cell.

Graves' disease—clinical syndrome in which thyrotoxicosis is associated with diffuse goiter, infiltrative exophthalmos, and sometimes infiltrative dermopathy; probably an autoimmune disease; accounts for 85% of cases of hyperthyroidism.

growth hormone—polypeptide hormone secreted by the anterior lobe of the pituitary gland that directly influences protein, carbohydrate, and lipid metabolism and controls the rate of skeletal and visceral growth; also called somatotropin.

growth hormone deficiency—includes a group of disorders of children characterized by subnormal growth velocity, delayed bone age, and subnormal growth hormone response to at least two stimuli for release of the hormone. In adults, the deficiency is characterized by general debility and increased mortality due to altered metabolism, strength, and body composition.

growth hormone–releasing hormone—somatocrinin; stimulates secretion of growth hormone.

growth hormone release–inhibiting hormone—somatostatin; released by the hypothalamus to inhibit the release of growth hormone and thyroid-stimulating hormone from the anterior pituitary. It is also released by the delta cells of the islets of Langerhans in the pancreas to inhibit the release of glucagon and insulin.

guanosine triphosphate (GTP)—nucleotide involved in energy metabolism and required for RNA synthesis.

Guillain-Barré syndrome—inflammatory demyelinating disorder of peripheral nerves.

hairy-cell leukemia (HCL)—variant of the chronic leukemias in which the transformed cell is probably an immunoglobulin-bearing B cell. The term *hairy* refers to the prominent cytoplasmic projections on these cells.

Haldane effect—enhanced affinity of hemoglobin for carbon dioxide when hemoglobin is deoxygenated.

hapten—small molecule, not antigenic in itself but able to induce antibody formation when complexed to a larger carrier molecule.

Hashimoto's thyroiditis—autoimmune condition resulting from a genetic defect in the function of thyroid-specific suppressor T cells; the most common cause of primary hypothyroidism.

health—state of complete physical, mental, and social well-being; more than the absence of disease or infirmity.

heat exhaustion—environmental hyperthermia characterized by symptomatic hypovolemia.

heat shock protein (HSP)—intracellular protein that is synthesized in increased amounts by cells subjected to heat stress.

heatstroke—most severe form of environmental hyperthermia, characterized by hypovolemia, neurological impairment, and permanent heat-induced injury of tissues.

HELLP syndrome—hemolysis, elevated liver enzymes, and low platelet count; may accompany preeclampsia.

hematemesis—vomiting of blood.

hematocele—effusion of blood into the tunica vaginalis testis as a result of traumatic, structural, or inflammatory disorders of the testis.

hematochezia—bright red blood in the stool.

hematocrit—volume percentage of erythrocytes in whole blood.

hematology—science pertaining to the blood and blood-forming tissues, or laboratory evaluation of the blood components.

hematoma—localized collection of clotted blood in an organ, space, or tissue.

hematopoiesis—differentiation and proliferation of blood cells from a single type of stem cell in the bone marrow.

hematuria—presence of blood in the urine. In gross hematuria, blood is evidenced by the color of the urine, while in microscopic hematuria blood cells are apparent only on magnification.

heme—component of hemoglobin consisting of a protoporphyrin ring into which an iron atom has been inserted; functions in oxygen transport, energy metabolism, and hepatic biotransformation of drugs.

hemiparesis—weakened or paralyzed muscles on one side of the body.

hemiplegia—paralysis of the muscles on one side of the body.

hemochromatosis—disorder characterized by the accumulation of excess iron in many organs, leading to cell damage and functional insufficiency.

hemodynamics—study of the movements of the blood and the forces concerned therein.

hemoglobin—iron-containing protein molecule found within erythrocytes that transports oxygen in the blood.

hemoglobinopathy—hematologic disorder due to genetic alteration in the molecular structure of hemoglobin.

hemolysis—rupture of erythrocytes with release of hemoglobin into the plasma.

hemolytic disease of the newborn—potentially fatal condition marked by excessive blood destruction in newborns in cases of Rh incompatibility.

hemolytic uremia syndrome (HUS)—childhood syndrome leading to acute renal failure due to damage to glomerular endothelial cells by a toxin (usually a verocytotoxin produced by *Escherichia coli*). The central nervous system may also be the target of toxic injury, and the hemostatic system is also involved. Fibrin is deposited on the walls of injured endothelial cells, creating thrombi that consume platelets and damage red cells as they pass through renal arterioles.

hemophilia—congenital bleeding disorder that results from deficiency or abnormal function of one or more components of the clotting cascade.

hemoptysis—coughing and spitting of blood originating from within the respiratory tract.

hemorrhagic shock—hypovolemic shock due to acute blood loss.

hemorrhoid—dilated vascular channel located beneath the lining of the anal canal; may be internal (originating in the upper anal canal above the pink dentate line and covered with mucosa) or external (originating in the lower canal, covered with skin).

hemostasis—process that defends against uncontrolled hemorrhage in the event of damage to blood vessels.

Henderson-Hasselbalch equation—equation demonstrating the 20:1 ratio of base to acid that must be present to yield a normal serum pH of 7.4; that is, pH = log pKc + $[HCO_3^-]/[H_2CO_3]$.

heparan sulfate—sulfated mucopolysaccharide structurally related to heparin; enhances the anticoagulant function of antithrombin III on the endothelial surface.

heparin—polysaccharide continuously produced by mast cells and basophils; combines with antithrombin III to enhance its anticoagulant activity.

hepatic coma—coma accompanying cerebral damage, resulting from degeneration of liver cells.

hepatic encephalopathy—condition, usually occurring secondary to advanced liver disease, that can progress to hepatic coma; marked by degeneration of handwriting ability, asterixis, increased disorientation, agitation, and combativeness.

hepatic failure—impairment of liver function to a degree resulting in a predictable syndrome of observable clinical effects; can also occur as an end-stage syndrome in patients with chronic, progressive liver diseases.

hepatic steatosis—accumulation of fat in hepatocytes due to faulty metabolism of fatty acids; may precede the development of cirrhosis.

hepatoblastoma—malignant intrahepatic tumor consisting chiefly of embryonic tissue, occurring in infants and young children.

hepatocellular carcinoma—malignant neoplasm originating from hepatocytes.

hepatomegaly—enlargement of the liver.

hepatopulmonary syndrome—disorder complicating hepatic failure; manifested by pulmonary microvascular dilation and oxygen diffusion impairment; can lead to acute respiratory failure.

hepatorenal syndrome—prerenal form of acute renal failure, occurring as a functional response to altered renal hemodynamics induced by hepatic failure.

hepatotoxicity—destruction of liver cells by toxins; can occur as a consequence of any drug or foreign substance that is metabolized by the liver.

hereditary spherocytosis—inherited defect of the red blood cell membrane, resulting in abnormal erythrocyte shape and anemia due to an increased rate of red blood cell hemolysis by the spleen.

herpes simplex—acute viral disease caused by herpes simplex virus type 1, marked by groups of vesicles on the lips, mouth, nose, eyes, and skin; and herpes simplex virus type 2, marked by groups of vesicles in the genital areas and classified as a sexually transmitted disease.

herpes zoster—shingles; acute disease caused by the highly contagious herpesvirus varicella-zoster; represents recurrence of infection due to activation of dormant virus.

heterozygous—possessing different genes at each locus of an allele.

hiatal hernia—protrusion of some part of the upper portion of the stomach through the esophageal hiatus into the thoracic cavity.

high-pressure pulmonary edema (HPPE)—fluid exudation into the pulmonary interstitium and alveoli; caused by abnormal permeability of pulmonary capillaries that may occur with brain tumors or serious head injuries.

Hirschsprung's disease—congenital obstruction of the colon due to absence of ganglion cells in the enteric nervous system.

Hodgkin's disease—malignant neoplasm originating in secondary lymphoid tissues in which the transformed cell is a Reed-Sternberg (RS) cell.

holism—view of the human or of health status as an integrated whole or totality.

homeostasis—state of internal balance or organization of function; the steady state.

homonymous hemianopsia—loss of half of the visual field in corresponding areas of both fields of vision.

homozygous—possessing identical genes at a given pair of alleles.

hormone—regulatory substance, secreted by an endocrine organ, which is transported in the bloodstream to target organs, where it exerts its effects by combining with specific receptors.

human leukocyte antigen (HLA)—human major histocompatibility genetic complex, located on the short arm of chromosome 6. Five loci have been identified: HLA-A, HLA-B, HLA-C, HLA-D, and HLA-DR (D-related). Each of these has multiple alleles, designated with numerals. Each of these genes encodes cell surface antigens on nucleated cells.
humoral immunity—immune response against circulating antigen, mediated by immunoglobulins synthesized by sensitized B lymphocytes.
Huntington's disease—autosomal dominant disorder characterized by delayed onset of progressive degeneration of neurons of the basal ganglia, cerebral cortex, and cerebellum.
hydatidiform mole—abnormal pregnancy resulting from a pathologic ovum in which initial trophoblastic cell division is abnormal and uncontrolled, resulting in rapid, neoplastic-like growth of grape-like clusters in the uterus; the most common form of gestational trophoblastic disease.
hydrocele—painless swelling of the scrotum caused by a collection of clear fluid in the tunica vaginalis testis.
hydrocephalus—excessive volume of cerebrospinal fluid, resulting in increased intracranial volume and/or pressure.
hydrogen ion (H^+)—cation that is the acidic component of body fluids.
hydrolysis—cleavage of a compound by the chemical addition of water, the hydroxyl group being incorporated into one fragment and the hydrogen atom in the other.
hydrostatic pressure—force for movement of fluid, derived from gravity or from mechanical pumping.
hyperaldosteronism—excessive secretion of aldosterone, which may occur as a primary condition, due to an aldosterone-secreting tumor, or may be secondary to extra-adrenal disease.
hyperalgesia—exaggerated or increased response to a noxious stimulus.
hyperandrogenism—syndrome of excess androgen secretion or enhanced androgen effect in females.
hyperbilirubinemia—elevation of total serum bilirubin above 1.2 mg/dL. Jaundice is apparent when levels rise above 2.0 to 2.5 mg/dL.
hypercalcemia—total serum calcium of more than 10.5 mg/dL.
hypercalcemia of malignancy—excess of calcium in the blood possibly resulting from increased resorption due to factors secreted at the site of metastasis, or release of factors such as parathyroid hormone-related peptide from tumor sites remote from bone.
hypercapnia—retention of carbon dioxide in the blood, manifested by a $Paco_2$ of 50 mm Hg or greater.
hypercarotenemia—excess of carotene in the blood, producing yellow-orange discoloration of the skin.
hyperchloremia—serum chloride greater than 103 mEq/L.
hypercoagulability—abnormally increased tendency of the blood to clot.
hyperemesis gravidarum—disorder of pregnant women in which extensive and prolonged vomiting leads to severe alteration in nutritional status and in fluid-electrolyte balance.
hyperemia—excess of blood within a tissue.
hyperglycemia—excess of glucose in the blood, associated with diabetes mellitus.
hyperhidrosis—increased sweating.
hyperinsulinemia—excess insulin in the blood.
hyperkalemia—elevation of serum potassium concentration above 5.5 mEq/L.
hyperkinesia—excessive and abnormal muscle movement; may manifest as tremors, tics, gait disturbances, and other involuntary movements.
hyperlipidemia—elevation of serum lipids, specifically cholesterol and triglycerides.
hyperlipoproteinemia—elevation of any class of lipoprotein in the blood either singly or, more usually, in combination; due to an acquired or a hereditary disorder of lipoprotein metabolism.
hypermagnesemia—serum level of magnesium greater than 2.5 mEq/L.
hypermetabolic state—clinical condition characterized by a sustained increase in metabolic rate.
hypernatremia—relative excess of sodium in the extracellular fluid; serum sodium greater than 147 mEq/L.
hyperopia—farsightedness.
hyperosmolar imbalance—fluid imbalance in which body fluids become more concentrated than normal, resulting in shrinkage of body cells.
hyperosmolar nonketotic state—acute complication of diabetes resulting from extreme hyperglycemia; manifested by severe dehydration due to osmotic diuresis, and absence of ketosis.
hyperparathyroidism—clinical syndrome resulting from excessive secretion of parathyroid hormone from the parathyroid gland.
hyperphosphatemia—serum phosphate level above 4.5 mg/dL.
hyperplasia—abnormal increase in volume of a tissue or organ caused by increased numbers of cells due to normal or abnormal mitotic activity.
hyperpolarization—increased voltage difference between resting membrane potential and threshold; decreased cellular excitability.
hyperreflexia—exaggeration of deep tendon reflexes (DTRs) and superficial reflexes.
hypersensitivity—state of altered reactivity in which the body reacts with an exaggerated immune response to a foreign antigen (e.g., allergy, anaphylaxis).
hypersomnia—sleep disorder characterized by excessive sleep.
hypertension—persistently high blood pressure.
hyperthermia—body temperature above 100°F or 37.8°C.
hyperthyroidism—hypermetabolic state induced by elevated levels of thyroid hormones in the blood, usually due to hyperfunction of the thyroid gland.
hypertonia—excessively increased muscle tone.
hypertonic—referring to a solution having greater osmolality than plasma or intracellular fluid.
hypertrophic cardiomyopathy—type of cardiomyopathy associated with familial inheritance, in which the walls of both ventricles become greatly thickened, obstructing aortic outflow and resulting in very small chamber sizes.
hypertrophic pyloric stenosis—congenital obstructive disorder of the gastric outlet resulting from hypertrophy of the circular musculature surrounding the pylorus.
hypertrophy—increase in muscle size due to structural enlargement of existing muscle cells.
hyperuricemia—excess of serum uric acid.
hyperventilation—increased rate and/or depth of breathing.
hypervolemia—abnormal increase in the volume of circulating plasma; fluid volume excess.
hypoaldosteronism—deficiency of aldosterone secretion due to an inherited metabolic defect, adrenal insufficiency, defect in renin secretion, or neurological disease.

hypocalcemia—total serum calcium of less than 8.5 mg/dL.
hypochloremia—serum chloride below 95 mEq/L.
hypocoagulability—abnormally increased bleeding tendency.
hypoglycemia—syndrome resulting from serum glucose levels below 60 mg/dL.
hypogonadism—decreased function of the male gonads causing testosterone deficiency, with retardation of growth and sexual development.
hypokalemia—serum potassium level below 3.5 mEq/L.
hypokinesia—decreased muscle movement; may manifest as muscle weakness or slowed movement.
hypomagnesemia—serum magnesium level less than 1.5 mEq/L.
hypometabolic state—clinical condition characterized by a sustained decrease in metabolic rate.
hyponatremia—serum sodium concentration of less than 135 mEq/L.
hypo-osmolar imbalance—fluid imbalance in which body fluids become more dilute than normal, resulting in swelling of body cells.
hypoparathyroidism—syndrome produced by greatly reduced function of the parathyroid glands or by removal of these bodies as a treatment for hyperparathyroidism; results from the effects of parathyroid hormone deficiency or resistance on calcium homeostasis.
hypophosphatemia—serum phosphate below 2.0 mg/dL.
hypopituitarism—deficiency of pituitary hormones that may be partial, affecting one or a few trophic hormones, or complete (panhypopituitarism), affecting all trophic hormones and their target endocrine organs.
hypoplasia—underdevelopment of an organ or tissue.
hypopolarization—decreased voltage difference between resting membrane potential and threshold; increased cellular excitability.
hypospadias—developmental anomaly in the male in which the urethra opens on the underside of the penis or on the perineum.
hypotension—low blood pressure.
hypothalamic-pituitary axis—negative feedback system that regulates the release of hormones from all major endocrine organs except the pancreas and parathyroids.
hypothermia—body temperature below 94°F or 34.4°C.
hypothyroidism—syndrome resulting from a deficiency of thyroid hormone or, less commonly, resistance to thyroid hormone effect; may be congenital or acquired.
hypotonia—decreased muscle tone.
hypotonic—referring to a solution with a lesser degree of osmolality than plasma or intracellular fluid.
hypovolemia—abnormal decrease in the volume of circulating plasma; fluid volume deficit.
hypovolemic shock—state of generalized deficit in tissue perfusion secondary to conditions that deplete blood volume (e.g., hemorrhage or third spacing).
hypoxemia—deficient oxygenation of the blood.
hypoxia—deficient oxygenation of body tissues.
hypoxic pulmonary vasoconstriction—adaptive response whereby the vessels perfusing unventilated or hypoventilated alveoli constrict, optimizing ventilation–perfusion matching.
iatrogenic—treatment-induced, adverse.
idiopathic—occurring without known cause.
idiopathic dilated cardiomyopathy—most common type of cardiomyopathy, characterized by uncertain cause and dilation of both ventricles. Congestive heart failure occurs when the Frank-Starling mechanism is exceeded.
idiopathic pulmonary fibrosis—disorder characterized by inflammation and fibrosis of the pulmonary interstitium and respiratory units; cause unknown.
idioventricular rhythm—slow rhythm paced by an ectopic focus in the ventricular myocardium.
immunity—security against a particular disease; nonsusceptibility to the invasive or pathogenic effects of foreign microorganisms or to the toxic effects of antigenic substances.
immunization—involves the injection or oral administration of vaccine, which usually consists of a small amount of killed or attenuated organism or its toxin.
immunodeficiency—reduction in either the humoral or cell-mediated immune response.
immunoglobulin—protein synthesized by B lymphocytes that mediates humoral immunity; antibody.
immunoglobulin superfamily—one of the four major categories of adhesion molecules, which includes neural cell adhesion molecules and intracellular adhesion molecules.
impaired glucose tolerance—condition in which serum glucose is elevated above normal but below the threshold for the diagnosis of diabetes mellitus.
impetigo—contagious, superficial, crust-forming bacterial infection of the skin, most often seen in children.
inborn errors of metabolism—clinical syndromes caused by deficiency or defective function of digestive enzymes as a result of genetic disorders such as galactosemia and phenylketonuria and others.
incidence—number of new cases of a specific disease occurring during a specified period.
inclusion-body myositis—type of inflammatory myopathy in which rimmed vacuoles and tubular filaments are seen in muscle cells.
incompetent cervix—short or funneled cervix that thins or dilates before termination of the normal period of gestation, resulting in premature expulsion of the fetus.
increased intracranial pressure (IICP)—clinical syndrome resulting from interstitial and intraventricular fluid pressure in excess of 15 mm Hg within the cranial vault; intracranial hypertension.
infant of a diabetic mother—newborn of a woman having diabetes mellitus during pregnancy; tends to be large for gestational age and is thus at higher risk for asphyxia and birth trauma at delivery; susceptible to hypoglycemia and at risk for congenital anomalies and neonatal complications.
infant respiratory distress syndrome—respiratory failure occurring occasionally in term infants but more commonly in premature infants, due to deficiency of surfactant production; formerly known as hyaline membrane disease. Increased surface tension results in difficulty of inflation of alveoli and terminal airways, complicated by decreased lung compliance and poor inspiratory muscle development. Hypoxic injury to the alveolar-capillary membrane results in thickening of this membrane, limiting gas exchange.
infection—inflammatory response initiated by invasion of microorganisms.
infectious mononucleosis—self-limited disorder characterized by proliferation of T lymphocytes in lymphoid tissues and non-neoplastic abnormality of circulating lymphocytes.
infective endocarditis (IE)—infection of the endocardial surface of the heart, including the valves.
infertility—failure of a couple to conceive after 1 year of unprotected sexual intercourse.

inflammation—nonspecific, usually localized protective response to any form of tissue injury, serving to destroy, dilute, or wall off both the injurious agent and the injured tissue and to prepare the area for healing.

inflammatory bowel disease—encompasses several chronic conditions of the intestine; the most common are Crohn's disease and ulcerative colitis.

inflammatory myopathy—disorder characterized by immune-mediated inflammation of skeletal muscle; includes dermatomyositis, polymyositis, and inclusion-body myositis.

inguinal hernia—protrusion of abdominal viscera, usually a loop of intestine, through a weakened area of the abdominal wall in the inguinal or groin region.

inhibin—peptide that participates in the regulation of gonadal, adrenal, and placental hormone production. Rising gonadotropin levels stimulate inhibin release from the pituitary; inhibin, in turn, inhibits gonadotropin release in a negative feedback mechanism. Inhibin is produced in the ovary, testis, and extragonadal tissues.

insomnia—sleep disorder characterized by insufficient sleep.

insulin—protein hormone formed in the β cells of the pancreatic islets of Langerhans; the major fuel-regulating hormone; secreted into the blood in response to a rise in concentration of blood glucose or amino acids; the only hormone that acts to lower blood glucose level.

insulin resistance—condition occurring in patients who have circulating anti-insulin antibodies in their blood or who produce specific insulin antagonists that are destructive to insulin. Insulin resistance is central to the major pathophysiologic effects of obesity; obese persons often have normal or elevated blood glucose levels despite hyperinsulinemia.

insulin-like growth factor (IGF)—peptide mediating growth hormone action; secreted by a variety of tissues including the liver and ovaries. The ovarian IGF system may act synergistically with follicle stimulating hormone and luteinizing hormone in regulation of the menstrual cycle.

integrin—membrane protein that binds one or more types of ligand in the matrix.

intercalated disk—gap junction that separates cardiac muscle cells, permitting syncytial function.

intermediate filament—the middle-sized type of protein fiber located in the cytoskeleton.

intermittent claudication—crampy pain of the lower extremities occurring first with exercise and later even at rest in those with arteriosclerosis obliterans. Pain is due to ischemia induced by peripheral atherosclerosis.

interstitial cystitis—idiopathic disorder characterized by chronic, unexplained irritative voiding symptoms, sterile urine, and specific changes within the bladder mucosa.

interstitial fluid—fluid found in the interstices between cells, the fluid phase of connective tissue, and the lymphatics.

intervertebral disk disease—condition of the spine that causes low back pain due to compression of a spinal nerve root by a herniated intervertebral disk.

intracellular adhesion molecule (I-CAM)—one of the immunoglobulin superfamily members, a category of adhesion molecule.

intracellular fluid (ICF)—fluid contained within body cells other than blood cells.

intracerebral hemorrhage—bleeding into the interstitium of the brain.

intrauterine growth retardation—deficient support of fetal growth in utero, resulting in birth of an infant who is small for gestational age.

intravascular fluid—plasma of the blood and fluid within blood cells.

intraventricular hemorrhage—bleeding within a cerebral ventricle.

intrinsic contractility—component of cardiac muscle contraction that is based on the rate of actin-myosin cross-bridge formation; inotropic state.

intromission—entry of the penis into the vagina.

ion—charged particle.

iron-deficiency anemia—disorder of oxygen transport due to deficiency of hemoglobin synthesis.

irritable bowel syndrome—chronic functional bowel disorder characterized by persistence or recurrence of the following symptoms for at least 3 months: abdominal pain or discomfort relieved with defecation or associated with a change in frequency or consistency of stool and irregular pattern of defecation at least 25% of the time with two or more of the following: altered stool frequency; hard, loose, or watery stool; straining or sense or urgency, feeling of incomplete evacuation; passage of mucus; and bloating or abdominal distention.

isoimmunity—immune attack against tissues originating from another human (e.g., ABO incompatibility, Rh incompatibility, and graft rejection).

isolated systolic hypertension—category of essential hypertension, common in the elderly, in which increased arterial stiffness is a primary etiologic factor. Systolic pressure is elevated while diastolic pressure is normal or low.

isotonic—referring to a solution having the same osmolality as the plasma or intracellular fluid.

jaundice—yellowness of skin, sclerae, mucous membranes, and excretions due to hyperbilirubinemia and deposition of bile pigments.

junctional rhythm—slow rhythm (40 to 60 beats per minute) originating in the atrioventricular junction.

Kaposi's sarcoma—multicentric, malignant neoplastic proliferation of the vascular endothelium in skin and other tissues, characterized by the development of bluish red cutaneous nodules, usually on the lower extremities; occurs in immunosuppressed patients such as transplant recipients and those with the acquired immunodeficiency syndrome.

karyotype—chromosomal composition of the cells of an individual.

Kawasaki disease—acute febrile illness of children that is the most common form of vasculitis and that may be complicated by the development of coronary artery aneurysms; mucocutaneous lymph node syndrome.

kernicterus—bilirubin-induced brain injury.

keto acid—carboxylic acid containing a carbonyl group; formed by the removal or rearrangement of carbon atoms from citric acid during the Krebs cycle.

ketoacidosis—accumulation of ketone bodies in the blood, which results in metabolic acidosis.

ketone body—acetone, acetoacetic acid, or β-hydroxybutyric acid; metabolic by-product of beta oxidation of lipids.

Krebs cycle—metabolic pathway by which carbon chains of sugars, fatty acids, and amino acids are converted to more stable forms, yielding energy, carbon dioxide, and water; also known as the tricarboxylic acid (TCA) cycle, citric acid cycle, and intermediary metabolism.

Kussmaul respiration—deep, gasping ventilation seen with respiratory compensation for metabolic acidosis; "air hunger."

kyphosis—abnormally increased convexity in the curvature of the thoracic spine as viewed from the side; also called hunchback.

lactic acid (lactate)—metabolic end product of glycolysis that may accumulate under anaerobic conditions, may be oxidized by the heart for energy, or may be converted to glucose by the liver.

lactic acidosis—severe elevation of blood lactate levels.

lactogenesis—milk production by mammary glands; inhibited by estrogen and progesterone during pregnancy but induced when removal of these hormones with delivery of the placenta allows prolactin to induce alveolar secretion and milk production.

lactose intolerance—impaired ability to absorb lactose due to lack of activity of the enzyme lactase, normally found in the brush border of the luminal surface of the small intestine.

Laennec's cirrhosis—cirrhosis of the liver closely associated with chronic excessive alcohol ingestion.

laryngeal cancer—presence of a malignant neoplasm on, immediately above, or immediately below the vocal cords.

laryngitis—inflammation of the mucosa of the larynx, resulting in sore throat and hoarseness.

latch-bridge—slow-cycling cross-bridge in smooth muscle that permits sustained contraction with minimal energy consumption.

Legg-Calvé-Perthes disease—osteochondrosis of the epiphysis of the femoral head.

letdown reflex—exocytotic transport of milk from the alveoli of the breast through the ducts to the nipple, triggered by sensory signals sent to the hypothalamus on suckling by the infant or by cortical stimulation of the hypothalamus; mediated by oxytocin, which induces contraction of smooth muscle surrounding milk-filled alveoli in the breasts.

leukemia—chronic or acute progressive malignant neoplasm of the blood-forming organs, marked by diffuse replacement of the bone marrow by abnormal leukocytes and their precursors. It is accompanied by a reduced number of erythrocytes and blood platelets, resulting in anemia and increased susceptibility to infection and hemorrhage. Leukemia is classified on the basis of its onset and course as acute or chronic and on the basis of its cell of origin as lymphoid or myeloid.

leukocyte—white blood cell.

leukocytosis—increase in circulating leukocytes; may represent either a normal proliferation of phagocytic cells in response to infection or allergy or a hematopoietic malignancy.

leukopenia—reduction in the number of circulating leukocytes; present in a variety of disorders that are manifested by a high risk of infection.

leukoplakia—disease marked by the development of white, thickened, precancerous patches on the mucous membranes of the cheeks, gums, or tongue.

leukopoiesis—white blood cell formation.

ligand-gated channel—membrane channel that opens or closes as a consequence of a conformational change in the membrane protein induced by binding of a specific substance (ligand).

light chain—small polypeptide chain associated with the myosin head and playing a regulatory role in muscle contraction.

lipodermatosclerosis—induration and fibrosis of the skin.

lipogenesis—formation of body fat from nonfat nutrients.

lipolysis—metabolic breakdown of fat, yielding glucose.

lobar pneumonia—lower respiratory tract infection beginning in one area of the lung and possibly progressing to involve an entire lobe; typical of aspiration pneumonia.

lordosis—forward curvature of the lumbar spine; also called swayback.

lower gastrointestinal bleeding—bleeding from the jejunum, ileum, colon, or rectum.

lower motor neuron disease—inhibition or interruption of lower motor neuron reflex arcs; results in diminished or absent motor activity.

lung cancer (bronchogenic carcinoma)—malignant neoplasm arising in lung tissue.

luteinizing hormone (LH)—gonadotropic hormone of the anterior pituitary gland that regulates the development and function of the female ovaries and male testes.

lymphedema—third spacing of protein-rich fluid as a result of lymphatic obstruction.

lymphocyte—mononuclear, nonphagocytic leukocyte found in the blood, lymph, and lymphoid tissues; comprises the body's immunologically competent cells and their precursors; differentiated into B and T lymphocytes.

lymphoma—neoplastic disorder of lymphoid tissue.

lymphoproliferative disorder—benign or malignant disorder characterized by excessive production of lymphocytes or their products.

macrosomia—large fetal size.

macrovascular disease—disorders of blood vessels that may manifest as coronary heart disease, cerebrovascular disease, or peripheral vascular disease; in diabetes, the vessels become atherosclerotic, and atherosclerosis progresses rapidly, owing to hypertension, possible glycosylation of vessel proteins, and dyslipidemia resulting from insulin resistance.

macular degeneration—common form of retinopathy producing loss of visual acuity secondary to destruction of the retinal area mediating central vision.

magnesium (Mg^{2+})—cation found primarily in intracellular fluid and bone that is a cofactor in many enzymatic reactions and is important in electrical activity of excitable cells.

malaise—subjective state of illness; general feeling of indisposition.

malignant—tending to become progressively worse and to result in death; with respect to neoplasms, having the capacity to invade and metastasize, as in cancer.

malignant hyperthermia—hypermetabolic disorder of skeletal muscle that is most often inherited as an autosomal dominant condition. Administration of a triggering agent (usually an inhalation anesthetic or muscle relaxant) results in sustained muscle contraction that produces extreme hyperthermia.

malignant melanoma—malignant neoplasm originating from melanocytes in the basal layer of the epidermis or, more commonly, in the aggregated melanocytes of an existing nevus; local invasion, regional lymph node metastasis, and distant metastasis are possible.

mastitis—inflammation of the mammary glands.

mastoiditis—inflammation of the mastoid antrum and cells.

mean arterial pressure (MAP)—average arterial pressure during the cardiac cycle, calculated by the following formula: MAP = (systolic pressure + 2 diastolic pressure)/3.

mechanically gated channel—membrane channel that opens in response to a deforming force such as pressure or friction.

mechanism (of disease)—combination of dynamic processes that cause disease, give rise to signs and symptoms, and signify the body's attempts to overcome disease.
meconium aspiration syndrome—inhalation of meconium by the fetus or newborn, which may result in atelectasis, emphysema, or pneumonia, and is commonly associated with persistent pulmonary hypertension of the newborn.
megakaryopoiesis—platelet formation.
meiosis—process of cell division in germ cells, which results in formation of four daughter cells, each with the diploid number of chromosomes; reduction division.
melanocyte-stimulating hormone (MSH)—hormone that stimulates production of the skin pigment melanin.
melasma—skin condition occurring in 50% to 75% of pregnant women; melanosis characterized by brownish pigmentation over the cheeks, forehead, upper lip, nose, or chin; fades in most women during the year after pregnancy.
melatonin—indoleamine hormone synthesized and released by the pineal body during the hours of darkness.
melena—black, tarry stools.
membrane potential—charge separation across a cell membrane.
menarche—initial onset of menstrual cycles, usually occurring between the ages of 11 and 15.
mendelian disorder—inherited genetic disorder that displays a pattern of inheritance consistent with principles of independent assortment and segregation (Mendel's laws).
Meniere's disease—auditory vertigo; chronic disorder of hearing and proprioception in which function of the auditory nerve (eighth cranial nerve) is impaired by excessive endolymphatic fluid pressure; often accompanied by nystagmus.
meningitis—inflammation of the meninges.
meningocele—form of spina bifida cystica in which only the meninges protrude in a fluid-filled sac.
menopause—cessation of menstruation, which occurs at an average age of 51; accompanies the depletion of oocytes.
menstrual cycle—regularly recurring physiologic changes in the endometrium that culminate in its shedding; varies in length of time between 21 and 35 days.
menstruation—cyclic shedding of cells of the endometrial lining of a nonpregnant uterus, evidenced as uterine contraction with crampy abdominal pain and vaginal bleeding; occurs every 28 days or so between puberty and menopause except during pregnancy, with flow lasting about 5 days.
mesoderm—embryonic tissue layer from which the connective tissues of the body differentiate.
metabolic acidosis—acidic pH resulting from accumulation of fixed acids or from loss of base from the blood and body tissues.
metabolic alkalosis—acid-base disorder in which an alkaline pH results from loss of fixed acid, from ingestion or retention of excess base, or from a compensatory renal and cellular response to hypokalemia.
metabolism—multiple processes by which cells acquire and use energy.
metastasize—to transfer disease from one part of the body to another.
methemoglobinemia—clinical disorder in which heme iron is oxidized from the normal ferrous (Fe^{2+}) state to the ferric (Fe^{3+}) state; increasing the affinity of any normal hemoglobin for oxygen. This shifts the oxyhemoglobin dissociation curve to the left, promoting tissue hypoxia.
microfilament—within the cytoplasm, the smallest type of protein fiber located in the cytoskeleton.
micropenis—congenitally small penis.
microtubule—the largest type of protein fiber located in the cytoskeleton.
microvascular disease—damage to small-diameter vessels; in diabetes contributes to hypertension, which worsens retinopathy and nephropathy and also promotes macrovascular disease; may play a role in neuropathy.
micturition—urination.
mineralocorticoid—any of a group of hormones elaborated by the cortex of the adrenal gland, so named because of their effects on sodium, chloride, and potassium concentrations in the extracellular fluid; aldosterone is the principal mineralocorticoid.
minimal lesion nephrotic syndrome (MLNS)—relatively benign idiopathic disorder characterized by proteinuria due to reversible loss of foot processes of otherwise-normal glomerular epithelial cells.
mitosis—process of cell division in body cells, which maintains the diploid number of chromosomes and forms two daughter cells that are exact replicas of the original.
mitral insufficiency—incomplete closure of the mitral valve during systole.
mitral stenosis—incomplete opening of the mitral valve during diastole.
mitral valve prolapse—abnormal enlargement of the mitral valve leaflets, with projection of the leaflets into the left atrium during systole.
mixed acid-base imbalance—combination of two or three primary acid-base imbalances. Respiratory acidosis and respiratory alkalosis cannot coexist, but all other combinations of respiratory acidosis, respiratory alkalosis, metabolic acidosis, and metabolic alkalosis are possible.
monocyte-macrophage—mononuclear phagocytic cell that functions similarly to a neutrophil in inflammation. Monocytes are inactive, circulating precursors to macrophages, which are the mature, active phagocytic cells. Macrophages are present for a longer period than neutrophils at sites of inflammation. They are important in phagocytosis of microorganisms and cellular debris, in preparation of the area for healing, and in processing and presentation of antigen for the cellular immune response.
Monro-Kellie doctrine—physiologic principle positing an equilibrium among the volumes of blood, brain tissue, and cerebrospinal fluid within the closed cranial vault. Should any one of these components increase in volume, a rise in intracranial pressure will occur unless another component is able to decrease its occupied space.
morbidity—occurrence of disease; state of being diseased.
morphogenesis—development of human shape and form.
morphology—form and structure.
mortality—rate of death due to a specific disease.
mosaicism—mixture of normal and abnormal cell lines in an individual in whom a genetic defect arises after initial cleavage of the zygote.
mottling—discoloration in irregular areas.
multifactorial inheritance—disorder resulting from the combined effects of one or more genetic mutations and environmental factors; familial or polygenetic inheritance.

multifetal pregnancy—gestation resulting from penetration of more than one ovum by sperm (fraternal twins) or from initial division of the zygote into daughter cells that then undergo separate development (monozygotic or identical twins); preterm delivery is usual.

multiple endocrine neoplasia (MEN)—rare familial syndrome of autonomous hyperfunction of more than one endocrine gland. Medullary thyroid carcinoma may be a component of MEN.

multiple myeloma—malignant neoplasm of bone marrow origin characterized by abnormal proliferation of a single clone of plasma cells that produce an immunoglobulin called the M protein; classified as a lymphoproliferative disorder.

multiple sclerosis—disorder of neurotransmission resulting from demyelination and ultimate destruction of axons of motor, sensory, and autonomic nerves.

murmur—vibratory (blowing or rushing) sound produced by increased turbulence of blood flow during the cardiac cycle.

muscle tone—resistance in a healthy muscle to passive elongation or stretch; possibly due to the elastic recoil of connectin.

muscular dystrophy—familial disorder characterized by progressive degeneration of skeletal muscle fibers.

mutagen—substance capable of inducing genetic mutation.

myalgia—muscle pain.

myasthenia gravis—autoimmune disorder characterized by progressive muscular weakness and fatigue with repetitive activity; believed to be caused by circulating antibodies that are directed against the postsynaptic acetylcholine receptors at the neuromuscular junction.

myasthenic crisis—extreme weakness of respiratory muscles in a patient with myasthenia gravis; can develop suddenly after a systemic infection, surgery, or other stressful event.

myelin—sheath derived from lipids and impermeable to ions; surrounds most large nerve fibers and speeds the conduction of nerve impulses.

myelomeningocele—form of spina bifida cystica in which the meninges, peripheral nerves, nerve roots, and possibly the spinal cord protrude in a fluid-filled sac.

myocardial infarction (MI)—death of myocardial cells due to prolonged ischemia secondary to occlusion of one or more coronary arteries.

myocarditis—inflammation and injury of the myocardium in the absence of ischemia.

myoglobinuria—myoglobin in the urine.

myopia—nearsightedness.

myosin—intracellular protein that, along with actin, is essential to muscle contraction.

myosin adenosine triphosphatase—enzyme on the myosin head in all muscle types. It cleaves adenosine triphosphate to adenosine diphosphate and inorganic phosphorus (P_i), providing energy for cross-bridge detachment.

myosin light chain kinase (MLCK)—enzyme in smooth muscle that phosphorylates the myosin head, dissociating the actin-myosin cross-bridge.

myosin phosphatase—enzyme in smooth muscle which dephosphorylates the myosin head, dissociating the actin–myosin cross-bridge.

myotonia—inability of muscle to relax completely after contraction.

myotonia congenita—congenital muscle disorder marked by tonic spasm and rigidity of certain muscles on attempts to move them.

myxedema—condition resulting from advanced hypothyroidism or deficiency of thyroxine, in which a mucopolysaccharide-rich fluid accumulates in connective tissues.

natriuresis—increased urinary output of sodium.

near-drowning—acute episode in which respiration is prevented by submersion in water for a sufficient length of time to lead to significant morbidity and possibly to mortality.

nebulin—nonelastic cytoskeletal protein associated with actin in striated muscle; regulates the length of actin strands.

necrosis—cell death due to injury-induced inflammatory degradation.

necrotizing enterocolitis—development of necrotic patches in the intestine that interfere with digestion and absorption and can lead to a paralytic ileus, perforation, and peritonitis; occurs most often in preterm and very immature neonates.

negative feedback loop—adaptive response system that counteracts perturbing forces, restoring homeostasis.

negative nitrogen balance—state in which more protein is utilized or lost from the body than is taken in.

neoplasia—new growth; process of accelerated or uninhibited growth of genetically abnormal cells.

neoplasm—mass of neoplastic cells; a tumor.

nephritic syndrome—clinical finding of red and white blood cells in the urine, along with casts of these cells. The nephritic syndrome indicates the presence of an inflammatory process within the glomerulus.

nephropathy—disease of the kidneys that commonly accompanies diabetes type 1 and type 2 and manifests as nodular lesions and thickening of the glomerular basement membrane.

nephrotic syndrome—clinical findings associated with proteinuria of greater than 3.5 g/day, low serum albumin, and, often, hyperlipoproteinemia.

Nernst potential—membrane voltage at which ion flux along an electrical gradient is offset by concentration-driven flux in the opposite direction; equilibrium potential.

neural tube—ectodermal embryonic structure that develops into the brain and spinal cord.

neural tube defect (NTD)—one of a group of congenital anomalies of the central nervous system arising from failure of dorsal induction of closure of the neural tube, an early embryonic structure that forms from folding of the ectodermal neural plate. The most common NTDs are anencephaly, encephalocele, spina bifida cystica, and spina bifida occulta.

neural-cell adhesion molecule (N-CAM)—one of the immunoglobulin superfamily members; a category of adhesion molecule.

neuroblastoma—malignant tumor of embryonic neural crest origin, usually arising in the autonomic nervous system or in the adrenal medulla.

neuroectoderm—subdivision of the ectodermal germ layer that gives rise to the organs of the central nervous system and some neuroendocrine organs.

neurogenic hyperthermia—category of conditions in which elevated body temperature is due to abnormal hypothalamic thermoregulation secondary to neurotrauma, toxicity, or idiosyncratic reaction to drugs.

neurogenic shock—distributive shock associated with head injury or strong stimuli that overwhelm the usual regulatory capacity of the nervous system. Blood pressure falls to the point where the supply of oxygen carried by the blood to the brain is insufficient.

neuroleptic malignant syndrome (NMS)—an idiosyncratic reaction to administration of, or withdrawal from, a neuroleptic drug, characterized by rigidity and hyperthermia due to blockade of dopaminergic receptors in the basal ganglia.

neuromuscular junction—specialized connection between a motor nerve and a skeletal muscle fiber; myoneural junction.

neuropathy—chronic symmetric sensory disease accompanying diabetes type 1 and type 2 involving the nerves of the lower limbs and often affecting autonomic nerves; results from neural hypoxia and demyelination secondary to microvascular disease and to hyperglycemia-induced metabolic derangement.

neurotransmitter—regulatory substance, secreted by neurons into synapses, that exerts effects by combining with postsynaptic receptors.

neutrophil—phagocytic granulocyte that can inactivate 5 to 20 bacteria. Neutrophils comprise more than half of the white blood cells in the peripheral circulation.

nevus—benign mole.

no-reflow phenomenon—continued decrease in blood flow in the microvasculature of the reperfused myocardium, possibly due to impaired endothelial function or to mechanical plugging of capillaries by neutrophils and red blood cells.

node of Ranvier—point of interruption in the myelin sheath of nerve fibers and characterized by voltage-gated channels; where action potentials are generated.

nonalcoholic steatohepatitis—hepatic disorder in which inflammation results from elevation of free fatty acids in the serum; histology resembles that of alcoholic liver disease but there is no history of alcohol abuse.

nondisjunction—mechanism leading to numerical chromosomal abnormality; failure of chromatid pairs to separate during mitosis, resulting in unequal numbers of chromosomes in daughter cells.

non-Hodgkin's lymphoma (NHL)—malignant neoplasm of secondary lymphoid tissue origin, in which the transformed cell is not a Reed-Sternberg cell.

nonshivering thermogenesis—production of heat in neonates by brown fat metabolism.

norepinephrine—major catecholamine hormone and neurotransmitter; secreted primarily by sympathetic neurons but also by the adrenal medulla.

normal pressure hydrocephalus (NPH)—idiopathic disorder characterized by increased volume but normal pressure of cerebrospinal fluid in intracranial ventricles; usually seen in elderly persons and accompanied by cortical atrophy.

normal sinus rhythm (NSR)—cardiac rhythm in which the rate, rhythm, and PQRST characteristics are all within normal parameters.

nystagmus—involuntary, rapid, rhythmic movement of the eyeball.

obesity—accumulation of an abnormally large quantity of adipose tissue; defined quantitatively with reference to ideal body weight, fraction of body fat, or body mass index.

obstetrics—biomedical specialty concerned with support of normal pregnancy and with prevention and treatment of associated disorders.

obstructive sleep apnea—syndrome of repeated episodes of obstructive cessation or reduction of ventilation during sleep; also called upper airway resistance syndrome.

occult bleeding—blood in stools that is not visible to the eye.

oligohydramnios—deficient amount of amniotic fluid.

oligomenorrhea—scanty, irregular, or infrequent menstruation.

oligospermia—deficient numbers of spermatozoa in the semen.

oliguria—decreased urine output relative to fluid intake.

oncogene—transformed proto-oncogene, capable of initiating or promoting malignant replication of cells.

oogenesis—development of ova from oogonia within the ovaries.

open system—system that exchanges matter, energy, and information with its environment.

ophthalmia neonatorum—hyperacute purulent infection of the conjunctiva of the neonate due to organisms acquired during vaginal delivery.

optic neuritis—inflammation of the optic nerve.

oral cancer—malignant neoplasms within the oral cavity; may involve the lips, cheek, gums, palate, floor of the mouth, and tongue; 90% are squamous cell carcinomas.

orchitis—inflammation of a testis; usually accompanies epididymitis.

organic osmolyte—small organic molecule present in all cells; its uptake or release by a cell protects the cell from extreme volume disturbances secondary to osmolar imbalances.

organomegaly—increase in organ size.

orthostatic (postural) hypotension—fall in blood pressure associated with dizziness, syncope, and blurred vision occurring on standing or when standing motionless in a fixed position.

Osgood-Schlatter disease—osteochondrosis of tibial tubercle, just below the knee.

osmolality—expression of the total concentration of solute per kilogram of water. In body fluids within the physiologic temperature range, osmolality is very similar to osmolarity, the solute concentration per liter.

osmolarity—concentration of solute per liter of solvent.

osmoreceptor—specialized cells that shrink or swell in response to altered osmolality of the extracellular fluid, initiating the thirst mechanism or antidiuretic hormone release from the posterior pituitary.

osmotic demyelination syndrome—clinical effects resulting from too-rapid correction of hyponatremia, in which osmotic injury to myelinated nerve fibers may cause paralysis or death.

osmotic pressure—a "pulling" force exerted by particles upon water, governing its movement across a semipermeable membrane from a more dilute solution to a more concentrated solution.

osteoarthritis (OA)—joint damage and inflammation secondary to biochemical alteration of the articular cartilage in one or a few joints; the most prevalent form of arthritis.

osteochrondrosis—disease characterized by avascular necrosis of the epiphyseal growth plates in growing children and adolescents, followed by regeneration or recalcification.

osteomalacia—adult rickets; bone disorder characterized by deficient mineralization of the bone matrix due to deficiency or abnormal metabolism of vitamin D; in adults, results in the formation of undermineralized bone during cyclic bone remodeling.

osteomyelitis—infectious disorder of bone characterized by progressive inflammatory destruction followed by new formation of bone; *Staphylococcus aureus* is the cause of 85% to 90% of cases.

osteoporosis—multifactorial disorder in which decreased bone mass and increased bone fragility result from disequilibrium of osteoblastic and osteoclastic activity.

osteosarcoma—malignant neoplasm of skeletal connective tissue often arising in epiphyseal sites; the most common malignant bone tumor of children.

otitis media—inflammation of the middle ear; common cause of conductive hearing loss.

otosclerosis—genetic disorder in which focal areas of the bony capsule of the inner ear remodel and harden; common cause of conductive hearing loss.

ovarian cancer—malignant neoplasm arising from ovarian surface epithelial cells, germ cells, and sex cord or stromal cells.

ovarian cyst—fluid-filled, non-neoplastic lesion within the ovary; classified as a functional cyst if it arises from some variation of the ovulatory process. Ovarian cysts may be single or multiple and involve one or both ovaries.

overflow incontinence—involuntary urination associated with urinary retention and bladder distention, in which bladder pressure overcomes the resistance of the external urinary sphincter.

ovulation—release of an ovum from the ovary.

oxidative phosphorylation—final common pathway of aerobic energy metabolism in which adenosine triphosphate formation is coupled with the transfer of electrons along coenzymes in the inner mitochondrial membrane; electron transport chain.

oxidative stress—particular form of cellular toxicity, related to oxidative phosphorylation, in which random errors in oxidation result in the formation of reactive oxygen species instead of water molecules.

oxygen debt—extra oxygen used in the oxidative energy processes after a period of strenuous exercise to reconvert lactic acid to glucose and reconvert decomposed adenosine triphosphate and creatine phosphate to their original states.

oxyhemoglobin dissociation curve—graphical representation (a sigmoid curve) of the relationship between the partial pressure of oxygen in arterial blood and the resulting saturation of hemoglobin with oxygen.

oxytocin—hypothalamic hormone stored in and released from the posterior pituitary in response to neural stimuli; its primary function is the stimulation of ejection of milk from the lactating mammary gland; it also stimulates rhythmic contraction of uterine smooth muscle.

pacemaker—excitable cell (cardiac, smooth muscle, or neuron) that is capable of self-generating an action potential. The term also refers to artificial pacemakers that may generate electrical impulses for stimulation of muscle contraction or neurotransmission.

pacemaker cell—excitable cell having an unstable resting membrane potential that renders it capable of initiating an action potential without external stimulation.

Paget's disease of bone—localized bone disorder characterized by lesions in the long bones and disturbance of the growth of new bone tissue with the result that the bones often thicken, become soft, and coarsen in texture; pathologic condition in which osteoclastic activity occurs in excess of bone formation.

palliation—relief of symptoms.

palpitations—perceptible "pounding" of the heart due to increased contractile force.

pancreatic cancer—carcinoma arising most commonly in the ductal epithelial cells of the exocrine pancreas. Carcinomas of the acinar cells of the exocrine pancreas and of the islet cells of the endocrine pancreas are rare.

pancreatic polypeptide hormone—hormone produced by the pancreatic polypeptide cells of the islets of Langerhans in the pancreas in response to hypoglycemia and to food ingestion; inhibits uptake of enzyme precursors by acinar cells.

pancreatitis—acute or chronic inflammation of the pancreas.

panhypopituitarism—complete hypopituitarism, affecting all trophic hormones and their target endocrine organs.

papilledema—edema of the optic disc of the retina.

paracrine—form of signaling that occurs when signaling molecules (neurotransmitters, cytokines, lipid mediators, and gases) bind to target cells located near the releasing cell.

paralysis—loss or impairment of motor function in a part due to a lesion of the neural or muscular mechanism.

paralytic ileus—transient form of functional bowel obstruction seen following general anesthesia.

paraphimosis—retraction of phimotic foreskin, causing swelling of the glans.

paraplegia—paralysis of both legs.

parasomnia—dysfunctional behavior associated with sleep (e.g., sleepwalking, night terrors).

parathyroid hormone (PTH)—polypeptide hormone secreted by the parathyroid glands that influences calcium and phosphorus metabolism and bone formation; regulates serum calcium levels.

parathyroid hormone–related protein—protein whose structure is similar enough to parathyroid hormone to bind to its receptor and mimic most of its actions; secreted by tumor cells as well as by many normal tissues.

paresis—muscle weakness; slight or incomplete paralysis.

paresthesia—abnormal sensation such as burning, itching, "pins and needles."

parity—the condition of a woman with respect to her having given birth to viable offspring.

Parkinson's disease—slowly progressive dyskinetic disorder caused by degeneration of dopaminergic neurons of the substantia nigra of the brain stem that project to the basal ganglia.

parkinsonism—condition in which the symptoms of Parkinson's disease occur secondarily to another disorder; characterized by muscle rigidity, gait disturbances, and a "pill-rolling" tremor of the hands.

paroxysmal supraventricular tachycardia (PSVT)—common form of tachycardia originating above the ventricles, occurring in brief episodes of sudden onset. PSVT often occurs in young, healthy individuals and may be associated with caffeine intake, tobacco use, fatigue, or stress.

passive transport—transport along a natural gradient, not requiring expenditure of energy.

patent ductus arteriosus—congenital heart defect in which the fetal channel between the pulmonary artery and the aorta fails to close; may precipitate congestive heart failure.

pathogenesis—development of disease.

pathologic jaundice—hyperbilirubinemia persisting beyond, or developing after, the neonatal period.

pathologic reflex—motor reflex that appears only with neurologic disease or trauma.

pathology—branch of medicine concerning the essential nature of disease, especially of the changes in body tissues and organs associated with disease.

pathophysiology—study of human physiologic function in disease.

peak expiratory flow rate—highest rate of air flow sustained for at least 10 msec with maximal expiratory effort.

pediculosis—cutaneous inflammation of the scalp, body, or groin secondary to infestation with lice.

pelvic inflammatory disease (PID)—infection of the uterus, fallopian tubes, and adjacent pelvic structures that is not associated with surgery or pregnancy.

pelvic support disorder—condition characterized by abnormal position or instability of pelvic organs due to decreased ligament support or weakness of pelvic outlet muscles.

penetrance—degree to which a genetic defect results in abnormality of the protein structure or function normally governed by the defective gene.

peptic ulcer disease—chronic inflammatory disorder resulting in deep erosion of the mucosa of the stomach or duodenum by acid and pepsin.

perfusion—passage of blood through tissues.

pericarditis—inflammation of the pericardial layers.

perimenopause—period of time just before and after menopause.

periodontal disease—inflammatory disorders of the gingiva, which can lead to tooth loss.

peripartum hemorrhage—excessive blood loss (more than 500 mL for a vaginal delivery) during the late prenatal period, labor, and delivery or during the postpartal period.

peripheral neuropathy—dysfunction of the peripheral nervous system.

peripheral pulse—point of palpable pulsation located at a point outside the heart and neck vessels; the temporal, radial, ulnar, brachial, femoral, popliteal, posterior tibial, and dorsalis pedis pulses.

peripheral vascular disease (PVD)—disorder of the veins, arteries, or lymphatics.

peristalsis—rhythmic contraction of visceral smooth muscle, serving to propel the contents of hollow organs such as the ureter or the bowel.

peritonitis—inflammation of the peritoneal membrane; may be sterile, resulting from noninfectious irritants, or infectious.

periventricular hemorrhage—bleeding around a cerebral ventricle.

periventricular leukomalacia—necrosis of white matter surrounding the ventricles of the brain, often caused by ischemic episodes early in gestation.

pernicious anemia—deficiency of vitamin B_{12} (cobalamin) resulting in impaired erythropoiesis and oxygen transport as well as in demyelination of peripheral nerves.

persistent pulmonary hypertension of the newborn—sustained elevation of pulmonary artery pressure; probably due to local imbalance in vasodilator and vasoconstrictor substances; contributing factors are meconium aspiration, surfactant deficiency, lung hypoplasia, and neonatal pneumonia.

persistent truncus arteriosus—uncommon congenital heart defect in which the embryologic common vessel fails to separate at its origin into the pulmonary artery and aorta.

petechiae—minute, pinpoint, nonraised, round, purplish red spots caused by intradermal or submucosal hemorrhage, which later turn blue or yellow.

Peyronie's disease—idiopathic disorder of the penis in which fibrous plaques develop on the dorsal surface of the shaft, resulting in a painful curvature of the penis when erect.

pH—expression of the degree of acidity or alkalinity of body fluids; the inverse of the hydrogen ion concentration.

phagocytosis—nonselective process by which certain white blood cells engulf and digest bacterial products and cellular debris; a form of endocytosis.

phantom pain—pain felt in a limb or organ that has been amputated or paralyzed.

pharyngitis—inflammation of the pharynx. Acute pharyngitis is due to viral or bacterial infection, while chronic pharyngitis is the result of continuous reinfection or chronic irritation of pharyngeal structures.

phenotype—outward, visible expression of the karyotype.

phenylketonuria—congenital error of metabolism in which the amino acid phenylalanine accumulates in the blood due to inadequate conversion of phenylalanine to tyrosine.

pheochromocytoma—catecholamine-secreting tumor originating in chromaffin cells. These cells are found primarily in the adrenal medulla and sympathetic ganglia. The condition is relatively rare and can be cured if diagnosed before there has been irreparable damage to the cardiovascular system; the primary symptom is hypertension.

phimosis—constriction of the orifice of the prepuce so that it cannot be drawn back over the glans.

phosphate (PO_4)—anion of variable valence, which is primarily intracellular and is found in large amounts in bones and teeth. Phosphate is an important component in buffer systems and in energy metabolism, with the high energy bonds of adenosine triphosphate serving as the primary energy currency of the cell.

photodermatitis—abnormal state of the skin due to either a photoallergic reaction (delayed hypersensitivity reaction to ultraviolet light) or a phototoxic reaction (irritant-induced inflammation).

photosensitivity—light-induced sensitivity of the skin.

physiologic jaundice—yellow tinge to the skin and sclerae, common in newborns due to lysis of fetal red blood cells and hepatic immaturity.

physiologic reflex—reflex that forms the basis of normal activity.

pickwickian syndrome—respiratory failure resulting from increased ventilatory work imposed by thoracic body fat in extremely obese individuals; can lead to secondary polycythemia and cor pulmonale.

piloerection—contraction of piloerector muscles at the base of hair follicles, creating "goose bumps," which decrease the surface area for radiant heat loss.

pinocytosis—nonselective process in which a small amount of extracellular fluid containing dissolved particles is surrounded by an invaginated portion of the cell membrane and taken into the cell; a form of endocytosis.

pituitary dwarfism—abnormally small stature due to deficiency of growth hormone or somatomedins.

pituitary giantism—height and weight greater than three standard deviations above the mean for age and sex; caused by a growth hormone-producing pituitary adenoma in which growth excess is present before closure of the epiphyseal plates.

pKa—dissociation constant for a buffer system; the pH at which 50% of the buffer's components are in acid form and 50% are in base form.

placenta accreta—placental complication in which the

chorionic villi penetrate beyond the endometrium into the myometrium; placental detachment is impaired and hemorrhage is likely.

placenta previa—low implantation of the placenta so that it partially or completely covers the cervical os; may result in the developing fetus obstructing its own placental blood supply and in peripartum hemorrhage.

placental insufficiency—inadequate placental function; may lead to deficient development of the fetus; has been implicated in the etiology of preeclampsia.

plasma colloid osmotic pressure (COP)—osmotic (oncotic) pressure attracting water to serum proteins, particularly albumin, favoring inward movement of tissue fluid into capillaries and promoting retention of fluid in the vascular space. The colloid osmotic pressure in capillary blood is normally about 28 mm Hg.

plasmin—active principle of the fibrinolytic system; a proteolytic enzyme with a high specificity for fibrin and the ability to dissolve fibrin clots.

plasminogen—inactive precursor of plasmin.

plateau—period during early repolarization when membrane potential is stable owing to offsetting calcium and potassium currents; present in cardiac tissue and in some types of smooth muscle.

platelet—disk-shaped, non-nucleated blood element with a very fragile membrane; formed in the red bone marrow by fragmentation of megakaryocytes.

platelet-activating factor (PAF)—lipid mediator of platelet aggregation.

pleural effusion—accumulation of fluid in the pleural space.

pleurisy—inflammation of the pleura; pleuritis.

pneumonia—inflammation of the respiratory unit tissues; may be either community-acquired or nosocomial.

pneumothorax—presence of air in the intrapleural space, leading to collapse of the lung due to loss of negative intrapleural pressure.

point mutation—base substitution at a single locus.

poliomyelitis—acute contagious viral disease that attacks the central nervous system, injuring or destroying the nerve cells that control the muscles and sometimes causing paralysis.

polycystic kidney disease—inherited disorder characterized by the development of multiple, bilateral, fluid-filled cysts throughout the kidneys as well as extrarenal manifestations.

polycystic ovary syndrome—metabolic disorder characterized by multiple ovarian cysts, insulin resistance, hyperandrogenism, and chronic anovulation in women without specific disease of the adrenal or pituitary glands.

polycythemia vera—myeloproliferative disorder of unknown etiology in which there is bone marrow hyperplasia and production of increased numbers of erythrocytes, leukocytes, and platelets.

polydipsia—increased thirst and compensatory water intake.

polyhydramnios—excessive amniotic fluid.

polymyositis—chronic, progressive inflammatory disease of skeletal muscle occurring in both children and adults; a type of inflammatory myopathy.

polyneuropathy—disorder of more than one category of peripheral nerve.

polyp—growth or mass protruding from a mucous membrane; usually an overgrowth of normal tissue.

porphyria—inherited enzyme disorder that affects the synthesis of heme and results in the accumulation of porphyrins. This accumulation may affect the skin, the nervous system, or both.

portal hypertension—abnormally increased pressure in the portal venous circulation due to narrowing of the capillary branches of the portal vessels; can be caused by inflammation or scarring of the liver; leads to impairment of the liver's ability to detoxify wastes and transport nutrients.

positive feedback loop—response system that amplifies forces perturbing a system, moving the system away from the steady state.

positive nitrogen balance—state in which more protein is taken into the body than is utilized or lost.

postabsorptive state—period in which no nutritional absorption is occurring; typically 4 hours or more after ingestion.

posthitis—inflammation of the prepuce or foreskin of the penis.

postmaturity—delivery of an infant after 42 weeks of gestation.

postnecrotic cirrhosis—disruption of hepatic architecture occurring as a complication of hepatitis, most often chronic hepatitis B virus or hepatitis C virus infection, but also seen occasionally with exposure to hepatotoxic drugs or chemicals.

postphlebitic syndrome—syndrome of chronic deep venous insufficiency after deep vein thrombosis; characterized by chronic pain, cellulitis, and stasis ulceration.

post-transcriptional processing—modification of the mRNA transcript before its diffusion from the nucleus.

post-translational processing—modification of a newly-transcribed peptide chain into its ultimate protein conformation.

potassium (K^+)—most abundant intracellular cation, important in action potential formation and acid-base homeostasis.

preeclampsia—most common form of pregnancy-induced hypertension; defined by the American College of Obstetricians and Gynecologists as elevation in blood pressure of more than 30 mm Hg (systolic) or 15 mm Hg (diastolic); blood pressure greater than 140/90 mm Hg after 20 weeks' gestation; proteinuria of more than 300 mg/24 hr; and clinically evident edema, especially of the face and hands.

preembryonic period—first 2 weeks of gestation.

pregnancy-induced hypertension—high blood pressure in pregnant women; most common form is preeclampsia.

preload—amount of stretch or tension of the ventricular myocardium just before contraction, determined primarily by fluid volume.

premature atrial contraction (PAC)—extrasystole of atrial origin.

premature junctional contraction (PJC)—extrasystole of atrioventricular junctional origin.

premature rupture of the membranes—unexpected rupture of the amnion before the onset of labor; constitutes a high risk of ascending infection and accounts for one third of cases of preterm labor.

premature ventricular contraction (PVC)—extrasystole of ventricular origin.

prematurity—delivery of a viable infant before the 37th week of gestation.

premenstrual syndrome (PMS)—predictable occurrence of distressing physical and psychological manifestations during the luteal phase of the menstrual cycle.

presbycusis—progressive, bilaterally symmetrical sensorineural hearing loss occurring with age; due to degenerative changes in the hair cells of the inner ear.

presbyopia—thickening and loss of elasticity of the lens with age.
pressure gradient—osmotic or hydrostatic force that governs the movement of fluid across biologic membranes.
preterm labor—labor occurring before 37 completed weeks of gestation; characterized by regular uterine contractions with progressive cervical dilation and effacement.
prevalence—number of cases of a specific disease in existence in a given population at a certain time.
prevention (of disease)—actions taken to avert the occurrence of disease.
priapism—prolonged, often painful erection in the absence of sexual stimulation; results from sludging of blood or arteriovenous shunting within the corpus cavernosum, leading to inefficient or obstructed venous outflow from the penis.
primary aging—process of physiologic aging attributable only to advancing age.
primary aldosteronism—adrenocortical hyperfunction disorder manifested primarily by mineralocorticoid excess.
primary biliary cirrhosis—disease characterized by the destruction of small intrahepatic bile ducts by an immune-mediated inflammatory reaction.
primary hypoalphalipoproteinemia—genetic disorder manifested by a deficiency of apoprotein A-I needed for the synthesis of high-density lipoproteins.
primary pulmonary hypertension—sustained elevation of pulmonary artery pressure in the absence of a specific cause such as congestive heart failure, congenital heart disease, or chronic respiratory disease.
primary sclerosing cholangitis—chronic cholestatic liver disease characterized by inflammation and fibrosis of both intrahepatic and extrahepatic bile ducts.
primary skin lesion—lesion arising from previously normal skin.
primitive reflex—motor reflex that is normally present during infancy but is suppressed later in life.
principle of electroneutrality—requirement that total anions equal total cations within the body.
procoagulant—substance favoring blood clotting.
progesterone—steroid sex hormone that is the principal progestational hormone; plays a major part in the menstrual cycle.
prognosis—probable course and outcome of a disease.
prolactin—polypeptide hormone secreted by the anterior pituitary gland that promotes growth of breast tissue, stimulates and sustains milk production in postpartum mammals, and affects libido and reproductive function in both males and females by inhibition of gonadotropin-releasing hormone. Prolactin secretion is inhibited by dopamine.
prostate cancer—malignant neoplasm of the prostate gland.
prostate-specific antigen—antigen that is elevated in all patients with prostatic cancer and in some males with inflammation of the prostate gland, as in benign prostatic hyperplasia.
prostatitis—inflammation of the prostate.
protein C—vitamin K–dependent protein, synthesized by the liver, which inactivates clotting factors V and VIII.
protein S—vitamin K–dependent protein that enhances protein C activity.
proteinuria—excretion of protein in the urine.
prothrombin—clotting factor II; serum glycoprotein that is the precursor of thrombin.
proto-oncogene—gene that normally induces cell proliferation and growth and that may be converted to a cancer-causing gene (oncogene) if mutated.
pruritus—itching.
pseudocyst—collection of pancreatic enzymes contained within fibrous walls of granulation tissue formed by the pancreas and other surrounding organs; occurs as a complication of acute pancreatitis.
pseudohyponatremia—artifactually low serum sodium level, resulting from excessive amounts of other solutes such as proteins or lipids, reducing the proportion of water in the serum.
pseudomembranous colitis—severe acute inflammation of the bowel mucosa, with the formation of pseudomembranous plaques.
psoriasis—chronic, recurrent inflammatory disorder of the skin characterized by episodes of excessively rapid turnover of keratinocytes and marked by discrete bright red macules, papules, or patches covered with lamellated silvery scales.
psychoneuroimmunology (PNI)—recently developed science that aims to clarify the relationships among the immune, nervous, and endocrine systems in regulation of human function.
psychosis—major mental disorder of organic or emotional origin, characterized by derangement of the personality and loss of contact with reality.
pulmonary edema—accumulation of fluid in the interstitial spaces of the lung.
pulmonary embolism—occlusion of one or more pulmonary arterial vessels by a bolus of material (usually a blood clot) arising from a source outside the lung.
pulmonary fibrosis—formation of fibrous tissue within the interstitium of the lungs.
pulmonary infarction—localized necrosis of lung tissue, due to obstruction of the arterial blood supply; occurs in about 10% of patients with massive pulmonary embolism.
pulmonary vascular resistance (PVR)—pressure within the pulmonary arterial system, constituting the afterload of the right ventricle. PVR is normally 20% of systemic vascular resistance (SVR).
pulmonic stenosis—narrowing or incomplete opening of the pulmonic valve.
pulse pressure—the difference between the systolic and diastolic pressures.
pulseless electrical activity (PEA)—state in which a discernible rhythm is evident on the electrocardiogram but there is no clinical evidence of perfusion.
purpura—hemorrhagic disease characterized by extravasation of blood into the tissues, under the skin, and through the mucous membranes and producing spontaneous ecchymoses and petechiae on the skin.
pyelonephritis—inflammation of the kidney and renal pelvis.
pyrogen—agent that causes fever.
pyrogenic hyperthermia—elevated body temperature induced by a pyrogen; fever.
pyruvic acid (pyruvate)—end product of aerobic glycolysis.
quadriplegia—paralysis of all extremities.
radiation—transfer of heat by electromagnetic waves from a warm object to cooler ambient air.
radiculopathy—disease of the spinal nerve roots, typically manifesting as shooting pains or paresthesias in the distribution of the affected nerve.
Raynaud's syndrome—condition characterized by excessive vasoconstriction in the fingers or, less commonly, the toes in response to cold, vibration, or stress.

reabsorption—return into the blood of a substance that has previously been secreted or filtered.

reactive airways dysfunction syndrome—development of asthma-like symptoms and airway hyperresponsiveness in a person with no previous respiratory problems after a single exposure to an inhaled toxin.

reactive oxygen species—toxic metabolite of oxygen that can damage cells; formed by random errors during oxidative metabolism, especially during reperfusion of hypoxic tissues; also called oxygen free radical.

reactive thrombocytosis—increase in platelets resulting from increased production of plasma platelet-stimulating factor; may occur in response to anemia, hemorrhage, malignancy, inflammation, or iron deficiency.

receptor—recognition-binding site, usually on a protein or glycoprotein located on the cell membrane, on an organelle membrane, or on an intracellular protein. Receptors bind specific ligands, with such binding serving as a regulatory signal. Cellular processes may then be altered or initiated by one of a number of signal transduction mechanisms.

receptor-mediated endocytosis—selective form of endocytosis in which binding of a ligand to a specific cell surface receptor results in both ligand and receptor being engulfed by the cell membrane and taken into the cell.

receptor tyrosine kinase (RTK)—receptor that has ligand-binding sites on the extracellular side of the plasma membrane as well as an intracellular component that is a kinase (phosphorylating) enzyme

recombinant DNA—technology whereby replacement of genes in cellular vehicles such as *Escherichia coli* results in production of a specific protein that is structurally and functionally identical to a natural human protein (e.g., insulin, erythropoietin, clotting factor VIII).

red cell indices—quantitative description of a typical red blood cell based on calculations made from measured hematology components including hematocrit, hemoglobin concentration, and erythrocyte count. The indices include mean corpuscular volume (MCV), mean corpuscular hemoglobin (MCH), and mean corpuscular hemoglobin concentration (MCHC) and are useful in classification of anemias.

reentry—most common mechanism of dysrhythmia, in which an abnormal short circuit develops within the cardiac conduction system. Because the complete system does not have to repolarize, very rapid generation of current wavefronts is permitted.

referred pain—pain originating in deep organs that is inaccurately perceived as originating from certain areas of the skin surface.

reflex arc—simplest neural pathway resulting in motor activity; consists of a sensory receptor, its sensory nerve, a synapse between the sensory nerve and an α-motoneuron, a motor nerve, and the neuromuscular junction between the motor nerve and a muscle fiber.

reflex incontinence—involuntary urination due to lack of normal inhibition of the micturition reflex.

refractory period—time following depolarization when an excitable cell is resistant to further stimulation.

regeneration—healing of injured tissue by replacement with cells identical in structure and function to the originals, occurring under optimal conditions in tissues capable of mitosis.

relative refractory period—time during repolarization when an excitable cell will depolarize only in response to a stronger-than-normal stimulus.

remission—temporary cessation of manifestations of a disease.

renal adenocarcinoma—most common type of renal cancer.

renal insufficiency—mild azotemia and possibly polyuria and nocturia due to impaired tubular transport and concentration of urine.

renal osteodystrophy—condition due to chronic kidney disease, marked by impaired kidney function, impaired vitamin D metabolism, elevated serum phosphorus levels, low or normal serum calcium levels, and stimulation of parathyroid function, resulting in various bone diseases, including osteitis fibrosa cystica, osteomalacia, osteoporosis, and osteosclerosis.

renal tubular acidosis (RTA)—variety of metabolic acidosis in which failure of renal reclamation or regeneration of bicarbonate results in proportional retention of chloride.

renin—hormone released from renal cells into the blood where it enzymatically converts the protein angiotensinogen to angiotensin I.

renin-angiotensin-aldosterone system (RAAS)—complex regulatory system governing fluid volume, electrolyte balance, and arterial blood pressure. Decreased renal blood flow, decreased serum sodium (or chloride), or increased sympathetic stimulation initiate renal release of renin, which triggers a cascade of enzymatic actions culminating in activation of the vasoconstrictor angiotensin II and release of the mineralocorticoid aldosterone from the adrenal cortex.

repair—healing of injured tissue by replacement with nonfunctional fibrous tissue.

repolarization—reestablishment of resting membrane potential after its discharge.

resolution—wound healing by recovery of cells sustaining nonlethal injury.

respiration—exchange of oxygen and carbon dioxide between the environment and the human system.

respiratory acidosis—acidic pH resulting from hypoventilation and subsequent retention of carbon dioxide in the extracellular fluid.

respiratory alkalosis—alkaline pH resulting from reduced carbon dioxide in the extracellular fluid, secondary to hyperventilation.

respiratory center—group of pacemaker neurons in the medulla oblongata of the brain stem in which the neural stimulus for ventilation originates, consisting of a dorsal inspiratory group and a ventral expiratory group.

respiratory failure—inability of the pulmonary system to maintain adequate oxygenation of the blood, manifested clinically as hypoxemia, and, if ventilation is impaired, hypercapnia.

respiratory quotient (RQ)—ratio of the volume of expired carbon dioxide to the volume of oxygen consumed in metabolism of a specific type of nutrient.

respiratory syncytial virus—virus isolated from children with bronchopneumonia and bronchitis, characteristically causing syncytium formation in tissue culture; the major cause of lower respiratory tract infections in infants and children younger than 3 years of age.

resting membrane potential—phase 4 of the action potential; inactive state in which voltage-gated sodium and calcium channels are closed. Gradients exist for inward flux of sodium and calcium and outward flux of potassium.

restrictive cardiomyopathy—rare condition associated with tropical infection in which the myocardium becomes very fibrous and noncompliant, although not hypertrophied. Congestive heart failure occurs due to decreased preload and decreased contractility.

reticulocyte—newly released red blood cell that still contains some RNA.

retinal detachment—noninflammatory disease of the retina; a form of retinopathy in which visual loss occurs secondary to separation of the neural and pigmented layers of the retina.

retinitis—inflammation of the retina.

retinopathy—noninflammatory visual deficit resulting from primary or secondary retinal disease.

retinopathy of prematurity (ROP)—overgrowth and tangling of retinal blood vessels of premature infants in response to prolonged exposure of retinal tissues to high oxygen concentrations, potentially causing retinal detachment and blindness; formerly known as retrolental fibroplasia.

retraction ring—complication of prolonged labor marked by failure of relaxation of the circular fibers at the internal opening of the cervix, obstructing delivery of the infant.

Rh incompatibility—condition in which the erythrocytes of an Rh+ fetus are lysed by anti-Rh antibodies forming in the blood of the Rh− mother. The Rh factor is one of many cell surface antigens on erythrocytes and is present in 85% of whites and 99% to 100% of nonwhite races.

rhabdomyolysis—syndrome resulting from the release of large quantities of muscle cell contents into the plasma in response to skeletal muscle injury.

rhabdomyosarcoma—malignant neoplasm arising from embryonic mesenchymal cells that differentiate into skeletal muscle; the most common muscle tumor.

rheumatoid arthritis (RA)—chronic systemic disorder in which connective tissues throughout the body (principally the joints) are damaged, probably by an autoimmune mechanism.

rheumatoid factor—serum antibodies directed against antigenic determinants on IgG, IgM, or IgA molecules; occurs in connective tissue diseases and infectious diseases.

rhonchus—continuous dry rattling sound in larger airways due to a partial obstruction, heard on auscultation.

rhythmicity—intrinsic, regular frequency of action potentials in an excitable cell.

ribonucleic acid (RNA)—single-stranded nucleic acid that functions in the transcription of the genetic code from deoxyribonucleic acid and translation of the code into protein.

rickets—bone disorder characterized by deficient mineralization of the bone matrix due to deficiency or abnormal metabolism of vitamin D; in children, results from abnormal growth of cartilage and bone.

rigor mortis—death-induced muscle stiffness due to cross-bridge persistence secondary to lack of adenosine triphosphate. The condition lasts for several hours after death, until contractile proteins degenerate.

risk factor—antecedent factor that is associated with subsequent development of disease but whose causative role may or may not be established.

rubella—communicable systemic viral infection characterized by fever and a rash; also called German measles.

rubeola—highly contagious systemic viral infection characterized by upper respiratory, ophthalmic, and integumentary manifestations; also called measles.

saltatory conduction—the leaping of current from one node of Ranvier to another along a myelinated nerve.

sarcoidosis—systemic disorder of unknown cause, characterized by noncaseating granulomatous lesions of multiple tissues, particularly the lungs and thoracic lymph nodes.

sarcolemma—elastic sheath covering every striated muscle fiber.

sarcoma—term applied to many malignant neoplasms of connective tissue origin.

sarcomere—functional unit of muscle.

scabies—communicable inflammatory disorder of the skin caused by mites.

scalded skin syndrome—infectious disease of infants and children occurring after infection with certain strains of *Staphylococcus aureus;* characterized by manifestations ranging from a localized bullous eruption to widespread development of easily ruptured fine vesicles and bullae resulting in exfoliation of large sheets of skin, leaving raw, denuded areas.

scarlet fever—acute contagious childhood disease caused by group A β-hemolytic streptococci; can be a complication of impetigo bullosa.

schizophrenia—psychosis characterized by dissociation or disruption of thought processes and a split among thought, emotion, and behavior; the most severe of mental illnesses.

sciatica—radiating pain down the buttock and leg along the course of the sciatic nerve.

scleroderma—connective tissue disorder characterized by fibrosis and degenerative changes in multiple organs, primarily in the skin, but also in the gastrointestinal tract, kidneys, heart, muscles, and lungs.

scoliosis—lateral sigmoid spinal curvature greater than 10 degrees; classified as nonstructural if there is no anatomic abnormality and structural if there are associated abnormalities of vertebral joints, bones, muscles, or ligaments.

seasonal affective disorder (SAD)—depressive illness that has been linked to lack of light exposure; may or may not be associated with melatonin imbalance.

seborrheic dermatitis—noninfectious, scaling inflammation of the skin appearing in areas of increased sebaceous gland activity.

second-degree atrioventricular block—conduction disturbance in which some, but not all, atrial impulses are blocked from transmission to the ventricles.

secondary active transport—transport in which a gradient created by active transport of one particle drives the passive transport of a second particle.

secondary aging—physiologic changes in the elderly due to diseases that may or may not accompany aging.

secondary skin lesion—lesion arising as a consequence of rupture, mechanical irritation, extension, invasion, normal healing, or abnormal healing of a primary lesion.

seizure—paroxysmal episode of spontaneous, uncontrolled neurotransmission evidenced on the electroencephalogram as well as by changes in motor, sensory, or behavioral activity.

selectin—one of the four major categories of adhesion molecules.

sensorineural hearing loss—hearing loss due to inner ear or neural pathway disorders.

sepsis—inflammatory response to systemic infection.

septic shock—subset of severe sepsis; sepsis-induced hypotension, persisting despite adequate fluid resuscitation, along with the presence of hypoperfusion abnormalities or organ dysfunction.

sex chromosome—chromosome responsible for determination of the sex of the individual, constituting an unequal pair—the female X and the male Y.

sex-linked—referring to an inherited disorder in which the defective trait is located on the X or Y chromosome. The X chromosome is the site of the defect in all significant sex-linked disorders.

sexually transmitted diseases—infections communicated primarily through sexual contact; in the United States the most prevalent are syphilis, gonorrhea, chlamydia, genital herpes, genital warts, trichomoniasis, and the acquired immunodeficiency syndrome.

Sheehan's syndrome—pituitary necrosis that follows postpartum hemorrhage and hypovolemia; a cause of hypopituitarism.

shivering thermogenesis—production of heat as a byproduct of rapid, fine muscle movements that are reflexly initiated by the hypothalamus.

shock—state of severe, generalized deficit in tissue perfusion.

sick sinus syndrome—abnormality of sinoatrial node automaticity resulting in inadequate cerebral blood flow and syncope (Stokes-Adams attacks).

sickle cell disease—autosomal recessive disorder resulting in formation of abnormal hemoglobin (Hb S), which causes erythrocytes to assume a crescent shape under certain conditions.

sign (of disease)—objective evidence of disease.

simple diffusion—movement of particles or fluid along natural gradients.

single gene mutation—abnormality of DNA limited to one gene locus (e.g., a point mutation or a frame shift).

sinus arrest—failure of the sinoatrial node to self-generate the cardiac impulse for one or more beats.

sinus arrhythmia—normal variant of normal sinus rhythm in which the heart rate and PQRST characteristics are normal but the rhythm is regularly irregular in synchrony with pulmonary ventilation.

sinus bradycardia—slow rhythm (less than 60 beats per minute) originating from the sinoatrial node.

sinus exit block—conduction disturbance in which the sinoatrial nodal impulse is prevented from leaving the sinoatrial node to excite atrial tissues.

sinus pause—failure of the sinoatrial node to generate the cardiac impulse for one beat.

sinus tachycardia—regular rhythm originating from the sinoatrial node with a rate between 100 and 180 beats per minute.

sinusitis—inflammation of one or more of the paranasal sinuses.

Sjögren's syndrome—immune-mediated triad of keratoconjunctivitis sicca, xerostomia, and the presence of a connective tissue disease, usually rheumatoid arthritis but sometimes systemic lupus erythematosus, scleroderma, or polymyositis; manifested by dry eyes and mouth.

sliding filament theory—best-accepted model of the molecular mechanism of muscle contraction, which proposes cross-bridge formation between actin and myosin. A conformational change in the myosin head then slides actin toward the center of the myosin molecule, shortening the sarcomere.

sodium (Na^+)—major cation in the extracellular fluid, constituting 90% to 95% of all cations and of primary importance in determining osmolality of the extracellular fluid.

solvent drag—movement of particles in association with movement of the fluid in which they are dissolved or suspended.

somatostatin—peptide hormone and neurotransmitter that inhibits the release of peptide hormones in many tissues; released by the hypothalamus to inhibit the release of growth hormone and thyroid-stimulating hormone from the anterior pituitary; also released by the delta cells of the islets of Langerhans in the pancreas to inhibit the release of glucagon and insulin; also called growth hormone release–inhibiting hormone.

spasticity—continuous involuntary, intense, and often painful resistance to muscle stretching due to abnormally increased tension associated with inappropriate neural stimulation.

specific gravity—the weight of a liquid compared with the weight of an equal amount of water, measured by means of a hydrometer.

spermatogenesis—development of mature spermatozoa from spermatogonia.

spina bifida cystica—incomplete fusion of one or more of the vertebrae, resulting in an external protrusion of the spinal tissue.

spina bifida occulta—incomplete fusion of one or more of the vertebrae, signaled only by an overlying dimple or tuft of hair.

spinal cord injury—traumatic complete or partial transection of the spinal cord.

spinal shock—distributive shock representing a functional disruption of neurotransmission in structurally intact reflex arcs below the level of spinal cord injury related to a lack of descending inputs from higher centers.

spinal stenosis—narrowing of the vertebral canal, nerve root canals, or intervertebral foramina of the lumbar spine, caused by encroachment of bone on the space; symptoms include low-back pain.

splenomegaly—enlargement of the spleen.

spontaneous abortion—unintended termination of pregnancy before fetal viability (usually 20 weeks' gestation or fetal weight less than 500 g); also called miscarriage.

spontaneous bacterial peritonitis—inflammation of the peritoneum in which there is no obvious intra-abdominal source of infection; bacteremia is probably the route of infection; commonly occurs in patients with ascites.

sprain—traumatic injury of one or more ligaments within a joint.

squamous cell carcinoma—malignant growth arising from squamous epithelium and having cuboid cells.

stasis ulcer—localized, deep area of tissue destruction overlying deep vein thrombosis and secondary to chronic edema and impaired perfusion.

static exercise—isometric contraction; the resisting force is greater than the force generated in the muscle fiber, and fiber shortening does not occur.

status asthmaticus—state of severe, sustained asthmatic attack that is not responsive to first-line treatment.

status epilepticus—medical emergency in which seizure activity is continuous for a prolonged period, potentially proving fatal due to cardiac failure or stroke induced by the resulting hypermetabolic state.

steatorrhea—fatty stools due to a malabsorption syndrome.

strain—localized injury of muscle or tendon fibers ranging from excessive stretch to tearing or rupture of a muscle.

streptokinase—enzyme produced by streptococci that catalyzes the conversion of plasminogen to plasmin; used therapeutically as a thrombolytic agent.

stress—nonspecific response of the body to any demand (Selye).
stress incontinence—involuntary urination induced by increased bladder pressure due to an external force.
stress ulcer—erosion of the gastric or duodenal mucosa resulting from stress-induced lack of perfusion and disruption of the protective mucus barrier.
stressor—force perturbing a system.
striae gravidarum—stretch marks in the skin of the enlarging breasts and abdomen, typically appearing at 6 to 7 months' gestation; caused by hormonally mediated changes in the skin structure and mechanical stretching by growth of underlying tissues.
stroke—persistent focal neurologic deficit of acute onset that is not associated with head trauma; cerebrovascular accident (CVA).
stroke volume (SV)—volume of blood ejected by the left ventricle during each systole.
subarachnoid hemorrhage (SAH)—bleeding into the subarachnoid space.
subdural hematoma—collection of clotted blood between the dura mater and the arachnoid.
subinvolution—failure of the uterus to decrease in size postpartum; characterized by persistent lochia.
subluxation—partial separation of the articulating surfaces of the bones; congenital or acquired.
sudden cardiac death (SCD)—death from cardiac cause (usually ventricular fibrillation but occasionally asystole, bradycardia, or heart block) that occurs within seconds to hours after the onset of symptoms.
sudden infant death syndrome (SIDS)—sudden death of an infant younger than 1 year of age that remains unexplained after a thorough case investigation, including performance of a complete autopsy, examination of the death scene, and review of the clinical history.
summation—mechanism by which rapid, sequential electrical impulses produce a sustained maximal increase in muscle tension (tetanus); spatial or temporal addition of ion currents across the membrane of an excitable cell.
superantigen—antigen that binds to T-cell regions other than those associated with a specific epitope.
supernormal period—period late in depolarization when a weaker-than-normal stimulus may trigger an action potential.
supraventricular tachycardia—rapid rhythm (150 to 250 beats per minute) originating from one or more atrial locations or from within the atrioventricular junction.
surfactant—lipoprotein produced by type II alveolar cells that separates the molecules of alveolar fluid, opposing surface tension.
symptom—indication of disease that is perceived by the patient
syncope—sudden loss of consciousness; fainting.
syndrome of inappropriate ADH secretion (SIADH)—syndrome in which the secretion of antidiuretic hormone is not inhibited by the hypo-osmolality of extracellular fluid, producing water retention and hyponatremia.
syndrome X—constellation of clinical manifestations of insulin resistance occurring concurrently in the same person, such as coronary heart disease, essential hypertension, hyperuricemia, and others.
synovitis—inflammation of the synovial membrane of a joint; may be caused by rheumatic fever, rheumatoid arthritis, gout, and others.
syphilis—contagious, usually sexually transmitted disease that leads to many structural and cutaneous lesions and is caused by a spirochete; can be treated with antibiotics. Congenital syphilis is a variety acquired from the mother by a fetus in utero.
syringomyelia—slowly progressive syndrome in which cavitation occurs in the central segments of the spinal cord; it may be of developmental origin, arise secondary to tumor, trauma, infarction, or hemorrhage, or be without known cause. It results in neurologic deficits consisting of muscular weakness and atrophy.
system—whole composed of interrelated, interacting parts.
systemic inflammatory response syndrome—most severe manifestation of inflammation, usually triggered by systemic infection. The syndrome is manifested as hypermetabolism and shock and often results in multiple organ failure.
systemic lupus erythematosus—chronic, multisystem, inflammatory disorder characterized by arthritis, dermatitis, and other systemic manifestations and by the presence in the blood of autoantibodies directed at one or more components of cell nuclei; generally considered a connective tissue disorder but may also be classified as an autoimmune disorder, a collagen vascular disorder, or a rheumatic disease.
systemic vascular resistance (SVR)—total resistance in the systemic circulation, ranging from 770 to 1500 dynes per second per cm^{-5}. SVR may be calculated from measurement of the cardiac output and mean arterial and central venous pressures, since CO = (MAP − CVP)/SVR.
systems theory—approach to unification of science; set of concepts that explain the interrelatedness of wholes.
systole—period of cardiac contraction during which blood is ejected into the aorta and pulmonary artery.
t-tubule—penetrating extension of the cell membrane (sarcolemma) that permits entry of extracellular calcium into cardiac and skeletal muscle cells.
tachycardia—heart rate greater than 100 beats per minute.
tachypnea—rapid breathing.
telomerase—enzyme that protects replicating germ cells and some cancer cells from the chromosomal shortening, which is a hallmark of cellular aging in body cells.
telomere—DNA sequence found at the end of a chromosome.
tendinitis—inflammation of tendons and of tendon-muscle attachments.
tension pneumothorax—condition in which the affected lung collapses and mediastinal structures shift due to rising positive intrapleural pressure resulting from a one-way valve created by chest wall injury. Atmospheric air enters during inspiration but cannot be expelled during exhalation.
teratogen—substance capable of inducing a defect in a developing embryo.
testicular cancer—malignant neoplasm of testicular tissue or germ cells.
testicular torsion—acute ischemic injury of the testis due to its rotation around the vascular pedicle of the spermatic cord.
testosterone—principal male sex hormone.
tetanus—continuous, maximal contractile state of skeletal muscle (tetany); also refers to a rare infectious disease caused by *Clostridium tetani* that is characterized by severe muscle spasm (lockjaw).
tetany—continuous, maximal contractile state of skeletal muscle.
tetralogy of Fallot—cyanotic heart defect characterized by

four abnormalities: pulmonic stenosis, ventricular septal defect, over-riding aorta, and right ventricular hypertrophy.

thermogenesis—production of heat.

thermoreceptor—specialized nerve ending that senses changes in tissue temperature and initiates afferent signals to the hypothalamic thermostat (preoptic nucleus).

thermoregulation—processes involved in regulation of body temperature (i.e., mechanisms of heat gain, heat conservation, and heat loss).

third spacing—development of excess fluid in the interstitial space (edema) or in a potential fluid space (effusion).

third-degree atrioventricular block—conduction disturbance in which all atrial impulses are prevented from entering the ventricles at the atrioventricular junction; complete heart block.

threshold—membrane voltage at which an excitable cell is committed to a full action potential.

thrombin—enzyme produced from activation of prothrombin; catalyzes the conversion of fibrinogen to fibrin during the clotting cascade.

thrombocyte—platelet.

thrombocytopenia—reduction in the number of circulating platelets to below 100,000/μL of blood, owing to diminished production, altered distribution, or increased destruction of these cells.

thromboembolism—obstruction of a blood vessel with thrombotic emboli carried by the blood.

thrombomodulin—protein expressed by endothelial cells that induces thrombin to activate protein C.

thrombophlebitis—inflammation of a vein associated with thrombus formation.

thrombotic thrombocytopenic purpura—syndrome of target organ dysfunction caused by marked platelet aggregation in the microcirculation.

thrombus—an aggregation of blood factors, primarily platelets and fibrin with entrapment of cellular elements, frequently causing vascular obstruction at the point of its formation.

thyroglobulin—glycoprotein that binds and stores thyroid hormones and their substrates.

thyroid cancer—malignant neoplasm of the thyroid gland. Of the thyroid cancers, papillary carcinomas account for 75% to 85%, follicular carcinomas comprise 10% to 20%, and medullary and anaplastic carcinomas are rare.

thyroid storm—sudden, massive output of thyroid hormones; occurs when the stress of trauma, serious illness, or thyroid manipulation is imposed on untreated hyperthyroidism present as a baseline state.

thyroid-stimulating hormone (TSH)—hormone secreted by the anterior lobe of the pituitary gland that has an affinity for and specifically stimulates the thyroid gland; also called thyrotropin.

thyroiditis—inflammation of the thyroid.

thyrotoxicosis—condition resulting from presentation to the tissues of excessive quantities of the thyroid hormones; may be due to hyperfunction of the thyroid gland or loss of storage function and leakage from the gland, or it may originate outside the thyroid.

thyrotropin-releasing hormone (TRH)—tripeptide hormone that stimulates release of stored thyroid-stimulating hormone (TSH) and induces accelerated synthesis of TSH by pituitary thyrotroph cells; synthesized in the hypothalamus.

thyroxine (T_4)—inactive thyroid hormone formed from coupling of two molecules of di-iodothyronine; serves as a precursor for formation of tri-iodothyronine.

thyroxine-binding globulin—transport protein to which thyroid hormones bind after their release into the blood.

tidal volume (TV or V_T)—volume of gas inspired and expired during a normal, relaxed breath.

tight junction—area in which the membrane proteins of adjacent cells are fused, preventing movement of molecules between the cells.

tinea—fungal infections of superficial skin layers, classified according to their body location.

tinnitus—noise in the ears such as ringing, buzzing, or roaring.

tissue factor pathway inhibitor—coagulation inhibitor that forms a complex with factors Xa, VIIa, and tissue factor in the presence of calcium, suppressing the extrinsic pathway of clotting.

tissue hydrostatic pressure (THP)—pressure exerted by excess fluid in the interstitial space (edema), favoring inward movement of fluid into capillaries.

tissue osmotic pressure (TOP)—slight osmotic (oncotic) pressure exerted by interstitial proteins on capillary fluid, promoting outward fluid movement from capillaries.

tissue plasminogen activator—substance released by vascular endothelial cells in the presence of thrombin and fibrin that activates plasminogen to plasmin during fibrinolysis.

titratable acid—urinary buffer in which weak acids containing ammonium or phosphate are formed when hydrogen ions are secreted into the urine, preventing acute changes in urine pH.

tonsillitis—inflammation and enlargement of a tonsil, especially the palatine tonsils of the throat.

toxic nodular goiter—hyperthyroidism arising in a nodular goiter; parts of the thyroid gland do not respond to normal negative feedback regulation by means of the hypothalamic-pituitary-thyroid axis.

toxin—substance capable of causing functional disturbance or structural damage within the body; a poison.

tracheoesophageal fistula—abnormal tube-like passage between the trachea and the esophagus.

transcellular fluid—fluid other than blood that is exchanged within the body (e.g., saliva, pleural fluid, peritoneal fluid, synovial fluid, intraocular fluid, and cerebrospinal fluid).

transfusion reaction—adverse clinical manifestations resulting from blood transfusion. Many different types of reactions are possible, mediated by immune and nonimmune mechanisms.

transient ischemic attack (TIA)—focal neurologic deficit that simulates the manifestations of stroke but that lasts less than 24 hours. TIAs often precede ischemic stroke.

translocation—form of chromosomal rearrangement; occurs when one chromosome breaks during cell division and part of it becomes attached to another chromosome.

transposition of the great vessels—cyanotic heart defect in which the pulmonary artery arises from the left ventricle and the aorta arises from the right ventricle, creating separate pulmonary and systemic circulations.

transudate—third-spaced fluid not containing protein, associated with hemodynamic, rather than inflammatory, etiologies.

trauma—injury, usually due to external force.

traumatic brain injury (TBI)—physical damage to, or functional impairment of, the cranial contents from acute mechanical energy exchange.

treatment (of disease)—intervention aimed at achievement of optimal outcome of disease.

tremor—repetitive movement resulting from abnormal

electrical stimulation of muscle secondary to stress, disease, or drug effects.

trichomoniasis—sexually transmitted disease caused by *Trichomonas vaginalis*.

trigeminal neuralgia—syndrome of excruciating facial pain due to disease of the fifth cranial nerve; also called tic douloureux.

triggered activity—propagated impulses initiated by afterdepolarizations; a mechanism of cardiac dysrhythmia.

triiodothyronine (T_3)—active thyroid hormone formed from coupling of di-iodothyronine and monoiodothyronine or from peripheral deiodination of thyroxine (T_4).

trisomy—chromosomal defect in which affected cells have three copies of a particular chromosome.

tropical sprue—bacterial infection of the small bowel that affects persons living in or visiting certain tropical countries.

tropomyosin—fibrous regulatory protein that may cover or uncover binding sites on actin in muscle.

troponin—regulatory protein in muscle that binds calcium and induces uncovering of binding sites on actin.

Trousseau's sign—classic indication of impending tetany, in which carpopedal (hand and wrist) spasm is stimulated with inflation of a blood pressure cuff.

Trousseau's syndrome—recurrent thrombophlebitis occurring in association with visceral carcinoma.

tubal ligation—sterilization of the female by constricting the fallopian tubes by means of ligatures.

tuberculosis (TB)—communicable infection of lung tissue (pulmonary tuberculosis) and potentially other tissues (extrapulmonary or miliary tuberculosis) caused by the bacillus *Mycobacterium tuberculosis*.

tumor—mass of abnormal cells; a neoplasm.

tumor-associated antigen—membrane protein marker that allows neoplastic cells to be recognized as abnormal by the immune system. Detection of such markers may be used in diagnosis or in development of immunotherapy against the tumor.

tumor suppressor gene—gene that normally suppresses cellular proliferation and growth.

turgor—condition of being turgid or full.

ulcerative colitis—inflammation of the mucosa and submucosa first involving the rectum and potentially ascending upward through the entire colon.

upper gastrointestinal bleeding—bleeding from the esophagus, stomach, or duodenum.

upper motor neuron disease—any disease of an upper motor neuron (neurons in the cerebral cortex that conduct impulses from the motor cortex to the motor nuclei of the cerebral nerves or to the ventral gray columns of the spinal cord), such as stroke or brain tumor.

uremia—syndrome resulting from imbalance in production of metabolic wastes and the efficacy of renal function in removing those wastes.

uremic acidosis—condition in chronic renal disease in which the ability to excrete acid is decreased.

ureteritis—inflammation of the ureter.

urethritis—inflammation of the urethra.

urge incontinence—involuntary urination associated with an unusually strong sensation of the need to void.

urinalysis—laboratory examination of a urine sample for physical characteristics (color, odor, opacity), specific gravity, pH, protein, glucose, ketone bodies, blood cells, casts, and crystals.

urinary buffer—renal tubular mechanism that permits the acceptance, in the tubular fluid, of large quantities of hydrogen ions with minimal changes in urine pH.

urinary incontinence—involuntary urination.

urinary tract infection—inflammatory conditions of the urethra, bladder, ureter, or kidney due to microorganisms.

urokinase—enzyme found in the urine of humans and other mammals that is secreted by kidney parenchymal cells and converts plasminogen to plasmin during fibrinolysis.

urolithiasis—formation of an obstructive solid mass of precipitates or "stones" in the tubules of the kidney or within the lower urinary tract.

urticaria—vascular reaction of the skin marked by transient appearance of slightly elevated patches that are redder or paler than the surrounding skin and often accompanied by severe itching; also called hives.

uterine fibroid tumor—benign tumor composed of myometrial smooth muscle and fibrous connective tissue; also called leiomyoma uteri.

uveitis—inflammation of part or all of the middle (vascular) tunic of the eye, the uvea.

vaginal candidiasis—infection of the vagina by fungi of the genus *Candida*.

varicella—chickenpox; acute, highly contagious disease caused by the herpesvirus varicella-zoster.

varicocele—scrotal swelling due to dilation of veins in the spermatic cord.

varicose veins—dilated and twisted superficial veins; varicosities.

vascular remodeling—an active process of structural alteration of the vascular wall mediated by angiogenic factors, vasoactive substances, and hemodynamic stimuli and involving changes in cell growth, cell death (apoptosis), cell migration, and alteration of the extracellular matrix.

vasculitis—inflammatory, destructive process affecting arteries, veins, or capillaries.

vasectomy—surgical sterilization of the male by interruption of the vas deferens with clipping, ligation, or cautery, preventing ascent of sperm from the testes.

vasogenic shock—category of shock due to maldistribution of circulating blood volume secondary to loss of vascular tone; also called distributive shock.

vasomotor center—neurons in the medulla oblongata that coordinate autonomic reflexes regulating blood vessel caliber.

vasovagal syncope—loss of consciousness, often induced by extreme emotional stress, secondary to an inappropriate excess of parasympathetic stimulation mediating vasodilation and deficient cerebral blood flow.

vegetative state—state of reduced consciousness in which the individual has sleep-wake cycles but lacks awareness of the environment.

venous stasis—stagnation of venous blood flow.

venous stasis ulcer—ulcer usually associated with secondary varicose veins and caused by abnormally high venous pressure.

ventilation—amount of air moved into and out of the alveoli during respiration.

ventilation–perfusion (V/Q) abnormality—suboptimal ratio of air delivery and capillary blood flow to the alveolus, impairing gas exchange.

ventricular fibrillation (VF)—dysrhythmia in which current flow within the ventricles is chaotic, resulting in mere quivering rather than effective contraction; most common dysrhythmia underlying sudden cardiac death.

ventricular flutter—very rapid rhythm (200 to 400 beats per minute) originating in the ventricles. Ventricular flutter often degenerates into ventricular fibrillation, a form of sudden cardiac death.

ventricular septal defect (VSD)—acyanotic congenital heart defect manifested by a hole in the interventricular septum.

ventricular tachycardia (VT)—rapid rhythm (100 to 200 beats per minute) originating from the ventricles.

verruca—wart; benign hyperplastic lesion of the skin or mucous membrane caused by the human papillomavirus.

vertigo—sensation of rotation or movement of one's self or of one's surroundings in any plane.

vesicle—a small sac that contains secretion such as protein hormones and mucus that is transported along cytoskeletal tracks to the plasma membrane.

viral hepatitis—inflammation of the liver with necrosis of liver cells, due to infection with one or more hepatitis viruses; classified as hepatitis A, B, C, D, or E.

vitamin D—steroid hormone that regulates calcium and phosphate metabolism in bone formation and growth.

voltage-gated channel—membrane channel that opens or closes as a consequence of a conformational change in the membrane protein induced by a change in membrane potential.

von Hippel-Lindau disease—autosomal dominant hereditary disorder characterized by angiomatosis of the retina and cerebellum, as well as by cystic lesions of the spinal cord and viscera. Neurologic symptoms and mental retardation may also be present. von Hippel-Lindau disease is associated with increased risk of renal cancer.

von Willebrand factor—subendothelial adhesive protein essential to platelet adhesion and platelet plug formation.

von Willebrand's disease—family of bleeding disorders caused by an abnormality of von Willebrand factor.

vulvovaginitis—inflammation of the vulva and vaginal tissues.

wandering atrial pacemaker—conduction disturbance caused by competition among one or more ectopic atrial or junctional pacemakers and the sinoatrial node, with all pacemakers having nearly the same intrinsic rate.

wellness—state characterized not only by absence of disease but also by minimization of modifiable risk factors.

Wenckebach phenomenon—most common form of second-degree atrioventricular block, in which there is a progressively greater delay of the atrial impulse with each beat, until one impulse is totally blocked from entering the ventricles.

Wilms' tumor—most common form of renal cancer in childhood, also known as nephroblastoma.

Wolff-Chaikoff effect—large increase in circulating iodine that inhibits synthesis of thyroid hormones by blocking the peroxidase enzyme.

Wolff-Parkinson-White (WPW) syndrome—most common form of disorder due to presence of a congenital accessory pathway for current flow between the atria and ventricles. WPW syndrome is usually seen in young males and manifests as supraventricular tachycardia due to macroreentry (preexcitation).

work of breathing—the amount of muscular effort required for inspiration and expiration, determining the oxygen consumption of the pulmonary system.

xanthoma—papule, nodule, or plaque in the skin and tendons formed from lipid deposits.

xerosis—abnormal dryness, as of the eye, skin, or mouth.

Zollinger-Ellison syndrome—comprises intractable atypical peptic ulcer, pathologically high secretion of gastric acid, and a gastrin-secreting tumor.

APPENDIX B: Abbreviations

AAA	abdominal aortic aneurysm
ABC	airway, breathing, and circulation
ABG	arterial blood gas
ABVD	Adriamycin, bleomycin, vinblastine, dacarbazine
ACE	angiotensin-converting enzyme
ACh	acetylcholine
ACLS	advanced cardiac life support
ACTH	adrenocorticotropic hormone
ADH	antidiuretic hormone
ADL	activities of daily living
ADP	adenosine diphosphate
AFP	alpha-fetoprotein
AGN	acute glomerulonephritis
AHCPR	Agency for Health Care Policy and Research
AIDS	acquired immunodeficiency syndrome
AIVR	accelerated idioventricular rhythm
AJCC	American Joint Committee on Cancer
ALG	antilymphocyte globulin
ALL	acute lymphocytic leukemia
ALP	alkaline phosphatase
ALS	amyotrophic lateral sclerosis
AML	acute myelocytic leukemia
ANA	antinuclear antibody
ANP	atrial natriuretic peptide
ANS	autonomic nervous system
AP	anteroposterior
APTT	activated partial thromboplastin time
Ara-A	adenine arabinoside
ARDS	adult respiratory distress syndrome
ARF	acute renal failure
ASA	acetylsalicylic acid
AST	aspartate aminotransferase
ATG	antithymocyte globulin
ATN	acute tubular necrosis
ATP	adenosine triphosphate
ATPase	adenosine triphosphatase
AV	atrioventricular; arteriovenous
AVM	arteriovenous malformation
AVN	avascular necrosis
AZT	azidothymidine (zidovudine)
BC	Bowman's capsule
BCG	bacille Calmette-Guérin
BMI	body mass index
BMT	bone marrow transplantation
BP	blood pressure
BPH	benign prostatic hyperplasia
BRM	biologic response modifier
BSE	breast self-examination
BSO	bilateral salpingo-oophorectomy
BUN	blood urea nitrogen
C & S	culture and sensitivity
CABG	coronary artery bypass graft
CAD	coronary artery disease
CAH	chronic active hepatitis
CAL	chronic airflow limitation
cAMP	cyclic adenosine monophosphate
CAPD	continuous ambulatory peritoneal dialysis
CAVH	continuous arteriovenous hemofiltration
CAVHD	continuous arteriovenous hemodialysis and filtration
CBC	complete blood count
CBD	common bile duct
CD4	cluster of differentiation 4
CDC	Centers for Disease Control and Prevention
CEA	carcinoembryonic antigen
CFU	colony-forming unit
CGN	chronic glomerulonephritis
CHF	congestive heart failure
CIN	cervical intraepithelial neoplasia
CIS	carcinoma in situ
CK	creatine kinase
CLL	chronic lymphocytic leukemia
cm	centimeter(s)
CML	chronic myelocytic leukemia
CMV	cisplatin, methotrexate, vinblastine; cytomegalovirus
CNS	central nervous system
CO	cardiac output
COLD	chronic obstructive lung disease
COPD	chronic obstructive pulmonary disease
CPAP	continuous positive airway pressure
CPK	creatine phosphokinase
CPR	cardiopulmonary resuscitation
CREST	calcium, Raynaud's phenomenon, esophageal dysmotility, sclerodactyly, telangiectasia

CRF	chronic renal failure
CRH	corticotropin-releasing hormone
CRI	chronic renal insufficiency
CSF	cerebrospinal fluid
CT	computed tomography
CTD	connective tissue disease
CTS	carpal tunnel syndrome
CVA	cerebrovascular accident (stroke)
CVP	central venous pressure
D&C	dilation and curettage
DCCT	Diabetes Control and Complications Trial
DCM	dilated cardiomyopathy
DCT	distal convoluted tubule
DDAVP	desmopressin acetate
ddI	dideoxyinosine (didanosine)
DES	diethylstilbestrol
DHT	dihydrotestosterone
DI	diabetes insipidus
DIC	disseminated intravascular coagulation
DIP	distal interphalangeal joint
DJD	degenerative joint disease
dL	deciliter(s)
DLE	discoid lupus erythematosus
DNA	deoxyribonucleic acid
DRE	digital rectal examination
DTR	deep tendon reflex
DVT	deep venous thrombosis
EBV	Epstein-Barr virus
ECF	extracellular fluid
ECG	electrocardiogram
EMD	electromechanical dissociation
EMG	electromyography
EOM	extraocular movement
EPO	erythropoietin
EPS	electrophysiologic study
ERCP	endoscopic retrograde cholangiopancreatography
ERS	erythrocyte sedimentation rate
ESR	erythrocyte sedimentation rate
ESRD	end-stage renal disease
FAM	fluorouracil, Adriamycin, and mitomycin C
FDA	(U.S.) Food and Drug Administration
FEF	forced expiratory flow
FEV	forced expiratory volume
FEV_1	forced expiratory volume in one second
FEV_1/FVC	ratio of expiratory volume in one second to forced vital capacity
F_IO_2	fraction of inspired oxygen
FRC	functional residual capacity
FSH	follicle-stimulating hormone

ft	foot (feet)
5-FU	5-fluorouracil
FVC	forced vital capacity
g/day	gram(s) per day
g	gram(s)
G6PD	glucose-6-phosphate dehydrogenase
GABA	gamma-aminobutyric acid
GAS	general adaptation syndrome
GBS	Guillain-Barré syndrome
GCS	Glasgow Coma Scale
GCSF	granulocyte colony-stimulating factor
GDM	gestational diabetes mellitus
GFR	glomerular filtration rate
GH	growth hormone
GHRIH	growth hormone–release inhibiting hormone
GHRH	growth hormone–releasing hormone
GI	gastrointestinal
GM-CSF	granulocyte-macrophage colony-stimulating factor
GnRH	gonadotropin-releasing hormone
GVHD	graft-versus-host disease
h	hour(s)
Hb	hemoglobin
HBIG	hepatitis B immune globulin
HBV	hepatitis B virus
hCG	human chorionic gonadotropin
HCM	hypertrophic cardiomyopathy
Hct	hematocrit
HCV	hepatitis C virus
HD	hemodialysis
HDL	high-density lipoprotein
HDV	hepatitis delta virus
HEV	hepatitis E virus
HLA	human leukocyte antigen
HPA	hypothalamic–pituitary axis
HPV	human papillomavirus
HR	heart rate
HSV	herpes simplex virus
5-HT	5-hydroxytryptamine (serotonin)
HTLV	human T-cell lymphotropic virus
Hz	Hertz
IABP	intra-aortic balloon pumping
IBS	irritable bowel syndrome
IBW	ideal body weight
ICD	implantable cardioverter-defibrillator
ICF	intracellular fluid
ICP	intracranial pressure
ICS	intercostal space
Ig	immunoglobulin
IHSS	idiopathic hypertrophic subaortic stenosis
IL	interleukin
IL-3	interleukin-3

IL-4	interleukin-4
IL-5	interleukin-5
IL-8	interleukin-8
IM	intramuscular
INR	international normalized ratio
IOP	intraocular pressure
ITP	idiopathic thrombocytopenic purpura
IU	International Unit(s)
IUD	intrauterine device
IU/L	International Unit(s) per liter
IV	intravenous
IVP	intravenous pyelography
kg	kilogram(s)
kJ	kilojoule(s)
KS	Kaposi's sarcoma
LAD	left anterior descending
LCA	left coronary artery
LDH	lactate dehydrogenase
LDL	low-density lipoprotein
LES	lower esophageal sphincter
LH	luteinizing hormone
LLQ	left lower quadrant
LMN	lower motor neuron
LOC	level of consciousness
LPS	lipopolysaccharide
LR	lactated Ringer's (solution)
LUQ	left upper quadrant
LVEDP	left ventricular end-diastolic pressure
M-CSF	monocyte-macrophage colony-stimulating factor
mA	milliampere(s)
MAC	*Mycobacterium avium* complex
MAO	monoamine oxidase
MAP	mean arterial pressure
MAST	military antishock trousers
MAT	multifocal atrial tachycardia
MCA	middle cerebral artery
MCH	mean corpuscular hemoglobin
MCHC	mean corpuscular hemoglobin concentration
MCL	modified chest lead
MCP	metacarpophalangeal
MCV	mean corpuscular volume
MD	muscular dystrophy
MDF	myocardial depressant factor
MEN	multiple endocrine neoplasia
mEq	milliequivalent(s)
mEq/L	milliequivalent(s) per liter
mg	milligram(s)
MG	myasthenia gravis
mg/dL	milligram(s) per deciliter
MHC	major histocompatibility complex
MI	myocardial infarction
min	minute(s)
mL	milliliter(s)
mL/kg	milliliter(s) per kilogram
mm	millimeter(s)
mm Hg	millimeter(s) of mercury
mmol	millimole(s)
mmol/L	millimoles per liter
MOPP	mechlorethamine, Oncovin, procarbazine, prednisone
mOsm	milliosmole(s)
mOsm/L	milliosmole(s) per liter
MRI	magnetic resonance imaging
MS	multiple sclerosis; morphine sulfate
msec	millisecond(s)
MSH	melanocyte-stimulating hormone
MTP	metatarsophalangeal
MTX	methotrexate
mU	milliunit(s)
mU/mL	milliunit(s) per milliliter
mV	millivolt(s)
MVAC	methotrexate, vinblastine, Adriamycin, cisplatin
NCI	National Cancer Institute
NE	norepinephrine
ng	nanogram(s)
NK	natural killer (cell)
NS	nephrotic syndrome; normal saline
NSAID	nonsteroidal anti-inflammatory drug
NSR	normal sinus rhythm
NYHA	New York Heart Association
OA	osteoarthritis
OBS	organic brain syndrome
OI	osteogenesis imperfecta
OSHA	(U.S.) Occupational Safety and Health Administration
OTC	over-the-counter
oz	ounce(s)
PA	posteroanterior
PAC	premature atrial contraction
$PaCO_2$	partial pressure of arterial carbon dioxide
PaO_2	partial pressure of arterial oxygen
Pap	Papanicolaou (test, smear)
PAP	pulmonary artery pressure
PAWP	pulmonary artery wedge pressure
PCP	*Pneumocystis carinii* pneumonia
PCT	proximal convoluted tubule
PE	pulmonary embolism
PEA	pulseless electrical activity
PEEP	positive end-expiratory pressure
PET	positron emission tomography
PFT	pulmonary function test
PGE_2	prostaglandin F_2
PGI_2	prostaglandin I_2 (prostacyclin)
pH	the negative logarithm of the hydrogen ion concentration

PID pelvic inflammatory disease
PIH prolactin-inhibiting hormone
PIP proximal interphalangeal, peak inspiratory pressure
PJC premature junctional contraction
PKD polycystic kidney disease
PMI point of maximal impulse
PMN polymorphonuclear cell
PMS premenstrual syndrome
PND paroxysmal nocturnal dyspnea
PNS parasympathetic nervous system
PO *per os* (by mouth)
PPD purified protein derivative
PRN *pro re nata* (as needed)
PSA prostate-specific antigen
PSE portal-systemic encephalopathy
PSS progressive systemic sclerosis
PSVT paroxysmal supraventricular tachycardia
PT prothrombin time
PTCA percutaneous transluminal coronary angioplasty
PTH parathyroid hormone (parathormone)
PTT partial thromboplastin time
PTU propylthiouracil
PUD peptic ulcer disease
PUVA psoralen and ultraviolet A
PV polycythemia vera
PVC premature ventricular contraction
PVD peripheral vascular disease
PVS persistent vegetative state
RA rheumatoid arthritis
RAI radioactive iodine
RAIU radioactive iodine uptake
RAS reticular activating system
RBC red blood cell
RCA right coronary artery
RDA recommended daily allowance; recommended dietary allowance
REM rapid eye movement
RLQ right lower quadrant
RNA ribonucleic acid
ROM range of motion
RPGN rapidly progressive glomerulonephritis
RSD reflex sympathetic dystrophy
RTA renal tubular acidosis
RUQ right upper quadrant
RV residual volume
SA sinoatrial
SaO_2 arterial oxygen saturation
SBE subacute bacterial endocarditis
SCD sequential compression device
SCI spinal cord injury
SCID severe combined immunodeficiency
sec second(s)
SGOT serum glutamic-oxaloacetic transaminase
SI Système International d'Unites
SIADH syndrome of inappropriate antidiuretic hormone
SLE systemic lupus erythematosus
SMX sulfamethoxazole
SNS sympathetic nervous system
SPF sunburn protection factor
SSKI saturated solution of potassium iodide
STD sexually transmitted disease
SV stroke volume
T_3 tri-iodothyronine
T_3RU tri-iodothyronine resin uptake
T_4 thyroxine
TAF tumor angiogenesis factor
TAH total abdominal hysterectomy
TB tuberculosis
TBSA total burn surface area
TEF tracheoesophageal fistula
TEN toxic epidermal necrolysis
TENS transcutaneous electrical nerve stimulation
TIA transient ischemic attack
TIBC total iron-binding capacity
TLC total lung capacity
TMJ temporomandibular joint
TMP trimethroprim
TNF tumor necrosis factor
TNM tumor, node, metastasis
t-PA tissue plasminogen activator
TPN total parenteral nutrition
TRH thyrotropin-releasing hormone
TSE testicular self-examination
TSH thyroid-stimulating hormone
tsp teaspoon(s)
TSS toxic shock syndrome
TTP thrombotic thrombocytopenic purpura
TURP transurethral resection of the prostate
μg microgram(s)
UGI upper gastrointestinal
UMN upper motor neuron
UTI urinary tract infection
UV ultraviolet
UVA ultraviolet A
UVB ultraviolet B
VC vital capacity
VDRL Venereal Disease Research Laboratory (test)
VF ventricular fibrillation

VMA	vanillylmandelic acid
V/Q	ventilation-perfusion
VT	ventricular tachycardia
V_T	tidal volume
VZV	varicella-zoster virus
WBC	white blood cell
WHO	World Health Organization
WHR	waist-to-hip ratio

Modified from Ignatavicius, D.D., Workman, M.L., and Mishler, M.A. *Medical-Surgical Nursing: A Nursing Process Approach.* (2nd ed.). Philadelphia: W.B. Saunders. (pp. 2320–2327).

APPENDIX C: Laboratory Values of Clinical Importance

REFERENCE VALUES FOR HEMATOLOGY

	Conventional Units	SI Units
Acid hemolysis (Ham test)	No hemolysis	No hemolysis
Alkaline phosphatase, leukocyte	Total score 14–100	Total score 14–100
Cell counts		
Erythrocytes		
Males	4.6–6.2 million/mm^3	4.6–6.2 × 10^{12}/L
Females	4.2–5.4 million/mm^3	4.2–5.4 × 10^{12}/L
Children (varies with age)	4.5–5.1 million/mm^3	4.5–5.1 × 10^{12}/L
Leukocytes, total	4500–11,000/mm^3	4.5–1.00 × 10^9/L
Leukocytes, differential counts*		
Myelocytes	0%	0/L
Band neutrophils	3–5%	150–400 × 10^6/L
Segmented neutrophils	54–62%	3000–5800 × 10^6/L
Lymphocytes	25–33%	1500–3000 × 10^6/L
Monocytes	3–7%	300–500 × 10^6/L
Eosinophils	1–3%	50–250 × 10^6/L
Basophils	0–1%	15–50 × 10^6/L
Platelets	150,000–400,000/mm^3	150–400 × 10^9/L
Reticulocytes	25,000–75,000/mm^3 (0.5–1.5% of erythrocytes)	25–75 × 10^9/L
Coagulation tests		
Bleeding time (template)	2.75–8.0 min	2.75–8.0 min
Coagulation time (glass tube)	5–15 min	5–15 min
D-Dimer	<0.5 μg/mL	<0.5 mg/L
Factor VIII and other coagulation factors	50–150% of normal	0.5–1.5 of normal
Fibrin split products (Thrombo-Welco test)	<10 μg/mL	<10 mg/L
Fibrinogen	200–400 mg/dL	2.0–4.0 g/L
Partial thromboplastin time (PTT)	20–35 sec	20–35 sec
Prothrombin time (PT)	12–14 sec	12–14 sec
Coombs' test		
Direct	Negative	Negative
Indirect	Negative	Negative
Corpuscular values of erythrocytes		
Mean corpuscular hemoglobin (MCH)	26–34 pg/cell	26–34 pg/cell
Mean corpuscular volume (MCV)	80–96 μm^3	80–96 fL
Mean corpuscular hemoglobin concentration (MCHC)	32–36 g/dL	320–360 g/L
Haptoglobin	20–165 mg/dL	0.20–1.65 g/L
Hematocrit		
Males	40–54 mL/dL	0.40–0.54
Females	37–47 mL/dL	0.37–0.47
Newborns	49–54 mL/dL	0.49–0.54
Children (varies with age)	35–49 mL/dL	0.35–0.49
Hemoglobin		
Males	13.0–18.0 g/dL	8.1–11.2 mmol/L
Females	12.0–16.0 g/dL	7.4–9.9 mmol/L
Newborns	16.5–19.5 g/dL	10.2–12.1 mmol/L
Children (varies with age)	11.2–16.5 g/dL	7.0–10.2 mmol/L
Hemoglobin, fetal	<1% of total	<0.01 of total
Hemoglobin A_{1C}	3–5% of total	0.03–0.05 of total
Hemoglobin A_2	1.5–3% of total	0.015–0.03 of total
Hemoglobin, plasma	0.0–5 mg/dL	0.0–3.2 μmol/L
Methemoglobin	30–130 mg/dL	19–80 μmol/L
Erythrocyte sedimentation rate (ESR)		
Wintrobe		
Males	0–5 mm/hr	0–5 mm/hr
Females	0–15 mm/hr	0–15 mm/hr
Westergren		
Males	0–15 mm/hr	0–15 mm/hr
Females	0–20 mm/hr	0–20 mm/hr

* Conventional units are percentages; SI units are absolute counts.

REFERENCE VALUES* FOR CLINICAL CHEMISTRY (BLOOD, SERUM, AND PLASMA)

	Conventional Units	SI Units
Acetoacetate plus acetone		
Qualitative	Negative	Negative
Quantitative	0.3–2.0 mg/dL	30–200 μmol/L
Acid phosphatase, serum (thymolphthalein monophosphate substrate)	0.1–0.6 U/L	0.1–0.6 U/L
ACTH (see corticotropin)		
Alanine aminotransferase (ALT, SGPT), serum	1–45 U/L	1–45 U/L
Albumin, serum	3.3–5.2 g/dL	33–52 g/L
Aldolase, serum	0.0–7.0 U/L	0.0–7.0 U/L
Aldosterone, plasma		
Standing	5–30 ng/dL	140–830 pmol/L
Recumbent	3–10 ng/dL	80–275 pmol/L
Alkaline phosphatase (ALP), serum		
Adult	35–150 U/L	35–150 U/L
Adolescent	100–500 U/L	100–500 U/L
Child	100–350 U/L	100–350 U/L
Ammonia nitrogen, plasma	10–50 μmol/L	10–50 μmol/L
Amylase, serum	25–125 U/L	25–125 U/L
Anion gap, serum, calculated	8–16 mEq/L	8–16 mmol/L
Ascorbic acid, blood	0.4–1.5 mg/dL	23–85 μmol/L
Aspartate aminotransferase (AST, SGOT), serum	1–36 U/L	1–36 U/L
Base excess, arterial blood, calculated	0 ± 2 mEq/L	0 ± 2 mmol/L
β-Carotene, serum	60–260 μg/dL	1.1–8.6 μmol/L
Bicarbonate		
Venous plasma	23–29 mEq/L	23–29 mmol/L
Arterial blood	21–27 mEq/L	21–27 mmol/L
Bile acids, serum	0.3–3.0 mg/dL	0.8–7.6 μmol/L
Bilirubin, serum		
Conjugated	0.1–0.4 mg/dL	1.7–6.8 μmol/L
Total	0.3–1.1 mg/dL	5.1–19.0 μmol/L
Calcium, serum	8.4–10.6 mg/dL	2.10–2.65 mmol/L
Calcium, ionized, serum	4.25–5.25 mg/dL	1.05–1.30 mmol/L
Carbon dioxide, total, serum or plasma	24–31 mEq/L	24–31 mmol/L
Carbon dioxide tension (P_{CO_2}), blood	35–45 mm Hg	35–45 mm Hg
Ceruloplasmin, serum	23–44 mg/dL	230–440 mg/L
Chloride, serum or plasma	96–106 mEq/L	96–106 mmol/L
Cholesterol, serum or EDTA plasma		
Desirable range	<200 mg/dL	<5.20 mmol/L
LDL cholesterol	60–180 mg/dL	1.55–4.65 mmol/L
HDL cholesterol	30–80 mg/dL	0.80–2.05 mmol/L
Copper	70–140 μg/dL	11–22 μmol/L
Corticotropin (ACTH), plasma, 8 A.M.	10–80 pg/mL	2–18 pmol/L
Cortisol, plasma		
8:00 A.M.	6–23 μg/dL	170–630 nmol/L
4:00 P.M.	3–15 μg/dL	80–410 nmol/L
10:00 P.M.	<50% of 8:00 A.M. value	<50% of 8:00 A.M. value
Creatine, serum		
Males	0.2–0.5 mg/dL	15–40 μmol/L
Females	0.3–0.9 mg/dL	25–70 μmol/L
Creatine kinase (CK), serum		
Males	55–170 U/L	55–170 U/L
Females	30–135 U/L	30–135 U/L
Creatine kinase MB isoenzyme, serum	<5% of total CK activity <5% ng/mL by immunoassay	<5% of total CK activity <5% ng/mL by immunoassay
Creatinine, serum	0.6–1.2 mg/dL	50–110 μmol/L
Estradiol-17β, adult		
Males	10–65 pg/mL	35–240 pmol/L
Females		
Follicular phase	30–100 pg/mL	110–370 pmol/L
Ovulatory phase	200–400 pg/mL	730–1470 pmol/L
Luteal phase	50–140 pg/mL	180–510 pmol/L
Ferritin, serum	20–200 ng/mL	20–200 μg/L
Fibrinogen, plasma	200–400 mg/dL	2.0–4.0 g/L
Folate, serum	3.0–18.0 ng/mL	6.8–41.0 nmol/L
erythrocytes	145–540 ng/mL	330–1220 nmol/L
Follicle-stimulating hormone (FSH), plasma		
Males	4–25 mU/mL	4–25 U/L
Females, premenopausal	4–30 mU/mL	4–30 U/L
Females, postmenopausal	40–250 mU/mL	40–250 U/L

Table continued on following page

REFERENCE VALUES* FOR CLINICAL CHEMISTRY (BLOOD, SERUM, AND PLASMA) *Continued*

	Conventional Units	SI Units
γ-Glutamyltransferase (GGT), serum	5–40 U/L	5–40 U/L
Gastrin, fasting, serum	0–110 pg/mL	0–110 mg/L
Glucose, fasting, plasma or serum	70–115 mg/dL	3.9–6.4 nmol/L
Growth hormone (hGH), plasma, adult, fasting	0–6 ng/mL	0–6 μg/L
Haptoglobin, serum	20–165 mg/dL	0.20–1.65 g/L
Immunoglobulins, serum (see Reference Values for Immunologic Procedures)		
Insulin, fasting, plasma	5–25 μU/mL	36–179 pmol/L
Iron, serum	75–175 μg/dL	13–31 μmol/L
Iron binding capacity, serum		
Total	250–410 μg/dL	45–73 μmol/L
Saturation	20–55%	0.20–0.55
Lactate		
Venous whole blood	5–20 mg/dL	0.6–2.2 mmol/L
Arterial whole blood	5–15 mg/dL	0.6–17 mmol/L
Lactate dehydrogenase (LD), serum	110–220 U/L	110–220 U/L
Lipase, serum	10–140 U/L	10–140 U/L
Lutropin (LH), serum		
Males	1–9 U/L	1–9 U/L
Females		
Follicular phase	2–10 U/L	2–10 U/L
Midcycle peak	15–65 U/L	15–65 U/L
Luteal phase	1–12 U/L	1–12 U/L
Postmenopausal	12–65 U/L	12–65 U/L
Magnesium, serum	1.3–2.1 mg/dL	0.65–1.05 mmol/L
Osmolality	275–295 mOsm/kg water	275–295 mOsmkg water
Oxygen, blood, arterial, room air		
Partial pressure (PaO_2)	80–100 mm Hg	80–100 mm Hg
Saturation (SaO_2)	95–98%	95–98%
pH, arterial blood	7.35–7.45	7.35–7.45
Phosphate, inorganic, serum		
Adult	3–4.5 mg/dL	1–1.5 mmol/L
Child	4–7 mg/dL	1.3–2.3 mmol/L
Potassium		
Serum	3.5–5 mEq/L	3.5–5 mmol/L
Plasma	3.5–4.5 mEq/L	3.5–4.5 mmol/L
Progesterone, serum, adult		
Males	0–0.4 ng/mL	0–1.3 mmol/L
Females		
Follicular phase	0.1–1.5 ng/mL	0.3–4.8 mmol/L
Luteal phase	2.5–28 ng/mL	8–89 mmol/L
Prolactin, serum		
Males	1–15 ng/mL	1–15 μg/L
Females	1–20 ng/mL	1–20 μg/L
Protein, serum, electrophoresis		
Total	6–8 g/dL	60–80 g/L
Albumin	3.5–5.5 g/dL	35–55 g/L
Globulins		
$Alpha_1$	0.2–0.4 g/dL	2–4 g/L
$Alpha_2$	0.5–0.9 g/dL	5–9 g/L
Beta	0.6–1.1 g/dL	6–11 g/L
Gamma	0.7–1.7 g/dL	6–17 g/L
Pyruvate, blood	0.3–0.9 mg/dL	0.03–0.10 mmol/L
Rheumatoid factor	0–30 IU/mL	0–30 kIU/L
Sodium, serum or plasma	135–145 mEq/L	135–145 mmol/L
Testosterone, plasma		
Males, adult	300–1200 ng/dL	10.4–41.6 nmol/L
Females, adult	20–75 ng/dL	0.7–2.6 nmol/L
Pregnant females	40–200 ng/dL	1.4–6.9 nmol/L
Thyroglobulin	3–42 ng/mL	3–42 μg/L
Thyrotropin (hTSH), serum	0.4–4.8 μIU/mL	0.4–4.8 mIU/L
Thyrotropin-releasing hormone (TRH)	5–60 pg/mL	5–60 ng/L
Thyroxine (FT_4), free, serum	0.9–2.1 ng/dL	12–27 pmol/L
Thyroxine (T_4), serum	4.5–12 μg/dL	58–154 nmol/L
Thyroxine-binding globulin (TBG)	15–34 μg/mL	15–34 mg/L
Transferrin	250–430 mg/dL	2.5–4.3 g/L
Triglycerides, serum, after 12-hr fast	40–150 mg/dL	0.4–1.5 g/L
Tri-iodothyronine (T_3), serum	70–190 ng/dL	1.1–2.9 nmol/L
Tri-iodothyronine uptake, resin (T_3RU)	25–38%	0.25–0.38

REFERENCE VALUES* FOR CLINICAL CHEMISTRY (BLOOD, SERUM, AND PLASMA) *Continued*

	Conventional Units	SI Units
Urate		
Males	2.5–8 mg/dL	150–480 μmol/L
Females	2.2–7 mg/dL	130–420 μmol/L
Urea, serum or plasma	24–49 mg/dL	4–8.2 nmol/L
Urea nitrogen, serum or plasma	11–23 mg/dL	8–16.4 nmol/L
Viscosity, serum	1.4–1.8 × water	1.4–1.8 × water
Vitamin A, serum	20–80 μg/dL	0.70–2.80 μmol/L
Vitamin B_{12}, serum	180–900 pg/mL	133–664 pmol/L

* Reference values may vary, depending on the method and sample source used.

REFERENCE VALUES FOR THERAPEUTIC DRUG MONITORING (SERUM)

	Therapeutic Range	Toxic Concentrations	Proprietary Names
Analgesics			
Acetaminophen	10–20 μg/mL	>250 μg/mL	Tylenol Datril
Salicylate	100–250 μg/mL	>300 μg/mL	Aspirin Bufferin
Antibiotics			
Amikacin	25–30 μg/mL	Peak >35 μg/mL Trough >10 μg/mL	Amikin
Chloramphenicol	10–20 μg/mL	>25 μg/mL	Chloromycetin
Gentamicin	5–10 μg/mL	Peak >10 μg/mL Trough >2 μg/mL	Garamycin
Tobramycin	5–10 μg/mL	Peak >10 μg/mL Trough >2 μg/mL	Nebcin
Vancomycin	5–10 μg/mL	Peak >40 μg/mL Trough >10 μg/mL	Vancocin
Anticonvulsants			
Carbamazepine	5–12 μg/mL	>15 μg/mL	Tegretol
Ethosuximide	40–100 μg/mL	>150 μg/mL	Zarontin
Phenobarbital	15–40 μg/mL	40–100 ng/mL (varies widely)	Luminal
Phenytoin	10–20 μg/mL	>20 μg/mL	Dilantin
Primidone	5–12 μg/mL	>15 μg/mL	Mysoline
Valproic acid	50–100 μg/mL	>100 μg/mL	Depakene
Antineoplastics and Immunosuppressives			
Cyclosporine	50–400 ng/mL	>400 ng/mL	Sandimmune
Methotrexate, high dose, 48 hr	Variable	>1 μmol/L 48 hr after dose	Mexate Folex
Tacrolimus (FK-506), whole blood	3–10 μg/L	>15 μg/L	Prograf
Bronchodilators and Respiratory Stimulants			
Caffeine	3–15 ng/mL	>30 ng/mL	
Theophylline (aminophylline)	10–20 μg/mL	>20 μg/mL	Elixophyllin Quibron
Cardiovascular Drugs			
Amiodarone (obtain specimen more than 8 hours after last dose)	1–2 μg/mL	>2 μg/mL	Cordarone
Digitoxin (obtain specimen 12–24 hours after last dose)	15–25 ng/mL	>35 ng/mL	Crystodigin
Digoxin (obtain specimen more than 6 hours after last dose)	0.8–2 ng/mL	>2.4 ng/mL	Lanoxin
Disopyramide	2–5 μg/mL	>7 μg/mL	Norpace
Flecainide	0.2–1 ng/mL	>1 ng/mL	Tambocor
Lidocaine	1.5–5 μg/mL	>6 μg/mL	Xylocaine
Mexiletine	0.7–2 ng/mL	>2 ng/mL	Mexitil
Procainamide	4–10 μg/mL	>12 μg/mL	Pronestyl
Procainamide plus NAPA	8–30 μg/mL	>30 μg/mL	
Propranolol	50–100 ng/mL	Variable	Inderal

Table continued on following page

REFERENCE VALUES FOR THERAPEUTIC DRUG MONITORING (SERUM) *Continued*

	Therapeutic Range	Toxic Concentrations	Proprietary Names
Quinidine	2–5 μg/mL	>6 μg/mL	Cardioquin Quinaglute
Tocainide	4–10 ng/mL	>10 ng/mL	Tonocard
Psychopharmacologic Drugs			
Amitriptyline	120–150 ng/mL	>500 ng/mL	Elavil Triavil
Bupropion	25–100 ng/mL	Not applicable	Wellbutrin
Desipramine	150–300 ng/mL	>500 ng/mL	Norpramin Pertofrane
Imipramine	125–250 ng/mL	>400 ng/mL	Tofranil Janimine
Lithium (obtain specimen 12 hours after last dose)	0.6–1.5 mEq/L	>1.5 mEq/L	Lithobid
Nortriptyline	50–150 ng/mL	>500 ng/mL	Aventyl Pamelor

REFERENCE VALUES FOR CLINICAL CHEMISTRY (URINE)

	Conventional Units	SI Units
Acetone and acetoacetate, qualitative	Negative	Negative
Albumin		
Qualitative	Negative	Negative
Quantitative	10–100 mg/24 hr	0.15–1.5 μmol/day
Aldosterone	3–20 μg/24 hr	8.3–55 nmol/day
δ-Aminolevulinic acid (δ-ALA)	1.3–7.0 mg/24 hr	10–53 μmol/day
Amylase	<17 U/hr	<17 U/hr
Amylase/creatinine clearance ratio	0.01–0.04	0.01–0.04
Bilirubin, qualitative	Negative	Negative
Calcium (regular diet)	<250 mg/24 hr	<6.3 nmol/day
Catecholamines		
Epinephrine	<10 μg/24 hr	<55 nmol/day
Norepinephrine	<100 μg/24 hr	<590 nmol/day
Total free catecholamines	4–126 μg/24 hr	24–745 nmol/day
Total metanephrines	0.1–1.6 mg/24 hr	0.5–8.1 μmol/day
Chloride (varies with intake)	110–250 mEq/24 hr	110–250 mmol/day
Copper	0–50 μg/24 hr	0.0–0.80 μmol/day
Cortisol, free	10–100 μg/24 hr	27.6–276 nmol/day
Creatine		
Males	0–40 mg/24 hr	0.0–0.30 mmol/day
Females	0–80 mg/24 hr	0.0–0.60 mmol/day
Creatinine	15–25 mg/kg/24 hr	0.13–0.22 mmol/kg/day
Creatinine clearance (endogenous)		
Males	110–150 mL/min/1.73 m^2	110–150 mL/min/1.73 m^2
Females	105–132 mL/min/1.73 m^2	105–132 mL/min/1.73 m^2
Cystine or cysteine	Negative	Negative
Dehydroepiandrosterone		
Males	0.2–2 mg/24 hr	0.7–6.9 μmol/day
Females	0.2–1.8 mg/24 hr	0.7–6.2 μmol/day
Estrogens, total		
Males	4–25 μg/24 hr	14–90 nmol/day
Females	5–100 μg/24 hr	18–360 nmol/day
Glucose (as reducing substance)	<250 mg/24 hr	<250 mg/day
Hemoglobin and myoglobin, qualitative	Negative	Negative
Homogentisic acid, qualitative	Negative	Negative
17-Hydroxycorticosteroids		
Males	3–9 mg/24 hr	8.3–25 μmol/day
Females	2–8 mg/24 hr	5.5–22 μmol/day
5-Hydroxyindoleacetic acid		
Qualitative	Negative	Negative
Quantitative	2–6 mg/24 hr	10–31 μmol/day
17-Ketogenic steroids		
Males	5–23 mg/24 hr	17–80 μmol/day
Females	3–15 mg/24 hr	10–52 μmol/day

REFERENCE VALUES FOR CLINICAL CHEMISTRY (URINE) *Continued*

	Conventional Units	SI Units
17-Ketosteroids		
Males	8–22 mg/24 hr	28–76 μmol/day
Females	6–15 mg/24 hr	21–52 μmol/day
Magnesium	6–10 mEq/24 hr	3–5 mmol/day
Metanephrines	0.05–1.2 ng/mg creatinine	0.03–0.70 mmol/mmol creatinine
Osmolality	38–1400 mOsm/kg water	38–1400 mOsm/kg water
pH	4.6–8.0	4.6–8.0
Phenylpyruvic acid, qualitative	Negative	Negative
Phosphate	0.4–1.3 g/24 hr	13–42 mmol/day
Porphobilinogen		
Qualitative	Negative	Negative
Quantitative	<2 mg/24 hr	<9 μmol/day
Porphyrins		
Coproporphyrin	50–250 μg/24 hr	77–380 nmol/day
Uroporphyrin	10–30 μg/24 hr	12–36 nmol/day
Potassium	25–125 mEq/24 hr	25–125 mmol/day
Pregnanediol		
Males	0.0–1.9 mg/24 hr	0.0–6.0 μmol/day
Females		
Proliferative phase	0.0–2.6 mg/24 hr	0.0–8.0 μmol/day
Luteal phase	2.6–10.6 mg/24 hr	8–33 μmol/day
Postmenopausal	0.2–1.0 mg/24 hr	0.6–3.1 μmol/day
Pregnanetriol	0.0–2.5 mg/24 hr	0.0–7.4 μmol/day
Protein, total		
Qualitative	Negative	Negative
Quantitative	10–150 mg/24 hr	10–150 mg/day
Protein/creatinine ratio	<0.2	<0.2
Sodium (regular diet)	60–260 mEq/24 hr	60–260 mmol/day
Specific gravity		
Random specimen	1.003–1.030	1.003–1.030
24-Hour collection	1.015–1.025	1.015–1.025
Urate (regular diet)	250–750 mg/24 hr	1.5–4.4 mmol/day
Urobilinogen	0.5–4 mg/24 hr	0.6–6.8 μmol/day
Vanillylmandelic acid (VMA)	1.0–8 mg/24 hr	5–40 μmol/day

REFERENCE VALUES FOR TOXIC SUBSTANCES

	Conventional Units	SI Units
Arsenic, urine	<130 μg/24 hr	<1.7 μmol/day
Bromides, serum, inorganic	<100 mg/dL	<10 mmol/L
Toxic symptoms	140–1000 mg/dL	14–100 mmol/L
Carboxyhemoglobin, blood	*% Saturation*	*Saturation*
Urban environment	<5%	<0.05
Smokers	<12%	<0.12
Symptoms		
Headache	>15%	>0.15
Nausea and vomiting	>25%	>0.25
Potentially lethal	>50%	>0.50
Ethanol, blood	<0.05 mg/dL <0.005%	<1.0 mmol/L
Intoxication	>100 mg/dL >0.1%	>22 mmol/L
Marked intoxication	300–400 mg/dL 0.3–0.4%	65–87 mmol/L
Alcoholic stupor	400–500 mg/dL 0.4–0.5%	87–109 mmol/L
Coma	>500 mg/dL >0.5%	>109 mmol/L
Lead, blood		
Adults	<25 μg/dL	<1.2 μmol/L
Children	<15 μg/dL	<0.7 μmol/L
Lead, urine	<80 μg/24 hr	<0.4 μmol/day
Mercury, urine	<30 μg/24 hr	<150 nmol/day

REFERENCE VALUES FOR CEREBROSPINAL FLUID

	Conventional Units	SI Units
Cells	<5 mm^3; all mononuclear	<5 × 10^6/L, all mononuclear
Protein electrophoresis	Albumin predominant	Albumin predominant
Glucose	50–75 mg/dL (20 mg/dL less than in serum)	2.8–4.2 mmol/L (1.1 mmol less than in serum)
IgG		
Children under 14	<8% of total protein	<0.08% of total protein
Adults	<14% of total protein	<0.14% of total protein
IgG index $\left(\frac{\text{CSF/serum IgG ratio}}{\text{CSF/serum albumin ratio}}\right)$	0.3–0.6	0.3–0.6
Oligoclonal banding on electrophoresis	Absent	Absent
Pressure, opening	70–180 mmH_2O	70–180 mmH_2O
Protein, total	15–45 mg/dL	150–450 mg/L

REFERENCE VALUES FOR TESTS OF GASTROINTESTINAL FUNCTION

Test Name	Conventional Units
Bentiromide	6-hr urinary arylamine excretion greater than 57% excludes pancreatic insufficiency
β-Carotene, serum	60–250 ng/dL
Fecal fat estimation	
Qualitative	No fat globules seen by high-power microscope
Quantitative	<6 g/24 hr (>95% coefficient of fat absorption)
Gastric acid output	
Basal	
Males	0.0–10.5 mmol/hr
Females	0.0–5.6 mmol/hr
Maximum (after histamine	9.0–48 mmol/hr
or pentagastrin)	6.0–31 mmol/hr
Males	
Females	0.0–0.31
Ratio: basal/maximum	0.0–0.29
Males	
Females	
Secretin test, pancreatic fluid	
Volume	>1.8 mL/kg/hr
Bicarbonate	>80 mEq/L
D-Xylose absorption test, urine	>20% of ingested dose excreted in 5 hr

REFERENCE VALUES FOR IMMUNOLOGIC PROCEDURES

	Conventional Units	SI Units
Complement, serum		
C3	85–175 mg/dL	0.85–1.75 g/L
C4	15–45 mg/dL	150–450 mg/L
Total hemolytic (CH_{50})	150–250 U/mL	150–250 U/mL
Immunoglobulins, serum, adult		
IgG	640–1350 mg/dL	6.4–13.5 g/L
IgA	70–310 mg/dL	0.70–3.1 g/L
IgM	90–350 mg/dL	0.90–3.5 g/L
IgD	0.0–6.0 mg/dL	0.0–60 mg/L
IgE	0.0–430 ng/dL	0.0–430 μg/L

Lymphocyte Subsets, Whole Blood, Heparinized

Antigen	*Cell Type**	*Percentage*	*Absolute*
CD3	Total T cells	56–77	860–1880
CD19	Total B cells	7–17	140–370
CD3 and CD4	Helper-inducer cells	32–54	550–1190
CD3 and CD8	Suppressor-cytotoxic cells	24–37	430–1060
CD3 and DR	Activated T cells	5–14	70–310
CD2	E rosette T cells	73–87	1040–2160
CD16 and CD56	Natural killer (NK) cells	8–22	130–500

* Helper/suppressor ratio: 0.8–1.8.

REFERENCE VALUES FOR SEMEN ANALYSIS

	Conventional Units	SI Units
Volume	2–5 mL	2–5 mL
Liquefaction	Complete in 15 min	Complete in 15 min
pH	7.2–8.0	7.2–8.0
Leukocytes	Occasional or absent	Occasional or absent
Spermatozoa		
Count	$60–150 \times 10^6$/mL	$60–150 \times 10^6$/mL
Motility	>80% motile	>0.80 motile
Morphology	80–90% normal forms	>0.80–0.90 normal forms
Fructose	>150 mg/dL	>8.33 mmol/L

From Conn, R.B., Borer, W.Z., and Snyder, J.W. (1997) *Current Diagnosis 9*. Philadelphia: W.B. Saunders, pp. 1235–1241.

APPENDIX D: AHCPR Guidelines

The following list presents Clinical Practice Guidelines, Quick Reference Guides for Clinicians, and Patient Guides published by the Agency for Health Care Policy and Research (AHCPR). An agency of the U.S. Department of Health and Human Services, Public Health Service, AHCPR was established in December 1989 to enhance the quality, appropriateness, and effectiveness of health care services and access to these services. AHCPR carries out its mission by conducting and supporting health research, developing Clinical Practice Guidelines, and disseminating research findings and guidelines to health care providers, policymakers, and the public.

Any of the following publications can be obtained by writing to the Center for Research Dissemination and Liaison, AHCPR Clearinghouse, P.O. Box 8547, Silver Spring, MD 20907, or by calling 1-800-358-9295. The Patient Guides are available in English and Spanish.

Recognition and initial assessment of Alzheimer's disease and related dementias. Clinical Practice Guideline. No. 19.

Early Alzheimer's disease. Patient and Family Guide. AHCPR Pub. No. 96–0704.

Unstable angina: Diagnosis and management. Clinical Practice Guideline. AHCPR Pub. No. 94–0602.

Diagnosing and managing unstable angina. Quick Reference Guide for Clinicians. AHCPR Pub. No. 94–0603.

Managing unstable angina. Patient and Family Guide. AHCPR Pub. No. 94–0604.

Acute low back problems in adults: Assessment and treatment. Quick Reference Guide for Clinicians. AHCPR Pub. No. 95–0643.

Management of cancer pain. Clinical Practice Guideline. AHCPR Pub. No. 94–0592.

Management of cancer pain: Adults. Quick Reference Guide for Clinicians. AHCPR Pub. No. 94–0593.

Managing cancer pain. Patient Guide. AHCPR Pub. No. 94–0595.

Cardiac rehabilitation. Clinical Practice Guideline. AHCPR Pub. No. 96–0672.

Cardiac rehabilitation as secondary prevention. Quick Reference Guide for Clinicians. AHCPR Pub. No. 96–0673.

Recovering from heart problems through cardiac rehabilitation. Patient Guide. AHCPR Pub. No. 96–0674.

Cataract in adults: Management of functional impairment. Clinical Practice Guideline. AHCPR Pub. No. 93–0542.

Management of cataract in adults. Quick Reference Guide for Clinicians. AHCPR Pub. No. 93–0543.

Cataract in adults. Patient Guide. AHCPR Pub. No. 93–0544.

Depression in primary care, vol 1: Detection and diagnosis. Clinical Practice Guideline. AHCPR Pub. No. 93–0550.

Depression in primary care, vol 2: Treatment of major depression. Clinical Practice Guideline. AHCPR Pub. No. 93–0551.

Depression in primary care: Detection, diagnosis, and treatment. Quick Reference Guide for Clinicians. AHCPR Pub. No. 93–0552.

Depression is a treatable illness. A Patient's Guide. AHCPR Pub. No. 93–0553.

Heart Failure: Evaluation and care of patients with left-ventricular systolic dysfunction. Clinical Practice Guideline. AHCPR Pub. No. 94–0612.

Heart failure: Management of patients with left-ventricular systolic dysfunction. Quick Reference Guide for Clinicians. AHCPR Pub. No. 94–0613.

Living with heart disease: Is it heart failure? Patient and Family Guide. AHCPR Pub. No. 94–0614.

Evaluation and management of early HIV infection. Clinical Practice Guideline. AHCPR Pub. No. 94–0572.

Managing early HIV infection. Quick Reference Guide for Clinicians. AHCPR Pub. No. 94–0573.

Understanding HIV. Consumer Guide. AHCPR Pub. No. 94–0574.

HIV and your child. Consumer Guide. AHCPR Pub. No. 94–0576.

Quality determinants of mammography. Clinical Practice Guideline. AHCPR Pub. No. 95–0632.

High-quality mammography: Information for referring providers. Quick Reference Guide for Clinicians. AHCPR Pub. No. 95–0633.

Things to know about quality mammograms. A Woman's Guide. AHCPR Pub. No. 95–0634.

Managing otitis media with effusion in young children. Quick Reference Guide for Clinicians. AHCPR Pub. No. 94–0623.

Middle ear fluid in young children. Parent Guide. AHCPR Pub. No. 94–0624.

Acute pain management: Operative or medical procedures and trauma. Clinical Practice Guideline. AHCPR Pub. No. 92–0032.

Acute pain management in adults: Operative procedures. Quick Reference Guide for Clinicians. AHCPR Pub. No. 92–0019.

Acute pain management in infants, children, and adolescents: Operative and medical procedures. Quick Reference Guide for Clinicians. AHCPR Pub. No. 92–0020.

Pain control after surgery. Patient Guide. AHCPR Pub. No. 92–0021.

Pressure ulcers in adults: Prediction and prevention. Clinical Practice Guideline. AHCPR Pub. No. 92–0047.

Pressure ulcers in adults: Prediction and prevention. Quick Reference Guide for Clinicians. AHCPR Pub. No. 92–0050.

Preventing pressure ulcers. Patient Guide. AHCPR Pub. No. 92–0048.

Pressure ulcer treatment. Quick Reference Guide for Clinicians. AHCPR Pub. No. 95–0653.

Benign prostatic hyperplasia: Diagnosis and treatment. Clinical Practice Guidelines. AHCPR Pub. No. 94–0582.

Benign prostatic hyperplasia: Diagnosis and treatment. Quick Reference Guide for Clinicians. AHCPR Pub. No. 94–0583.

Treating your enlarged prostate. Patient Guide. AHCPR Pub. No. 94–0584.

Sickle cell disease: Screening, diagnosis, management, and counseling in newborns and infants. Clinical Practice Guideline. AHCPR Pub. No. 93–0562.

Sickle cell disease: Comprehensive screening and management in newborns and infants. Quick Reference Guide for Clinicians. AHCPR Pub. No. 93–0563.

Sickle cell disease in newborns and infants. Guide for Parents. AHCPR Pub. No. 93–0564.

Smoking cessation. Clinical Practice Guideline. AHCPR Pub. No. 96–0692.

Helping smokers quit: A guide for primary care clinicians. Quick Reference Guide for Clinicians. AHCPR Pub. No. 96–0693.

Smoking cessation: Information for specialists. Quick Reference Guide for Clinicians. AHCPR Pub. No. 96–0694.
You can quit smoking. Patient Guide. AHCPR Pub. No. 96–0695.
Post-stroke rehabilitation. Clinical Practice Guideline. AHCPR Pub. No. 95–0662.
Post-stroke rehabilitation: Assessment, referral, and patient management. Quick Reference Guide for Clinicians. AHCPR Pub. No. 95–0663.
Recovering after a stroke. Patient and Family Guide. AHCPR Pub. No. 95–0664.
Urinary incontinence in adults. Clinical Practice Guideline. AHCPR Pub. No. 92–0038.
Urinary incontinence in adults. Quick Reference Guide for Clinicians. AHCPR Pub. No. 92–0041.
Urinary incontinence in adults. Patient Guide. AHCPR Pub. No. 92–0040.

From Black, J.M., and Matassarin-Jacobs, E. (1997). *Medical-Surgical Nursing: Clinical Management for Continuity of Care.* (5th ed.). Philadelphia: W.B. Saunders.

INDEX

Note: Page numbers in *italics* refer to illustrations; page numbers followed by b refer to boxed material, and those followed by t to tables.

A

B

G

J

K

L

M

N

O

P

Q

R

T

U

V

W

X

Y

Z